MOSBY'S

DRUG REFERENCE for HEALTH PROFESSIONS

THIRD EDITION

Writer and Consultant

MaryAnne Hochadel, PharmD, BCPS
Editor Emeritus
ELSEVIER/Gold Standard;
Clinical Pharmacist
Bayfront Medical Center
St. Petersburg, Florida;
Clinical Assistant Professor of Pharmacy Practice
University of Florida, College of Pharmacy
Gainesville, Florida

ELSEVIER
MOSBY

ELSEVIER
MOSBY

3251 Riverport Lane
St. Louis, Missouri 63043

MOSBY'S DRUG REFERENCE FOR HEALTH PROFESSIONS, THIRD EDITION
ISBN: 978-0-323-07736-1

Notice

Knowledge and best practice in this field are constantly changing. As new research and experience broaden our understanding, changes in research methods, professional practices, or medical treatment may become necessary.

Practitioners and researchers must always rely on their own experience and knowledge in evaluating and using any information, methods, compounds, or experiments described herein. In using such information or methods, they should be mindful of their own safety and the safety of others, including parties for whom they have a professional responsibility.

With respect to any drug or pharmaceutical products identified, readers are advised to check the most current information provided (i) on procedures featured or (ii) by the manufacturer of each product to be administered, to verify the recommended dose or formula, the method and duration of administration, and contraindications. It is the responsibility of practitioners, relying on their own experience and knowledge of their patients, to make diagnoses, to determine dosages and the best treatment for each individual patient, and to take all appropriate safety precautions.

To the fullest extent of the law, neither the Publisher nor the authors, contributors, or editors, assume any liability for any injury and/or damage to persons or property as a matter of products liability, negligence or otherwise, or from any use or operation of any methods, products, instructions, or ideas contained in the material herein.

International Standard Book Number: 978-0-323-07736-1

Vice President and Publisher: Linda Duncan
Executive Editor: Kellie White
Senior Developmental Editor: Jennifer Watrous
Publishing Services Manager: Pat Joiner-Myers
Design Direction: Kimberly Denando

Printed in the United States of America

Last digit is the print number: 9 8 7 6 5 4 3 2 1

DRUG INFORMATION REVIEWER PANEL

Laurel E. Ashworth, PharmD
Professor of Pharmacy Practice
Mercer University College of Pharmacy and Health Sciences
Atlanta, Georgia

Dana A. Brown, PharmD, BCPS
Assistant Dean for Academics
Assistant Professor of Pharmacy Practice
Lloyd L. Gregory School of Pharmacy
Palm Beach Atlantic University
West Palm Beach, Florida

Lindsay B. Curtin, PharmD, BCPS
Assistant Professor of Clinical Pharmacy
Philadelphia College of Pharmacy
University of the Sciences in Philadelphia
Philadelphia, Pennsylvania

Julie Phillips Karpinski, RPh, PharmD, BCPS
Assistant Professor, Pharmacy Practice
Director, Drug Information
Concordia University
Wisconsin School of Pharmacy
Mequon, Wisconsin

Donna Larson, EdD, MT(ASCP)DLM
Dean of Allied Health
Mt. Hood Community College
Gresham, Oregon

Terri L. Levien, PharmD
Clinical Associate Professor
College of Pharmacy
Washington State University Spokane
Spokane, Washington

Puja Patel, PharmD
Ambulatory/Managed Care Resident
Kaiser Permanente
Atlanta, Georgia

Tony Prosser, PharmD
Managing Editor, ToxED
Senior Editor, Clinical Pharmacology
ELSEVIER/Gold Standard
Tampa, Florida

Stephanie Schroeder, PharmD
Senior Editor, Clinical Content
ELSEVIER/Gold Standard
Wichita, Kansas

REVIEWERS

Karissa N. Dahlke, BS
Florida Society of Health System Pharmacists Council Member 2010–2011
Orlando, Florida

Deborah A. DeLuca, MS, JD
Assistant Professor
University School of Health and Medical Sciences
South Orange, New Jersey

Gautam J. Desai, DO, FACOFP, CPI
Associate Professor
Department of Family Medicine
Kansas City University of Medicine and Biosciences
College of Osteopathic Medicine
Kansas City, Missouri

Karen Drummond, CPC, CPC-H, CPC-I, CHA, MCMC, PCS, FCS, ACS-RA, ACS-OB/GYN, CIBS, CMC, CMBS-I
Instructor, Auditor, Consultant
AAPC Approved PMCC Instructor
Advisory Board Member for Board of Advanced Medical Specialty Coding
Board Member of American Institute for Healthcare Compliance On Line
Medical Coding and Billing Instructor for Health Care Consulting Services
Irmo, South Carolina

Sandy Fritz, MS, NCTMB
Owner and Head Instructor
Health Enrichment Center School of Therapeutic Massage
Lapeer, Michigan

Douglas S. Gardenhire, RRT-NPS
Director of Clinical Education
School of Health Professions
Division of Respiratory Therapy
Georgia State University
Atlanta, Georgia

Trisha LaPointe, PharmD, BCPS
Assistant Professor of Pharmacy Practice
Massachusetts College of Pharmacy and Health Sciences
School of Pharmacy
Boston Department of Pharmacy Practice
Boston, Massachusetts

Evie Mann, RMA
Associate Director of Education
The Medical Institute of Kentucky
Florence, Kentucky

Kim D. McKenna, MEd, RN, CEN, EMT-P
Director of Education
St. Charles County Ambulance District
St. Peters, Missouri

David Nissen, PharmD
Pharmacy Informatics
Missouri Baptist Medical Center
St. Louis, Missouri

Bernie R. Olin, PharmD
Associate Clinical Professor and Director of Drug Information
Auburn University
Harrison School of Pharmacy
Auburn, Alabama

Kazi Parvez, MBBS, RCT
Formerly:
Program Chair, Cardiology Technologist Program
Everest College
Toronto, Ontario, Canada

John J. Smith, EdD
AVP, Curriculum and Instruction
Corinthian Colleges, Inc.
Santa Ana, California

Linda M. Smith, CPC, CPC-I, CEMC, PCS, CAC, CMBS
Medical Billing and Coding Consultant Owner
MedOffice Resources
Greene, New York

Karen A. Vezina, RCT
Cardiology Technologist Program Chair
Everest College of Business, Technology and Health Care
Ottawa, Ontario, Canada

INTRODUCTION

INTRODUCTION

Mosby's Drug Reference for Health Professions is designed as an easy-to-use resource for current drug information for the busy health care professional. The information is provided in a standardized monograph format for ease of practical application. A number of important new medications have been introduced in the past few years, and these have been incorporated into this guide, which contains a concise overview of over 900 generic and over 2400 brand-name medications widely used in medical practice. This latest edition will be a welcome addition to any health care professional's drug reference library and will be used often for its practicality and quick summaries of essential drug facts.

DETAILS OF THE CONTENTS

Essential drug information in a user-friendly format. The bulk of this handbook contains an alphabetical listing of drug entries by generic name. Drug entries include the following:

- ***Generic and brand name.*** Drug entries are categorized by generic name alphabetically, followed by marketed U.S.- and Canadian-branded product names.

  ★ U. S. brand names
  🍁 Canadian brand names

  The star icon denotes the U.S. brand names, and the maple leaf icon denotes the Canadian brand names. The index provides both trade and brand-name listings for ease of lookup.
- ***Category and schedule.*** The U.S. FDA pregnancy risk category, as well as pertinent information regarding over-the-counter (OTC) status and U.S. DEA Controlled Substance Schedules, is listed.
- ***Classification.*** Each entry highlights important pharmacologic, chemical, and/or therapeutic use classifications.
- ***Mechanism of action.*** A brief pharmacologic description of the actions of the drug is given, followed by a brief statement of therapeutic effect.
- ***Pharmacokinetics.*** A relevant, yet concise, summary of the absorption, distribution, metabolism, and excretion characteristics is provided for each entry.
- ***Availability.*** Dosage forms currently approved for marketing in the United States are listed. Users should note that this information may change frequently. Users are encouraged to speak with their pharmacists regarding local drug availability, since marketing status and shortages of drug products may occur frequently in practice.
- ***Indications and dosages.*** Approved indications, routes, and dosages for approved populations of use are provided in a concise format. Pediatric and geriatric data are included when available. When specified, dosages for hepatic and renal impairment are also provided.
- ***Contraindications.*** Contraindications are listed as provided in manufacturer labeling, indicating circumstances under which a drug should not be used.
- ***Interactions.*** Common interactions with drugs, herbal and dietary supplements, and food are provided in a quick-reference format so that practitioners can easily screen medication profiles. New interaction data are often published as new drugs enter the market

are used widely in the intended populations, so the information presented may not always reflect the most current data. Practitioners are encouraged to use the information provided to screen for important interactions but also consider the need for other sources.

- ***Diagnostic test effects.*** This section provides a brief summary of both the expected and the potential effects that a drug has on commonly monitored laboratory testing (e.g., blood chemistry, renal function, liver function, and hematologic testing), as well as any known assay interference. When a therapeutic range is defined for a drug, it will also be presented in this section.
- ***IV incompatibilities and IV compatibilities.*** Medications that are used intravenously must be approached with caution, especially with respect to the use of other parenteral medications. In these sections, the user is presented common and well-known incompatibilities and published compatibilities with other medications at the Y-site. However, these data often depend on concentration and method of administration and are constantly updated. New incompatibility data may emerge at any time. The user is encouraged to always consult specialized resources for new incompatibility information before mixing or infusing any parenteral medication. The information provided is not meant to be inclusive but rather to be exemplary of the concerns with regard to IV incompatibility. This information is clarified with icons representing compatibilities and incompatibilities.
- ***Side effects.*** The health care professional will appreciate the prioritized presentation of side effects. This section provides an understanding of the published frequency of commonly reported side effects noted in clinical trials. Although the included frequencies are not always reflective of the frequencies seen once a drug is on the market, the guide provides a basic understanding of side effects that are expected, frequent, occasional, or rare, including basic percentage frequencies associated with the definitions. Although not meant to be absolutely inclusive, this guide includes the more commonly reported reactions in each category that are likely to be causally associated with a given drug.
- ***Serious reactions.*** Most practitioners would like to have a good understanding of those reactions that, because of their severity and potentially life-threatening nature, would require prompt intervention or lead to hospitalization. This section highlights those side effects, apart from other reactions, that often require specialized warnings or alerts. The practitioner is encouraged to always review these listings when reviewing an entry.
- ***Precautions and considerations.*** Using a practice-oriented format for health care professionals, this section very concisely summarizes the most relevant concepts in considerations for prescribing and monitoring a drug in given patient populations, including those who are pregnant or breastfeeding, as well as children and the elderly. The user of this guide will gain practical advice for monitoring drug effects during treatment and will appreciate the care-focused context of the information.

- ***Storage.*** The proper storage of medications, and their stability, is a concern in health care and patient home environments. Proper storage helps ensure that appropriate drug effects will be maintained. This section quickly summarizes proper storage for each entry.
- ***Administration.*** A concise summary of administering each dosage form is provided for the practitioner. Proper administration technique helps ensure that desired medication effects are attained. When known, techniques for limiting side effects during administration are highlighted. Alerts to hazards are also presented for important medications, such as chemotherapy.

Appendices. Quick reference guides to FDA pregnancy categories, normal laboratory values, and English-Spanish translations of common medication-related phrases are provided.

Electronic Resources. Register for free resources at www.mosbydrugref.com. The following assets are available:

- Audio drug name pronunciations and an audio glossary (including definitions) in MP3 format.
- Full-color pill atlas.
- Additional generic drug monographs.
- Monographs for herbal remedies, compound drugs, and OTC drugs.
- Generic-to-trade-name reference table.
- Medication math exercises.
- Information on drugs of abuse and general anesthetics.

SUMMARY

When it comes to providing quality information, *Mosby's Drug Reference for Health Professions* can be an important and practical resource. The spectrum of drug entries, the current information, and health care professional tips will be invaluable to providing patient and client care.

MaryAnne Hochadel
PharmD, BCPS

CONTENTS

For the glossary and other drug information resources, please visit www.mosbydrugref.com.

Abacavir

ah-bah'cah-veer

★ 🍁 Ziagen

CATEGORY AND SCHEDULE

Pregnancy Risk Category: C

Classification: Antiretroviral, nucleoside analog

MECHANISM OF ACTION

An antiretroviral that inhibits the activity of HIV-1 reverse transcriptase by competing with the natural substrate deoxyguanosine-5′-triphosphate (dGTP) and by its incorporation into viral DNA. *Therapeutic Effect:* Inhibits viral DNA growth.

PHARMACOKINETICS

Rapidly and extensively absorbed after PO administration. Protein binding: 50%. Widely distributed, including to CSF and erythrocytes. Metabolized in the liver to inactive metabolites. Excreted primarily in urine. Unknown whether removed by hemodialysis. *Half-life:* 1.5 h.

AVAILABILITY

Tablets: 300 mg.
Oral Solution: 20 mg/mL.

INDICATIONS AND DOSAGES

▸ **HIV infection (in combination with other antiretrovirals)**

PO

Adults. 300 mg twice a day or 600 mg once daily.
Children (3 mo and older). 8 mg/kg twice a day. Maximum: 300 mg twice a day.

▸ **Dosage in hepatic impairment**

Mild impairment

Adults: 200 mg twice a day.

Moderate to Severe Impairment

Contraindicated.

CONTRAINDICATIONS

Hypersensitivity to abacavir or its components.
Moderate to severe hepatic impairment.

INTERACTIONS

Drug

Ethanol: Increased abacavir levels.
Methadone: Methadone levels may be increased.

Herbal

None known.

Food

None known.

SIDE EFFECTS

Frequent

Adults: Nausea, nausea with vomiting, diarrhea, decreased appetite.
Children: Nausea with vomiting, fever, headache, diarrhea, rash.

Occasional

Adults: Insomnia.
Children: Decreased appetite.

SERIOUS REACTIONS

- A hypersensitivity reaction may be life threatening. Signs and symptoms include fever, rash, fatigue, intractable nausea and vomiting, severe diarrhea, abdominal pain, cough, pharyngitis, and dyspnea.
- Life-threatening hypotension may occur.
- Lactic acidosis and severe hepatomegaly may occur.

PRECAUTIONS & CONSIDERATIONS

Serious and sometimes fatal hypersensitivity reactions have been associated with abacavir therapy. Hypersensitivity reactions to abacavir may be characterized by constitutional symptoms such as achiness, fatigue, or generalized malaise; fever; GI symptoms, including abdominal pain, diarrhea, nausea, or vomiting; rash; and respiratory symptoms, including cough, dyspnea, or pharyngitis. Abacavir therapy should be discontinued if hypersensitivity is suspected. Abacavir therapy should never be restarted following a hypersensitivity reaction. A Med Guide and warning card that provide information about recognition of hypersensitivity reactions should be dispensed with each new prescription and refill. Screen all patients before initiation of abacavir therapy for the presence of the *HLA-B*5701* allele. Patients showing a positive result should have an abacavir allergy recorded and should **NOT** receive the medication; use in *HLA-B*5701*-positive patients is not recommended and is considered only with close medical supervision and under exceptional circumstances when the potential benefit outweighs the risk. Data are not conclusive, but one epidemiologic study suggested patients taking abacavir may have a greater risk of MI than do patients receiving other antiviral nucleosides. Use caution in patients with heart disease or heart risk factors. Lactic acidosis and severe hepatomegaly with steatosis, including fatal cases, have been reported with the use of nucleoside analogs alone or in combination, including abacavir and other antiretrovirals. Fat redistribution has also been observed in patients receiving antiretroviral therapy. It is unknown if abacavir is harmful in pregnancy. An Antiretroviral Pregnancy Registry is available at 1-800-258-4263. It is unknown if abacavir is excreted in human milk, but the drug is secreted into the milk of lactating rats. Because of both the potential for HIV transmission and the potential for serious adverse reactions in nursing infants, mothers should be instructed not to breastfeed.

Storage

Store at room temperature. Abacavir solution may also be stored in the refrigerator, but it should be protected from freezing.

Administration

Abacavir may be taken with or without food. Abacavir should always be used in combination with other antiretroviral agents. However, do not give with Epzicom or Trizivir, which both contain abacavir and result in duplication and overdosage.

Abciximab

ab-six'ih-mab

★ ReoPro

CATEGORY AND SCHEDULE

Pregnancy Risk Category: C

Classification: Monoclonal antibodies, platelet inhibitors, platelet glycoprotein IIb/IIIa inhibitor

MECHANISM OF ACTION

A glycoprotein IIb/IIIa receptor inhibitor that rapidly inhibits platelet aggregation by preventing the binding of fibrinogen to GP IIb/IIIa receptor sites on platelets. *Therapeutic Effect:* Prevents platelet aggregation. Prevents acute cardiac ischemic complications.

PHARMACOKINETICS

Rapidly cleared from plasma. Initial-phase half-life is < 10 min;

second-phase half-life is 30 min. Platelet function generally returns within 48 h.

AVAILABILITY

Injection: 2 mg/mL (5-mL vial).

INDICATIONS AND DOSAGES

▸ Percutaneous coronary intervention (PCI)

IV

Adults. 0.25 mg/kg IV bolus 10-60 min before PCI, then continuous IV infusion of 0.125 mcg/kg/min (maximum 10 mcg /min) for 12 h.

▸ Unstable angina when PCI is planned within 24 h

IV

Adults. 0.25 mg/kg, followed by 18- to 24-h infusion of 10 mcg/min, ending 1 h after procedure.

CONTRAINDICATIONS

Active internal bleeding, arteriovenous malformation or aneurysm, bleeding diathesis, history of cerebrovascular accident (CVA) within the past 2 yr or CVA with residual neurologic defect, hypersensitivity to any product component or to murine proteins, oral anticoagulant use within the past 7 days unless PT is ≤ 1.2 times control, history of vasculitis, intracranial neoplasm, prior IV dextran use before or intent to use during PTCA, recent surgery or trauma (within the past 6 wks), recent (within the past 6 wks or less) GI or genitourinary bleeding, thrombocytopenia (≤ 100,000 cells/μL), and severe uncontrolled hypertension.

INTERACTIONS

Drug

Anticoagulants, including heparin, and thrombolytics: May increase risk of hemorrhage.

Platelet aggregation inhibitors (such as aspirin, clopidogrel, dextran): May increase risk of bleeding.

Herbal

None known.

Food

None known.

DIAGNOSTIC TEST EFFECTS

Increases activated clotting time (ACT), aPTT, and PT. Decreases platelet count.

IV INCOMPATIBILITIES

Administer in separate line; no other medication should be added to infusion solution.

SIDE EFFECTS

Frequent (> 10%)

Nausea (16%), hypotension (12%), back pain (17%), chest pain (11%).

Occasional (4%-9%)

Vomiting, minor bleeding, headache.

Rare (< 4%)

Bradycardia, confusion, dizziness, pain, peripheral edema, thrombocytopenia, urinary tract infection.

SERIOUS REACTIONS

- Major bleeding complications may occur. If complications occur, stop the infusion immediately. Major bleeding can include intracranial hemorrhage and stroke.
- Hypersensitivity reaction may occur.
- Thrombocytopenia may be severe in up to 1% of patients.

PRECAUTIONS & CONSIDERATIONS

Caution is warranted with persons who weigh < 75 kg, those who are over age 65, those who have a history of GI disease, and those who are receiving aspirin, heparin, or thrombolytics. Also use abciximab cautiously in those who have had a PTCA within 12 h of the onset of signs and symptoms of acute myocardial infarction, who have had a prolonged PTCA (≥ 70 min), or who have had a failed PTCA because they are at increased risk for bleeding. It is unknown whether abciximab is distributed in breast milk. Safety and efficacy have not been established in children. There is an increased risk of bleeding in elderly patients. An electric razor and soft toothbrush should be used to prevent bleeding.

Notify the physician of signs of bleeding, including black or red stool, coffee-ground emesis, red or dark urine, or red-speckled mucus from cough. Assess for preexisting blood abnormalities, aPTT, platelet count, and PT before abciximab infusion, 2-4 h after treatment, and 24 h after treatment or before discharge, whichever is first. Signs and symptoms of hemorrhage, including a decrease in BP, increase in pulse rate, abdominal or back pain, and severe headache, should be monitored. Laboratory test results, including ACT, aPTT, platelet count, and PT, should also be assessed. Females' menstrual discharge should be determined and monitored for increase.

Storage

Store unopened vials refrigerated at 35.6-46.6° F. Do not freeze. Do not shake.

Administration

Solution for injection normally appears clear and colorless. Do not shake. Discard any unused portion or any preparation that contains opaque particles. Avoid IM injections and venipunctures; also avoid using indwelling urinary catheters and nasogastric tubes. Expect to discontinue heparin 4 h before the arterial sheath is removed. Stop abciximab and heparin infusion if serious bleeding uncontrolled by pressure occurs.

For the IV bolus, withdraw the necessary amount into a syringe. Filter the bolus injection using a sterile, nonpyrogenic, low protein-binding 0.25- or 5-μm syringe filter. For the IV infusion, withdraw the neccessary amount into a syringe. Inject into 250 mL of sterile 0.9% NaCl or D5W (for example, 10 mg in 250 mL equals a concentration of 40 mcg/mL). Filter either upon admixture using a sterile, nonpyrogenic, low protein-binding 0.2- or 5-μm syringe filter OR upon administration using an in-line, sterile, nonpyrogenic, low protein-binding 0.2- or 0.22-μm filter. Infuse at the calculated rate via a continuous infusion pump. Discard any unused portion at the end of the infusion. Give in separate IV line; do not add other medications to infusion. While femoral artery sheath is in position, maintain patient on complete bed rest with the head of bed elevated at 30 degrees. Maintain the affected limb in straight position. After the sheath has been removed, apply femoral pressure for 30 min, either manually or mechanically; then apply a pressure dressing. Bed rest should be maintained for 6-8 h after the sheath is removed or the drug is discontinued, whichever is later.

Acamprosate

ah-cam′pro-sate

Campral

CATEGORY AND SCHEDULE

Pregnancy Risk Category: C

Classification: Alcohol-abuse deterrent

MECHANISM OF ACTION

Actual mechanism unknown; may facilitate balance between GABA and glutamate neurotransmitter systems in the CNS to decrease alcohol craving.

PHARMACOKINETICS

Partially absorbed from the GI tract. Steady-state levels reached within 5 days of dosing; Protein binding negligible. *Half-life:* 20-33 h. Does not undergo metabolism; excreted unchanged in urine.

AVAILABILITY

Tablets, Enteric-Coated: 333 mg.

INDICATIONS AND DOSAGES

▸ **Maintenance of alcohol abstinence in alcohol-dependent patients who are abstinent at initiation of treatment**

PO

Adults, Elderly. 666 mg three times a day with or without food.

▸ **Dosage in renal impairment**

CrCl 30-49 mL/min: Decrease to 333 mg PO three times a day.

CrCl ≤ 30 mL/min: Contraindicated.

CONTRAINDICATIONS

Hypersensitivity.

Severe renal impairment (creatinine clearance of ≤ 30 mL/min).

INTERACTIONS

Drug

Antidepressants: May cause weight gain or loss.

Naltrexone: May increase acamprosate exposure, but no dose adjusment recommended.

Herbal

None known.

Food

None known.

DIAGNOSTIC TEST EFFECTS

None known.

SIDE EFFECTS

Frequent (17%)

Diarrhea.

Occasional (4%-6%)

Insomnia, asthenia, fatigue, anxiety, flatulence, nausea, depression, pruritus.

Rare (1%-3%)

Dizziness, anorexia, paraesthesia, diaphoresis, dry mouth.

SERIOUS REACTIONS

- Suicidal ideation/suicide attempts.

PRECAUTIONS & CONSIDERATIONS

Be aware that acamprosate does not eliminate or diminish withdrawal symptoms. Acamprosate helps maintain abstinence only when used as part of a treatment program that includes counseling and support. Use during pregnancy or breastfeeding only if benefit exceeds risk; drug has been teratogenic in animal studies and the drug is excreted in the milk of rats at concentrations similiar to those of blood; unknown if excreted in human milk. The safety and efficacy of acamprosate have not been established in children. Age-related renal impairment may require a dosage adjustment in elderly patients. Dizziness may occur. Avoid tasks that require mental alertness or motor skills until response to the drug has been established. Watch for unusual changes in mood or behavior as adverse events related to suicidal tendencies sometimes noted.

BUN and serum creatinine levels should be obtained before beginning treatment. Pattern of daily bowel activity should be assessed during therapy.

Storage

Store at room temperature.

Administration

Do not crush or break enteric-coated tablets. Take acamprosate without regard to food. However, persons who regularly eat three meals a day may be more compliant with the drug regimen if instructed to take acamprosate with food.

Treatment is initiated as soon as possible after the period of EtOH withdrawal, when the patient is abstinent, and is maintained even if the patient relapses.

Acarbose

a-car′bose

Precose Glucobay

Do not confuse Precose with PreCare.

CATEGORY AND SCHEDULE

Pregnancy Risk Category: B

Classification: Oral antidiabetic agents, α-glucosidase inhibitors

MECHANISM OF ACTION

An α-glucosidase inhibitor that delays digestion of carbohydrates, resulting in a smaller rise in blood glucose concentration after meals. *Therapeutic Effect:* Lowers postprandial hyperglycemia.

PHARMACOKINETICS

Limited (< 2%) oral absorption, absorbed dose excreted in urine, metabolized in the GI tract and major portion of dose excreted in feces; systemic exposure increased sixfold in subjects with severe renal impairment.

AVAILABILITY

Tablets: 25 mg, 50 mg, 100 mg.

INDICATIONS AND DOSAGES

▸ **Diabetes Mellitus Type 2**

Use as single drug or in combination with insulin or oral hypoglycemics (sulfonylureas, metformin) when diet is ineffective in controlling blood glucose levels.

PO

Adults, Elderly. Initially, 25 mg 3 times a day with first bite of each main meal. Increase at 4- to 8-wk intervals. Maximum: For patients weighing more than 60 kg, 100 mg 3 times a day; for patients weighing 60 kg or less, 50 mg 3 times a day.

CONTRAINDICATIONS

Chronic intestinal diseases associated with marked disorders of digestion or absorption, cirrhosis, colonic ulceration, conditions that may deteriorate as a result of increased gas formation in the intestine, diabetic ketoacidosis, hypersensitivity to acarbose, inflammatory bowel disease, partial intestinal obstruction or predisposition to intestinal obstruction, significant renal dysfunction (serum creatinine level ≥ 2 mg/dL).

INTERACTIONS

Drug

Digestive enzymes, intestinal absorbents (such as charcoal): Reduces effects of acarbose; avoid concomitant use.

Digoxin: May affect bioavailability of oral digoxin, and dose adjustment may be needed.

Herbal

None known.

Food

None known.

DIAGNOSTIC TEST EFFECTS

May increase AST (SGOT) and ALT levels (SGPT).

SIDE EFFECTS

Side effects diminish in frequency and intensity over time.

Frequent

Transient GI disturbances: flatulence (77%), diarrhea (33%), abdominal pain (21%).

SERIOUS REACTIONS

- Elevated liver transaminases may occur. May cause jaundice.

PRECAUTIONS & CONSIDERATIONS

Caution is warranted with fever or infection and in those who have had surgery or trauma because these states may cause loss of glycemic control. Acarbose use is not recommended during pregnancy. It is unknown if acarbose is distributed in breast milk. Safety and efficacy have not been established in children. Hypoglycemia may be difficult to recognize in the elderly.

Food intake and blood glucose should be monitored before and during therapy. A 1-h postprandial glucose may be helpful in optimizing dosage during initial treatment. Glycosylated hemoglobin and AST (SGOT) levels should also be assessed. Consult the physician when glucose demands are altered (such as with fever, heavy physical activity, infection, stress, trauma). Exercise, good personal hygiene (including foot care), not smoking, and weight control are essential parts of therapy. Patients should be advised to have oral glucose (dextrose) available to treat hypoglycemia if also treated with a sulfonylurea or insulin, since, acarbose delays/inhibits breakdown of table sugar, making it ineffective for the rapid treatment of hypoglycemia.

Storage

Do not store above 25° C (77° F). Protect from moisture. Keep container tightly closed.

Administration

Take acarbose with the first bite of each main meal. Do not skip or delay meals. If a meal is skipped, then the acarbose dose for that meal should be omitted.

Acebutolol

a-se-byoo'toe-lole

Sectral

Novo-Acebutolol, Rhotral

CATEGORY AND SCHEDULE

Pregnancy Risk Category: B (D if used in second or third trimester)

Classification: Antiadrenergics, β-blocking antihypertensives, antiarrhythmics, class II

MECHANISM OF ACTION

A β_1-adrenergic blocker that competitively blocks β_1-adrenergic receptors in cardiac tissue. Reduces the rate of spontaneous firing of the sinus pacemaker and delays AV conduction. *Therapeutic Effect:* Slows heart rate, decreases cardiac output, decreases BP, and exhibits antiarrhythmic activity.

PHARMACOKINETICS

Route	Onset	Peak	Duration
PO (hypotensive)	1-1.5 h	2-8 h	24 h

Well absorbed from the GI tract. Protein binding: 26%. Undergoes extensive first-pass liver metabolism to active metabolite. Eliminated via bile, secreted into GI tract via intestine, and excreted in urine. Removed by hemodialysis. *Half-life:* 3-4 h; metabolite, 8-13 h.

AVAILABILITY
Capsules: 200 mg, 400 mg.

INDICATIONS AND DOSAGES
▸ **Mild to moderate hypertension**
PO
Adults. Initially, 400 mg/day in 1 or 2 divided doses. Range: Up to 1200 mg/day in 2 divided doses. Usual maintenance: 400-800 mg/day.
Elderly. Initially, 200-400 mg/day. Maximum: 800 mg/day.
▸ **Ventricular arrhythmias**
PO
Adults. Initially, 200 mg q12h. Increase gradually to 600-1200 mg/day in 2 divided doses.
Elderly. Initially, 200-400 mg/day. Maximum: 800 mg/day.
▸ **Dosage in renal impairment**
Dosage is modified based on creatinine clearance.

Creatinine % Clearance (mL/min)	Usual Dosage
25-49	Reduce dose by 50%
< 25	Reduce dose by 75%

OFF-LABEL USES
Treatment of chronic angina pectoris, post-myocardial infarction.

CONTRAINDICATIONS
Cardiogenic shock, second- and third-degree heart block, overt heart failure, severe bradycardia.

INTERACTIONS
Drug
Diuretics, other antihypertensives, especially catecholamine-depleting drugs: May increase hypotensive effect of acebutolol.
Antidiabetic agents: May mask symptoms of hypoglycemia and prolong hypoglycemic effect of insulin and oral hypoglycemics.
α-adrenergic agonists: Increased risk of hypertensive reaction.
NSAIDs: May blunt antihypertensive response.
Herbal
None known.
Food
None known.

DIAGNOSTIC TEST EFFECTS
May increase antinuclear antibody titer and alkaline phosphatase, bilirubin, BUN, serum creatinine, HDL, lipoproteins, potassium, AST (SGOT), ALT (SGPT), triglyceride, and uric acid levels.

SIDE EFFECTS
Frequent
Hypotension manifested as dizziness, nausea, diaphoresis, headache, cold extremities, fatigue, constipation, or diarrhea.
Occasional
Insomnia, urinary frequency, impotence or decreased libido.
Rare
Rash, arthralgia, myalgia, confusion (especially in elderly patients), altered taste.

SERIOUS REACTIONS
- Overdose may produce profound bradycardia and may cause heart failure symptoms.
- Abrupt withdrawal may result in diaphoresis, palpitations, headache, and tremors.
- Abrupt withdrawal may cause severe effects such as to precipitate CHF or MI in patients with heart disease; thyroid storm in those with thyrotoxicosis.
- Hypoglycemia may occur in patients with previously controlled diabetes. May mask select symptoms of hypoglycemia such as tachycardia.
- Thrombocytopenia, with unusual bleeding or bruising, occurs rarely.

PRECAUTIONS & CONSIDERATIONS

Caution is warranted with bronchospastic disease, diabetes, hyperthyroidism, impaired renal or hepatic function, inadequate cardiac function, and peripheral vascular disease. Acebutolol readily crosses the placenta and is distributed in breast milk. Acebutolol use should be avoided in pregnant women after the first trimester because it may result in low-birth-weight infants. The drug may also produce apnea, bradycardia, hypoglycemia, or hypothermia during childbirth. No age-related precautions have been noted in children, and dosages have not been established. Use cautiously in elderly patients, who may have age-related peripheral vascular disease. Beta-blockade can precipitate or aggravate the symptoms of arterial insufficiency in patients with peripheral or mesenteric vascular disease.
Be aware that salt and alcohol intake should be restricted. Nasal decongestants or OTC cold preparations (stimulants) should not be used without physician approval.

Monitor BP for hypotension; respiratory status for shortness of breath; pattern of daily bowel activity and stool consistency; ECG for arrhythmias; and pulse for quality, rate, and rhythm during treatment. If pulse rate is 60 beats/min or lower or systolic BP is < 90 mm Hg, withhold the medication and cantact the physician. Sings and symptoms of CHF, such as excessive fatigue, prolonged dizziness, decreased urine output, distended neck veins, dyspnea (particularly on exertion or lying down), night cough, peripheral edema, and sudden weight gain should also be assessed. Notify physician if these occur.

Storage
Store at room temperature.
Administration
Acebutolol may be taken without regard to meals. Do not abruptly discontinue the drug.

Acetaminophen

ah-seet'ah-min-oh-fen
★ Apra, Feverall, Genapap, Mapap, Tylenol, Tylenol Extra Strength, Tylenol Arthritis Pain, Tylenol Meltaways 🍁 Atasol, Tempra
Do not confuse with Fiorinal, Hycodan, Indocin, Percodan, or Tuinal.

CATEGORY AND SCHEDULE

Pregnancy Risk Category: B
OTC

Classification: Analgesics, nonnarcotic, antipyretics

MECHANISM OF ACTION

A central analgesic whose exact mechanism is unknown but appears to inhibit prostaglandin synthesis in the CNS and, to a lesser extent, block pain impulses through peripheral action. Acetaminophen acts centrally on the hypothalamic heat-regulating center, producing peripheral vasodilation (heat loss, sweating). *Therapeutic Effect:* Results in antipyresis. Produces analgesic effect.

PHARMACOKINETICS

Route	Onset	Peak	Duration
PO	15-30 min	1-1.5 h	4-6 h

Rapidly, completely absorbed from GI tract; rectal absorption variable.

Protein binding: 20%-50%. Widely distributed to most body tissues. Metabolized in liver; excreted in urine. Removed by hemodialysis. *Half-life:* 1-4 h (half-life is increased in those with liver disease, elderly, neonates; decreased in children).

AVAILABILITY

Caplet: 500 mg.
Caplet, Extended Release: 650 mg.
Capsule: 500 mg.
Oral Solution: 160 mg/5 mL
Oral Solution, Extra Strength: 500 mg/15 mL.
Oral Solution, Infant Drops: 80 mg/0.8 mL
Rectal Suppository: 80 mg, 120 mg, 325 mg, 650 mg.
Oral Suspension: 160 mg/5 mL.
Oral Suspension, Infant Drops: 80 mg/0.8 mL.
Tablet: 325 mg, 500 mg.
Tablet, Chewable: 80 mg, 160 mg.
Tablet, Disintegrating: 80 mg, 160 mg.

INDICATIONS AND DOSAGES

▸ **Analgesia and antipyresis**

PO

Adults, Elderly. 325-650 mg q4-6h or 1 g 3-4 times/day. Maximum: 4 g/day.
Children. 10-15 mg/kg/dose q4-6h as needed. Maximum: 5 doses/24 h.
Neonates. 10-15 mg/kg/dose q6-8h as needed.

Rectal

Adults. 650 mg q4-6h. Maximum: 6 doses/24 h.
Children. 10-15 mg/kg/dose q4-6h as needed. Maximum: no more than 6 doses/24 h and not to exceed 75 mg/kg/day.
Neonates. 10-15 mg/kg/dose q6-8h as needed.

CONTRAINDICATIONS

Hypersensitivity. Also, self-treatment is not recommended by those with active alcoholism, liver disease, or viral hepatitis, all of which increase the risk of hepatotoxicity.

INTERACTIONS

Drug

Alcohol (chronic use), hepatotoxic medications (e.g., phenytoin), liver-enzyme inducers (e.g., cimetidine): May increase risk of hepatotoxicity with prolonged high dose or single toxic dose.
Warfarin: Most data indicate significant interaction not likely; however, any time a new medication, such as acetaminophen, is added and taken regularly, INR monitoring is recommended.

Herbal

Chaparral: Potential hepatotoxicity; avoid use.
Comfrey: Potential hepatotoxicity; avoid use.

DIAGNOSTIC TEST EFFECTS

May increase serum bilirubin, SGOT (AST), and SGPT (ALT). Therapeutic serum level: 10-30 mcg/mL; toxic serum level: > 200 mcg/mL at 4 h post acute ingestion. Must use nomogram to determine risk of toxicity. During chronic supratherapeutic use, toxicity is usually assumed if level is > 10 mcg/mL and AST or ALT elevated.

SIDE EFFECTS

Rare

Hypersensitivity reaction.

SERIOUS REACTIONS

Hepatotoxicity

- Acetaminophen toxicity is the primary serious reaction.
- Early signs and symptoms of acetaminophen toxicity include

anorexia, nausea, diaphoresis, and generalized weakness within the first 12 to 24 h.

• Later signs of acetaminophen toxicity include vomiting, right upper quadrant tenderness, and elevated liver function tests within 48-72 h after ingestion.

• The antidote to acute acetaminophen toxicity is acetylcysteine (Mucomyst), and it should be administered as soon as possible following toxic dose.

PRECAUTIONS & CONSIDERATIONS

While acute overdose may cause severe hapatic toxicity, chronic overuse of acetaminophen may also cause significant liver injury. Caution is warranted with liver disease, G6PD deficiency, phenylketonuria, sensitivity to acetaminophen, and severe impaired renal function. Adult dose should not exceed 4 g per day. Chronic alcoholics should limit intake to 2 g or less per day. Acetaminophen crosses the placenta and is distributed in breast milk. Acetaminophen is routinely used in all stages of pregnancy and appears safe for short-term use. There are no age-related precautions noted in children or in elderly patients. Be aware that children may receive repeat doses 4-5 times a day to a maximum of 5 doses in 24 h. Withhold the drug and contact the physician if respirations are 12/min or lower (20/min or lower in children).

Consult with the physician before using acetaminophen in children under 2 yr of age; oral use for more than 5 days in children, more than 10 days in adults, or fever lasting more than 3 days. Severe or recurrent pain or high, continuous fever, which may indicate a serious illness, should be monitored.

Storage

Store at room temperature. Avoid high heat, excessive humidity, and freezing. Suppositories may be refrigerated if needed; do not freeze.

Administration

Take oral acetaminophen without regard to meals. Tablets may be crushed.

For rectal use, remove wrapper and moisten suppository with cold water before inserting well up into the rectum.

Acetazolamide

ah-seat-ah-zole′ah-myd

Diamox, Diamox Sequels

Acetazolam

Do not confuse with acetohexamide.

CATEGORY AND SCHEDULE

Pregnancy Risk Category: C

Classification: Diuretic, anticonvulsant, carbonic anhydrase inhibitors

MECHANISM OF ACTION

A carbonic anhydrase inhibitor that reduces formation of hydrogen and bicarbonate ions from carbon dioxide and water by inhibiting, in proximal renal tubule, the enzyme carbonic anhydrase, thereby promoting renal excretion of sodium, potassium, bicarbonate, water. *Ocular:* Reduces rate of aqueous humor formation, lowers intraocular pressure. *Therapeutic Effect:* Produces anticonvulsant activity by retarding neuronal conduction in the brain; produces a diuretic effect generally.

PHARMACOKINETICS

SR: Absorption 3-6 h; onset 2 h; peak activity attained 3-6 h; duration 18-24 h.
IR: Absorption 1-4 h; onset 1-1.5 h; peak activity attained 1-4 h; duration 8-12 h.
IV: Onset 2 min; peak activity attained 15 min; duration 4-5 h. Excreted unchanged in urine. Removed by hemodialysis. *Half-life:* 2.4-5.8 h.

AVAILABILITY

Capsules, Sustained Release: 500 mg (Diamox Sequels).
Powder for Injection; Lyophilized: 500 mg.
Tablets: 125 mg, 250 mg.

INDICATIONS AND DOSAGES

▸ **Chronic simple (open-angle) glaucoma**

PO

Adults. 250 mg 1-4 times/day, not to exceed 1 g/day. *Extended-Release:* 500 mg 1-2 times/day usually given in morning and evening, not to exceed 1 g/day.

▸ **Secondary glaucoma, preop treatment of closed-angle glaucoma (short term)**

PO

Adults. Initially 500 mg; then 125-250 mg q4h.

IV

Adults. 500 mg IV for acute lowering of IOP in patients unable to take PO. If needed, may repeat the dose in 2-4 h.

▸ **Drug-induced edema**

PO/IV

Adults. 250-375 mg daily for 1-2 days, alternating with a day of rest.

▸ **Epilepsy**

PO

Adults. Optimum range is 375-1000 mg/day in 1-4 divided doses, unless given with another anticonvulsant therapy where initial dosage should be 250 mg/day.

▸ **Acute mountain sickness**

PO

Adults. 500-1000 mg/day in divided doses using tablets or sustained release capsules. If possible, begin 24-48 h before ascent; continue at least 48 h at high altitude.

▸ **Diuresis in CHF**

PO/IV

Adults. Initially 250-375 mg (5 mg/kg) every morning, then given on alternate days or for 2 days alternating with 1 day of rest. Use lowest effective dosage.

▸ **Dosage in renal impairment (immediate release products only)**

Creatinine Clearance (mL/min)	Dosage Interval
10-50	q12h
Less than 10	Avoid use

CONTRAINDICATIONS

Hypersensitivity to acetazolamide, product components, or to other sulfonamides; severe renal disease, hepatic cirrhosis, decreased sodium or potassium serum levels, adrenal insufficiency, hypochloremic acidosis, severe pulmonary obstruction with increased risk of acidosis. Long-term use is contraindicated in patients with chronic noncongestive angle-closure glaucoma.

INTERACTIONS

Drug (not limited to the following)

Phenytoin: May increase serum concentrations of phenytoin.
Primidone: May decrease serum concentrations of primidone.
Quinidine: May decrease urinary excretion of quinidine and increase effects.
Salicylates: May increase risk of acetazolamide accumulation and toxicity including CNS depression and metabolic acidosis.

Herbal and Food
None known.

DIAGNOSTIC TEST EFFECTS

May increase ammonia, bilirubin, glucose, chloride, uric acid, calcium. May decrease bicarbonate, potassium. May cause false-positive results for urinary protein with Albustix®, Labstix®, Albutest®, Bumintest®; interferes with HPLC theophylline assay and uric acid assay.

IV INCOMPATIBILITIES

Multivitamin injection, TPN.

IV COMPATIBILITIES

Dextran, pantoprazole (Protonix), ranitidine (Zantac).

SIDE EFFECTS

Frequent
Drowsiness, dizziness; loss of appetite; transient myopia; unusually tired/weak; increased urination/frequency; altered taste (metallic); nausea; numbness or tingling in extremities, lips, mouth.
Occasional
Depression, drowsiness, skin rash; uticaria.
Rare
Photosensitivity, confusion, tinnitus, severe muscle weakness, bruising; hearing disturbances.

SERIOUS REACTIONS

- Long-term therapy may result in acidosis.
- Nephrotoxicity/hepatotoxicity occurs occasionally, manifested as dark urine/stools, pain in lower back, jaundice, dysuria, crystalluria, renal colic/calculi.
- Bone marrow depression may be manifested as aplastic anemia, thrombocytopenia, thrombocytopenic purpura, leukopenia, agranulocytosis, hemolytic anemia.
- Rare but serious hypersensitivity reactions similar to sulfonamides; Stevens–Johnson syndrome; toxic epidermal necrolysis and anaphylaxis.

PRECAUTIONS & CONSIDERATIONS

Advise patient to stop taking acetazolamide immediately and to contact his or her health care provider if any of the following symptoms occur: sore throat, unexplained fever, pallor, purpura, hematuria, unusual bleeding or bruising; blood in urine; tingling or tremors in hands or feet; hearing changes; flank or loin pain.

Caution is warranted in patients being treated for glaucoma; intraocular pressures should be measured and documented in the patient's record before starting therapy and periodically during therapy. When the patient is using acetazolamide to prevent symptoms from high altitude sickness, advise patient that if rapid ascent causes high altitude sickness, rapid descent is necessary.

It is unknown if acetazolamide crosses the placenta or is distributed in the breast milk. Safety and efficacy have not been established in children. Acetazolamide may cause drowsiness. Avoid alcohol and performing tasks that require mental alertness or motor skills. Patient should avoid unnecessary exposure to sunlight and artificial tanning.
Storage
Store oral dosage forms and unopened injection at room temperature. Reconstituted solution for injection may be stored up to 12 h at room temperature and for 3 days under refrigeration.
Administration
IM administration is not recommended because of pain secondary to the alkaline pH. Reconstitute with at least 5 mL of sterile water to provide a solution containing not more than

100 mg/mL. The preferred route is direct IV injection. Recommended rate of administration is 100-500 mg/min for IV push; not to exceed 500 mg/min. May further dilute if necessary in 50 mL of either D5W or 0.9% NaCl for IV infusion administration over 15-30 min. Do not administer if particulate matter, cloudiness, or discoloration is noted.

Give oral acetazolamide with food. Do not crush, chew, or swallow contents of long-acting capsule. Capsules may be opened and the contents sprinkled on soft food.

Acetic Acid

a-cee'tik as'id

★ Borofair, VoSol

Do not confuse with salicylic acid.

Classification: Anti-infectives, otics, dermatologic and bladder irrigation

MECHANISM OF ACTION

The mechanism by which acetic acid exerts its antibacterial and antifungal actions is unknown. *Therapeutic Effect:* Antibacterial and antifungal.

PHARMACOKINETICS

Unknown.

AVAILABILITY

Solution (Irrigation): 0.25%.
Solution (Otic): 2%.

INDICATIONS AND DOSAGES

▸ Superficial infections of the external auditory canal

TOPICAL (EXTERNAL OTIC)

Adults, Elderly, Children. Carefully remove all cerumen and debris to allow acetic acid to contact infected surfaces directly. To promote continuous contact, insert a wick saturated with acetic acid into the ear canal; the wick may also be saturated after insertion. Instruct the patient to keep the wick in for at least 24 h and to keep it moist by adding 3-5 drops of acetic acid every 4-6 h. The wick may be removed after 24 h, but the patient should continue to instill 5 drops of acetic acid 3 or 4 times daily thereafter, for as long as indicated. Dosing should be tapered gradually after apparent response to avoid relapse.

▸ Dermatologic irrigation

For irrigation of skin sites as required, usually a 0.25% solution used 2 or 3 times per day.

▸ Bladder irrigation

For continuous irrigation of the urinary bladder with 0.25% irrigation, the rate approximates urine flow rates or 500-1500 mL/24 h; for periodic irrigation of an indwelling catheter to maintain patency, about 50 mL of 0.25% irrigation is required.

CONTRAINDICATIONS

Hypersensitivity to acetic acid or any of the ingredients. Perforated tympanic membrane is frequently considered a contraindication to the use of any medication in the external ear canal.

DIAGNOSTIC TEST EFFECTS

None known.

SIDE EFFECTS

Occasional

Stinging or burning.

Rare

Local irritation, superinfection, hematuria.

SERIOUS REACTIONS

- Superinfection with prolonged use.
- Discontinue promptly if sensitization or irritation occurs.

PRECAUTIONS & CONSIDERATIONS
Acidosis may occur with systemic absorption of irrigation solution. It is unknown whether acetic acid crosses the placenta or is distributed into breast milk. No age-related precautions have been noted in children or the elderly. Discontinue otic solution if sensitization or irritation occurs.

Transient burning or stinging may be noted when first instilled into acutely inflamed areas.

Storage
Unopened irrigations and otic solution may be stored at room temperature. Once irrigation opened, use contents promptly. Policies usually dictate discarding open irrigation solution within 24-28 h.

Administration
Insert saturated wick of cotton into the ear canal and leave for at least 24 h, keeping moist by adding 3-5 drops every 4-6 h. For maintenance, instill drops as long as indicated.

Acetylcysteine
a-see-til-sis′tay-een
Acetadote, Mucomyst
Parvolex
Do not confuse acetylcysteine with acetylcholine.

CATEGORY AND SCHEDULE
Pregnancy Risk Category: B

Classification: Antidotes, mucolytics

MECHANISM OF ACTION
An intratracheal respiratory inhalant that splits the linkage of mucoproteins, reducing the viscosity of pulmonary secretions. Protects against acetaminophen-induced hepatotoxicity by maintaining or restoring glutathione levels or by acting as an alternate substrate for conjugation with, and thus detoxification of, the toxic acetaminophen reactive metabolite. *Therapeutic Effect:* Facilitates the removal of pulmonary secretions by coughing, postural drainage, mechanical means. Protects against acetaminophen overdose-induced hepatotoxicity.

PHARMACOKINETICS
Low oral bioavailability. *Half-life:* 11 h (newborns), 5.6 h (adults).

AVAILABILITY
Injection (Acetadote): 20% (200 mg/mL).
Inhalation Solution (Mucomyst): 10% (100 mg/mL), 20% (200 mg/mL).

INDICATIONS AND DOSAGES
▸ **Adjunctive treatment of viscid mucus secretions from chronic bronchopulmonary disease and for pulmonary complications of cystic fibrosis**

Nebulization
Adults, Elderly, Children. 3-5 mL (20% solution) 3-4 times a day or 6-10 mL (10% solution) 3-4 times a day. Range: 1-10 mL (20% solution) q2-6h or 2-20 mL (10% solution) q2-6h.
Infants. 1-2 mL (20%) or 2-4 mL (10%) 3-4 times a day.

▸ **Treatment of viscid mucus secretions in patients with a tracheostomy**

INTRATRACHEAL
Adults, Children. 1-2 mL of 10% or 20% solution instilled into tracheostomy q1-4h.

▸ **Acetaminophen overdose**

PO (ORAL SOLUTION 5%)
Adults, Elderly, Children. Loading dose of 140 mg/kg, followed in 4 h by maintenance dose of 70 mg/kg q4h for 17 additional doses (unless acetaminophen assay reveals nontoxic level). Repeat

dose if emesis occurs within 1 h of administration.
IV (ACETADOTE)
Adults, Elderly, Children. 150 mg/kg infused over 60 min, then 50 mg/kg infused over 4 h, then 100 mg/kg infused over 16 h.

OFF-LABEL USES

Prevention of renal damage from dyes given during certain diagnostic tests (such as CT scans).
PO or IV
Adults, Elderly. 600-1200 mg twice a day for 4 doses starting the day before the procedure.

CONTRAINDICATIONS

None known.

DIAGNOSTIC TEST EFFECTS

None known.

SIDE EFFECTS

Frequent
Inhalation: Stickiness on face, transient unpleasant odor.
Occasional
Inhalation: Increased bronchial secretions, throat irritation, nausea, vomiting, rhinorrhea.
IV: Nausea, vomiting, flushing, pruritus, rash, tachycardia.
Rare
Inhalation: Rash.
Oral: Facial edema, bronchospasm, wheezing.

SERIOUS REACTIONS

- Large doses may produce severe nausea and vomiting.
- Anaphylactoid reactions with flushing and erythema reported.

PRECAUTIONS & CONSIDERATIONS

Caution is warranted with bronchial asthma and in elderly or debilitated patients with severe respiratory insufficiency. Maintain adequate hydration. A disagreeable color may emanate from the solution during initial administration, but it disappears quickly.

If bronchospasm occurs, discontinue treatment; notify the physician. A bronchodilator may be needed. Assess respiratory rate, depth, rhythm, and type (such as abdominal or thoracic) and color, consistency, and amount of sputum.

Storage
Injectable solution: Store at room temperature. Following reconstitution with D5W, solution is stable for 24 h at room temperature. A color change may occur in opened vials (light purple) but does not affect the safety or efficacy.

Inhalation solution: Store at room temperature; once opened, store under refrigeration and use within 96 h. Use diluted solutions within 1 h. A color change may occur in opened vials (light purple) but does not affect the safety or efficacy.

Administration
To create the oral solution, dilute 20% solution with water or soft drinks to create a 5% concentration. Use within 1 h. Soft drinks and the use of a straw will best enhance palatability; water is best used if given via NG tube. When administering the solution by nebulizer, avoid contact with those parts of the equipment that contain copper, iron, or rubber because the drug will react with these materials on contact. For inhalation, may administer either undiluted or diluted with 0.9% NaCl.

For adults ≥ 40 kg: For IV use, give 3 infusions of different strengths: first dose (150 mg/kg) in 200 mL D5W and infused over 15 min, second dose (50 mg/kg) in 500 mL D5W and infused over 4 h, third dose (100 mg/kg) in 1000 mL D5W and infused over 16 h.

For children and adults < 40 kg: Dilutions are adjusted. Consult prescribing information.

Acitretin

a-si-tre′tin

Soriatane

CATEGORY AND SCHEDULE

Pregnancy Risk Category: X

Classification: Dermatologics, systemic retinoids, antipsoriatics

MECHANISM OF ACTION

A second-generation retinoid that adjusts factors influencing epidermal proliferation, RNA/DNA synthesis, controls glycoprotein, and governs immune response. *Therapeutic Effect:* Regulates keratinocyte growth and differentiation.

PHARMACOKINETICS

Well absorbed from the GI tract. Food increases the rate of absorption. Protein binding: > 99%. Metabolized in liver. Excreted in bile and urine. Not removed by hemodialysis. *Half-life:* 49 h. With alcohol consumption, acitretin is converted to etretinate, which has a half-life of 120 days.

AVAILABILITY

Capsules: 10 mg, 17.5 mg, 22.5 mg, 25 mg (Soriatane).

INDICATIONS AND DOSAGES

▸ Psoriasis

PO

Adults, Elderly. 25-50 mg/day as a single dose with main meal. Maintenance: 25-50 mg/day after the initial response is noted. Lower doses are required in patients receiving phototherapy. Continue until lesions have resolved.

OFF-LABEL USES

Treatment of nonpsoriatic dermatoses, keratinization disorders, Darier's disease, palmoplantar keratoses, lichen planus; children with lamellar ichthyosis, nonbullous and bullous ichthyosiform erythroderma, Sjögren-Larsson syndrome; should be prescribed only by physicians knowledgeable in the use of systemic retinoids.

CONTRAINDICATIONS

Pregnancy or those who intend to become pregnant within 3 yr following discontinuation of therapy, severely impaired liver or kidney function, chronic abnormal elevated lipid levels, concomitant use of methotrexate or tetracyclines, ingestion of alcohol (in females of reproductive potential), hypersensitivity to acitretin, etretinate, or other retinoids, sensitivity to parabens (used as preservative in gelatin capsule).

INTERACTIONS

Drug

Alcohol: May prevent elimination of acitretin by conversion of drug to etretinate. Females must *not* drink alcohol during or for 2 mo after stopping treatment with acitretin.
"Minipill" oral contraceptive: May interfere with contraceptive effect.
Methotrexate: May increase risk of hepatotoxicity. Contraindicated.
Tetracyclines: May increase risk of increased intracranial pressure. Contraindicated.
Sulfonylureas: May potentiate blood glucose lowering.
Phenytoin: May increase phenytoin free levels via decreased protien binding.
Vitamin A: May increase risk of vitamin A toxicity.

Herbal

St. John's wort: May increase risk of unplanned pregnancy as a result of lessening of effects of hormonal contraceptives.

Food
None known.

DIAGNOSTIC TEST EFFECTS

May increase triglycerides, SGOT (AST), SGPT (ALT). May decrease HDL (high density lipoprotein). May alter blood glucose control. Triglycerides and LFTs should be monitored at 1- to 2-wk intervals until response to drug is estabilished.

SIDE EFFECTS

Frequent
Lip inflammation, alopecia, skin peeling, shakiness, dry eyes, rash, hyperesthesia, paresthesia, sticky skin, dry mouth, epistaxis, dryness/thickening of conjunctiva.
Occasional
Eye irritation, brow and lash loss, sweating, chills, sensation of cold, flushing, edema, blurred vision, diarrhea, nausea, thirst.

SERIOUS REACTIONS

• Benign intracranial hypertension (pseudotumor cerebri) occurs rarely.
• Hepatotoxicity with clinical jaundice.
• Teratogen
• Ossification abnormalities.
• Thromboembolic risk.
• Hepatotoxicity with clinical jaundice.
• Night blindness.
• Potential for severe emotional lability or depression.

PRECAUTIONS & CONSIDERATIONS

Caution is warranted with impaired hepatic or renal function and in those with elevated cholesterol/triglycerides. Safety and efficacy have not been established in children. Be aware that acitretin should be avoided in elderly patients with renal impairment. Decreased tolerance to contact lenses may develop. Follow a cholesterol-free diet for best results. Depression and other psychiatric symptoms such as aggression or thoughts of self-harm have occurred during therapy with systemic retinoids, including acitretin. Significant changes in liver function tests occur in up to 1/3 of patients; monitor closely. Photosensitivity may occur.

Be aware that acitretin is contraindicated in pregnant women. Women should not take acitretin if pregnant or planning to become pregnant within the next 3 yr. Two pregnancy tests with negative results must be obtained before starting treatment. Two forms of birth control must be used for 1 mo before beginning with acitretin, during treatment, and 3 yr after treatment. Acitretin has teratogenic effects. An agreement/informed consent must be signed before treatment begins. Patients should not donate blood during and for at least 3 yr after completing acitretin therapy so that women of childbearing potential do not receive blood from patients receiving acetretin.
Storage
Store at room temperature. Protect from light and high humidity.
Administration
Give with main meal of the day or milk.

Acyclovir

ay-sye′kloe-ver
🍁 Zovirax
Do not confuse with Zostrix, Zyvox.

CATEGORY AND SCHEDULE

Pregnancy Risk Category: B

Classification: Antivirals

MECHANISM OF ACTION

A synthetic nucleoside that converts to acyclovir triphosphate, becoming part of the DNA chain. *Therapeutic Effect:* Interferes with DNA synthesis and viral replication. Virustatic.

PHARMACOKINETICS

Poorly absorbed from the GI tract; minimal absorption following topical application. Protein binding: 9%-36%. Widely distributed. Penetrates CSF levels roughly 13%-52% those of plasma. Partially metabolized unchanged in liver. Excreted primarily unchanged in urine. Removed by hemodialysis. *Half-life:* 2.5 h (increased in impaired renal function).

AVAILABILITY

Capsules: 200 mg.
Tablets: 400 mg, 800 mg.
Injection (lyophilized powder for reconstitution): 50 mg/mL once reconstituted.
Oral Suspension: 200 mg/5 mL.
Injection, Solution: 25 mg/mL.
Cream: 5%.
Ointment: 5%.

INDICATIONS AND DOSAGES

▸ **Genital herpes (initial episode)**
IV
Adults, Elderly, Children 12 yr and older. 5 mg/kg q8h for 5 days.
PO
Adults, Elderly, Children 12 yr and older. 200 mg q4h 5 times a day.
TOPICAL (OINTMENT)
Cover all lesions every 3 h, 6 times a day for 7 days. Begin as soon as signs and symptoms appear.

▸ **Genital herpes (recurrent)**
Less than 6 episodes per year:
PO
Adults, Elderly, Children 12 yr and older. 200 mg q4h 5 times a day for 5 days.
6 episodes or more per year:
PO
Adults, Elderly, Children 12 yr and older. 400 mg 2 times a day or 200 mg 3-5 times a day for up to 12 mo.

▸ **Herpes labialis (cold sores), recurrent**
TOPICAL (CREAM)
Adults, Children 12 yr and older. Apply 5 times per day for 4 days (i.e., during the prodrome or when lesions appear).

▸ **Herpes simplex mucocutaneous**
IV
Adults, Elderly, Children 12 yr and older. 5 mg/kg/dose q8h for 7 days.
Children younger than 12 yr. 10 mg/kg q8h for 7 days.

▸ **Herpes simplex neonatal**
IV
Children younger than 4 mo. 10 mg/kg q8h for 10 days.

▸ **Herpes simplex encephalitis**
IV
Adults, Elderly, Children 12 yr and older. 10 mg/kg q8h for 10 days.
Children 3 mo to younger than 12 yr. 20 mg/kg q8h for 10 days.

▸ **Herpes zoster (caused by varicella)**
IV
Adults, Elderly, Children 12 yr and older. 10 mg/kg q8h for 7 days.
Children younger than 12 yr. 20 mg/kg q8h for 7 days.

▸ **Herpes zoster (shingles)**
PO
Adults, Elderly, Children 12 yr and older. 800 mg q4h 5 times a day for 7-10 days.

▸ **Varicella (chickenpox)**
PO
Adults, Elderly, Children older than 12 yr or children 2-12 yr, weighing 40 kg or more. 800 mg 4 times a day for 5 days.
Children 2-12 yr, weighing < 40 kg. 20 mg/kg 4 times a day for 5 days. Maximum: 800 mg/dose.

▸ **Dosage in renal impairment**
Dosage and frequency are modified based on severity of infection and degree of renal impairment.
PO
If normal dose is 800 mg 5 times/day, decrease to 800 mg q12h. If normal dose is 200 mg 5 times/day or 400 mg q12h, decrease dose to 200 mg q12h.
IV

Creatinine Clearance (mL/min)	Dosage %	Dosage Interval
> 50	100	8 h
25-50	100	12 h
10-25	100	24 h
< 10	50	24 h

OFF-LABEL USES
Treatment of herpes simplex ocular infections, infectious mononucleosis.

CONTRAINDICATIONS
Hypersensitivity to acyclovir or valacyclovir.

INTERACTIONS
Drug
Nephrotoxic medications (such as aminoglycosides): May increase the risk of drug-induced nephrotoxicity.
Probenecid: May increase acyclovir half-life.

DIAGNOSTIC TEST EFFECTS
May increase BUN and serum creatinine concentrations.

IV INCOMPATIBILITIES
In general, do not mix any other drugs in an acyclovir syringe. Acyclovir has as many incompatibilities as compatibilities. Caution should be used with *any* administration at a Y-site. Ampicillin/Sulbactam (Unasyn), aztreonam (Azactam), caffeine citrate (Cafcit), cefepime (Maxipime), ciprofloxacin (Cipro), diazepam (Valium), diltiazem (Cardizem), dobutamine (Dobutrex), dopamine (Intropin), haloperidol lactate, hydroxyzine, levofloxacin (Levaquin), meropenem (Merrem IV), midazolam (Versed), nitroprusside, ondansetron (Zofran), pentamidine, phenytoin (Dilantin), piperacillin, potasium phosphate, quinupristin-dalfopristin (Synercid), tacrolimus (Prograf), tazobactam (Zosyn), TPN verapamil.

IV COMPATIBILITIES
Allopurinol (Alloprim), amikacin (Amikin), ampicillin, cefazolin (Ancef), cefotaxime (Claforan), ceftazidime (Fortaz), ceftriaxone (Rocephin), cimetidine (Tagamet), clindamycin (Cleocin), famotidine (Pepcid), fluconazole (Diflucan), gentamicin, heparin, hydromorphone (Dilaudid), imipenem (Primaxin), lorazepam (Ativan), magnesium sulfate, methylprednisolone (Solu-Medrol), metoclopramide (Reglan), metronidazole (Flagyl), morphine, multivitamins, potassium chloride, propofol (Diprivan), ranitidine (Zantac), vancomycin.

SIDE EFFECTS
Frequent
Parenteral (7%-9%): Phlebitis or inflammation at IV site, nausea, vomiting.
Topical ointment (28%): Burning, stinging.
Occasional
Parenteral (3%): Pruritus, rash, urticaria.
Oral (6%-12%): Malaise, nausea.
Topical ointment (4%): Pruritus.
Rare
Oral (1%-3%): Vomiting, rash, diarrhea, headache.
Parenteral (1%-2%): Confusion, hallucinations, seizures, tremors.
Topical (< 1%): Rash.

SERIOUS REACTIONS

- Rapid parenteral administration, excessively high doses, or fluid and electrolyte imbalance may produce renal failure exhibited by such signs and symptoms as abdominal pain, decreased urination, decreased appetite, increased thirst, nausea, and vomiting.
- Extravasation may cause tissue necrosis.

PRECAUTIONS & CONSIDERATIONS

Caution is warranted with concurrent use of nephrotoxic agents, dehydration, fluid and electrolyte imbalance, neurologic abnormalities, or renal or hepatic impairment. Acyclovir crosses the placenta and is distributed in breast milk. In the elderly, age-related renal impairment may require dosage adjustment. Females should have a Pap smear at least annually because of the increased risk of cervical cancer in women with genital herpes. Avoid touching lesions with fingers to prevent spreading infection to new sites.

History of allergies, particularly to acyclovir, should be obtained before treatment. Herpes simplex lesions should be assessed before treatment to compare baseline with treatment effect. IV site should be assessed for signs and symptoms of phlebitis, including heat, pain, or red streaking over the vein. Cutaneous lesions should be evaluated for signs of effective drug treatment. Adequate ventilation as well as hydration should be maintained. Appropriate isolation precautions should be maintained in persons with chickenpox and disseminated herpes zoster.

Storage

Store capsules, tablets, cream, ointment, suspension at room temperature. Store vials at room temperature. Reconstituted vial solutions of 50 mg/mL will remain stable for 12 h at room temperature. Refrigeration of reconstituted solution may cause a precipitate that will redissolve at room temperature. IV infusion (piggyback) is stable for 24 h at room temperature. Yellow discoloration does not affect potency.

Administration

Oral: Shake suspension well before administration. Take without regard to food.

Topical: Use finger cot or rubber glove to apply topical acyclovir. Avoid eye contact.

IV: Add 10 mL sterile water for injection to each 500-mg vial or 20 mL sterile water for injection to each 1000-mg vial for final concentration of 50 mg/mL. Do not use bacteriostatic water for injection containing benzyl alcohol or parabens because this will cause a precipitate to form. Shake well until solution is clear. Further dilute with at least 100 mL D5W or 0.9% NaCl. Final concentration should be ≤ 7 mg/mL. Neonatal doses are usually diluted in preservative-free NS, to a concentration of 5 mg/mL.

Infuse over at least 1 h because renal tubular damage may occur with too-rapid administration. Maintain adequate hydration during infusion and for 2 h following IV administration. Use syringe pump for neonatal administration.

Adalimumab

Ah-dah-lim′you-mab

★ 🍁 Humira

Do not confuse with Humulin

CATEGORY AND SCHEDULE

Pregnancy Risk Category: B

Classification: Disease-modifying antirheumatic drugs, immunomodulators, monoclonal antibodies, tumor necrosis factor (TNF) modulators

MECHANISM OF ACTION

A monoclonal antibody that binds specifically to TNF-α, blocking its interaction with cell surface TNF receptors. *Therapeutic Effect:* Reduces inflammation, tenderness, and swelling for various inflammatory diseases; slows or prevents progressive destruction of joints in rheumatoid arthritis.

PHARMACOKINETICS

Time to peak serum concentration 131 h. *Half-life:* 10-20 days.

AVAILABILITY

Pediatric Injection: 20 mg/0.4 mL in prefilled syringes.
Injection: 40 mg/0.8 mL in prefilled syringes or prefilled pens.

INDICATIONS AND DOSAGES

▸ Ankylosing spondylitis

SC

Adults. 40 mg every other week.

▸ Crohn's disease

SC

Adults. 160 mg initially on day 1 (given as four 40-mg injections in 1 day or as two 40-mg injections per day for 2 consecutive days), followed by 80 mg 2 wks later (day 15). Two weeks later (day 29), begin a maintenance dosage of 40 mg every other week.

▸ Juvenile idiopathic arthritis

SC

Children 4-17 yr of age. Weight-based dosing. For patients weighing 15 kg to < 30 kg, the dose is 20 mg every other week. For patients weighing 30 kg or more, the dose is 40 mg every other week.

▸ Plaque psoriasis

SC

Adults. 80 mg initial dose (given as two 40-mg injections on day 1), followed by 40 mg every other week starting 1 wk after the initial dose.

▸ Psoriatic arthritis

SC

Adults. 40 mg every other week.

▸ Rheumatoid arthritis

SC

Adults, Elderly. 40 mg every other week. Dose may be increased to 40 mg/wk in those not taking methotrexate.

CONTRAINDICATIONS

Active infections.

INTERACTIONS

Drug

Abatacept: Concomitant use not recommended. Increased risk of serious infections with combined use.
Anakinra: Concomitant use not recommended. Increased risk of serious infections with combined use.
Methotrexate: Reduces the absorption of adalimumab by 29%-40%, but dosage adjustment is unnecessary if given concurrently.
Rilonacept: Concomitant use not recommended. Increased risk of serious infections with combined use.
Vaccines, live: Use not recommended. Altered immune response. Increased risk of secondary transmission of infection from vaccine.

DIAGNOSTIC TEST EFFECTS

May increase levels of blood cholesterol, other lipids, liver aminotransferases, creatine phosphokinase, and serum alkaline phosphatase.

SIDE EFFECTS

Frequent (20%)
Injection site reactions: erythema, pruritus, pain, and swelling.
Occasional (9%-12%)
Headache, rash, sinusitis, nausea.

Rare (5%-7%)
Abdominal or back pain, hypertension.

SERIOUS REACTIONS

- Rare reactions include hypersensitivity reactions, malignancies, neurologic events, respiratory tract infections, bronchitis, UTIs, and more serious infections (such as pneumonia, tuberculosis, cellulitus, pyelonephritis, and septic arthritis).

PRECAUTIONS & CONSIDERATIONS

Serious infections, sepsis, tuberculosis, and opportunistic infections have occurred during therapy with TNF blockers, including adalimumab. Patients should be screened for active or recent infection, tuberculosis risk factors, and latent tuberculosis infection before initiating therapy. Closely monitor patients developing an infection during therapy. Use of adalimumab may increase the risk of reactivation of hepatitis B virus in patients who are chronic carriers of the virus. Caution is warranted with cardiovascular disease, demyelinating disorders, history of sensitivity to monoclonal antibodies, preexisting or recent onset of CNS disturbances, in elderly patients, and in pregnant women. It is unknown whether adalimumab is excreted in breast milk. The safety and efficacy of adalimumab have not been established in children younger than 4 yr of age. Cautious use in the elderly is necessary because they are at increased risk for serious infection and malignancy. Avoid receiving live vaccines during adalimumab treatment. Syringe needle cover contains latex; avoid contact if sensitive to latex.

Laboratory values, particularly serum alkaline phosphatase levels, should be monitored before and during therapy. Therapeutic response, such as improved grip strength, increased joint mobility, reduced joint tenderness, and relief of pain, stiffness, and swelling, should also be assessed.

Storage
Refrigerate adalimumab. Do not freeze. Protect from light; store in original carton until administration.

Administration
For subcutaneous use, rotate injection sites on thighs and abdomen. Do not shake the injection. Administer each injection at least 1 inch from previous site. Never inject drug into bruised, hard, red, or tender areas. Do not inject within 2 inches of the navel. Discard any unused portion. Injection site reactions generally occur in the first month of treatment and decrease with continued therapy.

Adapalene

a-dap′ah-leen
★ 🍁 Differin

CATEGORY AND SCHEDULE

Pregnancy Risk category: C

Classification: Dermatologics, retinoids

MECHANISM OF ACTION

Binds to retinoic acid receptors in cell nuclei modulating cell differentiation, keratinization. Possesses anti-inflammatory properties. *Therapeutic Effect:* Normalizes differentiation of follicular epithelial cells.

PHARMACOKINETICS

Absorption through the skin is low. Trace amount found in plasma following topical application. Excreted primarily by biliary route.

AVAILABILITY

Gel: 0.1%, 0.3%.
Cream: 0.1%.

INDICATIONS AND DOSAGES

▸ **Acne vulgaris**

TOPICAL

Adults, Elderly, Children > 12 yr. Apply to affected area once daily at bedtime after washing.

CONTRAINDICATIONS

Hypersensitivity to adapalene, vitamin A, or any components. Do not use if patient has current sunburn. Wait until fully recovered.

INTERACTIONS

Drug

Quinolones, phenothiazines, sulfonamides, sulfonylureas, tetracyclines, thiazide diuretics: Adapalene may increase the effects of these photosensitizing agents.

Benzoyl peroxide, salicylic acid, sulfur, resorcinol, alcohol: Additive local irritation when used with adapalene.

DIAGNOSTIC TEST EFFECTS

None known.

SIDE EFFECTS

Frequent

Erythema, scaling, dryness, pruritus, burning (likely to occur first 2-4 wks, lessens with continued use).

Occasional

Skin irritation, stinging, sunburn, acne flares, erythema, photosensitivity, xerosis.

SERIOUS REACTIONS

• Concurrent use of other potential irritating topical products (soaps, cleansers, aftershave, cosmetics) may produce severe topical irritation.

PRECAUTIONS & CONSIDERATIONS

Caution is warranted for patients with eczema and seborrheic dermatitis. Adapalene has not been studied in pregnant women. It is unknown whether adapalene enters the breast milk. Safety and efficacy have not been established in children younger than 12 yr or in elderly patients.

A burning sensation, stinging, dryness, itching, or redness of the skin may occur, especially during the first month of use. Other skin products such as hair-removal products, shaving creams with a large amount of alcohol, other acne medications, and certain soaps and cleansers may irritate the skin while using adapalene. Minimize sun exposure.

Storage

Store at room temperature.

Administration

Apply a small amount as a thin film once a day, at least 1 h before bedtime. Apply the medicine to dry, clean areas affected by acne. Rub in gently and well. Avoid contact with eyes, lips, angles of the nose, and mucous membranes. Do not apply to cuts, abrasions, eczematous skin, or sunburned skin.

Adefovir Dipivoxil

ah-deh′foh-veer dye-piv-ox′-il

☆ 🍁 Hepsera

CATEGORY AND SCHEDULE

Pregnancy Risk Category: C

Classification: Antiretroviral, nucleoside reverse transcriptase inhibitor

MECHANISM OF ACTION

An antiviral that inhibits the enzyme DNA polymerase in the hepatitis B virus, causing DNA chain termination after its incorporation into viral DNA. *Therapeutic Effect:* Prevents replication of the hepatitis B virus.

PHARMACOKINETICS

Prodrug converted to adefovir. Excreted in urine. *Half-life:* 7 h (increased in impaired renal function).

AVAILABILITY

Tablets: 10 mg.

INDICATIONS AND DOSAGES

▸ **Chronic hepatitis B in patients with normal renal function**

PO

Adults, Elderly. 10 mg once a day.

▸ **Chronic hepatitis B in patients with impaired renal function (adults)**

Adults, Elderly with creatinine clearance 20-49 mL/min. 10 mg q48h.

Adults, Elderly with creatinine clearance 10-19 mL/min. 10 mg q72h.

Adults, Elderly on hemodialysis. 10 mg every 7 days following dialysis.

CONTRAINDICATIONS

Hypersensitivity.

INTERACTIONS

Drug

Ibuprofen: Increases adefovir bioavailability and plasma concentration.

Dofetilide, tenofovir: Adefovir competes for renal elimination, raising levels of these drugs. Do not use together,

Metformin: Adefovir may compete for renal elimination. May increase risk of lactic acidosis.

Nephrotoxic drugs: Watch for increased risk of renal effects.

DIAGNOSTIC TEST EFFECTS

May increase serum amylase, serum creatinine, AST (SGOT) and ALT (SGPT) levels.

SIDE EFFECTS

Frequent (13%)

Asthenia.

Occasional (4%-9%)

Headache, abdominal pain, nausea, flatulence.

Rare (3%)

Diarrhea, dyspepsia.

SERIOUS REACTIONS

- Nephrotoxicity (characterized by increased serum creatinine and decreased serum phosphorus levels) is a treatment-limiting toxicity of adefovir therapy.
- Lactic acidosis and severe hepatomegaly occur rarely, particularly in those who are overweight, in combination with other antiretrovirals, or in female patients.

PRECAUTIONS & CONSIDERATIONS

Caution is warranted with impaired renal function and known risk factors for liver disease and in elderly patients. Baseline renal function laboratory values should be obtained before therapy begins and routinely thereafter. Adjust adefovir dosage with preexisting renal insufficiency. Obtain HIV antibody assay before adefovir therapy begins because unrecognized or untreated HIV infection may result in an emergence of HIV resistance. Not approved for use in children less than 12 yr. It is not known if adefovir causes fetal harm during pregnancy. In general, breastfeeding while on treatment is not recommended.

! Notify the physician immediately if unusual muscle pain, stomach pain with nausea and vomiting, cold feeling in arms and legs, or dizziness occurs. These signs and symptoms may signal the onset of lactic acidosis. Notify physician if yellow skin color or yellowing of the whites of the eyes or other unusual signs or symptoms occur. Reliable forms of contraception should be used.

Storage

Store at room temperature.

Administration

Give adefovir without regard to food. Give as prescribed because there is a risk for developing serious hepatitis if the drug is stopped abruptly.

Adenosine

ah-den'oh-seen

Adenocard, Adenoscan

CATEGORY AND SCHEDULE

Pregnancy Risk Category: C

Classification: Antiarrhythmics, diagnostics, nonradioactive

MECHANISM OF ACTION

A cardiac agent that slows impulse formation in the SA node and conduction time through the AV node. Adenosine also acts as a diagnostic aid in myocardial perfusion imaging or stress echocardiography. *Therapeutic Effect:* Depresses left ventricular function and restores normal sinus rhythm.

PHARMACOKINETICS

Rapidly cleared from blood after IV administration, metabolized to cyclic AMP and inosine primarily by red blood cells and vascular endothelial cells. *AMP half-life:* < 10 seconds.

AVAILABILITY

Injection (Adenocard): 3 mg/mL in 2-mL, 4-mL syringes.

Injection (Adenoscan): 3 mg/mL in 20-mL, 30-mL vials.

INDICATIONS AND DOSAGES

▸ **Paroxysmal supraventricular tachycardia (PSVT)**

RAPID IV BOLUS

Adults, Elderly. Initially, 6 mg given over 1-2 seconds. If first dose does not convert within 1-2 min, give 12 mg; may repeat 12-mg dose in 1-2 min if no response has occurred.

Children. Initially 0.1 mg/kg (maximum: 6 mg). If ineffective, may give 0.2 mg/kg (maximum 12 mg).

▸ **Diagnostic testing**

IV INFUSION

Adults. 140 mcg/kg/min for 6 min.

CONTRAINDICATIONS

Atrial fibrillation or flutter, second- or third-degree AV block or sick sinus syndrome (except with functioning pacemaker), ventricular tachycardia.

INTERACTIONS

Drug

Carbamazepine: May increase degree of heart block caused by adenosine.

Dipyridamole: May increase effect of adenosine.

Methylxanthines (e.g., caffeine, theophylline): May decrease the effect of adenosine.

Food

Caffeine: May decrease effect of adenosine. Avoid dietary caffeine 12-24 h before adenosine stress testing.

DIAGNOSTIC TEST EFFECTS

None known.

IV INCOMPATIBILITIES

Any solution other than 0.9% NaCl lactated Ringer's, D5LR, or D5W.

IV COMPATIBILITIES

Abciximab (ReoPro).

SIDE EFFECTS

Frequent (12%-18%)

Facial flushing, dyspnea.

Occasional (2%-7%)
Headache, nausea, light-headedness, chest pressure.
Rare (≤ 1%)
Numbness or tingling in arms; dizziness; diaphoresis; hypotension; palpitations; chest, jaw, or neck pain.

SERIOUS REACTIONS

- May produce short-lasting heart block.

PRECAUTIONS & CONSIDERATIONS

Caution is warranted with arrhythmias at the time of conversion, asthma, heart block, and hepatic and renal failure. Additional caution is advised in elderly patients who may be at increased risk for severe bradycardia or AV block.

Facial flushing, headache, and nausea may occur, but these symptoms will resolve. Notify the physician if chest pain, pounding, or palpitations or difficulty breathing or shortness of breath occurs.
Before administering adenosine, the arrhythmia should be identified on a 12-lead EKG. Heart rate and rhythm on a continuous cardiac monitor and the apical pulse rate, rhythm, and quality should be assessed. BP, respirations, intake and output, and electrolytes should also be monitored.
Storage
Solution may be stored at room temperature and normally appears clear. Crystallization occurs if solution is refrigerated. If crystallization occurs, dissolve crystals by warming to room temperature. Discard unused portion.
Administration
Administer undiluted very rapidly, over 1-2 seconds, directly into vein, or if using an IV line, use the port closest to the insertion site. If the IV line is infusing fluid other than 0.9% NaCl, flush the line first before administering adenosine. Follow the rapid bolus injection with a rapid 0.9% NaCl flush.

IV infusion (diagnostic use): Administer undiluted using a syringe pump or volumetric infusion pump.

Agalsidase-β

a-gal′si-daze bay′tah
Fabrazyme
Fabrazyme, Replagal

CATEGORY AND SCHEDULE

Pregnancy Risk Category: B

Classification: Enzymes, metabolic

MECHANISM OF ACTION

An enzyme that treats Fabry disease, an X-linked genetic disorder, by catalyzing the hydrolysis of glycosphingolipids, reducing their accumulation in the kidneys' capillary endothelium and other body tissues. *Therapeutic Effect:* Provides an exogenous source of α-galactosidase A, an enzyme, missing in those with Fabry disease.

PHARMACOKINETICS

Nonlinear pharmacokinetics. *Half-life:* 45-102 min, dose-dependent.

AVAILABILITY

Powder for Injection: 5 mg, 35 mg (5 mg/mL when reconstituted).

INDICATIONS AND DOSAGES

▸ **Fabry disease**

IV INFUSION
Adults, Elderly. 1 mg/kg q2wk.

CONTRAINDICATIONS

None known.

DIAGNOSTIC TEST EFFECTS

None known.

IV INCOMPATIBILITIES

Do not mix any other medications with agalsidase-β.

SIDE EFFECTS

Expected (45%-52%)
Infusion reactions (rigors, fever, headache).
Frequent (21%-38%)
Rhinitis, nausea, anxiety, pharyngitis, edema, skeletal pain.
Occasional (14%-17%)
Temperature change sensation, hypotension, pallor, paresthesia, pruritus, urticaria, bronchitis.
Rare (7%-10%)
Depression, arthralgia, dyspepsia, laryngitis, sinusitis.

SERIOUS REACTIONS

- Serious infusion reactions, such as tachycardia, hypertension, throat tightness, chest pain, dyspnea, vomiting, lip edema, and rash, occur frequently.
- Other serious reactions include bradycardia, arrhythmias, vertigo, nephrotic syndrome, CVA, and cardiac arrest.

PRECAUTIONS & CONSIDERATIONS

Caution is warranted with fever, compromised cardiac function, moderate to severe hypertension, and renal impairment. The product contains mannitol, so caution should be observed in patients stating a mannitol hypersensitivity.
Storage
Store vials in the refrigerator. Allow them to reach room temperature before reconstitution, which takes about 30 min. The reconstituted and diluted solution should be used immediately; if this is not possible, the solution may be stored in the refrigerator for 24 h.
Administration
Pretreatment antipyretics should be administered. Reconstitute each 37-mg vial by slowly injecting 7.2 mL of sterile water for injection. Roll and tilt gently. Do not shake or agitate. Before adding the reconstituted solution to 500 mL 0.9% NaCl, remove an equal volume from the 500-mL infusion bag, and then add the agalsidase-β to the 500-mL 0.9% NaCl infusion bag. Administer at a rate of no more than 0.25 mg/min (15 mg/h). Expect to decrease the infusion rate if an infusion reaction occurs. If no reaction occurs, the infusion rate may be increased in increments of 0.05-0.08 mg/min (3-5 mg/h). Plan to decrease the infusion rate or temporarily stop the infusion if a reaction occurs. As prescribed, give additional antipyretics, antihistamines, or steroids to alleviate symptoms. Patients with compromised cardiac function should be closely monitored because they are at increased risk for severe complications from infusion reactions.

Albendazole

all-ben′dah-zole
★ Albenza

CATEGORY AND SCHEDULE

Pregnancy Risk Category: C

Classification: Anthelmintic, systemic

MECHANISM OF ACTION

A benzimidazole carbamate anthelmintic that degrades parasite cytoplasmic microtubules, irreversibly blocks cholinesterase secretion and glucose uptake in helminth and larvae (depletes glycogen, decreases ATP production, depletes energy). Vermicidal. *Therapeutic Effect:* Immobilizes and kills worms.

PHARMACOKINETICS
Poorly and variable absorbed GI tract. Widely distributed, cyst fluid, including CSF. Protein binding: 70%. Extensively metabolized in liver. Primarily excreted in bile. Not removed by hemodialysis. *Half-life:* 8-12 h (prolonged in impaired heptatic function).

AVAILABILITY
Tablets: 200 mg (Albenza).

INDICATIONS AND DOSAGES
▸ **Neurocysticercosis**

PO

Adults, Elderly weighing ≥ 60 kg. 400 mg 2 times/day. Give for 8 to 30 days.

Adults, Elderly weighing < 60 kg. 15 mg/kg/day, given in two divided doses (maximum 800 mg/day). Give for 8 to 30 days.

▸ **Cystic hydatid**

PO

Adults, Elderly weighing ≥ 60 kg. 400 mg 2 times/day for 28 days, rest 14 days, repeat for 2 more cycles.

Adults, Elderly weighing < 60 kg. 15 mg/kg/day given in two divided doses (maximum 800 mg/day) for 28 days, rest 14 days, repeat for 2 more cycles.

OFF-LABEL USES
Giardiasis, microsporidiosis, taeniasis, gnathostomiasis, liver flukes, trichuriasis.

CONTRAINDICATIONS
Hypersensitivity to albendazole, benzimidazoles, or any component of the formulation.

INTERACTIONS
Drug

Cimetidine, dexamethasone, praziquantel: May increase albendazole concentration.

Theophylline: Active treatment may decrease theophylline levels, and levels may rise when albendazole discontinued.

Herbal

Ginseng: May increase intestinal elimination of albendazole. Leads to decreased intestinal effectiveness.

Food

Grapefruit juice: May increase risk of albendazole adverse effects.

DIAGNOSTIC TEST EFFECTS
May decrease total white blood cell (WBC) count. Monitor liver function tests.

SIDE EFFECTS
Frequent

Neurocysticercosis: Nausea, vomiting, headache.

Hydatid: Abnormal liver function tests, abdominal pain, nausea, vomiting.

Occasional

Neurocysticercosis: Increased intracranial pressure, meningeal signs.

Hydatid: Headache, dizziness, alopecia, fever.

SERIOUS REACTIONS
- Granulocytopenia or pancytopenia occurs rarely.
- In the presence of cysticercosis, drug may produce retinal damage in presence of retinal lesions.
- Hepatoxicity is rare.

PRECAUTIONS & CONSIDERATIONS
Caution is warranted in patients with liver impairment or biliary obstruction. Bone marrow suppression may occur. It is unknown whether albendazole is excreted in breast milk. Safety and efficacy data are limited for children, particularly children younger than 6 yr. Expect to use the smallest dose necessary to achieve optimal

results. There are no age-related precautions noted in elderly patients. Fecal specimens should be obtained 3 wks after treatment. Patients being treated for neurocysticercosis should receive corticosteroid and anticonvulsant therapy, as indicated.

If fever, chills, sore throat, unusual bleeding or bruising, rash, or hives occurs, notify the physician. All patients should have monitoring of CBC and transaminases before therapy and every 2 wks during therapy. Patients should be advised to avoid becoming pregnant while on therapy and for 1 mo after completing therapy. Therapy should be initiated after a negative pregnancy test. Use in pregnancy only if no alternative therapy is appropriate.

Administration

Take albendazole with meals. Fatty meals are preferred. For young children, the tablets should be crushed or chewed and swallowed with a drink of water. Mixing the dose with applesauce or pudding may help ease administration.

Albumin, Human

al-byew'min

★ Albuminar, Albutein, Buminate, Plasbumin

🍁 Alburex

Do not confuse with albuterol.

CATEGORY AND SCHEDULE

Pregnancy Risk Category: C

Classification: Plasma expanders

MECHANISM OF ACTION

A plasma protein fraction that acts as a blood volume expander. *Therapeutic Effect:* Provides temporary increase in blood volume; reduces hemoconcentration and blood viscosity.

PHARMACOKINETICS

Distributed throughout extracellular fluid. *Half-life:* 15-20 days.

AVAILABILITY

Injection: 5%, 20%, 25%.

INDICATIONS AND DOSAGES

▸ **Hypovolemia**

IV

Adults, Elderly. Initially, 25 g; may repeat in 15-30 min. Maximum: 250 g within 48 h.

Children. 0.5-1 g/kg/dose (10-20 mL/kg/dose of 5% albumin). Maximum: 6 g/kg/day.

▸ **Hypoproteinemia**

IV

Adults, Elderly. 25 g IV. May repeat in 15-30 min. Maximum: 250 g in 48 h.

Children. 0.5-1 g/kg/dose (10-20 mL/kg/dose of 5% albumin). Repeat in 1-2 days.

▸ **Burns**

IV

Adults, Elderly, Children. Initially, give large volumes of crystalloid infusion to maintain plasma volume. After 24 h, give 25 g, then adjust dosage to maintain plasma albumin concentration of 2-2.5 g/100 mL.

▸ **Cardiopulmonary bypass**

IV

Adults, Elderly. 5% or 25% albumin with crystalloid to maintain plasma albumin concentration of 2.5 g/100 mL.

▸ **Acute nephrosis, nephrotic syndrome**

IV

Adults, Elderly. 25 g of 25% injection, with diuretic once a day for 7-10 days.

▸ **Hemodialysis**

IV

Adults, Elderly. 100 mL (25 g) of 25% albumin.

▸ **Hyperbilirubinemia, erythroblastosis fetalis**
IV
Infants. 1 g/kg 1-2 h before transfusion.

CONTRAINDICATIONS

Heart failure, history of allergic reaction to albumin level, hypervolemia, normal serum albumin, pulmonary edema, severe anemia.

DIAGNOSTIC TEST EFFECTS

May increase serum alkaline phosphatase concentration.

IV INCOMPATIBILITIES

Intravenous lipid emulsion (Liposyn), micafungin (Mycamine), midazolam (Versed), vancomycin (Vancocin), verapamil, protein hydrolysates, amino acid solutions, alcohol-containing solutions.

IV COMPATIBILITIES

Diltiazem (Cardizem), lorazepam (Ativan), whole blood, plasma, 0.9% NaCl, D5W, sodium lactate.

SIDE EFFECTS

Rare

High dose in repeated therapy: altered vital signs, chills, fever, increased salivation, nausea, vomiting, urticaria, tachycardia.

SERIOUS REACTIONS

- Fluid overload may occur, marked by increased BP and distended neck veins. Neurologic changes that may occur include headache, weakness, blurred vision, behavioral changes, incoordination, and isolated muscle twitching. Pulmonary edema may also occur, evidenced by rapid breathing, rales, wheezing, and coughing.

PRECAUTIONS & CONSIDERATIONS

Caution is warranted with hepatic or renal impairment, hypertension, normal serum albumin level, poor heart function, and pulmonary disease. It is unknown whether albumin crosses the placenta or is distributed in breast milk. No age-related precautions have been noted in children or in elderly patients.

Notify the physician of difficulty breathing, itching, or rash. BP for hypertension or hypotension, intake and output, and skin for flushing and urticaria should be monitored. Signs and symptoms of fluid overload, hypovolemia, and pulmonary edema should be assessed frequently.

Storage

Store at room temperature. Albumin normally appears as a clear, brownish, odorless, and moderately viscous fluid. Do not use if the solution has been frozen, appears turbid, or contains sediment or if the vial has been open 4 h or longer.

Administration

! Dosage is based on the condition; duration of administration is based on the response. Make a 5% solution from 25% solution by adding 1 part 25% solution to 4 parts 0.9% NaCl (preferred) or D5W. Do not use sterile water for injection because life-threatening acute renal failure and hemolysis can occur. Give by IV infusion. Rate varies depending on therapeutic use, blood volume, and concentration of the solute. Give 5% solution at 5-10 mL/min. Give 25% at a usual rate of 2-3 mL/min. A slower rate (1 mL/min) is recommended in patients with normal blood volume. Administer 5% solution undiluted; administer 25% solution undiluted or diluted with 0.9% NaCl (preferred) or D5W. May give without regard to patient's blood group or Rh factor type.

Albuterol

al-byoo′ter-ole

★ AccuNeb, Proair HFA, Proventil HFA, Ventolin HFA, VoSpire ER 🍁 Airomir, Apo-Salvent, Ventodisk

Do not confuse albuterol with Albutein or atenolol, or Proventil with Prinivil.

Also known as salbutamol.

CATEGORY AND SCHEDULE

Pregnancy Risk Category: C

Classification: Adrenergic β_2 agonist, bronchodilator

MECHANISM OF ACTION

A sympathomimetic that stimulates β_2-adrenergic receptors in the lungs, resulting in relaxation of bronchial smooth muscle. *Therapeutic Effect:* Relieves bronchospasm and reduces airway resistance.

PHARMACOKINETICS

Route	Onset (min)	Peak (h)	Duration (h)
PO	15-30	2-3	4-6
PO (extended-release)	30	2-4	12
Inhalation	5-15	0.5-2	2-5

Rapidly, well absorbed from the GI tract; gradually absorbed from the bronchi after inhalation. Metabolized in the liver. Primarily excreted in urine. *Half-life:* 2.7-5 h (PO); 3.8 h (inhalation).

AVAILABILITY

Syrup: 2 mg/5 mL.
Tablet: 2 mg, 4 mg.
Tablets (Extended-Release [VoSpire ER]): 4 mg, 8 mg.
Inhalation (HFA Aerosol [Proventil, Ventolin]): 90 mcg/spray.
Inhalation Solution (AccuNeb): 0.63 mg/3 mL, 1.25 mg/3 mL.
Inhalation Solution: 0.021%, 0.042%, 0.083%, 0.5%.

INDICATIONS AND DOSAGES

▸ **Bronchospasm**

PO

Adults, Children older than 12 yr. 2-4 mg 3-4 times a day. Maximum: 8 mg 4 times/day.
Elderly. 2 mg 3-4 times a day. Maximum: 8 mg 4 times a day.
Children 6-12 yr. 2 mg 3-4 times a day. Maximum: 24 mg/day.

PO (EXTENDED-RELEASE)

Adults, Children older than 12 yr. 4-8 mg q12h.
Children 6-12 yr. 4 mg q12h.

INHALATION

Adults, Elderly, Children older than 12 yr. 1-2 puffs by metered dose inhaler q4-6h as needed.
Children 4-12 yr. 1-2 puffs 4 times a day.

NEBULIZATION

Adults, Elderly, Children older than 12 yr. 2.5 mg 3-4 times a day.
Children 2-12 yr. 0.63-1.25 mg 3-4 times a day.

▸ **Exercise-induced bronchospasm**

INHALATION

Adults, Elderly, Children 4 yr and older. 2 puffs 15-30 min before exercise.

OFF-LABEL USES

Acute treatment of hyperkalemia.

CONTRAINDICATIONS

History of hypersensitivity to sympathomimetics, particularly albuterol or levalbuterol.

INTERACTIONS

Drug

β-blockers: Antagonize effects of albuterol.
Digoxin: May increase the risk of arrhythmias.

Diuretics: Hypokalemia associated with diuretic may worsen with albuterol. Monitor potassium levels.
MAOIs, tricyclic antidepressants: May potentiate cardiovascular effects. Potential for hypertensive crisis.
Food
Caffeine: Limit use of caffeine, increased CNS stimulation.

DIAGNOSTIC TEST EFFECTS

May increase blood glucose level. May decrease serum potassium level.

SIDE EFFECTS

Frequent
Headache (27%); nausea (15%); restlessness, nervousness, tremors (20%); dizziness (< 7%); throat dryness and irritation, pharyngitis (< 6%); BP changes, including hypertension (3%-5%); heartburn, transient wheezing (< 5%).
Occasional (2%-3%)
Insomnia, asthenia, altered taste. Inhalation: Cough, bronchial irritation.
Rare
Somnolence, diarrhea, dry mouth, flushing, diaphoresis, anorexia.

SERIOUS REACTIONS

- Excessive sympathomimetic stimulation may produce palpitations, extrasystole, tachycardia, chest pain, a slight increase in BP followed by a substantial decrease, chills, diaphoresis, and blanching of skin.
- Too-frequent or excessive use may lead to decreased bronchodilating effectiveness and severe, paradoxical bronchoconstriction.

PRECAUTIONS & CONSIDERATIONS

Caution is warranted in patients with cardiovascular disease, diabetes mellitus, hypertension, glaucoma, seizure disorders, and hyperthyroidism. Albuterol appears to cross the placenta; it is unknown whether albuterol is distributed in breast milk. Albuterol may inhibit uterine contractility. The safety and efficacy of this drug have not been established in children < 2 yr of age (syrup, nebulizer solution), < 4 yr of age (inhaler), or < 6 yr of age (tablets). Elderly patients may be more prone to tremors and tachycardia because of increased sensitivity to sympathomimetics. Drink plenty of fluids to decrease the thickness of lung secretions. Avoid excessive use of caffeinated products, such as chocolate, cocoa, cola, coffee, and tea.

Pulse rate and quality, 12-lead ECG, respiratory rate, depth, rhythm and type, ABG, and serum potassium levels should be monitored.
Storage
Store at room temperature. Use nebulization solution within 1 wk of opening foil pouch.
Administration
Do not crush or break extended-release tablets. Take albuterol without regard to food.

For inhalation, shake the container well before inhalation. Prime before first use or if inhaler has not been used for 2 wks. Wait 2 min before inhaling the second dose to allow for deeper bronchial penetration. Rinse mouth with water immediately after inhalation to prevent mouth and throat dryness. Take no more than 2 inhalations at any one time because excessive use may decrease the drug's effectiveness or produce paradoxical bronchoconstriction.

For nebulizer use, dilute 0.5 mL of 0.5% solution to a final volume of 3 mL with 0.9% NaCl to provide 2.5 mg. Administer over 5-15 min. The nebulizer should be used with compressed air or oxygen (O_2) at a rate of 6-10 L/min.

NOTE: Lower concentrations of nebulization solution require no dilution before nebulizer administration.

Alclometasone

al-kloe-met'a-sone

★ Aclovate

Do not confuse with Accolate.

CATEGORY AND SCHEDULE

Pregnancy Risk Category: C

Classification: Corticosteroids, topical, dermatologics

MECHANISM OF ACTION

Topical corticosteroids exhibit anti-inflammatory, antipruritic, and vasoconstrictive properties. Clinically, these actions correspond to decreased edema, erythema, pruritus, plaque formation, and scaling of the affected skin. Low- to medium-potency topical corticosteroid.

PHARMACOKINETICS

Approximately 3% is absorbed during an 8-h period. Metabolized in the liver. Excreted in the urine.

AVAILABILITY

Cream, as Dipropionate: 0.05% (Aclovate).
Ointment, as Diproprionate: 0.05% (Aclovate).

INDICATIONS AND DOSAGES

▸ **Corticosteroid-responsive dermatoses: atopic dermatitis, contact dermatitis, dermatitis, discoid lupus erythematosus, eczema, exfoliative dermatitis, granuloma annulare, lichen planus, lichen simplex, polymorphous light eruption, pruritus, psoriasis, Rhus dermatitis, seborrheic dermatitis, xerosis**

TOPICAL

Adults, Elderly, Children 1 yr and older. Apply a thin film to the affected area 2-3 times a day.

CONTRAINDICATIONS

Hypersensitivity to alclometasone, other corticosteroids, or any of its components.

DIAGNOSTIC TEST EFFECTS

None known.

SIDE EFFECTS

Frequent
The most common side effect is transient mild skin irritation consisting of mild burning, pruritus, or erythema. Others include, maculopapular rash, xerosis.
Occasional
Acneiform rash, contact dermatitis, folliculitis, glycosuria, growth inhibition, headache, hyperglycemia, infection, miliaria, papilledema, skin atrophy, skin hypopigmentation, skin ulcer, striae, telangiectasia.
Rare
Adrenocortical insufficiency, increased intracranial pressure, pseudotumor cerebri, impaired wound healing, Cushing syndrome, HPA suppression, skin ulcers, tolerance, withdrawal, visual impairment, ocular hypertension, cataracts.

PRECAUTIONS & CONSIDERATIONS

Caution is warranted with pregnancy. It is unknown whether alclometasone is distributed in breast milk. Alclometasone should not be used for diaper dermatitis. Children are more susceptible to HPA axis suppression than adults. There are no age-related precautions noted

for elderly patients. Avoid use on herpetic lesions; avoid use as monotherapy on sites with bacterial or fungal infections.
Storage
Store at room temperature.
Administration
Do not use occlusive dressings unless directed by physician. Apply a thin film topically to affected area 2-3 times daily. Massage gently until medication disappears.

Aldesleukin

Al-des-lew'kin
Proleukin
Also known as interleukin-2 or IL-2. Do not confuse interleukin-2 with interferon 2.

CATEGORY AND SCHEDULE

Pregnancy Risk Category: C

Classification: Antineoplastics, biologic response modifier

MECHANISM OF ACTION

A biological response modifier that acts like human recombinant interleukin-2, promoting proliferation, differentiation, and recruitment of T and B cells, lymphokine-activated and natural cells, and thymocytes. *Therapeutic Effect:* Enhances cytolytic activity in lymphocytes.

PHARMACOKINETICS

Primarily distributed into plasma, lymphocytes, lungs, liver, kidney, and spleen. Metabolized to amino acids in the cell lining the kidneys. *Half-life:* 85 min.

AVAILABILITY

Powder for Injection, 22 million units (1.3 mg).

INDICATIONS AND DOSAGES

▸ **Metastatic melanoma, metastatic renal cell carcinoma**
IV
Adults. 600,000 units/kg q8h for 14 doses; followed by 9 days of rest, then another 14 doses for a total of 28 doses per course. Course may be repeated after rest period of at least 7 wks from date of hospital discharge.

OFF-LABEL USES

Treatment of colorectal cancer, Kaposi sarcoma, non-Hodgkin lymphoma.

CONTRAINDICATIONS

Abnormal pulmonary function or thallium stress test results, organ allografts, retreatment in those who experience any of the following toxicities: bowel ischemia or perforation, coma, or toxic psychosis lasting longer than 48 h, GI bleeding requiring surgery, intubation lasting more than 72 h, pericardial tamponade, renal dysfunction requiring dialysis for longer than 72 h, repetitive or difficult-to-control seizures; angina, MI, recurrent chest pain with ECG changes, sustained ventricular tachycardia, uncontrolled or unresponsive cardiac rhythm disturbances.

INTERACTIONS

Drug
Antihypertensives: May increase hypotensive effect.
Cardiotoxic, hepatotoxic, myelotoxic, or nephrotoxic medications: May increase the risk of toxicity.
Glucocorticoids: May decrease the effects of aldesleukin.
Interferon-α: May increase the risk of myocardial injury, including myocardial infarction, myocarditis, ventricular hypokinesia, and severe rhabdomyolysis.

Iodinated contrast media: Administration subsequent to aldesleukin associated with acute, atypical adverse reactions within hours of contrast media.
Herbal
None known.
Food
None known.

DIAGNOSTIC TEST EFFECTS

May increase BUN and serum alkaline phosphatase, bilirubin, creatinine, AST (SGOT), and ALT (SGPT) levels. May decrease serum calcium, magnesium, phosphorus, potassium, and sodium levels.

IV INCOMPATIBILITIES

5-fluorouracil (5-FU), ganciclovir (Cytovene), lorazepam (Ativan), pentamidine (Pentam), prochlorperazine (Compazine), promethazine (Phenergan), rituximab (Rituxan), trastuzumab (Herceptin).

IV COMPATIBILITIES

Amikacin, calcium gluconate, fluconazole (Diflucan), gentamicin, lorazepam (Ativan), magnesium sulfate, metoclopramide, morphine, ondansetron (Zofran), ranitidine (Zantac), tobramycin, vancomycin.

SIDE EFFECTS/ADVERSE REACTIONS

Side effects are generally self-limiting and reversible within 2-3 days after discontinuing therapy.
Frequent (48%-89%)
Fever, chills, nausea, vomiting, hypotension, diarrhea, oliguria or anuria, mental status changes, irritability, confusion, depression, sinus tachycardia, pain (abdominal, chest, back), fatigue, dyspnea, pruritus.
Occasional (17%-47%)
Edema, erythema, rash, stomatitis, anorexia, weight gain, infection (urinary tract infection, injection site, catheter tip), dizziness.
Rare (4%-15%)
Dry skin, sensory disorders (vision, speech, taste), dermatitis, headache, arthralgia, myalgia, weight loss, hematuria, conjunctivitis, proteinuria.

SERIOUS REACTIONS

- Anemia, thrombocytopenia, and leukopenia occur commonly.
- GI bleeding and pulmonary edema occur occasionally.
- Capillary leak syndrome results in hypotension (systolic pressure < 90 mm Hg or a 20-mm Hg drop from baseline systolic pressure), extravasation of plasma proteins and fluid into extravascular space, and loss of vascular tone. It may result in cardiac arrhythmias, angina, MI, and respiratory insufficiency.
- Other rare reactions include fatal malignant hyperthermia, cardiac arrest, CVA, pulmonary emboli, bowel perforation, gangrene, and severe depression leading to suicide.

PRECAUTIONS & CONSIDERATIONS

Restrict aldesleukin therapy to patients with normal cardiac and pulmonary function as determined by thallium stress testing and pulmonary function testing. Extreme caution should be used in patients with a history of cardiac or pulmonary disease even if they have normal thallium stress and pulmonary function test results. Also use the drug cautiously with fixed requirements for large volumes of fluid (such as those with hypercalcemia) or a history of seizures. Aldesleukin use should be avoided in patients of either sex who do not practice effective contraception. The safety and efficacy of aldesleukin have not been established in children. Elderly patients may require cautious use of the drug because of age-related renal impairment. They are also less able to tolerate drug-related toxicities.

Notify the physician of difficulty urinating, black tarry stools, pinpoint red spots on skin, bruising, fever, signs of local infection, sore throat, or unusual bleeding from any site. Treat persons with bacterial infection and those with indwelling central lines with antibiotic therapy before beginning aldesleukin therapy. A negative CT scan for CNS metastasis must be obtained before beginning therapy. Immediately report any symptoms of depression or suicidal ideation. CBC, electrolytes, liver and renal function, amylase concentration, BP, mental status, intake and output, extravascular fluid accumulation, platelet count, pulse oximetry values, and weight should be assessed. Notify physician of somnolence or lethargy, as drug may need to be withheld.

Consider the use of medications to reduce aldesleukin side effects: NSAIDs/antipyretics starting before first dose to reduce fever, meperidine to control rigors associated with fever, H_2 antagonists/PPIs to reduce gastrointestinal (GI) bleeding/irritation, antiemetics and antidiarrheals, hydroxyzine or diphenhydramine for pruritic rashes, and antibiotic prophylaxis.

Storage

Refrigerate—do not freeze—unopened vials. The reconstituted solution is stable for 48 h at room temperature or refrigerated (refrigerated is preferred).

Administration

! Withhold the drug in patients who exhibit moderate to severe lethargy or somnolence because continued administration may result in coma. Protocols are available from the manufacturer to hold doses for multiple types of organ dysfunction, including oliguria, hepatic dysfunction, respiratory or cardiac compromise, CNS changes, GI irritation or bleeding, or skin rashes. The protocols also indicate when treatment courses may be continued. Aldesleukin should be administered only in a hospital setting with availability of an intensive care facility and specialists skilled in cardiopulmonary or intensive care medicine.

For IV use, reconstitute the 22-million-unit vial with 1.2 mL sterile water for injection to provide a concentration of 18 million units/mL. Do not use bacteriostatic water for injection or 0.9% NaCl. During reconstitution, direct the diluent at the side of the vial. Swirl the content gently; do not shake to avoid foaming. Further dilute the dose in 50 mL D5W and infuse over 15 min. Do not use an in-line filter. Warm the solution to room temperature before infusion. Closely monitor the patient for a drop in mean arterial BP, a sign of capillary leak syndrome. Continued treatment may result in edema, pleural effusion, mental status changes, and significant hypotension (systolic pressure < 90 mm Hg or a 20 mm Hg drop from baseline systolic pressure).

Alefacept

ale′fah-cept

★ 🍁 Amevive

CATEGORY AND SCHEDULE

Pregnancy Risk Category: B

Classification:

Immunosuppressives

MECHANISM OF ACTION

An immunologic agent that interferes with the activation of T lymphocytes by binding to the lymphocyte antigen, thus reducing the number of circulating T lymphocytes. *Therapeutic Effect:* Prevents T cells from becoming overactive, which may help reduce symptoms of chronic plaque psoriasis.

PHARMACOKINETICS

Bioavailability 63% with IM administration. *Half-life:* 270 h.

AVAILABILITY

Powder for Injection: 15 mg. Alefacept is distributed to physicians' offices and specialty pharmacies, with administration intended in the physician's office.

INDICATIONS AND DOSAGES

▸ Plaque psoriasis

IM

Adults, Elderly. 15 mg once weekly for 12 wks. Retreatment for one additional cycle acceptable after 12 wks of rest.

CONTRAINDICATIONS

HIV infection, history of systemic malignancy, concurrent use of immunosuppressive agents or phototherapy, active serious infection or sepsis. Hypersensitivity to drug or hamster proteins.

INTERACTIONS

Drug

Live-virus vaccines: Avoid concurrent use.

DIAGNOSTIC TEST EFFECTS

Decreases serum T-lymphocyte levels. Monitor CD4+ T-lymphocyte counts before and weekly during the 12-wk treatment period. Withhold the dose if the CD4+ count is < 250 cells/μL. Discontinue treatment if the count remains below 250 cells/μL for 1 mo. May increase serum AST (SGOT) and ALT (SGPT) levels.

IV INCOMPATIBILITIES

Do not mix alefacept with any other medications. Do not reconstitute it with any diluent other than that supplied by the manufacturer.

SIDE EFFECTS

Frequent (16%)

Injection site pain and inflammation.

Occasional (5%)

Chills.

Rare (2% or less)

Pharyngitis, dizziness, cough, nausea, myalgia.

SERIOUS REACTIONS

- Rare reactions include hypersensitivity reactions, infusion reactions, liver injury, lymphopenia, malignancies, and serious infections requiring hospitalization (such as abscess, pneumonia, and postoperative wound infection).
- Coronary artery problems or disorder and MI occur in fewer than 1% of patients.

PRECAUTIONS & CONSIDERATIONS

Caution is warranted in patients with chronic infections, history of recurrent infections, high risk for malignancy, and in elderly patients. It is unknown whether alefacept crosses the placenta or is distributed in breast milk. The safety and efficacy of this drug have not been established in children. Cautious use is necessary in elderly patients because they are at increased risk for infections and certain malignancies. Avoid contact with infected individuals and situations that might increase the risk for infection.

Notify the physician of any signs of infection or malignancy.

Storage

Store unopened vials in the refrigerator protected from light. Do not freeze. Use the drug immediately after reconstitution or within 4 h if refrigerated. Discard unused portion within 4 h of reconstitution.

Administration

For IM administration, withdraw 0.6 mL of the supplied diluent and, with the needle pointed at the sidewall of the vial, slowly inject the diluent into the vial of alefacept. Swirl the vial gently to dissolve the contents; do not shake or vigorously agitate the vial to avoid excessive foaming. The reconstituted solution should be clear and colorless to slightly yellow. Do not use if it becomes discolored or cloudy or contains undissolved material.

For IM use, final concentration is 15 mg/0.5 mL. Inject the full 0.5 mL of solution. Use a different IM site for each new IM injection at least 1 inch from an old site, avoiding tender, bruised, red, or hard areas.

Alemtuzumab

Al-em-two′zoo-mab

★ Campath 🍁 MabCampath

CATEGORY AND SCHEDULE

Pregnancy Risk Category: C

Classification: Antineoplastics, monoclonal antibodies

MECHANISM OF ACTION

Binds to CD52, a cell surface glycoprotein, found on the surface of all B and T lymphocytes, most monocytes, macrophages, natural killer cells, and granulocytes. *Therapeutic Effect:* Produces cytotoxicity, reducing tumor size.

PHARMACOKINETICS

Half-life: 11 h after the first dose and 6 days after the last dose. Peak and trough levels rise during first few weeks of therapy and approach steady state by about wk 6.

AVAILABILITY

Solution for Injection: 30 mg/3 mL.

INDICATIONS AND DOSAGES

▸ **B-cell chronic lymphocytic leukemia in patients who have been treated with alkylating agents and failed fludarabine therapy**

IV INFUSION

Adults, Elderly. Initially, 3 mg/day as a 2-h infusion. When the 3-mg daily dose is tolerated (with only low-grade or no infusion-related toxicities), increase daily dose to 10 mg. When the 10 mg/day dose is tolerated, maintenance dose may be initiated. Ability to go to maintenance dose usually achieved in 3-7 days. *Maintenance:* 30 mg given 3 times/wk on alternate days (such as Monday, Wednesday, and Friday or Tuesday, Thursday, and Saturday) for up to 12 wks.

CONTRAINDICATIONS

Active systemic infections, history of hypersensitivity or anaphylactic reaction to the drug, or hamster proteins.

INTERACTIONS

Drug

Live-virus vaccines: May potentiate viral replication, increase side effects, and decrease the patient's antibody response to the vaccine.

Herbal

None known.

Food

None known.

DIAGNOSTIC TEST EFFECTS

May decrease hemoglobin level, platelet count, and WBC count.

IV INCOMPATIBILITIES

Do not mix alemtuzumab with any other medications.

SIDE EFFECTS

Frequent

Rigors (86%-89%), tremors (86%), fever (85%), nausea (54%), vomiting (41%), rash (40%), fatigue (34%), hypotension (32%), urticaria (30%), pruritus (14%-24%), skeletal pain, headache (24%), diarrhea (22%), anorexia (20%).

Occasional (< 10%)

Myalgia, dizziness, abdominal pain, throat irritation, vomiting, neutropenia, rhinitis, bronchospasm, urticaria.

SERIOUS REACTIONS

- Neutropenia occurs in 85% of patients, anemia occurs in 80% of patients, and thrombocytopenia occurs in 72% of patients.
- Serious infection risk due to bone marrow suppression.
- Serious infusion-related reactions may occur.
- A rash occurs in 40% of patients.
- Respiratory toxicity, manifested as dyspnea, cough, bronchitis, pneumonitis, and pneumonia, occurs in 16%-26% of patients.

PRECAUTIONS & CONSIDERATIONS

Alemtuzumab has the potential to cause depletion of B- and T-lymphocytes in the fetus. Effective contraception is recommended during and for 6 mo after treatment for women of childbearing potential and men of reproductive potential. Discontinue breastfeeding during treatment and for at least 3 mo after the last dose. The safety and efficacy of alemtuzumab have not been established in children. No age-related precautions have been noted in the elderly. Vaccinations and contact with anyone who has recently received a live-virus vaccine should be avoided. Crowds and those with known infection should also be avoided.

Infusion-related reactions, including chills, fever, hypotension, and rigors, which usually occur 30 min to 2 h after starting the first infusion, should be monitored; these reactions may resolve by slowing the drip rate. Signs and symptoms for hematologic toxicity, including excessive fatigue or weakness, ecchymosis, fever, signs of local infection, sore throat, or unusual bleeding from any site, should be assessed. CBC should be monitored frequently during and after therapy to assess for anemia, neutropenia, and thrombocytopenia. Prophylactic therapy against PCP pneumonia and herpes viral infections is recommended upon initiation of therapy and for at least 2 mo following the last dose or until CD4+ counts are ≥ 200 cells/μL (whichever is later).

Storage

Refrigerate ampules before dilution. Do not freeze. Use the solution within 8 h after dilution. The diluted solution may be stored at room temperature or refrigerated. Discard the solution if it becomes discolored or contains particulate matter.

Administration

! Expect to pretreat with 650 mg of acetaminophen and 50 mg of diphenhydramine before each infusion to prevent infusion-related side effects.

Withdraw the needed amount from the vial into a syringe. Inject it into 100-mL 0.9% NaCl or D5W. Gently invert the bag to mix the contents; do not shake it. Give the 100-mL solution as a 2-h IV infusion. Do not give alemtuzumab by IV push or bolus.

Alendronate

ah-len′dro-nate

Fosamax

Do not confuse Fosamax with Flomax.

CATEGORY AND SCHEDULE

Pregnancy Risk Category: C

Classification: Bisphosphonates

MECHANISM OF ACTION

A bisphosphonate that inhibits normal and abnormal bone resorption, without retarding mineralization. *Therapeutic Effect:* Leads to significantly increased bone mineral density; reverses the progression of osteoporosis.

PHARMACOKINETICS

Poorly absorbed after oral administration; oral bioavailability < 1%. Protein binding: 78%. After oral administration, rapidly taken into bone, with uptake greatest at sites of active bone turnover. Excreted in urine. *Terminal half-life:* > 10 yr (reflects release from skeleton as bone is resorbed).

AVAILABILITY

Tablets: 5 mg, 10 mg, 35 mg, 40 mg, 70 mg.
Oral Solution: 70 mg/75 mL.

INDICATIONS AND DOSAGES

▸ **Osteoporosis (in men)**

PO

Adults, Elderly. 10 mg once a day in the morning, or 70 mg once weekly.

▸ **Glucocorticoid-induced osteoporosis**

PO

Adults, Elderly. 5 mg once a day in the morning.
Postmenopausal women not receiving estrogen. 10 mg once a day in the morning.

▸ **Postmenopausal osteoporosis**

PO (TREATMENT)

Adults, Elderly. 10 mg once a day in the morning or 70 mg once weekly.

PO (PREVENTION)

Adults, Elderly. 5 mg once a day in the morning or 35 mg once weekly.

▸ **Paget disease**

PO

Adults, Elderly. 40 mg once a day in the morning for 6 mo; then wait 6 mo before considering retreatment.

CONTRAINDICATIONS

Abnormalities of the esophagus that delay esophageal emptying, such as stricture or achalasia; hypocalcemia; inability to stand or sit upright for at least 30 min; renal impairment (CrCl < 35 mL/min); sensitivity to alendronate or phosphonates; patients with aspiration risk.

INTERACTIONS

Drug

Aspirin: May increase GI disturbances.
IV ranitidine: May double the bioavailability of alendronate.

Herbal

None known.

Food

Beverages other than plain water, dietary supplements, food: May interfere with absorption of alendronate.

DIAGNOSTIC TEST EFFECTS

Reduces serum calcium and serum phosphate concentrations. Significantly decreases serum alkaline phosphatase level in patients with Paget disease.

SIDE EFFECTS

Frequent (7%-8%)
Back pain, abdominal pain.
Occasional (2%-3%)
Nausea, abdominal distention, constipation, diarrhea, flatulence.
Rare (< 2%)
Rash.

SERIOUS REACTIONS

- Overdose causes hypocalcemia, hypophosphatemia, and significant GI disturbances.
- Esophageal irritation occurs if alendronate is not given with 6-8 oz of plain water or if the patient lies down within 30 min of drug administration.
- Severe and occasionally debilitating bone, joint, or muscle pain. Rare reports of atypical femur fractures.
- Osteonecrosis of the jaw.

PRECAUTIONS & CONSIDERATIONS

Caution is warranted with hypocalcemia or vitamin D deficiency and in patients with GI disease, including dysphagia, frequent heartburn, GI reflux disease, hiatal hernia, and ulcers. Alendronate may cause decreased maternal weight gain and incomplete fetal ossification and delay delivery. It is unknown whether alendronate is excreted in breast milk. Do not give to women who are breastfeeding. Safety and efficacy of alendronate have not been established in children. No age-related precautions have been noted for elderly patients.

Consider beginning weight-bearing exercises and modifying behavioral factors, such as reducing alcohol consumption and stopping cigarette smoking. Plan to correct hypocalcemia and vitamin D deficiency, if present, before starting alendronate therapy. Patients should be taking adequate calcium and vitamin D supplementation during treatment. Serum electrolytes, including serum alkaline phosphatase and serum calcium levels, should be monitored.

Administration

! Give at least 30 min before the first food, beverage, or medication of the day.

Expected benefits occur only when alendronate is taken with a full glass (6-8 oz) of plain water first thing in the morning and at least 30 min before the first food, beverage, or medication of the day. Taking alendronate with beverages other than plain water, including mineral water, orange juice, and coffee, significantly reduces absorption of the medication.

! Do not lie down for at least 30 min after taking the medication. Remaining upright helps the drug move quickly to the stomach and reduces the risk of esophageal irritation.

Alfuzosin

al-few-zoe′sin
Uroxatral Xatral

CATEGORY AND SCHEDULE

Pregnancy Risk Category: B; however, this drug is not indicated for use in women.

Classification: Antiadrenergics, α-blocking, peripheral

MECHANISM OF ACTION

An α-1 antagonist that targets receptors around bladder neck and prostate capsule. *Therapeutic*

Effect: Relaxes smooth muscle and improves urinary flow and symptoms of prostatic hyperplasia.

PHARMACOKINETICS

Bioavailability 49% following meal; reduced 50% in fasting state. Peak levels reached in 8 h. Protein binding: 90%. Extensively metabolized in the liver. Primarily excreted in urine. *Half-life:* 3-9 h.

AVAILABILITY

Tablets (Extended-Release): 10 mg.

INDICATIONS AND DOSAGES

▸ **Benign prostatic hyperplasia**

PO

Adult men. 10 mg once a day, approximately 30 min after same meal each day.

CONTRAINDICATIONS

History of hypersensitivity to alfuzosin; moderate to severe hepatic insufficiency (Child Pugh Class B and C); potent CYP3A4 inhibitors (itraconazole, ketoconazole, ritonavir).

INTERACTIONS

Drug

Antihypertensive agents, nitrates: Increased potential for hypotension.

Cimetidine: May increase alfuzosin blood concentration.

CYP3A4 inducers: May reduce alfuzosin levels, decrease effect.

CYP3A4 inhibitors: May increase alfuzosin levels and increase side effects; potent inhibitors (e.g., itraconazole, ketoconazole, ritonavir) are contraindicated.

Other α-blockers, such as doxazosin, prazosin, tamsulosin, and terazosin: May increase the α-blockade effects of both drugs.

Herbal

None known.

Food

Food increases extent of absorption.

DIAGNOSTIC TEST EFFECTS

None known.

SIDE EFFECTS

Frequent (6%-7%)

Dizziness, headache, malaise.

Occasional (4%)

Dry mouth.

Rare (2%-3%)

Nausea, dyspepsia (such as heartburn and epigastric discomfort), diarrhea, orthostatic hypotension, tachycardia, drowsiness.

SERIOUS REACTIONS

- Ischemia-related chest pain may occur rarely.
- Alpha-blockers associated with Intraoperative Floppy Iris Syndrome during cataract surgery.
- Priapism (very rare).
- Toxic skin eruptions (very rare).

PRECAUTIONS & CONSIDERATIONS

Caution is warranted for patients with coronary artery disease, hepatic impairment, known history of QT-interval prolongation, orthostatic hypotension, severe renal impairment, or under general anesthesia. Alfuzosin is not indicated for use in women and children. No age-related precautions have been noted for elderly patients.

Dizziness and light-headedness may occur. Tasks that require mental alertness or motor skills should be avoided until response to the drug is established. Notify the physician if headache occurs.

Administration

Take after the same meal each day. The extended-release tablet should not be crushed or chewed.

Aliskiren

a-lis-kye′ren

★ Tekturna 🍁 Rasilez

CATEGORY AND SCHEDULE

Pregnacy Risk Category: C (first trimester) and D (second and third trimesters)

Classification: Antihypertensive, renin inhibitor

MECHANISM OF ACTION

A direct renin inhibitor that decreases plasma renin activity and inhibits the conversion of angiotensinogen to angiotensin I. *Therapeutic Effect:* Reduced blood pressure.

PHARMACOKINETICS

Poorly absorbed; oral bioavailability 2.5%; high-fat meal reduced extent of absorption 71%. Metabolized by CYP3A4. *Half-life:* 24 h.

AVAILABILITY

Tablets: 150 mg, 300 mg.

INDICATIONS AND DOSAGES

▸ **Hypertension**

PO

Adults. 150 mg once daily, may increase to 300 mg once daily after 2 wks.

CONTRAINDICATIONS

Previous hypersensitivity or angioedema from the drug.

INTERACTIONS

Drug

Cyclosporine: May increase aliskiren concentrations; concomitant use not recommended.

Furosemide: May reduce furosemide concentrations, reducing furosemide activity.

Potassium-sparing diuretics, potassium supplements, salt substitutes containing potassium, or other drugs that increase potassium: Caution is advised.

Herbal

None known.

Food

High-fat meal reduces the extent of absorption; aliskiren should be administered consistently with regard to meals.

DIAGNOSTIC TEST EFFECTS

May increase serum creatinine and BUN, serum potassium, serum uric acid, and creatine kinase; may reduce hemoglobin and hematocrit.

SIDE EFFECTS

Occasional (> 2%)

Diarrhea.

Rare (< 2%)

Abdominal pain, angioedema, cough, dyspepsia, edema, GI reflux, gout, hypotension, hyperkalemia, rash, renal stones.

SERIOUS REACTIONS

• Angioedema, seizures.

PRECAUTIONS & CONSIDERATIONS

Use in pregnancy can cause injury and death to the developing fetus. Discontinue as soon as possible if pregnancy occurs. Safety and effectiveness have not been established in pediatric patients. No age-related precautions noted in elderly patients. Use with caution in patients with severe renal impairment.

Storage

Store at room temperature; protect from moisture.

Administration

Administer consistently with regard to meals. Antihypertensive effect at a given dose generally observed by 2 wks. May be taken with other antihypertensives.

Alitretinoin

ah-lee-tret'ih-noyn

Panretin

Panretin, Toctino

CATEGORY AND SCHEDULE

Pregnancy Risk Category: D

Classification: Topical retinoid

MECHANISM OF ACTION

Binds to and activates all known retinoid receptors. Once activated, receptors act as transcription factors, regulating genes that control cellular differentiation and proliferation. *Therapeutic Effect:* Inhibits growth of Kaposi sarcoma (KS) cells.

PHARMACOKINETICS

Minimally absorbed following topical administration; plasma concentrations not detectable.

AVAILABILITY

Gel: 0.1%.

INDICATIONS AND DOSAGES

▸ **Kaposi Sarcoma skin lesions**

TOPICAL

Adults. Initially, apply twice a day to lesions. May increase to 3 or 4 times a day.

OFF LABEL USES

Cutaneous T-cell lymphomas.

CONTRAINDICATIONS

Hypersensitivity to retinoids or alitretinoin ingredients; when systemic therapy is required (more than 10 new KS lesions in the previous month, symptomatic pulmonary KS, symptomatic visceral involvement, symptomatic lymphedema).

INTERACTIONS

Drug

DEET insect repellant: Alitretinoin increases DEET systemic absorption; do not use DEET products.

DIAGNOSTIC TEST EFFECTS

None known.

SIDE EFFECTS

Frequent (3%-77%)

Rash (erythema, scaling, irritation, redness, dermatitis), itching, exfoliative dermatitis (flaking, peeling, desquamation, exfoliation), stinging, tingling, edema, skin disorders (scabbing, crusting, drainage).

SERIOUS REACTIONS

- Severe local skin reaction (intense erythema, edema, vesiculation) may limit treatment.

PRECAUTIONS & CONSIDERATIONS

Avoid pregnancy, and discontinue breastfeeding when used. Safety and efficacy are unknown for children and patients older than 65 yr, do not use products containing DEET. May cause photosensitivity; minimize exposure of treated areas to sunlight and sunlamps.

Storage

Store at room temperature.

Administration

Apply sufficient gel to cover the lesion with a generous coating. Allow gel to dry for 3-5 min before covering with clothing. Do not cover with occlusive dressings. Avoid bathing, showering, and swimming for 3 h after application. Because unaffected skin may become irritated, avoid application of the gel to healthy skin surrounding the lesions. In addition, do not apply the gel on or near mucosal surfaces of the body. If application site toxicity occurs, the application frequency can be reduced. If severe irritation occurs, application of drug can be discontinued for a few days until the symptoms subside.

A response of KS lesions may be seen as soon as 2 wks after initiation of therapy, but most patients require longer application. With continued application, further benefit may be attained. Some patients have required more than 14 wks to respond. Continue alitretinoin gel as long as the patient is benefiting.

Allopurinol

al-oh-pure′ih-nole

★ Aloprim, Zyloprim

🍁 Alloprin

Do not confuse Zyloprim with ZORprin.

CATEGORY AND SCHEDULE

Pregnancy Risk Category: C

Classification: Antigout agents, purine analogs, antihyperuricemic

MECHANISM OF ACTION

A xanthine oxidase inhibitor that decreases uric acid production by inhibiting xanthine oxidase, an enzyme. *Therapeutic Effect:* Reduces uric acid concentrations in both serum and urine.

PHARMACOKINETICS

Route	Onset	Peak	Duration
PO/IV	2-3 days	1-3 wks	1-2 wks

Well absorbed from the GI tract. Widely distributed. Metabolized in the liver to active metabolite. Excreted primarily in urine. Removed by hemodialysis. *Half-life:* 1-3 h; metabolite, 12-30 h.

AVAILABILITY

Tablets (Zyloprim): 100 mg, 300 mg.
Powder for Injection (Aloprim): 500 mg.

INDICATIONS AND DOSAGES

▸ **For primary or secondary gout (tophi, arthritis, uric acid, lithiasis, etc.)**

PO

Adults, Children older than 10 yr. Initially, 100 mg/day; may increase by 100 mg/day at weekly intervals. Maximum: 800 mg/day. Maintenance: 100-200 mg 2-3 times a day or 300 mg/day.

▸ **To prevent uric acid nephropathy during chemotherapy**

PO

Adults. Initially, 600-800 mg/day, given in divided doses, starting 2-3 days before initiation of chemotherapy or radiation therapy.
Children 6-10 yr. 100 mg 3 times a day or 300 mg once a day. Reassess at 48 h.
Children < 6 yr. 50 mg 3 times a day.

IV

Adults. 200-400 mg/m^2/day beginning 24-48 h before initiation of chemotherapy.
Children. 200 mg/m^2/day. Maximum: 600 mg/day.

▸ **Recurrent calcium oxalate calculi**

PO

Adults. 200-300 mg/day.
Elderly. Initially, 100 mg/day, gradually increased until optimal uric acid level is reached.

▸ **Dosage in renal impairment (adults)**

Dosage is modified based on creatinine clearance.

Creatinine Clearance (mL/min)	Dosage Adjustment
10-20	200 mg/day
3-9	100 mg/day
< 3	100 mg at extended intervals

CONTRAINDICATIONS

Asymptomatic hyperuricemia, history of severe hypersensitivity reactions to allopurinol.

INTERACTIONS

Drug

ACE inhibitors: May increase risk of hypersensitivity reactions.
Amoxicillin, ampicillin: May increase incidence of rash.
Azathioprine, mercaptopurine: May increase therapeutic effect and toxicity of azathioprine and mercaptopurine.
Cyclophosphamide: May increase cyclophosphamide myelosuppressive effect, increasing risk of bleeding and infection.
Warfarin: May increase anticoagulant effect of coumarins.
Thiazide diuretics: May decrease renal elimination of allopurinol. Monitor need for dose adjustment.

Herbal

None known.

Food

None known.

DIAGNOSTIC TEST EFFECTS

May increase BUN, serum creatinine, serum alkaline phosphatase, AST (SGOT), and ALT (SGPT) levels.

IV INCOMPATIBILITIES

Amikacin (Amikin), amphotericin B, carmustine (BiCNU), cefotaxime (Claforan), chlorpromazine (Thorazine), cimetidine (Tagamet), clindamycin (Cleocin), cytarabine (Ara-C), dacarbazine (DTIC), daunorubicin, diphenhydramine (Benadryl), doxorubicin (Adriamycin), doxycycline (Vibramycin), droperidol (Inapsine), floxuridine, fludarabine (Fludara), gentamicin (Garamycin), haloperidol (Haldol), hydroxyzine (Vistaril), idarubicin (Idamycin), imipenem-cilastatin (Primaxin), mechlorethamine, meperidine (Demerol), methylprednisolone (Solu-Medrol), metoclopramide (Reglan), minocycline, nalbuphine, netilmicin, ondansetron (Zofran), prochlorperazine (Compazine), promethazine (Phenergan), sodium bicarbonate, streptozocin (Zanosar), tobramycin (Nebcin), vinorelbine (Navelbine).

IV COMPATIBILITIES

Bumetanide (Bumex), calcium gluconate, furosemide (Lasix), heparin, hydromorphone (Dilaudid), lorazepam (Ativan), morphine, potassium chloride.

SIDE EFFECTS

Occasional

Oral: Somnolence, unusual hair loss.
IV: Rash, nausea, vomiting.

Rare

Diarrhea, headache.

SERIOUS REACTIONS

! Pruritic maculopapular rash possibly accompanied by malaise, fever, chills, joint pain, nausea, and vomiting should be considered a toxic reaction.
• Severe hypersensitivity may follow appearance of rash.
• Bone marrow depression, hepatic toxicity, peripheral neuritis, and acute renal failure occur rarely.

PRECAUTIONS & CONSIDERATIONS

Caution is warranted with CHF, diabetes mellitus, hypertension, and impaired renal or hepatic function. It is unknown whether allopurinol crosses the placenta. Allopurinol is excreted in breast milk; use only when clearly needed in nursing women. No age-related precautions have been noted in children or in elderly patients. The drug should be discontinued if rash or other evidence of allergic reaction appears. Avoid tasks that require mental alertness or motor skills until response to the drug has been established.

High fluid intake (3000 mL/day) should be encouraged; intake and output should be monitored; output should be at least 2000 mL/day, urine for cloudiness and unusual color and odor, CBC, liver function tests, and serum uric acid levels should also be assessed. Signs and symptoms of a therapeutic response, including improved joint range of motion and reduced redness, swelling, and tenderness, should be evaluated.

Storage

Store unreconstituted vials at room temperature. Store reconstituted infusion at room temperature; give within 10 h. Do not refrigerate. Do not use if precipitate forms or solution is discolored.

Administration

May take with or immediately after meals or milk. Drink enough fluid daily to maintain a urine output of 2 L/day, if possible. Administer dosages > 300 mg/day in divided doses. It may take 1 wk or longer for the full therapeutic effect of the drug to be evident.

For IV use, reconstitute 500-mg vial with 25 mL sterile water for injection, which produces a clear, almost colorless solution (concentration of 20 mg/mL). Further dilute with 0.9% NaCl or D5W as desired, with a final maximum concentration of 6 mg/mL. Infuse over 30-60 min.

Almotriptan

al-moe-trip'tan

★ 🍁 Axert

Do not confuse Axert with Antivert.

CATEGORY AND SCHEDULE

Pregnancy Risk Category: C

Classification: Selective serotonin receptor agonists, antimigraine agents

MECHANISM OF ACTION

A serotonin receptor agonist that binds selectively to vascular receptors, producing a vasoconstrictive effect on cranial blood vessels. *Therapeutic Effect:* Produces relief of migraine headache.

PHARMACOKINETICS

Well absorbed after PO administration; bioavailability 70%. Metabolized by MAO type A and CYP3A4 and 2D6, excreted in urine (40% as unchanged drug). *Half-life:* 3-4 h.

AVAILABILITY

Tablets: 6.5 mg, 12.5 mg.

INDICATIONS AND DOSAGES

▸ Migraine headache

PO

Adults, Elderly, and Children ≥ 12 yr. 6.25-12.5 mg. If headache improves but then returns, dose may be repeated after 2 h. Maximum: 25 mg/24 h.

▸ Dosage in hepatic or renal impairment (CrCl < 30 mL/min)

Recommended initial dose is 6.25 mg and maximum daily dose is 12.5 mg.

CONTRAINDICATIONS

Arrhythmias associated with conduction disorders, hemiplegic or basilar migraine, ischemic heart disease (including angina pectoris, history of MI, silent ischemia, and Prinzmetal's angina), uncontrolled hypertension, use within 24 h of ergotamine-containing preparation or another serotonin receptor agonist; use within 14 days of MAOIs,Wolff-Parkinson-White syndrome.

INTERACTIONS

Drug

Ergotamine-containing medications: May produce a vasospastic reaction. Do not use triptan within 24 h of ergot drug.
Erythromycin, itraconazole, ketoconazole, ritonavir: May increase the almotriptan plasma level.
MAOIs: Risk of serotonin syndrome. Do not take within 2 wks of MAOI treatment.
SSRIs/SNRIs (citalopram, desvenlafaxine, duloxetine, escitalopram, fluoxetine, fluvoxamine, paroxetine, sertraline, venlafaxine): May produce weakness, hyperreflexia, and incoordination; serotonin syndrome.

DIAGNOSTIC TEST EFFECTS

None known.

SIDE EFFECTS

Frequent (> 1%)

Nausea, dry mouth, paresthesia, flushing.

Occasional (< 1%)

Changes in temperature sensation, asthenia, dizziness, chest pain, neck pain, back pain.

SERIOUS REACTIONS

- Excessive dosage may produce tremor, red extremities, reduced respirations, cyanosis, seizures, chest pain, and serotonin syndrome.
- Serious arrhythmias occur rarely in patients with hypertension or diabetes, obese patients, smokers, and those with a strong family history of coronary artery disease.
- Hypertensive crisis.

PRECAUTIONS & CONSIDERATIONS

Caution is warranted with controlled hypertension, a history of CVA, mild to moderate hepatic or renal impairment, and cardiovascular risk factors. It is unknown whether almotriptan is distributed in breast milk. The safety and efficacy of almotriptan have not been established in children younger than 12 yr. No age-related precautions have been noted in elderly patients. Tasks that require mental alertness or motor skills should be avoided.

Notify the physician immediately if palpitations, pain or tightness in the chest or throat, or pain or weakness in the extremities occurs. Migraines and associated symptoms, including nausea and vomiting, photophobia, and phonophobia (sound sensitivity), should be assessed before and during treatment.

Storage

Store at room temperature.

Administration

If headache comes back after the first dose, give a second dose as long as 2 h or more have elapsed since initial dose. If pain unrelieved after first dose, do not give a second dose; check with prescriber. Do not exceed dose limits per each 24 h.

Alosetron

a-low'seh-tron

★ Lotronex

Do not confuse Lotronex with Lovenox

CATEGORY AND SCHEDULE

Pregnancy Risk Category: B

Classification: Selective serotonin receptor antagonist, neuroenteric modulator

A

MECHANISM OF ACTION

A serotonin ($5\text{-}HT_3$) receptor antagonist that mediates abdominal pain, bloating, nausea, vomiting, peristalsis, and secretory reflexes. *Therapeutic Effect:* Alleviates diarrhea, reduces gastric pain.

PHARMACOKINETICS

Rapidly absorbed after PO administration. Extensively metabolized in liver. Excreted primarily in urine and, to a lesser extent, in feces. *Half-life:* 1.5 h.

AVAILABILITY

Tablets: 0.5 mg, 1 mg.

INDICATIONS AND DOSAGES

▸ Irritable bowel syndrome (IBS), diarrhea predominant

PO

Adult women. 0.5 mg twice a day. If after 4 wks the dose is well tolerated but does not adequately control IBS symptoms, may increase to 1 mg twice a day. Maximum: 2 mg/day. Discontinue in patients without an adequate response after 4 wks of treatment at a dose of 1 mg twice daily.

CONTRAINDICATIONS

Constipation; concomitant fluvoxamine; diverticulitis (active or history of); GI bleeding, obstruction, or perforation; history of ischemic colitis, ulcerative colitis, or Crohn disease; history of severe or chronic constipation or sequelae from constipation; severe hepatic impairment; thrombophlebitis; unable to understand or comply with required patient-physician agreement.

INTERACTIONS

Drug

Apomorphine: May enhance hypotensive effect of apomorphine; contraindicated.

Fluvoxamine: Substantially increases alosetron concentrations; contraindicated.

CYP1A2 inhibitors: May increase levels and effects of alosetron; use with caution. Potent CYP1A2 inhibitors (e.g., enoxacin, mexilitene, zileuton) should be avoided unless clinically necessary.

CYP3A4 inhibitors: May increase levels and effects of alosetron; use with caution.

Hydralazine, isoniazid, procainamide: Alosetron might inhibit metabolism of these drugs.

DIAGNOSTIC TEST EFFECTS

None.

SIDE EFFECTS

Frequent (29%)

Constipation.

Occasional (2%-10%)

Nausea, GI or abdominal discomfort or pain, abdominal distention, hemorrhoids, regurgitation and reflux.

Rare (< 1%)

Sedation, abnormal dreams, anxiety, hypertension, clinical depression.

SERIOUS REACTIONS

- Acute ischemic colitis and serious complications of constipation have resulted in the rare need for blood transfusions and surgery or have caused death.

PRECAUTIONS & CONSIDERATIONS

Caution is warranted with hepatic function impairment. Be aware alosetron is indicated for use in women only. The safety and efficacy of this drug have not been established in men. It is unknown whether alosetron is excreted in breast milk. The safety and efficacy of alosetron have not been established in children. Caution is advised for elderly patients, who may be at greater risk for complications of constipation.

Urgency and diarrhea may be reduced within 1 wk of treatment, but the drug's full therapeutic effects may not occur for up to 4 wks. Persistent constipation may require interruption of treatment or drug management. Notify the physician or nurse if bloody diarrhea, severe constipation, or a sudden worsening of stomach pain occurs. Therapy should be discontinued immediately in patients developing constipation or symptoms of ischemic colitis; therapy should not be resumed in patients developing ischemic colitis. Pattern of daily bowel activity and stool consistency should be monitored. Adequate hydration should be maintained.

Only physicians enrolled in the manufacturer's prescribing program may prescribe alosetron. Program stickers must be affixed to all prescriptions. A Med Guide must be distributed with alosetron each time an outpatient prescription or refill is dispensed.

Storage

Store at room temperature. Protect from light and moisture.

Administration

Take alosetron without regard to food.

Alprazolam

al-pray'zoe-lam

★ Alprazolam Intensol, Niravam, Xanax, Xanax XR

🍁 Apo-Alpraz, Xanax TS

Do not confuse alprazolam with lorazepam, or Xanax with Tenex or Zantac.

CATEGORY AND SCHEDULE

Pregnancy Risk Category: D
Controlled Substance Schedule: IV

Classification: Anxiolytics, benzodiazepines, sedatives/hypnotics

MECHANISM OF ACTION

A benzodiazepine that enhances the action of the inhibitory neurotransmitter γ-aminobutyric acid in the brain. *Therapeutic Effect:* Produces anxiolytic effect from its CNS depressant action.

PHARMACOKINETICS

Well absorbed from GI tract. Protein binding: 80%. Metabolized in the liver primarily by CYP3A4. Primarily excreted in urine. Minimal removal by hemodialysis. *Half-life:* 11-16 h.

AVAILABILITY

Oral Solution: 1 mg/mL.
Tablets: 0.25 mg, 0.5 mg, 1 mg, 2 mg.
Tablets (Extended-Release): 0.5 mg, 1 mg, 2 mg, 3 mg.
Tablets (Orally Disintegrating): 0.25 mg, 0.5 mg, 1 mg, 2 mg.

INDICATIONS AND DOSAGES

▸ **Anxiety disorders**

PO

Adults (immediate release). Initially, 0.25-0.5 mg 3 times a day. May titrate q3-4 days. Maximum: 4 mg/day in divided doses.

Elderly, Debilitated Patients. Patients with hepatic disease or low serum albumin. Initially, 0.25 mg 2-3 times a day. Gradually increase to optimum therapeutic response.

▸ **Anxiety with depression**

PO

Adults. 2.5-3 mg/day in divided doses.

▸ **Panic disorder**

PO, IMMEDIATE RELEASE

Adults. Initially, 0.5 mg 3 times a day. May increase at 3- to 4-day intervals. Range: 5-6 mg/day.

Elderly. Initially, 0.125-0.25 mg 2 times a day; may increase in 0.125-mg increments until desired effect attained.

PO, EXTENDED RELEASE
Alert to switch from immediate-release to extended-release form, give total daily dose (immediate release) as a single daily dose of extended-release form.
Adults. Initially, 0.5-1 mg once a day. May titrate at 3- to 4-day intervals. Range: 3-6 mg/day.
Elderly. Initially, 0.5 mg once a day.

CONTRAINDICATIONS

Hypersensitivity to alprazolam or other benzodiazepines. Acute alcohol intoxication with depressed vital signs, acute angle-closure glaucoma, concurrent use of itraconazole or ketoconazole.

INTERACTIONS

Drug
Alcohol, other CNS depressants: Potentiate effects of alprazolam and may increase sedation.
CYP3A4 inhibitors, cimetidine, erythromycin, fluvoxamine, nefazodone, oral contraceptives, propoxyphene, protease inhibitors (e.g., ritonavir): May inhibit metabolism and increase serum concentrations of alprazolam; use with caution.
CYP3A4 inducers, carbamazepine: May induce metabolism and decrease serum concentration of alprazolam.
Indinavir itraconazole, ketoconazole: Increase alprazolam serum concentration; contraindicated.
Imipramine, desipramine: Alprazolam may increase serum concentrations of these drugs; clinical effects uncertain.
Herbal
Gotu kola, kava kava, valerian: May increase CNS depressant effect of alprazolam.
St. John's wort: Increases alprazolam clearance; decreases alprazolam half-life from 12 h to 6 h.
Food
Grapefruit, grapefruit juice: May inhibit alprazolam's metabolism.
High-fat meal: May alter the rate, but not extent, of absorption.

DIAGNOSTIC TEST EFFECTS

None known.

SIDE EFFECTS

Frequent (> 10%)
Ataxia; light-headedness; somnolence; headache, dry mouth.
Occasional
Confusion, blurred vision, hypotension, nausea, syncope.
Rare
Behavioral problems such as anger, impaired memory, depressed mood, paradoxical reactions such as insomnia, nervousness, or irritability.

SERIOUS REACTIONS

- Abrupt or too-rapid withdrawal may result in pronounced restlessness, irritability, insomnia, hand tremors, abdominal and muscle cramps, diaphoresis, vomiting, and seizures.
- Overdose results in somnolence, confusion, diminished reflexes, and coma.
- Blood dyscrasias have been reported rarely.

PRECAUTIONS & CONSIDERATIONS

Caution is warranted with impaired renal or hepatic function or in patients with severe debilitating illness such as myasthenia gravis or severe COPD. Dizziness and drowsiness may occur. Change positions slowly from recumbent, to sitting, before standing to prevent dizziness. Alcohol, tasks that require mental alertness or motor skills, and smoking should also be avoided. Women on long-term therapy should use effective contraception during therapy and notify the physician immediately if they become or may be pregnant. Breastfeeding is not recommended; benzodiazepines are excreted in human milk and infant can become lethargic.

Storage

Store at room temperature.

Keep tightly closed. Keep orally disintegrating tablet in bottle until time of administration and protect from moisture.

Administration

Take alprazolam without regard to food. Crush tablets as needed. Mix concentrated oral solution with liquids or semisolid foods (e.g., water, juice, soda or soda-like beverages, applesauce, pudding). Use the calibrated dropper to measure doses.

Handle orally disintegrating tablets with dry hands. If only half an orally disintegrating tablet is used, the other half should be discarded because it might not remain stable.

Take extended-release tablets once a day; swallow tablets whole and do not break, chew, or crush tablets.

Alprostadil

al-pros′ta-dil

🇨🇦 Caverject, Caverject Impulse, Edex, Muse, Prostin VR Pediatric

Do not confuse alprostadil with alprazolam.

CATEGORY AND SCHEDULE

Pregnancy Risk Category: X

Classification: Naturally occurring prostaglandin (E1, PGE1)

MECHANISM OF ACTION

A prostaglandin that directly affects vascular and ductus arteriosus smooth muscle and relaxes trabecular smooth muscle. *Therapeutic Effect:* Causes vasodilation; dilates cavernosal arteries, allowing blood flow to and entrapment in the lacunar spaces of the penis.

PHARMACOKINETICS

Rapidly metabolized and cleared from the body by urinary excretion. *Half-life:* 5-10 min.

AVAILABILITY

Injection (Prostin VR Pediatric): 500 mcg/mL.
Injection, Aqueous (Caverject): 10 mcg/mL, 20 mcg/mL, 40 mcg/mL.
Powder for Injection (Caverject, Edex): 5 mcg, 10 mcg, 20 mcg, 40 mcg.
Powder for Injection (Caverject Impulse): 10 mcg, 20 mcg.
Urethral Pellet (Muse): 125 mcg, 250 mcg, 500 mcg, 1000 mcg.

INDICATIONS AND DOSAGES

▸ **Maintain patency of ductus arteriosus**

IV INFUSION (PROSTIN VR PEDIATRIC ONLY)

Neonates. Initially, 0.05-0.1 mcg/kg/min. Maintenance: 0.01-0.4 mcg/kg/min. Use lowest possible dose that maintains response. Maximum: 0.4 mcg/kg/min.

▸ **Impotence**

URETHRAL PELLET (MUSE)

Adult. Initial dose 125-250 mcg, maintenance dose individualized. Maximum: 2 systems per 24 h.

INTRACAVERNOSAL (CAVERJECT, EDEX)

Adults. Dosage is individualized. Initial dose titrated in physician's office. Initial dose is 1.25 or 2.5 mcg.

CONTRAINDICATIONS

Hypersensitivity. Not for use in women. Conditions predisposing to priapism (sickle cell anemia, multiple myeloma, leukemia, venous thrombosis); anatomic deformation of penis, penile implants. The intracavernosal injection is if penile angulation, cavernosal fibrosis, or Peyronie disease is present. The urethral suppository is contraindicated in urethral stricture, balanitis, Peyronie disease, or acute or chronic urethritis. There are no specific contraindications to use of alprostadil in neonates.

INTERACTIONS

Drug

Anticoagulants, including heparin, thrombolytics: May increase the risk of bleeding.
Sympathomimetics: May decrease the effect of alprostadil.
Vasodilators: May increase risk of hypotension.

Herbal

None known.

Food

None known.

DIAGNOSTIC TEST EFFECTS

May increase blood bilirubin levels. May decrease glucose, serum calcium, and serum potassium levels.

IV INCOMPATIBILITIES

Do not mix with any other drugs.

SIDE EFFECTS

Frequent

Intracavernosal (1%-4%): Penile pain (37%), prolonged erection, hypertension, localized pain, penile fibrosis, injection site hematoma or ecchymosis, headache, respiratory infection, flu-like symptoms.
Intraurethral (3%): Penile pain (36%), urethral pain or burning, testicular pain, urethral bleeding, headache, dizziness, respiratory infection, flu-like symptoms.
Systemic (> 1%): Fever, seizures, flushing, bradycardia, hypotension, tachycardia, apnea, diarrhea.

Occasional

Intracavernosal (< 1%): Hypotension, pelvic pain, back pain, dizziness, cough, nasal congestion.
Intraurethral (< 3%): Fainting, sinusitis, back and pelvic pain.
Systemic (< 1%): Anxiety, lethargy, myalgia, arrhythmias, respiratory depression, anemia, bleeding, thrombocytopenia, hematuria.

SERIOUS REACTIONS

- Systemic overdose is manifested as apnea, flushing of the face and arms, and bradycardia. Occurs in neonates often (10%), especially in those of low birth weight (< 2 kg).
- Cardiac arrest and sepsis occur rarely.

PRECAUTIONS & CONSIDERATIONS

Caution is warranted with coagulation defects, polycythemia, severe hepatic disease, and thrombocythemia. Be aware that erection should occur within 2-5 min of administration. Notify the physician if erection lasts for longer than 4 h or becomes painful. Alprostadil should not be used if sexual partner is pregnant unless a condom barrier is being used.

Use with caution in neonates with bleeding tendencies. Arterial pressure by auscultation, Doppler transducer, or umbilical artery catheter should be monitored with ductus arteriosus. Infusion rate should be decreased immediately if a significant decrease in arterial pressure occurs. Continuous cardiac monitoring should be performed. Heart sounds, femoral pulse (to monitor lower extremity circulation), and respiratory status should be assessed. In addition, signs and symptoms of hypotension should be monitored and BP, ABG values, and temperature should be assessed. Apnea usually appears during the first hour of infusion. If apnea or bradycardia occurs, infusion should be discontinued immediately and the physician should be notified.

Storage
Store aqueous injection (Caverject) in the freezer until dispensed; once dispensed store in freezer up to 3 mo. May be kept in refrigerator for up to 7 days; once refrigerated, it must be used within 7 days or discarded; do not refreeze. Once the ampule is removed from the foil wrapper, it must be used immediately after allowing to warm to room temperature or discarded. Open ampules of alprostadil injection must be used immediately. Alprostadil lyophilized powder (Caverject) should be stored in a refrigerator until dispensed. Once dispensed it can be stored at room temperature for up to 3 mo. Reconstituted solution should be used within 24 h when stored at room temperature. Do not refrigerate or freeze reconstituted solution. Alprostadil dual-chamber system (Caverject Impulse) and cartridges (Edex) should be stored at room temperature. Refrigerate Muse pellet unless used within 14 days. Store the pediatric parenteral form in refrigerator. Dilute drug before administration. Prepare fresh dose every 24 h and discard unused portions.

Administration
! Doses > 40 mcg (Edex) or 60 mcg (Caverject) are not recommended.
! *Pediatric injection:* Give by continuous IV infusion or through umbilical artery catheter placed at ductal opening. Prepare continuous IV infusion by diluting 1 mL of alprostadil containing 500 mcg, with D5W or 0.9% NaCl to yield a solution containing 2-20 mcg/mL. Diluting volumes can range from 25 to 250 mL, depending on the patient and the available infusion device. Infuse the lowest possible dose over the shortest possible time. Decrease the infusion rate immediately if a significant decrease in arterial pressure is noted via auscultation, Doppler transducer, or umbilical artery catheter. Discontinue the infusion immediately if signs and symptoms of overdose, such as apnea and bradycardia, occur.

Alteplase
al'te-plase
Activase, Activase Cathflo
Do not confuse alteplase or Activase with Altace.

CATEGORY AND SCHEDULE
Pregnancy Risk Category: C

Classification: Thrombolytics, tissue plasminogen activator

MECHANISM OF ACTION
A tissue plasminogen activator that acts as a thrombolytic by binding to the fibrin in a thrombus and converting entrapped plasminogen to plasmin. This process initiates fibrinolysis. *Therapeutic Effect:* Degrades fibrin clots, fibrinogen, and other plasma proteins.

PHARMACOKINETICS
Rapidly metabolized in the liver. Primarily excreted in urine. Approximately 80% present in plasma cleared within 10 min.

AVAILABILITY
Powder for Injection (Activase Cathflo): 2 mg.
Powder for Injection (Activase): 50 mg, 100 mg.

INDICATIONS AND DOSAGES

▸ Acute MI

IV INFUSION

Adults weighing > 67 kg. 100 mg over 90 min, starting with 15-mg bolus over 1-2 min, then 50 mg over 30 min, then 35 mg over 60 min. Or a 3-h infusion, giving 60 mg over first hour (6-10 mg as bolus over 1-2 min), 20 mg over second hour, and 20 mg over third hour.

Adults weighing 67 kg or less. 100 mg over 90 min, starting with 15-mg bolus, then 0.75 mg/kg over 30 min (maximum: 50 mg), then 0.5 mg/kg over 60 min (maximum: 35 mg). Or 3-h infusion of 1.25 mg/kg giving 60% of dose over first hour (6%-10% as 1- to 2-min bolus), 20% over second hour, and 20% over third hour.

▸ Acute pulmonary emboli

IV INFUSION

Adults. 100 mg over 2 h. Institute or reinstitute heparin near end or immediately after infusion when aPTT or thrombin time (TT) returns to twice normal or less.

▸ Acute ischemic stroke

IV INFUSION

Adults. 0.9 mg/kg over 60 min (10% total dose as initial IV bolus over 1 min). Administered within 3-4.5 h of symptoms onset.

▸ Central venous catheter clearance

IV

Adults, Elderly, Children (weighing 30 kg or more). 2 mg; may repeat after 2 h if catheter function not restored.

Children weighing 10-30 kg. Instill 110% of the internal lumen volume of the catheter, not to exceed 2 mg in 2 mL. May repeat after 2 h if catheter function is not restored.

OFF-LABEL USES

Coronary thrombolysis.

CONTRAINDICATIONS

Active internal bleeding, AV malformation or aneurysm, bleeding diathesis, intracranial neoplasm, intracranial or intraspinal surgery or trauma, recent (within past 2 mo) cerebrovascular accident, severe uncontrolled hypertension; additional contraindication in acute stroke includes evidence of intracranial hemorrhage on pretreatment evaluation, suspicion of subarachnoid hemorrhage, history of intracranial hemorrhage, seizure at onset of stroke.

INTERACTIONS

Drug

Anticoagulants, including heparin: May increase risk of hemorrhage.
Nitroglycerin: May decrease alteplase concentrations, thereby reducing alteplase effect.
Platelet aggregation inhibitors, including aspirin, NSAIDs, abciximab, ticlopidine: May increase the risk of bleeding.

Herbal

Cat's claw, dong quai, evening primrose, feverfew, red clover, horse chestnut, garlic, green tea, ginseng, ginkgo: Can have antiplatelet activity, may increase risk of bleeding.

Food

None known.

DIAGNOSTIC TEST EFFECTS

Decreases plasminogen and fibrinogen levels during infusion, which decreases clotting time (and confirms the presence of lysis).

IV INCOMPATIBILITIES

Do not add other medications to the container of alteplase solution or administer other medications through the same IV line. Incompatible with dobutamine, dopamine, heparin, nitroglycerin.

IV COMPATIBILITIES

Eptifibatide (Integrelin), lidocaine, metoprolol (Lopressor), propranolol (Inderal).

SIDE EFFECTS

Frequent

Superficial bleeding at puncture sites, decreased BP.

Occasional

Allergic reaction, such as rash or wheezing; bruising. GI bleeding (5%), GU bleeding (4%), and ecchymosis (1%). Retroperitoneal bleeds, epistaxis, and gingival bleeding reported in < 1%.

SERIOUS REACTIONS

- Severe internal hemorrhage may occur. Intracranial hemorrhage may cause death. Do not use doses > 150 mg due to increased risk.
- Lysis of coronary thrombi may produce atrial or ventricular arrhythmias or stroke.

PRECAUTIONS & CONSIDERATIONS

Caution is warranted with recent (within past 10 days) major surgery or GI bleeding, organ biopsy, trauma, cerebrovascular disease, cardiopulmonary resuscitation, diabetic retinopathy, endocarditis, left heart thrombus, occluded AV cannula at infected site, severe hepatic or renal disease, thrombophlebitis, in elderly patients, and in pregnant women or within the first 10 postpartum days. Alteplase is used only when the benefit to the mother outweighs the risk to a fetus. Also, it is unknown whether alteplase crosses the placenta or is distributed in breast milk. Safety and efficacy have not been established in children (Activase) or in children < 2 yr or weighing < 10 kg (Activase Cathflo). In elderly patients, there is an increased risk of bleeding. Patients must be carefully selected and monitored. An electric razor and a soft toothbrush should be used to reduce the risk of bleeding.

Immediately report signs of bleeding, such as oozing from cuts or gums. Serum creatine kinase (CK), CK-MB concentrations, 12-lead ECG, electrolyte levels, hematocrit, platelet count, TT, aPTT, PT, and fibrinogen levels should be evaluated before therapy starts. BP and pulse and respiration rates should be checked every 15 min until stable; then check hourly. Continuous cardiac monitoring should be performed.

Storage

Store 50-mg and 100-mg vials at room temperature or in refrigerator. Protect from light. Solution is stable for 8 h after reconstitution. Discard unused portion. Store 2-mg vials in refrigerator.

Administration

Reconstitute immediately before use with sterile water for injection. Reconstitute 100-mg vial with 100 mL sterile water for injection (50-mg vial with 50 mL sterile water for injection) without preservative to provide a concentration of 1 mg/mL. May dilute further with equal volume of D5W or 0.9% NaCl to provide a concentration of 0.5 mg/mL. Gently swirl or slowly invert vial; avoid excessive agitation. After reconstitution, solution normally appears colorless to pale yellow. Give by IV infusion via infusion pump. (See individual dosages above.) If minor bleeding occurs at puncture site, apply pressure for 30 seconds; if unrelieved, apply a pressure dressing. If uncontrolled hemorrhage occurs, discontinue the infusion immediately. Slowing the rate of infusion may worsen the hemorrhage. Avoid undue pressure when injecting the drug into the catheter because the catheter can rupture or expel a clot into circulation.

See manufacturer's directions for reconstitution and catheter instillation of Activase Cathflo.

Aluminum Chloride Hexahydrate

a-loo'mi-num klor'ide heks-a-hye'drate

★ Drysol, Hypercare

CATEGORY AND SCHEDULE

Pregnancy Risk Category: C

Classification: Antiperspirants

MECHANISM OF ACTION

Aluminum salts cause an obstruction of the distal sweat gland. This obstruction causes metal ions to precipitate with mucopolysaccharides, damaging epithelial cells along the lumen of the duct and forming a plug to block sweat output. *Therapeutic Effect:* Results in decreased secretion of the sweat glands.

PHARMACOKINETICS

Not known.

AVAILABILITY

Topical Solution: 20% (Drysol, Hypercare).

INDICATIONS AND DOSAGES

▸ **Antiperspirant**

TOPICAL

Adults, Elderly, Children 12 yr and older. Apply to each underarm once a day at bedtime.

▸ **Hyperhidrosis**

TOPICAL

Adults, Elderly, Children 12 yr and older. Apply to affected areas once a day at bedtime.

CONTRAINDICATIONS

Hypersensitivity to aluminum chloride or any one of its components.

INTERACTIONS

Drug

None known.

Herbal

None known.

Food

None known.

DIAGNOSTIC TEST EFFECTS

None known.

SIDE EFFECTS

Frequent

Itching, burning, tingling sensation.

Occasional

Rash.

SERIOUS REACTIONS

- Hypersensitivity reaction, such as rash, may occur.

PRECAUTIONS & CONSIDERATIONS

It is unknown whether aluminum chloride hexahydrate crosses the placenta or is distributed in breast milk. These products may be harmful to cotton fibers and certain metals.

Skin may become irritated during use. Aluminum chloride hexahydrate should not be applied to broken, irritated, or recently shaved skin. Do not use other antiperspirants or deodorants during treatment.

Administration

Aluminum chloride hexahydrate is for external use only. It should be applied to dry skin. The treated area should be covered with a sheet of plastic wrap held in place with a snug T-shirt to avoid aluminum chloride hexahydrate rubbing off at night. The next morning, discard the plastic wrap if used and wash the skin with a mild soap. Excessive sweating may be stopped after 2 or more treatments; thereafter, apply 1-2 times/wk or as needed.

Aluminum Hydroxide

a-loo′mi-num hye-drox′ide

★ Alternagel

CATEGORY AND SCHEDULE

Pregnancy Risk Category: C

OTC

Classification: Gastrointestinals, vitamins/minerals

MECHANISM OF ACTION

An antacid that reduces gastric acid by binding with phosphate in the intestine and is then excreted as aluminum carbonate in feces; decreased serum phosphate levels may result in increased absorption of calcium. The drug also has astringent and adsorbent properties. *Therapeutic Effect:* Neutralizes or increases gastric pH; reduces phosphate levels in urine, preventing formation of phosphate urinary calculi; reduces the serum phosphate level; decreases the fluidity of stools.

AVAILABILITY

Suspension: 600 mg/5 mL (Alternagel), 320 mg/5 mL.

INDICATIONS AND DOSAGES

▸ **Antacid**

PO

Adults, Elderly. 500-1500 mg 3-6 times daily, between meals and at bedtime.

▸ **Hyperphosphatemia**

PO

Adults, Elderly. Initially, 300-600 mg 3 times a day with meals.

Children. 50-150 mg/kg/day in divided doses q4-6h.

CONTRAINDICATIONS

Hypophosphatemia.

INTERACTIONS

Drug

Bisphosphonates, iron preparations, isoniazid, ketoconazole, phenytoin, quinolones, tetracyclines, alumimun hydroxide: May decrease absorption of this drug.

Methenamine: May decrease effects of the methenamine.

Salicylate: May increase salicylate excretion.

Herbal

None known.

Food

None known.

DIAGNOSTIC TEST EFFECTS

May increase the serum gastrin level and systemic and urinary pH. May decrease the serum phosphate level.

SIDE EFFECTS

Frequent

Chalky taste, mild constipation, abdominal cramps.

Occasional

Nausea, vomiting, speckling, or whitish discoloration of stools.

SERIOUS REACTIONS

- Prolonged constipation may result in intestinal obstruction.
- Excessive or chronic use may produce hypophosphatemia manifested as anorexia, malaise, muscle weakness, or bone pain, which may result in osteomalacia and osteoporosis.
- Prolonged use may produce urinary calculi.
- Prolonged or excessive use, especially in neonates or those with renal failure, may produce aluminum toxicity encephalopathy.

PRECAUTIONS & CONSIDERATIONS

Caution is warranted with Alzheimer disease, chronic diarrhea, cirrhosis, constipation, dehydration, edema, fecal impaction, fluid restrictions, gastric outlet obstruction, GI or rectal bleeding, heart failure, impaired renal function, low sodium diets, symptoms of appendicitis, and in elderly patients. Aluminum hydroxide is rarely used as an antacid or phosphate binder in children; other agents are considered safer. Elderly patients may be at increased risk of constipation and fecal impaction.

Stool discoloration may occur but will resolve when the drug is discontinued. Adequate hydration should be maintained. Pattern of daily bowel activity and stool consistency and serum aluminum, calcium, phosphate, and uric acid levels should be monitored.

Administration

Take aluminum hydroxide 1-3 h after meals and at bedtime when used as an antacid. Expect the dosage to be individualized based on the antacid's neutralizing or phosphate-binding capacity. Shake the suspension well before use. Do not take other oral drugs within 1-2 h of antacid administration.

Alvimopan

al-vi-moe'pan

★ 🍁 Entereg

CATEGORY AND SCHEDULE

Pregnancy Risk Category: B

Classification: Gastrointestinal agents, peripheral μ-opioid receptor antagonist

MECHANISM OF ACTION

Antagonizes the peripheral effects of opioids on GI motility and secretion by competitively binding to GI tract μ-opioid receptors. Achieves this effect without reversing the central analgesic effects of μ-opioid agonists. *Therapeutic Effect:* Reduces physiologic ileus postoperatively and helps maintain GI motility to enhance surgical recovery and diet tolerance, and can reduce time to discharge.

PHARMACOKINETICS

Limited systemic bioavailability (roughly 6%) and does not cross the blood-brain barrier. Protein binding: 80%. Mostly excreted by biliary secretion and via unabsorbed drug passing in the feces. Some drug hydrolyzed by gut microflora to a metabolite. Metabolite is excreted in feces and urine. *Half-life:* 10-18 h (range for alvimopan and metabolite). Accumulation may occur with chronic dosing in hepatic or severe renal impairment.

AVAILABILITY

Capsules: 12 mg.

INDICATIONS AND DOSAGES

▸ **Postoperative ileus: to accelerate GI recovery time following partial large or small bowel resection with primary anastomosis**

PO

Adults. 12 mg PO for 1 dose within 30 min and up to 5 h before surgery; then 12 mg twice daily beginning the day after surgery. Maximum duration of 7 days or until hospital discharge (e.g., maximum total therapy = 15 doses).

CONTRAINDICATIONS

Patients who have taken therapeutic doses of opioids for more than 7 consecutive days immediately prior to this drug.

INTERACTIONS

Drug

Methylnaltrexone: Shares similar mechanism of action to alvimopan; potential for additive GI effects.

Drugs that strongly inhibit p-glycoprotein (e.g., verapamil, cyclosporine, amiodarone, itraconazole, quinine, spirinolactone, quinidine, diltiazem): Alvimopan has not been studied with these drugs; potential for altered alvimopan activity.

Herbal and Food

None known.

DIAGNOSTIC TEST EFFECTS

None known.

SIDE EFFECTS

Frequent (3%-10%)

Constipation, flatulence, dyspepsia, anemia, hypokalemia, back pain, urinary retention.

Occasional (1%-2%)

Diarrhea, abdominal pain, cramping.

Rare (< 1%)

Nausea and vomiting. See Serious Reactions.

SERIOUS REACTIONS

- There were more reports of MI (usually 1-4 mo after treatment) in those treated with alvimopan (0.5 mg twice daily) compared with placebo in 1 study of patients receiving opioids for chronic pain. The results have not been noted in other controlled studies. A causal relationship with the drug has not been established.

PRECAUTIONS & CONSIDERATIONS

Alvimopan is available only to hospitals that enroll in the ENTEREG Access Support and Education (E.A.S.E.) program. The program limits use of alvimopan to short-term, inpatient use; patients will not receive more than 15 doses and the drug will not be dispensed to patients after they have been discharged from the hospital. Not recommended for use in patients undergoing surgery for complete bowel obstruction. Those who have received opiates in the days prior to surgery are likely to be more sensitive to the effects of this drug. Use caution in patients with mild or moderate hepatic or renal impairment; not recommended in those with severe hepatic impairment (Child-Pugh class C) or end-stage renal disease (CrCl < 10 mL/min or ESRD) is present. There are no data in pregnant women; animal studies do not show teratogenic effects. It is unknown if the drug is excreted in human breast milk, but it is detected in the milk of lactating rats. The safety and efficacy of alvimopan have not been established in children.

Monitor bowel sounds, stool frequency, serum potassium, hemoglobin/hematocrit, and patient pain scales. Watch for reduction in bloating, abdominal distention, and for the passage of flatus, which are signs of therapeutic effectiveness. Report diarrhea, nausea, vomiting, or increased abdominal pain to physician.

Storage

Store capsules at controlled room temperature, in the original carton.

Administration

Preoperative dose usually given in fasting state. May administer subsequent doses without regard to meals.

Amantadine Hydrochloride

a-man′ta-deen hi-droh-klor′ide

★ Symmetrel 🍁 Med-Amantadine, PMS-Amantadine

CATEGORY AND SCHEDULE

Pregnancy Risk Category: C

Classification: Antiparkinsonian agents, antivirals

MECHANISM OF ACTION

A dopaminergic agonist that blocks the uncoating of influenza A virus, preventing penetration into the host and inhibiting M2 protein in the assembly of progeny virions. Amantadine also blocks the reuptake of dopamine into presynaptic neurons and causes direct stimulation of postsynaptic receptors. *Therapeutic Effect:* Antiviral and antiparkinsonian activity.

PHARMACOKINETICS

Rapidly and completely absorbed from the GI tract. Protein binding: 67%. Widely distributed. Primarily excreted in urine. Minimally removed by hemodialysis. *Half-life:* 16 h (increased in the elderly and in impaired renal function).

AVAILABILITY

Capsule: 100 mg.
Syrup: 50 mg/5 mL.
Tablets: 100 mg.

INDICATIONS AND DOSAGES

▸ **Prevention and symptomatic treatment of respiratory illness due to influenza A virus**

NOTE: Due to increased resistance, the CDC recommends that amantadine no longer be used for treatment or prophylaxis of influenza A in the United States until susceptibility is reestablished.

PO

Adults ≥ 65 yr. 100 mg/day.
Adults and children 13-64 yr. 200 mg/day or 100 mg twice a day.
Children 10-12 yr. 5 mg/kg/day up to 200 mg/day in 2 divided doses.
Children 1-9 yr. 5 mg/kg/day in 2 divided doses (up to 150 mg/day).

▸ **Parkinson's disease, extrapyramidal symptoms**

PO

Adults, Elderly. Initially, 100 mg once daily. May increase to 100 mg twice daily, if necessary, after at least 1 wk. Occasionally, patient might need 300-400 mg/day in divided doses, but this is rare.

▸ **Dosage in renal impairment**

Dose and frequency are modified based on creatinine clearance.

Creatinine Clearance (mL/min)	Dosage
30-50	200 mg first day; 100 mg/day thereafter
15-29	200 mg first day; 100 mg on alternate days
< 15	200 mg every 7 days

CONTRAINDICATIONS

Hypersensitivity to amantadine, rimantadine, or any product ingredients.

INTERACTIONS

Drug

Alcohol: May increase CNS effects, including dizziness, confusion, light-headedness, and orthostatic hypotension.

Anticholinergics, antihistamines, phenothiazine, tricyclic antidepressants: May increase anticholinergic effects of amantadine.

Hydrochlorothiazide, triamterene: May increase amantadine blood concentration and risk for toxicity.

Live attenuated influenza vaccine: Avoid use of vaccine within 2 wks before or 48 h after amantadine; may reduce vaccine response.

Herbal

None known.

Food

None known.

DIAGNOSTIC TEST EFFECTS

None known.

SIDE EFFECTS

Frequent (5%-10%)

Nausea, dizziness, poor concentration, insomnia, nervousness.

Occasional (1%-5%)
Orthostatic hypotension, anorexia, headache, livedo reticularis (reddish blue, netlike blotching of skin), blurred vision, urine retention, dry mouth or nose, depression, anxiety and irritability, hallucinations, somnolence, abnormal dreams, agitation.
Rare
Vomiting, irritation or swelling of eyes, rash, visual disturbances.

SERIOUS REACTIONS

- CHF, leukopenia, and neutropenia occur rarely.
- Hyperexcitability, seizures, and ventricular arrhythmias may occur.
- Neuroleptic malignant syndrome has occurred upon rapid dose reduction or withdrawal.
- Suicide, suicidal ideation or attempt.

PRECAUTIONS & CONSIDERATIONS

Caution is warranted with cerebrovascular disease, CNS depression, impulse control disorder, CHF, history of seizures, liver disease, orthostatic hypotension, peripheral edema, psychosis, recurrent eczematoid dermatitis, renal dysfunction, and those receiving CNS stimulants. Avoid use in patients with untreated angle-closure glaucoma. There have been reports of suicidal ideation and suicide attempts in patients with and without a history of psychiatric illness. May exacerbate psychiatric symptoms in patients with a history of psychiatric illness. Teratogenic effects observed in animal studies and impaired fertility observed in animal studies and humans. It is distributed into breast milk; use is not recommended in breastfeeding. There are no safety or efficacy data in children < 1 yr of age. Elderly patients may exhibit increased sensitivity to amantadine's anticholinergic effects. In elderly patients, age-related decreased renal function may require dosage adjustment. Avoid alcohol and taking any medications, including over-the-counter (OTC) drugs without first consulting the physician.

Skin should be monitored for peripheral edema, blotching, or rash. Dizziness should be monitored. Food tolerance and episodes of nausea and vomiting should be evaluated. If new symptoms, especially blurred vision, dizziness, nausea or vomiting, and skin blotching or rash, occur, notify the physician. Get up slowly from a sitting or lying position. Do not drive, use machinery, or engage in other activities that require mental acuity if dizziness or blurred vision occurs.
Administration
Use of 2 divided doses may reduce CNS side effects. May take without regard to food. Administer nighttime dose several hours before bedtime to prevent insomnia. Continue therapy for the full length of treatment and evenly space drug doses around the clock.

Ambenonium

am-be-noe'nee-um
★ Mytelase

CATEGORY AND SCHEDULE

Pregnancy Risk Category: C

Classification: Cholinesterase inhibitors

MECHANISM OF ACTION

A cholinesterase inhibitor that enhances and prolongs cholinergic function by increasing the concentration of acetylcholine through inhibition of the hydrolysis of acetylcholine. *Therapeutic Effect:* Increases muscle strength in myasthenia gravis.

PHARMACOKINETICS

Poorly absorbed after PO administration. Onset of action observed within 20-30 min.

AVAILABILITY

Tablets: 10 mg (Mytelase).

INDICATIONS AND DOSAGES

▸ **Myasthenia gravis**

PO

Adults. Initially, 5 mg PO 3 or 4 times per day; gradually increase at intervals of 48 h or more to individual response. Usual maintenance dose 5-25 mg 3 or 4 times a day; however, some rare patients may require 50-75 mg PO 3 or 4 times per day; watch for cholinergic effects.

CONTRAINDICATIONS

Known hypersensitivity to ambenonium. Not recommended in patients receiving routine administration of atropine or other belladonna derivatives. Not recommended in patients receiving mecamylamine.

INTERACTIONS

Drug

Atropine: Suppresses GI side effects; may mask the symptoms of ambenonium overdose.

Herbal

None known.

Food

None known.

DIAGNOSTIC TEST EFFECTS

None known.

SIDE EFFECTS

Frequent

Abdominal pain, diarrhea, increased salivation, miosis, sweating, and vomiting.

Occasional

Anxiety, blurred vision, and urinary urgency.

Rare

Trembling, difficulty moving or controlling movement of the tongue, neck, or arms.

SERIOUS REACTIONS

- Overdosage may result in cholinergic crisis, characterized by severe nausea, vomiting, diarrhea, increased salivation, diaphoresis, bradycardia, hypotension, flushed skin, stomach pain, respiratory depression, seizures, and paralysis of muscles.
- Increasing muscle weakness of myasthenia gravis may occur.

Antidote: 0.5-1 mg IV atropine sulfate with other supportive treatment.

PRECAUTIONS & CONSIDERATIONS

Not recommended if mechanical GI obstruction is present. Caution is warranted in patients with asthma, bladder outflow obstruction, bradycardia, COPD, recent coronary occlusion, vagotonia, hyperthyroidism, cardiac arrhythmias, Parkinson disease, and a history of peptic ulcer disease. It is unknown whether ambenonium crosses the placenta or is excreted in breast milk. Safety and efficacy of ambenonium have not been established in children.

Anticholinergic insensitivity may develop; reduce or withhold ambenonium until the patient becomes sensitive again. Cholinergic reaction, such as diaphoresis, dizziness, excessive salivation, feeling of facial warmth, GI cramping or discomfort, lacrimation, pallor, trembling or difficulty moving or controlling movement of the tongue, neck, or arms, and urinary urgency should be reported.

Storage

Store at room temperature away from light and moisture.

Administration
Ambenonium should be given after food in divided doses at the same times each day.

Ambrisentan

am-bri-sen'tan
★ Letairis
🍁 Volibris

CATEGORY AND SCHEDULE

Pregnancy Risk Category: X

Classification: Endothelin antagonist, vasodilator

MECHANISM OF ACTION

Endothelin receptor antagonist with greater selectivity for the endothelin A receptor than the endothelin B receptor. Stimulation of endothelin receptors is associated with vasoconstriction. Endothelin levels are increased in pulmonary arterial hypertension and correlate with increased mean right arterial pressure and disease severity. *Therapeutic Effect:* Symptomatic improvement in pulmonary artery hypertension and reduced rate of clinical worsening.

PHARMACOKINETICS

Rapidly absorbed; peak concentrations reached within 2 h. Highly plasma protein bound: 99%. Nonrenal elimination. *Half-life:* 9 h.

AVAILABILITY

Tablets: 5 mg, 10 mg.

INDICATIONS AND DOSAGES

▸ **Pulmonary Arterial Hypertension**
PO
Adult. Initiate at 5 mg once daily, consider increasing to 10 mg once daily if 5 mg tolerated.

CONTRAINDICATIONS

Pregnancy.

INTERACTIONS

Drug
Cyclosporine: May increase ambrisentan concentrations and effects; use with caution.
CYP3A4 potent inhibitors (e.g., itraconazole, ketoconazole): May increase ambrisentan concentrations and effects; use with caution.
CYP2C19 potent inhibitors (e.g., omeprazole): May increase ambrisentan concentrations and effects; use with caution.
Herbal
St. John's wort: May reduce abrisentan concentrations and effects; avoid concomitant use.
Food
Grapefruit juice: May increase ambrisentan concentrations and effects.

DIAGNOSTIC TEST EFFECTS

Decreased hemoglobin, increased liver aminotransferases (ALT, AST).

SIDE EFFECTS

Frequent (> 10%)
Peripheral edema, headache.
Occasional (1%-10%)
Nasal congestion, sinusitis, flushing, palpitations, abdominal pain, constipation, decreased hemoglobin, increased hepatic transaminases, dyspnea.

SERIOUS REACTIONS

• Serious liver injury, fluid retention with decompensated heart failure.

PRECAUTIONS & CONSIDERATIONS

Ambrisentan is only available through a restricted distribution system because of the risks of serious liver toxicity and birth defects. The name of the program is Letairis Education and Access Program (LEAP). A Med

Guide must be dispensed with every prescription and refill.

Treat women of childbearing potential only after a negative pregnancy test. Women of childbearing potential must use two reliable methods of contraception unless a nonhormonal IUD is in place. Monthly pregnancy tests are required. It is not known whether ambrisentan is distributed in breast milk; breastfeeding is not recommended.

Ambrisentan is not recommended in patients with moderate or severe hepatic impairment. Liver aminotransferases should be monitored monthly; discontinue therapy if elevated to 5 times the upper limit of normal or if elevations are accompanied by increases in bilirubin or signs or symptoms of liver dysfunction.

Monitor hemoglobin at initiation, 1 mo after initiation, and periodically thereafter; reductions in hemoglobin levels have been observed within the first few weeks of therapy.

Safety and efficacy have not been established in pediatric patients. Peripheral edema occurs more frequently in elderly patients.

Storage

Store at room temperature in the original blister packaging.

Administration

May be taken with or without food. Tablets should not be split, crushed, or chewed. Take at about the same time each day.

Amcinonide

am-sin'oh-nide

🍁 Cyclocort

CATEGORY AND SCHEDULE

Pregnancy Risk Category: C

Classification: Anti-inflammatory, steroidal, topical

MECHANISM OF ACTION

Topical corticosteroids have anti-inflammatory, antipruritic, and vasoconstrictive properties. The exact mechanism of the anti-inflammatory process is unclear. Amcinonide is categorized as a high-potency topical corticosteroid. *Therapeutic Effect:* Reduces or prevents tissue response to inflammatory process. High-potency fluorinated corticosteroid.

PHARMACOKINETICS

Well absorbed systemically. Large variation in absorption among sites: forearm 1%, scalp 4%, forehead 7%, scrotum 36%. Greatest penetration occurs at groin, axillae, and face. Protein binding in varying degrees. Metabolized in liver. Primarily excreted in urine.

AVAILABILITY

Cream: 0.1%.
Lotion: 0.1%.
Ointment: 0.1%.

INDICATIONS AND DOSAGES

▸ **Corticosteroid-responsive dermatoses**

TOPICAL

Adults, Elderly. Apply sparingly 2-3 times/day.

CONTRAINDICATIONS

History of hypersensitivity to amcinonide or other corticosteroids; use on face, groin, or axilla.

INTERACTIONS

Drug

None known.

Herbal

None known.

Food

None known.

DIAGNOSTIC TEST EFFECTS

Uncommon under usual use.

SIDE EFFECTS

Frequent
Itching, redness, irritation, burning.
Occasional
Dryness, folliculitis, hypertrichosis, acneiform eruptions, hypopigmentation, perioral dermatitis.
Rare
Allergic contact dermatitis, maceration of the skin, secondary infection, skin atrophy.
Systemic: Absorption more likely with occlusive dressings or extensive application in young children.

SERIOUS REACTIONS

- The serious reactions of long-term therapy and the addition of occlusive dressings are reversible hypothalamic-pituitary-adrenal (HPA) axis suppression, manifestations of Cushing syndrome, hyperglycemia, and glucosuria.
- Abruptly withdrawing the drug after long-term therapy may require supplemental systemic corticosteroids.

PRECAUTIONS & CONSIDERATIONS

Caution is necessary when using amcinonide over large surface areas, prolonged use, and the addition of occlusive dressings. Long-term therapy and the addition of occlusive dressings can lead to reversible hypothalamic-pituitary-adrenal (HPA) axis suppression, manifestations of Cushing syndrome, hyperglycemia, and glucosuria. Children may absorb larger amounts and may be more susceptible to toxicity. It is unknown whether amcinonide is distributed in breast milk.

Signs of a rash in addition to fever and sore throat should be reported. Sunlight should be avoided.

Administration
Amcinonide should be applied sparingly to the skin and rubbed gently into affected area. Apply after bath or shower for best absorption, and do not cover the area with any coverings, plastic pants, or tight diapers unless instructed. Occlusive dressings may be used in the management of psoriasis or recalcitrant conditions. Avoid contact with eyes.

Amifostine

am-ih-fos′teen
★ Ethyol
Do not confuse Ethyol with ethanol.

CATEGORY AND SCHEDULE

Pregnancy Risk Category: C

Classification: Cytoprotective, radioprotective

MECHANISM OF ACTION

An antineoplastic adjunct and cytoprotective agent that is converted to an active metabolite by alkaline phosphatase in tissues. The active metabolite binds to and detoxifies metabolites of cisplatin. These actions occur more readily in normal tissues than in tumor tissue. *Therapeutic Effect:* Reduces the toxic effect of the chemotherapeutic agent cisplatin.

PHARMACOKINETICS

Rapidly cleared from plasma. Converted in tissue to active free thiol metabolite. Tissue uptake highest in bone marrow, skin, GI mucosa, salivary glands. *Half-life:* Distribution half-life < 1 min; elimination half-life 8 min. Less than

10% remains in plasma 6 min after drug administration.

AVAILABILITY

Lyophilized Powder for Injection: 500 mg.

INDICATIONS AND DOSAGES

▸ **To reduce cumulative renal toxicity from repeated administration of cisplatin in patients with advanced ovarian cancer**

IV

Adults. 910 mg/m² once a day as 15-min infusion, beginning 30 min before chemotherapy. A 15-min infusion is better tolerated than extended infusions. If the full dose cannot be administered, dose for subsequent cycles should be 740 mg/m².

▸ **Treatment of postoperative radiation-induced xerostomia in patients with head and neck cancer**

IV

Adults. 200 mg/m² once a day as 3-min infusion, starting 15-30 min before radiation therapy.

CONTRAINDICATIONS

Sensitivity to aminothiol compounds or mannitol.

INTERACTIONS

Drugs

Antihypertensives: Increased risk of hypotension; interrupt antihypertensive therapy for at least 24 h before amifostine administration.

DIAGNOSTIC TEST EFFECTS

May lower serum calcium levels with multiple doses.

IV INCOMPATIBILITIES

Do not mix with any other drugs or solutions except those with established compatibility. Acyclovir, amphotericin B, cefoperazone, cisplatin, ganciclovir, hydroxyzine HCl, mycophenolate mofetil, prochlorperazine, quinupristin-dalfopristin (Synercid).

IV COMPATIBILITIES

Per manufacturer, compatibility only established with 0.9% NaCl and NaCl with other additives.

SIDE EFFECTS

Frequent (> 10%)

Transient reduction in BP (usually starts 14 min into infusion, lasts about 6 min and returns to normal in 5–15 min); severe nausea, vomiting.

Occasional

Flushing or feeling of warmth or chills or feeling of coldness; dizziness, hiccups, sneezing, somnolence.

Rare

Clinically relevant hypocalcemia, mild rash.

SERIOUS REACTIONS

- A pronounced drop in BP may require temporary cessation of amifostine and fluid resuscitation.
- Serious cutaneous reactions, including erythema multiforme, Stevens-Johnson syndrome, toxic epidermal necrolysis, toxoderma, and exfoliative dermatitis.
- Anaphylaxis, arrhythmias, seizures, syncope.

PRECAUTIONS & CONSIDERATIONS

Patients should be well hydrated. Monitor BP frequently during infusion and as clinically indicated following completion of infusion. Safety not established in patients with cardiovascular disease, in elderly patients, in lactating women, or in children. Antiemetic medications should be administered before and in conjunction with amifostine. Interrupt antihypertensive therapy 24 h preceding amifostine administration. Amifostine does not negate the chemotherapeutic effect of the treatments for which it is indicated to accompany; the drug should not be used in other situations for other chemotherapy or radiation except in a clinical trial.

Patients should be closely assessed for cutaneous reactions before each dose. Therapy should be permanently discontinued for serious or severe cutaneous reactions or cutaneous reactions associated with fever or other constitutional symptoms.

Storage

Store unreconstituted vials at room temperature. Reconstituted solution is stable for up to 5 h at room temperature or up to 24 h in the refrigerator. The infusion solution prepared in polyvinylchloride bags at concentrations of 5-40 mg/mL is stable for up to 5 h at room temperature or 24 h in the refrigerator.

Administration

Reconstitute each vial with 9.7 mL normal saline. The concentration in the vial is 500 mg/10 mL. The needed drug dose is then further diluted with 0.9% NaCl injection in PVC bags at concentrations ranging from 5-40 mg/mL. Before chemotherapy, amifostine should be administered as a 15-min infusion. Before radiation therapy, amifostine should be administered as a 3-min infusion.

Amikacin

am-i-kay'sin

★ Amikin

Do not confuse with Amicar.

CATEGORY AND SCHEDULE

Pregnancy Risk Category: C

Classification: Antibiotics, aminoglycosides

MECHANISM OF ACTION

An aminoglycoside antibiotic that irreversibly binds to protein on bacterial ribosomes. *Therapeutic Effect:* Interferes with protein synthesis of susceptible bacterial microorganisms.

PHARMACOKINETICS

Rapid, complete absorption after IM administration. Protein binding: 0%-10%. Widely distributed (does not cross the blood-brain barrier, low concentrations in CSF). Excreted unchanged in urine. Removed by hemodialysis. *Half-life:* 2-4 h (increased in impaired renal function and neonates; decreased in cystic fibrosis and burn or febrile patients).

AVAILABILITY

Injection. 50 mg/mL, 250 mg/mL.

INDICATIONS AND DOSAGES

▸ Uncomplicated urinary tract infections

IV, IM

Adults, Elderly. 250 mg q12h.

▸ Moderate to severe infections

IV, IM

Adults, Elderly. 15 mg/kg/day in divided doses q8-12h. Maximum 1.5 g/day.

Children, Infants. 15 mg/kg/day in divided doses q8h.

Neonates. 10 mg/kg loading dose, followed by 7.5 mg/kg q12h.

▸ Dosage in renal impairment

Dosage and frequency are modified based on the degree of renal impairment and serum drug concentration. After a loading dose of 5-7.5 mg/kg, the maintenance dose and frequency are based on serum creatinine levels and creatinine clearance and are adjusted based on therapeutic drug monitoring. Common off-label dosing strategies use a "once daily" dose of 15 mg/kg and then adjust the frequency of administration according to serum levels and medically accepted dosing nomograms.

CONTRAINDICATIONS

Hypersensitivity to amikacin, other aminoglycosides (cross-sensitivity), or their components.

INTERACTIONS

Drug

Loop diuretics: May increase the risk of ototoxicity because both agents have the potential to cause ototoxicity and potent diuretics may alter amikacin concentrations.
Nephrotoxic medications, other aminoglycosides, ototoxic medications: May increase the risk of nephrotoxicity or ototoxicity.
Neuromuscular blockers: May enhance neuromuscular blockade.

DIAGNOSTIC TEST EFFECTS

May increase serum bilirubin, BUN, serum creatinine, serum LDH, SGOT (AST), and SGPT (ALT) levels. May decrease serum calcium, magnesium, potassium, and sodium concentrations. Therapeutic peak serum level is 15-35 mcg/mL, and therapeutic trough is < 4-8 mcg/mL, depending on infection severity and site of infection. Toxic peak concentration is > 35 mcg/mL, and toxic trough serum level is > 10 mcg/mL.

IV INCOMPATIBILITIES

Amphotericin B, ampicillin, azathioprine (Imuran), azithromycin (Zithromax IV), cefazolin (Ancef), diazepam, folic acid, ganciclovir, heparin, Hetastarch 6%, indomethacin, pentobarbital, phenytoin (Dilantin), propofol (Diprivan), sulfamethoxazole/trimethoprim, thiopental, trastuzumab (Herceptin).

IV COMPATIBILITIES

Amiodarone (Cordarone), aztreonam (Azactam), calcium gluconate, cefepime (Maxipime), cimetidine (Tagamet), ciprofloxacin (Cipro), clindamycin (Cleocin), diltiazem (Cardizem), enalapril (Vasotec), esmolol (BreviBloc), fluconazole (Diflucan), furosemide (Lasix), levofloxacin (Levaquin), lorazepam (Ativan), magnesium sulfate, midazolam (Versed), morphine, ondansetron (Zofran), potassium chloride, ranitidine (Zantac), vancomycin.

SIDE EFFECTS

Frequent

IM: Pain, induration.
IV: Phlebitis, thrombophlebitis.

Occasional

Hypersensitivity reactions (rash, fever, urticaria, pruritus).

Rare

Neuromuscular blockade (difficulty breathing, drowsiness, weakness).

SERIOUS REACTIONS

- Serious reactions may include nephrotoxicity (as evidenced by reduced urine output, decreased appetite, nausea, vomiting, increased BUN and serum creatinine levels, and decreased creatinine clearance); and ototoxicity (as evidenced by tinnitus, dizziness, and loss of hearing).
- Neuromuscular blockade and weakness occur rarely.

PRECAUTIONS & CONSIDERATIONS

Caution is warranted with patients with 8th cranial nerve (vestibulocochlear nerve) impairment, decreased renal function, myasthenia gravis, and Parkinson disease. Amikacin readily crosses the placenta, and small amounts are distributed in breast milk. It may produce fetal nephrotoxicity. Neonates and premature infants may be more susceptible to amikacin toxicity because of their immature renal function. Elderly patients are at increased risk for amikacin toxicity because of age-related renal impairment as well as an increased risk for hearing loss. Signs and symptoms of superinfection, particularly changes in the oral mucosa, diarrhea, and genital or anal pruritus, should be monitored. Safety for treatment periods exceeding 14 days has not been established.

Determine the history of allergies, especially to aminoglycosides and sulfites. Expect to correct dehydration before beginning aminoglycoside therapy. Establish the baseline hearing acuity before beginning therapy. Obtain a specimen for culture and sensitivity testing before giving the first dose. Therapy may begin before test results are known. Urinalysis results to detect casts, RBCs, WBCs, and decreased specific gravity should be monitored. Expect to monitor peak and trough serum amikacin levels. Be alert for ototoxic and neurotoxic side effects.

Storage
Store vials at room temperature. Solutions normally appear clear but may become pale yellow; the yellow color does not affect the drug's potency. Discard the solution if a precipitate forms or dark discoloration occurs. Intermittent IV infusion (piggyback) is stable for 24 h at room temperature.

Administration
For intermittent IV infusion (piggyback), dilute each 500 mg with 100 mL of 0.9% NaCl or D5W. Infuse over 30-60 min for adults and older children. Dilution volumes for younger children and infants must be individualized. Infuse over 60-120 min for infants and young children.

For IM injection, administer slowly to minimize patient discomfort. Injections administered into the gluteus maximus are less painful than those given in the lateral aspect of the thigh.

Amiloride Hydrochloride

a-mill′oh-ride hi-droh-klor′ide
Midamor
Do not confuse with amiodarone or amlodipine.

CATEGORY AND SCHEDULE
Pregnancy Risk Category: B

Classification: Diuretics, potassium sparing

MECHANISM OF ACTION
A guanidine derivative that acts as a potassium-sparing diuretic, antihypertensive, and antihypokalemic by directly interfering with sodium reabsorption in the distal tubule. *Therapeutic Effect:* Increases sodium and water excretion and decreases potassium excretion.

PHARMACOKINETICS

Route	Onset	Peak	Duration
PO	2 h	6-10 h	24 h

Incompletely absorbed from GI tract. Protein binding: Minimal. Primarily excreted in urine; partially eliminated in feces. *Half-life:* 6-9 h.

AVAILABILITY
Tablets: 5 mg.

INDICATIONS AND DOSAGES

▸ To treat hypertension and congestive heart failure and to counteract potassium loss induced by other diuretics

PO

Adults. 5-10 mg/day, up to 20 mg/day.
Elderly. Initially, 5 mg/day or every other day.

▸ Dosage in renal impairment

Creatinine Clearance (mL/min)	Dosage
10-50	50% of normal
< 10	Avoid use

OFF-LABEL USES

Liver cirrhosis and nephrotic syndrome.

CONTRAINDICATIONS

Hypersensitivity; use of potassium supplements except if serious hypokalemia present, acute or chronic renal insufficiency, anuria, diabetic nephropathy, patients on other potassium-sparing diuretics, serum potassium > 5.5 mEq/L.

INTERACTIONS

Drug

ACE inhibitors, including captopril, and potassium-sparing diuretics: May increase potassium levels.
Anticoagulants, including heparin: May decrease effect of anticoagulants, including heparin.
Drospirenone: May increase potassium levels.
Lithium: May decrease lithium clearance and increase risk of lithium toxicity.
NSAIDs: May decrease antihypertensive effect.

Herbal

Licorice: May cause potassium loss.

Food

None known.

DIAGNOSTIC TEST EFFECTS

May increase BUN, calcium excretion, and glucose, serum creatinine, serum magnesium, serum potassium, and uric acid levels. May decrease serum sodium levels.

SIDE EFFECTS

Frequent (3%-8%)

Headache, nausea, diarrhea, vomiting, decreased appetite.

Occasional (1%-3%)

Dizziness, constipation, abdominal pain, weakness, fatigue, cough, impotence, hyperkalemia.

Rare (< 1%)

Tremors, vertigo, confusion, nervousness, insomnia, thirst, dry mouth, heartburn, shortness of breath, increased urination, hypotension, rash.

SERIOUS REACTIONS

- Severe hyperkalemia may produce irritability, anxiety, a feeling of heaviness in the legs, paresthesia of hands, face, and lips, hypotension, bradycardia, tented T waves, widening of QRS, and ST depression.

PRECAUTIONS & CONSIDERATIONS

Caution is warranted with cardiopulmonary disease, diabetes mellitus, or liver insufficiency, BUN > 30 mg/dL or serum creatinine > 1.5 mg/dL, and in elderly and debilitated patients. Be aware that it is unknown whether amiloride crosses the placenta or is distributed in breast milk. There are no age-related precautions noted in children. In elderly patients, age-related decreased renal function increases the risk of hyperkalemia and may require caution. Incidence of hyperkalemia is increased when administered without a kaliuretic diuretic. Be aware a high-potassium diet and potassium supplements can be dangerous, especially with liver or kidney problems.

Notify the physician of signs and symptoms of hyperkalemia: confusion; difficulty breathing; irregular heartbeat; nervousness; numbness of the hands, feet, or lips; unusual tiredness; and weakness in the legs. BP, vital signs, electrolytes, intake and output, weight, and potassium levels should be monitored before and during treatment. A baseline 12-lead ECG should also be obtained.

Storage

Store at controlled room temperature; protect from light and moisture

Administration

Take with food. Therapeutic effect of the drug takes several days to begin and can last for several days after the drug is discontinued.

Aminocaproic Acid

a-mee-noe-ka-proe′ik as′id

★ Amicar

Do not confuse Amicar with amikacin or Amikin.

CATEGORY AND SCHEDULE

Pregnancy Risk Category: C

Classification: Hemostatic

MECHANISM OF ACTION

A systemic hemostatic that acts as an antifibrinolytic and antihemorrhagic by inhibiting the activation of plasminogen activator substances. *Therapeutic Effect:* Prevents fibrinolysis.

PHARMACOKINETICS

Mean peak concentration reached within 1-2 h. Primarily excreted unchanged in the urine (65%). *Half-life:* 2 h.

AVAILABILITY

Tablets: 500 mg, 1000 mg.
Injection: 250 mg/mL.

INDICATIONS AND DOSAGES

▸ **Acute bleeding**

PO, IV INFUSION

Adults, Elderly. 4-5 g over first hour; then 1-1.25 g/h. Continue for 8 h or until bleeding is controlled. Maximum: 30 g/24 h.

Children. 3 g/m^2 over first hour; then 1 g/m^2/h. Maximum: 18 g/m^2/24 h.

OFF-LABEL USES

Prevention of recurrence of subarachnoid hemorrhage, prevention of hemorrhage in hemophiliacs following dental surgery.

CONTRAINDICATIONS

Evidence of active intravascular clotting process, disseminated intravascular coagulation without concurrent heparin therapy, hematuria of upper urinary tract origin (unless benefit outweighs risk); newborns (parenteral form).

INTERACTIONS

Drug

Oral contraceptives, estrogens: May increase clotting factors leading to a hypercoagulable state.

DIAGNOSTIC TEST EFFECTS

May elevate serum potassium level.

IV INCOMPATIBILITIES

Sodium lactate. Do not mix with other medications. Do not give with Factor IX complexes or anti-inhibitor coagulant complexes.

SIDE EFFECTS

Occasional

Nausea, diarrhea, cramps, decreased urination, decreased BP, dizziness, headache, muscle fatigue and weakness, myopathy, bloodshot eyes.

SERIOUS REACTIONS

- Too-rapid IV administration produces hypotension, tinnitus, rash, arrhythmias, unusual fatigue, and weakness.
- Rarely, a grand mal seizure occurs, generally preceded by weakness, dizziness, and headache.

PRECAUTIONS & CONSIDERATIONS

Caution is warranted with hyperfibrinolysis, skeletal muscle weakness, and impaired cardiac, hepatic, or renal function. No information is available concerning the distribution of aminocaproic acid in breast milk. There is no documented evidence of age-related problems in children; however, injectable contains benzyl alcohol and is not recommended for use in newborns. Although no elderly-related problems have been noted, cautious use is advised because of the risk of age-related renal impairment, which may require dosage reduction. Women may experience an increase in menstrual flow.

Notify the physician of red or dark urine, muscular pain or weakness, abdominal or back pain, gingival bleeding, black or red stool, coffee-ground vomitus, or blood-tinged mucus from cough. BP, heart rate and rhythm, and pulse rate, serum creatine kinase, and AST (SGOT) levels should be monitored.

Storage

Store tablets and solution at room temperature; keep tightly closed. Do not freeze solution.

Store injection at room temperature.

Administration

! Expect to administer a reduced dose if the patient has cardiac, renal, or hepatic impairment.

For IV use, dilute each 1 g in up to 50 mL 0.9% NaCl, D5W, Ringer's solution, or sterile water for injection. Do not use sterile water for injection in those with subarachnoid hemorrhage. Do not give by direct injection. Give only by IV infusion. Infuse 5 g or less over the first hour in 250 mL of solution. Give each succeeding 1 g over 1 h in 50-100 mL of solution. Monitor for hypotension during the infusion. Be aware that rapid infusion may produce arrhythmias, including bradycardia.

Aminophylline

am-in-off'i-lin

Phyllocontin

Do not confuse aminophylline with amitriptyline or ampicillin.

CATEGORY AND SCHEDULE

Pregnancy Risk Category: C

Classification: Bronchodilators, xanthine derivatives

MECHANISM OF ACTION

A xanthine derivative that acts as a bronchodilator by directly relaxing smooth muscle of the bronchial airways and pulmonary blood vessels. *Therapeutic Effect:* Relieves bronchospasm and increases vital capacity.

PHARMACOKINETICS

Aminophylline is rapidly converted to theophylline. See theophylline monograph.

AVAILABILITY

Tablets: 100 mg, 200 mg.
Injection (aminophylline): 25 mg/mL.

INDICATIONS AND DOSAGES

Note that aminophylline dose equals theophylline dose divided by 0.8. Doses should be calculated based on ideal body weight.

Theophylline is usually preferred for oral dosages.

▸ **Chronic bronchospasm**

PO

Adults, Elderly, Children weighing more than 45 kg. Aminophylline 380 mg/day divided every 6-8 h, after 3 days if tolerated may increase to aminophylline 507 mg/day divided every 6-8 h, and after 3 additional days if tolerated and increased dose is necessary may increase to aminophylline 760 mg/day divided every 6-8 h. Maximum dose is theophylline 400 mg/day in adults with risk factors for reduced clearance or when concentration monitoring is not feasible.

▸ **Acute bronchospasm in patients not currently taking theophylline**

PO

Adults, children older than 1 yr. Initially, loading dose of aminophylline 6.25 mg/kg, then maintenance dosage of oral theophylline based on patient group (shown below).

Patient Group	Maintenance Theophylline Dosage*
Healthy, nonsmoking adults	3 mg/kg q8h
Elderly patients, patients with cor pulmonale	2 mg/kg q8h
Patients with CHF or hepatic disease	1-2 mg/kg q12h
Children 9-16 yr, young adult smokers	3 mg/kg q6h
Children 1-8 yr	4 mg/kg q6h

*Convert dose to aminophylline equivalent if using aminophylline. Aminophylline dose equals theophylline dose divided by 0.8.

IV INFUSION

Adults, Children older than 1 yr. Initially, loading dose of 6 mg/kg (aminophylline); maintenance dosage of aminophylline based on patient group (shown next).

Patient Group	Maintenance Aminophylline Dosage
Healthy, nonsmoking adults	0.7 mg/kg/h
Elderly patients, patients with cor pulmonale, CHF, or hepatic impairment	0.25 mg/kg/h
Children 13-16 yr	0.7 mg/kg/h
Children 9-12 yr, young adult smokers	0.9 mg/kg/h
Children 1-8 yr	1-1.2 mg/kg/h
Children 6 mo to 1 yr	0.6-0.7 mg/kg/h
Children 6 wks to 6 mo	0.5 mg/kg/h
Neonates	5 mg/kg q12h

▸ **Acute bronchospasm in patients currently taking theophylline**

PO, IV

Adults, children older than 1 yr. Obtain serum theophylline level. If not possible and patient is in respiratory distress and not experiencing toxic effects, may give theophylline 2.5 mg/kg dose. Maintenance: Dosage based on peak serum theophylline concentration, clinical condition, and presence of toxicity.

CONTRAINDICATIONS

History of hypersensitivity to caffeine or xanthine.

INTERACTIONS

Drug

β-blockers: May decrease the effects of aminophylline.

Cimetidine, ciprofloxacin, erythromycin, fluvoxamine, norfloxacin, tacrine, zileuton: May increase theophylline blood concentration and risk of aminophylline toxicity.

Phenytoin, primidone, rifampin: May increase theophylline metabolism.
Smoking: May decrease theophylline blood concentration.
Food
Charcoal-broiled foods; high-protein, low-carbohydrate diet: May decrease the theophylline blood level.

DIAGNOSTIC TEST EFFECTS

None known. Measure serum theophylline level to guide all dosage adjustments.

IV INCOMPATIBILITIES

Amiodarone (Cordarone), ciprofloxacin (Cipro), dobutamine (Dobutrex), epinephrine, hydroxyzine, magnesium sulfate, norepinephrine, ondansetron (Zofran).

IV COMPATIBILITIES

Aztreonam (Azactam), ceftazidime (Fortaz), dopamine, fluconazole (Diflucan), heparin, morphine, potassium chloride.

SIDE EFFECTS

Frequent
Altered smell (during IV administration) nausea, restlessness, tachycardia, tremor.
Occasional
Heartburn, vomiting, headache, mild diuresis, insomnia.

SERIOUS REACTIONS

- Too-rapid IV administration or excessive dosage may produce marked hypotension with accompanying faintness, light-headedness, palpitations, tachycardia, hyperventilation, nausea, vomiting, angina-like pain, seizures, ventricular fibrillation, and cardiac standstill.

PRECAUTIONS & CONSIDERATIONS

Monitor signs and symptoms of theophylline toxicity, as well as serum drug levels, often to ensure appropriate dosage. Caution is warranted with diabetes mellitus; glaucoma; hypertension; hyperthyroidism; cardiac, renal, or hepatic impairment; peptic ulcer disease; and seizure disorder. Aminophylline crosses the placenta and small amounts of the drug may be distributed in breast milk and cause irritability in the breastfeeding infant. Use the drug cautiously in children < 1 yr. Drink plenty of fluids to decrease the thickness of lung secretions. Avoid excessive use of caffeinated products, such as chocolate, cocoa, cola, coffee, and tea. Smoking, charcoal-broiled foods, and a high-protein, low-carbohydrate diet may decrease the theophylline level.

Pulse rate and quality; respiratory rate, depth, rhythm, and type; ABG levels; and serum potassium levels should be monitored. Peak serum concentration should be obtained 1 h after an IV dose, 1-2 h after an immediate-release dose, and 3-8 h after a sustained-release dose. Serum trough level should be obtained just before the next dose. Lips and fingernails should be assessed for signs of hypoxemia, such as a blue or gray color in light-skinned patients and a gray color in dark-skinned patients.

Storage
Store injection vials at room temperature. Do not use if crystals are present.

Store tablets and oral solution at room temperature. Protect from light and moisture.

Administration
Take oral aminophylline with food to avoid GI distress.

Discard the solution for injection if it contains a precipitate. For IV use, give loading dose diluted in 100-200 mL of D5W or 0.9% NaCl. Prepare maintenance dose in larger-volume parenteral infusion. Usual concentration for maintenance infusion is 1 mg/mL. Do not exceed a flow rate of 25 mg/min for either piggyback or infusion. Administer loading dose over 20-30 min. Use an infusion pump or microdrip to regulate IV administration.

Aminosalicylic Acid

a-mee-noe-sal-i-sil′ik as′id

★ Paser

CATEGORY AND SCHEDULE

Pregnancy Risk Category: C

Classification: Antitubercular anti-infective

MECHANISM OF ACTION

An antitubercular agent active against *M. tuberculosis.* Thought to exhibit competitive antagonism of folic acid synthesis. *Therapeutic Effect:* Bacteriostatic activity in susceptible microorganisms.

PHARMACOKINETICS

Readily absorbed from the GI tract. Protein binding: 50%-60%. Widely distributed (including CSF). Metabolized in liver. Primarily excreted in urine. Removed by hemodialysis. *Half-life:* 1.1-1.62 h.

AVAILABILITY

Packet Granules: 4 g/packet granules (Paser).

INDICATIONS AND DOSAGES

▸ **Tuberculosis in combination with other agents; most commonly used for Multi-drug Resistant TB (MDR-TB)**

PO

Adults, Elderly. 4 g in divided doses 3 times/day.

Children. 150 mg/kg/day in divided doses 3 times/day. Maximum: 12 g/day.

OFF-LABEL USES

Crohn disease, hyperlipidemia, ulcerative colitis.

CONTRAINDICATIONS

End-stage renal disease, hypersensitivity to aminosalicylic acid products.

INTERACTIONS

Drug

Cyanocobalamin: May decrease cyanocobalamin absorption.

Digoxin: May decrease digoxin absorption.

Isoniazid: May increase isoniazid serum levels.

DIAGNOSTIC TEST EFFECTS

May alter bilirubin levels in urinalysis.

SIDE EFFECTS

Occasional

Abdominal pain, diarrhea, nausea, vomiting.

Rare

Hypersensitivity reactions, hepatotoxicity, thrombocytopenia.

SERIOUS REACTIONS

• Liver toxicity and hepatitis, blood dyscrasias occur rarely.

• Agranulocytosis, methemoglobinemia, thrombocytopenia have been reported.

PRECAUTIONS & CONSIDERATIONS

Patients with aspirin-sensitive asthma and nasal polyps may be more likely to experience sensitivity reactions. Precaution is necessary with liver insufficiency, peptic ulcer disease, impaired renal function, and congestive heart failure. It is unknown whether aminosalicylic acid crosses the placenta or is excreted in breast milk. There are no age-related precautions noted in children or in elderly patients. Be aware that skeleton of the granules may appear in the stool.

Liver function should be monitored during therapy. Symptoms of hepatitis as evidenced by anorexia, dark urine, fatigue, jaundice, nausea, vomiting, and weakness should be assessed. If hepatitis is suspected, withhold the drug and notify the physician promptly.

Storage

Store in refrigerator or freezer.

Administration

May sprinkle granules on acidic food such as applesauce or yogurt or mix with acidic drink such as tomato, orange, grapefruit, grape, cranberry, or apple juice or fruit punch. Granules must be swirled in drink since they will not dissolve. Care must be taken to maintain the enteric coating; in the presence of gastric acid, unprotected aminosalicylic acid is converted to a known hepatotoxin. Discard medication if the package is swollen or the granules are dark brown or purple.

Amiodarone

a-mee′oh-da-rone

☆ Cordarone, Pacerone

Do not confuse amiodarone with amiloride or Cordarone with Cardura.

CATEGORY AND SCHEDULE

Pregnancy Risk Category: D

Classification: Antiarrhythmics, class III

MECHANISM OF ACTION

A cardiac agent that prolongs duration of myocardial cell action potential and refractory period by acting directly on all cardiac tissue. Decreases AV and sinus node function. *Therapeutic Effect:* Suppresses arrhythmias.

PHARMACOKINETICS

Route	Onset	Steady State	Duration
PO	3 days to 3 wks	1 wk to 5 mo	7-50 days after discontinuation

Slowly, variably absorbed from GI tract; oral bioavailability is 35%-65%. Protein binding: 96%. Extensively metabolized by CYP3A4 and CYP2C8 to active metabolite. Excreted via bile; not removed by hemodialysis. *Half-life:* 26-107 days; metabolite, 61 days.

AVAILABILITY

Tablets (Cordarone): 200 mg.
Tablets (Pacerone): 100 mg, 200 mg, 400 mg.
Injection (Cordarone): 50 mg/mL.

INDICATIONS AND DOSAGES

▸ **Life-threatening recurrent ventricular fibrillation or hemodynamically unstable ventricular tachycardia**

PO

Adults, Elderly. Initially, load with (unless patient has been on IV treatment) 800-1600 mg/day in 2-4 divided doses for 1-3 wks. After arrhythmia is controlled or side effects occur, reduce to 600-800 mg/day for about 4 wks. Maintenance: 200-600 mg/day with a usual maintenance dose of 400 mg/day.

IV INFUSION
Adults. Initially, 150 mg over 10 min, then 360 mg over 6 h; then 540 mg over 18 h. May continue at 0.5 mg/min for up to 2-3 wks regardless of age or renal or left ventricular function.

OFF-LABEL USES

ACLS protocol for ventricular arrhythmias. Treatment and prevention of supraventricular arrhythmias and symptomatic atrial flutter refractory to conventional treatment.

CONTRAINDICATIONS

Bradycardia-induced syncope (except in the presence of a pacemaker), cardiogenic shock, second- and third-degree AV block, severe hepatic disease, severe sinus-node dysfunction; hypersensitivity to amiodarone or its components, including iodine.

INTERACTIONS

Drug
Antiarrhythmics: May increase cardiac effects.
Azole antifungals, fluoroquinolones, macrolides, ranolazine, thioridazine, vardenafil, ziprasidone: Risk of cardiac arrhythmias, including torsades de pointes, may be increased.
β-blockers, oral anticoagulants: May increase effect of β-blockers and oral anticoagulants.
Cyclosporine: Increased cyclosporine concentrations.
Digoxin, phenytoin: May increase drug concentration and risk of toxicity of digoxin and phenytoin.
Protease inhibitors: Increased amiodarone concentrations/toxicity; ritonavir and nelfinavir are contraindicted with amiodarone.
Simvastatin: May increase risk of myopathy/rhabdomyolysis.
Warfarin: Increased anticoagulant effect; closely monitor International Normalized Ratio.
Herbal
St. John's wort: May reduce amiodarone concentrations.
Food
All foods: Food increases the rate and extent of absorption. Dose consistently with regard to meals.
Grapefruit juice: Increased amiodarone concentrations; avoid grapefruit juice.

DIAGNOSTIC TEST EFFECTS

May increase antinuclear antibody titers and AST (SGOT), ALT (SGPT), and serum alkaline phosphatase levels. May cause changes in ECG and thyroid function test results. Therapeutic serum level is 0.5-2.5 mcg/mL, but is not well correlated with efficacy as a result of long half-life of drug.

IV INCOMPATIBILITIES

Aminophylline, ampicillin/sulbactam (Unasyn), argatroban, atenolol, cefamandole, cefazolin (Ancef), ceftazidime (Fortaz), digoxin (Lanoxin), doxorubicin, ertapenem (Invanz), heparin, imipenem/cilastatin (Primaxin), levofloxacin, (Levaquin), mezlocillin, micafungin (Mycamine), paclitaxel, piperacillin/tazobactam (Zosyn), potassium phosphate, sodium acetate, sodium bicarbonate, sodium phosphate

IV COMPATIBILITIES

Dobutamine (Dobutrex), dopamine (Intropin), furosemide (Lasix), insulin (regular), labetalol (Normodyne), lidocaine, midazolam (Versed), morphine, nitroglycerin, norepinephrine (Levophed), phenylephrine (Neo-Synephrine), potassium chloride, vancomycin.

SIDE EFFECTS

Expected
Corneal microdeposits are noted in almost all patients treated for more than 6 mo (can lead to blurry vision).

Frequent (> 3%)
Parenteral: Hypotension, nausea, fever, bradycardia.
Oral: Constipation, headache, decreased appetite, nausea, vomiting, paresthesias, photosensitivity, muscular incoordination, hypothyroidism, malaise, fatigue, tremor, abnormal liver function tests.

Occasional (< 3%)
Oral: Bitter or metallic taste, decreased libido, dizziness, facial flushing, blue-gray coloring of skin (face, arms, and neck), blurred vision, bradycardia, asymptomatic corneal deposits, hyperthyroidism.

Rare (< 1%)
Oral: Rash, vision loss, blindness, peripheral neuropathy.

SERIOUS REACTIONS

- Serious, potentially fatal pulmonary toxicity (alveolitis, pulmonary fibrosis, pneumonitis, acute respiratory distress syndrome) may begin with progressive dyspnea and cough with crackles, decreased breath sounds, pleurisy, CHF.
- Amiodarone may worsen existing arrhythmias or produce new arrhythmias (called proarrhythmias).
- Hepatotoxicity may occur.
- May induce hyper- or hypothyroidism.

PRECAUTIONS & CONSIDERATIONS

A Med Guide must be dispensed with every prescription and refill.

Caution is warranted with thyroid disease. Amiodarone crosses the placenta and is distributed in breast milk; it adversely affects fetal development. Safety and efficacy of amiodarone have not been established in children. Elderly patients may be more sensitive to amiodarone's effects on thyroid function and may experience increased incidence of ataxia or other neurotoxic effects. Amiodarone may cause photosensitivity; wear sunscreen and sun-protective clothing.

! Signs and symptoms of pulmonary toxicity, including progressively worsening cough and dyspnea, should be assessed. Dosage should be discontinued or reduced if toxicity occurs.

Chest x-ray, ECG, pulmonary function tests, liver enzyme tests, AST, ALT, and serum alkaline phosphatase level should be obtained at baseline and during therapy. Apical pulse and BP should be assessed immediately before giving amiodarone. Withhold the medication and notify the physician if the pulse rate is 60 beats/min or lower or the systolic BP is < 90 mm Hg. Pulse rate for bradycardia, an irregular rhythm, and quality should be monitored. ECG for changes such as widening of the QRS complex and prolonged PR and QT intervals should be assessed; notify the physician of significant interval changes. Signs and symptoms of hyperthyroidism, such as difficulty breathing, bulging eyes (exophthalmos), eyelid edema, frequent urination, hot and dry skin, and weight loss, and signs and symptoms of hypothyroidism, such as cool and pale skin, lethargy, night cramps, periorbital edema, and pudgy hands and feet should also be monitored.

Storage
Store unopened vials at room temperature. Protect from light.

Store tablets at room temperature.

Administration
For oral use, take with meals to reduce GI distress. Dose consistently with regard to meals. Tablets may be crushed if necessary.
! IV infusion concentrations > 3 mg/mL can cause peripheral vein phlebitis.
For IV administration, use glass or polyolefin containers for dilution. Avoid evacuated glass containers. Dilute the loading dose of 150 mg in 100 mL D5W to yield a solution of 1.5 mg/mL. Dilute the maintenance dose of 900 mg in 500 mL D5W to yield a solution of 1.8 mg/mL. Avoid a concentration exceeding 2 mg/mL unless a central venous catheter is used. Administer with a volumetic infusion pump. When possible, administer through central venous catheter used only for amiodarone. Use an in-line filter.

Amitriptyline

a-mee-trip'ti-leen
★ Elavil 🍁 Levate, Novo-Triptyn
Do not confuse amitriptyline with aminophylline or nortriptyline, or Elavil with Equanil or Mellaril.

CATEGORY AND SCHEDULE

Pregnancy Risk Category: C

Classification: Antidepressants, tricyclic

MECHANISM OF ACTION

A tricyclic antidepressant that blocks the reuptake of neurotransmitters, including norepinephrine and serotonin, at presynaptic membranes, thus increasing their availability at postsynaptic receptor sites. Also has strong anticholinergic activity. *Therapeutic Effect:* Relieves depression.

PHARMACOKINETICS

Rapidly and well absorbed from the GI tract. Protein binding: 90%. Undergoes first-pass metabolism in the liver. Nortriptyline is an active metabolite. Metabolites excreted in urine. Minimal removal by hemodialysis. *Half-life:* 10-26 h.

AVAILABILITY

Tablets: 10 mg, 25 mg, 50 mg, 75 mg, 100 mg, 150 mg.

INDICATIONS AND DOSAGES

▸ **Depression**
PO
Adults. Initially, 25-75 mg/day as a single dose at bedtime or in divided doses. May gradually increase up to 300 mg/day. Titrate to lowest effective dosage.
Elderly. Initially, 10-25 mg at bedtime. May increase by 10-25 mg at weekly intervals. Range: 25-150 mg/day.

OFF-LABEL USES

Relief of neuropathic pain, such as that experienced by patients with diabetic neuropathy or postherpetic neuralgia; treatment of bulimia nervosa.

CONTRAINDICATIONS

Acute recovery period after MI; use within 14 days of MAOIs, hypersensitivity.

INTERACTIONS

Drug
Antithyroid agents: May increase the risk of agranulocytosis.
Cimetidine, valproic acid: May increase amitriptyline blood concentration and risk of toxicity.

Clonidine, guanadrel: May decrease the effects of these drugs.
CNS depressants (including alcohol, anticonvulsants, barbiturates, phenothiazines, and sedative-hypnotics): May increase CNS and respiratory depression and the hypotensive effects of amitriptyline.
CYP2D6 inhibitors: May increase amitriptyline blood concentrations and risk of toxicity.
MAOIs: May increase the risk of neuroleptic malignant syndrome, seizures, hypertensive crisis, and hyperpyresis. Contraindicated for concomitant use. Make sure at least 14 days elapse between the use of MAOIs and amitriptyline.
Phenothiazines: May increase the sedative and anticholinergic effects of amitriptyline.
Sympathomimetics: May increase the risk of cardiac effects.
Herbal
St. John's wort: May decrease amitriptyline concentration.

DIAGNOSTIC TEST EFFECTS

May alter blood glucose levels and ECG readings. Therapeutic serum drug level is 120-250 ng/mL; toxic serum drug level is > 500 ng/mL.

SIDE EFFECTS

Frequent
Dizziness, somnolence, dry mouth, orthostatic hypotension, headache, increased appetite, weight gain, nausea, unusual fatigue, unpleasant taste.
Occasional
Blurred vision, confusion, constipation, hallucinations, delayed micturition, eye pain, arrhythmias, fine muscle tremors, parkinsonian syndrome, anxiety, diarrhea, diaphoresis, heartburn, insomnia.
Rare
Hypersensitivity, alopecia, tinnitus, breast enlargement, photosensitivity.

SERIOUS REACTIONS

- Overdose may produce confusion, seizures, severe somnolence, arrhythmias, fever, hallucinations, agitation, dyspnea, vomiting, and unusual fatigue or weakness.
- Abrupt discontinuation after prolonged therapy may produce headache, malaise, nausea, vomiting, and vivid dreams.
- Blood dyscrasias and cholestatic jaundice occur rarely.

PRECAUTIONS & CONSIDERATIONS

A Med Guide should be dispensed with every prescription and refill.

Caution is warranted with cardiovascular disease, diabetes mellitus, angle-closure glaucoma, hiatal hernia, history of seizures, history of urine retention or urinary obstruction, hyperthyroidism, increased intraocular pressure, hepatic or renal disease, benign prostatic hyperplasia, and schizophrenia. Amitriptyline crosses the placenta and is minimally distributed in breast milk. Not approved for use in children < 12 yrs of age. Children are more sensitive to an acute overdose and are at increased risk for amitriptyline toxicity. In addition, antidepressants have been associated with an increased risk of suicidal thinking and behavior in children, adolescents, and young adults with major depressive disorder and other psychiatric disorders. Elderly patients are more sensitive to the drug's anticholinergic effects and are at increased risk for amitriptyline toxicity.

Anticholinergic, sedative, and hypotensive effects may occur, but tolerance usually develops to these effects. Because dizziness may occur, change positions slowly, and avoid alcohol and tasks that require alertness or motor skills. CBC and blood chemistry profile should be obtained before and periodically during therapy, especially with long-term use. BP and pulse rate should be monitored to detect for arrhythmias and hypotension.

Administration

Take oral amitriptyline tablets with food or milk if GI distress occurs. Do not abruptly discontinue the drug. Full therapeutic effect may be noted in 2-4 wks.

Bedtime once-daily administration may increase compliance and limit side effects.

Amlodipine

am-low′di-peen

★ 🍁 Norvasc

Do not confuse amlodipine with amiloride, or Norvasc with Navane or Vascor.

CATEGORY AND SCHEDULE

Pregnancy Risk Category: C

Classification: Calcium channel blockers, antianginal, antihypertensive

MECHANISM OF ACTION

A calcium channel blocker that inhibits calcium movement across cardiac and vascular smooth-muscle cell membranes. *Therapeutic Effect:* Relieves angina by dilating coronary arteries, peripheral arteries, and arterioles. Decreases total peripheral vascular resistance and BP by vasodilation.

PHARMACOKINETICS

Route	Onset	Peak	Duration
PO	0.5-1 h	6-12 h	24 h

Slowly absorbed from the GI tract. Protein binding: 93%. Extensively metabolized in the liver; active drug and metabolites excreted primarily in urine. Not removed by hemodialysis. *Half-life:* 30-50 h (increased in elderly patients and in those with liver cirrhosis).

AVAILABILITY

Tablets: 2.5 mg, 5 mg, 10 mg.

INDICATIONS AND DOSAGES

▸ Hypertension

PO

Adults. Initially, 5 mg/day as a single dose. Maximum: 10 mg/day.

Elderly and Debilitated Patients. Initially, 2.5 mg/day as a single dose. Titrate to 5 mg/day if needed.

Children 6-17 yr. 2.5-5 mg/day as a single dose.

▸ Angina (chronic stable or vasospastic)

PO

Adults. 5-10 mg/day as a single dose.

Elderly. 5 mg/day as a single dose. Maximum: 10 mg.

▸ Dosage in hepatic impairment

For adults and elderly patients, give 2.5 mg/day for hypertension; 5 mg/day for angina.

CONTRAINDICATIONS

Severe hypotension, known sensitivity to amlodipine.

INTERACTIONS

Drug

None known.

Herbal

St. John's wort: May decrease amlodipine levels.

DIAGNOSTIC TEST EFFECTS
None known.

SIDE EFFECTS
Frequent (> 5%)
Peripheral edema, headache, flushing.
Occasional (1%-5%)
Dizziness, palpitations, nausea, unusual fatigue or weakness (asthenia).
Rare (< 1%)
Chest pain, bradycardia, orthostatic hypotension.

SERIOUS REACTIONS
• Overdose may produce excessive peripheral vasodilation and marked hypotension with reflex tachycardia.

PRECAUTIONS & CONSIDERATIONS
Caution is warranted with aortic stenosis, CHF, and impaired hepatic function. Expect to adjust dosage in hepatic impairment. It is unknown whether amlodipine crosses the placenta or is distributed in breast milk. The safety and efficacy of amlodipine have not been established in children younger than 6 yr of age. Elderly patients are more sensitive to amlodipine's hypotensive effects, and its half-life may be increased in these patients. Tasks that require alertness and motor skills should be avoided until drug effects are known.

Asthenia or headache may occur. Apical pulse, BP, and renal and liver function test results should be monitored before and during therapy. Skin should be assessed for flushing and peripheral edema, especially behind the medial malleolus and the sacral area.
Administration
Amlodipine may be taken without regard to food. Do not abruptly discontinue amlodipine.

Ammonium Lactate
ah-moe′nee-um lack′tate
★ Amlactin, Lac-Hydrin, Lac-Hydrin Five, LAC-Lotion
🍁 Dermalac

CATEGORY AND SCHEDULE
Pregnancy Risk Category: B

Classification: Dermatologics

MECHANISM OF ACTION
Lactic acid is an α-hydroxy acid that influences hydration, decreases corneocyte cohesion, reduces excessive epidermal keratinization in hyperkeratotic conditions, and induces synthesis of mucopolysaccharides and collagen in photodamaged skin. The exact mechanism is not known. *Therapeutic Effect:* Increases hydration of the skin.

PHARMACOKINETICS
Not known.

AVAILABILITY
Cream: 12% (Amlactin).
Lotion: 5% (Lac-Hydrin Five), 12% (Amlactin, Lac-Hydrin. LAC-Lotion).

INDICATIONS AND DOSAGES
▸ Treatment of ichthyosis vulgaris and xerosis
PO
Adults, Elderly, Children. Apply sparingly and rub into area thoroughly twice daily.

CONTRAINDICATIONS
Hypersensitivity to ammonium lactate.

INTERACTIONS
Drug
Calcipotriene: May decrease the effects of calcipotriene.

DIAGNOSTIC TEST EFFECTS
None known.

SIDE EFFECTS
Occasional (2%-15%)
Burning, stinging, rash, itching, dry skin.

PRECAUTIONS & CONSIDERATIONS
Ammonium lactate should not be used on broken skin or in areas of infection, and do not apply to the face, inguinal areas, or abraded skin. It is not known whether ammonium lactate is distributed in breast milk. Safety and efficacy have not been established in children younger than 2 yr of age. Treated skin areas may be sensitive to sunlight (UV) exposure.

Storage
Store at room temperature.

Administration
Gently cleanse area before application. Shake lotion well before application. Use occlusive dressings only as ordered. Apply sparingly and rub into area thoroughly. Avoid contact with the eyes and mucous membranes.

Amobarbital
am-oh-bar'bi-tal
★ Amytal Sodium

CATEGORY AND SCHEDULE
Pregnancy Risk Category: D
Controlled Substance Schedule: II

Classification: Barbiturates, preanesthetics, sedatives/hypnotics

MECHANISM OF ACTION
A barbiturate that depresses the sensory cortex, decreases motor activity, and alters cerebellar function. *Therapeutic Effect:* Produces drowsiness, sedation, and hypnosis.

PHARMACOKINETICS
Protein binding: 60%. Metabolized in liver primarily by the hepatic microsomal enzyme system. Primarily excreted in urine. *Half-life:* 16-40 h.

AVAILABILITY
Powder for Injection: 500 mg (Amytal Sodium).

INDICATIONS AND DOSAGES
▸ **Preanesthetic sedative**
IM/IV
Adults, Children 6 yr and older. 65-200 mg single dose. Alternatively, use a weight-based dose: 3-5 mg/kg/dose.

▸ **Short-term treatment of insomnia**
IM/IV
Adults. 65-200 mg at bedtime.
Elderly. Not recommended.
Children older than 6 yr. 2-3 mg/kg/dose at bedtime.

OFF-LABEL USES
Refractory seizures.

CONTRAINDICATIONS
History of manifest or latent porphyria, marked liver dysfunction, marked respiratory disease in which dyspnea or obstruction is evident, and hypersensitivity to amobarbital products.

INTERACTIONS
Drug
Anticoagulants, steroids: May decrease the effects of anticoagulants and steroids.
Anticonvulsants, barbiturates, benzodiazepines, valproic acid: May increase the metabolism of anticonvulsants, barbiturates, benzodiazepines, and valproic acid.
CNS depressants: May increase respiratory depression and hypotension.

Corticosteroids, doxycycline, griseofulvin: May decrease the effect of corticosteroids, doxycycline, and griseofulvin.
MAOIs: Increased hypotensive or prolonged activity of barbiturate.
Herbal
Kava kava, Valerian: May increase CNS depression.
St. John's wort: May decrease the effects of amobarbital sodium.
Food
Ethanol: May increase CNS depression.

DIAGNOSTIC TEST EFFECTS

May falsely elevate phenobarbital levels when measured with EMIT(R) system.

IV INCOMPATIBILITIES

Atracurium, cefazolin (Ancef), cephalothin, chlorpromazine (Thorazine), cimetidine (Tagamet), clindamycin (Cleocin), codeine, dimenhydrinate, diphenhydramine (Benadryl), droperidol, hydrocortisone, hydroxyzine (Vistaril), insulin, isoproterenol (Isuprel), levorphanol (Levo-Dromaron), meperidine (Demerol), methadone (Dolophine), methyldopa (Aldomet), morphine, norepinephrine (Levophed), pancuronium, penicillin G (Bicillin), pentazocine (Talwin), phytonadione (AquaMEPHYTON), procaine (Novocain), prochlorperazine (Compazine), streptomycin, succinylcholine (Anectine), vancomycin.

IV COMPATIBILITIES

Amikacin, aminophylline.

SIDE EFFECTS

Frequent
Somnolence, headache, confusion, dizziness.
Occasional
Nausea, vomiting, visual abnormalities, such as spots before eyes, difficulty focusing, blurred vision, dry mouth or pharynx, tongue irritation, water retention, increased sweating, constipation, or diarrhea.

SERIOUS REACTIONS

- Overdosage results in severe respiratory depression, skeletal muscle flaccidity, bronchospasm, cardiovascular disturbances, such as congestive heart failure (CHF), hypotension or hypertension, arrhythmias, cold and clammy skin, cyanosis, and coma.
- Tolerance may occur with repeated use.
- Extravasation may cause local tissue damage.

PRECAUTIONS & CONSIDERATIONS

Caution is necessary in patients with impaired cardiac, liver, or renal function. Amobarbital crosses the placenta and is distributed in breast milk. Teratogenic effects have been reported after first-trimester exposure; withdrawal reactions have been observed in infants following third-trimester exposure. Behavioral changes are more likely to occur in children and elderly patients. Monitor BP for hypotension, level of sedation, and pulse for bradycardia as well as respiratory rate and rhythm. Change positions slowly to avoid orthostatic hypotension. Tasks that require mental alertness or motor skills should be avoided.
Storage
Store at room temperature. Once reconstituted, no more than 30 min should pass from the time the vial is opened and the contents are used as the drug/solution hydrolyzes upon exposure to air. Discard any unused portion.

Administration
IM: Administer deeply into a large muscle. Reconstitute 500 mg with 2.5 mL of sterile water for injection to give a solution of 200 mg/mL for IM use. Do not use more than 5 mL at any single site (may cause tissue damage). Maximum: 500 mg.
IV: Use only when IM administration is not feasible; reserve IV route for hospitalized patients with close observation. Administer by slow IV injection. For IV use, reconstitute 500 mg with 5 mL of sterile water for injection to give a concentration of 100 mg/mL. Do not use solution that has not become clear within 5 min of addition of diluent. The rate of IV injection should not exceed 50 mg/min in adults to prevent sudden respiratory depression, apnea, and hypotension.

Amoxapine
a-moks'a-peen
Do not confuse with atomoxetine or atropine.

CATEGORY AND SCHEDULE
Pregnancy Risk Category: C

Classification: Antidepressants, cyclic

MECHANISM OF ACTION
A cyclic antidepressant that blocks the reuptake of neurotransmitters, such as norepinephrine and serotonin, at CNS presynaptic membranes, increasing their availability at postsynaptic receptor sites. The metabolite 7-OH-amoxapine has significant dopamine receptor blocking activity similar to that of haloperidol. *Therapeutic Effect:* Produces antidepressant effects.

PHARMACOKINETICS
Rapidly, well absorbed from the GI tract. Protein binding: 90%. Metabolized in liver. Excreted in urine and feces. *Half-life:* 8 h.

AVAILABILITY
Tablets: 25 mg, 50 mg, 100 mg, 150 mg.

INDICATIONS AND DOSAGES
▸ **Depression**
PO
Adults. 50 mg 2-3 times/day. May increase to 100 mg 2-3 times/day. Maximum: 300 mg/day (outpatient); higher doses have been used rarely (inpatient).
Elderly. Initially, 25 mg at bedtime. May increase by 25 mg/day q3-7 days.

CONTRAINDICATIONS
Acute recovery period following myocardial infarction (MI), within 14 days of MAOI ingestion, hypersensitivity to dibenzoxazepine compounds.

INTERACTIONS
Drug
Alcohol, CNS depressants: May increase CNS and respiratory depression and amoxapine's hypotensive effects.
CYP2D6 inhibitors, such as cimetidine, quinidine, fluoxetine, sertraline, paroxetine: May increase amoxapine blood concentration and risk of side effects. Sufficient time must elapse before initiating amoxapine in a patient withdrawing from fluoxetine treatment (at least 5 wks may be necessary).
Clonidine, guanadrel: May decrease the effects of clonidine and guanadrel.
Fluoroquinolones, sympathomimetics: May increase cardiac effects.

MAOIs: May increase the risk of convulsions, hyperpyresis, and hypertensive crisis. Contraindicated.
Nefopam: May increase risk of seizures.
Phenothiazines: Similar metabolic pathways and clinical activity, increased CNS, anticholinergic, and hypotensive effects.
Herbal
St. John's wort: May increase risk of serotonin syndrome.
Food
None known.

DIAGNOSTIC TEST EFFECTS

May increase serum glucose levels.

SIDE EFFECTS

Frequent
Drowsiness, fatigue, xerostomia, constipation, weight gain.
Occasional
Nausea, dizziness, headache, confusion, nervousness, restlessness, insomnia, edema, tremor, blurred vision, aggressiveness, muscle weakness.
Rare
Paradoxical reactions (agitation, restlessness, nightmares, insomnia, extrapyramidal symptoms, particularly fine hand tremor), laryngitis, seizures.

SERIOUS REACTIONS

- High dosage may produce cardiovascular effects, including severe postural hypotension, dizziness, tachycardia, palpitations, arrhythmias, and seizures. High dosage may also result in altered temperature regulation, such as hyperpyrexia or hypothermia.
- Abrupt withdrawal from prolonged therapy may produce headache, malaise, nausea, vomiting, and vivid dreams.
- Extrapyramidal reactions, neuroleptic malignant syndrome, and tardive dyskinesia may occur as a result of the dopamine receptor blocking activity of the metabolite.

PRECAUTIONS & CONSIDERATIONS

Caution is warranted with cardiac conduction disturbances, cardiovascular disease, hyperthyroidism, seizure disorders, and urinary retention and in persons taking thyroid replacement therapy. Be aware that amoxapine is distributed in breast milk. Safety and effectiveness have not been established in children < 16 yr of age. Antidepressants have been associated with an increased risk of suicidal thinking and behavior in children, adolescents, and young adults with major depressive disorder and other psychiatric disorders.

Expect to use lower dosages in elderly patients. Higher dosages are not tolerated well and increase the risk of toxicity in elderly patients. Blurred vision, drowsiness, constipation, and dry mouth may occur during therapy. Change positions slowly to avoid postural hypotension. Avoid alcohol and tasks that require mental alertness or motor skills. Tolerance usually develops to amoxapine's anticholinergic effects, postural hypotension, and sedative effects. The risk of tardive dyskinesia must be considered when contemplating chronic use.
Storage
Store at room temperature.
Administration
Once dose is established, may be taken as a single dose usually at bedtime, usually without food. May be taken with food to improve GI tolerability. Doses > 300 mg/day should be taken in divided doses.

Amoxicillin

a-mox'i-sill-in

Amoxil, Moxatag

Apo-Amoxi, Novamoxin, Nu-Amoxi

Do not confuse amoxicillin with amoxapine, Diamox, Trimox, or Tylox.

CATEGORY AND SCHEDULE

Pregnancy Risk Category: B

Classification: Antibiotics, penicillins, aminopenicillins

MECHANISM OF ACTION

A penicillin that inhibits bacterial cell wall synthesis. *Therapeutic Effect:* Bactericidal in susceptible microorganisms.

PHARMACOKINETICS

Well absorbed from the GI tract. Protein binding: 20%. Partially metabolized in the liver. Primarily excreted in urine. Removed by hemodialysis. *Half-life:* 1-1.3 h (increased in impaired renal function).

AVAILABILITY

Capsules: 250 mg, 500 mg.
Powder for Oral Suspension: 125 mg/5 mL, 200 mg/5 mL, 250 mg/5 mL, 400 mg/5 mL.
Tablets: 250 mg, 500 mg, 875 mg.
Tablets, Chewable: 125 mg, 200 mg, 250 mg, 400 mg.
Tablets, Extended-Release (Moxatag): 775 mg.

INDICATIONS AND DOSAGES

▸ **Ear, nose, throat, genitourinary, skin, and skin-structure infections**

PO

Adults, Elderly, Children weighing more than 40 kg. 250-500 mg q8h or 500-875 mg (tablets) twice a day.
Adults, Children 12 yr of age and older. 775 mg once daily (tonsillitis/pharyngitis due to *Streptococcus pyogenes*).
Children weighing < 40 kg. 20-45 mg/kg/day in divided doses q8-12h.

▸ **Lower respiratory tract infections**

PO

Adults, Elderly, Children weighing more than 40 kg. 500 mg q8h or 875 mg (tablets) twice a day.
Children weighing < 40 kg. 40 mg/kg/day in divided doses q8h or 45 mg/kg/day in divided doses q12h.

▸ **Acute, uncomplicated gonorrhea**

PO

Adults. 3 g one time with 1 g probenecid. Follow with tetracycline or erythromycin therapy.
Prepubertal children 2 yr and older. 50 mg/kg plus probenecid 25 mg/kg as a single dose. Do not use in children < 2 yr old.

▸ **Acute otitis media**

PO

Children. 80-90 mg/kg/day in divided doses q12h.

▸ ***Helicobacter pylori* infection**

PO

Adults, Elderly. 1 g given two or three times per day for 14 days (in combination with other antibiotics).

▸ **Prevention of endocarditis**

PO

Adults, Elderly. 2 g 1 h before procedure.
Children. 50 mg/kg 1 h before procedure.

▸ **Usual neonatal and young infant dosage**

Children younger than 3 mo, Neonates. 20-30 mg/kg/day in divided doses q12h.

▸ **Dosage in renal impairment (adults)**

Dosage interval is modified based on creatinine clearance.
Creatinine clearance 10-30 mL/min. 250-500 mg q12h.

Creatinine clearance < 10 mL/min. 250-500 mg q24h.

OFF-LABEL USES

Treatment of dental-related infection, Lyme disease, and typhoid fever.

CONTRAINDICATIONS

Hypersensitivity to any penicillin.

INTERACTIONS

Drug

Allopurinol: May increase incidence of rash.
Methotrexate: May reduce the renal clearance of methotrexate.
Oral contraceptives: May decrease effectiveness of oral contraceptives.
Probenecid: Increase amoxicillin blood concentration.

DIAGNOSTIC TEST EFFECTS

May increase BUN and serum LDH, bilirubin, creatinine, AST (SGOT), and ALT (SGPT) levels. May cause a positive direct Coombs' test.

SIDE EFFECTS

Frequent

GI disturbances (mild diarrhea, nausea, or vomiting), headache, oral or vaginal candidiasis.

Occasional

Generalized rash, urticaria.

SERIOUS REACTIONS

- Antibiotic-associated colitis and other superinfections may result from altered bacterial balance.
- Severe hypersensitivity reactions, including anaphylaxis and acute interstitial nephritis, occur rarely.

PRECAUTIONS & CONSIDERATIONS

Caution is warranted with antibiotic-associated colitis or a history of allergies, especially to cephalosporins. Amoxicillin crosses the placenta, appears in cord blood and amniotic fluid, and is distributed in breast milk in low concentrations. Amoxicillin administration may lead to allergic sensitization, candidiasis, diarrhea, and skin rash in infants. Immature renal function in neonates and young infants may delay renal excretion of amoxicillin. Age-related renal impairment may require dosage adjustment in elderly patients.

History of allergies, especially to cephalosporins or penicillins, should be determined before giving the drug. Withhold amoxicillin and promptly notify the physician if rash or diarrhea occurs. A high percentage of patients with infectious mononucleosis have developed rash during amoxicillin therapy. Severe diarrhea with abdominal pain, blood or mucus in stool, and fever may indicate antibiotic-associated colitis. Signs and symptoms of superinfection, including anal or genital pruritus, black hairy tongue, diarrhea, increased fever, sore throat, ulceration or changes of oral mucosa, and vomiting, should be monitored.

Storage

Store capsules or tablets at room temperature. After reconstitution, the oral suspension is stable for 14 days either at room temperature or refrigerated. Refrigeration is preferred.

Administration

Chew or crush chewable tablets thoroughly before swallowing. Take amoxicillin capsules, tablets, chewable tablets, and suspension without regard to food; extended-release tablets should be taken within 1 h of finishing a meal. Take evenly around the clock and continue for the full course of treatment. Suspension may be mixed with formula, milk, fruit juice, ginger ale, or cold drinks; administered immediately after mixing. Consume the entire dose.

Amoxicillin/ Clavulanate

a-mox'i-sill-in clav-u-lan'ate

★ AmoClan, Augmentin, Augmentin ES 600, Augmentin XR 🍁 Apo-Amoxi Clav, Clavulin

Do not confuse with amoxapine.

CATEGORY AND SCHEDULE

Pregnancy Risk Category: B

Classification: Antibiotics, penicillins, aminopenicillins, plus a beta-lactamase inhibitor.

MECHANISM OF ACTION

Amoxicillin inhibits bacterial cell wall synthesis, while clavulanate inhibits bacterial β-lactamase. *Therapeutic Effect:* Amoxicillin is bactericidal in susceptible microorganisms. Clavulanate protects amoxicillin from enzymatic degradation.

PHARMACOKINETICS

Well absorbed from the GI tract. Protein binding: 20%. Partially metabolized in the liver. Primarily excreted in urine. Removed by hemodialysis. *Half-life:* 1-1.3 h (increased in impaired renal function).

AVAILABILITY

Powder for Oral Suspension: 125 mg/31.25 mg per 5 mL, 200 mg/28.5 mg per 5 mL, 250 mg/62.5 mg per 5 mL, 400 mg/57 mg per 5 mL, 600 mg/42.9 mg per 5 mL.
Tablets: 250 mg/125 mg, 500 mg/ 125 mg, 875 mg/125 mg.
Tablets (Extended-Release, Augmentin XR): 1000 mg/62.5 mg.
Tablets (Chewable): 200 mg/28.5 mg, 250 mg/62.5 mg, 400 mg/57 mg.

INDICATIONS AND DOSAGES

NOTE: Weight-based dosing is based on amoxicillin component.

▸ **Mild to moderate infections**

PO:

Adults, Elderly, Children weighing more than 40 kg. 250 mg q8h or 500 mg q12h.

Children weighing < 40 kg. 20 mg/kg/day in divided doses q8h or 25 mg/kg/day in divided doses q12h.

▸ **Respiratory tract, sinusitis, and other severe infections**

PO

Adults, Elderly, Children weighing more than 40 kg. 500 mg q8h or 875 mg q12h.

Children weighing < 40 kg. 40 mg/kg/day in divided doses q8h or 45 mg/kg/day in divided doses q12h.

PO (AUGMENTIN XR)

Adults. Usual dose 2 tablets q12h for community acquired pneumonia.

▸ **Otitis media**

PO

Children. 90 mg/kg/day in divided doses q12h for 10 days.

▸ **Usual neonate dosage**

PO

Neonates, Infants younger than 3 mo. 30 mg/kg/day in divided doses q12h.

▸ **Dosage in renal impairment (adults)**

Dosage and frequency are modified based on creatinine clearance.
Creatinine clearance 10-30 mL/min: 250-500 mg q12h.
Creatinine clearance < 10 mL/min: 250-500 mg q24h.

OFF-LABEL USES

Treatment of dental-related infections, periodontitis.

CONTRAINDICATIONS

Hypersensitivity to any penicillins, history of cholestatic jaundice/hepatic function impairment associated with amoxicillin/clavulanate; extended-release formulation also contraindicated in severe renal impairment (CrCl < 30 mL/min) and in hemodialysis patients.

INTERACTIONS

Drug

Allopurinol: May increase incidence of rash.
Methotrexate: May reduce the renal clearance of methotrexate.
Oral contraceptives: May decrease effects of oral contraceptives.
Probenecid: May increase amoxicillin and clavulanate blood concentration.

DIAGNOSTIC TEST EFFECTS

May increase serum AST (SGOT) and ALT (SGPT) levels. May cause a positive direct Coombs' test.

SIDE EFFECTS

Frequent

GI disturbances (mild diarrhea, nausea, vomiting), headache, oral or vaginal candidiasis.

Occasional

Generalized rash, urticaria.

SERIOUS REACTIONS

- Antibiotic-associated colitis and other superinfections may result from altered bacterial balance.
- Severe hypersensitivity reactions, including anaphylaxis and acute interstitial nephritis, occur rarely.
- Hepatotoxicity (rare).

PRECAUTIONS & CONSIDERATIONS

Caution is warranted with antibiotic-associated colitis or a history of allergies, especially to cephalosporins. Amoxicillin and clavulanate cross the placenta, appear in cord blood and amniotic fluid, and are distributed in breast milk in low concentrations. Amoxicillin and clavulanate may lead to allergic sensitization, candidiasis, diarrhea, and skin rash in infants. Immature renal function in neonates and young infants may delay renal excretion of amoxicillin and clavulanate. Age-related renal impairment may require dosage adjustment in elderly patients.

History of allergies, especially to cephalosporins or penicillins, should be determined before giving the drug. Withhold and promptly notify the physician if rash or diarrhea occurs. Severe diarrhea with abdominal pain, blood or mucus in stool, and fever may indicate antibiotic-associated colitis. Signs and symptoms of superinfection, including anal or genital pruritus, black hairy tongue, diarrhea, increased fever, sore throat, ulceration or changes of oral mucosa, and vomiting, should be monitored.

Storage

Store capsules or tablets at room temperature. After reconstitution, the oral suspension is stable for 10 days refrigerated.

Administration

! Drug dosage is expressed in terms of amoxicillin. Dosage forms cannot be interchanged based on amoxicillin component alone; must also consider clavulanate content.

May be taken without regard to meals; however, absorption is enhanced and tolerability improved when taken at the start of a meal. Chew or crush chewable tablets thoroughly before swallowing. Shake oral suspension well prior to each use. Extended-release tablets should not be crushed or chewed. Space doses evenly around the clock and continue for the full course of treatment.

Amphetamine; Dextroamphetamine

am-fet'ah-meen

Adderall, Adderall XR

CATEGORY AND SCHEDULE

Pregnancy Risk Category: C
Controlled Substance Schedule: II

Classification: Adrenergic agonists, amphetamines, anorexiants, central nervous system stimulants, ADHD agents

MECHANISM OF ACTION

A sympathomimetic amine that produces CNS and respiratory stimulation, mydriasis, bronchodilation, a pressor response, and contraction of the urinary sphincter. Directly affects α and β receptor sites in peripheral system. Enhances release of norepinephrine by blocking reuptake, inhibiting monoamine oxidase. May also modulate serotonergic pathways. *Therapeutic Effect:* Increases motor activity, mental alertness; decreases drowsiness, fatigue. Improves attention span, decreases distractability, and decreases impulsivity.

PHARMACOKINETICS

Well absorbed from the GI tract. Protein binding: 20%. Widely distributed (including CSF). Metabolized in liver. Excreted in urine. Unknown if removed by hemodialysis. *Half-life:* 9-14 h.

AVAILABILITY

Adderall XR Capsules (Extended-Release): 5 mg, 10 mg, 15 mg, 20 mg, 25 mg, 30 mg.
Tablets: 5 mg, 7.5 mg, 10 mg, 12.5 mg, 15 mg, 20 mg, 30 mg.

INDICATIONS AND DOSAGES

▸ **ADHD**

PO

Adults. 5-20 mg 1-3 times/day.

Adults, Children older than 12 yr. Initially, 5 mg twice a day. Increase by 10 mg at weekly intervals until therapeutic response achieved. Usual maximum: 60 mg/day.

Children 6-12 yr. Initially, 5 mg twice a day. Increase by 5 mg/day at weekly intervals until therapeutic response achieved. Usual maximum: 40 mg/day.

Children 3-6 yr. Initially, 5 mg once or twice a day. Increase by 5 mg/day at weekly intervals until therapeutic response achieved.

▸ **Extended-release capsules**

NOTE: Patients (adults and children) already taking divided doses of Adderall immediate-release tablets may switch to Adderall XR once daily at the same total daily dose.

Adults. Usual 5-20 mg once daily. Maximum: 30 mg/day.

Children 6 yr and older. Initially, 5-10 mg once daily. Increase by 5 or 10 mg weekly to effective dose. Maximum: 30 mg/day.

Children < 6 yr. Do not use extended release.

▸ **Narcolepsy**

PO

Adults. 5-20 mg 1-3 times/day.

Children older than 12 yr. Initially, 5 mg twice a day. Increase by 10 mg at weekly intervals until therapeutic response achieved. Usual maximum: 60 mg/day.

Children 6-12 yr. Initially, 5 mg once or twice a day. Increase by 5 mg/day at weekly intervals until therapeutic response achieved. Usual maximum: 60 mg/day.

OFF-LABEL USES

Depression, obsessive-compulsive disorder.

CONTRAINDICATIONS

Advanced arteriosclerosis, agitated states, glaucoma, history of drug abuse, history of hypersensitivity to sympathomimetic amines, hyperthyroidism, moderate to severe hypertension, symptomatic cardiovascular disease, during use of an MAOI or within 14 days following discontinuation of an MAOI.

INTERACTIONS

Drug

β-blockers: May increase risk of bradycardia, heart block, and hypertension.
CNS stimulants: May increase the effects of amphetamine. Concurrent use of other CNS stimulants not recommended.
Digoxin: May increase the risk of arrhythmias with this drug.
MAOIs: May prolong and intensify the effects of amphetamine. May cause hypertensive crisis. Contraindicated.
Meperidine: May increase the risk of hypotension, respiratory depression, seizures, and vascular collapse.
Tricyclic antidepressants: May increase cardiovascular effects.
GI antacids and sodium bicarbonate and urinary alkalinizers: Increase amphetamine absorption and decrease urinary elimination, respectively. Avoid concurrent use.
Methenamine and urinary acidifiers: Increase amphetamine elimination.
Lithium: Antagonize effect of amphetamines; concurrent use not recommended.

Dietary Supplement

Melatonin: Potential for additive neurologic and cardiac effects.

DIAGNOSTIC TEST EFFECTS

May increase plasma corticosteroid concentrations.

SIDE EFFECTS

Frequent

Irregular pulse, increased motor activity, talkativeness, nervousness, mild euphoria, insomnia.

Occasional

Headache, chills, dry mouth, GI distress, worsening depression in patients who are clinically depressed, tachycardia, palpitations, chest pain.

SERIOUS REACTIONS

- Overdose may produce skin pallor or flushing, arrhythmias, and psychosis.
- Abrupt withdrawal following prolonged administration of high dosage may produce lethargy (may last for weeks).
- Prolonged administration to children with ADHD may produce a temporary suppression of normal weight and height patterns.
- Any cardiac symptoms should prompt immediate evaluation.

PRECAUTIONS & CONSIDERATIONS

Med Guide is required with each prescription and refill. Sudden cardiac death has been reported at usual doses in those with structural cardiac abnormalities and should generally not be used in such patients. Even those with mild hypertension should be approached cautiously. Precaution is necessary with acute stress reaction, emotional instability, history of drug dependence, seizures, and in elderly and debilitated patients and those who are tartrazine-sensitive. Amphetamine crosses the placenta and is distributed in breast milk. Use in pregnancy may be associated with teratogenic effects, premature delivery, low birthweight, and infant withdrawal symptoms. Children may be more susceptible to develop abdominal pain, anorexia, decreased weight, and insomnia. A thorough cardiovascular assessment is recommended before initiation of therapy in pediatric patients; assessment should include medical history, family history, and physical examination with consideration of ECG testing. There are no age-related precautions noted for elderly patients.

Decreased appetite, dizziness, dry mouth, or pronounced nervousness may be experienced. Tasks that require mental alertness or motor skills should be avoided until the effects of the drug are determined.

Storage

Store at room temperature. Protect from light. Keep tightly closed.

Administration

Do not take in late afternoon or evening because the drug can cause insomnia. The first dose is given upon awakening.

Do not crush, chew, or cut XR form. XR form may be opened and sprinkled on 1 tsp of applesauce; entire dose is swallowed immediately without chewing the beads.

Amphotericin B/ Amphotericin B Cholesteryl/ Amphotericin B Lipid Complex/ Liposomal Amphotericin B

am-foe-ter'i-sin bee

★ Abelcet, AmBisome, Amphocin, Amphotec

CATEGORY AND SCHEDULE

Pregnancy Risk Category: B

Classification: Antifungals

MECHANISM OF ACTION

An antifungal and antiprotozoal that is generally fungistatic but may become fungicidal with high dosages or very susceptible microorganisms. This drug binds to sterols in the fungal cell membrane. Lipid-based formulations deliver higher drug concentrations to sites of infection and reduced levels in normal tissues. *Therapeutic Effect:* Increases fungal cell-membrane permeability, allowing loss of potassium and other cellular components. Fungicidal.

PHARMACOKINETICS

Protein binding: 90%. Widely distributed. Metabolic fate unknown. Excreted slowly over weeks to months by the kidneys. Approximately 40% of a given dose is excreted in the first 7 days. Minimal removal by hemodialysis. Amphotec and Abelcet are not dialyzable. *Half-life:* amphotericin B desoxycholate, 24 h (increased in neonates and children); Amphotec, 26-28 h; Abelcet, 7.2 days; AmBisome, 100-153 h.

AVAILABILITY

Injection, Powder for Reconstitution: (Amphotec): 50 mg, 100 mg.
Injection, Powder for Reconstitution (AmBisome, Amphocin, amphotericin B desoxycholate): 50 mg.
Injection, Suspension (Abelcet): 5 mg/mL.

INDICATIONS AND DOSAGES

NOTE: Amphotericin B products are not interchangeable.

▸ **Cryptococcosis; blastomycosis; systemic candidiasis; disseminated forms of moniliasis, coccidioidomycosis, and histoplasmosis; zygomycosis; sporotrichosis; aspergillosis**

IV INFUSION (AMPHOTERICIN B DESOXYCHOLATE)
Adults, Elderly. Dosage based on patient tolerance and severity of infection. Initially, 1-mg test dose is given over 20-30 min. If test dose is tolerated, 5-mg dose may be given the same day. Subsequently, dosage is increased by 5 mg q12-24h until desired daily dose is reached. Alternatively, if test dose is tolerated, 0.25 mg/kg is given on same day and 0.5 mg/kg on second day; then dosage is increased until desired daily dose is reached. Common dose: 1 mg/kg/day up to 1.5 mg/kg every other day. Maximum: 1.5 mg/kg/day.
Children. Test dose of 0.1 mg/kg/dose (maximum 1 mg) is infused over 20-60 min. If test dose is tolerated, initial dose of 0.4 mg/kg may be given on same day; dosage is then increased in 0.25-mg/kg increments as needed. Maintenance dose: 0.25-1 mg/kg/day.

▸ **Invasive fungal infections unresponsive to or intolerant of amphotericin B.**
IV INFUSION (ABELCET)
Adults, Children. 5 mg/kg once daily at rate of 2.5 mg/kg/h.

▸ **Empiric treatment of fungal infections in patients with febrile neutropenia; aspergillosis, candidiasis, or cryptococcosis in patients with renal impairment and those who have experienced toxicity or treatment failure with amphotericin B desoxycholate**
IV INFUSION (AMBISOME)
Adults, Children. 3-5 mg/kg once daily over 2 h. Doses up to 6 mg/kg/day used for cryptococcal meningitis.

▸ **Invasive aspergillosis in patients with renal impairment and those who have experienced toxicity or treatment failure with amphotericin B desoxycholate**
IV INFUSION (AMPHOTEC)
Adults, Children. 3-4 mg/kg once daily over 2-4 h.

CONTRAINDICATIONS
Hypersensitivity to amphotericin B or specific components of the various products.

INTERACTIONS
Drug
Bone marrow depressants: May increase the risk of anemia.
Digoxin: May increase the risk of digoxin toxicity from hypokalemia.
Nephrotoxic medications: May increase the risk of nephrotoxicity.
Steroids: May cause severe hypokalemia.

DIAGNOSTIC TEST EFFECTS
May increase BUN, serum alkaline phosphatase, serum creatinine, serum SGOT (AST), and SGPT (ALT) levels. May decrease serum calcium, magnesium, and potassium levels.

IV INCOMPATIBILITIES
NOTE: Many drugs are incompatible with Amphotericin B. Always check specialized references for compatibility. Some incompatibilities include:

Abelcet, AmBisome, Amphotec: Do not mix with any other drug, diluent, or solution.

Amphotericin B desoxycholate: Allopurinol (Aloprim), amifostine (Ethyol), aztreonam (Azactam), calcium gluconate, cefepime (Maxipime), cimetidine (Tagamet), ciprofloxacin (Cipro), docetaxel (Taxotere), dopamine (Intropin), doxorubicin (Adriamycin), enalapril (Vasotec), etoposide (VP-16), filgrastim (Neupogen), fluconazole (Diflucan), fludarabine (Fludara), foscarnet (Foscavir), gemcitabine (Gemzar), magnesium sulfate, meropenem (Merrem IV), ondansetron (Zofran), paclitaxel (Taxol), piperacillin and tazobactam (Zosyn), potassium chloride, propofol (Diprivan), vinorelbine (Navelbine).

IV COMPATIBILITIES

Do not mix with saline solutions, other medications, or electrolytes or preservatives.

SIDE EFFECTS

Frequent (>10%)

Abelcet: Chills, fever, increased serum creatinine level, multiple organ failure.

AmBisome: Hypokalemia, hypomagnesemia, hyperglycemia, hypocalcemia, edema, abdominal pain, back pain, chills, chest pain, hypotension, diarrhea, nausea, vomiting, headache, fever, rigors, insomnia, dyspnea, epistaxis, increased hepatic or renal function test results.

Amphotec: Chills, fever, hypotension, tachycardia, increased serum creatinine level, hypokalemia, bilirubinemia.

Amphotericin B desoxycholate: Fever, chills, headache, anemia, hypokalemia, hypomagnesemia, anorexia, malaise, generalized pain, nephrotoxicity.

SERIOUS REACTIONS

- Cardiovascular toxicity (as evidenced by hypotension, ventricular fibrillation, and anaphylaxis) occurs rarely.
- Altered vision and hearing, seizures, hepatic failure, coagulation defects, multiple organ failure, and sepsis may be noted.

PRECAUTIONS & CONSIDERATIONS

Due to potential toxicities, reserved for serious and potentially life-threatening fungal infections. Caution is warranted with renal impairment and in combination with antineoplastic therapy. Drug is prescribed only for progressive, potentially fatal fungal infection. Keep in mind that conventional amphotericin, amphotericin B desoxycholate, is more nephrotoxic than the alternative formulations of amphotericin B, including Albecet, AmBisome, and Amphotec. Amphotericin B crosses the placenta, and it is unknown whether amphotericin B is distributed in breast milk. There are no age-related precautions noted in children or in elderly patients.

History of allergies, especially to amphotericin B and sulfites, should be determined before giving the drug. Be aware that other nephrotoxic medications should be avoided, if possible. Antiemetics, antihistamines, antipyretics, or small doses of corticosteroids may be given before or during amphotericin administration to help control adverse reactions.

BP, pulse, respirations, and temperature should be monitored twice every 15 min, then every 30 min for the initial 4 h of the infusion to assess for adverse reactions. Adverse reactions include abdominal pain, anorexia, chills, fever, nausea, shaking, and vomiting. If signs and symptoms of adverse reactions occur, slow the infusion and give prescribed drugs to provide symptomatic relief. For a severe reaction or for patients without orders for symptomatic relief, stop the infusion and notify the physician.

Storage

Refrigerate Albecet as unreconstituted solution. Albecet reconstituted solution is stable for 48 h if refrigerated and 6 h at room temperature.

Refrigerate AmBisome as unreconstituted solution. AmBisome reconstituted solution of 4 mg/mL is stable for 24 h. AmBisome reconstituted solution concentration of 1-2 mg/mL is stable for 6 h.

Store Amphotec as unreconstituted solution at room temperature. Amphotec reconstituted solution and solution diluted for infusion are stable for 24 h if refrigerated.

Refrigerate Conventional Amphotericin B as unreconstituted solution. The reconstituted solution is stable for 24 h at room temperature or 7 days if refrigerated. Diluted solution ≤ 0.1 mg/mL should be used promptly. Do not use the solution if it is cloudy or contains a precipitate. Protect from light.

Administration

! Amphotericin products are not interchangeable. To prevent inadvertent overdose with amphotericin B, verify product name and dosage if dose exceeds 1.5 mg/kg. For IV use, observe strict aseptic technique because no bacteriostatic agent or preservative is present. For all products: Do not mix with saline solutions. Use dextrose solutions only for preparing infusions. All products should be infused using controlled infusion devices.

Shake Abelcet 20-mL (100-mg) vial gently until contents are dissolved. Withdraw required Abelcet dose using a 5-µm filter needle supplied by manufacturer. Inject Abelcet dose into D5W; 4 mL D5W is required for each 1 mL (5 mg) to obtain final concentration of 1 mg/mL. Double concentration for pediatric and fluid-restricted patients (2 mg/mL). Infuse Abelcet over 2 h by slow IV infusion. Shake the contents if the infusion is > 2 h. Reconstitute each 50-mg AmBisome vial with 12 mL sterile water for injection to provide concentration of 4 mg/mL. Shake AmBisome vial vigorously for 30 seconds. Then withdraw the required AmBisome dose and empty the syringe contents through a 5-µm filter into an infusion of D5W to provide final concentration of 1-2 mg/mL. Infuse AmBisome over 2 h by slow IV infusion.

Add 10 mL sterile water for injection to each 50-mg Amphotec vial to provide a concentration of 5 mg/mL. Shake the Amphotec vial gently. Further dilute Amphotec vial only with D5W using specific amount recommended by manufacturer to provide concentration of 0.16-0.83 mg/mL. Infuse Amphotec over 2-4 h by slow IV infusion.

Rapidly inject 10 mL sterile water for injection to each 50-mg amphotericin B desoxycholate vial to provide concentration of 5 mg/mL. Immediately shake amphotericin B desoxycholate vial until the solution is clear. Further dilute each 1 mg amphotericin B desoxycholate in at least 10 mL D5W to provide a concentration of 0.1 mg/mL. Be aware that the potential for thrombophlebitis may be less with the use of pediatric scalp vein needles or by adding dilute heparin solution, as prescribed. Infuse conventional amphotericin over 2-6 h by slow IV infusion.

Ampicillin Sodium

am-pi-sill′in soe′dee-um

🍁 Novo-Ampicillin, Apo-Ampi, Nu-Ampi

Do not confuse ampicillin with aminophylline, Imipenem, or Unipen.

CATEGORY AND SCHEDULE

Pregnancy Risk Category: B

Classification: Antibiotics, penicillins, aminopenicillins

MECHANISM OF ACTION

A penicillin that inhibits cell wall synthesis in susceptible microorganisms. *Therapeutic Effect:* Bactericidal.

PHARMACOKINETICS

Moderately absorbed from the GI tract. Protein binding: 28%. Widely distributed. Partially metabolized in the liver. Primarily excreted in urine. Removed by hemodialysis. *Half-life:* 1-1.5 h (increased in impaired renal function).

AVAILABILITY

Capsules: 250 mg, 500 mg.
Powder for Oral Suspension: 125 mg/5 mL, 250 mg/5 mL.
Powder for Injection: 125 mg, 250 mg, 500 mg, 1 g, 2 g.

INDICATIONS AND DOSAGES

▸ **Respiratory tract, skin, and skin-structure infections**

PO

Adults, Elderly, Children weighing more than 40 kg. 250-1000 mg q6h.
Children weighing < 20 kg. 50-100 mg/kg/day in divided doses q6h.

IV, IM

Adults, Elderly, Children weighing more than 40 kg. 500-1000 mg q6h.
Children weighing < 40 kg. 25-50 mg/kg/day in divided doses q6h.

▸ **Bacterial meningitis, septicemia**

IV, IM

Adults, Elderly. 2 g q4h or 3 g q6h.
Children. 100-200 mg/kg/day in divided doses q3-4h.

▸ **Uncomplicated gonococcal infections**

PO

Adults. 3.5 g one time with 1 g probenecid.

▸ **Perioperative prophylaxis**

IV, IM

Adults, Elderly. 2 g 30 min before procedure. May repeat in 8 h.
Children. 50 mg/kg 30 min before procedure. May repeat in 8 h.

▸ **Usual neonatal dosage**

Neonates 7-28 days old. 75 mg/kg/day in divided doses q8h up to 200 mg/kg/day in divided doses q6h.
Neonates 0-7 days old. 50 mg/kg/day in divided doses q12h up to 150 mg/kg/day in divided doses q8h.

▸ **Dosage in renal impairment (adults)**

Creatinine Clearance (mL/min)	% of Normal Dosage
10-30	Give q6-12h
< 10	Give q12h

CONTRAINDICATIONS

Hypersensitivity to any penicillin.

INTERACTIONS

Drug

Allopurinol: May increase incidence of rash.
Oral contraceptives: May decrease effectiveness of oral contraceptives.
Probenecid: May increase ampicillin blood concentration.

Herbal

None known.

Food

None known.

DIAGNOSTIC TEST EFFECTS

May increase AST (SGOT) and ALT (SGPT) levels. May cause a positive direct Coombs' test.

IV INCOMPATIBILITIES

Amikacin (Amikin), aminophylline, amphotericin B, caspofungin (Cancidas), codeine, diazepam, diltiazem, dobutamine, dopamine, fluconazole (Diflucan), gentamicin, lansoprazole (Prevacid), lorazepam, midazolam (Versed), nitroprusside, ondansetron (Zofran), phenytoin, promethazine (Phenergan), sodium bicarbonate, tobramycin, verapamil.

IV COMPATIBILITIES

Calcium gluconate, cefepime (Maxipime), famotidine (Pepcid), furosemide (Lasix), heparin, hydromorphone (Dilaudid), insulin (regular), levofloxacin (Levaquin), magnesium sulfate, morphine, multivitamins, potassium chloride, propofol (Diprivan).

SIDE EFFECTS

Frequent
Pain at IM injection site, GI disturbances (mild diarrhea, nausea, vomiting), oral or vaginal candidiasis.
Occasional
Generalized rash, urticaria, phlebitis or thrombophlebitis (with IV administration), headache.
Rare
Dizziness, seizures (especially with IV therapy).

SERIOUS REACTIONS

• Antibiotic-associated colitis and other superinfections may result from altered bacterial balance.
• Severe hypersensitivity reactions, including anaphylaxis and acute interstitial nephritis, occur rarely.

PRECAUTIONS & CONSIDERATIONS

Caution is warranted with antibiotic-associated colitis or a history of allergies, especially to cephalosporins. Ampicillin readily crosses the placenta, appears in cord blood and amniotic fluid, and is distributed in breast milk in low concentrations. Ampicillin may lead to allergic sensitization, candidiasis, diarrhea, and skin rash in infants. Immature renal function in neonates and young infants may delay renal excretion of ampicillin. Keep in mind that high dosages may be needed for neonatal meningitis. Age-related renal impairment may require dosage adjustment for elderly patients.

History of allergies, especially to cephalosporins or penicillins, should be determined before giving the drug. Withhold and promptly notify the physician if rash or diarrhea occurs. A high incidence of rash has been observed in patients with infectious mononucleosis treated with ampicillin. Severe diarrhea with abdominal pain, blood or mucus in stool, and fever may indicate antibiotic-associated colitis. Signs and symptoms of superinfection, including anal or genital pruritus, black hairy tongue, diarrhea, increased fever, sore throat, ulceration or changes in oral mucosa, and vomiting, should be monitored. Intake and output, renal function tests, urinalysis, and the injection sites should be assessed.

Storage
Store capsules at room temperature. After reconstitution, the oral solution is stable for 7 days at room temperature or 14 days if refrigerated. Refrigeration is preferred. An IV solution diluted with 0.9% NaCl is stable for 2-8 h at room temperature or 3 days if refrigerated. An IV solution diluted with D5W is stable for 2 h at room temperature or 3 h if refrigerated. Discard the IV solution if a precipitate forms. The reconstituted solution for IM injection is stable for 1 h.

Administration
Give oral forms 1 h before or 2 h after meals for maximum absorption. Shake oral solution well before use.

For IV injection, dilute each 250- or 500-mg vial with 5 mL sterile water for injection and each 1- or 2-g vial with 10 mL. For intermittent IV infusion (piggyback), further dilute with 50-100 mL 0.9% NaCl or D5W. Administer each 125-, 250-, or 500-mg dose over 3-5 min and each

1- to 2-g dose over 10-15 min. Infuse intermittent IV infusion (piggyback) over 20-30 min. Because of the potential for hypersensitivity and anaphylaxis, start the initial dose at a few drops per minute, increase the dosage slowly to the prescribed rate, and stay with the patient for the first 10-15 min. Then assess every 10 min during the infusion for signs and symptoms of hypersensitivity or anaphylaxis. Expect to switch to the oral route as soon as possible.

For IM use, reconstitute each vial with sterile water for injection or bacteriostatic water for injection. Consult individual ampicillin vials or package insert for specific volumes of diluent. Inject the drug deep into a large muscle mass.

Ampicillin/ Sulbactam

am'pi-sill-in/sul-bac'tam

★ Unasyn

CATEGORY AND SCHEDULE

Pregnancy Risk Category: B

Classification: Antibiotics, penicillins, aminopenicillins, plus a beta-lactamase inhibitor

MECHANISM OF ACTION

Ampicillin inhibits bacterial cell wall synthesis, whereas sulbactam inhibits bacterial β-lactamase. *Therapeutic Effect:* Ampicillin is bactericidal in susceptible microorganisms. Sulbactam protects ampicillin from enzymatic degradation.

PHARMACOKINETICS

Protein binding: 28%-38%. Widely distributed. Partially metabolized in the liver. Primarily excreted in urine. Removed by hemodialysis. *Half-life:* 1 h (increased in impaired renal function).

AVAILABILITY

Powder for Injection: 1.5 g (ampicillin 1 g/sulbactam 500 g), 3 g (ampicillin 2 g/sulbactam 1 g).

INDICATIONS AND DOSAGES

▸ **Skin/skin-structure, intra-abdominal, and gynecologic infections**

IV, IM

Adults, Elderly, Children > 40 kg. 1.5 g (1 g ampicillin/500 mg sulbactam) to 3 g (2 g ampicillin/1 g sulbactam) q6h.

Children 1-12 yr and < 40 kg. 150-300 mg/kg/day in divided doses q6h.

▸ **Dosage in renal impairment**

Dosage and frequency are modified based on creatinine clearance and the severity of the infection.

Creatinine Clearance (mL/min)	Adult Dosage
> 30	1.5-3 g q6-8h
15-29	1.5-3 g q12h
5-14	1.5-3 g q24h
< 5	Not recommended

OFF-LABEL USES

Treatment of pneumonia or aspiration pneumonia; alternative for pelvic inflammatory disease.

CONTRAINDICATIONS

Hypersensitivity to any penicillin.

INTERACTIONS

Drug

Allopurinol: May increase incidence of rash.

Oral contraceptives: May decrease effectiveness of oral contraceptives.

Probenecid: May increase ampicillin blood concentration.

Herbal

None known.

Food

None known.

DIAGNOSTIC TEST EFFECTS

May increase serum LDH, alkaline phosphatase, creatinine, AST (SGOT), and ALT (SGPT) levels. May cause a positive direct Coombs' test.

IV INCOMPATIBILITIES

Acyclovir, aminophylline, amphotericin B, caspofungin (Cancidas), ciprofloxacin (Cipro), diazepam, diltiazem (Cardizem), dobutamine, dopamine, fluconazole (Diflucan), idarubicin (Idamycin), lansoprazole (Prevacid), lorazepam, midazolam (Versed), nitroprusside, ondansetron (Zofran), phenytoin, promethazine (Phenergan), sargramostim (Leukine), sodium bicarbonate, tobramycin, verapamil.

SIDE EFFECTS

Frequent

Diarrhea and rash (most common), urticaria, pain at IM injection site, thrombophlebitis with IV administration, oral or vaginal candidiasis.

Occasional

Nausea, vomiting, headache, malaise, urine retention.

SERIOUS REACTIONS

- Severe hypersensitivity reactions, including anaphylaxis, acute interstitial nephritis, and blood dyscrasias, may occur.
- Antibiotic-associated colitis and other superinfections may result from altered bacterial balance.
- Overdose may produce seizures.

PRECAUTIONS & CONSIDERATIONS

Caution is warranted with antibiotic-associated colitis or a history of allergies, especially to cephalosporins. Ampicillin and sulbactam readily cross the placenta, appear in cord blood and amniotic fluid, and are distributed in breast milk in low concentrations. Ampicillin and sulbactam may lead to allergic sensitization, candidiasis, diarrhea, and skin rash in infants. The safety and efficacy of ampicillin and sulbactam have not been established in children younger than 1 yr. Age-related renal impairment may require dosage adjustment in elderly patients.

History of allergies, especially to cephalosporins or penicillins, should be determined before giving the drug. Withhold and promptly notify the physician if rash or diarrhea occurs. A high incidence of rash has been observed in patients with infectious mononucleosis treated with ampicillin. Severe diarrhea with abdominal pain, blood or mucus in stool, and fever may indicate antibiotic-associated colitis. Signs and symptoms of superinfection, including anal or genital pruritus, black hairy tongue, diarrhea, increased fever, sore throat, ulceration or changes of oral mucosa, and vomiting, should be monitored. Intake and output, renal function tests, urinalysis, and the injection sites should be assessed.

Storage

Store at room temperature prior to reconstitution. When reconstituted with 0.9% NaCl, the IV solution is stable for 8 h at room temperature or 48 h if refrigerated. Stability may differ with other diluents. Discard the IV solution if a precipitate forms.

Administration

For IV injection, dilute with 10-20 mL sterile water for injection. For intermittent IV infusion (piggyback), further dilute with 50-100 mL D5W or 0.9% NaCl. Administer IV injection slowly, over 10-15 min. Administer intermittent IV infusion (piggyback) over 15-30 min. Because of the potential for hypersensitivity and anaphylaxis, start the initial dose at a few drops per minute and then increase the dose slowly to the ordered rate. Stay with the patient for the first 10-15 min; then check every 10 min during the infusion for signs and symptoms of hypersensitivity or anaphylaxis.

For IM use, reconstitute each 1.5-g vial with 3.2 mL or each 3-g vial with 6.4 mL of sterile water for injection to provide a concentration of 250 mg ampicillin/125 mg sulbactam per milliliter. Administer the injection deep into a large muscle mass within 1 h of preparation.

Amyl Nitrite

am'il nye'trite

★ Amyl Nitrite

Do not confuse with nitrates or inhaled ammonia spirits.

CATEGORY AND SCHEDULE

Pregnancy Risk Category: C

Classification: Antianginal; nitrates, vasodilators

MECHANISM OF ACTION

A nitrite vasodilator that relaxes smooth muscles. Reduces afterload and improves vascular supply to the myocardium. *Therapeutic Effect:* Dilates coronary arteries, improves blood flow to ischemic areas within myocardium. Following inhalation, systemic vasodilation occurs.

PHARMACOKINETICS

The vapors are absorbed rapidly through the pulmonary alveoli and metabolized rapidly. Partially excreted in the urine.

AVAILABILITY

Inhalation: 0.3 mL glass ampule (amyl nitrite).

INDICATIONS AND DOSAGES

▸ **Acute relief of angina pectoris**

NASAL INHALATION

Adults, Elderly. Place crushed ampule to nostrils for 0.18-0.3 mL inhalation of vapors. Repeat at 5- to 10-min intervals. No more than 3 doses in 30-min period. Call emergency if pain is not relieved after 1 dose, even though repeat dose will be given.

OFF-LABEL USES

Cyanide toxicity.

CONTRAINDICATIONS

Closed-angle glaucoma, cerebral hemorrhage or recent head injury, postural hypotension, hypersensitivity to nitrites.

INTERACTIONS

Drug

Sildenafil and other phosphodiesterase inhibitors (e.g., tadalafil, vardenafil): May increase hypotensive effects. Contraindicated.

Herbal

None known.

Food

Ethanol: May increase hypotensive effects.

DIAGNOSTIC TEST EFFECTS

None known.

SIDE EFFECTS

Frequent

Headache (may be severe) occurs mostly in early therapy, diminishes rapidly in intensity, usually disappears during continued treatment; transient flushing of face and neck; dizziness (especially if patient is standing immobile or is in a warm environment); weakness; postural hypotension.

Occasional

Nausea, rash, vomiting.

Rare

Involuntary passage of urine and feces, restlessness, weakness.

SERIOUS REACTIONS

- Large doses may produce hemolytic anemia or methemoglobinemia.
- Severe postural hypotension manifested by fainting, pulselessness, cold or clammy skin, and profuse sweating may occur.
- Tolerance may occur with repeated, prolonged therapy.
- High dose tends to produce severe headache.

PRECAUTIONS & CONSIDERATIONS

Caution is warranted in patients with acute MI, blood volume depletion from diuretic therapy, glaucoma (contraindicated in closed-angle glaucoma), liver or renal disease, severe anemia, and systolic BP < 90 mm Hg. Test for apical pulse and blood pressure before amyl nitrite is administered and periodically after dose. Facial or neck flushing should be reported.

It is unknown whether amyl nitrite crosses the placenta or is distributed in breast milk. Safety and efficacy of amyl nitrite have not been established in children. Elderly patients are more susceptible to the hypotensive effects of amyl nitrite, and age-related renal impairment may require cautious use.

Storage

Store at room temperature and protect from light. Keep the drug container away from heat and moisture.

Administration

Ampules for inhalation should be used at the first sign of angina. Wrap ampule in woven sterile gauze. Crush amyl nitrite ampule with fingers and hold to the nostrils for inhalation of vapors. Wave under the nose; patient should inhale 1-6 times. May repeat in 3-5 min.

Anagrelide

ah-na'greh-lide

★ 🍁 Agrylin

CATEGORY AND SCHEDULE

Pregnancy Risk Category: C

Classification: Platelet count-reducing agent

MECHANISM OF ACTION

A hematologic agent that reduces platelet production and prevents platelet shape changes caused by platelet-aggregating agents. *Therapeutic Effect:* Inhibits platelet aggregation.

PHARMACOKINETICS

After oral administration, plasma concentration peaks within 1 h. Extensively metabolized. Primarily excreted in urine. *Half-life:* 1.3 h.

AVAILABILITY

Capsules: 0.5 mg, 1 mg.

INDICATIONS AND DOSAGES

▸ **Thrombocythemia secondary to myeloproliferative disorders**

PO

Adults, Elderly. Initially, 0.5 mg 4 times a day or 1 mg twice a day. Adjust to lowest effective dosage, increasing by up to 0.5 mg/day or

less in any 1 wk. Maximum: 10 mg/day or 2.5 mg/dose.
Children 7 yr of age or older. Initially 0.5 mg/day. Adjust to lowest effective dose, increasing by up to 0.5 mg/day or less in any 1 wk. Maximum: 10 mg/day or 2.5 mg/dose.

▸ **Dose in hepatic impairment.**
PO
Initially 0.5 mg/day. Adjust to lowest effective dose, increasing by up to 0.5 mg/day or less in any 1 wk. Do not use in severe hepatic impairment.

CONTRAINDICATIONS

Severe hepatic impairment.

INTERACTIONS

Drug
Other platelet inhibitors: May increase risk for bleeding.
Rasagiline: Anagrelide may theoretically reduce rasagiline metabolism.
Herbal
None known.
Food
None known.

DIAGNOSTIC TEST EFFECTS

May increase liver enzymes (ASR, ALT) (rare). Will lower platelet count; monitor every 2 days during the first week of treatment and at least weekly thereafter until maintenance reached.

SIDE EFFECTS

Frequent (≥ 10%)
Headache, palpitations, diarrhea, abdominal pain, nausea, flatulence, bloating, asthenia, pain, dizziness.
Occasional (5% to < 10%)
Tachycardia, chest pain, vomiting, paresthesia, peripheral edema, anorexia, dyspepsia, rash.
Other (< 5%)
Confusion, insomnia, hemorrhage, increased liver enzymes, bruising, vision changes, constipation, GI distress.

SERIOUS REACTIONS

- Angina, heart failure, and arrhythmias occur rarely.
- Progressive dyspnea with pulmonary infiltrates may indicate interstitial lung disease (e.g., allergic alveolitis, interstitial pneumonitis) that may require drug discontinuation.

PRECAUTIONS & CONSIDERATIONS

Caution is warranted with cardiac disease and hepatic or renal impairment. It is unknown whether anagrelide crosses the placenta or is distributed in breast milk. Anagrelide may cause fetal harm; it is not recommended in pregnant women. Strongly urge women to use contraceptives while taking anagrelide. Age-related precautions have not been observed in pediatric patients. Use anagrelide cautiously in elderly patients, who may have age-related cardiac disease and decreased renal and hepatic function.

Hemoglobin, hematocrit, and platelet and WBC counts should be obtained before treatment. Skin should be monitored for bruises or petechiae, and catheter and needle sites should be inspected for bleeding. Persons with suspected heart disease should be assessed for tachycardia, palpitations, and signs and symptoms of CHF, such as dyspnea. If progressive dyspnea and/or pulmonary infiltrates occur, these may indicate interstitial lung disease.

Storage
Store at room temperature. Protect from light.
Administration
Take without regard to food. Platelet count should respond within 7-14 days of beginning therapy.

Anakinra

an-a-kin'ra

Kineret

Do not confuse with amikacin.

CATEGORY AND SCHEDULE

Pregnancy Risk Category: B

Classification: Disease-modifying antirheumatic drugs, interleukin-receptor antagonists

MECHANISM OF ACTION

An interleukin-1 (IL-1) receptor antagonist that blocks the binding of IL-1, a protein that is a major mediator of joint disease and is present in excess amounts in patients with rheumatoid arthritis. *Therapeutic Effect:* Inhibits the inflammatory response.

PHARMACOKINETICS

No accumulation of anakinra in tissues or organs was observed after daily subcutaneous doses. Excreted in urine. *Half-life:* 4-6 h.

AVAILABILITY

Pre-filled injection: 100 mg/0.67 mL syringe.

INDICATIONS AND DOSAGES

▸ **Rheumatoid arthritis**

SC

Adults, Elderly. 100 mg/day, given at same time each day.

▸ **Renal impairment**

Creatinine clearance < 30 mL/min: Consider decreasing the dose to q48h (every other day).

CONTRAINDICATIONS

Known hypersensitivity to *Escherichia coli*–derived proteins, anakinra, or product components; do not initiate if active infection.

INTERACTIONS

Drug

Live-virus vaccines: Avoid because of potential risk of infection.

DIAGNOSTIC TEST EFFECTS

May decrease WBC, platelet, and absolute neutrophil counts.

SIDE EFFECTS

Frequent (> 10%)

Injection site ecchymosis, erythema, and inflammation; infection; headache.

Occasional

Nausea, diarrhea, abdominal pain, neutropenia.

SERIOUS REACTIONS

- Infections, including upper respiratory tract infection, sinusitis, flu-like symptoms, and cellulitis, have been noted.
- Neutropenia may occur, particularly when anakinra is used in combination with tumor necrosis factor-blocking agents.
- Hypersensitivity and anaphylactoid reactions.

PRECAUTIONS & CONSIDERATIONS

Caution is warranted with asthma and renal impairment. Asthmatics are at increased risk for serious infection, and those with renal impairment are at increased risk for a toxic reaction. It is unknown whether anakinra is distributed in breast milk. The safety and efficacy of anakinra have not been established in children. Use anakinra cautiously in elderly patients, who may experience age-related renal impairment. Avoid contact with infected individuals and situations that might increase risk for infection.

Neutrophil count should be monitored before therapy begins, monthly for 3 mo during therapy, and then quarterly for up to 1 yr. Evaluate for inflammatory reactions, especially during the first 4 wks of therapy. Inflammation is uncommon after the first month of therapy.

Storage

Keep the drug refrigerated. Do not freeze or shake it. Protect from light.

Administration

There may be trace amounts of small, translucent/white protein particles in the solution. Do not use if solution is discolored or cloudy. If particles appear excessive in a syringe, do not use it. Give by subcutaneous injection; recommended sites are outer upper arms, abdomen (except within 2 inches of navel), front middle thigh, or outer buttocks. Use a new site for each injection and do not inject into an area that is tender, red, bruised, scarred, or hard. Do not inject close to a vein.

Anastrozole

an-as'troe-zole

★ 🍁 Arimidex

Do not confuse Arimidex with Imitrex.

CATEGORY AND SCHEDULE

Pregnancy Risk Category: D

Classification: Aromatase inhibitors, hormones/hormone modifiers

MECHANISM OF ACTION

Decreases the circulating estrogen level by inhibiting aromatase, the enzyme that catalyzes the final step in estrogen production. *Therapeutic Effect:* Inhibits the growth of breast cancers that are stimulated by estrogens.

PHARMACOKINETICS

Well absorbed into systemic circulation (absorption not affected by food). Protein binding: 40%. Extensively metabolized in the liver. Eliminated by biliary system and, to a lesser extent, kidneys. *Mean half-life:* 50 h in postmenopausal women. Steady-state plasma levels reached in about 7 days.

AVAILABILITY

Tablets: 1 mg.

INDICATIONS AND DOSAGES

▸ **First-line, second-line, and adjuvant treatment of hormonally responsive breast cancer**

PO

Adults, Elderly. 1 mg once a day.

CONTRAINDICATIONS

Hypersensitivity to drug. Pregnancy.

INTERACTIONS

Drug

Estrogen-containing products: May reduce anastrozole therapeutic effect.

Tamoxifen: May reduce anastrozole concentrations.

Herbal

Black cohosh, hops, licorice, red clover, thyme, and dong quai: Avoid herbals with potential estrogenic activity.

Food

None known.

DIAGNOSTIC TEST EFFECTS

May elevate serum GGT level in patients with liver metastasis. May increase serum LDL, serum alkaline phosphate, AST (SGOT), ALT (SGPT), and total cholesterol levels. May reduce bone mineral density.

SIDE EFFECTS

Frequent (8%-16%)
Asthenia, nausea, headache, hot flashes, back pain, vomiting, cough, diarrhea.
Occasional (4%-6%)
Constipation, abdominal pain, anorexia, bone pain, pharyngitis, dizziness, rash, dry mouth, peripheral edema, pelvic pain, depression, chest pain, paresthesia.
Rare (1%-2%)
Weight gain, diaphoresis, persistent vaginal bleeding.

SERIOUS REACTIONS

- Thrombophlebitis and thromboembolism occur rarely.
- Hypersensitivity, including anaphylactoid reactions and Stevens-Johnson syndrome.
- Ischemic cardiovascular events (rare).
- Hepatitis with jaundice.

PRECAUTIONS & CONSIDERATIONS

Anastrozole is indicated only for postmenopausal women. Women who are or may be pregnant should not use anastrozole because the drug crosses the placenta and may cause fetal harm. Pregnancy should be excluded before therapy begins. It is unknown whether anastrozole is excreted in breast milk. The safety and efficacy of anastrozole have not been established in children. No age-related precautions have been noted in elderly patients.

Potential side effects, including dizziness and weakness, may occur. Notify the physician if asthenia, hot flashes, and nausea or diarrhea become unmanageable.
Storage
Store at room temperature.
Administration
Take orally without regard to food.

Anidulafungin

ann-id-yoo-la-fun'jin
★ 🍁 Eraxis

CATEGORY AND SCHEDULE

Pregnancy Risk Category: C

Classification: Antifungal, echinocandins

MECHANISM OF ACTION

An antifungal that inhibits the synthesis of 1,3-β-D-glucan, an essential component of the fungal cell wall. *Therapeutic Effect:* Fungicidal.

PHARMACOKENETICS

Protein binding: 84%. Metabolism in the liver has not been observed. Approximately 30% eliminated in feces; < 1% excreted in the urine. *Half-life:* 26.5 h.

AVAILABILITY

Lyophilized Powder for Injection: 50 mg, 100 mg.

INDICATIONS AND DOSAGES

▸ **Candidemia**
IV
Adults. 200 mg loading dose on day 1, followed by 100 mg daily thereafter. Continue for at least 14 days after the last positive culture.
▸ **Esophageal candidiasis**
IV
Adults. 100 mg loading dose on day 1, followed by 50 mg daily for a minimum of 14 days and for at least 7 days following resolution of symptoms.
Children. Safety and efficacy have not been established.

CONTRAINDICATIONS

Hypersensitivity to anidulafungin or its components.

INTERACTIONS

Drug

Cyclosporine: May increase anidulafungin concentrations, but no dose adjustment needed.

DIAGNOSTIC TEST EFFECTS

Increased liver function test values.

IV INCOMPATIBILITIES

Do not mix with other medications. Specific known incompatibilities include diazepam, ertapenem (Invanz), magnesium sulfate, pemetrexed (Alimta), phenytoin, potassium phosphate, sodium bicarbonate, sodium phosphate.

SIDE EFFECTS

Occasional (2%-10%)

Diarrhea, hypokalemia, abnormal liver function.

Rare (< 2%)

Rash, urticaria, flushing, pruritus, dyspnea, hypotension, deep vein thrombosis.

SERIOUS REACTIONS

- Histamine-mediated symptoms, including rash, urticaria, flushing, pruritus, dyspnea, and hypotension, have been reported.

PRECAUTIONS & CONSIDERATIONS

Caution in patients with preexisting hepatic impairment and neutropenia. Abnormal liver function test results have been observed in patients treated with anidulafungin. Clinical hepatic abnormalities have been observed in patients with preexisting hepatic impairment or concomitant medical conditions. Teratogenic effects observed in animal studies; use in pregnancy only if clearly needed. Use with caution in breastfeeding. Safety and effectiveness have not been established in pediatric patients.

Storage

Store unopened vials in refrigerator. After reconstitution, vial solution may be kept up to 1 h in refrigerator prior to preparing infusion. Infusion solution may be kept refrigerated but should be used within 24 h of preparation. Do not freeze.

Administration

For IV infusion only after appropriate dilution. Reconstitute each 50-mg vial with 15 mL of sterile water for injection (SWI) or each 100-mg vial with 30 mL of SWI. Concentration will be 3.33 mg/mL. Further dilute vial contents with D5W or 0.9 NaCl to a final infusion concentration of 0.77 mg/mL. Infuse IV at a rate not to exceed 1.1 mg/min.

Anthralin

anth-rah'lin

★ Dritho-Creme HP, Dritho-Scalp, Micanol, Psoriatec

Do not confuse with Antagon, Antabuse, or Andriol.

CATEGORY AND SCHEDULE

Pregnancy Risk Category: C

Classification: Dermatologic agents, antipsoriatic

MECHANISM OF ACTION

A topical agent that binds DNA, inhibiting synthesis of nucleic protein, and reduces mitotic activity.

PHARMACOKINETICS

Poorly absorbed systemically but excellent epidermal absorption. Auto-oxidized to inactive metabolites—danthrone and dianthrone. Rapid urinary excretion, so significant levels do not accumulate in the blood or other tissues. *Half-life:* 6 h.

AVAILABILITY

Cream: 0.5% (Dritho-Scalp), 1% (Dritho-Creme HP, Micanol, Psoriatec).

INDICATIONS AND DOSAGES

▸ **Psoriasis**

TOPICAL

Adults, Elderly. Apply in a thin layer to affected areas once daily. For conventional therapy, the treatment is left on 8-12 h (preferably overnight) before showering/bathing. Short-contact therapy has application time that is gradually increased from 5-10 min to 20-30 min daily before bathing.

OFF-LABEL USES

Inflammatory linear verrucous epidermal nevus.

CONTRAINDICATIONS

Acute psoriasis where inflammation is present, erythroderma, hypersensitivity to anthralin.

INTERACTIONS

Drug

Topical corticosteroids: Because psoriasis may worsen upon discontinuation of long-term topical corticosteroid therapy, allow 1 wk between discontinuation of corticosteroid therapy and initiation of anthralin therapy.

Herbal

None known.

Food

None known.

SIDE EFFECTS

Frequent

Irritation.

Rare

Staining of the skin or fingernails.

SERIOUS REACTIONS

- Hypersensitivity reaction, such as burning, erythema, and dermatitis, may occur.

PRECAUTIONS & CONSIDERATIONS

Caution should be used in renal disease. Patch test should be obtained to rule out the possibility of allergy versus an irritation reaction. It is unknown whether anthralin crosses the placenta and is detected in breast milk. Safety and effectiveness have not been determined for use in children. Severe irritation or edema should be reported.

Administration

For external use only. Apply only to the skin affected with psoriasis. Do not apply to face or genitalia areas. For skin application, apply sparingly only to psoriatic lesions and rub gently and carefully into the skin until absorbed. For scalp application, comb hair to remove scalar debris, wet hair, and, after suitably parting, rub cream well into the lesions, taking care to prevent the cream from spreading onto the forehead or neck. Wash hands thoroughly after using because anthralin may stain skin, hair, and fabric. After prescribed time, rinse area where applied with cool or lukewarm water only. Avoid hot water and soap or shampoo as they could cause product to stain or irritate. Following anthralin removal, the area can be cleaned with usual soap or shampoo.

Antihemophilic Factor (Factor VIII, AHF)

★ Advate, Alphanate, Helixate FS, Hemofil M, Humate-P, Koate DVI, Kogenate FS, Monarc M, Monoclate-P, Recombinate

Do not confuse with Alfenta.

CATEGORY AND SCHEDULE

Pregnancy Risk Category: C

Classification: Antihemophilic agents, blood clotting factors

MECHANISM OF ACTION

An antihemophilic agent that assists in conversion of prothrombin to thrombin, essential for blood coagulation. Replaces missing clotting factor. *Therapeutic Effect:* Produces hemostasis; corrects or prevents bleeding episodes.

AVAILABILITY

Injection: Actual number of AHF units is listed on each vial and varies from brand to brand.

INDICATIONS AND DOSAGES

▸ **Treatment and prevention of bleeding in patients with hemophilia A factor VIII deficiency, hypofibrinogenemia, von Willebrand disease**

IV

Adults, Elderly, Children. Dosage is highly individualized and is based on patient's weight, severity of bleeding, and coagulation studies.

OFF-LABEL USES

Treatment of disseminated intravascular coagulation.

CONTRAINDICATIONS

Hypersensitivity to mouse, hamster, or bovine protein, or to porcine or murine factor, depending on product source.

INTERACTIONS

Drug

None known.

Herbal

None known.

Food

None known.

DIAGNOSTIC TEST EFFECTS

None known.

IV INCOMPATIBILITIES

Do not mix with other IV solutions or medications.

SIDE EFFECTS

Occasional

Allergic reaction, including fever, chills, urticaria, wheezing, hypotension, nausea, feeling of chest tightness; stinging at injection site; dizziness; dry mouth; headache; altered taste.

SERIOUS REACTIONS

- There is a risk of transmitting viral hepatitis and other viral illnesses with product derived from pooled human plasma.
- Intravascular hemolysis may occur if large or frequent doses are used with blood group A, B, or AB.

PRECAUTIONS & CONSIDERATIONS

Caution is warranted with hepatic disease and in those with blood type A, B, or AB. If large doses are given with these blood types, expect to monitor Hct and direct Coombs' test to check for hemolytic anemia. If hemolytic anemia occurs, expect to give transfusions with type O blood. Avoid overinflating cuff when monitoring BP. Take BP manually, avoiding automatic BP cuffs. Electric razor and soft toothbrush should be used to prevent bleeding.

Notify the physician of abdominal or back pain, gingival bleeding, black or red stool, coffee-ground emesis, dark or red urine, or red-speckled mucus from cough. IV site should be monitored for oozing. Vital signs should also be monitored throughout therapy.

Storage

Store in the refrigerator. Do not freeze. Some products allow storage at room temperature for up to 6 mo.

Administration

For IV use, refer to individual products for reconstitution and IV infusion requirements, as products vary. Warm concentrate and diluent to room temperature. Gently agitate or rotate to dissolve. Do not shake vigorously.

Complete dissolution may take 5-10 min. Filter before administering. Use plastic syringes. A controlled infusion device is often used. Administer IV at a rate of approximately 2 mL/min. Some products allow infusion up to 10 mL/min.

Antithymocyte Globulin, Equine

an'tye-thye'moe-site glob'yoo-lin

Atgam

Do not confuse Atgam with Ativan.

CATEGORY AND SCHEDULE

Pregnancy Risk Category: C

Classification: Immune globulins, immunosuppressant

MECHANISM OF ACTION

A biological response modifier that acts as a lymphocyte selective immunosuppressant, reducing the number and altering the function of T lymphocytes, which are responsible for cell-mediated and humoral immunity. Lymphocyte immune globulin N also stimulates the release of hematopoietic growth factors. *Therapeutic Effect:* Prevents allograft rejection; treats aplastic anemia.

PHARMACOKINETICS

Onset rapid, absorption T_{max} is 5 days. Elimination mean half-life is 5.7 days. *Half-life:* 2.7-8.7 days.

AVAILABILITY

Injection: 250 mg/5 mL.

INDICATIONS AND DOSAGES

▸ **To delay onset of renal graft allograft rejection**

IV

Adults, Elderly, Children. 15 mg/kg/day for 14 days, then every other day for a total of 21 doses in 28 days. First dose within 24 h before or after transplantation.

▸ **Treatment of renal allograft rejection**

IV

Adults, Elderly, Children. First dose can be delayed until the diagnosis of the first rejection episode. Then give 10-15 mg/kg/day for 14 days, then every other day for a total of 21 doses. Maximum: 21 doses.

▸ **Renal allograft recipients**

IV

Adults, Elderly. 10-30 mg/kg/day.
Children. 5-25 mg/kg/day.

▸ **Aplastic anemia**

IV

Adults, Elderly, Children. 10-20 mg/kg once a day for 8-14 days, then every other day for a total of 21 doses.

OFF-LABEL USES

Immunosuppressant in bone marrow, heart, and liver transplants, treatment of pure red cell aplasia, multiple sclerosis, myasthenia gravis, and scleroderma.

CONTRAINDICATIONS

Systemic hypersensitivity reaction to previous injection of lymphocyte immune globulin N or other equine gamma globulin preparations.

INTERACTIONS

Drug

Immunosuppressants: May increase risk of infection developing.

Herbal

None known.

Food

None known.

DIAGNOSTIC TEST EFFECTS

May alter renal function test results.

IV INCOMPATIBILITIES

No information is available for Y-site administration.

SIDE EFFECTS

Frequent

Fever (51%), thrombocytopenia (30%), rash, chills (16%), leukopenia (14%), systemic infection (13%).

Occasional (5%-10%)

Serum sickness-like reaction, dyspnea, apnea, arthralgia, chest pain, back pain, flank pain, nausea, vomiting, diarrhea, phlebitis.

SERIOUS REACTIONS

- Thrombocytopenia may occur but is generally transient.
- A severe hypersensitivity reaction, including anaphylaxis, occurs rarely.

PRECAUTIONS & CONSIDERATIONS

! Lymphocyte immune globulin should be administered by physicians experienced in immunosuppressive treatment of renal transplant or aplastic anemia. Adequate laboratory and support equipment should be available.

Although rare, there is a risk of transmitting human and equine blood-based infections, particularly Creutzfeld-Jakob disease.

Caution is warranted with concurrent immunosuppressive therapy. Immediately notify the physician of chest pain, rapid or irregular heartbeat, shortness of breath, wheezing, or swelling of the face or throat, which may occur during the IV infusion. Avoid exposure to people with colds or infections, and notify the physician as soon as signs or symptoms of infection, thrombocytopenia, or leukopenia develop. Dosage adjustments should be considered in patients with profound bone marrow suppression.

Although risk of hypersensitivity is rare, hypersensitivity can occur at any time during therapy. Serum sickness, although rare, could occur within the first 6-18 days of therapy.

Experience with children is limited; it has been administered safely to a small number of renal allograft pediatric recipients and aplastic anemia pediatric patients at dosages comparable to those used in adults.

Before administration, test the patient with an intradermal injection of 0.1 mL of a freshly prepared 1:1000 dilution of lymphocyte immune globulin in normal saline and a contralateral NaCl injection as control.

Storage

Keep the drug refrigerated before and after dilution. Discard the diluted solution after 24 h. Protect from freezing.

Administration

Do not use intradermally, subcutaneously, intramuscularly, intra-arterially, or by IV bolus.

An intradermal test dose is recommended prior to beginning treatment (see prescribing information from manufacturer).

For IV use, dilute the total daily dose with 0.9% NaCl, as prescribed, to a final concentration of no more than 4 mg/mL. Gently rotate the diluted solution; avoid shaking it. Use a 0.2- to 1-micron filter, and infuse the total daily dose over at least 4 h. To prevent chemical phlebitis, avoid using a peripheral vein for IV infusion. Instead, expect to use a central venous catheter, a Groshong catheter, or a peripherally inserted central catheter. Avoid contact of the undiluted lymphocyte immune globulin with air. Expect to monitor frequently for chills, fever, erythema, and pruritus. An order for prophylactic antihistamines or corticosteroids should be obtained to treat these potential side effects.

Apomorphine

aye-poe-more′feen

★ Apokyn

CATEGORY AND SCHEDULE

Pregnancy Risk Category: C

Classification: Antiparkinsonian agents, dopaminergics

MECHANISM OF ACTION

An antiparkinson agent that stimulates postsynaptic dopamine receptors in the brain. *Therapeutic Effect:* Relieves signs and symptoms of Parkinson disease and improves motor function.

PHARMACOKINETICS

Rapidly absorbed after subcutaneous administration. Protein binding: 99.9%. Widely distributed. Rapidly eliminated from plasma. Not detected in urine or secretions. *Half-life:* 41-45 min.

AVAILABILITY

Injection: 10 mg/mL in cartridges to be used with injection pen.

INDICATIONS AND DOSAGES

▸ **Acute, intermittent treatment of hypomobility ("off" episodes) associated with advanced Parkinson disease**

SC

Adults, Elderly. Initially, 0.2 mL (2 mg) used "as needed" to treat an acute "off" episode; may be increased in 0.1-mL (1-mg) increments every few days. Maximum: 0.6 mL (6 mg). Initial doses are determined by administering test doses in-clinic where a medical professional can closely monitor BP pre-dose and at 20, 40, and 60 min post dose. No more than 1 dose per "off" episode should be administered. Doses > 0.6 mL (6 mg), total daily doses > 2 mL (20 mg), and dosing more than 5 times per day are not recommended. Rotate injection sites.

NOTE: Apomorphine should be given with an antinauseant but NOT a serotonin 5-HT3 antagonist (contraindicated). Trimethobenzamide is recommended for nausea at a dose of 300 mg 3 times daily started 3 days before the initial dose of apomorphine and continued for at least the first 2 mo of therapy to combat nausea.

▸ **Dose in renal impairment.**

Test dose and starting dose should be reduced to 0.1 mL (1 mg).

CONTRAINDICATIONS

Concurrent use of 5-HT3 antagonists such as alosetron, dolasetron, granisetron, ondansetron, or palonosetron; hypersensitivity to apomorphine or any of the product ingredients (sodium metabisulfite); IV administration.

INTERACTIONS

Drug

Alosetron, dolasetron, granisetron, ondansetron, palonosetron: May produce profound hypotension and loss of consciousness. Contraindicated.

Butyrophenones, metoclopramide, phenothiazines, thioxanthenes: Decrease the effectiveness of apomorphine.

CNS depressants: May increase CNS depressant effects.

Antihypertensives, vasodilators: Increased risk of hypotension and adverse events.

Drugs that prolong QT interval: Increased risk of QT interval prolongation and torsades de pointes.
Food
Alcohol: Can worsen side effects; avoid.

DIAGNOSTIC TEST EFFECTS

May increase serum alkaline phosphatase level.

SIDE EFFECTS

Common (≥ 2%)
Injection site discomfort, nausea, vomiting, headache, dizziness, falls, syncope, hypersalivation, pallor, yawning, diaphoresis, somnolence, chest pain, rhinorrhea, orthostatic hypotension, dyskinesia or worsening dyskinesia, frequent erections, hallucinations.
Rare (< 2%)
Psychosis, stomatitis, altered taste, intense urges, such as gambling or inappropriate sexual urges.

SERIOUS REACTIONS

- Respiratory depression or CNS stimulation (characterized by tachypnea, bradycardia, or persistent vomiting) may occur.
- Cardiovascular events, such as prolonged QT interval, angina, ischemic events.
- Falling asleep suddenly during activities of daily living, which can be potentially dangerous.
- Priapism.
- Hallucinations.

PRECAUTIONS & CONSIDERATIONS

Caution is warranted with asthma, cardiac decompensation, cardiovascular or cerebrovascular disease, concomitant use of alcohol, antihypertensives or vasodilators, hypotension, sleep disorders, and renal impairment. Caution should also be used in persons prone to nausea and vomiting and those susceptible to QT/QTc prolongation, such as persons with hypokalemia, hypomagnesemia, bradycardia, genetic predisposition, or concomitant use of drugs that prolong the QTc interval. It is unknown whether apomorphine is distributed in breast milk. The safety and efficacy of apomorphine have not been established in children. Elderly patients are more likely to develop hallucinations and confusion and to experience falls, cardiovacular events, and respiratory disorders. Patients should use caution when driving or operating machinery until the effects of the drug are known.

Monitor BP; be alert for postural instability due to orthostasis or dyskinesia. If patients falls asleep during activities where they would normally be alert, notify prescriber.

Storage
Store at room temperature.

Administration
! Do not use intravenously. The manufacturer recommends expressing the dose of apomorphine in milliliters (mL) not milligrams (mg) to avoid confusion.

When initiating treatment, except patient to be receiving an appropriate antiemetic (trimethobenzamide) to curb nausea and vomiting. A test dose is given initially, with both supine and standing BP checked per-dose and at 20-, 40-, and 60-min post dose. Apomorphine is administered subcutaneously via use of a multidose-containing dosing pen. Follow directions carefully for use of the dosing pen and cartridges.

Apraclonidine Hydrochloride

ap-ra-kloe′ni-deen hi-droh-klor′-ide

Iopidine

Do not confuse with, clomiphene, Klonopin, Lodine, or quinidine.

CATEGORY AND SCHEDULE

Pregnancy Risk Category: C

Classification: Selective α_2-adrenergic agonist

MECHANISM OF ACTION

An ocular α-adrenergic agent that is relatively selective for α_2 receptor agonist. *Therapeutic Effect:* Reduces intraocular pressure.

PHARMACOKINETICS

Onset of action occurs within 1 h. The duration of a single dose is about 12 h. *Half-life:* 8 h.

AVAILABILITY

Ophthalmic Solution: 0.5%, 1%.

INDICATIONS AND DOSAGES

▸ **Glaucoma**

OPHTHALMIC

Adults, Elderly. Instill 1 drop of 0.5% solution to affected eye(s) 3 times a day.

▸ **Intraocular hypertension post laser surgery**

OPHTHALMIC

Adults, Elderly. Instill 1 drop of 1% solution in operative eye(s) 1 h before surgery and 1 drop postoperatively.

CONTRAINDICATIONS

Hypersensitivity to apraclonidine or clonidine or any component of the formulation; MAO inhibitor therapy.

DRUG INTERACTIONS

Drugs

MAO inhibitors: Concomitant use contraindicated.

DIAGNOSTIC TEST EFFECTS

None known.

SIDE EFFECTS/ADVERSE REACTIONS

Frequent (5%-15%)

Eye discomfort, hyperemia, pruritus, dry mouth.

Occasional (1%-5%)

Headache, constipation, dizziness, somnolence, conjunctivitis, changes in visual acuity, mydriasis, ocular inflammation.

Rare

Nasal decongestion.

SERIOUS REACTIONS

- Allergic reaction occurs rarely.
- Peripheral edema and arrhythmias have been reported.

PRECAUTIONS & CONSIDERATIONS

Tachyphylaxis frequently develops. Use with caution in patients with impaired renal or liver function, depression, cardiovascular disease, cerebrovascular disease, Raynaud disease, or thromboangiitis obliterans and in patients receiving concomitant cardiovascular drugs. Safety and effectiveness have not been established in pediatric patients. No unique precautions have been identified in elderly patients.

Storage

Store at room temperature.

Administration

Wait 5 min between instillation of other ophthalmic agents. Use nasolacrimal occlusion to reduce systemic exposure.

Aprepitant

ap-re'pi-tant

Emend

Do not confuse aprepitant with fosaprepitant.

CATEGORY AND SCHEDULE

Pregnancy Risk Category: B

Classification: Antiemetics/antivertigo, substance P antagonists

MECHANISM OF ACTION

A selective human substance P and neurokinin-1 (NK1) receptor antagonist that inhibits chemotherapy-induced nausea and vomiting centrally in the chemoreceptor trigger zone. *Therapeutic Effect:* Prevents the acute and delayed phases of chemotherapy-induced emesis, including vomiting caused by high-dose cisplatin.

PHARMACOKINETICS

Crosses the blood-brain barrier. Extensively metabolized in the liver. Eliminated primarily by liver metabolism (not excreted renally). *Half-life:* 9-13 h.

AVAILABILITY

Capsules: 80 mg, 125 mg.

INDICATIONS AND DOSAGES

▸ Prevention of chemotherapy-induced nausea and vomiting

PO

Adults, Elderly. 125 mg 1 h before chemotherapy on day 1 and 80 mg once a day in the morning on days 2 and 3. Given as part of regimens that include a steroid and a 5-HT3 antagonist.

▸ Prevention of postoperative nausea and vomiting

PO

Adults, Elderly. 40 mg within 3 h before induction of anesthesia.

CONTRAINDICATIONS

Hypersensitivity, concurrent use of pimozide (Orap), cisapride.

INTERACTIONS

Drug

Alprazolam, docetaxel, etoposide, ifosfamide, imatinib, irinotecan, midazolam, paclitaxel, triazolam, vinblastine, vincristine, vinorelbine: May increase the plasma concentrations of these drugs.

Antifungals, clarithromycin, diltiazem, nefazodone, nelfinavir, ritonavir: Increase aprepitant plasma concentration.

Carbamazepine, phenytoin, rifampin: Decrease aprepitant plasma concentration.

Contraceptives: May decrease the effectiveness of estrogen or progestin contraceptives. Alternative or back-up methods of contraception should be used during treatment and for 1 mo following the last dose of aprepitant.

Corticosteroids: Increase levels of systemic corticosteroids. If the patient is also receiving a steroid, expect to reduce the IV steroid dose by 25% and the oral dose by 50%.

Paroxetine: May decrease the effectiveness of either drug.

Warfarin: May decrease the effectiveness of warfarin.

Herbal

St. John's wort: May decrease aprepitant levels.

Food

Grapefruit juice: May increase aprepitant concentrations.

DIAGNOSTIC TEST EFFECTS
May increase BUN level and serum creatinine, AST (SGOT), and ALT (SGPT) levels. May produce proteinuria.

SIDE EFFECTS
Frequent (10%-17%)
Fatigue, nausea, hiccups, diarrhea, constipation, anorexia.
Occasional (4%-8%)
Headache, dizziness, dehydration, heartburn.
Rare (≤ 3%)
Abdominal pain, epigastric discomfort, gastritis, tinnitus, insomnia.

SERIOUS REACTIONS
- Neutropenia and mucous membrane disorders occur rarely.

PRECAUTIONS & CONSIDERATIONS
Caution in hepatic impairment. It is unknown whether aprepitant crosses the placenta or is distributed in breast milk. The safety and efficacy of aprepitant have not been established in children. No age-related precautions have been noted in elderly patients.

Nausea and vomiting should be relieved shortly after drug administration. Notify the physician if headache or persistent vomiting occurs. Pattern of daily bowel activity and stool consistency should be assessed.

Storage
Store at room temperature in original package.

Administration
As prescribed prior to chemotherapy, aprepitant is given with corticosteroids and a serotonin (5-HT3) antagonist.

Take aprepitant orally without regard to food.

Arformoterol Tartrate

ar-for-moe'ter-ole tar'trate

★ Brovana

CATEGORY AND SCHEDULE
Pregnancy Risk Category: C

Classification: β_2 agonist

MECHANISM OF ACTION
A long-acting β_2 agonist that stimulates adrenergic receptors in bronchial smooth muscle, causing relaxation of smooth muscle. *Therapeutic Effect:* Produces bronchodilation.

PHARMACOKENETICS
Primarily absorbed by the pulmonary system following inhalation. Protein binding: 52%-65%. Primarily metabolized by glucuronidation. Primarily excreted in urine; partial elimination in feces. *Half-life:* 26 h.

AVAILABILITY
Solution for Nebulization: 15 mcg/2 mL.

INDICATIONS AND DOSAGES
▸ **COPD**

ORAL INHALATION

Adults. 15 mcg (2 mL) twice a day by nebulization.

Children. Safety and efficacy have not been established in children.

CONTRAINDICATIONS
Hypersensitivity to arformoterol, racemic formoterol, or its components.

DRUG INTERACTIONS
Drug

β-blockers: May interfere with each other's effects.

Methylxanthines (e.g., aminophylline, theophylline), steroids, diuretics: May potentiate hypokalemic effects.
Tricyclic antidepressants, drugs that prolong QT interval: May potentiate cardiovascular effects.

DIAGNOSTIC TEST EFFECTS

None known.

SIDE EFFECTS/ADVERSE REACTIONS

Occasional (2%-10%)
Pain, chest pain, back pain, sinusitis, rash, leg cramps, dyspnea, peripheral edema.
Rare (< 2%)
Oral candidiasis, pulmonary congestion.

SERIOUS REACTIONS

- May increase the risk of asthma-related death.
- May exacerbate cardiovascular conditions including arrhythmias and hypertension.
- Hypersensitivity reactions including urticaria, angioedema, rash, bronchospasm, and anaphylaxis may occur.

PRECAUTIONS & CONSIDERATIONS

Use with caution in patients with acutely deteriorating COPD, cardiovascular disorders, convulsive disorders, diabetes mellitus, hypokalemia, thyrotoxicosis. Do not coadminister with other long-acting β_2 agonists.
Storage
Before dispensing, store in protective foil pouch in the refrigerator. After dispensing, unopened foil pouches may be stored at room temperature up to 6 wks. Remove from foil pouch immediately before use. Solution should be colorless; discard any vial that is not.
Administration
Administered with a standard jet nebulizer connected to an air compressor. May be administered with mouthpiece or face mask. Administer undiluted; do not mix with other medications in nebulizer.

Argatroban

ar-gat'tro-ban
★ Acova
Do not confuse with Aggrestat or Orgaran.

CATEGORY AND SCHEDULE

Pregnancy Risk Category: B

Classification: Anticoagulants, thrombin inhibitors

MECHANISM OF ACTION

A direct thrombin inhibitor that reversibly binds to thrombin-active sites. Inhibits thrombin-catalyzed or thrombin-induced reactions, including fibrin formation, activation of coagulant factors V, VIII, and XIII; also inhibits protein C formation and platelet aggregation. *Therapeutic Effect:* Produces anticoagulation.

PHARMACOKINETICS

Following IV administration, distributed primarily in extracellular fluid. Protein binding: 54%. Metabolized in the liver. Primarily excreted in the feces, presumably through biliary secretion. *Half-life:* 39-51 min.

AVAILABILITY

Injection: 100 mg/mL.

INDICATIONS AND DOSAGES

▸ **To prevent and treat heparin-induced thrombocytopenia**

IV INFUSION
Adults, Elderly. Initially, 2 mcg/kg/min administered as a continuous infusion. After initial infusion, dose may be adjusted until steady state aPTT is 1.5-3 times initial baseline value, not to exceed 100 seconds. Maximum dose: 10 mcg/kg/min.

▸ **During percutaneous coronary intervention**
IV INFUSION
Adults, Elderly. Initially, give a loading dose of 350 mcg/kg by slow IV injection over 3-5 min, *follow* with IV infusion of 25 mcg/kg/min. ACT checked in 5-10 min following bolus. If ACT is < 300 seconds, give additional bolus 150 mcg/kg, increase infusion to 30 mcg/kg/min. If ACT is > 450 seconds, decrease infusion to 15 mcg/kg/min. Once ACT of 300-450 seconds achieved, proceed with procedure.

▸ **Dosage in hepatic impairment**
Adults (HIT). Decrease initial dose to 0.5 mcg/kg/min; adjust as indicated.
Adults (PCI) with significant hepatic impairment (AST or ALT ≥ 3× ULN): Do not use.

CONTRAINDICATIONS

Overt major bleeding, hypersensitivity.

INTERACTIONS

Drug
Antiplatelet agents, thrombolytics, other anticoagulants: May increase the risk of bleeding. All parenteral anticoagulants should be discontinued before administration of argatroban. There is an increased risk of intracranial bleeding when used concomitantly with thrombolytic therapy.
Herbal
Feverfew, red clover, horse chestnut, garlic, green tea, ginseng, ginkgo: Can have antiplatelet activity, may increase risk of bleeding.

DIAGNOSTIC TEST EFFECTS

Increases aPTT, International Normalized Ratio, and PT. Also increases activated clotting time (ACT).

IV INCOMPATIBILITIES

Do not mix with other medications or solutions. Specific incompatibilities include amiodarone.

SIDE EFFECTS

Frequent (3%-8%)
Dyspnea, hypotension, chest pain, fever, diarrhea, nausea, pain, vomiting, infection, cough, minor bleeding.

SERIOUS REACTIONS

- Ventricular tachycardia and atrial fibrillation occur occasionally.
- Major bleeding and sepsis occur rarely.

PRECAUTIONS & CONSIDERATIONS

Caution is warranted with congenital or acquired bleeding disorders, hepatic impairment, severe hypertension, and ulcerations. Also, use argatroban cautiously immediately following administration of spinal anesthesia, lumbar puncture, and major surgery. It is unknown whether argatroban is excreted in breast milk; use in breastfeeding is not recommended. Safety and efficacy of argatroban have not been established in children younger than 18 yr of age. No age-related precautions have been noted in elderly patients. An electric razor and soft toothbrush should be used to prevent bleeding.

Notify the physician of abdominal pain, bleeding at surgical site, black or red stool, coffee-ground vomitus, red or dark urine, or blood-tinged mucus from cough. Activated clotting time, aPTT, PT, platelet count, BP, pulse rate, and menstrual flow should be monitored.

Storage

Before reconstitution, store at room temperature. Following reconstitution, the solution is stable for 24 h at room temperature and for 48 h if refrigerated. Avoid exposing the solution to direct sunlight. Discard the solution if it appears cloudy or has an insoluble precipitate.

Administration

Before infusion, dilute the solution 100-fold in 0.9% NaCl, D5W, or lactated Ringer's solution to provide a final concentration of 1 mg/mL. Mix the solution by repeatedly inverting the bag for 1 min. Following reconstitution, the solution may briefly appear hazy because of formation of microprecipitates. These rapidly dissolve when the solution is mixed. Administer as an IV infusion.

Aripiprazole

ara-pip'rah-zole

★ 🍁 Abilify

Do not confuse Abilify with Ambien.

CATEGORY AND SCHEDULE

Pregnancy Risk Category: C

Classification: Antipsychotics

MECHANISM OF ACTION

An antipsychotic agent that provides partial agonist activity at dopamine and serotonin (5-HT_{1A}) receptors and antagonist activity at serotonin (5-HT_{2A}) receptors. *Therapeutic Effect:* Diminishes schizophrenic behavior.

PHARMACOKINETICS

Well absorbed through the GI tract. Protein binding: 99% (primarily albumin). Reaches steady levels in 2 wks. Metabolized in the liver. Eliminated primarily in feces and, to a lesser extent, in urine. Not removed by hemodialysis. *Half-life:* 75 h (increased in CYP2D6 poor metabolizers).

AVAILABILITY

Injection Solution: 7.5 mg/mL.
Oral Solution: 1 mg/mL.
Tablets, Orally Disintegrating: 10 mg, 15 mg.
Tablets: 2 mg, 5 mg, 10 mg, 15 mg, 20 mg, 30 mg.

INDICATIONS AND DOSAGES

▸ Acute agitation associated with schizophrenia or bipolar disorder

IM

Adults. 9.75 mg as a single dose (range 5.25-15 mg); repeated doses may be given at intervals of at least 2 h to a maximum of 30 mg/day.

▸ Bipolar disorder

PO

Adults, Elderly. 15 mg once daily. May increase to 30 mg once daily.
Children 10 yr of age and older: 2 mg daily for 2 days, followed by 5 mg daily for 2 days with a further increase to a target dose of 10 mg daily; subsequent dose increases may be made in 5-mg increments up to a maximum dose of 30 mg/day.

▸ Depression, adjunctive therapy

PO

Adults, Elderly. Initial dose of 2-5 mg/day, with adjustments of 5 mg/day at intervals of at least 1 wk. Usual dose range 2-15 mg/day.

▸ Schizophrenia

PO

Adults, Elderly. Initially, 10-15 mg once a day. May increase up to 30 mg/day. At least 2 wks should elapse between dosage adjustments.

Adolescents 13 yr of age and older: 2 mg daily for 2 days, followed by 5 mg daily for 2 days with a further increase to a target dose of 10 mg daily; subsequent dose increases may be made in 5-mg increments up to a maximum of 30 mg/day.

▸ **Irritabillity associated with autistic disorder**

PO

Children 6 yr of age and older. Initially, 2 mg once daily. Increase to 5 mg/day, with subsequent increases to 10 mg/day or a maximum of 15 mg/day if needed. Increase by no more than 5 mg/wk.

OFF-LABEL USES

Schizoaffective disorder.

CONTRAINDICATIONS

Hypersensitivity.

INTERACTIONS

Drug

Carbamazepine: May decrease the aripiprazole blood concentration.

Strong CYP3A4, CY2D6 inhibitors, such as fluoxetine, ketoconazole, quinidine, paroxetine: May increase the aripiprazole blood concentration.

Herbal

St. John's wort: May decrease aripiprazole levels.

Kava kava, valerian: May incease CNS depression.

DIAGNOSTIC TEST EFFECTS

None known.

SIDE EFFECTS

Frequent (5%-11%)

Weight gain, headache, insomnia, vomiting.

Occasional (3%-4%)

Light-headedness, nausea, akathisia, somnolence.

Rare (2% or less)

Blurred vision, constipation, asthenia or loss of energy and strength, anxiety, fever, rash, cough, rhinitis, orthostatic hypotension, hyperglycemia.

SERIOUS REACTIONS

• Extrapyramidal symptoms and neuroleptic malignant syndrome occur rarely.

• Serious allergic reactions (e.g., anaphylaxis) occur rarely.

PRECAUTIONS & CONSIDERATIONS

Caution is warranted with cardiovascular or cerebrovascular diseases (because it may induce hypotension), dementia-related psychosis (increased risk of death with use of atypical antipsychotics), history of seizures or conditions that may lower the seizure threshold (such as Alzheimer disease), hepatic or renal impairment, and Parkinson disease (because of potential for exacerbation). Use with caution in patients with diabetes or with risk factors for diabetes. CNS depressants and alcohol should be avoided during therapy. It is unknown whether aripiprazole crosses the placenta. Because this drug may be distributed in breast milk, female patients should avoid breastfeeding during therapy. The safety and efficacy of aripiprazole have not been established in children < 6 yr of age. Antidepressants have been observed to increase the risk of suicidal thinking and behavior in children, adolescents, and young adults with major depressive disorder and other psychiatric disorders. Elderly patients with dementia-related psychosis treated with antipsychotic drugs are at an increased risk of death. Most deaths appear to be either CV (e.g., heart failure, sudden death) or infectious (e.g., pneumonia) in nature.

Extrapyramidal symptoms and tardive dyskinesia, manifested as chewing or puckering of the mouth, puffing of the cheeks, or tongue protrusion, should be monitored. BP, pulse rate, weight, and therapeutic response should also be monitored. Hydration and hypovolemia should be corrected before beginning therapy.

Storage

Store at room temperature.

Administration

Take oral aripiprazole without regard to food. For Discmelt tablets, keep in blister package until time of use; remove tablet with dry hands. Place on tongue and let dissolve; may be taken with liquid only if needed. Use a calibrated device to measure the oral solution.

Injection is for IM use only. Inject slowly into deep muscle mass.

Armodafinil

are-moe-daf'i-nil

★ Nuvigil

CATEGORY AND SCHEDULE

Pregnancy Risk Category: C

Controlled Substance Schedule: IV

Classification: Central nervous system (CNS) stimulants

MECHANISM OF ACTION

An α_1-agonist (R-enantiomer of modafinil) that may bind to dopamine reuptake carrier sites, increasing α activity and decreasing ω, τ, and β brain wave activity. Effects appear to be similar to sympathomimetics, such as the amphetamines. *Therapeutic Effect:* Promotes wakefulness, although, exact mechanism is unknown.

PHARMACOKINETICS

Well absorbed. Widely distributed. Hydrolyzed and metabolized in the liver. Less than 10% excreted in the urine. Unknown if removed by hemodialysis. *Half-life:* 15 h.

AVAILABILITY

Tablets: 50 mg, 150 mg, 250 mg.

INDICATIONS AND DOSAGES

▸ **Narcolepsy and obstructive sleep apnea/hypopnea syndrome (OSAHS)**

PO

Adults, Elderly, Adolescents 17 yr and older. 150-250 mg once daily in the morning. Consider lower doses in the elderly.

▸ **Shift-work sleep disorder**

PO

Adults. Give 150 mg once daily roughly 1 hr prior to the scheduled work shift.

▸ **Dosage in hepatic impairment**

Reduce normal dosage (usually by up to 50%) in those with moderate to severe liver disease.

CONTRAINDICATIONS

Hypersensitivity to modafinil or armodafinil.

INTERACTIONS

Drug

Antifungals, erythromycins, other CYP3A4 isoenzyme inhibitors: Increase armodafinil concentrations and may necessitate armodafinil dose reduction.

Cyclosporine, hormonal contraceptives, theophylline: May decrease plasma concentrations of these drugs; nonhormonal contraception is recommended during treatment.

Diazepam, phenytoin, propranolol, clomipramine, warfarin, and other CYP2C19 substrates: May increase plasma concentrations of these drugs. For warfarin, monitor INR closely.
Other CNS stimulants: May increase CNS stimulation.
Herbal
None known.
Food
Alcohol: Manufacturer recommends avoidance.

DIAGNOSTIC TEST EFFECTS

None known.

SIDE EFFECTS

Frequent
Anxiety, insomnia, nausea, dizziness, headache, nervousness.
Occasional
Anorexia, diarrhea, dry mouth or skin, muscle stiffness, polydipsia, rhinitis, paresthesia, tremor, vomiting, palpitations. Agitation, excitation, hypertension, and insomnia may occur.

SERIOUS REACTIONS

- Psychiatric symptoms such as hallucinations, delusions, unusual moods or behaviors, and aggression may occur.
- Serious rash, including Stevens-Johnson syndrome, TEN, and eosinophilia.
- Serious hypersensitivity including angioedema (rare).

PRECAUTIONS & CONSIDERATIONS

Those with hepatic or renal impairment or physiologic changes due to aging may require decreased dosage. Caution is warranted in patients with a history of clinically significant mitral valve prolapse, left ventricular hypertrophy, psychiatric illness, substance abuse, or seizures. Nonhormonal contraceptive methods should be used during therapy and 1 mo afterward because armodafinil decreases the effectiveness of hormonal contraceptives. It is unknown whether the drug is excreted in breast milk; caution is warranted in lactation. Use caution when giving the drug to pregnant women. The safety and efficacy of this drug have not been established in children younger than 17 yr; children may have an increased risk of serious rash.

Dizziness may occur, so tasks that require mental alertness and motor skills should be avoided until response to the drug is established. Sleep pattern should be assessed throughout therapy.
Storage
Store tablets at room temperature.
Administration
Take armodafinil without regard to food once daily. If treating narcolepsy, dose is taken as single dose in the morning. In patients with shift-work sleep disorder, the dose is taken 1 h before the start of the work shift.

Arsenic Trioxide

ar′sen-ik try-ox′ide
★ Trisenox
Do not confuse with Trimox.

CATEGORY AND SCHEDULE

Pregnancy Risk Category: D

Classification: Antineoplastics, miscellaneous

MECHANISM OF ACTION

An antineoplastic that produces morphologic changes and DNA fragmentation in promyelocytic leukemia cells. *Therapeutic Effect:* Produces cell death.

AVAILABILITY

Injection: 1 mg/mL in glass ampules.

INDICATIONS AND DOSAGES

▸ Acute promyelocytic leukemia

IV INFUSION

Adults, Elderly, Children 5 yr of age and older. Induction: 0.15 mg/kg/day until bone marrow remission. Begin consolidation treatment. Do not exceed 60 induction doses. 3-6 wks after completion of induction therapy, 0.15 mg/kg/day for 25 doses over a period of up to 5 wks.

CONTRAINDICATIONS

Hypersensitivity to arsenic.

INTERACTIONS

Drug

Amphotericin B, diuretics: May produce electrolyte imbalances.

Antiarrhythmics, thioridazine: May prolong QT interval.

DIAGNOSTIC TEST EFFECTS

May decrease hemoglobin levels, serum calcium and magnesium levels, and platelet and WBC counts. May increase AST (SGOT) and ALT (SGPT) levels.

IV INCOMPATIBILITIES

Do not mix arsenic trioxide with any other medications.

SIDE EFFECTS

Expected (50%-75%)

Nausea, cough, fatigue, fever, headache, vomiting, abdominal pain, tachycardia, diarrhea, dyspnea.

Frequent (30%-43%)

Dermatitis, insomnia, edema, rigors, prolonged QT interval, sore throat, pruritus, arthralgia, paresthesia, anxiety.

Occasional (20%-28%)

Constipation, myalgia, hypotension, epistaxis, anorexia, dizziness, sinusitis.

Occasional (8%-15%)

Ecchymosis, nonspecific pain, weight gain, herpes simplex, wheezing, flushing, diaphoresis, tremor, hypertension, palpitations, dyspepsia, eye irritation, blurred vision, asthenia, diminished breath sounds, crackles.

Rare

Confusion, petechiae, dry mouth, oral candidiasis, incontinence, rhonchi.

SERIOUS REACTIONS

- Seizures, GI hemorrhage, renal impairment or failure, pleural or pericardial effusion, hemoptysis, and sepsis occur rarely.
- Prolonged QT interval, complete AV block, unexplained fever, dyspnea, weight gain, and effusion are evidence of arsenic toxicity. If arsenic toxicity is apparent, stop arsenic trioxide treatment and begin steroid treatment as ordered.

PRECAUTIONS & CONSIDERATIONS

Caution is warranted with cardiac abnormalities and renal impairment. Arsenic trioxide is distributed in breast milk and may cause fetal harm. It should not be used by pregnant or breastfeeding women.

Notify the physician if confusion, muscle weakness, fever, vomiting, difficulty breathing, or rapid pulse rate occurs. CBC, creatinine, 12-lead ECG, liver function test results, blood chemistry values, serum electrolyte levels (hypokalemia is more common than hyperkalemia), and blood glucose levels (hyperglycemia is more common than hypoglycemia) should be assessed before and during therapy.

Storage
Store the drug at room temperature. The diluted solution is stable for 24 h at room temperature and 48 h if refrigerated.
Administration
CAUTION: Observe usual procedures for preparation, administration, and disposal of cytotoxic drugs.
! A central venous line is not required for administration of arsenic; the drug may be infused through a peripheral line.

After withdrawing the drug from ampule, dilute it with 100-250 mL D5W or 0.9% NaCl. Infuse the solution intravenously over 1-2 h. The duration of the infusion may be extended up to 4 h.

Artemether/ Lumefantrine

ar-tem′e-ther/loo-me-fan′treen

★ 🍁 CoArtem

CATEGORY AND SCHEDULE

Pregnancy Risk Category: C

Classification: Antimalarial, antiprotozoal

MECHANISM OF ACTION

Both drugs are active against the erythrocytic stages of *P. falciparum* and *P. vivax*. The antimalarial activity of artemether may involve free radical damage to membrane systems in the parasite during the asexual developmental states. Both inhibit nucleic acid and protein synthesis. Synergistic effects limit parasite resistance. *Therapeutic Effect:* Rapid clearance of most *Plasmodium* species from the blood. In the treatment of *P. vivax*, additional agents are required to ensure cure.

PHARMACOKINETICS

Both drugs highly bound to human serum proteins. Artemether is rapidly eliminated from plasma with a half-life of 2-3 h. The main route of metabolism is via the CYP3A4/5 isoenzymes. The biologically active metabolite, DHA, is formed primarily via CYP3A4/5. The half-life of lumefantrine is 3-6 days. Due to this slow elimination, lumefantrine exposure increases after each dose and reaches a peak on day 3 of therapy. Lumefantrine metabolism is mainly catalyzed by the CYP3A4 isoenzyme, and glucuronidation occurs after oxidative biotransformation.

AVAILABILITY

Tablets: Artemether 20 mg/ lumefantrine 120 mg.

INDICATIONS AND DOSAGES

▸ **Treatment of malaria:**

PO

Adults, Adolescents, and Children weighing > 35 kg. 4 tablets as a single dose PO upon diagnosis, then again after 8 h, and then 4 tablets PO twice daily (am and pm) for the next 2 days (total course of 24 tablets).
Adults, Adolescents, and Children weighing ≥ 25 kg and < 35 kg. 3 tablets per dose PO upon diagnosis, then again after 8 h, and then 3 tablets PO twice daily (am and pm) for the next 2 days (total course of 18 tablets).
Children weighing ≥ 15 kg and < 25 kg. 2 tablets per dose PO upon diagnosis, then again after 8 h, and then 2 tablets PO twice daily (am and pm) for the next 2 days (total course of 12 tablets). *Children and Infants 2 mo of age and older and*

≥ 5 kg and < 15 kg. 1 tablet per dose PO upon diagnosis, then again after 8 h, and then 1 tablet PO twice daily (morning and evening) for the next 2 days (total course of 6 tablets).

CONTRAINDICATIONS

Hypersensitivity to artemether, lumefantrine, or any components of the product.

INTERACTIONS

Drug

Drugs that prolong the QT interval (e.g., class IA [quinidine, procainamide, disopyramide] or class III [amiodarone, sotalol] antiarrhythmics; antipsychotics (pimozide, ziprasidone); macrolide antibiotics; fluoroquinolones; azole antifungals; terfenadine; astemizole; or cisapride: Additive risk of cardiac effects; avoid use of artemether/lumefantrine.

Hormonal contraceptives: Artemether/lumefantrine may reduce contraceptive effect; nonhormonal methods are recommended.

CYP3A4 inhibitors: May increase the levels and effects of artemether/ lumefantrine.

Antiretroviral therapy: Variable effects; may reduce antiretroviral activity; may increase levels of artemether/lumefantrine. Caution advised.

CYP2D6 substrates (selected β-blockers, flecainide, fluoxetine, paroxetine, risperidone, thioridazine, tricyclic antidepressants, venlafaxine): Lumefantrine may increase the levels and effects of CYP2D6 substrates.

Halofantrine: May increase risk of cardiac effects; do not administer within 1 mo of each other.

Herbal

None known.

Food

Grapefruit juice: Avoid grapefruit juice as it may increase drug levels in the blood.

DIAGNOSTIC TEST EFFECTS

Increase in LFTs, increased hematocrit, changes in platelet count or white blood cell count may occasionally occur. May prolong QTc interval of EKG.

SIDE EFFECTS

Frequent

Mild transient headaches, nausea, dizziness, weakness, loss of appetite, arthralgia, myalgia, fatigue, chills, fever.

Occasional

Vomiting, diarrhea, tinnitus, dyspepsia, tremor, ataxia, somnolence, mood changes.

Rare

Urticaria, bullous skin rashes.

SERIOUS REACTIONS

- QT prolongation resulting in ECG changes and risk for torsade de pointes.
- Allergic reactions including serious skin rashes, anaphylaxis, angioedema.

PRECAUTIONS & CONSIDERATIONS

Avoid use in patients with known QT prolongation or cardiac arrhythmia, those with hypokalemia or hypomagnesemia, and those taking other drugs that prolong the QT interval. Other antimalarials should not be given concomitantly, unless there is no other treatment option, due to limited safety data. Do NOT give with halofantrine or within 1 mo of each other, due to potential cardiac risks. The drugs have not been studied in patients with renal or hepatic impairment. Use with caution in the elderly. Use with caution during lactation, as the drug may pass to breast milk. Avoid administration in pregnancy if possible as use of the drug may result in fetal loss or a potential for birth defects, especially in the first trimester. Fetal defects have been reported when artemisinins are administered to animals. Females should be advised to use nonhormonal contraception during the month of administration, due to a potential to decrease the efficacy of hormonal birth control methods.

Monitor the patient for resolution of signs and symptoms and drug tolerance; if the patient vomits up a dose twice, then the prescriber should be contacted for a change in orders. Adequate food intake is a must to avoid recrudescence. This drug combination has not been studied for effectiveness to prevent malaria.

Storage

Store tablets at room temperature; close tightly and protect from moisture.

Administration

Take the tablets with food. Patients with acute malaria are frequently averse to food. Encourage patient to resume normal eating as soon as possible as this improves absorption of the drugs and limits the chance for treatment failure and relapse. For patients who are unable to swallow the tablets such as infants and children, the tablets may be crushed and mixed with a small amount of water (1 to 2 tsp) immediately prior to use. Follow dose whenever possible by food/drink (e.g., milk, formula, pudding, broth, etc.). In the event of vomiting within 1 to 2 h of administration, give a repeat dose. If the repeat dose is vomited, switch to an alternative antimalarial for treatment.

Ascorbic Acid (Vitamin C)

a-skor′bic as′id

★ 🍁 Acerola C, Ascor-L, Cenolate, Vicks Vitamin C Orange Drops

CATEGORY AND SCHEDULE

Pregnancy Risk Category: A (C if used in doses above recommended daily allowance, or if injectable forms used)

OTC, injectable, Rx only

Classification: Vitamins, water-soluble vitamins

MECHANISM OF ACTION

Assists in collagen formation and tissue repair and is involved in oxidation-reduction reactions and other metabolic reactions. *Therapeutic Effect:* Involved in carbohydrate use and metabolism, as well as synthesis of carnitine, lipids, and proteins. Preserves blood vessel integrity.

PHARMACOKINETICS

Readily absorbed from the GI tract. Protein binding: 25%. Oxidation is the primary method of metabolism to inactive metabolites; drug and metabolites excreted in the urine. Removed by hemodialysis.

AVAILABILITY

Capsules: 500 mg, 1 g.
Capsules (Controlled-Release): 500 mg, 1 g.
Oral Solution: 500 mg/5 mL.
Lozenge: 25 mg.
Tablets: 100 mg, 250 mg, 500 mg, 1 g.
Tablets (Chewable): 100 mg, 250 mg, 500 mg, 1000 mg.

Tablets (Controlled-Release): 500 mg, 1 g, 1500 mg.
Injection: 500 mg/mL.

INDICATIONS AND DOSAGES

▸ Dietary supplement

PO

Adults, Elderly. 50-200 mg/day.
Children. 35-100 mg/day.

▸ Scurvy

PO

Adults, Elderly. 100-250 mg 1-2 times a day.
Children. 100-300 mg/day in divided doses.

OFF-LABEL USES

Control of idiopathic methemoglobinemia acidification of urine.

CONTRAINDICATIONS

None known.

INTERACTIONS

Drug

Deferoxamine: Vitamin C often used adjunctively with deferoxamine; however, to avoid interaction, must not be started until at least 1 mo of initial deferoxamine treatment for iron toxicity. See manufacturer recommendations.
Warfarin: No interaction unless high doses of vitamin C given (e.g., grams per day); if high doses given, then may interfere with anticoagulant effect.

Herbal

None known.

Food

None known.

DIAGNOSTIC TEST EFFECTS

May decrease urinary pH. May increase urine, uric acid, and urine oxalate levels. Patients with diabetes may obtain false reading of urinary glucose test. Interferes with amine-dependent stool occult blood tests and may cause false negative results. Avoid using within 72 h of testing.

IV INCOMPATIBILITIES

Aminophylline, azathioprine, ceftazidime (Fortaz), ceftriaxone (Rocephin), dantrolene, diazepam, erythromycin, hydralazine, inamrinone, midazolam, nitroprusside, pentobarbital, phenytoin.

IV COMPATIBILITIES

Calcium gluconate, heparin, TPN.

SIDE EFFECTS

Rare

Abdominal cramps, nausea, vomiting, diarrhea, increased urination with doses exceeding 1 g. Parenteral: Flushing, headache, dizziness, sleepiness or insomnia, soreness at injection site.

SERIOUS REACTIONS

- Ascorbic acid may acidify urine, leading to crystalluria.
- Large doses of IV ascorbic acid may lead to deep vein thrombosis.
- Abrupt discontinuation after prolonged use of large doses may produce rebound ascorbic acid deficiency.

PRECAUTIONS & CONSIDERATIONS

Caution is warranted in patients with diabetes mellitus, patients with a history of renal calculi, and persons on sodium-restricted diet. Ascorbic acid crosses the placenta and is excreted in breast milk. Large doses of ascorbic acid taken during pregnancy may produce rebound scurvy in neonates. No age-related precautions have been noted in children or in elderly patients.

Eating foods rich in vitamin C, including citrus fruits, green peppers, brussels sprouts, rose hips, spinach, strawberries, and watercress, is encouraged.

Clinical improvement, such as improved wound healing, should be assessed. Signs and symptoms of recurring vitamin C deficiency, including bleeding gums, digestive difficulties, gingivitis, poor wound healing, and arthralgia, should also be monitored.

Storage
Oral dosage forms: Store at room temperature. Protect from moisture.

Refrigerate injection vials and protect them from freezing and sunlight.

Administration
Take oral ascorbic acid without regard to food. Reduce the dosage gradually because abrupt discontinuation may produce rebound deficiency.

Injection used only when oral route not amenable. Injection may be given undiluted or may be diluted in D5W, 0.9% NaCl, or lactated Ringer's solution. For IV push, dilute with an equal volume of D5W or 0.9% NaCl and infuse over 10 min. For IV solution, infuse over 4-12 h.

May also be given IM or SC.

Asenapine

a-sen′a-peen

★ 🍁 Saphris

CATEGORY AND SCHEDULE

Pregnancy Risk Category: C

Classification: Antipsychotics, atypical

MECHANISM OF ACTION

A dibenzepin derivative that antagonizes dopamine (D2) and serotonin (5-HT2A) receptors. No affinity for muscarinic receptors. Produces central nervous system (CNS) depressant effects. *Therapeutic Effect*: Diminishes manifestations of psychotic symptoms.

PHARMACOKINETICS

Bioavailability approx. 35% after SL administration. Food and water interfere with absorption. Protein binding: 95%. Extensively distributed throughout the body. Direct glucuronidation by UGT1A4 and oxidative metabolism by predominantly CYP1A2 are the primary metabolic pathways. Undergoes extensive metabolism in the liver. Excreted in urine and feces. *Half-life:* Roughly 24 h.

AVAILABILITY

Sublingual Tablets (Saphris): 5 mg, 10 mg.

INDICATIONS AND DOSAGES

▸ **Schizophrenia**

SL

Adults. 5 mg twice daily

▸ **Bipolar mania**

SL

Adults. 10 mg twice daily. May reduce to 5 mg twice daily if target dose not tolerated.

▸ **Patients with hepatic impairment**

Do not use in patients with severe hepatic impairment.

CONTRAINDICATIONS

Hypersensitivity to the drug.

INTERACTIONS

Drug

Alcohol, other CNS depressants: May increase CNS depressant effects.

Antihypertensives: May increase the hypotensive effects of these drugs.
Fluvoxamine and other strong CYP1A2 inhibitors: May increase the asenapine blood concentration; coadminister with caution.
Paroxetine: Asenapine may increase paroxetine concentrations; coadminister with caution.
Dopamine agonists, levodopa: Asenapine may antagonize the effects of these drugs.
Drugs that prolong the QT interval (e.g., class IA [quinidine, procainamide, disopyramide] or class III [amiodarone, sotalol] antiarrhythmics; antipsychotics (pimozide, ziprasidone); macrolide antibiotics; fluoroquinolones; azole antifungals; terfenadine; astemizole; or cisapride: Potential additive risk of cardiac effects; avoid co-use when possible.
Herbal
None known.
Food
Taking food or drink within the first 10 min of taking asenapine will reduce absorption significantly.
Alcohol: Avoidance is recommended.

DIAGNOSTIC TEST EFFECTS

May significantly increase serum GGT, prolactin, AST (SGOT), and ALT (SGPT) levels, cholesterol or triglycerides, blood glucose. Reductions in WBC count (rare).

SIDE EFFECTS

Frequent (5%-11%)
Weight gain, headache, insomnia, vomiting, constipation, dizziness, somnolence.
Occasional (3%-4%)
Nausea, akathisia, alterations in taste, anxiety, fatigue, arthralgia.
Rare (2% or less)
Blurred vision, asthenia, fever, rash, cough, rhinitis, orthostatic hypotension, hyperglycemia, dysphagia, indigestion, irritability.

SERIOUS REACTIONS

- Extrapyramidal symptoms and neuroleptic malignant syndrome occur rarely.
- Seizures occur rarely.
- Development of diabetes.
- QT prolongation (rare).
- Agranulocytosis, leukopenia, neutropenia (rare).

PRECAUTIONS & CONSIDERATIONS

Caution is warranted with cardiovascular or cerebrovascular diseases, hypotension, history of seizures or conditions that may lower the seizure threshold (such as Alzheimer's disease), hepatic or renal impairment, and Parkinson disease. Use with caution in patients with diabetes or with risk factors for diabetes. CNS depressants and alcohol should be avoided during therapy. It is unknown whether asenapine crosses the placenta. Because this drug may be distributed in breast milk, female patients should avoid breastfeeding during therapy. The safety and efficacy of asenapine have not been established in children. Elderly patients with dementia-related psychosis treated with antipsychotic drugs are at an increased risk of death. Most deaths appear to be either CV (e.g., heart failure, sudden death) or infectious (e.g., pneumonia) in nature.

Extrapyramidal symptoms and tardive dyskinesia, manifested as chewing or puckering of the mouth, puffing of the cheeks, or tongue protrusion, should be monitored. BP, pulse rate, weight, and therapeutic response should also be monitored.

Dehydration, electrolyte disturbances, and hypovolemia should be corrected before beginning therapy.

Drowsiness may occur. Tasks requiring mental alertness or motor skills should be avoided until the effects of the drug are known. Dehydration, particularly during exercise; exposure to extreme heat; and concurrent use of medications that cause dry mouth or other drying effects should also be avoided. A healthy diet and exercise program should be maintained to prevent weight gain. Notify the physician of extrapyramidal symptoms. BP, CBC, and therapeutic response should be assessed. Rapid postural changes should be avoided due to possible development of orthostatic hypotension. Symptoms including sore tongue, problems eating or swallowing, fever, or infection need to be reported immediately.

Storage

Store at room temperature. Keep sublingual tablets in blister package until time of use.

Administration

Tablets are fragile, so do not push them through the blister packaging. Place under tongue without water and allow to completely dissolve, without swallowing. Do not crush or chew the tablets. Patients should be instructed to not eat or drink for 10 min after administration.

Asparaginase

a-spare′a-gi-nase

★ Elspar 🍁 Erwinase, Kidrolase

Do not confuse with pegaspargase.

CATEGORY AND SCHEDULE

Pregnancy Risk Category: C

Classification: Antineoplastics, enzymes

MECHANISM OF ACTION

An enzyme that inhibits DNA, RNA, and protein synthesis by breaking down asparagine, thus depriving tumor cells of this essential amino acid. Cell cycle-specific for G_1 phase of cell division. *Therapeutic Effect:* Kills leukemic cells.

PHARMACOKINETICS

Metabolized by the reticuloendothelial system through slow sequestration. *Half-life:* 39-49 h IM; 8-30 h IV.

AVAILABILITY

Powder for Injection: 10,000 International Units.

INDICATIONS AND DOSAGES

▸ **Acute lymphocytic leukemia (usual dosages)**

IV OR IM

Adults, Elderly, Children. 6000 International Units/m^2 IM or IV 3 times a week, usually as part of multi-agent chemotheraphy.

CONTRAINDICATIONS

History of hypersensitivity to asparaginase, history of pancreatitis, serious thrombosis, or serious hemorrhagic events with prior asparaginase treatment.

INTERACTIONS

Drug

Antigout medications: May decrease the effects of these drugs.

Anticoagulants: Additive bleeding risk.

Live-virus vaccines: May potentiate virus replication, increase vaccine side effects, and decrease the patient's antibody response to the vaccine.

Methotrexate: May block effects of methotrexate if doses are not timed appropriately.

Steroids, vincristine: May increase the risk of neuropathy and disturbances of erythropoiesis; may enhance hyperglycemic effect of asparaginase.

Herbal and Food

None known.

DIAGNOSTIC TEST EFFECTS

May increase BUN, blood ammonia, and blood glucose levels; serum alkaline phosphatase, bilirubin, uric acid, AST (SGOT), and ALT (SGPT) levels; platelet count; PT; activated partial thromboplastin time; and thrombin time. May decrease blood-clotting factors (including antithrombin, plasma fibrinogen, and plasminogen) as well as serum albumin, calcium, and cholesterol levels.

IV INCOMPATIBILITIES

Not widely studied; Y-site administrations with other medications not recommended.

SIDE EFFECTS

Frequent

Allergic reaction (rash, urticaria, arthralgia, facial edema, hypotension, respiratory distress) pancreatitis (severe stomach pain, nausea, and vomiting).

Occasional

CNS effects (confusion, drowsiness, depression, anxiety, and fatigue), stomatitis, hypoalbuminemia or uric acid nephropathy (manifested as edema of feet or lower legs), hyperglycemia.

Rare

Hyperthermia (including fever or chills), thrombosis, seizures.

SERIOUS REACTIONS

- CNS thrombosis and other serious thrombotic events; discontinue drug if occurs.
- Pancreatitis may be fulminant or fatal and requires drug discontinuation.
- Coagulopathy and bleeding.
- Hepatotoxicity usually occurs within 2 wks of initial treatment.
- The risk of an allergic reaction, including anaphylaxis, increases after repeated therapy.
- Myelosuppression may be severe.

PRECAUTIONS & CONSIDERATIONS

Caution is warranted with diabetes mellitus, current or recent chickenpox, gout, herpes zoster, infection, hepatic or renal impairment, and in those who have recently had cytotoxic or radiation therapy. Asparaginase use should be avoided during pregnancy, especially during the first trimester and during breastfeeding. No age-related precautions have been noted in children or the elderly. Immunizations and coming in contact with those who have recently received a live-virus vaccine should be avoided.

! Expect to discontinue asparaginase at the first sign or symptom of renal failure (oliguria, anuria) or pancreatitis (abdominal pain, nausea and vomiting, elevated serum amylase and lipase levels). Adequate hydration should be maintained to help prevent kidney problems.

Signs and symptoms of hematologic toxicity, such as excessive fatigue and weakness, ecchymosis, fever, signs of local infection, sore throat, and unusual bleeding from any site, should be assessed. Baseline CNS function should be assessed and a comprehensive blood chemistry should be obtained before therapy begins and whenever more than 1 wk has elapsed between doses.

Storage
Refrigerate unopened vials; do not freeze. Reconstituted solutions are stable for 8 h if refrigerated.

Administration
CAUTION: Observe and exercise usual cautions for handling and preparing solutions of cytotoxic drugs.

! Asparaginase dosage is individualized based on clinical response and the tolerance of the drug's adverse effects. When administering this drug in combination therapy, consult specific protocols for optimum dosage and sequence of drug administration.

Keep antihistamines, epinephrine, IV corticosteroid, and oxygen equipment readily available before administering asparaginase. Observe patients for 1 h after administration of the drug, especially during repeat doses, in case allergic reaction occurs.

If gelatinous, fiber-like particles develop in the solution, remove them by using a 5-μm filter during administration. For IV use, reconstitute the 10,000-unit vial with 5 mL sterile water for injection or 0.9% NaCl to provide a concentration of 2000 International Units/mL. Shake gently to ensure complete dissolution. Vigorous shaking will produce foam and cause some loss of potency. For IV injection, administer asparaginase solution into the tubing of free-flowing IV solution of D5W or 0.9% NaCl over at least 30 min. For IV infusion, further dilute with up to 1000 mL D5W or 0.9% NaCl.

For IM use, add 2 mL 0.9% NaCl to 10,000-unit vial to provide a concentration of 5000 International Units/mL. Administer no more than 2 mL at any one site.

Aspirin/ Acetylsalicylic Acid

as'pir-in/ah-seet'il-sill-ic as'id

★ Bayer, Bufferin, Ecotrin, Halfprin, St. Joseph's 🍁 Asaphen, Entrophen, Lowprin, Rivasa

Do not confuse with aspirin with Aricept, Afrin, or Asendin, or Ecotrin with Edecrin.

CATEGORY AND SCHEDULE

Pregnancy Risk Category: C (D if full dose used in third trimester)
OTC

Classification: Analgesics, non-narcotic, antipyretics, salicylates

MECHANISM OF ACTION

A nonsteroidal salicylate that inhibits prostaglandin synthesis, acts on the hypothalamus heat-regulating center, and interferes with the production of thromboxane A, a substance that stimulates platelet aggregation. *Therapeutic Effect:* Reduces inflammatory response and intensity of pain; decreases fever; inhibits platelet aggregation.

PHARMACOKINETICS

Route	Onset	Peak	Duration
PO	1 h	2-4 h	24 h

Rapidly and completely absorbed from GI tract; enteric-coated absorption delayed; rectal absorption delayed and incomplete. Protein binding: High. Widely distributed. Rapidly hydrolyzed to salicylate. *Half-life:* 15-20 min (aspirin); 2-3 h (salicylate at low dose); more than 20 h (salicylate at high dose).

AVAILABILITY

Chewing Gum: 227 mg.
Tablets: 162 mg, 325 mg, 500 mg, 650 mg.

Tablets, Chewable: 81 mg.
Tablets, Enteric-Coated: 81 mg, 325 mg, 500 mg, 650 mg.
Suppository: 300 mg, 600 mg.

INDICATIONS AND DOSAGES

▸ Analgesia, fever
PO, RECTAL
Adults, Elderly. 325-1000 mg q4-6h.
Children. 10-15 mg/kg/dose q4-6h. Maximum: 4 g/day.

▸ Anti-inflammatory
PO
Adults, Elderly. Initially, 2.4-3.6 g/day in divided doses; then 3.6-5.4 g/day.

▸ Juvenile rheumatoid arthritis
Children. Initially, 60-90 mg/kg/day in divided doses; then 80-100 mg/kg/day. Adjust to target salicylate concentration of 15-30 mg/dL.

▸ Suspected myocardial infarction (MI)
PO
Adults, Elderly. 160-325 mg as soon as the MI is suspected, then daily for 30 days after the MI.

▸ Prevention of MI
PO
Adults, Elderly. 75-325 mg/day.

▸ Prevention of stroke after transient ischemic attack
PO
Adults, Elderly. 50-325 mg/day.

▸ Kawasaki disease
PO
Children. 80-100 mg/kg/day in divided doses during acute phase, then decrease to 3-5 mg/kg/day for maintenance. Discontinue after 6 wks if no cardiac abnormalities; otherwise continue.

▸ Coronary artery bypass graft
PO
Adults, Elderly. 75-325 mg/day starting 6 h following procedure.

▸ Percutaneous transluminal coronary angioplasty
PO
Adults, Elderly. 80-325 mg/day starting 2 h before procedure.

▸ Stent implantation
PO
Adults, Elderly. 325 mg 2 h before implantation and 160-325 mg daily thereafter.

▸ Carotid endarterectomy
Adults, Elderly. 81-325 mg/day preoperatively and daily thereafter.

▸ Acute ischemic stroke
PO
Adults, Elderly. 160-325 mg/day, initiated within 48 h in patients who are not candidates for thrombolytics and are not receiving systemic anticoagulation.

OFF-LABEL USES

Prevention of thromboembolism, treatment of Kawasaki disease.

CONTRAINDICATIONS

Allergy to tartrazine dye, bleeding disorders, GI bleeding or ulceration, hepatic impairment, history of hypersensitivity to aspirin or NSAIDs, children/teenagers with chicken pox or flu-like symptoms.

INTERACTIONS

Drug

Alcohol, NSAIDs: May increase the risk of adverse GI effects, including ulceration. NSAIDs may negate cardioprotective effects of ASA.
Antacids, urinary alkalinizers: Increase the excretion of aspirin.
Anticoagulants, heparin, thrombolytics: Increase the risk of bleeding.
Insulin, oral antidiabetics: May increase the effects of these drugs (with large doses of aspirin).
Methotrexate, zidovudine: May increase the risk of toxicity of these drugs.
Nephrotoxic medications, vancomycin: May increase the risk of toxicity.

Platelet aggregation inhibitors, valproic acid: May increase the risk of bleeding.
Probenecid, sulfinpyrazone: May decrease the effects of these drugs.
Herbal
None known.
Food
None known.

DIAGNOSTIC TEST EFFECTS

May alter serum alkaline phosphatase, uric acid, AST (SGOT), and ALT (SGPT) levels. May prolong PT and bleeding time. May decrease serum cholesterol, serum potassium, and T3 and T4 levels. The therapeutic aspirin level for antiarthritic effect is 20-30 mg/dL; the toxic level is > 30 mg/dL.

SIDE EFFECTS

Occasional
GI distress (including abdominal distention, cramping, heartburn, and mild nausea); allergic reaction (including bronchospasm, pruritus, and urticaria).

SERIOUS REACTIONS

- High doses of aspirin may produce GI bleeding and gastric mucosal lesions.
- Dehydrated, febrile children may experience aspirin toxicity quickly. Reye syndrome may occur in children with chickenpox or the flu.
- Low-grade toxicity characterized by tinnitus, generalized pruritus (possibly severe), headache, dizziness, flushing, tachycardia, hyperventilation, diaphoresis, and thirst.
- Marked toxicity is characterized by hyperthermia, restlessness, seizures, abnormal breathing patterns, respiratory failure, and coma.

PRECAUTIONS & CONSIDERATIONS

Caution is warranted with chronic renal insufficiency, vitamin K deficiency, and the "aspirin triad" of asthma, nasal polyps, and rhinitis. Aspirin readily crosses the placenta and is distributed in breast milk. Pregnant women should not take aspirin during the last trimester of pregnancy because the drug may prolong gestation and labor and cause adverse effects in the fetus, such as premature closure of the ductus arteriosus, low birth weight, hemorrhage, stillbirth, and death. Caution should be used giving aspirin to children with acute febrile illness. Do not give aspirin to children with chickenpox or the flu because this increases their risk of developing Reye's syndrome. Know that behavioral changes and vomiting may be early signs of Reye's syndrome. Lower aspirin dosages are recommended for elderly patients because they are more susceptible to aspirin toxicity. Withhold the drug and contact the physician if respirations are 12/min or lower (20/min or lower in children). Alcohol and NSAIDs should be avoided because of increased risk of GI bleeding.

Notify the physician if ringing in the ears (tinnitus) or persistent abdominal or GI pain occurs. Temperature should be taken just before and 1 h after giving the drug. Urine pH should be monitored for signs of sudden acidification, indicated by a pH of 5.5-6.5: sudden acidification may cause the serum salicylate level to greatly increase, leading to toxicity. Be aware the anti-inflammatory effect should occur within 1-3 wks.

Storage
Store tablets at room temperature, tightly closed. Protect from moisture. Refrigerate suppositories.
Administration
Do not give aspirin to children or teenagers with chickenpox or the flu because this increases their risk of developing Reye's syndrome. Do not use aspirin that smells of vinegar because this odor indicates chemical breakdown of the drug. Do not crush or break enteric-coated or extended-release tablets. Take aspirin with water, milk, or meals if GI distress occurs.

For rectal use, if the suppository is too soft, refrigerate it for 30 min or run cold water over the foil wrapper. Remove foil wrapper before use. Moisten the suppository with cold water before inserting it well into the rectum.

Atazanavir Sulfate

ah-tah-zan'ah-veer sul'fate
Reyataz
Do not confuse Reyataz with Retavase.

CATEGORY AND SCHEDULE

Pregnancy Risk Category: B

Classification: Antiretroviral, HIV-1 protease inhibitor

MECHANISM OF ACTION

An antiviral that acts as an HIV-1 protease inhibitor, selectively preventing the processing of viral precursors found in cells infected with HIV-1. *Therapeutic Effect:* Prevents the formation of mature HIV virions.

PHARMACOKINETICS

Rapidly absorbed after PO administration. Protein binding: 86%. Extensively metabolized in the liver. Excreted primarily in urine and, to a lesser extent, in feces. *Half-life:* 5-8 h.

AVAILABILITY

Capsules: 100 mg, 150 mg, 200 mg, 300 mg.

INDICATIONS AND DOSAGES

▸ **HIV-1 infection (therapy-naïve)**
PO
Adults, Elderly. 400 mg once a day with food. If given with ritonavir, dosage is 300 mg once daily.
Children 6-17 yr of age (15 kg to < 25 kg). 150 mg with ritonavir; 80 mg once a day with food.
Children 6-17 yr of age (25 to < 32 kg). 200 mg with ritonavir; 100 mg once a day with food.
Children 6-17 yr of age (32 to <39 kg). 250 mg with ritonavir; 100 mg once a day with food.
Children 6-17 yr of age (at least 39 kg). 300 mg with ritonavir; 100 mg once a day with food.
▸ **HIV-1 infection (therapy-naïve; concurrent therapy with efavirenz, tenofovir, H_2 receptor antagonist, or proton pump inhibitor)**
PO
Adults, Elderly. 300 mg atazanavir with 100 mg ritonavir as a single daily dose with food.
▸ **HIV-1 infection (treatment-experienced)**
PO
Adults, Elderly. 300 mg with ritonavir (Norvir) 100 mg once a day.
Children 6-17 yr of age (25 to < 32 kg). 200 mg with ritonavir; 100 mg once a day with food.
Children 6-17 yr of age (32 to < 39 kg). 250 mg with ritonavir; 100 mg once a day with food.

Children 6-17 yr of age (at least 39 kg). 300 mg with ritonavir; 100 mg once a day with food.

▸ **HIV-1 infection (treatment-experienced; concurrent therapy with H_2 receptor antagonist)**

PO

Adults, Elderly. 300 mg with ritonavir; 100 mg as a single daily dose with food.

▸ **HIV-1 infection (treatment-experienced; concurrent therapy with H_2 receptor antagonist and tenofovir)**

PO

Adults, Elderly. 400 mg with ritonavir; 100 mg as a single daily dose with food.

▸ **HIV-1 infection in patients with moderate hepatic impairment**

PO

Adults, Elderly. 300 mg once a day with food.

▸ **HIV-1 infection in treatment-naïve patients with end-stage renal disease managed with hemodialysis**

PO

Adults, Elderly. 300 mg with ritonavir; 100 mg once a day with food.

CONTRAINDICATIONS

Hypersensitivity, concurrent use with cisapride, ergot derivatives, indinavir, irinotecan, lovastatin, midazolam, pimozide, rifampin, simvastatin, triazolam, and St. John's wort.

INTERACTIONS

Drugs

Antacids, didanosine, buffered medications: Take atazanavir 2 h before or 1 h after.

Amiodarone, clarithromycin, cyclosporine, ergot derivatives, fentanyl, fluticasone, irinotecan, lapatinib, lovastatin, midazolam, rifabutin, sildenafil, simvastatin, sirolimus, tacrolimus, tadalafil, tenofovir, trazodone, triazolam, vardenafil: May increase concentrations of these drugs and increase risk of toxicity.

H_2 receptor antagonists: Take atazanavir with or 10 h after the H_2 antagonist.

Nevirapine, tenofovir: May reduce atazanavir concentrations.

Proton pump inhibitor: Take 12 h prior to atazanavir in therapy naïve; avoid use with atazanavir in treatment-experienced patients.

β-blockers, calcium channel blockers, cisapride, clarithromycin, pimozide, ranolazine: Increased risk of arrhythmias.

Warfarin: Increased risk of bleeding; monitor INR.

Herbal

St. John's wort: May reduce atazanavir concentrations. Contraindicated.

Food

All foods: Atazanavir bioavailability increased when taken with food.

DIAGNOSTIC TEST EFFECTS

Increased amylase, bilirubin, cholesterol, CPK, glucose, hepatic transaminases, lipase, triglycerides; decreased hemoglobin, neutrophils.

SIDE EFFECTS

Frequent (> 10%)

Nausea, rash, cough, headache.

Occasional (2%-10%)

Dizziness, jaundice, vomiting, depression, diarrhea, abdominal pain, fever, lipodystrophy, peripheral neuropathy, hyperbilirubinemia.

Rare

Insomnia, fatigue, back pain.

SERIOUS REACTIONS

• A severe hypersensitivity reaction (marked by angioedema and chest pain) and jaundice may occur.

- Nephrolithiasis.
- Lactic acidosis.
- Hepatotoxicity.
- Hypersensitivity reactions with serious rashes.
- AV conduction problems.
- Hyperbilirubinemia.

PRECAUTIONS & CONSIDERATIONS

Prolongs PR interval. Use with caution in preexisting conduction disorders, diabetes mellitus, hyperglycemia, hepatic impairment, and renal impairment. Monitor liver function, HBV infection, and redistribution of body fat. It is not known if atazanavir is harmful in pregnancy. Because of the potential HIV transmission, instruct mothers not to breastfeed. Safety and efficacy not established in children < 6 yr. Avoid use in infants < 3 mo due to risk of kernicterus.

Storage

Store at room temperature.

Administration

Administer with food. Swallow capsules whole.

Atenolol

a-ten′oh-lol

Tenormin Tenormin, Apo-Atenol

Do not confuse atenolol with albuterol or timolol.

CATEGORY AND SCHEDULE

Pregnancy Risk Category: D

Classification: Antiadrenergics, β-blocking

MECHANISM OF ACTION

A β_1-adrenergic blocker that acts as an antianginal, antiarrhythmic, and antihypertensive agent by blocking β_1-adrenergic receptors in cardiac tissue. *Therapeutic Effect:* Slows sinus node heart rate, decreasing cardiac output and BP. Decreases myocardial oxygen demand.

PHARMACOKINETICS

Route	Onset	Peak	Duration
PO	1 h	2-4 h	24 h

Incompletely absorbed from the GI tract. Protein binding: 6%-16%. Minimal liver metabolism. Primarily excreted unchanged in urine. Removed by hemodialysis. *Half-life:* 6-7 h (increased in impaired renal function).

AVAILABILITY

Tablets: 25 mg, 50 mg, 100 mg.

INDICATIONS AND DOSAGES

▸ **Hypertension**

PO

Adults. Initially, 25-50 mg once a day. May increase dose up to 100 mg once a day.

Elderly. Usual initial dose, 25 mg a day.

Children. Initially, 0.5-1 mg/kg/dose given once a day. Range: 0.5-1.5 mg/kg/day. Maximum: 2 mg/kg/day or 100 mg/day.

▸ **Angina pectoris**

PO

Adults. Initially, 50 mg once a day. May increase dose up to 200 mg once a day.

Elderly. Usual initial dose, 25 mg a day. Range same as for adults.

▸ **Dosage in renal impairment**

Dosage interval is modified based on creatinine clearance.

Creatinine Clearance (mL/min)	Maximum Dosage and Interval
15-35	50 mg a day
< 15	25 mg/day

OFF-LABEL USES

Improved survival in diabetics with heart disease; treatment of hypertrophic cardiomyopathy, pheochromocytoma, and syndrome of mitral valve prolapse; prevention of migraine, thyrotoxicosis, and tremors.

CONTRAINDICATIONS

Cardiogenic shock, overt heart failure, second- or third-degree heart block, severe bradycardia.

INTERACTIONS

Drug

Cimetidine: May increase atenolol blood concentration.

Diuretics, other antihypertensives: May increase hypotensive effect of atenolol.

Insulin, oral hypoglycemics: May mask symptoms of hypoglycemia and prolong hypoglycemic effect of insulin and oral hypoglycemics.

NSAIDs: May decrease antihypertensive effect of atenolol.

Sympathomimetics, xanthines: May mutually inhibit effects.

Herbal

None known.

Food

None known.

DIAGNOSTIC TEST EFFECTS

May increase serum antinuclear antibody titer and BUN, glucose, serum creatinine, potassium, lipoprotein, triglyceride, and uric acid levels.

SIDE EFFECTS

Atenolol is generally well tolerated, with mild and transient side effects.

Frequent

Hypotension manifested as cold extremities, constipation or diarrhea, diaphoresis, dizziness, fatigue, headache, and nausea.

Occasional

Insomnia, flatulence, urinary frequency, impotence or decreased libido, mental depression.

Rare

Rash, arthralgia, myalgia, confusion (especially in the elderly), altered taste.

SERIOUS REACTIONS

- Overdose may produce profound bradycardia and hypotension.
- Abrupt atenolol withdrawal may result in diaphoresis, palpitations, headache, and tremors.
- Atenolol administration may precipitate CHF or MI in patients with cardiac disease; thyroid storm in those with thyrotoxicosis; and peripheral ischemia in those with existing peripheral vascular disease.
- Hypoglycemia may occur in patients with previously controlled diabetes.
- Thrombocytopenia, manifested as unusual bruising or bleeding, occurs rarely.

PRECAUTIONS & CONSIDERATIONS

Caution is warranted with bronchospastic disease, diabetes, hyperthyroidism, impaired renal or hepatic function, inadequate cardiac function, and peripheral vascular disease. Atenolol readily crosses the placenta and is distributed in breast milk. Atenolol use should be avoided in pregnant women after the first trimester because it may result in low-birth-weight infants. The drug may also produce apnea, bradycardia, hypoglycemia, and hypothermia during childbirth. No age-related precautions have been noted in children. Use cautiously in elderly patients, who may have age-related peripheral vascular disease and impaired renal function. Be aware that salt and alcohol intake should be restricted. Nasal decongestants or OTC cold preparations (stimulants) should not be used without physician approval.

Orthostatic hypotension may occur, so rise slowly from a lying to sitting position and dangle the legs from the bed momentarily before standing. Notify the physician of confusion, depression, dizziness, rash, or unusual bruising or bleeding. BP for hypotension, respiratory status for shortness of breath, and pulse for quality, rate, and rhythm should be monitored during treatment. If pulse rate is 60 beats/min or lower or systolic BP is < 90 mm Hg, withhold the medication and contact the physician. Signs and symptoms of CHF, such as decreased urine output, distended neck veins, dyspnea (particularly on exertion or lying down), night cough, peripheral edema, and weight gain should also be assessed.

Storage

Store at room temperature.

Administration

Take oral atenolol without regard to meals. Crush tablets if necessary. Do not abruptly discontinue the drug. Compliance is essential to control angina and hypertension.

Atomoxetine

at′o-mox-e-teen

★ 🍁 Strattera

Do not confuse atomoxetine with atorvastatin.

CATEGORY AND SCHEDULE

Pregnancy Risk Category: C

Classification: Selective norepinephrine reuptake inhibitors, ADHD agents

MECHANISM OF ACTION

A norepinephrine reuptake inhibitor that enhances noradrenergic function by selective inhibition of the presynaptic norepinephrine transporter. *Therapeutic Effect:* Improves attention span, decreases distractability, and decreases impulsivity.

PHARMACOKINETICS

Rapidly absorbed after PO administration. Protein binding: 98% (primarily to albumin). Metabolized in the liver by CYP2D6. Eliminated primarily in urine and, to a lesser extent, in feces. Not removed by hemodialysis. *Half-life:* 4-5 h in general population. Patients with poor metabolizer status for CYP2D6 and those with liver disease have increased AUC and half-life, up to 24 h.

AVAILABILITY

Capsules: 10 mg, 18 mg, 25 mg, 40 mg, 60 mg, 80 mg, 100 mg.

INDICATIONS AND DOSAGES

▸ **ADHD**

PO

Adults, Children weighing 70 kg and more. 40 mg once a day. May increase after at least 3 days to 80 mg as a single daily dose or in divided doses. Maximum: 100 mg.

Children weighing < 70 kg. Initially, 0.5 mg/kg/day. May increase after at least 3 days to 1.2 mg/kg/day. Maximum: 1.4 mg/kg/day or 100 mg.

▸ **ADHD with concomitant therapy with CYP2D6 strong inhibitors (fluoxetine, paroxetine, quinidine) or in known poor CYP2D6 metabolizers**

PO

Adults, Children weighing 70 kg and more. 40 mg once a day. Only increase to usual target dose of 80 mg/day if symptoms fail to improve after 4 wks and initial dose is well tolerated. *Children weighing < 70 kg.* Initially, 0.5 mg/kg/day. Only increase to usual target dose of 1.2 mg/kg/day if symptoms fail to improve after 4 wks and initial dose is well tolerated.

▸ **Dosage in hepatic impairment**

Expect to administer 50% of normal atomoxetine dosage to patients with moderate hepatic impairment and 25% of normal dosage to those with severe hepatic impairment.

CONTRAINDICATIONS

Angle-closure glaucoma, hypersensitivity, use with or within 14 days of MAOIs.

INTERACTIONS

Drug

Albuterol: Cardiovascular effects of albuterol may be potentiated.

CYP2D6 inhibitors, such as fluoxetine, paroxetine, quinidine: May increase atomoxetine blood concentration. Adjust dose.

MAOIs: May increase the risk of toxic effects. Contraindicated.

Herbal

None known.

Food

None known.

DIAGNOSTIC TEST EFFECTS

Rarely may cause laboratory abnormalities consistent with liver injury, such as markedly increased LFTs and bilirubin levels.

SIDE EFFECTS

Frequent

Headache, dyspepsia, nausea, vomiting, fatigue, decreased appetite, dizziness, altered mood.

Occasional

Tachycardia, hypertension, weight loss, delayed growth in children, irritability.

Rare

Insomnia, sexual dysfunction in adults, fever, aggressiveness, hostility.

SERIOUS REACTIONS

- Hepatotoxicity.
- Priapism.
- Urine retention or urinary hesitance may occur.

PRECAUTIONS & CONSIDERATIONS

Caution is warranted with cardiovascular disease, tachycardia, hypertension, moderate or severe hepatic impairment, and a risk of urine retention. Be aware that concurrent use of pressor medications that can increase heart rate or BP should be avoided. It is unknown whether atomoxetine is excreted in breast milk. The safety and efficacy of atomoxetine have not been established in children younger than 6 yr. A thorough cardiovascular assessment is recommended before initiation of therapy in pediatric patients; assessment should include medical history, family history, and physical examination with consideration of ECG testing. Atomoxetine increased the risk of suicidal ideation in short-term studies in children or adolescents with ADHD. Age-related cardiovascular or cerebrovascular disease and hepatic or renal impairment may increase the risk of side effects in elderly patients.

Dizziness may occur, so avoid tasks that require mental alertness and motor skills. Notify the physician if fever, irritability, palpitations, or vomiting occurs. BP, pulse rate, mood changes, urine output, and fluid and electrolyte status should be monitored.

Storage

Store at room temperature.

Administration
Take atomoxetine without regard to food. Take the last daily dose of atomoxetine early in the evening to avoid insomnia. Swallow capsules whole. Do not chew, crush, or open.

Atorvastatin

a-tor'va-sta-tin
★🍁 Lipitor
Do not confuse Lipitor with Levatol.

CATEGORY AND SCHEDULE
Pregnancy Risk Category: X

Classification:
Antihyperlipidemics, HMG CoA reductase inhibitors

MECHANISM OF ACTION
An antihyperlipidemic that inhibits HMG-CoA reductase, the enzyme that catalyzes the early step in cholesterol synthesis. *Therapeutic Effect:* Decreases LDL and VLDL cholesterol and plasma triglyceride levels; increases HDL cholesterol concentration.

PHARMACOKINETICS
Poorly absorbed from the GI tract. Protein binding is > 98%. Metabolized in the liver. Minimally eliminated in urine. Plasma levels are markedly increased in chronic alcoholic hepatic disease but are unaffected by renal disease. *Half-life:* 14 h.

AVAILABILITY
Tablets: 10 mg, 20 mg, 40 mg, 80 mg.

INDICATIONS AND DOSAGES
▸ **Hyperlipidemia, reduction of risk of myocardial infarction (MI), angina revascularization procedures, or stroke in patients with certain risk factors**
PO
Adults, Elderly. Initially, 10-40 mg a day given as a single dose. Dose range: 10-80 mg/day. Increase at 2- to 4-wk intervals to maximum of 80 mg/day.
Children 10-17 yr. Initially, 10 mg/day, may increase to 20 mg/day.
▸ **Familial hypercholesterolemia**
PO
Children 10-17 yr. Initially, 10 mg/day. May increase to 20 mg/day.
▸ **Dosages in patients taking cyclosporine, clarithromycin, or taking a combination of ritonavir plus saquinavir or lopinavir**
Limit initial dose to 10 mg/day.

CONTRAINDICATIONS
Active hepatic disease, lactation, pregnancy, unexplained elevated liver function test results, rhabdomyolysis, hypersensitivity.

INTERACTIONS
Drug
Antacids, colestipol: Decrease atorvastatin absorption.
Gemfibrozil, nicotinic acid: Increase the risk of myopathy or rhabdomyolysis.
Cyclosporine, erythromycin, itraconazole, protease inhibitors, clarithromycin, diltiazem: CYP3A4 inhibitors increase atorvastatin blood concentration and increase the risk of myopathy or rhabdomyolysis.
Digoxin: Increased digoxin levels.
Herbal
St. John's wort: May reduce atorvastatin concentrations.
Food
Fiber, oat bran, pectin: May reduce atorvastatin absorption; separate time of administration.
Grapefruit juice: May increase the bioavailability of atorvastatin

resulting in an increased risk of myopathy or rhabdomyolysis. Avoid.

DIAGNOSTIC TEST EFFECTS

May increase serum CK and transaminase concentrations.

SIDE EFFECTS

Atorvastatin is generally well tolerated. Side effects are usually mild and transient.

Frequent (16%)

Headache.

Occasional (2%-5%)

Myalgia, rash or pruritus, allergy.

Rare (1%-2%)

Flatulence, dyspepsia.

SERIOUS REACTIONS

- Cataracts may develop, and photosensitivity may occur.
- Hepatotoxicity or rhabdomyolysis occur rarely.

PRECAUTIONS & CONSIDERATIONS

Caution is warranted with a history of hepatic disease, hypotension, major surgery, severe acute infection, substantial alcohol consumption, trauma, those receiving anticoagulant therapy, and those with severe acute infection, uncontrolled seizures, or severe endocrine, electrolyte, or metabolic disorders. Atorvastatin is distributed in breast milk and is contraindicated during lactation. It is contraindicated during pregnancy because it may produce skeletal malformation. Pregnancy should be determined before beginning therapy. Safety and efficacy of atorvastatin have not been established in children younger than 10 yr of age. No age-related precautions have been noted in elderly patients.

Notify the physician of headache, malaise, pruritus, or rash. Laboratory results and serum cholesterol and triglyceride levels and hepatic function test results should be documented before therapy. Serum cholesterol and triglyceride levels should be monitored periodically during therapy. Be aware that diet is an important part of treatment.

Storage

Store at room temperature.

Administration

May be taken without regard to food. Do not break film-coated tablets. Administer at any time of day but at a consistent time daily.

Atovaquone

a-toe'va-kwone

Mepron

CATEGORY AND SCHEDULE

Pregnancy Risk Category: C

Classification: Antiprotozoals

MECHANISM OF ACTION

A systemic anti-infective that inhibits the mitochondrial electron-transport system at the cytochrome bc1 complex (complex III), which interrupts nucleic acid and adenosine triphosphate synthesis. *Therapeutic Effect:* Antiprotozoal and antipneumocystic activity.

PHARMACOKINETICS

Absorption increased with a high-fat meal. Protein binding: > 99%. Metabolized in liver. Primarily excreted in feces. *Half-life:* 2-3 days.

AVAILABILITY

Oral Suspension: 750 mg/5 mL.

INDICATIONS AND DOSAGES

▸ ***Pneumocystis carinii* pneumonia (PCP)**

PO

Adults, adolescents 13 yr of age and older. 750 mg twice a day with food for 21 days.

▸ **Prevention of PCP**

PO

Adults, adolescents 13 yr of age and older. 1500 mg once a day with food.

OFF-LABEL USES

Malaria, babesiosis, toxoplasmosis.

CONTRAINDICATIONS

Development or history of potentially life-threatening allergic reaction to the drug.

INTERACTIONS

Drug

Rifampin or rifabutin: May decrease atovaquone blood concentration and increase rifampin blood concentration.

Herbal

None known.

Food

Ingestion with a fatty meal increases absorption.

DIAGNOSTIC TEST EFFECTS

May increase serum alkaline phosphatase, amylase, AST (SGOT), and ALT (SGPT) levels. May decrease serum sodium levels.

SIDE EFFECTS

Frequent (> 10%)

Rash, nausea, diarrhea, headache, vomiting, fever, insomnia, cough.

Occasional (< 10%)

Abdominal discomfort, thrush, pruritus, dizziness, asthenia, anemia, neutropenia.

SERIOUS REACTIONS

- Anemia occurs rarely.

PRECAUTIONS & CONSIDERATIONS

Caution is warranted with chronic diarrhea, hepatic disease, malabsorption syndromes, and severe PCP and in elderly patients, who require close monitoring because of age-related cardiac, hepatic, and renal impairment. Safety and effectiveness have not been established in pediatric patients < 13 yr of age.

Notify the physician if diarrhea, rash, or other new symptoms occur. Pattern of daily bowel activity and stool consistency and skin for rash should be monitored. Hemoglobin levels, intake and output, and renal function should be assessed. Medical history for problems that may interfere with the drug's absorption, such as GI disorders, (e.g., significant diarrhea,vomiting), should be determined before beginning therapy.

Storage

Store at room temperature. Do not freeze.

Administration

Shake suspension well before using. Administer with meals. Failure to administer with meals may cause lack of response to treatment. Take atovaquone for the full course of treatment.

Atropine

a'troe-peen

★ Atreza, Atropen, Atropine Sulfate, Isopto-Atropine, SalTropine

Do not confuse with Akarpine or Aplisol.

CATEGORY AND SCHEDULE

Pregnancy Risk Category: C

Classification: Antiarrhythmics, anticholinergics, antidotes, cycloplegics, mydriatics, ophthalmics, preanesthetics

MECHANISM OF ACTION

An acetylcholine antagonist that inhibits the action of acetylcholine by competing with acetylcholine for common binding sites on muscarinic receptors, which are located on exocrine glands, cardiac and smooth-muscle ganglia, and intramural neurons. This action blocks all muscarinic effects. *Therapeutic Effect:* Decreases GI motility and secretory activity and genitourinary muscle tone (ureter, bladder); produces ophthalmic cycloplegia and mydriasis.

PHARMACOKINETICS

Rapidly absorbed after oral administration. Crosses blood-brain barrier. Renally eliminated. Not removed by hemodialysis. *Half-life:* 2.5 h.

AVAILABILITY

Injection: 0.05 mg/mL, 0.1 mg/mL, 0.4 mg/mL, 1 mg/mL.
Injection (Autoinjectors): 0.25 mg, 0.5 mg, 1 mg, 2 mg.
Ophthalmic Ointment: 1%.
Ophthalmic Solution: 1%.
Tablets: 0.4 mg.

INDICATIONS AND DOSAGES

▸ **Asystole, slow pulseless electrical activity**

IV

Adults, Elderly. 1 mg; may repeat q3-5min up to total dose of 0.04 mg/kg. Normal maximum: 3 mg total.

▸ **Preanesthetic**

IV/IM/SC

Adults, Elderly. 0.4-0.6 mg 30-60 min preoperatively.
Children weighing 5 kg or more. 0.01-0.02 mg/kg/dose to maximum of 0.4 mg/dose.
Children weighing < 5 kg. 0.02 mg/kg/dose 30-60 min preoperatively.

▸ **Bradycardia**

IV

Adults, Elderly. 0.5-1 mg q5min not to exceed 2 mg or 0.04 mg/kg.
Children. 0.02 mg/kg with a minimum of 0.1 mg to a maximum of 0.5 mg in children and 1 mg in adolescents. May repeat in 5 min. Maximum total dose: 1 mg in children, 2 mg in adolescents.

▸ **Reduction salivation and bronchial secretions**

PO

Adults. 0.4 mg.
Children. Weight-based doses: 7-16 lb, 0.1 mg; 17-24 lb, 0.15 mg; 24-40 lb, 0.2 mg; 40-65 lb, 0.3 mg; 65-90 lb, 0.4 mg; over 90 lb, 0.4 mg.

▸ **Cycloplegia/mydriasis**

OPHTHALMIC

Adults. 1 drop of solution in the eye 3 times a day or small amount of ointment in the eye once or twice daily.

▸ **Organophosphate nerve agent or insecticide poisoning**

IM (AUTO-INJECTOR)

Adults, Elderly, and Children > 41kg or over 10 yr of age. 2 mg; may repeat up to 3 doses as directed until under medical care.
Children 18-41 kg or roughly 4-10 yr of age. 1 mg; may repeat up to 3 doses as directed.
Children 7-18 kg or roughly 6 mo-4 yr of age. 0.5 mg; may repeat up to 3 doses as directed.
Infants < 7 kg or < 6 mo of age. 0.25 mg; may repeat up to 3 doses as directed.

CONTRAINDICATIONS

Generally contraindicated in patients with glaucoma, pyloric stenosis, or prostatic hypertrophy, except in doses usually used for preanesthesia or when emergency exists (e.g., nerve agent poisoning or ACLS protocol).

INTERACTIONS

Drug

Antacids, antidiarrheals: May decrease absorption of atropine.

Anticholinergics: May increase effects of atropine.

Ketoconazole: May decrease absorption of ketoconazole.

Potassium chloride: May increase severity of GI lesions (wax matrix) due to slowing DI transit.

Herbal and Food

None known.

DIAGNOSTIC TEST EFFECTS

None known.

IV INCOMPATIBILITIES

Pantoprazole, phenytoin, thiopental sodium.

IV COMPATIBILITIES

Diphenhydramine (Benadryl), droperidol (Inapsine), fentanyl (Sublimaze), glycopyrrolate (Robinul), heparin, hydromorphone (Dilaudid), midazolam (Versed), morphine, potassium chloride.

SIDE EFFECTS

Frequent

Dry mouth, nose, and throat that may be severe; decreased sweating, constipation, irritation at subcutaneous or IM injection site.

Occasional

Swallowing difficulty, blurred vision, bloated feeling, impotence, urinary hesitancy.

Rare

Allergic reaction, including rash and urticaria; mental confusion or excitement, particularly in children, fatigue.

SERIOUS REACTIONS

- Overdosage may produce tachycardia; palpitations; hot, dry, or flushed skin; absence of bowel sounds; increased respiratory rate; nausea; vomiting; confusion; somnolence; slurred speech; dizziness; and CNS stimulation.
- Overdosage may also produce psychosis as evidenced by agitation, restlessness, rambling speech, visual hallucinations, paranoid behavior, and delusions, followed by depression.

PRECAUTIONS & CONSIDERATIONS

Extreme caution should be used with autonomic neuropathy, diarrhea, known and suspected GI infections, and mild to moderate ulcerative colitis. Caution is also warranted with CHF, COPD, coronary artery disease, esophageal reflux or hiatal hernia associated with reflux esophagitis, gastric ulcer, hepatic or renal disease, hypertension, hyperthyroidism, and tachyarrhythmias. Use atropine cautiously in the elderly and in infants.

Warm, dry, flushing feeling may occur upon administration. The patient should urinate before taking this drug to reduce the risk of urine retention. BP, pulse rate, temperature, pattern of daily bowel activity and stool consistency, intake and output, and skin turgor and mucous membranes should be assessed.

Storage

Store at room temperature.

Administration

! Notify physician and expect to discontinue atropine immediately if blurred vision, dizziness, or increased pulse rate occurs.

For IV use, give the drug rapidly, to prevent paradoxical slowing of the heart rate. Give undiluted or diluted in 10 mL of sterile water for injection. Atropine may also be given by IM or subcutaneous injection.

Auto-injectors are used for emergency field use; remove victim from contraminated area and then follow manufacturer instructions for IM use.

Oral tablets are usually given 30 min prior to meals.

Auranofin

ah-ran′oh-fin

★ 🍁 Ridaura

Do not confuse Ridaura with Cardura.

CATEGORY AND SCHEDULE

Pregnancy Risk Category: C

Classification: Disease-modifying antirheumatic drugs, gold compounds

MECHANISM OF ACTION

Gold compounds that alter cellular mechanisms, collagen biosynthesis, enzyme systems, and immune responses. *Therapeutic Effect:* Suppress synovitis in the active stage of rheumatoid arthritis.

PHARMACOKINETICS

Auranofin (29% gold): Moderately absorbed from the GI tract. Protein binding: 60%. Rapidly metabolized. Primarily excreted in urine. *Half-life:* 21-31 days.

AVAILABILITY

Capsules (Ridaura): 3 mg.

INDICATIONS AND DOSAGES

▸ **Rheumatoid arthritis**

PO

Adults, Elderly. 6 mg/day as a single or 2 divided doses. If there is no response in 6 mo, may increase to 9 mg/day in 3 divided doses. If response is still inadequate, discontinue.

CONTRAINDICATIONS

Bone marrow aplasia, history of gold-induced pathologies (including blood dyscrasias, exfoliative dermatitis, necrotizing enterocolitis, and pulmonary fibrosis), severe blood dyscrasias.

INTERACTIONS

Drug

Bone marrow depressants; hepatotoxic and nephrotoxic medications: May increase the risk of aurothioglucose toxicity.

Penicillamine: May increase the risk of hematologic or renal adverse effects.

Herbal

None known.

Food

None known.

DIAGNOSTIC TEST EFFECTS

May decrease hemoglobin level, hematocrit, and WBC and platelet counts. May increase urine protein level. May alter liver function test results.

SIDE EFFECTS

Frequent

Diarrhea (50%), pruritic rash (26%), abdominal pain (14%), stomatitis (13%), nausea (10%).

SERIOUS REACTIONS

• Signs and symptoms of gold toxicity, the primary serious reaction, include decreased hemoglobin level, decreased granulocyte count

(< 150,000/mm^3), proteinuria, hematuria, stomatitis, blood dyscrasias (anemia, leukopenia [WBC count < 4000/mm^3], thrombocytopenia, and eosinophilia), glomerulonephritis, nephrotic syndrome, and cholestatic jaundice.

PRECAUTIONS & CONSIDERATIONS

Caution is warranted with blood dyscrasias, compromised cerebral or cardiovascular circulation, eczema, a history of sensitivity to gold compounds, marked hypertension, renal or liver impairment, severe debilitation, Sjögren syndrome in rheumatoid arthritis, and systemic lupus erythematosus. Auranofin crosses the placenta and is distributed in breast milk. These drugs should be used only when their benefits outweigh the possible risks to the fetus. Safety and effectiveness have not been established in children. Use these drugs cautiously in patients who may have age-related renal impairment. Avoid exposure to sunlight, which may turn skin gray or blue. Oral hygiene should be diligently maintained to help prevent stomatitis.

Notify the physician if GI symptoms (nausea, vomiting, or abdominal cramps), metallic taste, sore mouth, pruritus, or rash occurs. Pattern of daily bowel activity and stool consistency, urine for hematuria and proteinuria, CBC (particularly hemoglobin level, hematocrit, and WBC and platelet counts), renal and liver function tests (especially BUN level and serum alkaline phosphatase, creatinine, AST [SGOT], and ALT [SGPT] levels), skin for rash, and oral mucous membranes for stomatitis should be monitored. Therapeutic response, including improved grip strength, increased joint mobility, reduced joint tenderness, and relief of pain, stiffness, and swelling, should also be assessed.

Storage

At controlled room temperature.

Administration

Take without regard to food. Taking with food may help GI tolerance. Therapeutic response to the drug may occur in 3-6 mo.

Azacitidine

ay-zah-sigh′tih-deen

Vidaza

Do not confuse azacitidine with azathioprine.

CATEGORY AND SCHEDULE

Pregnancy Risk Category: D

Classification: Antineoplastics, antimetabolites

MECHANISM OF ACTION

An antineoplastic agent that exerts a cytotoxic effect on rapidly dividing cells by causing demethylation of DNA in abnormal hematopoietic cells in the bone marrow. *Therapeutic Effect:* Restores normal function to tumor-suppressor genes regulating cellular differentiation and proliferation.

PHARMACOKINETICS

Rapidly absorbed after subcutaneous administration. Metabolized by the liver. Eliminated in urine. *Half-life:* 4 h.

AVAILABILITY

Powder for Injection: 100 mg.

INDICATIONS AND DOSAGES

▸ **Myelodysplastic syndrome**

IV, SC

Adults, Elderly. 75 mg/m^2/day for 7 days every 4 wks. Dosage may be increased after 2 cycles to 100 mg/m^2

if initial dose is insufficient and toxicity is manageable.

OFF-LABEL USES

Acute myelogenous leukemia, chronic myelogenous leukemia.

CONTRAINDICATIONS

Advanced malignant hepatic tumors, hypersensitivity to the drug or to mannitol.

INTERACTIONS

Drug

Bone marrow suppressants: May increase myelosuppression.
Live-virus vaccines: May potentiate virus replication, increase vaccine side effects, and decrease the patient's antibody response to the vaccine.

DIAGNOSTIC TEST EFFECTS

May decrease hemoglobin level, hematocrit, and WBC, RBC, and platelet counts. May increase serum creatinine and potassium levels.

SIDE EFFECTS

Frequent (29%-71%)

Nausea, vomiting, fever, diarrhea, fatigue, injection site erythema, constipation, ecchymosis, cough, dyspnea, weakness.

Occasional (16%-26%)

Rigors, petechiae, injection site pain, pharyngitis, arthralgia, headache, limb pain, dizziness, peripheral edema, back pain, erythema, epistaxis, weight loss, myalgia.

Rare (8%-13%)

Anxiety, abdominal pain, rash, depression, tachycardia, insomnia, night sweats, stomatitis.

SERIOUS REACTIONS

- Hematologic toxicity, manifested most commonly as anemia, leukopenia, neutropenia, and thrombocytopenia, is a common adverse effect.
- Hepatotoxicity.
- Nephrotoxicity.

PRECAUTIONS & CONSIDERATIONS

Caution is warranted with hepatic or renal impairment. Azacitidine may be embryotoxic, causing developmental abnormalities in the fetus. Barrier contraception should be used while receiving azacitidine. Men should not try to father a child while on treatment. Women of childbearing age should avoid becoming pregnant while taking azacitidine. Breastfeeding while taking azacitidine should be avoided. The safety and efficacy of azacitidine have not been established in children. Age-related renal impairment may increase the risk of renal toxicity in elderly patients.

Notify the physician of nausea and vomiting, bleeding, and any signs of infection, including fever and flulike symptoms. Blood counts should be obtained before each dosing cycle to monitor the response and assess for drug toxicity.

Storage

Store vials at room temperature. The reconstituted solution may be stored for up to 1 h at room temperature or up to 8 h if refrigerated. After removing from refrigeration, allow the drug suspension to return to room temperature and use it within 30 min.

Administration

CAUTION: Observe usual precautions for preparations, handling, administration, and disposal of cytotoxic drugs. For subcutaneous administration, use strict aseptic technique when preparing the drug. Reconstitute azacitidine with 4 mL sterile water for injection. The reconstituted suspension will appear cloudy. Divide doses

> 4 mL equally into two syringes. To resuspend the contents, invert the syringe 2 or 3 times and roll it between your palms for 30 seconds immediately before administration. For SC injection, rotate injection sites among the abdomen, upper arm, and thigh for each injection. Administer each new injection at least 1 inch from a previous injection site. If azacitidine comes into contact with skin, immediately wash with soap and water.

For IV infusion: Dilute the appropriate dose in 50-100 mL of 0.9% NaCl or lactated Ringer's injection. Administer IV infusion over 10-40 min; infusion must be completed within 1 h of reconstitution.

Azathioprine

ay-za-thye′oh-preen

★ Azasan, Imuran

🍁 Apo-Azathioprine, Teva-Azathioprine

Do not confuse azathioprine with azacitidine or Azulfidine, or Imuran with Elmiron or Imferon.

CATEGORY AND SCHEDULE

Pregnancy Risk Category: D

Classification: Disease-modifying antirheumatic drugs, immunosuppressives

MECHANISM OF ACTION

An immunologic agent that antagonizes purine metabolism and inhibits DNA, protein, and RNA synthesis. *Therapeutic Effect:* Suppresses cell-mediated hypersensitivities; alters antibody production and immune response in transplant recipients; reduces the severity of arthritis symptoms.

AVAILABILITY

Tablets (Azasan): 75 mg, 100 mg.
Tablets (Imuran): 50 mg.
Injection: 100-mg vial.

INDICATIONS AND DOSAGES

▸ **Adjunct in prevention of renal allograft rejection**

PO, IV

Adults, Elderly, Children.
3-5 mg/kg/day on day of transplant, then 1-3 mg/kg/day as maintenance dose.

▸ **Rheumatoid arthritis**

PO

Adults. Initially, 1 mg/kg/day as a single dose or in 2 divided doses. May increase by 0.5 mg/kg/day after 6-8 wks at 4-wk intervals up to maximum of 2.5 mg/kg/day. Maintenance: Lowest effective dosage. May decrease dose by 0.5 mg/kg or 25 mg/day q4wk (while other therapies, such as rest, physiotherapy, and salicylates, are maintained).

Elderly. Initially, 1 mg/kg/day (50-100 mg); may increase by 25 mg/day until response or toxicity.

▸ **Dosage in renal impairment**

Dosage is modified based on creatinine clearance.

Creatinine Clearance (mL/min)	Dose
10-50	75% of usual dose
< 10	50% of usual dose

OFF-LABEL USES

Treatment of biliary cirrhosis, chronic active hepatitis, glomerulonephritis, inflammatory bowel disease, inflammatory myopathy, multiple sclerosis, myasthenia gravis, nephrotic syndrome, pemphigoid, pemphigus, polymyositis, systemic lupus erythematosus.

CONTRAINDICATIONS
Pregnant patients with rheumatoid arthritis.

INTERACTIONS
Drug
ACE inhibitors: May increase risk of anemia and severe leukopenia.
Allopurinol: May increase activity and risk of toxicity of azathioprine.
Anticoagulants: May decrease anticoagulant activity.
Bone marrow depressants: May increase myelosuppression.
Live-virus vaccines: May potentiate virus replication, increase the vaccine's side effects, and decrease the patient's antibody response to the vaccine.
Other immunosuppressants: May increase the risk of infection.
Herbal
None known.
Food
None known.

DIAGNOSTIC TEST EFFECTS
May decrease serum albumin, Hgb, and serum uric acid levels. May increase serum alkaline phosphatase, amylase, bilirubin, AST (SGOT), and ALT (SGPT) levels.

IV INCOMPATIBILITIES
Aminoglycosides, ampicillin, ampicillin-sulbacatam (Unasyn), bumetanide (Bumex), calcium chloride, cephalosporins, diazepam, diphenhydramine, dopamine, dobutamine, epinephrine, hydrocortisone, imipenem-cilastatin (Primaxin), magnesium sulphate, meperidine, methylparabens, midazolam (Versed), ondansetron (Zofran), phenol, phenytoin, propylparabens, promethazine, vancomycin, and many others.

SIDE EFFECTS
Frequent
Nausea, vomiting, anorexia (particularly during early treatment and with large doses).
Occasional
Rash.
Rare
Severe nausea and vomiting with diarrhea, abdominal pain, hypersensitivity reaction.

SERIOUS REACTIONS
- Azathioprine use increases the risk of developing neoplasia (new abnormal-growth tumors).
- Significant leukopenia and thrombocytopenia may occur, particularly in those undergoing kidney transplant rejection. Increased risk of serious infection.
- Hepatotoxicity occurs rarely.

PRECAUTIONS & CONSIDERATIONS
Azathioprine should be used cautiously in immunosuppressed patients, those who have undergone previous treatment for rheumatoid arthritis with alkylating agents (such as chlorambucil, cyclophosphamide, and melphalan), and patients with current or recent chickenpox. Avoid pregnancy during treatment.

Notify the physician if abdominal pain, fever, mouth sores, sore throat, or unusual bleeding occurs. CBC (especially platelet count) and liver function tests should be monitored weekly during the first month of therapy, twice monthly during the second and third months of treatment, and monthly thereafter. The dosage should be reduced or discontinued if the WBC count falls rapidly. Therapeutic response, including improved grip strength, increased joint mobility, reduced joint tenderness, and relief of pain, stiffness, and swelling, should be assessed in rheumatoid arthritis patients.

Storage

Store the tablets at room temperature. Store the parenteral form at room temperature. After reconstitution, the IV solution is stable for 24 h at room temperature.

Administration

Take oral azathioprine during or after meals to reduce the risk of GI disturbances. The drug's therapeutic response may take up to 12 wks to appear.

For IV use, reconstitute the 100-mg vial with 10 mL sterile water for injection to provide a concentration of 10 mg/mL. Swirl the vial gently to dissolve the solution. The solution may be further diluted in 50 mL or more of either D5W or 0.9% NaCl. Infuse the solution over 30-60 min (range is 5 min to 8 h).

Azelaic Acid

aye-zeh-lay′ick as′id

★ Azelex, Finacea, Finevin

🍁 Finacea

CATEGORY AND SCHEDULE

Pregnancy Risk Category: B

Classification: Topical antimicrobial, antiacne

MECHANISM OF ACTION

The exact mechanism of action of azelaic acid is not known. Possesses antimicrobial activity against *Propionibacterium acnes* and *Staphylococcus epidermidis*. *Therapeutic Effect:* Inhibits microbial cellular protein synthesis.

PHARMACOKINETICS

Minimal absorption after topical administration. Metabolized in liver. Excreted in urine as unchanged drug. *Half-life:* 12 h.

AVAILABILITY

Cream: 20%.
Gel: 15%.

INDICATIONS AND DOSAGES

▸ **Mild to moderate acne**

TOPICAL

Adults, Adolescents. Apply cream to affected area twice daily (morning and evening).

▸ **Mild to moderate rosacea**

TOPICAL

Adults. Apply gel to affected area twice daily (morning and evening).

CONTRAINDICATIONS

Hypersensitivity to azelaic acid or any component of the formulation.

DRUG INTERACTIONS

Drug

None known.

Herbal

None known.

Food

None known.

DIAGNOSTIC TEST EFFECTS

None known.

SIDE EFFECTS

Occasional

Pruritus, stinging, burning, tingling, erythema, dryness, rash, peeling, irritation, contact dermatitis.

Rare

Worsening of asthma, vitiligo depigmentation, small depigmented spots, hypertrichosis, reddening (signs of keratosis pilaris), exacerbation of recurrent cold sore, fever blister, or oral herpes simplex.

SERIOUS REACTIONS

- None reported.

PRECAUTIONS & CONSIDERATIONS

Monitor for early signs of hypopigmentation, particularly in patients with dark complexions.

Storage

Store at room temperature.

Administration

For external use only. Massage a thin layer into the affected area. Avoid contact with the eyes, mouth, and mucous membranes. Cosmetics may be applied after the gel has dried.

Azelastine

a'zel-ah-steen

★ Astelin, Astepro, Optivar

Do not confuse Optivar with Optiray.

CATEGORY AND SCHEDULE

Pregnancy Risk Category: C

Classification: Antihistamines, H1, inhalation, ophthalmics

MECHANISM OF ACTION

An antihistamine that competes with histamine for histamine receptor sites on cells in the blood vessels, GI tract, and respiratory tract. *Therapeutic Effect:* Relieves symptoms associated with seasonal allergic rhinitis such as increased mucus production and sneezing and symptoms associated with allergic conjunctivitis, such as redness, itching, and excessive tearing.

PHARMACOKINETICS

Route	Onset	Peak	Duration
Nasal spray	0.5-1 h	2-3 h	12 h
Ophthalmic	N/A	3 min	8 h

Well absorbed through nasal mucosa. Primarily excreted in feces. *Half-life:* 22 h.

AVAILABILITY

Nasal Spray (Astelin): 137 mcg/spray.
Ophthalmic Solution (Optivar): 0.05%.
Nasal Spray (Astepro): 205.5 mcg/spray.

INDICATIONS AND DOSAGES

▸ **Allergic rhinitis**

NASAL

Adults, Elderly, Children 12 yr and older. 1-2 sprays in each nostril twice a day.

Children 5-11 yr. 1 spray in each nostril twice a day.

▸ **Allergic conjunctivitis**

OPHTHALMIC

Adults, Elderly, Children 3 yr or older. 1 drop into affected eye twice a day.

CONTRAINDICATIONS

History of hypersensitivity.

INTERACTIONS

Drug

Alcohol, other CNS depressants: May increase CNS depression.

Cimetidine: May increase azelastine blood concentration but only when azelastine given orally.

Herbal

None known.

Food

None known.

DIAGNOSTIC TEST EFFECTS

May suppress flare and wheal reactions to antigen skin testing unless drug is discontinued 4 days before testing.

SIDE EFFECTS

Frequent (15%-20%)

Headache, bitter taste.

Rare
Nasal burning, paroxysmal sneezing. Ophthalmic: Transient eye burning or stinging, bitter taste, headache.

SERIOUS REACTIONS

- Epistaxis occurs rarely with nasal administration.

PRECAUTIONS & CONSIDERATIONS

Caution is warranted with renal impairment. It is unknown whether azelastine crosses the placenta or is distributed in breast milk. Azelastine has been shown to cause developmental toxicity when given orally to mice, rats, and rabbits; use in pregnancy only if necessary. The safety and efficacy of azelastine have not been established in children younger than 3 yr. No age-related precautions have been noted in elderly patients. Avoid drinking alcoholic beverages during therapy.

Storage
Store at room temperature.

Administration
For intranasal use, prime the pump with 4 sprays or until a fine mist appears before using the nasal spray the first time. After the first use and if the pump has not been used for 3 or more days, prime the pump with 2 sprays or until a fine mist appears. To administer the spray, clear nasal passages as much as possible before use. Tilt head slightly forward. Insert the applicator tip into one nostril, pointing the tip toward the nasal passage and away from the nasal septum. While holding the other nostril closed, spray into the nostril and inhale at the same time to deliver the drug as high into the nasal passages as possible. Repeat in the other nostril. Wipe the applicator tip with a clean, damp tissue and replace cap immediately after use. Avoid spraying nasal drug into the eyes.

For ophthalmic use, tilt head back and instill the solution in the conjunctival sac of the affected eye. Close the eye; then press gently on the lacrimal sac for 1 min.

Azithromycin

ay-zi-thro-mye′sin
Zithromax, Zithromax TRI-PAK, Zithromax Z-PAK, Zmax
Do not confuse azithromycin with erythromycin.

CATEGORY AND SCHEDULE

Pregnancy Risk Category: B

Classification: Antibiotics, macrolides

MECHANISM OF ACTION

A macrolide antibiotic that binds to ribosomal receptor sites of susceptible organisms, inhibiting RNA-dependent protein synthesis. *Therapeutic Effect:* Bacteriostatic or bactericidal, depending on the drug dosage.

PHARMACOKINETICS

Rapidly absorbed from the GI tract. Protein binding: 7%-50%. Widely distributed. Eliminated primarily unchanged by biliary excretion. *Half-life:* 68 h.

AVAILABILITY

Ophthalmic Solutions: 1%.
Oral Suspension: 100 mg/5 mL, 200 mg/5 mL.
Oral Suspension, Extended-Release Zmax: 2 g.
Tablets: 250 mg, 500 mg, 600 mg. *Tri-Pak:* 500 mg (3 tablets), Z-Pak: 250 mg (6 tablets).
Injection: 500 mg.

INDICATIONS AND DOSAGES

▸ **Respiratory tract, skin, and skin-structure infections**

PO

Adults, Elderly. 500 mg once, then 250 mg/day for 4 days.

Children 6 mo and older. 10 mg/kg once (maximum 500 mg), then 5 mg/kg/day for 4 days (maximum 250 mg).

▸ **Single-dose treatment of community-acquired pneumonia**

PO (EXTENDED RELEASE SUSPENSION ONLY)

Adults and Children ≥ 34 kg. 2g single dose; give at least 1 h before or 2 h after a meal. May also use for adults (only) for sinusitis.

Children weighing 5 to < 34 kg. 60 mg/kg single dose; give at least 1 h before or 2 h after a meal. See manufacturer-specific dosing table.

▸ **Acute bacterial exacerbations of COPD**

PO

Adults. 500 mg/day for 3 days.

▸ **Otitis media**

PO

Children 6 mo and older. 10 mg/kg once (maximum 500 mg), then 5 mg/kg/day for 4 days (maximum 250 mg). Single dose: 30 mg/kg. Maximum: 1500 mg. Three-day regimen: 10 mg/kg/day as single daily dose. Maximum: 500 mg/day.

▸ **Pharyngitis, tonsillitis**

PO

Children older than 2 yr. 12 mg/kg/day (maximum 500 mg) for 5 days.

▸ **Chancroid**

PO

Adults, Elderly. 1 g as single dose.

Children. 20 mg/kg as single dose. Maximum: 1 g.

▸ **Treatment of *Mycobacterium avium* complex (MAC)**

PO

Adults, Elderly. 500 mg/day in combination.

Children. 5 mg/kg/day (maximum 250 mg) in combination.

▸ **Prevention of MAC**

PO

Adults, Elderly. 1200 mg/wk alone or with rifabutin.

Children. 5 mg/kg/day (maximum 250 mg) or 20 mg/kg/wk (maximum 1200 mg) alone or with rifabutin.

▸ **Nongonococcal urethritis and cervicitis due to *Chlamydia trachomatis***

PO

Adults. 1 g as a single dose.

▸ **Gonococcal urethritis**

PO

Adults. 2 g as a single dose, but CDC does not recommend due to severe GI distress.

▸ **Bacterial conjunctivitis**

OPHTHALMIC

Adults, Elderly, Children 1 yr and older. 1 drop in the affected eye twice daily, 8-12 h apart for the first 2 days, then instill 1 drop in the affected eye once daily for the next 5 days.

▸ **Usual pediatric dosage**

PO

Children older than 6 mo. 10 mg/kg once (maximum 500 mg) then 5 mg/kg/day for 4 days (maximum 250 mg).

▸ **Usual parenteral dosage (community-acquired pneumonia, PID)**

IV

Adults. 500 mg/day, followed by oral therapy to complete the course of treatment. Usually IV given for at least 2 days.

OFF-LABEL USES

Chlamydial infections, gonococcal pharyngitis, uncomplicated gonococcal infections of the cervix, urethra, and rectum, dental-related infections, pertussis, alternative for ophthalmia neonatorum prophylaxis (Azasite).

CONTRAINDICATIONS
Hypersensitivity to azithromycin or other macrolide antibiotics.

INTERACTIONS
Drug
Aluminum- or magnesium-containing antacids: May decrease azithromycin blood concentration.
Carbamazepine, cyclosporine, theophylline, warfarin: May rarely increase the plasma concentrations of these drugs.
Herbal
None known.
Food
None known.

DIAGNOSTIC TEST EFFECTS
May increase serum CK, AST (SGOT), and ALT (SGPT) levels.

IV INCOMPATIBILITIES
Amikacin, aztreonam (Azactam), cephalosporins, clindamycin (Cleocin), famotidine (Pepcid), fentanyl, furosemide, gentamicin, imipenem-cilastin (Primaxin), morphine, potassium chloride, quinupristin-dalfopristin (Synercid), ticarcillin-claculanate (Timentin), tobramycin.

IV COMPATIBILITIES
None known; don't mix with other medications.

SIDE EFFECTS
Occasional
PO, IV: Nausea, vomiting, diarrhea, abdominal pain.
Ophthalmic: eye irritation, burning, staining.
Rare
PO, IV: Headache, dizziness, allergic reaction.

SERIOUS REACTIONS
- Antibiotic-associated colitis and other superinfections may result from altered bacterial balance.
- Acute interstitial nephritis and hepatotoxicity occur rarely.

PRECAUTIONS & CONSIDERATIONS
Caution is warranted with hepatic or renal dysfunction. Determine whether there is a history of hepatitis or allergies to azithromycin or other macrolides before beginning therapy. It is unknown whether azithromycin is distributed in breast milk. The safety and efficacy of azithromycin have not been established in children younger than 16 yr for IV use and younger than 6 mo for oral use. No age-related precautions have been noted in elderly patients with normal renal function.

GI discomfort, nausea, or vomiting should be assessed. Evaluate for signs and symptoms of superinfection, including genital or anal pruritus, sore mouth or tongue, and moderate to severe diarrhea. Assess for signs and symptoms of hepatotoxicity, such as abdominal pain, fever, GI disturbances, and malaise. Liver function tests should be monitored.
Storage
Store the oral suspension at room temperature. The immediate-release suspension is stable for 10 days after reconstitution. The extended-release suspension should be consumed within 12 h of reconstitution. Store injection vials at room temperature. After reconstitution, the injectable solution is stable for 24 h at room temperature or 7 days if refrigerated. Store unopened ophthalmic solution in refrigerator. Once opened, store in refrigerator or at room temperature for up to 14 days.
Administration
Give immediate-release tablets without regard to food; tolerability may be improved by administration with food. Do not administer the oral suspension with food. Give it at least 1 h before or 2 h after a meal. Take the oral suspension with 8 oz of water at least 1 h before or 2 h after consuming

any food or beverages. Azithromycin should be taken 1 h before or 2 h after antacids. Space doses evenly around the clock and continue taking for the full course of treatment.

For IV use, reconstitute each 500-mg vial with 4.8 mL sterile water for injection to provide a concentration of 100 mg/mL. Shake well to ensure dissolution. Further dilute the solution with 250 or 500 mL 0.9% NaCl or D5W to provide a final concentration of 2 mg/mL or 1 mg/mL, respectively. Infuse the drug over 60 min.

Shake ophthalmic solution before each use.

Aztreonam

az-tree'oo-nam

Azactam, Cayston

Cayston

CATEGORY AND SCHEDULE

Pregnancy Risk Category: B

Classification: Antibacterial, monobactams

MECHANISM OF ACTION

A monobactam antibiotic that inhibits bacterial cell wall synthesis. *Therapeutic Effect:* Bactericidal.

PHARMACOKINETICS

Completely absorbed after IM administration. Protein binding: 56%-60%. Partially metabolized by hydrolysis. Primarily excreted unchanged in urine. Removed by hemodialysis. *Half-life:* 1.4-2.2 h (increased in impaired renal or hepatic function).

AVAILABILITY

Injection Powder for Reconstitution: 500 mg, 1 g, 2 g.

Injection Powder Inhalation Solution: 75 mg.

INDICATIONS AND DOSAGES

▸ **Urinary tract infections**

IV, IM

Adults, Elderly. 500 mg to 1 g q8-12h.

▸ **Moderate to severe systemic infections**

IV, IM

Adults, Elderly. 1-2 g q8-12h.

▸ **Severe or life-threatening infections**

IV

Adults, Elderly. 2 g q6-8h.

▸ **Cystic fibrosis**

IV

Children. 50 mg/kg/dose q6-8hr up to 200 mg/kg/day. Maximum: 8g/day.

NEBULIZER INHALATION

Adults and Children 7 years and older: 75 mg nebulized 3 times daily for 28 days then 28 days off. Give each dose at least 4 h apart; administer a bronchodilator before nebulizing aztreonam.

▸ **Mild to severe infections in children**

IV

Children. 30 mg/kg q6-8hr. Maximum: 120 mg/kg/day.

Neonates. 60-120 mg/kg/day q6-12h.

▸ **Dosage in renal impairment**

Dosage and frequency are modified based on creatinine clearance and the severity of the infection.

Creatinine Clearance (mL/min)	Adult Dosage
10-30	1-2 g initially, then ½ usual dose at usual intervals
< 10	1-2 g initially; then ¼ usual dose at usual intervals

OFF-LABEL USES
Treatment of bone and joint infections.

CONTRAINDICATIONS
Hypersensitivity.

INTERACTIONS
Drug
None known.
Herbal
None known.
Food
None known.

DIAGNOSTIC TEST EFFECTS
May increase serum alkaline phosphatase, creatinine, LDH, AST (SGOT), and ALT (SGPT) levels. Produces a positive direct Coombs' test.

IV INCOMPATIBILITIES
Acyclovir (Zovirax), amphotericin (Fungizone), azithromycin (Zithromax), daunorubicin (Cerubidine), ganciclovir (Cytovene), lorazepam (Ativan), metronidazole (Flagyl), nafcillin, vancomycin (Vancocin).

IV COMPATIBILITIES
Aminophylline, ampicillin, bumetanide (Bumex), calcium gluconate, cefazolin, cimetidine (Tagamet), clindamycin, diltiazem (Cardizem), dobutamine (Dobutrex), dopamine (Intropin), famotidine (Pepcid), furosemide (Lasix), gentamicin, heparin, hydromorphone (Dilaudid), insulin (regular), magnesium sulfate, morphine, potassium chloride, propofol (Diprivan), tobramycin.

SIDE EFFECTS
Occasional (< 3%)
Discomfort and swelling at IM injection site, nausea, vomiting, diarrhea, rash.
Rare (< 1%)
Phlebitis or thrombophlebitis at IV injection site, abdominal cramps, headache, hypotension.

SERIOUS REACTIONS
- Antibiotic-associated colitis and other superinfections may result from altered bacterial balance.
- Severe hypersensitivity reactions, including anaphylaxis, occur rarely.
- Nebulized soultion may cause bronchospasm; therefore pretreat with bronchodilator.

PRECAUTIONS & CONSIDERATIONS
Caution is warranted with hepatic or renal impairment or a history of allergies, especially to antibiotics. Aztreonam crosses the placenta and is distributed in amniotic fluid and in low concentrations in breast milk. The safety and efficacy of aztreonam have not been established in children < 9 mo old. Age-related renal impairment may require a dosage adjustment in the elderly. History of allergies, especially to antibiotics, should be determined before giving aztreonam. Cross-reactivity of aztreonam is extremely rare, but give with caution if a history of serious hypersensitivity to beta-lactams.

GI discomfort, nausea, and vomiting may occur. Pattern of daily bowel activity and stool consistency and skin for rash should be assessed. Signs and symptoms of phlebitis, such as heat, pain, red streaking over the vein, and pain at the IM injection site, should also be assessed. Be alert for signs and symptoms of superinfection, including anal or genital pruritus, black hairy tongue, vomiting, diarrhea, fever, sore throat, and ulceration or changes of oral mucosa.

Storage
Store vials at room temperature. The solution normally appears colorless to light yellow. After reconstitution, the solution is stable for 48 h at room temperature and 7 days if refrigerated. Discard the solution if a precipitate forms. Discard unused portions of solution. After reconstitution for IM injection, the solution is stable for 48 h at room temperature and 7 days if refrigerated.

Administration
For IV push, dilute each gram with 6-10 mL of sterile water for injection. Administer IV push, over 3-5 min. For intermittent IV infusion, further dilute with 50-100 mL of D5W or 0.9% NaCl. Administer IV infusion over 20-60 min.

For IM use, shake the vial immediately and vigorously after adding the diluent. Inject the drug deep into a large muscle mass.

Do not reconstitute aztreonam for inhalation until ready to use. Use the diluent supplied by manufacturer and squeeze contents into the aztreonam vial. Gently swirl until dissolved. Give bronchodilator prior to aztreonam nebulizer. For patients taking multiple inhaled therapies, use bronchodilator first, then mucolytic, and then aztreonam. Administer via an Altera Nebulizer System only. Do not mix any with any other drugs. Administration typically takes 2-3 min.

Bacitracin

bass-i-tray'sin

★ Baci-IM 🍁 Baciject, Bacitin

Do not confuse bacitracin with Bactrim or Bactroban.

CATEGORY AND SCHEDULE

Pregnancy Risk Category: C

Rx/OTC

Classification: Anti-infective, polypeptide antibiotics

MECHANISM OF ACTION

An antibiotic that interferes with plasma membrane permeability and inhibits bacterial cell wall synthesis in susceptible bacteria. *Therapeutic Effect:* Bacteriostatic. Primarily active against gram-positive organisms.

PHARMACOKINETICS

Poorly absorbed from mucous membranes or intact or denuded skin. Rapidly and completely absorbed following IM administration. Not absorbed with bladder irrigation but can be absorbed with mediastinal or peritoneal lavage. Excreted slowly by glomerular filtration.

AVAILABILITY

Powder for Injection: 50,000 units.
Ophthalmic Ointment: 500 units/g.
Topical Ointment: 500 units/g.

INDICATIONS AND DOSAGES

▸ **Superficial ocular infections**

OPHTHALMIC

Adults: ½-inch ribbon in conjunctival sac q3-4h.

▸ **Skin abrasions, superficial skin infections**

TOPICAL

Adults, Children. Apply to affected area 1-5 times/day.

▸ **Surgical treatment and prophylaxis**

IRRIGATION (OFF-LABEL USE)

Adults, Elderly. 50,000-150,000 units, as needed; typically dissolved in 1000 mL sterile NS or sterile water for irrigation.

▸ **Pneumonia and empyema caused by susceptible staphylococci**

IM

Infants weighing < 2500 g. 900 units/kg/24 h in 2-3 divided doses.
Infants weighing more than 2500 g. 1000 units/kg/24 h in 2-3 divided doses.

CONTRAINDICATIONS

None known.

INTERACTIONS

Drug

Aminoglycosides, polymyxin B, colistin, cisplatin, amphotericin B, foscarnet, vancomycin, others: Avoid concurrent use of other nephrotoxic medications when possible when bacitracin is given systemically.

Neuromuscular blockers: Systemic use during surgery may increase or prolong skeletal muscle relaxation of neuromuscular blockers.

Herbal

None known.

Food

None known.

DIAGNOSTIC TEST EFFECTS

None known.

SIDE EFFECTS

Rare

IM: Rash, nausea, vomiting, pain at injection site.
Ophthalmic: Burning, itching, redness, swelling, pain.
Topical: Hypersensitivity reaction (allergic contact dermatitis, burning, inflammation, pruritus).

B

SERIOUS REACTIONS

- Severe hypersensitivity reactions, including apnea and hypotension, occur rarely.
- Renal failure due to glomerular and tubular necrosis (occurs commonly with systemic use but may also occur with topical irrigation).

PRECAUTIONS & CONSIDERATIONS

! When administering a fixed-combination product containing bacitracin, be familiar with the side effects of each of the product's drug components. History of allergies, especially to bacitracin, should be determined before giving the drug.

Burning, itching, increased irritation, and rash should be reported immediately. Be alert for signs and symptoms of hypersensitivity, such as burning, inflammation, and pruritus. When using preparations containing corticosteroids, closely monitor the patient for any unusual signs or symptoms because corticosteroids may mask clinical signs.

Monitor renal function closely with use of the injectable. Maintain adequate hydration. Discontinue therapy if renal toxicity occurs.

Storage

Topical and ophthalmic products may be stored at room temperature. Store unreconstituted powder for injection in refrigerator. Reconstituted solutions are stable for 1 wk when stored in the refrigerator. Topical irrigations may be stored for up to 3 days.

Administration

For ophthalmic use, place a gloved finger on the lower eyelid and pull it out until a pocket is formed between the eye and lower lid. Place ¼ to ½ inch of the ointment in the pocket. Close the eye gently for 1-2 min and roll the eyeball to increase the drug's contact with the eye. Remove excess ointment around the eye with a tissue.

For IM use, dilute powder for injection with NS containing 2% procaine HCl to a concentration between 5000 and 10,000 units/mL. Diluents containing parabens should not be used as they cause cloudy solutions or precipitate formation. IM injections should be given in the upper outer quadrant of the buttocks, alternating right and left and avoiding multiple injections in the same region.

Baclofen

bak'loe-fen

Lioresal

Do not confuse baclofen with Bactroban or Beclovent.

CATEGORY AND SCHEDULE

Pregnancy Risk Category: C

Classification: Skeletal muscle relaxant, central acting

MECHANISM OF ACTION

A direct-acting skeletal muscle relaxant that inhibits transmission of reflexes at the spinal cord level. *Therapeutic Effect:* Relieves muscle spasticity.

PHARMACOKINETICS

Well absorbed from the GI tract. Protein binding: 30%. Partially metabolized in the liver. Primarily excreted in urine. *Half-life:* 2.5-4 h; intrathecal: 1.5 h.

AVAILABILITY

Tablets: 10 mg, 20 mg.
Intrathecal Injection: 50 mcg/mL, 500 mcg/mL, 2000 mcg/mL.

INDICATIONS AND DOSAGES

▸ **Spasticity**

PO

Adults. Initially, 5 mg 3 times/day. May increase by 15 mg/day at 3-day intervals. Range: 40-80 mg/day. Maximum: 80 mg/day.

Elderly. Initially, 5 mg 2-3 times/day. May gradually increase dosage.

USUAL MAINTENANCE INTRATHECAL DOSAGE

NOTE: Initial titration and close monitoring are required. Maintenance doses vary, these represent general ranges only.

Adults, Elderly, Children older than 12 yr. 100-700 mcg/day.

Children 12 yr and younger. 100-300 mcg/day.

OFF-LABEL USES

Treatment of trigeminal neuralgia, hiccups.

CONTRAINDICATIONS

Hypersensitivity.

INTERACTIONS

Drug

Alcohol, other CNS depressants: May increase CNS depression.

Morphine epidural (when intrathecal baclofen used): Increased risk for hypotension or dyspnea.

Herbal

None known.

Food

None known.

DIAGNOSTIC TEST EFFECTS

May increase blood glucose level and serum alkaline phosphatase, AST (SGOT), and ALT (SGPT) levels.

SIDE EFFECTS

Frequent (> 10%)

Transient somnolence, asthenia, dizziness, light-headedness, nausea, vomiting.

Occasional (2%-10%)

Headache, paresthesia, constipation, anorexia, hypotension, confusion, nasal congestion.

Rare (< 1%)

Paradoxical CNS excitement or restlessness, slurred speech, tremor, dry mouth, diarrhea, nocturia, impotence.

SERIOUS REACTIONS

- Abrupt discontinuation of baclofen may produce hallucinations and seizures and rebound spasticity (may be severe on abrupt withdrawal of intrathecal).
- Overdose results in blurred vision, seizures, myosis, mydriasis, severe muscle weakness, strabismus, respiratory depression, and vomiting.

PRECAUTIONS & CONSIDERATIONS

Caution is warranted with diabetes mellitus, epilepsy, impaired renal function, preexisting psychiatric disorders, and a history of CVA. Baclofen is distributed in breast milk; avoidance of breastfeeding is recommended. Due to a potential for adverse fetal effects, use is not recommended during pregnancy. The safety and efficacy of baclofen have not been established in children younger than 12 yr for the oral, and 4 yr for intrathecal, forms. Elderly patients may require decreased dosage because of age-related renal impairment. They are also at increased risk for CNS toxicity, manifested as confusion, hallucinations, depression, and sedation.

Drowsiness may occur but is usually diminished with continued therapy. Avoid alcohol, CNS depressants, and tasks that require mental alertness or motor skills. Blood counts and liver and renal function tests should be obtained periodically for those on long-term therapy. Therapeutic response, such as decreased intensity of skeletal muscle pain, should be assessed. For patients receiving intrathecal baclofen, watch for symptoms that may indicate overdose; the patient should be taken immediately to a hospital for assessment and emptying of the pump reservoir and appropriate management if such symptoms occur.

Storage

Oral: Room temperature. Keep tightly closed.
Intrathecal: Do not freeze. Do not heat sterilize.

Administration

Take baclofen without regard to food. Crush tablets as needed. Do not abruptly discontinue the drug after long-term therapy.

Prior to pump implantation and initiation of chronic infusion of baclofen intrathecal, patients must demonstrate a positive clinical response to a bolus dose administered intrathecally in a screening trial. After the screening trial, a pump specifically approved for baclofen intrathecal injection administration is implanted and filled. Physicians must be adequately trained/educated in chronic intrathecal infusion therapy.

For patients requiring dilutions of medication other than the available manufacturer concentrations, the drug must be diluted with preservative-free NS. During periodic refills of the pump, the daily dose may be increased by no more than 5%-20% to maintain adequate symptom control. The daily dose may be reduced by 10%-20% if side effects occur.

Balsalazide

ball-sal'a-zide

★ Colazal

Do not confuse Colazal with Clozaril.

CATEGORY AND SCHEDULE

Pregnancy Risk Category: B

Classification: GI anti-inflammatory, 5-aminosalicylates

MECHANISM OF ACTION

A 5-aminosalicylic acid derivative that changes intestinal microflora, altering prostaglandin production and inhibiting function of natural killer cells, mast cells, neutrophils, and macrophages. *Therapeutic Effect:* Diminishes inflammatory effect in colon.

PHARMACOKINETICS

Drug reaches colon intact; bacterial azoreductases release 5-aminobenzyl-*B*-analine and mesalamine (active metabolite); low, variable systemic absorption; peak concentration 1-2 h, protein binding ≈99%; < 1% renal excretion; most excreted in feces (65%).

AVAILABILITY

Capsules: 750 mg.

INDICATIONS AND DOSAGES

▸ **Ulcerative colitis**

PO

Adults, Elderly. Three 750-mg capsules 3 times/day for 8-12 wks.
Children 5-17 yr. Three 750-mg capsules 3 times/day or one 750-mg capsule 3 times/day for 8 wks.

CONTRAINDICATIONS

Hypersensitivity to 5-aminosalicylates, and salicylates.

INTERACTIONS

Drug

6-mercaptopurine or thioguanine: Balsalazide may inhibit action of TPMT, an enzyme that metabolizes these chemotherapies, and may increase risk of bone marrow suppression/toxicity.

Warfarin: Rare reports of increased INR; monitor.

Herbal

None known.

Food

None known.

SIDE EFFECTS

Frequent (6%-8%)

Headache, abdominal pain, nausea, diarrhea.

Occasional (2%-4%)

Vomiting, arthralgia, rhinitis, insomnia, fatigue, flatulence, coughing, dyspepsia.

SERIOUS REACTIONS

• Liver toxicity occurs rarely.

PRECAUTIONS & CONSIDERATIONS

Caution is warranted with renal disease or renal impairment. Notify the physician if abdominal pain, severe headache or chest pain, or unresolved diarrhea occurs. Watch for any worsening of ulcerative colitis symptoms. Patients with pyloric stenosis may have prolonged gastric retention of the drug. Serum chemistry laboratory values, including BUN, alkaline phosphatase, bilirubin, creatinine, AST (SGOT), and ALT (SGPT) levels, should be obtained before treatment.

Storage

Store at room temperature.

Administration

May administer without regard to food. For patients with difficulty swallowing, the capsules may be opened and the contents sprinkled on applesauce and immediately consumed. The contents may be chewed if necessary. Teeth and tongue staining may occur in some patients taking balsalazide sprinkled on applesauce.

Basiliximab

bay-zul-ix'ah-mab

★ 🍁 Simulect

Do not confuse with daclizumab.

CATEGORY AND SCHEDULE

Pregnancy Risk Category: B

Classification:

Immunosuppressives, monoclonal antibodies

MECHANISM OF ACTION

A monoclonal antibody that binds to and blocks the receptor of interleukin-2, a protein that stimulates the proliferation of T lymphocytes, which play a major role in organ transplant rejection. *Therapeutic Effect:* Prevents lymphocytic activity and impairs response of the immune system to antigens, which prevents acute renal transplant rejection.

PHARMACOKINETICS

Half-life: Adults, 4-10 days; children, 5-17 days.

AVAILABILITY

Powder for Injection: 10 mg, 20 mg.

B

INDICATIONS AND DOSAGES

▸ **Prevention of acute organ rejection in patients receiving a kidney transplant, with cyclosporine and corticosteriods**

IV

Adults, Elderly, Children weighing 35 kg or more. 20 mg within 2 h before transplant surgery and 20 mg 4 days after transplant.

Children weighing < 35 kg. 10 mg within 2 h before transplant surgery and 10 mg 4 days after transplant.

OFF-LABEL USES

Prevention of acute organ rejection following liver transplant.

CONTRAINDICATIONS

Hypersensitivity to basiliximab, murine proteins, or any component of the formulation such as mannitol hypersensitivity.

INTERACTIONS

Drug

Live-virus vaccines: Defer until immune function improves.

DIAGNOSTIC TEST EFFECTS

May increase BUN and serum cholesterol, creatinine, and uric acid levels. May decrease platelet count and serum magnesium and phosphate levels. May increase or decrease blood glucose, hematocrit, hemoglobin level, and serum calcium and potassium levels.

IV INCOMPATIBILITIES

Specific information is not available. Do not infuse other drugs through the same IV line.

SIDE EFFECTS

Frequent (> 10%)

GI disturbances (constipation, diarrhea, dyspepsia), CNS effects (dizziness, headache, insomnia, tremor), respiratory tract infection, dysuria, acne, leg or back pain, peripheral edema, hypertension.

Occasional (3%-10%)

Angina, neuropathy, abdominal distention, tachycardia, rash, hypotension, urinary disturbances (urinary frequency, genital edema, hematuria), arthralgia, hirsutism, myalgia.

SERIOUS REACTIONS

- Serious hypersensitivity, including anaphylactic shock; risk increases with repeat cycles.
- Capillary-leak syndrome.

PRECAUTIONS & CONSIDERATIONS

Caution is warranted in patients with infection and a history of malignancy. It is unknown whether basiliximab crosses the placenta or is distributed in breast milk. Basiliximab is not recommended for breastfeeding or pregnant women; avoid pregnancy. No age-related precautions have been noted in children or in elderly patients.

Notify the physician of fever, sore throat, unusual bleeding or bruising, difficulty breathing or swallowing, itching, rapid heartbeat, rash, swelling of lower extremities, or weakness. BUN, blood glucose, serum calcium, creatinine, alkaline phosphatase, potassium, uric acid levels, vital signs, particularly BP and pulse rate, should be assessed before and during therapy. Patients previously administered basiliximab should only be reexposed with extreme caution.

Storage

Refrigerate unopened vials. Do not freeze. Use drug within 4 h after reconstitution (within 24 h if refrigerated).

Administration

Discard the solution if a precipitate forms. Reconstitute 10-mg vial with

2.5 mL, and 20-mg vial with 5 mL, of sterile water for injection. Shake gently to dissolve. If administered as injection, further dilution is not needed. Dilute 10 mg in 25 mL or 20 mg in 50 mL of 0.9% NaCl or D5W if going to give as IV infusion. Gently invert to avoid foaming. Infuse over 20-30 min.

BCG, Intravesical

bee cee jee in'tra-ves-i-cal
★ TheraCys, Tice BCG
🍁 OncoTICE, ImmuCyst

CATEGORY AND SCHEDULE

Pregnancy Risk Category: C

Classification: Antineoplastics, biological response modifiers

MECHANISM OF ACTION

An antineoplastic that produces a local inflammatory reaction with histiocytic and leukocytic infiltration in the urinary bladder. *Therapeutic Effect:* Decreases superficial cancerous lesions in the urinary bladder.

AVAILABILITY

Vials: 50 mg (Tice BCG), 81 mg (TheraCys).

INDICATIONS AND DOSAGES

▸ **Treatment and prevention of bladder carcinoma in situ; prophylaxis of primary or recurrent stage Ta and/or T1 papillary tumors following transurethral resection**

INTRAVESICAL (THERACYS)

Adults, Elderly. One dose in 50 mL 0.9% NaCl once weekly for 6 wks, then repeated 3, 6, 12, 18, and 24 mo after initial treatment. Begin 7-14 days after biopsy or transurethral resection.

INTRAVESICAL (TICE BCG)

Adults, Elderly. One dose in 50 mL 0.9% NaCl once weekly for 6 wks; may repeat once. Thereafter, continue monthly for 6-12 mo.

CONTRAINDICATIONS

Hypersensitivity. Compromised immune system, concurrent corticosteroid or immunosuppressive therapy, fever from infection or undetermined cause, HIV infection, active tuberculosis, or urinary tract infection.

INTERACTIONS

Drug

Bone marrow depressants, immunosuppressants: May decrease the immune response and increase the risk of osteomyelitis and disseminated BCG infection.

Live-virus vaccines: May potentiate virus replication, increase vaccine side effects, and decrease the patient's antibody response to the vaccine.

DIAGNOSTIC TEST EFFECTS

Falsely positive tuberculin reaction.

SIDE EFFECTS

Frequent

Dysuria, urinary frequency, hematuria, hypersensitivity reaction (manifested as malaise, fever, chills).

Occasional

Cystitis, urinary urgency, nausea, vomiting, anorexia, diarrhea, myalgia, arthralgia.

SERIOUS REACTIONS

- Disseminated BCG infection is usually characterized by a fever higher than 103° F (or persistently higher than 101° F for more than 2 days), chills, and severe malaise.

PRECAUTIONS & CONSIDERATIONS

BCG is an infectious agent. Instillation of the drug with an actively bleeding mucosa may promote systemic BCG infection.

Postpone for at least 1 wk following transurethral resection, biopsy, traumatic catheterization, or gross hematuria.

Before beginning treatment, establish renal status; obtain a urine specimen for culture and sensitivity tests to rule out a urinary tract infection; determine medications the person is taking concurrently, especially corticosteroids and immunosuppressants; and determine whether the person has compromised immune system, has a fever, or is HIV positive. Immunizations and coming in contact with those who have recently received a live-virus vaccine should be avoided during BCG treatment. Use is not recommended during pregnancy, and it is advisable to discontinue breastfeeding during treatment.

Notify the physician if blood in urine, chills, fever, frequent or painful urination, joint pain, or nausea or vomiting occurs. Renal status should be diligently monitored. Dysuria, hematuria, urinary frequency, and urinalysis should be assessed to check for urinary tract infection.

Storage

Store vials in refrigerator. Store reconstituted solution in refrigerator and use within 2 h.

Administration

! Be aware that BCG contains live, attenuated mycobacteria. Treat the drug as infectious material, and use protective gear when reconstituting it. Avoid contact with the drug if immunocompromised. Prepare intravesical product in a biological safety cabinet and handle using aseptic technique. All equipment and supplies used should be disposed of as biohazards. Do not prepare parenteral drugs in areas where BCG has been prepared.

For intravesical use, reconstitute the powder immediately before administration. Discard any unused portion within 2 h of reconstitution. After adding diluent to the powder, gently swirl the solution, or repeatedly inject and withdraw the solution from the vial until the solution is mixed. Avoid vigorous shaking, which could cause foaming.

Wear gloves, gown, and mask to avoid inadvertent exposure to BCG organisms while administering the solution. Patients should not drink liquids for 4 h prior to treatment and should empty their bladder prior to BCG administration.

The drug is instilled via gravity flow through a urethral catheter. During the first hour of drug administration, the patient should lie in different positions (supine, prone, and both sides) for 15 min each to allow the drug to come in contact with all parts of the bladder. The patient should try to retain the solution for 2 h after instillation to avoid spraying or splashing the infected urine. All urine should be disinfected when expelled within 6 h of drug instillation with an equal volume of 5% hypochlorite solution (undiluted household bleach) and allowed to stand 15 min before flushing.

Becaplermin

beh-cap′lear-min

★ 🍁 Regranex

Do not confuse Regranex with Repronex or Granulex.

CATEGORY AND SCHEDULE

Pregnancy Risk Category: C

Classification: Topical wound repair, recombinant human platelet-derived growth factor

MECHANISM OF ACTION

A platelet-derived growth factor that heals open wounds. *Therapeutic Effect:* Promotes chemotactic recruitment and proliferation of cells involved in wound repair and enhances the formation of granulation tissue.

PHARMACOKINETICS

Minimal systemic absorption when applied to wounds; bioavailability roughly 3%.

AVAILABILITY

Gel: 0.01% (Regranex).

INDICATIONS AND DOSAGES

▸ **Diabetic foot ulcer and decubitus ulcers**

TOPICAL

Adults, Elderly. Apply once daily and leave in place for 12 h before removal (see Administration). Amount to be applied is calculated in cm according to ulcer size; each square cm of ulcer surface will require roughly a 0.25-cm length of gel squeezed from a 15-g tube.

CONTRAINDICATIONS

Neoplasms at site of application, hypersensitivity to becaplermin or any component of the formulation.

INTERACTIONS

Drug

None known.

Herbal

None known.

Food

None known.

DIAGNOSTIC TEST EFFECTS

None known.

SIDE EFFECTS

Occasional

Local rash near ulcer.

SERIOUS REACTIONS

• An increase in mortality due to secondary malignancy; risk increased in those treated with > 3 tubes.

PRECAUTIONS & CONSIDERATIONS

Caution should be used on wounds showing exposed joints, tendons, ligaments, or bones. It is unknown whether becaplermin crosses the placenta or is distributed in breast milk. Safety and efficacy have not been established in children < 16 yr of age. There are no age-related precautions noted in elderly patients.

Storage

Refrigerate gel. Do not freeze.

Administration

Measure gel on a clean, nonabsorbable surface. Transfer to ulcer and spread as a thin, continuous layer onto the ulcer. Cover site with saline-moistened dressing for approx. 12 h. Remove and wash any residual gel from ulcer and replace with new gauze pad moistened with 0.9% NaCl until next application. Dose requires recalculation weekly or biweekly, depending on the rate of change in the width and length of ulcer.

Beclomethasone Dipropionate

be-kloe-meth′a-sone di-pro′-pi-o-nate

★ Beconase AQ, QVAR

🍁 Rivanase AQ

Do not confuse Beconase AQ with baclofen.

CATEGORY AND SCHEDULE

Pregnancy Risk Category: C

Classification: Corticosteroids, halogenated

MECHANISM OF ACTION

An adrenocorticosteroid that prevents or controls inflammation by controlling the rate of protein synthesis, decreasing migration of polymorphonuclear leukocytes and fibroblasts, and reversing capillary permeability.
Therapeutic Effect: Inhalation: Inhibits bronchoconstriction, produces smooth muscle relaxation, decreases mucus secretion. Intranasal: Decreases response to seasonal and perennial allergens.

PHARMACOKINETICS

Rapidly absorbed from pulmonary, nasal, and GI tissue. Undergoes extensive first-pass metabolism in the liver. Protein binding: 87%. Primarily eliminated in feces. *Half-life:* 15 h.

AVAILABILITY

Oral Inhalation (QVAR): 40 mcg per inhalation, 80 mcg/inhalation.
Nasal spray (Beconase AQ): 42 mcg/spray.

INDICATIONS AND DOSAGES

▸ Long-term control of bronchial asthma, reduces need for oral corticosteroid therapy for asthma

ORAL INHALATION

Adults, Elderly, Children 12 yr and older. 40-160 mcg twice a day. Maximum: 320 mcg twice a day.
Children 5-11 yr. 40 mcg twice a day. Maximum: 80 mcg twice a day.

▸ Relief of seasonal or perennial rhinitis, prevention of nasal polyp recurrence after surgical removal, treatment of nonallergic rhinitis

NASAL INHALATION

Adults, Children older than 12 yr. 1-2 sprays in each nostril twice a day.
Children 6-12 yr. 1 spray in each nostril twice a day. May increase up to 2 sprays in each nostril twice a day.

CONTRAINDICATIONS

Hypersensitivity to beclomethasone, status asthmaticus.

INTERACTIONS

Drug
None known.
Herbal
None known.
Food
None known.

DIAGNOSTIC TEST EFFECTS

None known.

SIDE EFFECTS

Frequent
Inhalation (4%-14%): Throat irritation, dry mouth, hoarseness, cough.
Intranasal: Nasal burning, mucosal dryness.
Occasional
Inhalation (2%-3%): Localized fungal infection (thrush).
Intranasal: Nasal-crusting epistaxis, sore throat, ulceration of nasal mucosa.
Rare
Inhalation: Transient bronchospasm, esophageal candidiasis.
Intranasal: Nasal and pharyngeal candidiasis, eye pain.

SERIOUS REACTIONS

- An acute hypersensitivity reaction, as evidenced by urticaria, angioedema, and severe bronchospasm, occurs rarely.
- A transfer from systemic to local steroid therapy may unmask previously suppressed bronchial asthma condition.

• Potential adrenal insufficiency if used to replace systemic corticosteriod use.
• Signs and symptoms of hypercorticism.
• Nasal septum perforation with chronic use and improper technique.

PRECAUTIONS & CONSIDERATIONS

Caution is warranted with cirrhosis, glaucoma, hypothyroidism, osteoporosis, tuberculosis, and untreated systemic infections. Avoid nasal corticosteroid use in patients with recent nasal septal ulcers, nasal surgery, or nasal trauma until healing has occurred. It is unknown whether beclomethasone crosses the placenta or is distributed in breast milk. In children, prolonged treatment and high doses may decrease cortisol secretion and the short-term growth rate. No age-related precautions have been noted in elderly patients.

Those receiving beclomethasone by inhalation should maintain fastidious oral hygiene; notify the physician or nurse if sore throat or mouth develops. If using a bronchodilator inhaler concomitantly with a steroid inhaler, use the bronchodilator several minutes before using the corticosteroid to help the steroid penetrate into the bronchial tree. Those using beclomethasone intranasally should notify the physician if nasal irritation occurs or if symptoms, such as sneezing, fail to improve. Persons who are using drugs that suppress the immune system are more susceptible to infections than healthy individuals are.

Storage

Store respiratory inhalation and nasal spray at room temperature.

Administration

For inhalation, first shake the container well. Exhale completely and place the mouthpiece between the lips. Inhale and hold the breath for as long as possible before exhaling. Allow at least 1 min between inhalations. Rinse mouth after each use. Do not change the beclomethasone dosage schedule or stop taking the drug abruptly; taper dosage gradually under medical supervision.

For intranasal use, clear nasal passages as much as possible. The first time the nasal spray is used, or if it has not been used for 7 days, prime the pump by spraying away from others into the air; press down and release 6 times or until a fine mist appears. Insert the spray tip into the nostril, pointing toward the nasal passages, away from the nasal septum. Spray beclomethasone into the nostril while holding the other nostril closed, and at the same time, inhale through the nose to deliver the medication as high into the nasal passages as possible. Do not change the beclomethasone dosage schedule or stop taking the drug abruptly; taper dosage gradually under medical supervision.

Belladonna Alkaloids; Phenobarbital

bell-a-don′a al′kuh-loydz

★ 🍁 Donnatal, Donnatal Extentabs, Medi-Tal, Antispasmodic Elixir

CATEGORY AND SCHEDULE

Pregnancy Risk Category: C

Classification: Anticholinergic, antispasmodic, gastrointestinal

MECHANISM OF ACTION

Competitive inhibitors of the muscarinic actions of acetylcholine act at receptors located in exocrine glands, smooth and cardiac muscle, and intramural neurons. Composed of 3 main constituents: atropine, scopolamine, and hyoscyamine. Scopolamine exerts greater effects on the CNS, eye, and secretory glands than the constituents atropine and hyoscyamine. Atropine exerts more activity on the heart, intestine, and bronchial muscle and exhibits a more prolonged duration of action compared with scopolamine. Hyoscyamine exerts similar actions to atropine but has more potent central and peripheral nervous system effects. *Therapeutic Effect:* Peripheral anticholinergic and antispasmodic action, mild sedation.

PHARMACOKINETICS

None known.

AVAILABILITY

Combination products:

Tablets: Hyoscyamine sulfate 0.1037 mg, atropine sulfate 0.0194 mg, scopolamine hydrobromide 0.0065 mg, and phenobarbital 16.2 mg (Donnatal).

Tablets, Extended Release: Hyoscyamine sulfate 0.3111 mg, atropine sulfate 0.0582 mg, scopolamine hydrobromide 0.0195 mg, and phenobarbital 48.6 mg (Donnatal Extentabs).

Elixir: Hyoscyamine sulfate 0.1037 mg, atropine sulfate 0.0194 mg, scopolamine hydrobromide 0.0065 mg, and phenobarbital 16.2 mg per 5 mL (Antispasmodic, Donnatal).

INDICATIONS AND DOSAGES

▸ Irritable bowel syndrome, acute enterocolitis

NOTE: FDA has not evaluated for safety and efficacy; it is "possibly effective." No children's dose is presented here, despite manufacturer labeling, due to lack of FDA approval.

PO (IMMEDIATE-RELEASE DOSAGE FORMS)

Adults. 1-2 tablets 3-4 times daily or 1-2 tsp of elixir 3-4 times daily according to conditions and severity of symptoms.

PO (EXTENDED-RELEASE TABLETS)

Adults. 1 tablet every 12 h; may give every 8 h if needed.

CONTRAINDICATIONS

Narrow-angle glaucoma, obstructive uropathy, obstructive disease of tract, paralytic ileus, intestinal atony of the elderly or debilitated patient, tachycardia, acute myocardial ischemia, unstable cardiovascular status in acute hemorrhage, severe ulcerative colitis, especially if complicated by toxic megacolon, myasthenia gravis, hiatal hernia associated with reflux esophagitis, hypersensitivity to any component of the formulation, acute intermittent porphyria.

INTERACTIONS

Drug

NOTE: Phenobarbital increases the metabolism of many medications, including hormonal contraceptives, antiretroviral medications for HIV, theophylline, warfarin, and other narrow-therapeutic index drugs.

Oral medications: Belladonna decreases gastric emptying time therefore affecting absorption of orally administered agents.

Anticholinergic drugs: May enhance anticholinergic effect.

Tricyclic antidepressants: May enhance anticholinergic effect.

Cisapride: Atropine may decrease effects of cisapride.

Antiarrhythmics: May result in additive antivagal effects on atrioventricular nodal conduction.

Alcohol: May result in additive CNS depression.

Cholinesterase inhibitors for dementia: Belladonna alkaloids may counteract the actions of these drugs.
Herbal
Anticholinergic herbs: May enhance anticholinergic effect.
Food
None known.

DIAGNOSTIC TEST EFFECTS
None known.

SIDE EFFECTS
Frequent
Dry mouth, urinary retention, flushing, pupillary dilation, constipation, confusion, redness of the skin, flushing, dry skin, allergic contact dermatitis, headache, excitement, agitation, dizziness, light-headedness, drowsiness, unsteadiness, confusion, slurred speech, sedation, hyperreflexia, convulsions, vertigo, coma, mydriasis, photophobia, blurred vision, dilation of pupils.
Rare
Hallucinations, acute psychosis, Stevens-Johnson syndrome, photosensitivity.

SERIOUS REACTIONS
• Signs and symptoms of overdose include headache, nausea, vomiting, blurred vision, dilated pupils, hot and dry skin, dizziness, dryness of the mouth, difficulty in swallowing, and CNS stimulation, coma.

PRECAUTIONS & CONSIDERATIONS
Caution is warranted with ulcerative colitis or intestinal disease, coronary artery disease, dehydration, diarrhea caused by poisoning, Down syndrome, acute dysentery, glaucoma, hepatic and renal function impairment, hiatal hernia, prostatic hyperplasia, urinary retention, asthma, COPD, and brain damage. Belladonna alkaloids cross the placenta and are distributed into breast milk. Consider additional or alternative methods of contraception or higher-dose hormonal contraceptives since phenobarbital may interfere with hormonal contraceptive efficacy. Safety and efficacy have not been established in children younger than 6 yr. Infants and young children may be more susceptible to adverse effects of belladonna alkaloids. Elderly patients may be more susceptible to the anticholinergic effects; avoid use in this population.

Constipation, difficulty urinating, decreased sweating, drowsiness, dry mouth, increased heart rate, headache, orthostatic hypotension may occur. Change positions slowly to avoid light-headedness. Avoid alcohol, CNS depressants, and tasks that require mental alertness.
Storage
Store at room temperature.
Administration
Dose should be adjusted to the needs of the individual to assume symptomatic control with minimum adverse effects. Do not crush, cut, or chew extended-release tablets.

Belladonna and Opium
bell-a-don'a

CATEGORY AND SCHEDULE
Pregnancy Risk Category: C
Controlled Substance Schedule: II

Classification: Analgesics, narcotic, anticholinergics

MECHANISM OF ACTION
Anticholinergic alkaloids that inhibit the action of acetylcholine at postganglionic (muscarinic) receptor

B

sites. Opium contains more than 20 alkaloids, such as morphine (10%), narcotine (6%), papaverine (1%), and codeine (0.5%). Morphine depresses cerebral cortex, hypothalamus, and medullary centers. *Therapeutic Effect:* Decreases digestive secretions, increases GI muscle tone, reduces GI force, reduces ureteral spasm, and alters pain perception and emotional response to pain.

PHARMACOKINETICS

Onset of action occurs within 30 min. Absorption is dependent on body hydration. Oxidative dealkylation produces active compounds that impart analgesia. Morphine is conjugated in the liver to form the 3-glucuronide, which passes into the bile and is reabsorbed and excreted in the urine.

AVAILABILITY

Suppository: 16.2 mg belladonna extract/30 mg opium, 16.2 mg belladonna extract/60 mg opium.

INDICATIONS AND DOSAGES

▸ **Pain associated with ureteral spasm not responsive to conventional analgesics**

RECTAL

Adults, Elderly. 1 suppository 1-2 times/day. Maximum: 4 doses/day.

CONTRAINDICATIONS

Glaucoma, severe renal or hepatic disease, bronchial asthma, respiratory depression, convulsive disorders, acute alcoholism, premature labor, hypersensitivity to belladonna or opium or product components.

INTERACTIONS

Drug

Alcohol, CNS depressants: May increase CNS or respiratory depression, hypotension.

Anticholinergics: May increase the effects of belladonna and opium.

Phenothiazines: May decrease the antipsychotic effects of these drugs.

Cholinesterase inhibitors for dementia: Belladonna alkaloids may counteract the actions of these drugs.

Herbal

None known.

Food

None known.

DIAGNOSTIC TEST EFFECTS

May increase serum SGOT (AST) and SGPT (ALT) levels.

SIDE EFFECTS

Frequent

Dry mouth, nose, skin, and throat; decreased sweating; constipation; irritation at site of administration; drowsiness; urinary retention; dizziness.

Occasional

Blurred vision, decreased flow of breast milk, bloated feeling, drowsiness, headache, intolerance to light, nervousness, and flushing.

Rare

Dizziness, faintness, pruritus, urticaria.

SERIOUS REACTIONS

- Respiratory depression, increased intraocular pain, loss of memory, orthostatic hypotension, tachycardia, and ventricular fibrillation rarely occur.
- Tolerance to the drug's analgesic effect and physical dependence may occur with repeated use.

PRECAUTIONS & CONSIDERATIONS

True addiction may result from opium usage. Extreme caution should be used with acute alcoholism, anoxia, CNS depression, hypercapnia, respiratory depression or dysfunction, seizures, shock, and untreated myxedema. Caution is also warranted with acute abdominal conditions, Addison disease, chronic obstructive pulmonary disease (COPD), hypothyroidism, impaired liver function, increased intracranial pressure, prostatic hypertrophy, and urethral stricture. It is unknown whether belladonna and opium cross the placenta or are distributed in breast milk. Children may be more susceptible to respiratory depression; not recommended for use in children < 12 yr of age. Elderly patients may also be more susceptible to respiratory depression, and the drug may cause paradoxical excitement. Age-related prostatic hypertrophy or obstruction and renal impairment may increase the risk of urinary retention, and dosage adjustment is recommended for elderly patients. Alcohol, tasks that require mental alertness and motor skills, hot baths, and saunas should be avoided.

Storage

Store at room temperature. Do not refrigerate and protect from moisture.

Administration

Remove wrapper. Moisten finger and suppository before rectal insertion.

Benazepril

be-naze'a-pril

Lotensin

Do not confuse benazepril with Benadryl, or Lotensin with Loniten or lovastatin

CATEGORY AND SCHEDULE

Pregnancy Risk Category: C (D if used in second or third trimester)

Classification: Antihypertensive agents, Angiotensin-converting enzyme inhibitors

MECHANISM OF ACTION

An ACE inhibitor that decreases the rate of conversion of angiotensin I to angiotensin II, a potent vasoconstrictor. Reduces peripheral arterial resistance. *Therapeutic Effect:* Lowers BP.

PHARMACOKINETICS

Route	Onset	Peak	Duration
PO	1 h	2-4 h	24 h

Partially absorbed from the GI tract. Protein binding: 97%. Metabolized in the liver to active metabolite. Primarily excreted in urine. Minimal removal by hemodialysis. *Half-life:* 35 min; metabolite 10-11 h.

AVAILABILITY

Tablets: 5 mg, 10 mg, 20 mg, 40 mg.

INDICATIONS AND DOSAGES

▸ **Hypertension (monotherapy)**

PO

Adults. Initially, 10 mg/day. Maintenance: 20-40 mg/day as single dose or in 2 divided doses. Maximum: 80 mg/day.

Elderly. Initially, 5-10 mg/day. Range: 20-40 mg/day.

Children 6 yr of age and older. Initially 0.2 mg/kg once daily (maximum: initially 5 mg/day). Maintenance: 0.1-0.6 mg/kg once daily. Maximum: 0.6 mg/kg (40 mg)/day.

▸ **Hypertension (combination therapy)**

PO

Adults. May discontinue diuretic 2-3 days before initiating benazepril, then dose as noted above. Diuretic can be reinitiated if needed. If unable to discontinue diuretic, begin benazepril at reduced dose of 5 mg/day.

▸ **Dosage in renal impairment**

For adult patients with creatinine clearance < 30 mL/min, initially, 5 mg/day titrated up to maximum

B

of 40 mg/day. Not recommended in children with creatinine clearance < 30 mL/min.

OFF-LABEL USES

Treatment of congestive heart failure, diabetic nephropathy.

CONTRAINDICATIONS

History of angioedema or allergy from previous treatment with ACE inhibitors. Also contraindicated in those experiencing angioedema in past from other causes (e.g., hereditary angioedema).

INTERACTIONS

Drug

Alcohol, antihypertensives, diuretics: May increase the effects of benazepril.

Lithium: May increase the lithium blood concentration and risk of lithium toxicity.

NSAIDs: May decrease the effects of benazepril.

Potassium-sparing diuretics, potassium supplements: May cause hyperkalemia. Avoid when possible.

Drospirenone-ethinyl estradiol: May cause hyperkalemia; monitor potassium carefully for the first month in which OC is instituted.

Herbal

None known.

Food

None known.

DIAGNOSTIC TEST EFFECTS

May increase BUN, serum alkaline phosphatase, serum bilirubin, serum potassium, AST (SGOT), and ALT (SGPT) levels. May decrease serum sodium levels. May cause positive antinuclear antibody titer.

SIDE EFFECTS

Frequent (3%-6%)

Cough, headache, dizziness.

Occasional (1-2%)

Fatigue, somnolence or drowsiness, nausea, hyperkalemia.

Rare (< 1%)

Rash, fever, myalgia, diarrhea, loss of taste.

SERIOUS REACTIONS

- Excessive hypotension ("first-dose syncope") may occur in patients with CHF and in those who are severely salt or volume depleted.
- Angioedema (swelling of the face and lips) and hyperkalemia occur rarely.
- Agranulocytosis and neutropenia may be noted in those with collagen vascular disease, including scleroderma and systemic lupus erythematosus, and impaired renal function.
- Nephrotic syndrome may be noted in patients with history of renal disease.
- Hyperkalemia.

PRECAUTIONS & CONSIDERATIONS

Patients with renal artery stenosis should not receive ACE inhibitors because renal insufficiency can result. Caution is warranted with cerebrovascular and coronary insufficiency, diabetes mellitus, hypovolemia, renal impairment, and sodium depletion as well as persons on dialysis and in those receiving diuretics. Benazepril crosses the placenta, and it is unknown whether it is distributed in breast milk. Benazepril may cause fetal or neonatal morbidity or mortality with exposure during the second or third trimesters. Discontinue use as soon as possible once pregnancy is detected. Safety and efficacy of benazepril have not been established in children < 6 yr of age. Elderly patients may be more sensitive to the hypotensive effects of benazepril.

Dizziness and orthostatic hypotension may occur. Rise slowly from lying to sitting position, and permit legs to dangle from the bed momentarily before standing to reduce the hypotensive effect of benazepril. Full therapeutic effect of benazepril may take 2-4 wks. BP should be obtained immediately before giving each benazepril dose, in addition to regular monitoring. Be alert to fluctuations in BP. If an excessive reduction in BP occurs, place the person in the supine position with legs elevated. CBC and blood chemistry should be obtained before beginning benazepril therapy, then every 2 wks for the next 3 mo, and periodically thereafter in patients with autoimmune disease or renal impairment and in those who are taking drugs that affect immune response or leukocyte count.

Storage

May store tablets at room temperature. Compounded oral suspension is stable for up to 30 days under refrigeration.

Administration

May take without regard to food. Do not skip doses. For those with swallowing diffculty, an oral suspension may be prepared by a pharmacist, in accordance with manufacturer recommendations. Shake well before each use and measure dose with a calibrated oral syringe or spoon.

Bendamustine

ben-da-muss'teen

★🍁 Treanda

CATEGORY AND SCHEDULE

Pregnancy Risk Category: D

Classification: Antineoplastic, alkylating agent, nitrogen mustard derivative

MECHANISM OF ACTION

An alkylating and antimetabolite agent that causes DNA strand breaks, resulting in apoptosis. Also inhibits several mitotic checkpoints, causing a necrotic form of cell death morphologically distinct from the alkylating actions. Cell cycle–phase nonspecific. *Therapeutic Effect:* Results in cancer cell death.

PHARMACOKINETICS

Drug is 95% protein-bound. Metabolism occurs primarily by hydrolysis via CYP1A2 isoenzyme to slightly active metabolites, γ-hydroxy bendamustine (M3) and N-desmethyl-bendamustine (M4). The parent compound is primarily responsible for cytotoxicity. Approximately 90% of any given dose is excreted in the feces. *Half-life:* 40 min after single dose (active metabolites: M3 half-life 3 h, M4 half-life 30 min).

AVAILABILITY

Powder for Injection: 25 mg, 100 mg.

INDICATIONS AND DOSAGES

NOTE: Dosages and regimens may depend on type of cancer and use in combination with other agents. See prescribing information.

▸ **Chronic lymphocytic leukemia (CLL)**

IV INFUSION

Adults, Elderly. 100 mg/m^2 IV over 30 min on days 1 and 2 of a 28-day cycle, up to 6 cycles. Hematologic or nonhematologic toxicities may require a reduction of dose to 25-50 mg/m^2, or a delay in treatment.

▸ **Indolent B-cell non-Hodgkin lymphoma**

IV INFUSION

Adults, Elderly. 120 mg/m^2 IV over 60 min on days 1 and 2 of a 21-day cycle, up to 8 cycles.

B

Hematologic or nonhematologic toxicities may require a reduction of dose to 60-90 mg/m^2 or a delay in treatment.

▸ **Moderate to severe hepatic impairment or renal impairment (CrCl < 40 mL/min)**

Use not recommended due to lack of clinical data.

IV INCOMPATIBILITIES

Do not mix with or infuse with other medications.

CONTRAINDICATIONS

Hypersensitivity to the drug or to mannitol.

INTERACTIONS

Drug

Allopurinol: May increase risk of serious skin reactions; monitor closely.

CYP1A2 inhibitors (e.g., fluvoxamine, ciprofloxacin): May increase concentrations and toxic effects of bendamustine.

CYP1A2 inducers (e.g., omeprazole, cigarette smoking): May alter therapeutic response to bendamustine by reducing bendamustine concentrations.

Digoxin: May reduce digoxin concentrations.

Herbal

None known.

Food

None known.

DIAGNOSTIC TEST EFFECTS

Increases in bilirubin, AST, ALT, uric acid; decreases in leukocyte, platelet, and RBC counts.

SIDE EFFECTS

Frequent (> 30%)

Nausea and vomiting, myelosuppression, pyrexia, diarrhea, fatigue or asthenia.

Occasional

Esophagitis, stomatitis, anorexia, dysphagia, weight loss, male infertility and azospermia, pneumonia, hypokalemia, dehydration, infusion-related reactions.

Rare

Thrombophlebitis.

SERIOUS REACTIONS

- Hematologic toxicity due to myelosuppression occurs frequently and includes thrombocytopenia and neutropenia. Neutropenia may lead to infection.
- Hyperbilirubinemia occurs frequently.
- Infusion-related reactions are common and may include anaphylactoid events; premedication with antihistamines, antipyretics, and corticosteroids may help attenuate.
- Hyperuricemia and tumor lysis syndrome.
- Skin reactions may be serious, and extravasation may lead to hospitalization for management.

PRECAUTIONS & CONSIDERATIONS

Administer with caution to patients with depressed platelet, leukocyte, or erythrocyte counts or with renal or hepatic impairment. Women of childbearing potential should be advised to avoid pregnancy, as the drug may cause fetal harm. Not recommended for use in breastfeeding. Safety and efficacy in children have not been established.

Nausea and vomiting occur frequently; prophylactic antiemetics are advised. Observe patient closely for signs of infusion-related reactions, skin reactions, immunosuppression, or infection. Advise patients to report shortness of breath, significant fatigue, bleeding, fever, or other signs of infection. Because patients may experience significant fatigue, they should use care in driving or other potentially hazardous tasks. Premedication may be necessary in subsequent cycles if infusion reactions occur. Follow good oral hygiene and be alert for mouth ulceration. Doses will be reduced, withheld, or delayed if significant hematologic or nonhematologic toxicities occur.

Storage

Store powder for injection at room temperature protected from light. Once reconstituted, the vial contents should be further diluted within 30 min. Infusion solutions may be stored at room temperature for up to 3 h. If refrigerated, the infusion solution must be used within 24 h.

Administration

CAUTION: Observe and exercise usual precautions for handling, preparing, and administering cytotoxic drugs.

To prepare injectable: dilute 25-mg vial with 5 mL of sterile water for injection (SWI) or 100-mg vial with 20 mL of SWI. Shake well; vial concentration will be 5 mg/mL. Draw up the required dose and transfer to 500 mL of either 0.9% NaCl infusion or 500 mL of dextrose2.5%/0.45%NaCl infusion. The final concentration should be within 0.2 mg/mL and 0.6 mg/mL. Thoroughly mix bag contents. Infuse IV over 30 or 60 min, dependent on protocol recommendations (see dosage). Precautions should be taken to avoid extravasation.

Bentoquatam

ben'toe-kwa-tam

★ IvyBlock

CATEGORY AND SCHEDULE

Pregnancy Risk Category: NR

Classification: Rhus dermatitis protectant

MECHANISM OF ACTION

An organoclay substance that absorbs and binds to urushiol, the active principle in poison oak, ivy, and sumac. *Therapeutic Effect:* Blocks urushiol skin contact and absorption.

PHARMACOKINETICS

None reported.

AVAILABILITY

Lotion: 5% (IvyBlock).

INDICATIONS AND DOSAGES

▸ **Prophylaxis of contact dermatitis caused by poison oak, ivy, or sumac**

TOPICAL

Adults, Elderly, Children 6 yr and older. Apply thin film over skin at least 15 min before potential exposure. Reapply q4hr or sooner if needed.

CONTRAINDICATIONS

Hypersensitivity to bentoquatam or any of its components such as methylparabens.

INTERACTIONS

Drug

None known.

Herbal

None known.

Food

None known.

DIAGNOSTIC TEST EFFECTS

None known.

SIDE EFFECTS

Occasional

Erythema.

SERIOUS REACTIONS

• None reported.

PRECAUTIONS & CONSIDERATIONS

Caution is necessary in patients with a history of allergic-type

B

responses to medications, especially topical formulations, open wounds, psoriatic lesions, or other cutaneous conditions. The use of bentoquatam has not been studied in pregnancy. There are no age-related precautions noted in children or in elderly patients.

Storage

Store at room temperature.

Administration

Bentoquatam is for external use only. Bentoquatam is a protectant, not a treatment, for poison oak, ivy, or sumac. Shake well before use. Apply 15 min before exposure. Do not apply after exposure. Reapply every 4 h or sooner if needed to maintain protection.

Benzocaine

ben′zoe-kane

★ Americaine Anesthetic Lubricant, Americaine Otic, Anbesol, Anbesol Baby Gel, Anbesol Maximum Strength, Babee Teething, Benzodent, Cepacol, Cetacaine, Chiggerex, Chiggertox, Cylex, Dermoplast, Detaine, Foille, Foille Medicated First Aid, Foille Plus, HDA Toothache, Hurricane, Lanacane, Mycinettes, Omedia, Orabase-B, Orajel, Orajel Baby, Orajel Baby Nighttime, Orajel Maximum Strength, Orasol, Oticaine, Otocain, Retre-Gel, Solarcaine, Trocaine, Zilactin, Zilactin-B, Zilactin Baby

CATEGORY AND SCHEDULE

Pregnancy Risk Category: C

Classification: Topical ester local anesthetic

MECHANISM OF ACTION

A local anesthetic that blocks nerve conduction in the autonomic, sensory, and motor nerve fibers. Competes with calcium ions for membrane binding. Reduces permeability of resting nerves to potassium and sodium ions. *Therapeutic Effect:* Produces local analgesic effect.

PHARMACOKINETICS

Poorly absorbed by topical administration. Well absorbed from mucous membranes and traumatized skin. Metabolized in liver and by hydrolysis with cholinesterase. Minimal excretion in urine.

AVAILABILITY

Cream: 5%, 20% (Lanacane).
Lozenge: 10 mg (Cepacol, Trocaine), 15 mg (Cyclex, Mycinettes).
Oral Aerosol: 14% (Cetacaine), 20% (Hurricane).
Oral Gel: 6.3% (Anbesol), 6.5% (HDA Toothache), 7.5% (Anbesol Baby, Detaine, Orajel Baby), 10% (Orajel, Orajel Baby Nighttime, Zilactin-B, Zilactin Baby), 20% (Anbesol Maximum Strength, Hurricane).
Oral Liquid: 6.3% (Anbesol), 7.5% (Orajel Baby), 10% (Orajel), 20% (Anbesol Maximum Strength, Hurricane).
Oral Lotion: 2.5% (Babee Teething).
Oral Ointment: 20% (Benzodent).
Otic Solution: 20% (Americaine Otic, Omedia, Oticaine, Otocain).
Paste: 20% (Orabase-B).
Topical Aerosol: 5% (Foille, Foille Plus), 20% (Dermoplast, Solarcaine).
Topical Gel: 5% (Retre-Gel), 20% (Americaine Anesthetic Lubricant).
Topical Liquid: 2% (Chiggertox).
Topical Ointment: 2% (Chiggerex), 5% (Foille Medicated First Aid).

INDICATIONS AND DOSAGES

▸ Canker sores

TOPICAL

Adults, Elderly, Children older than 2 yr. Apply gel, liquid, or ointment to affected area. Maximum: 4 times/day.

▸ Denture srritation

TOPICAL

Adults, Elderly. Apply a thin layer of gel to affected area up to 4 times/day or until pain is relieved.

▸ General lubrication

TOPICAL

Adults, Elderly, Children older than 2 yr. Apply gel to exterior of tube or instrument before use.

▸ Otitis externa, otitis media

OTIC

Adults, Elderly, Children older than 1 yr. Instill 4-5 drops into external ear canal of affected ears. Repeat q1-2h as needed.

▸ Pain and itching associated with sunburn, insect bites, minor cuts, scrapes, minor burns, minor skin irritations

TOPICAL

Adults, Elderly, Children older than 2 yr. Apply to affected area 3-4 times/day.

▸ Pharyngitis

PO

Adults, Elderly. 1 lozenge q2hr. Maximum: 8 lozenges/day.

▸ Toothache/teething pain

TOPICAL

Adults, Elderly, Children older than 2 yr. Apply gel, liquid, or ointment to affected areas. Maximum: 4 times/day. Do not use for more than 7 days.

▸ Anesthesia

TOPICAL

Adults, Elderly. Apply aerosol, gel, ointment, liquid q4-12h as needed.

CONTRAINDICATIONS

Hypersensitivity to benzocaine or ester-type local anesthetics, perforated tympanic membrane or ear discharge (otic preparations).

INTERACTIONS

Drug

Hyaluronidase: May increase the incidence of systemic reaction to benzocaine, when used at same sites.

Herbal

None known.

Food

None known.

DIAGNOSTIC TEST EFFECTS

None known.

SIDE EFFECTS

Occasional

Burning, stinging, angioedema, contact dermatitis, taste disorders.

SERIOUS REACTIONS

• Methemoglobinemia occurs rarely in infants and young children.

PRECAUTIONS & CONSIDERATIONS

Caution should be used with children younger than 2 yr and infants and with inflamed skin or open wounds. It is unknown whether benzocaine crosses the placenta or is distributed in breast milk. Safety and efficacy of this drug have not been established in children younger than 2 yr for topical preparations and younger than 1 yr for otic solutions. There are no age-related precautions for elderly patients. Avoid contact with eyes.

An allergic reaction with blue color around mouth, fingers, or toes; fast breathing; redness; pain or swelling; or unusual tiredness or weakness should be reported immediately (may signal methemoglobinemia).

Storage

Store at room temperature. Topical sprays are flammable and contents are under pressure. Do not use near fire or flame or expose to high heat.

Administration

Oral or dental use: Do not eat 1 h before topical oral administration. Rinse mouth well before reinserting dentures. Do not use for more than 1 wk.

Topical dermal use: Follow manufacturer's product-specific directions for use. Clean area before applying topical benzocaine. For external use only. If using aerosol, hold can 6-12 inches away from affected area. If applying to face, spray in palm of hand and then apply to affected area. Do not spray for longer than 2 seconds.

Benzonatate

ben-zoe'na-tate

★ Tessalon Perles, Zonatuss

CATEGORY AND SCHEDULE

Pregnancy Risk Category: C

Classification: Antitussive, nonnarcotic, ester, local anesthetic

MECHANISM OF ACTION

A nonnarcotic antitussive that anesthetizes stretch receptors in respiratory passages, lungs, and pleura. *Therapeutic Effect:* Reduces cough.

PHARMACOKINETICS

PO onset 15-20 min; duration 3-8 h; metabolized by liver, excreted in urine.

AVAILABILITY

Capsules: 100 mg, 200 mg.

INDICATIONS AND DOSAGES

▸ **Antitussive**

PO

Adults, Elderly, Children older than 10 yr. 100 mg 3 times/day only if needed, may give up to q4h (maximum 600 mg/day).

OFF-LABEL USES

Intractable hiccups.

CONTRAINDICATIONS

Hypersensitivity to benzonatate or other ester local anesthetics.

INTERACTIONS

Drug

CNS depressants: May increase the effects of benzonatate.

Herbal

None known.

Food

None known.

DIAGNOSTIC TEST EFFECTS

None known.

SIDE EFFECTS

Occasional

Mild somnolence, mild dizziness, constipation, GI upset, skin eruptions, nasal congestion.

SERIOUS REACTIONS

- A paradoxical reaction, including restlessness, insomnia, euphoria, nervousness, and tremor, has been noted, especially in overdose.
- Severe hypersensitivity (rare).
- Bizarre behavior, confusion, visual hallucinations (rare) more likely when given with other CNS medications.

PRECAUTIONS & CONSIDERATIONS

Caution is warranted with a productive cough. Dizziness and drowsiness are common side effects. Safety and efficacy not established in children under 10 yr. Unknown if the drug may cause fetal harm or if excreted in breast milk; caution advised. Avoid tasks that require mental alertness or motor skills until response to the drug has been established. Fluid intake and environmental humidity should be increased to lower the viscosity of secretions.

Storage
Store at room temperature. Protect from moisture and light; keep tightly closed.
Administration
Take benzonatate without regard to food. Swallow the capsules whole; chewing them or dissolving them in the mouth may produce temporary local anesthesia or choking, which may compromise the airway.

Benzoyl Peroxide

ben′zoe-ill per-ox′ide

Benprox, Benzac, Benzac AC, Benzac W, Benzagel, BenzeFoam, Benziq, Brevoxyl, Clearasil, Clearplex, Clinac BPO, Del-Aqua, Desquam-E, Desquam-X, Inova, Lavoclen, NeoBenz, PanOxyl, Peroderm, Triaz, Zaclir, Zoderm

CATEGORY AND SCHEDULE

Pregnancy Risk Category: C
OTC

Classification: Antiacne agent, topical; keratolytic, topical

MECHANISM OF ACTION

A keratolytic agent that releases free-radical oxygen, which oxidizes bacterial proteins in the sebaceous follicles, decreasing the number of anaerobic bacteria and decreasing irritating-type free fatty acids. *Therapeutic Effect:* Bactericidal action against *Propionibacterium acnes* and *Staphylococcus epidermidis.*

PHARMACOKINETICS

Minimal absorption through skin. Gel is more penetrating than cream. Metabolized to benzoic acid in skin. Excreted in urine as benzoate.

AVAILABILITY

Cream, Topical: 2.5%, 3.5%, 5%, 5.5%, 8.5%, 10%.
Gel, Topical: 2.5%, 4%, 4.5%, 5%, 6%, 6.5%, 7%, 8%, 8.5%, 9%, 10%.
Liquid, Topical: 2.5%, 3%, 4%, 5%, 6%, 8%, 9%, 10%.
Lotion, Topical: 3%, 4%, 5%, 5.5%, 6%, 8%, 10%.
Cleanser Suspension/Wash: 2.5%, 4%, 4.5%, 5%, 5.25%, 5.75%, 6%, 6.5%, 7%, 8%, 8.5%, 10%.
Soap Bar, Topical: 5%, 10%.

INDICATIONS AND DOSAGES

▸ **Acne**

TOPICAL

Adults. Apply 2.5%-10% concentration 1-2 times/day; cleansers used 1-2 times/day. If applied just once a day, then bedtime application after gentle cleansing is recommended.

OFF-LABEL USES

Dermal ulcers, seborrheic dermatitis, surgical wounds, tinea pedis, tinea versicolor.

CONTRAINDICATIONS

Hypersensitivity to benzoyl peroxide or any component of the formulation.

INTERACTIONS

Drug
Sunscreens containing PABA: May cause skin to change color when both agents are used concomitantly.
Retinoids: May increase skin irritation.
Herbal
None known.
Food
None known.

DIAGNOSTIC TEST EFFECTS

None known.

B

SIDE EFFECTS

Occasional

Irritation, dryness, burning, peeling, stinging, contact dermatitis, bleaching of hair.

SERIOUS REACTIONS

- Hypersensitivity reactions have been reported with benzoyl peroxide use.

PRECAUTIONS & CONSIDERATIONS

Caution should be used on skin because benzoyl peroxide may cause contact dermatitis, hair bleaching, and seborrhea. Caution should also be used around the eyes, lips, mucous membranes, and highly inflamed skin. Sun exposure may increase skin irritation. Be aware that cross-sensitization may occur with benzoic acid derivatives such as cinnamon and other topical anesthetics. It is unknown whether benzoyl peroxide crosses the placenta or is distributed in breast milk. Safety and efficacy of benzoyl peroxide have not been established in children younger than 12 yr. There are no age-related precautions noted for elderly patients.

Mild stinging and redness may occur. Be aware that benzoyl peroxide may bleach hair and fabric.

Storage

Store at room temperature.

Administration

For topical use only. If excessive dryness or peeling occurs, decrease concentration of product used or frequency of application. Avoid eyes and mucous membranes. Follow directions for specific product type.

Benztropine

benz'troe-peen

★ Cogentin 🍁 Apo-Benztropine

Do not confuse benztropine with bromocriptine.

CATEGORY AND SCHEDULE

Pregnancy Risk Category: C

Classification: Anticholinergic, antidyskinetic

MECHANISM OF ACTION

An antiparkinsonian agent that selectively blocks central cholinergic receptors, helping to balance cholinergic and dopaminergic activity. *Therapeutic Effect:* Reduces the incidence and severity of akinesia, rigidity, and tremor.

PHARMACOKINETICS

IM/IV: Onset 15 min, duration 6-10 h. PO: onset 1 h, duration 6-10 h.

AVAILABILITY

Tablets: 0.5 mg, 1 mg, 2 mg.
Injection: 1 mg/mL.

INDICATIONS AND DOSAGES

▸ **Parkinsonism**

PO

Adults. 0.5-6 mg/day as a single dose or in 2 divided doses. Titrate by 0.5 mg at 5- to 6-day intervals.

Elderly. Initially, 0.5 mg once or twice a day. Titrate by 0.5 mg at 5- to 6-day intervals. Maximum: 4 mg/day.

▸ **Drug-induced extrapyramidal symptoms**

PO, IM

Adults. 1-4 mg once or twice a day.

Children older than 3 yr. 0.02-0.05 mg/kg/dose once or twice a day.

▸ **Acute dystonic reactions**

IM, IV (IM PREFERRED)

Adults. Initially, 1-2 mg; then 1-2 mg PO twice a day to prevent recurrence.

IV INCOMPATIBILITIES

Diazepam, furosemide, phenytoin.

CONTRAINDICATIONS

Angle-closure glaucoma, benign prostatic hyperplasia, children younger than 3 yr, GI obstruction, intestinal atony, megacolon, myasthenia gravis, paralytic ileus, severe ulcerative colitis.

INTERACTIONS

Drug

Alcohol, other CNS depressants: May increase sedation.

Amantadine, anticholinergics, MAOIs: May increase the effects of benztropine.

Antacids, antidiarrheals: May decrease the absorption and effects of benztropine.

Phenothiazines, tricyclic antidepressants: May increase the risk of heat intolerance, hyperthermia, and heatstroke.

DIAGNOSTIC TEST EFFECTS

None known.

SIDE EFFECTS

Frequent

Somnolence, dry mouth, blurred vision, constipation, decreased sweating or urination, GI upset, photosensitivity.

Occasional

Headache, memory loss, muscle cramps, anxiety, peripheral paresthesia, orthostatic hypotension, abdominal cramps, tachycardia.

Rare

Rash, confusion, eye pain.

SERIOUS REACTIONS

- Overdose may produce severe anticholinergic effects, such as unsteadiness, somnolence, tachycardia, dyspnea, skin flushing, and severe dryness of the mouth, nose, or throat.
- Severe paradoxical reactions, marked by hallucinations, tremor, seizures, and toxic psychosis, may occur.

PRECAUTIONS & CONSIDERATIONS

Caution is warranted with arrhythmias, heart disease, hypertension, hepatic or renal impairment, obstructive diseases of the GI or genitourinary tracts, urine retention, benign prostatic hyperplasia, tachycardia, and treated open-angle glaucoma. Caution is advised in hot weather; benztropine may increase risk of hyperthermia and heatstroke. Elderly (older than 60 yr) patients are more likely to develop agitation, disorientation, confusion, and psychotic-like symptoms.

Dizziness, drowsiness, and dry mouth are expected responses to the drug. Alcohol and tasks that require mental alertness or motor skills should be avoided. Notify the physician of agitation, headache, somnolence, or confusion.

Storage

Store at room temperature.

Administration

Oral: May give without regard to meals. Initial doses usually given at bedtime or dose may be divided throughout the day to treat tremors. Improvement usually occurs in 1-2 days.

Benzyl Alcohol

ben′zil al′co-hol

Ulesfia

CATEGORY AND SCHEDULE

Pregnancy Risk Category: B

Classification:

Anti-infectives, topical, pediculicides

MECHANISM OF ACTION

Inhibits lice from closing their respiratory spiracles, obstructing the spiracles and causing the lice to asphyxiate. *Therapeutic Effect:* Pediculocidal; product is NOT ovocidal.

PHARMACOKINETICS

Minimal absorption after topical application. Slight amounts detected in plasma in infants and children after 3 times the normal exposure period.

AVAILABILITY

Lotion: 5% (Ulesfia).

INDICATIONS AND DOSAGES

▸ **Head lice**

TOPICAL

Adults, Children 6 mo and older. Apply sufficient lotion to dry hair and leave on for 10 min before rinsing off. The amount of lotion needed for each application is dependent on the length of the hair; the manufacturer provides guidelines based on hair length. Repeat application in 7 days after initial treatment.

CONTRAINDICATIONS

None specifically noted by manufacturer. Recommended not to use in infants younger than 6 months; benzyl alcohol may cause a "gasping syndrome" in neonates. Hypersensitivity to any component of the formulation.

INTERACTIONS

Drug

None known.

Herbal

None known.

Food

None known.

DIAGNOSTIC TEST EFFECTS

None known.

SIDE EFFECTS

Occasional

Skin irritation, eye stinging or irritation, contact sensitization (itching, redness), hypoesthesia at application site, pruritus, erythema.

Rare (< 1%)

Application site dryness, paresthesia, dermatitis, dandruff, skin exfoliation, rash.

SERIOUS REACTIONS

- None reported.

PRECAUTIONS & CONSIDERATIONS

No age-related precautions have been noted for suspension or topical use in children over 6 mo of age. Not recommended for use in children under 6 mo, especially in neonates, who are susceptible to benzyl alcohol toxicity. The drug has not been studied in elderly patients older than 60 yr.

Keep out of reach of children; children receiving treatment should be in direct supervision of an adult during each treatment application period. Use care to avoid eye exposure during use. If the eyes come in contact with the lotion, flush the eyes immediately for several minutes with water. If irritation persists, contact physician. Watch for signs of contact/allergy during applications. Because lice are contagious, use caution to avoid infecting others. To help prevent the spread of lice from one patient to another: Avoid head-to-head contact at school (e.g., playground, in physical education or sports activities, and any play with other children). Avoid sleepovers. Do not share combs, brushes, hats, towels, pillows, bedding, helmets, or other hair-related personal items with anyone else, whether they have lice or not. After finishing treatment, check everyone in the family for lice after 1 wk. Machine wash any bedding and clothing used by anyone having lice or thought to have been exposed to lice. Machine wash at high temperatures (150° F) and tumble in a hot dryer for 20 min.

Storage

Store in a dry place at room temperature; do not freeze.

Administration

For external use only. Shake well before use. Caregivers may wish to wear gloves for application. Patient should cover face and eyes with a towel and keep eyes tightly closed during application. Apply to dry hair using enough lotion to completely saturate the scalp and hair and leave on for 10 min. Use care to avoid contact with eyes and mucous membranes. After 10 min, rinse with water. Patient may shampoo hair immediately after use if desired. Wash hands after application. Remove nits with nit comb. Repeat application in 7 days after initial treatment. The lotion will not kill the nits, so the repeat application in 7 days is essential for curing infestation.

Bepotastine

bep'oh-tas'teen

Bepreve

CATEGORY AND SCHEDULE

Pregnancy Risk Category: C

Classification:

Ophthalmic, antihistamine

MECHANISM OF ACTION

An ophthalmic H_1 receptor antagonist that inhibits histamine-stimulated vascular permeability in the conjunctiva and stabilizes mast cells. *Therapeutic Effect:* Relieves ocular itching associated with allergic conjunctivitis.

PHARMACOKINETICS

Minimal absorption after ophthalmic administration; concentration peaks at 1-2 h after instillation. Any drug absorbed is metabolized by liver. Metabolites are excreted in urine.

AVAILABILITY

Ophthalmic Solution: 1.5%.

INDICATIONS AND DOSAGES

▸ **Allergic conjunctivitis**

OPHTHALMIC

Adults, Elderly, Children 2 yr and older. 1 drop in affected eye(s) twice daily.

CONTRAINDICATIONS

Hypersensitivity to bepotastine or any other component of the formulation.

INTERACTIONS

Drug

None reported.

Herbal and Food

None known.

B

SIDE EFFECTS

Frequent (> 5%)
Mild taste disturbance immediately after instillation, temporary eye stinging right after use.
Occasional (2%-5%)
Headache, nasopharyngitis.

SERIOUS REACTIONS

• None known. Allergic reactions occur rarely.

PRECAUTIONS & CONSIDERATIONS

This product should not be used to treat eye irritation associated with contact lenses. Do not wear contact lenses while instilling the solution. The preservative in the solution can be absorbed by soft contact lenses. Safety and efficacy have not been established in children < 2 yr of age. Not known to what extent bepotastine is distributed in breast milk; use with caution during lactation and pregnancy due to lack of data. There are no specific precautions in the elderly.
Storage
Store at room temperature. Do not use if solution becomes discolored. Tightly close after each use.
Administration
For topical ophthalmic use only. Remove any contact lenses prior to use. Wash hands prior to administration. Be careful not to touch dropper tip to any surface to avoid contamination. Tilt the head back and place the solution in the conjunctival sac of the affected eye(s). Close the eye and then press gently on the lacrimal sac for 1 min. Wait at least 10 min after use before inserting contact lenses.

Beractant

ber-akt'ant
★ 🍁 Survanta
Do not confuse Survanta with Sufenta.

CATEGORY AND SCHEDULE

Pregnancy Risk Category: This drug is not indicated for use in pregnant women.

Classification: Surfactants, lung

MECHANISM OF ACTION

A natural bovine lung extract that reduces alveolar surface tension, stabilizing alveoli. *Therapeutic Effect:* Improves lung compliance and respiratory gas exchange.

PHARMACOKINETICS

Not absorbed systemically.

AVAILABILITY

Intratracheal Suspension for Inhalation: 25 mg/mL vials.

INDICATIONS AND DOSAGES

▸ **Prevention and rescue treatment of respiratory distress syndrome (RDS) or hyaline membrane disease in premature infants**
ENDOTRACHEAL
Infants. 100 mg of phospholipids/kg birth weight (4 mL/kg).
Give within 15 min of birth if infant weighs < 1250 g and has evidence of surfactant deficiency; give within 8 h when RDS is confirmed by x-ray and requires mechanical ventilation. May repeat 6 h or longer after preceding dose. Maximum: 4 doses in the first 48 h of life.

CONTRAINDICATIONS

None known.

INTERACTIONS

Drug
None known.
Herbal
None known.
Food
None known.

DIAGNOSTIC TEST EFFECTS

None known.

SIDE EFFECTS

Frequent
Transient bradycardia, oxygen (O_2) desaturation, increased carbon dioxide (CO_2) retention.
Occasional
Endotracheal tube reflux.
Rare
Apnea, endotracheal tube blockage, hypotension or hypertension, pallor, vasoconstriction.

SERIOUS REACTIONS

• Life-threatening nosocomial sepsis may occur but is a risk factor for the population in general.

PRECAUTIONS & CONSIDERATIONS

Caution should be used in persons at risk for circulatory overload. This drug is for use only in neonates. No age-related precautions have been noted.

The infant should be monitored with arterial or transcutaneous measurement of systemic O_2 and CO_2. Visitors should be limited during treatment. Handwashing and other infection control measures should be monitored to minimize the risk of nosocomial infections.

Storage
Refrigerate vials. Unopened, unused vials may be returned to the refrigerator only once and within 8 h after having been warmed to room temperature.

Administration
Administer beractant in a highly supervised setting. Clinicians caring for the neonate must be experienced with intubation and ventilator management.

Warm the vial by letting it stand at room temperature for 20 min or warming in your hand for 8 min. Gently swirl the vial, if needed, to redisperse contents. Do not shake it. The solution normally appears off-white to light brown. Enter each single-use vial only once; discard unused suspension. Use a 20-gauge or larger needle to withdraw the proper dose from the vial. Do not filter.

Instill the drug through a catheter inserted into the infant's endotracheal tube in 4 quarter doses, with the infant in a different position for each quarter dose. Do not instill it into the mainstem bronchus. Monitor the infant for bradycardia and decreased arterial O_2 saturation during administration. Stop the procedure, as prescribed, if the infant experiences these effects, and take appropriate measures before reinstituting therapy.

Besifloxacin

be'si-flox'a-sin
Besivance
Do not confuse Besivance with Glucovance.

CATEGORY AND SCHEDULE

Pregnancy Risk Category: C

Classification:
Ophthalmic anti-infectives, quinolones

B

MECHANISM OF ACTION
A fluoroquinolone that inhibits the enzyme DNA gyrase and topoisomerase IV in susceptible bacteria, interfering with bacterial cell replication. *Therapeutic Effect:* Bactericidal.

PHARMACOKINETICS
Minimally absorbed systemically during ophthalmic administration. *Half-life:* 7 h.

AVAILABILITY
Ophthalmic Suspension (Besivance): 0.6%.

INDICATIONS AND DOSAGES
▸ **Bacterial conjunctivitis**
OPHTHALMIC
Adults, Elderly, and Children 1 yr or older. Instill 1 drop in the affected eye(s) 3 times a day, 4-12 h apart, for 7 days.

CONTRAINDICATIONS
Hypersensitivity to besifloxacin or other quinolones.

INTERACTIONS
Drug
None reported.
Herbal and Food
None known.

SIDE EFFECTS
Frequent (≥ 2%)
Conjunctival redness.
Occasional (1%-2%)
Blurred vision, eye pain or sensation of something in eye, itching, headache.
Rare (< 1%)
Hypersensitivity reaction.

SERIOUS REACTIONS
None known.

PRECAUTIONS & CONSIDERATIONS
For topical ophthalmic use only. Patients should not wear contact lenses if they have bacterial conjunctivitis and should not wear them during the course of treatment with besifloxacin. This drug will not treat vaccinia, varicella, herpes simplex, mycobacterial infection, or fungal disease of an ocular structure. Safety and effectiveness have not been established in children < 1 yr of age. The extent the drug is distributed in breast milk is not known; use with caution during lactation and during pregnancy due to lack of data. There are no specific precautions in the elderly. As with other anti-infectives, prolonged use may result in overgrowth of nonsusceptible organisms, including fungi. If superinfection occurs, discontinue use and institute alternative therapy after appropriate evaluation and ophthalmic examination.
Storage
Store at controlled room temperature. Protect from light.
Administration
Shake bottle well before each use. Wash hands prior to administration. Remove any contact lenses prior to use. Be careful not to touch dropper tip to any surface to avoid contamination. Tilt the head back and place the solution in the conjunctival sac of the affected eye(s). Close the eye and then press gently on the lacrimal sac for 1 min. Wait at least 10 min after use before instilling other eyedrops.

Betamethasone

bay-ta-meth'a-sone

Betaderm, Betanate, Celestone, Celestone Soluspan, Del-Beta, Diprolene, Diprolene AF, Luxiq

CATEGORY AND SCHEDULE

Pregnancy Risk Category: C

Classification: Corticosteroid

MECHANISM OF ACTION

An adrenocortical steroid that controls the rate of protein synthesis, depresses the migration of polymorphonuclear leukocytes and fibroblasts, reduces capillary permeability, and prevents or controls inflammation. *Therapeutic Effect:* Decreases tissue response to inflammatory process.

PHARMACOKINETICS

PO: Onset 1-2 h, peak 1 h, duration 3 days. IM/IV: Onset 10 min, peak 4-8 h, duration 1-1.5 days. Metabolized in liver, excreted in urine as steroids, crosses the placenta.

AVAILABILITY

Cream (Betamethasone, dipropionate, Betanate, Del-Beta): 0.05%.
Cream (Betamethasone, dipropionate, [augmented], Diprolene AF): 0.05%.
Gel (Betamethasone, dipropionate, [augmented]: 0.05%.
Lotion: (Betamethasone dipropionate, Del-Beta): 0.05%.
Cream (Betamethasone dipropionate, [augmented], Diprolene): 0.05%.
Lotion (Betamethasone dipropionate, Del-Beta): 0.05%.
Ointment: 0.05%.
Cream (Betamethasone valerate, Betaderm, Beta-Val): 0.1%.
Foam (Betamethasone valerate, Luxiq): 0.12%.
Lotion (Betamethasone valerate, Beta-Val): 0.1%
Ointment (Betamethasone valerate): 0.1%
Syrup (Celestone): 0.6 mg/5 mL.
Injection Suspension (Celestone, Soluspan): 6 mg/mL.

INDICATIONS AND DOSAGES

▸ **Anti-inflammation, immunosuppression, corticosteroid replacement therapy**

PO

Adults, Elderly. 0.6-7.2 mg/day.
Children. 0.063-0.25 mg/kg/day in 3-4 divided doses.

IM

Adults. 0.6-9 mg/day (generally, ⅓ to ½ of oral dose) divided every 12-24 h.
Children. 0.0175-0.125 mg/kg/day divided every 6-12 h or 0.5-7.5 mg base/m^2/day divided every 6-12 h.

▸ **Relief of inflamed and pruritic dermatoses**

TOPICAL

Adults, Elderly. 1-2 times a day.
Foam: Apply twice a day.

INTRADERMAL

Adults. 0.2 mL/cm^2/dose. Maximum dose 1 mL/wk.

▸ **Rheumatoid arthritis/osteoarthritis**

INTRA-ARTICULAR

Adults. 0.5-2 mL; 1-2 mL in very large joints (hip), 1 mL in large joints (knee, ankle, or shoulder), 0.5-1 mL in medium joints (wrist, elbow), and 0.25-0.5 mL in small joints (hand, chest).

▸ **Bursitis**

INTRABURSAL

Adult. 0.5-1 mL depending on affected area.

B

OFF-LABEL USES

Fetal lung maturation to prophylax against anticipated neonatal respiratory immaturity (IM dosage).

CONTRAINDICATIONS

Hypersensitivity to betamethasone, systemic fungal infections.

INTERACTIONS

Drug

Amphotericin; diuretics: May increase hypokalemia.
Digoxin: May increase digoxin toxicity secondary to hypokalemia.
Insulin, oral hypoglycemics: May decrease the effects of these drugs (example: rifampin).
Hepatic enzyme inducers: May decrease the systemic effect of betamethasone.
Live-virus vaccines: May decrease the patient's antibody response to vaccine, and potentiate virus replication.

DIAGNOSTIC TEST EFFECTS

May increase blood glucose levels and serum lipids, amylase, and sodium levels. May decrease serum calcium, potassium, and thyroxine levels.

SIDE EFFECTS

Frequent

Systemic: Increased appetite, abdominal distention, nervousness, insomnia, false sense of well-being.
Topical: Burning, stinging, pruritus.

Occasional

Systemic: Dizziness, facial flushing, diaphoresis, decreased or blurred vision, mood swings.
Topical: Allergic contact dermatitis, purpura or blood-containing blisters, thinning of skin with easy bruising, telangiectases or raised dark red spots on skin.

SERIOUS REACTIONS

• Systemic hypercorticism and adrenal suppression.

PRECAUTIONS & CONSIDERATIONS

Caution is warranted with persons at increased risk for peptic ulcer disease and in those with cirrhosis, diabetes, heart failure, hypothyroidism, myasthenia gravis, osteoporosis, renal impairment, or nonspecific ulcerative colitis. Monitor the growth and development of children receiving long-term steroid therapy.

Mood swings, ranging from euphoria to depression, may occur. Initially, tuberculosis skin test, x-rays, and ECG should be evaluated. Blood glucose level, BP, serum electrolyte levels, height, and weight should be monitored before and during therapy. Injectable form should not be given intravenously.

Storage

Store all forms at room temperature. Protect injection from light.

Administration

Give oral betamethasone with milk or food to decrease GI upset. Give single doses in the morning before 9 AM; give multiple doses at evenly spaced intervals. Do not abruptly discontinue the drug.

For topical use, gently cleanse area before applying drug. Apply sparingly and rub into area thoroughly. Use occlusive dressings only as ordered. Do not use topical form on broken skin or in areas of infection, and do not apply to the face or inguinal areas or to wet skin.

Celestone Soluspan is NOT for intravenous use. The injection is given intradermally, intrabursal, intra-articular, or intramascually. Each route requries specific techniques and needle/syringe types for injection. Shake well before using. If coadministration of a local

B

anesthetic is desired, betamethasone sodium phosphate/betamethasone acetate injectable suspension may be mixed with 1% or 2% lidocaine hydrochloride or similar local anesthetics, using the formulations that do not contain parabens. The drug dose is first withdrawn into a syringe, and then the anesthetic is drawn into the syringe. Briefly shake to mix.

Betaxolol

bay-tax'oh-lol

★ Betoptic, Betoptic-S, Kerlone

Do not confuse betaxolol with bethanechol.

CATEGORY AND SCHEDULE

Pregnancy Risk Category: C (D if used in second or third trimester)

Classification: Antihypertensive, selective β_1-blocker

MECHANISM OF ACTION

An antihypertensive and antiglaucoma agent that blocks β_1-adrenergic receptors in cardiac tissue. Reduces aqueous humor production. *Therapeutic Effect:* Slows sinus heart rate, decreases BP, and reduces intraocular pressure (IOP).

PHARMACOKINETICS

PO: Peak 3-4 h. *Half-life:* 14-22 h. Protein binding: 50%; some hepatic metabolism; excreted in urine mostly unchanged.

AVAILABILITY

Tablets (Kerlone): 10 mg, 20 mg.
Ophthalmic Solution (Betoptic): 0.5%.
Ophthalmic Suspension (Betoptic-S): 0.25%.

INDICATIONS AND DOSAGES

▸ **Hypertension**

PO

Adults. Initially, 5-10 mg/day. May increase to 20 mg/day after 7-14 days. Maximum: 40 mg/day.
Elderly. Initially, 5 mg/day, then titrate as per adult dose.

▸ **Chronic open-angle glaucoma and ocular hypertension**

SOLUTION-EYEDROPS

Adults, Elderly: 1-2 drop(s) twice a day in affected eye(s).

SUSPENSION EYEDROPS (BETOPTIC-S)

1 drop twice a day in affected eyes.

▸ **Oral dosage in renal impairment**

Adult and elderly patients on dialysis. Initially give 5 mg/day; increase by 5 mg/day q2wk. Maximum: 20 mg/day.

OFF-LABEL USES

Treatment of angle-closure glaucoma during or after iridectomy, malignant glaucoma, secondary glaucoma; with miotics, to decrease IOP in acute and chronic angle-closure glaucoma.

CONTRAINDICATIONS

Cardiogenic shock, overt cardiac failure, second- or third-degree heart block, sinus bradycardia, hypersensitivity.

INTERACTIONS

Drug

Cimetidine: May increase betaxolol blood concentration.
Diuretics, other antihypertensives: May increase hypotensive effect of betaxolol.
Insulin, oral hypoglycemics: May mask signs and symptoms of hypoglycemia from these drugs.
NSAIDs: May decrease antihypertensive effect.

B

Sympathomimetics, xanthines: May mutually inhibit hypotensive effects and may mask symptoms of hypoglycemia.

DIAGNOSTIC TEST EFFECTS

May increase serum antinuclear antibody titer and BUN, serum lipoprotein, creatinine, potassium, uric acid, and triglyceride levels.

SIDE EFFECTS

Betaxolol is generally well tolerated, with mild and transient side effects.

Frequent

Systemic: Hypotension manifested as dizziness, nausea, diaphoresis, headache, fatigue, constipation or diarrhea, dyspnea.
Ophthalmic: Eye irritation, visual disturbances.

Occasional

Systemic: Insomnia, flatulence, urinary frequency, impotence or decreased libido, bradycardia, bronchospasm.
Ophthalmic: Increased light sensitivity, watering of eye.

Rare

Systemic: Rash, arrhythmias, arthralgia, myalgia, confusion, altered taste, increased urination, alopecia.
Ophthalmic: Dry eye, conjunctivitis, eye pain.

SERIOUS REACTIONS

- Overdose may produce profound bradycardia, hypotension, and bronchospasm.
- Abrupt withdrawal may result in diaphoresis, palpitations, headache, and tremors.
- Betaxolol administration may precipitate CHF or MI in patients with cardiac disease; thyroid storm in those with thyrotoxicosis; and peripheral ischemia in those with existing peripheral vascular disease.
- Hypoglycemia may occur in patients with previously controlled diabetes.
- Ophthalmic overdose may produce bradycardia, hypotension, bronchospasm, and acute cardiac failure.

PRECAUTIONS & CONSIDERATIONS

Caution is warranted with diabetes, hyperthyroidism, impaired hepatic or renal function, inadequate cardiac function, and peripheral vascular disease. Betaxolol is excreted in breast milk; use with caution in nursing mothers.

Orthostatic hypotension may occur, so rise slowly from a lying to sitting position and dangle the legs from the bed momentarily before standing. Notify the physician of fatigue, headache, prolonged dizziness, and shortness of breath. BP for hypotension, respiratory status for shortness of breath, pattern of daily bowel activity and stool consistency, and pulse for quality, rate, and rhythm should be monitored during treatment. If pulse rate is 60 beats/min or lower or systolic BP is < 90 mm Hg, withhold the medication and contact the physician. Signs and symptoms of CHF, such as decreased urine output, distended neck veins, dyspnea (particularly on exertion or lying down), night cough, peripheral edema, and weight gain should also be assessed.

Storage

Store at room temperature (all forms).

Administration

To assess tolerance for betaxolol, obtain a standing systolic BP 1 h after giving the drug. Do not abruptly discontinue betaxolol. Compliance is essential to control glaucoma and hypertension.

Shake ophthalmic suspension well before using. After administration, perform nasolacrimal occlusion to reduce systemic absorption. Remove contact lens before administration and wait 15 min before reinserting. If other ophthalmic solutions are being used concurrently, administer at least 10 min before instilling the suspension.

Oral: May give without regard to food.

Bethanechol

be-than′e-kole

★ Urecholine 🍁 Duvoid, Myotonachol

Do not confuse bethanechol with betaxolol.

CATEGORY AND SCHEDULE

Pregnancy Risk Category: C

Classification: Cholinergic stimulant

MECHANISM OF ACTION

A cholinergic that acts directly at cholinergic receptors in the smooth muscle of the urinary bladder and GI tract. Increases detrusor muscle tone. *Therapeutic Effect:* May initiate micturition and bladder emptying. Improves gastric and intestinal motility.

PHARMACOKINETICS

PO onset 30-90 min, duration 1-6 h. SC onset 5-15 min, duration 2 h; excreted by kidneys.

AVAILABILITY

Tablets: 5 mg, 10 mg, 25 mg, 50 mg.

INDICATIONS AND DOSAGES

▸ Postoperative and postpartum urine retention, neurogenic atony of bladder with retention

PO

Adults, Elderly. 10-50 mg 3-4 times a day. Minimum effective dose determined by giving 5-10 mg initially, then repeating same amount at 1-h intervals until desired response is achieved, or maximum of 50 mg is reached.

OFF-LABEL USES

Treatment of congenital megacolon, gastroesophageal reflux, postoperative gastric atony.

CONTRAINDICATIONS

Active or latent bronchial asthma, acute inflammatory GI tract conditions, anastomosis, bladder wall instability, cardiac or coronary artery disease, epilepsy, hypertension, hyperthyroidism, hypotension, GI or urinary tract obstruction, parkinsonism, peptic ulcer, pronounced bradycardia, recent GI resection, vasomotor instability.

INTERACTIONS

Drug

Cholinesterase inhibitors: May increase the effects and risk of toxicity of bethanechol.

Procainamide, quinidine: May decrease the effects of bethanechol.

Herbal

None known.

Food

None known.

DIAGNOSTIC TEST EFFECTS

May increase serum amylase, lipase, and AST (SGOT) levels.

SIDE EFFECTS

Occasional

Belching, blurred or changed vision, diarrhea, urinary urgency.

B

SERIOUS REACTIONS

- Overdosage produces CNS stimulation (including insomnia, anxiety, and orthostatic hypotension) and cholinergic stimulation (such as headache, increased salivation, diaphoresis, nausea, vomiting, flushed skin, abdominal pain, and seizures).

PRECAUTIONS & CONSIDERATIONS

Notify the physician of difficulty breathing, irregular heartbeat, muscle weakness, nausea and vomiting, diarrhea, severe abdominal pain, and increased salivation or sweating. Intake and output and vital signs should be monitored. Not recommended in nursing mothers. Use with caution in patients with hypertension, urinary retention. Safety and effectiveness not established in children.

Administration

Take 1 h before meals or 2 h after meals to reduce nausea.

Bevacizumab

beh-vah-siz′oo-mab

Avastin

Do not confuse Avastin with Astelin.

CATEGORY AND SCHEDULE

Pregnancy Risk Category: C

Classification: Antineoplastics, monoclonal antibody; vascular endothelial growth factor (VEGF) inhibitor

MECHANISM OF ACTION

An antineoplastic that binds to and inhibits vascular endothelial growth factor, a protein that plays a major role in the formation of new blood vessels to tumors. *Therapeutic Effect:* Inhibits metastatic disease progression.

PHARMACOKINETICS

Clearance varies by body weight, gender, and tumor burden. *Half-life:* 20 days (range, 11-50 days).

AVAILABILITY

Injection: 100 mg/4 mL or 400 mg/16 mL vials.

INDICATIONS AND DOSAGES

▸ **First-line treatment of metastatic carcinoma of the colon or rectum in combination with 5-fluorouracil (5-FU)**

IV INFUSION

Adults, Elderly. 5 mg/kg once every 14 days when used with bolus irinotecan/5-FU/leucovorin; 10 mg/kg once every 14 days when used with 5-FU/leucovorin/oxaliplatin.

▸ **Nonsquamous non–small cell lung cancer**

IV INFUSION

Adults, Elderly. 15 mg/kg once every 3 wks in combination with carboplatin and paclitaxel.

▸ **Metastatic HER2-negative breast cancer**

IV INFUSION

Adults, Elderly. 10 mg/kg once every 14 days. Used in a regimen with paclitaxel.

▸ **Renal cell cancer**

IV INFUSION

Adults, Elderly. 10 mg/kg once every 2 wks in combination with interferon alfa.

▸ **Gliobiastoma**

IV INFUSION

Adults, Elderly. 10 mg/kg once every 2 wks.

OFF-LABEL USES

Age-related macular degeneration, ovarian cancer.

CONTRAINDICATIONS

Bevacizumab therapy should be permanently discontinued in patients developing GI perforation, hypertensive crisis, nephrotic syndrome, fistula, serious bleeding, wound dehiscence requiring medical intervention.

INTERACTIONS

Drug

Sunitinib: May cause hemolytic anemia; avoid combination.

Herbal

None known.

Food

None known.

DIAGNOSTIC TEST EFFECTS

May decrease serum potassium, sodium, and hemoglobin levels; hematocrit; and WBC and platelet counts.

IV INCOMPATIBILITIES

Do not mix bevacizumab with dextrose solutions.

SIDE EFFECTS

Frequent (25%-73%)

Asthenia, vomiting, anorexia, hypertension, epistaxis, stomatitis, constipation, headache, dyspnea, urinary tract infections manifested as urinary frequency or urgency and proteinuria.

Occasional (15%-21%)

Altered taste, dry skin, exfoliative dermatitis, dizziness, flatulence, excessive lacrimation, skin discoloration, weight loss, myalgia.

Rare (6%-8%)

Nail disorder, skin ulcer, alopecia, confusion, abnormal gait, dry mouth.

SERIOUS REACTIONS

- Congestive heart failure, deep vein thrombosis, GI perforation, hypertensive crisis, nephrotic syndrome, and severe hemorrhage are the most serious reactions that occur.
- Anemia, neutropenia, and thrombocytopenia occur occasionally.
- Hypersensitivity reactions occur rarely.
- Wound dehiscence and wound healing complications.

PRECAUTIONS & CONSIDERATIONS

Caution is warranted with congestive heart failure, epistaxis, hypertension, proteinuria, and renal insufficiency. Bevacizumab should be permanently discontinued in patients developing GI perforation, fistula formation, wound dehiscence, serious bleeding, a severe arterial thromboembolic event, nephrotic syndrome, hypertensive crisis, or hypertensive encephalopathy. Therapy should be temporarily suspended in patients with moderate to severe proteinuria, with severe hypertension, or undergoing surgery. Bevacizumab is teratogenic and has the potential to impair fertility. Its use by pregnant women may decrease maternal and fetal body weight and increase the risk of fetal skeletal abnormalities. Breastfeeding women should not take bevacizumab. The safety and efficacy of bevacizumab have not been established in children. Patients older than 65 yr have a higher incidence of serious adverse reactions. Avoid receiving immunizations without the physician's approval and avoid contact with crowds, people with known infections, and anyone who has recently received a live-virus vaccine.

Notify the physician if asthenia (loss of energy), abdominal pain, chills, fever, or nausea and vomiting occur. BP, CBC, serum potassium, and sodium levels should be

B

monitored before and regularly during bevacizumab treatment. Urine should be assessed for proteinuria. Persons with a urine dipstick reading of 2+ or more should have a 24-h urine collection. Pattern of daily bowel activity and stool consistency should be monitored.

Storage

Refrigerate vials. Do not freeze. The diluted infusion solution may be refrigerated for up to 8 h.

Administration

! Do not give bevacizumab by IV push or IV bolus. Withdraw the amount of bevacizumab needed for a dose and dilute it in 100 mL 0.9% NaCl. Do not administer or mix with dextrose solutions. Discard any unused portion. Infuse the initial dose of bevacizumab over 90 min after chemotherapy. If the person tolerates the first infusion well, the second infusion may be administered over 60 min. If 60-min infusion is tolerated, subsequent infusions may be given over 30 min.

Bexarotene

beks-air′oh-teen

★ 🍁 Targretin

CATEGORY AND SCHEDULE

Pregnancy Risk Category: X

Classification: Antineoplastic, retinoids

MECHANISM OF ACTION

This retinoid antineoplastic agent binds to and activates retinoid X receptor subtypes, which regulate the genes that control cellular differentiation and proliferation. *Therapeutic Effect:* Inhibits growth of tumor cell lines of hematopoietic and squamous cell origin and induces tumor regression.

PHARMACOKINETICS

Moderately absorbed from the GI tract. Protein binding: > 99%. Metabolized in the liver. Primarily eliminated through the hepatobiliary system. *Half-life:* 7 h.

AVAILABILITY

Capsules, Soft Gelatin: 75 mg.
Gel, Topical: 1%.

INDICATIONS AND DOSAGES

▸ Cutaneous T-cell lymphoma refractory to at least one prior systemic therapy

PO

Adults. 300 mg/m²/day. If no response and initial dose is well tolerated, may be increased to 400 mg/m²/day. If not tolerated, may decrease to 200 mg/m²/day, then to 100 mg/m²/day. Round doses to nearest 75 mg.

TOPICAL

Adults. Initially apply once every other day. May increase at weekly intervals up to 4 times/day. Most patients tolerate and maintain 2-4 times/day application.

OFF-LABEL USES

Treatment of non–small cell lung cancer; breast cancer; Kaposi sarcoma.

CONTRAINDICATIONS

Retinoid hypersensitivity, pregnancy.

INTERACTIONS

Drug

Antidiabetics: May enhance the effects of these drugs.

Erythromycin, itraconazole, ketoconazole: May increase bexarotene blood concentrations.

Phenytoin, rifampin: May decrease bexarotene blood concentrations.

Oral contraceptives: May reduce efficacy of hormonal contraceptive contraceptives.
Vitamin A supplements and other retinoids: Increased toxicity; avoid concurrent use.
DEET-containing insect repellents: Should not be used with bexarotene gel because of increased risk of DEET toxicity.
Food
Grapefruit juice: May increase bexarotene blood concentration and risk of toxicity.

DIAGNOSTIC TEST EFFECTS

May increase serum cholesterol, triglyceride, and LDL levels. May increase CA-125 assay value in patients with ovarian cancer. May decrease serum HDL cholesterol levels, total thyroxine, and thyroid-stimulating hormone levels. May produce elevated liver function test results.

SIDE EFFECTS

Frequent
Hyperlipidemia (79%), headache (30%), hypothyroidism (29%), asthenia (20%).
Occasional
Rash (17%); nausea (15%); peripheral edema (13%); dry skin, abdominal pain (11%); chills, exfoliative dermatitis (10%); diarrhea (7%); changes in mood or behaviour (< 10%).

SERIOUS REACTIONS

• Pancreatitis, hepatic failure, and pneumonia occur rarely.

PRECAUTIONS & CONSIDERATIONS

Caution is warranted with diabetes mellitus, lipid abnormalities, and hepatic impairment. Bexarotene use should be avoided during pregnancy because the drug may cause fetal harm. Pregnancy should be determined before beginning oral or topical treatment. Two reliable contraceptive methods (one nonhormonal) should be used during therapy and for 1 mo afterward. Women should notify their physician if they plan to become or become pregnant. It is unknown if bexarotene is distributed in breast milk; however, breastfeeding is not recommended. The safety and efficacy of bexarotene have not been established in children. No age-related precautions have been noted in the elderly. Abrasive, drying, or medicated soaps should be avoided during therapy.

Baseline lipid profile, liver function, thyroid function, and WBC count should be determined. Cholesterol and triglyceride levels, CBC, and liver and thyroid function test results should be monitored during therapy.
Storage
Store at room temperatures.
Protect from light and moisture.
Avoid high temperatures.
Administration
Take oral bexarotene with a fat-containing meal. Avoid application of topical bexarotene to normal skin. Cover lesion with generous coating; avoid occlusive dressings. Allow to dry before applying clothing. Wait 20 min after bathing before applying gel. Avoid bathing or swimming for at least 3 h after applying.

Bicalutamide

bye-ka-loo′ta-mide
Casodex

CATEGORY AND SCHEDULE

Pregnancy Risk Category: X

Classification: Nonsteroidal antiandrogen, antineoplastic

MECHANISM OF ACTION
An antiandrogen antineoplastic agent that competitively inhibits androgen action by binding to androgen receptors in target tissue. *Therapeutic Effect:* Decreases growth of prostatic carcinoma.

PHARMACOKINETICS
Well absorbed from the GI tract. Protein binding: 96%. Metabolized in the liver to inactive metabolite. Excreted in urine and feces. Not removed by hemodialysis. *Half-life:* 5.8 days (prolonged in severe liver disease).

AVAILABILITY
Tablets: 50 mg.

INDICATIONS AND DOSAGES
▸ Prostatic carcinoma
PO
Adults, Elderly. 50 mg once a day in morning or evening, given concurrently with a luteinizing hormone-releasing hormone (LHRH) analogue or after surgical castration.

CONTRAINDICATIONS
Pregnancy, use in women, hypersensitivity to any component of the formulation.

INTERACTIONS
Drug
Potent CYP3A4 inhibitors: May increase bicalutamide exposure.
Warfarin: May increase warfarin's effects.
Herbal
St. John's wort: May decrease bicalutamide concentrations.

DIAGNOSTIC TEST EFFECTS
May increase BUN level and serum alkaline phosphatase, bilirubin, AST (SGOT), and ALT (SGPT) levels. May decrease blood hemoglobin level and WBC count.

SIDE EFFECTS
Frequent
Hot flashes (49%), breast pain (38%), muscle pain (27%), constipation (17%), diarrhea (10%), asthenia (15%), nausea (11%).
Occasional (8%-9%)
Nocturia, abdominal pain, peripheral edema.
Rare (3%-7%)
Vomiting, weight loss, dizziness, insomnia, rash, impotence, gynecomastia.

SERIOUS REACTIONS
- Sepsis, CHF, hypertension, hepatotoxicity, and iron deficiency anemia may occur.

PRECAUTIONS & CONSIDERATIONS
Caution is warranted with moderate to severe hepatic impairment. Liver function test results should be obtained before beginning therapy. Bicalutamide may inhibit spermatogenesis; this drug is not used in women, but is expected to cause fetal harm if a woman is exposed in pregnancy. The safety and efficacy of bicalutamide have not been established in children. No age-related precautions have been noted in elderly patients.

Notify the physician if nausea and vomiting persist.

Storage
Store at controlled room temperature.
Administration
Give oral bicalutamide at the same time each day and without regard to food. Avoid abruptly discontinuing the drug. Both bicalutamide and the LHRH analogue must be continued to achieve the desired therapeutic effect.

Bimatoprost

bye-mat'oh-prost

Lumigan, Latisse

CATEGORY AND SCHEDULE

Pregnancy Risk Category: C

Classification: Ophthalmic agents, prostaglandin analogues

MECHANISM OF ACTION

A synthetic analogue of prostaglandin with ocular hypotensive activity. *Therapeutic Effect:* Reduces intraocular pressure (IOP) by increasing the outflow of aqueous humor, increases eyelash growth.

PHARMACOKINETICS

Absorbed through the cornea and hydrolyzed to the active free acid form. Protein binding: 88%. Moderately distributed into body tissues. Metabolized in liver. Primarily excreted in urine; some elimination in feces. *Half-life:* 45 min.

AVAILABILITY

Ophthalmic solution: 0.03%

INDICATIONS AND DOSAGES

▸ **Glaucoma, Ocular Hypertension**

OPHTHALMIC

Adults, Elderly. 1 drop in affected eye(s) once daily, in the evening.

▸ **Hypotrichosis of eyelashes**

TOPICAL (LATISSE ONLY)

Adults. 1 drop at night, applied to the upper eyelid margin.

CONTRAINDICATIONS

Hypersensitivity to bimatoprost or any other component of the formulation.

DIAGNOSTIC TEST EFFECTS

None known.

SIDE EFFECTS

Frequent

Conjunctival hyperemia, growth of eyelashes, increased iris pigmentation, and ocular pruritus.

Occasional

Ocular dryness, visual disturbance, ocular burning, foreign body sensation, eye pain, pigmentation of the periocular skin, blepharitis, cataract, superficial punctate keratitis, eyelid erythema, ocular irritation, and eyelash darkening.

Rare

Intraocular inflammation (iritis).

SERIOUS REACTIONS

- Systemic adverse events, including infections (colds and upper respiratory tract infections), headaches, asthenia, and hirsutism, have been reported.

PRECAUTIONS & CONSIDERATIONS

May permanently increase pigmentation in iris and eyelid and produce changes in eye color and changes in eyelashes (color, length, shape). Use with caution in patients with uveitis or risk factors for macular edema. Effects in pregnancy and lactation not known; use with caution and only if clearly needed in women who are pregnant or breastfeeding. Safety and effectiveness have not been established in children. Remove contact lenses to apply; wait 15 min after administration to reinsert.

Storage

Store at room temperature.

Administration

For Lumigan: Tilt the head back slightly and pull the lower eyelid down with the index finger to form a pouch. Instill drop(s) and gently

B

close the eyes for 1-2 min. Do not blink. Do not touch the tip of the dropper to any surface to avoid contamination. If more than 1 topical ophthalmic agent is being used, wait at least 5 min between administration of each.
For Latisse: Patient's face should be clean; remove all makeup. Use only the disposable sterile applicator provided. Each applicator should be used for 1 eye only; dispose of after use. Apply 1 drop of solution to the applicator, then place along the skin of the upper eyelid margin at the base of the eyelashes. Blot excess runoff with a tissue. Do not apply to the lower eyelash line.

Bisacodyl

bis-ah-koe'dill
★ Alophen, Bisac-Evac, Biscolax, Correctol, Dacodyl, Dulcolax, Ex-Lax Ultra, Fematrol, Femilax, Fleets Bisacodyl, Verocolate
🍁 Apo-Biscodyl, Carters
Do not confuse bisacodyl with bisoprolol or Visicol, or Veracolate with Accolate.

CATEGORY AND SCHEDULE

Pregnancy Risk Category: C
OTC

Classification: Laxative, stimulant

MECHANISM OF ACTION

A GI stimulant that has a direct effect on colonic smooth musculature by stimulating the intramural nerve plexi. *Therapeutic Effect:* Promotes fluid and ion accumulation in the colon, increasing peristalsis and producing a laxative effect.

PHARMACOKINETICS

Route	Onset	Peak	Duration
PO	6-12 h	N/A	N/A
Rectal	15-60 min	N/A	N/A

Minimal absorption following oral and rectal administration. Absorbed drug is excreted in urine; remainder is eliminated in feces.

AVAILABILITY

Tablets, Enteric Coated: 5 mg.
Suppositories, Rectal: 10 mg.
Enema: 10 mg.

INDICATIONS AND DOSAGES

▸ **For use in bowel preparation regimens**
PO
Adults, Children older than 12 yr. 10-mg single dose. Following the 1st bowel movement (or after a max of 6 h after bisacodyl dose), give the prepared bowel prep solution as directed until consumed.
▸ **Treatment of constipation**
PO
Adults, Children older than 12 yr. 5-15 mg as needed.
Children 6-12 yr. 5-10 mg or 0.3 mg/kg at bedtime or after breakfast.
RECTAL
Adults, Children 12 yr and older. 10 mg to induce bowel movement.
Children 6-11 yr. 5-10 mg as a single dose.

CONTRAINDICATIONS

Hypersensitivity, GI obstruction, bowel perforation, toxic colitis, toxic megacolon, undiagnosed rectal bleeding. Tablets should not be given if dysphagia is present.

INTERACTIONS

Drug
Antacids, H_2-blockers, proton-pump inhibitors: May cause rapid

dissolution of bisacodyl tablets, producing gastric irritation or dyspepsia, possible vomiting.
Oral medications: May decrease transit time of concurrently administered oral medications.
Food
Milk: May cause rapid dissolution of bisacodyl tablets, increasing stomach irritation.

DIAGNOSTIC TEST EFFECTS

None known.

SIDE EFFECTS

Frequent
Some degree of abdominal discomfort, nausea, mild cramps, and faintness.
Occasional
Rectal administration: burning of rectal mucosa, mild proctitis.

SERIOUS REACTIONS

• Long-term use may result in laxative dependence, chronic constipation, and loss of normal bowel function.
• Prolonged use or overdose may result in electrolyte or metabolic disturbances (such as hypokalemia, hypocalcemia, and metabolic acidosis or alkalosis) as well as persistent diarrhea, vomiting, muscle weakness, malabsorption, and weight loss.

PRECAUTIONS & CONSIDERATIONS

Excessive use of bisacodyl may lead to fluid and electrolyte imbalance. It is unknown whether bisacodyl crosses the placenta or is distributed in breast milk. Avoid oral bisacodyl use in children younger than 6 yr of age. Rectal use ok in younger children with medical supervision. Repeated use of bisacodyl in elderly patients may cause orthostatic hypotension and weakness because of electrolyte loss.

In the treatment of constipation, increasing fluid intake, exercising, and eating a high-fiber diet should be instituted to promote defecation. Notify the physician if unrelieved constipation, dizziness, muscle cramps or pain, rectal bleeding, or weakness occurs. Electrolyte levels, hydration status, daily bowel activity, and stool consistency should be assessed.

When used for bowel preparation, carefully follow prescribed regimen to get best result for colon cleansing.
Storage
Store at room temperature; suppositories may be stored in refrigerator.
Administration
Take oral bisacodyl on an empty stomach for faster action. Offer 6-8 glasses of water a day to aid in stool softening. Administer tablets whole; do not chew or crush them. Avoid taking within 1 h of antacids, milk, or other oral medications.

For rectal use, if suppository is too soft, chill for 30 min in refrigerator or run cold water over wrapper. Unwrap and moisten suppository with cold water before inserting deep into rectum.

Bismuth Subsalicylate

bis′muth sub-sal-ih′sah-late
★ Bismatrol, Kaopectate, Maalox Total Stomach Relief, Peptic Relief, Pepto-Bismol
🍁 Stomak-Care, Pepto-Bismol

CATEGORY AND SCHEDULE

Pregnancy Risk Category: C
OTC

Classification: Antidiarrheal, salicylates

MECHANISM OF ACTION

An antinauseant and antiulcer agent that absorbs water and toxins in the large intestine and forms a protective coating in the intestinal mucosa. Also possesses antisecretory and antimicrobial effects. *Therapeutic Effect:* Prevents diarrhea. Helps treat *Helicobacter pylori*–associated peptic ulcer disease.

AVAILABILITY

Caplet: 262 mg.
Liquid: 262 mg/15 mL, 524 mg/15 mL, 525 mg/15 mL.
Tablet (Chewable): 262 mg.

INDICATIONS AND DOSAGES

▸ Diarrhea, gastric distress

PO

(Doses based on 262 mg/15 mL liquid or 262 mg tablets)

Adults, Children over 12 yrs of age. 2 tablets (30 mL) q30-60 min. Maximum: 8 doses in 24 h.

▸ *H. pylori*–associated duodenal ulcer, gastritis

PO

Adults, Elderly. 525 mg 4 times a day, for 14 days. Combined with metronidazole, tetracycline, and acid-suppressive therapy.

OFF-LABEL USES

Prevention of traveler's diarrhea.

CONTRAINDICATIONS

Salicylate hypersensitivity.
Bleeding ulcers, gout, hemophilia, hemorrhagic states, renal impairment, pregnancy (third trimester); children and teenagers who have or are recovering from chickenpox, influenza symptoms, or influenza because of the risk of Reye syndrome. Not a suitable treatment for dysentery.

INTERACTIONS

Drug

Anticoagulants, heparin, thrombolytics: May increase the risk of bleeding.
Aspirin, other salicylates: May increase the risk of salicylate toxicity.
Insulin, oral antidiabetics: Large dose may increase the effects of insulin and oral antidiabetics.
Tetracyclines: May decrease the absorption of tetracyclines.

Herbal

Willow bark: May increase risk of salicylate toxicity.

Food

None known.

DIAGNOSTIC TEST EFFECTS

May alter serum alkaline phosphatase, AST (SGOT), ALT (SGPT), and uric acid levels. May decrease serum potassium level. May prolong PT.

SIDE EFFECTS

Frequent

Grayish black stools.

Rare

Constipation.

SERIOUS REACTIONS

• Debilitated patients may develop impaction.
• Symptoms of salicylate toxicity include abdominal pain, diaphoresis, dizziness, rapid respirations, drowsiness, headache, hearing loss or tinnitus, nausea/vomiting, metabolic acidosis. Encephalopathy including confusion, myasthenia, tremor or unusal body movements may be present.
• Hypersensitivity reactions may include anaphylaxis, angioedema, hives or other rashes, or acute asthma.

PRECAUTIONS & CONSIDERATIONS

Caution is warranted with diabetes and in elderly patients. Avoid bismuth if taking aspirin or other salicylates because of increased risk of toxicity. Also, inform the physician if taking anticoagulants because this drug combination can dangerously prolong bleeding time. Be aware that stool may appear black or gray; may cause darkening of the tongue. Pattern of daily bowel activity and stool consistency should be monitored. Due to risk of Reye syndrome and lack of clinical data to support use, do not use in infants and children < 12 yr of age. In general, avoid use in pregnancy, especially in third trimester. Use with caution during breastfeeding.

Storage

Store in a dry place at room temperature.

Administration

Shake liquid/suspension well before administration. Measure suspension dosage with calibrated spoon or cup.

Caplets should be swallowed whole.

Chew the chewable tablet before swallowing. Alternatively, allow the chewable tablet to dissolve before swallowing.

Bisoprolol

bis-ope′pro-lal

★ Zebeta

🍁 Apo-Bisoprolol, Monocor

Do not confuse Zebeta with DiaBeta.

CATEGORY AND SCHEDULE

Pregnancy Risk Category: C

Classification: Antihypertensive, selective β_1-blocker

MECHANISM OF ACTION

An antihypertensive that blocks β_1-adrenergic receptors in cardiac tissue. *Therapeutic Effect:* Slows sinus heart rate and decreases BP.

PHARMACOKINETICS

Well absorbed from the GI tract. Protein binding: roughly 30%. Eliminated equally by renal and nonrenal pathways with about 50%. of the dose appearing unchanged in the urine and the remainder appearing in the form of inactive metabolites. Not removed by hemodialysis. *Half-life:* 9-12 h (increased in impaired renal function).

AVAILABILITY

Tablets: 5 mg, 10 mg.

INDICATIONS AND DOSAGES

▸ **Hypertension**

PO

Adults. Initially, 5 mg/day. May increase up to 20 mg/day.

Elderly. Initially, 2.5-5 mg/day. May increase by 2.5-5 mg/day. Maximum: 20 mg/day.

▸ **Dosage in renal or hepatic impairment**

For adults and elderly patients with cirrhosis or hepatitis or whose creatinine clearance is < 40 mL/min; initially give 2.5 mg/day, then titrate.

OFF-LABEL USES

Angina pectoris, heart failure, premature ventricular contractions, supraventricular arrhythmias.

CONTRAINDICATIONS

Cardiogenic shock, overt cardiac failure, second- or third-degree heart block (except in patients with functioning artificial pacemaker), marked sinus bradycardia.

B

INTERACTIONS

Drug

Cimetidine: May increase bisoprolol blood concentration.

Diuretics, other antihypertensives: May increase the hypotensive effect of bisoprolol.

Insulin, oral hypoglycemics: May mask symptoms of hypoglycemia and prolong the hypoglycemic effect of these drugs.

NSAIDs: May decrease antihypertensive effect.

Sympathomimetics, xanthines: May mutually inhibit effects.

Rifampin: May decrease bisoprolol blood concentration.

Herbal

None known.

Food

None known.

DIAGNOSTIC TEST EFFECTS

May increase antinuclear antibody titer and BUN, serum lipoprotein, creatinine, potassium, uric acid, and triglyceride levels.

SIDE EFFECTS

Frequent

Hypotension manifested as dizziness, nausea, diaphoresis, headache, cold extremities, fatigue, constipation, or diarrhea.

Occasional

Insomnia, flatulence, urinary frequency, impotence, or decreased libido.

Rare

Rash, arthralgia, myalgia, confusion (especially in the elderly), altered taste.

SERIOUS REACTIONS

- Overdose may produce profound bradycardia and hypotension.
- Abrupt withdrawal may result in diaphoresis, palpitations, headache, and tremulousness.
- Bisoprolol administration may precipitate congestive heart failure and myocardial infarction in patients with heart disease; thyroid storm in those with thyrotoxicosis; and peripheral ischemia in those with existing peripheral vascular disease.
- Hypoglycemia may occur in patients with previously controlled diabetes.
- Thrombocytopenia, including unusual bruising and bleeding, occurs rarely.

PRECAUTIONS & CONSIDERATIONS

Caution is warranted with bronchospastic disease, diabetes, hyperthyroidism, impaired hepatic or renal function, inadequate cardiac function, and peripheral vascular disease. Bisoprolol readily crosses the placenta and is distributed in breast milk. Bisoprolol use should be avoided in pregnant women after the first trimester because it may result in low-birth-weight infants. The drug may also produce apnea, bradycardia, hypoglycemia, or hypothermia at birth. The safety and efficacy of bisoprolol have not been established in children. In elderly patients, age-related peripheral vascular disease may increase the risk of decreased peripheral circulation. Be aware that salt and alcohol intake should be restricted. Nasal decongestants or OTC cold preparations (stimulants) should not be used without physician approval.

Orthostatic hypotension may occur, so rise slowly from a lying to sitting position and dangle the legs from the bed momentarily before standing. Tasks that require mental alertness or motor skills should be avoided. BP for hypotension, respiratory status for shortness of breath, pattern of daily bowel activity and stool consistency, and pulse for quality, rate, and rhythm should be monitored. If pulse rate is 60 beats/min or lower or systolic BP is < 90 mm Hg, withhold the medication and contact the physician. Signs and symptoms of CHF, such as decreased urine output, distended neck veins, dyspnea (particularly on exertion or lying down), night cough, peripheral edema, and weight gain, should also be assessed.

Storage

Store at controlled room temperature and protect from moisture.

Administration

Bisoprolol may be taken without regard to food. Do not abruptly discontinue. Compliance is essential to control hypertension.

Bivalirudin

bye-val'i-roo-din

Angiomax

CATEGORY AND SCHEDULE

Pregnancy Risk Category: B

Classification: Anticoagulants, thrombin inhibitors

MECHANISM OF ACTION

An anticoagulant that specifically and reversibly inhibits thrombin by binding to its receptor sites. *Therapeutic Effect:* Decreases acute ischemic complications in patients with unstable angina pectoris.

PHARMACOKINETICS

Route	Onset	Peak	Duration
IV	Immediate	N/A	1 h

Primarily eliminated by kidneys. A total of 25% removed by hemodialysis. *Half-life:* 25 min (increased in moderate to severe renal impairment).

AVAILABILITY

Injection, Lyophilized Powder: 250 mg.

INDICATIONS AND DOSAGES

▸ Anticoagulant in patients with unstable angina who are undergoing percutaneous transluminal coronary angioplasty (PTCA) or percutaneous coronary intervention (PCI); patients undergoing pci with (or at risk of) heparin-induced thrombocytopenia/thrombosis syndrome (HIT/HITTS)

IV

Adults, Elderly. 0.75 mg/kg as IV bolus, followed by continuous infusion of 1.75 mg/kg/h for the duration of the procedure and up to 4 h postprocedure. NOTE: In patients without HIT/HITTS, 5 min after the initial bolus dose an activated clotting time (ACT) is performed and an additional bolus of 0.3 mg/kg is given if needed. Infusion may be continued beyond the initial 4 h at a lower rate of 0.2 mg/kg/h for up to 20 h.

▸ Dosage in renal impairment

GFR	Infusion Dose Reduced to
10-29 mL/min	1 mg/kg/h
Dialysis	0.25 mg/kg/h

OFF-LABEL USE

Alternative to heparin during acute MI (STEMI).

CONTRAINDICATIONS

Active major bleeding, hypersensitivity.

INTERACTIONS

Drug

Platelet aggregation inhibitors thrombolytics, warfarin: May increase the risk of bleeding complications.

Herbal

Ginkgo biloba: May increase the risk of bleeding.

Food

None known.

DIAGNOSTIC TEST EFFECTS

Prolongs aPTT and PT.

IV INCOMPATIBILITIES

Do not mix with other medications. Specific Y-site incompatibilities include alteplase (tPA, Activase), amiodarone, amphotericin B, caspofungin (Cancidas), chlorpromazine, diazepam, lansoprazole (Prevacid), phenytoin, prochlorperazine, quinidine gluconate, quinupristin-dalfopristin (Synercid), reteplase (Retavase), streptokinase, vancomycin.

SIDE EFFECTS

Frequent (42%)

Back pain.

Occasional (12%-15%)

Nausea, headache, hypotension, generalized pain.

Rare (4%-8%)

Injection site pain, bleeding (e.g., epistaxis, hematoma), insomnia, hypertension, anxiety, vomiting, pelvic or abdominal pain, bradycardia, nervousness, dyspepsia, fever, urine retention.

SERIOUS REACTIONS

- A serious hemorrhagic event occurs rarely and is characterized by a fall in BP or hematocrit.

PRECAUTIONS & CONSIDERATIONS

Caution is warranted with conditions associated with increased risk of bleeding, including bacterial endocarditis, cerebrovascular accident, hemorrhagic diathesis, intracerebral surgery, recent major bleeding, recent major surgery, stroke, severe hypertension, and severe hepatic or renal impairment. It is unknown whether bivalirudin is distributed in breast milk or crosses the placenta. Safety and efficacy of bivalirudin have not been established in children. In elderly patients, age-related renal impairment may require dosage adjustment. Elderly patients experience more bleeding events than younger patients. Women should be aware that menstrual flow may be heavier than usual.

Notify the physician of bleeding from femoral vein site, blood in urine or stool, or discomfort or pain (especially chest pain) after treatment. Pulse rate, BP, aPTT, hematocrit, BUN and serum creatinine levels, and stool or urine cultures for occult blood should be monitored.

Storage

Store unreconstituted vials at room temperature.

Administration

! Bivalirudin is intended for use with aspirin, 300-325 mg PO daily. Treatment should be initiated immediately before angioplasty.

To each 250-mg vial, add 5 mL sterile water for injection. Gently swirl until all material is dissolved. For the initial IV bolus and infusion, further dilute each vial in 50 mL D5W or 0.9% NaCl to yield final concentration of 5 mg/mL: 1 vial in 50 mL, 2 vials in 100 mL, 5 vials in 250 mL. If low-rate (e.g., the 0.2-mg/kg/h infusion) is used after the initial infusion, reconstitute a vial as directed and dilute in 500 mL D5W or 0.9% NaCl to yield a final concentration of 0.5 mg/mL. Diluting produces a clear, colorless solution; do not use solution if it is cloudy or contains a precipitate.

Bleomycin Sulfate

blee-oh-my'sin sull'fate

Blenoxane

CATEGORY AND SCHEDULE

Pregnancy Risk Category: D

Drug Class: Antineoplastic, natural antineoplastics

MECHANISM OF ACTION

A glycopeptide antibiotic whose mechanism of action is unknown. Is most effective in the G2 phase of cell division. *Therapeutic Effect:* Appears to inhibit DNA synthesis and, to a lesser extent, RNA and protein synthesis.

PHARMACOKINETICS

Half-life: 2 h; when creatinine clearance is > 35 mL/min, half-life is increased in lower clearance; metabolized in liver, 50% excreted in urine (unchanged).

AVAILABILITY

Powder for Injection: 15 units, 30 units.

INDICATIONS AND DOSAGES

▸ **For monotherapy or in combination therapy for testicular carcinoma; lymphomas (including Hodgkin disease, choriocarcinoma, reticulum cell sarcoma, and lymphosarcoma); and squamous cell carcinomas of the head and neck (including mouth, tongue, tonsil, nasopharynx, oropharynx, sinus, palate, lip, buccal mucosa, gingiva, epiglottis, and larynx)**

IV, IM, SC

Adults, Elderly. 10-20 units/m^2 (0.25-0.5 unit/kg) 1-2 times/wk. For Hodgkin disease, after a 50% response is obtained, the maintenance dose is usually 1 unit/day or 5 units/week. NOTE: Other dosing regimens have been used for selected cancers, and bleomycin dosing in such regimens varies with the concurrent usage of other chemotherapy along with bleomycin.

▸ **As a sclerosing agent to treat malignant pleural effusions and prevent recurrent pleural effusions**

INTRAPLEURAL

Adults, Elderly. 60 units as a single injection.

▸ **General dose in renal impairment (Adults)**

IV/IM/SC

CrCl 40-50 mL/min. 70% of normal dose.

CrCl 30-40 mL/min. 60% of normal dose.

CrCl 20-30 mL/min. 55% of normal dose.

CrCl 10-20 mL/min. 45% of normal dose.

CrCl 5-10 mL/min. 40% of normal dose.

CONTRAINDICATIONS

Hypersensitivity.

INTERACTIONS

Drug

Digoxin: May reduce digoxin serum concentrations.

Phenytoin: May reduce phenytoin serum concentrations.

Tobacco: Smoking increases pulmonary toxicity risk.

Herbal

None known.

Food

None known.

B

DIAGNOSTIC TEST EFFECTS
None known.

SIDE EFFECTS
Frequent
Anorexia, weight loss, erythematous skin swelling, urticaria, rash, striae, vesiculation, hyperpigmentation (particularly at areas of pressure, skinfolds, cuticles, IM injection sites, and scars), stomatitis (usually evident 1-3 wks after initial therapy); may also be accompanied by decreased skin sensitivity followed by skin hypersensitivity, nausea, vomiting, alopecia, and (with parenteral form) fever or chills (typically occurring a few hours after large single dose and lasting 4-12 h).

SERIOUS REACTIONS
• Interstitial pneumonitis occurs in 10% of patients and occasionally progresses to pulmonary fibrosis. This condition appears to be dose or age related, occurring more often in patients receiving a total dose > 400 units and those older than 70 yr.
• Nephrotoxicity and hepatotoxicity occur infrequently.
• Idiosyncratic reaction consisting of hypertension, mental confusion, fever, chills, and wheezing has been reported in 1% of lymphoma patients treated with bleomycin.

PRECAUTIONS & CONSIDERATIONS
Use with caution in patients with renal impairment, compromised pulmonary function. Avoid use in pregnant or lactating women.
Storage
Store unreconstituted powder for injection in the refrigerator. Diluted solution stable for 24 h at room temperature.
Administration
CAUTION: Observe and exercise usual cautions for handling and preparing solutions of cytotoxic drugs.

Do not reconstitute or dilute with D5W or other dextrose-containing diluents.

When reconstituting for IM or subcutaneous use, the 15-unit vial should be dissolved with 1-5 mL of sterile water for injection or 0.9% NaCl injection, or bacteriostatic water for injection. The 30-unit vial may be reconstituted with 2-10 mL of the listed diluents.

For IV Use, 15 units or 30 units should be dissolved in 5 mL or 10 mL respectively, of 0.9% NaCl and given slowly over a period of 10 min.

For intrapleural use, 60 units is dissolved in 50-100 mL NaCl 0.9% and administered through a thoracostomy tube after drainage of excess pleural fluid and confirmation of complete lung expansion.

Bortezomib
bor-teh'zoe-mib
★ 🍁 Velcade

CATEGORY AND SCHEDULE
Pregnancy Risk Category: D

Classification: Antineoplastics, proteasome inhibitors, signal transduction inhibitors

MECHANISM OF ACTION
A proteasome inhibitor and antineoplastic agent that degrades conjugated proteins required for cell-cycle progression and mitosis, disrupting cell proliferation.
Therapeutic Effect: Produces antitumor and chemosensitizing activity and cell death.

PHARMACOKINETICS

Distributed to tissues and organs, with highest level in the GI tract and liver. Protein binding: 83%. Primarily metabolized by CYP enzymes 3A4, 2C19, and 1A2. Deboronated metabolites are not active. The pathways of elimination are not characterized in humans. *Half-life:* The mean elimination half-life upon multiple dosing ranged from 40-193 h after the 1-mg/m^2 dose and 76-108 h after the 1.3-mg/m^2 dose.

AVAILABILITY

Powder for Injection: 3.5 mg.

INDICATIONS AND DOSAGES

▸ **Previously untreated multiple myeloma**

IV

Adults, Elderly: Administered in combination with oral melphalan and prednisone for nine 6-wk treatment cycles. Treatment cycles 1-4 consist of 1.3 mg/m^2 twice weekly on days 1, 4, 8, 11, 22, 25, 29 and 32. Treatment cycles 5-9 consist of 1.3 mg/m^2 once weekly on days 1, 8, 22, and 29. Consecutive doses are separated by at least 72 h.

▸ **Relapsed multiple myeloma or for mantle cell lymphoma**

IV

Adluts Elderly. Treatment cycle consists of 1.3 mg/m^2 twice weekly on days 1, 4, 8, and 11 followed by a 10-day rest priod (days 12-21). Therapy beyond 8 cycles may be given once weekly for 4 wks (days 1, 8, 15, and 22) followed by a 13-day rest (day 23-35). Consecutive doses are separated by at least 72h.

▸ **Moderate or severe hepatic impairment (all indications)**

Reduce to 0.7 mg/m^2 in first cycle. Consider escalation to 1 mg/m^2 or further reduction to 0.5 mg/m^2 in other cycles based on patient tolerance.

▸ **Dosage adjustment guidelines**

Therapy is withheld at onset of grade 3 nonhematologic or grade 4 hematologic toxicities, excluding neuropathy.

See manufacturer's recommendations for adjustments based on disease state, grade of toxicity, and toxicity type.

CONTRAINDICATIONS

Hypersensitivity to bortezomib, boron, or mannitol.

INTERACTIONS

Drug

Oral antidiabetics: May alter the response of these drugs.

Potent CYP3A4 inhibitors (e.g., ketoconazole, ritonavir): May increase bortezomib exposure. Closely monitor.

Herbal

St. John's wort: May decrease bortezomib levels, may significantly decrease blood hemoglobin and hematocrit levels and neutrophil, platelet, and WBC counts.

SIDE EFFECTS

Expected (36%-65%)

Fatigue, malaise, asthenia, nausea, diarrhea, anorexia, constipation, fever, vomiting.

Frequent (21%-28%)

Headache, insomnia, arthralgia, limb pain, edema, paresthesia, dizziness, rash.

Occasional (11%-18%)

Dehydration, cough, anxiety, bone pain, muscle cramps, myalgia, back pain, abdominal pain, taste alteration, dyspepsia, pruritus, hypotension (including orthostatic hypotension), rigors, blurred vision.

B

SERIOUS REACTIONS

- Thrombocytopenia occurs in 40% of patients. Platelet count peaks at day 11 and returns to baseline by day 21. GI and intracerebral hemorrhage are associated with drug-induced thrombocytopenia.
- Anemia occurs in 32% of patients.
- New-onset or worsening neuropathy occurs in 37% of patients. Symptoms may improve in some patients when bortezomib is discontinued.
- Reversible posterior leukoencephalopathy syndrome.
- Pneumonia occurs occasionally; rare reports of pneumonitis, interstitial pneumonia, lung infiltration, and acute respiratory distress syndrome.
- New onset or exacerbation of heart failure, new onset of decreased left ventricular ejection fraction.
- Tumor lysis syndrome, acute hepatic failure (rare).

PRECAUTIONS & CONSIDERATIONS

Caution is warranted with history of syncope, risk factors for heart disease, diabetes, hepatic impairment. Caution should also be used with any medication that increases the risk of dehydration, hypotension, and hepatic or renal function impairment. Bortezomib may induce degenerative effects in the ovaries and testes and may affect male and female fertility. Breastfeeding is not recommended. The safety and efficacy of bortezomib have not been established in children. Elderly patients are at increased risk for grade 3 and 4 thrombocytopenia.

Notify the physician of orthostatic hypotension, fever, pregnancy, nausea, vomiting, or diarrhea. Tasks that require mental alertness or motor skills should be avoided until response to the drug is established. Signs and symptoms of peripheral neuropathy, including a burning sensation, hyperesthesia, neuropathic pain, and paresthesia of the extremities, should be assessed. CBC, especially platelet count, should be monitored before and throughout bortezomib treatment. Intake and output and BP should also be monitored. Adequate hydration should be maintained to prevent dehydration. IM injections or rectal medications and performing other procedures that may induce trauma and bleeding should be avoided.

Storage

Store unopened vials at room temperature. Protect from light. The reconstituted solution is stable at room temperature for up to 8 h.

Administration

CAUTION: Observe and exercise usual cautions for handling and preparing solutions of cytotoxic drugs.

Reconstitute the vial with 3.5 mL 0.9% NaCl. The solution will have a final concentration of 1 mg/mL and will be clear and colorless. Take care to withdraw the correct dose. Give bortezomib as a 3- to 5-second bolus IV injection.

Bosentan

bo′sen-tan

★ 🍁 Tracleer

Do not confuse with Tricor.

CATEGORY AND SCHEDULE

Pregnancy Risk Category: X

Classification: Antihypertensive; endothelin receptor antagonist

MECHANISM OF ACTION

An endothelin receptor antagonist that blocks endothelin-1, the neurohormone that constricts pulmonary arteries. *Therapeutic Effect:* Improves exercise ability and slows clinical worsening of pulmonary arterial hypertension (PAH).

PHARMACOKINETICS

Highly bound to plasma proteins, mainly albumin. Metabolized in the liver. Eliminated by biliary excretion. *Half-life:* Approximately 5 h.

AVAILABILITY

Tablets: 62.5 mg, 125 mg.

INDICATIONS AND DOSAGES

▸ **PAH in those with World Health Organization Class III or IV symptoms**

PO

Adults, Elderly weighing more than 40 kg. 62.5 mg twice a day for 4 wks; then increase to maintenance dosage of 125 mg twice a day.

Adults, Elderly, weighing < 40 kg. 62.5 mg twice a day.

CONTRAINDICATIONS

Administration with cyclosporine or glyburide, pregnancy, hypersensitivity, moderate or severe liver impairment.

INTERACTIONS

NOTE: Bosentan may interact with many drugs, as it induces drug metabolism. Review prescribing information carefully with any new prescription.

Drug

Atorvastatin, hormonal contraceptives (including oral, injectable, and implantable), lovastatin, simvastatin, warfarin: May decrease the plasma concentrations of these drugs.

Cyclosporine, ketoconazole, tacrolimus: Increases plasma concentration of bosentan. Cyclosporine is contraindicated.

Glyburide: Increased risk of liver injury. Bosentan also decreases glyburide concentrations. Glyburide is contraindicated.

Ritonavir: Increased bosentan levels and decreased ritonavir levels.

Herbal

St. John's wort: May decrease bosentan serum concentrations.

Food

Grapefruit juice: May increase bosentan serum concentrations.

DIAGNOSTIC TEST EFFECTS

May increase serum bilirubin, AST (SGOT), and ALT (SGPT) levels. May decrease blood hemoglobin and hematocrit levels.

SIDE EFFECTS

Occasional

Headache, nasopharyngitis, flushing.

Rare

Dyspepsia (heartburn, epigastric distress), fatigue, pruritus, hypotension, lower extremity edema, low sperm counts.

SERIOUS REACTIONS

- Abnormal hepatic function, with significant liver enzyme elevations; rare cases of unexplained hepatic cirrhosis.
- Major birth defects.

PRECAUTIONS & CONSIDERATIONS

Bosentan administration may induce atrophy of seminiferous tubules of the testes, cause male infertility, or reduced sperm count. Bosentan causes fetal harm and has teratogenic effects on the fetus, including malformations of the face, head, large vessels, and mouth.

B

Breastfeeding is not recommended. The safety and efficacy of bosentan use in children have not been established. Use cautiously in elderly patients because the higher frequency of decreased cardiac, hepatic, and renal function is more common in this age group.

Because pregnancy must be avoided during bosentan therapy, it should be ruled out before the start of therapy. A negative result from a urine or serum pregnancy test should be obtained during the first 5 days of a normal menstrual period and at least 11 days after the last act of sexual intercourse before drug therapy begins. Monthly pregnancy tests should be performed during bosentan therapy. Female patients should not rely on hormonal contraceptives as sole birth control method.

Liver function tests (serum aminotransferase, serum alkaline phosphatase, bilirubin, AST [SGOT], and ALT [SGPT]) should be monitored before bosentan therapy begins and monthly thereafter. Changes in monitoring and treatment should be initiated if an elevation in liver enzymes occurs. Treatment should be stopped if clinical symptoms of hepatic injury, including abdominal pain, fatigue, jaundice, nausea, and vomiting, occur or if bilirubin level increases. Blood hemoglobin level at 1 and 3 mo should also be obtained after treatment begins and every 3 mo thereafter; a decrease in blood hematocrit and hemoglobin levels signifies anemia.

Storage
Store tablets at room temperature.

Administration
Take bosentan in the morning and evening, with or without food. Do not break or crush film-coated tablets. Swallow the film-coated tablets whole, and avoid chewing them.

Botulism A/B Immune Globulin Intravenous (Human)

bot′ue-lizm ih′mewn glob′yoo-lin

BabyBIG

CATEGORY AND SCHEDULE

Pregnancy Risk Category: Not assigned.

Classification: Immune globulins

MECHANISM OF ACTION

Contains IgG antibodies from immunized donors who contributed to the plasma pool from which the product was derived. The titer of antibodies in the reconstituted product against type A botulinum toxin is at least 15 IU/mL and against type B toxin is at least 2 IU/mL. These antibodies bind and neutralize the target toxin. *Therapeutic effect:* In the case of infants exposed to botulinum neurotoxin type A or B, this product is expected to provide antibodies at levels sufficient to neutralize the circulating neurotoxin, decreasing ICU time, related support, and overall hospitalization.

PHARMACOKINETICS

Traditional pharmacokinetic studies have not been done. The half-life is roughly 28 days in infants and is similar to other IVIG products. A single IV infusion is expected to provide a protective antibody level for up to 6 months.

AVAILABILITY

Lyophilized Powder for Injection: 100-mg single-dose vial, supplied with 2 mL sterile water for injection diluent.

INDICATIONS AND DOSAGES

▸ **Treatment of infant botulism caused by types A or B**

IV

Infants. Recommended dose is 2 mL/kg (roughly 75 mg/kg) given as a single IV infusion.

▸ **Dosage in renal impairment:** Administer at minimum concentration and rate of infusion.

CONTRAINDICATIONS

Allergies to human immune globulins or IgA deficiency with anti-IgA antibodies.

INTERACTIONS

Drug

Live-virus vaccines: Immune globulin administration may blunt immune response to live viral vaccines. Defer immunization with live vaccines until 3 mo after administration.

Nephrotoxic drugs: If receiving other nephrotoxic drugs, may be at increased risk of renal deterioration.

Herbal

None known.

Food

None known.

DIAGNOSTIC TEST EFFECTS

Increases in serum creatinine and BUN have been observed as soon as 1-2 days following treatment with other IGIV products.

SIDE EFFECTS

Occasional (≥ 5%)

Mild, transient erythematous rash of the face or trunk.

Less frequent (< 5%)

Chills, muscle cramps, back pain, fever, nausea, vomiting, and wheezing.

SERIOUS REACTIONS

- Anaphylactic reactions are rare. Keep epinephrine readily available.
- Renal dysfunction/failure (especially with sucrose-containing products) as a result of osmotic nephrosis; BabyBIG contains sucrose.
- An aseptic meningitis syndrome has occurred with use of other IVIG products.
- Hemolysis.
- Noncardiogenic pulmonary edema.
- Overdose may produce chills, diaphoresis, dizziness, facial flushing, nausea, vomiting, fever, and hypotension.

PRECAUTIONS & CONSIDERATIONS

Live vaccine administration should be deferred for 3 mo after this immune globulin. Caution is warranted with cardiovascular disease, a history of thrombosis, impaired renal function, sepsis, or volume depletion and concurrent use of nephrotoxic drugs. This drug has been used in pediatric patients under 1 yr of age only; data relating to use in any other population are not available.

Patients should be well hydrated prior to the initiation of the infusion. Assess renal function, including BUN or serum creatinine, prior to the initial infusion and periodically thereafter, especially for infants at risk of developing acute renal failure. Monitor the patient's vital signs continuously and observe for any associated symptoms. If a patient develops an infusion reaction, slow the rate of infusion immediately or temporarily interrupt the infusion.

Storage

Refrigerate unopened vials; do not freeze. Reconstituted vials should be used within 2 h. Do not use the injection if the solution is turbid.

B

Administration
Reconstitute the vial with 2 mL of sterile water for injection to obtain a 50-mg/mL concentration. When using a double-ended transfer needle for reconstitution, insert one end first into the vial of water. The lyophilized powder is supplied in an evacuated vial; therefore, the water should transfer by suction (the jet of water should be aimed to the side of the vial). After the diluent is transferred, the residual vacuum should be released to hasten the dissolution. Rotate gently to wet all the powder. It will take roughly 30 min to dissolve the powder. Do not shake, as this will cause foaming. Use the solution only if it is colorless, particulate-free, and not turbid. Begin infusion within 2 h after reconstitution. Conclude within 4 h of reconstitution, unless infusion is temporarily interrupted for adverse reaction.

Monitor vital signs continuously during IV infusion. Administer using low-volume tubing and a constant infusion pump (i.e., an IVAC pump or equivalent) through a separate IV line. If a separate line is not possible, it may be "piggybacked" into a preexisting line if that line contains either 0.9% NaCl, or one of the following dextrose solutions (with or without NaCl added): D2.5W, D5W, D10W, or D20W. If a preexisting line must be used, do not dilute BabyBIG more than 1:2 with any of the above-named solutions. Use an in-line or syringe-tip sterile, disposable filter (18 μm). Begin infusion slowly. Administer IV at 0.5 mL/kg/h (25 mg/kg/h). If no untoward reactions occur after 15 min, may increase to 1 mL/kg/h (50 mg/kg/h). Do not exceed this rate. Monitor the patient closely during and after each rate change. At the recommended rates, infusion of the indicated dose should take 127.5 min total elapsed time.

If untoward reactions occur, slowing the infusion rate or temporarily interrupting infusion may resolve them. If anaphylaxis or a serious drop in blood pressure occurs, discontinue the infusion and administer epinephrine.

Brimonidine

bry-mo'nih-deen

★🍁 Alphagan P

Do not confuse with bromocriptine.

CATEGORY AND SCHEDULE

Pregnancy Risk Category: B

Classification: Ophthalmic agents, antiglaucoma agents, α_2-adrenergic receptor agonist

MECHANISM OF ACTION

An ophthalmic agent that is a selective α_2-adrenergic agonist. *Therapeutic Effect:* Reduces intraocular pressure (IOP).

PHARMACOKINETICS

There is some systemic absorption following opthalmic use. Plasma concentrations peak within 0.5-2.5 h after ocular administration. Distributed into aqueous humor. Metabolized in liver. Primarily excreted in urine. *Half-life:* 3 h.

AVAILABILITY

Ophthalmic Solution (Alphagan P): 0.1%, 0.15%.
Ophthalmic Solution: 0.2%.

B

INDICATIONS AND DOSAGES

▸ **Glaucoma, Ocular Hypertension**

OPHTHALMIC

Adults, Elderly, Children 2 yr and older. 1 drop in affected eye(s) 3 times a day.

CONTRAINDICATIONS

Concurrent use of MAOI therapy, hypersensitivity to brimonidine tartrate or any other component of the formulation.

INTERACTIONS

Drug

CNS depressants: Potential additive effects.

Antihypertensives, β-blockers, cardiac glycosides: Caution because brimonidine may also reduce heart rate and blood pressure.

MAOIs: Contraindicated due to potential risk of sympathomimetic interaction with MAOI and risk of hypertensive crisis.

SIDE EFFECTS

Occasional

Allergic conjunctivitis, conjunctival hyperemia, eye pruritus, burning sensation, conjunctival folliculosis, oral dryness, visual disturbances.

SERIOUS REACTIONS

- Bradycardia; hypotension; iritis; miosis; skin reactions, including erythema, eyelid, pruritus, rash; vasodilation; and tachycardia have been reported.

PRECAUTIONS & CONSIDERATIONS

Brimonidine should be used with caution in patients with severe cardiovascular disease, depression, cerebral or coronary insufficiency, Raynaud phenomenon, orthostatic hypotension, or thromboangiitis obliterans. Use not recommended in children younger than 2 yr. Somnolence occurs more frequently in children 2-6 yr of age than in older children.

Storage

Store at room temperature.

Administration

Care should be taken to avoid contamination; do not touch the tip of the dropper to any other surface. Wash hands before and after use. Tilt the head back slightly and pull lower eyelid down with index finger to form a pouch. Squeeze drop into the pouch and gently close eyes for 1 to 2 min. Do not blink. Nasolacrimal occlusion is advised to reduce systemic exposure. If more than 1 topical ophthalmic product is to be used, administration should be separated by at least 5 min. Wait 15 min after using before inserting contact lenses.

Brinzolamide

brin-zol′ah-mide

Azopt

CATEGORY AND SCHEDULE

Pregnancy Risk Category: C

Classification: Ophthalmic agents, antiglaucoma agents, carbonic anhydrase inhibitor

MECHANISM OF ACTION

An ophthalmic agent that inhibits carbonic anhydrase. Decreases aqueous humor secretion. *Therapeutic Effect:* Reduces intraocular pressure (IOP).

PHARMACOKINETICS

Systemically absorbed to some degree. Protein binding: 60%. Distributed extensively in red blood cells. Site of metabolism has not been established. Metabolized to active and inactive metabolites.

Primarily excreted unchanged in urine.

AVAILABILITY

Ophthalmic Suspension: 1%.

INDICATIONS AND DOSAGES

▸ **Glaucoma, ocular hypertension**

OPHTHALMIC

Adults, Elderly. Instill 1 drop in affected eye(s) 3 times a day.

CONTRAINDICATIONS

Hypersensitivity to brinzolamide, sulfonamides, or any of the product ingredients.

INTERACTIONS

Drug

Carbonic anhydrase inhibitors: Concurrent use with oral carbonic anhydrase inhibitors may lead to additive toxicity.

Herbal

None known.

Food

None known.

DIAGNOSTIC TEST EFFECTS

None known.

SIDE EFFECTS

Frequent (5%-10%)

Temporary blurred vision; bitter, sour, or unusual taste.

Occasional (1%-5%)

Blepharitis, dermatitis, dry eye, ocular discharge, ocular discomfort and pain, ocular pruritus, headache, rhinitis, hyperemia.

Rare (< 1%)

Allergic reactions, alopecia, chest pain, conjunctivitis, diarrhea, diplopia, dizziness, dry mouth, dyspnea, dyspepsia, eye fatigue, hypertonia, keratoconjunctivitis, keratopathy, kidney pain, lid margin crusting or sticky sensation, nausea, pharyngitis, tearing, urticaria.

SERIOUS REACTIONS

- Electrolyte imbalance, development of acidosis, and possible CNS effects may occur.
- Systemic hypersensitivity effects including blood dyscrasias, Stevens-Johnson syndrome, toxic epidermal necrolysis, and fulminant hepatic necrosis possible.

PRECAUTIONS & CONSIDERATIONS

Use with caution in patients with renal impairment, hepatic impairment. Safety and effectiveness have not been established in children or during pregnancy or lactation.

Storage

Store at room temperature.

Administration

Shake well before using. Care should be taken to avoid contamination; do not touch the tip of the dropper to any other surface. Wash hands before use. Tilt the head back slightly and pull lower eyelid down with index finger to form a pouch. Squeeze 1 drop into the pouch and gently close eyes. If more than one ophthalmic agent is being used, separate administration by at least 10 min. The preservative, benzalkonium chloride, may be absorbed by soft contact lenses. Remove contact lenses before instillation; may reinsert 15 min after instillation.

Bromfenac

brom'fen-ak

★ 🍁 Xibrom

Do not confuse bromfenac with diclofenac.

CATEGORY AND SCHEDULE

Pregnancy Risk Category: C

Classification: Nonsteroidal anti-inflammatory drugs, ophthalmic

MECHANISM OF ACTION

An NSAID that inhibits prostaglandin synthesis, reducing the intensity of pain and inflammation. In animal eyes, prostaglandins have been shown to produce disruption of the blood-aqueous humor barrier, vasodilatation, increased vascular permeability, leukocytosis, and increased intraocular pressure. *Therapeutic Effect:* Produces analgesic and anti-inflammatory effects in the eye.

PHARMACOKINETICS

Pharmacokinetics following ocular administration in humans are unknown. Based on the dose of 1 drop to each eye (0.09 mg) and information from other routes of administration, the systemic concentration is estimated to be negligible (< 50 ng/mL) at steady state in humans.

AVAILABILITY

Ophthalmic Solution (Xibrom): 0.09%.

INDICATIONS AND DOSAGES

▸ **Relief of ocular pain and inflammation in patients who have had cataract extraction**

OPHTHALMIC

Adults, Elderly. Apply 1 drop to affected eye(s) twice daily beginning 24 h after surgery and continuing for 2 wks.

CONTRAINDICATIONS

Hypersensitivity to bromfenac or any formulation ingredient.

INTERACTIONS

Drug

Ophthalmic corticosteroids: Co-use may increase risk of delay in healing.

Herbal

None known.

Food

None known.

DIAGNOSTIC TEST EFFECTS

None known.

SIDE EFFECTS

Frequent (2%-7%)

Abnormal sensation in eye; conjunctival hyperemia; eye irritation (including burning/stinging); ocular pain, pruritus, or redness; headache; and iritis.

SERIOUS REACTIONS

- Rare hypersensitivity reactions.
- Corneal adverse events such as thinning, erosion, or perforation.

PRECAUTIONS & CONSIDERATIONS

Use with caution in those with sulfite sensitivity, or previous allergic reactions to other NSAIDS; cross-reactivity may occur. There have been reports that ocularly applied NSAIDs may cause increased bleeding of ocular tissues following ocular surgery. Topical NSAIDS may slow or delay healing, or may cause keratitis. Use with caution in patients with known bleeding tendencies or who are on medications affecting bleeding times. Patients with complicated ocular surgeries, corneal denervation, corneal epithelial defects, diabetes mellitus, dry eye syndrome, or repeat

B

ocular surgeries may be at increased risk for corneal adverse events, which may become sight threatening. Use more than 24 h prior to surgery or use beyond 14 days post surgery may increase patient risk for the occurrence and severity of corneal adverse events. Patients should not wear contact lenses during treatment. The safety and efficacy of bromfenac have not been established in children. Use during pregnancy or lactation only if clearly needed due to lack of data. No particular precautions needed in elderly patients.

Therapeutic response, such as decreased pain, surgical healing, and inflammation, should be assessed.

Storage

Store at controlled room temperature.

Administration

Take care to avoid contamination; do not allow dropper tip to touch any surface. Wash hands before use. Place index finger on the lower eyelid and pull gently until a pouch is formed. Place the prescribed number of drops in the pouch. Gently close the eye, and apply digital pressure to the lacrimal sac for 1-2 min to minimize the risk of systemic effects. Blot excess solution with a tissue.

Bromocriptine

broe-moe-krip′teen

★ Cycloset, Parlodel

🍁 Apo-Bromocriptine

Do not confuse bromocriptine with benztropine, or Parlodel with pindolol.

CATEGORY AND SCHEDULE

Pregnancy Risk Category: C

Classification: Antiparkinsonian agents, antidiabetic agents, dopamine receptor agonist

MECHANISM OF ACTION

A dopamine agonist that directly stimulates dopamine receptors in the corpus striatum and inhibits prolactin secretion. Also suppresses secretion of growth hormone. *Therapeutic Effect:* Improves symptoms of parkinsonism; suppresses galactorrhea and reduces serum growth hormone concentrations in acromegaly; lowers blood glucose and improves glucose tolerance in diabetes mellitus.

PHARMACOKINETICS

Indication	Onset	Peak	Duration
Prolactin lowering	2 h	8 h	24 h
Antiparkinsonian	0.5-1.5 h	2 h	N/A
Growth hormone suppressant	1-2 h	4-8 wks	4-8 h

Minimally absorbed from the GI tract. Protein binding: 90%-96%. Metabolized in the liver. Excreted in feces by biliary secretion. *Half-life:* 15 h.

AVAILABILITY

Capsules: 5 mg.
Tablets: 2.5 mg.
Tablets: 0.8 mg (Cycloset).

INDICATIONS AND DOSAGES

▸ **Hyperprolactinemia**

PO

Adults, Elderly. Initially, 1.25-2.5 mg/day. May increase by 2.5 mg/day at 3- to 7-day intervals. Range: 2.5 mg 2-3 times a day.

▸ **Parkinson disease**

PO

Adults, Elderly. Initially, 1.25 mg twice a day. May increase by 2.5 mg/day every 14-28 days. Range: 30-90 mg/day.

▸ **Acromegaly**
PO
Adults, Elderly. Initially, 1.25-2.5 mg. May increase at 3-7 day intervals. Usual dose 20-30 mg/day. Maximum: 100 mg/day.
▸ **Diabetes mellitus type 2**
PO (CYCLOSET ONLY)
Adults, Elderly. Intially, 0.8 mg/day. May increase weekly by 0.8 mg to an effective range of 1.6-4.8 mg/day.

OFF-LABEL USES
Treatment of cocaine addiction, hyperprolactinemia associated with pituitary adenomas, neuroleptic malignant syndrome.

CONTRAINDICATIONS
Hypersensitivity to ergot alkaloids, peripheral vascular disease, pregnancy, severe ischemic heart disease, uncontrolled hypertension.

INTERACTIONS
Drug
Alcohol: May produce a disulfiram-like reaction (chest pain, confusion, flushed face, nausea, vomiting).
Erythromycin, clarithromycin, ritonavir, protease inhibitors, itraconazole, ketoconazole: May increase bromocriptine blood concentration and risk of toxicity.
Ergot alkaloids: Concurrent use is not recommended as it may increase ergot-related side effects.
Estrogens, progestins: May decrease the effects of bromocriptine.
Haloperidol, MAOIs, phenothiazines, risperidone: May decrease bromocriptine's prolactin-lowering effect.
Hypotension-producing medications: May increase hypotension.
Levodopa: May increase the effects of bromocriptine.
Sibutramine: May increase the risk of serotonin syndrome.
Sympathomimetics: Do not use together for more than 10 days, as this may increase risk of hypertension and tachycardia.
Herbal
St. John's wort: May reduce bromocriptine levels.
Food
None known.

DIAGNOSTIC TEST EFFECTS
May increase plasma growth hormone concentration.

SIDE EFFECTS
Frequent
Nausea (49%), headache (19%), dizziness (17%).
Occasional (3%-7%)
Fatigue, light-headedness, vomiting, abdominal cramps, diarrhea, constipation, nasal congestion, somnolence, dry mouth.
Rare
Muscle cramps, urinary hesitancy.

SERIOUS REACTIONS
- Visual or auditory hallucinations have been noted in patients with Parkinson disease.
- Somnolence and sudden sleep onset.
- Long-term, high-dose therapy may produce continuing rhinorrhea, syncope, GI hemorrhage, peptic ulcer, and severe abdominal pain.
- Rare cases of pleural or retroperitoneal fibrosis.
- Some antiprakinsonian medications associated with melanoma development.

PRECAUTIONS & CONSIDERATIONS
Caution is warranted with cardiac, renal, or hepatic function

B

impairment, hypertension, and psychiatric disorders. Be aware the incidence of side effects is high, especially at the beginning of therapy and with high dosages. Bromocriptine use is not recommended during pregnancy or breastfeeding. Nonhormonal contraceptives are recommended to women during treatment. When used in the treatment of hyperprolactinemia, bromocriptine should be withdrawn when pregnancy is diagnosed. The safety and efficacy of bromocriptine have not been established in children. Elderly patients are more prone to CNS adverse effects.

Dizziness, drowsiness, and dry mouth are expected responses to the drug. Alcohol and tasks that require mental alertness or motor skills should be avoided. Also, change positions slowly and dangle the legs momentarily before standing to avoid light-headedness. Notify the physician if watery nasal discharge occurs. Constipation should be assessed during treatment.

Storage

Store at room temperature. Protect from light.

Administration

Lie down after taking the first dose to avoid light-headedness. Take with food to decrease the incidence of nausea.

For Cycloset: Take with food within 2 h after waking in the morning.

Brompheniramine

brome-fen-ir'a-meen

★ Bidhist, BPM, J-Tan PD, Lodrane 24, LoHist-12, Respa-BR, TanaCof-XR, Vazol

CATEGORY AND SCHEDULE

Pregnancy Risk Category: B

Rx

Classification: Antihistamines, H_1-receptor antagonist

MECHANISM OF ACTION

An alkylamine that competes with histamine at histaminic receptor sites. Inhibits central acetylcholine. *Therapeutic Effect:* Results in anticholinergic, antipruritic, antitussive, antiemetic effects. Produces antidyskinetic, sedative effect.

PHARMACOKINETICS

Rapidly absorbed after PO administration. Widely distributed. Metabolized in liver. Primarily excreted in urine. *Half-life:* 25 h.

AVAILABILITY

Capsule, Extended Release: 12 mg (Lodrane 24).
Tablets, Extended Release: 6 mg (Bidhist, LoHist).
Elixir: 2 mg/5 mL (Vazol).
Oral Suspension: 4 mg/5 mL (J-Tan), 8 mg/5 mL (TanaCof-XR).

INDICATIONS AND DOSAGES

▸ **Allergic rhinitis, anaphylaxis, urticarial transfusion reactions, urticaria**

PO

Adults, Elderly, Children 12 yr and older. Extended-release tablets: 6-12 mg every 12 h; extended-release

capsules: 12-24 mg once daily; oral suspension: 12-24 mg every 12 h (up to 48 mg/24 h); oral liquid: 4 mg 4 times daily.
Children 6-12 yr. Extended-release tablets: 6 mg every 12 h; extended-release capsules: 12 mg once daily; oral suspension: 12 mg every 12 h (up to 24 mg/24 h); oral liquid: 2 mg 4 times daily.
Children 2-6 yr. Chewable tablets: 6 mg every 12 h (up to 12 mg/24 h); oral suspension: 6 mg every 12 h (up to 12 mg/24 h); oral liquid: 1 mg 4 times daily.
Children 12 mo to 2 yr. Oral suspension 3 mg every 12 h (up to 6 mg/24 h); oral liquid 0.5 mg/kg/day in divided doses 4 times daily.

CONTRAINDICATIONS

Concurrent MAOI therapy, focal CNS lesions, newborn or premature infants, nursing mothers, hypersensitivity to brompheniramine or related drugs.

INTERACTIONS

Drug
Alcohol and CNS depressants: May increase sedative effects.
Anticholinergics: May increase anticholinergic effects.
MAOIs: May increase anticholinergic and CNS depressant effects.
Procarbazine: May increase CNS depressant effects.
Herbal
None known.
Food
None known.

DIAGNOSTIC TEST EFFECTS

May suppress wheal and flare reactions to antigen skin testing unless antihistamines are discontinued 4 days before testing.

SIDE EFFECTS

Frequent
Drowsiness; dizziness; dry mouth, nose, or throat; urinary retention; thickening of bronchial secretions.
Elderly: Sedation, dizziness, hypotension.
Occasional
Epigastric distress, flushing, blurred vision, tinnitus, paresthesia, sweating, chills.

SERIOUS REACTIONS

- Children may experience dominant paradoxical reactions, including restlessness, insomnia, euphoria, nervousness, and tremors.
- Overdosage in children may result in hallucinations, seizures, and death.
- Hypersensitivity reactions, such as eczema, pruritus, rash, cardiac disturbances, and photosensitivity, may occur.

PRECAUTIONS & CONSIDERATIONS

Caution is warranted with asthma, narrow-angle glaucoma, increased intraocular pressure, hyperthyroidism, cardiovascular disease, hypertension, pyloroduodenal or bladder neck obstruction, glucose-6-phosphate dehydrogenase (G6PD) deficiency, or prostatic hypertrophy. It is unknown whether brompheniramine crosses the placenta or is detected in breast milk. There is an increased risk of seizures in neonates and premature infants if the drug is used during the third trimester of pregnancy. Brompheniramine use is not recommended in newborns or premature infants because these groups are at an increased risk of experiencing paradoxical reaction. Elderly patients are at an increased risk of developing confusion,

B

dizziness, hyperexcitability, hypotension, and sedation.

Dizziness, drowsiness, and dry mouth are expected side effects of brompheniramine. Avoid alcohol during therapy.

Storage

Store at room temperature. Protect from light to prevent discoloration.

Administration

Give oral brompheniramine with meals to minimize GI upset. Shake oral suspensions well before each use. Do not crush, cut, or chew extended-release dosage forms.

Budesonide

bu-dess'ah-nide

★ Entocort EC, Pulmicort Flexhaler, Pulmicort Respules, Rhinocort Aqua

CATEGORY AND SCHEDULE

Pregnancy Risk Category: B

Classification: Corticosteroids, inhalation

MECHANISM OF ACTION

A glucocorticoid that inhibits the accumulation of inflammatory cells and decreases and prevents tissues from responding to the inflammatory process. *Therapeutic Effect:* Relieves symptoms of asthma, allergic rhinitis, or Crohn disease.

PHARMACOKINETICS

Minimally absorbed from nasal tissue; moderately absorbed from inhalation. Protein binding: 88%. Primarily metabolized in the liver. *Half-life:* 2-3 h.

AVAILABILITY

Capsules (Entocort EC): 3 mg.
Powder for Oral Inhalation (Pulmicort Flexhaler): 90 mcg/inhalation, 180 mcg/inhalation.
Suspension for Oral Inhalation (Pulmicort Respules): 0.25 mg/2 mL, 0.5 mg/2 mL, 1 mg/2 mL.
Nasal Spray (Rhinocort Aqua): 32 mcg/spray.

INDICATIONS AND DOSAGES

▸ **Allergic or vasomotor rhinitis**

INTRANASAL (RHINOCORT AQUA)

Adults, Elderly, Children 6 yr and older. 1 spray in each nostril once a day. Maximum: 4 sprays/nostril for adults and children 12 yr and older; 2 sprays/nostril for children younger than 12 yr.

▸ **Bronchial asthma**

NEBULIZATION

Children 12 mo to 8 yr. 0.25-1 mg/day titrated to lowest effective dosage.

INHALATION

Adults, Elderly, Children 6 yr and older. Flexhaler: Initially 180-360 mcg twice daily. Maximum: Adults: 720 mcg twice a day. Children: 360 mcg twice a day.

▸ **Crohn disease**

PO

Adults, Elderly. 9 mg once a day for up to 8 wks.

CONTRAINDICATIONS

Hypersensitivity to any corticosteroid or its components, persistently positive sputum cultures for *Candida albicans,* primary treatment of status asthmaticus, systemic fungal infections, untreated localized infection involving nasal mucosa.

INTERACTIONS

Drug

Cimetidine: May increase the serum concentrations of budesonide.

CYP3A4 inhibitors: May increase the serum level and toxicity of budesonide.

Herbal

St. John's wort: May decrease levels of budesonide.

Food

Grapefruit juice: May double systemic exposure to oral budesonide.

DIAGNOSTIC TEST EFFECTS

None known.

SIDE EFFECTS

Frequent (≥ 3%)

Nasal: Mild nasopharyngeal irritation, burning, stinging, or dryness; headache; cough.
Inhalation: Flu-like symptoms, headache, pharyngitis.

Occasional (1%-3%)

Nasal: Dry mouth, dyspepsia, rebound congestion, rhinorrhea, loss of taste.
Inhalation: Back pain, vomiting, altered taste, voice changes, abdominal pain, nausea, dyspepsia.

SERIOUS REACTIONS

- An acute hypersensitivity reaction marked by urticaria, angioedema, and severe bronchospasm; occurs rarely.
- Nasal septum perforation with chronic use or improper technique.

PRECAUTIONS & CONSIDERATIONS

Caution is warranted with adrenal insufficiency, cirrhosis, glaucoma, hypothyroidism, osteoporosis, tuberculosis, and untreated infection. It is unknown whether budesonide crosses the placenta or is distributed in breast milk. In children, prolonged treatment and high doses may decrease cortisol secretion and short-term growth rate. No age-related precautions have been noted in elderly patients.

Symptoms should improve in 24 h, but the drug's full effect may take 3-7 days to appear. Those using budesonide intranasally should notify the physician if nasal irritation occurs or if symptoms, such as sneezing, fail to improve.

Storage

Store all budesonide dosage forms at room temperature. Once foil envelope for inhalation suspension has been opened, all ampules must be used within 2 wks. Discard Flexhaler when dose indicator displays zero. Discard nasal spray after 120 sprays.

Administration

Oral capsule should be swallowed whole. Do not crush or chew.
For inhalation, prime inhaler before first use. Exhale completely and place the mouthpiece between the lips. Inhale and hold breath for as long as possible before exhaling. Allow at least 1 min between inhalations. Rinse mouth after each use to decrease dry mouth and hoarseness and prevent fungal infection of the mouth.
Inhalation suspension for nebulization should be shaken well before using. Administer with jet nebulizer connected to an air compressor; do not use ultrasonic nebulizer. Do not mix with other medications in nebulizer. Rinse mouth after each use; wash face if using face mask.

For intranasal use, clear nasal passages as much as possible. Shake gently before use. Prime before first use by actuating 8 times. If not used for 2 consecutive days, reprime with 1 spray or until a fine spray appears. If not used for 14 days, rinse applicator and reprime with 2 sprays or until a fine spray appears. Tilt the head slightly forward. Insert the spray tip into the nostril, pointing toward the nasal passages,

B

away from the nasal septum. Spray budesonide into the nostril while holding the other nostril closed, and at the same time inhale through the nose to deliver the medication as high into the nasal passages as possible.

Bumetanide

byoo-met′a-nide

Bumex, Burinex

CATEGORY AND SCHEDULE

Pregnancy Risk Category: C (D if used in pregnancy-induced hypertension)

Classification: Diuretics, loop

MECHANISM OF ACTION

A loop diuretic that enhances excretion of sodium, chloride, and, to lesser degree, potassium, by direct action at the ascending limb of the loop of Henle and in the proximal tubule. *Therapeutic Effect:* Produces diuresis.

PHARMACOKINETICS

Route	Onset	Peak	Duration
PO	30-60	60-120 min	4-6 h
IV	Rapid	15-30 min	2-3 h
IM	40	60-120 min	4-6 h

Completely absorbed from the GI tract (absorption decreased in CHF and nephrotic syndrome). Protein binding: 94%-96%. Partially metabolized in the liver. Primarily excreted in urine. Not removed by hemodialysis. *Half-life:* 1-1.5 h in adults; prolonged in neonates and infants.

AVAILABILITY

Tablets: 0.5 mg, 1 mg, 2 mg.
Injection: 0.25 mg/mL.

INDICATIONS AND DOSAGES

▸ **Edema**

PO

Adults. 0.5-2 mg as a single dose in the morning. May repeat q4-5h.
Elderly. 0.5 mg/day, increased as needed.

IV, IM

Adults, Elderly. 0.5-2 mg/dose; may repeat in 2-3 hr. Or 0.5-1 mg/h by continuous IV infusion. Maximum: 10 mg/day.

▸ **Hypertension**

PO

Adults, Elderly. Initially, 0.5 mg/day. Range: 1-4 mg/day. Maximum: 5 mg/day. Larger doses may be given 2-3 doses/day.

▸ **Usual pediatric dosage**

PO, IV, IM

Children. 0.015-0.1 mg/kg/dose q6-24h. Maximum: 10 mg/day.

OFF-LABEL USES

Treatment of hypercalcemia.

CONTRAINDICATIONS

Anuria, hepatic coma, severe electrolyte depletion, hypersensitivity to bumetanide.

INTERACTIONS

Drug

Amphotericin B, nephrotoxic and ototoxic medications: May increase the risk of nephrotoxicity and ototoxicity.
Anticoagulants, heparin: May decrease the effects of these drugs.
Lithium: May increase the risk of lithium toxicity.
Other hypokalemia-causing medications: May increase the risk of hypokalemia.

Herbal
None known.
Food
None known.

DIAGNOSTIC TEST EFFECTS

May increase blood glucose, BUN, serum uric acid, and urinary phosphate levels. May decrease serum calcium, chloride, magnesium, potassium, and sodium levels.

IV INCOMPATIBILITIES

Amphotericin B, chlorpromazine, diazepam, haloperidol, inamrinone, midazolam (Versed), nesiritide (Natrecor), ofloxacin (Floxin), phenytoin, quinupristin-dalfopristin (Synercid).

IV COMPATIBILITIES

Aztreonam (Azactam), cefepime (Maxipime), diltiazem (Cardizem), dobutamine (Dobutrex), furosemide (Lasix), lorazepam (Ativan), milrinone (Primacor), morphine, piperacillin and tazobactam (Zosyn), propofol (Diprivan).

SIDE EFFECTS

Expected
Increased urinary frequency and urine volume.
Frequent
Orthostatic hypotension, dizziness.
Occasional
Blurred vision, diarrhea, headache, anorexia, premature ejaculation, impotence, dyspepsia.
Rare
Rash, urticaria, pruritus, asthenia, muscle cramps, nipple tenderness.

SERIOUS REACTIONS

• Vigorous diuresis may lead to profound water and electrolyte depletion, resulting in hypokalemia, hyponatremia, dehydration, coma, and circulatory collapse.
• Ototoxicity, manifested as deafness, vertigo, or tinnitus, may occur, especially in patients with severe renal impairment and those taking other ototoxic drugs.
• Blood dyscrasias and acute hypotensive episodes have been reported.

PRECAUTIONS & CONSIDERATIONS

Caution is warranted with diabetes mellitus, hypersensitivity to sulfonamides, hepatic or renal impairment, and in elderly and debilitated patients. It is unknown whether bumetanide is distributed in breast milk. The safety and efficacy of bumetanide have not been established in children. Bumetanide is a potent displacer of bilirubin; avoid use in neonates at risk for kernicterus. Elderly patients are at increased risk for circulatory collapse or thromboembolic episodes and may be more sensitive to the drug's hypotensive and electrolyte effects. Age-related renal impairment may require reduced dosage or an extended dosage interval in older patients. Consuming foods high in potassium such as apricots, bananas, legumes, meat, orange juice, raisins, whole grains, including cereals, and white and sweet potatoes, is encouraged.

An increase in the frequency and volume of urination and hearing abnormalities, such as a sense of fullness or ringing in the ears, may occur. BP, vital signs, electrolytes, intake and output, and weight should be monitored before and during treatment. Be aware of signs of electrolyte disturbances such as hypokalemia or hyponatremia. Hypokalemia may cause arrhythmias, altered mental status, muscle cramps, asthenia, and tremor. Hyponatremia may result in cold and clammy skin, confusion, and thirst.

B

Storage
Store vials at room temperature. Protect from light.
Administration
Take bumetanide with food to avoid GI upset, preferably with breakfast to help prevent nocturia.

Bumetanide is compatible with D5W, 0.9% NaCl, and lactated Ringer's solution, but it may also be given undiluted. The solution remains stable for 24 h if diluted. Administer the drug by IV push over 1-2 min. Bumetanide may also be given as a continuous infusion.

Bupivacaine

byoo-piv'a-caine
★ Marcaine, Marcaine Spinal, Sensorcaine, Sensorcaine-MPF

CATEGORY AND SCHEDULE

Pregnancy Risk Category: C

Classification: Anesthetics, local

MECHANISM OF ACTION

An amide-type anesthetic that stabilizes neuronal membranes and prevents initiation and transmission of nerve impulses, thereby effecting local anesthetic actions. *Therapeutic Effect:* Produces local analgesia.

PHARMACOKINETICS

Onset of action occurs within 4-10 min, depending on route of administration. Duration is 1.5-8.5 h. Well absorbed. Protein binding: 95%. Metabolized in liver. Excreted in urine. *Half-life:* 1.5-5.5 h (adults), 8.1 h (neonates).

AVAILABILITY

Injection: 0.25% (Marcaine, Sensorcaine-MPF), 0.5% (Marcaine, Sensorcaine-MPF), 0.75% (Marcaine, Marcaine Spinal, Sensorcaine-MPF).

INDICATIONS AND DOSAGES

Dose varies with procedure, depth of anesthesia, vascularity of tissues, duration of anesthesia, and condition of patient.

▸ **Analgesic, epidural (partial to moderate motor blockade)**

Adults, Elderly. 10-20 mL (25-50 mg) of a 0.25% solution. Repeat once q3hr as needed.
Children > 10 kg. 1-2.5 mg/kg single dose as a 0.125% or 0.25% solution or 0.2-0.4 mg/kg/h continuous infusion as a 0.1%, 0.125%, or 0.25% solution. Maximum: 0.4 mg/kg/h.
Children < 10 kg. 1-1.25 mg/kg single dose as a 0.125% or 0.25% solution or 0.1-0.2 mg/kg/h continuous infusion as a 0.1%, 0.125%, or 0.25% solution. Maximum: 0.2 mg/kg/h.

▸ **Analgesic, epidural (moderate to complete motor blockade)**

Adults, Elderly. 10-20 mL (50-100 mg) as a 0.5% solution. Repeat once q3h as needed.
Children > 10 kg. 1-2.5 mg/kg single dose as a 0.125% or 0.25% solution or 0.2-0.4 mg/kg/h continuous infusion as a 0.1%, 0.125%, or 0.25% solution. Maximum: 0.4 mg/kg/h.
Children < 10 kg. 1-1.25 mg/kg single dose as a 0.125% or 0.25% solution or 0.1-0.2 mg/kg/h continuous infusion as a 0.1%, 0.125%, or 0.25% solution. Maximum: 0.2 mg/kg/h.

▸ **Analgesic, epidural (complete motor blockade)**
Adults. 10-20 mL (75-150 mg) as a 0.75% solution. Repeat once q3h as needed.
Children weighing >10 kg. 1-2.5 mg/kg single dose as a 0.125% or 0.25% solution or 0.2-0.4 mg/kg/h continuous infusion as a 0.1%, 0.125%, or 0.25% solution. Maximum: 0.4 mg/kg/h.
Children weighing < 10 kg. 1-1.25 mg/kg single dose as a 0.125% or 0.25% solution or 0.1-0.2 mg/kg/h continuous infusion as a 0.1%, 0.125%, or 0.25% solution. Maximum: 0.2 mg/kg/h.

▸ **Analgesic, intrapleural**
Adults, Elderly. 10-30 mL bolus of 0.25%, 0.375%, or 0.5% q4-8h or 0.375% solution with epinephrine continuous infusion at 6 mL/h after 20 mL loading dose.

▸ **Analgesic, caudal (moderate to complete blockade)**
Adults, Elderly. 15-30 mL of 0.5% solution (75-150 mg) or 0.25% solution (37.5-75 mg), repeated once every 3 h as needed.
Children weighing > 10 kg. 1-2.5 mg/kg single dose as a 0.125% or 0.25% solution or 0.2-0.4 mg/kg/h continuous infusion as a 0.1%, 0.125%, or 0.25% solution. Maximum: *0.4 mg/kg/h.*
Children weighing < 10 kg. 1-1.25 mg/kg single dose as a 0.125% or 0.25% solution or 0.1-0.2 mg/kg/h continuous infusion as a 0.1%, 0.125%, or 0.25% solution. Maximum: 0.2 mg/kg/h.

▸ **Analgesic, dental**
Adults, Elderly. 1.8-3.6 mL of 0.5% solution (9-18 mg) with epinephrine. A second dose of 9 mg may be administered. Maximum: 90 mg total dose.

▸ **Analgesic, peripheral nerve block (moderate to complete motor blockade)**
Adults, Elderly. 5-37.5 mL (25-175 mg) of 0.5% solution or 5-70 mL (12.5-175 mg) of 0.25% solution. Repeat q3h as needed. Maximum: up to 400 mg/day.
Children 12 yr and older. 0.3-2.5 mg/kg as a 0.25% or 0.5% solution. Maximum: 1 mL/kg of 0.25% solution or 0.5 mL/kg of 0.5% solution.

▸ **Analgesic, retrobulbar (complete motor blockade)**
Adults, Elderly. 2-4 mL (15-30 mg) of 0.75% solution.

▸ **Analgesic, sympathetic blockade**
Adults, Elderly. 20-50 mL (50-125 mg) of 0.25% (no epinephrine) solution. Repeat once q3h as needed.

▸ **Analgesic, hyperbaric spinal (obstetric, normal vaginal delivery)**
Adults, Elderly. 0.8 mL (6 mg) bupivacaine in dextrose as 0.75% solution.

▸ **Analgesic, hyperbaric spinal (obstetrical, cesarean section)**
Adults, Elderly. 1-1.4 mL (7.5-10.5 mg) bupivacaine in dextrose as 0.75% solution.

▸ **Anesthesia, hyperbaric spinal (surgical, lower extremity, and perineal procedures)**
Adults, Elderly. 1 mL (7.5 mg) bupivacaine in dextrose as 0.75% solution.
Children 12 yr and older. 0.3-0.6 mg/kg bupivacaine in dextrose as a 0.75% solution.

▸ **Anesthesia, spinal (surgical, lower abdominal procedures)**
Adults, Elderly. 1.6 mL (12 mg) bupivacaine in dextrose as 0.75% solution.
Children 12 yr and older. 0.3-0.6 mg/kg bupivacaine in dextrose as a 0.75% solution.

B

▸ **Anesthesia, spinal (surgical, hyperbaric, upper abdominal procedures)**
Adults, Elderly. 2 mL (15 mg) bupivacaine in dextrose administered in horizontal position.
Children 12 yr and older. 0.3-0.6 mg/kg bupivacaine in dextrose as a 0.75% solution.
▸ **Analgesic, local infiltration**
Adults, Elderly. 0.25% solution. Maximum: 225 mg with epinephrine or 175 mg without epinephrine.
Children 12 yr and older. 0.5-2.5 mg/kg as a 0.25% or 0.5% solution. Maximum: 1 mL/kg of 0.25% solution or 0.5 mL/kg of 0.5% solution.

CONTRAINDICATIONS

Local infection at the site of proposed lumbar puncture (spinal anesthesia), obstetric paracervical block anesthesia, septicemia (spinal anesthesia), severe hemorrhage, severe hypotension or shock, arrhythmias such as complete heart block, which severely restrict cardiac output (spinal anesthesia), sulfite allergy (epinephrine-containing solutions only), hypersensitivity to bupivacaine products or to other amide-type anesthetics.

INTERACTIONS

Drug
Angiotensin-converting enzyme inhibitors: May increase risk of bradycardia and hypotension as well as loss of consciousness.
β-Blockers, ergot-type drugs, MAOIs, TCAs, phenothiazines, vasopressors: May increase the risk of bupivacaine toxicity.
Cisatracurium, rapacuronium: May increase neuromuscular blocking action.
Hyaluronidase: May increase incidence of systemic reaction to bupivacaine.
Propofol: May increase hypnotic effect of propofol.
Ropivacaine: May prolong effect of intrathecal bupivacaine.
Verapamil: May increase risk of heart block.
Herbal
St. John's wort: May increase risk of cardiovascular collapse and/or delay emergence from anesthesia.
Food
None known.

DIAGNOSTIC TEST EFFECTS

None known.

SIDE EFFECTS

Occasional
Hypotension, bradycardia, palpitations, respiratory depression, dizziness, headache, vomiting, nausea, restlessness, weakness, blurred vision, tinnitus, apnea.

SERIOUS REACTIONS

- Arterial hypotension, bradycardia, ventricular arrhythmias, CNS depression and excitation, convulsions, respiratory arrest, tinnitus have been reported.
- Solutions with epinephrine contain metabisulfite, a sulfite that may cause allergic-type reactions, including anaphylaxis.

PRECAUTIONS & CONSIDERATIONS

Caution is warranted with pregnancy as well as obstetrical epidural anesthesia. Only concentrations lower than 0.75% should be used for obstetrical anesthesia. Caution should be used with regional anesthesia (Bier block), hyperthyroidism, hepatic disease, impaired cardiovascular function, hypertension, and heart block because there is a higher risk for developing bupivacaine toxicity. Solutions containing vasoconstrictors should be used cautiously in areas with limited blood supply, in the presence of disease that may adversely affect the cardiovascular system, or with peripheral vascular disease. Caution should also be used with retrobulbar blocks because bupivacaine has caused respiratory arrest.

Solutions containing epinephrine or other vasopressors should not be used concomitantly with ergot-type oxytocic drugs. Use in extreme caution in persons receiving MAOIs or tricyclic antidepressants because severe hypertension can occur. Spinal anesthetics should not be injected during uterine contractions. Local anesthetic solutions containing antimicrobial preservatives should not be used for caudal or epidural anesthesia. Reduced doses should be given to debilitated, elderly, acutely ill, and young people. It is unknown if bupivacaine is a triggering agent for malignant hyperthermia. Bupivacaine may cause severe disturbances of cardiac rhythm, shock, or heart block after spinal anesthesia. Severe dose-related cardiac arrhythmias may occur if preparations containing a vasoconstrictor such as epinephrine are used during or following the administration of chloroform, cyclopropane, halothane, trichloroethylene, or other related agents.

Bupivacaine is distributed in breast milk. Fetal bradycardia frequently follows obstetrical paracervical block with some amide-type local anesthetics and may be associated with fetal acidosis. Bupivacaine spinal with dextrose is not recommended in children younger than 18 yr. Some elderly may require dosage adjustment.

Storage

Store at room temperature. Protect from light. Bupivacaine 1.25 mg/mL in 0.9% NaCl injection is stable for up to 32 days when refrigerated.

Administration

Only preservative-free injection should be used for epidural or caudal blocks. Dosage varies with anesthetic procedure, area to be anesthetized, vascularity of the tissues, number of neuronal segments to be blocked, depth of anesthesia and degree and muscle relaxation required, duration of anesthesia desired, individual tolerance, and physical condition of the person. The 0.75% solutions should not used for obstetric epidural anesthesia due to reports of cardiac arrest and death occurring with this concentration. Repeated doses of bupivacaine may cause significant increases in blood levels with each repeated dose due to accumulation of the drug or its metabolites or to slow metabolic degradation. Concentrated solutions (0.5%-0.75%) should be given in incremental doses of 3-5 mL with sufficient time between doses to detect toxic manifestations of unintentional intravascular or intrathecal injection during epidural administration. Bupivacaine should be used in dextrose only for spinal analgesia. The lowest bupivacaine dosage that gives effective anesthesia should be used to avoid high plasma levels and serious systemic side effects.

B

Buprenorphine

byoo-pre-nor′feen

Buprenex, Butrans, Subutex.

Butrans

Do not confuse Buprenex with Bumex.

CATEGORY AND SCHEDULE

Pregnancy Risk Category: C
Controlled Substance Schedule: III

Classification: Opioid agonist-antagonist

MECHANISM OF ACTION

An opioid agonist-antagonist that binds with opioid receptors in the CNS. *Therapeutic Effect:* Alters the perception of and emotional response to pain; produces minimal opioid withdrawal symptoms.

PHARMACOKINETICS

IM onset 15-30 min, duration 4-6 h; absorption 90%-100%; hepatic metabolism; excreted in feces (68%-71%); also renal excretion.

AVAILABILITY

Tablets, Sublingual: 2 mg, 8 mg.
Injection: 0.3 mg/mL.
Transdermal Patch: 5 mcg/hr, 10 mcg/hr, 20 mcg/hr.

INDICATIONS AND DOSAGES

▸ Analgesia

IV, IM

Adults, Children older than 12 yr. 0.3 mg q6-8h as needed. May repeat once in 30-60 min. Range: 0.15-0.6 mg q4-8h as needed.

Children 2-12 yr. 2-6 mcg/kg q4-6h as needed.

Elderly. 0.15 mg q6h as needed.

TRANSDERMAL PATCH

Adults. For opioid-naïve patients, apply a 5 mcg/h patch q 7 days. After a minimum of 72 h for each dose, may titrate to analgesia. Use close supervision during titration every 3 days. Do not exceed 20 mcg/h patch every 7 days.

▸ Opioid dependence

SUBLINGUAL

NOTE: Under the Drug Addiction Treatment Act of 2000 (DATA), only physicians who meet certain criteria may prescribe buprenorphine tablets for opioid dependence.

Adults, Elderly, Children older than 16 yr. Initially, 12-16 mg/day, beginning at least 4 h after last use of heroin or short-acting opioid. Maintenance: 16 mg/day. Range: 4-24 mg/day. Patients should be switched to buprenorphine and naloxone combination, which is preferred for maintenance treatment to defer abuse.

CONTRAINDICATIONS

Hypersensitivity to buprenorphine; hypersensitivity to naloxone for those receiving the fixed combination product containing naloxone (Suboxone).

INTERACTIONS

Drug

CNS depressants, MAOIs: May increase CNS or respiratory depression and hypotension.

Other opioid analgesics: May decrease the effects of other opioid analgesics.

Herbal

Kava kava, St. John's wort, valerian: May increase CNS depression.

Food

None known.

DIAGNOSTIC TEST EFFECTS

May increase serum amylase and lipase levels.

SIDE EFFECTS

Frequent

Tablet: Headache, pain, insomnia, anxiety, depression, nausea, abdominal pain, constipation, back pain, weakness, rhinitis, withdrawal syndrome, infection, diaphoresis. Injection (more than 10%): Sedation.

Occasional

Injection: Hypotension, respiratory depression, dizziness, headache, vomiting, nausea, vertigo.

SERIOUS REACTIONS

- Overdose results in cold and clammy skin, weakness, confusion, severe respiratory depression, cyanosis, pinpoint pupils, and extreme somnolence progressing to seizures, stupor, and coma.

PRECAUTIONS & CONSIDERATIONS

Caution is warranted with hepatic impairment and possible neurologic injury. Dizziness may occur, so change positions slowly and avoid tasks that require mental alertness or motor skills. BP, pulse rate, respiratory status, and clinical improvement should be monitored.

Storage

Store all dosage forms at controlled room temperature. Avoid excessive heat.

Administration

Place the sublingual tablet under the tongue until dissolved. If two or more tablets are needed, all may be placed under the tongue at the same time. Do not chew or swallow whole.

For IV use, administer buprenorphine slowly, over at least 2 min. No dilution is necessary for either IV or IM.

Apply transdermal patch to the left or right upper outer arm, upper chest, upper back, or the side of the chest, on a clean, dry and nearly hairless area. Do not apply to broken or irritated skin; rotate sites. Wear for 7 days. After removal, wait a minimum of 21 days before reapplying to the same skin site again. If a patch falls off, apply new patch to a different site.

Bupropion

byoo-proe′pee-on

★ 🍁 Aplenzin, Budeprion, Buproban, Wellbutrin, Wellbutrin SR, Wellbutrin XL, Zyban

Do not confuse bupropion with buspirone, Wellbutrin with Wellcovorin or Wellferon, or Zyban with Zagam.

CATEGORY AND SCHEDULE

Pregnancy Risk Category: C

Classification: Antidepressant

MECHANISM OF ACTION

An aminoketone that blocks the reuptake of neurotransmitters, including serotonin and norepinephrine at CNS presynaptic membranes, increasing their availability at postsynaptic receptor sites. Also reduces the firing rate of noradrenergic neurons. *Therapeutic Effect:* Relieves depression and nicotine withdrawal symptoms.

PHARMACOKINETICS

Rapidly absorbed from the GI tract. Protein binding: 84%. Crosses the blood-brain barrier. Undergoes extensive first-pass metabolism in the liver to active metabolite. Primarily excreted in urine. *Half-life:* 14 h.

AVAILABILITY

Tablets (Wellbutrin): 75 mg, 100 mg.
Tablets, Sustained Release (Wellbutrin SR, Zyban): 100 mg, 150 mg.
Tablets, Extended Release (Wellbutrin XL): 150 mg, 300 mg.

Tablets, Extended Release (Aplenzin): 174 mg, 348 mg, 522, mg.

INDICATIONS AND DOSAGES

▸ Depression

PO (IMMEDIATE RELEASE)

Adults. Initially, 100 mg twice a day. May increase to 100 mg 3 times a day no sooner than 3 days after beginning therapy. Maximum: 450 mg/day.

Elderly. 37.5 mg twice a day. May increase by 37.5 mg q3-4 days. Maintenance: Lowest effective dosage.

PO (SUSTAINED RELEASE)

Adults, Elderly. Initially, 150 mg/day as a single dose in the morning. May increase to 150 mg twice a day as early as day 4 after beginning therapy. Maximum: 400 mg/day.

PO (EXTENDED RELEASE WELLBUTRIN XL ONLY)

Adults. 150 mg once a day. May increase to 300 mg once a day. Maximum: 450 mg once a day.

PO (EXTENDED RELEASE, APLENZIN ONLY)

Adluts, 174 mg once a day in the morning. May increase to 348 mg once a day on day 4 of treatment. Maximum: 522 mg once a day.

▸ Smoking cessation

PO (ZYBAN)

Adults. Initially, 150 mg a day for 3 days; then 150 mg twice a day for 7-12 wks. Longer duration of maintenance therapy may be considered. Do not exceed 300 mg/day.

CONTRAINDICATIONS

Hypersensitivity. Current or prior diagnosis of anorexia nervosa or bulimia, seizure disorder, use within 14 days of MAOIs.

INTERACTIONS

! NOTE: It is important for a patient taking one product of bupropion to avoid other products containing the drug.

Drug

Carbamazepine, nevirapine, phenobarbital, phenytoin, rifampin: Decreased bupropion levels.

Desipramine, paroxetine, sertraline: May increase bupropion levels.

MAOIs: Concurrent use or use within 14 days contraindicated.

Tricyclic antidepressants, phenothiazines, benzodiazepines, alcohol, haloperidol, and trazodone: Increased seizure risk.

Herbal

None known.

Food

None known.

DIAGNOSTIC TEST EFFECTS

None known.

SIDE EFFECTS

Frequent

Constipation, weight gain or loss, nausea, vomiting, anorexia, dry mouth, headache, diaphoresis, tremors, sedation, insomnia, dizziness, agitation.

Occasional

Diarrhea, akinesia, blurred vision, tachycardia, confusion, hostility, fatigue.

SERIOUS REACTIONS

- The risk of seizures increases in patients taking more than 150 mg/dose of bupropion, in patients with a history of bulimia or seizure disorders, and in patients discontinuing drugs that may lower the seizure threshold.

PRECAUTIONS & CONSIDERATIONS

Bupropion should be used with caution in patients with renal and hepatic disease, bipolar disorder, recent myocardial infarction, cranial trauma, undergoing electroconvulsive therapy, and in elderly patients. Initial and maximum doses are reduced in patients with severe hepatic cirrhosis. Use in pregnancy only if the potential benefit outweighs the possible risks. Is excreted in breast milk; use is not recommended in nursing mothers. Bupropion is not FDA approved for use in children. A thorough cardiovascular assessment is recommended before initiation of therapy in pediatric patients; assessment should include medical history, family history, and physical examination with consideration of ECG testing. In addition, antidepressants have been associated with an increased risk of suicidal thinking and behavior in children, adolescents, and young adults with major depressive disorder and other psychiatric disorders. Elderly patients may be at greater risk of accumulation with chronic dosing.

Storage

Store at controlled room temperature.

Administration

May take without regard to food. Swallow sustained release and extended-release tablets whole; do not crush or chew.

Buspirone

byoo-spir′own

★ BuSpar 🍁 Bustab

Do not confuse buspirone with bupropion.

CATEGORY AND SCHEDULE

Pregnancy Risk Category: B

Classification: Anxiolytics

MECHANISM OF ACTION

Although its exact mechanism of action is unknown, this nonbarbiturate is thought to bind to serotonin and dopamine receptors in the CNS. The drug may also increase norepinephrine metabolism in the locus ceruleus. *Therapeutic Effect:* Produces anxiolytic effect.

PHARMACOKINETICS

Rapidly and completely absorbed from the GI tract. Protein binding: 95%. Undergoes extensive first-pass metabolism. Metabolized in the liver to active metabolite. Primarily excreted in urine. Not removed by hemodialysis. *Half-life:* 2-3 h.

AVAILABILITY

Tablets: 5 mg, 7.5 mg, 10 mg, 15 mg, 30 mg.

INDICATIONS AND DOSAGES

▸ **Generalized Anxiety Disorders**

PO

Adults. 5 mg 2-3 times a day or 7.5 mg twice a day. May increase by 5 mg/day every 2-4 days. Maintenance: 15-30 mg/day in 2-3 divided doses. Maximum: 60 mg/day.

Elderly. Initially, 5 mg twice a day. May increase by 5 mg/day every 2-3 days. Maximum: 60 mg/day.

Children 6 yr and older. Initially, 2.5-5 mg/day. May increase by 5 mg/day at weekly intervals. Usual maintenance dose: 15-30 mg/day in divided doses.

OFF-LABEL USES

Management of panic attack.

CONTRAINDICATIONS

Concurrent use of MAOIs, severe hepatic or renal impairment, hypersensitivity.

B

INTERACTIONS

Drug

Erythromycin, itraconazole: May increase buspirone blood concentration and risk of toxicity.

MAOIs: May increase BP. Contraindicated.

Other CNS depressants: Potentiates effects of buspirone and may increase sedation.

Herbal

Kava kava: May increase sedation.

St. John's wort: May decrease buspirone levels.

Food

Alcohol: Potentiates effects of buspirone and may increase sedation.

Grapefruit, grapefruit juice: May increase buspirone blood concentration and risk of toxicity. Avoid concurrent use.

DIAGNOSTIC TEST EFFECTS

None known.

SIDE EFFECTS

Frequent (6%-12%)

Dizziness, somnolence, nausea, headache.

Occasional (2%-5%)

Nervousness, fatigue, insomnia, dry mouth, light-headedness, mood swings, blurred vision, poor concentration, diarrhea, paresthesia.

Rare

Muscle pain and stiffness, nightmares, chest pain, involuntary movements.

SERIOUS REACTIONS

- Overdose may produce severe nausea, vomiting, dizziness, drowsiness, abdominal distention, and excessive pupil contraction.

PRECAUTIONS & CONSIDERATIONS

Caution is warranted with impaired renal or hepatic function. It is unknown whether buspirone crosses the placenta or is distributed in breast milk. The safety and efficacy of buspirone have not been established in children under 6 yr of age. No age-related precautions have been noted in children. No age-related precautions have been noted in elderly patients.

Drowsiness may occur but usually disappears with continued therapy. Change positions slowly from recumbent, to sitting, before standing to prevent dizziness. Alcohol and tasks that require mental alertness or motor skills should also be avoided. Autonomic responses, such as cold, clammy hands and diaphoresis, and motor responses, such as agitation, trembling, and tension, should be assessed. Hepatic and renal function should be monitored in long-term therapy.

Administration

Take buspirone consistently either with or without food. Crush tablets if needed. Improvement may be noticed within 7-10 days of starting therapy, but optimum therapeutic effect generally takes 3-4 wks to appear.

Busulfan

byoo-sull′fan

Busulfex, Myleran

Do not confuse Myleran with Alkeran, Leukeran, or Mylicon.

CATEGORY AND SCHEDULE

Pregnancy Risk Category: D

Classification: Antineoplastic, alkylating agent

MECHANISM OF ACTION

An alkylating agent that interferes with DNA replication and RNA synthesis. Cell cycle-phase nonspecific. *Therapeutic Effect:* Disrupts nucleic acid function and causes myelosuppression.

PHARMACOKINETICS

Completely absorbed from the GI tract. Protein binding: 33%. Metabolized in the liver. Primarily excreted in urine. Minimally removed by hemodialysis. *Half-life:* 2.5 h.

AVAILABILITY

Tablets: 2 mg.
Injection solution: 6 mg/mL.

INDICATIONS AND DOSAGES

▸ Remission induction in chronic myelogenous leukemia (CML)

PO

Adults, Elderly. 4-8 mg/day; up to 12 mg/day. Maintenance: 1-4 mg/day to 2 mg/wks. Continue until WBC count is 10,000-20,000/mm^3, and resume when WBC count reaches 50,000/mm^3.

Children. 0.06-0.12 mg/kg/day. Maintenance: Titrate to maintain leukocyte count above 40,000/mm^3, reduce dose by 50% if count is 30,000-40,000/mm^3, and discontinue if the count is 20,000/mm^3 or less.

▸ Marrow ablative conditioning for bone marrow transplantation

IV

Adults, Elderly, Children weighing more than 12 kg. 0.8 mg/kg/dose q6h for total of 16 doses. (Use IBW or ABW, whichever is lower.)

Children weighing 12 kg or less. 1.1 mg/kg/dose (ABW) q6h for 16 doses.

PO

Adults, Elderly. 1 mg/kg/dose (IBW) q6h for 16 doses.

IV INCOMPATIBILITIES

Do *not* dilute in dextrose 5% because it is incompatible.

CONTRAINDICATIONS

Disease resistance to previous therapy with this drug; hypersensitivity to any component of the formulation.

INTERACTIONS

Drug

Acetaminophen: Reduced busulfan clearance if used within 72 h before or concurrently with busulfan.

Itraconazole, ketoconazole: Increased busulfan levels.

Metronidazole: Increased busulfan trough concentrations and increased toxicity.

Herbal

St. John's wort: May decrease busulfan levels.

Food

Alcohol: May increase GI irritation.

DIAGNOSTIC TEST EFFECTS

Therapy associated with severe myelosuppression; AST elevation; increased creatinine, bilirubin, glucose; reduced calcium, potassium, magnesium.

SIDE EFFECTS

Expected

Nausea, stomatitis, vomiting, anorexia, insomnia, diarrhea, fever, abdominal pain, anxiety.

Frequent

Headache, rash, asthenia, infection, chills, tachycardia, dyspepsia.

Occasional

Constipation, dizziness, edema, pruritus, cough, dry mouth, depression, abdominal enlargement, pharyngitis, hiccups, back pain, alopecia, myalgia.

Rare

Injection site pain, arthralgia, confusion, hypotension, lethargy.

B

SERIOUS REACTIONS

- Busulfan's major adverse effect is myelosuppression, resulting in hematologic toxicity, as evidenced by anemia, severe leukopenia, and severe thrombocytopenia.
- Very high busulfan dosages may produce blurred vision, muscle twitching, and tonic-clonic seizures. High concentrations are also associated with increased risk of hepatic veno-occlusive disease.
- Long-term therapy (more than 4 yr) may produce pulmonary syndrome ("busulfan lung"), characterized by persistent cough, congestion, crackles, and dyspnea.
- Hyperuricemia may produce uric acid nephropathy, renal calculi, and acute renal failure.

PRECAUTIONS & CONSIDERATIONS

Severe bone marrow suppression is common; may result in prolonged pancytopenia and severe neutropenia, thrombocytopenia, and/or anemia. Secondary malignancies have been observed following busulfan therapy. Seizures have been associated with use; initiate prophylactic anticonvulsant therapy before high-dose treatment. Solvent in the IV formulation has been associated with impaired fertility, hepatotoxicity, hallucinations, somnolence, lethargy, and confusion. Busulfan may cause fetal harm if administered during pregnancy. Women of childbearing potential should avoid pregnancy while receiving busulfan. Breastfeeding is not recommended during busulfan therapy.

Storage

Store unopened injectable in refrigerator. Final solution stable 8 h at room temperature; complete infusion within the 8 h. Dilution in NS is stable for 12 h in refrigerator; infusion must be completed within the 12 h. Store tablet at room temperature.

Administration

CAUTION: Observe and exercise usual cautions for handling and preparing solutions of cytotoxic drugs. Dilute injectable with NS or D5W. Final concentration usually 0.5 mg/mL. IV dose should be administered as a 2-h infusion via a central line.

Administer oral tablets 1 h before or 2 h after meals.

Butabarbital Sodium

byoo-tah-bar′bi-tal so′dee-uhm

★ Butisol

CATEGORY AND SCHEDULE

Pregnancy Risk Category: D

Controlled Substance Schedule: III

Classification: Sedative-hypnotic, barbiturates

MECHANISM OF ACTION

A barbiturate and nonselective CNS depressant that binds at GABA receptor complex, enhancing GABA activity. *Therapeutic Effect:* Produces hypnotic effect due to CNS depression.

PHARMACOKINETICS

Widely distributed. Metabolized in liver. Minimally excreted unchanged in urine. *Half-life:* 34-100 h.

AVAILABILITY

Tablets: 30 mg, 50 mg.
Elixir: 30 mg/5 mL.

INDICATIONS AND DOSAGES

▸ **Insomnia, short-term**

PO

Adults. 50-100 mg at bedtime.

▸ **Preoperative sedation**

PO
Adults. 50-100 mg, 60-90 min before surgery.
Children. 2-6 mg/kg. Maximum: 100 mg.

▸ **Sedation, daytime**
PO
Adults. 15-30 mg 3-4 times a day.

CONTRAINDICATIONS

Porphyria, barbiturate sensitivity.

INTERACTIONS

Drug
Alcohol, CNS depressants: May be increased sedative and respiratory depressant effects.
Corticosteroids, cyclosporine, doxycyline, lamotrigine, methadone, oral contraceptives, quinidine, theophylline, tricyclic antidepressants, warfarin: Increased metabolism of these agents may reduce their therapeutic effects.
Herbal
Valerian, kava, kava: May increase sedative effects.
Food
Alcoholic beverages: Increased sedative and respiratory depressant effects.

DIAGNOSTIC TEST EFFECTS

None known.

SIDE EFFECTS

Occasional (1%-3%)
Somnolence.
Rare (< 1%)
Confusion, dizziness, agitation, nausea, vomiting, constipation, headache, hypotension, acne.

SERIOUS REACTIONS

• Skin eruptions appear as hypersensitivity reaction.
• Blood dyscrasias, liver disease, and hypocalcemia occur rarely.

PRECAUTIONS & CONSIDERATIONS

Use with caution in patients with depression, a history of drug abuse, hepatic or renal impairment, respiratory disease, and in elderly patients and children. Avoid use in pregnancy; may cause fetal harm. Acute withdrawal symptoms may occur in neonates following in utero exposure near term. Excreted in breast milk; use with caution in nursing mothers. Paradoxical reactions, including agitation and hyperactivity, have been observed in patients with pain and pediatric patients.
Administration
May take orally without regard to food.

Butenafine

byoo-ten′a-feen
★ Lotrimin Ultra, Mentax

CATEGORY AND SCHEDULE

Pregnancy Risk Category: B
OTC/Rx

Classification: Antifungals, topical, dermatologics

MECHANISM OF ACTION

An antifungal agent that locks biosynthesis of ergosterol, essential for fungal cell membrane. Fungicidal. *Therapeutic Effect:* Relieves dermatophytic infections.

PHARMACOKINETICS

Total amount absorbed into systemic circulation has not been determined. Metabolized in liver. Excreted in urine. *Half-life:* Biphasic decline with half-lives of 35 h and > 150 h.

AVAILABILITY

Cream: 1% (Lotrimin Ultra, Mentax).

B

INDICATIONS AND DOSAGES

▸ **Tinea corporis, tinea cruris, tinea versicolor**

TOPICAL

Adults, Elderly, Children 12 yr and older. Apply to affected area and immediate surrounding skin once daily for 2 wks.

▸ **Tinea pedis**

TOPICAL

Adults, Elderly, Children 12 yr and older. Apply to affected area and immediate surrounding skin twice daily for 7 days or once daily for 4 wks.

CONTRAINDICATIONS

Hypersensitivity to butenafine or any component of the formulation.

INTERACTIONS

Drug

None known.

Herbal

None known.

Food

None known.

DIAGNOSTIC TEST EFFECTS

None known.

SIDE EFFECTS

Occasional (2%)

Contact dermatitis, burning/stinging, worsening of the condition.

Rare (≤ 2%)

Erythema, irritation, pruritus.

SERIOUS REACTIONS

• None known.

PRECAUTIONS & CONSIDERATIONS

Caution should be used with sensitivity to naftifine or other allylamine antifungals. It is unknown whether butenafine is excreted in breast milk. Safety and efficacy of butenafine have not been established in children younger than 12 yr. There are no age-related precautions noted for elderly patients. Avoid contact with eyes, nose, mouth, or other mucous membranes.

Storage

Store products at room temperature.

Administration

For external use only. Gently cleanse and dry area prior to application. Use occlusive dressings only as ordered. Apply sparingly and rub into area thoroughly. Use for full course of treatment.

Butoconazole

byoo-toe-ko′na-zole

★ 🍁 Gynazole-1

CATEGORY AND SCHEDULE

Pregnancy Risk Category: C

Classification: Antifungals, vaginal azole antifungals

MECHANISM OF ACTION

An antifungal imidazole derivatives that inhibits the steroid synthesis, a vital component of fungal cell formation, thereby damaging the fungal cell membrane. *Therapeutic Effect:* Fungistatic.

PHARMACOKINETICS

Following vaginal use, roughly 1.7% of the dose was absorbed. Peak plasma levels of the drug and its metabolites occur between 12 and 24 h after vaginal administration.

AVAILABILITY

Cream: 2% (Gynazole-1, Rx).

INDICATIONS AND DOSAGES

▸ **Treatment of vaginal candidiasis**

VAGINAL

Adults, Elderly. Insert one applicatorful (5 g cream, or 100 mg of butoconazole) intravaginally as a single dose.

CONTRAINDICATIONS
Hypersensitivity to butoconazole or any of its components.

INTERACTIONS
Drug
Spermicides (e.g., nonoxynol-9): May inactivate spermicide; use other form of contraception.
Herbal
Not known.
Food
Not known.

SIDE EFFECTS
Occasional
Vaginal itching, burning, irritation.

SERIOUS REACTIONS
- Soreness, swelling, pelvic pain, or cramping rarely occurs.

PRECAUTIONS & CONSIDERATIONS
Be aware that butoconazole contains mineral oil, which may weaken latex or rubber products such as condoms. Tampons should not be used while using butoconazole because tampons can absorb and decrease the efficacy of the medication. It is unknown whether butoconazole crosses the placenta or is distributed in breast milk. Limit use during pregnancy to the second and third trimesters. Safety and efficacy not established in females under 12 yrs of age.
Storage
Store at room temperature and avoid temperatures above 86° F. Do not use product if applicator tip is missing or broken.
Administration
Peel back the protective foil and remove the prefilled applicator. Applicator is designed to be used with the tip in place.
Insert one applicatorful intravaginally as a single dose.

Butorphanol

byoo-tor′fa-nole
Stadol, Stadol NS
Apo-Butorphanol
Do not confuse butorphanol with butabarbital or Stadol with Haldol or sotalol.

CATEGORY AND SCHEDULE
Pregnancy Risk Category: C, (D if used for prolonged time, high dose at term)
Controlled Substance Schedule: IV

Classification: Analgesics, narcotic agonist-antagonist

MECHANISM OF ACTION
An opioid that binds to opiate receptor sites in the central nervous system (CNS). Reduces the intensity of pain stimuli incoming from sensory nerve endings. *Therapeutic Effect:* Alters pain perception and emotional response to pain.

PHARMACOKINETICS

Route	Onset (min)	Peak	Duration (h)
IM	10-30	30-60 min	3-4
IV	< 1	30 min	2-4
Nasal	15	1-2 h	4-5

Rapidly absorbed after IM injection. Protein binding: 80%. Extensively metabolized in the liver. Primarily excreted in urine. *Half-life:* 2.5-4 h.

AVAILABILITY
Injection: 1 mg/mL, 2 mg/mL.
Nasal Spray: 1 mg/spray.

B

INDICATIONS AND DOSAGES

▸ **Analgesia**

IM

Adults. 1-4 mg q3-4h as needed.
Elderly. 1 mg q4-6h as needed.

IV

Adults. 0.5-2 mg q3-4h as needed.
Elderly. 1 mg q4-6h as needed.

▸ **Migraine**

NASAL

Adults. 1 mg or 1 spray in one nostril. May repeat in 60-90 min. May repeat 2-dose sequence q3-4h as needed. Alternatively, 2 mg (one spray each nostril) if patient remains recumbent; may repeat in 3-4 h.

▸ **Patients with hepatic or renal impairment:**

NASAL

Limit intial dose to 1 mg, followed by 1 mg in 90-120 min if needed. Follow patient response rather than repeat at fixed times, at no less than q6h.

IM/IV

Initial dose should generally be half the normal dose, that is, 0.5 mg IV or 1 mg IM. Repeat no less than q6h, as indicated by patient response.

CONTRAINDICATIONS

Hypersensitivity to butorphanol tartrate or the preservation benzethonium chloride, which is found in some products (nasal spray and multidose injection vials).

INTERACTIONS

Drug

Alcohol, CNS depressants: May increase CNS or respiratory depression and hypotension.
Buprenorphine: Effects may be decreased with buprenorphine.
MAOIs: May produce severe, fatal reaction unless dose is reduced by one fourth.
Sumatriptan nasal spray: May reduce butorphanol levels; may increase risk of transient high BP.

Herbal

None known.

Food

None known.

DIAGNOSTIC TEST EFFECTS

None known.

IV INCOMPATIBILITIES

Amphotericin B complex (Abelcet, AmBisome, Amphotec).

IV COMPATIBILITIES

Atropine, diphenhydramine (Benadryl), droperidol, hydroxyzine (Vistaril), morphine, promethazine (Phenergan), propofol (Diprivan).

SIDE EFFECTS

Frequent

Parenteral: Somnolence (43%), dizziness (19%).
Nasal: Nasal congestion (13%), insomnia (11%).

Occasional

Parenteral (3%-9%): Confusion, diaphoresis, clammy skin, lethargy, headache, nausea, vomiting, dry mouth.
Nasal (3%-9%): Vasodilation, constipation, unpleasant taste, dyspnea, epistaxis, nasal irritation, upper respiratory tract infection, tinnitus.

Rare

Parenteral: Hypotension, pruritus, blurred vision, sensation of heat, CNS stimulation, insomnia.
Nasal: Hypertension, tremor, ear pain, paresthesia, depression, sinusitis.

SERIOUS REACTIONS

- Abrupt withdrawal after prolonged use may produce symptoms of narcotic withdrawal, such as abdominal cramping, rhinorrhea, lacrimation, anxiety, increased temperature, and piloerection or goose bumps.

• Overdose results in severe respiratory depression, skeletal muscle flaccidity, cyanosis, and extreme somnolence progressing to seizures, stupor, and coma.

• Tolerance to analgesic effect and physical dependence may occur with chronic use.

PRECAUTIONS & CONSIDERATIONS

Because of its opioid antagonist properties, butorphanol is not recommended for use in opioid-dependent patients. The use of butorphanol in patients with head injury may be associated with CO_2 retention and secondary elevation of CSF pressure, and alterations in mental state. The drug may produce respiratory depression, especially in patients suffering from CNS diseases or respiratory impairment.

Caution is warranted with hypertension, impaired liver or renal function, or myocardial infarction, before biliary tract surgery (because the drug produces spasm of sphincter of Oddi), and in elderly or debilitated patients. During labor, assess fetal heart tones and uterine contractions. Be aware that the safety and efficacy of butorphanol have not been established in children younger than 18 yr of age. Be aware that elderly patients may be more sensitive to effects. Adjust drug dose and interval for elderly patients.

Dizziness and drowsiness may occur, so change positions slowly and avoid alcohol, CNS depressants, and tasks that require mental alertness or motor skills until response to the drug is established. BP, pulse rate and quality, respirations, and clinical improvement of pain should be monitored.

Storage

Store at room temperature.

Administration

Injection may be given by IM or IV push. For IV use, butorphanol may be given undiluted. Administer over 3-5 min.

For intranasal use, blow nose to clear nasal passages as much as possible. Before first use, prime pump 7-8 times. If unit not used for > 48 h, then reprime by pumping 1-2 times. Spray into nostril while holding other nostril closed and concurrently inspire through nose to permit medication as high into nasal passages as possible. Alternate nostrils when repeat doses are given.

Cabergoline

ca-ber'goe-leen

★ 🍁 Dostinex

CATEGORY AND SCHEDULE

Pregnancy Risk Category: B

Classification: Dopamine agonist; antihyperprolactinemic

MECHANISM OF ACTION

Agonist at dopamine D_2 receptors, suppressing prolactin secretion. *Therapeutic Effects:* Shrinks prolactinomas, restores gonadal function.

PHARMACOKINETICS

Cabergoline is administered orally and undergoes significant first-pass metabolism following systemic absorption. Extensively metabolized in the liver. Elimination is primarily in the feces. *Half-life:* 80 h.

AVAILABILITY

Tablet: 0.5 mg.

INDICATIONS AND DOSAGES

▸ **Hyperprolactemia (idiopathic or due to primary pituitary adenomas)**

PO

Adults, Elderly. 0.25 mg 2 times per wk, titrate by 0.25 mg/dose no more than every 4 wks up to 1 mg 2 times/wk. Serum prolactin level guides dose adjustment.

OFF-LABEL USES

Parkinson disease, restless leg syndrome (RLS).

CONTRAINDICATIONS

Hypersensitivity to cabergoline, ergot alkaloids. Uncontrolled hypertension.

INTERACTIONS

Drug

Antihypertensives: May increase hypotensive effect.

Cimetidine, haloperidol, loxapine, MAOIs, methyldopa, metoclopramide, molindone, olanzapine, phenothiazines, pimozide, reserpine, risperidone, thiothixene, tricyclic antidepressants: Antagonizes the prolactin-lowering effect of cabergoline.

Antipsychotics, phenothiazine-type antiemetics: Cabergoline may diminish the effects of these dopamine agonists.

Levodopa: Additive neurologic effects are possible.

Ergot alkaloids: May lead to ergot toxicity.

Antiretroviral drugs: May lead to ergot toxicity.

Imatinib: May increase the risk of ergot-related side effects.

Herbal

None known.

Food

None known.

DIAGNOSTIC TEST EFFECTS

None known.

SIDE EFFECTS

Frequent

Nausea, orthostatic hypotension, confusion, dyskinesia, hallucinations, peripheral edema.

Occasional

Headache, vertigo, dizziness, dyspepsia, postural hypotension, constipation, asthenia, fatigue, abdominal pain, drowsiness.

Rare

Vomiting, dry mouth, diarrhea, flatulence, anxiety, depression, dysmenorrhea, dyspepsia, mastalgia, paresthesias, vertigo, visual impairment, peptic ulcer.

SERIOUS REACTIONS

- Overdosage may produce nasal congestion, syncope, or hallucinations.
- Cardiac valvulopathy or pleuropulmonary or pulmonary fibrotic changes occur rarely.

PRECAUTIONS & CONSIDERATIONS

Dopamine agonist use is not recommended for postpartum lactation inhibition or suppression. Caution is advised in patients with hepatic impairment. Orthostatic hypotension frequently reported; risk increased with initial doses > 1 mg and concurrent use of other blood pressure–lowering medications. It is unknown whether cabergoline crosses the placenta or is distributed into breast milk. In general, dopamine agonists like cabergoline are not used in pregnant women. Safety and efficacy have not been established in children or in elderly patients.

Nausea, headache, constipation, and dizziness may occur during therapy.

Storage

Store at room temperature.

Administration

Take without regard to meals.

Caffeine Citrate

kaf′een sit′rate

★ Cafcit

CATEGORY AND SCHEDULE

Pregnancy Risk Category: C

Classification: CNS stimulants, xanthine derivatives

MECHANISM OF ACTION

A methylxanthine and competitive inhibitor of phosphodiesterase that blocks antagonism of adenosine receptors. *Therapeutic Effect:* Stimulates respiratory center, increases minute ventilation, decreases threshold of or increases response to hypercapnia, increases skeletal muscle tone, decreases diaphragmatic fatigue, increases metabolic rate, and increases oxygen consumption.

PHARMACOKINETICS

Protein binding: 36%. Widely distributed through the tissues and CSF. Metabolized in liver; limited metabolism in preterm neonates. Excreted in urine. *Half-life:* 4-5 h in adults, children, and older infants; 3-4 days in neonates.

AVAILABILITY

Intravenous Solution: 20 mg/mL (Cafcit).

Oral Solution: 20 mg/mL (Cafcit).

INDICATIONS AND DOSAGES

▸ **Neonatal apnea**

IV/PO

Dosage listed as caffeine citrate. *Infants between 28 and 33 wks gestational age.* Loading dose: 20 mg/kg IV over 30 min. Maintenance: 5 mg/kg/day IV over 10 min or orally beginning 24 h after loading dose.

CONTRAINDICATIONS

Hypersensitivity to caffeine, xanthines, or any other component of the formulation.

INTERACTIONS

Drug

Cimetidine: May increase effects of caffeine citrate.

Ketoconazole: May increase effects of caffeine citrate.

MAOIs: Increased risk for cardiac arrhythmia or hypertension.

Phenobarbital: May decrease effects of caffeine citrate.

C

Phenytoin: May decrease effects of caffeine citrate.
Theophylline: May increase caffeine concentrations and toxicity.
Herbal
None known.
Food
None known.

DIAGNOSTIC TEST EFFECTS

May alter blood glucose concenration. Therapeutic caffeine level: 8-40 mg/L. Serious toxicity may occur at 50 mg/L.

IV INCOMPATIBILITIES

Furosemide, lorazepam, nitroglycerin, pantoprazole.

IV COMPATIBILITIES

Amino acid solutions, D5W, IV fat emulsion, antipyrine, calcium, dopamine, fentanyl, heparin, D50W.

SIDE EFFECTS

Occasional
Feeding intolerance, irritability, restlessness.
Rare
Necrotizing enterocolitis, rash, tachycardia, increased ventricular output, increased stroke volume, GI intolerance, hypo/hyperglycemia, increased creatinine clearance, increased sodium and calcium excretion.

SERIOUS REACTIONS

- Accidental injury, sepsis, hemorrhage, gastritis, GI hemorrhage, disseminated intravascular coagulation, acidosis, abnormal healing, cerebral hemorrhage, dyspnea, lung edema, dry skin, retinopathy, and kidney failure have been reported.
- Overdosage includes symptoms of fever, tachypnea, jitteriness, insomnia, fine tremor of the extremities, hypertonia, opisthotonos, tonic-clonic movements, nonpurposeful jaw and lip movements, vomiting, hyperglycemia, elevated blood urea nitrogen, and elevated total leukocyte concentration.

PRECAUTIONS & CONSIDERATIONS

Caution should be used in infants with cardiovascular disorders, hepatic or renal impairment, and seizure disorders. Use with caution in adult patients with tremor, anxiety, agitation, or heart arrhythmias. Caffeine readily crosses the placenta and is excreted in breast milk. Safety and efficacy in long-term treatment of infants have not been established. Be aware that necrotizing enterocolitis may occur in infants. There are no age-related precautions noted in elderly patients.
Storage
Store at room temperature.
Administration
! Be aware that 20 mg of caffeine citrate = 10 mg caffeine base. Take care in calculating dosage. Do not administer if particulate matter or discoloration is visible; discard vial. Discard unused portion. Administer IV using a syringe pump over 30 min for loading dose and over 10 min for maintenance doses. Oral administration: May give with formula feedings.

Calcipotriene

kal-sip′oh-tri-een
Dovonex

CATEGORY AND SCHEDULE

Pregnancy Risk Category: C

Classification: Dermatologics, topical vitamin D analogues

C

MECHANISM OF ACTION
A synthetic vitamin D_3 analogue that regulates skin cell (keratinocyte) production and development. *Therapeutic Effect:* Preventing abnormal growth and production of psoriasis (abnormal keratinocyte growth).

PHARMACOKINETICS
Minimal absorption through intact skin. Metabolized in liver.

AVAILABILITY
Cream: 0.005% (Dovonex).
Ointment: 0.005% (Dovonex).
Topical Solution: 0.005% (Dovonex).

INDICATIONS AND DOSAGES
▸ **Psoriasis**
TOPICAL
Adults, Elderly, Children 12 yr and older. Apply thin layer to affected skin twice daily (morning and evening); rub in gently and completely.
▸ **Scalp psoriasis**
TOPICAL SOLUTION
Adults, Elderly, Children 12 yr and older. Apply to lesions twice daily after combing hair.

CONTRAINDICATIONS
Hypercalcemia or evidence of vitamin D toxicity, use on face, hypersensitivity to calcipotriene or any component of the formulation. Scalp solution also contraindicated in patients with acute psoriatic eruptions.

INTERACTIONS
Drug
None known.
Herbal
None known.
Food
None known.

DIAGNOSTIC TEST EFFECTS
Excessive use may increase serum calcium level.

SIDE EFFECTS
Frequent
Burning, itching, skin irritation.
Occasional
Erythema, dry skin, peeling, rash, worsening of psoriasis, dermatititis.
Rare
Skin atrophy, hyperpigmentation, folliculitis.

SERIOUS REACTIONS
- Potential for hypercalcemia may occur.

PRECAUTIONS & CONSIDERATIONS
Caution should be used with history of nephrolithiasis. It is unknown whether calcipotriene crosses the placenta or is distributed in breast milk. Be aware that children and elderly patients are at greater risk for skin reactions. Improvement is usually noted after 2 wks of therapy and marked improvement after 8 wks of therapy.
Storage
Store at room temperature. Avoid sunlight; do not freeze.
Administration
Apply cream or ointment by rubbing gently into the affected and surrounding area twice daily (in morning and in the evening). Wash hands after application.

Apply scalp solution after combing hair to remove scaly debris and part the hair. Apply solution only to lesions and rub in gently and completely. Avoid spread of solution to the forehead.

C

Calcitonin

kal-si-toe′nin
★ Calcimar, Fortical, Miacalcin
🍁 Caltine, Calcimar, Miacalcin
Do not confuse calcitonin with calcitriol.

CATEGORY AND SCHEDULE

Pregnancy Risk Category: C

Classification: Hormones/hormone modifiers, calcium modifiers, bone resorption

MECHANISM OF ACTION

A synthetic hormone that decreases osteoclast activity in bones, decreases tubular reabsorption of sodium and calcium in the kidneys, and increases absorption of calcium in the GI tract. *Therapeutic Effect:* Regulates serum calcium concentrations and inhibits bone resorption, lowering fracture risk.

PHARMACOKINETICS

Injection rapidly metabolized (primarily in kidneys); primarily excreted in urine. Nasal form rapidly absorbed. *Half-life:* 70-90 min (injection); 43 min (nasal).

AVAILABILITY

Injection: 200 international units/mL (calcitonin-salmon).
Nasal Spray: 200 international units/spray (calcitonin-salmon).

INDICATIONS AND DOSAGES

▸ **Skin testing before treatment in patients with suspected sensitivity to calcitonin-salmon**

Adults, Elderly. Prepare a 10-international units/mL dilution; withdraw 0.05 mL from a 200-international units/mL vial in a tuberculin syringe; fill up to 1 mL with 0.9% NaCl. Take 0.1 mL and inject intracutaneously on inner aspect of forearm. Observe after 15 min; a positive response is the appearance of more than mild erythema or wheal.

▸ **Paget disease**

IM, SUBCUTANEOUS
Adults, Elderly. Initially, 100 international units/day. Maintenance: 50 international units/day or 50-100 international units every 1-3 days.
INTRANASAL
Adults, Elderly. 200-400 international units/day.

▸ **Postmenopausal osteoporosis**

IM, SUBCUTANEOUS
Adults, Elderly. 100 international units every other day with adequate calcium and vitamin D intake.
INTRANASAL
Adults, Elderly. 200 international units/day as a single spray, alternating nostrils daily.

▸ **Hypercalcemia**

IM, SUBCUTANEOUS
Adults, Elderly. Initially, 4 international units/kg q12h; may increase to 8 international units/kg q12h if no response in 2 days; may further increase to 8 international units/kg q6h if no response in another 2 days.

OFF-LABEL USES

Treatment of secondary osteoporosis due to drug therapy or hormone disturbance, phantom limb pain.

CONTRAINDICATIONS

Hypersensitivity to calcitomin-salmon or salmon protein.

INTERACTIONS

Drug
Lithium: May decrease lithium levels by increasing renal clearance.
Herbal
None known.

C

Food
None known.

DIAGNOSTIC TEST EFFECTS
None known.

SIDE EFFECTS
Frequent
IM, Subcutaneous (10%): Nausea (may occur 30 min after injection, usually diminishes with continued therapy), inflammation at injection site.
NASAL (10%-12%): Rhinitis, nasal irritation, redness, sores.
Occasional
IM, Subcutaneous (2%-5%): Flushing of face or hands.
NASAL (3%-5%): Back pain, arthralgia, epistaxis, headache.
Rare
IM, Subcutaneous: Epigastric discomfort, dry mouth, diarrhea, flatulence.
Nasal: Itching of earlobes, edema of feet, rash, diaphoresis.

SERIOUS REACTIONS
- Patients with a protein allergy may develop a hypersensitivity reaction.
- Severe nasal ulceration is rare with nasal form.

PRECAUTIONS & CONSIDERATIONS
Caution is warranted with history of allergy. Calcitonin does not cross the placenta, and it is unknown whether the drug is distributed in breast milk; its safety in breastfeeding women has not been established. The safety and efficacy of this drug have not been established in children. Elderly patients may experience a higher incidence of nasal adverse events with the nasal spray.

Nausea may occur but usually decreases with continued therapy. Notify the physician if itching, rash, shortness of breath, or significant nasal irritation occurs. Electrolyte levels should be checked. Improvement in biochemical abnormalities and bone pain usually occurs in the first few months of treatment; with neurologic lesions, improvement may take more than a year.

Storage
Refrigerate the unopened nasal spray and injection; do not freeze. Nasal spray may be stored at room temperature 30-35 days once the pump has been activated.

Administration
Patients should have adequate intake of calcium and vitamin D during treatment. Calcitonin may be administered as IM or subcutaneous injection. No more than 2 mL should be given IM at any one site. Bedtime administration may reduce flushing and nausea. Rotate injection sites.

Given as single spray to one nostril only per day; alternate nostrils used daily. For intranasal use, clear nasal passages as much as possible. Tilt head slightly forward and insert the spray tip into the nostril, pointing toward the nasal passages and away from the septum. Spray into the nostril while holding the other nostril closed, and at the same time inhale through the nose to deliver the drug as high into the nasal passage as possible. Bring to room temperature and prime pump before first use.

Calcitriol
kal-si-trye′ole
★ 🍁 Calcijex, Rocaltrol, Vectical

CATEGORY AND SCHEDULE
Pregnancy Risk Category: C

Classification: Vitamin D analogues, bone resorption inhibitors, dermatologic antipsoriatic agents

C

MECHANISM OF ACTION

A fat-soluble vitamin that is essential for absorption, utilization of calcium phosphate, and normal calcification of bone. *Therapeutic Effect:* Stimulates calcium and phosphate absorption from small intestine, promotes secretion of calcium from bone to blood, promotes renal tubule phosphate resorption, and acts on bone cells to stimulate skeletal growth and on parathyroid gland to suppress hormone synthesis and secretion. In the skin, calcitriol reduces T-helper function, and thymocyte and lymphocyte proliferation. The exact role of these immunologic mechanisms in the reduction of psoriatic lesions is unknown.

PHARMACOKINETICS

Rapidly absorbed from small intestine. Extensive metabolism in kidneys. Primarily excreted in feces; minimal excretion in urine. *Half-life:* 5-8 h (prolonged in children and patients on hemodialysis). Approximately 6% of a topical dose is absorbed when applied to psoriatic skin.

AVAILABILITY

Capsule: 0.25 mcg, 0.5 mcg (Rocaltrol).
Injection: 1 mcg/mL, 2 mcg/mL (Calcijex).
Oral Solution: 1 mcg/mL (Rocaltrol).
Ointment (Vectical): 3 mcg/g.

INDICATIONS AND DOSAGES

▸ **Renal failure on dialysis**

PO

Adults, Elderly. 0.25 mcg/day or every other day; increase dose at 4- to 8-wk intervals. Usual range 0.5-1 mcg/day.

Children. 0.25-2 mcg/day with hemodialysis.

IV

Adults, Elderly. 0.5 mcg/day (0.01 mcg/kg) 3 times/wk. Dose range: 0.5-3 mcg (0.01-0.05 mcg/kg) 3 times/wk. Adjust dose at 2- to 4-wk intervals.

Children. 0.01-0.05 mcg/kg 3 times/wk with hemodialysis.

▸ **Renal failure predialysis**

PO

Adults, Children 3 yr and older. Initially 0.25 mcg daily, may increase to 0.5 mcg daily.

Children < 3 yr of age. Initially 0.01-0.015 mcg/kg once daily.

▸ **Hypoparathyroidism/pseudohypoparathyroidism**

PO

Adults, Elderly, Children 6 yr and older. Initial dose 0.25 mcg/day, range 0.5-2 mcg once daily.

Children 1-5 yr. 0.25-0.75 mcg once daily.

Children < 1 yr. 0.04-0.08 mcg/kg once daily.

▸ **Vitamin D–dependent rickets**

PO

Adults, Elderly, Children. 1 mcg once daily.

▸ **Vitamin D–resistant rickets**

PO

Adults, Elderly, Children. 0.015-0.02 mcg/kg once daily. Maintenance: 0.03-0.06 mcg/kg once daily. Maximum: 2 mcg once daily.

▸ **Psoriasis**

TOPICAL

Adults: Apply ointment twice daily to affected areas. Maximum: 200 g/wk.

CONTRAINDICATIONS

Hypercalcemia, vitamin D toxicity, hypersensitivity to other vitamin D products or analogues.

INTERACTIONS

Drug

Aluminum-containing antacid (long-term use): May increase aluminum concentration and aluminum bone toxicity.

Calcium-containing preparations, thiazide diuretics: May increase the risk of hypercalcemia.

Magnesium-containing antacids: May increase magnesium concentration.

Herbal

None known.

Food

None known.

DIAGNOSTIC TEST EFFECTS

May increase serum cholesterol, calcium, magnesium, and phosphate levels. May decrease serum alkaline phosphatase.

SIDE EFFECTS

Occasional

Hypercalcemia, headache, irritability, constipation, metallic taste, nausea, polyuria. With topical use, pruritus (3%), erythema, skin discomfort, and contact dermatitis have been reported.

SERIOUS REACTIONS

- Early signs of overdosage are manifested as weakness, headache, somnolence, nausea, vomiting, dry mouth, constipation, muscle and bone pain, and metallic taste sensation.
- Later signs of overdosage are evidenced by polyuria, polydipsia, anorexia, weight loss, nocturia, photophobia, rhinorrhea, pruritus, disorientation, hallucinations, hyperthermia, hypertension, and cardiac arrhythmias.
- Hypersensitivity may include serious skin rashes, such as erythema multiforme.

PRECAUTIONS & CONSIDERATIONS

Caution is warranted with coronary artery disease, kidney stones, malabsorption syndrome, and renal impairment.

It is unknown whether calcitriol crosses the placenta. It is distributed in breast milk; breastfeeding is not recommended. Children may be more sensitive to the effects of calcitriol. Unique age-related precautions have not been observed in elderly patients. Serum alkaline phosphatase, BUN, serum calcium, serum creatinine, serum magnesium, serum phosphate, and urinary calcium levels should be monitored. Therapeutic serum calcium level is 9-10 mg/dL. Daily dietary calcium intake should be estimated; minimum intake should be 600 mg daily. Maintain adequate fluid intake.

Storage

Store at room temperature. Protect from light.

Administration

IV may be administered undiluted as bolus through catheter at the end of hemodialysis.

Give oral calcitriol without regard to food. Swallow the drug whole and avoid crushing, chewing, or opening the capsules.

For topical use, apply thin film to affected area(s) and rub in gently and completely.

Calcium Acetate

kal′see-um as′e-tate

★ 🍁 Calphron, Eliphos, PhosLo

Do not confuse PhosLo with PhosChol.

CATEGORY AND SCHEDULE

Pregnancy Risk Category: C Rx

Classification: Minerals and electrolytes, phosphate-binding agents

C

MECHANISM OF ACTION
Calcium is a mineral that is essential for the function and integrity of the nervous, muscular, and skeletal systems. Calcium acetate combines with dietary phosphate to form insoluble calcium phosphate. Does not promote aluminum absorption. *Therapeutic Effect:* Controls hyperphosphatemia in end-stage renal disease.

PHARMACOKINETICS
Moderately absorbed from the small intestine (absorption depends on product solubility, the presence of vitamin D, and patient's pH). When taken orally at meals, much of the calcium in calcium acetate is readily soluble and combines with phosphate from the diet in the proximal small intestine. The calcium phosphate product is primarily eliminated in feces.

AVAILABILITY
Gelcap (PhosLo): 667 mg.
Tablet (Calphron, Eliphos): 667 mg.

INDICATIONS AND DOSAGES
▸ To control hyperphosphatemia in end-stage renal disease
PO
Adults, Elderly. 2 tablets or gelcaps 3 times a day with meals. May increase gradually to bring serum phosphate below 6 mg/dL, as long as hypercalcemia does not develop. Most patients require 3-4 gelcaps or tablets with each meal.

CONTRAINDICATIONS
Patients with hypercalcemia.

INTERACTIONS
Drug
Digoxin: May increase the risk of arrhythmias if hypercalcemia occurs.
Fluoroquinolones bisphosphonates, thyroid hormones, phenytoin, tetracyclines: May decrease the oral absorption of these drugs; separate times of administration.
Herbal
None known.
Food
None known.

DIAGNOSTIC TEST EFFECTS
May increase blood pH and serum calcium levels. May decrease serum phosphate levels.

SIDE EFFECTS
Occasional
Nausea, mild constipation.
Rare
Skin rash, pruritus, or allergic reaction, fecal impaction, metabolic alkalosis.

SERIOUS REACTIONS
- Mild hypercalcemia ($Ca^{++} > 10.5$ mg/dL) may be asymptomatic, or may cause constipation, nausea and vomiting, headache, increased thirst, irritability, decreased appetite, metallic taste, fatigue, or weakness and may respond to a reduction in dosage or a temporary discontinuation of medicine. Severe hypercalcemia may cause confusion, somnolence, arrhythmias, increased painful urination, and coma.
- Chronic hypercalcemia may lead to vascular or soft-tissue calcification.

PRECAUTIONS & CONSIDERATIONS
The serum calcium level should be monitored twice weekly during the early dose adjustment period to avoid overdosage acutely or chronically. The serum calcium times phosphate (CaxP) product should not be allowed to exceed 66. A reduction in dose will often resolve mild hypercalcemia.

Caution is warranted with patients on digitalis glycosides; avoidance of calcium acetate in these patients is recommended. Calcium is normally distributed in breast milk. Use in pregnancy only when clearly needed. Safety and effectiveness have not been established in children. Patients should be counseled regarding dietary restrictions and adherence and the need to avoid over-the-counter antacids. Adequate hydration should be maintained. BP, ECG, serum magnesium, phosphate and potassium levels, urine calcium concentrations, and renal function test results should be monitored.

Storage

Store at room temperature.

Administration

Take with meals.

Calcium Salts

★ Calciject, Calcionate, Calcitrate, Caltrate, Citracal, Dicarbosil, Oscal, PhosLo, Titralac, Tums 🍁 PhosLo, Calcijet

Do not confuse OsCal with Asacol, Citracal with Citrucel, or PhosLo with PhosChol.

CATEGORY

Pregnancy Risk Category: C

OTC (carbonate, citrate, glubionate, gluconate [oral forms only])

Classification: Minerals

MECHANISM OF ACTION

An electrolyte that is essential for the function and integrity of the nervous, muscular, and skeletal systems. Calcium plays an important role in normal cardiac and renal function, respiration, blood coagulation, and cell membrane and capillary permeability. It helps to regulate the release and storage of neurotransmitters and hormones, and it neutralizes or reduces gastric acid (increased pH). Calcium combines with dietary phosphate to form insoluble calcium phosphate. *Therapeutic Effect:* Replaces calcium in deficiency states; controls hyperphosphatemia in end-stage renal disease.

PHARMACOKINETICS

Moderately absorbed from the small intestine (absorption depends on presence of vitamin D metabolites and patient's pH). Primarily eliminated in feces. Urinary excretion plays a minor role. Roughly 99% of filtered calcium is reabsorbed by the kidney with less than 1% excreted. Parathyroid hormone, calcitonin, and 1,25 dihydroxycholecalciferol help control calcium equilibrium.

AVAILABILITY

NOTE: There are a variety of calcium supplements available in the U.S. market; the following represent familiar dosage forms and brands.

Calcium carbonate

Tablets (Caltrate 600): Equivalent to 600 mg elemental calcium.

Tablets (OsCal 500): Equivalent to 500 mg elemental calcium.

Tablets (Chewable [OsCal 500]): Equivalent to 500 mg elemental calcium.

Tablets (Chewable [Tums]): Equivalent to 200 mg elemental calcium.

Calcium Chloride

Injection: 10% (100 mg/mL) equivalent to 27.2 mg (1.36 mEq) elemental calcium per mL.

Calcium Citrate

Tablets (Calcitrate): 250 mg (equivalent to 53 mg elemental calcium).

C

Tablets (Citracal): 950 mg (equivalent to 200 mg elemental calcium).
Calcium Glubionate
Syrup: 1.8 g/5 mL (equivalent to 115 mg of elemental calcium per 5 mL).
Calcium Gluconate
Injection: 10% (equivalent to 9 mg [0.45-0.48 mEq] elemental calcium per mL).

INDICATIONS AND DOSAGES

▸ **Hyperphosphatemia**
PO (CALCIUM CARBONATE)
Adults, Elderly. 2 tablets 3 times a day with meals. May increase gradually to bring serum phosphate below 6 mg/dL, as longs as hypercalcemia does not develop. Most patients require 3-4 Tums tablets with each meal.
▸ **Hypocalcemia**
PO (CALCIUM CARBONATE)
Adults, Elderly. 1-2 g/day in 3-4 divided doses.
Children. 45-65 mg/kg/day in 3-4 divided doses.
PO (CALCIUM GLUBIONATE)
Adults, Elderly. 16-18 g/day in 4-6 divided doses.
Children, Infants. 0.6-2 g/kg/day in 4 divided doses.
Neonates. 1.2 g/kg/day in 4-6 divided doses.
IV (CALCIUM CHLORIDE)
Adults, Elderly. 0.5-1 g repeated q4-6h as needed.
Children. 2.5-5 mg/kg/dose q4-6h.
IV (CALCIUM GLUCONATE)
Adults, Elderly. 2-15 g/24 h.
Children. 200-500 mg/kg/day.
▸ **Antacid**
PO (CALCIUM CARBONATE)
Adults, Elderly. 1-2 tablets (5-10 mL) q2h as needed.
▸ **Osteoporosis**
PO (CALCIUM CARBONATE)
Adults, Elderly. 1200 mg/day.
▸ **Cardiac arrest**
IV (CALCIUM CHLORIDE)
Adults, Elderly. 2-4 mg/kg. May repeat q10min.
Children. 20 mg/kg. May repeat in 10 min.
▸ **Hypocalcemia tetany**
IV (CALCIUM CHLORIDE)
Adults, Elderly. 1 g. May repeat in 6 h.
Children. 10 mg/kg over 5-10 min. May repeat in 6-8 h.
IV (CALCIUM GLUCONATE)
Adults, Elderly. 1-3 g until therapeutic response achieved.
Children. 100-200 mg/kg/dose q6-8h.

CONTRAINDICATIONS

Hypercalcemia. Contraindicated for cardiac resuscitation in the presence of ventricular fibrillation or in patients with the risk of existing digitalis toxicity. Not recommended in the treatment of asystole and electromechanical dissociation.

INTERACTIONS

Drug
Digoxin: May increase the risk of arrhythmias if hypercalcemia occurs.
Fluroquinolones bisphosphonates, thyroid hormones, phenytoin, tetracyclines: May decrease the oral absorption of these drugs; separate times of administration.
Herbal
None known.
Food
None known.

DIAGNOSTIC TEST EFFECTS

May increase blood pH and serum gastrin and calcium levels. May decrease serum phosphate and potassium levels.

IV INCOMPATIBILITIES

Calcium chloride: Amphotericin B complex (Abelcet, AmBisome, Amphotec), some cephalosporins, dexamethasone, diazepam, haloperidol, lansoprazole, magnesium sulfate, pantoprazole, phenytoin, propofol (Diprivan), quinupristin-dalfopristin (Synercid), sodium or potassium phosphate (concentration dependent).

Calcium gluconate: Amphotericin B complex (Abelcet, AmBisome, Amphotec), some cephalosporins, dexamethasone, diazepam, fluconazole (Diflucan), haloperidol, lansoprazole, magnesium sulfate, pantoprazole, phenytoin, quinupristin-dalfopristin (Synercid), sodium or potassium phosphate (concentration dependent).

IV COMPATIBILITIES

Calcium chloride: Amikacin (Amikin), dobutamine (Dobutrex), lidocaine, milrinone (Primacor), morphine, norepinephrine (Levophed). Calcium gluconate: Ampicillin, aztreonam (Azactam), cefazolin (Ancef), cefepime (Maxipime), ciprofloxacin (Cipro), dobutamine (Dobutrex), enalapril (Vasotec), famotidine (Pepcid), furosemide (Lasix), heparin, lidocaine, magnesium sulfate, meropenem (Merrem IV), midazolam (Versed), milrinone (Primacor), norepinephrine (Levophed), piperacillin and tazobactam (Zosyn), potassium chloride, propofol (Diprivan).

SIDE EFFECTS

Frequent

PO: Chalky taste.

Parenteral: Hypotension; flushing; feeling of warmth; nausea; vomiting; pain, rash, redness, or burning at injection site; diaphoresis.

Occasional

PO: Mild constipation, fecal impaction, peripheral edema, metabolic alkalosis (muscle pain, restlessness, slow breathing).

Rare

Difficult or painful urination.

SERIOUS REACTIONS

- Hypercalcemia. Early signs include constipation, headache, dry mouth, increased thirst, irritability, decreased appetite, metallic taste, fatigue, weakness, and depression. Later signs include confusion, somnolence, hypertension, photosensitivity, arrhythmias, nausea, vomiting, and increased painful urination.

PRECAUTIONS & CONSIDERATIONS

Caution is warranted with chronic renal impairment, decreased cardiac function, dehydration, history of renal calculi, and patients with sarcoidosis. Calcium distributed in breast milk. Injectable products contain aluminum that may be toxic if kidney function is impaired; premature neonates are particularly at risk. Restrict IV use in children because their small vasculature increases the risk of developing extreme irritation and possible tissue necrosis or sloughing. Oral absorption may be decreased in the elderly. Avoid consuming excessive amounts of alcohol, caffeine, and tobacco.

Adequate hydration should be maintained. BP, ECG, serum magnesium, phosphate and potassium levels, urine calcium concentrations, and renal function test results should be monitored.

Storage

Store vials and oral products at room temperature. If crystallization of calcium gluconate injection occurs during storage, warming vial in a 140° F water bath for 15-30 min with occasional shaking may dissolve the precipitate. Cool to body temperature before use. All injections must be clear at the time of use. Discard any unused portions once opened.

C

Storage
Store at room temperature; do not freeze.
Administration
Take tablets with a full glass of water 30 min to 1 h after meals. Dilute the syrup in juice or water and administer it before meals to increase absorption. Chew the chewable tablets well before swallowing them. Do not take calcium within 2 h of consuming other oral drugs or fiber-containing foods.

Injections of calcium should be made slowly through a small needle into a large vein to minimize venous irritation and avoid undesirable reactions.

Calcium chloride may be given undiluted or may be diluted with an equal amount 0.9% NaCl or sterile water for injection. Give calcium chloride 10% by slow IV push (0.5-1 mL/min). Rapid administration may produce bradycardia, hypotension, peripheral vasodilation, a chalky or metallic taste, and a feeling of warmth.

Calcium gluconate may be given undiluted or may be diluted in up to 1000 mL 0.9% NaCl. When administering calcium gluconate by intermittent IV infusion, the maximum rate is 200 mg/min. Rapid administration may produce arrhythmias, hypotension, and vasodilation.

Calfactant

cal-fac'tant
★ Infasurf

CATEGORY AND SCHEDULE

Pregnancy Risk Category: This drug is not indicated for use in pregnant women.

Classification: Surfactants, lung

MECHANISM OF ACTION

A natural lung extract that reduces alveolar surface tension, stabilizing the alveoli. *Therapeutic Effect:* Restores surface activity to infant lungs, improves lung compliance and respiratory gas exchange.

PHARMACOKINETICS

No studies have been performed.

AVAILABILITY

Intratracheal Suspension: 35-mg/mL vials.

INDICATIONS AND DOSAGES

▸ **Respiratory distress syndrome (RDS)**

INTRATRACHEAL

Neonates. 3 mL/kg of birth weight administered as soon as possible after birth in 2 doses of 1.5 mL/kg. Repeat 3-mL/kg doses, up to a total of 4 doses each given 12 h apart.

CONTRAINDICATIONS

None known.

INTERACTIONS

Drug
None known.
Herbal
None known.
Food
None known.

DIAGNOSTIC TEST EFFECTS

None known.

SIDE EFFECTS

Frequent
Cyanosis (65%), airway obstruction (39%), bradycardia (34%), reflux of surfactant into endotracheal tube (21%), need for manual ventilation (16%).
Occasional
Need for reintubation (3%).

SERIOUS REACTIONS

- Cyanosis, airway obstruction, bradycardia, and reflux of surfactant into endotracheal tube may occur.

PRECAUTIONS & CONSIDERATIONS

Caution is warranted with a hypersensitivity to calfactant. This drug is for use only in neonates. No age-related precautions have been noted.

The neonate's oxygenation and ventilation should be monitored using arterial or transcutaneous measurement of systemic oxygen (O_2) and carbon dioxide (CO_2). Visitors should be limited during treatment. Handwashing and other infection control measures should be monitored to minimize the risk of nosocomial infections.

Storage

Refrigerate vials. Unopened, unused vials may be returned to refrigerator within 24 h after having been warmed to room temperature. Repeated warming to room temperature should be avoided. Warming before administration is not necessary.

Administration

Gently swirl the vial, if needed, to redisperse contents. Do not shake it. Enter each single-use vial only once; discard unused suspension. Instill the drug intratracheally through a side port adapter into the infant's endotracheal tube. Give each aliquot over 20-30 ventilatory breaths. Administer only during the inspiratory cycle. Between aliquot dosages, turn the infant so that the opposite lung is in the dependent position.

Candesartan

kan-de-sar'tan

★ 🍁 Atacand

CATEGORY AND SCHEDULE

Pregnancy Risk Category: C (D if used in second or third trimester)

Classification: Antihypertensive agents, angiotensin II receptor

MECHANISM OF ACTION

An angiotensin II receptor, type AT1, antagonist that blocks the vasoconstrictor and aldosterone-secreting effects of angiotensin II, inhibiting the binding of angiotensin II to the AT1 receptors. *Therapeutic Effect:* Causes vasodilation, decreases peripheral resistance, and decreases BP.

PHARMACOKINETICS

Route	Onset	Peak	Duration
PO	2-3 h	6-8 h	24 h

Rapidly, completely absorbed. Protein binding: > 99%. Undergoes minor hepatic metabolism to inactive metabolite. Excreted unchanged in urine and in the feces through the biliary system. Not removed by hemodialysis. *Half-life:* 9 h.

AVAILABILITY

Tablets: 4 mg, 8 mg, 16 mg, 32 mg.

INDICATIONS AND DOSAGES

▸ **Hypertension as monotherapy or in combination with other antihypertensives**

PO

Adults, Elderly. Initially, 16 mg once a day in those who are not volume depleted. Can be given once or twice a day with total daily doses of

8-32 mg. Give lower initial dosage in those treated with diuretics or with impaired renal function or moderate hepatic disease.
Children 6-17 yr. If < 50 kg, the dose range is 2-16 mg per day. The recommended starting dose is 4-8 mg. For those ≥ 50 kg, the dose range is 4-32 mg per day. The starting dose is 8-16 mg.
Children 1 to < 6 yr. The starting dose is 0.20 mg/kg (oral suspension). The dose range is 0.05-0.4 mg/kg per day.
NOTE: Children with GFR < 30 mL/min/1.73 m^2 should not receive the drug.

▸ **Heart failure**
PO
Adults, Elderly. Initially 4 mg once daily. Target dose of 32 mg once daily can be reached by doubling dose approximately every 2 wks as tolerated.

CONTRAINDICATIONS
Hypersensitivity to candesartan.

INTERACTIONS
Drug
Lithium: May increase serum lithium levels; monitor lithium levels.
Pottassium-sparing diuretics, eplerenone, drospirenone: May increase serum potassium; monitor potassium levels.
Herbal
None known.
Food
None known.

DIAGNOSTIC TEST EFFECTS
May increase BUN, serum alkaline phosphatase, serum bilirubin, serum creatinine, potassium, AST (SGOT), and ALT (SGPT) levels. May decrease blood hemoglobin and hematocrit levels.

SIDE EFFECTS
Occasional (3%-6%)
Upper respiratory tract infection, dizziness, back and leg pain.
Rare (1%-2%)
Pharyngitis, rhinitis, headache, fatigue, diarrhea, nausea, dry cough, peripheral edema, mild hyperkalemia.

SERIOUS REACTIONS
- Overdosage may manifest as hypotension and tachycardia. Bradycardia occurs less often. Institute supportive measures.

PRECAUTIONS & CONSIDERATIONS
Caution is warranted with hepatic and renal impairment, renal artery stenosis, severe congestive heart failure, and dehydration. It is unknown whether candesartan is distributed in breast milk. Candesartan may cause fetal or neonatal morbidity or mortality. If pregnancy is detected, discontinue use. Safety and efficacy of candesartan have not been established in children < 1 yr of age. No age-related precautions have been noted in elderly patients.

Apical pulse and BP should be assessed immediately before each candesartan dose and regularly throughout therapy. Be alert to fluctuations in apical pulse and BP. If an excessive reduction in BP occurs, place the patient in the supine position with feet slightly elevated and notify the physician. Tasks that require mental alertness or motor skills should be avoided. Blood hemoglobin and hematocrit and BUN, serum alkaline phosphatase, serum bilirubin, serum creatinine, AST (SGOT), and ALT (SGPT) levels should be obtained before and during therapy. Also monitor potassium in heart failure patients. Maintain adequate hydration;

exercising outside during hot weather should be avoided to decrease the risk of dehydration and hypotension.

Storage

Store at room temperature. The compounded suspension will expire 30 days after first opened; do not freeze.

Administration

Take candesartan without regard to food.

The manufacturer has provided instructions for a pharmacist to compound an oral suspension if needed. Shake well before each use.

Capecitabine

ka-pe-site'a-been

★ 🍁 Xeloda

Do not confuse Xeloda with Xenical.

CATEGORY AND SCHEDULE

Pregnancy Risk Category: D

Classification: Antineoplastics, antimetabolites

MECHANISM OF ACTION

An antimetabolite that is enzymatically converted to 5-fluorouracil. Inhibits enzymes necessary for synthesis of essential cellular components. *Therapeutic Effect:* Interferes with DNA synthesis, RNA processing, and protein synthesis.

PHARMACOKINETICS

Readily absorbed from the GI tract. Protein binding: < 60%. Metabolized in the liver. Primarily excreted in urine. *Half-life:* 45 min.

AVAILABILITY

Tablets: 150 mg, 500 mg.

INDICATIONS AND DOSAGES

▸ **Metastatic breast cancer, colon cancer**

PO

Adults, Elderly. Initially, 2500 mg/m^2/day in 2 equally divided doses approximately q12h for 2 wks. Follow with a 1-wk rest period; given in 3-wk cycles. Expect dosages to be modified during the treatment course depending on the grade and type of any toxicities that appear.

▸ **Dosage in moderate renal impairment (CrCl 30-50 mL/min)**

PO

Adults, Elderly. Initally 950 mg/m^2 twice daily. If creatinine clearance is less than 30 mL/min, contraindicated.

CONTRAINDICATIONS

Severe renal impairment, hypersensitivity to capecitabine, fluorouracil, or any component of the formulation; known deficiency of dihydropyrimidine dehydrogenase.

INTERACTIONS

Drug

Phenytoin: May increase phenytoin levels.

Warfarin: May increase the effects of warfarin. Monitor INR frequently and watch for bleeding.

Herbal

None known.

Food

None known.

DIAGNOSTIC TEST EFFECTS

May increase serum alkaline phosphatase, bilirubin, AST (SGOT), and ALT (SGPT) levels. May decrease blood hematocrit, hemoglobin level, and WBC count.

SIDE EFFECTS

Frequent (> 5%)

Diarrhea (sometimes severe), nausea, vomiting, stomatitis, hand and foot syndrome (painful palmar-plantar swelling with paresthesia, erythema, and blistering), fatigue, anorexia, dermatitis.

Occasional (< 5%)

Constipation, dyspepsia, nail disorder, headache, dizziness, insomnia, edema, myalgia.

SERIOUS REACTIONS

- Serious reactions may include myelosuppression (evidenced by neutropenia, thrombocytopenia, and anemia), cardiovascular toxicity (marked by angina, cardiomyopathy, and deep vein thrombosis), respiratory toxicity (marked by dyspnea, epistaxis, and pneumonia), and lymphedema.

PRECAUTIONS & CONSIDERATIONS

Use cautiously in patients with a history of coronary artery disease, concomitant coumarin-derived anticoagulant therapy, concomitant phenytoin therapy, renal impairment, or liver dysfunction due to liver metastases. Caution is also warranted in elderly patients. Avoid use in pregnant women. It is unknown whether capecitabine is distributed in breast milk. Safety and efficacy of capecitabine have not been established in children. Monitor for signs of infection. Monitor for symptoms of hand-and-foot syndrome, diarrhea, nausea, vomiting, and stomatitis. Also watch for fever, and monitor CBC for hematologic changes.

Storage

Store at room temperature; keep tightly closed.

Administration

Take capecitabine within 30 min after a meal; take with water. Be aware that the prescription may require the patient to take tablets of different strengths to get the correct dose.

Capreomycin

kap-ree-oh-mye′sin

Capastat

Do not confuse with Captopril, Capsaicin, or Kanamycin.

CATEGORY AND SCHEDULE

Pregnancy Risk Category: C

Classification: Antimycobacterials

MECHANISM OF ACTION

A cyclic polypeptide antimicrobial but the mechanism of action is not well understood. *Therapeutic Effect:* Suppresses mycobacterial multiplication.

PHARMACOKINETICS

Not well absorbed from the gastrointestinal (GI) tract. Undergoes little metabolism. Primarily excreted unchanged in urine. *Half-life:* 4-6 h (half-life is increased with impaired renal function).

AVAILABILITY

Injection: 100 mg/mL (Capastat).

INDICATIONS AND DOSAGES

▸ **Tuberculosis**

IM/IV

Adults, Elderly. 1 g daily (not to exceed 20 mg/kg/day) for 60-120 days, followed by 1 g 2-3 times/wk.

▸ **Dosage in renal impairment**

CrCl > 100 mL/min: 13-15 mg/kg every 24 h.

CrCl 80-100 mL/min: 10-13 mg/kg every 24 h.

CrCl 60-80 mL/min: 7-10 mg/kg every 24 h.

CrCl 40-60 mL/min: 11-14 mg/kg every 48 h.

CrCl 20-40 mL/min: 10-14 mg/kg every 72 h.

CrCl < 20 mL/min: 4-7 mg/kg every 72 h.

OFF-LABEL USES

Treatment of atypical mycobacterial infections.

CONTRAINDICATIONS

Hypersensitivity to capreomycin.

INTERACTIONS

Drug

Aminoglycosides: May increase the risk of aminoglycoside toxicity.

Nondepolarizing neuromuscular blocking agents: May increase neuromuscular blockade.

Herbal

None known.

Food

None known.

DIAGNOSTIC TEST EFFECTS

None known.

SIDE EFFECTS

Frequent

Ototoxicity, nephrotoxicity.

Occasional

Eosinophilia.

Rare

Rash, fever, urticaria, hypokalemia, thrombocytopenia, vertigo.

SERIOUS REACTIONS

- Renal failure, ototoxicity, and thrombocytopenia can occur.

PRECAUTIONS & CONSIDERATIONS

Cautiously use with preexisting hearing impairment, renal dysfunction, or concurrent use of other ototoxic or nephrotoxic drugs. It is unknown whether capreomycin crosses the placenta and is excreted in breast milk. Safety and efficacy are not established in children. Age-related renal impairment may require dosage adjustment in elderly patients. Complete blood count (CBC) and renal and liver function test results should be obtained before the initiation of therapy. Hearing changes must be reported immediately. Renal function, electrolytes, and acid-base balance should be monitored during therapy.

Storage

Unopened vials are stored at room temperature. After reconstitution, solutions may be stored for up to 24 h under refrigeration. The solution for injection may acquire a pale straw color and darken with time. This is not associated with a loss of potency or development of toxicity.

Administration

Reconstitute by dissolving the vial contents (1 g) in 2 mL of 0.9% NaCl injection or sterile water for injection. Allow 2-3 min for complete dissolution. Further dilute in NS 100 mL for IV administration. Administer IV over 60 min. Administer deep IM into large muscle mass.

Capsaicin

cap-say'sin

★ Qutenza, Trixaicin, Zostrix, Zostrix HP, Zostrix Neuropathy

Do not confuse Zostrix with Zovirax.

CATEGORY AND SCHEDULE

Pregnancy Risk Category: B

OTC (topical creams), Rx (dermal patch)

Classification: Analgesics, topical

C

MECHANISM OF ACTION

A topical analgesic that depletes and prevents reaccumulation of the chemomediator of pain impulses (substance P) from peripheral sensory neurons to CNS.
Therapeutic Effect: Relieves pain.

PHARMACOKINETICS

Transient, low systemic exposure following topical use. Highest plasma level detected during patch use was 4.6 ng/mL immediately upon removal. Levels below the limit of detection 3-6 h after removal.

AVAILABILITY

Cream: 0.025%, 0.035%, 0.075%, 0.1%, 0.25%.
Gel: 0.025%, 0.05%.
Lotion: 0.025%, 0.075%.
Patch: 8% (Qutenza).
Roll-on: 0.075%.

INDICATIONS AND DOSAGES

▸ **Treatment of neuralgia, osteoarthritis, rheumatoid arthritis**

TOPICAL

Adults, Elderly, Children older than 2 yr. Apply directly to affected area 3-4 times/day. Continue for optimal clinical response.

▸ **Post-herpetic Neuralgia**

PATCH (QUTENZA)

Adults, Elderly. Up to 4 patches per treatment applied for 60 min and repeated no more frequently than q3mo.

CONTRAINDICATIONS

Hypersensitivity to capsaicin or any component of the formulation.

INTERACTIONS

Drug

Anticoagulants, antiplatelet agents, low-molecular-weight heparins, thrombolytic agents: May increase risk of bleeding.

Herbal

None known.

Food

None known.

DIAGNOSTIC TEST EFFECTS

None known.

SIDE EFFECTS

Frequent

Burning, stinging, erythema at site of application.

SERIOUS REACTIONS

• Pain during topical patch application may require analgesics.

PRECAUTIONS & CONSIDERATIONS

Caution is warranted with concurrent use of nephrotoxic agents, dehydration, fluid and electrolyte imbalance, neurologic abnormalities, and renal or hepatic impairment. It is unknown whether capsaicin crosses the placenta or is distributed in breast milk. Safety and efficacy have not been established in children < 2 yr of age. There are no age-related precautions noted for elderly patients.

Transient burning may occur on application and usually disappears after 72 h with continued use. If Qutenza patch is used, the patient may require pain relievers during the procedure to minimize discomfort. Inform the patient that the treated area may be sensitive to heat for a few days, including bathing and exercise.

Storage

Store at room temperature.

Administration

Capsaicin is for external use only. Avoid eye or mucous membrane contact. Wash hands immediately after application, unless used on arthritic hands, then wait 30 min, then wash.

If there is no improvement or condition deteriorates after 28 days, discontinue use and consult physician.

For Qutenza patch, administered only by health care personnel; do not apply at home. Pretreat with local anesthetic to treatment area plus 1-2 cm of surrounding area (e.g., lidocaine 4% cream used 60 min prior to patch application). Use only nitrile gloves when handling and when cleaning capsaicin residue. Latex gloves do not provide adequate protection. Have provider mark area to be treated. Do not apply to the face. The patch can be cut to match the size and the shape of the treatment area. Use only on dry, intact (unbroken) skin. Apply the patch to dry, intact skin within 2 h of opening the pouch. Dispose of used and unused patches, cleansing gel, and other treatment materials in accordance with the local biomedical waste procedures.

Captopril

cap'toe-pril

★ 🍁 Capoten

Do not confuse captopril with Capitrol.

CATEGORY AND SCHEDULE

Pregnancy Risk Category: C (D if used in second or third trimester)

Classification: Antihypertensive agents, angiotensin-converting enzyme (ACE) inhibitors

MECHANISM OF ACTION

An ACE inhibitor that suppresses the renin-angiotensin-aldosterone system and prevents conversion of angiotensin I to angiotensin II, a potent vasoconstrictor; may also inhibit angiotensin II at local vascular and renal sites. Decreases plasma angiotensin II, increases plasma renin activity, and decreases aldosterone secretion. *Therapeutic Effect:* Reduces peripheral arterial resistance, pulmonary capillary wedge pressure; improves cardiac output and exercise tolerance.

PHARMACOKINETICS

Route	Onset	Peak	Duration
PO	0.25 h	0.5-1.5 h	Dose related

Rapidly, well absorbed from the GI tract (absorption is decreased in the presence of food). Protein binding: 25%-30%. Metabolized in the liver. Primarily excreted in urine. Removed by hemodialysis. *Half-life:* < 3 h (increased in those with impaired renal function).

AVAILABILITY

Tablets: 12.5 mg, 25 mg, 50 mg, 100 mg.

INDICATIONS AND DOSAGES

▸ **Hypertension**

PO

Adults, Elderly. Initially, 12.5-25 mg 2-3 times a day. After 1-2 wks, may increase to 50 mg 2-3 times a day. Diuretic may be added if no response in additional 1-2 wks. If taken in combination with diuretic, may increase to 100-150 mg 2-3 times a day after 1-2 wks. Maintenance: 25-150 mg 2-3 times a day. Maximum: 450 mg/day.

▸ **Congestive heart failure**

PO

Adults, Elderly. Initially, 6.25-25 mg 3 times a day. Increase to 50 mg 3 times a day. After at least 2 wks, may

C

increase to 50-100 mg 3 times a day. Maximum: 450 mg/day.

▸ **Post-myocardial infarction, left ventricular dysfunction**

PO

Adults, Elderly. 6.25 mg a day, then 12.5 mg 3 times a day. Increase to 25 mg 3 times a day over several days up to 50 mg 3 times a day over several weeks.

▸ **Diabetic nephropathy**

PO

Adults, Elderly. 25 mg 3 times a day.

▸ **Usual pediatric dose**

Children. Initially 0.3-0.5 mg/kg/dose titrated up to a maximum of 6 mg/kg/day in 2-4 divided doses.

Neonates. Initially, 0.05-0.1 mg/kg/dose q8-24h titrated up to 0.5 mg/kg/dose given q6-24h. Maximum: 2 mg/kg/day.

▸ **Dosage in renal impairment (adults)**

Creatinine clearance 10-50 mL/min. 75% of normal dosage.

Creatinine clearance < 10 mL/min. 50% of normal dosage.

OFF-LABEL USES

Diagnosis of anatomic renal artery stenosis, hypertensive urgency.

CONTRAINDICATIONS

History of angioedema from previous treatment with ACE inhibitors. Also contraindicated in those experiencing angioedema in past from other causes (e.g., hereditary angioedema).

INTERACTIONS

Drug

Alcohol, antihypertensives, diuretics: May increase the effects of captopril.

Lithium: May increase lithium blood concentration and risk of lithium toxicity.

NSAIDs: May decrease the effects of captopril.

Potassium-sparing diuretics, drospirenone, eplerenone, potassium supplements: May cause hyperkalemia.

Herbal

None known.

Food

All food: Food significantly reduces drug absorption by 30%-40%.

DIAGNOSTIC TEST EFFECTS

May increase BUN, serum alkaline phosphatase, serum bilirubin, serum creatinine, serum potassium, AST (SGOT), and ALT (SGPT) levels. May decrease serum sodium levels. May cause positive antinuclear antibody titer.

SIDE EFFECTS

Frequent (4%-7%)

Rash.

Occasional (2%-4%)

Pruritus, dysgeusia (change in sense of taste), hyperkalemia.

Rare (0.5% to < 2%)

Headache, cough, insomnia, dizziness, fatigue, paresthesia, malaise, nausea, diarrhea or constipation, dry mouth, tachycardia.

SERIOUS REACTIONS

- Excessive hypotension (first-dose syncope) may occur in patients with CHF and in those who are severely salt and volume depleted.
- Angioedema (swelling of face and lips) occurs rarely.
- Agranulocytosis and neutropenia may be noted in those with collagen vascular disease, including scleroderma and systemic lupus erythematosus, and impaired renal function.
- Nephrotic syndrome may be noted in those with history of renal disease.

PRECAUTIONS & CONSIDERATIONS

Caution is warranted with cerebrovascular or coronary insufficiency, hypovolemia, renal impairment, sodium depletion, those on dialysis and/or receiving diuretics, and in elderly patients. Captopril crosses the placenta, is distributed in breast milk, and may cause fetal or neonatal morbidity or mortality. Safety and efficacy of captopril have not been established in children. Elderly patients may be more sensitive to the hypotensive effects of captopril.

Dizziness may occur. BP should be obtained immediately before giving each captopril dose, in addition to regular monitoring. Be alert to fluctuations in BP. If an excessive reduction in BP occurs, place the person in the supine position with legs elevated. CBC and blood chemistry should be obtained before beginning captopril therapy, then every 2 wks for the next 3 mo, and periodically thereafter in patients with autoimmune disease or renal impairment and in those who are taking drugs that affect immune response or leukocyte count. Skin for rash and urinalysis for proteinuria should also be assessed. CBC, BUN, serum creatinine, and serum potassium should be monitored in those who are receiving a diuretic. Full therapeutic effect of captopril may take several weeks.

Storage

Store at room temperature. Keep tightly closed to protect from moisture.

Administration

Give captopril 1 h before meals for maximum absorption because food significantly decreases drug absorption.

Crush tablets if necessary. Do not skip doses.

Carbachol

kar'ba-kole

★ 🍁 Isopto Carbachol, Miostat

CATEGORY AND SCHEDULE

Pregnancy Risk Category: C

Classification: Antiglaucoma agent, ophthalmic; miotic

MECHANISM OF ACTION

A direct-acting parasympathomimetic agent that stimulates cholinergic receptors resulting in muscarinic and nicotinic effects. Indirectly promotes release of acetylcholine. *Therapeutic Effect:* Produces contraction of the iris sphincter muscle, resulting in miosis and reduction in intraocular pressure associated with decreased resistance to aqueous humor outflow.

PHARMACOKINETICS

None reported.

AVAILABILITY

Ophthalmic Solution: 1.5%, 3%.
Solution for Intraocular Administration: 0.01%.

INDICATIONS AND DOSAGES

▸ Glaucoma

OPHTHALMIC

Adults, Elderly. Instill 1–2 drops of 0.75%–3% solution in affected eye(s) up to 3 times a day.

▸ Miosis, ophthalmic surgery

OPHTHALMIC

Adults, Elderly. Instill 0.5 mL of 0.01% solution into anterior chamber before or after securing sutures.

CONTRAINDICATIONS

Acute iritis, hypersensitivity to carbachol or any component of the formulation.

C

INTERACTIONS

Drugs
None known.
Herbal
None known.
Food
None known.

DIAGNOSTIC TEST EFFECTS

None known.

SIDE EFFECTS

Occasional
Blurred vision, burning/irritation of eye, decreased night vision, headache.
Rare
Diaphoresis, abdominal cramps.

SERIOUS REACTIONS

Retinal detachment.

PRECAUTIONS & CONSIDERATIONS

Intraocular carbachol 0.01% should be used with caution in patients with acute cardiac failure, bronchial asthma, peptic ulcer, hyperthyroidism, GI spasm, urinary tract obstruction, and Parkinson disease. Safety and effectiveness have not been established in children.
Storage
Store at room temperature.
Administration
Tilt the head back slightly and pull the lower eyelid down with the index finger to form a pouch. Instill drop(s) and gently close the eyes for 1-2 min. Do not blink. Use nasolacrimal occlusion to reduce systemic absorption. Do not touch the tip of the dropper to any surface to avoid contamination.

Sterile technique must be used for intraocular administration. Instill no more than 0.5 mL into the anterior chamber. Discard unused portion.

Carbamazepine

kar-ba-maz'e-peen
★ Carbatrol, Epitol, Equetro, Tegretol, Tegretol XR
🍁 Apo-Carbamazepine, Mazepine
Do not confuse Tegretol with Cartrol, Toradol, or Trental.
Do not confuse carbamazepine with oxcarbazepine.

CATEGORY AND SCHEDULE

Pregnancy Risk Category: D

Classification: Anticonvulsants, antipsychotics

MECHANISM OF ACTION

An iminostilbene derivative that decreases sodium and calcium ion influx into neuronal membranes, reducing posttetanic potentiation at synapses. *Therapeutic Effect:* Reduces seizure activity.

PHARMACOKINETICS

Slowly and completely absorbed from the GI tract. Protein binding: 75%. Metabolized in the liver to active metabolite. Primarily excreted in urine. Not removed by hemodialysis. *Half-life:* 25-65 h (decreased with chronic use).

AVAILABILITY

Capsules (Extended Release [Carbatrol, Equetro]): 100 mg, 200 mg, 300 mg.
Suspension (Tegretol): 100 mg/5 mL.
Tablets (Epitol, Tegretol): 200 mg.
Tablets (Chewable [Tegretol]): 100 mg.
Tablets (Extended Release [Tegretol XR]): 100 mg, 200 mg, 400 mg.

INDICATIONS AND DOSAGES

NOTE: Extended-release dosage forms are given twice daily, while immediate-release dosage forms may be given twice, 3 times, or 4 times per day.

▸ **Seizure control**

PO

Adults, Children older than 12 yr. Initially, 200 mg twice a day. May increase dosage by 200 mg/day at weekly intervals. Range: 400-1200 mg/day in 2-4 divided doses. Maximum: 1.6-2.4 g/day.

Children 6-12 yr. Initially, 100 mg twice a day. May increase by 100 mg/day at weekly intervals. Range: 20-30 mg/kg/day. Maxiumum: 1000 mg/day.

Children younger than 6 yr. Initially 5 mg/kg/day. May increase at weekly intervals to 10 mg/kg/day up to 20 mg/kg/day. Do not use extended-release forms.

Elderly. Initially 100 mg 1-2 times a day. May increase by 100 mg/day at weekly intervals. Usual dose 400-1000 mg/day.

▸ **Trigeminal neuralgia, diabetic neuropathy**

PO

Adults. Initially, 100 mg twice a day. May increase by 100 mg twice a day up to 400-800 mg/day. Maxiumum: 1200 mg/day.

Elderly. Initially 100 mg 1-2 times a day. May increase by 100 mg/day at weekly intervals. Usual dose 400-1000 mg/day.

▸ **Bipolar disorder**

PO

Adults. Initially 200 mg twice a day. May increase by 200 mg/day. Maximum: 1600 mg/day.

OFF-LABEL USES

Diabetes insipidus, agitation associated with dementia.

CONTRAINDICATIONS

Concomitant use of MAOIs, history of myelosuppression, hypersensitivity to carbamazepine or tricyclic antidepressants. Carbamazepine renders nefazodone ineffective; do not given with nefazodone.

INTERACTIONS

Drug

NOTE: Carbamazepine induces the metabolism of many drugs, which can lessen their efficacy.

Anticoagulants, clarithromycin, diltiazem, erythromycin, estrogens, propoxyphene, quinidine, steroids: May decrease the effects of these drugs.

Antipsychotics, haloperidol, tricyclic antidepressants: May increase CNS depressant effects.

Cimetidine: May increase carbamazepine blood concentration and risk of toxicity.

Isoniazid: May increase metabolism of isoniazid; may increase carbamazepine blood concentration and risk of toxicity.

MAOIs: May cause seizures and hypertensive crisis. Contraindicated.

Etravirine, nefazodone, delavirdine: Decreases concentrations of these to negligible; do not give.

Other anticonvulsants, barbiturates, benzodiazepines, valproic acid: May increase the metabolism of these drugs.

Verapamil: May increase the toxicity of carbamazepine.

Herbal

None known.

Food

Grapefruit: May increase the absorption and blood concentration of carbamazepine.

C

DIAGNOSTIC TEST EFFECTS

May increase BUN and blood glucose levels and serum alkaline phosphatase, bilirubin, AST (SGOT), ALT (SGPT), protein, cholesterol, HDL, and triglyceride levels. May decrease serum calcium and thyroid hormone (T3, T4, T4 index) levels. Therapeutic serum level is 4-12 mcg/mL; toxic serum level is > 12 mcg/mL.

SIDE EFFECTS

Frequent

Drowsiness, dizziness, nausea, vomiting.

Occasional

Visual abnormalities (spots before eyes, difficulty focusing, blurred vision), dry mouth or pharynx, tongue irritation, headache, fluid retention, diaphoresis, constipation or diarrhea, behavioral changes in children.

SERIOUS REACTIONS

- Toxic and serious multiorgan hypersensitivity reactions may include blood dyscrasias (such as aplastic anemia, agranulocytosis, thrombocytopenia, leukopenia, leukocytosis, and eosinophilia), cardiovascular disturbances (such as CHF, hypotension or hypertension, thrombophlebitis and arrhythmias), and dermatologic effects (such as rash, urticaria, pruritus, photosensitivity, Stevens-Johnson syndrome, and toxic epidermal necrolysis).
- Abrupt withdrawal may precipitate status epilepticus.

PRECAUTIONS & CONSIDERATIONS

Caution is warranted with impaired cardiac, hepatic, and renal function. AEDs increase the risk of suicidal thoughts or behavior in patients taking these drugs for any indication. Monitor for the emergence or worsening of depression, suicidal thoughts, or unusual behavior or moods. Be aware that carbamazepine crosses the placenta and accumulates in fetal tissue and is associated with fetal defects. It is also distributed in breast milk. Children are more likely than adults to develop behavioral changes. Elderly patients are more susceptible to agitation, AV block, bradycardia, confusion, and syndrome of inappropriate antidiuretic hormone secretion. Individuals who possess a genetic susceptibility marker known as the *HLA-B*1502* allele have an increased risk of developing Stevens-Johnson syndrome and/or toxic epidermal necrolysis compared with persons without this genotype. The presence of this genetic variant exists in up to 15% of people of Asian descent, varying from < 1% in Japanese and Koreans, to 2%-4% of South Asians and Indians, to 10%-15% of populations from China, Taiwan, Malaysia, and the Philippines. This variant is virtually absent in those of white, African-American, Hispanic, or European ancestry. Genetic testing is recommended before initiation of therapy in most patients of Asian ancestry for the presence of this genetic marker. A positive result should preclude use of carbamazepine unless the benefit exceeds risk. An increased risk of suicidal behavior and suicidal ideation has been observed in patients receiving antiepileptic therapies. Monitor for anxiety, depression, or changes in behavior.

Drowsiness may occur but disappears with continued therapy, so tasks that require mental alertness or motor skills should be avoided. Notify the physician if visual disturbances, fever, joint pain, mouth ulcerations, sore throat, or unusual bleeding occur. Seizure disorder, including the duration, frequency, and intensity of seizures, should be assessed before and during therapy. BUN level, CBC, serum iron determination, and urinalysis should be obtained before and periodically during carbamazepine therapy.

Storage

Store the tablets, capsules, and oral suspension at room temperature.

Administration

! If the patient must change to another anticonvulsant, plan to decrease the carbamazepine dose gradually as therapy begins with a low dose of the replacement drug. When transferring from tablets to suspension, expect to divide the total daily tablet dose into smaller, more frequent doses of suspension. Also plan to administer extended-release tablets in 2 divided doses.

Take carbamazepine with meals to reduce the risk of GI distress. Shake the oral suspension well. Do not administer it simultaneously with any other liquid medicine. Do not crush extended-release tablets. May open extended-release capsules and administer beads sprinkled on applesauce; however, do not crush or chew.

Carbamide Peroxide

car′bah-mide per-ox-ide

★ Auro Ear Drops, Debrox, Gly-Oxide, Murine Ear Drops, Orajel Perioseptic

CATEGORY AND SCHEDULE

Pregnancy Risk Category: C

Classification: Cerumenolytic; topical oral anti-inflammatory

MECHANISM OF ACTION

A cerumenolytic that releases oxygen on contact with moist mouth tissues to provide cleansing effects, reduce inflammation, relieve pain, and inhibit odor-forming bacteria. In the ear, oxygen is released and hydrogen peroxide is reduced to water, which enables the chemical reaction.

Therapeutic Effect: Relieves inflammation of gums and lips. Emulsifies and disperses earwax.

PHARMACOKINETICS

Not known.

AVAILABILITY

Solution, Oral: 10% (Gly-Oxide), 15% (Orajel Perioseptic).

Solution, Otic: 6.5% (Auro Ear Drops, Debrox, Murine Ear Drops).

INDICATIONS AND DOSAGES

▸ **Earwax removal**

OTIC SOLUTION

Adults, Elderly, Children 12 yr or older. Tilt head and administer 5-10 drops twice a day for up to 4 days.

Children 12 yr or younger. Tilt head and administer 1-5 drops twice a day for up to 4 days.

▸ **Oral lesions**

TOPICAL, SOLUTION

Adults, Elderly, Children. Apply several drops undiluted on affected area 4 times a day after meals and at bedtime. Expectorate after 1-3 min.

CONTRAINDICATIONS

Dizziness, ear discharge or drainage, recent ear surgery or tympanic membrane perforation, ear pain, irritation, or rash, hypersensitivity to carbamide peroxide or any one of its components.

C

INTERACTIONS

Drug
None known.
Herbal
None known.
Food
None known.

DIAGNOSTIC TEST EFFECTS

Not known.

SIDE EFFECTS

Occasional
Oral: Gingival sensitivity.

SERIOUS REACTIONS

• Opportunistic infections caused by organisms like *Candida albicans* are possible with prolonged use.

PRECAUTIONS & CONSIDERATIONS

With prolonged use of oral carbamide peroxide, there is a potential for overgrowth of opportunistic organisms, damage to periodontal tissues, and delayed wound healing; should not be used for longer than 7 days. Otic solution should not be used for longer than 4 days. It is unknown whether carbamide peroxide crosses the placenta or is distributed in breast milk. There are no age-related precautions noted in elderly patients.
Administration
Oral topical use: Use several drops after a meal or at bedtime. Mix with saliva, swish for several minutes, and expectorate. Do not rinse mouth after use.

Otic product use: For use in the ear only. Tilt the patient's head sideways to instill in ear. Keep drops in ear for several minutes by keeping head tilted and placing cotton in ear. Tip of the applicator should not enter the ear canal. Any wax remaining after treatment may be removed by gently flushing the ear with warm water, using a soft rubber bulb ear syringe.

Carbidopa and Levodopa

kar-bi-doe′pa; lee-voe-doe′pa
★ Parcopa, Sinemet, Sinemet CR
🍁 DuoDopa, Levocarb SR, Sinemet, Sinemet CR
Do not confuse Sinemet with Serevent.

CATEGORY AND SCHEDULE

Pregnancy Risk Category: C

Classification: Antiparkinsonian agents, dopaminergics

MECHANISM OF ACTION

Levodopa is converted to dopamine in the basal ganglia, thus increasing dopamine concentration in the brain and inhibiting hyperactive cholinergic activity. Carbidopa prevents peripheral breakdown of levodopa, allowing more levodopa to be available for transport into the brain.
Therapeutic Effect: Reduces tremor.

PHARMACOKINETICS

Carbidopa is rapidly and completely absorbed from the GI tract. Widely distributed. Excreted primarily in urine. Levodopa is converted to dopamine. Excreted primarily in urine. *Half-life:* 1-2 h (carbidopa); 1-3 h (levodopa).

AVAILABILITY

Tablets: 10 mg carbidopa/100 mg levodopa, 25 mg carbidopa/100 mg levodopa, 25 mg carbidopa/250 mg levodopa.
Tablets (Extended Release): 25 mg carbidopa/100 mg levodopa, 50 mg carbidopa/200 mg levodopa.

Tablets (Orally Disintegrating Parcopa): 10 mg carbidopa/100 mg levodopa, 25 mg carbidopa/100 mg levodopa, 25 mg carbidopa/250 mg levodopa.

INDICATIONS AND DOSAGES

▸ **Parkinsonism**

PO

Adults. Initially, 25/100 mg 2-4 times a day. May increase up to 200/2000 mg daily in divided doses.

Elderly. Initially, 25/100 mg twice a day. May increase as necessary.

When converting a patient from Sinemet to Sinemet CR (50 mg/200 mg), dosage is based on the total daily dose of levodopa:

Sinemet (mg)	Sinemet CR
300-400	1 tablet twice a day
500-600	1.5 tablets twice a day or 1 tablet 3 times a day
700-800	4 tablets in 3 or more divided doses
900-1000	5 tablets in 3 or more divided doses

Intervals between doses of Sinemet CR should be 4-8 h while awake.

CONTRAINDICATIONS

Angle-closure glaucoma, use within 14 days of MAOIs, history of melanoma.

INTERACTIONS

Drug

Anticonvulsants, benzodiazepines, haloperidol, phenothiazines: May decrease the effects of carbidopa and levodopa.

MAOIs: May increase the risk of hypertensive crisis. Contraindicated.

Selegiline: May increase levodopa-induced dyskinesias, nausea, orthostatic hypotension, confusion, and hallucinations.

Iron salts: May reduce levodopa absorption.

Herbal

None known.

Food

Protein: Avoid high-protein diet. Distribute dietary protein throughout the day to avoid fluctuations in levodopa absorption.

Pyridoxine/vitamin B_6: May reduce levodopa's effect at high doses.

DIAGNOSTIC TEST EFFECTS

May increase BUN level and serum LDH, alkaline phosphatase, bilirubin, AST (SGOT), and ALT (SGPT) levels.

SIDE EFFECTS

Frequent (10%-90%)

Uncontrolled movements of the face, tongue, arms, or upper body; nausea and vomiting (80%); anorexia (50%).

Occasional

Depression, anxiety, confusion, nervousness, urine retention, palpitations, dizziness, light-headedness, decreased appetite, blurred vision, constipation, dry mouth, flushed skin, headache, insomnia, diarrhea, unusual fatigue, darkening of urine and sweat.

Rare

Hypertension, ulcer, hemolytic anemia (marked by fatigue).

SERIOUS REACTIONS

- Patients on long-term therapy have a high incidence of involuntary choreiform, dystonic, and dyskinetic movements.
- Numerous mild to severe CNS and psychiatric disturbances may occur, including reduced attention span, anxiety, nightmares, daytime somnolence, euphoria, fatigue, paranoia, psychotic episodes, depression, and hallucinations.

C

- Increased risk of melanoma noted in Parkinson patients.
- Orthostasis, syncope.

PRECAUTIONS & CONSIDERATIONS

Caution is warranted with active peptic ulcer, severe cardiac, endocrine, hepatic, pulmonary, or renal impairment, treated open-angle glaucoma, a history of myocardial infarction, bronchial asthma (because of tartrazine sensitivity), and emphysema. It is unknown whether carbidopa and levodopa cross the placenta or are distributed in breast milk. However, this drug may inhibit lactation. Women should not breastfeed while taking this drug. The safety and efficacy of carbidopa and levodopa have not been established in children younger than 18 yr. Elderly patients are more sensitive to levodopa's effects. Elderly patients receiving anticholinergics are at increased risk for adverse CNS effects, such as anxiety, confusion, and nervousness.

Dizziness, drowsiness, dry mouth, and darkened urine may occur. Alcohol and tasks that require mental alertness or motor skills should be avoided. Notify the physician if agitation, headache, lethargy, or confusion occurs. Relief of symptoms, such as improvement of masklike facial expression, muscular rigidity, shuffling gait, and resting tremors of the hands and head, should be assessed.

Storage

Store at room temperature.

Administration

! Plan to discontinue levodopa at least 12 h before giving carbidopa and levodopa. Expect the initial dose to provide at least 25% of the previous levodopa dose. Void before giving carbidopa and levodopa to reduce the risk of urine retention.

Take carbidopa and levodopa without regard to food. If GI upset occurs, take with food. Scored tablets may be crushed as needed. Extended-release tablets may be cut in half but not crushed. Orally disintegrating tablets should be allowed to dissolve on the tongue and then swallowed with saliva.

Carboplatin

car-bow'play-tin

Do not confuse carboplatin with Cisplatin or Platinol.

CATEGORY AND SCHEDULE

Pregnancy Risk Category: D

Classification: Antineoplastics, platinum agents

MECHANISM OF ACTION

A platinum coordination complex that inhibits DNA synthesis by cross-linking with DNA strands, preventing cell division. Cell cycle-phase nonspecific. *Therapeutic Effect:* Interferes with DNA function.

PHARMACOKINETICS

Protein binding: Low. Hydrolyzed in solution to active form. Primarily excreted in urine. *Half-life:* 2.6-5.9 h.

AVAILABILITY

Powder for Injection: 50 mg, 150 mg, 450 mg.
Injection Solution: 10 mg/mL.

INDICATIONS AND DOSAGES

▸ **Ovarian carcinoma (monotherapy)**

IV INFUSION

Adults. 360 mg/m^2 on day 1, every 4 wks. Do not repeat dose until neutrophil and platelet counts are within acceptable levels. Adjust drug dosage in previously treated patients based on lowest posttreatment platelet or neutrophil count. Increase dosage only once to no more than 125% of starting dose.

▸ **Ovarian carcinoma (combination therapy)**

IV INFUSION

Adults. 300 mg/m² (with cyclophosphamide) on day 1, every 4 wks. Do not repeat dose until neutrophil and platelet counts are within acceptable levels.

▸ **Calvert formula for AUC-based dosing in adults as an alternative method of dosing for ovarian cancer: Total dose (mg) = Target AUC × (GFR + 25)**

▸ **Adult dosage in renal impairment**

Initial dosage is based on creatinine clearance; subsequent dosages are based on the patient's tolerance and degree of myelosuppression.

Creatinine Clearance (mL/min)	Dosage Day 1 (mg/m²)
≥ 60	No adjustment
41-59	250
16-40	200

OFF-LABEL USES

Treatment of bony and soft tissue sarcoma; germ cell tumor; neuroblastoma pediatric brain tumor; small-cell lung cancer; solid tumors of the bladder, cervix, and testes; squamous cell carcinoma of the esophagus.

CONTRAINDICATIONS

History of severe allergic reaction to cisplatin, platinum compounds, or mannitol; severe bleeding; severe myelosuppression.

INTERACTIONS

Drug

Bone marrow depressants: May increase myelosuppression.

Live-virus vaccines: May potentiate virus replication and decrease the patient's antibody response to the vaccine.

Nephrotoxic, ototoxic medications: May increase the risk of nephrotoxicity/ototoxicity.

Phenytoin: Phenytoin levels may be reduced.

Warfarin: The effects of warfarin may be increased.

Herbal and Food

None known.

DIAGNOSTIC TEST EFFECTS

May decrease serum electrolyte levels, including calcium, magnesium, potassium, and sodium. High dosages (more than 4 times the recommended dosage) may elevate BUN and serum alkaline phosphatase, bilirubin, creatinine, and AST SGOT levels.

IV INCOMPATIBILITIES

Amphotericin B complex (Abelcet, AmBisome, Amphotec), diazepam, lansoprazole, leucovorin calcium, phenytoin.

IV COMPATIBILITIES

Etoposide (VePesid), granisetron (Kytril), ondansetron (Zofran), paclitaxel (Taxol).

SIDE EFFECTS

Frequent

Nausea (75%-80%), vomiting (65%).

Occasional

Generalized pain (17%), diarrhea or constipation (6%), peripheral neuropathy (4%).

Rare (2%-3%)

Alopecia, asthenia, hypersensitivity reaction (erythema, pruritus, rash, urticaria, and rarely bronchospasm and hypotension).

C

SERIOUS REACTIONS

- Myelosuppression may be severe, resulting in anemia, infection (sepsis, pneumonia), and bleeding.
- Prolonged treatment may result in peripheral neurotoxicity.
- High doses may be associated with reversible vision loss.
- Serious hypersensitivity reactions (rare).

PRECAUTIONS & CONSIDERATIONS

Caution is warranted in renal impairment. Be aware that prior aminoglycoside therapy may potentiate carboplatin-induced renal toxicity. Use cautiously in elderly patients who were previously treated with cisplatin; they are at an increased risk of developing carboplatin-induced peripheral neuropathy. Avoid using carboplatin in pregnant women. The use of a contraceptive is recommended during therapy. It is unknown whether carboplatin is distributed in breast milk. Safety and efficacy have not been established in children. Tell the patient of the possibility of hair loss and that normal hair growth should resume after treatment has ended.

Storage

Store at room temperature. Protect from light. Diluted solutions are stable for 8 h at room temperature.

Administration

CAUTION: Observe and exercise usual cautions for handling and preparing solutions of cytotoxic drugs.

Be aware that aluminum reacts with carboplatin to form an inactive precipitate; intravenous sets and needles containing aluminum that may come in contact with carboplatin should not be used.

Given as an IV infusion. Carboplatin injection can be diluted to concentrations as low as 0.5 mg/mL with D5W or 0.9% NaCl injection. Infusion may be given over 15 min or longer.

Carboprost

kar'boe-prost

Hemabate

CATEGORY AND SCHEDULE

Pregnancy Risk Category: C

Classification: Abortifacients, oxytocics, prostaglandins, stimulants, uterine

MECHANISM OF ACTION

A prostaglandin similar to prostaglandin F2α (dinoprost) that directly acts on myometrium and stimulates contraction in gravid uterus. *Therapeutic Effect:* Produces cervical dilation and softening.

PHARMACOKINETICS

None reported.

AVAILABILITY

Injection: 250 mcg carboprost and 83 mcg tromethamine/mL (Hemabate).

INDICATIONS AND DOSAGES

▸ Pregnancy termination between 13 and 20 wks, gestation under select circumstances

IM

Adults. Initially, 100-250 mcg, may repeat at 1.5- to 3.5-h intervals. May increase up to 500 mcg if uterine contractility inadequate. Maximum: 12-mg total dose or continuous administration for more than 2 days.

▸ **Postpartum uterine hemorrhage**
IM
Adults. Initially, 250 mcg, may repeat at 15- to 90-min intervals. Maximum: 2 mg total dose.

OFF-LABEL USES

Treatment of incomplete abortion.

CONTRAINDICATIONS

Acute pelvic inflammatory disease, active cardiac disease, pulmonary disease, renal disease, hepatic disease, hypersensitivity to carboprost or other prostaglandins.

INTERACTIONS

Drug
Oxytocin, oxytocics: May cause uterine hypertonus leading to uterine rupture or cervical lacerations.
Herbal
None known.
Food
None known.

DIAGNOSTIC TEST EFFECTS

None known.

SIDE EFFECTS

Frequent
Nausea, transient pyrexia, vomiting, diarrhea.
Occasional
Facial flushing.
Rare
Endometritis.

SERIOUS REACTIONS

• Excessive dosing may cause uterine hypertonicity with spasm and tetanic contraction, leading to cervical laceration/perforation and uterine rupture and hemorrhage.

PRECAUTIONS & CONSIDERATIONS

Caution is warranted in patients with a history of hypotension or hypertension, anemia, jaundice, diabetes mellitus, epilepsy, compromised (scarred) uterus, cardiovascular disease, adrenal disease, or hepatic disease.
NOTE: Use is not indicated if the fetus has reached a stage of viability in utero. Be aware that carboprost tromethamine use is contraindicated during later pregnancy and that small amounts of the drug are found in breast milk. There is no information available on carboprost tromethamine use in children or in elderly patients. Avoid smoking because of added effects of vasoconstriction.

Strength, duration, and frequency of contractions as well as vital signs should be monitored every 15 min until stable, then hourly until abortion is complete. Fever, chills, foul-smelling/increased vaginal discharge, and uterine cramps/pain should be reported immediately.
Storage
Refrigerate ampules. Do not freeze.
Administration
Administer by deep IM injection. Be aware that carboprost tromethamine should not be injected IV because it may result in bronchospasm, hypertension, vomiting, and anaphylaxis.

Carisoprodol

kar'i-so-pro'dol
★ Soma

CATEGORY AND SCHEDULE

Pregnancy Risk Category: C

Classification: Skeletal muscle relaxant, central acting

MECHANISM OF ACTION

A centrally acting skeletal muscle relaxant whose exact mechanism is unknown. Effects may be due to its

C

CNS depressant actions. *Therapeutic Effect:* Relieves muscle spasms and pain.

PHARMACOKINETICS

Onset 2 h; duration 4-6 h. *Half-life:* 2.5 h. *Meprobamate half-life:* 10 h. Metabolized in liver to meprobamate by the CYP2C19 isoenzyme; excreted by kidneys.

AVAILABILITY

Tablets: 250 mg, 350 mg.

INDICATIONS AND DOSAGES

▸ Adjunct to rest, physical therapy, analgesics, and other measures for relief of discomfort from acute, painful musculoskeletal conditions

PO

Adults, Elderly, Adolescents over 16 yr of age. 250-350 mg 4 times a day. Duration of therapy should be limited to 2-3 wks.

CONTRAINDICATIONS

Acute intermittent porphyria, sensitivity to meprobamate or other carbanates.

INTERACTIONS

Drug

Alcohol, other CNS depressants: May increase CNS depression.

Herbal

None known.

Food

None known.

DIAGNOSTIC TEST EFFECTS

None known.

SIDE EFFECTS

Frequent (> 10%)

Somnolence.

Occasional (1%-10%)

Tachycardia, facial flushing, dizziness, headache, light-headedness, dermatitis, nausea, vomiting, abdominal cramps, dyspnea.

SERIOUS REACTIONS

- Overdose may cause CNS and respiratory depression, shock, and coma.
- Rarely idiosyncratic reaction appears within minutes or hours of the first dose. Symptoms reported include extreme weakness, transient quadriplegia, dizziness, ataxia, temporary loss of vision, diplopia, mydriasis, dysarthria, agitation, euphoria, confusion, and disorientation.
- Seizures (rare).

PRECAUTIONS & CONSIDERATIONS

Caution is warranted in patients with hepatic and renal impairment and addictive personalities and in elderly patients. Drowsiness or dizziness may occur. Avoid alcohol, CNS depressants, and tasks that require mental alertness or motor skills. Liver and renal function tests should be obtained at baseline and periodically for those on long-term therapy. Therapeutic response, such as relief of muscle spasm and pain, should be assessed.

Storage

Store at room temperaure.

Administration

Take carisoprodol without regard to food. Take the last dose of the day at bedtime.

Carmustine

kar-muss'teen

★ 🍁 BiCNU, Gliadel

CATEGORY AND SCHEDULE

Pregnancy Risk Category: D

Classification: Antineoplastic, nitrosureas, alkylating agent

MECHANISM OF ACTION

An alkylating agent and nitrosourea that inhibits DNA and RNA synthesis by cross-linking with DNA and RNA strands, preventing cell division. Cell cycle–phase nonspecific. *Therapeutic Effect:* Interferes with DNA and RNA function.

PHARMACOKINETICS

Degraded within 15 min; crosses blood-brain barrier; 70% excreted in urine within 96 h; 10% excreted as CO_2; fate of 20% is unknown. *Half-life:* 20 min (active metabolites half-life 67 h).

AVAILABILITY

Powder for Injection: 100 mg.
Wafer: 7.7 mg.

INDICATIONS AND DOSAGES

▸ **Disseminated Hodgkin disease, non-Hodgkin lymphoma, multiple myeloma, and primary and metastatic brain tumors in previously untreated patients (monotherapy)**

IV (BiCNU) INFUSION

NOTE: Dosages and regimens depend on type of cancer and use in combination with other agents. See prescribing information.

Adults, Elderly. 150-200 mg/m² as a single dose or 75-100 mg/m² on 2 successive days.

Children with brain tumors. 200-250 mg/m² every 4-6 wks as a single dose.

IMPLANTATION (GLIADEL) FOR BRAIN TUMOR INDICATIONS

Adults, Elderly, Children. Up to 8 wafers may be placed in resection cavity.

CONTRAINDICATIONS

Hypersenstivity to carmustine.

INTERACTIONS

Drug

Cimetidine: May increase concentrations and toxic effects of carmustine.

Digoxin: May reduce digoxin concentrations.

Phenytoin: May reduce phenytoin concentrations.

DIAGNOSTIC TEST EFFECTS

Increases in bilirubin, alkaline phosphatase, AST; decreases in leukocytes, platelets.

SIDE EFFECTS

Frequent

Nausea and vomiting within min to 2 h after administration (may last up to 6 h); myelosuppression.

Occasional

Diarrhea, esophagitis, anorexia, dysphagia.

Rare

Thrombophlebitis.

SERIOUS REACTIONS

- Hematologic toxicity due to myelosuppression occurs frequently. Thrombocytopenia occurs about 4 wks after carmustine treatment begins and lasts 1-2 wks.
- Leukopenia is evident 5-6 wks after treatment begins and lasts 1-2 wks. Anemia occurs less frequently and is less severe.
- Mild, reversible hepatotoxicity also occurs frequently.
- Prolonged high-dose carmustine therapy may produce impaired renal function and pulmonary toxicity (pulmonary infiltrate or fibrosis).

PRECAUTIONS & CONSIDERATIONS

Administer with caution to patients with depressed platelet, leukocyte, or erythrocyte counts or with renal or hepatic impairment. Pretreatment pulmonary function testing is

C

advised. Nausea and vomiting occur frequently with carmustine therapy; prophylactic antiemetics are advised. Women of childbearing potential should be advised to avoid pregnancy. Not recommended for use in breastfeeding.

Storage

Store powder for injection in refrigerator. Reconstituted and diluted solutions may be stored at room temperature for up to 8 h. Store wafers in freezer. Unopened foil pouches may be held at room temperature for up to 6 h.

Administration

CAUTION: Observe and exercise usual cautions for handling and preparing solutions of cytotoxic drugs.

To prepare injectable, dilute powder with 3 mL of absolute alcohol. Further dilute with 27 mL of sterile water for injection to a concentration of 3.3 mg/mL. May further dilute with D5W. Displays significant absorption to PVC containers; administer in glass or polyolefin containers. Infuse over 1-2 h using polyethylene tubing. Protect from light.

For wafers: Wear surgical gloves to handle. See specialized instructions to avoid loss of sterility or unintended exposure, which may cause burns and depigmentation of skin.

Carteolol

kar-tee′oh-lole

Do not confuse with carvedilol.

CATEGORY AND SCHEDULE

Pregnancy Risk Category: C

Classification: Ophthalmic agents, antiglaucoma agents, β-adrenergic blocker

MECHANISM OF ACTION

An antihypertensive that blocks β_1-adrenergic receptors at normal doses and β_2-adrenergic receptors at large doses. Predominantly blocks β_1-adrenergic receptors in cardiac tissue if given orally. Reduces aqueous humor production. *Therapeutic Effect:* Decreases intraocular pressure (IOP).

PHARMACOKINETICS

Carteolol has not been detected in plasma following ocular use; however, systemic absorption has been reported with use of other ocular β-blockers. Minimally metabolized in liver. Primarily excreted unchanged in urine. Not removed by hemodialysis. *Half-life:* 6 h (increased in decreased renal function).

AVAILABILITY

Ophthalmic Solution: 1%.

INDICATIONS AND DOSAGES

▸ **Open-angle glaucoma, ocular hypertension**

OPHTHALMIC

Adults, Elderly. 1 drop 2 times a day to affected eye(s).

OFF-LABEL USES

Combination with miotics decreases IOP in acute/chronic angle-closure glaucoma, treatment of secondary glaucoma, malignant glaucoma, angle-closure glaucoma during or after iridectomy.

CONTRAINDICATIONS

Bronchial asthma, COPD, bronchospasm, overt cardiac failure, cardiogenic shock, heart block greater than first degree, persistently severe bradycardia.

INTERACTIONS

Drug

Other hypotensives: May increase hypotensive effect.

DIAGNOSTIC TEST EFFECTS

May increase serum ANA titer, BUN, serum LDH, lipoprotein, alkaline phosphatase, bilirubin, creatinine, potassium, triglyceride, uric acid, SGOT (AST), and SGPT (ALT) levels.

SIDE EFFECTS

Frequent

Transient eye irritation, burning, tearing, conjunctival hypermia, and edema of eyelids.

Occasional

Blurred or cloudy vision, photophobia, decreased night vision, ptosis, blepharoconjunctivitis, corneal sensitivity.

Rare

Bradycardia, decreased BP, cardiac arrhythmia, heart palpitation, dyspnea, asthenia, headache, dizziness, insomnia, sinusitis, and taste perversion.

SERIOUS REACTIONS

- Abrupt withdrawal (particularly in those with coronary artery disease) may produce angina or precipitate myocardial infarction. (systemic)
- May precipitate thyroid crisis in those with thyrotoxicosis. (systemic)
- β-blockers may mask signs and symptoms of acute hypoglycemia (tachycardia, BP changes) in diabetic patients.

PRECAUTIONS & CONSIDERATIONS

Caution is warranted with impaired renal, cardiac, or liver function; thyrotoxicosis, diminished pulmonary function, myasthenia. Be aware that carteolol crosses the placenta and is distributed in small amounts in breast milk. Safety and efficacy of carteolol have not been established in children. In patients with angle-closure glaucoma, carteolol should be used with a miotic and not alone.

Storage

Store ophthalmic solution at room temperature.

Administration

Tilt the head back slightly and pull the lower eyelid down with the index finger to form a pouch. Instill drop(s) and gently close the eyes for 1-2 min. Do not blink. Use nasolacrimal occlusion to reduce systemic absorption. Do not touch the tip of the dropper to any surface to avoid contamination. Wait several minutes before use of other eyedrops.

Carvedilol

kar-vea'die-lole

★ Coreg

Do not confuse carvedilol with carteolol.

CATEGORY AND SCHEDULE

Pregnancy Risk Category: C

Classification: Antihypertensives, β-adrenergic blocker

MECHANISM OF ACTION

An antihypertensive that possesses nonselective β-blocking and α-adrenergic blocking activity. Causes vasodilation. *Therapeutic Effect:* Reduces cardiac output, exercise-induced tachycardia, and reflex orthostatic tachycardia; reduces peripheral vascular resistance.

C

PHARMACOKINETICS

Route	Onset	Peak	Duration
PO	30 min	1-2 h	24 h

Rapidly and extensively absorbed from the GI tract. Protein binding: 98%. Metabolized in the liver. Excreted primarily via bile into feces. Minimally removed by hemodialysis. *Half-life:* 7-10 h. Food delays rate of absorption.

AVAILABILITY

Capsules (Extended Release): 10 mg, 20 mg, 40 mg, 80 mg.
Tablets: 3.125 mg, 6.25 mg, 12.5 mg, 25 mg.

INDICATIONS AND DOSAGES

▸ **Hypertension**
PO (IMMEDIATE RELEASE)
Adults, Elderly. Initially, 6.25 mg twice a day. May double at 7- to 14-day intervals to highest tolerated dosage. Maximum: 50 mg/day.
PO (EXTENDED RELEASE)
Adults, Elderly. Initially 20 mg once daily. May double at 7- to 14-day intervals to highest tolerated dosage. Maximum 80 mg/day.
▸ **Congestive heart failure**
PO (IMMEDIATE RELEASE)
Adults, Elderly. Initially, 3.125 mg twice a day. May double at 2-wk intervals to highest tolerated dosage. Maximum: For patients weighing more than 85 kg, give 50 mg twice a day; for those weighing 85 kg or less, give 25 mg twice a day.
PO (EXTENDED RELEASE)
Adults, Elderly. Initially 10 mg once daily for 2 wks. May double at 2-wk intervals to highest tolerated dosage. Maximum 80 mg/day.
▸ **Left ventricular dysfunction**
PO (IMMEDIATE RELEASE)
Adults, Elderly. Initially, 3.125-6.25 mg twice a day. May increase at intervals of 3-10 days up to 25 mg twice a day.
PO (EXTENDED RELEASE)
Adults, Elderly. Initially 10-20 mg once daily. May increase at intervals of 3-10 days up to 80 mg once daily.
▸ **Patients can be converted from immediate release to extended-release carvedilol at the following doses:**

Twice-Daily Dose (mg)	Once-Daily Dose (mg) (Coreg-CR)
3.125	10
6.25	20
12.5	40
25	80

OFF-LABEL USES

Treatment of angina pectoris, idiopathic cardiomyopathy.

CONTRAINDICATIONS

Hypersensitivity. Bronchial asthma or related bronchospastic conditions, cardiogenic shock, pulmonary edema, second- or third-degree AV block, severe bradycardia, clinical hepatic impairment.

INTERACTIONS

Drug
Alcohol: Alcohol may affect the extended-release properties, resulting in fasting absorption and a higher peak. Avoid alcohol, including alcohol in prescription and nonprescription medications, for at least 2 h after carvedilol extended-release administration.
Calcium blockers: Increase risk of conduction disturbances.
Clonidine: May potentiate BP effects.
Cimetidine: May increase carvedilol blood concentration.
Digoxin: Increases concentrations of this drug.
Diuretics, other antihypertensives: May increase hypotensive effect.

Insulin, oral hypoglycemics: May mask symptoms of hypoglycemia and prolong hypoglycemic effect of these drugs.
Rifampin: Decreases carvedilol blood concentration.
Herbal
None known.
Food
None known.

DIAGNOSTIC TEST EFFECTS
Increases in AST and ALT.

SIDE EFFECTS
Carvedilol is generally well tolerated, with mild and transient side effects.
Frequent (4%-6%)
Fatigue, dizziness.
Occasional (2%)
Diarrhea, bradycardia, rhinitis, back pain.
Rare (< 2%)
Orthostatic hypotension, somnolence, urinary tract infection, viral infection.

SERIOUS REACTIONS
- Overdose may produce profound bradycardia, hypotension, bronchospasm, cardiac insufficiency, cardiogenic shock, and cardiac arrest.
- Abrupt withdrawal may result in diaphoresis, palpitations, headache, and tremors.
- Carvedilol administration may precipitate congestive heart failure (CHF) and myocardial infarction (MI) in patients with heart disease, thyroid storm in those with thyrotoxicosis, and peripheral ischemia in those with existing peripheral vascular disease.
- Hypoglycemia may occur in patients with previously controlled diabetes.

PRECAUTIONS & CONSIDERATIONS
Caution should be used in those undergoing anesthesia and in those with CHF controlled with ACE inhibitor, digoxin, or diuretics; diabetes mellitus; hypoglycemia; impaired hepatic function; peripheral vascular disease; and thyrotoxicosis. It is unknown whether carvedilol crosses the placenta or is distributed in breast milk. Carvedilol use should be avoided in pregnant women after the first trimester because it may result in low-birth-weight infants. The drug may also produce apnea, bradycardia, hypoglycemia, or hypothermia during childbirth. The safety and efficacy of carvedilol have not been established in children. In elderly patients, the incidence of dizziness may be increased. Be aware that salt and alcohol intake should be restricted. Nasal decongestants or OTC cold preparations (stimulants) should not be used without physician approval.

Orthostatic hypotension may occur, so rise slowly from a lying to sitting position and dangle the legs from the bed momentarily before standing. Tasks that require mental alertness or motor skills should be avoided. Apical pulse and BP should be assessed immediately before giving carvedilol. BP for hypotension; respiratory status for shortness of breath, pattern of daily bowel activity and stool consistency; ECG for arrhythmias; and pulse for quality, rate, and rhythm should be monitored during treatment. If pulse rate is 55 beats/min or lower or systolic BP is < 90 mm Hg, withhold the medication and contact the physician. Signs and symptoms of CHF, such as decreased urine output, distended neck veins, dyspnea (particularly on exertion or lying down), night cough, peripheral edema, and weight gain, should also be assessed.

Storage
Store at room temperature. Protect from light and moisture.

C

Administration
Take carvedilol tablets with food to slow the rate of absorption and reduce the risk of orthostatic hypotension. Carvedilol extended-release capsules should be taken once daily in the morning with food. Swallow extended-release capsules whole, without crushing or chewing. Capsules may be opened and the contents sprinkled on applesauce.

Caspofungin Acetate

kas-poe-fun′jin as′e-tate
Cancidas

CATEGORY AND SCHEDULE

Pregnancy Risk Category: C

Classification: Antifungal, systemic, echinocandins

MECHANISM OF ACTION

An antifungal that inhibits the synthesis of glucan, a vital component of fungal cell formation, thereby damaging the fungal cell membrane. *Therapeutic Effect:* Fungicidal.

PHARMACOKINETICS

Distributed in tissue. Extensively bound to albumin. Protein binding: 97%. Slowly metabolized in liver to active metabolite. Excreted primarily in urine and to a lesser extent in feces. Not removed by hemodialysis. *Half-life:* 40-50 h.

AVAILABILITY

Powder for Injection: 50-mg, 70-mg vials.

INDICATIONS AND DOSAGES

▸ **Aspergillosis**
IV INFUSION
Adults, Elderly, Children older than 12 yr. Give single 70-mg loading dose on day 1, followed by 50 mg/day thereafter.

▸ **Invasive candidiasis**
IV INFUSION
Adults, Elderly. Initially, 70 mg followed by 50 mg daily.

▸ **Esophageal candidiasis**
IV INFUSION
Adult, Elderly. 50 mg a day.

▸ **Empirical therapy, neutropenic patients**
IV INFUSION
Adults, Elderly. Give single 70-mg loading dose on day 1, followed by 50 mg/day thereafter. If 50-mg dose is tolerated, but does not provide adequate clinical response, dose can be increased to 70 mg/day.

▸ **Dosage in hepatic impairment**
IV INFUSION
Adults, Elderly with moderate hepatic impairment. Reduce daily dose to 35 mg. Loading dose, when indicated, remains 70 mg.

CONTRAINDICATIONS

Hypersensitivity to any of the product ingredients.

INTERACTIONS

Drug
Carbamazepine, dexamethasone, efavirenz, nelfinavir, nevirapine, phenytoin, rifampin: May decrease blood concentration of caspofungin.
Cyclosporine: May increase caspofungin concentrations and increase incidence of hepatic transaminase elevations.
Tacrolimus: May decrease the effect of tacrolimus.
Herbal
None known.
Food
None known.

DIAGNOSTIC TEST EFFECTS

May increase PT as well as serum alkaline phosphatase, serum bilirubin, serum creatinine, LDH, SGOT (AST), SGPT (ALT), serum uric acid, urine pH, urine protein, urine RBC, and urine WBC levels. May decrease hemoglobin, hematocrit, platelet count, and serum albumin, serum bicarbonate, serum protein, and serum potassium levels.

IV INCOMPATIBILITIES

Do not mix caspofungin with any other medication or use dextrose as a diluent.

SIDE EFFECTS

Frequent (26%)
Fever.
Occasional (4%-11%)
Headache, nausea, phlebitis.
Rare (3% or less)
Paresthesia, vomiting, diarrhea, abdominal pain, myalgia, chills, tremor, insomnia.

SERIOUS REACTIONS

- Hypersensitivity reactions (characterized by rash, facial swelling, pruritus, and a sensation of warmth, hypotension, tachycardia) may occur.

PRECAUTIONS & CONSIDERATIONS

Caution is warranted for patients with liver function impairment. Be aware that caspofungin crosses the placental barrier, may be embryotoxic, and is distributed in breast milk. Be aware that the safety and efficacy of caspofungin have not been established in children. In elderly patients, age-related moderate renal impairment may require dosage adjustment.

Baseline temperature, liver function test results, and history of allergies should be obtained before giving the drug. Signs and symptoms of liver function should be assessed. If increased shortness of breath, itching, facial swelling, or a rash occurs, notify the physician. Report pain, burning, or swelling at the IV infusion site.

Storage
Refrigerate but warm it to room temperature before preparing it with the diluent. The reconstituted solution, before it is prepared as the patient infusion solution, may be stored at room temperature for 1 h. The final infusion solution can be stored at room temperature for 24 h or up to 48 h under refrigeration. Discard the solution if it contains particulate or is discolored.

Administration
For IV infusion only. For a 50- to 70-mg loading dose, add 10.5 mL 0.9% NaCl to the 50- or 70-mg vial. Transfer 10 mL of the reconstituted solution to 250 mL 0.9% NaCl or other compatible solution (see manufacturer's recommendations). Do not use dextrose solutions to prepare or infuse the drug. For 35-mg dose in persons with moderate liver insufficiency, add 10.5 mL 0.9% NaCl to the 50-mg vial. Transfer 7 mL to 100 or 250 mL 0.9% NaCl. Infuse over 60 min.

Castor Oil

cass'ter-oil

CATEGORY AND SCHEDULE

Pregnancy Risk Category: X
OTC

Classification: Laxative, stimulant

MECHANISM OF ACTION

A laxative prepared from the bean of the castor plant; the exact mechanism of action is unknown.

C

Acts primarily in the small intestine. May be hydrolyzed to ricinoleic acid, which reduces net absorption of fluid and electrolytes and stimulates peristalsis. *Therapeutic Effect:* Increases peristalsis, promotes laxative effect.

PHARMACOKINETICS
Minimal absorption by the GI tract. May be metabolized like other fatty acids within the gut.

AVAILABILITY
Oral liquid: 95%, 100%.

INDICATIONS AND DOSAGES
▸ **Constipation**
PO
Adults, Elderly, Children 12 yr and older. 15-60 mL as a single dose.
Children 2-12 yr. 5-15 mL as a single dose.
Children < 2 yr. 1-2 mL as a single dose. Maximum: 5 mL as a single dose.

CONTRAINDICATIONS
Abdominal pain, appendicitis, intestinal obstruction, nausea, vomiting, pregnancy.

INTERACTIONS
Drug
None known
Herbal
Licorice: May increase risk of hypokalemia.
Food
None known.

DIAGNOSTIC TEST EFFECTS
None known.

SIDE EFFECTS
Occasional
Some degree of abdominal discomfort, nausea, mild cramps, griping, faintness.

SERIOUS REACTIONS
• Long-term use may result in laxative dependence, chronic constipation, and loss of normal bowel function.
• Chronic use or overdosage may result in electrolyte disturbances, such as hypokalemia, hypocalcemia, metabolic acidosis or alkalosis, persistent diarrhea, malabsorption, and weight loss. Electrolyte disturbance may produce vomiting and muscle weakness.

PRECAUTIONS & CONSIDERATIONS
Caution should be used for extended periods (> 1 wk) of castor oil use. Be aware that castor oil is contraindicated in pregnancy. It is unknown whether castor oil is distributed in breast milk. Safety and efficacy of castor oil have not been established in children younger than 2 yr of age. No age-related precautions have been noted in elderly patients, but monitor for signs of dehydration and electrolyte loss. Avoid taking within 1 h of other oral medication because it decreases drug absorption.
Storage
Store at room temperature.
Administration
Take castor oil on an empty stomach for faster results. Drink at least 6-8 glasses of water a day to aid in stool softening.

Cefaclor
sef'a-klor
🍁 Apo-Cefaclor, Ceclor

CATEGORY AND SCHEDULE
Pregnancy Risk Category: B

Classification: Antibiotics, cephalosporin (second generation)

MECHANISM OF ACTION

A second-generation cephalosporin that binds to bacterial cell membranes and inhibits cell wall synthesis. *Therapeutic Effect:* Bactericidal.

PHARMACOKINETICS

Well absorbed from the GI tract. Protein binding: 25%. Widely distributed. Primarily excreted unchanged in urine. Moderately removed by hemodialysis. *Half-life:* 0.6-0.9 h (increased in impaired renal function).

AVAILABILITY

Capsules: 250 mg, 500 mg.
Oral Suspension: 125 mg/ 5 mL, 187 mg/5 mL, 250 mg/5 mL, 375 mg/5 mL.
Tablets, Extended Release: 500 mg.

INDICATIONS AND DOSAGES

▸ Bronchitis

PO

Adults, Elderly (extended release). 500 mg q12h for 7 days.

▸ Lower respiratory tract infections

PO

Adults, Elderly. 250-500 mg q8h.

▸ Otitis media

PO

Children. 20-40 mg/kg/day in 2-3 divided doses. Maximum: 1 g/day.

▸ Pharyngitis, skin/skin structure infections, tonsillitis

PO

Adults, Elderly (extended release). 375 mg q12h.

Adults, Elderly (regular release). 250-500 mg q8h.

Children. 20-40 mg/kg/day in 2-3 divided doses. Maximum: 1 g/day.

▸ Urinary tract infections

PO

Adults, Elderly. 250-500 mg q8h.

Children. 20-40 mg/kg/day in 2-3 divided doses q8h. Maximum: 1 g/day.

PO (EXTENDED-RELEASE TABLETS)

Adults, Children older than 16 yr. 375-500 mg q12h.

▸ Otitis media

PO

Children older than 1 mo. 40 mg/kg/day in divided doses q8h. Maximum: 1 g/day.

CONTRAINDICATIONS

History of anaphylactic reaction to penicillins or hypersensitivity to cephalosporins.

INTERACTIONS

Drug

Probenecid: May increase cefaclor blood concentration.

Herbal

None known.

Food

None known.

DIAGNOSTIC TEST EFFECTS

May increase BUN level and serum alkaline phosphatase, bilirubin, creatinine, LDH, AST (SGOT), and ALT (SGPT) levels. May cause a positive direct or indirect Coombs' test.

SIDE EFFECTS

Frequent

Oral candidiasis, mild diarrhea, mild abdominal cramping, vaginal candidiasis.

Occasional

Nausea, serum sickness-like reaction (marked by fever and joint pain; usually occurs after the second course of therapy and resolves after the drug is discontinued).

Rare

Allergic reaction (pruritus, rash, and urticaria).

SERIOUS REACTIONS

- Antibiotic-associated colitis and other superinfections may result from altered bacterial balance.

C

• Nephrotoxicity may occur, especially in patients with preexisting renal disease.
• Patients with a history of allergies, especially to penicillin, are at increased risk for developing a severe hypersensitivity reaction, marked by severe pruritus, angioedema, bronchospasm, and anaphylaxis.

PRECAUTIONS & CONSIDERATIONS

Caution is warranted with a history of GI disease (especially antibiotic-associated colitis or ulcerative colitis), renal impairment, and concurrent use of nephrotoxic medications. Be aware that cefaclor readily crosses the placenta and is distributed in breast milk. No age-related precautions have been noted in children older than 1 mo. In elderly patients, age-related renal impairment may require dosage adjustment.

Although mild GI effects may be tolerable, an increase in their severity may indicate the onset of antibiotic-associated colitis. Assess the mouth for white patches on the mucous membranes and tongue, the pattern of daily bowel activity and stool consistency, signs and symptoms of superinfection including abdominal pain, moderate to severe diarrhea, severe anal or genital pruritus, and severe mouth soreness. Renal function should be assessed.

Storage

Store capsules, extended-release tablets, and powder for suspension at room temperature. After reconstitution, oral suspension is stable for 14 days if refrigerated.

Administration

Take without regard to meals; if GI upset occurs, give with food or milk. Do not cut, crush, or chew extended-release tablets.

Shake oral suspension well before using.

Cefadroxil

sef-a-drox′ill

CATEGORY AND SCHEDULE

Pregnancy Risk Category: B

Classification: Antibiotics, cephalosporin (first generation)

MECHANISM OF ACTION

A first-generation cephalosporin that binds to bacterial cell membranes and inhibits cell wall synthesis. *Therapeutic Effect:* Bactericidal.

PHARMACOKINETICS

Well absorbed from the GI tract. Protein binding: 15%-20%. Widely distributed. Primarily excreted unchanged in urine. Removed by hemodialysis. *Half-life:* 1.2-1.5 h (increased in impaired renal function).

AVAILABILITY

Capsules: 500 mg.
Oral Suspension: 250 mg/5 mL, 500 mg/5 mL.
Tablets: 1000 mg.

INDICATIONS AND DOSAGES

▸ **Urinary tract infection**

PO

Adults, Elderly. 1-2 g/day as a single dose or in 2 divided doses.
Children. 30 mg/kg/day in 2 divided doses. Maximum: 2 g/day.

▸ **Skin and skin-structure infections, group A β-hemolytic streptococcal pharyngitis, tonsillitis**

PO

Adults, Elderly. 1-2 g in 2 divided doses.
Children. 30 mg/kg/day in 2 divided doses. Maximum: 2 g/day.

▸ **Impetigo**

PO

Children. 30 mg/kg/day as a single dose or in 2 divided doses. Maximum: 2 g/day.

▸ **Dosage in renal impairment (adults)**

After an initial 1-g dose, dosage and frequency are modified based on creatinine clearance and the severity of the infection.

Creatinine Clearance (mL/min)	Dosage Interval
25-50	500 mg q12h
10-25	500 mg q24h
0-10	500 mg q36h

CONTRAINDICATIONS

History of anaphylactic reaction to penicillins or hypersensitivity to cephalosporins.

INTERACTIONS

Drug

Probenecid: Increases cefadroxil blood concentration.

Herbal

None known.

Food

None known.

DIAGNOSTIC TEST EFFECTS

May increase BUN level and serum alkaline phosphatase, bilirubin, creatinine, LDH, AST (SGOT), and ALT (SGPT) levels. May cause a positive direct or indirect Coombs' test.

SIDE EFFECTS

Frequent

Oral candidiasis, mild diarrhea, mild abdominal cramping, vaginal candidiasis.

Occasional

Nausea, unusual bruising or bleeding, serum sickness-like reaction (marked by fever and joint pain; usually occurs after the second course of therapy and resolves after the drug is discontinued).

Rare

Allergic reaction (rash, pruritus, urticaria), thrombophlebitis (pain, redness, swelling at injection site).

SERIOUS REACTIONS

- Antibiotic-associated colitis and other superinfections may result from altered bacterial balance.
- Nephrotoxicity may occur, especially in patients with preexisting renal disease.
- Patients with a history of allergies, especially to penicillin, are at increased risk for developing a severe hypersensitivity reaction, marked by severe pruritus, angioedema, bronchospasm, and anaphylaxis.

PRECAUTIONS & CONSIDERATIONS

Caution is warranted for patients with a history of GI disease (especially antibiotic-associated colitis or ulcerative colitis), renal impairment, and concurrent use of nephrotoxic medications. Be aware that cefadroxil readily crosses the placenta and is distributed in breast milk. No age-related precautions have been noted for children. In elderly patients, age-related renal impairment may require dosage adjustment.

Although mild GI effects may be tolerable, an increase in their severity may indicate the onset of antibiotic-associated colitis. Assess the mouth for white patches on the mucous membranes and tongue, pattern of daily bowel activity and stool consistency, signs and symptoms of superinfection including abdominal pain, moderate to severe diarrhea, severe anal or genital pruritus, and severe mouth soreness. Renal function should be assessed.

Storage
Store capsules, extended-release tablets, and powder for suspension at room temperature. After reconstitution, oral suspension is stable for 14 days if refrigerated.

Administration
Take without regard to meals; if GI upset occurs, give with food or milk. Shake oral suspension well before using.

Cefazolin

sef-a'zoe-lin

Ancef

Do not confuse cefazolin with cefprozil or Cefzil.

CATEGORY AND SCHEDULE

Pregnancy Risk Category: B

Classification: Antibiotics, cephalosporin (first generation)

MECHANISM OF ACTION

A first-generation cephalosporin that binds to bacterial cell membranes and inhibits cell wall synthesis. *Therapeutic Effect:* Bactericidal.

PHARMACOKINETICS

Widely distributed. Protein binding: 85%. Primarily excreted unchanged in urine. Moderately removed by hemodialysis. *Half-life:* 1.4-1.8 h (increased in impaired renal function).

AVAILABILITY

Powder for Injection: 500 mg, 1 g, 5 g, 10 g, 20 g.

INDICATIONS AND DOSAGES

▸ **Uncomplicated UTIs**
IV, IM
Adults, Elderly. 1 g q12h.

▸ **Mild to moderate infections**
IV, IM
Adults, Elderly. 250-500 mg q8-12h.

▸ **Severe infections**
IV, IM
Adults, Elderly. 0.5-1 g q6-8h.

▸ **Life-threatening infections**
IV, IM
Adults, Elderly. 1-1.5 g q6h. Maximum: 12 g/day.

▸ **Perioperative prophylaxis**
IV, IM
Adults, Elderly. 1 g 30-60 min before surgery, 0.5-1 g during surgery, and q6-8h for up to 24 h postoperatively.

▸ **Usual pediatric dosage**
Children. 50-100 mg/kg/day in divided doses q8h. Maximum: 6 g/day.
Neonates older than 7 days. 40-60 mg/kg/day in divided doses q8-12h.
Neonates 7 days and younger. 40 mg/kg/day in divided doses q12h.

▸ **Dosage in renal impairment (adults)**
Dosing frequency is modified based on creatinine clearance.

Creatinine Clearance (mL/min)	Dosage Interval
10-30	Usual dose q12h
< 10	Usual dose q24h

CONTRAINDICATIONS

History of anaphylactic reaction to penicillins or hypersensitivity to cephalosporins.

INTERACTIONS

Drug
Probenecid: Increases cefazolin blood concentration.
Warfarin: May increase response to warfarin.

Herbal
None known.

Food
None known.

DIAGNOSTIC TEST EFFECTS

May increase INR, BUN level, and serum alkaline phosphatase, bilirubin, creatinine, LDH, AST (SGOT), and ALT (SGPT) levels. May cause a positive direct or indirect Coombs' test.

IV INCOMPATIBILITIES

Amikacin (Amikin), amiodarone (Cordarone), calcium chloride, caspofungin (Cancidas), diazepam, diphenhydramine, dobutamine, dopamine, erythromycin, haloperidol, hydromorphone (Dilaudid), inamrinone, lansoprazole (Prevacid), levofloxacin (Levaquin), pantoprazole (Protonix), phenytoin, tobramycin.

IV COMPATIBILITIES

Calcium gluconate, diltiazem (Cardizem), famotidine (Pepcid), heparin, insulin (regular), lidocaine, midazolam (Versed), morphine, multivitamins, potassium chloride, propofol (Diprivan), vecuronium (Norcuron).

SIDE EFFECTS

Frequent

Discomfort with IM administration, oral candidiasis, mild diarrhea, mild abdominal cramping, vaginal candidiasis.

Occasional

Nausea, serum sickness-like reaction (marked by fever and joint pain; usually occurs after the second course of therapy and resolves after the drug is discontinued).

Rare

Allergic reaction (rash, pruritus, urticaria), thrombophlebitis (pain, redness, swelling at injection site).

SERIOUS REACTIONS

- Antibiotic-associated colitis and other superinfections may result from altered bacterial balance.
- Nephrotoxicity may occur, especially in patients with pre-existing renal disease.
- Patients with a history of allergies, especially to penicillin, are at increased risk for developing a severe hypersensitivity reaction, marked by severe pruritus, angioedema, bronchospasm, and anaphylaxis.

PRECAUTIONS & CONSIDERATIONS

Caution is warranted with a history of GI disease (especially antibiotic-associated colitis or ulcerative colitis), seizure disorder, renal impairment, and concurrent use of nephrotoxic medications. May be associated with increased INR, especially in nutritionally deficient patients, prolonged treatment, hepatic or renal disease. Be aware that cefazolin readily crosses the placenta and is distributed in breast milk. No age-related precautions have been noted in children. In elderly patients, age-related renal impairment may require dosage adjustment.

Although mild GI effects may be tolerable, an increase in their severity may indicate the onset of antibiotic-associated colitis. Assess the mouth for white patches on the mucous membranes and tongue, pattern of daily bowel activity and stool consistency, signs and symptoms of superinfection including abdominal pain, moderate to severe diarrhea, severe anal or genital pruritus, and severe mouth soreness. Renal function should be assessed.

Storage

Store unreconstituted vials at room temperature protected from light. Solution normally appears light yellow to yellow. IV infusion (piggyback) is stable for 24 h at room temperature and 10 days if refrigerated. Discard solution if precipitate forms.

C

Administration
To minimize discomfort, give IM injection deep and slowly. To minimize injection site discomfort, give the IM injection in the gluteus maximus rather than lateral aspect of thigh. Administer cefazolin for the full length of treatment and evenly space doses around the clock.

For IV use, reconstitute each 1 g with at least 10 mL sterile water for injection. May further dilute in 50-100 mL D5W or 0.9% NaCl to decrease the incidence of thrombophlebitis. For IV push, maximum concentration should be 100 mg/mL and administer over 3-5 min. For intermittent IV infusion (piggyback), infuse over 20-30 min.

Cefdinir

sef'di-neer
★ Omnicef

CATEGORY AND SCHEDULE
Pregnancy Risk Category: B

Classification: Antibiotics, cephalosporin (third generation)

MECHANISM OF ACTION
A third-generation cephalosporin that binds to bacterial cell membranes and inhibits cell wall synthesis. *Therapeutic Effect:* Bactericidal.

PHARMACOKINETICS
Moderately absorbed from the GI tract. Protein binding: 60%-70%. Widely distributed. Not appreciably metabolized. Primarily excreted unchanged in urine. Minimally removed by hemodialysis. *Half-life:* 1-2 h (increased in impaired renal function).

AVAILABILITY
Capsules: 300 mg.
Oral Suspension: 125 mg/5 mL, 250 mg/5 mL.

INDICATIONS AND DOSAGES
▸ **Community-acquired pneumonia**
PO
Adults, Elderly, Children 13 yr and older. 300 mg q12h for 10 days.

▸ **Acute exacerbation of chronic bronchitis**
PO
Adults, Elderly. 300 mg q12h for 5-10 days.

▸ **Acute maxillary sinusitis**
PO
Adults, Elderly, Children 13 yr and older. 300 mg q12h or 600 mg q24h for 10 days.
Children 6 mo to 12 yr. 7 mg/kg q12h or 14 mg/kg q24h for 10 days.

▸ **Pharyngitis or tonsillitis**
PO
Adults, Elderly, Children 13 yr and older. 300 mg q12h for 5-10 days or 600 mg q24h for 10 days.
Children 6 mo to 12 yr. 7 mg/kg q12h for 5-10 days or 14 mg/kg q24h for 10 days.

▸ **Uncomplicated skin or skin-structure infections**
PO
Adults, Elderly, Children 13 yr and older. 300 mg q12h for 10 days.
Children 6 mo to 12 yr. 7 mg/kg q12h for 10 days.

▸ **Acute bacterial otitis media**
PO (CAPSULES)
Children 6 mo to 12 yr. 7 mg/kg q12h or 14 mg/kg q24h for 10 days.

▸ **Usual pediatric dosage for oral suspension**
Children weighing 81-95 lb (37-43 kg). 12.5 mL (2.5 tsp) q12h or 25 mL (5 tsp) q24h.
Children weighing 61-80 lb (28-36 kg). 10 mL (1.5 tsp) q12h or 20 mL (4 tsp) q24h.

Children weighing 41-60 lb (19-27 kg). 7.5 mL (1 tsp) q12h or 15 mL (3 tsp) q24h.
Children weighing 20-40 lb (9-18 kg). 5 mL (1 tsp) q12h or 10 mL (2 tsp) q24h.
Infants weighing < 20 lb (9 kg). 2.5 mL (1/2 tsp) q12h or 5 mL (1 tsp) q24h.

▸ **Dosage in renal impairment (adults)**

For patients with creatinine clearance < 30 mL/min, dosage is 300 mg/day as single daily dose. For hemodialysis patients, dosage is 300 mg every other day.

CONTRAINDICATIONS

History of anaphylactic reaction to penicillins or hypersensitivity to cephalosporins.

INTERACTIONS

Drug

Antacids: Decrease cefdinir blood concentration.
Magnesium or iron supplements: Decrease cefdinir blood concentration.
Probenecid: Increases cefdinir blood concentration.

Herbal

None known.

Food

None known.

DIAGNOSTIC TEST EFFECTS

May increase serum alkaline phosphatase, bilirubin, LDH, AST (SGPT), and ALT (SGOT) levels. May produce a false-positive reaction for ketones in urine.

SIDE EFFECTS

Frequent

Oral candidiasis, mild diarrhea, mild abdominal cramping, vaginal candidiasis.

Occasional

Nausea, serum sickness-like reaction (marked by fever and joint pain; usually occurs after the second course of therapy and resolves after the drug is discontinued).

Rare

Allergic reaction (rash, pruritus, urticaria).

SERIOUS REACTIONS

- Antibiotic-associated colitis and other superinfections may result from altered bacterial balance.
- Nephrotoxicity may occur, especially in patients with preexisting renal disease.
- Patients with a history of allergies, especially to penicillin, are at increased risk for developing a severe hypersensitivity reaction, marked by severe pruritus, angioedema, bronchospasm, and anaphylaxis.

PRECAUTIONS & CONSIDERATIONS

Caution is warranted for patients with hypersensitivity to penicillins or other drugs, a history of GI disease (especially antibiotic-associated colitis or ulcerative colitis), and liver or renal impairment. Be aware that cefdinir readily crosses the placenta and is not detected in breast milk. Be aware that infants and newborns may have lower renal clearance of cefdinir. In elderly patients, age-related decreases in renal function may require decreased cefdinir dosage or increased dosing interval.

Although mild GI effects may be tolerable, an increase in their severity may indicate the onset of antibiotic-associated colitis. Assess the mouth for white patches on the mucous membranes and tongue, pattern of daily bowel activity and stool consistency, signs and symptoms of superinfection including abdominal pain, moderate to severe diarrhea, severe anal or genital pruritus, and severe mouth soreness. Renal function should be assessed.

Storage

Capsules and unreconstituted powder for oral suspension are stored at room temperature. Store mixed suspension at room temperature. Discard unused portion after 10 days.

Administration

Take without regard to meals; if GI upset occurs, give with food or milk. Reconstitute oral suspension according to package label. Shake oral suspension well before administering. Continue therapy for the full length of treatment and evenly space doses around the clock.

Cefditoren

seff-di-tore′en

★ Spectracef

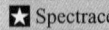

CATEGORY AND SCHEDULE

Pregnancy Risk Category: B

Classification: Antibiotics, cephalosporin (third generation)

MECHANISM OF ACTION

A third-generation cephalosporin that binds to bacterial cell membranes and inhibits cell wall synthesis. *Therapeutic Effect:* Bactericidal.

PHARMACOKINETICS

Moderately absorbed from the GI tract. Protein binding: 88%. Not metabolized. Excreted in the urine. Minimally removed by hemodialysis. *Half-life:* 1.6 h (half-life increased with impaired renal function).

AVAILABILITY

Tablets: 200 mg, 400 mg.

INDICATIONS AND DOSAGES

▸ **Pharyngitis, tonsillitis, skin infections**

PO

Adults, Elderly, Children older than 12 yr. 200 mg twice a day for 10 days.

▸ **Acute exacerbation of chronic bronchitis**

PO

Adults, Elderly, Children older than 12 yr. 400 mg twice a day for 10 days.

▸ **Community-acquired pneumonia**

PO

Adults, Elderly, Children older than 12 yr. 400 mg twice a day for 14 days.

▸ **Dosage in renal impairment**

Dosage and frequency are modified based on creatinine clearance.

Creatinine Clearance (mL/min)	Dosage
50-80	No adjustment necessary
30-49	200 mg twice a day
< 30	200 mg once a day

CONTRAINDICATIONS

Carnitine deficiency or inborn errors of metabolism that may result in carnitine deficiency, known allergy to cephalosporins, or anaphylactic reactions to penicillins, hypersensitivity to milk protein.

INTERACTIONS

Drug

Antacids containing magnesium or aluminum, H_2 receptor antagonists: May decrease the absorption of cefditoren.

Probenecid: May increase the absorption of cefditoren.

Warfarin: May increase response to warfarin.

Herbal
None known.
Food
High-fat meals: Increase the cefditoren plasma concentration.

DIAGNOSTIC TEST EFFECTS
May cause a positive direct or indirect Coombs' test and a false-positive urine glucose testing. May increase INR, alkaline phosphatase, bilirubin, LDH, creatinine. May cause pancytopenia, neutropenia, and agranulocytosis.

SIDE EFFECTS
Occasional (11%)
Diarrhea.
Rare (1%-4%)
Nausea, headache, abdominal pain, vaginal candidiasis, dyspepsia, vomiting. Carnitine deficiency might occur if the drug is used for long periods of time (months).

SERIOUS REACTIONS
- Antibiotic-associated colitis and other superinfections may occur.
- Patients with a history of allergies, especially to penicillin, are at increased risk for developing a severe hypersensitivity reaction, marked by severe pruritus, angioedema, bronchospasm, and anaphylaxis.

PRECAUTIONS & CONSIDERATIONS
Caution is warranted with allergies, renal impairment, seizure disorder, a history of GI disease, and hypersensitivity to penicillins or other drugs. May be associated with increased INR, especially in nutritionally deficient patients, prolonged treatment, hepatic or renal disease. It is unknown whether cefditoren is distributed in breast milk. The safety and efficacy of cefditoren have not been established in children younger than 12 yr. Age-related renal impairment may require a dosage adjustment in elderly patients.

Although mild GI effects may be tolerable, an increase in their severity may indicate the onset of antibiotic-associated colitis. Assess the mouth for white patches on the mucous membranes and tongue; also check the pattern of daily bowel activity and stool consistency, signs and symptoms of superinfection including abdominal pain, moderate to severe diarrhea, severe anal or genital pruritus, and severe mouth soreness. Renal function should be assessed.
Storage
Store at room temperature. Protect from light and moisture.
Administration
Take with meals to enhance drug absorption. Take for the full length of treatment. Do not skip doses.

Cefepime
sef′e-peem
Maxipime
Do not confuse with ceftidine.

CATEGORY AND SCHEDULE
Pregnancy Risk Category: B

Classification: Antibiotics, cephalosporin (fourth generation)

MECHANISM OF ACTION
A fourth-generation cephalosporin that binds to bacterial cell membranes and inhibits cell wall synthesis. *Therapeutic Effect:* Bactericidal.

PHARMACOKINETICS
Well absorbed after IM administration. Protein binding: 20%. Widely distributed. Primarily

excreted unchanged in urine. Removed by hemodialysis. *Half-life:* 2-2.3 h (increased in impaired renal function and in elderly patients).

AVAILABILITY

Powder for Injection: 1 g, 2 g.

INDICATIONS AND DOSAGES

▸ **Pneumonia**

IV

Adults, Elderly. 1-2 g q12h for 7-10 days.

Children 2 mo and older. 50 mg/kg q12h. Maximum: 2 g/dose.

▸ **Intra-abdominal infections**

IV

Adults, Elderly. 2 g q12h for 10 days.

▸ **Skin and skin-structure infections**

IV

Adults, Elderly. 2 g q12h for 10 days.

Children 2 mo and older. 50 mg/kg q12h. Maximum: 2 g/dose.

▸ **Urinary tract infections**

IV/IM

Adults, Elderly. 0.5-2 g q12h for 7-10 days.

Children 2 mo and older. 50 mg/kg q12h. Maximum: 2 g/dose.

▸ **Febrile neutropenia**

IV

Adults, Elderly. 2 g q8h.

Children 2 mo and older. 50 mg/kg q8h. Maximum: 2 g/dose.

▸ **Dosage in renal impairment**

Dosage and frequency are modified based on creatinine clearance and the severity of the infection, and the initial dosage given.

CONTRAINDICATIONS

History of anaphylactic reaction to penicillins or hypersensitivity to cephalosporins.

INTERACTIONS

Drug

Aminoglycosides, loop diuretics: Increased risk of nephrotoxicity.

Probenecid: May increase cefepime blood concentration.

Warfarin: May increase response to warfarin.

Herbal

None known.

Food

None known.

DIAGNOSTIC TEST EFFECTS

May increase serum alkaline phosphatase, bilirubin, INR, LDH, AST (SGOT), and ALT (SGPT) levels. May cause a positive direct or indirect Coombs' test.

IV INCOMPATIBILITIES

Acyclovir (Zovirax), amphotericin (Fungizone), cimetidine (Tagamet), ciprofloxacin (Cipro), cisplatin (Platinol), dacarbazine (DTIC), daunorubicin (Cerubidine), diazepam (Valium), diphenhydramine (Benadryl), dobutamine (Dobutrex), dopamine (Intropin), doxorubicin (Adriamycin), droperidol (Inapsine), famotidine (Pepcid), ganciclovir (Cytovene), haloperidol (Haldol), magnesium, magnesium sulfate, mannitol, meperidine (Demerol), metoclopramide (Reglan), morphine, ofloxacin (Floxin), ondansetron (Zofran), vancomycin (Vancocin).

IV COMPATIBILITIES

Bumetanide (Bumex), calcium gluconate, furosemide (Lasix), hydromorphone (Dilaudid), lorazepam (Ativan), propofol (Diprivan).

SIDE EFFECTS

Frequent

Discomfort with IM administration, oral candidiasis, mild diarrhea, mild abdominal cramping, vaginal candidiasis.

C

Occasional
Nausea, serum sickness-like reaction (marked by fever and joint pain; usually occurs after the second course of therapy and resolves after the drug is discontinued).
Rare
Allergic reaction (rash, pruritus, urticaria), thrombophlebitis (pain, redness, swelling at injection site).

SERIOUS REACTIONS

• Antibiotic-associated colitis manifested and other superinfections may result from altered bacterial balance.
• Nephrotoxicity may occur, especially in patients with preexisting renal disease.
• Patients with a history of allergies, especially to penicillin, are at increased risk for developing a severe hypersensitivity reaction, marked by severe pruritus, angioedema, bronchospasm, and anaphylaxis.

PRECAUTIONS & CONSIDERATIONS

Caution is warranted with renal impairment, seizure disorder. May be associated with increased INR, especially in nutritionally efficient patients, prolonged treatment, hepatic or renal disease. It is unknown whether cefepime is distributed in breast milk. No age-related precautions have been noted in children older than 2 mo. Age-related renal impairment may require dosage adjustment in elderly patients.

Although mild GI effects may be tolerable, an increase in their severity may indicate the onset of antibiotic-associated colitis. Assess the pattern of daily bowel activity and stool consistency, the mouth for white patches on the mucous membranes and tongue, signs and symptoms of superinfection including abdominal pain, moderate to severe diarrhea, severe anal or genital pruritus, and severe mouth soreness. Renal function should also be assessed.
Storage
Store unreconstituted vials at room temperature and protect from light. Solution is stable for 24 h at room temperature or 7 days if refrigerated.
Administration
For IM use, add 1.3 mL sterile water for injection, 0.9% NaCl, or D5W to 500-mg vial (2.4 mL for 1-g and 2-g vials). To minimize the pain experienced by the patient, give IM injection slowly and deeply into a large muscle mass (e.g., upper gluteus maximus) instead of the lateral aspect of the thigh.

For IV use, add 5 mL to 500-mg vial (10 mL for 1-g and 2-g vials). Further dilute with 50-100 mL 0.9% NaCl, or D5W. For IV push, administer over 3-5 min. For intermittent IV infusion (piggyback), infuse over 30 min.

Cefixime

sef-ix'ime
★ 🍁 Suprax
Do not confuse Suprax with Sporanox, Surbex, or Surfak.

CATEGORY AND SCHEDULE

Pregnancy Risk Category: B

Classification: Antibiotics, cephalosporin (third generation)

MECHANISM OF ACTION

A third-generation cephalosporin that binds to bacterial cell membranes and inhibits cell wall synthesis. *Therapeutic Effect:* Bactericidal.

C

PHARMACOKINETICS

Moderately absorbed from the GI tract. Protein binding: 65%-70%. Widely distributed. Primarily excreted unchanged in urine. Minimally removed by hemodialysis. *Half-life:* 3-4 h (increased in renal impairment).

AVAILABILITY

Oral Suspension: 100 mg/5 mL, 200 mg/5 mL.
Tablets: 400 mg.

INDICATIONS AND DOSAGES

▸ **Otitis media, acute bronchitis, acute exacerbations of chronic bronchitis, pharyngitis, tonsillitis, and uncomplicated urinary tract infections**

PO

Adults, Elderly, Children weighing more than 50 kg. 400 mg/day as a single dose or in 2 divided doses.
Children 6 mo to 12 yr weighing < 50 kg. 8 mg/kg/day as a single dose or in 2 divided doses.
Maximum: 400 mg/day.

▸ **Uncomplicated gonorrhea**

PO

Adults. 400 mg as a single dose.

▸ **Dosage in renal impairment**

Dosage is modified based on creatinine clearance.

Creatinine Clearance (mL/min)	% of Usual Dose
20-60	75
< 20	50

CONTRAINDICATIONS

History of anaphylactic reaction to penicillins, hypersensitivity to cephalosporins.

INTERACTIONS

Drug

Aminoglycosides, loop diuretics: May increase risk of nephrotoxicity.
Carbamazepine: May increase carbamazepine concentrations.
Probenecid: Increases serum concentration of cefixime.
Warfarin: Increases prothrombin time.

Herbal

None known.

Food

None known.

DIAGNOSTIC TEST EFFECTS

May increase BUN and serum alkaline phosphatase, bilirubin, creatinine, AST (SGOT), and ALT (SGPT) levels. May increase LDH level. May cause a positive direct or indirect Coombs' test.

SIDE EFFECTS

Frequent

Oral candidiasis, mild diarrhea, mild abdominal cramping, vaginal candidiasis.

Occasional

Nausea, serum sickness-like reaction (marked by arthralgia and fever; usually occurs after second course of therapy and resolves after drug is discontinued).

Rare

Allergic reaction (rash, pruritus, urticaria).

SERIOUS REACTIONS

- Antibiotic-associated colitis and other superinfections may result from altered bacterial balance.
- Nephrotoxicity may occur, especially in patients with preexisting renal disease.
- Patients with a history of allergies, especially to penicillin, are at increased risk for developing a severe hypersensitivity reaction, marked by severe pruritus, angioedema, bronchospasm, and anaphylaxis.

C

PRECAUTIONS & CONSIDERATIONS

Caution is warranted with hypersensitivity to penicillin, history of gastrointestinal disease (particularly colitis), and renal impairment. Cefixime crosses the placenta. It is not known whether it is distributed in breast milk. No age-related precautions have been noted in children. Age-related renal impairment in elderly may require dose adjustment.

Stool changes, abdominal cramps, diarrhea, nausea, vomiting, headache, sore mouth or tongue may occur. If fever, skin itching, rash, or swelling occurs, notify the physician immediately.

Storage

Suspension is stable at room temperature or under refrigeration for 14 days. Flavor improves with refrigeration.

Store tablets at room temperature.

Administration

NOTE: When treating otitis media, the suspension is preferred due to higher serum concentrations achieved compared to the tablets. Shake well before using. Take tablets or suspension with food if GI irritation occurs. Continue for the full length of treatment.

Cefotaxime

sef-oh-taks'eem

Claforan

Do not confuse cefotaxime with cefoxitin, ceftizoxime, cefuroxime, or Claritin.

CATEGORY AND SCHEDULE

Pregnancy Risk Category: B

Classification: Antibiotics, cephalosporin (third generation)

MECHANISM OF ACTION

A third-generation cephalosporin that binds to bacterial cell membranes and inhibits cell wall synthesis. *Therapeutic Effect:* Bactericidal.

PHARMACOKINETICS

Widely distributed, including to CSF. Protein binding: 30%-50%. Partially metabolized in the liver to active metabolite. Primarily excreted in urine. Moderately removed by hemodialysis. *Half-life:* 1 h (increased in impaired renal function).

AVAILABILITY

Powder for Injection: 500 mg, 1 g, 2 g, 10 g.
Injection: 1 g, 2 g.

INDICATIONS AND DOSAGES

▸ **Uncomplicated infections**

IV, IM

Adults, Elderly. 1 g q12h.

▸ **Mild to moderate infections**

IV, IM

Adults, Elderly. 1-2 g q8h.

▸ **Severe infections**

IV, IM

Adults, Elderly. 2 g q6-8h.

▸ **Life-threatening infections**

IV

Adults, Elderly. 2 g q4h.

▸ **Gonorrhea**

IM

Adults. (Male): 1 g as a single dose. (Female): 0.5 g as a single dose.

▸ **Perioperative prophylaxis**

IV, IM

Adults, Elderly. 1 g 30-90 min before surgery.

▸ **Cesarean section**

IV

Adults. 1 g as soon as umbilical cord is clamped, then 1 g 6 and 12 h after first dose.

▸ **Usual pediatric dosage**

Children weighing 50 kg or more.

C

1-2 g q6-8h; May give q4h for life-threatening infection.
Children 1 mo to 12 yr weighing < 50 kg. 100-200 mg/kg/day in divided doses q6-8h.

▸ **Dosage in renal impairment**
For patients with creatinine clearance < 20 mL/min, give half of dose at usual dosing intervals.

OFF-LABEL USES
Treatment of Lyme disease.

CONTRAINDICATIONS
History of anaphylactic reaction to penicillins or hypersensitivity to cephalosporins.

INTERACTIONS
Drug
Aminoglycosides, loop diuretics: May increase risk of nephrotoxicity.
Probenecid: May increase cefotaxime blood concentration.
Herbal
None known.
Food
None known.

DIAGNOSTIC TEST EFFECTS
May increase liver function test results and produce a positive direct or indirect Coombs' test.

IV INCOMPATIBILITIES
Allopurinol (Aloprim), filgrastim (Neupogen), fluconazole (Diflucan), hetastarch (Hespan), pentamidine (Pentam IV), vancomycin (Vancocin).

IV COMPATIBILITIES
Diltiazem (Cardizem), famotidine (Pepcid), hydromorphone (Dilaudid), lorazepam (Ativan), magnesium sulfate, midazolam (Versed), morphine, propofol (Diprivan).

SIDE EFFECTS
Frequent
Discomfort with IM administration, oral candidiasis, mild diarrhea, mild abdominal cramping, vaginal candidiasis.
Occasional
Nausea, serum sickness-like reaction (marked by fever and joint pain; usually occurs after the second course of therapy and resolves after the drug is discontinued).
Rare
Allergic reaction (rash, pruritus, urticaria), thrombophlebitis (pain, redness, swelling at injection site).

SERIOUS REACTIONS
• Antibiotic-associated colitis and other superinfections may result from altered bacterial balance.
• Nephrotoxicity may occur, especially in patients with preexisting renal disease.
• Patients with a history of allergies, especially to penicillin, are at increased risk for developing a severe hypersensitivity reaction, marked by severe pruritus, angioedema, bronchospasm, and anaphylaxis.
• Granulocytopenia and rarely granulocytosis have occurred with prolonged therapy (i.e., longer than 10 days).

PRECAUTIONS & CONSIDERATIONS
Caution is warranted with history of GI disease (especially antibiotic-associated or ulcerative colitis) and renal impairment. Cefotaxime readily crosses the placenta and is distributed in breast milk. No age-related precautions have been noted for use in children. Age-related renal impairment may require dosage adjustment in elderly patients.

Although mild GI effects may be tolerable, an increase in their severity may indicate the onset of antibiotic-associated colitis. The pattern of daily bowel activity and stool consistency, the mouth for white patches on the mucous membranes and tongue, signs and symptoms of superinfection including abdominal pain, moderate to severe diarrhea, severe anal or genital pruritus, and severe mouth soreness should be assessed. Renal function should be assessed.

Storage

Store powder for injection at room temperature and premixed solutions in the freezer. The solution for IV use normally appears light yellow to amber. The IV infusion (piggyback) may become darker, but this does not affect potency. The IV infusion (piggyback) prepared from the powder for injection is stable for 24 h at room temperature, 5 days if refrigerated, and 13 wks if frozen. Thawed previously frozen premixed bags are stable for 24 h at room temperature or 10 days if refrigerated. Discard the solution if a precipitate forms.

Administration

For IV use, add 10 mL of sterile water for injection to each 500-mg, 1-g, or 2-g vial to provide a concentration of 50, 95, or 180 mg/mL, respectively. The resulting solution may be further diluted with 50-100 mL of 0.9% NaCl or D5W. Administer the IV push over 3-5 min. More rapid IV administration through a central line has been associated with a high incidence of cardiac arrhythmias. Administer the intermittent IV infusion (piggyback) over 20-30 min.

For IM use, reconstitute the drug with sterile water for injection or bacteriostatic water for injection. Add 2, 3, or 5 mL to each 500-mg, 1-g, or 2-g vial, respectively, to yield a concentration of 230, 300, or 330 mg/mL, respectively. To minimize patient discomfort, slowly inject the drug deep into the gluteus maximus rather than the lateral aspect of the thigh. Administer a 2-g IM dose at two separate sites.

Cefotetan

sef'oh-tee-tan

★ Cefotan

Do not confuse cefotetan with cefoxitin or Ceftin.

CATEGORY AND SCHEDULE

Pregnancy Risk Category: B

Classification: Antibiotics, cephalosporin (second generation)

MECHANISM OF ACTION

A second-generation cephalosporin that binds to bacterial cell membranes and inhibits cell wall synthesis. *Therapeutic Effect:* Bactericidal.

PHARMACOKINETICS

Protein binding: 78%-91%. Primarily excreted unchanged in urine. Minimally removed by hemodialysis. *Half-life:* 3-4.6 h (increased in impaired renal function).

AVAILABILITY

Powder for Injection: 1 g, 2 g, 10 g.
Premixed IVPB, Frozen: 1 g, 2 g.

INDICATIONS AND DOSAGES

▸ **Urinary tract infections**

IV, IM

Adults, Elderly. 1-2 g in divided doses q12-24h.

▸ **Mild to moderate infections**

IV, IM

Adults, Elderly. 1-2 g q12h.

C

▸ **Severe infections**
IV
Adults, Elderly. 2 g q12h.
▸ **Life-threatening infections**
IV
Adults, Elderly. 3 g q12h.
▸ **Perioperative prophylaxis**
IV
Adults, Elderly. 1-2 g 30-60 min before surgery.
▸ **Cesarean section**
IV
Adults. 1-2 g as soon as umbilical cord is clamped.
▸ **Usual pediatric dosage**
Children. 40-80 mg/kg/day in divided doses q12h. Maximum: 6 g/day.
▸ **Dosage in renal impairment**
Dosing frequency is modified based on creatinine clearance and the severity of the infection.

Creatinine Clearance (mL/min)	Dosage Interval
10-30	Usual dose q24h
< 10	Usual dose q48h

CONTRAINDICATIONS

History of anaphylactic reaction to penicillins or hypersensitivity to cephalosporins.

INTERACTIONS

Drug

Alcohol: May produce a disulfiram-like reaction (facial flushing, headache, nausea, pruritus, tachycardia).

Heparin, warfarin, other anticoagulants: May increase the risk of bleeding.

Herbal

None known.

Food

None known.

DIAGNOSTIC TEST EFFECTS

May increase BUN level and serum alkaline phosphatase, creatinine, AST (SGOT), and ALT (SGPT) levels. May prolong PT and produce a positive direct or indirect Coombs' test.

IV INCOMPATIBILITIES

Amphotericin B, caspofungin (Cancidas), diazepam, dobutamine, doxycycline, erythromycin, haloperidol, lansoprazole (Prevacid), pantoprazole, phenobarbital, phenytoin, sodium bicarbonate, tobramycin, vancomycin (Vancocin).

IV COMPATIBILITIES

Diltiazem (Cardizem), famotidine (Pepcid), heparin, insulin (regular), morphine, propofol (Diprivan).

SIDE EFFECTS

Frequent

Discomfort with IM administration, oral candidiasis, mild diarrhea, mild abdominal cramping, vaginal candidiasis.

Occasional

Nausea, unusual bleeding or bruising, serum sickness-like reaction (marked by fever and joint pain; usually occurs after the second course of therapy and resolves after the drug is discontinued).

Rare

Allergic reaction (rash, pruritus, urticaria), thrombophlebitis (pain, redness, swelling at injection site).

SERIOUS REACTIONS

- Antibiotic-associated colitis and other superinfections may result from altered bacterial balance.
- Nephrotoxicity may occur, especially in patients with preexisting renal disease.
- Patients with a history of allergies, especially to penicillin, are at increased risk for developing a severe hypersensitivity reaction, marked by severe pruritus, angioedema, bronchospasm, and anaphylaxis.
- Hemolytic anemia.

PRECAUTIONS & CONSIDERATIONS

Caution is warranted with history of GI disease (especially antibiotic-associated or ulcerative colitis), renal impairment, and concurrent use of nephrotoxic drugs. May be associated with increased INR, especially in nutritionally deficient patients, prolonged treatment, hepatic or renal disease. Cefotetan readily crosses the placenta and is distributed in breast milk. The safety and efficacy have not been established in children. Age-related renal impairment may require dosage adjustment in elderly patients.

Although mild GI effects may be tolerable, an increase in their severity may indicate the onset of antibiotic-associated colitis. Assess the pattern of daily bowel activity and stool consistency, the mouth for white patches on the mucous membranes and tongue, signs and symptoms of superinfection including abdominal pain, moderate to severe diarrhea, severe anal or genital pruritus, and severe mouth soreness. Renal function should also be assessed.

Storage

The solution normally appears colorless to light yellow. A deeper yellow does not indicate loss of potency. The IV infusion (piggyback) is stable for 24 h at room temperature, 96 h if refrigerated, and 12 wks if frozen. Discard the solution if a precipitate forms.

Administration

For IV use, reconstitute each 1-g vial with 10 mL of sterile water for injection to provide a concentration of 95 mg/mL. The resulting solution may be further diluted with 50-100 mL of 0.9% NaCl or D5W. Administer IV push over 3-5 min. Administer intermittent IV infusion (piggyback) over 20-30 min.

For IM use, add 2 mL of sterile water for injection or other appropriate diluent to each 1-g vial, or 3 mL to each 2-g vial, to provide a concentration of 400 mg/mL or 500 mg/mL, respectively. To minimize discomfort, slowly inject the drug deep into the gluteus maximus rather than the lateral aspect of the thigh.

Cefoxitin

se-fox′i-tin

★ Mefoxin

Do not confuse cefoxitin with cefotaxime, cefotetan, or Cytoxan.

CATEGORY AND SCHEDULE

Pregnancy Risk Category: B

Classification: Antibiotics, cephalosporin (second generation)

MECHANISM OF ACTION

A second-generation cephalosporin that binds to bacterial cell membranes and inhibits cell wall synthesis. *Therapeutic Effect:* Bactericidal.

AVAILABILITY

Powder for Injection: 1 g, 2 g, 10 g.
Premixed IVPB, Frozen: 1 g, 2 g.

INDICATIONS AND DOSAGES

▸ **Mild to moderate infections**

IV

Adults, Elderly. 1-2 g q6-8h.

▸ **Severe infections**

IV

Adults, Elderly. 1 g q4h or 2 g q6-8h up to 2 g q4h.

C

▸ **Perioperative prophylaxis**
IV
Adults, Elderly. 2 g 30-60 min before surgery, then q6h for up to 24 h after surgery.
Children older than 3 mo. 30-40 mg/kg 30-60 min before surgery, then q6h for up to 24 h after surgery.
▸ **Cesarean section**
IV
Adults. 2 g as soon as umbilical cord is clamped, then 2 g 4 and 8 h after first dose, then q6h for up to 24 h.
▸ **Usual pediatric dosage**
Children older than 3 mo. 80-160 mg/kg/day in 4-6 divided doses. Maximum: 12 g/day.
Neonates. 90-100 mg/kg/day in divided doses q8h.
▸ **Dosage in renal impairment (adults)**
After a loading dose of 1-2 g, dosage and frequency are modified based on creatinine clearance and the severity of the infection.

Creatinine Clearance (mL/min)	Dosage
30-50	1-2 g q8-12h
10-29	1-2 g q12-24h
5-9	500 mg-1 g q12-24h
< 5	500 mg-1 g q24-48h

CONTRAINDICATIONS
History of anaphylactic reaction to penicillins or hypersensitivity to cephalosporins.

INTERACTIONS
Drug
Aminoglycosides, loop diuretics: May increase risk of nephrotoxicity.
Probenecid: Increases serum concentration of cefoxitin.
Herbal
None known.
Food
None known.

DIAGNOSTIC TEST EFFECTS
May increase BUN level and serum alkaline phosphatase, creatinine, AST (SGOT), and ALT (SGPT) levels. May produce a positive direct or indirect Coombs' test.

IV INCOMPATIBILITIES
Filgrastim (Neupogen), pentamidine (Pentam IV), vancomycin (Vancocin).

IV COMPATIBILITIES
Diltiazem (Cardizem), famotidine (Pepcid), heparin, hydromorphone (Dilaudid), magnesium sulfate, morphine, multivitamins, propofol (Diprivan).

SIDE EFFECTS
Frequent
Oral candidiasis, mild diarrhea, mild abdominal cramping, vaginal candidiasis.
Occasional
Nausea, serum sickness-like reaction (marked by fever and joint pain; usually occurs after the second course of therapy and resolves after the drug is discontinued).
Rare
Allergic reaction (pruritus, rash, urticaria), thrombophlebitis (pain, redness, swelling at injection site).

SERIOUS REACTIONS
- Antibiotic-associated colitis and other superinfections may result from altered bacterial balance.
- Nephrotoxicity may occur, especially in patients with preexisting renal disease.
- Patients with a history of allergies, especially to penicillin, are at increased risk for developing a severe hypersensitivity reaction, marked by severe pruritus, angioedema, bronchospasm, and anaphylaxis.

PRECAUTIONS & CONSIDERATIONS

Caution is warranted with history of GI disease (especially antibiotic-associated or ulcerative colitis), renal impairment, and concurrent use of nephrotoxic drugs.

Although mild GI effects may be tolerable, an increase in their severity may indicate the onset of antibiotic-associated colitis. Assess the pattern of daily bowel activity and stool consistency, the mouth for white patches on the mucous membranes and tongue, signs and symptoms of superinfection including abdominal pain, moderate to severe diarrhea, severe anal or genital pruritus, and severe mouth soreness. Renal function should also be assessed.

Storage

The solution normally appears colorless to light amber; a darker color does not indicate loss of potency. Reconstituted solution is stable for 6 h at room temperature and 7 days if refrigerated. The IV infusion (piggyback) is stable for 24 h at room temperature and 48 h if refrigerated. Thawed, previously frozen premixed solution is stable for 24 h at room temperature or 21 days if refrigerated. Discard the solution if a precipitate forms.

Administration

! Give by intermittent IV infusion (piggyback) or IV push. Space doses evenly around the clock.

For IV use, reconstitute each 1-g vial with 10 mL of sterile water for injection to provide a concentration of 95 mg/mL. The resulting solution may be further diluted with 50-100 mL of sterile water for injection, 0.9% NaCl, or D5W. Administer IV push over 3-5 min. Administer intermittent IV infusion (piggyback) over 10-60 min.

Cefpodoxime

sef-pod′ox-ime

★ Vantin

Do not confuse Vantin with Ventolin.

CATEGORY AND SCHEDULE

Pregnancy Risk Category: B

Classification: Antibiotics, cephalosporin (third generation)

MECHANISM OF ACTION

A third-generation cephalosporin that binds to bacterial cell membranes and inhibits cell wall synthesis. *Therapeutic Effect:* Bactericidal.

PHARMACOKINETICS

Well absorbed from the GI tract (food increases absorption). Protein binding: 21%-40%. Widely distributed. Primarily excreted unchanged in urine. Partially removed by hemodialysis. *Half-life:* 2.3 h (increased in impaired renal function and elderly patients).

AVAILABILITY

Oral Suspension: 50 mg/5 mL, 100 mg/5 mL.
Tablets: 100 mg, 200 mg.

INDICATIONS AND DOSAGES

▸ **Chronic bronchitis, pneumonia**

PO

Adults, Elderly, Children older than 13 yr. 200 mg q12h for 10-14 days.

▸ **Gonorrhea (men and women), rectal gonococcal infection (female patients only)**

PO

Adults, Children older than 13 yr. 200 mg as a single dose.

▸ **Skin and skin-structure infections**

PO

C

Adults, Elderly, Children older than 13 yr. 400 mg q12h for 7-14 days.

▸ **Pharyngitis, tonsillitis**

PO

Adults, Elderly, Children older than 13 yr. 100 mg q12h for 5-10 days.

Children 6 mo to 13 yr.
5 mg/kg q12h for 5-10 days. Maximum: 100 mg/dose.

▸ **Acute maxillary sinusitis**

PO

Adults, Children older than 13 yr. 200 mg twice a day for 10 days.

Children 2 mo to 13 yr. 5 mg/kg q12h for 10 days. Maximum: 400 mg/day.

▸ **Urinary tract infection**

PO

Adults, Elderly, Children older than 13 yr. 100 mg q12h for 7 days.

▸ **Acute otitis media**

PO

Children 6 mo to 13 yr. 5 mg/kg q12h for 5 days. Maximum: 400 mg/dose.

▸ **Dosage in renal impairment**

For patients with creatinine clearance < 30 mL/min, usual dose is given q24h. For patients on hemodialysis, usual dose is given 3 times/wk after dialysis.

CONTRAINDICATIONS

History of anaphylactic reaction to penicillins or hypersensitivity to cephalosporins.

INTERACTIONS

Drug

Antacids, H_2 antagonists: May decrease cefpodoxime absorption.

Probenecid: May increase cefpodoxime blood concentration.

Herbal

None known.

Food

None known.

DIAGNOSTIC TEST EFFECTS

May increase BUN level and serum alkaline phosphatase, bilirubin, creatinine, LDH, AST (SGOT), and ALT (SGPT) levels. May produce a positive direct or indirect Coombs' test.

SIDE EFFECTS

Frequent

Oral candidiasis, mild diarrhea, mild abdominal cramping, vaginal candidiasis.

Occasional

Nausea, serum sickness-like reaction (marked by fever and joint pain; usually occurs after the second course of therapy and resolves after the drug is discontinued).

Rare

Allergic reaction (pruritus, rash, urticaria).

SERIOUS REACTIONS

• Antibiotic-associated colitis and other superinfections may result from altered bacterial balance.

• Nephrotoxicity may occur, especially in patients with preexisting renal disease.

• Patients with a history of allergies, especially to penicillin, are at increased risk for developing a severe hypersensitivity reaction, marked by severe pruritus, angioedema, bronchospasm, and anaphylaxis.

PRECAUTIONS & CONSIDERATIONS

Caution is warranted with history of GI disease (especially antibiotic-associated or ulcerative colitis), renal impairment, and concurrent use of nephrotoxic drugs. Cefpodoxime readily crosses the placenta and is distributed in breast milk. The safety and efficacy of cefpodoxime have not been established in children younger than 6 mo. Age-related renal impairment may require a dosage adjustment in elderly patients.

Although mild GI effects may be tolerable, an increase in their severity may indicate the onset of antibiotic-associated colitis. Assess the pattern of daily bowel activity and stool consistency, the mouth for white patches on the mucous membranes and tongue, signs and symptoms of superinfection including abdominal pain, moderate to severe diarrhea, severe anal or genital pruritus, and severe mouth soreness. Renal function should also be assessed.

Storage

Store tablets and unreconstituted suspension powder at room temperature. After reconstitution, the oral suspension is stable for 14 days if refrigerated.

Administration

Administer cefpodoxime tablets with food to enhance drug absorption; suspension may be taken without regard to food. Shake suspension well before each use.

Cefprozil

sef-pro′zil

★ Cefzil

Do not confuse cefprozil with Cefazolin, Cefol, Ceftin, or Kefzol.

CATEGORY AND SCHEDULE

Pregnancy Risk Category: B

Classification: Antibiotics, cephalosporin (second generation)

MECHANISM OF ACTION

A second-generation cephalosporin that binds to bacterial cell membranes and inhibits cell wall synthesis. *Therapeutic Effect:* Bactericidal.

PHARMACOKINETICS

Well absorbed from the GI tract. Protein binding: 36%-45%. Widely distributed. Primarily excreted unchanged in urine. Moderately removed by hemodialysis. *Half-life:* 1.3 h (increased in impaired renal function).

AVAILABILITY

Oral Suspension: 125 mg/5 mL, 250 mg/5 mL.
Tablets: 250 mg, 500 mg.

INDICATIONS AND DOSAGES

▸ **Pharyngitis, tonsillitis**

PO

Adults, Elderly. 500 mg q24h for 10 days.

Children 2-12 yr. 7.5 mg/kg q12h for 10 days.

▸ **Acute bacterial exacerbation of chronic bronchitis, secondary bacterial infection of acute bronchitis**

PO

Adults, Elderly. 500 mg q12h for 10 days.

▸ **Skin and skin-structure infections**

PO

Adults, Elderly. 250-500 mg q12h for 10 days.

Children. 20 mg/kg q24h for 10 days.

▸ **Acute sinusitis**

PO

Adults, Elderly. 250-500 mg q12h for 10 days.

Children 6 mo to 12 yr. 7.5-15 mg/kg q12h for 10 days.

▸ **Otitis media**

PO

Children 6 mo to 12 yr. 15 mg/kg q12h for 10 days. Maximum: 1 g/day.

▸ **Dosage in renal impairment**

Patients with creatinine clearance < 30 mL/min receive 50% of usual dose at usual interval.

CONTRAINDICATIONS

History of anaphylactic reaction to penicillins or hypersensitivity to cephalosporins.

INTERACTIONS

Drug

Probenecid: Increases serum concentration of cefprozil.

Herbal

None known.

Food

None known.

DIAGNOSTIC TEST EFFECTS

May increase liver function test results. May produce a positive direct or indirect Coombs' test.

SIDE EFFECTS

Frequent

Oral candidiasis, mild diarrhea, mild abdominal cramping, vaginal candidiasis.

Occasional

Nausea, serum sickness reaction (marked by fever and joint pain; usually occurs after the second course of therapy and resolves after the drug is discontinued).

Rare

Allergic reaction (pruritus, rash, urticaria).

SERIOUS REACTIONS

- Antibiotic-associated colitis and other superinfections may result from altered bacterial balance.
- Nephrotoxicity may occur, especially in patients with preexisting renal disease.
- Patients with a history of allergies, especially to penicillin, are at increased risk for developing a severe hypersensitivity reaction, marked by severe pruritus, angioedema, bronchospasm, and anaphylaxis.

PRECAUTIONS & CONSIDERATIONS

Caution is warranted with history of GI disease (especially antibiotic-associated or ulcerative colitis), renal impairment, and concurrent use of nephrotoxic drugs. Cefprozil readily crosses the placenta and is distributed in breast milk. The safety and efficacy of cefprozil have not been established in children younger than 6 mo. Avoid use of suspension in patients with phenylketonuria. Age-related renal impairment may require a dosage adjustment in elderly patients.

Although mild GI effects may be tolerable, an increase in their severity may indicate the onset of antibiotic-associated colitis. Assess the pattern of daily bowel activity and stool consistency, the mouth for white patches on the mucous membranes and tongue, signs and symptoms of superinfection including abdominal pain, moderate to severe diarrhea, severe anal or genital pruritus, and severe mouth soreness. Renal function should be assessed.

Storage

After reconstitution, the oral suspension is stable for 14 days if refrigerated.

Administration

Shake the oral suspension well before using. Take cefprozil without regard to meals; however, if GI upset occurs, give it with food or milk.

Ceftazidime

sef-taz'i-deem

★ Ceptaz, Fortaz, Tazicef, Tazidime 🍁 Fortaz

Do not confuse ceftazidime with ceftizoxime.

CATEGORY AND SCHEDULE

Pregnancy Risk Category: B

Classification: Antibiotic, cephalosporin (third generation)

MECHANISM OF ACTION

A third-generation cephalosporin that binds to bacterial cell membranes and inhibits cell wall synthesis. *Therapeutic Effect:* Bactericidal.

PHARMACOKINETICS

Widely distributed (including to CSF). Protein binding: 5%-17%. Primarily excreted unchanged in urine. Removed by hemodialysis. *Half-life:* 2 h (increased in impaired renal function).

AVAILABILITY

Powder for Injection (Fortaz, Tazicef, Tazidime): 500 mg, 1 g, 2 g, 6 g.
Premixed IVPB, Frozen: 1 g, 2 g.

INDICATIONS AND DOSAGES

▸ **Urinary tract infection**

IV, IM

Adults. 250-500 mg q8-12h.

▸ **Mild to moderate infections**

IV, IM

Adults. 1 g q8-12h.

▸ **Uncomplicated pneumonia, skin and skin-structure infections**

IV, IM

Adults. 0.5-1 g q8h.

▸ **Bone and joint infections**

IV

Adults. 2 g q12h.

▸ **Meningitis, serious gynecologic and intra-abdominal infections**

IV

Adults. 2 g q8h.

▸ **Pseudomonal pulmonary infections in patients with cystic fibrosis**

IV

Adults. 30-50 mg/kg q8h. Maximum: 6 g/day.

▸ **Usual elderly dosage**

Elderly (with normal renal function). 500 mg-1 g q12h.

▸ **Usual pediatric dosage**

Children 1 mo to 12 yr. 100-150 mg/kg/day in divided doses q8h. Maximum: 6 g/day.

Neonates 0-4 wks. 100-150 mg/kg/day in divided doses q8-12h.

▸ **Dosage in renal impairment**

After an initial 1-g dose, dosage and frequency are modified based on creatinine clearance and the severity of the infection.

Creatinine Clearance (mL/min)	Adult Dosage
30-50	1 g q12h
16-30	1 g q24h
6-15	500 mg q24h
<5	500 mg q48h

CONTRAINDICATIONS

History of anaphylactic reaction to penicillins or hypersensitivity to cephalosporins.

INTERACTIONS

Drug

Probenecid: May increase ceftazidime blood concentration.

Warfarin: May increase warfarin effect.

Herbal

None known.

Food

None known.

DIAGNOSTIC TEST EFFECTS

May increase BUN level and serum alkaline phosphatase, creatinine, INR, LDH, AST (SGOT), and ALT (SGPT) levels. May produce a positive direct or indirect Coombs' test. Interferes with crossmatching procedures and hematologic tests.

IV INCOMPATIBILITIES

Acetylcysteine (Acetadote), amphotericin B complex (Abelcet, AmBisome, Amphotec), acetylcysteine (Acetadote), caspofungin (Cancidas), diazepam, diphenhydramine, dobutamine, doxorubicin liposomal (Doxil), fluconazole (Diflucan), haloperidol, idarubicin (Idamycin), lansoprazole (Prevacid), midazolam (Versed), nitroprusside, pentamidine (Pentam IV), phenytoin, thiamine, vancomycin (Vancocin), verapamil, warfarin (Coumadin).

IV COMPATIBILITIES

Diltiazem (Cardizem), famotidine (Pepcid), heparin, hydromorphone (Dilaudid), morphine, propofol (Diprivan).

SIDE EFFECTS

Frequent

Discomfort with IM administration, oral candidiasis, mild diarrhea, mild abdominal cramping, vaginal candidiasis.

Occasional

Nausea, serum sickness-like reaction (marked by fever and joint pain; usually occurs after the second course of therapy and resolves after the drug is discontinued).

Rare

Allergic reaction (pruritus, rash, urticaria), thrombophlebitis (pain, redness, swelling at injection site).

SERIOUS REACTIONS

- Antibiotic-associated colitis and other superinfections may result from altered bacterial balance.
- Nephrotoxicity may occur, especially in patients with preexisting renal disease.
- Patients with a history of allergies, especially to penicillin, are at increased risk for developing a severe hypersensitivity reaction, marked by severe pruritus, angioedema, bronchospasm, and anaphylaxis.

PRECAUTIONS & CONSIDERATIONS

Caution is warranted with history of GI disease (especially antibiotic-associated or ulcerative colitis), seizure disorder, renal impairment, and concurrent use of nephrotoxic drugs. May be associated with increased INR, especially in nutritionally deficient patients, prolonged treatment, and hepatic or renal disease. Ceftazidime readily crosses the placenta and is distributed in breast milk. No age-related precautions have been noted in children. Age-related renal impairment may require a dosage adjustment in elderly patients.

Although mild GI effects may be tolerable, an increase in their severity may indicate the onset of antibiotic-associated colitis. Assess the pattern of daily bowel activity and stool consistency, the mouth for white patches on the mucous membranes and tongue, signs and symptoms of superinfection including abdominal pain, moderate to severe diarrhea, severe anal or genital pruritus, and severe mouth soreness.
Renal function should also be assessed.

Storage

The solution normally appears light yellow to amber, but it tends to darken; color change does not indicate loss of potency. Reconstituted solution is stable for 24 h at room temperature, 7 days if refrigerated, or 12 wks if frozen. The IV infusion (piggyback) is stable for 24 h at room temperature and 7 days if refrigerated. Thawed premixed frozen solutions are stable for 24 h at room temperature and 7 days if refrigerated. Discard the solution if a precipitate forms.

Administration
For IV use, add 10 mL of sterile water for injection to each 1-g vial to provide a concentration of 90 mg/mL. The resulting solution may be further diluted with 50-100 mL of 0.9% NaCl, D5W, or another compatible diluent. Administer IV push over 3-5 min. Administer intermittent IV infusion (piggyback) over 15-30 min.

For IM use, to reconstitute, add 1.5 mL of sterile water for injection or lidocaine 1% to 500-mg vial, if prescribed, or 3 mL to 1-g vial to provide a concentration of 280 mg/mL. To minimize patient discomfort, slowly inject the drug deep into the gluteus maximus rather than into the lateral aspect of the thigh.

Ceftibuten

cef'te-bute-in
☒ Cedax

CATEGORY AND SCHEDULE

Pregnancy Risk Category: B

Classification: Antibiotic, cephalosporin (third generation)

MECHANISM OF ACTION

A third-generation cephalosporin that binds to bacterial cell membranes and inhibits cell wall synthesis. *Therapeutic Effect:* Bactericidal.

PHARMACOKINETICS

Rapidly absorbed from the gastrointestinal tract. Excreted primarily in urine. *Half-life:* 2-3 h.

AVAILABILITY

Capsules: 400 mg.
Oral Suspension: 90 mg/5 mL.

INDICATIONS AND DOSAGES

▸ **Chronic bronchitis**
PO
Adults, Elderly. 400 mg/day once a day for 10 days.

▸ **Pharyngitis, tonsillitis**
PO
Adults, Elderly. 400 mg once a day for 10 days.
Children 6 mo of age and older. 9 mg/kg once a day for 10 days. Maximum: 400 mg/day.

▸ **Otitis media**
PO
Children 6 mo of age and older. 9 mg/kg once a day for 10 days. Maximum: 400 mg/day.

▸ **Dosage in renal impairment**
Dosage is modified based on creatinine clearance.

Creatinine Clearance (mL/min)	Dosage
50 (and higher)	400 mg or 9 mg/kg q24h
30-49	200 mg or 4.5 mg/kg q24h
< 30	100 mg or 2.25 mg/kg q24h

CONTRAINDICATIONS

History of anaphylactic reaction to penicillins or hypersensitivity to cephalosporins.

INTERACTIONS

Drug
Aminoglycosides: Increased risk of nephrotoxicity.

C

Probenecid: Increases serum ceftibuten level.

Herbal
None known.

Food
None known.

DIAGNOSTIC TEST EFFECTS

May increase BUN level and serum alkaline phosphatase, bilirubin, creatinine, LDH, AST (SGOT), and ALT (SGPT) levels. May produce a positive direct or indirect Coombs' test.

SIDE EFFECTS

Frequent
Oral candidiasis, mild diarrhea (discharge, itching).

Occasional
Nausea, serum sickness-like reaction (marked by fever and joint pain; usually occurs after the second course of therapy and resolves after the drug is discontinued).

Rare
Allergic reaction (rash, pruritus, urticaria).

SERIOUS REACTIONS

- Antibiotic-associated colitis and other superinfections may result from altered bacterial balance.
- Nephrotoxicity may occur, especially in patients with preexisting renal disease.
- Patients with a history of allergies, especially to penicillin, are at increased risk for developing a severe hypersensitivity reaction, marked by severe pruritus, angioedema, bronchospasm, and anaphylaxis.

PRECAUTIONS & CONSIDERATIONS

Caution is warranted with history of GI disease (especially antibiotic-associated or ulcerative colitis), renal impairment, and allergies to penicillins or other drugs.

Although mild GI effects may be tolerable, an increase in their severity may indicate the onset of antibiotic-associated colitis. Assess the pattern of daily bowel activity and stool consistency, the mouth for white patches on the mucous membranes and tongue, signs and symptoms of superinfection including abdominal pain, moderate to severe diarrhea, severe anal or genital pruritus, and severe mouth soreness. Renal function should also be assessed.

Storage
Reconstituted suspension is stable for 14 days if refrigerated.

Administration
Take capsule without regard to food; may take with food or milk if GI upset occurs. Take suspension 1 h before or 2 h after a meal. Take a full course of treatment, and space drug doses evenly around the clock. Shake suspension well before each use.

Ceftizoxime

sef-ti-zox'eem

★ Cefizox

Do not confuse ceftizoxime with cefotaxime or ceftazidime.

CATEGORY AND SCHEDULE

Pregnancy Risk Category: B

Classification: Antibiotics, cephalosporin (third generation)

MECHANISM OF ACTION

A third-generation cephalosporin that binds to bacterial cell membranes and inhibits cell wall synthesis. *Therapeutic Effect:* Bactericidal.

PHARMACOKINETICS

Widely distributed (including to CSF). Protein binding: 30%. Primarily excreted unchanged in urine.

Moderately removed by hemodialysis. *Half-life:* 1.7 h (increased in impaired renal function).

AVAILABILITY

Premixed IVPB, Frozen: 1 g, 2 g.

INDICATIONS AND DOSAGES

▸ **Uncomplicated urinary tract infection**

IV

Adults, Elderly. 500 mg q12h.

▸ **Mild, moderate, or severe infections of the biliary, respiratory, and genitourinary tracts; skin, bone, and intra-abdominal infections; meningitis; and septicemia**

IV

Adults, Elderly. 1-2 g q8-12h.

▸ **Life-threatening infections of the biliary, respiratory, and genitourinary tracts; skin, bone, and intra-abdominal infections; meningitis; and septicemia**

IV

Adults, Elderly. 3-4 g q8h, up to 2 g q4h.

▸ **Pelvic inflammatory disease (PID)**

IV

Adults. 2 g q4-8h.

▸ **Usual pediatric dosage**

Children older than 6 mo. 50 mg/kg q6-8h. Maximum: 12 g/day.

▸ **Dosage in renal impairment**

After a loading dose of 0.5-1 g, dosage and frequency are modified based on creatinine clearance and the severity of the infection.

Creatinine Clearance (mL/min)	Adult Dosage
50-79	0.5 g-1.5 g q8h
5-49	0.25 g-1 g q12h
< 5	0.25-0.5 g q24h or 0.5 g-1 g q48h

CONTRAINDICATIONS

History of anaphylactic reaction to penicillins or hypersensitivity to cephalosporins.

INTERACTIONS

Drug

Aminoglycosides: May increase risk of nephrotoxicity.

Probenecid: Increases serum concentration of ceftizoxime.

Herbal

None known.

Food

None known.

DIAGNOSTIC TEST EFFECTS

May increase BUN level and serum alkaline serum phosphatase, creatinine, AST (SGOT), and ALT (SGPT) levels. May produce a positive direct or indirect Coombs' test.

IV INCOMPATIBILITIES

Diazepam, dobutamine, erythromycin, filgastrim (Neupogen), haloperidol, lansoprazole (Prevacid), phenytoin, thiamine.

IV COMPATIBILITIES

Hydromorphone (Dilaudid), morphine, propofol (Diprivan).

SIDE EFFECTS

Frequent

Discomfort with IM administration, oral candidiasis, mild diarrhea, mild abdominal cramping, vaginal candidiasis.

Occasional

Nausea, serum sickness-like reaction (fever, joint pain; usually occurs after the second course of therapy and resolves after the drug is discontinued).

Rare

Allergic reaction (rash, pruritus, urticaria), thrombophlebitis (pain, redness, swelling at injection site).

C

SERIOUS REACTIONS

- Antibiotic-associated colitis manifested and other superinfections may result from altered bacterial balance.
- Nephrotoxicity may occur, especially in patients with preexisting renal disease.
- Patients with a history of allergies, especially to penicillin, are at increased risk for developing a severe hypersensitivity reaction, marked by severe pruritus, angioedema, bronchospasm, and anaphylaxis.

PRECAUTIONS & CONSIDERATIONS

Caution is warranted with history of GI disease (especially antibiotic-associated or ulcerative colitis) and hepatic or renal impairment. Ceftizoxime readily crosses the placenta and is distributed in breast milk. Ceftizoxime use in children is associated with transient elevations of blood eosinophil count and serum CK, AST (SGOT), and ALT (SGPT) levels. Age-related renal impairment may require a dosage adjustment in elderly patients.

Although mild GI effects may be tolerable, an increase in their severity may indicate the onset of antibiotic-associated colitis. Assess the pattern of daily bowel activity and stool consistency, the mouth for white patches on the mucous membranes and tongue, signs and symptoms of superinfection including abdominal pain, moderate to severe diarrhea, severe anal or genital pruritus, and severe mouth soreness. Renal function should also be assessed.

Storage

The solution normally appears clear to pale yellow. A change from yellow to amber does not indicate loss of potency. Thawed premixed frozen solution is stable for 24 h at room temperature and 10 days if refrigerated. Discard the solution if a precipitate forms.

Administration

For IV use, infuse intermittent IV infusion (piggyback) over 15-30 min.

Ceftriaxone

sef-try-ax'one

Rocephin

CATEGORY AND SCHEDULE

Pregnancy Risk Category: B

Classification: Antibiotics, cephalosporin (third generation)

MECHANISM OF ACTION

A third-generation cephalosporin that binds to bacterial cell membranes and inhibits cell wall synthesis. *Therapeutic Effect:* Bactericidal.

PHARMACOKINETICS

Widely distributed (including to CSF). Protein binding: 83%-96%. Primarily excreted unchanged in urine. Not removed by hemodialysis. *Half-life:* 4.3-4.6 h IV; 5.8-8.7 h IM (increased in impaired renal function).

AVAILABILITY

Powder for Injection: 250 mg, 500 mg, 1 g, 2 g, 10 g.
Premixed IVPB, Frozen: 1 g, 2 g.

INDICATIONS AND DOSAGES

▸ **Mild to moderate infections**

IV, IM

Adults, Elderly. 1-2 g as a single dose or in 2 divided doses.

▸ **Serious infections**

IV, IM

Adults, Elderly. Up to 4 g/day in 2 divided doses.

Children. 50-75 mg/kg/day in divided doses q12h. Maximum: 2 g/day.

▸ **Skin and skin-structure infections**
IV, IM
Children. 50-75 mg/kg/day as a single dose or in 2 divided doses. Maximum: 2 g/day.

▸ **Meningitis**
IV
Children. Initially 100 mg/kg, then 100 mg/kg/day as a single dose or in divided doses q12h. Maximum: 4 g/day.

▸ **Lyme disease**
IV
Adults, Elderly. 2-4 g a day for 10-14 days.

▸ **Acute bacterial otitis media**
IM
Children. 50 mg/kg as a single dose.

▸ **Perioperative prophylaxis**
IV, IM
Adults, Elderly. 1 g 0.5-2 h before surgery.

▸ **Uncomplicated gonorrhea**
IM
Adults. 250 mg plus azithromycin or doxycycline one time.

▸ **Dosage in renal impairment**
Dosage modification is usually unnecessary, but liver and renal function test results should be monitored in persons with both renal and liver impairment or severe renal impairment.

CONTRAINDICATIONS

History of anaphylactic reaction to penicillins or hypersensitivity to cephalosporins; hyperbilirubinemic neonates; concomitant use with calcium-containing solutions or products.

INTERACTIONS

Drug
Calcium-containing solutions: Ceftriaxone may precipitate with calcium when mixed. Avoid coadministration, even via separate infusion lines or at different times. Do not administer calcium-containing solutions or products within 48 h after the last dose of ceftriaxone.
Warfarin: May increase the effects of warfarin.
Herbal
None known.
Food
None known.

DIAGNOSTIC TEST EFFECTS

May increase BUN level, INR, and serum alkaline phosphatase, bilirubin, creatinine, AST (SGOT), and ALT (SGPT) levels. May produce a positive direct or indirect Coombs' test. Interferes with crossmatching procedures and hematologic tests.

IV INCOMPATIBILITIES

! NOTE: Do NOT use diluents containing calcium (e.g., Ringer's solution) to reconstitute or for further dilution for IV use. Precipitation can also occur when mixed with calcium-containing solutions in the same IV line, including continuous calcium-containing infusions (i.e., parenteral nutrition), via a Y-site.

Aminophylline, amphotericin B complex (Abelcet, AmBisome, Amphotec), calcium, filgrastim (Neupogen), fluconazole (Diflucan), labetalol (Normodyne), pentamidine (Pentam IV), vancomycin (Vancocin).

IV COMPATIBILITIES

Diltiazem (Cardizem), heparin, lidocaine, morphine, propofol (Diprivan).

SIDE EFFECTS

Frequent
Discomfort with IM administration, oral candidiasis, mild diarrhea,

mild abdominal cramping, vaginal candidiasis.

Occasional

Nausea, serum sickness-like reaction (marked by fever and joint pain; usually occurs after the second course of therapy and resolves after the drug is discontinued).

Rare

Allergic reaction (rash, pruritus, urticaria), thombophlebitis (pain, redness, swelling at injection site).

SERIOUS REACTIONS

- Antibiotic-associated colitis and other superinfections may result from altered bacterial balance.
- Nephrotoxicity may occur, especially in patients with preexisting renal disease.
- Patients with a history of allergies, especially to penicillin, are at increased risk for developing a severe hypersensitivity reaction, marked by severe pruritus, angioedema, bronchospasm, and anaphylaxis.
- Renal and pulmonary ceftriaxone-calcium precipitations, including some fatalities in neonates.

PRECAUTIONS & CONSIDERATIONS

Caution is warranted in patients with a history of GI disease (especially antibiotic-associated or ulcerative colitis), hepatic or renal impairment, and concurrent use of nephrotoxic drugs. May be associated with increased INR, especially in nutritionally deficient patients or those who have undergone prolonged treatment or have hepatic or renal disease. Ceftriaxone readily crosses the placenta and is distributed in breast milk. Ceftriaxone use in children may displace serum bilirubin from serum albumin. Use ceftriaxone cautiously in neonates, who may become hyperbilirubinemic; use is contraindicated in neonates with hyperbilirubinemia. Age-related renal impairment may require a dosage adjustment in elderly patients.

Although mild GI effects may be tolerable, an increase in their severity may indicate the onset of antibiotic-associated colitis. Assess the pattern of daily bowel activity and stool consistency, the mouth for white patches on the mucous membranes and tongue, signs and symptoms of superinfection including abdominal pain, moderate to severe diarrhea, severe anal or genital pruritus, and severe mouth soreness. Renal function should also be assessed.

Storage

Store unreconstituted vials at room temperature. The solution normally appears light yellow to amber. The IV infusion (piggyback) is stable for 3 days at room temperature and 10 days if refrigerated. Thawed premixed frozen solutions are stable for 3 days at room temperature or 21 days if refrigerated. Discard the solution if a precipitate forms.

Administration

For IV use, add 2.4 mL of sterile water for injection to each 250-mg vial, 4.8 mL to each 500-mg vial, 9.6 mL to each 1-g vial, and 19.2 mL to each 2-g vial to provide a concentration of 100 mg/mL. The resulting solution may be further diluted with 50-100 mL of 0.9% NaCl or D5W. Infuse the intermittent IV infusion (piggyback) over 15-30 min for adults and over 10-30 min for children or neonates. Alternate IV sites and use large veins to reduce the risk of phlebitis.

For IM use, add 0.9 mL of sterile water for injection, 0.9% NaCl, D5W, bacteriostatic water and 0.9% benzyl alcohol, or 1% lidocaine to each 250-mg vial; 1.8 mL to each 500-mg vial; 3.6 mL to each 1-g vial; and 7.2 mL to each 2-g vial to provide a concentration of 250 mg/mL. To minimize patient discomfort, slowly inject the drug deep into the gluteus maximus rather than the lateral aspect of the thigh.

Cefuroxime

sef-yoor-ox'eem

★ Ceftin, Zinacef

Do not confuse cefuroxime with cefotaxime, Cefzil, or deferoxamine.

CATEGORY AND SCHEDULE

Pregnancy Risk Category: B

Classification: Antibiotics, cephalosporin (second generation)

MECHANISM OF ACTION

A second-generation cephalosporin that binds to bacterial cell membranes and inhibits cell wall synthesis. *Therapeutic Effect:* Bactericidal.

PHARMACOKINETICS

Rapidly absorbed from the GI tract. Protein binding: 33%-50%. Widely distributed (including to CSF). Primarily excreted unchanged in urine. Moderately removed by hemodialysis. *Half-life:* 1.3 h (increased in impaired renal function).

AVAILABILITY

Oral Suspension: 125 mg/5 mL, 250 mg/5 mL.
Tablets: 125 mg, 250 mg, 500 mg.
Powder for Injection: 750 mg, 1.5 g, 7.5 g.
Premixed IVPB, Frozen: 750 mg, 1.5 g.

INDICATIONS AND DOSAGES

▸ **Ampicillin-resistant influenza; bacterial meningitis; early Lyme disease; genitourinary tract, gynecologic, skin, and bone infections; septicemia; gonorrhea; and other gonococcal infections**

IV, IM

Adults, Elderly. 750 mg-1.5 g q8h.
Children. 75-100 mg/kg/day divided q8h. Maximum: 8 g/day.
Neonates. 50-100 mg/kg/day divided q12h.

PO

Adults, Elderly. 125-500 mg twice a day, depending on the infection. For uncomplicated gonorrhea, give a 1-g single dose.

▸ **Pharyngitis, tonsillitis**

PO

Children 3 mo to 12 yr. 125 mg (tablets) q12h or 20 mg/kg/day (suspension) in 2 divided doses.

▸ **Acute otitis media, acute bacterial maxillary sinusitis, impetigo**

PO

Children 3 mo to 12 yr. 250 mg (tablets) q12h or 30 mg/kg/day (suspension) in 2 divided doses.

▸ **Bacterial meningitis**

IV

Children 3 mo to 12 yr. 200-240 mg/kg/day in divided doses q6-8h.

▸ **Perioperative prophylaxis**

IV

Adults, Elderly. 1.5 g 30-60 min before surgery and 750 mg q8h after surgery.

▸ **Dosage in renal impairment**

Adult dosage and frequency are modified based on creatinine clearance and the severity of the infection. The usual initial (loading dose) is given, followed by maintenance as follows:

C

Creatinine Clearance (mL/min)	Adult Dosage
> 20	Use usual dose
10-20	750 mg q12h
< 10	750 mg q24h

CONTRAINDICATIONS

History of anaphylactic reaction to penicillins or hypersensitivity to cephalosporins.

INTERACTIONS

Drug

Antacids, H_2 antagonists: May reduce cefuroxime absorption.

Probenecid: Increases serum concentration of cefuroxime.

Herbal

None known.

Food

None known.

DIAGNOSTIC TEST EFFECTS

May increase serum alkaline phosphatase, bilirubin, LDH, AST (SGOT), and ALT (SGPT) levels. May produce a positive direct or indirect Coombs' test.

IV INCOMPATIBILITIES

Azithromycin (Zithromax IV), calcium chloride, caspofungin (Cancidas), diazepam, diphenhydramine, dobutamine, doxycycline, filgrastim (Neupogen), fluconazole (Diflucan), haloperidol, magnesium sulfate, midazolam (Versed), phenobarbital, phenytoin, promethazine, sodium bicarbonate, vancomycin (Vancocin).

IV COMPATIBILITIES

Diltiazem (Cardizem), hydromorphone (Dilaudid), morphine, propofol (Diprivan).

SIDE EFFECTS

Frequent

Discomfort with IM administration, oral candidiasis, mild diarrhea, mild abdominal cramping, vaginal candidiasis.

Occasional

Nausea, serum sickness-like reaction (marked by fever and joint pain; usually occurs after the second course of therapy and resolves after the drug is discontinued).

Rare

Allergic reaction (rash, pruritus, urticaria), thrombophlebitis (pain, redness, swelling at injection site).

SERIOUS REACTIONS

- Antibiotic-associated colitis and other superinfections may result from altered bacterial balance.
- Nephrotoxicity may occur, especially in patients with preexisting renal disease.
- Patients with a history of allergies, especially to penicillin, are at increased risk for developing a severe hypersensitivity reaction, marked by severe pruritus, angioedema, bronchospasm, and anaphylaxis.

PRECAUTIONS & CONSIDERATIONS

Caution is warranted for patients with a history of GI disease (especially antibiotic-associated or ulcerative colitis), renal impairment, and concurrent use of nephrotoxic drugs. May be associated with increased INR, especially in nutritionally deficient patients, prolonged treatment, hepatic or renal disease. Cefuroxime readily crosses the placenta and is distributed in breast milk. No age-related precautions have been noted in children. Age-related renal impairment may require a dosage adjustment in elderly patients.

Although mild GI effects may be tolerable, an increase in their severity may indicate the onset of antibiotic-associated colitis. Assess the pattern of daily bowel activity and stool consistency, the mouth for white patches on the mucous membranes and tongue, signs and symptoms of superinfection including abdominal pain, moderate to severe diarrhea, severe anal or genital pruritus, and severe mouth soreness. Renal function should also be assessed.

Storage

Reconstituted oral suspension is stable for 10 days refrigerated. The injection solution normally appears light yellow to amber; a darker color does not indicate loss of potency. Reconstituted solution is stable for 24 h at room temperature and 48 h if refrigerated. The IV infusion (piggyback) is stable for 24 h at room temperature, 7 days if refrigerated, and 26 wks if frozen. Thawed previously frozen premixed solution is stable for 24 h at room temperature or 21 days if refrigerated. Discard the solution if a precipitate forms.

Administration

Cefuroxime axetil tablets and powder for oral suspension are not bioequivalent and are therefore not substitutable on a mg/mg basis; bioavailability is greater with the tablets. Take cefuroxime tablets without regard to food. However, if GI upset occurs, give with food or milk. Avoid crushing tablets because they have a bitter taste. Give the oral suspension with food. Shake suspension well prior to each use.

For IV use, to reconstitute, add 8 mL of sterile water for injection to each 750-mg vial, or 14 mL to each 1.5-g vial to provide a concentration of 100 mg/mL. For intermittent IV infusion (piggyback), further dilute with 50-100 mL of 0.9% NaCl or D5W. Administer the IV push over 3-5 min. Infuse the intermittent IV infusion (piggyback) over 15-60 min.

For IM use, to minimize patient discomfort, slowly inject the drug deep into the gluteus maximus rather than the lateral aspect of the thigh.

Celecoxib

sel-eh-cox'ib

★ 🍁 Celebrex

Do not confuse Celebrex with Cerebyx or Celexa.

CATEGORY AND SCHEDULE

Pregnancy Risk Category: C (D if used in third trimester or near delivery)

Classification: Nonsteroidal anti-inflammatory, analgesic, COX-2 inhibitor

MECHANISM OF ACTION

An NSAID that inhibits cyclooxygenase-2, the enzyme responsible for prostaglandin synthesis. Mechanism of action in treating familial adenomatous polyposis is unknown. *Therapeutic Effect:* Reduces inflammation and relieves pain.

PHARMACOKINETICS

Widely distributed. Protein binding: 97%. Metabolized in the liver. Primarily eliminated in feces. *Half-life:* 11.2 h.

AVAILABILITY

Capsules: 50 mg, 100 mg, 200 mg, 400 mg.

C

INDICATIONS AND DOSAGES

▸ **Osteoarthritis**

PO

Adults, Elderly. 200 mg/day as a single dose or 100 mg twice a day.

▸ **Rheumatoid arthritis**

PO

Adults, Elderly. 100-200 mg twice a day.

▸ **Acute pain, primary dysmenorrhea**

PO

Adults, Elderly. Initially, 400 mg with additional 200 mg on day 1, if needed. Maintenance: 200 mg twice a day as needed.

▸ **Familial adenomatous polyposis**

PO

Adults, Elderly. 400 mg twice daily (with food).

▸ **Juvenile rheumatoid arthritis**

PO

Children 2 yr and older and weighing 10-25 kg. 50 mg twice daily.

Children 2 yr and older and weighing more than 25 kg. 100 mg twice daily.

▸ **Ankylosing spondylitis**

PO

Adults. 200 mg once daily or 100 mg twice daily. May increase to 400 mg/day.

▸ **Dose in moderate hepatic impairment**

Reduce dose 50%.

▸ **Dose in renal impairment**

Not recommended for patients with advanced renal disease.

CONTRAINDICATIONS

Hypersensitivity to aspirin, NSAIDs, or sulfonamides; perioperative pain in the setting of coronary artery bypass graft surgery.

INTERACTIONS

Drug

Fluconazole: May increase celecoxib blood level.

Lithium: May increase lithium blood levels.

Warfarin: May increase the risk of bleeding.

Herbal

None known.

Food

None known.

DIAGNOSTIC TEST EFFECTS

May increase AST (SGOT) and ALT (SGPT) levels.

SIDE EFFECTS

Frequent (> 5%)

Diarrhea, dyspepsia, headache, hypertension, upper respiratory tract infection.

Occasional (1%-5%)

Abdominal pain, flatulence, nausea, back pain, peripheral edema, dizziness, rash.

SERIOUS REACTIONS

• None known.

PRECAUTIONS & CONSIDERATIONS

Be aware of the potential for increased risk of cardiovascular events and GI bleeding associated with celecoxib use. Caution is warranted with smokers and patients with active alcoholism, who have a history of peptic ulcer disease, who are receiving anticoagulant or steroid therapy, and who are elderly. It is unknown whether celecoxib crosses the placenta or is distributed in breast milk. Celecoxib should not be used during the third trimester of pregnancy because it may cause adverse effects in the fetus, such as premature closure of the ductus arteriosus. The safety and efficacy of celecoxib have not been established in children younger than 18 yr. No age-related precautions have been noted in elderly patients. Alcohol and aspirin should be avoided during celecoxib therapy because these substances increase the risk of GI bleeding.

Therapeutic response, such as decreased pain, stiffness, swelling, and tenderness, improved grip strength, and increased joint mobility, should be evaluated.

Storage

Store at room temperature.

Administration

Celecoxib at dosages up to 200 mg twice daily can be administered without regard to timing of meals. Administer higher dosages (400 mg twice daily) with food to improve absorption. For patients with difficulty swallowing, the capsules may be opened and the contents sprinkled on applesauce.

Cephalexin

sef-a-lex'in

★ Keflex, Panixine Disperdose

🍁 Apo-Cephalex, Keflex, Novo-Lexin, Nu-Cephalex

CATEGORY AND SCHEDULE

Pregnancy Risk Category: B

Classification: Antibiotics, cephalosporin (first generation)

MECHANISM OF ACTION

A first-generation cephalosporin that binds to bacterial cell membranes and inhibits cell wall synthesis. *Therapeutic Effect:* Bactericidal.

PHARMACOKINETICS

Rapidly absorbed from the GI tract. Protein binding: 10%-15%. Widely distributed. Primarily excreted unchanged in urine. Moderately removed by hemodialysis. *Half-life:* 0.9-1.2 h (increased in impaired renal function).

AVAILABILITY

Powder for Oral Suspension: 125 mg/5 mL, 250 mg/5 mL.
Capsules or Tablets: 250 mg, 500 mg.
Tablets for Oral Suspension: 125 mg, 250 mg.

INDICATIONS AND DOSAGES

▸ Bone infections, prophylaxis of rheumatic fever, follow-up to parenteral therapy

PO

Adults, Elderly. 250-500 mg q6h up to 4 g/day.

▸ Streptococcal pharyngitis, skin and skin-structure infections, uncomplicated cystitis

PO

Adults, Elderly. 500 mg q12h.

▸ Usual pediatric dosage

Children. 25-100 mg/kg/day in 2-4 divided doses.

▸ Otitis media

PO

Children. 75-100 mg/kg/day in 4 divided doses.

▸ Dosage in renal impairment

After usual initial dose, dosing frequency is modified based on creatinine clearance and the severity of the infection.

Creatinine Clearance (mL/min)	Dosage Interval
10-40	Usual dose q8-12h
< 10	Usual dose q12-24h

CONTRAINDICATIONS

History of anaphylactic reaction to penicillins or hypersensitivity to cephalosporins.

INTERACTIONS

Drug

Probenecid: Increases serum concentration of cephalexin.

C

Herbal
None known.
Food
None known.

DIAGNOSTIC TEST EFFECTS
May increase INR, serum alkaline phosphatase, AST (SGOT), and ALT (SGPT) levels. May produce a positive direct or indirect Coombs' test.

SIDE EFFECTS
Frequent
Oral candidiasis, mild diarrhea, mild abdominal cramping, vaginal candidiasis.
Occasional
Nausea, serum sickness-like reaction (marked by fever and joint pain; usually occurs after the second course of therapy and resolves after the drug is discontinued).
Rare
Allergic reaction (rash, pruritus, urticaria).

SERIOUS REACTIONS
- Antibiotic-associated colitis and other superinfections may result from altered bacterial balance.
- Nephrotoxicity may occur, especially in patients with preexisting renal disease.
- Patients with a history of allergies, especially to penicillin, are at increased risk for developing a severe hypersensitivity reaction, marked by severe pruritus, angioedema, bronchospasm, and anaphylaxis.

PRECAUTIONS & CONSIDERATIONS
Caution is warranted with history of GI disease (especially antibiotic-associated or ulcerative colitis), renal impairment, and concurrent use of nephrotoxic drugs. May be associated with increased INR, especially in nutritionally deficient patients, those undergoing prolonged treatment, and patients with hepatic or renal disease. Cephalexin readily crosses the placenta and is distributed in breast milk. No age-related precautions have been noted in children. Age-related renal impairment may require a dosage adjustment in elderly patients.

Although mild GI effects may be tolerable, an increase in their severity may indicate the onset of antibiotic-associated colitis. Assess the pattern of daily bowel activity and stool consistency, the mouth for white patches on the mucous membranes and tongue, signs and symptoms of superinfection including abdominal pain, moderate to severe diarrhea, severe anal or genital pruritus, and severe mouth soreness. Renal function should be assessed.

Storage
Keep tablets, capsules, unreconstituted powder for oral suspension, and tablets for dispersion at room temperature in tightly closed containers. After reconstitution, the oral suspension is stable for 14 days if refrigerated.

Administration
Space drug doses evenly around the clock.

Shake the oral suspension well before using. Take oral cephalexin without regard to meals. However, if GI upset occurs, give with food or milk.

For dispersible tablets for suspension: Do not chew or swallow the tablets. Mix tablet in about 10 mL of water. Drink entire mixture. Rinse container with additional water and drink the contents to ensure the whole dose is taken.

Certolizumab Pegol

sir-toe-liz'oo-mab peg'ol

Cimzia

Do not confuse Cimzia with Cymbalta.

CATEGORY AND SCHEDULE

Pregnancy Risk Category: B

Classification: Disease-modifying antirheumatic drugs, gastrointestinal anti-inflammatory agents, biologic response modifiers, monoclonal antibodies, tumor necrosis factor (TNF) modulators

MECHANISM OF ACTION

A monoclonal antibody that binds to tumor necrosis factor (TNF), inhibiting functional activity of TNF-α. Reduces infiltration of inflammatory cells. *Therapeutic Effect:* Decreases intestinal inflammation, decreases synovitis and joint erosion.

PHARMACOKINETICS

Peak plasma concentrations are attained 54-171 h after subcutaneous injection. The bioavailability is approximately 80%. There is a linear relationship between the dose and the maximum serum concentration and the area under the certolizumab pegol plasma concentration versus time curve (AUC). *Terminal Half-life:* Roughly 14 days.

AVAILABILITY

Powder for Injection: 200 mg.
Prefilled Injection Syringes: 200 mg/mL.

INDICATIONS AND DOSAGES

▸ **Moderate to severe Crohn disease**

SUBCUTANEOUS

Adults, Elderly. 400 mg initially and at wks 2 and 4. If response occurs, follow with 400 mg every 4 wks.

▸ **Rheumatoid arthritis (RA), moderate to severe**

SUBCUTANEOUS

Adults, Elderly. 400 mg initially and at wks 2 and 4. Follow with 200 mg every other week; consider a dose of 400 mg every 4 wks for maintenance regimens.

CONTRAINDICATIONS

Hypersensitivity to certolizumab.

INTERACTIONS

Drug

Abatacept, rilonacept, anakinra, natalizumab, and other TNF-modulating drugs: May increase the risk of adverse effects such as infection risk. Concurrent use not recommended.
Immunosuppressants: May increase risk of serious infection.
Live vaccines: May decrease immune response to vaccine. Deferral of live vaccination may be necessary; consult CDC guidelines.

Herbal

Echinacea: In theory, may alter effect of certolizumab.

Food

None known.

DIAGNOSTIC TEST EFFECTS

May cause erroneously elevated activated partial thromboplastin time (aPTT) results even though the drug does not affect coagulation.

SIDE EFFECTS

Frequent (≥ 5%)

Upper respiratory infections (e.g., nasopharyngitis, laryngitis), urinary tract infections, rash, arthralgia.

C

Occasional (3%-5%)
Injection site reactions, headache, fatigue, fever, increased blood pressure, myalgia, back pain.
Rare (< 3%)
Urticaria, psoriasis, optic neuritis or vision change, stomatitis, mood changes, vasculitis, changes in blood counts, alopecia, menstrual changes, anxiety. Autoantibody production may produce a lupus-like syndrome.

SERIOUS REACTIONS

- Hypersensitivity reactions may occur, including angioedema or serum-sickness-like syndromes.
- Severe hepatic reactions or reactivation of hepatitis B.
- Anemia, leukopenia, pancytopenia, or aplastic anemia (rare).
- Potential for lymphoma or other malignancy in young adults or children.
- New or worsening heart failure or other heart changes.
- Reactivation of latent tuberculosis has occurred.
- Serious infections, such as bacteremia or pneumonia.
- Demyelinating disorders, exacerbation or new onset

PRECAUTIONS & CONSIDERATIONS

Certolizumab should not be initiated in patients with an active infection, including clinically important localized infections. Weigh risks and benefits in patients (1) with chronic or recurrent infection; (2) who have been exposed to tuberculosis; (3) who have resided or traveled in areas of endemic TB or endemic mycoses, such as histoplasmosis, coccidioidomycosis, or blastomycosis with underlying conditions that may predispose them to infection. A PPD and/or chest x-ray should be obtained prior to use. Caution is warranted in patients with a history of recurrent infections and in patients on concomitant immunosuppresant agents, especially those receiving corticosteroids. Use with caution in patients with hypertension, existing history of heart failure, or other significant heart disease or in those with hepatic disease or a history of hepatitis. There are no data regarding use in pregnant women. It is unknown whether certolizumab is distributed in breast milk; discontinuation of breast-feeding is recommended. Safety and efficacy of the drug have not been established in children. Use cautiously in elderly patients.

Notify the physician of signs of infection, such as fever or sore throat, or if there are signs of allergic reaction. Monitor BP. Persons with rheumatoid arthritis should report increase in pain, stiffness, or swelling of joints. Persons with Crohn disease should report changes in stool color, consistency, abdominal complaints, or elimination pattern.

Storage
Refrigerate powder for injection and prefilled syringes in the original carton. Do not freeze. Protect from light. Once powder is reconstituted, can store in the vial in the refrigerator for up to 24 h prior to injection. Do not freeze. The syringes are glass and may break if dropped or mishandled. Inspect product before use once in solution. The solution will be clear to opalescent, colorless to pale yellow liquid and free from particulates; if cloudy or discolored or if has large particles, do not use.

Administration
For subcutaneous use only.

Reconstitute each lyophilized vial with 1 mL of sterile water for injection and a syringe with a 20-gauge needle. Gently swirl without shaking. Leave vials undisturbed; full dissolution may take as long as 30 min. Concentration will be 200 mg/mL. Let come to room temperature before injecting, but for no more than 2 h. Using a new 20-gauge needle for each vial, withdraw the reconstituted solution into a separate syringe for each vial, so that each syringe contains 1 mL. Switch to a 23-gauge (dosing) needle before administration and inject the full contents of each syringe subcutaneously into the thigh or abdomen. Where a 400-mg dose is required, separate sites should be used for each 200-mg (1-mL) injection. A patient may be taught to use the prefilled syringes.

Cetirizine

si-tear′a-zeen

Zyrtec Reactine

Do not confuse Zyrtec with Zantac or Zyprexa.

CATEGORY AND SCHEDULE

Pregnancy Risk Category: B

OTC

Classification: Antihistamines, H_1, low sedating

MECHANISM OF ACTION

A second-generation piperazine that competes with histamine for H_1-receptor sites on effector cells in the GI tract, blood vessels, and respiratory tract. *Therapeutic Effect:* Prevents allergic response, produces mild bronchodilation, and blocks histamine-induced bronchitis.

PHARMACOKINETICS

Route	Onset	Peak	Duration
PO	< 4-8 h	< 1 h	24 h

Rapidly and almost completely absorbed from the GI tract (absorption not affected by food). Protein binding: 93%. Undergoes low first-pass metabolism; not extensively metabolized. Primarily excreted in urine (more than 80% as unchanged drug). *Half-life:* 6.5-10 h.

AVAILABILITY

Oral Solution: 5 mg/5 mL.
Tablets: 5 mg, 10 mg.
Tablets (Chewable): 5 mg, 10 mg.

INDICATIONS AND DOSAGES

▸ Allergic rhinitis, urticaria

PO

Adults, Elderly, Children older than 5 yr. Initially, 5-10 mg/day as a single dose or in 2 divided doses.
Children 2-5 yr. 2.5 mg/day. May increase up to 5 mg/day as a single dose or in 2 divided doses.
Children 12-23 mo. Initially, 2.5 mg/day. May increase up to 5 mg/day in 2 divided doses.
Children 6-11 mo. 2.5 mg once a day.

▸ Dosage in renal or hepatic impairment (adults)

For creatinine clearance of 11-31 mL/min, receiving hemodialysis (creatinine clearance of < 7 mL/min), and those with hepatic impairment, dosage is decreased to 5 mg once a day.

CONTRAINDICATIONS

Hypersensitivity to cetirizine or hydroxyzine.

INTERACTIONS

Drug

Alcohol, other CNS depressants: May increase CNS depression.

Herbal

None known.

Food

None known.

C

DIAGNOSTIC TEST EFFECTS

May suppress wheal and flare reactions to antigen skin testing, unless drug is discontinued 4 days before testing.

SIDE EFFECTS

Occasional (2%-10%)

Pharyngitis; dry mucous membranes, nose, or throat; nausea and vomiting; abdominal pain; headache; dizziness; fatigue; thickening of mucus; somnolence; photosensitivity; urine retention.

SERIOUS REACTIONS

• Children may experience paradoxical reactions, including restlessness, insomnia, euphoria, nervousness, and tremor.
• Dizziness, sedation, and confusion are more likely to occur in elderly patients.

PRECAUTIONS & CONSIDERATIONS

Caution is warranted with renal or hepatic impairment. Cetirizine use is not recommended during the early months of pregnancy. It is unknown whether cetirizine is excreted in breast milk. Breastfeeding is not recommended. Cetirizine is less likely to cause anticholinergic effects in children. Elderly patients are more likely to experience anticholinergic effects, such as dry mouth and urine retention, as well as dizziness, sedation, and confusion. Avoid drinking alcoholic beverages, prolonged exposure to sunlight, and tasks that require alertness or motor skills until response to the drug is established.

Drowsiness may occur at dosages > 10 mg/day. Therapeutic response should be monitored.

Storage

All dosage forms can be stored at room temperature.

Administration

Take cetirizine without regard to food. Chewable tablets should be throughly chewed. May take chewable tablets with or without water.

Cetuximab

ceh-tux'ih-mab

Erbitux

CATEGORY AND SCHEDULE

Pregnancy Risk Category: C

Classification: Antineoplastics, monoclonal antibodies

MECHANISM OF ACTION

A monoclonal antibody that binds to the epidermal growth factor receptor (EGFR), a glycoprotein on normal and tumor cells, thus inhibiting cell growth and inducing apoptosis. *Therapeutic Effect:* Inhibits the growth and survival of tumor cells that overexpress EGFR.

PHARMACOKINETICS

Reaches steady-state levels by the third weekly infusion. Clearance decreases as dose increases. *Half-life:* 112 h (range, 63-230 h).

AVAILABILITY

Injection: 2 mg/mL.

INDICATIONS AND DOSAGES

▸ **Metastatic colorectal carcinoma, squamous cell carcinoma of the head and neck**

IV INFUSION

Adults, Elderly. Initially, 400 mg/m^2 over 2 h as a loading dose. Maintenance: 250 mg/m^2 infused over 60 min weekly.

Expect to reduce the infusion rate by 50% for infusion-related reactions and to adjust dose based on the degree (grade) of dermatologic toxicity during treatment. Serious infusion reactions may require discontinuation of treatment.

CONTRAINDICATIONS

None known.

INTERACTIONS

Drug

None known.

Herbal

None known.

Food

None known.

DIAGNOSTIC TEST EFFECTS

May decrease WBC count, magnesium, calcium, potassium, hematocrit, and hemoglobin level.

IV INCOMPATIBILITIES

Do not mix cetuximab with any other medications.

SIDE EFFECTS

Frequent (25%-90%)

Acneiform rash, malaise, fever, nausea, diarrhea, constipation, headache, abdominal pain, anorexia, vomiting.

Occasional (10%-16%)

Nail disorder, back pain, stomatitis, peripheral edema, pruritus, cough, insomnia.

Rare (5%-9%)

Weight loss, depression, dyspepsia, conjunctivitis, alopecia.

SERIOUS REACTIONS

- Anemia occurs in 10% of patients.
- A severe infusion reaction, characterized by rapid onset of airway obstruction, a precipitous drop in blood pressure, and severe urticaria, occurs rarely.
- Dermatologic toxicity, pulmonary embolus, interstitial lung disease, leukopenia, and renal failure occur rarely.
- Cardiopulmonary arrest has been reported in patients receiving cetuximab in conjunction with radiation therapy.

PRECAUTIONS & CONSIDERATIONS

Caution is warranted with hypersensitivity to murine proteins and in patients with a history of coronary artery disease, heart failure, arrhythmias, or lung disease. Cetuximab crosses the placental barrier and may cause fetal harm or spontaneous abortion. Use adequate contraception in both males and females during and for 6 mo following the last dose. Women should not breastfeed while taking cetuximab or for 2 mo after completion of treatment. The safety and efficacy of cetuximab have not been established in children. No age-related precautions have been noted in elderly patients. Vaccinations and contact with crowds, persons with a known infection, and anyone who has recently received a live-virus vaccine should be avoided. Sun exposure should be limited and sunscreen should be worn outdoors during and for 2 mo after treatment completion because sunlight can exacerbate skin reactions.

Signs and symptoms of an infusion reaction, such as rapid onset of bronchospasm, hoarseness, hypotension, stridor, and urticaria, should be monitored for at least 1 h after each infusion. The severe infusion reaction may occur during subsequent infusions. Skin should be assessed for evidence of dermatologic toxicity, such as dry skin, exfoliative

C

dermatitis or rash, and inflammatory sequelae. Electrolytes, hemoglobin levels, and hematocrit levels should be monitored.

Storage

Refrigerate vials. Do not freeze. Preparations in infusion containers are stable for up to 8 h at room temperature or 12 h if refrigerated. Discard any unused portion. The solution should appear clear and colorless; it may contain a small amount of visible white particulates.

Administration

! Premedicate the patient with 50 mg diphenhydramine IV. Cetuximab may be used as monotherapy or in combination with irinotecan. Do not give cetuximab by IV push or bolus. For IV infusion only, use a controlled rate IV pump or an IV syringe pump.

Do not shake or dilute the vials. The undiluted injection is placed either in appropriate empty IV containers or syringes prior to infusion. Affix the line and prime it with solution before starting the infusion. Administer through a low-protein-binding 0.22-μm in-line filter. Repeat until total dose is given. Use 0.9% NaCl solution to flush line at the end of infusion. Give the first dose as a 120-min IV infusion. Administer maintenance infusions over 60 min. The maximum infusion rate is 5 mL/min. When administered in conjunction with radiation therapy in head and neck carcinoma, first dose is given 1 wk before initiation of radiation therapy and maintenance therapy is administered for the duration of radiation therapy with each infusion completed 1 h before radiation. Patient should be monitored closely for 1 h after each infusion.

Cevimeline

sev-im′el-ine

★ Evoxac

Do not confuse Evoxac with Eurax or cevimeline with Savella.

CATEGORY AND SCHEDULE

Pregnancy Risk Category: C

Classification: Cholinergic (muscarinic) agonist

MECHANISM OF ACTION

A cholinergic agonist that binds to muscarinic receptors of effector cells, thereby increasing secretion of exocrine glands, such as salivary glands. *Therapeutic Effect:* Relieves dry mouth.

PHARMACOKINETICS

Rapid absorption after oral administration, peak levels 1.5-2 h. Protein binding: 20%. Metabolized in liver by CYP2D6 and CYP3A4 isoenzymes. *Half-life:* 5 h. 84% excreted in urine within 24 h.

AVAILABILITY

Capsules: 30 mg.

INDICATIONS AND DOSAGES

▸ **Dry mouth associated with Sjögren syndrome**

PO

Adults. 30 mg 3 times a day.

CONTRAINDICATIONS

Acute iritis, angle-closure glaucoma, uncontrolled asthma.

INTERACTIONS

Drug

Amiodarone, diltiazem, erythromycin, fluoxetine, itraconazole, ketoconazole,

paroxetine, quinidine, ritonavir, verapamil: May increase the effects of cevimeline.
Atropine, phenothiazines, tricyclic antidepressants: May decrease the effects of cevimeline.
β-Blockers: May increase the risk of conduction disturbances.
Herbal
None known.
Food
All foods: Decreases the absorption rate of cevimeline.

DIAGNOSTIC TEST EFFECTS
None known.

SIDE EFFECTS
Frequent (11%-19%)
Diaphoresis, headache, nausea, sinusitis, rhinitis, upper respiratory tract infection, diarrhea.
Occasional (3%-10%)
Dyspepsia, abdominal pain, cough, urinary tract infection, vomiting, back pain, rash, dizziness, fatigue.
Rare (1%-2%)
Skeletal pain, insomnia, hot flashes, excessive salivation, rigors, anxiety.

SERIOUS REACTIONS
- Cevimeline use may result in decreased visual acuity, especially at night, and impaired depth perception.

PRECAUTIONS & CONSIDERATIONS
Caution is warranted in patients with cardiovascular disease, congestive heart failure, asthma, chronic bronchitis, COPD, cholecystitis, biliary obstruction, cholelithiasis, GI ulcers, seizure disorders, Parkinson disease, urinary tract or bladder obstruction, and a history of nephrolithiasis. Avoid driving at night or performing hazardous duties in reduced lighting because cevimeline use may decrease visual acuity or impair depth perception. Adequate hydration should be maintained to prevent dehydration. Vital signs should be monitored.
Storage
Store at room temperature.
Administration
Take cevimeline without regard to food. Administration with food may decrease GI upset.

Charcoal, Activated
★ Actidose-Aqua, Actidose with Sorbitol, Aqueous Charcodote, Charcoal Plus DS, Charcocaps, EZ-Char, Liqui-Char
🍁 Aqueous Charcodote

CATEGORY AND SCHEDULE
Pregnancy Risk Category: C

Classification: Antidote

MECHANISM OF ACTION
An antidote that adsorbs (detoxifies) ingested toxic substances, irritants, intestinal gas. *Therapeutic Effect:* Inhibits GI absorption and absorbs intestinal gas.

PHARMACOKINETICS
Not orally absorbed from the GI tract. Not metabolized. Excreted in feces as charcoal. *Half-life:* Unknown.

AVAILABILITY
Capsules, Activated: 260 mg (Charcocaps).
Liquid, Activated: 15 g, 25 g, 50 g (Actidose-Aqua).
Liquid, Activated: 25 g, 50 g (Actidose with Sorbitol).
Pellets, Activated: 25 g (EZ-Char).

C

INDICATIONS AND DOSAGES

▸ **Acute poisoning**

PO ACTIDOSE SUSPENSION, EZ-CHAR

Adults, Elderly, Children 12 yr and older. Give 30-100 g as slurry (30 g in at least 8 oz H_2O) or 12.5-50 g in aqueous or sorbitol suspension. Usually given as single dose.

Children more than 1 yr and < 12 yr. 25-50 g as a single dose. Smaller doses (10-25 g) may be used in children aged 1-5 yr because of smaller gut lumen capacity.

OFF-LABEL USES

Antiflatulent, antidiarrheal (dietary supplements marketed in capsules/ tablets).

CONTRAINDICATIONS

Intestinal obstruction, GI tract that is not anatomically intact, patients at risk of hemorrhage or GI perforation. If use would increase risk and severity of aspiration; not effective for cyanide, mineral acids, caustic alkalis, organic solvents, iron, ethanol, methanol poisoning, lithium. Do not use charcoal with sorbitol in patients with fructose intolerance; charcoal with sorbitol not recommended in children younger than 1 yr of age or in persons with hypersensitivity to charcoal or any component of the formation.

INTERACTIONS

Drug

Orally administered medications: May decrease absorption of orally administered medications.

Ipecac: May decrease the effect of ipecac.

Herbal

None known.

Food

Ice cream, chocolate syrup, sherbet, marmalade, milk: May reduce the absorptive properties of charcoal.

DIAGNOSTIC TEST EFFECTS

None known.

SIDE EFFECTS

Occasional

Diarrhea, GI discomfort, intestinal gas.

SERIOUS REACTIONS

• Hypernatremia, hypokalemia, and hypermagnesemia may occur with coadministration of cathartics.

PRECAUTIONS & CONSIDERATIONS

Caution should be used with decreased peristalsis. It is unknown whether charcoal crosses the placenta or is distributed in breast milk. Safety and efficacy of charcoal have not been established in children < 1 yr old. There are no age-related precautions noted for elderly patients. Be aware that charcoal causes the stools to turn black.

Be aware that charcoal may cause vomiting, which is hazardous in petroleum distillate and caustic ingestions. Be aware that if charcoal and sorbitol are administered, doses should be limited to prevent excessive fluid and electrolyte loss.

Storage

Store at controlled room temperature. Do not freeze. Keep tightly closed.

Administration

Charcoal is most effective when administered within 1 h of ingestion for most ingestions. It is common to administer via an NG or gastric tube.

Be aware that about 10 g of activated charcoal for each 1 g of toxin is considered adequate but may require multiple doses. If sorbitol is also used, sorbitol dose should not exceed 1.5 g/kg. When using multiple doses of charcoal, sorbitol should be given with every other dose (not to exceed 2 doses/day).

Be aware that if treatment includes ipecac syrup, vomiting should be induced before administration of charcoal.

Chloral Hydrate

klor-al hye′drate

★ Somnote

🍁 Chloral Hydrate Odan

CATEGORY AND SCHEDULE

Pregnancy Risk Category: C

Controlled Substance Schedule: IV

Classification: Sedatives/hypnotics

MECHANISM OF ACTION

A nonbarbiturate chloral derivative that produces CNS depression. *Therapeutic Effect:* Induces quiet, deep sleep, with only a slight decrease in respiratory rate and BP.

PHARMACOKINETICS

Rapid absorption after oral administration, peak levels 30-45 min. Duration: 2-5 h. Metabolized to trichloroethanol in liver and other tissues and, to a lesser extent, trichloroacetic acid, in liver. Glucuronide conjugate excreted in urine. *Half-life:* 7-9.5 h.

AVAILABILITY

Capsules (Somnote): 500 mg.
Syrup: 500 mg/5 mL.
Suppositories: 500 mg.

INDICATIONS AND DOSAGES

▸ Premedication for anesthesia, medical procedures, or diagnostics, such as EEG or CT scan

PO, RECTAL

Adults. 0.5-1.5 g. Maximum: 2 g.

Children. 25-50 mg/kg/dose 30-60 min prior to event. Use PO form only. May repeat in 30 min. The total dose should not exceed 100 mg/kg or 2 g, whichever is less. Normally, do not need to exceed 1.5 g in children.

CONTRAINDICATIONS

Marked hepatic or renal impairment, hypersensitivity, or an idiosyncratic reaction to the drug.

INTERACTIONS

Drug

Alcohol, other CNS depressants: May increase the effects of chloral hydrate.

Furosemide (IV): May alter BP and cause diaphoresis if given within 24 h after chloral hydrate.

Warfarin: May increase the effect of warfarin.

Herbal

None known.

Food

None known.

DIAGNOSTIC TEST EFFECTS

None known.

SIDE EFFECTS

Occasional

Gastric irritation (nausea, vomiting, flatulence, diarrhea), rash, sleepwalking.

Rare

Headache, paradoxical CNS hyperactivity or nervousness in children, excitement or restlessness in elderly patients, particularly in patients with pain.

SERIOUS REACTIONS

- Overdose may produce somnolence, confusion, slurred speech, severe incoordination, respiratory depression, and coma.

C

PRECAUTIONS & CONSIDERATIONS

Caution is warranted in patients with clinical depression, patients with a history of drug abuse, patients with porphyria, gastritis, cardiac disease, and in neonates. Do not drive if taking chloral hydrate before a procedure. BP, pulse rate, and respiratory rate, rhythm, and depth should be assessed immediately before and during chloral hydrate use. Elderly patients should be monitored for paradoxical reactions, such as excitability.

Storage

Store suppositories at room temperature; do not refrigerate them. Store capsules and syrup at room temperature.

Administration

! Only trained health care workers (not parents or care providers) should administer this drug to children in preparation for a procedure and only AFTER the child has arrived at the facility to ensure proper monitoring of neurologic and respiratory status, and availability of resuscitation equipment in the event of respiratory depression.

! Always verify a child's mg/kg dosage to avoid serious overdose. Take chloral hydrate capsules with a full glass of water or fruit juice. Swallow the capsules whole and do not chew them. Dilute the dose of syrup in water to minimize gastric irritation. May dilute in juice to mask unpleasant taste.

For rectal use, if the suppository is too soft to insert, chill in the refrigerator for 30 min or run cold water over it before removing the foil wrapper. First remove the foil wrapper and moisten the suppository with cold water. Lie down on side and use finger to push the suppository well up into the rectum.

Chloramphenicol

klor-am-fen'i-kole

★ 🍁 Chloromycetin

Do not confuse chloramphenicol with chlorambucil.

CATEGORY AND SCHEDULE

Pregnancy Risk Category: C

Classification: Anti-infectives, ophthalmics, otics, antibiotics, chloramphenicol and derivatives

MECHANISM OF ACTION

A dichloroacetic acid derivative that inhibits bacterial protein synthesis by binding to bacterial ribosomal receptor sites. *Therapeutic Effect:* Bacteriostatic (may be bactericidal in high concentrations).

PHARMACOKINETICS

Widely distributed, crosses blood-brain barrier. Extensively metabolized to inactive metabolites, primarily via glucuronidation. *Half-life:* 1.6-3.3 h (prolonged in renal and hepatic impairment).

AVAILABILITY

Powder for Injection: 1-g vial.

INDICATIONS AND DOSAGES

▸ **Mild to moderate infections caused by organisms resistant to other less toxic antibiotics**

IV

Adults, Elderly. 50-100 mg/kg/day in divided doses q6h. Maximum: 4 g/day.

Children older than 1 mo.
50-75 mg/kg/day in divided doses q6h. Maximum: 4 g/day.

▸ **Meningitis**

IV

Adults, Children older than 1 mo.
75-100 mg/kg/day in divided doses q6h.

CONTRAINDICATIONS

Hypersensitivity to chloramphenicol. Due to toxicity risk, do not use in treatment of trivial infections or where it is not indicated, or as a prophylactic agent to prevent bacterial infections.

INTERACTIONS

Drug

Anticonvulsants, bone marrow depressants: May increase myelosuppression.
Clindamycin, erythromycin: May antagonize the effects of these drugs.
Iron supplements: May antagonize hematopoietic response to iron therapy.
Oral antidiabetics: May increase the effects of these drugs.
Phenobarbital, phenytoin, warfarin: May increase blood concentrations of these drugs.
Vitamin B_{12}: May decrease the effects of vitamin B_{12} in patients with pernicious anemia.

Herbal

None known.

Food

None known.

DIAGNOSTIC TEST EFFECTS

Therapeutic blood level: 10-20 mcg/mL; toxic blood level: > 25 mcg/mL.

IV INCOMPATIBILITIES

In general, do not mix chloramphenicol with other medications.

SIDE EFFECTS

Occasional

Systemic: Nausea, vomiting, diarrhea.

Rare

"Gray baby" syndrome in neonates (abdominal distention, blue-gray skin color, cardiovascular collapse, unresponsiveness), rash, shortness of breath, confusion, headache, optic neuritis (blurred vision, eye pain), peripheral neuritis (numbness and weakness in feet and hands).

SERIOUS REACTIONS

- Superinfection from bacterial or fungal overgrowth may occur.
- There is a narrow margin between effective therapy and toxic levels producing blood dyscrasias.
- Myelosuppression, with resulting aplastic anemia, hypoplastic anemia, and pancytopenia, may occur weeks or months later.
- Optic neuritis may cause blindness.

PRECAUTIONS & CONSIDERATIONS

Caution is warranted with myelosuppression, glucose-6-phosphate dehydrogenase deficiency, or renal or hepatic impairment and in those who have previously undergone cytotoxic drug therapy or radiation therapy. Caution should be used in children younger than 2 yr and in children of any age with impaired or immature metabolic processes, especially neonates and premature neonates.

Concurrent use of other drugs that cause myelosuppression should be determined before therapy because chloramphenicol should not be given concurrently with these drugs, if possible. Baseline blood studies should also be determined before beginning chloramphenicol therapy.

Nausea, vomiting, and visual disturbances should be reported. Pattern of daily bowel activity and stool consistency, mental status, and skin for rash should be assessed. Be alert for signs and symptoms of superinfection, such as anal or genital pruritus, a change in the oral mucosa, diarrhea, and increased fever. Know and monitor the drug's therapeutic blood level, which is

C

10-20 mcg/mL; toxic blood level is > 25 mcg/mL. Monitor complete blood counts at baseline and a minimum of every 2 days during treatment.

Storage

Store vials at room temperature.

Administration

Space drug doses evenly around the clock and continue for the full course of treatment.

Expect to change therapy to an antibiotic of less risk as soon as possible. Prepare IV injection by adding 10 mL of sterile water for injection on dextrose 5% into the 1-g vial (concentration: 100 mg/mL). Withdraw correct dose. Inject dose over at least a 1-min interval.

Chlordiazepoxide

klor-dye-az-e-pox′ide

★ Librium

🍁 Apo-Chlordiazepoxide

Do not confuse Librium with Librax.

CATEGORY AND SCHEDULE

Pregnancy Risk Category: D

Controlled Substance Schedule: IV

Classification: Anxiolytics, benzodiazepines

MECHANISM OF ACTION

A benzodiazepine that enhances the action of the inhibitory neurotransmitter γ-aminobutyric acid in the CNS. *Therapeutic Effect:* Produces anxiolytic effect.

PHARMACOKINETICS

Slow onset after oral administration, peak levels 2 h. Metabolized in liver (active metabolites). *Half-life:* 24-48 h. Metabolites excreted in urine.

AVAILABILITY

Capsules: 5 mg, 10 mg, 25 mg.

INDICATIONS AND DOSAGES

▸ **Alcohol withdrawal symptoms**

PO

Adults, Elderly. 50-100 mg. May repeat q2-4h. Maximum: 300 mg/24 h.

▸ **Anxiety**

PO

Adults. 15-100 mg/day in 3-4 divided doses.

Elderly. 5 mg 2-4 times a day.

▸ **Preoperative apprehension and anxiety**

PO

Adults. 5-10 mg 3-4 times/day on days preceding surgery.

▸ **Usual pediatric dose (anxiety)**

Children 6 yr of age and older. 5 mg 2-4 times/daily, may increase to 10 mg 2-3 times/daily.

▸ **Adjustment for renal impairment**

If creatinine clearance is less than 10 mL/min, reduce usual dose by 50%.

▸ **Adjustment for hepatic impairment**

Use with caution; drug may accumulate with repeat dosing.

CONTRAINDICATIONS

Hypersensitivity to the drug.

INTERACTIONS

Drug

Other CNS depressants: May increase CNS depression.

Herbal

Kava kava, valerian: May increase CNS depression.

Food

Alcohol: May increase CNS depression.

DIAGNOSTIC TEST EFFECTS

None known. Therapeutic serum drug level is 1-3 mcg/mL; toxic serum drug level is > 5 mcg/mL.

SIDE EFFECTS

Frequent

Somnolence, ataxia, dizziness, confusion (particularly in elderly or debilitated patients).

Occasional

Rash, peripheral edema, GI disturbances, anterograde amnesia.

Rare

Paradoxical CNS reactions, such as hyperactivity or nervousness in children and excitement or restlessness in elderly patients (generally noted during first 2 wks of therapy, particularly in presence of uncontrolled pain).

SERIOUS REACTIONS

- Abrupt or too-rapid withdrawal may result in pronounced restlessness, irritability, insomnia, hand tremors, abdominal or muscle cramps, diaphoresis, vomiting, and seizures.
- Overdosage results in somnolence, confusion, diminished reflexes, and coma.

PRECAUTIONS & CONSIDERATIONS

Caution is warranted with impaired renal or hepatic function. Caution is also warranted in patients with CNS depression or in those with severe pulmonary disease or respiratory depression. Avoid use in first trimester of pregnancy. Use during pregnancy may cause fetal harm. Use during lactation is not recommended as the drug is distributed to breast milk. Safety and effectiveness in children under the age of 6 yr have not been established. Drowsiness may occur. Change positions slowly from recumbent to sitting before standing to prevent dizziness. Alcohol and tasks that require mental alertness or motor skills should also be avoided. Autonomic responses, such as cold, clammy hands and diaphoresis, and motor responses, such as agitation, trembling, and tension, should be assessed. BP, pulse rate, and respiratory rate, rhythm, and depth should be monitored immediately before giving the drug.

Storage

Store capsules at room temperature.

Administration

Take orally without regard to meals. Do not abruptly discontinue after long-term therapy.

Chlorhexidine Gluconate

klor-hex′ih-deen gloo′ko-nate

★ 🍁 Betasept Surgical Scrub, Oro-Clense, Peridex, PerioChip, PerioGard, PerioRx, Perisol

CATEGORY AND SCHEDULE

Pregnancy Risk Category: C

Classification: Anti-infective

MECHANISM OF ACTION

An antiseptic and antimicrobial agent that is active against a broad spectrum of microbes. The chlorhexidine molecule, due to its positive charge, reacts with the microbial cell surface, destroys the integrity of the cell membrane, penetrates the cell, and precipitates the cytoplasm, and the cell dies. *Therapeutic Effect:* Causes cell death.

PHARMACOKINETICS

Initially, the chlorhexidine gluconate dental chip releases approximately 40% of the drug within the first 24 h, then releases the remainder in an almost linear fashion for 7-10 days.

Approximately 30% of the active ingredient, chlorhexidine gluconate, is retained in the oral cavity following oral rinsing. This retained drug is slowly released into the oral fluids. Poorly absorbed from the GI tract.

Primarily excreted in feces. *Half-life:* Unknown.

C

AVAILABILITY
Chip: 2.5 mg.
Oral Rinse: 0.12%.
Topical Solution: 2%, 4%.
Topical Rinse: 0.5%.
Topical Wipes: 0.5%.
Topical Sponge: 4%.

INDICATIONS AND DOSAGES
▸ **Gingivitis**
ORAL RINSE
Adults, Elderly. Swish and spit for 30 seconds twice daily.
▸ **Periodontitis**
DENTAL IMPLANT (PERIOCHIP)
Adults, Elderly. One chip is inserted into a periodontal pocket; insert a new chip q3mo; maximum of 8 chips per dental visit.
▸ **Topical cleansing of skin**
CLEANSER
Rinse with water, apply chlorhexidine and wash, rinse with water.
PREOPERATIVE SKIN PREPARATION
Apply to site and swab for 2 min. Dry with sterile towel. Repeat.

OFF-LABEL USES
Acute aphthous ulcers and denture stomatitis (dental rinse).

CONTRAINDICATIONS
Hypersensitivity to chlorhexidine gluconate or any component of the formulation.

INTERACTIONS
Drug
None known.
Herbal and Food
None known.

DIAGNOSTIC TEST EFFECTS
None known.

SIDE EFFECTS
Occasional
Oral rinse: Altered taste, staining of teeth, toothache, increased tartar on teeth.
Topical: Skin erythema and roughness, dryness, sensitization, allergic reactions.

SERIOUS REACTIONS
- Anaphylaxis has been reported.

PRECAUTIONS & CONSIDERATIONS
Oral rinse not intended for periodontitis. Avoid use of topical solution in children < 2 yr of age.
Storage
Store oral rinse, dental implant, and topical solutions at room temperature. Protect from light and freezing.
Administration
Dental implant: Avoid flossing for 10 days after chip insertion.

Dental rinse: Swish dose in mouth for 30 seconds, then expectorate. Do not rinse with water, use other mouthwashes, brush teeth, or eat immediately after using. Do not swallow the rinse.

Use topical solutions and scrubs as advised for each individual product; keep topical products out of the ears, mouth, and eyes.

Chloroquine/ Chloroquine Phosphate
klor′oh-kwin
★ Aralen
🍁 Novo-Chloroquine

CATEGORY AND SCHEDULE
Pregnancy Risk Category: C

Classification: Antimalarial, antiprotozoal

MECHANISM OF ACTION
An amebecide that concentrates in parasite acid vesicles and may interfere with parasite protein synthesis. *Therapeutic Effect:* Inhibits parasite growth.

PHARMACOKINETICS
Rate of absorption is variable. Chloroquine is almost completely absorbed from the GI tract. Protein binding: 50%-65%. Widely distributed into body tissues such as eyes, heart, kidneys, liver, and lungs. Partially metabolized to active de-ethylated metabolites (principal metabolite is desethylchloroquine). Excreted in urine. Removed by hemodialysis. *Half-life:* 1-2 mo.

AVAILABILITY
Tablets: 250 mg, 500 mg (Aralen).

INDICATIONS AND DOSAGES
▸ **Chloroquine phosphate**

Treatment of malaria (acute attack): Dose (mg base)

PO

Dose	Time	Adults (mg)	Children (mg/kg)
Initial	Day 1	600	10
Second	6 h later	300	5
Third	Day 2	300	5
Fourth	Day 3	300	5

▸ **Malaria prophylaxis**

PO

Adults. 300 mg (base)/wk on same day each week beginning 2 wks before exposure; continue for 6-8 wks after leaving endemic area.
Children. 5 mg (base)/kg/wk with start duration as for adults.

▸ **Amebiasis**

PO

Adults. 1 g (600 mg base) daily for 2 days; then 500 mg (300 mg base)/ day for at least 2-3 wks.

OFF-LABEL USES
Treatment of rheumatoid arthritis, discoid lupus erythematosus, solar urticaria.

CONTRAINDICATIONS
Hypersensitivity to 4-aminoquinoline compounds, retinal or visual field changes.

INTERACTIONS
Drug

Alcohol: May increase GI irritation.
Ampicillin: May reduce the absorption of ampicillin. Separate administration by 2 h.
Antacids and kaolin: May be decreased due to GI binding with kaolin or magnesium trisilicate.
Cimetidine: May increase levels of chloroquine.
Cyclosporine: May increase cyclosporine concentrations.
CYP2D6 inhibitors (chlorpromazine, delavirdine, fluoxetine, miconazole, paroxetine, pergolide, quinidine, quinine, ritonavir, ropinirole): May increase the levels and effects of chloroquine.
CYP2D6 substrates (amphetamines, selected β-blockers, dextromethorphan, fluoxetine, lidocaine, mirtazapine, nefazodone, paroxetine, risperidone, ritonavir, thioridazine, tricyclic antidepressants, venlafaxine): May increase the levels and effects of CYP2D6 substrates.
CYP2D6 prodrug substrates: Chloroquine may decrease the levels and effects of CYP2D6 prodrug substrates.
CYP3A4 inducers (aminoglutethimide, carbamazepine, nafcillin, nevirapine, phenobarbital, phenytoin, and rifamycins): CYP3A4 inducers may decrease the levels and effects of chloroquine.

C

CYP3A4 inhibitors (azole antifungals, ciprofloxacin, clarithromycin, diclofenac, doxycycline, erythromycin, imatinib, isoniazid, nefazodone, nicardipine, propofol, protease inhibitors, quinidine, and verapamil): May increase the levels and effects of chloroquine.
Mefloquine: May increase risk of convulsions.
Penicillamine: May increase concentration of penicillamine and increase risk of hematologic, renal, or severe skin reaction.
Praziquantel: May decrease praziquantel concentrations.
Herbal and Food
None known.

DIAGNOSTIC TEST EFFECTS

Acute decrease in hematocrit, hemoglobin, and RBC count may occur.

SIDE EFFECTS

Frequent
Mild transient headache, anorexia, nausea, vomiting.
Occasional
Visual disturbances (blurring, difficulty focusing); nervousness; fatigue; pruritus, especially of palms, soles, scalp; bleaching of hair; irritability; personality changes; diarrhea; skin eruptions.
Rare
Abdominal cramps, headache, hypotension.

SERIOUS REACTIONS

- Ocular toxicity and ototoxicity have been reported.
- Prolonged therapy: Peripheral neuritis and neuromyopathy, hypotension, ECG changes, agranulocytosis, aplastic anemia, thrombocytopenia, convulsions, psychosis.
- Overdosage includes symptoms of headache, vomiting, visual disturbance, drowsiness, convulsions, hypokalemia followed by cardiovascular collapse, and death.

PRECAUTIONS & CONSIDERATIONS

Caution is warranted with alcoholism, severe blood disorders, liver disease, neurologic disorders, auditory damage, porphyria, psoriasis, and G6PD deficiency. It is unknown whether chloroquine crosses the placenta or is distributed in breast milk. Be aware that children are especially susceptible to chloroquine effects. There are no age-related precautions noted in elderly patients.

History of allergies, especially to antibiotics, should be determined before giving chloroquine.

Visual disturbances should be reported immediately.
Storage
Store tablets at room temperature.
Administration
Chloroquine PO_4 500 mg = 300 mg base.

Give oral chloroquine with food or milk to minimize GI irritation. May mix with chocolate syrup or enclose in gelatin capsules to mask the bitter taste.

Chlorothiazide

klor-oh-thye′a-zide
★ Diuril

CATEGORY AND SCHEDULE

Pregnancy Risk Category: C

Classification: Diuretics, thiazide

MECHANISM OF ACTION

A sulfonamide derivative that acts as a thiazide diuretic and antihypertensive. As a diuretic, it blocks the reabsorption of water and the electrolytes sodium and potassium at the cortical diluting segment of the distal tubule. As an antihypertensive, it reduces plasma; extracellular fluid volume decreases peripheral vascular resistance (PVR) by direct effect on blood vessels. *Therapeutic Effect:* Promotes diuresis, reduces BP.

PHARMACOKINETICS

Poorly absorbed from the GI tract. Not metabolized. Primarily excreted unchanged in urine. Not removed by hemodialysis. *Half-life:* 45-120 min.

AVAILABILITY

Powder for Injection, Lyophilized: 0.5 g.
Oral Suspension: 250 mg/5 mL (Diuril).
Tablets: 250 mg, 500 mg.

INDICATIONS AND DOSAGES

▸ Edema, hypertension

PO

Adults. 0.5-1 g 1-2 times/day for hypertension. For edema, may give every other day or 3-5 days/wk.
Children 12 yr and older. 10-20 mg/kg/dose in divided doses q8-12h. Maximum: 2 g/day.
Children 2-12 yr. 10-20 mg/kg/day in divided doses q12-24 h; not to exceed 1 g/day.
Children 6 mo to 2 yr. 10-20 mg/kg/day in divided doses q12-24h. Maximum: 375 mg/day.
Children younger than 6 mo. 20-30 mg/kg/day in divided doses q12h. Maximum: 375 mg/day.

▸ Hypertension/edema

IV

Adults. 0.5-1 g in divided doses q12-24h. For edema, may give every other day or 3-5 days/wk.

OFF-LABEL USES

Treatment of diabetes insipidus, prevention of calcium-containing renal stones.

CONTRAINDICATIONS

Anuria, history of hypersensitivity to sulfonamides or thiazide diuretics, renal decompensation.

INTERACTIONS

Drug

Cholestyramine, colestipol: May decrease the absorption and effects of chlorothiazide.
Digoxin: May increase the risk of toxicity of digoxin caused by hypokalemia.
Lithium: May increase the risk of toxicity of lithium.
NSAIDs: May decrease the absorption and effects of chlorothiazide.
Probenecid: May increase concentrations of chlorothiazide.

Herbal

Ginkgo biloba: May increase BP.
Licorice: May increase risk of hypokalemia and decrease effectiveness of chlorothiazide.
Ma huang: May decrease hypotensive effect of chlorothiazide.
Yohimbe: May decrease effects of chlorothiazide.

Food

None known.

DIAGNOSTIC TEST EFFECTS

None known.

C

SIDE EFFECTS

Expected. Increase in urine frequency and volume.

Frequent

Potassium depletion.

Occasional

Postural hypotension, headache, GI disturbances, photosensitivity reaction, muscle spasms, alopecia, rash, urticaria.

SERIOUS REACTIONS

- Vigorous diuresis may lead to profound water loss and electrolyte depletion, resulting in hypokalemia, hyponatremia, and dehydration.
- Acute hypotensive episodes may occur.
- Hyperglycemia may be noted during prolonged therapy.
- GI upset, pancreatitis, dizziness, paresthesias, headache, blood dyscrasias, pulmonary edema, allergic pneumonitis, and dermatologic reactions occur rarely.
- Overdosage can lead to lethargy and coma without changes in electrolytes or hydration.

PRECAUTIONS & CONSIDERATIONS

Caution should be used with diabetes mellitus, electrolyte imbalance, hyperuricemia or gout, hypotension, systemic lupus erythematosus, hypercholesterolemia, impaired liver function, and severe renal disease. Chlorothiazide crosses the placenta, and a small amount is distributed in breast milk. Breastfeeding is not recommended in this patient population. Safety and efficacy of IV chlorothiazide have not been established in children and infants. Be aware that elderly patients may be more sensitive to the drug's electrolyte and hypotensive effects. Age-related renal impairment may require caution in elderly patients.

Frequency and volume of urination are expected to increase. Be aware that chlorothiazide may aggravate digitalis toxicity. Be aware that sensitivity reactions may occur with or without history of allergy or asthma. Skin should be protected from sunlight.

Hypokalemia may result in change in mental status, muscle cramps, nausea, tachycardia, tremor, vomiting, and weakness.

Hyponatremia may result in clammy and cold skin, confusion, and thirst. Be especially alert for potassium depletion in persons taking digoxin, such as cardiac arrhythmias. Foods high in potassium, such as apricots, bananas, legumes, meat, orange juice, white and sweet potatoes, and raisins, and whole grains, such as cereals, should be eaten during treatment.

Storage

Store at room temperature.

Administration

May take with food or milk if GI upset occurs, preferably with breakfast to help prevent nocturia. Shake oral suspension well before use.

Prepare injection just before each administration because chlorothiazide does not contain preservatives. Discard unused portion. Do not administer subcutaneously or intramuscularly. May be given slowly by direct IV injection or infusion. Reconstitute with 18 mL sterile water for injection for a final concentration of 28 mg/mL. For IV infusion, may add to dextrose 5% or 0.9% NaCl injection solutions.

Chlorpheniramine

klor-fen-ir'a-meen

★ Aller-Chlor, Chlor-Trimeton, Chlor-Trimeton Allergy, Chlor-Trimeton Allergy 12 Hour, Diabetic Tussin Allergy Relief, TanaHist-PD 🍁 Chlor-Tripolon, Novo-Pheniran

Do not confuse with chlorpromazine or chlorpropamide.

CATEGORY AND SCHEDULE

Pregnancy Risk Category: C

OTC (tablets, syrup)

Classification: Antihistamines, H_1, sedating

MECHANISM OF ACTION

A propylamine derivative antihistamine that competes with histamine for histamine receptor sites on cells in the blood vessels, GI tract, and respiratory tract. *Therapeutic Effect:* Inhibits symptoms associated with seasonal allergic rhinitis such as increased mucus production and sneezing.

PHARMACOKINETICS

Well absorbed after PO administration. Food delays absorption. Widely distributed. Metabolized in liver. Primarily excreted in urine. Not removed by dialysis. *Half-life:* 20 h.

AVAILABILITY

Syrup: 2 mg/5 mL (Aller-Chlor, Diabetic Tussin Allergy Relief [sugar free]).
Tablets: 4 mg (Aller-Chlor, Chlor-Trimeton).
Tablets (Sustained Release): 12 mg (Chlor-Trimeton Allergy 12 Hour).
Capsules (Extended Release): 8 mg.
Suspension: 8 mg/5 mL.
Oral Drops Suspension: 2 mg/mL.

INDICATIONS AND DOSAGES

▸ **Allergic rhinitis, common cold**

PO

Adults, Elderly. 4 mg q6-8h, or 8-12 mg (sustained release) q8-12h, or 16 mg (sustained release) q24h. Maximum: 24 mg/day.
Children 12 yr and older. 4 mg q6-8h or 8 mg (sustained release) q12h. Maximum: 24 mg/day.
Children 6-11 yr. 2 mg q4-6h. Maximum: 12 mg/day.

CONTRAINDICATIONS

Hypersensitivity to chlorpheniramine or its components; MAOI therapy; breastfeeding; newborn or premature infants.

INTERACTIONS

Drug

Alcohol, central nervous system (CNS) depressants: May increase CNS depressant effects.
Anticholinergics: May increase anticholinergic effects.
MAOIs: May increase anticholinergic and CNS depressant effects.
Phenytoin, fosphenytoin: May increase the risk of phenytoin toxicity.
Procarbazine: May increase CNS depressant effects.

Herbal and Food

None known.

DIAGNOSTIC TEST EFFECTS

None known.

SIDE EFFECTS

Frequent

Drowsiness; dizziness; muscular weakness; hypotension; dry mouth, nose, throat, and lips; urinary

retention; thickening of bronchial secretions.
Elderly: Sedation, dizziness, hypotension.
Occasional
Epigastric distress, flushing, visual or hearing disturbances, paresthesia, diaphoresis, chills.

SERIOUS REACTIONS

- Children may experience dominant paradoxical reactions, including restlessness, insomnia, euphoria, nervousness, and tremors.
- Overdosage in children may result in hallucinations, seizures, and death.
- Hypersensitivity reactions, such as eczema, pruritus, rash, cardiac disturbances, and photosensitivity, may occur.
- Overdosage may vary from CNS depression, including sedation, apnea, hypotension, cardiovascular collapse, and death, to severe paradoxical reaction, such as hallucinations, tremor, and seizures.

PRECAUTIONS & CONSIDERATIONS

Caution is warranted with asthma, cardiovascular disease, chronic obstructive pulmonary disease (COPD), hypertension, hyperthyroidism, narrow-angle glaucoma, increased intraocular pressure (IOP), peptic ulcer disease, prostatic hypertrophy, pyloroduodenal or bladder neck obstruction, and seizure disorders. It is unknown whether chlorpheniramine crosses the placenta or is detected in breast milk. Be aware that chlorpheniramine use is not recommended in newborns or premature infants since these groups are at an increased risk of experiencing paradoxical reaction. Be aware that elderly patients are at an increased risk of developing confusion, dizziness, hyperexcitability, hypotension, and sedation.

Dizziness, drowsiness, and dry mouth are expected side effects. Tasks that require mental alertness or motor skills should be avoided. Tolerance to the drug's sedative effects can occur.
Storage
Store at room temperature.
Administration
Give oral chlorpheniramine without regard to meals. Do not crush, break, or chew sustained-release tablets. Shake suspensions well before use.

Chlorpromazine

klor-proe′ma-zeen
Do not confuse chlorpromazine with chlorpropamide, clomipramine, or prochlorperazine.

CATEGORY AND SCHEDULE

Pregnancy Risk Category: C

Classification: Phenothiazine, antiemetic, antipsychotic

MECHANISM OF ACTION

A phenothiazine that blocks dopamine neurotransmission at postsynaptic dopamine receptor sites. Possesses strong anticholinergic, sedative, and antiemetic effects; moderate extrapyramidal effects; and slight antihistamine action. *Therapeutic Effect:* Relieves nausea and vomiting; improves psychotic conditions; controls intractable hiccups and porphyria.

PHARMACOKINETICS

Rapidly absorbed after oral or IM administration. Protein binding: 92%-97%. Metabolized in the liver. Excreted in urine. *Half-life:* 6 h.

AVAILABILITY

Tablets: 10 mg, 25 mg, 50 mg, 100 mg, 200 mg.
Injection: 25 mg/mL.

INDICATIONS AND DOSAGES

▸ **Severe nausea or vomiting**

PO

Adults, Elderly. 10-25 mg q4-6h.
Children. 0.55 mg/kg q4-6h.

IM

Adults, Elderly. 25 mg; may repeat 25-50 mg q3-4h as needed until vomiting stops. Then switch to oral dosage.
Children. 0.55 mg/kg q6-8h.

▸ **Psychotic disorders**

PO

Adults, Elderly. 75-800 mg/day 3-4 divided doses.
Children older than 6 mo. 0.55 mg/kg q4-6h.

IM, IV

Adults, Elderly. Initially, 25 mg; may repeat in 1-4 h. May gradually increase to 400 mg q4-6h. Maximum: 300-800 mg/day.
Children older than 6 mo. 0.5-1 mg/kg q6-8h. Maximum: 75 mg/day for children 5-12 yr; 40 mg/day for children younger than 5 yr.

▸ **Intractable hiccups**

PO, IM, Or IV

Adults. 25-50 mg PO 3 times a day. If symptoms persist after 2-3 days, try a single 25-50 mg IM or IV dose.

▸ **Acute intermittent porphyria**

PO

Adults. 25-50 mg 3-4 times a day.

IM

Adults, Elderly. 25 mg 3-4 times a day.

▸ **Preoperative apprehension and anxiety**

PO

Adults. 25-50 mg, single dose 2-3 h before surgery.
Children. 0.5 mg/kg, single dose 2-3 h before surgery.

▸ **Tetanus**

IM Or IV

Adults: 25-50 mg 3-4 times/day; in conjunction with barbiturates.
Children: 0.55 mg/kg q6-8h. If <23 kg, do not exceed 40 mg/day. If 23-45 kg, do not exceed 75 mg/day.

OFF-LABEL USES

Symptomatic treatment of Huntington disease.

CONTRAINDICATIONS

Comatose states and hypersensitivity to phenothiazine. Do not use in the presence of large amounts of CNS depressants (alcohol, barbiturates, narcotics, etc.).

INTERACTIONS

Drug

Alcohol, other CNS depressants: May increase respiratory depression and the hypotensive effects of chlorpromazine.
Extrapyramidal symptom-producing medications (e.g., metoclopramide): Increased risk of extrapyramidal symptoms.
Hypotensives: May increase hypotension. May counteract guanethidine and related drugs.
Levodopa: May decrease the effects of levodopa.
Lithium: May decrease the absorption of chlorpromazine and produce adverse neurologic effects.
MAOIs, tricyclic antidepressants: May increase the anticholinergic and sedative effects of chlorpromazine.
Metrizamide: Discontinue phenothiazine 48 h before myelography and do not start until 24 h after, due to seizure risk.

C

QT-prolonging drugs: May have additive effect on QT interval.
Warfarin: Effectiveness of warfarin may be decreased; monitor INR.
Herbal
None known.
Food
None known.

DIAGNOSTIC TEST EFFECTS

May produce false-positive pregnancy and phenylketonuria (PKU) test results. May cause ECG changes, including Q- and T-wave disturbances. Therapeutic serum drug level is 50-300 mcg/mL; toxic serum drug level is > 750 mcg/mL.

SIDE EFFECTS

Frequent
Somnolence, blurred vision, hypotension, color vision or night vision disturbances, dizziness, decreased sweating, constipation, dry mouth, nasal congestion.
Occasional
Urinary retention, photosensitivity, rash, decreased sexual function, swelling or pain in breasts, weight gain, nausea, vomiting, abdominal pain, tremors.

SERIOUS REACTIONS

- Extrapyramidal symptoms appear to be dose related and are divided into three categories: akathisia (including inability to sit still, tapping of feet), parkinsonian symptoms (such as mask-like face, tremors, shuffling gait, hypersalivation), and acute dystonias (including torticollis, opisthotonos, and oculogyric crisis). A dystonic reaction may also produce diaphoresis and pallor.
- Tardive dyskinesia, including tongue protrusion, puffing of the cheeks, and puckering of the mouth, is a rare reaction that may be irreversible.
- Abrupt discontinuation after long-term therapy may precipitate nausea, vomiting, gastritis, dizziness, and tremors.
- Blood dyscrasias, particularly agranulocytosis and mild leukopenia, may occur.
- Chlorpromazine may lower the seizure threshold.

PRECAUTIONS & CONSIDERATIONS

Possible risk factors for leukopenia/neutropenia include preexisting low WBC or history of drug-induced neutropenia. Monitor CBC frequently during the first few months of therapy. The injection contains sodium metabisulfite and sodium sulfite, sulfites that may cause allergic-type reactions in those with sulfite sensitivity. Safety in pregnancy has not been established, and there is evidence for excretion into breast milk. Use with caution in children less than 12 yr of age.

Caution is warranted with alcoholism; glaucoma; history of seizures; hypocalcemia (increases susceptibility to dystonias); impaired cardiac, hepatic, renal, or respiratory function; benign prostatic hyperplasia; and urine retention. Increased mortality has been observed in elderly patients with dementia-related psychosis treated with antipsychotics. Alcohol, tasks that require mental alertness or motor skills, and excessive exposure to sunlight and heat should be avoided. Skin should not come in contact with the injection solution because it can cause contact dermatitis.

Drowsiness may occur, and urine may darken. Notify the physician of visual disturbances. CBC, calcium, hydration status, and skin should

be assessed. Be alert for signs of neutropenia (fever), movement disorders, or hypotension.
Storage
All products should be stored at room temperature. Do not freeze. A slight yellow color to injection is acceptable.
Administration
! Do not give chlorpromazine by the subcutaneous route because severe tissue necrosis may occur.

For IM use, to prevent irritation at the injection site, dilute the injection solution with sodium chloride for injection or add 2% procaine, as prescribed. Inject IM slowly deep into upper outer quadrant of buttock; keep point recumbent for at least 30 min after injection.
! The IV route is reserved for severe hiccups, tetanus, and surgery. Never administer IV undiluted; the drug is given as an IV infusion diluted in 0.9% NaCl injection to a final concentration of at least 1 mg/mL and infused no faster than 1 mg/min (adults) or 0.5 mg/min (children). The patient should be supine and carefully monitored for hypotension before and after the infusion.

Give oral tablets with food, milk, or a full glass of water to minimize GI irritation.

Chlorpropamide

klor-pro′pa-mide
Do not confuse with chlorpromazine.

CATEGORY AND SCHEDULE

Pregnancy Risk Category: C

Classification: Antidiabetic agents, sulfonylureas, first generation

MECHANISM OF ACTION

A first-generation sulfonylurea that promotes release of insulin from β cells of pancreas. *Therapeutic Effect:* Lowers blood glucose concentration.

PHARMACOKINETICS

Rapidly absorbed from the gastrointestinal (GI) tract. Protein binding: 60%-90%. Extensively metabolized in liver. Drugs and metabolites excreted primarily in urine. Removed by hemodialysis. *Half-life:* 30-62 h.

AVAILABILITY

Tablets: 100 mg, 250 mg.

INDICATIONS AND DOSAGES

▸ **Diabetes mellitus, type 2**
PO
Adults. Initially, 250 mg once a day. Maintenance: 250-500 mg once a day. Maximum: 750 mg/day.
Elderly. Initially, 100-125 mg once a day. Maintenance: 100-250 mg once a day. Increase or decrease by 50-125 mg/day at 3- to 5-day intervals.
▸ **Renal function impairment**
Creatinine clearance 50-80 mL/min: Reduce dosage by 50%.
Creatinine clearance is less than 50 mL/min: do not use.

OFF-LABEL USES

Neurogenic diabetes insipidus.

CONTRAINDICATIONS

Diabetic complications, such as ketosis, acidosis, and diabetic coma, severe liver or renal impairment, therapy for type 1 diabetes mellitus, or hypersensitivity to sulfonylureas.

INTERACTIONS

Drug
Alcohol: Disulfiram-like reactions may occur. Symptoms of low blood sugar, including sweating, shaking,

weakness, drowsiness, and trouble concentrating, will occur.
β-Blockers, MAOIs, NSAIDs, salicylates: May increase hypoglycemic effect.
Fluoroquinolone antibiotics: May increase the risk of hypoglycemia.
Glucocorticoids, thiazide diuretics: May increase blood glucose.
Oral contraceptives: May increase blood glucose.
Herbal
Bitter melon: May increase the risk of hypoglycemia.
St. John's wort: May increase the risk of hypoglycemia.
Food
None known.

DIAGNOSTIC TEST EFFECTS
None known.

SIDE EFFECTS
Frequent
Headache, upper respiratory tract infection.
Occasional
Sinusitis, myalgia (muscle aches), pharyngitis, aggravated diabetes mellitus.

SERIOUS REACTIONS
- Possible increased risk of cardiovascular mortality with this class of drugs.
- Overdosage can cause severe hypoglycemia prolonged by extended half-life.

PRECAUTIONS & CONSIDERATIONS
Caution is necessary with elderly patients and those with liver function impairment. Chlorpropamide should be avoided in elderly patients because of the high risk of hypoglycemia. Blood glucose should be checked before giving chlorpropamide. Chlorpropamide crosses the placenta and is distributed in breast milk and is not recommended in pregnant or breastfeeding women. Abdominal or chest pain, dark urine or light stool, hypoglycemic reactions, fever, nausea, palpitations, rash, vomiting, or yellowing of the eyes or skin should be reported immediately.

Be alert to conditions that alter blood glucose requirements, such as fever, increased activity, stress, or a surgical procedure. Hypoglycemia, such as anxiety, cool, wet skin, diplopia, dizziness, headache, hunger, numbness in mouth, tachycardia, and tremors, and hyperglycemia, including deep, rapid breathing, dim vision, fatigue, nausea, polydipsia, polyphagia, polyuria, and vomiting, can occur. Blood glucose levels, hemoglobin levels, and liver function tests should be monitored during therapy. Because of the long half-life of chlorpropamide, hypoglycemia may be prolonged. Careful monitoring and frequent feedings may be required for several days. Candy or a source of glucose for immediate response to hypoglycemia should be carried.
Storage
Store at room temperature in a well-closed container.
Administration
Give chlorpropamide with or without regard to meals. Usually given in the morning with breakfast.

Chlorthalidone
klor-thal'i-doan
★ Thalitone
🍁 Apo-Chlorthalidone

CATEGORY AND SCHEDULE
Pregnancy Risk Category: B

Classification: Antihypertensive agents, diuretics, thiazide, and derivatives

MECHANISM OF ACTION
A thiazide diuretic that blocks reabsorption of sodium, potassium, and water at the distal convoluted tubule; also decreases plasma and extracellular fluid volume and peripheral vascular resistance. *Therapeutic Effect:* Produces diuresis; lowers BP.

PHARMACOKINETICS

Route	Onset	Peak	Duration
PO (diuretic)	2 h	2-6 h	Up to 36 h

Rapidly absorbed from the GI tract. Excreted unchanged in urine. *Half-life:* 35-50 h. Onset of antihypertensive effect: 3-4 days. *Optimal Therapeutic Effect:* 3-4 wks.

AVAILABILITY
Tablets: 15 mg, 25 mg, 50 mg, 100 mg.

INDICATIONS AND DOSAGES
▸ **Hypertension**

PO

Adults. Initially 15-25 mg once daily; may increase to 45-50 mg once daily. Titrate as needed. Maximum: 100 mg/day.

▸ **Edema**

PO

Adults. Initially 50-100 mg once daily or 100 mg on alternate days. Some patients may require increase to 150 mg/day or every other day. Maximum: 200 mg/day.

CONTRAINDICATIONS
Anuria, history of hypersensitivity to sulfonamides or thiazide diuretics, renal decompensation.

INTERACTIONS
Drug

Cholestyramine, colestipol: May decrease the absorption and effects of chlorthalidone.

Digoxin: May increase the risk of digoxin toxicity associated with chlorthalidone-induced hyperkalemia.

Lithium: May increase the risk of lithium toxicity.

Herbal

None known.

Food

None known.

DIAGNOSTIC TEST EFFECTS
May increase blood glucose and serum cholesterol, LDL, bilirubin, calcium, creatinine, uric acid, and triglyceride levels. May decrease urinary calcium and serum magnesium, potassium, and sodium levels.

SIDE EFFECTS
Expected

Increase in urinary frequency and urine volume.

Frequent

Potassium depletion (rarely produces symptoms).

Occasional

Anorexia, impotence, diarrhea, orthostatic hypotension, GI disturbances, photosensitivity.

Rare

Rash.

SERIOUS REACTIONS
- Vigorous diuresis may lead to profound water and electrolyte depletion, resulting in hypokalemia, hyponatremia, and dehydration.
- Acute hypotensive episodes may occur.
- Hyperglycemia may occur during prolonged therapy.
- Overdose can lead to lethargy and coma without changes in electrolytes or hydration.

PRECAUTIONS & CONSIDERATIONS
Caution is warranted with diabetes mellitus, gout, hypercholesterolemia, hepatic

impairment, and severe renal disease and in elderly and debilitated patients. Chlorthalidone crosses the placenta, and a small amount is distributed in breast milk. Breastfeeding is not recommended for patients taking this drug. Safety and efficacy have not been established in children. Elderly patients may be more sensitive to the drug's hypotensive and electrolyte effects. Consuming foods high in potassium, such as apricots, bananas, legumes, white and sweet potatoes, meat, orange juice, and raisins, and whole grains, including cereals, and is encouraged. Avoid prolonged exposure to sunlight.

Dizziness or light-headedness may occur, so change positions slowly to reduce the drug's hypotensive effect. An increase in the frequency and volume of urination may also occur. BP, vital signs, electrolytes, intake and output, and weight should be monitored before and during treatment. Blood glucose levels should be checked after prolonged therapy, because hyperglycemia may occur. Be aware of the signs of electrolyte disturbances, such as hypokalemia. Hypokalemia may cause arrhythmias, altered mental status, muscle cramps, asthenia, and tremor.

Storage

Store at room temperature in a well-closed container. Protect from light.

Administration

Take chlorthalidone with food or milk, preferably with breakfast to help prevent nocturia. Crush tablets if needed.

Chlorzoxazone

klor-zox'a-zone

★ Parafon Forte DSC, Relax-DS

Do not confuse with chlorthalidone.

CATEGORY AND SCHEDULE

Pregnancy Risk Category: C

Classification: Skeletal muscle relaxant, centrally acting

MECHANISM OF ACTION

A skeletal muscle relaxant that inhibits transmission of reflexes at the spinal cord level. *Therapeutic Effect:* Relieves muscle spasticity.

PHARMACOKINETICS

Readily absorbed from the GI tract. Metabolized in liver. Primarily excreted in urine. *Half-life:* 1.1 h.

AVAILABILITY

Tablets: 500 mg.

INDICATIONS AND DOSAGES

▸ **Musculoskeletal pain**

PO

Adults, Elderly. 250-500 mg 3-4 times/day. Maximum: 750 mg 3-4 times/day.

CONTRAINDICATIONS

Hypersensitivity to chlorzoxazone or any one of its components.

INTERACTIONS

Drug

Alcohol CNS depressants: May increase CNS depression.

Herbal

Garlic: May inhibit metabolism of chlorzoxazone.

Kava kava: May increase CNS depression.

St. John's wort: May decrease the effectiveness of chlorzoxazone.
Food
None known.

DIAGNOSTIC TEST EFFECTS
False-positive for serum aprobarbital when using Toxi-Lab Screen. May cause elevated LFTs.

SIDE EFFECTS
Frequent
Drowsiness, fever, headache.
Occasional
Nausea, vomiting, stomach cramps, rash.

SERIOUS REACTIONS
- Overdosage results in nausea, vomiting, diarrhea, and hypotension.
- Serious hepatocellular toxicity has been reported rarely; it is idiosyncratic and unpredictable. Report early signs/symptoms such as anorexia, nausea, vomiting, right upper quadrant pain, dark urine, or jaundice. Discontinue drug immediately.

PRECAUTIONS & CONSIDERATIONS
Caution is necessary with liver impairment. Blood counts and liver and renal function tests should be performed periodically for those on long-term therapy. There is an increased risk of CNS toxicity, manifested as confusion, hallucinations, mental depression, and sedation in elderly patients.

Drowsiness may occur during treatment but usually diminishes with continued therapy. Tasks that require mental alertness or motor skills should be avoided until response to drug is established. Alcohol and CNS depressants should be avoided.
Storage
Store at room temperature.
Administration
Take without regard to meals. Scored tablets may be divided.

Cholestyramine Resin
koe-less-tir′a-meen
★ Prevalite, Questran, Questran Lite 🍁 Olestyr

CATEGORY AND SCHEDULE
Pregnancy Risk Category: B

Classification: Antihyperlipidemics, bile acid sequestrants

MECHANISM OF ACTION
An antihyperlipoproteinemic that binds with bile acids in the intestine, forming an insoluble complex. Binding results in partial removal of bile acid from enterohepatic circulation. *Therapeutic Effect:* Removes LDL cholesterol from plasma.

PHARMACOKINETICS
Not absorbed from the GI tract. Decreases in serum LDL apparent in 5-7 days and in serum cholesterol in 1 mo. Serum cholesterol returns to baseline levels about 1 mo after drug is discontinued.

AVAILABILITY
Powder for Oral Suspension: 4 g.

INDICATIONS AND DOSAGES
▸ **Primary hypercholesterolemia**
PO
Adults, Elderly. 3-4 g 3-4 times a day. Maximum: 24 g/day in 2-4 divided doses.

Children older than 10 yr. 2 g/day. Maximum: 8 g/day in 2 or more divided doses.

▸ **Pruritis associated with biliary stasis**

PO

Adults, Elderly. 4 g 1-2 times a day. Maintenance: Up to 16 g/day in divided doses.

OFF-LABEL USES

Treatment of diarrhea (due to bile acids), hyperoxaluria.

CONTRAINDICATIONS

Complete biliary obstruction, hypersensitivity to cholestyramine or tartrazine.

INTERACTIONS

Drug

NOTE: To minimize drug interactions, given other drugs at least 1 h before or at least 4-6 h after cholestyramine.

Anticoagulants: May increase effects of these drugs by decreasing level of vitamin K.

Digoxin, folic acid, penicillins, propranolol, tetracyclines, thiazides, thyroid hormones, other medications: May bind and decrease absorption of these drugs.

Oral vancomycin: Binds and decreases the effects of oral vancomycin.

Warfarin: May decrease warfarin absorption.

Herbal

None known.

Food

Vitamins A, D, E, K: Cholestyramine may interfere with absorption.

DIAGNOSTIC TEST EFFECTS

May increase serum alkaline phosphatase, serum magnesium, AST (SGOT), and ALT (SGPT) levels. May decrease serum calcium, potassium, and sodium levels. May prolong prothrombin time.

SIDE EFFECTS

Frequent

Constipation (may lead to fecal impaction), nausea, vomiting, abdominal pain, indigestion.

Occasional

Diarrhea, belching, bloating, headache, dizziness.

Rare

Gallstones, peptic ulcer disease, malabsorption syndrome. Sipping or holding the resin suspension in the mouth for prolonged periods may cause tooth discoloration, erosion of enamel or decay; maintain good oral hygiene.

SERIOUS REACTIONS

- GI tract obstruction, hyperchloremic acidosis, and osteoporosis secondary to calcium excretion may occur.
- High dosage may interfere with fat absorption, resulting in steatorrhea.

PRECAUTIONS & CONSIDERATIONS

Caution is warranted with bleeding disorders, GI dysfunction (especially constipation), hemorrhoids, and osteoporosis. Cholestyramine is not systemically absorbed and may interfere with maternal absorption of fat-soluble vitamins. Phenylketonurics should not use light formulations, which contain phenylalanine. No age-related precautions have been noted in children. Cholestyramine use is limited in children younger than 10 yr of age. Elderly patients are at increased risk for experiencing adverse nutritional effects and GI side effects.

Notify the physician of abdominal discomfort, flatulence, and food intolerance. Pattern of daily bowel activity and stool consistency should be assessed. High-fiber foods, such as fruits, whole grain cereals, and vegetables, will reduce the risk of constipation. History of hypersensitivity to aspirin, cholestyramine, and tartrazine should be determined before beginning cholestyramine therapy. Serum cholesterol and triglyceride levels should be checked at baseline and periodically thereafter.

Storage

Store powder at room temperature in a well-closed container.

Administration

Do not take cholestyramine in its dry form because it is highly irritating and may cause choking. Place the dose in a glass or cup. Mix with 2-6 oz noncarbonated fruit juice, milk, or water. Mix thoroughly. May also mix with highly fluid soups or pulpy fruits with a high moisutre content such as applesauce or crushed pineapple. Usually take at mealtimes, but may adjust time to avoid drug interactions.

Choline Magnesium Trisalicylate

koe′leen mag-nees′ee-um tri-sal′eh-cye′late

CATEGORY AND SCHEDULE

Pregnancy Risk Category: C (D if full dose used in third trimester of pregnancy)

Classification: Analgesics, nonnarcotic, salicylates

MECHANISM OF ACTION

A nonsteroidal salicylate that inhibits prostaglandin synthesis and acts on the hypothalamus heat-regulating center. *Therapeutic Effect:* Reduces inflammatory response and intensity of pain stimulus reaching sensory nerve endings.

PHARMACOKINETICS

Rapidly absorbed from the GI tract. Oral route onset 1 h, peak 2 h, and duration 9-17 h. Protein binding: High. Widely distributed. Excreted in the urine. *Half-life:* 2-3 h.

AVAILABILITY

Tablets: 500 mg, 750 mg, 1000 mg.
Liquid: 500 mg/5 mL.

INDICATIONS AND DOSAGES

▸ **Osteoarthritis, rheumatoid arthritis, analgesia, antipyretic, anti-inflammatory**

PO

Adults, Elderly. Initially, 500-1500 mg q8-12h or 3g at bedtime.
Children weighing < 37 kg. 50 mg/kg/day in divided doses.

CONTRAINDICATIONS

History of hypersensitivity to choline magnesium trisalicylate, aspirin, or other salicylates.

INTERACTIONS

Drug

Alcohol, NSAIDs: May increase the risk of adverse GI effects, including ulceration and GI bleeding. Concurrent use with other salicylates may cause salicylate toxicity.
Antacids, urinary alkalinizers: Increase the excretion of choline magnesium trisalicylate.
Anticoagulants, heparin, thrombolytics: Increase the risk of bleeding.
Methotrexate: Salicylates inhibit renal methotrexate excretion.
Sulfonylureas: Enhanced hypoglycemic effect.
Platelet aggregation inhibitors, valproic acid: May increase the risk of bleeding.

C

Probenecid: May decrease the effect of these drugs.
Herbal
Cat's claw, dong quai, evening primrose, feverfew, garlic, ginger, ginkgo, red clover, horse chestnut, green tea, ginseng: May increase the risk of bleeding.
Food
Curry powder, paprika, licorice, Benedictine liqueur, prunes, raisins, tea, gherkins: May increase the risk of salicylate accumulation.

DIAGNOSTIC TEST EFFECTS

Free T4 values may be increased due to competitive plasma protein binding; may see a concurrent decrease in total plasma T4. Thyroid function is not affected. *Plasma salicylate therapeutic level*: 150-300 mcg/mL. Toxic level > 300 mcg/mL.

SIDE EFFECTS

Occasional
Nausea, dyspepsia (heartburn, indigestion, epigastric pain), tinnitus.
Rare
Anorexia, headache, vomiting, flatulence, dizziness, somnolence, insomnia, fatigue, hearing impairment.

SERIOUS REACTIONS

- High doses may produce GI bleeding.
- Overdosage may be characterized by ringing in ears, generalized pruritus (may be severe), headache, dizziness, flushing, tachycardia, hyperventilation, sweating, and thirst.

PRECAUTIONS & CONSIDERATIONS

Caution should be used with dehydration, erosive gastritis, peptic ulcer disease, and chronic renal insufficiency. Caution is also warranted in children with acute viral febrile illness because choline magnesium trisalicylate increases the risk of developing Reye syndrome. Choline magnesium trisalicylate crosses the placenta and is distributed in breast milk. It should be avoided during the last trimester of pregnancy because the drug may adversely affect the fetal cardiovascular system, causing premature closure of ductus arteriosus. Lower choline magnesium trisalicylate dosages are recommended in elderly patients because this age group may be more susceptible to toxicity.
Storage
Store all products at room temperature.
Administration
Take choline magnesium trisalicylate with meals to avoid GI upset. Liquid may be mixed with fruit juice or water just before drinking.

Ciclesonide

Sye-kles′oh-nide
Alvesco, Omnaris

CATEGORY AND SCHEDULE

Pregnancy Risk Category: C

Classification: Respiratory agent, anti-inflammatory, corticosteroid

MECHANISM OF ACTION

Corticosteroid prodrug, activated by esterases in the respiratory tract, to active des-ciclesonide. Des-ciclesonide is a glucocorticoid that inhibits the accumulation of inflammatory cells and decreases and prevents tissues from responding to the inflammatory process. *Therapeutic*

Effect: Inhalation: Inhibits bronchoconstriction, produces smooth muscle relaxation, decreases mucus secretion. Intranasal: Decreases response to seasonal and perennial allergies.

PHARMACOKINETICS

Oral bioavailability < 1%; extensive first-pass metabolism. Primarily excreted in the feces. *Half-life:* 0.71 h ciclesonide; 6-7 h des-ciclesonide.

AVAILABILITY

Nasal Spray: 50 mcg per spray.
Inhalation Aerosol: 80 mcg per actuation, 160 mcg per actuation.

INDICATIONS AND DOSAGES

▸ **Maintenance treatment of asthma**
ORAL INHALATION
Adults, Elderly, Children 12 yr and older. Starting dose 80 mcg twice daily in patients previously treated with bronchodilators alone or previously treated with another inhaled corticosteroid, with titration as needed. Lowest effective dose should be used. Maximum recommended dose is 160 mcg twice daily in patients previously treated with bronchodilators alone and 320 mcg twice daily in patients previouly treated with inhaled corticosteroids. In patients receiving oral corticosteroids, ciclesonide dose is 320 mcg twice daily.

▸ **Perennial allergic rhinitis**
INTRANASAL
Adults, Elderly, Children 12 yr and older. 200 mcg per day administered as two 50-mcg sprays per nostril once daily.

▸ **Seasonal allergic rhinitis**
INTRANASAL
Adults, Elderly, Children 6 yr and older. 200 mcg per day administered as two 50-mcg sprays per nostril once daily.

CONTRAINDICATIONS

Hypersensitivity to ciclesonide or any of the product ingredients, status asthmaticus (inhaled).

INTERACTIONS

Drug
Ketoconazole: May increase concentrations of des-ciclesonide.
Herbal
None known.
Food
None known.

DIAGNOSTIC TEST EFFECTS

None known.

SIDE EFFECTS

Frequent (> 3%)
Oral inhalation: Headache, nasopharyngitis, sinusitis, pharyngolaryngeal pain, upper respiratory infection, arthralgia, nasal congestion, pain in extremity, back pain.
Nasal: Headache, epistaxis, nasopharyngitis, pharyngolaryngeal pain.
Occasional
Nasal: ear pain.

SERIOUS REACTIONS

- An acute hypersensitivity reaction, as evidenced by urticaria, angioedema, and severe bronchospasm, occurs rarely.
- A transfer from systemic to local steroid therapy may unmask previously suppressed bronchial asthma condition.
- Potential adrenal insufficiency if used to replace systemic corticosteroid.
- Signs and symptoms of hypercorticism.
- Nasal septal perforation has been reported in association with nasal corticosteroid use.

C

PRECAUTIONS & CONSIDERATIONS

Caution is warranted for patients with glaucoma, hypothyroidism, osteoporosis, tuberculosis, and untreated systemic infections. Avoid nasal corticosteroid use in patients with recent nasal septal ulcers, nasal surgery, or nasal trauma until healing has occurred. It is unknown whether ciclesonide or des-ciclesonide crosses the placenta or is distributed in breast milk. In children, prolonged treatment and high doses may decrease cortisol secretion and the short-term growth rate. Safety and effectiveness have not been established in children under the age of 12 yr for the inhalation or under the age of 6 yr for the nasal spray. No age-related precautions have been noted in elderly patients.

Those receiving by inhalation should maintain fastidious oral hygiene; notify the physician or nurse if sore throat or mouth develops. Those using intranasally should notify the physician if nasal irritation occurs or if symptoms, such as sneezing, fail to improve. Persons who are using drugs that suppress the immune system are more susceptible to infections than healthy individuals.

Storage

Store at room temperature. Discard inhaler when dose indicator displays zero. Discard nasal spray after 120 sprays after initial priming or 4 mo after removal from the foil pouch.

Administration

For inhalation, prime before first use and when not used for more than 10 days by actuating 3 times. If also using a bronchodilator inhaler, use the bronchodilator several minutes before using ciclesonide to help the steroid penetrate into the bronchial tree. Exhale completely and place the mouthpiece between the lips. Inhale and hold breath for as long as possible before exhaling. If more than one inhalation is necessary, allow at least 1 min between inhalations. Rinse mouth after each use to decrease dry mouth and hoarseness and prevent fungal infection of the mouth.

For intranasal use, clear nasal passages as much as possible. Prime before first use by actuating 8 times. Prime if not used for more than 4 consecutive days by actuating once or until a fine spray appears. Shake gently before use. Insert the spray tip into the nostril, pointing toward the nasal passages, away from the nasal septum. Spray into the nostril while holding the other nostril closed, and at the same time, inhale through the nose to deliver the medication as high into the nasal passages as possible.

Ciclopirox

sye-kloe-peer′ox

★ 🍁 Loprox, Penlac

Do not confuse ciclopirox with ciprofloxacin or Loprox with Lonox.

CATEGORY AND SCHEDULE

Pregnancy Risk Category: B

Classification: Antifungals, topical

MECHANISM OF ACTION

An antifungal that inhibits the transport of essential elements in the fungal cell, thereby interfering with biosynthesis in fungi. *Therapeutic Effect:* Results in fungal cell death.

PHARMACOKINETICS

Absorbed through intact skin but only about 1% is absorbed systemically. Distributed to epidermis and dermis, including hair, hair follicles, and sebaceous glands. Protein binding: 98%. Primarily excreted in urine and to a lesser extent in feces. *Half-life:* 1.7 h.

AVAILABILITY

Cream: 0.77% (Loprox).
Gel: 0.77% (Loprox).
Lotion: 0.77% (Loprox TS).
Shampoo: 1% (Loprox).
Topical Solution, Nail Lacquer: 8% (Penlac).

INDICATIONS AND DOSAGES

▸ **Tinea pedis**

TOPICAL

Adults, Elderly, Children 10 yr and older. Apply 2 times a day until signs and symptoms significantly improve. Usually for 4 wks.

▸ **Tinea cruris, tinea corporis**

TOPICAL

Adults, Elderly, Children 10 yr and older. Apply 2 times a day until signs and symptoms significantly improve. Usually 2-4 wks.

▸ **Onychomycosis**

TOPICAL (NAIL LACQUER SOLUTION)

Adults, Elderly, Children 10 yr and older. Apply to the affected area (nails) daily. Remove with alcohol every 7 days. May require months of treatment.

▸ **Seborrheic dermatitis**

GEL

Adults, Elderly, Children 10 yr and older. Apply to affected scalp areas 2 times a day, in the morning and evening for 4 wks.

SHAMPOO

Adults, Elderly, Children 10 yr and older. Apply 5 mL (1 tsp) to wet hair; lather, and leave in place about 3 min; rinse. May use up to 10 mL for longer hair. Repeat twice weekly for 4 wks; allow a minimum of 3 days between applications.

CONTRAINDICATIONS

Hypersensitivity to ciclopirox or any one of its components.

INTERACTIONS

Drug
Not known.
Herbal
Not known.
Food
Not known.

DIAGNOSTIC TEST EFFECTS

None known.

SIDE EFFECTS

Rare
Topical: Irritation, burning, redness, pain at the site of application.

SERIOUS REACTIONS

- None known.

PRECAUTIONS & CONSIDERATIONS

Avoid use of occlusive wrappings or dressings. Avoid contact with eyes. If local irritation occurs, ciclopirox should be discontinued. It is unknown whether ciclopirox crosses the placenta or is distributed in breast milk. Safety and efficacy have not been established in children younger than 10 yr old. No age-related precautions have been noted for elderly patients.

Storage
Store products at room temperature. Nail lacquer solution should be protected from light. Nail solution is flammable and should be stored away from heat and flame.

Administration
Apply topical formulation by rubbing gently into the affected and surrounding area twice daily until signs and symptoms improve.

Apply nail lacquer once daily, preferably at bedtime or 8 h before washing, to the affected nails with the applicator brush provided. Cover evenly over the entire nail plate. Ciclopirox should not be removed on a daily basis. Daily applications should be made over the previous coat. Remove with alcohol every 7 days. Repeat cycle throughout the duration of therapy. File away with emery board loose nail material, and trim nails every 7 days after ciclopirox is removed with alcohol.

Apply gel to affected scalp areas twice daily, in the morning and evening for 4 wks, or use the shampoo twice weekly for 4 wks. Clinical improvement usually occurs within the first week, with continuing resolution of signs and symptoms through the fourth week of treatment.

Cidofovir

ci-dah'fo-veer

★ Vistide

CATEGORY AND SCHEDULE

Pregnancy Risk Category: C

Classification: Antivirals

MECHANISM OF ACTION

An anti-infective that inhibits viral DNA synthesis by incorporating itself into the growing viral DNA chain. *Therapeutic Effect:* Suppresses replication of cytomegalovirus (CMV).

PHARMACOKINETICS

Protein binding: < 6%. Excreted primarily unchanged in urine. Effect of hemodialysis unknown. *Elimination Half-life:* 1.4-3.8 h.

AVAILABILITY

Injection: 75 mg/mL (5-mL vial).

INDICATIONS AND DOSAGES

▸ **CMV retinitis in patients with AIDS (in combination with probenecid)**

IV INFUSION

Adults. Induction: 5 mg/kg at constant rate over 1 h once weekly for 2 consecutive weeks. Give 2 g of PO probenecid 3 h before cidofovir dose, and then give 1 g 2 h and 8 h after completion of the 1-h cidofovir infusion (total of 4 g). In addition, give 1 L of 0.9% NaCl over 1-2 h immediately before the cidofovir infusion. If tolerated, a second liter may be infused over 1-3 h at the start of the infusion or *immediately* afterward. *Maintenance:* 5 mg/kg cidofovir at constant rate over 1 h once every 2 wks.

▸ **Dosage in renal impairment**

Patients with CrCl ≤ 55 mL/min before treatment must not receive cidofovir. Once treatment starts in other patients, decrease dose to 3 mg/kg if Scr increases 0.3-0.4 mg/dL above baseline. Discontinue if a rise in Scr is 0.5 mg/dL or more.

OFF-LABEL USES

Treatment of ganciclovir-resistant cytomegalovirus (CMV), foscarnet-resistant CMV, adenovirus, and acyclovir-resistant herpes simplex virus or progressive vaccinia infection.

CONTRAINDICATIONS

Direct intraocular injection, history of clinically severe hypersensitivity to probenecid or other sulfa-containing drugs, hypersensitivity to cidofovir, renal impairment (serum creatinine level > 1.5 mg/dL, creatinine clearance of 55 mL/min or less, or urine protein level > 100 mg/dL), use with or within 7 days of other nephrotoxic medications.

INTERACTIONS

Drug

Nephrotoxic medications (such as aminoglycosides, amphotericin B, foscarnet, tacrolimus IV pentamidine): Increase the risk of nephrotoxicity. Discontinue these at least 7 days before cidofovir treatment.

Tenofovir: Cidofovir may increase tenofovir serum concentrations.

Zidovudine: For persons also taking zidovudine (AZT), expect to discontinue zidovudine administration temporarily or to decrease AZT dose by 50% on days of cidofovir infusion. Be aware that concurrent probenecid use reduces the metabolic clearance of zidovudine.

Herbal

None known.

Food

None known.

DIAGNOSTIC TEST EFFECTS

May decrease neutrophil count and serum bicarbonate, phosphate, and uric acid levels. May elevate serum creatinine levels.

IV INCOMPATIBILITIES

No information available for Y-site administration. Do not mix or infuse with other medications.

SIDE EFFECTS

Frequent

Nausea, vomiting (65%), fever (57%), asthenia (46%), rash (30%), diarrhea (27%), headache (27%), alopecia (25%), chills (24%), anorexia (22%), dyspnea (22%), abdominal pain (17%).

SERIOUS REACTIONS

- Serious adverse reactions may include proteinuria (80%), nephrotoxicity (53%), neutropenia (31%), elevated serum creatinine levels (29%), infection (24%), anemia (20%), ocular hypotony (a decrease in intraocular pressure, 12%), and pneumonia (9%).
- Concurrent use of probenecid may produce a hypersensitivity reaction characterized by a rash, fever, chills, and anaphylaxis.
- Acute renal failure occurs rarely.
- Metabolic acidosis.

PRECAUTIONS & CONSIDERATIONS

Caution is warranted with preexisting diabetes. Be aware that cidofovir is embryotoxic and results in reduced fetal body weight in animals. Females of childbearing age should use effective contraception during and for 1 mo after cidofovir treatment; male patients should practice barrier contraceptive methods during and for 3 mo after treatment. Be aware that it is unknown whether cidofovir is excreted in breast milk. Do not administer to breastfeeding women. Breastfeeding is not recommended in this population because of the possibility of HIV transmission. Be aware that the safety and efficacy of cidofovir have not been established in children. In elderly patients, age-related renal impairment may require dosage adjustment.

Renal function should be closely monitored through serum creatinine levels and urinalysis during therapy. Urine protein and white blood cell (WBC) count should also be monitored. Visual acuity and ocular symptoms should be evaluated.

Storage

Store cidofovir at room temperature. Refrigerate admixtures for no longer than 24 h. Allow refrigerated

C

admixtures to warm to room temperature before use. Discard any unused solution.

Administration

CAUTION: Expect to prepare in a biological safety cabinet. Use the same cautions for preparing and administering as are used for chemotherapy.

! Do not exceed the recommended dosage, frequency, or infusion rate. Dilute in 100 mL 0.9% NaCl and infuse over 1 h. Prepare to administer IV hydration with 0.9% NaCl and give oral probenecid with each cidofovir infusion to minimize the risk of nephrotoxicity. Eat food before each dose of probenecid to help reduce nausea and vomiting. As prescribed, administer an antiemetic to reduce the risk of nausea. Give cidofovir IV infusion over 60 min.

Cilostazol

sil-os'tah-zol

★ Pletal

Do not confuse Pletal with Plendil.

CATEGORY AND SCHEDULE

Pregnancy Risk Category: C

Classification: Platelet inhibitors

MECHANISM OF ACTION

A phosphodiesterase III inhibitor that inhibits platelet aggregation. Dilates vascular beds with greatest dilation in femoral beds. *Therapeutic Effect:* Improves walking distance in patients with intermittent claudication.

PHARMACOKINETICS

Moderately absorbed from the GI tract. Protein binding: 95%-98%. Extensively metabolized in the liver. Excreted primarily in the urine and, to a lesser extent, in the feces. Not removed by hemodialysis. *Half-life:* 11-13 h. Therapeutic effect is usually noted in 2-4 wks but may take as long as 12 wks.

AVAILABILITY

Tablets: 50 mg, 100 mg.

INDICATIONS AND DOSAGES

▸ **Intermittent claudication**

PO

Adults, Elderly. 100 mg twice a day at least 30 min before or 2 h after meals. Reduce dose to 50 mg twice a day with concurrent CYP3A4 or CYP2C19 inhibitors.

CONTRAINDICATIONS

Congestive heart failure of any severity, hemostatic disorders or active bleeding, (e.g., such as intracranial bleeding or bleeding peptic ulcer), hypersensitivity to cilostazol or any of the product ingredients.

INTERACTIONS

Drug

CYP3A4 inhibitors (azole antifungals, clarithromycin, diltiazem, erythromycin, fluoxetine, nefazodone, protease inhibitors, quinidine, sertraline, telithromycin, and verapamil): May increase cilostazol concentration.

CYP2C19 inhibitors (delavirdine, fluconazole, fluvoxamine, omeprazole, and ticlopidine): May increase cilostazol concentration.

Aspirin: May potentiate inhibition of platelet aggregation.

Clopidogrel, ticlopidine: Ticlopidine may decrease cilostazol metabolism. Effects of clopidogrel with cilostazol unknown; may potentiate platelet effects.

Herbal

None known.

Food
Grapefruit juice: May increase blood concentration and risk of toxicity of cilostazol. Do not give with grapefruit juice.
High-fat meal: May increase cilostazol peak concentration up to 90%.

DIAGNOSTIC TEST EFFECTS
May increase BUN and serum creatinine levels. May decrease hemoglobin and hematocrit.

SIDE EFFECTS
Frequent (10%-34%)
Headache, diarrhea, palpitations, dizziness, pharyngitis.
Occasional (3%-7%)
Nausea, rhinitis, back pain, peripheral edema, dyspepsia, abdominal pain, tachycardia, cough, flatulence, myalgia.
Rare (1%-2%)
Leg cramps, paresthesia, rash, vomiting.

SERIOUS REACTIONS
- Signs and symptoms of overdose are noted by severe headache, diarrhea, hypotension, and cardiac arrhythmias.
- Leukopenia and thrombocytopenia, with progression to agranulocytosis when cilostazol was not immediately discontinued.

PRECAUTIONS & CONSIDERATIONS
Use with caution in patients with heart disease and renal or hepatic impairment. There are no adequate studies of use in pregnant women. The drug may be distributed to breast milk and use during lactation not recommended. Safety and efficacy of cilostazol have not been established in children. No age-related precautions have been noted in elderly patients. Hemoglobin, hematocrit, and platelet counts should be obtained before and periodically during treatment.

Effect of treatment on symptoms during walking or other activities should be assessed periodically.

Storage
Store at room temperature.
Administration
Take cilostazol at least 30 min before or 2 h after meals. Do not give with grapefruit juice. Doses are usually given before breakfast and dinner.

Cimetidine
sye-met′i-deen
★ Tagamet, Tagamet HB
🍁 Nu-Cimet
Do not confuse cimetidine with simethicone.

CATEGORY AND SCHEDULE
Pregnancy Risk Category: B
OTC 200 mg tablets; other forms Rx only

Classification: Gastrointestinal agents, antiulcer agents, H_2 histamine receptor antagonist

MECHANISM OF ACTION
An antiulcer agent and gastric acid reducer that inhibits histamine action at H_2 receptor sites of parietal cells. *Therapeutic Effect:* Inhibits gastric acid secretion during fasting, at night, or when stimulated by food, caffeine, or insulin.

PHARMACOKINETICS
Well absorbed from the GI tract. Protein binding: 15%-20%. Widely distributed. Metabolized in the liver. Primarily excreted in urine. Not removed by hemodialysis. *Half-life:* 2 h; increased with impaired renal function.

C

AVAILABILITY

Tablets (Tagamet HB): 200 mg.
Tablets (Tagamet): 300 mg, 400 mg, 800 mg.
Liquid: 300 mg/5 mL.
Injection: 150 mg/mL.

INDICATIONS AND DOSAGES

▸ **Active gastric or duodenal ulcer**

PO

Adults, Elderly. 300 mg 4 times a day or 400 mg twice a day or 800 mg at bedtime.

IM, IV

Adults, Elderly. 300 mg q6h or 150 mg IV as single dose followed by 37.5 mg/h continuous infusion.

▸ **Prevention of duodenal ulcer**

PO

Adults, Elderly. 400-800 mg at bedtime.

▸ **Gastric hypersecretory secretions**

PO, IV, IM

Adults, Elderly. 300-600 mg q6h. Maximum: 2400 mg/day.

Children. 20-40 mg/kg/day in divided doses q6h.

Infants. 10-20 mg/kg/day in divided doses q6-12h.

Neonates. 5-10 mg/kg/day in divided doses q8-12h.

▸ **Gastrointestinal reflux disease**

PO

Adults, Elderly. 800 mg twice a day or 400 mg 4 times a day for 12 wks.

▸ **OTC use**

PO

Adults, Elderly. 200 mg up to 30 min before meals. Maximum: 2 doses/ day.

▸ **Prevention of upper GI bleeding**

IV INFUSION

Adults, Elderly. 50 mg/h. If CrCl < 30 mL/min, give 25 mg/h.

▸ **Dosage in renal impairment**

Dosage is based on a 300-mg dose in adults. Dosage interval is modified based on creatinine clearance.

Creatinine Clearance (mL/min)	Dosage Interval
> 40	q6h
20-40	q8h or decrease dose by 25%
< 20	q12h or decrease dose by 50%

Give after hemodialysis and q12h between dialysis sessions.

OFF-LABEL USES

Prevention of aspiration pneumonia; treatment of acute urticaria, common warts.

CONTRAINDICATIONS

Hypersensitivity to cimetidine or other H_2 antagonists.

INTERACTIONS

Drug

Antacids: May decrease the absorption of cimetidine if administered at the same time.

Calcium channel blockers, cyclosporine, lidocaine, metoprolol, metronidazole, oral anticoagulants, oral antidiabetics, phenytoin, propranolol, theophylline, tricyclic antidepressants: May decrease the metabolism and increase the blood concentrations of these drugs.

CYP 1A2, 2C19, 2D6, 3A4, 2C9, and 2E1 substrates: Cimetidine inhibits these isoenzymes and may decrease the metabolism and increase the blood concentrations of substrates of these isoenzymes.

Ketoconazole: May decrease the absorption of ketoconazole.

Herbal

St. John's wort: May decrease cimetidine levels.

Food

None known.

DIAGNOSTIC TEST EFFECTS

Interferes with skin tests using allergen extracts. May increase prolactin, serum creatinine, and transaminase levels. May decrease parathyroid hormone concentration.

IV INCOMPATIBILITIES

Allopurinol (Aloprim), amphotericin B complex (Abelcet, AmBisome, Amphotec), ampicillin, cefepime (Maxipime), diazepam, furosemide, phenobarbital, phenytoin, warfarin.

IV COMPATIBILITIES

Aminophylline, diltiazem (Cardizem), heparin, hydromorphone (Dilaudid), insulin (regular), lidocaine, lorazepam (Ativan), midazolam (Versed), morphine, potassium chloride, propofol (Diprivan).

SIDE EFFECTS

Occasional (2%-4%)

HEADACHE: Elderly and severely ill patients, patients with impaired renal function: Confusion, agitation, psychosis, depression, anxiety, disorientation, hallucinations. Effects reverse 3-4 days after discontinuance.

Rare (< 2%)

Diarrhea, dizziness, somnolence, nausea, vomiting, gynecomastia, rash, impotence.

SERIOUS REACTIONS

- Rapid IV administration may produce cardiac arrhythmias and hypotension.
- Rare cases of neutropenia, agranulocytosis, or thrombocytopenia.
- Rare severe hypersensitivity reactions.

PRECAUTIONS & CONSIDERATIONS

Caution is warranted for patients with impaired hepatic or renal function and in elderly patients. Cimetidine crosses the placenta and is distributed in breast milk. Cimetidine use in infants may suppress gastric acidity, inhibit drug metabolism, and produce CNS stimulation. Long-term use in children may induce cerebral toxicity and affect the hormonal system. Elderly patients are more likely to experience confusion, especially those with impaired renal function. Tasks that require mental alertness or motor skills should also be avoided until response to the drug has been established.

Notify the physician if blood in emesis or stool or dark, tarry stool occurs. Pattern of daily bowel activity and stool consistency, electrolytes, and hydration status should be monitored. Patients should avoid or reduce lifestyle factors contributing to GI distress, such as smoking.

Storage

Store at room temperature. Reconstituted IV solution is stable for 48 h at room temperature.

Administration

For IV push, do not administer larger than a 300-mg dose. Dilute each 300 mg (2 mL) with 18 mL 0.9% NaCl, (NS) to a total volume of 20 mL. Administer over not < 5 min to prevent arrhythmias and hypotension.

For intermittent IV (piggyback) administration, dilute 300 mg in at least 50 mL of D5W or NS and infuse over 15-20 min.

For continuous IV infusion, dilute the 24-h dose with 100-1000 mL 0.9% NaCl, D5W, or other compatible solution and infuse over 24 h. Use a volumetric pump if volume is less than 250 mL.

For IM use, administer undiluted. Inject deep into large muscle mass, such as the gluteus maximus. IM administration may produce transient discomfort at the injection site.

Take oral cimetidine without regard to food. Antacid therapy may be used along with oral cimetidine, but administration times should be separate to avoid interference with cimetidine absorption.

C

Cinacalcet

sin-a-cal′set

★ 🍁 Sensipar

CATEGORY AND SCHEDULE

Pregnancy Risk Category: C

Classification: Calcimimetic agent

MECHANISM OF ACTION

A calcium receptor agonist that increases the sensitivity of the calcium-sensing receptor on the parathyroid gland to extracellular calcium, thus lowering the parathyroid hormone (PTH) level. *Therapeutic Effect:* Decreases serum calcium and PTH levels.

PHARMACOKINETICS

Extensively distributed after PO administration. Protein binding: 93%-97%. Rapidly and extensively metabolized by hepatic enzymes. Metabolites primarily eliminated in urine with a lesser amount excreted in feces. *Half-life:* 30-40 h.

AVAILABILITY

Tablets: 30 mg, 60 mg, 90 mg.

INDICATIONS AND DOSAGES

▸ **Hypercalcemia in parathyroid carcinoma**

PO

Adults, Elderly. Initially, 30 mg twice a day. Titrate dosage sequentially (60 mg twice a day, 90 mg twice a day, and 90 mg 3-4 times a day) every 2-4 wks as needed to normalize serum calcium levels.

▸ **Secondary hyperparathyroidism in patients on dialysis**

PO

Adults, Elderly. Initially, 30 mg once a day. Titrate dosage sequentially (60, 90, 120, and 180 mg once a day) every 2-4 wks to target intact PTH levels of 150-300 pg/mL.

CONTRAINDICATIONS

Hypersensitivity.

INTERACTIONS

Drug

CYP2D6 substrates (e.g., dextromethorphan, flecainide, fluoxetine, lidocaine, mirtazapine, nefazodone, paroxetine, propafenone risperidone, ritonavir, thioridazine, tricyclic antidepressants, venlafaxine): Increased concentrations of CYP2D6 substrates. Cinacalcet is a strong CYP2D6 inhibitor; thioridazine may be contraindicated.

CYP3A4 inhibitors (e.g., azole antifungals, clarithromycin, erythromycin, nefazodone, protease inhibitors, telithromycin, and verapamil): Increase cinacalcet plasma concentration.

Herbal

None known.

Food

High-fat meals: Increase cinacalcet plasma concentration.

DIAGNOSTIC TEST EFFECTS

Reduces serum calcium level and reduces intact PTH levels.

SIDE EFFECTS

Frequent (21%-31%)

Nausea, vomiting, diarrhea.

Occasional (10%-15%)

Myalgia, dizziness.

Rare (5%-7%)

Asthenia, hypertension, anorexia, noncardiac chest pain.

SERIOUS REACTIONS

- Overdose may lead to hypocalcemia.

- Hypotension and heart failure have been reported in patients with cardiovascular disease.

PRECAUTIONS & CONSIDERATIONS

Caution is warranted in patients with cardiovascular disease, seizure disorder, chronic kidney disease not on hemodialysis, or hepatic impairment. Cinacalcet may cross the placental barrier. Cinacalcet's safe use during breastfeeding has not been established. The safety and efficacy of cinacalcet have not been established in children. No age-related precautions have been noted in elderly patients.

Notify the physician if diarrhea or vomiting occurs. Serum electrolyte levels and pattern of daily bowel activity and stool consistency should be monitored.

Storage

Store tablets at room temperature.

Administration

Do not break or crush film-coated tablets. Take the drug with food or shortly after a meal.

Ciprofloxacin

sip-ro-floks′a-sin

★ Cetraxal, Ciloxan, Cipro, Cipro XR, Proquin XR

🍁 Ciloxan, Cipro, Cipro XR

Do not confuse ciprofloxacin with Cytoxan, or Cetraxal with Celexa or Trexall.

CATEGORY AND SCHEDULE

Pregnancy Risk Category: C

Classification: Anti-infectives, ophthalmics, antibiotics, quinolones

MECHANISM OF ACTION

A fluoroquinolone that inhibits the enzyme DNA gyrase in susceptible bacteria, interfering with bacterial cell replication. *Therapeutic Effect:* Bactericidal.

PHARMACOKINETICS

Well absorbed from the GI tract (food delays absorption). Protein binding: 20%-40%. Widely distributed (including to CSF). Metabolized in the liver to active metabolite. Primarily excreted in urine. Minimal removal by hemodialysis. *Half-life:* 4-6 h (increased in patients with impaired renal function and in elderly patients).

AVAILABILITY

Tablets (Cipro): 100 mg, 250 mg, 500 mg, 750 mg.
Tablets, Extended Release (Cipro XR, Proquin XR): 500 mg, 1000 mg.
Infusion: 200 mg/100 mL, 400 mg/200 mL.
Injection Solution: 10 mg/mL.
Ophthalmic Ointment (Ciloxan): 0.3%.
Ophthalmic Suspension (Ciloxan): 0.3%.
Oral Suspension: 250 mg/5 mL, 500 mg/5 mL.
Otic Suspension (Cetraxal): 0.2%

INDICATIONS AND DOSAGES

▸ **Mild to moderate urinary tract infection (UTI)**

PO

Adults, Elderly. 250 mg q12h.

IV

Adults, Elderly. 200 mg q12h.

▸ **Complicated UTIs, mild to moderate respiratory tract, bone, joint, skin, and skin-structure infections; infectious diarrhea**

PO

Adults, Elderly. 500 mg q12h.

IV

Adults, Elderly. 400 mg q12h.

▸ **Severe, complicated infections**

PO

Adults, Elderly. 750 mg q12h.

IV

Adults, Elderly. 400 mg q12h.

C

▸ **Prostatitis**
PO
Adults, Elderly. 500 mg q12h for 28 days.
▸ **Uncomplicated bladder infection**
PO
Adults. 100 mg twice a day for 3 days.
▸ **Acute sinusitis**
PO
Adults. 500 mg q12h.
▸ **Uncomplicated gonorrhea**
PO
Adults. 250 mg as a single dose.
NOTE: CDC does not recommend due to resistant *N. gonorrhoeae.*
▸ **Cystic fibrosis**
IV
Children. 30 mg/kg/day in 2-3 divided doses. Maximum: 1.2 g/day.
PO
▸ **Corneal ulcer**
OPHTHALMIC
Adults, Elderly. 2 drops q15min for 6 h, then 2 drops q30min for the remainder of first day, 2 drops q1h on second day, and 2 drops q4h on days 3-14.
▸ **Bacterial conjunctivitis**
OPHTHALMIC DROPS
Adults, Elderly, and Children ≥ 1 yr. 1-2 drops q2h for 2 days, then 2 drops q4h for next 5 days.
OPHTHALMIC OINTMENT
Adults, Elderly, and Children ≥ 1 yr. ½-inch ribbon 3 times daily for 2 days, then twice daily for next 5 days.
▸ **Otitis externa**
OTIC
Adults, Elderly, and Children > 1 yr. Instill 0.5 mg (0.25 mL single-use drops) into affected ear(s) q12h for 7 days.
▸ **Dosage in renal impairment**
Dosage and frequency are modified based on creatinine clearance and the severity of the infection.

Creatinine Clearance	Dosage Interval
< 30 mL/min	Usual dose q18-24h

▸ **Hemodialysis**
250-500 mg q24h (after dialysis).
▸ **Peritoneal dialysis**
250-500 mg q24h (after dialysis).

OFF-LABEL USES

Treatment of chancroid.

CONTRAINDICATIONS

Hypersensitivity to ciprofloxacin or other quinolones, concurrent tizanidine; for ophthalmic administration: vaccinia, varicella, epithelial herpes simplex, keratitis, mycobacterial infection, fungal disease of ocular structure, use after uncomplicated removal of a foreign body.

INTERACTIONS

Drug
Antacids, iron preparations, calcium or magnesium supplement, sucralfate: May decrease ciprofloxacin absorption. Separate times of administration.
Caffeine, oral anticoagulants: May increase the effects of these drugs.
Theophylline: Decreases clearance and may increase blood concentration and risk of toxicity of theophylline.
Tizanidine: Decreases clearance and increases toxicity of tizanidine substantially. Contraindicated.
Herbal
None known.
Food
Enteral feedings: Reduce ciprofloxacin absorption.

DIAGNOSTIC TEST EFFECTS

May increase BUN and serum alkaline phosphatase, bilirubin, creatinine, LDH, AST (SGOT), and ALT (SGPT) levels.

IV INCOMPATIBILITIES

Acyclovir, aminophylline, ampicillin and sulbactam (Unasyn), azithromycin (Zithromax), cefepime (Maxipime), dexamethasone (Decadron), dotrecogin alfa (Xigris), furosemide (Lasix), heparin, hydrocortisone (Solu-Cortef), lansoprazole (Prevacid IV), magnesium sulfate, methylprednisolone (Solu-Medrol), pantoprazole (Protonix), phenytoin (Dilantin), piperacillin-tazobactam (Zosyn), potassium or sodium phosphates, propofol (Diprivan), rituximab (Rituxan), sodium bicarbonate, warfarin (Coumadin).

IV COMPATIBILITIES

Calcium gluconate, diltiazem (Cardizem), dobutamine (Dobutrex), dopamine (Intropin), lidocaine, lorazepam (Ativan), midazolam (Versed), potassium chloride.

SIDE EFFECTS

Frequent (2%-5%)
Nausea, diarrhea, dyspepsia, vomiting, constipation, flatulence, confusion, crystalluria.
Ophthalmic: Burning, crusting in corner of eye.
Occasional (<2%)
Abdominal pain or discomfort, headache, rash.
Ophthalmic: Bad taste, sensation of something in eye, eyelid redness or itching.
Rare (< 1%)
Dizziness, confusion, tremors, hallucinations, hypersensitivity reaction, insomnia, dry mouth, paresthesia.
Ophthalmic: Crystal precipitates that generally resolve in 1-7 days.

SERIOUS REACTIONS

- Superinfection (especially enterococcal or fungal), nephropathy, cardiopulmonary arrest, chest pain, tendon inflammation/rupture, and cerebral thrombosis may occur.
- Hypersensitivity reactions, including photosensitivity (as evidenced by rash, pruritus, blisters, edema, and burning skin), have occurred in patients receiving fluoroquinolones.
- Arthropathy may occur if the drug is given to children younger than 18 yr.
- Sensitization to the ophthalmic form of the drug may contraindicate later systemic use of ciprofloxacin.
- Tendonitis or tendon rupture.

PRECAUTIONS & CONSIDERATIONS

History of hypersensitivity to ciprofloxacin and other quinolones should be determined before therapy.

Caution is warranted in patients with CNS disorders, renal impairment, seizures, risk factors for QT prolongation, and those taking caffeine or theophylline. It is unknown whether ciprofloxacin is distributed in breast milk. If possible, pregnant or breastfeeding women should avoid taking the drug because of the risk of arthropathy in the fetus or infant. The safety and efficacy of ciprofloxacin have not been established in children younger than 18 yr except for select indications. Age-related renal impairment may require a dosage adjustment in elderly patients.

Dizziness, headache, tremors, visual problems, and chest and joint pain should be reported. Food tolerance and pattern of daily bowel activity and stool consistency should be assessed. If tendon pain is reported, evaluate; tendon rupture may require surgical repair and extended disability.

Storage
Store all products at room temperature. Once reconstituted, the oral suspension and diluted IVPB are stable for up to 14 days at room temperature. The solution normally appears clear and colorless or slightly yellow.

C

Administration
Oral ciprofloxacin may be taken without regard to food, but the preferred administration time is 2 h after a meal. Shake the oral suspension well before taking it, and do not chew the microcapsules in the suspension. Do not administer antacids containing aluminum or magnesium within 2 h of ciprofloxacin. Take full course of therapy, and do not skip doses.

For IV use, after withdrawing the drug from a 200- or 400-mg vial, further dilute it with D5W or 0.9% NaCl for injection to a final concentration of 1-2 mg/mL. Infuse the drug over 60 min. Also available prediluted in ready-to-use infusion containers.

For ophthalmic use, tilt the head back and place the solution in the conjunctival sac of the affected eye. Close the eye and then press gently on the lacrimal sac for 1 min.

For otic use, warm container in hands for approx. 1 min. Patient should lie with the affected ear upward and maintain position least 1 min after instillation. Instill 1 single-use container (0.25 mL) into affected ear canal.

Cisplatin

sis-plah'tin

Do not confuse cisplatin with carboplatin or oxaliplatin.

CATEGORY AND SCHEDULE

Pregnancy Risk Category: D

Classification: Antineoplastic, platinum compounds

MECHANISM OF ACTION

A platinum coordination complex that inhibits DNA and, to a lesser extent, RNA, protein synthesis by cross-linking with DNA strands, preventing cell division. Cell cycle–phase nonspecific. *Therapeutic Effect:* Causes cell-cycle arrest in G2 phase and induces programmed cancer cell death (apoptosis).

PHARMACOKINETICS

Widely distributed. Protein binding: > 90%. Undergoes rapid nonenzymatic conversion to inactive metabolite. Excreted in urine. Removed by hemodialysis. *Half-life:* 58-73 h (increased with impaired renal function).

AVAILABILITY

Injection Solution: 1 mg/mL.

INDICATIONS AND DOSAGES

NOTE: Regimens vary widely with indication for use, other medications employed. Consult specialized references to confirm protocols.

▸ **Advanced bladder carcinoma, metastatic ovarian tumors, lung cancer, metastatic testicular tumors**

IV INFUSION

Adults, Elderly. For intermittent dosage schedule, 37-75 mg/m^2 once every 2-3 wks or 50-100 mg/m^2 over 4-8 h once every 21-28 days. For daily dosage schedule, 15-20 mg/m^2/day for 5 days every 3-4 wks.

OFF LABEL USES

Use in children for various cancers, use in adults for many different solid tumor protocols.

CONTRAINDICATIONS

Hearing impairment; myelosuppression; hypersensitivity to cisplatin or other platinum compounds, creatinine clearance less than 50 mL/min, preexisting renal impairment.

INTERACTIONS

Drug

Nephrotoxic, ototoxic medications: May increase the risk of nephrotoxicity/ototoxicity.

Herbal and Food

None known.

DIAGNOSTIC TEST EFFECTS

Increased hepatic transaminases, BUN, serum creatinine; decreased serum sodium, calcium, magnesium, uric acid.

IV INCOMPATIBILITIES

Amphotericin B, cefepime, dantrolene, diazepam, gallium, insulin, lansoprazole, mesna, pantoprazole, piperacillin-tazobactam, thiotepa, TPN. Refer to specialized references to check compatibility with other medications and solutions.

SIDE EFFECTS

Frequent

Nausea, vomiting (generally beginning 1-4 h after administration and lasting up to 24 h); myelosuppression (25%-30% of patients, with recovery generally in 18-23 days); mild alopecia; ototoxicity; nephrotoxicity.

Occasional

Peripheral neuropathy (with prolonged therapy [4-7 mo]). Pain or redness at injection site, loss of taste or appetite.

Rare

Hemolytic anemia, blurred vision, stomatitis.

SERIOUS REACTIONS

- An anaphylactic reaction manifested as angioedema, wheezing, tachycardia, and hypotension may occur in the first few minutes of IV administration in patients previously exposed to cisplatin.
- Nephrotoxicity occurs in 28%-36% of patients.
- Ototoxicity, including tinnitus and hearing loss, occurs in 31% of patients of cisplatin. It may be more severe in children or more frequent or severe with repeated doses.

PRECAUTIONS & CONSIDERATIONS

Cisplatin therapy is highly emetogenic; all patients must receive prophylactic antiemetic therapy. Caution with renal impairment and in elderly patients, who may be more susceptible to peripheral neuropathy and nephrotoxicity. Avoid use in pregnant women. Do not breastfeed during treatment.

Storage

Store at room temperature. Do not refrigerate. Protect from light. The amber vial, following initial entry, is stable for 28 days protected from light or 7 days under fluorescent room light. If IV infusion is not used within 6 h, protect solution from light. Diluted infusion is stable for up to 24 h at room temperature. Do not refrigerate (precipitates).

Administration

CAUTION: Observe and exercise usual cautions for handling and preparing solutions of cytotoxic drugs. Verify any cisplatin doses > 100 mg/m2 per course; such high doses are rarely used.

Hydration with 0.9% NaCl is usually begun before the infusion and continued after. Expect pretreatment with a 5HT-3 antagonist and corticosteroids.

Give by slow IV infusion only. Cisplatin may be diluted in 0.9% NaCl to a final concentration of 50-500 mg/L. Needles or IV sets containing aluminum parts should not be used for preparation or administration. Aluminum reacts with cisplatin, causing a precipitate and a loss of potency. Infuse IV no faster than 1 mg/min.

Citalopram

sye-tal′oh-pram

Celexa

Do not confuse Celexa with Celebrex, Zyprexa, or Cerebyx.

CATEGORY AND SCHEDULE

Pregnancy Risk Category: C

Classification: Antidepressants, selective serotonin reuptake inhibitors (SSRIs)

MECHANISM OF ACTION

A selective serotonin reuptake inhibitor that blocks the uptake of the neurotransmitter serotonin at CNS presynaptic neuronal membranes, increasing its availability at postsynaptic receptor sites. *Therapeutic Effect:* Relieves depression.

PHARMACOKINETICS

Well absorbed after PO administration. Protein binding: 80%. Primarily metabolized in the liver. Primarily excreted in feces with a lesser amount eliminated in urine. *Half-life:* 35 h.

AVAILABILITY

Oral Solution: 10 mg/5 mL.
Tablets: 10 mg, 20 mg, 40 mg.

INDICATIONS AND DOSAGES

▸ Depression

PO

Adults. Initially, 20 mg once a day in the morning or evening. May increase in 20-mg increments at intervals of no less than 1 wk. Maximum: 60 mg/day.
Elderly, Patients with hepatic impairment. 20 mg/day. May titrate to 40 mg/day only for nonresponding patients.

OFF-LABEL USES

Treatment of anxiety, obsessive-compulsive disorder, hot flashes, premenstrual dysphoric disorder, panic disorder, post-traumatic stress.

CONTRAINDICATIONS

Sensitivity to citalopram, use within 14 days of MAOIs.

INTERACTIONS

Drug

Antifungals, cimetidine, macrolide antibiotics: May increase the citalopram plasma level.
Carbamazepine: May decrease the citalopram plasma level.
MAOIs: May cause serotonin syndrome. Contraindicated.
Metoprolol: Increases the metoprolol plasma level.
Anticoagulants, antiplatelet agents, NSAIDs, aspirin: May increase bleeding risk.
Nefazodone, triptans, sibutramine, trazodone, venlafaxine: May increase risk of serotonin syndrome.

Herbal

Valerian, St. John's wort, SAM-e, kava kava: May alter psychotropic response. St. John's wort may increase serotonin activity.

Food

None known.

DIAGNOSTIC TEST EFFECTS

May reduce serum sodium level.

SIDE EFFECTS

Frequent (11%-21%)

Nausea, dry mouth, somnolence, insomnia, diaphoresis.

Occasional (4%-8%)

Tremor, diarrhea, abnormal ejaculation, dyspepsia, fatigue, anxiety, vomiting, anorexia.

Rare (2%-3%)
Sinusitis, sexual dysfunction, menstrual disorder, abdominal pain, agitation, decreased libido, platelet dysfunction with or without bleeding.

SERIOUS REACTIONS

- Overdose is manifested as serotonin syndrome and symptoms may include nausea, vomiting, sedation, dizziness, sweating, facial flushing, mental status changes, myoclonia, restlessness, shivering, and hypertension.
- SIADH and hyponatremia have been reported rarely, most commonly in elderly patients.

PRECAUTIONS & CONSIDERATIONS

Caution is warranted in patients with hepatic and renal impairment and in those with a history of hypomania, mania, and seizures. Citalopram is distributed in breast milk. Citalopram use in children may increase anticholinergic effects and hyperexcitability. Antidepressants have been reported to increase the risk of suicidal thinking and behavior in children, adolescents, and young adults (18-24 yr of age) with major depressive disorder (MDD) and other psychiatric disorders. Patients should be closely monitored for clinical worsening, suicidality, or unusual changes in behavior, particularly during the initial 1-2 mo of therapy or following dosage adjustments. Elderly patients are more sensitive to the drug's anticholinergic effects, such as dry mouth, and are more likely to experience confusion, dizziness, hyperexcitability, and sedation.

Alcohol and tasks that require mental alertness or motor skills should be avoided. CBC and blood chemistry tests should be performed before and periodically during therapy, especially with long-term use.

Administration
Take citalopram without regard to food. Crush scored tablets, if necessary. Do not abruptly discontinue citalopram.

Clarithromycin

clare-i-thro-mye'sin
★ 🍁 Biaxin, Biaxin XL

CATEGORY AND SCHEDULE

Pregnancy Risk Category: C

Classification: Antibiotics, macrolides

MECHANISM OF ACTION

A macrolide that binds to ribosomal receptor sites of susceptible organisms, inhibiting protein synthesis of the bacterial cell wall. *Therapeutic Effect:* Bacteriostatic; may be bactericidal with high dosages or very susceptible microorganisms.

PHARMACOKINETICS

Well absorbed from the GI tract. Protein binding: 65%-75%. Widely distributed. Metabolized in the liver to active metabolite. Primarily excreted in urine. Not removed by hemodialysis. *Half-life:* 3-7 h; metabolite 5-7 h (increased in impaired renal function).

AVAILABILITY

Oral Suspension: 125 mg/5 mL, 250 mg/5 mL.
Tablets: 250 mg, 500 mg.
Tablets (Extended Release): 500 mg.

C

INDICATIONS AND DOSAGES

▸ Bronchitis

PO

Adults, Elderly. 500 mg q12h for 7-14 days or extended-release tablets 1g q24h for 7 days.

▸ Skin, soft-tissue infections

PO

Adults, Elderly. 250 mg q12h for 7-14 days.

Children.
7.5 mg/kg q12h for 10 days.

▸ MAC prophylaxis

PO

Adults, Elderly. 500 mg 2 times/day.

Children.
7.5 mg/kg q12h. Maximum: 500 mg 2 times/day.

▸ MAC treatment

PO

Adults, Elderly. 500 mg 2 times/day in combination with other effective drugs.

Children. 7.5 mg/kg q12h in combination. Maximum: 500 mg 2 times/day.

▸ Pharyngitis, tonsillitis

PO

Adults, Elderly. 250 mg q12h for 10 days.

Children. 7.5 mg/kg q12h for 10 days.

▸ Pneumonia

PO

Adults, Elderly. 250 mg q12h for 7-14 days or extended-release tablets 1g q24h for 7 days.

Children. 7.5 mg/kg q12h.

▸ Maxillary sinusitis

PO

Adults, Elderly. 500 mg q12h for 14 days or extended-release tablets 1g q24h for 14 days.

Children. 7.5 mg/kg q12h.
Maximum: 500 mg 2 times/day.

▸ *Helicobacter pylori*

PO

Adults, Elderly. 500 mg q12h for 10-14 days in combination with amoxicillin or metronidazole, and a PPI.

▸ Acute otitis media

PO

Children. 7.5 mg/kg q12h for 10 days.

▸ Dosage in renal impairment

CrCl 30-60 mL/min: In patients receiving ritonavir, reduce recommended clarithromycin dose by 50%.

CrCl < 30 mL/min: Reduce recommended dose by 50%. In patients receiving ritonavir, decrease recommended clarithromycin dose by 75%.

CONTRAINDICATIONS

Hypersensitivity to clarithromycin or other macrolide antibiotics; concurrent use of any of the following drugs: cisapride, pimozide, astemizole, terfenadine, and ergotamine or dihydroergotamine.

INTERACTIONS

Drug

Cisapride, pimozide, astgemizole, terfenadine, and ergot alkaloids: Clarithromycin increases blood levels and toxicity. Contraindicated.

Lovastatin, other HMG-CoA reductase inhibitors: May increase risk for rhabdomyolysis. Temporary halt of statin recommended.

Carbamazepine, digoxin, theophylline: May increase blood concentration and toxicity of these drugs.

Rifampin: May decrease clarithromycin blood concentration.

Ritonavir: Increases clarithromycin concentrations; reduce clarithromycin dose.

Warfarin: May increase warfarin effects.

Zidovudine: May decrease blood concentration of zidovudine.

Herbal

St. John's wort: May decrease clarithromycin blood concentration.

Red yeast rice: May cause rhabdomyolysis. Avoid.
Food
None known.

DIAGNOSTIC TEST EFFECTS

May (rarely) increase BUN, AST (SGOT), and ALT (SGPT) levels.

SIDE EFFECTS

Occasional (3%-6%)
Diarrhea, nausea, altered (metallic) taste, abdominal pain.
Rare (1%-2%)
Headache, dyspepsia.

SERIOUS REACTIONS

- Antibiotic-associated colitis and other superinfections may result from altered bacterial balance.
- Hepatotoxicity, QT prolongation, and thrombocytopenia occur rarely.

PRECAUTIONS & CONSIDERATIONS

Caution is warranted in patients with hepatic or renal dysfunction and in elderly patients with severe renal impairment. Determine whether there is a history of hepatitis or allergies to clarithromycin or other macrolides before beginning therapy. Macrolides have been associated with QTc prolongation; use with caution in patients with risk factors for QT prolongation. It is unknown whether clarithromycin is distributed in breast milk. The safety and efficacy of clarithromycin have not been established in children younger than 6 mo. Age-related renal impairment may require a dosage adjustment in older patients.

Daily bowel activity and stool consistency should be assessed. Mild GI effects may be tolerable, but severe symptoms may indicate the onset of antibiotic-associated colitis. Be alert for signs and symptoms of superinfection, including abdominal pain, anal or genital pruritus, moderate to severe diarrhea, and mouth soreness.

Storage
Store at room temperature. Reconstituted oral suspension is stable for 14 days at room temperature. Do not refrigerate; suspension may gel.
Administration
Shake suspension well before use, Take tablets and oral suspension with or without food; take extended-release tablets with food. Take clarithromycin tablets with 8 oz of water. Do not crush or break extended-release tablets. Space doses evenly around the clock, and continue taking clarithromycin for the full course of therapy.

Clemastine

klem′as-teen
★ Dayhist Allergy, Tavist Allergy
🍁 Tavist

CATEGORY AND SCHEDULE

Pregnancy Risk Category: B
OTC (1.34-mg tablet)

Classification: Antihistamines, H_1 receptor antagonist, sedating

MECHANISM OF ACTION

An ethanolamine that competes with histamine on effector cells in the GI tract, blood vessels, and respiratory tract. *Therapeutic Effect:* Relieves allergy symptoms, including urticaria, rhinitis, and pruritus.

PHARMACOKINETICS

Route	Onset	Peak	Duration
PO	15-60 min	5-7 h	10-12 h

Well absorbed from the GI tract. Metabolized in the liver. Excreted primarily in urine.

C

AVAILABILITY

Syrup. 0.5 mg/5 mL.
Tablets (Dayhist Allergy, Tavist Allergy): 1.34 mg (OTC), 2.68 mg.

INDICATIONS AND DOSAGES

▸ **Allergic rhinitis, urticaria**

PO

Adults, Children 12 years and older: 1.34 mg twice a day up to 2.68 mg 3 times a day. Maximum: 8.04 mg/day.
Children 6-11 yr. 0.5-1 mg twice a day (use syrup). Maximum: 3 mg/day.
Elderly. 1.34 mg 1-2 times a day.

CONTRAINDICATIONS

Angle-closure glaucoma, hypersensitivity to clemastine, use within 14 days of MAOIs.

INTERACTIONS

Drug

Alcohol, other CNS depressants: May increase CNS depression.
MAOIs: May increase the anticholinergic and CNS depressant effects of clemastine.

Herbal and Food

None known.

DIAGNOSTIC TEST EFFECTS

May suppress wheal and flare reactions to antigen skin testing unless drug is discontinued 4 days before testing.

SIDE EFFECTS

Frequent

Somnolence; dizziness; urine retention; thickening of bronchial secretions; dry mouth, nose, or throat; in elderly, sedation, dizziness, hypotension.

Occasional

Epigastric distress, flushing, blurred vision, tinnitus, paresthesia, diaphoresis, chills.

SERIOUS REACTIONS

- A hypersensitivity reaction, marked by eczema, pruritus, rash, cardiac disturbances, angioedema, and photosensitivity, may occur.
- Overdose symptoms may vary from CNS depression, including sedation, apnea, cardiovascular collapse, and death, to severe paradoxical reaction, such as hallucinations, tremor, and seizures.
- Children may experience paradoxical reactions, such as restlessness, insomnia, euphoria, nervousness, and tremors.
- Overdose in children may result in hallucinations, seizures, and death.

PRECAUTIONS & CONSIDERATIONS

Caution is warranted with increased intraocular pressure, renal disease, cardiac disease, hypertension, seizure disorder, hyperthyroidism, asthma, GI or genitourinary obstruction, peptic ulcer disease, and benign prostatic hyperplasia. Clemastine is excreted in breast milk and should not be used in breastfeeding women. The safety and efficacy of clemastine have not been established in children younger than 6 yr. Age-related renal impairment may require a dosage adjustment in elderly patients. Avoid drinking alcoholic beverages and tasks that require alertness or motor skills until response to the drug is established.

Drowsiness, dizziness, and dry mouth may occur; tolerance may develop to the sedative effects. BP and therapeutic response should be monitored.

Administration
Take clemastine without regard to food. Crush scored tablets as needed.

Clevidipine

kle-vid'a-peen
Cleviprex
Do not confuse clevidipine with clonidine or cladribine.

CATEGORY AND SCHEDULE

Pregnancy Risk Category: C

Classification: Antihypertensives, calcium channel blockers (dihydropyridine group)

MECHANISM OF ACTION

A dihydropyridine antihypertensive agent that inhibits calcium ion movement across cell membranes during depolarization, and is primarily selective for vascular smooth muscle. *Therapeutic Effect:* Decreases systemic vascular resistance and BP.

PHARMACOKINETICS

Rapidly distributed and metabolized. Blood concentration declines in a multiphasic pattern following end of the infusion. > 99.5% bound to plasma proteins. Rapidly metabolized via hydrolysis by blood and extravascular esterases; elimination unlikely to be affected by hepatic or renal dysfunction. The primary metabolites are carboxylic acid metabolite (inactive) and formaldehyde. Of parent drug and metabolite, 63%-74% is excreted in the urine, 7%-22% excreted in the feces. *Half-life:* The initial phase half-life is ultrashort, approx 1 min; the terminal half-life is 15 min.

AVAILABILITY

Injection (Cleviprex): 0.5 mg/mL, in either 50-mL or 100-mL vials.

INDICATIONS AND DOSAGES

▸ **Short-term treatment of hypertension when oral therapy is not feasible or desirable**
IV INFUSION
Adults, Elderly. Initiate IV infusion at 1-2 mg/h. Double the dose at short (90-sec) intervals. As BP reaches goal, increase the dose by less than doubling and lengthen the time between adjustments to q 5-10 min. A 1-2 mg/h increase will generally produce an additional 2-4 mm Hg decrease in SBP. Maintenance dose usually 4-6 mg/h. Severe hypertension may require higher doses. Maximum: 16 mg/h; limited use of short-term doses of 32 mg/h. Give no more than 1000 mL or an average of 21 mg/h per 24 h, due to lipid in emulsion formulation. Usually, infusions do not exceed 72 h total.

▸ **Dosage in hepatic or severe renal impairment**
IV INFUSION
Initiate IV infusion at 1-2 mg/h, titrate as above.

CONTRAINDICATIONS

Hypersensitivity to clevidipine; allergies to soybeans, soy products, eggs, or egg products; defective lipid metabolism (e.g., pathologic hyperlipemia, lipoid nephrosis, or acute pancreatitis if it is accompanied by hyperlipidemia); and severe aortic stenosis.

INTERACTIONS

Drug
Antihypertensives: Would be expected to have additive effects on BP.
Herbal
None.

C

Food
None.

DIAGNOSTIC TEST EFFECTS
None known.

IV INCOMPATIBILITIES
Do not mix or dilute with any other medications, as these will interfere with stability of the emulsion. Do not administer in the same line as other medications.

IV COMPATIBILITIES
Cleviprex should not be diluted, but it can be administered with the following: Water for injection, 0.9% NaCl, D5W, D5NS, D5LR, LR, and 10% amino acid.

SIDE EFFECTS
Frequent (> 2%)
Headache, nausea, vomiting.
Rare (< 1%)
Palpitations, angina, syncope, dyspnea.

SERIOUS REACTIONS
- Hypotension and reflex tachycardia are potential consequences of rapid upward titration. If overdose occurs, discontinuation of the infusion leads to a reduction in antihypertensive effects within 5-15 min.
- Unstable angina, MI, cardiac arrest (rare).

PRECAUTIONS & CONSIDERATIONS
Caution is warranted in patients with cardiomyopathy, heart failure, severe left ventricular dysfunction, and in those concurrently receiving β-blockers; the drug will not protect against β-blocker withdrawal symptoms. Cleviprex contains approximately 0.2 g of lipid per milliliter (2 kcal). Lipid intake restrictions may be necessary for some patients. It is unclear whether the drug crosses the placenta. It should be administered only when the benefit to the mother exceeds the risk to the fetus. It is unknown whether it is distributed in breast milk. The safety and efficacy of clevidipine have not been established in children. There are no particular cautions in the elderly or in those with hepatic or renal impairment.

Notify the physician if anginal pain, dizziness, irregular heartbeat, nausea, shortness of breath, swelling, or symptoms of hypotension occur. Assess BP for hypotension and monitor heart rate and pulse continuously during infusion and until vital signs are stable. Also watch skin for dermatitis, facial flushing, and monitor ECG. Use caution with postural changes.

Storage
Store unopened vials refrigerated in the original carton protected from light. Do not freeze. Vials in cartons may be transferred to controlled room temperature for a period not to exceed 2 mo. Drug vials contain phospholipids and can support microbial growth. Do not use if contamination is suspected. The injection is a milky-white emulsion.

Administration
For IV use, no premixing is required, and the drug may be given by peripheral or central line. Commercially available standard plastic cannulae may be used to administer the infusion. Use strict aseptic technique. Once the infusion is spiked, use and discard within 4 h. Invert vial gently several times before use to ensure uniformity of the emulsion prior to administration. If contamination is suspected, discard. Titrate drug to achieve the desired blood pressure reduction. Monitor for the possibility of rebound hypertension for at least 8 h

after the infusion is stopped if not on other antihypertensives.

Clindamycin

klin-da-mye′sin

★ Cleocin, Cleocin-T, Clindamax, Clindesse 🍁 Dalacin

CATEGORY AND SCHEDULE

Pregnancy Risk Category: B

Classification: Lincomycin derivative anti-infective

MECHANISM OF ACTION

A lincosamide antibiotic that inhibits protein synthesis of the bacterial cell wall by binding to bacterial ribosomal receptor sites. Topically, it decreases fatty acid concentration on the skin. *Therapeutic Effect:* Bacteriostatic. Prevents outbreaks of acne vulgaris.

PHARMACOKINETICS

Rapidly absorbed from the GI tract. Protein binding: 92%-94%. Widely distributed. Metabolized in the liver to some active metabolites. Primarily excreted in urine. Not removed by hemodialysis. *Half-life:* 2.4-3 h (increased in impaired renal function and premature infants).

AVAILABILITY

Capsules: 75 mg, 150 mg, 300 mg.
Oral Solution: 75 mg/5 mL.
Injection: 150 mg/mL.
Injection Solution Premixed: 300 mg, 600 mg, 900 mg.
Topical Gel: 1%.
Topical Foam: 1%.
Topical Lotion: 1%.
Topical Solution: 1%.
Vaginal Cream: 2%.
Vaginal Suppository: 100 mg.

INDICATIONS AND DOSAGES

▸ **Chronic bone and joint, respiratory tract, skin and soft-tissue, intra-abdominal, and female genitourinary infections; endocarditis; septicemia**

PO

Adults, Elderly. 150-450 mg/dose q6-8h.
Children. 10-30 mg/kg/day in 3-4 divided doses. Maximum: 1.8 g/day.

IV, IM

Adults, Elderly. 1.2-1.8 g/day in 2-4 divided doses. Maximum: 4.8 g/day.
Children. 25-40 mg/kg/day in 3-4 divided doses.

▸ **Bacterial vaginosis**

PO

Adults, Elderly. 300 mg twice a day for 7 days.

INTRAVAGINAL

Adults. One applicatorful at bedtime for 3-7 days or 1 suppository at bedtime for 3 days. A 1-dose regimen is also available (Clindesse).

▸ **Acne vulgaris**

TOPICAL

Adults. Apply thin layer to affected area twice a day; foam once daily.

OFF-LABEL USES

Treatment of malaria, otitis media, *Pneumocystis carinii* pneumonia, toxoplasmosis, dental abscess.

CONTRAINDICATIONS

History of antibiotic-associated colitis, regional enteritis, or ulcerative colitis; hypersensitivity to clindamycin or lincomycin; known allergy to tartrazine dye.

INTERACTIONS

Drug

Adsorbent antidiarrheals: May delay absorption of clindamycin.
Chloramphenicol, erythromycin: May antagonize the effects of clindamycin.

C

Cyclosporine: May alter cyclosporine levels with systemic use; monitor closely.
Neuromuscular blockers: May increase the effects of these drugs.
Herbal and Food
None known.

DIAGNOSTIC TEST EFFECTS
May increase serum alkaline phosphatase, AST (SGOT), and ALT (SGPT) levels.

IV INCOMPATIBILITIES
Allopurinol (Aloprim), caspofungin (Cancidas), diazepam, filgrastim (Neupogen), fluconazole (Diflucan), haloperidol, idarubicin (Idamycin), lansoprazole (Prevacid IV), phenytoin, promethazine, quinupristin-dalfopristin (Synercid), traztuzumab (Herceptin).

IV COMPATIBILITIES
Amiodarone (Cordarone), diltiazem (Cardizem), heparin, hydromorphone (Dilaudid), magnesium sulfate, midazolam (Versed), morphine, multivitamins, propofol (Diprivan).

SIDE EFFECTS
Frequent
Systemic: Abdominal pain, nausea, vomiting, diarrhea.
Topical: Dry, scaly skin.
Vaginal: Vaginitis, pruritus.
Occasional
Systemic: Phlebitis or thrombophlebitis with IV administration, pain and induration at IM injection site, allergic reaction, urticaria, pruritus.
Topical: Contact dermatitis, abdominal pain, mild diarrhea, burning or stinging.
Vaginal: Headache, dizziness, nausea, vomiting, abdominal pain.
Rare
Vaginal: Hypersensitivity reaction.

SERIOUS REACTIONS
- Antibiotic-associated colitis and other superinfections may occur during and several weeks after clindamycin therapy (including the topical form).
- Blood dyscrasias (leukopenia, thrombocytopenia) and nephrotoxicity (proteinuria, azotemia, oliguria) occur rarely.

PRECAUTIONS & CONSIDERATIONS
Caution is warranted with severe renal or hepatic dysfunction and in patients using neuromuscular blockers concurrently. Do not apply topical preparations to abraded areas or near the eyes. Systemic clindamycin readily crosses the placenta and is distributed in breast milk. It is unknown whether the topical and vaginal forms of clindamycin are distributed in breast milk. Use clindamycin cautiously in children < 1 mo old. No age-related precautions have been noted in elderly patients. Use caution when applying topical clindamycin concurrently with abrasive, peeling acne agents, soaps, or alcohol-containing cosmetics to avoid a cumulative effect. Sexual intercourse during treatment with the vaginal form of clindamycin should be avoided.

Diarrhea should be reported promptly to the physician because of the potential for developing serious colitis (even with topical or vaginal clindamycin). Pattern of daily bowel activity and stool consistency should be assessed. Skin should be assessed for dryness, irritation, and rash. Be alert for signs and symptoms of superinfection, such as anal or genital pruritus, a change in oral mucosa, increased fever, and severe diarrhea. History of allergies, particularly to clindamycin or lincomycin, should be determined before beginning drug therapy.

Storage
Store capsules and topical formulations at room temperature. After reconstitution, the oral solution is stable for 2 wks at room temperature. Do not refrigerate the oral solution to avoid thickening it. The pre-mixed IV infusion is stable at room temperature for up to 16 days or up to 32 days under refrigeration.

Administration
Take capsules and solution with water and without regard to food.

For IV infusion, dilute 300-600 mg with 50 mL D5W or 0.9% NaCl (900-1200 mg with 100 mL). Never exceed a concentration of 18 mg/mL. Infuse 50-mL (300- to 600-mg) piggyback solution over 10-20 min; infuse 100-mL (900-mg to 1.2-g) piggyback solution over 30-40 min. Be aware that severe hypotension or cardiac arrest can occur with too-rapid administration. Do not administer more than 1.2 g in a single infusion.

For IM use, do not exceed 600 mg/dose. Give by deep IM injection.

Do not apply topical or intravaginal preparations near the eyes or on abraded areas. Rinse eyes with copious amounts of cool tap water if these forms of clindamycin accidentally come in contact with eyes. For intravaginal use, use provided applicators to insert dosage.

Clioquinol, Hydrocortisone

klee-oh-kwee′nole, hye-dro-kor′ti-sone

★ Ala-Quin, Dofscort

CATEGORY AND SCHEDULE

Pregnancy Risk Category: C

Classification: Anti-infectives, topical; antifungals, topical; corticosteroids, topical; dermatologics

MECHANISM OF ACTION

Clioquinol is a broad-spectrum antibacterial agent, but the mechanism of action is unknown. Hydrocortisone is a corticosteroid that diffuses across cell membranes, forms complexes with specific receptors, and further binds to DNA and stimulates transcription of mRNA (messenger RNA) and subsequent protein synthesis of various enzymes thought to be ultimately responsible for the anti-inflammatory effects of corticosteroids applied topically to the skin. *Therapeutic Effect:* Alters membrane function and produces antibacterial activity.

PHARMACOKINETICS

Clioquinol is absorbed through the skin; absorption may be increased with use of an occlusive dressing.

AVAILABILITY

Cream: 3% clioquinol and 0.5% hydrocortisone (Ala-Quin), 3% clioquinol and 1% hydrocortisone (Dofscort).

INDICATIONS AND DOSAGES

▸ **Antibacterial, antifungal skin conditions**

TOPICAL

Adults, Elderly, Children 12 yr and older. Apply to skin 3-4 times/day. Typical duration is 2-4 wks.

CONTRAINDICATIONS

Lesions of the eye, tuberculosis of skin, diaper rash, children < 2 yr of age; hypersensitivity to clioquinol or hydrocortisone or any other component of the formulation.

INTERACTIONS

Drug
None known.

Herbal
None known.
Food
None known.

DIAGNOSTIC TEST EFFECTS

May alter thyroid function tests. Clioquinol may produce false-positive ferric chloride test results for phenylketonuria (PKU).

SIDE EFFECTS

Occasional
Blistering, burning, itching, peeling, skin rash, redness, swelling.

SERIOUS REACTIONS

- Thinning of skin with easy bruising may occur with prolonged use.

PRECAUTIONS & CONSIDERATIONS

Caution is warranted with herpes simplex, eczema vaccinatum, varicella, or other viral infections of the skin as well as intolerance to chloroxine, iodine, or iodine-containing preparations. It is unknown whether clioquinol and hydrocortisone cross placenta or are distributed in breast milk. No age-related precautions have been noted in children or elderly patients.

This medication may stain fabrics, skin, hair, and nails yellow. The affected area should be kept clean and dry. Light clothing should be worn to promote ventilation.
Storage
Store at room temperature.
Administration
Before applying, wash affected area with soap and water and dry thoroughly. Apply a thin layer to affected area. Wash hands after application.

Clobetasol

klo-bet'a-sol
★ Clobex, Cormax, Olux, Olux-E, Temovate, Temovate E, Temovate Scalp
🍁 Clobex, Cormax, Dermovate, Olux, Olux-E, Temovate, Temovate E, Temovate Scalp

CATEGORY AND SCHEDULE

Pregnancy Risk Category: C

Classification: Topical corticosteroid, very high potency

MECHANISM OF ACTION

A corticosteroid that inhibits accumulation of inflammatory cells at inflammation sites, phagocytosis, lysosomal enzyme release, and synthesis or release of mediators of inflammation. *Therapeutic Effect:* Decreases or prevents tissue response to inflammatory process.

PHARMACOKINETICS

May be absorbed from intact skin. Metabolized in liver. Excreted in the urine.

AVAILABILITY

Cream: 0.05% (Temovate).
Cream, in Emollient Base: 0.05% (Temovate E).
Foam: 0.05% (Olux, Olux-E).
Gel: 0.05% (Temovate).
Lotion: 0.05% (Clobex).
Ointment: 0.05% (Cormax, Temovate).
Shampoo: 0.05% (Clobex).
Topical Solution: 0.05% (Cormax, Temovate).
Topical Spray: 0.05% (Clobex).

INDICATIONS AND DOSAGES

▸ **Corticosteroid-responsive dermatoses, such as eczema, psoriasis**
TOPICAL

Adults, Elderly, Children 12 yr and older. Apply 2 times/day for 2 wks.
FOAM
Adults, Elderly, Children 12 yr and older. Apply 2 times/day for 2 wks.
SHAMPOO
Adults, Elderly. Apply thin film to dry scalp once daily; leave in place for 15 min, and then add water, lather; rinse thoroughly.
Maximum dose: For any use, do not exceed 50 g or mL per week. Treatment often cycles for 2 wks, off for 2 wks, then begins again if needed.

CONTRAINDICATIONS

Hypersensitivity to clobetasol or other corticosteroids.

INTERACTIONS

Drug
None known.
Herbal
None known.
Food
None known.

DIAGNOSTIC TEST EFFECTS

None known.

SIDE EFFECTS

Frequent
Local irritation, dry skin, itching, redness.
Occasional
Skin atrophy.
Rare
Allergic contact dermatitis, Cushing syndrome, numbness of fingers.

SERIOUS REACTIONS

- Overdosage can occur from topically applied clobetasol propionate absorbed in sufficient amounts to produce systemic effects producing reversible adrenal suppression, manifestations of Cushing syndrome, hyperglycemia, and glucosuria in some patients.

PRECAUTIONS & CONSIDERATIONS

Avoid use of occlusive dressings on affected area. Skin irritation should be reported. HPA axis suppression should be evaluated by ACTH stimulation test, AM plasma cortisol test, or urinary free cortisol test. It is unknown whether clobetasol propionate crosses the placenta or is distributed in breast milk. Safety and efficacy of clobetasol have not been established in children less than 12 yr of age. No age-related precautions have been noted in elderly patients.
Storage
Store all products at room temperature. Do not refrigerate or freeze. Topical spray and foam must be kept away from heat; spray is flammable.
Administration
Apply sparingly to skin or scalp and rub into area thoroughly. Use for 2 wks. If using for the scalp, part the hair and apply to the area.

Clocortolone

klo-kort′o-lone
★ Cloderm
Do not confuse clocortolone or Cloderm with Clocort.

CATEGORY AND SCHEDULE

Pregnancy Risk Category: C

Classification: Corticosteroids, topical low potency

MECHANISM OF ACTION

A topical corticosteroid that inhibits accumulation of inflammatory cells at inflammation sites, suppresses mitotic activity, and causes vasoconstriction. *Therapeutic Effect:* Decreases or prevents tissue response to inflammatory process.

PHARMACOKINETICS

Absorption is variable and dependent upon many factors, including the integrity of skin, dose, vehicle used, and use of occlusive dressings. Small amounts may be absorbed from the skin. Metabolized in liver. Excreted in the urine and feces.

AVAILABILITY

Cream: 0.1%.

INDICATIONS AND DOSAGES

▸ **Corticosteroid-responsive dermatoses**

TOPICAL

Adults, Elderly, Children 12 yr and older. Apply 1-4 times/day.

CONTRAINDICATIONS

Hypersensitivity to clocortolone pivalate or other corticosteroids; viral, fungal, or tubercular skin lesions.

INTERACTIONS

Drug, Herbal, and Food

None known.

DIAGNOSTIC TEST EFFECTS

None known.

SIDE EFFECTS

Occasional

Local irritation, burning, itching, redness, allergic contact dermatitis.

Rare

Hypertrichosis, hypopigmentation, maceration of skin, miliaria, perioral dermatitis, skin atrophy, striae.

SERIOUS REACTIONS

- Overdosage can occur from topically applied clocortolone pivalate absorbed in sufficient amounts to produce systemic effects in some patients.

PRECAUTIONS & CONSIDERATIONS

Avoid use of occlusive dressings on affected area. Skin irritation should be reported. HPA axis suppression should be evaluated by ACTH stimulation test, AM plasma cortisol test, or urinary free cortisol test. It is unknown whether clocortolone crosses the placenta or is distributed in breast milk. Safety and efficacy of clocortolone have not been established in children under 12 yr. No age-related precautions have been noted in elderly patients.

Storage

Store at room temperature, do not freeze.

Administration

Apply topical preparation sparingly. Do not use on broken skin. Avoid use of occlusive dressings.

Clofarabine

kloe-far′ah-been

★ 🍁 Clolar

Do not confuse clofarabine with cladribine or clevidipine.

CATEGORY AND SCHEDULE

Pregnancy Risk Category: D

Classification: Antineoplastic, antimetabolites, purine analogs

MECHANISM OF ACTION

An antineoplastic agent that inhibits DNA synthesis by decreasing deoxynucleotide triphosphate pools. It inhibits ribonucleoside reductase, terminates elongation of the DNA chain, and inhibits repair through incorporation into the DNA chain by competitive inhibition of DNA polymerases. *Therapeutic Effect:* Inhibits synthesis of DNA.

PHARMACOKINETICS

Protein binding: 47%. Negligible liver metabolism. Primarily excreted in urine. *Half-life:* 5.2 h.

AVAILABILITY

Injection Solution: 1 mg/mL.

INDICATIONS AND DOSAGES

▸ **ALL**

IV

Young Adults and Children 1-21 yr. 52 mg/m2 over 2 h daily for 5 consecutive days. Repeat every 2–6 wks following recovery or return to baseline organ function.

CONTRAINDICATIONS

Hypersensitivity to clofarabine or its components.

INTERACTIONS

Drug, Herbal, and Food

None known.

Live-virus vaccines: Defer vaccination due to potential virus replication, adverse reactions to the virus, immunosuppression.

DIAGNOSTIC TEST EFFECTS

Increased AST, ALT, potassium, uric acid, creatinine.

IV INCOMPATIBILITIES

Do not administer with any other medications through the same IV line.

IV COMPATIBILITIES

Dextrose 5%, 0.9% NaCl. No other information available.

SIDE EFFECTS

Frequent

Infection, vomiting, nausea, febrile neutropenia, diarrhea, pruritus, headache, ALT increased, dermatitis, pyrexia, AST increased, rigors, abdominal pain, fatigue, pericardial effusion, tachycardia, epistaxis, anorexia, petechiae, hypotension, pain in limb, left ventricular systolic dysfunction, anxiety, constipation, edema, pain, cough, erythema, flushing, mucosal inflammation, hematuria, dizziness, bilirubin increased, jaundice, gingival bleeding, hepatomegaly, injection site pain, myalgia, respiratory distress, palmar-plantar sore throat, back pain, dyspnea, erythrodysesthesia syndrome, staphylococcal infection, oral candidiasis, appetite decreased, cellulitis, depression, irritability, arthralgia, herpes simplex, hypertension, lethargy.

Occasional

Somnolence, weight gain, tremor, pleural effusion, pneumonia, systemic inflammatory response syndrome (SIRS)/capillary leak syndrome, transfusion reaction, bacteremia, creatinine increased.

SERIOUS REACTIONS

- Tumor lysis syndrome may occur.
- Severe bone marrow suppression, including neutropenia, anemia, and thrombocytopenia, has been observed.
- Risk of serious infections due to bone marrow suppression.

PRECAUTIONS & CONSIDERATIONS

Use with caution in renal or hepatic impairment. Safety and effectiveness have not been established in patients over 21 yr of age. High emetic potential; all patients should receive prophylactic antiemetics. Prophylactic corticosteroids should be considered to SIRS/capillary leak syndrome; prophylactic allopurinol may be considered if tumor lysis is anticipated. Avoid clofarabine use in pregnancy and breastfeeding. Women of childbearing potential should be advised to use adequate contraception.

Storage

Store vials at room temperature. Reconstituted solution must be used within 24 h at room temperature.

Administration

CAUTION: Observe and exercise usual cautions for handling and preparing solutions of cytotoxic drugs.

Injection should be filtered through a 0.2 μm syringe filter and then diluted with D5W or 0.9% NaCl (final concentration: 0.15-0.4 mg/mL.)

Infused IV over 2 h; expect continuous intravenous fluid therapy and supportive measures to prophylax potential side effects.

Clomiphene

kloe'mi-feen

Serophene

Do not confuse clomiphene with clomipramine or clonidine.

CATEGORY AND SCHEDULE

Pregnancy Risk Category: X

Classification: Nonsteroidal ovulatory stimulant, antiestrogen

MECHANISM OF ACTION

An ovulation stimulator that promotes release of pituitary gonadotropins. *Therapeutic Effect:* Stimulates ovulation.

PHARMACOKINETICS

Readily absorbed. Time to peak occurs within 6.5 h. Undergoes enterohepatic recirculation. Primarily excreted in feces. *Half-life:* 5-7 days.

AVAILABILITY

Tablets: 50 mg (Clomid, Milophene, Serophene).

INDICATIONS AND DOSAGES

▸ Infertility in females due to anovulation or irregular ovulation

PO

Adults. 50 mg/day for 5 days (first course); start the regimen on the fifth day of cycle. Increase dose only if unresponsive to cyclic 50 mg. Maximum: 100 mg/day for 5 days. Do not exceed 6 courses of treatment.

OFF-LABEL USES

Infertility in men.

CONTRAINDICATIONS

Liver dysfunction, abnormal uterine bleeding, enlargement or development of ovarian cyst, uncontrolled thyroid or adrenal dysfunction in the presence of an organic intracranial lesion such as pituitary tumor, pregnancy, hypersensitivity to clomiphene.

INTERACTIONS

Drug

Danazol: May decrease the response of clomiphene.

Estradiol: May decrease estradiol.

Herbal

Black cohosh chasteberry, DHEA: Possible interference with fertility treatment.

Food

None known.

DIAGNOSTIC TEST EFFECTS

Altered levels of thyroid function tests.

SIDE EFFECTS

Frequent (10%-13%)
Hot flashes, ovarian enlargement.
Occasional (2%-5%)
Abdominal/pelvic discomfort, bloating, nausea, vomiting, breast discomfort (females).
Rare (< 1%)
Vision disturbances, abnormal menstrual flow, breast enlargement (males), headache, mental depression, ovarian cyst formation, thromboembolism, uterine fibroid enlargement.

SERIOUS REACTIONS

- Thrombophlebitis, alopecia, and polyuria occur rarely.
- Ectopic pregnancy is possible; bilateral tubal pregnancy is rare.
- While not necessarily an adverse event, multiparity rates are 3%-5%, most commonly twins.
- Ovarian hyperstimulation syndrome/enlargement
- Visual changes.

PRECAUTIONS & CONSIDERATIONS

Caution should be used with liver dysfunction, polycystic ovary disease, and multiple pregnancies. Clomiphene use should be avoided during pregnancy, and it is distributed in breast milk. Safety and efficacy have not been established in children or in elderly patients. Pregnancy should be immediately reported. Visual disturbances, dizziness, light-headedness may occur.

Administration
Take clomiphene without regard to meals. Encourage coitus to coincide with ovulation.

Clomipramine

klom-ip′ra-meen

★ Anafranil 🍁 Anafranil, Apo-Clomipramine, Novo-Clopamine

Do not confuse clomipramine with chlorpromazine or clomiphene, or Anafranil with alfentanil, enalapril, or nafarelin.

CATEGORY AND SCHEDULE

Pregnancy Risk Category: C

Classification: Antidepressants, tricyclic

MECHANISM OF ACTION

A tricyclic antidepressant that blocks the reuptake of neurotransmitters, such as norepinephrine and serotonin, at CNS presynaptic membranes, increasing their availability at postsynaptic receptor sites. *Therapeutic Effect:* Reduces obsessive-compulsive behavior.

PHARMACOKINETICS

Well absorbed from GI tract. Protein binding: 97%. Principally bound to albumin. Distributed into cerebrospinal fluid. Metabolized in the liver. Undergoes extensive first-pass effect. Excreted in urine and feces. *Half-life:* 19-37 h.

AVAILABILITY

Capsules: 25 mg, 50 mg, 75 mg.

INDICATIONS AND DOSAGES

▸ **Obsessive-compulsive disorder**

PO

Adults, Elderly. Initially, 25 mg/day. May gradually increase to 100 mg/day in the first 2 wks. Maximum: 250 mg/day.

Children 10 yr and older.

Initially, 25 mg/day. May gradually increase up to maximum of 200 mg/day.

OFF-LABEL USES

Treatment of bulimia nervosa, cataplexy associated with narcolepsy, mental depression.

CONTRAINDICATIONS

Acute recovery period after MI, use within 14 days of MAOIs, hypersensitivity to TCAs.

INTERACTIONS

Drug

Antithyroid agents: May increase the risk of agranulocytosis.
Cimetidine: May increase clomipramine concentration and risk of toxicity.
Clonidine, guanadrel: May decrease the effects of these drugs.
MAOIs: May increase the risk of neuroleptic malignant syndrome, seizures, hyperpyresis, and hypertensive crisis. Contraindicated.
Other CNS depressants: May increase CNS and respiratory depression and the hypotensive effects of clomipramine.
SSRIs: Fluoxetine, sertraline, paroxetine, fluvoxamine inhibit CYP2D6 and may decrease TCA metabolism.
QT-prolonging drugs: Effects on QT interval may be additive.
Phenothiazines: May increase the anticholinergic and sedative effects of clomipramine.
Sympathomimetics: May increase the risk of cardiac effects.

Herbal

None known.

Food

Alcohol: May increase CNS and respiratory depression and the hypotensive effects of clomipramine.
Grapefruit juice: May increase clomipramine concentrations.

DIAGNOSTIC TEST EFFECTS

May alter the blood glucose level and ECG readings.

SIDE EFFECTS

Frequent

Somnolence, fatigue, dry mouth, blurred vision, constipation, sexual dysfunction (42%), ejaculatory failure (20%), impotence, weight gain (18%), delayed micturition, orthostatic hypotension, diaphoresis, impaired concentration, increased appetite, urine retention.

Occasional

GI disturbances (such as nausea, GI distress, and metallic taste), asthenia, aggressiveness, muscle weakness.

Rare

Paradoxical reactions (agitation, restlessness, nightmares, insomnia), extrapyramidal symptoms, (particularly fine hand tremor), laryngitis, seizures.

SERIOUS REACTIONS

- Overdose may produce seizures; cardiovascular effects, such as severe orthostatic hypotension, dizziness, tachycardia, palpitations, and arrhythmias; and altered temperature regulation, including hyperpyrexia or hypothermia.
- Abrupt discontinuation after prolonged therapy may produce headache, malaise, nausea, vomiting, and vivid dreams.
- Anemia and agranulocytosis have been noted.

PRECAUTIONS & CONSIDERATIONS

Caution is warranted in patients with cardiac disease, diabetes mellitus, glaucoma, hiatal hernia, history of seizures, history of urinary obstruction or urine retention, hyperthyroidism, increased intraocular pressure, benign prostatic hyperplasia, renal or hepatic disease, and schizophrenia. Clomipramine is minimally distributed in breast milk. Clomipramine use is not recommended for children younger than 10 yr. Antidepressants have been reported to increase the risk of suicidal thinking and behavior in children, adolescents, and young adults (18-24 yr of age) with major depressive disorder (MDD) and other psychiatric disorders. Patients should be closely monitored for clinical worsening, suicidality, or unusual changes in behavior, particularly during the initial 1-2 mo of therapy or following dosage adjustments. A lower dosage should be given to elderly patients, who are at increased risk for drug toxicity.

Dizziness may occur, so change positions slowly and avoid alcohol and tasks that require mental alertness or motor skills. CBC to detect signs of anemia and agranulocytosis and ECG to detect arrhythmias should be performed before and periodically during therapy.

Storage

Store at room temperature and protect from moisture.

Administration

Take clomipramine with food or milk if GI distress occurs. Administer in divided doses with food during dose titration; final dose may be administered once daily at bedtime to minimize daytime sedation. Full therapeutic effect may be noted in 2-4 wks. Do not abruptly discontinue clomipramine.

Clonazepam

kloe-na'zi-pam

Klonopin Apo-Clonazepam, Clonapam, Rivotril

Do not confuse clonazepam with clonidine or lorazepam.

CATEGORY AND SCHEDULE

Pregnancy Risk Category: D

Controlled Substance Schedule: IV

Classification: Anxiolytic, anticonvulsant, benzodiazepines

MECHANISM OF ACTION

A benzodiazepine that depresses all levels of the CNS, inhibits nerve impulse transmission in the motor cortex, and suppresses abnormal discharge in petit mal seizures. *Therapeutic Effect:* Produces anxiolytic and anticonvulsant effects.

PHARMACOKINETICS

Well absorbed from the GI tract. Protein binding: 85%. Metabolized in the liver. Excreted in urine. Not removed by hemodialysis. *Half-life:* 18-50 h.

AVAILABILITY

Tablets: 0.5 mg, 1 mg, 2 mg.

Tablets (Disintegrating): 0.125 mg, 0.25 mg, 0.5 mg, 1 mg, 2 mg.

INDICATIONS AND DOSAGES

▸ **Adjunctive treatment of Lennox-Gastaut syndrome (petit mal variant) and akinetic, myoclonic, and absence (petit mal) seizures**

PO

Adults, Elderly, Children 10 yr and older. 1.5 mg/day; may be increased in 0.5- to 1-mg increments every 3 days until seizures are controlled.

Do not exceed maintenance dosage of 20 mg/day.
Infants, Children < 10 yr or weighing < 30 kg. 0.01-0.03 mg/kg/day in 2-3 divided doses; may be increased by up to 0.5 mg every 3 days until seizures are controlled. Do not exceed maintenance dosage of 0.2 mg/kg/day.

▸ **Panic disorder**

PO

Adults, Elderly. Initially, 0.25 mg twice a day; increased in increments of 0.125-0.25 mg twice a day every 3 days. Maximum: 4 mg/day.

OFF-LABEL USES

Adjunctive treatment of seizures; treatment of simple, complex partial, and tonic-clonic seizures.

CONTRAINDICATIONS

Narrow-angle glaucoma, significant hepatic disease.

INTERACTIONS

Drug

Alcohol, other CNS depressants: May increase CNS depressant effect.
Ketoconazole, itraconazole, fluconazole, protease inhibitors, nefazodone: May increase clonazepam serum levels.

Herbal

Kava kava: May increase sedation.
St. John's wort: May decrease clonazepam concentrations.

Food

None known.

DIAGNOSTIC TEST EFFECTS

None known.

SIDE EFFECTS

Frequent

Mild, transient drowsiness; ataxia; behavioral disturbances (aggression, irritability, agitation), especially in children.

Occasional

Rash, ankle, or facial edema, nocturia, dysuria, change in appetite or weight, dry mouth, sore gums, nausea, blurred vision.

Rare

Paradoxical CNS reactions, including hyperactivity or nervousness in children and excitement or restlessness in elderly patients (particularly in the presence of uncontrolled pain).

SERIOUS REACTIONS

- Abrupt withdrawal may result in pronounced restlessness, irritability, insomnia, hand tremors, abdominal or muscle cramps, diaphoresis, vomiting, and status epilepticus.
- Overdose results in somnolence, confusion, diminished reflexes, and coma.

PRECAUTIONS & CONSIDERATIONS

Caution is warranted with chronic respiratory disease and impaired renal and hepatic function. Clonazepam crosses the placenta and may be distributed in breast milk. Chronic clonazepam use during pregnancy may produce withdrawal symptoms and CNS depression in neonates. Long-term clonazepam use may adversely affect the mental and physical development of children. Elderly patients are usually more sensitive to clonazepam's CNS effects, such as ataxia, dizziness, and oversedation. Expect to give them a lower dosage and increase it gradually. Alcohol, smoking, and tasks that require mental alertness or motor skills should be avoided.

Drowsiness and dizziness may occur. History of the seizure disorder, including the duration, frequency, and intensity of seizures, should be assessed. Autonomic responses, such as cold or clammy hands and diaphoresis, and motor responses, such as agitation, trembling, and tension, in those with panic disorder should also be assessed. CBC and blood chemistry tests and hepatic and renal function should be periodically monitored.

Storage

Store at room temperature; keep disintegrating tablet in package until time of use.

Administration

If the patient must switch to another anticonvulsant, expect to decrease the clonazepam dose gradually as therapy begins with a low dose of the replacement drug.

Do not abruptly discontinue the drug after long-term therapy. Strict maintenance of drug therapy is essential for seizure control.

Swallow the tablet whole with water. For the orally disintegrating tablet (ODT): After opening, peel back the foil on the blister. Do not push ODT through foil. Immediately, using dry hands, place ODT in the mouth. ODT will dissolve quickly and can be easily swallowed with or without water.

Clonidine

klon′ih-deen

★ Catapres, Catapres TTS, Duraclon, Kapvay 🍁 Dixarit

Do not confuse clonidine with clomiphene, Klonopin, or quinidine, or Catapres with Cetapred.

CATEGORY AND SCHEDULE

Pregnancy Risk Category: C

Classification: Antihypertensive, central α-adrenergic agonist

MECHANISM OF ACTION

An antiadrenergic, sympatholytic agent that prevents pain signal transmission to the brain and produces analgesia at pre- and post-α-adrenergic receptors in the spinal cord. *Therapeutic Effect:* Reduces peripheral resistance; decreases BP and heart rate.

PHARMACOKINETICS

Route	Onset	Peak	Duration
PO	0.5-1 h	2-4 h	Up to 8 h

Well absorbed from the GI tract. Transdermal best absorbed from the chest and upper arm; least absorbed from the thigh. Protein binding: 20%-40%. Metabolized in the liver. Primarily excreted in urine. Minimally removed by hemodialysis. *Half-life:* 12-16 h (increased with impaired renal function).

AVAILABILITY

Tablets (Catapres): 0.1 mg, 0.2 mg, 0.3 mg.
Tablets, Extended Release (Kapvay): 0.1 mg.
Transdermal Patch (Catapres TTS): 2.5 mg (release at 0.1 mg/24 h), 5 mg (release at 0.2 mg/24 h), 7.5 mg (release at 0.3 mg/24 h).
Injection (Duraclon): 100 mcg/mL, 500 mcg/mL.

INDICATIONS AND DOSAGES

▸ **Hypertension**

PO

Adults. Initially, 0.1 mg twice a day. Increase by 0.1-0.2 mg q2-4 days. Maintenance: 0.2-1.2 mg/day in 2-4 divided doses up to maximum of 2.4 mg/day.
Elderly. Initially, 0.1 mg at bedtime. May increase gradually.

C

Children. 5-25 mcg/kg/day in divided doses q6h. Increase at 5- to 7-day intervals. Maximum: 0.9 mg/day.
TRANSDERMAL
Adults, Elderly. System delivering 0.1 mg/24 h up to 0.6 mg/24 h q7 days.

▸ **Severe pain**
EPIDURAL
Adults, Elderly. 30-40 mcg/h.
Children. Initially, 0.5 mcg/kg/h, not to exceed adult dose.

▸ **ADHD**
PO (KAPVAY EXTENDED RELEASE TABLETS)
Children 6-18 yr. Initially 0.1 mg/day PO at bedtime. Increase weekly by 0.1 mg/day increments, up to 0.4 mg/day PO as needed to attain the desired response. Divide dose > 0.1 mg/day into 2 doses, morning and at bedtime. If the divided doses are not equal, give the larger dose at bedtime.

OFF-LABEL USES

Diagnosis of pheochromocytoma, alcohol or opioid withdrawal, treatment of menopausal flushing.

CONTRAINDICATIONS

Hypersensitivity to clonidine or any product component, epidural contraindicated with bleeding diathesis or infection at the injection site, or anticoagulation therapy.

INTERACTIONS

Drug
β-Blockers: Potential for additive effects on BP or heart rate.
Tricyclic antidepressants: May decrease effect of clonidine.
Herbal
None known.
Food
Alcohol: Potentiate CNS effects.

DIAGNOSTIC TEST EFFECTS

None known.

SIDE EFFECTS

Frequent
Dry mouth (40%), somnolence (33%), dizziness (16%), sedation, constipation (10%).
Occasional (1%-5%)
Depression, swelling of feet, loss of appetite, decreased sexual ability, itching eyes, dizziness, nausea, vomiting, nervousness. Decreases in blood pressure or heart rate.
Transdermal: Itching, reddening or darkening of skin.
Rare (< 1%)
Nightmares, vivid dreams, cold feeling in fingers and toes.

SERIOUS REACTIONS

- Overdose produces profound hypotension, irritability, bradycardia, respiratory depression, hypothermia, miosis (pupillary constriction), arrhythmias, and apnea.
- Abrupt withdrawal may result in rebound hypertension, nervousness, agitation, anxiety, insomnia, hand tingling, tremor, flushing, and diaphoresis.

PRECAUTIONS & CONSIDERATIONS

Caution is warranted with cerebrovascular disease, chronic renal failure, Raynaud disease, recent myocardial infarction, severe coronary insufficiency, and thromboangiitis obliterans. Clonidine crosses the placenta and is distributed in breast milk. Children are more sensitive to clonidine's effects. A thorough cardiovascular assessment is recommended before initiation in pediatric patients; include medical history, family history, and physical examination, and consider ECG testing. Elderly patients may be more sensitive.

Dizziness and light-headedness may occur. Rise slowly from a lying to a sitting position and permit legs to dangle momentarily. BP should be obtained immediately before giving each dose. Be alert for BP fluctuations. Daily bowel activity and stool consistency should also be assessed. Expect concurrent β-blocker therapy to be discontinued several days before discontinuing clonidine therapy to prevent clonidine withdrawal hypertensive crisis; and clonidine dosage should be reduced over 2-4 days.

Administration
Take oral clonidine without regard to food. Do not chew, crush, or break extended release tablets. Take last dose of the day just before bedtime. Avoid skipping doses or voluntarily discontinuing clonidine because it can produce severe, rebound hypertension.

For transdermal use, apply the system to dry, hairless area of intact skin on upper arm or chest. Rotate sites to prevent skin irritation. Do not trim patch to adjust dose.

Epidural injection must be diluted in 0.9% NaCl injection to a concentration of 100 mcg/mL before use. Administered using a continuous epidural device.

Clopidogrel

clo-pid′o-grill
★ 🍁 Plavix
Do not confuse Plavix with Paxil.

CATEGORY AND SCHEDULE
Pregnancy Risk Category: B

Classification: Platelet aggregation inhibitor

MECHANISM OF ACTION
A thienopyridine derivative that inhibits binding of the enzyme adenosine phosphate (ADP) to its platelet receptor and subsequent ADP-mediated activation of a glycoprotein complex. *Therapeutic Effect:* Inhibits platelet aggregation.

PHARMACOKINETICS

Route	Onset	Peak	Duration
PO	1 h	2 h	N/A

Rapidly absorbed. Protein binding: 98%. Extensively metabolized by the liver. Eliminated equally in the urine and feces. *Half-life:* 8 h.

AVAILABILITY
Tablets: 75 mg, 300 mg.

INDICATIONS AND DOSAGES
▸ **Recent MI, recent stroke, or established peripheral arterial disease**
PO
Adults, Elderly. 75 mg once a day.
▸ **Acute coronary syndrome (unstable angina or non-Q-wave acute MI), including those who have PCI or CABG:**
PO
Adults, Elderly. Initially, 300 mg loading dose, then 75 mg once a day (in combination with aspirin).

CONTRAINDICATIONS
Hypersensitivity to clopidogrel, active pathological bleeding such as peptic ulcer or intracranial hemorrhage.

INTERACTIONS
Drug
Anticoagulants: May increase the risk of bleeding.
Clarithromycin, erythromycin: May reduce the effects of clopidogrel.

C

Fluvastatin, NSAIDs, phenytoin, tamoxifen, tolbutamide, torsemide, warfarin: May interfere with metabolism of these drugs.
Omeprazole, possibly other PPIs with CYP2C19 inhibiting activity: Reduce conversion of clopidogrel to active metabolite; may result in cardiovascular events due to decreased efficacy. Avoid when possible.
Herbal
Ginger, ginkgo biloba, white willow: May increase the risk of bleeding.
Food
None known.

DIAGNOSTIC TEST EFFECTS
Prolongs bleeding time.

SIDE EFFECTS
Frequent (15%)
Skin disorders.
Occasional (6%-8%)
Upper respiratory tract infection, chest pain, flu-like symptoms, headache, dizziness, arthralgia.
Rare (3%-5%)
Fatigue, edema, hypertension, abdominal pain, dyspepsia, diarrhea, nausea, epistaxis, dyspnea, rhinitis.

SERIOUS REACTIONS
- Thrombotic thrombocytopenic purpura.
- GI hemorrhage.

PRECAUTIONS & CONSIDERATIONS
Caution is warranted with hematologic disorders, history of bleeding, hypertension, hepatic or renal impairment, and in preoperative persons. Be aware that it may take longer to stop bleeding during drug therapy.

Notify the physician of unusual bleeding. Also, notify dentists and other physicians before surgery is scheduled or when new drugs are prescribed. Platelet count for thrombocytopenia, hemoglobin level, WBC count, and BUN, serum bilirubin, creatinine, AST (SGOT) and ALT (SGPT) levels should be monitored. Platelet count should be obtained before clopidogrel therapy, every 2 days during the first week of treatment, and weekly thereafter until therapeutic maintenance dose is reached. Be aware that abrupt discontinuation of clopidogrel produces an elevated platelet count within 5 days.
Storage
Store at room temperature.
Administration
Take clopidogrel without regard to food. Do not crush coated tablets.

Clorazepate
klor-az'e-pate
★ Tranxene
Do not confuse clorazepate with clofibrate or clonazepam.

CATEGORY AND SCHEDULE
Pregnancy Risk Category: D
Controlled Substance Schedule: IV

Classification: Anticonvulsants, anxiolytic, benzodiazepine

MECHANISM OF ACTION
A benzodiazepine that depresses all levels of the CNS, including limbic and reticular formation, by binding to benzodiazepine receptor sites on the γ-aminobutyric acid (GABA) receptor complex. Modulates GABA, a major inhibitory neurotransmitter in the brain. *Therapeutic Effect:* Produces anxiolytic effect, suppresses seizure activity.

PHARMACOKINETICS

Well absorbed after oral administration. Rapidly metabolized by liver to nordiazepam, which is slowly eliminated. *Half-life:* 40-50 h. Protein binding of nordiazepam: 97%-98%. Metabolites (nordiazepam, oxazepam, and glucuronide conjugates) excreted in urine.

AVAILABILITY

Tablets: 3.75 mg, 7.5 mg, 15 mg.

INDICATIONS AND DOSAGES

▸ **Anxiety**

PO

Adults, Elderly. (Regular release): 7.5-15 mg 2-4 times a day. (Sustained release): 11.25 mg or 22.5 mg once a day at bedtime.

▸ **Anticonvulsant (adjunct)**

PO

Adults, Elderly, Children older than 12 yr. Initially, 7.5 mg 2-3 times a day. May increase by 7.5 mg at weekly intervals. Maximum: 90 mg/day.

Children 9-12 yr. Initially, 3.75-7.5 mg twice a day. May increase by 2.75 mg at weekly intervals. Maximum: 60 mg/day.

▸ **Alcohol withdrawal**

PO

Adults, Elderly. Initially, 30 mg, then 15 mg 2-4 times a day on first day. Gradually decrease dosage over subsequent days. Maximum: 90 mg/day.

CONTRAINDICATIONS

Hypersensitivity, acute narrow-angle glaucoma.

INTERACTIONS

Drug

Other CNS depressants: May increase CNS depressant effects.

Herbal

Kava kava, St. John's wort, valerian: May increase CNS depression.

Food

Alcohol: May increase CNS depressant effects.

Grapefruit juice: Clorazepate concentrations may be increased.

DIAGNOSTIC TEST EFFECTS

Decreased hematocrit; abnormal liver and renal function tests. Therapeutic serum drug level is 0.12-1.5 mcg/mL; toxic serum drug level is > 5 mcg/mL.

SIDE EFFECTS

Frequent

Somnolence.

Occasional

Dizziness, GI disturbances, nervousness, blurred vision, dry mouth, headache, confusion, ataxia, rash, irritability, slurred speech.

Rare

Paradoxical CNS reactions, such as hyperactivity or nervousness in children and excitement or restlessness in elderly or debilitated patients (generally noted during first 2 wks of therapy, particularly in the presence of uncontrolled pain).

SERIOUS REACTIONS

- Abrupt or too-rapid withdrawal may result in pronounced restlessness, irritability, insomnia, hand tremors, abdominal or muscle cramps, diaphoresis, vomiting, and seizures.
- Overdose results in somnolence, confusion, diminished reflexes, and coma.

PRECAUTIONS & CONSIDERATIONS

Caution is warranted in patients with acute alcohol intoxication and renal and hepatic impairment. Women should use effective contraception during therapy and notify their physician immediately if they become or may be pregnant.

C

Drowsiness and dizziness may occur. Change positions slowly from recumbent to sitting, before standing, to prevent dizziness. Alcohol, smoking, and tasks that require mental alertness or motor skills should also be avoided. Autonomic responses, such as cold, clammy hands and diaphoresis, and motor responses, such as agitation, trembling, and tension, should be assessed. Seizure frequency and intensity should be assessed.

Storage

Store at controlled room temperature, protect from heat and moisture.

Administration

If the person must change to another anticonvulsant, plan to decrease clorazepate dosage gradually as low-dose therapy begins with the replacement drug.

Do not abruptly discontinue the medication after long-term use, because this may precipitate seizures. Strict compliance with the drug regimen is essential for seizure control.

May take without regard to food.

Clotrimazole

kloe-try'mah-zole

★ Cruex, Gyne-Lotrimin-3, Gyne-Lotrimin-7, Lotrimin, Lotrimin AF 🍁 Canesten, Clotrimaderm

CATEGORY AND SCHEDULE

Pregnancy Risk Category: B (topical), C (troches)

OTC/Rx

Classification: Azole antifungal, topical, vaginal

MECHANISM OF ACTION

An antifungal that binds with phospholipids in fungal cell membrane. Alters cell membrane permeability. *Therapeutic Effect:* Inhibits yeast growth.

PHARMACOKINETICS

Poorly, erratically absorbed from GI tract. Bound to oral mucosa. Absorbed portion metabolized in liver. Eliminated in feces. Topical: Minimal systemic absorption (highest concentration in stratum corneum). Intravaginal: Small amount systemically absorbed. *Half-life:* 3.5-5 h.

AVAILABILITY

Combination Pack: Vaginal tablet 100 mg and vaginal cream 1%.
Lotion: 1% (Lotrimin).
Topical Cream: 1% (Cruex, Lotrimin, Lotrimin AF).
Topical Solution: 1% (Lotrimin, Lotrimin AF).
Troches: 10 mg.
Vaginal Cream: 1% (Gyne-Lotrimin-7), 2% (Gyne-Lotrimin-3).
Vaginal Tablets: 100 mg, 500 mg (Gyne-Lotrimin).

INDICATIONS AND DOSAGES

▸ **Oropharyngeal candidiasis treatment**

TROCHE

Adults, Elderly. 10 mg 5 times/day for 14 days.

▸ **Oropharyngeal candidiasis prophylaxis**

TROCHE

Adults, Elderly. 10 mg 3 times/day.

▸ **Cutaneous candidiasis or tinea corporis; tinea cruris; tinea pedis**

TOPICAL

Adults, Elderly. Apply to affected area 2 times/day. Therapeutic effect may take up to 8 wks.

▸ **Vulvovaginal candidiasis**

VAGINAL (CREAM, 7-Day regimen)

Adults, Elderly. 1 applicatorful at bedtime for 7-14 days.
VAGINAL (CREAM, 3-day regimen)
Adults, Elderly. 1 applicatorful at bedtime for 3 days.

OFF-LABEL USES

Topical: Treatment of paronychia, tinea barbae, tinea capitis.

CONTRAINDICATIONS

Hypersensitivity to clotrimazole or any component of the formulation.

INTERACTIONS

Drug
Vaginal spermicides: Clotrimazole vaginal may inactivate contraceptive effect.
Tacrolimus: Troche use may increase risk of tacrolimus toxicity.
Herbal
None known.
Food
None known.

DIAGNOSTIC TEST EFFECTS

May increase SGOT (AST).

SIDE EFFECTS

Frequent
Oral: Nausea, vomiting, diarrhea, abdominal pain.
Occasional
Topical: Itching, burning, stinging, erythema, urticaria.
Vaginal: Mild burning, irritation, cystitis.
Rare
Vaginal: Itching, rash, lower abdominal cramping, headache.

SERIOUS REACTIONS

- None reported.

PRECAUTIONS & CONSIDERATIONS

Caution is warranted in patients with hepatic disorder with oral therapy. It is unknown whether clotrimazole crosses the placenta or is distributed in breast milk. Troche use is not recommended in children < 3 yr of age; use of intravaginal and topical products not established in those < 12 yr. There are no special precautions for the elderly. During vaginal treatment, patients should refrain from sexual intercouse and not use tampons; do not use condoms or diaphragms or cervical cap, as product may damage them and make them unreliable. For any OTC use, the patient should seek advice for any condition not responding after 1 wk, or if condition is associated with fever, rash, or complicated by potential immunosuppression. Separate personal items and linens.
Storage
Store at room temperature. Do not freeze.
Administration
Lozenges must be dissolved in mouth more than 15-30 min for oropharyngeal therapy. Do not chew. Swallow saliva.

When using topical preparation, rub well into affected, surrounding areas. Do not apply occlusive covering or other preparations. Keep area clean and dry. Wear light clothing to promote ventilation.

To use vaginally, use vaginal applicator and insert high in vagina. Continue to use during menses.

Clozapine

klo'za-peen
Clozaril, FazaClo
Do not confuse clozapine with Cloxapen or clofazimine, or Clozaril with Clinoril or Colazal.

CATEGORY AND SCHEDULE

Pregnancy Risk Category: B

Classification: Antipsychotic, atypical

C

MECHANISM OF ACTION

A dibenzodiazepine derivative that mainly blocks dopamine D_1 and D_4 receptors and also blocks serotonin type 2 receptors. Increases turnover of GABA in the nucleus accumbens. Some side effects occur due to α_1-adrenergic blockage and anticholinergic effects. One exception is M4 muscarinic receptor agonism, which causes hypersalivation. Drug lowers seizure threshold. *Therapeutic Effect:* Diminishes schizophrenic behavior.

PHARMACOKINETICS

Absorbed rapidly and almost completely. Distributed rapidly and extensively. Crosses the blood-brain barrier. Protein binding: 95%. Metabolized in the liver. Excreted in urine and feces. *Half-life:* 8 h.

AVAILABILITY

Tablets (Clozaril): 25 mg, 50 mg, 100 mg, 200 mg.
Oral disintegrating tablets (FazaClo): 12.5 mg, 25 mg, 100 mg.

INDICATIONS AND DOSAGES

▸ **Schizophrenic disorders, reduce suicidal behavior**

PO

Adults. Initially, 25 mg once or twice a day. May increase by 25-50 mg/day over 2 wks until dosage of 300-450 mg/day is achieved. May further increase by 50-100 mg/day no more than once or twice a week.
Range: 200-600 mg/day. Maximum: 900 mg/day.
Elderly. Initially, 25 mg/day. May increase by 25 mg/day. Maximum: 450 mg/day.

CONTRAINDICATIONS

Coma, concurrent use of other drugs that may suppress bone marrow function, history of clozapine-induced agranulocytosis or severe granulocytopenia, myeloproliferative disorders, severe CNS depression, uncontrolled epilepsy, paralytic ileus.

INTERACTIONS

Drug

Alcohol, other CNS depressants: May increase CNS depressant effects.
Bone marrow depressants: May increase myelosuppression.
Lithium: May increase the risk of confusion, dyskinesia, and seizures.
Phenobarbital: Decreases clozapine blood concentration.

Herbal

St. John's wort: May decrease clozapine levels.
Kava kava, gotu kola, valerian, St. John's wort: May increase CNS depression.

Food

None known.

DIAGNOSTIC TEST EFFECTS

May increase serum glucose levels.

SIDE EFFECTS

Frequent

Somnolence (39%), salivation (31%), tachycardia (25%), dizziness (19%), constipation (14%).

Occasional

Hypotension (9%); headache (7%); tremor, syncope, diaphoresis, dry mouth (6%); nausea, visual disturbances (5%); nightmares, restlessness, akinesia, agitation, hypertension, abdominal discomfort or heartburn, weight gain (4%).

Rare

Rigidity, confusion, fatigue, insomnia, rash, fecal impaction.

SERIOUS REACTIONS

- Seizures occur in about 3% of patients.

- Overdose produces CNS depression (including sedation, coma, and delirium), respiratory depression, and hypersalivation.
- Blood dyscrasias, particularly agranulocytosis and mild leukopenia, may occur. If WBC < 2000/mm^3 or ANC < 1000/mm^3, do not rechallenge.
- Myocarditis.
- Paralytic ileus.

PRECAUTIONS & CONSIDERATIONS

Caution is warranted in patients with alcohol withdrawal and in those with cardiovascular disease, glaucoma, diabetes, history of seizures, benign prostatic hyperplasia, myocarditis, myasthenia gravis, urine retention, and impaired hepatic, renal, or respiratory function.

Drowsiness may occur but generally subsides with continued therapy. Increased mortality has been observed in elderly patients with dementia-related psychosis treated with antipsychotics. Alcohol and tasks that require mental alertness or motor skills should be avoided. BP for hypertension or hypotension, heart rate for tachycardia, and CBC for blood dyscrasias (particularly agranulocytosis and mild leukopenia) should be assessed.

Clozapine is available only through a distribution system that ensures monitoring of WBC count and ANC. WBC count should be monitored every week for the first 6 mo of continuous therapy, then biweekly when WBC counts are acceptable.

Storage

Store tablets at room temperature. Orally disintegrating tablet (ODT) should be left in the unopened blister until time of use. Protect from moisture.

Administration

Take clozapine without regard to food. Do not abruptly discontinue. Expect to monitor blood work before prescription can be filled.

For ODT: Just prior to use, peel the foil from the blister and gently remove. Do not push through the blister foil. Immediately place the tablet in the mouth and allow to disintegrate and swallow with saliva, or chew as desired. No water is needed. If a partial tablet is needed for the dose, discard the unused portion.

Co-Trimoxazole (Sulfamethoxazole and Trimethoprim)

koe-trye-mox′a-zole

★ Bacter-Aid DS, Bactrim, Bactrim DS, Sulfatrim Pediatric, Septra, Septra DS, Sultrex Pediatric 🍁 Novo-Trimel, Nu-Cotrimox, Trisulfa, Trisulfa DS

Do not confuse Bactrim with bacitracin, co-trimoxazole with clotrimazole, or Septra with Sectral or Septa.

CATEGORY AND SCHEDULE

Pregnancy Risk Category: C

Classification: Antibiotics, folate antagonists, sulfonamides

MECHANISM OF ACTION

A sulfonamide and folate antagonist that blocks bacterial synthesis of essential nucleic acids. *Therapeutic Effect:* Bactericidal in susceptible microorganisms.

C

PHARMACOKINETICS

Rapidly and well absorbed from the GI tract. Protein binding: 45%-60%. Widely distributed. Metabolized in the liver. Excreted in urine. Minimally removed by hemodialysis. *Half-life:* Sulfamethoxazole 6-12 h, trimethoprim 8-10 h (increased in impaired renal function).

AVAILABILITY

! All dosage forms have same 5:1 ratio of sulfamethoxazole (SMX) to trimethoprim (TMP).

Oral Suspension (Sultrex Pediatric, Sulfatrim Pediatric): SMX 200 mg/5 mL and TMP 40 mg/5 mL.

Tablets (Bactrim, Septra): SMX 400 mg and TMP 80 mg.

Tablets, double strength (Bacter-Aid DS, Bactrim DS, Septra DS): SMX 800 mg and TMP 160 mg.

Injection: SMX 80 mg/mL and TMP 16 mg/mL.

INDICATIONS AND DOSAGES

▸ **Mild to moderate infections**

PO

Adults, Elderly. 160 mg TMP/800 mg SMX q12hr.

Children older than 2 mo. 8-12 mg/kg/day based on the TMP component in divided doses q12hr.

IV

Adults, Elderly, Children older than 2 mo. 8-12 mg/kg/day based on the TMP component in divided doses q6-12h.

▸ **Serious infections, *Pneumocystis carinii* pneumonia (PCP)**

PO, IV

Adults, Elderly, Children older than 2 mo. 15-20 mg/kg/day based on the TMP component in divided doses q6-8h.

▸ **Prevention of PCP**

PO

Adults. 160 mg TMP/800 mg SMX each day.

Children. 150 mg/m^2/day based on the TMP component in 2 divided doses on 3 consecutive days/wk.

▸ **Traveler's diarrhea**

PO

Adults, Elderly. 160 mg TMP/800 mg SMX q12h for 5 days.

▸ **Acute exacerbation of chronic bronchitis**

PO

Adults, Elderly. 160 mg TMP/800 mg SMX q12h for 14 days.

▸ **Prevention of urinary tract infection**

PO

Adults, Elderly, Children older than 2 mo. 2 mg/kg/dose once a day.

▸ **Dosage in renal impairment**

Dosage and frequency are modified based on creatinine clearance, the severity of the infection, and the serum concentration of the drug. For those with creatinine clearance of 15-30 mL/min, a 50% dosage reduction is recommended.

OFF-LABEL USES

Treatment of bacterial endocarditis; gonorrhea; meningitis; septicemia; sinusitis; and biliary tract, bone, joint, chancroid, chlamydial, intra-abdominal, skin, and soft-tissue infections.

CONTRAINDICATIONS

Known hypersensitivity to trimethoprim or sulfonamides, a history of drug-induced immune thrombocytopenia with these drugs; megaloblastic anemia due to folate deficiency, marked hepatic damage, or several renal insufficiency if patient cannot be closely monitored. Do not use in pregnancy or breast feeding because sulfonamides may cause kernicterus. Do not use in infants < 2 mo of age.

INTERACTIONS

Drug

Cyclosporine: May decrease cyclosporine levels and increase risk of nephrotoxicity.
Hemolytics: May increase the risk of toxicity.
Hepatotoxic medications: May increase the risk of hepatotoxicity.
Hydantoin anticonvulsants, oral antidiabetics, warfarin: May increase or prolong the effects of these drugs and increase their risk of toxicity.
Methenamine: May form a precipitate.
Methotrexate: May increase the effects of methotrexate.
Warfarin: Potentiates anticoagulant effect of warfarin.

Herbal and Food

None known.

DIAGNOSTIC TEST EFFECTS

May increase BUN and serum alkaline phosphatase, creatinine, potassium, AST (SGOT), and ALT (SGPT) levels; decreases glucose.

IV INCOMPATIBILITIES

NOTE: SMZ-TMP incompatible with many drugs at Y-site. Consult specialized resources prior to infusing. Incompatibilities include alfentanil, amikacin, aminophylline, ampicillin, ampicillin-sulbactam (Unasyn), aztreonam, bumetanide, butorphanol, calcium glucnonate, caspofungin (Cancidas), most cephalosporins, cimetidine, clindamycin (Cleocin), codeine, dexamethasone, diazepam, digoxin (Lanoxin), dobutamine, dopamine, famotidine (Pepcid), fluconazole (Diflucan), foscarnet (Foscavir), furosemide, gentamicin, haloperidol, hydrocortisone, imipenem-cilastatin (Primaxin), regular insulin, lactaged Ringer's, mannitol, methylprednisolone, metoclopramide, midazolam (Versed), nitroglycerin, nitroprusside, ondansetron (Zofran), promethazine, quinupristin-dalfopristin (Synercid), sodium bicarbonate.

SIDE EFFECTS

Frequent

Anorexia, nausea, vomiting, rash (generally 7-14 days after therapy begins), urticaria.

Occasional

Diarrhea, abdominal pain, pain or irritation at the IV infusion site.

Rare

Headache, vertigo, insomnia, seizures, hallucinations, depression.

SERIOUS REACTIONS

- Rash, fever, sore throat, pallor, purpura, cough, and shortness of breath may be early signs of serious adverse reactions.
- Fatalities have occasionally occurred after Stevens-Johnson syndrome, toxic epidermal necrolysis, fulminant hepatic necrosis, agranulocytosis, aplastic anemia, and other blood dyscrasias in patients taking sulfonamides.
- Myelosuppression, decreased platelet count, and severe dermatologic reactions may occur, especially in elderly patients.

PRECAUTIONS & CONSIDERATIONS

Caution is warranted with impaired renal or hepatic function or glucose-6-phosphate dehydrogenase deficiency. Co-trimoxazole use is contraindicated during pregnancy at term and during breastfeeding. Co-trimoxazole readily crosses the placenta and is distributed in breast milk. Co-trimoxazole use is contraindicated in children younger than 2 mo old; if given to newborns,

C

it may produce kernicterus. Elderly patients have an increased risk of developing myelosuppression, decreased platelet count, and severe skin reactions.

History of bronchial asthma, hypersensitivity to trimethoprim or any sulfonamide, or sulfite sensitivity should be determined before beginning drug therapy. Report any new symptoms, especially bleeding, bruising, fever, sore throat, and a rash or other skin changes. Intake and output, pattern of daily bowel activity and stool consistency, skin for rash, renal and liver function, CNS symptoms such as hallucinations, headache, insomnia, and vertigo should be assessed. Vital signs should be monitored at least twice a day.

Storage

Store tablets and oral suspension at room temperature. Store unopened vials at room temperature; do not refrigerate or freeze. Be aware that the IV infusion solution is stable for 2-6 h. Discard the solution if it is cloudy or contains a precipitate.

Administration

! Be aware that drug dosing is expressed in terms of trimethoprim content.

Take the oral form with 8 oz water on an empty stomach. Have the patient drink several additional glasses of water each day. Shake oral suspension well before each use.

For piggyback IV infusion, dilute each 5-mL vial with 75-125 mL D5W. Do not mix co-trimoxazole with other drugs or solutions. Infuse the solution over 60-90 min. Avoid bolus or rapid infusion and IM injection. Ensure that the patient is adequately hydrated.

Codeine

koe'deen

🍁 Codeine, Contin

Do not confuse codeine with Cardene or Lodine.

CATEGORY AND SCHEDULE

Pregnancy Risk Category: C (D if used for prolonged periods or at high dosages at term)

Controlled Substance Schedule: II (analgesic), III (fixed-combination form)

Classification: Analgesics, narcotic, antitussives

MECHANISM OF ACTION

An opioid agonist that binds to opioid receptors at many sites in the CNS, particularly in the medulla. This action inhibits the ascending pain pathways. *Therapeutic Effect:* Alters the perception of and emotional response to pain, suppresses cough reflex.

PHARMACOKINETICS

Well absorbed after oral administration. Rapidly metabolized by liver/10% methylated to the active analgesic morphine; the conversion is mediated by CYP2D6. *Half-life:* 2.5-3 h. Metabolites excreted in urine.

AVAILABILITY

Tablets: 15 mg, 30 mg, 60 mg.

INDICATIONS AND DOSAGES

▸ **Analgesia**

PO

Adults, Elderly. 30 mg q4-6h. Range: 15-60 mg.

Children. 0.5-1 mg/kg q4-6h. Maximum: 60 mg/dose.

▸ **Cough**

PO

Adults, Elderly, Children 12 yr and older. 10-20 mg q4-6h.
Children 6-11 yr. 5-10 mg q4-6h.
Children 2-5 yr. 2.5-5 mg q4-6h.

▸ Dosage in renal impairment

Dosage is modified based on creatinine clearance.

Creatinine Clearance (mL/min)	Dosage
10-50	75% of usual dose
< 10	50% of usual dose

OFF-LABEL USES

Treatment of noninfectious diarrhea.

CONTRAINDICATIONS

Hypersensitivity to codeine.
Some products list paralytic ileus, presence of respiratory depression in absence of resuscitative equipment, and severe bronchial asthma or hypercarbia as additional contraindications.

INTERACTIONS

Drug

Alcohol, other CNS depressants: May increase hypotension and CNS or respiratory depression.
MAOIs: May produce a severe, sometimes fatal reaction; plan to administer a test dose, which is one-quarter of usual codeine dose.
CYP2D6 inhibitors (chlorpromazine, delavirdine, fluoxetine, miconazole, paroxetine, pergolide, quinidine, quinine, ritonavir, and ropinirole): May decrease the effects of codeine.

Herbal

St. John's wort, valerian, kava kava, gotu kola: Increase CNS depression.
St. John's wort: May reduce codeine concentrations; speed conversion to the metabolite.

Food

None known.

DIAGNOSTIC TEST EFFECTS

May increase serum amylase and lipase levels.

SIDE EFFECTS

Frequent

Constipation, somnolence, nausea, vomiting.

Occasional

Paradoxical excitement, confusion, palpitations, facial flushing, decreased urination, blurred vision, dizziness, dry mouth, headache, hypotension (including orthostatic hypotension), decreased appetite.

Rare

Hallucinations, depression, abdominal pain, insomnia.

SERIOUS REACTIONS

- Too-frequent use may result in paralytic ileus.
- Overdose may produce cold and clammy skin, confusion, seizures, decreased BP, restlessness, pinpoint pupils, bradycardia, respiratory depression, decreased LOC, and severe weakness.
- The patient who uses codeine repeatedly may develop a tolerance to the drug's analgesic effect as well as physical dependence.

PRECAUTIONS & CONSIDERATIONS

Extreme caution should be used in patients with acute alcoholism, anoxia, CNS depression, hypercapnia, respiratory depression or dysfunction, seizures, shock, and untreated myxedema. Caution is also warranted in patients with acute abdominal conditions, Addison disease, COPD, hypothyroidism, hepatic impairment, increased intracranial pressure, benign prostatic hyperplasia, and urethral

C

stricture. Codeine crosses the placenta and is distributed in breast milk. Regular use of opioids during pregnancy may produce withdrawal symptoms in the neonate. Codeine may prolong labor if it is administered in the latent phase of the first stage of labor or before the cervix is dilated 4-5 cm. The neonate may develop respiratory depression if the mother receives codeine during labor. Nursing infants may be exposed to high levels of the codeine metabolite, morphine, in breast milk. Caution is advised with use in breastfeeding. Infant should be closely monitored for signs of toxicity. Children and elderly patients are more prone to paradoxical excitement and respiratory depression. In elderly patients, age-related renal impairment may increase the risk of codeine-induced urine retention.

Dizziness and drowsiness may occur, so change positions slowly and avoid alcohol, CNS depressants, and tasks that require mental alertness or motor skills until response to the drug is established. Vital signs, pattern of daily bowel activity and stool consistency, and clinical improvement of pain should be monitored.

Administration

Be aware that ambulatory patients and patients not in severe pain may be more prone to dizziness, hypotension, nausea, and vomiting than patients in the supine position and those in severe pain.

For oral use, take codeine with food or milk to minimize adverse GI effects.

Colchicine

kol'chi-seen

★ 🍁 Colcrys

CATEGORY AND SCHEDULE

Pregnancy Risk Category: D

Classification: Antigout agents

MECHANISM OF ACTION

An alkaloid that decreases leukocyte motility, phagocytosis, and lactic acid production. *Therapeutic Effect:* Decreases urate crystal deposits and reduces inflammatory process.

PHARMACOKINETICS

Rapidly absorbed from the GI tract. Highest concentration is in the liver, spleen, and kidney. Protein binding: 30%-50%. Reenters the intestinal tract by biliary secretion and is reabsorbed from the intestines. Partially metabolized in the liver. Eliminated primarily in feces.

AVAILABILITY

Tablets: 0.6 mg.

INDICATIONS AND DOSAGES

▸ Acute gout flare

PO

Adults, Elderly. 1.2 mg (2 tablets) at the first sign of the flare then 0.6 mg (1 tablet) 1 h later. Higher doses are not more effective. Maximum: 1.8 mg over a 1-h period. May also give in patients already receiving colchicine prophylaxis, with first dose not to exceed 1.2 mg, then 0.6 mg at 1 h later. Wait 12 h and then resume the prophylactic dose.

▸ **Prophylaxis of gout flares**
PO
Adults, Elderly, and Children > 16 yr. 0.6 mg once or twice daily. Maximum: 1.2 mg/day.

▸ **Familial Mediterranean fever (FMF)**
PO
Adults, Elderly on no interacting drugs. 1.2-2.4 mg PO daily in 1 to 2 divided doses; start at lower dose and titrate by increments of 0.3 mg/day.
Children > 12 yr. 1.2-2.4 mg PO daily in 1 to 2 divided doses; titrate within this range by increments of 0.3 mg/day.
Children 6-12 yr. 0.9-1.8 mg PO daily in 1 to 2 divided doses.
Children 4-6 yr. 0.3-1.8 mg PO daily in 1 to 2 divided doses.

FOR ANY INDICATION: Patients on a strong CYP3A4 inhibitor, moderate CYP3A4 inhibitor, or a P-gp inhibitor in past 14 days or patients with renal or hepatic impairment
Recommendations for dosage adjustment are dependent on indication for use, age of patient, and the concomitant use of interacting drugs. See specific prescribing information; dosages MUST be adjusted downward. Patients with renal or hepatic impairment on interacting drugs must NOT receive colchicine.

OFF-LABEL USES

Amyloidosis, biliary cirrhosis, recurrent pericarditis, sarcoid arthritis.

CONTRAINDICATIONS

Hypersensitivity. Do not use in patients with renal or hepatic impairment in conjunction with P-gp or strong CYP3A4 inhibitors. In these patients, life-threatening and fatal colchicine toxicity has been reported with colchicine taken in therapeutic doses.

INTERACTIONS

Drug
Bone marrow depressants: May increase the risk of blood dyscrasias.
P-gp (e.g., cyclosporine, ranolazine) or strong CYP3A4 inhibitors (this includes all protease inhibitors [except when fosamprenavir is used without ritonavir], clarithromycin, ketoconazole, itraconazole, nefazodone; moderate inhibitors include aprepitant, fluconazole, erythromycin, diltiazem, verapamil): May decrease colchicine metabolism, resulting in increased colchicine toxicity.
NSAIDs: May increase the risk of bone marrow depression, neutropenia, and thrombocytopenia.
Herbal
None known.
Food
Vitamin B_{12}: Vitamin B_{12} absorption may be reduced.
Grapefruit juice: May decrease colchicine metabolism and increase risk of toxicity; avoid use or adjust dosage downward.

DIAGNOSTIC TEST EFFECTS

May increase serum alkaline phosphatase and AST (SGOT) levels. May decrease platelet count.

SIDE EFFECTS

Frequent
Nausea, vomiting, abdominal discomfort.
Occasional
Anorexia.
Rare
Hypersensitivity reaction, including angioedema.

C

SERIOUS REACTIONS

- Bone marrow depression, including aplastic anemia, agranulocytosis, and thrombocytopenia, may occur with long-term therapy.
- Overdose initially causes a burning feeling in the skin or throat, severe diarrhea, and abdominal pain. The patient then experiences fever, seizures, delirium, and renal impairment, marked by hematuria and oliguria. The third stage of overdose causes hair loss, leukocytosis, and stomatitis.

PRECAUTIONS & CONSIDERATIONS

Caution is warranted with impaired hepatic function and in elderly or debilitated patients. It is unknown whether colchicine crosses the placenta. The drug appears to be excreted in breast milk, and due to potential adverse events, particularly in premature infants, breastfeeding is not advised. Safety and efficacy of colchicine have not been established in children less than 4 yr old for FMF, and the drug has not been fully tested to treat acute gout flares in children. Elderly patients may be more susceptible to cumulative toxicity, and age-related renal impairment may increase the risk.

The drug should be discontinued immediately if GI symptoms occur. If taken for gout, limit intake of high-purine foods, such as fish and organ meats, and drink 8-10 eight-oz glasses of fluid daily while taking colchicine.

Notify the physician if fever, numbness, skin rash, sore throat, fatigue, unusual bleeding or bruising, or weakness occurs. The drug should be discontinued as soon as gout pain is relieved or at the first appearance of diarrhea, nausea, or vomiting. High fluid intake (3000 mL/day) should be encouraged; intake and output should be monitored; output should be at least 2000 mL/day. Signs and symptoms of a therapeutic response, including improved joint range of motion and reduced joint tenderness, redness, and swelling, should be evaluated.

Storage

Store at room temperature.

Administration

Take colchicine without regard to meals. Do not administer with grapefruit juice unless prescriber has reduced daily dosage.

Colesevelam

koh-le-sev′e-lam

★ Welchol

CATEGORY AND SCHEDULE

Pregnancy Risk Category: B

Classification: Antihyperlipidemics, bile acid sequestrants

MECHANISM OF ACTION

A bile acid sequestrant and nonsystemic polymer that binds with bile acids in the intestines, preventing their reabsorption and removing them from the body. *Therapeutic Effect:* Decreases LDL cholesterol.

PHARMACOKINETICS

Insignificant absorption. 0.05% of dose excreted in urine after 1 mo of chronic use.

AVAILABILITY

Tablets: 625 mg.

Powder for Suspension: 1.875 g per packet; 3.75 g per packet.

INDICATIONS AND DOSAGES

▸ **To decrease LDL cholesterol level in primary hypercholesterolemia (Fredrickson**

type IIa); adjunctive therapy for type 2 diabetes mellitus
PO (TABLETS)
Adults, Elderly. 3 tablets with meals twice a day or 6 tablets once a day with a meal.
PO (POWDER FOR SUSPENSION)
Adults, Elderly. 1.875-g packet with meals twice a day or 3.75-g packet once a day with a meal.

CONTRAINDICATIONS

Complete biliary obstruction, hypersensitivity to colesevelam serum TG > 500 mg/dL.

INTERACTIONS

Drug

NOTE: Oral drugs, especially those with a narrow therapeutic index, should be administered at least 4 h prior to colesevelam to help avoid interactions whenever possible. Monitor response to and/or drug levels of other drugs.

Aspirin, clindamycin, digoxin, furosemide, glipizide, hydrocortisone, imipramine, NSAIDs, phenytoin, propranolol, tetracyclines, thiazide diuretics, vitamin A, vitamin D, vitamin E, vitamin K: May decrease the absorption of these drugs.

Herbal

None known.

Food

None known.

DIAGNOSTIC TEST EFFECTS

Can increase serum triglycerides.

SIDE EFFECTS

Frequent (8%-12%)

Flatulence, constipation, infection, dyspepsia (heartburn, epigastric distress).

SERIOUS REACTIONS

- GI tract obstruction may occur.

PRECAUTIONS & CONSIDERATIONS

Caution is warranted in patients with dysphagia, patients with severe GI motility disorders, patients who have had major GI tract surgery, and those susceptible to fat-soluble vitamin deficiency. Colesevelam is not absorbed systemically. It may decrease proper maternal vitamin absorption and may affect breastfeeding infants. Safety and efficacy of colesevelam have not been established in children. No age-related precautions have been noted in elderly patients.

Pattern of daily bowel activity and stool consistency should be assessed. Serum cholesterol and triglyceride levels should be checked at baseline and periodically thereafter.

Storage

Store at room temperature and protect from moisture. Mix powder for suspension just prior to administration.

Administration

Take tablets with a meal and a full glass of liquid.

Do not take powder for suspension in dry form; this will cause esophageal distress and choking. To prepare, empty 1 packet into a glass or cup. Add 4-8 oz of water. Stir well and drink. Take with meals.

Colestipol

koe-les'ti-pole

Colestid

CATEGORY AND SCHEDULE

Pregnancy Risk Category: C

Classification: Antihyperlipidemics, bile acid sequestrants

C

MECHANISM OF ACTION

An antihyperlipoproteinemic that binds with bile acids in the intestine, forming an insoluble complex. Binding results in partial removal of bile acid from enterohepatic circulation. *Therapeutic Effect:* Removes low-density lipoproteins (LDLs) and cholesterol from plasma.

PHARMACOKINETICS

Not absorbed from the GI tract. Excreted in the feces.

AVAILABILITY

Granules: 5-g packet (Colestid).
Tablet: 1 g (Colestid).

INDICATIONS AND DOSAGES

▸ **Primary hypercholesterolemia**

PO, GRANULES

Adults, Elderly. Initially, 5 g 1-2 times/day. Range: 5-30 g/day once or in divided doses.

PO, TABLETS

Adults, Elderly. Initially, 2 g 1-2 times/day. Range: 2-16 g/day.

OFF-LABEL USES

Treatment of diarrhea (due to bile acids); hyperoxaluria.

CONTRAINDICATIONS

Complete biliary obstruction, hypersensitivity to bile acid sequestering resins, pancreatitis due to high triglycerides.

INTERACTIONS

Drug

Anticoagulants: May increase effects of these drugs by decreasing vitamin K.

Digoxin, folic acid, penicillins, propranolol, tetracyclines, thiazides, thyroid hormones, and other medications: May bind and decrease absorption of these drugs.

Oral vancomycin: Binds and decreases the effects of oral vancomycin.

Warfarin: May decrease warfarin absorption.

Herbal

Vitamin A, vitamin E: May decrease vitamin A and vitamin E absorption.

Food

None known.

DIAGNOSTIC TEST EFFECTS

May decrease serum calcium, potassium, and sodium levels. May prolong prothrombin time or INR.

SIDE EFFECTS

Frequent

Constipation (may lead to fecal impaction), nausea, vomiting, stomach pain, indigestion.

Occasional

Diarrhea, belching, bloating, headache, dizziness.

Rare

Gallstones, peptic ulcer, malabsorption syndrome.

SERIOUS REACTIONS

- GI tract obstruction, hyperchloremic acidosis, and osteoporosis secondary to calcium excretion may occur.
- High dosage may interfere with fat absorption, resulting in steatorrhea.

PRECAUTIONS & CONSIDERATIONS

Caution is warranted in patients with bleeding disorders, GI dysfunction (especially constipation), hemorrhoids, and osteoporosis. Abdominal discomfort, flatulence, and food tolerance may occur during therapy. Colestipol may interfere with maternal absorption of fat-soluble vitamins. No age-related precautions have been noted in children. Elderly patients are at an increased risk of experiencing adverse nutritional effects and GI side effects. Electrolytes and serum cholesterol and triglyceride levels should be monitored during therapy.

Storage

Store at room temperature and protect from moisture. Mix just prior to administration.

Administration

Take other drugs at least 1 h before or 4-6 h after colestipol because this drug is capable of binding drugs in the GI tract. Do not take granules dry because they are highly irritating. Mix with 3-6 oz fruit juice, milk, soup, or water. May add to pulpy fruits such as crushed pineapple, pears, peaches, or fruit cocktail. Place powder on the surface of the liquid for 1-2 min to prevent lumping, and then mix thoroughly. When mixing the powder with carbonated beverages, use an extra large glass and stir the liquid slowly to avoid excessive foaming. Take before meals to reduce the risk of constipation.

Conivaptan

con-ih-vap'tan

★ Vaprisol

CATEGORY AND SCHEDULE

Pregnancy Risk Category: C

Classification: Vasopressin antagonist

MECHANISM OF ACTION

An arginine vasopressin (AVP) V1A and V2 selective antagonist that inhibits vasopressin binding V1A in the liver and V1 and V2 sites in renal collecting ducts. Results in excretion of free water. *Therapeutic Effect:* Restores normal fluid and electrolyte status.

PHARMACOKINETICS

Protein binding: 99%. Metabolized in liver; CYP450 3A4 is responsible for primary metabolism. Primarily eliminated in feces (approximately 83%); minimal excretion in urine (about 12%). *Half-life:* 3.6–8.6 h.

AVAILABILITY

Premixed IV Infusion: 20 mg/100 mL D5W.

INDICATIONS AND DOSAGES

▸ **Hyponatremia**

IV

Adults. Initially, a loading dose of 20 mg given over 30 min. Maintenance: 20 mg/day as continuous infusion over 24 h for an additional 1-3 days. May titrate to maximum dose of 40 mg/day; total duration should not exceed 4 days after loading dose.

Children. Safety and efficacy have not been established in children.

▸ **Renal impairment**

Dose adjustments not necessary in those with CrCl > 60 mL/min. If CrCl < 30 mL/min, use is not recommended. Contraindicated in anuria.

CONTRAINDICATIONS

Known allergy to conivaptan, corn or corn products; anuria (no benefit can be expected), use with strong CYP3A4 inhibitors (see interactions), hypovolemic hyponatremia.

INTERACTIONS

Drug

CYP3A4 inducers: May decrease the levels and effects of conivaptan.

C

CYP3A4 inhibitors (e.g., erythromycin): May increase the levels and effects of conivaptan. Use with strong CYP3A4 inhibitors is contraindicated, including ketoconazole, itraconazole, clarithromycin, ritonavir, and indinavir.
CYP3A4 substrates: Conivaptan may increase the levels and effects of CYP3A4 substrates, including midazolam and amlodipine, simvastatin, and other "statins." Avoid use of these agents during and for 1 wk after conclusion of treatment.
Digoxin: May increase the levels of digoxin.
Herbal
St. John's wort: May reduce conivaptan levels.

IV INCOMPATIBILITIES
Lactated Ringer's. Do not mix or infuse with other medications, since no other information available.

IV COMPATIBILITIES
Dextrose 5%, per manufacturer compatible with 0.9% NaCl (NS) for up to 22 h when coadministered via Y-site at a rate of 4.2 mL/h for conivaptan and 2.1 mL/h or 6.3 mL/h for NS.

DIAGNOSTIC TEST EFFECTS
Increased sodium.

SIDE EFFECTS
Frequent
Injection site reaction, headache.
Occasional
Hypokalemia, thirst, vomiting, diarrhea, hypertension, orthostatic hypotension, polyuria, phlebitis, constipation, dry mouth, anemia, fever, nausea, confusion, erythema, insomnia, hyperglycemia or hypoglycemia, hyponatremia, pneumonia, urinary tract infection, hypomagnesemia, pain, dehydration, oral candidiasis, hematuria.

SERIOUS REACTIONS
- Atrial fibrillation has been reported.

PRECAUTIONS & CONSIDERATIONS
Use with caution in patients with hyponatremia with underlying congestive heart failure or renal or hepatic impairment. Monitor neurologic status and sodium concentrations closely to avoid overly rapid correction of serum Na+ concentration (> 12 mEq/L over 24 h) during treatment. Monitor for signs of heart decompensation, orthostatic hypotension, and infusion site reactions, which may be frequent and uncomfortable.
Storage
Store premixed infusion at controlled room temperature. Protect from light. Do not remove overwrap until time of use. Do not freeze. Discard any unused portion.
Administration
! Only given in settings where serum Na concentrations, volume status, and blood pressure can be monitored closely.

Loading dose: Administer 20 mg/100 mL premixed flexible infusion over 30 min. Maintenance: For patients receiving 20 mg/day, administer one 20 mg/100 mL premixed flexible container over 24 h. For patients requiring a maintenance dose of 40 mg/day, administer 2 consecutive 20 mg/100 mL premixed flexible containers over 24 h.
! Do NOT use premixed flexible containers in series connections as they may result in the formation of air embolism.

C

Cortisone

kor'ti-sone

Cortone

Do not confuse cortisone with Cort-Dome.

CATEGORY AND SCHEDULE

Pregnancy Risk Category: D

Classification: Glucocorticoid, short-acting

MECHANISM OF ACTION

An adrenocortical steroid that inhibits the accumulation of inflammatory cells at inflammation sites, phagocytosis, lysosomal enzyme release and synthesis, and release of mediators of inflammation. *Therapeutic Effect:* Prevents or suppresses cell-mediated immune reactions. Decreases or prevents tissue response to inflammatory process.

PHARMACOKINETICS

Slowly absorbed. Hepatic metabolism to inactive metabolites. *Half-life:* 0.5-2 h.

AVAILABILITY

Tablets: 25 mg.

INDICATIONS AND DOSAGES

Dosage is dependent on the condition being treated and patient response.

▸ **Anti-inflammation, immunosuppression**

PO

Adults, Elderly. 25-300 mg/day in divided doses q12-24h.

Children. 2.5-10 mg/kg/day in divided doses q6-8h.

▸ **Physiologic replacement**

PO

Adults, Elderly. 25-35 mg/day.

Children. 0.5-0.75 mg/kg/day in divided doses q8h.

CONTRAINDICATIONS

Hypersensitivity to corticosteroids, administration of live-virus vaccine, peptic ulcers (except in life-threatening situations), systemic fungal infection.

INTERACTIONS

Drug

Amphotericin: May increase hypokalemia.

Digoxin: May increase digoxin toxicity caused by hypokalemia.

Diuretics, insulin, oral hypoglycemics, potassium supplements: May decrease the effects of these drugs.

Hepatic enzyme inducers: May decrease the effects of cortisone.

Live-virus vaccines: May decrease the patient's antibody response to vaccine, increase vaccine side effects, and potentiate virus replication.

Herbal

None known.

Food

None known.

DIAGNOSTIC TEST EFFECTS

May increase blood glucose and serum lipid, amylase, and sodium levels. May decrease serum calcium, potassium, and thyroxine levels.

SIDE EFFECTS

Frequent

Insomnia, heartburn, anxiety, abdominal distention, increased diaphoresis, acne, mood swings, increased appetite, facial flushing, delayed wound healing, increased susceptibility to infection, diarrhea or constipation.

Occasional

Headache, edema, change in skin color, frequent urination.

Rare
Tachycardia, allergic reaction (such as rash and hives), psychologic changes, hallucinations, depression.

SERIOUS REACTIONS

- Long-term therapy may cause hypocalcemia, hypokalemia, muscle wasting in arms and legs, osteoporosis, spontaneous fractures, amenorrhea, cataracts, glaucoma, peptic ulcer disease, and congestive heart failure.
- Abrupt withdrawal following long-term therapy may cause anorexia, nausea, fever, headache, joint pain, rebound inflammation, fatigue, weakness, lethargy, dizziness, and orthostatic hypotension.

PRECAUTIONS & CONSIDERATIONS

Caution is warranted with diabetes, cirrhosis, congestive heart failure, glaucoma, history of tuberculosis (cortisone may reactivate tuberculosis disease), hypertension, hypothyroidism, nonspecific ulcerative colitis, osteoporosis, psychosis, seizure disorders, and thromboembolic disorders. Monitor growth and development of children receiving long-term corticosteroid therapy. Dentist or other physicians should be informed of cortisone therapy if taken within the past 12 mo.

Not recommended for use during pregnancy or breastfeeding; other corticosteroids normally employed if needed.

Mood swings, ranging from euphoria to depression, may occur. Notify the physician of fever, muscle aches, sore throat, and sudden weight gain or swelling. Blood glucose level, BP, serum electrolyte levels, height, and weight should be monitored before and during therapy. Be alert to signs and symptoms of infection caused by reduced immune response, including fever, sore throat, and vague symptoms. In long-term therapy, signs and symptoms of hypocalcemia should be assessed.

Storage
Store at room temperature. Protect from light and moisture.

Administration
Do not abruptly discontinue the drug; the drug must be withdrawn gradually under medical supervision. May be taken with food to reduce GI irritation.

Cosyntropin

kos-syn-troe′pin

★ 🍁 Cortrosyn

CATEGORY AND SCHEDULE

Pregnancy Risk Category: C

Classification: Hormones/hormone modifiers

MECHANISM OF ACTION

A glucocorticoid that stimulates initial reaction in synthesis of adrenal steroids from cholesterol. *Therapeutic Effect:* Increases endogenous corticoid synthesis.

PHARMACOKINETICS

Time to peak for IM and IV push dose about 1 h. Plasma cortisol levels rise within 5 min; peak plasma cortisol levels are reached within 45-60 min.

AVAILABILITY

Powder for Reconstitution: 0.25 mg (Cortrosyn).

INDICATIONS AND DOSAGES

▸ **Screening test for adrenal function**

IM

Adults, Elderly, Children 2 yr and older. 0.25-0.75 mg one time.
Children < 2 yr. 0.125 mg one time.

Neonates. 0.015 mg/kg/dose.
IV, INFUSION
Adults. 0.25 mg in D5W or 0.9% NaCl infused at rate of 0.04 mg/h.

CONTRAINDICATIONS

Hypersensitivity to cosyntropin or corticotrophin.

INTERACTIONS

Drug
Bupropion: May lower seizure threshold.
Fluoroquinolones: May increase risk for tendon rupture.
Itraconazole: May increase cosyntropin plasma concentrations and side effects.
Rotavirus vaccine: May increase risk of infection by live vaccine.
Herbal
Echinacea, ma huang: May decrease effectiveness of cosyntropin.
Licorice: May increase risk of corticosteroid side effects.
Saiboku-to: May increase and prolong effect of cosyntropin.
Food
None known.

DIAGNOSTIC TEST EFFECTS

None known.

SIDE EFFECTS

Occasional
Nausea, vomiting.
Rare
Hypersensitivity reaction (fever, pruritus).

SERIOUS REACTIONS

- None reported.

PRECAUTIONS & CONSIDERATIONS

Be aware that short duration for diagnostic use does not produce effects of long-term cosyntropin therapy. It is unknown whether cosyntropin crosses the placenta or is distributed in breast milk. No age-related precautions have been noted in children or in elderly patients.

If an allergic reaction with itching, hives, swelling in face or hands, swelling or tingling in mouth or throat, tightness in chest, and trouble breathing occurs, notify the physician.

The following criteria may be used as guidelines to determine whether there has been a normal response to cosyntropin:

- Morning control plasma cortisol concentration exceeds 5 mcg (0.005 mg) per 100 mL.
- 30-min cortisol concentration shows an increase of at least 7 mcg (0.007 mg) per 100 mL above the control level.
- 30-min cortisol concentration exceeds 18 mcg (0.018 mg) per 100 mL.
- If a 60-min test interval is used, a normal response to cosyntropin is shown by a plasma cortisol concentration that is approximately 2 times the baseline concentration.

Storage
Store unreconstituted product at room temperature.

When constituted with 0.9% NaCl, cosyntropin is stable for 24 h at room temperature.

Administration
Each 0.25 mg of cosyntropin is equivalent to 25 units of corticotrophin. Peak plasma cortisol concentrations usually occur 45-60 min after cosyntropin administration.

For IM injection, 1 mL of diluent provided (0.9% NaCl injection) should be added to the vial containing 250 mcg (0.025 mg) of cosyntropin. The resultant solution contains 250 mcg (0.025 mg) of cosyntropin per mL.

For IV infusion, cosyntropin may be further diluted with D5W or 0.9% NaCl injection. Administer 0.25 mg in D5W or 0.9% NaCl infused at rate of 0.04 mg/h.

Cromolyn

kroe′moe-lin

★ Crolom, Gastrocrom, Intal, Nasalcrom 🍁 Apo-Cromolyn, Nalcrom, Opticrom, Rhinaris-CS

CATEGORY AND SCHEDULE

Pregnancy Risk Category: B

Classification: Antiasthmatic, mast cell stabilizer, ophthalmic anti-inflammatory, respiratory anti-inflammatory

MECHANISM OF ACTION

An antiasthmatic and antiallergic agent that prevents mast cell release of histamine, leukotrienes, and slow-reacting substances of anaphylaxis by inhibiting degranulation after contact with antigens. *Therapeutic Effect:* Helps prevent symptoms of asthma, allergic rhinitis, mastocytosis, and exercise-induced bronchospasm.

PHARMACOKINETICS

Minimal absorption after PO, inhalation, or nasal administration. Absorbed portion excreted in urine or by biliary system. *Half-life:* 80-90 min.

AVAILABILITY

Oral Concentrate (Gastrocrom): 100 mg/5 mL.
Nasal Spray (Nasalcrom): 5.2 mg/actuation.
Solution for Nebulization: 10 mg/mL.
Ophthalmic Solution (Crolom): 4%.

INDICATIONS AND DOSAGES

▸ Asthma

INHALATION (NEBULIZATION)
Adults, Elderly, Children older than 2 yr. 20 mg 3-4 times a day.

▸ Prevention of bronchospasm

INHALATION (NEBULIZATION)
Adults, Elderly, Children older than 2 yr. 20 mg within 1 h before exercise or exposure to allergens.

▸ Food allergy, inflammatory bowel disease

PO
Adults, Elderly, Children older than 12 yr. 200-400 mg 4 times a day.
Children 2-12 yr. 100-200 mg 4 times a day. Maximum: 40 mg/kg/day.
If patient has renal or hepatic impairment, consider dose reduction.

▸ Allergic rhinitis

INTRANASAL
Adults, Elderly, Children older than 6 yr. 1 spray each nostril 3-4 times a day. May increase up to 6 times a day.

▸ Systemic mastocytosis

PO
Adults, Elderly, Children older than 12 yr. 200 mg 4 times a day.
Children 2-12 yr. 100 mg 4 times a day. Maximum: 40 mg/kg/day.
Children younger than 2 yr. 20 mg/kg/day in 4 divided doses. Maximum: 30 mg/kg/day (children 6 mo to 2 yr).

▸ Allergic-type conjunctivitis

OPHTHALMIC
Adults, Elderly, Children older than 4 yr. 1-2 drops in both eyes 4-6 times a day.

CONTRAINDICATIONS

Hypersensitivity; drug has no role in treatment of status asthmaticus.

INTERACTIONS

Drug

None known.

Herbal
None known.
Food
None known.

DIAGNOSTIC TEST EFFECTS
None known.

SIDE EFFECTS
Frequent
PO: Headache, diarrhea.
Inhalation: Cough, dry mouth and throat, stuffy nose, throat irritation, unpleasant taste.
Nasal: Nasal burning, stinging, or irritation; increased sneezing.
Ophthalmic: Eye burning or stinging.
Occasional
PO: Rash, abdominal pain, arthralgia, nausea, insomnia.
Inhalation: Bronchospasm, hoarseness, lacrimation.
Nasal: Cough, headache, unpleasant taste, postnasal drip.
Ophthalmic: Lacrimation and itching of eye.
Rare
Inhalation: Dizziness, painful urination, arthralgia, myalgia, rash.
Nasal: Epistaxis, rash.
Ophthalmic: Chemosis or edema of conjunctiva, eye irritation.

SERIOUS REACTIONS
- Anaphylaxis occurs rarely when cromolyn is given by the inhalation, nasal, or oral route.

PRECAUTIONS & CONSIDERATIONS
Caution is warranted with arrhythmias and coronary artery disease. When discontinuing the drug, taper the dosage cautiously because symptoms may recur. It is unknown whether cromolyn crosses the placenta or is distributed in breast milk. No age-related precautions have been noted in children. Age-related hepatic and renal impairment may require a dosage adjustment in elderly patients. Drink plenty of fluids to decrease the thickness of lung secretions.

Baseline exercise and activity tolerance should be established. Pulse rate and quality and respiratory rate, depth, rhythm, and type should be monitored. Observe for cyanosis manifested as lips and fingernails with a blue or dusky color in light-skinned patients, a gray color in dark-skinned patients.
Storage
Oral concentrate ampules should be kept in foil packet and protected from light at room temperature until time of use. Do not use if it contains a precipitate (particles or cloudiness) or becomes discolored. All other dosage forms are kept at room temperature.
Administration
Take oral cromolyn at least 30 min before meals. Pour contents of capsule into water and stir until completely dissolved. Do not mix the drug with food, fruit juice, or milk.

For inhalation, do not mix with other drugs in the nebulizer.

For intranasal use, clear nasal passages as much as possible; a nasal decongestant may be required. Tilt the head slightly forward. Insert the spray tip into the nostril, pointing toward the nasal passages, away from the nasal septum. Spray into the nostril while holding the other nostril closed, and at the same time, inhale through the nose to deliver the medication as high into the nasal passages as possible.

For ophthalmic use, place a finger on the lower eyelid and pull it down until a pocket is formed between the eye and lower lid. Hold the dropper above the pocket and instill the prescribed number of drops into the pocket. Close the eyes gently. Apply gentle finger pressure to the lacrimal sac after instillation to lessen systemic absorption.

C

Crotamiton

kroe-tam′i-ton

Eurax

Do not confuse Eurax with Euflex, Eulexin, or Evoxac.

CATEGORY AND SCHEDULE

Pregnancy Risk Category: C

Classification: Anti-infectives, topical, scabicides/pediculicides

MECHANISM OF ACTION

A scabicidal agent whose exact mechanism is unknown. *Therapeutic Effect:* Scabicidal activity against *Sarcoptes scabiei.*

PHARMACOKINETICS

Not known.

AVAILABILITY

Cream: 10% (Eurax).
Lotion: 10% (Eurax).

INDICATIONS AND DOSAGES

▸ Treatment of scabies

TOPICAL

Adults, Elderly, Children. Wash and scrub away loose scales and towel dry. Apply a thin layer and massage into the skin over the entire body with special attention to skinfolds, creases, and interdigital spaces. Repeat application in 24 h. Take a cleansing bath 48 h after the final application. Treatment may be repeated after 7-10 days if live mites are still present.

▸ Pruritus due to a variety of skin conditions

TOPICAL

Adults, Elderly, Children. Massage into affected areas until medication is completely absorbed. Repeat as needed. Most find relief with 2-3 applications per day. The need to use may resolve by about 5 days unless prescriber prolongs course.

OFF-LABEL USES

Pediculosis capitis.

CONTRAINDICATIONS

Hypersensitivity to crotamiton or any one of its components.

INTERACTIONS

Drug
None known.
Herbal
None known.
Food
None known.

DIAGNOSTIC TEST EFFECTS

None known.

SIDE EFFECTS

Occasional
Itching, burning, irritation, warm sensation, contact dermatitis.

SERIOUS REACTIONS

- None known.

PRECAUTIONS & CONSIDERATIONS

It is unknown whether crotamiton crosses the placenta or is distributed in breast milk. Safety and efficacy of crotamiton have not been established in children. No age-related precautions have been noted in elderly patients.
Storage
Store at room temperature.

Administration
Avoid contact with eyes and mucous membranes; do not apply to inflamed skin. Shake lotion well before use.

For scabies: After bathing, massage gently and well into the skin from the chin to the toes, including folds and creases and under fingernails after trimming fingernails short. Apply again 24 h later. A 60-g tube/bottle is sufficient for the 2 applications. Clothing and bed linen should be changed the next day and may be dry-cleaned, or washed in the hot cycle of the washing machine. A cleansing bath should be taken 48 h after the last application.

Cyanocobalamin (Vitamin B_{12})

sye-an-oh-koe-bal′a-min

★ 🍁 Nutri-Twelve Injection, Nascobal

CATEGORY AND SCHEDULE

Pregnancy Risk Category: A (C if used in doses above recommended daily allowance)

Classification: Vitamin B_{12}, water-soluble vitamin

MECHANISM OF ACTION

Acts as a coenzyme for various metabolic functions, including fat and carbohydrate metabolism and protein synthesis. *Therapeutic Effect:* Necessary for cell growth and replication, hematopoiesis, and myelin synthesis.

PHARMACOKINETICS

In the presence of calcium, absorbed systemically in lower half of ileum. Initially, bound to intrinsic factor; this complex passes down intestine, binding to receptor sites on ileal mucosa. Protein binding: High. Metabolized in the liver. Primarily eliminated unchanged in urine. *Half-life:* 6 days.

AVAILABILITY

Lozenge: 50 mcg, 100 mcg, 250 mcg, 500 mcg.
Tablets: 50 mcg, 100 mcg, 250 mcg, 500 mcg, 1000 mcg, 5000 mcg.
Tablet (Extended Release): 1000 mcg, 1500 mcg.
Tablet (Sublingual): 1000 mcg, 2500 mcg, 5000 mcg.
Injection: 1000 mcg/mL.
Nasal Solution: 500 mcg/0.1 mL actuation.

INDICATIONS AND DOSAGES

▸ **Pernicious anemia**

IM, SUBCUTANEOUS

Adults, Elderly. 100 mcg/day for 7 days, then every other day for 7 days, then every 3-4 days for 2-3 wks. Maintenance: 100 mcg/mo.
Children. 30-50 mcg/day for 2 or more weeks. Maintenance: 100 mcg/mo.
Neonates. 1000 mcg/day for 2 or more weeks. Maintenance: 50 mcg/mo.

▸ **Uncomplicated vitamin B_{12} deficiency**

PO

Adults, Elderly. 1000-2000 mcg/day.

IM, SUBCUTANEOUS

Adults, Elderly. 100 mcg/day for 5-10 days, followed by 100-200 mcg/mo.

NASAL (NASCOBAL)

Adults. 500 mcg in one nostril once weekly.

▸ **Complicated vitamin B_{12} deficiency**

IM, SUBCUTANEOUS

Adults, Elderly. 1000 mcg (with IM or IV folic acid 15 mg) as a single dose, then 1000 mcg/day plus oral folic acid 5 mg/day for 7 days.

C

CONTRAINDICATIONS

Folic acid deficiency anemia, hereditary optic nerve atrophy, history of allergy to cobalamins.

INTERACTIONS

Drug

Alcohol, colchicines, metformin, proton-pump inhibitors: May decrease the absorption of cyanocobalamin.

Octreotide: May decrease cyanocobalamin blood concentration.

Herbal

None known.

Food

None known.

DIAGNOSTIC TEST EFFECTS

None known.

SIDE EFFECTS

Occasional

Diarrhea, pruritus.

SERIOUS REACTIONS

- Impurities in preparation may cause a rare allergic reaction.
- Peripheral vascular thrombosis, pulmonary edema, hypokalemia, and congestive heart failure may occur.

PRECAUTIONS & CONSIDERATIONS

Cyanocobalamin crosses the placenta and is excreted in breast milk. No age-related precautions have been noted in children or in elderly patients. Eating foods rich in vitamin B_{12}, including clams, dairy products, egg yolks, fermented cheese, herring, muscle and organ meats, oysters, and red snapper, is encouraged.

Notify the physician of symptoms of infection. Serum potassium level, which normally ranges from 3.5 to 5 mEq/L, and serum cyanocobalamin level, which normally ranges from 200 to 800 mcg/mL, should be monitored. Also, watch for a rise in the blood reticulocyte count, which peaks in 5-8 days. Reversal of deficiency symptoms (anorexia, ataxia, fatigue, hyporeflexia, insomnia, irritability, loss of positional sense, pallor, and palpitations on exertion) should also be assessed. A therapeutic response to treatment usually occurs within 48 h.

Administration

Take oral cyanocobalamin with meals to increase absorption.

Before the initial dose, activate Nascobal spray nozzle by pumping until first appearance of spray, and then prime twice more. The unit must be reprimed once immediately before each subsequent use. Administer 1 h before or after ingestion of hot foods or liquids.

Injection is administrered IM or by deep subcutaneous injection; intravenous (IV) injection is not usually recommended as it is excreted more readily by that route. However, cyanocobalamin may be mixed with TPN solutions.

Cyclobenzaprine

sye-kloe-ben′za-preen

Amrix, Fexmid, Flexeril

Do not confuse cyclobenzaprine with cycloserine or cyproheptadine, or Flexeril with Floxin, or Amrix with Arixtra.

CATEGORY AND SCHEDULE

Pregnancy Risk Category: B

Classification: Skeletal muscle relaxant, centrally acting tricyclic

MECHANISM OF ACTION
A centrally acting skeletal muscle relaxant that reduces tonic somatic muscle activity at the level of the brainstem. *Therapeutic Effect:* Relieves local skeletal muscle spasm.

PHARMACOKINETICS

Route	Onset	Peak	Duration
PO	1 h	3-4 h	12-24 h

Well but slowly absorbed from the GI tract. Protein binding: 93%. Metabolized in the GI tract and the liver. Primarily excreted in urine. *Half-life:* 1-3 days.

AVAILABILITY
Capsule (Extended Release, Amrix): 15 mg, 30 mg.
Tablets: 5 mg, 7.5 mg, 10 mg.

INDICATIONS AND DOSAGES
▸ **Acute, painful musculoskeletal conditions**
PO
Adults. Initially, 5 mg 3 times a day. May increase to 10 mg 3 times a day OR 15 mg extended-release capsule once daily. May increase to 30 mg once daily.
Elderly. 5 mg 3 times a day; extended-release capsules not recommended in elderly patients.
▸ **Dosage in hepatic impairment**
Mild: 5 mg 3 times a day; extended-release capsules not recommended in hepatic impairment.
Moderate and severe: Not recommended.

OFF-LABEL USES
Treatment of fibromyalgia.

CONTRAINDICATIONS
Hypersensitivity, acute recovery phase of MI, arrhythmias, congestive heart failure, heart block, conduction disturbances, hyperthyroidism, use within 14 days of MAOIs.

INTERACTIONS
Drug
Alcohol, other CNS depression–producing medications (such as tricyclic antidepressants): May increase CNS depression.
MAOIs: May increase the risk of hypertensive crisis and severe seizures. Contraindicated.
Herbal
Valerian, kava kava, gotu kola: May increase CNS depression.

DIAGNOSTIC TEST EFFECTS
None known.

SIDE EFFECTS
Frequent
Somnolence (39%), dry mouth (27%), dizziness (11%).
Rare (1%-3%)
Fatigue, asthenia, blurred vision, headache, nervousness, confusion, nausea, constipation, dyspepsia, unpleasant taste.

SERIOUS REACTIONS
• Overdose may result in visual hallucinations, hyperactive reflexes, muscle rigidity, vomiting, and hyperpyrexia.

PRECAUTIONS & CONSIDERATIONS
Caution is warranted with angle-closure glaucoma, impaired hepatic or renal function, increased intraocular pressure, and history of urine retention. It is unknown whether cyclobenzaprine crosses the placenta or is distributed in breast milk. The safety and efficacy of cyclobenzaprine have not been established in children. Elderly patients have an increased sensitivity to the drug's anticholinergic effects, such as confusion and urine retention.

C

Drowsiness may occur but usually diminishes with continued therapy. Avoid alcohol, CNS depressants, and tasks that require mental alertness or motor skills. Change positions slowly to help avoid the drug's hypotensive effects. Therapeutic response, such as decreased skeletal muscle pain, stiffness, and tenderness and improved mobility, should be assessed.

Storage

Store all products at room temperature. Keep tightly closed.

Administration

Do not administer cyclobenzaprine for longer than 2-3 wks without reevaluation. Take cyclobenzaprine without regard to food. Take extended-release capsules at roughly the same time daily; do not crush or chew.

Cyclophosphamide

sye-kloe-foss'fa-mide

★ 🍁 Procytox

CATEGORY AND SCHEDULE

Pregnancy Risk Category: D

Classification: Antineoplastic alkylating agent

MECHANISM OF ACTION

An alkylating agent that inhibits DNA and RNA protein synthesis by cross-linking with DNA and RNA strands, preventing cell growth. Cell cycle-phase nonspecific. *Therapeutic Effect:* Potent immunosuppressant.

PHARMACOKINETICS

Well absorbed from the GI tract. Protein binding: Low. Crosses the blood-brain barrier. Metabolized in the liver to active metabolites. Primarily excreted in urine. Removed by hemodialysis. *Half-life:* 3-12 h.

AVAILABILITY

Injection, Powder for Solution: 500 mg, 1 g, 2 g.
Tablets: 25 mg, 50 mg.

INDICATIONS AND DOSAGES

NOTE: Regimens vary widely with indication for use, other medications employed. Consult specialized references to confirm protocols.

▸ **Ovarian adenocarcinoma, breast carcinoma, Hodgkin disease, non-Hodgkin lymphoma, multiple myeloma, leukemia (acute lymphoblastic, acute myelogenous, acute monocytic, chronic granulocytic, chronic lymphocytic), mycosis fungoides, disseminated neuroblastoma, retinoblastoma**

PO

Adults. 1-5 mg/kg/day.
Children. Initially, 2-8 mg/kg/day. Maintenance: 2-5 mg/kg twice a week.

IV

Adults. 40-50 mg/kg in divided doses over 2-5 days, 10-15 mg/kg every 7-10 days, or 3-5 mg/kg twice a week.
Children. 2-8 mg/kg/day for 6 days or total dose for 7 days once a week.

▸ **Biopsy-proven minimal-change nephrotic syndrome**

PO

Adults, Children. 2.5-3 mg/kg/day for 60-90 days.

CONTRAINDICATIONS

Severely depressed bone marrow function; hypersensitivity to cyclophosphamide.

INTERACTIONS

Drug

Allopurinol: Increased cyclophosphamide levels.
Cyclosporine: Decreased cyclosporine levels.
Succinylcholine: Prolonged succinylcholine effects.

Vaccines, Live: Increased risk of infection by live vaccine.
Warfarin: Increased risk elevated INR and bleeding.
Herbal
St. John's wort: Reduced cyclophosphamide effectiveness.

DIAGNOSTIC TEST EFFECTS

Myelosuppression risk, monitor CBC with differential and platelets; nephrotoxicity risk, monitor BUN, urinalysis, and serum creatinine.

IV INCOMPATIBILITIES

Amphotericin B cholesteryl sulfate complex , diazepam, lansoprazole (Prevacid IV), phenytoin.

SIDE EFFECTS

Expected
Marked leukopenia 8-15 days after initial therapy.
Frequent
Nausea, vomiting (beginning about 6 h after administration and lasting about 4 h), alopecia.
Occasional
Diarrhea, darkening of skin and fingernails, stomatitis, headache, diaphoresis.
Rare
Pain or redness at injection site.

SERIOUS REACTIONS

- Cyclophosphamide's major toxic effect is myelosuppression resulting in blood dyscrasias, such as leukopenia, anemia, thrombocytopenia, and hypoprothrombinemia.
- Expect leukopenia to resolve in 17-28 days. Anemia generally occurs after large doses or prolonged therapy. Thrombocytopenia may occur 10-15 days after drug initiation.
- Hemorrhagic cystitis occurs commonly in long-term therapy, especially in pediatric patients.
- Pulmonary fibrosis and cardiotoxicity have been noted with high doses.
- Amenorrhea, azoospermia, and hyperkalemia may also occur. Permanent or long-standing sterility is a possibility.
- Anaphylactoid reactions may rarely occur.

PRECAUTIONS & CONSIDERATIONS

Ensure adequate fluid intake and frequent voiding to reduce occurrence of hemorrhagic cystitis. Use with caution in patients with leukopenia, thrombocytopenia, tumor cell infiltration of bone marrow, previous radiation therapy, previous therapy with other cytotoxic agents, impaired hepatic function, or impaired renal function. Emetic potential ranges from very high with high doses to moderate with oral therapy. Women of childbearing potential should be advised to avoid becoming pregnant. Avoid use in nursing mothers. No unique precautions in pediatric patients or in elderly patients.
Storage
Store unopened vials and tablets at room temperature, but protect against temperatures > 86° F, which cause melting. The injection (when prepared for either direct injection or infusion) is stable for 24 h at room temperature or for 6 days in the refrigerator. Extemporaneous oral liquids are prepared by dissolving the oral drug in Aromatic Elixir, N.F. and may be stored under refrigeration in glass containers and used within 14 days.
Administration
CAUTION: Observe and exercise usual cautions for handling and preparing cytotoxic drugs.

Administer orally during or after meals. Do not crush or cut tablets. To reduce risk of bladder irritation, do not administer tablets at bedtime.

Parenteral product is most commonly given by either direct IV injection or by IV infusion. When given by direct IV injection, ONLY dilute with 0.9% NaCl; dilution with water creates a hypotonic solution that cannot be directly injected.

For IV infusion, may reconstitute with sterile water for injection, OR 0.9% NaCl, and then FURTHER dilute in one of the following: D5W, D5NS, D5LR, LR, 0.45% NaCl, or $\frac{1}{6}$M sodium lactate injection. Infusions are typically given over 1 hr.

Cycloserine

sye-kloe-ser′een

★ Seromycin

CATEGORY AND SCHEDULE

Pregnancy Risk Category: C

Classification:
Antimycobacterials

MECHANISM OF ACTION

An antitubercular that inhibits cell wall synthesis by competing with the amino acid, D-alanine, for incorporation into the bacterial cell wall. *Therapeutic Effect:* Causes disruption of bacterial cell wall. Bactericidal or bacteriostatic.

PHARMACOKINETICS

Readily absorbed from the GI tract. No protein binding. Widely distributed (including cerebrospinal fluid [CSF]). Metabolized in liver. Primarily excreted in urine. Removed by hemodialysis. *Half-life:* 10 h.

AVAILABILITY

Capsules: 250 mg (Seromycin).

INDICATIONS AND DOSAGES

▸ Tuberculosis

Adults, Elderly. 250 mg q12h for 14 days, then 500 mg to 1g/day in 2 divided doses for 18-24 mo. Maximum: 1 g as a single daily dose. Adjust dose to keep levels < 30 mcg/mL.
Children. 10-20 mg/kg/day in 2 divided doses. Maximum: 1000 mg/day for 18-24 mo.

▸ Dosage in renal impairment

Creatinine Clearance (mL/min)	Dosage Interval
10-50	q24h
< 10	q36-48h

OFF-LABEL USES

Gaucher disease, acute urinary tract infections.

CONTRAINDICATIONS

Epilepsy, depression, severe anxiety, psychosis, severe renal insufficiency, excessive concurrent use of alcohol, history of hypersensitivity reactions with previous cycloserine therapy.

INTERACTIONS

Drug

Alcohol: May increase CNS effects.
Isoniazid, ethionamide: May increase cycloserine toxicity.
Phenytoin: May increase the risk of epileptic seizures.

Herbal

Vitamin B_{12}: May decrease vitamin B_{12}.
Folic acid: May decrease folic acid.

DIAGNOSTIC TEST EFFECTS

Toxic cycloserine concentrations: > 30 mcg/mL.

SIDE EFFECTS

Occasional

Drowsiness, headache, dizziness, vertigo, seizures, confusion, psychosis, paresis, tremor, vitamin B_{12} deficiency, folate deficiency, cardiac arrhythmias, increased liver enzymes.

SERIOUS REACTIONS

- Neurotoxicity, as evidenced by confusion, agitation, CNS depression, psychosis, coma, and seizures, occurs rarely.
- Neurotoxic effects of cycloserine may be treated and prevented with the administration of 200-300 mg of pyridoxine daily.

PRECAUTIONS & CONSIDERATIONS

Caution is warranted with epilepsy, depression, severe anxiety, psychosis, severe renal disease, and chronic alcoholism. Hypersensitivity reactions to cycloserine should be determined before starting treatment. Cycloserine crosses the placenta and is excreted in breast milk. No age-related precautions have been noted in children or in elderly patients. Cycloserine concentrations should be monitored. Toxicity is greatly increased at levels more than 30 mcg/mL.

Drowsiness, mental confusion, dizziness, or tremors may occur during treatment. Excessive amounts of alcoholic beverages should be avoided.

Storage

Store at room temperature.

Administration

May be taken with food.

Pyridoxine (vitamin B_6) may be coadministered to help prevent neurotoxicity.

Cyclosporine

sye-kloe-spor′in

★ 🍁 Gengraf, Neoral, Restasis, Sandimmune

Do not confuse cyclosporine with cycloserine, cyclophosphamide, or Cyklokapron.

CATEGORY AND SCHEDULE

Pregnancy Risk Category: C

Classification:

Immunosuppressant

MECHANISM OF ACTION

A cyclic polypeptide that inhibits both cellular and humoral immune responses by inhibiting interleukin-2, a proliferative factor needed for T-cell activity. *Therapeutic Effect:* Prevents organ rejection and relieves symptoms of psoriasis and arthritis.

PHARMACOKINETICS

Variably absorbed from the GI tract. Protein binding: 90%. Widely distributed. Metabolized in the liver. Eliminated primarily by biliary or fecal excretion. Not removed by hemodialysis. *Half-life:* Adults, 10-27 h; children, 7-19 h.

AVAILABILITY

Capsules, Softgel (Sandimmune): 25 mg, 100 mg.
Capsules, Softgel [modified] (Gengraf, Neoral): 25 mg, 100 mg.
Oral Solution (Sandimmune): 100 mg/mL in 50-mL bottle with calibrated liquid measuring device.
Oral Solution [modified] (Gengraf, Neoral): 100 mg/mL.
Injection (Sandimmune): 50 mg/mL.
Ophthalmic Emulsion (Restasis): 0.05%.

C

INDICATIONS AND DOSAGES

! Sandimmune capsules and oral solution have decreased bioavailability compared with the Gengraf and Neoral modified capsules and oral solution. Gengraf, Neoral, and generic modified cyclosporine formulations are not bioequivalent to Sandimmune. Blood concentration monitoring should be used to guide dosing changes and conversion between formulations.

▸ **Transplantation, prevention of organ rejection**

PO

Adults, Elderly, Children. 10-18 mg/ kg/dose given 4-12h before organ transplantation. Maintenance: 5-15 mg/kg/day in divided doses, then tapered to 3-10 mg/kg/day.

IV

Adults, Elderly, Children. Initially, 5-6 mg/kg/dose given 4-12h before organ transplantation. Maintenance: 2-10 mg/kg/day in divided doses.

▸ **Rheumatoid arthritis**

PO

Adults, Elderly. Initially, 2.5 mg/kg/ day in 2 divided doses. May increase by 0.5-0.75 mg/kg/day. Maximum: 4 mg/kg/day.

▸ **Psoriasis**

PO

Adults, Elderly. Initially, 2.5 mg/kg/ day in 2 divided doses. May increase by 0.5 mg/kg/day. Maximum: 4 mg/ kg/day.

▸ **Dry eye**

OPHTHALMIC

Adults, Elderly. Instill 1 drop in each affected eye q12h.

OFF-LABEL USES

Treatment of alopecia areata, aplastic anemia, atopic dermatitis, Behçet syndrome, biliary cirrhosis, prevention of corneal transplant rejection.

CONTRAINDICATIONS

History of hypersensitivity to cyclosporine or polyoxyethylated castor oil; contraindicated in psoriasis and rheumatoid arthritis patients with abnormal renal function, uncontrolled hypertension, or malignancies; contraindicated with concurrent PUVA or UVB therapy, methotrexate or other immunosuppressives, coal tar, or radiation therapy in psoriasis patients; ophthalmic contraindicated in patients with active ocular infection.

Check for contraindicated drugs due to serious interactions.

INTERACTIONS

NOTE: Many drugs may cause serious drug interactions with cyclosporine; check carefully. Notable interactions are listed here.

Drug

ACE inhibitors, potassium-sparing diuretics, potassium supplements: May cause hyperkalemia.

Bosentan: Cyclosporine greatly increases bosentan concentrations. Contraindicated.

Cimetidine, danazol, diltiazem, erythromycin, ketoconazole, itraconazole, methotrexate, protease inhibitors, voriconazole: May increase cyclosporine concentration and risk of hepatotoxicity and nephrotoxicity.

Immunosuppressants: May increase risk of infection and lymphoproliferative disorders.

Live-virus vaccines: May increase vaccine side effects, potentiate virus replication, and decrease the patient's antibody response to the vaccine.

HMG-CoA reductase inhibitors: Cyclosporine may increase statin levels and increase the risk of acute

renal failure and rhabdomyolysis. Pitavastatin is contraindicated; many other statin agents require dose reduction.
Carbamazepine, oxcarbazepine, phenobarbital, phenytoin, rifampin, sulfasalazine, ticlopidine: May decrease cyclosporine levels.
Herbal
St. John's wort: May decrease cyclosporine plasma levels. Contraindicated.
Food
Grapefruit, grapefruit juice: May increase the absorption and risk of toxicity of cyclosporine. Avoid.

DIAGNOSTIC TEST EFFECTS

May increase BUN and serum alkaline phosphatase, amylase, bilirubin, creatinine, potassium, uric acid, AST (SGOT), and ALT (SGPT) levels. May decrease serum magnesium level. Therapy is usually guided by trough concentrations, with desired whole blood trough 150-400 ng/mL; plasma trough 50-125 ng/mL.

IV INCOMPATIBILITIES

Amphotericin B complex (Abelcet, AmBisome, Amphotec), diazepam, drotecogin alfa (Xigris), magnesium, phenobarbital, phenytoin, voriconazole (VFend).

SIDE EFFECTS

Frequent
Mild to moderate hypertension (26%), hirsutism (21%), tremor (12%).
Occasional (2%-4%)
Acne, leg cramps, gingival hyperplasia (marked by red, bleeding, and tender gums), paresthesia, diarrhea, nausea, vomiting, headache.
Rare (< 1%)
Hypersensitivity reaction, abdominal discomfort, gynecomastia, sinusitis.

SERIOUS REACTIONS

- Mild nephrotoxicity occurs in 25% of renal transplant patients, 38% of cardiac transplant patients, and 37% of liver transplant patients, generally 2-3 mo after transplantation (more severe toxicity generally occurs soon after transplantation). Hepatotoxicity occurs in 4% of renal transplant patients, 7% of cardiac transplant patients, and 4% of liver transplant patients, generally within the first month after transplantation. Both toxicities usually respond to dosage reduction.
- Severe hyperkalemia and hyperuricemia occur occasionally.
- Increased infection risk due to immunosuppression.
- Use may increase risk of non-melanoma skin cancers.

PRECAUTIONS & CONSIDERATIONS

Caution is warranted in patients with cardiac impairment, chickenpox, herpes zoster infection, hypokalemia, malabsorption syndrome, renal or hepatic impairment, and pregnant women. Cyclosporine readily crosses the placenta and is distributed in breast milk. Women taking this drug should not breastfeed. No age-related precautions have been noted in transplant children. Elderly patients are at increased risk for hypertension and an increased serum creatinine level.

Headache, excessive hair growth, gum disease, and tremor may occur. Good oral hygiene should be maintained to prevent gingivitis. Renal function studies, liver function tests, and drug levels should be monitored before beginning cyclosporine therapy and regularly during treatment. Mild toxicity is characterized by a slow rise in serum levels; more overt toxicity, by a rapid rise in serum levels. Hematuria is

C

also noted in nephrotoxicity. Serum potassium level for hyperkalemia and BP for hypertension should also be assessed.

Storage

The capsules should be kept in original foil wrapping and stored in a dry, cool environment, away from direct light. Do not refrigerate the oral solution because it may separate. The liquid form should be kept in the amber-colored glass container. Discard the oral solution 2 mo after the bottle has been opened. Store the parenteral form at room temperature and protect it from light. After diluted, solution is stable for 24 h. Store ophthalmic emulsion at room temperature.

Administration

! Always confirm the formulation prescribed, as the different cyclosporine formulas are not interchangeable.

For the oral solutions, always measure dose with calibrated device that comes with the bottle. In a glass container, mix Sandimmune oral solution with room-temperature milk, chocolate milk, or orange juice or mix Neoral or Gengraf oral solution with room temperature orange or apple juice. Stir the mixture well, and have the patient drink it immediately. Avoid using Styrofoam containers because the liquid form of the drug may adhere to the wall of the container. Add more diluent to the glass container and mix it with the remaining solution to ensure that the total amount of cyclosporine is swallowed. Dry the outside of the measuring device before replacing it in its cover. Do not rinse it with water. Take the drug at the same time each day.

All oral cyclosporine dosage forms should be taken consistently with regard to time of day and relation to meals. Do not give with grapefruit juice.

For IV use, dilute each milliliter of injection with 20-100 mL 0.9% NaCl or D5W. Infuse the solution over 2-6 h. Monitor continuously for the first 30 min of the infusion and frequently thereafter for a hypersensitivity reaction, marked by facial flushing and dyspnea.

For ophthalmic use, invert vial several times to obtain a uniform suspension. Remove any contact lenses before administration. May reinsert lenses 15 min after drug administration. May use with artificial tears. Single-use vial; discard after use.

Cyproheptadine

si-proe-hep′ta-deen

Do not confuse with cyclobenzaprine.

CATEGORY AND SCHEDULE

Pregnancy Risk Category: B

Classification: Antihistamines, H_1 receptor antagonist, sedating

MECHANISM OF ACTION

An antihistamine that competes with histamine at histaminic receptor sites. Anticholinergic effects cause drying of nasal mucosa. Competes with serotonin at receptor sites in intestinal smooth muscle and other locations. Antagonism of serotonin on the appetite center of the hypothalamus may account for cyproheptadine's ability to stimulate appetite and counteract some effects of SSRI antidepressants. *Therapeutic Effect*: Relieves allergic conditions (urticaria, pruritus).

PHARMACOKINETICS

Well absorbed from GI tract. Metabolized in liver. Primarily eliminated in feces. *Half-life:* 16 h.

AVAILABILITY

Syrup: 2 mg/5 mL.
Tablets: 4 mg.

INDICATIONS AND DOSAGES

▸ **Allergic condition**

PO

Adults, Children older than 15 yr. 4 mg 3 times/day. May increase dose but do not exceed 0.5 mg/kg/day.
Children 7-14 yr. 4 mg 2-3 times/day, or 0.25 mg/kg daily in divided doses.
Children 2-6 yr. 2 mg 2-3 times/day, or 0.25 mg/kg daily in divided doses.
Elderly. Initially, 4 mg 2 times/day.

OFF-LABEL USES

Stimulation of appetite; treatment of anorgasmy secondary to SSRI use; treatment of serotonin-syndrome.

CONTRAINDICATIONS

Acute asthmatic attack, patients receiving MAOIs, history of hypersensitivity to antihistamines.

INTERACTIONS

Drug

Alcohol, central nervous system (CNS) depressants: May increase CNS depression.
SSRI antidepressants: May antagonize SSRI effects if used chronically.
MAOIs: May increase anticholinergic and CNS depressant effects.
Protirelin: May decrease TSH response.

Herbal

None known.

Food

None known.

DIAGNOSTIC TEST EFFECTS

May suppress flare and wheal reaction to antigen skin testing unless drug is discontinued 4 days before testing. May increase SGPT (AST) levels.

SIDE EFFECTS

Frequent

Drowsiness, dizziness, muscular weakness, dry mouth/nose/throat/lips, urinary retention, thickening of bronchial secretions.

▸ **Elderly**

Frequent

Sedation, dizziness, hypotension.

Occasional

Epigastric distress, flushing, visual disturbances, hearing disturbances, paresthesia, sweating, chills.

SERIOUS REACTIONS

• Children may experience dominant paradoxical reaction (restlessness, insomnia, euphoria, nervousness, tremors).
• Overdosage in children may result in hallucinations, convulsions, death.
• Hypersensitivity reaction (eczema, pruritus, rash, cardiac disturbances, angioedema, photosensitivity) may occur.
• Overdosage may vary from CNS depression (sedation, apnea, cardiovascular collapse, death) to severe paradoxical reaction (hallucinations, tremor, seizures).

PRECAUTIONS & CONSIDERATIONS

Caution is warranted with narrow-angle glaucoma, peptic ulcer, prostatic hypertrophy, pyloroduodenal or bladder neck obstruction, asthma, COPD, increased intraocular pressure, cardiovascular disease,

C

hyperthyroidism, hypertension, and seizure disorders. It is unknown whether cyproheptadine crosses the placenta or is distributed in breast milk. Safety and efficacy of cyproheptadine have not been established in newborns. Be aware that elderly patients are more likely to experience dizziness, sedation, confusion, and hypotension.

Dry mouth, drowsiness, and dizziness are expected side effects. Tolerance to sedative effects may occur. Avoid alcohol and tasks that require alertness and motor skills.

Storage

Store at room temperature.

Administration

Give without regard to meals. Scored tablets may be crushed.

Cytarabine

sye-tare′a-been

★ Ara-C 🍁 Cytosar

Do not confuse cytarabine with Cytadren, Cytovene, or vidarabine. Do not confuse conventional Ara-C with DepoCyt, a liposomal form of cytarabine not discussed in this monograph.

CATEGORY AND SCHEDULE

Pregnancy Risk Category: D

Classification: Antineoplastics, antimetabolites

MECHANISM OF ACTION

An antimetabolite that is converted intracellularly to a nucleotide. Cell cycle-specific for S phase of cell division. *Therapeutic Effect:* May inhibit DNA synthesis. Potent immunosuppressive activity.

PHARMACOKINETICS

Widely distributed; moderate amount crosses the blood-brain barrier. Protein binding: 15%. Primarily excreted in urine. *Half-life:* 1-3 h.

AVAILABILITY

Injection Powder: 100 mg, 500 mg, 1 g, 2 g.
Injection Solution: 20 mg/mL, 100 mg/mL.

INDICATIONS AND DOSAGES

▸ To induce remission in acute lymphocytic leukemia, acute and chronic myelocytic leukemia, or meningeal leukemia

IV

Adults, Elderly, Children.

For acute non-lymphocytic leukemia, the usual dose in combination with other anticancer drugs is 100 mg/m^2 per day by continuous IV infusion (days 1-7) OR 100 mg/m^2 IV q12h (days 1-7). For acute lymphocytic leukemia, consult specialized resources for current protocols.

INTRATHECAL

Adults, Elderly, Children.

The usual dose range is 5-75 mg/m^2. The frequency of administration varies from once a day for 4 days, to once every 4 days. The most frequently used dose is 30 mg/m^2 every 4 days.

OFF-LABEL USES

Treatment of Hodgkin disease, myelodysplastic syndrome, non-Hodgkin lymphorna.

CONTRAINDICATIONS

None known.

INTERACTIONS

Drug

Antigout medications: May decrease the effects of these drugs.

Bone marrow depressants: May increase myelosuppression.
Cyclophosphamide: May increase the risk of cardiomyopathy.
Digoxin: May decrease levels of digoxin.
Flucytosine: May decrease therapeutic effect of flucytosine.
Live-virus vaccines: May potentiate virus replication, increase vaccine side effects, and decrease the patient's antibody response to the vaccine.
Herbal
None known.
Food
None known.

DIAGNOSTIC TEST EFFECTS

May increase serum alkaline phosphatase, bilirubin, uric acid, and AST (SGOT) levels.

IV INCOMPATIBILITIES

Amphotericin B complex (Abelcet, AmBisome, Amphotec), ganciclovir (Cytovene), insulin (regular).

IV COMPATIBILITIES

Dexamethasone (Decadron), diphenhydramine (Benadryl), filgrastim (Neupogen), granisetron (Kytril), hydromorphone (Dilaudid), lorazepam (Ativan), morphine, ondansetron (Zofran), potassium chloride, propofol (Diprivan).

SIDE EFFECTS

Frequent
IV, Subcutaneous (16%-33%): Asthenia, fever, pain, altered taste and smell, nausea, vomiting (risk greater with IV push than with continuous IV infusion).

Intrathecal (11%-28%): Headache, asthenia, altered taste and smell, confusion, somnolence, nausea, vomiting.

Occasional
IV, subcutaneous (7%-11%): Abnormal gait, somnolence, constipation, back pain, urinary incontinence, peripheral edema, headache, confusion.

Intrathecal (3%-7%): Peripheral edema, back pain, constipation, abnormal gait, urinary incontinence.

SERIOUS REACTIONS

- Myelosuppression may result in blood dyscrasias, such as leukopenia, anemia, thrombocytopenia, megaloblastosis, and reticulocytopenia, after a single IV dose.
- Leukopenia, anemia, and thrombocytopenia should be expected with daily or continuous IV therapy.
- Cytarabine syndrome (as evidenced by fever, myalgia, rash, conjunctivitis, malaise, and chest pain) and hyperuricemia/tumor lysis syndrome may occur.
- Acute pancreatitis has been reported in patients receiving continuous infusions.
- High-dose cytarabine therapy may produce severe CNS, GI, and pulmonary toxicity.

PRECAUTIONS & CONSIDERATIONS

Caution is warranted in cardiomyopathy, hepatic impairment, and preexisting drug-induced bone marrow suppression. Caution should also be used in women of childbearing age. The use of contraception should be advised. It is unknown whether cytarabine is distributed in breast milk. Monitor leukocyte and platelet counts daily during the induction phase. Perform bone marrow examinations and liver and kidney function tests periodically. Monitor uric acid serum concentrations.

C

Storage
Unopened vials may be stored at room temperature. Reconstituted solutions are stable at room temperature for 48 h. However, it is recommended to use the prepared injections or infusions as soon as possible after they are prepared.

Administration
CAUTION: Observe and exercise usual cautions for handling and preparing solutions of cytotoxic drugs.

The drug can be administered by IV injection or infusion, as a continuous IV infusion, subcutaneously (rarely used), or intrathecally. The correct dose and route and time of administration of cytarabine will vary from protocol to protocol. Clinicians should consult the appropriate references to verify ordered dilutions and rates of infusion.

Intrathecal use of cytarabine requires the use of single-dose, *unpreserved* solutions only. Do not use bulk injection to prepare intrathecal doses. Avoid using diluents containing benzyl alcohol; preservative-free 0.9% NaCL is usually used. Note that DepoCyt, a liposomal, intrathecal cytarabine, is not discussed in this monograph; consult specialized references for information.

For IV infusion, the dose is commonly diluted in 100-250 mL of D5W or 0.9% NaCl and infused over 0.5-2 hrs. Continuous infusions have also been employed for select indications.

Dacarbazine

da-kar'ba-zeen

★ DTIC-Dome 🍁 DTIC

Do not confuse dacarbazine with Dicarbosil or procarbazine.

CATEGORY AND SCHEDULE

Pregnancy Risk Category: C

Classification: Antineoplastics, alkylating agents

MECHANISM OF ACTION

An alkylating antineoplastic agent that forms methyldiazonium ions, which attack nucleophilic groups in DNA. Cross-links DNA strands. *Therapeutic Effect:* Inhibits DNA, RNA, and protein synthesis.

PHARMACOKINETICS

Minimally crosses the blood-brain barrier. Protein binding: 5%. Metabolized in the liver. Excreted in urine. *Half-life:* 5 h (increased in impaired renal function).

AVAILABILITY

Powder for Injection: 100-mg vials, 200-mg vials.

INDICATIONS AND DOSAGES

▸ **Malignant melanoma**

IV

Adults, Elderly. 2-4.5 mg/kg/day for 10 days, repeated q4wk; or 250 mg/m^2/day for 5 days, repeated q3wk.

▸ **Hodgkin disease**

IV

Adults, Elderly. 150 mg/m^2/day for 5 days, repeated q4wk; or 375 mg/m^2 once, repeated every 15 days (as combination therapy).

OFF-LABEL USES

Treatment of islet cell carcinoma, neuroblastoma, soft tissue sarcoma.

CONTRAINDICATIONS

Demonstrated hypersensitivity to dacarbazine.

INTERACTIONS

Drug

Bone marrow depressants: May enhance myelosuppression.

Live-virus vaccines: May potentiate virus replication, and decrease the patient's antibody response to the vaccine.

Herbal

None known.

Food

None known.

DIAGNOSTIC TEST EFFECTS

May increase BUN, serum alkaline phosphatase, AST (SGOT), and ALT (SGPT) levels.

IV INCOMPATIBILITIES

Allopurinol (Aloprim), amphotericin B (including liposomal forms), cefepime (Maxipime), heparin, pantoprazole (Protonix), pemetrexed (Alimta), piperacillin/tazobactam (Zosyn).

IV COMPATIBILITIES

Etoposide (VePesid), granisetron (Kytril), ondansetron (Zofran), paclitaxel (Taxol).

SIDE EFFECTS

Frequent (90%)

Nausea, vomiting, (occurs within 1 h of initial dose, may last up to 12 h), anorexia.

Occasional

Facial flushing, paresthesia, alopecia, flu-like symptoms (fever, myalgia, malaise), dermatologic reactions, confusion, blurred vision, headache, lethargy.

Rare

Diarrhea, stomatitis, photosensitivity.

D

SERIOUS REACTIONS

- Myelosuppression is frequent and may result in blood dyscrasias, such as leukopenia and thrombocytopenia, generally 2-4 wks after the last dacarbazine dose.
- Hepatotoxicity occurs rarely.
- Anaphylaxis.
- Extravasation may cause tissue damage and severe pain.

PRECAUTIONS & CONSIDERATIONS

Caution is warranted with hepatic or renal impairment. Because dacarbazine is highly emetogenic, antiemetic therapy for the prevention of acute and delayed emesis is recommended. Because of the risk of fetal harm, pregnant women should not take dacarbazine, especially during the first trimester. Breastfeeding should be avoided while receiving treatment. The safety and efficacy of dacarbazine have not been established in children. In elderly patients, age-related renal impairment may require a dosage adjustment. Immunizations and coming in contact with those who have recently received a live-virus vaccine should be avoided during treatment.

Notify the physician if easy nausea and vomiting, bruising, fever, signs of local infection, sore throat, or unusual bleeding from any site occurs. Adequate hydration should be maintained to avoid dehydration from vomiting. Erythrocyte, leukocyte, and platelet counts for evidence of myelosuppression should be monitored. Restricting the patient's oral intake of food for 4-6 h prior to treatment may help reduce nausea. Expect toleration of GI symptoms after the first 1 or 2 days.

Storage

Refrigerate unopened vials and protect them from light. The reconstituted solution containing 10 mg/mL is stable for up to 8 h at room temperature or up to 72 h if refrigerated. Solutions further diluted with D5W or 0.9% NaCl are stable for up to 8 h at room temperature or up to 24 h if refrigerated.

Administration

CAUTION: Observe and exercise appropriate precautions for handling, preparing, and administering cytotoxic drugs.

Dacarbazine dosage is individualized based on clinical response and tolerance of the drug's adverse effects. When administering this drug in combination therapy, consult specific protocols for optimum dosage and sequence of drug administration.

Give dacarbazine by IV push or IV infusion, as prescribed. For IV use, reconstitute the 100-mg vial with 9.9 mL (or the 200-mg vial with 19.7 mL) sterile water for injection to provide a concentration of 10 mg/mL. Give by IV push over 2-3 min. Because IV push administration may cause severe pain along the injected vein, IV infusion may be preferred. For IV infusion, further dilute in 250 mL D5W or 0.9% NaCl. Infuse the drug over 15-30 min. Discard it if the color changes from ivory to pink, because this indicates decomposition. Apply hot packs if the patient develops a burning sensation, irritation, or local pain at the injection site. Monitor the injection site for signs and symptoms of extravasation, including coolness, stinging, swelling, and slight or no blood return.

Dalfampridine

dal-fam′pri-dine

Ampyra

CATEGORY AND SCHEDULE

Pregnancy Risk Category: C

Classification:

Neurologic agents, potassium channel blockers

MECHANISM OF ACTION

Broad-spectrum potassium channel blocker; mechanism not fully understood. In animals, inhibition of potassium channels increases the action potential conduction in demyelinated axons. *Therapeutic Effect:* Improves motor function for walking.

PHARMACOKINETICS

Well absorbed; largely unbound to plasma proteins. Clearance significantly correlated with renal function. Mostly excreted unchanged; 90.3% of the drug in the urine is parent drug. The CYP2E1 isoenzyme is the major enzyme responsible for the 3-hydroxylation of the drug to 2 inactive metabolites, also excreted in the urine. *Half-life:* 5.2-6.5 h.

AVAILABILITY

Tablets, Extended Release: 10 mg.

INDICATIONS AND DOSAGES

▸ **To improve walking for patients with multiple sclerosis**

PO

Adults. 10 mg twice daily.

▸ **Dosage in renal impairment**

CrCl 51-80 mL/min: No dose adjustment is needed, but elimination is decreased, and may have increased seizure risk. CrCl ≤ 50 mL/min: Contraindicated.

CONTRAINDICATIONS

Hypersensitivity, moderate to severe renal impairment, history of seizure.

INTERACTIONS

Drug

Other aminopyridine (e.g., 4-aminopyridine, fampridine): Do not take together. These represent duplicate medications and may increase seizure risk.

Herbal

None known.

Food

Alcohol: Manufacturer recommends avoidance, although specific drug interactions not known.

DIAGNOSTIC TEST EFFECTS

None known.

SIDE EFFECTS

Common (≥ 2%)

Urinary tract infection, insomnia, dizziness, headache, nausea, asthenia, back pain, paresthesia, nasopharyngitis, constipation, dyspepsia, pharyngeal pain.

Occasional

Balance disorders, relapse of multiple sclerosis, confusional state.

SERIOUS REACTIONS

- Seizures.
- Serious bladder or urinary tract infections.

PRECAUTIONS & CONSIDERATIONS

Those with renal impairment or physiologic changes due to aging may require decreased dosage. It is unknown whether the drug is excreted in breast milk; the manufacturer does not recommend use during breastfeeding. Use caution when giving the drug to pregnant women; use only when benefit outweighs risk to fetus. The safety and efficacy of this drug have not been established in children. Age-related renal impairment may require precautions for use in elderly patients. Use caution in driving or other hazardous tasks until the effects of the drug are known.

MS symptoms and gait should be assessed throughout therapy; monitor for neurologic excitability, such as tremor. If seizures occur, notify physician immediately and discontinue use.

Storage

Store at room temperature.

Administration

Take without regard to food. Do not crush, cut, or chew the extended-release tablet. The twice daily doses should be evenly spaced, approximately 12 h apart.

Dalteparin

doll'teh-pare-in

★ 🍁 Fragmin

CATEGORY AND SCHEDULE

Pregnancy Risk Category: B

Classification: Anticoagulants, low-molecular-weight heparins

MECHANISM OF ACTION

A low-molecular-weight heparin that enhances inhibition of factor Xa and thrombin by antithrombin. Only slightly influences platelet aggregation, PT, and aPTT. *Therapeutic Effect:* Produces anticoagulation.

PHARMACOKINETICS

Route	Onset	Peak	Duration
Subcutaneous	1-2 h	4 h	12 h

Protein binding: < 10%. *Half-life:* 3-5 h.

AVAILABILITY

Single-Dose Syringe: 2500 IU/0.2 mL, 5000 IU/0.2 mL, 7500 IU/0.3 mL, 10,000 IU/0.4 mL, 10,000 IU/1 mL, 12,500 IU/0.5 mL, 15,000 IU/0.6 mL, 18,000 IU/0.72 mL.

Multiple-Dose Vial: 10,000 IU/1 mL, 25,000 IU/mL.

INDICATIONS AND DOSAGES

▸ Prophylaxis of deep vein thrombosis (DVT), low- to moderate-risk abdominal surgery

SUBCUTANEOUS

Adults, Elderly. 2500 international units 1-2 h before surgery, then daily for 5-10 days.

▸ Prophylaxis of DVT, high-risk abdominal surgery

SUBCUTANEOUS

Adults, Elderly. 5000 international units the evening before surgery, then 5000 international units/day for 5-10 days. In patients with malignancy, 2500 international units 1-2 h before surgery, then 2500 international units 12 h later, then 5000 international units daily for 5-10 days.

▸ Prophylaxis of DVT, total hip surgery

SUBCUTANEOUS

Adults, Elderly. 2500 international units 1-2 h before surgery, then 2500 units 4-8 h after surgery, then 5000 units/day for 5-10 days; or 2500 international units 4-8 h after surgery, then 5000 international units/day for 5-10 days; or 5000 international units 10-12 h before surgery, then 5000 international units 4-8 h after surgery, then 5000 units/day for 5-10 days.

▸ Unstable angina, non–Q-wave MI

SUBCUTANEOUS

Adults, Elderly. 120 international units/kg q12h (maximum: 10,000 international units/dose) given with aspirin until clinically stable; usual duration 5-8 days.

▸ **Prophylaxis of DVT or pulmonary embolism in the acutely ill patient**
SUBCUTANEOUS
Adults, Elderly. 5000 international units once a day. Usual duration 12-14 days.

▸ **Extended treatment of symptomatic venous thromboembolism (VTE) in patients with cancer**
SUBCUTANEOUS
Adults, Elderly. 200 international units/kg once daily (maximum 18,000 international units/day for first 30 days). 150 international units/kg once daily (maximum 18,000 international units/day for months 2-6).
Doses for patients with cancer and symptomatic VTE with platelet counts 50,000-100,000/mm^3: Reduce dose by 2500 international units daily until platelet count recovers to 100,000/mm^3. Discontinue if platelet count < 50,000/mm^3.
Dose for renal insufficiency in patients with cancer and symptomatic VTE: Target anti-Xa range 0.5-1.5 international units/mL (sample 4-6 h after dose after patient has received 3-4 doses).

CONTRAINDICATIONS

Active major bleeding, history of heparin-induced thrombocytopenia (HIT or HITT), hypersensitivity to dalteparin, heparin, or pork products, AND do not use in patients undergoing epidural/neuraxial anesthesia as (1) a treatment of unstable angina and non–Q-wave MI or (2) for prolonged VTE prophylaxis.

INTERACTIONS

Drug
Anticoagulants, platelet inhibitors, thrombolytics, NSAIDs: May increase risk of bleeding.

Herbal
Supplements with antiplatelet or anticoagulant effects (e.g., feverfew, garlic, ginger, ginkgo biloba, ginseng, red clover, sweet clover, white willow, etc.).
Food
None known.

DIAGNOSTIC TEST EFFECTS

Increases (reversible) LDH, serum alkaline phosphatase, AST (SGOT), and ALT (SGPT) levels. Anti-factor Xa level may be useful to monitor anticoagulant effect in patients with severe renal impairment or if abnormal coagulation parameters occur. Routinely monitor CBC (drug can reduce platelet counts).

SIDE EFFECTS

Occasional (3%-7%)
Hematoma at injection site.
Pain at injection site.
Rare (< 1%)
Hypersensitivity reaction (chills, fever, pruritus, urticaria, asthma, rhinitis, lacrimation, headache); mild, local skin irritation; skin necrosis; alopecia, mild bleeding (e.g., ecchymosis).

SERIOUS REACTIONS

- Major bleeding occurs rarely.
- Overdose may lead to bleeding complications ranging from local ecchymoses to major hemorrhage.
- Thrombocytopenia occurs rarely.
- Epidural or spinal hematoma may cause paralysis.

PRECAUTIONS & CONSIDERATIONS

Caution is warranted with neuraxial (spinal/epidural) anesthesia or spinal puncture, bacterial endocarditis, conditions with increased risk of hemorrhage, history of heparin-induced thrombocytopenia, recent GI ulceration and hemorrhage, hypertensive or diabetic retinopathy, impaired hepatic or renal function, and uncontrolled arterial hypertension. Dalteparin should be used with caution in pregnant women, particularly during the last trimester and immediately postpartum because it increases the risk of maternal hemorrhage. It is unknown whether dalteparin is distributed in breast milk. Safety and efficacy of dalteparin have not been established in children. The drug contains benzyl alcohol and may cause a "gasping syndrome" in exposed neonates. No age-related precautions have been noted in elderly patients. Other medications, including OTC drugs, should be avoided.

Notify the physician of signs of bleeding, breathing difficulty, bruising, dizziness, fever, itching, light-headedness, rash, or swelling. Report any tingling, numbness in the lower limbs, or muscular weakness immediately, as this may indicate spinal/epidural hematoma. Serious bleeding is treated with protamine (see protamine). Baseline CBC and BP should be established. CBC and stool for occult blood should be monitored throughout therapy.

Storage

Store drug at room temperature.

Administration

Administer subcutaneously. Do not inject intramuscularly. The patient should sit or lie down before deep subcutaneous injection. Inject into U-shaped area around the navel, upper outer side of thigh, or upper outer quadrangle of buttock. Use a fine needle (25- to 26-gauge) to minimize tissue trauma. Introduce the entire length of the needle (1/2-inch) into skinfold held between the thumb and forefinger, holding the needle during injection at a 45- to 90-degree angle. Do not rub the injection site after administration to avoid bruising. Alternate administration site with each injection. The usual length of dalteparin therapy is 5-10 days. Perform an ice massage at the injection site shortly before injection to prevent excessive bruising.

Danazol

da'na-zole

🍁 Cyclomen

CATEGORY AND SCHEDULE

Pregnancy Risk Category: X

Classification: Hormones/hormone modifiers, androgenic anti-estrogenic

MECHANISM OF ACTION

A weakly androgenic testosterone derivative that suppresses the pituitary-ovarian axis. Follicle-stimulating hormone (FSH) and luteinizing hormone (LH) output are reduced, and there is lowered estrogen production and hypothalamic-pituitary response. Recent evidence suggests a direct inhibitory effect at target sites by the binding to gonadal steroid receptors at target organs. The drug also decreases IgG, IgM, and IgA levels, as well as phospholipid and IgG isotope autoantibodies. Also increases the levels of the deficient C1 esterase inhibitor (C1EI) in patients with hereditary angioedema. *Therapeutic Effect:* Produces anovulation and amenorrhea, reduces the production of estrogen, corrects biochemical deficiency as seen in hereditary angioedema.

PHARMACOKINETICS
Well absorbed from the GI tract. Metabolized in liver, primarily to 2-hydroxymethylethisterone. Excreted in urine. *Half-life:* 4.5 h.

AVAILABILITY
Capsules: 50 mg, 100 mg, 200 mg.

INDICATIONS AND DOSAGES
▸ **Endometriosis**
PO
Adults. Initially, 200-400 mg/day in 2 divided doses; usual maintenance 800 mg/day in 2 divided doses for 3-9 mo.
▸ **Fibrocystic breast disease**
PO
Adults. 100-400 mg/day in 2 divided doses. Usual duration is 4-6 mo.
▸ **Hereditary angioedema**
PO
Adults. Initially, 200 mg 2-3 times/day. Decrease dose by 50% or less at 1- to 3-mo intervals. If attack occurs, increase dose by up to 200 mg/day.

OFF-LABEL USES
Treatment of gynecomastia, menorrhagia, precocious puberty, premenstrual syndrome.

CONTRAINDICATIONS
Cardiac impairment, pregnancy, breastfeeding, severe liver or renal disease, undiagnosed genital bleeding, porphyria.

INTERACTIONS
Drug
Carbamazepine, cyclosporine, tacrolimus, and warfarin: May increase levels and increase risk of toxicity of these drugs.
HMG-CoA reductase inhibitors: May increase chance of developing myopathy or rhabdomyolysis.
Hormonal contraceptives: May decrease effectiveness of contraceptives.
Hypoglycemic agents: May increase the risk of hypoglycemia.
Herbal
None known.
Food
All foods: May delay time to peak.
High-fat meal: Increases plasma concentration.

DIAGNOSTIC TEST EFFECTS
May increase blood hemoglobin and hematocrit levels, LDL concentrations, serum alkaline phosphatase, bilirubin, calcium, potassium, SGOT (AST) levels, and sodium levels. May decrease HDL concentrations. May alter levels of testosterone, androstenedione, and dehydroepiandrosterone.

SIDE EFFECTS
Frequent
Females: Amenorrhea, breakthrough bleeding/spotting, decreased breast size, increased weight, irregular menstrual periods.
Males: Semen abnormalities, spermatogenesis reduction.
Occasional
Males/females: Edema, rhabdomyolysis (muscle cramps, unusual fatigue), virilism (acne, oily skin), flushed skin, altered moods.
Rare
Males/females: Hematuria, gingivitis, carpal tunnel syndrome, cataracts, severe headache, vomiting, rash, photosensitivity, anxiety, depression, sleep disorders.
Females: Enlarged clitoris, hoarseness, deepening voice, hair growth, monilial vaginitis.
Males: Decreased testicle size.

D

SERIOUS REACTIONS

• Jaundice may occur in those receiving 400 mg/day or more. Liver dysfunction, eosinophilia, thrombocytopenia, pancreatitis occur rarely.
• Peliosis and benign hepatic adenoma have occurred with long-term use.
• Benign intracranial hypertension (pseudotumor cerebri) occurs rarely. Monitor for papilledema, headache, nausea and vomiting, and visual disturbances.
• Thromboembolism, thrombotic, and thrombophlebitic events have occurred, including fatal strokes.

PRECAUTIONS & CONSIDERATIONS

Caution should be used with seizure disorder, migraine, or conditions influenced by edema. Be aware that danazol use is contraindicated during pregnancy and lactation. Exclude pregnancy prior to initiating treatment in femals. If pregnancy is suspected, notify the physician. Nonhormonal contraceptives should be used during therapy. Safety and efficacy of danazol have not been established in children. Be aware that danazol should be used with caution in elderly patients. Breast cancer should be ruled out before starting therapy for fibrocystic breast disease. Monitor liver function.

If masculinizing effects, weight gain, muscle cramps, or fatigue occurs, notify the physician. Spotting or bleeding may occur in the first months of therapy.

Storage

Store at room temperature.

Administration

Take full course of treatment as prescribed by the physician. Administration with meals may lessen GI upset.

Dantrolene

dan'troe-leen

★ Dantrium, Revonto

🍁 Dantrium

Do not confuse Dantrium with Daraprim.

CATEGORY AND SCHEDULE

Pregnancy Risk Category: C

Classification: Skeletal muscle relaxant

MECHANISM OF ACTION

A skeletal muscle relaxant that reduces muscle contraction by interfering with release of calcium ion. Reduces calcium ion concentration. *Therapeutic Effect:* Dissociates excitation-contraction coupling. Interferes with catabolic process associated with malignant hyperthermic crisis.

PHARMACOKINETICS

Poorly absorbed from the GI tract. Protein binding: High. Metabolized in the liver. Primarily excreted in urine. *Half-life:* IV 4-8 h; PO 8.7 h.

AVAILABILITY

Capsules: 25 mg, 50 mg, 100 mg.
Powder for Injection: 20-mg vial.

INDICATIONS AND DOSAGES

▸ **Spasticity**

PO

Adults, Elderly. Initially, 25 mg/day. Increase to 25 mg 2-4 times a day, then by 25-mg increments every 4-7 days up to 100 mg 2-4 times a day.
Children 5 yr and older. Initially, 0.5 mg/kg twice a day. Increase to 0.5 mg/kg 3-4 times a day, then in increments of 0.5 mg/kg/day up to 3 mg/kg 2-4 times a day. Maximum: 100 mg 4 times a day.

▸ **Prevention of malignant hyperthermic crisis**

PO

Adults, Elderly. 4-8 mg/kg/day in 3-4 divided doses 1-2 days before surgery; give last dose 3-4 h before surgery.

IV

Adults, Elderly, Children. 2.5 mg/kg about 1.25 h before surgery.

▸ **Management of malignant hyperthermic crisis**

IV

Adults, Elderly, Children. Initially a minimum of 1 mg/kg rapid IV; may repeat up to total cumulative dose of 10 mg/kg. May follow with 4-8 mg/kg/day PO in 4 divided doses up to 3 days after crisis.

OFF-LABEL USES

Relief of exercise-induced pain in patients with muscular dystrophy, treatment of flexor spasms and neuroleptic malignant syndrome, heatstroke.

CONTRAINDICATIONS

Active hepatic disease, hypersensitivity; do not use where spasticity is utilized to sustain upright posture and balance or to maintain increased function.

INTERACTIONS

Drug

Calcium channel blockers: Use together not recommended for hyperthermia due to rare risk for cardiovascular collapse.

Vecuronium: Dantrolene may potentiate neuromuscular blockade.

CNS depressants: May increase CNS depression with short-term use.

Liver toxic medications, estrogens: May increase the risk of liver toxicity with chronic use.

CYP3A4 inducers/inhibitors: May alter dantrolene plasma levels.

Herbal

St. John's wort: May decrease plasma level of dantrolene.

Food

None known.

DIAGNOSTIC TEST EFFECTS

May alter liver function test results.

IV INCOMPATIBILITIES

Dantrolene is incompatible with most medications. Do not infuse with other medications. Not compatible with D5W or 0.9% NaCl.

SIDE EFFECTS

Frequent (> 10%)

Drowsiness, dizziness, weakness, general malaise, diarrhea (mild), rash, nausea.

Occasional

Confusion, diarrhea (may be severe), headache, insomnia, constipation, urinary frequency.

Rare

Paradoxical CNS excitement or restlessness, paresthesia, tinnitus, slurred speech, tremor, blurred vision, dry mouth, nocturia, impotence, rash, pruritus.

SERIOUS REACTIONS

- There is a risk of liver toxicity, most notably in women, those 35 yr of age and older, those taking other medications concurrently, or those taking ≥ 800 mg per day.
- Overt hepatitis noted most frequently between 3rd and 12th mo of therapy.
- Overdosage results in vomiting, muscular hypotonia, muscle twitching, respiratory depression, and seizures.

PRECAUTIONS & CONSIDERATIONS

Caution is warranted for patients with a history of previous liver disease and impaired cardiac or pulmonary function. Be aware that dantrolene readily crosses the placenta and should not be used in breastfeeding mothers.

Drowsiness may occur but usually diminishes with continued therapy. Avoid alcohol, CNS depressants, and tasks that require mental alertness or motor skills. Notify the physician if bloody or tarry stools, continued weakness, diarrhea, fatigue, itching, nausea, or skin rash occurs. Blood tests, such as liver and renal function tests, should be performed before and during therapy. Therapeutic response, such as decreased intensity of skeletal muscle pain or spasm, should be assessed.

Storage

Store at room temperature. Protect from light. Use infusion within 6 h after reconstitution. Discard if cloudy or a precipitate is present.

Administration

Take oral dantrolene without regard to meals.

For IV use, reconstitute 20-mg vial with 60 mL sterile water for injection to provide a concentration of 0.33 mg/mL. Transfer dose to an IV infusion bag, but do NOT use glass bottle (precipitates). For IV infusion, administer over 1 h. Diligently monitor for extravasation because of high pH of IV preparation and risk for severe complications.

Dapsone

dap′sone

★ Aczone

Do not confuse with Diprosone.

CATEGORY AND SCHEDULE

Pregnancy Risk Category: C

Classification: Antiprotozoal

MECHANISM OF ACTION

An antibiotic that is a competitive antagonist of para-aminobenzoic acid (PABA); it prevents normal bacterial utilization of PABA for synthesis of folic acid. *Therapeutic Effect:* Inhibits bacterial growth.

AVAILABILITY

Tablets: 25 mg, 100 mg.
Topical Gel: 5%

INDICATIONS AND DOSAGES

▸ **Leprosy**

PO

Adults, Elderly. 50-100 mg/day for 3-10 yr.
Children. 1-2 mg/kg/24 h. Maximum: 100 mg/day.

▸ **Dermatitis herpetiformis**

PO

Adults, Elderly. Initially, 50 mg/day. May increase up to 300 mg/day.

▸ ***Pneumocystis carinii* pneumonia (PCP) (off-label)**

PO

Adults, Elderly. 100 mg/day in combination with trimethoprim for 21 days.

▸ **Prevention of PCP (off-label)**

PO

Adults, Elderly. 100 mg/day.
Children older than 1 mo. 2 mg/kg/day. Maximum: 100 mg/day. Alternate dosing: 4 mg/kg/dose once weekly. Maximum: 200 mg/dose.

▸ **Acne**

TOPICAL GEL

Adults and children 12 yr and older: Apply thin layer twice daily to affected areas.

OFF-LABEL USES

Malaria prophylaxis, PCP prophylaxis and treatment, toxoplasmosis prophylaxis.

CONTRAINDICATIONS

Hypersensitivity to the drug or product components.

INTERACTIONS

Drug

CYP2C9 and CYP3A4 inhibitors: May increase levels and effects of dapsone.

CYP2C9 and CYP3A4 inducers: May decrease levels and effects of dapsone.

Methotrexate: May increase hematologic reactions.

Probenecid: May decrease the excretion of dapsone.

Protease inhibitors (including ritonavir): May increase dapsone blood concentration.

Rifampin: May decrease rifampin blood concentration.

Trimethoprim: May increase the risk of toxic effects of both drugs.

Herbal

St. John's wort: May decrease dapsone blood concentration.

Food

None significant.

DIAGNOSTIC TEST EFFECTS

Decreases hemoglobin.

SIDE EFFECTS

Frequent (> 10%)

Hemolytic anemia, methemoglobinemia, rash.

Occasional (1%-10%)

Hemolysis, photosensitivity reaction, tachycardia, headache, insomnia, dermatitis, abdominal pain, nausea.

SERIOUS REACTIONS

- Agranulocytosis, aplastic anemia, and blood dyscrasias may occur.
- Stevens-Johnson syndrome has occurred rarely.
- Drug-induced hepatitis.

PRECAUTIONS & CONSIDERATIONS

Caution is warranted with agranulocytosis, severe anemia, aplastic anemia, glucose-6-phosphate dehydrogenase deficiency, hemoglobin M deficiency, or a hypersensitivity to dapsone or its derivatives (such as sulfoxone sodium). Overexposure to sun or ultraviolet light should be avoided.

Baseline CBC should be obtained. Hypersensitivity to dapsone or its derivatives should be determined before therapy. Skin should be assessed for a dermatologic reaction. Signs and symptoms of hemolysis, such as jaundice, should be monitored. Persistent fatigue, fever, or sore throat should be reported.

Storage

Store at room temperature; protect from light; do not freeze.

Administration

Take dapsone without regard to food.

Topical gel: Apply thin layer to affected areas; rub in gently and completely. Gel is gritty. Wash hands after applying.

Daptomycin

dap'toe-my-sin

★🍁 Cubicin

CATEGORY AND SCHEDULE

Pregnancy Risk Category: B

Classification: Anti-infectives lipopeptides

MECHANISM OF ACTION

A lipopeptide antibacterial agent that binds to bacterial membranes and causes a rapid depolarization of the membrane potential. The loss of membrane potential leads to inhibition of protein, DNA, and RNA synthesis. *Therapeutic Effect:* Bactericidal.

PHARMACOKINETICS
Widely distributed. Protein binding: 90%. Primarily excreted unchanged in urine. Moderately removed by hemodialysis. *Half-life:* 7-8 h (increased in impaired renal function).

D

AVAILABILITY
Powder for Injection: 500 mg/vial.

INDICATIONS AND DOSAGES
▸ **Complicated skin and skin-structure infections**
IV INFUSION
Adults, Elderly. 4 mg/kg every 24 h for 7-14 days.
▸ **Bacteremia from *Staphylococcus aureus* (MSSA or MRSA), including right-sided endocarditis**
IV INFUSION
Adults, Elderly. 6 mg/kg every 24 h for 2-6 wks.
▸ **Dosage in renal impairment**
For patients with creatinine clearance of < 30 mL/min, dosage is 4 mg/kg q48h for 7-14 days for skin infections. For patients with creatinine clearance of < 30 mL/min, dosage is 6 mg/kg q48h for 2-6 wks for bacteremia.

OFF-LABEL USES
Nonpulmonary infections caused by vancomycin-resistant enterococci (VRE).

CONTRAINDICATIONS
Hypersensitivity.

INTERACTIONS
Drug
HMG-CoA reductase inhibitors (e.g., "statins"): May cause myopathy.
Tobramycin: Increases the serum concentration of daptomycin.
Herbal
None known.
Food
None known.

DIAGNOSTIC TEST EFFECTS
May increase serum CPK levels. May alter liver function test results. May alter serum potassium levels.

IV INCOMPATIBILITIES
Because only limited data are available on the compatibility of daptomycin injection with other intravenous substances, additives or other medications should not be added to daptomycin vials or infusions. Diluents containing dextrose. If the same IV line is used to administer different drugs, the line should be flushed with 0.9% NaCl. Acyclovir (Zovirax), allopurinol (Aloprim), amphotericin B cholesteryl sulfate complex (Amphotec), amphotericin B lipid complex (Abelcet), gemcitabine (Gemzar), impipenem/cilastatin (Primaxin), methotrexate, metronidazole (Flagyl), minocycline (Minocin), mitomycin (Mutamycin), nesiritide (Natrecor), nitroglycerin, pantoprazole (Protonix), pentobarbital, phenytoin, remifentanil (Ultiva), streptozocin, sufentanil (Sufenta), thiopental (Thioplex).

IV COMPATIBILITIES
0.9% NaCl or lactated Ringer's injection.

SIDE EFFECTS
Frequent (5%-13%)
Constipation, nausea, peripheral injection site reactions, headache, diarrhea, vomiting, anemia, peripheral edema, chest pain, hypertension, hypotension, insomnia.
Occasional (3%-4%)
Insomnia, rash, vomiting, abdominal pain, injection site reaction.
Rare (< 3%)
Pruritus, dizziness.

SERIOUS REACTIONS

- Skeletal muscle myopathy, characterized by muscle pain and weakness, particularly of the distal extremities, occurs rarely.
- Antibiotic-associated colitis and other superinfections may result from altered bacterial balance.
- Renal failure has occurred.
- Hypersensitivity.

PRECAUTIONS & CONSIDERATIONS

Daptomycin should not be used to treat pneumonia as the drug is inactivated by pulmonary surfactant. Caution is warranted with pregnancy, musculoskeletal disorders, and renal impairment. Avoid concurrent use of HMG-CoA reductase inhibitors because they may cause myopathy. It is unknown whether daptomycin is distributed in breast milk. The safety and efficacy of this drug have not been established in children younger than 18 yr of age. No age-related precautions have been noted in elderly patients.

Report headache, dizziness, nausea, rash, severe diarrhea, new muscle weakness, or any other new symptoms. Mild GI effects may be tolerable, but severe symptoms may indicate the onset of antibiotic-associated colitis. Pattern of daily bowel activity and stool consistency should be monitored. Culture and sensitivity tests should be obtained before giving the first dose of daptomycin; therapy may begin before the test results are known. Check for white patches on the mucous membranes and tongue. Be alert for signs and symptoms of superinfection, including abdominal pain, moderate to severe diarrhea, severe anal or genital pruritus, and severe mouth soreness.

Storage

Store the unopened vials in the refrigerator. The reconstituted and diluted solutions are stable for 12 h at room temperature and up to 48 h if refrigerated.

Administration

Do not mix with dextrose-containing solutions. Reconstitute the 250-mg vial with 5 mL 0.9% NaCl and the 500-mg vial with 10 mL 0.9% NaCl. Do not shake. The vial concentration will be 50 mg/mL. Prepared dose may be given by IV injection over a period of 2 min, or may dilute further for infusion. Further dilute in 50 mL 0.9% NaCl. Infuse the intermittent IV infusion over 30 min.

Daptomycin should not be used in conjunction with ReadyMED elastomeric infusion pumps (Cardinal Health, Inc.) due to the leaching of an impurity, 2-mercaptobenzothiazole (MBT), from this pump system into the daptomycin solution.

Darbepoetin Alfa

dar-beh-poe′ee-tin

Aranesp

Do not confuse Aranesp with Aricept.

CATEGORY AND SCHEDULE

Pregnancy Risk Category: C

Classification: Hematopoietic agents, erythropoiesis-stimulating agents (ESAs)

MECHANISM OF ACTION

A glycoprotein that stimulates formation of red blood cells in bone marrow; increases the serum half-life of epoetin. *Therapeutic Effect:*

Induces erythropoiesis and release of reticulocytes from bone marrow.

PHARMACOKINETICS

Well absorbed after subcutaneous (SC) administration. *Half-life (CRF):* IV 21 h, SC 48.5 h. *Half-life (cancer):* SC adults 74 h, children 49 h.

AVAILABILITY

Injection, Single-Dose Vials: 25 mcg/mL, 40 mcg/mL, 60 mcg/mL, 100 mcg/mL, 150 mcg/mL, 200 mcg/mL, 300 mcg/mL.
Injection, Prefilled Syringes: 25 mcg/0.42 mL, 40 mcg/0.4 mL, 60 mcg/0.3 mL, 100 mcg/0.5 mL, 150 mcg/0.3 mL, 200 mcg/0.4 mL, 300 mcg/0.6 mL, 500 mcg/1 mL.

INDICATIONS AND DOSAGES

▸ Anemia in chronic renal failure

IV BOLUS, SUBCUTANEOUS

Adults, Elderly. Initially, 0.45 mcg/kg once weekly. Adjust dosage to achieve and maintain a target hemoglobin level not to exceed 12 g/dL (target 10-12 g/dL). Do not increase dosage more frequently than once monthly. Limit increases in hemoglobin level by < 1 g/dL over any 2-wk period. IV route preferred in hemodialysis patients.
Children >1 yr. Convert from epoetin alfa based on manufacturer dosing table.
Dosage adjustment: If hemoglobin level approaches 12 g/dL or increases >1 g/dL in any 2-wk period, decrease dose by 25%. If it continues to rise, discontinue therapy temporarily, then resume with 25% reduction. If hemoglobin level does not increase by 1 g/dL after 4 wks, increase dose by 25%.

▸ Anemia associated with chemotherapy

IV, SUBCUTANEOUS

Adults, Elderly. 2.25 mcg/kg/dose once a week or 500 mcg every 3 wks. Adjust dosage to achieve and maintain a target hemoglobin level not to exceed 12 g/dL.
Dosage adjustment: If hemoglobin exceeds 12 g/dL, withhold dose and then restart at 40% dose reduction. If hemoglobin increases 1 g/dL in any 2-wk period, decrease dose by 40%. If hemoglobin does not increase by 1 g/dL after 6 wks, increase dose up to 4.5 mcg/kg once a week.

CONTRAINDICATIONS

History of sensitivity to hamster cell-derived products or human albumin, uncontrolled hypertension.

INTERACTIONS

Drug, Herbal, Food

None known.

DIAGNOSTIC TEST EFFECTS

May increase BUN, serum phosphorus, serum potassium, serum creatinine, serum uric acid, and serum sodium levels. May decrease bleeding time, serum iron concentration, and serum ferritin.

IV INCOMPATIBILITIES

Do not mix with other medications.

SIDE EFFECTS

Frequent (11%-33%)

Myalgia, fatigue, edema, fever, dizziness, constipation, vomiting, nausea, abdominal pain, arthralgia, infection, hypertension or hypotension, headache, diarrhea.

Occasional (3%-10%)

Angina, rash, injection site pain, vascular access infection, flu-like syndrome, reaction at administration site, asthenia, dizziness.

SERIOUS REACTIONS

• Vascular access thrombosis, congestive heart failure (CHF), sepsis, arrhythmias, thrombosis, myocardial infarction (MI), stroke, transient ischemic attack (TIA), and anaphylactic reaction occur rarely.

• Pure red blood cell aplasia and severe anemia, with or without other cytopenias, associated with neutralizing antibodies to erythropoietin have occurred, predominantly in patients with CRF receiving darbepoetin by subcutaneous administration.

• Erythropoiesis-stimulating agents (ESAs) increase the risk for death and serious cardiovascular events in controlled clinical trials when administered to target a hemoglobin of more than 12 g/dL and in cancer patients receiving chemotherapy. There is an increased risk of serious arterial and venous thromboembolic reactions, including MI, stroke, CHF, and hemodialysis graft occlusion. To reduce cardiovascular risks, use the lowest dose of ESAs that will gradually increase the hemoglobin concentration to a level sufficient to avoid the need for red blood cell (RBC) transfusion. The hemoglobin concentration should not exceed 12 g/dL; the rate of hemoglobin increase should not exceed 1 g/dL in any 2-wk period.

• ESAs have shortened time to tumor progression and reduced survival time in solid tumor patients with target hemoglobin > 12 g/dL.

PRECAUTIONS & CONSIDERATIONS

Caution is warranted with hemolytic anemia, a history of seizures, known porphyria (impairment of erythrocyte formation in bone marrow), sickle cell anemia, and thalassemia. It is unknown whether darbepoetin alfa crosses the placenta or is distributed in breast milk. Safety and efficacy of darbepoetin alfa have not been established in children. In elderly patients, age-related renal impairment may require dosage adjustment. Avoid tasks that require mental alertness or motor skills until response to the drug is established. Prefilled syringe needle covers contain dry natural rubber, which may cause allergic reactions in individuals with latex hypersensitivity.

Notify the physician of severe headache. Hematocrit level should be monitored diligently. The dosage should be reduced if hematocrit level increases more than 4 points in 2 wks. CBC with differential, hemoglobin, reticulocyte count, BUN, phosphorus, potassium, serum creatinine, and serum ferritin levels should also be monitored before and during therapy. In addition, BP must be monitored aggressively for an increase because 25% of persons taking darbepoetin alfa require antihypertensive therapy and dietary restrictions. Keep in mind that most patients will eventually need supplemental iron therapy.

Storage

Refrigerate vials. Do not shake vials vigorously because doing so may denature medication, rendering it inactive. Do not freeze. Protect from light.

Administration

For IV use, further dilution is not necessary. May be given as an IV bolus. IV administration is preferred route for patients with renal failure.

For subcutaneous administration, use one dose per vial; do not reenter vial. Discard unused portion. Also available in prefilled syringes or auto-injectors. Do not inject into an area that is red, bruised, hard, or tender. Rotate sites of SC administration with each injection.

D

Darifenacin Hydrobromide

dare-ih-fen′ah-sin

☆ 🍁 Enablex

CATEGORY AND SCHEDULE

Pregnancy Risk Category: C

Classification: Antimuscarinics, urinary incontinence agents, bladder antispasmodics

MECHANISM OF ACTION

A urinary antispasmodic agent that acts as a direct antagonist at muscarinic receptor sites in cholinergically innervated organs. Blockade of the receptors limits bladder contractions. *Therapeutic Effect:* Reduces symptoms of bladder irritability and overactivity; improves bladder capacity.

AVAILABILITY

Tablets (Extended Release): 7.5 mg, 15 mg.

INDICATIONS AND DOSAGES

▸ **Overactive bladder**

PO

Adults, Elderly. Initially, 7.5 mg once daily. If response is not adequate after at least 2 wks, dosage may be increased to 15 mg once daily. Dose should not exceed 7.5 mg once daily with concomitant CYP3A4 inhibitors.

▸ **Dosage in hepatic impairment**

For patients with moderate hepatic impairment, maximum dosage is 7.5 mg once daily.

CONTRAINDICATIONS

GI or gastrourinary obstruction, paralytic ileus, severe hepatic impairment, uncontrolled angle-closure glaucoma, urine retention.

INTERACTIONS

Drug

Aminoglutethimide, carbamazepine, nafcillin, nevirapine, phenobarbital, phenytoin, rifamycins, CYP3A4 inducers: May decrease the effects and blood level of darifenacin.

Amphetamines, β-blockers (selected), dextromethorphan, fluoxetine, lidocaine, mirtazapine, nefazodone, paroxetine, risperidone, ritonavir, thioridazine, tricyclic antidepressants, venlafaxine, CYP2D6 substrates: May increase the effects and blood levels of these drugs.

Anticholinergic agents: Anticholinergic side effects may be increased.

Azole antifungals, ciprofloxacin, clarithromycin, diclofenac, doxycycline, erythromycin, imatinib, isoniazid, nefazodone, nicardipine, propofol, protease inhibitors, quinidine, verapamil, CYP3A4 inhibitors: May increase the effects and blood level of darifenacin. Maximum dose 7.5 mg daily with potent CYP3A4 inhibitors.

Codeine, hydrocodone, oxycodone, tramadol, CYP2D6 prodrug substrates: May decrease the effects and blood levels of these drugs.

Digoxin: Increased digoxin levels.

Herbal

St. John's wort: May decrease effects and blood level of darifenacin.

Food

None known.

DIAGNOSTIC TEST EFFECTS

None known.

SIDE EFFECTS

Frequent (21%-35%)

Dry mouth, constipation.

Occasional (4%-8%)
Dyspepsia, headache, hypertension, peripheral edema, nausea, abdominal pain.
Rare (2%-3%)
Asthenia, diarrhea, dizziness, dry eyes.

SERIOUS REACTIONS

- Urinary tract infection occurs occasionally.
- Heat prostration may occur.
- Acute urinary retention requiring treatment.
- Rare cases of hypersensitivity, such as angioedema.

PRECAUTIONS & CONSIDERATIONS

Caution is warranted with bladder outflow obstruction, constipation, controlled angle-closure glaucoma, decreased GI motility, GI obstructive disorders, hiatal hernia, myasthenia gravis, nonobstructive prostatic hyperplasia, reflux esophagitis, ulcerative colitis, moderate hepatic dysfunction, and urine retention. Safety and efficacy have not been established in pediatric patients. Effects in pregnancy and breastfeeding are unknown.
Storage
Store at room temperature; protect from light.
Administration
Take darifenacin without regard to food. Swallow extended-release tablets whole; do not cut or crush them.

Darunavir

da-roon'ah-veer
★ 🍁 Prezista
Do not confuse darunavir with Denavir.

CATEGORY AND SCHEDULE

Pregnancy Risk Category: C

Classification:
Antiretrovirals, protease inhibitors

MECHANISM OF ACTION

A protease inhibitor that suppresses HIV protease, an enzyme necessary for splitting viral polyprotein precursors into mature and infectious viral particles. *Therapeutic Effect:* Interrupts HIV replication, slowing the progression of HIV infection.

PHARMACOKINETICS

A single 600-mg dose of darunavir exhibits an absolute bioavailability of 37%. Coadministration with ritonavir (100 mg twice daily) increases bioavailability to 82%. Coadministration with ritonavir increases darunavir concentrations approximately 14-fold. Roughly 95% bound to plasma proteins, specifically α-1-acid glycoprotein. Primarily metabolized in liver via CYP3A; 80% of a single dose is excreted in the feces and approximately 14% is recovered in the urine. Unchanged darunavir accounted for approximately 41% and 8% of the administered dose in feces and urine, respectively. *Half-life:* 15 h (increased in very impaired hepatic function).

AVAILABILITY

Tablets: 75 mg, 150 mg, 300 mg, 400 mg, 600 mg.

INDICATIONS AND DOSAGES

▸ **HIV infection (in combination with other antiretrovirals)**
PO
Adults. Treatment-naïve: 800 mg (two 400-mg tablets) with ritonavir (100 mg) once daily with food. Treatment-experienced: 600 mg (600-mg tablet or two 300-mg tablets) with ritonavir (100 mg) twice daily with food.
Children 6 to < 18 yr. Do not use once-daily dosing; dose is weight based and should not exceed adult dosing:

Body Weight (kg)	Darunavir Dose
20 to < 30 kg	375 mg with ritonavir (50 mg) BID
30 to < 40 kg	450 mg with ritonavir (60 mg) BID
≥ 40 kg	600 mg with ritonavir (100 mg) BID

CONTRAINDICATIONS

Hypersensitivity to darunavir; coadministration with alfuzosin, ergot alkaloids, cisapride, pimozide, oral midazolam, triazolam, St. John's wort, lovastatin, simvastatin, rifampin, and sildenafil. Also, since darunavir is boosted with ritonavir, review ritonavir contraindications. The manufacturer recommends against use of darunavir in patients with severe hepatic impairment.

INTERACTIONS

Drug

Alfuzosin: Increases alfuzosin levels and significantly increases hypotension risk. Contraindicated.
Antifungal agents, delavirdine, NNRTIs: May increase levels of darunavir.
Calcium channel blockers: Darunavir may increase concentrations of calcium channel blockers. Monitor BP and heart rate.
Clarithromycin: May increase levels of clarithromycin.
Colchicine: May increase levels of colchicine and resultant risk of toxicity.
CYP3A4 inducers: May decrease effects of darunavir.
CYP3A4 inhibitors: May increase effects of darunavir.
CYP3A4 substrates: Levels of CYP3A4 substrates may be increased by darunavir. Contraindicated with cisapride and pimozide.
Ergot alkaloids: Effects of ergot alkaloids may be increased. Contraindicated.
HMG CoA reductase inhibitors: Darunavir may increase side effects. Use contraindicated with lovastatin, simvastatin.
Sildenafil (when given routinely for pulmonary HTN): Levels may be increased by darunavir. Contraindicated.
Alprazolam, oral midazolam: Increases the risk of prolonged sedation. Contraindicated.
Rifamycins: Decrease darunavir concentrations. Avoid.
Warfarin: Decreased anticoagulant effect. Monitor INR.

Herbal

St. John's wort: May decrease darunavir blood concentration and effect. Contraindicated.

Food

All food: Enhances darunavir blood concentration; give with food.

DIAGNOSTIC TEST EFFECTS

May increase serum AST (SGOT) and ALT (SGPT), serum amylase, lipase, triglyceride or cholesterol levels, blood glucose.

SIDE EFFECTS

Frequent (≥ 5%)

Diarrhea, abdominal pain, headache, rash.

Occasional (2%-5%)

Nausea, insomnia, vomiting, anorexia, accumulation of fat in waist, abdomen, or back of neck.

Rare (< 2%)

Fatigue, abnormal dreams, asthenia, heartburn, flatulence, hyperglycemia, myalgia, urticaria and other hypersensitivity.

SERIOUS REACTIONS

- Pancreatitis.
- Stevens-Johnson syndrome and other serious skin rashes.

- Hepatitis/liver failure.
- Reports of bleeding in patients with hemophilia.

PRECAUTIONS & CONSIDERATIONS

Darunavir contains a sulfonamide moiety. Use with caution in patients with a known sulfonamide allergy. Use with caution in mild to moderate liver function impairment, hemophilia, or diabetes mellitus. Be aware that it is unknown whether darunavir is excreted in breast milk. Breastfeeding is not recommended in this population because of the possibility of HIV transmission. Use with caution during pregnancy due to lack of data. The safety and efficacy of this drug have not been established in children under the age of 6 yr and the drug should not be used in those < 3 yr.

Establish baseline lab values (chemistry, CBC, HIV status, etc.) and monitor hepatic function before and during therapy. Assess the pattern of GI side effects and stool consistency. Evaluate for abdominal discomfort or headache.

Storage

Store drug at room temperature.

Administration

Take darunavir with food; administration with ritonavir is essential to therapeutic effectiveness. If dose is missed and less than 12 h have elapsed since it was due, the patient may take the missed dose. If dose is missed and there is less than 12 h before the next dose is due, take the next dose at the regularly scheduled time; do not double the dose.

Dasatinib

da-sa'ti-nib

Sprycel

CATEGORY AND SCHEDULE

Pregnancy Risk Category: D

Classification: Antineoplastic, signal transduction inhibitors (STIs)

MECHANISM OF ACTION

Inhibits BCR-ABL tyrosine kinase, an enzyme created by the Philadelphia chromosome abnormality found in patients with chronic myeloid leukemia (CML). Also inhibits SRC family kinases. *Therapeutic Effect:* Suppresses tumor growth during the three stages of CML: blast crisis, accelerated phase, and chronic phase.

PHARMACOKINETICS

Protein binding: 96%. Metabolized in liver, primarily by CYP450 3A4. Primarily eliminated in feces (85%, 19% as unchanged); minimal excretion in urine (4%, 0.1% unchanged). *Half-life:* 3-5 h.

AVAILABILITY

Tablets: 20 mg, 50 mg, 70 mg, 100 mg.

INDICATIONS AND DOSAGES

▸ **ALL, Philadelphia chromosome–positive, resistant or intolerant to prior therapy**

PO

Adults. Initially, 140 mg once per day. In clinical studies, dose escalation to 180 mg once daily was allowed in patients who did not achieve a hematologic or cytogenetic response at the recommended starting dosage.

▸ **CML, accelerated, or myeloid, or lymphoid blast phase**
Adults. Initially, 140 mg once per day. In clinical studies, dose escalation to 180 mg once daily was allowed in patients who did not achieve a hematologic or cytogenetic response at the recommended starting dosage.
▸ **CML, chronic phase**
Adults. 100 mg PO once daily. In clinical studies, dose escalation to 140 mg once daily was allowed in patients who did not achieve a hematologic or cytogenetic response at the recommended starting doseage.

CONTRAINDICATIONS
Hypersensitivity to dasatinib or its components.

INTERACTIONS
Drug
H_2 antagonists, proton pump inhibitors: Decreased dasatinib absorption.
Anticoagulants, NSAIDs: Increased risk of bleeding.
CYP3A4 inhibitors (e.g., clarithromycin, erythromycin, azole antifungals): May increase the levels and adverse effects of dasatinib. Consider dasatinib dose reduction.
CYP3A4 substrates (midazolam, triazolam): Increased plasma concentrations of these drugs with increased CNS depression.
QTc-prolonging medications (e.g., class Ia or III antiarrhythmics): Additive effects on QT interval.
Herbal
St. John's wort: Decrease dasatinib levels.
Food
Grapefruit juice: May increase dasatinib levels and adverse effects. Do not drink grapefruit juice while taking dasatinib.

DIAGNOSTIC TEST EFFECTS
Myelosuppression, QTc prolongation.

SIDE EFFECTS
Frequent
Neutropenia, thrombocytopenia, diarrhea, headache, musculoskeletal pain, fatigue, fever, superficial edema, rash, nausea, dyspnea, upper respiratory infection, abdominal pain, pleural effusion, vomiting, arthralgia, asthenia, loss of appetite, inflammatory disease of mucous membrane, GI hemorrhage, constipation, weight loss, dizziness, chest pain, neuropathy, myalgia, weight increase, cardiac dysrhythmia, pruritus, pneumonia, swollen abdomen, pneumonia, shivering.
Occasional
Febrile neutropenia, CHF, pericardial effusion, pulmonary edema, prolonged QT interval, anemia.
Rare
Pulmonary hypertension, CNS hemorrhage, ascites.

SERIOUS REACTIONS
• Severe CNS hemorrhage, including fatalities, have been reported.
• Dasatinib may cause severe bone marrow suppression (thrombocytopenia, neutropenia, anemia).
• Fluid retention, including pleural and pericardial effusion, severe ascites, and generalized edema, has been reported.

PRECAUTIONS & CONSIDERATIONS
Use with caution in patients with impaired hepatic function, cardiovascular disease, pulmonary disease, and patients with QTc prolongation or at risk for QT prolongation including those with hypokalemia, hypomagnesemia, congenital long QT syndrome,

taking other medications known to prolong QTc, or receiving cumulative high-dose anthracycline therapy. Safety and effectiveness have not been established in children. Fluid retention may occur more often in the elderly. Men and women of childbearing potential should be advised to use adequate contraception as the drug may cause fetal harm. Breast milk excretion unknown; do not breastfeed.

Storage

Store at room temperature.

Administration

Tablets should be swallowed whole, not crushed or cut. May be taken without regard to food. Dosage adjustments are recommended based on tolerability and potential drug interactions.

Daunorubicin

daw-noe-roo′bi-sin

★ Cerubidine, DaunoXome

Do not confuse daunorubicin with dactinomycin or doxorubicin. Do NOT confuse conventional daunorubicin with daunorubicine liposomal (DaunoXome) due to different indications and dosage regimens.

CATEGORY AND SCHEDULE

Pregnancy Risk Category: D

Classification: Antineoplastics, anthracyclines

MECHANISM OF ACTION

An anthracycline antibiotic that inhibits DNA and DNA-dependent RNA synthesis by binding with DNA strands. Liposomal encapsulation increases uptake by tumors, prolongs drug action, and may decrease toxicity. *Therapeutic Effect:* Prevents cell division.

PHARMACOKINETICS

Widely distributed. Protein binding: High. Does not cross the blood-brain barrier. Metabolized in the liver to active metabolite. Excreted in urine; eliminated by biliary excretion. *Half-life:* 18.5 h; metabolite: 26.7 h.

AVAILABILITY

Cerubidine (daunorubicin hydrochloride)

Powder for Injection: 20 mg.

Solution for Injection: 5 mg/mL.

DaunoXome (liposomal daunorubicin)

Injection: 2 mg/mL.

INDICATIONS AND DOSAGES

▸ **Acute lymphocytic leukemia (ALL)**

IV

Adults. 45 mg/m^2 on days 1-3 of induction course.

Children < 2 or BSA < 0.5. Give 2.1 mg/kg/dose per protocol.

Children > 2 and BSA > 0.5. Give .25 mg/m^2 on day 1 each week for 4-6 cycles.

▸ **Acute myeloid leukemia (AML)**

IV

Adults < 60 yr. 45 mg/m^2 on days 1-3 of first cycle and on days 1 and 2 of subsequent courses.

Adults > 60 yr. 30 mg/m^2 on days 1-3 of induction course and on days 1 and 2 of subsequent cycles.

Children < 2 or BSA < 0.5. Give 2.1 mg/kg/dose per protocol.

Children > 2 and BSA > 0.5. Give 30-60 mg/m^2 on days 1-3 of cycle.

▸ **Acute nonlymphocytic leukemia (ANLL)**

IV

Adults < 60 yr. 45 mg/m^2 on days 1-3 of first cycle and on days 1 and 2 of subsequent courses.

Adults > 60 yr. 30 mg/m^2 on days 1-3 of induction course and on days 1 and 2 of subsequent cycles.

▸ **Kaposi sarcoma (DaunoXome only)**

IV

Adults. 40 mg/m^2 (DaunoXome) over 1 h repeated q2wk.

▸ **Dosage in renal impairment**

ALL, AML, ANLL

Adults, Children. Serum creatinine > 3 mg/dL. 50% of normal dose.

Kaposi sarcoma (DaunoXome)

Serum creatinine > 3 mg/dL. 50% of normal dose.

▸ **Dosage in hepatic impairment**

ALL, AML, ANLL

Bilirubin 1.2-3 mg/dL. 75% of normal dose.

Bilirubin 3.1-5 mg/dL. 50% of normal dose.

Bilirubin > 5 mg/dL. Daunorubicin is not recommended for use in this patient population.

Kaposi sarcoma (DaunoXome).

Bilirubin 1.2-3 mg/dL. 75% of normal dose.

Bilirubin > 3 mg/dL. 50% of normal dose.

OFF-LABEL USES

Treatment of chronic myelocytic leukemia, Ewing sarcoma, neuroblastoma, non-Hodgkin lymphoma, Wilms tumor.

CONTRAINDICATIONS

Hypersensitivity to daunorubicin.

INTERACTIONS

Drug

Antigout medications: May decrease the effects of these drugs.

Bevacizumab, trastuzumab, cyclophosphamide: May increase cardiotoxic effects.

Bone marrow depressants: May enhance myelosuppression.

Live-virus vaccines: May potentiate virus replication, increase vaccine side effects, and decrease the patient's antibody response to the vaccine.

Killed vaccines: May decrease the patient's antibody response to the vaccine.

Herbal and Food

None known.

DIAGNOSTIC TEST EFFECTS

May increase serum alkaline phosphatase, bilirubin, uric acid, and AST (SGOT) levels.

IV INCOMPATIBILITIES

Daunorubicin hydrochloride: Allopurinol (Aloprim), amphotericin B liposomal (AmBisome), aztreonam (Azactam), cefepime (Maxipime), dexamethasone sodium phosphate, heparin, ertapenem (Invanz), fludarabine (Fludara), lanosprazole (Prevacid), levofloxacin (Levaquin), pantoprazole (Protonix), pemetrexed (Alimta), piperacillin/tazobactam (Zosyn).

DaunoXome: Do not mix with any other solution, especially NaCl or bacteriostatic agents (such as benzyl alcohol).

Rituximab (Rituxan), tigecycline (Tygacil).

IV COMPATIBILITIES

Daunorubicin hydrochloride: Amifostine (Ethyol), anidulafungin (Eraxis), bivalirudin (Angiomax), carboplatin, caspofungin (Cancidas), cisplatin, cyclophosphamide (Cytoxan), cytarabine (Cytosar), dactinomycin (Cosmegen), daptomycin (Cubicin), dexmedetomidine (Precedex), etoposide (VePesid), etoposide phosphate (EtopoPhos), fenoldopam (Corlopam), filgrastim (Neupogen), gemcitabine (Gemzar), granisetron (Kytril), hydrocortisone sodium succinate, melphalan (Alkeran), meperidine (Demerol), methotrexate, ondansetron (Zofran), oxaliplatin (Eloxatin), paclitaxel (Taxol), palonosetron (Aloxi), quinupristin/dalfopristin (Synercid), rituximab (Rituxan), sodium acetate, sodium bicarbonate, teniposide (Vumon), thiotepa (Thioplex), tigecycline (Tygacil), trastuzumab (Herceptin), vincristine (Vincasar), vinorelbine (Navelbine), voriconazole (Vfend). **DaunoXome:** Bivalirudin (Angiostat), meperidine (Demerol), sodium acetate, tirofibran (Aggrastat), trastuzumab (Herceptin).

SIDE EFFECTS

Frequent (> 15%)
Complete alopecia (scalp, axillary, pubic), nausea, vomiting (beginning a few hours after administration and lasting 24-48 h), discoloration of bodily fluids.
DaunoXome: Mild to moderate nausea, fatigue, diarrhea, fever, abdominal pain, anorexia, headache, rigors, back pain, cough, dyspnea, mild alopecia.
Occasional (5%-14%)
Diarrhea, abdominal pain, esophagitis, stomatitis, transverse pigmentation of fingernails and toenails.
Rare (< 5%)
Transient fever, chills, hypertension, palpitation, tachycardia, anxiety, confusion.

SERIOUS REACTIONS

- Myelosuppression may cause hematologic toxicity, manifested as severe leukopenia, anemia, and thrombocytopenia. Platelet and WBC counts typically nadir in 10-14 days and return to normal levels by the third week of daunorubicin treatment. Neutropenic fever commonly occurs.
- Allergic reactions (DanuoXome) in 25% of patients.
- The risk of cardiotoxicity (either acute, manifested as transient ECG abnormalities, or chronic, manifested as congestive heart failure [CHF]) increases when the total cumulative dose exceeds 550 mg/m^2 in adults, 400 mg/m^2 in adults receiving chest radiation, 300 mg/m^2 in children older than 2 yr, or 10 mg/kg in children younger than 2 yr. Monitor LV function at baseline and periodically.
- Severe, local tissue damage leading to ulceration and necrosis can occur with extravasation.
- Secondary malignancy may occur when used in combination with chemotherapy or radiation.

PRECAUTIONS & CONSIDERATIONS

Caution is warranted in elderly patients, preexisting cardiac disease, CHF, hepatic or renal function impairment, myelosuppression, hyperuricemia, and concomitant radiation. Avoid using daunorubicin in pregnant women. It is unknown whether daunorubicin is distributed in breast milk. Cardiac, hepatic, and renal function should be monitored prior to each cycle.
Storage
Daunorubicin hydrochloride: Store vials of powder at room temperature, vials of solution in refrigerator. Reconstituted solutions are stable for 4 days at room temperature. Protect from light. **Daunorubicin liposomal (DaunoXome):** Store vials in refrigerator. Protect from light. Diluted solution stable in refrigerator for 6 h.
Administration
CAUTION: Observe and exercise appropriate precautions

for handling, preparing, and administering cytotoxic drugs. Do not administer IM or SC. Avoid extravasation, potent vesicant.
Daunorubicin hydrochloride: Reconstitute by adding 4 mL of sterile water for injection to the vial and shaking gently to dissolve to produce 5 mg of daunorubicin per mL. The desired dose is withdrawn into a syringe containing 10-15 mL of 0.9% NaCl and then given IV over 3-5 min into the tubing or sidearm in a rapidly flowing IV infusion of D5W or 0.9% NaCl injection.
Daunorubicin liposomal (DaunoXome): Only dilute with D5W to 1 mg/mL. Do not filter. Administered IV over 1-2 h.

Decitabine

de-sye′ta-been
★ 🍁 Dacogen

CATEGORY AND SCHEDULE

Pregnancy Risk Category: D

Classification: Antineoplastic, pyrimidine analogues

MECHANISM OF ACTION

A pyrimidine antimetabolite that is incorporated into DNA and inhibits DNA methyltransferase causing hypomethylation and subsequent cell death. *Therapeutic Effect:* Restores normal function to tumor-suppressor genes regulating cellular differentiation and proliferation.

PHARMACOKINETICS

Few pharmacokinetic data available; *Half life:* less than 1 h.

AVAILABILITY

Powder for Injection: 50 mg.

INDICATIONS AND DOSAGES

▸ **Myelodysplastic Syndrome (MDS)**

IV

Adults. 15 mg/m^2 over 3 h; repeat every 8 h for 3 days; repeat cycle every 6 wks for a minimum of 4 cycles.
Alternatively, 20 mg/m^2 over 1 h once daily for 5 days; repeat cycle every 4 wks. Dose may be adjusted or delayed based on tolerability.

CONTRAINDICATIONS

Hypersensitivity to decitabine or its components.

INTERACTIONS

Drug

Live-virus vaccines: May potentiate virus replication, increase vaccine side effects, and decrease the patient's antibody response to the vaccine.

Herbal and Food

None known.

DIAGNOSTIC TEST EFFECTS

Myelosuppression, hyperglycemia, increased liver enzymes.

IV COMPATIBILITIES

Stable in NS, D5W, and lactated Ringer's.

SIDE EFFECTS

Common (> 30%)

Neutropenia, thrombocytopenia, anemia, fatigue, fever, nausea, cough, petechiae, constipation or diarrhea, hyperglycemia.

Less Common (10%-30%)

Headache, insomnia, swelling, altered albumin, magnesium or potassium, bruising, chills, dizziness, rash, general myalgia, poor appetite, mouth sores/stomatitis, pharyngitis, drowsiness, confusion, altered liver function tests, confusion, pruritus, heartburn.

Rare (< 10%)
Mental status changes, serious bleeding, gingival disorders, serious infections of various sites, allergic reactions, injection site reactions, acute febrile neutrophilic dermatosis.

SERIOUS REACTIONS

- Neutropenia and thrombocytopenia are expected to occur.
- Anaphylactic reactions are rare.
- Opportunistic infection risks.

PRECAUTIONS & CONSIDERATIONS

Use with caution in patients with bone marrow depression, or renal or hepatic impairment. Safety and effectiveness have not been established in children. No unique precautions were observed in the elderly. Advise women of childbearing potential to avoid becoming pregnant while receiving treatment. Advise men not to father a child while receiving decitabine or for 2 mo after discontinuation of therapy. Not known if excreted in breast milk; do not breastfeed.

Storage
Store vials at room temperature. Use within 15 min of reconstitution. Solution prepared with cold infusion fluids may be stored in the refrigerator for up to 7 h.

Administration
CAUTION: Observe and exercise appropriate precautions for handling, preparing, and administering cytotoxic drugs.

Reconstitute vial with 10 mL sterile water for injection and further dilute with NS, D5W, or Ringer's lactate injection to final concentration of 0.1-1 mg/mL. Administer by IV infusion for duration specified by dose protocol.

Moderately emetogenic; consider antiemetic pretreatment. Dosing may be delayed or reduced based on tolerability.

Deferasirox

de-fer'a-si-rox
Exjade
Do not confuse deferasirox with deferoxamine.

CATEGORY AND SCHEDULE

Pregnancy Risk Category: C

Classification: Antidotes, chelators

MECHANISM OF ACTION

An orally active chelator that binds selectively with iron to form a complex. One oral dose of deferasirox appears to be 4-5 times more effective than parenteral deferoxamine in promoting the excretion of chelatable iron from hepatocellular iron stores. Deferasirox chelates excess iron that enters the reticuloendothelial system as insoluble ferritin rather than iron required for enzyme activity. At recommended doses, drug is able to prevent net iron accumulation in most patients receiving frequent transfusions. *Therapeutic Effect:* Promotes urine excretion of iron.

PHARMACOKINETICS

Bioavailability roughly 70%. Food variably increases absorption. Protein binding: 99%, mostly to albumin. Glucuronidation via UGT is the main metabolic pathway, with subsequent biliary excretion. CYP450 (oxidative) metabolism is minor (8%). Drug undergoes enterohepatic recycling. Parent drug and metabolites are primarily (84%) excreted in the feces. Renal excretion is minimal. *Half-life:* 8-16 h.

AVAILABILITY

Tablets for Oral Suspension: 125 mg, 250 mg, 500 mg.

D

INDICATIONS

▸ **Chronic iron toxicity secondary to transfusional iron overload**

PO

Adults, Children > 2 yr. Initially, give 20 mg/kg daily (round to the nearest whole tablet strength). Following initial dosing, adjust q 3-6 mo by 5 to 10 mg/kg (to the nearest whole tablet strength) based on serum ferritin. Maximum recommended: 40 mg/kg/day.

▸ **Adjustment if taking a potent UGT inducer or cholestyramine.**

Adults, Children > 2 yr. Consider increase to 30 mg/kg daily initially; round to the nearest whole tablet strength.

CONTRAINDICATIONS

Hypersensitivity to drug or product components, severe renal disease (CrCl < 40 mL/min or serum creatinine > 2 times upper limit of normal); poor performance status and high-risk myelodysplastic syndromes or advanced malignancies; thrombocytopenia.

INTERACTIONS

Drug

Aluminum-containing antacids: May interfere with absorption of deferasirox and iron-chelating action; avoid.

Anticoagulants (e.g., warfarin): There may be increased risk of hemorrhage; monitor INR and patient status closely.

Cholestyramine and UGT inducers (rifampin, phenytoin, phenobarbital, ritonavir): Avoid if possible, as they significantly reduce deferasirox efficacy. If used together, increase deferasirox dose.

Nephrotoxic Drugs (e.g., aminoglycosides, platinum compounds, vancomycin): May increase risk for renal dysfunction; monitor renal function closely.

Substrates of CYP3A4 (e.g., cyclosporine, simvastatin, hormonal contraceptive agents): Potential for reduced efficacy of these drugs.

Substrates of CYP2C8 (e.g., repaglinide, paclitaxel): Potential for increased levels of these drugs.

Herbal and Food

None known.

DIAGNOSTIC TEST EFFECTS

May increase liver transaminases, serum creatinine. May lower blood cell counts.

SIDE EFFECTS

Frequent (≥ 8%)

Nausea, vomiting, skin rash, diarrhea, abdominal pain, increased serum creatinine.

Occasional

Edema, gastritis, glycosuria, increased blood glucose, proteinuria, purpura, dizziness, insomnia, restlessness or anxiety, drug fever, elevated liver enzymes.

SERIOUS REACTIONS

- Serious allergic reactions (which include angioedema) have been reported, usually within the first month of treatment.
- Acute renal failure.
- Hepatitis and hepatic failure, possible pancreatitis.
- GI bleeding in at-risk patients.
- Agranulocytosis, neutropenia, and thrombocytopenia.
- Ocular (optic neuritis) or hearing disturbances/loss occur rarely.

PRECAUTIONS & CONSIDERATIONS

Use caution in patients with multiple comorbidities and who have preexisting renal conditions, are elderly, or are receiving medicines that reduce renal function. Closely monitor the renal function of patients with creatinine clearances between 40 and less than 60 mL/min. Maintain adequate hydration. Monitor serum creatinine and other renal parameters at baseline and monthly after initiation of treatment. Consider dose reduction, interruption, or discontinuation for increases in serum creatinine. Monitor hepatic function before the initiation of treatment, every 2 wks during the first month and monthly thereafter. Consider dose modifications or interruption of treatment for severe or persistent LFT elevations. Remain alert for signs and symptoms of GI ulceration and hemorrhage during therapy. Monitor blood counts regularly. Be alert for signs of allergic reactions, such as severe skin rash. Auditory and ophthalmic testing (including slit lamp examinations and dilated fundoscopy) are recommended before starting treatment and at regular intervals (every 12 mo). If disturbances are noted, consider dose reduction or interruption. Measure serum ferritin monthly to assess response to therapy and to evaluate for the possibility of overchelation of iron. It is unknown whether drug crosses the placenta or is distributed in breast milk. Use only when absolutely necessary. Safety and efficacy have not been evaluated in children < 2 yr of age. Monitor children for growth and development.

Storage

Store dispersible tablets at room temperature; keep tightly closed; and protect from moisture.

Administration

Take on an empty stomach at least 30 min before food, at the same time each day. Do not chew tablets or swallow them whole. Do not take with aluminum-containing antacid products. Disperse tablet by stirring in water, orange juice, or apple juice until a fine suspension is obtained. Disperse doses of < 1 g in 3.5 oz of liquid and doses of ≥ 1 g in 7 oz of liquid. After swallowing the suspension, resuspend any residue in a small volume of liquid and swallow.

Deferoxamine

de-fer-ox'a-meen

Desferal

CATEGORY AND SCHEDULE

Pregnancy Risk Category: C

Classification: Antidotes, chelators

MECHANISM OF ACTION

An antidote that binds with iron to form complex. *Therapeutic Effect:* Promotes urine excretion of acute iron poisoning or chronic iron overload.

PHARMACOKINETICS

Well absorbed after IM or SC administration. Widely distributed. Rapidly metabolized in tissues, plasma. Excreted in urine, eliminated in feces via biliary excretion. Removed by hemodialysis. *Half-life:* 6 h.

AVAILABILITY

Injection: 500 mg, 2 g.

INDICATIONS AND DOSAGES

▸ **Acute iron intoxication**

IM (PREFERRED)

Children > 3yr. 90 mg/kg/dose every 8 h. Maximum: 6 g/day.

Adults. 1000 mg initially, then 500 mg q4h for up to 2 doses. Subsequent doses have been given every 4-12 h. Maximum: 6 g/day.
IV (FOR PATIENTS IN SHOCK)
Adults. 1000 mg initially, then 500 mg q4h for up to 2 doses. Subsequent doses have been given. Every 4-12 h. Maximum: 6 g/day.
Children. 15 mg/kg/h. Maximum: 6 g/day.

▸ **Chronic iron overload**
SUBCUTANEOUS (VIA SC INFUSION PUMP)
Adults. 1-2 g/day (20-40 mg/kg) over 8-24 h.
Children. 20-40 mg/kg/day over 8-24 h. Maximum 1000-2000 mg/24 h.
IM/IV
Adults. 0.5-1 g/day IM. In addition to IM, 2 g infused at rate not to exceed 15 mg/kg/h for each unit of blood transfused. Maximum: 1 g/day if not transfused; 6 g/day on transfusion days.
Children (IV). 15 mg/kg/h.

OFF-LABEL USES

Diagnosis and treatment of aluminum toxicity in chronic kidney disease.

CONTRAINDICATIONS

Severe renal disease, anuria, primary hemochromatosis, hypersensitivity to deferoxamine mesylate or any component of the formulation.

INTERACTIONS

Drug
Vitamin C: May increase effect of deferoxamine.
Prochlorperazine: May cause loss of consciousness, mechanism unclear.
Herbal and Food
None known.

DIAGNOSTIC TEST EFFECTS

May cause a falsely high total iron-binding capacity (TIBC).

IV INCOMPATIBILITIES

Do not mix with any other intravenous medications.

SIDE EFFECTS

Frequent
Pain, induration at injection site, urine color change (to orange-rose).
Occasional
Abdominal discomfort, diarrhea, leg cramps, impaired vision.

SERIOUS REACTIONS

- Neurotoxicity, including high-frequency hearing loss, and seizures have been reported.
- Adult respiratory distress syndrome with high doses.
- Infusion reactions (flushing, hypotension, urticaria, shock) with rapid infusion.
- Ocular disturbances with prolonged or high doses.

PRECAUTIONS & CONSIDERATIONS

Caution should be used with aluminum overload or aluminum-related encephalopathy.

It is unknown whether drug crosses the placenta or is distributed in breast milk. Use only when absolutely necessary. Be aware that skeletal anomalies may present in neonate. Safety and efficacy have not been evaluated in children < 3 yr of age. Monitor children for growth retardation. Be aware that age-related renal impairment may require caution. Reddish urine may occur.

Storage
Store unopened vials at room temperature. After reconstitution, use within 3 h. If prepared aseptically, the manufacturer states the product may be stored at room temperature

for a maximum of 24 h. Do not refrigerate reconstituted solution.

Administration

In general, IM route is preferred unless in shock. Reconstitute each 500-mg vial with 2 mL sterile water for injection to provide a concentration of 250 mg/mL or dilute each 2-g vial with 8 mL of sterile water for injection.

For IM administration, inject deeply into upper outer quadrant of buttock. May give undiluted.

For subcutaneous injection, administer very slowly. May give undiluted. An SC infusion pump is utilized.

For IV administration, further dilute with 0.9% NaCl, D5W, or lactated Ringer's and administer at maximum rate of 15 mg/kg/h for the first 1000 mg given. Use a slower rate for any subsequent doses, not to exceed 125 mg/h. A too-rapid IV administration may produce skin flushing, urticaria, hypotension, or shock.

Delavirdine

deh-la′ver-deen

★ 🍁 Rescriptor

Do not confuse Rescriptor with Retrovin or Ritonavir.

CATEGORY AND SCHEDULE

Pregnancy Risk Category: C

Classification: Antiretrovirals, nonnucleoside reverse transcriptase inhibitors

MECHANISM OF ACTION

A nonnucleoside reverse transcriptase inhibitor that binds directly to HIV-1 reverse transcriptase and blocks RNA- and DNA-dependent DNA polymerase activities. *Therapeutic Effect:* Interrupts HIV replication, slowing the progression of HIV infection.

PHARMACOKINETICS

Rapidly absorbed after PO administration. Protein binding: 98%. Primarily distributed in plasma. Metabolized in the liver. Eliminated in feces and urine. *Half-life:* 2-11 h.

AVAILABILITY

Tablets: 100 mg, 200 mg.

INDICATIONS AND DOSAGES

▸ **HIV infection (in combination with other antiretrovirals)**

PO

Adults. 400 mg 3 times a day.

CONTRAINDICATIONS

Hypersensitivity. Concomitant use with alprazolam, cisapride, ergot alkaloids, midazolam, pimozide, rifampin, or triazolam.

INTERACTIONS

NOTE: Please see detailed manufacturer's information regarding the management of drug interactions. In some cases, dosage adjustment or an alternate agent is recommended.

Drug

Antacids, H_2 blockers, proton pump inhibitors: May reduce absorption. Separate antacids by at least 1 h. Concurrent use with H_2 blockers and proton pump inhibitors is not recommended.

Benzodiazepines: May cause life-threatening adverse reactions. See contraindications.

Carbamazepine, phenobarbital, phenytoin, CYP3A4: May decrease delavirdine blood concentration.

Corticosteroids, inhaled: May increase systemic effects of corticosteroids.

CYP2C9, CYP2C19, CYP2D6, CYP3A4 substrates: Levels and effects of substrates may be increased by delavirdine.

Didanosine: Decreased concentrations of both drugs. Separate administration by 1 h.

Protease inhibitors: Delavirdine has been reported to increase the serum concentrations of amprenavir, indinavir, nelfinavir, ritonavir, and saquinavir. Decreased delavirdine concentrations may occur when used with amprenavir and nelfinavir. Dose reduction of indinavir and saquinavir should be considered.

Rifabutin, rifampin: May decrease delavirdine blood concentrations. Contraindicated.

Antiarrhythmics, calcium channel blockers, clarithromycin, methadone, immunosuppressants, sildenafil, lovastatin, simvastatin: Increased levels and side effects of these medications may occur.

Herbal

St. John's wort: May decrease delavirdine levels and efficacy. Avoid.

Food

None known.

DIAGNOSTIC TEST EFFECTS

May increase AST (SGOT) and ALT (SGPT), bilirubin, and amylase levels. Prothrombin time may increase. May decrease neutrophil count or hemoglobin.

SIDE EFFECTS

Frequent (> 18%)

Rash, pruritus, headache, nausea.

Occasional (> 2%)

Vomiting, fever, depression, diarrhea, fatigue, anorexia, anxiety.

SERIOUS REACTIONS

- Severe skin rashes, including Stevens-Johnson syndrome, have been reported.

PRECAUTIONS & CONSIDERATIONS

Caution should be used with impaired liver function. It is unknown whether delavirdine crosses the placenta or is distributed in breast milk. Breastfeeding is not recommended due to risk of HIV transmission. Be aware that safety and efficacy have not been established in children younger than 16 yr and elderly patients. Delavirdine is not a cure for HIV infection, nor does it reduce the risk of transmission to others. Must give in combination with other antiretrovirals to adequately treat HIV and reduce chance of resistance.

Expect to obtain baseline laboratory testing, especially liver function tests, before beginning therapy and at periodic intervals during therapy. Assess for any nausea or vomiting and for skin rash. Determine the pattern of bowel activity and stool consistency. Monitor eating pattern and weight loss. Consume small, frequent meals to help offset anorexia and nausea. Medications, including OTC drugs, should not be taken without consulting the physician.

Storage

Store at room temperature, tightly closed. Protect from high humidity.

Administration

May take without regard to food. May disperse 100-mg tablets in water before consumption. Add 4 tablets to at least 3 oz of water and allow to stand for a few minutes, then stir well. Drink promptly. Refill glass with water, and swallow to ensure full dose. Do not dissolve 200-mg tablets. Persons with achlorhydria should take delavirdine with orange juice or cranberry juice. Do not administer within 1 h of antacids or didanosine.

Demeclocycline

dem-e-kloe-sye′kleen

★ Declomycin

CATEGORY AND SCHEDULE

Pregnancy Risk Category: D

Classification: Antibiotics, tetracyclines

MECHANISM OF ACTION

A broad-spectrum tetracycline antibiotic that inhibits bacterial protein synthesis by binding to ribosomal receptor sites; also inhibits ADH-induced water reabsorption. *Therapeutic Effect:* Bacteriostatic; also produces water diuresis.

AVAILABILITY

Tablets: 150 mg, 300 mg.

INDICATIONS AND DOSAGES

▸ Mild to moderate infections, including acne, pertussis, chronic bronchitis, and urinary tract infection

PO

Adults, Elderly. 150 mg 4 times a day or 300 mg 2 times a day.

Children older than 8 yr. 8-12 mg/kg/day in 2-4 divided doses.

▸ Uncomplicated gonorrhea

PO

Adults. Initially, 600 mg, then 300 mg q12hr for 4 days for total of 3 g.

▸ Syndrome of inappropriate ADH secretion (SIADH)

PO

Adults, Elderly. Initially, 900-1200 mg/day in 3-4 divided doses, then decrease dose to 600-900 mg/day in divided doses.

CONTRAINDICATIONS

Children 8 yr and younger, pregnancy, hypersensitivity to tetracyclines.

INTERACTIONS

Drug

Acitretin: Contraindicated due to potential for increased intracranial pressure (ICP).

Antacids or supplements containing aluminum, calcium, or magnesium; laxatives containing magnesium; oral iron preparations; zinc: Impair the absorption of demeclocycline. Take demeclocycline 1 h before or 2 h after these cations.

Cholestyramine, colestipol: May decrease demeclocycline absorption.

Methotrexate: May increase methotrexate levels.

Methoxyflurane: Combination may increase risk of nephrotoxicity.

Oral contraceptives: May decrease the effects of oral contraceptives.

Penicillins: Concomitant therapy may decrease efficacy. Avoid.

Warfarin: Tetracyclines may depress plasma prothrombin activity, may increase INR; monitor INR.

Herbal

None known.

Food

Dairy products: May decrease demeclocycline absorption. Take demeclocycline 1 h before or 2 h after meals.

DIAGNOSTIC TEST EFFECTS

May increase BUN and serum alkaline phosphatase, amylase, bilirubin, AST (SGOT), and ALT (SGPT) levels. With prolonged use, brown-black microscopic discolaration of thyroid gland; very rare reports of abnormal thyroid function.

SIDE EFFECTS

Frequent

Anorexia, nausea, vomiting, diarrhea, dysphagia, possibly severe photosensitivity (with moderate to high demeclocycline dosage).

D

Occasional
Urticaria; rash; diabetes insipidus syndrome, marked by polydipsia, polyuria, and weakness (with long-term therapy).

D

SERIOUS REACTIONS

- Superinfection (especially fungal), anaphylaxis, and benign intracranial hypertension occur rarely.
- Bulging fontanelles occur rarely in infants.
- Nephropathy can occur if expired.
- Pseudotumor cerebri has been reported rarely.
- May induce nephrogenic diabetes insipidus.

PRECAUTIONS & CONSIDERATIONS

Caution is warranted with renal and hepatic impairment, and in those who can't avoid sun or ultraviolet exposure, because such exposure may produce a severe photosensitivity reaction. Should be avoided in children < 8 yr because can cause permanent tooth discoloration, damage to tooth enamel. Do not use during pregnancy because of effects on fetal bone and tooth development. Tetracyclines are excreted in breast milk and are generally not recommended during breastfeeding.

History of allergies, especially to tetracyclines, should be determined before drug therapy. Pattern of daily bowel activity, stool consistency, food intake and tolerance, renal function, and skin for rash should be assessed. Be alert for signs and symptoms of superinfection, such as anal or genital pruritus, diarrhea, and ulceration or changes of the oral mucosa or tongue. BP and mental alertness should be monitored because of the potential for increased intracranial pressure.

Storage
Store at room temperature.

Administration
Take demeclocycline doses on an empty stomach with a full glass of water. Space drug doses evenly around the clock and continue taking for the full course of treatment. Take antacids containing aluminum, calcium, or magnesium; laxatives containing magnesium;
or oral iron preparations 1-2 h before or after demeclocycline because they may impair the drug's absorption.

Desipramine

dess-ip'ra-meen

Norpramin Apo-Desipramine

Do not confuse desipramine with disopyramide or imipramine.

CATEGORY AND SCHEDULE

Pregnancy Risk Category: C

Classification: Antidepressants, tricyclic

MECHANISM OF ACTION

A tricyclic antidepressant that blocks the reuptake of neurotransmitters, such as norepinephrine and serotonin, at presynaptic membranes, increasing their availability at postsynaptic receptor sites. Also has strong anticholinergic activity. *Therapeutic Effect:* Relieves depression.

PHARMACOKINETICS

Rapidly and well absorbed from the GI tract. Protein binding: 90%. Metabolized in the liver. Primarily excreted in urine. Minimally removed by hemodialysis. *Half-life:* 12-27 h.

AVAILABILITY

Tablets: 10 mg, 25 mg, 50 mg, 75 mg, 100 mg, 150 mg.

INDICATIONS AND DOSAGES

▸ **Depression**

PO

Adults. 75 mg/day. May gradually increase to 150-200 mg/day. Maximum: 300 mg/day.

Elderly. Initially, 10-25 mg/day. May gradually increase to 75-100 mg/day. Maximum: 300 mg/day.

Children older than 12 yr. Initially, 25-50 mg/day. May gradually increase to 100 mg/day. Maximum: 150 mg/day.

OFF-LABEL USES

Treatment of bulimia nervosa, cataplexy associated with narcolepsy, neurogenic pain, panic disorder, social phobia.

CONTRAINDICATIONS

Angle-closure glaucoma, use within 14 days of MAOIs, use in postmyocardial infarction period, hypersensitivity to desipramine.

INTERACTIONS

Drug

Alcohol, other CNS depressants: May increase CNS and respiratory depression and the hypotensive effects of desipramine.

Anticholinergic agents: May increase toxicity.

Antithyroid agents: May increase the risk of agranulocytosis.

Carbamazepine: May decrease desipramine levels. Desipramine may increase carbamazepine levels.

Cimetidine, ritonavir: May increase desipramine blood concentration and risk of toxicity.

Clonidine, guanadrel: May decrease the effects of these drugs.

CYP2D6 inhibitors: May increase effects of desipramine.

Fluoxetine: May increase desipramine levels and toxicity. Reduce desipramine dose by 75%.

MAOIs: May increase the risk of neuroleptic malignant syndrome, hyperpyrexia, hypertensive crisis, and seizures. Contraindicated.

Phenothiazines: May increase the anticholinergic and sedative effects of desipramine.

Phenytoin: May decrease the desipramine blood concentration.

Sympathomimetics: May increase the risk of cardiac effects.

Serotonergic agents, SSRIs, sibutramine: Concomitant use may increase serotonergic effects and risk for serotonin syndrome.

Herbal

St. John's wort: May increase desipramine's pharmacologic effects and risk of toxicity, specifically serotonin syndrome.

Food

None known.

DIAGNOSTIC TEST EFFECTS

May alter blood glucose level and ECG readings. Therapeutic serum drug level is 50-300 ng/mL; toxic serum drug level is > 400 ng/mL.

SIDE EFFECTS

Frequent

Somnolence, fatigue, dry mouth, blurred vision, constipation, delayed micturition, orthostatic hypotension, diaphoresis, impaired concentration, increased appetite, urine retention.

Occasional

GI disturbances (such as nausea, GI distress, metallic taste).

Rare

Paradoxical reactions (agitation, restlessness, nightmares, insomnia), extrapyramidal symptoms (particularly fine hand tremor).

SERIOUS REACTIONS

• Overdose may produce confusion, seizures, somnolence, arrhythmias, fever, hallucinations, dyspnea, vomiting, and unusual fatigue or weakness.
• Abrupt discontinuation after prolonged therapy may produce severe headache, malaise, nausea, vomiting, and vivid dreams.
• Tricyclics may cause bone marrow suppression (rare).
• Orthostatic hypotension may occur.

PRECAUTIONS & CONSIDERATIONS

Cross-sensitivity to other dibenzazepines. Antidepressants increase the risk of suicidal thinking and behavior in children, adolescents, and young adults (18-24 yr of age) with major depressive disorder (MDD) and other psychiatric disorders. Caution is warranted with cardiac conduction disturbances, cardiovascular disease, hyperthyroidism, diabetes, hepatic and renal dysfunction, seizure disorders, urine retention, and in those taking thyroid replacement therapy. Desipramine crosses the placenta and is minimally distributed in breast milk. Desipramine use is not recommended for children younger than 6 yr. Expect to administer lower dosages to elderly patients because they are at increased risk for drug toxicity.

Anticholinergic, sedative, and hypotensive effects may occur during early therapy, but tolerance to these effects usually develops. Because dizziness may occur, change positions slowly and avoid alcohol and avoid tasks that require mental alertness or motor skills. CBC and blood chemistry tests to assess hepatic and renal function and ECG to detect arrhythmias should be performed before and periodically during therapy.

Administration

Take desipramine with food or milk if GI distress occurs. Full therapeutic effect may be noted in 2-4 wks. Do not abruptly discontinue desipramine. Once titrated, maintenance dose may be given once per day, at bedtime.

Desloratadine

des-loer-at'ah-deen

★ Clarinex, Clarinex Reditabs

🍁 Aerius

Do not confuse with Claritin or loratadine.

CATEGORY AND SCHEDULE

Pregnancy Risk Category: C

Classification: Antihistamines, nonsedating

MECHANISM OF ACTION

A nonsedating antihistamine that exhibits selective peripheral histamine H_1 receptor blocking action. Competes with histamine at receptor sites. *Therapeutic Effect:* Prevents allergic responses mediated by histamine, such as rhinitis and urticaria.

PHARMACOKINETICS

Rapidly and almost completely absorbed from the GI tract. Distributed mainly in liver, lungs, GI tract, and bile. Metabolized in the liver to active metabolite and undergoes extensive first-pass metabolism. Eliminated in urine and feces. *Half-life:* 27 h (increased in elderly patients and in those with renal or hepatic impairment).

D

AVAILABILITY

Syrup: 0.5 mg/mL.
Tablets: 5 mg.
Tablets (Orally Disintegrating [Reditabs]): 2.5 mg, 5 mg.

INDICATIONS AND DOSAGES

▸ **Urticaria**
PO
Adults, Elderly, Children 12 yr and older. 5 mg once a day.
Children 6-11 mo. 1 mg once a day.
Children 12 mo to 5 yr. 1.25 mg once a day.
Children 6-11 yr. 2.5 mg once a day.

▸ **Seasonal or perennial allergic rhinitis**
PO
Adults, Elderly, Children 12 yr and older. 5 mg once a day.
Children 2-5 years. 1.25 mg once a day.
Children 6-11 yr. 2.5 mg once a day.

▸ **Dosage in hepatic or renal impairment**
Adult dosage is decreased to 5 mg every other day.

CONTRAINDICATIONS

None known.

INTERACTIONS

Drug
Erythromycin, ketoconazole: May increase desloratadine blood concentration. But dosage adjustment not recommended.
Herbal
None known.
Food
None known.

DIAGNOSTIC TEST EFFECTS

May suppress wheal and flare reactions to antigen skin testing unless the drug is discontinued 4 days before testing.

SIDE EFFECTS

Frequent (> 10%)
Headache.
Occasional (9%-39%)
Dry mouth, fatigue, dizziness, nausea.
Rare (< 3%)
Dysmenorrhea, myalgia, diarrhea, somnolence.

SERIOUS REACTIONS

• None known.

PRECAUTIONS & CONSIDERATIONS

Caution is warranted in patients with hepatic and renal impairment. Desloratadine is excreted in breast milk and should not be used by breastfeeding women. The safety and efficacy of desloratadine have not been established in children younger than 6 mo. Children and elderly patients are more sensitive to the drug's anticholinergic effects, such as dry mouth, nose, and throat. Avoid drinking alcoholic beverages and performing tasks that require alertness or motor skills until response to the drug is established. Desloratadine orally disintegrating tablets contain phenylalanine 1.75 mg per tablet.

Drowsiness may occur. Increase fluid intake with upper respiratory allergies to decrease the viscosity of secretions, offset thirst, and replace fluids lost from diaphoresis. Therapeutic response should be monitored.

Storage
Store at room temperature. Keep disentegrating tablets in blister packaging until ready to use.

Administration
Do not crush or break film-coated tablets. Place rapidly disintegrating tablets on the tongue immediately after opening the blister; tablet disintegration occurs rapidly. Administer with or without water. Oral solution often used for children's doses.

D

Desmopressin

des-moe-press'in

★ DDAVP, Stimate 🍁 Minirin, Octostim

CATEGORY AND SCHEDULE

Pregnancy Risk Category: B

Classification: Antidiuretics, hormones/hormone modifiers

MECHANISM OF ACTION

A synthetic pituitary hormone that increases reabsorption of water by increasing permeability of collecting ducts of the kidneys. Also serves as a plasminogen activator. *Therapeutic Effect:* Increases plasma factor VIII (antihemophilic factor). Decreases urinary output.

PHARMACOKINETICS

Route	Onset	Peak	Duration
PO	1 h	2-7 h	6-8 h
IV	15-30 min	1.5-3 h	N/A
Intranasal	15 min to 1 h	1-5 h	5-21 h

Poorly absorbed after oral or nasal administration. Metabolism: Unknown. *Half-life:* Oral: 1.5-2.5 h. Intranasal: 3.3-3.5 h. IV: 0.4-4 h.

AVAILABILITY

Tablets (DDAVP): 0.1 mg, 0.2 mg.
Injection (DDAVP): 4 mcg/mL.
Nasal Solution (DDAVP Rhinal tube): 100 mcg/mL.
Nasal Spray (Stimate): 1.5 mg/mL (150 mcg/spray).
Nasal Spray (DDAVP): 100 mcg/mL (10 mcg/spray).

INDICATIONS AND DOSAGES

▸ **Primary nocturnal enuresis**

PO

Children 6 yr and older. 0.2-0.6 mg once before bedtime.

▸ **Central cranial diabetes insipidus**

PO

Adults, Elderly, Children 12 yr and older. Initially, 0.05 mg twice a day. Range: 0.1-1.2 mg/day in 2-3 divided doses.

Children at least 4 yr. Initially, 0.05 mg; then twice a day. Range: 0.1-1.2 mg daily in 2-3 divided doses.

INTRANASAL

Adults, Elderly, Children older than 12 yr. 5-40 mcg (0.05-0.4 mL) in 1-3 doses/day.

Children 3 mo to 12 yr. Initially, 5 mcg (0.05 mL)/day in 1-2 divided doses. Range: 5-30 mcg (0.05-0.3 mL)/day.

IV, SUBCUTANEOUS

Adults, Elderly, Children older than 12 yr. 2-4 mcg/day in 2 divided doses or 1/10 of maintenance intranasal dose.

▸ **Hemophilia A, von Willebrand disease (type I)**

IV INFUSION

Adults, Elderly, Children 3 mo and older weighing 10 kg or more. 0.3 mcg/kg diluted in 50 mL 0.9% NaCl.

Children weighing < 10 kg. 0.3 mcg/kg diluted in 10 mL 0.9% NaCl.

INTRANASAL (STIMATE)

Adults, Elderly, Children 11 mo and older weighing 50 kg or more. 300 mcg; use 1 spray in each nostril.

Adults, Elderly, Children 11 mo and older weighing < 50 kg. 150 mcg as a single spray.

CONTRAINDICATIONS

Hypersensitivity. Hyponatremia, moderate to severe renal dysfunction. (Creatinine clearance less than 50 mL/min).

INTERACTIONS

Drug

Carbamazepine, chlorpropamide, clofibrate: May increase the effects of desmopressin.

Demeclocycline, lithium, norepinephrine: May decrease effects of desmopressin.

Herbal

None known.

Food

None known.

DIAGNOSTIC TEST EFFECTS

May increase AST and ALT.

SIDE EFFECTS

Occasional

IV: Pain, redness, or swelling at injection site; headache; abdominal cramps; vulval pain; flushed skin; mild BP elevation or decrease; nausea with high dosages.

Nasal: Rhinorrhea, nasal congestion, slight BP elevation, dizziness, rhinitis.

SERIOUS REACTIONS

- Water intoxication or hyponatremia, marked by headache, somnolence, confusion, decreased urination, rapid weight gain, seizures, and coma, may occur in overhydration. Children, elderly patients, and infants are especially at risk. As a result of FDA review, intranasal desmopressin is no longer indicated for treatment of primary nocturnal enuresis. Tablets may be used, but treatment should be stopped during acute illness or conditions with increased water consumption.

PRECAUTIONS & CONSIDERATIONS

Caution is warranted with fluid or electrolyte imbalances, coronary artery disease, hypertensive cardiovascular disease, and predisposition to thrombus formation. Use cautiously in neonates younger than 3 mo because this age group is at increased risk for fluid balance problems. Hemophilia A with factor VIII levels < 5%; hemophilia B; severe type I, type IIB, or platelet-type von Willebrand disease are precautions for use. Careful fluid restrictions are recommended in infants. Fluid intake should be restricted for 1 h prior to dose and for 8 h after administration. Caution should be used in patients with polydipsia or SIADH. Elderly patients are at increased risk for hyponatremia and water intoxication. Avoid overhydration.

Notify the physician of abdominal cramps, headache, heartburn, nausea, or shortness of breath. Signs and symptoms of diabetes insipidus should be monitored. Also, serum electrolyte levels, fluid intake, serum osmolality, urine volume, urine specific gravity, and weight should be assessed. Factor VIII antigen level, aPTT, and factor VIII activity level should be assessed for hemophilia.

Storage

Store oral desmopressin away from light and excessive heat. Refrigerate desmopressin for injection. Refrigerate DDAVP nasal solution and Stimate nasal spray. DDAVP nasal solution and Stimate nasal spray are stable for 3 wks at room temperature if unopened; DDAVP nasal spray is stable at room temperature. Store in upright position.

Administration

For IV infusion, dilute in 10-50 mL 0.9% NaCl and prepare to infuse over 15-30 min. For preoperative use, administer 30 min before procedure, as prescribed. Monitor BP and pulse during infusion.

For subcutaneous use, estimate therapeutic response by adequacy of sleep duration. Expect to adjust morning and evening dosages separately.

! Stimate Nasal spray and DDAVP nasal spray are not exchangeable because of significant differences in concentration. Follow patient package insert for correct administration techniques.

To administer nasal solution, draw up a measured quantity of desmopressin with a calibrated catheter (Rhinal tube). Insert one end in nose and blow on the other end to deposit the solution deep in the nasal cavity. For infants, young children, and obtunded patients, an air-filled syringe may be attached to the catheter to deposit the solution.

Desonide

dess'oh-nide

★ Desonate, DesOwen, LoKara, Verdeso 🍁 Desocort

CATEGORY AND SCHEDULE

Pregnancy Risk Category: C

Classification: Corticosteroids, low potency, topical, dermatologics

MECHANISM OF ACTION

A topical corticosteroid that has anti-inflammatory, antipruritic, and vasoconstrictive properties. The exact mechanism of the anti-inflammatory process is unclear. *Therapeutic Effect:* Reduces or prevents tissue response to the inflammatory process.

PHARMACOKINETICS

Large variation in absorption determined by many factors. Metabolized in the liver. Primarily excreted by the kidneys and small amounts in the bile.

AVAILABILITY

Lotion: 0.05% (DesOwen, LoKara).
Cream: 0.05% (DesOwen).
Ointment: 0.05% (DesOwen).
Foam: 0.05% (Verdeso).
Gel: 0.05% (Desonate).

INDICATIONS AND DOSAGES

▸ **Corticosteroid-responsive dermatoses**

TOPICAL

Adults, Elderly. Apply sparingly 2-4 times/day.

▸ **Atopic dermatitis**

TOPICAL (AEROSOL/GEL)

Adults, Elderly, Children > 3 mo. Apply sparingly 2-4 times/day.

CONTRAINDICATIONS

History of hypersensitivity to desonide.

INTERACTIONS

Drug

None known.

Herbal

None known.

Food

None known.

DIAGNOSTIC TEST EFFECTS

None known.

SIDE EFFECTS

Occasional

Burning and stinging at site of application, dryness, skin peeling, contact dermatitis.

SERIOUS REACTIONS

• The serious reactions of long-term therapy and the addition of occlusive dressings are reversible hypothalamic-pituitary-adrenal (HPA) axis suppression, manifestations of Cushing syndrome, hyperglycemia, and glucosuria.

PRECAUTIONS & CONSIDERATIONS

Caution should be used over large surface areas, with prolonged use, and in addition to occlusive dressings as well as uncontrolled or untreated infections. Avoid use of occlusive dressings on affected area. Skin irritation should be reported. It is unknown whether desonide crosses the placenta or is distributed in the breast milk. Children may absorb larger amounts of the topical form and may be more susceptible to toxicity. No age-related precautions have been noted in elderly patients. Treatment should not exceed 4 consecutive weeks.

Storage

Store at room temperature; protect foam from excessive heat, fire, or smoking; foam aerosol is flammable.

Administration

Gently cleanse area before topical application. Use occlusive dressings only as directed. Apply sparingly and rub into area gently and thoroughly. Do not apply foam directly to face; dispense into hands and apply. Shake lotion well before use.

Desoximetasone

des-ox-i-met′a-sone

★ Topicort, Topicort-LP

🍁 Desoxi, Topicort

Do not confuse desoximetasone with dexamethasone.

CATEGORY AND SCHEDULE

Pregnancy Risk Category: C

Classification: Corticosteroids, medium-high potency, topical, dermatologics

MECHANISM OF ACTION

A medium to high potency, fluorinated topical corticosteroid that has anti-inflammatory, antipruritic, and vasoconstrictive properties. The exact mechanism of the anti-inflammatory process is unclear. *Therapeutic Effect:* Reduces tissue response to the inflammatory process.

PHARMACOKINETICS

Large variation in absorption among sites. Overall, roughly 5%-7% systemically absorbed. Metabolized in liver. Primarily excreted in urine.

AVAILABILITY

Cream: 0.25% (Topicort), 0.05% (Topicort-LP).
Gel: 0.05% (Topicort).
Ointment: 0.25% (Topicort).

INDICATIONS AND DOSAGES

▸ **Corticosteroid-responsive dermatoses**

Topical

Adults, Elderly. Apply sparingly 2 times/day.
Children >10 yr. Apply sparingly 1-2 times/day.

CONTRAINDICATIONS

History of hypersensitivity to desoximetasone, topical fungal infections.

INTERACTIONS

Drug

None known.

Herbal

None known.

Food

None known.

DIAGNOSTIC TEST EFFECTS

None known.

SIDE EFFECTS

Frequent
Itching, redness, irritation, burning at site of application.
Occasional
Dryness, folliculitis, hypertrichosis, acneiform eruptions, hypopigmentation, perioral dermatitis.
Rare
Allergic contact dermatitis, adrenal suppression, atrophy, striae, miliaria, photosensitivity.

SERIOUS REACTIONS

- Serious reactions of long-term therapy and addition of occlusive dressings are reversible hypothalamic-pituitary-adrenal (HPA) axis suppression, manifestations of Cushing syndrome, hyperglycemia, and glucosuria.
- Abruptly withdrawing the drug after long-term therapy may require supplemental systemic corticosteroids.

PRECAUTIONS & CONSIDERATIONS

Urinary free cortisol test and ACTH stimulation test should be evaluated before therapy. It is unknown whether desoximetasone is excreted in breast milk. No age-related precautions have been established for elderly patients. Pediatric patients may absorb larger amounts and may be more susceptible to toxicity. Safety and efficacy have not been evaluated in children younger than 10 yr.

Caution should be used over large surface areas, with prolonged use, and addition of occlusive dressings.
Storage
Store at room temperature.
Administration
Gently cleanse area before application. Use occlusive dressings only as directed. Apply sparingly. Rub into area gently and thoroughly.

Desvenlafaxine

Des-ven'la-fax'een
★ 🍁 Pristiq

CATEGORY AND SCHEDULE

Pregnancy Risk Category: C

Classification: Antidepressants, serotonin and norepinephrine reuptake inhibitors

MECHANISM OF ACTION

A phenethylamine derivative and major active metabolite of venlafaxine that potentiates central nervous system (CNS) neurotransmitter activity by inhibiting the reuptake of serotonin, and norepinephrine. *Therapeutic Effect:* Relieves depression.

PHARMACOKINETICS

Well absorbed from the GI tract. Protein binding: 30%. Primarily metabolized by conjugation (UGT) and, to a minor extent, oxidative metabolism via CYP3A4. Roughly 45% excreted unchanged in urine. Not removed by hemodialysis. *Half-life:* range, 9-13 h (increased in hepatic or renal impairment).

AVAILABILITY

Tablets, extended-release: 50 mg, 100 mg.

INDICATIONS AND DOSAGES

▸ **Depression**
PO
Adults, Elderly. Initially, 50 mg/day. May increase to 100 mg/day if needed. Up to 400 mg/day given in clinical trials, but additional

benefit versus 100 mg/day is uncertain.

▸ **Dosage in renal impairment**

Moderate renal impairment: 50 mg/day.

Severe renal impairment and end-stage renal disease (ESRD): 50 mg every other day.

▸ **Dosage in hepatic impairment**

Dose escalation above 100 mg/day is not recommended.

CONTRAINDICATIONS

Hypersensitivity to desvenlafaxine or venlafaxine; use within 14 days of MAOIs.

INTERACTIONS

Drug

MAOIs: Contraindicated. May cause neuroleptic malignant syndrome, autonomic instability (including rapid fluctuations of vital signs), extreme agitation, hyperthermia, mental status changes, myoclonus, rigidity, and coma.

NSAIDs, aspirin, anticoagulants: Desvenlafaxine may affect platelet function; effects may be additive to these drugs, with potential increase in bleeding risk.

Serotonergic agents (e.g., linezolid, SSRIs, triptans): May increase risk of serotonin syndrome.

Herbal

St. John's wort: Increased risk of serotonin syndrome.

Food

None known.

DIAGNOSTIC TEST EFFECTS

May decrease serum sodium levels. May increase LDL, total cholesterol and triglyceride levels. May rarely increase BUN level and serum alkaline phosphatase, bilirubin, cholesterol, uric acid, AST (SGOT), and ALT (SGPT) levels.

SIDE EFFECTS

Frequent (> 20%)

Nausea, headache, dry mouth.

Occasional (5%-20%)

Dizziness, insomnia, constipation, diarrhea, vomiting, hyperhydrosis, somnolence, fatigue, tremor, mydriasis, nervousness, ejaculatory disturbance, anorexia.

Rare (< 5%)

Anxiety, asthenia, blurred vision, irritability, tremor, abnormal dreams, impotence, weight loss, increased blood pressure.

SERIOUS REACTIONS

- A sustained increase in diastolic BP of 10-15 mmHg occurs occasionally. May increase intraocular pressure.
- Serotonin syndrome and reactions similar to neuroleptic malignant syndrome (NMS).
- Platelet dysfunction and bleeding.
- Hyponatremia.
- Interstitial lung disease or eosinophilic pneumonia is very rare.

PRECAUTIONS & CONSIDERATIONS

Caution is warranted in patients with suicidal tendencies and those with abnormal platelet function, pre-existing hypertension, cardiac disease or recent myocardial infarction, cerebrovascular disease, hyperlipidemia, volume depletion, hyperthyroidism, mania, angle-closure glaucoma, hepatic and renal impairment, and seizure disorder. Notify the physician if pregnant or planning to become pregnant. Complications have been observed in neonates exposed to related drugs in the third trimester; consider tapering in the third trimester. Desvenlafaxine is excreted in breast milk; breastfeeding is not recommended during treatment. The safety and efficacy of desvenlafaxine have not been established in children.

Antidepressants have been reported to increase the risk of suicidal thinking and behavior in children, adolescents, and young adults (18-24 yr of age) with major depressive disorder (MDD) and other psychiatric disorders. Mania or hypomania may be activated. Age-related renal dysfunction may prompt need for dose reduction in elderly patients.

Drowsiness, dizziness, and light-headedness may occur, so avoid alcohol and tasks that require mental alertness or motor skills until the effects of the drug are known. Monitor for clinical worsening, suicidality, and unusual changes in behavior. BP, pulse rate, and weight should be assessed during therapy.

Storage

Store at room temperature.

Administration

May take without regard to food. Tablets are taken whole; do not divide, crush, chew, or dissolve. When discontinuing, plan to taper the dosage slowly to avoid a discontinuation syndrome.

Dexamethasone

dex-a-meth′a-sone

★ Baycadron, Decadron, DexPak Taperpak, Maxidex, Ozurdex, Zema-Pak 🍁 Dexasone, Diodex

Do not confuse dexamethasone with desoximetasone or dextromethorphan, or Maxidex with Maxzide, or Zema-Pak with ZPak.

CATEGORY AND SCHEDULE

Pregnancy Risk Category: C (D if used in the first trimester)

Classification: Corticosteroids, ophthalmic, dermatologics

MECHANISM OF ACTION

A long-acting glucocorticoid that inhibits accumulation of inflammatory cells at inflammation sites, phagocytosis, lysosomal enzyme release and synthesis, and release of mediators of inflammation. *Therapeutic Effect:* Prevents and suppresses cell and tissue immune reactions and inflammatory process.

PHARMACOKINETICS

Rapidly, completely absorbed from the GI tract after oral administration. Widely distributed. Protein binding: High. Metabolized in the liver. Primarily excreted in urine. Minimally removed by hemodialysis. *Half-life:* 3-4.5 h.

AVAILABILITY

Elixir: 0.5 mg/5 mL.
Ophthalmic Suspension, Solution: 0.1% drops.
Oral Solution: 0.5 mg/5 mL, 1 mg/mL.
Tablets: 0.5 mg, 0.75 mg, 1 mg, 1.5 mg, 2 mg, 4 mg, 6 mg.
Injection: 4 mg/mL, 10 mg/mL.
Intravitreal Implant (Ozurdex): 0.7 mg.

INDICATIONS AND DOSAGES

▸ **Anti-inflammatory**

PO/IV/IM

Adults, Elderly. 0.75-9 mg/day in divided doses q6-12h.

Children. 0.08-0.3 mg/kg/day in divided doses q6-12h.

▸ **Cerebral edema**

IV

Adults, Elderly. Initially, 10 mg, then 4 mg (IM/IV) q6h.

IV/IM

Children. Loading dose of 1-2 mg/kg, then 1-1.5 mg/kg/day in divided doses q4-6h.

▸ **Nausea and vomiting in chemotherapy patients**
IV
Adults, Elderly. 8-20 mg once, then 4 mg (PO) q4-6hr or 8 mg q8h. Many dosage regimens available.
*Children.*10 mg/m^2/dose (maximum: 20 mg), then 5 mg/m^2/dose q6h.
▸ **Physiologic replacement**
PO/IV/IM
Children, Adults. 0.03-0.15 mg/kg/day in divided doses q6-12h.
▸ **Usual ophthalmic dosage, ocular inflammatory conditions**
SUSPENSION/SOLUTION
Adults, Elderly, Children. Initially, 2 drops q1h while awake and q2h at night for 1 day, then reduce to 1 drop q4h, then 3-4 times/day.
▸ **Ocular inflammation due to macular edema following retinal vein occlusion**
INTRAVITREAL IMPLANT
Adults. 0.7 mg implant is injected surgically via a specialized application system. Monitor the patient for elevated IOP.

CONTRAINDICATIONS

Active untreated systemic infections; fungal, tuberculosis, or viral diseases of the eye.

INTERACTIONS

Drug
Amphotericin B: May increase hypokalemia.
Aprepitant: May increase levels and effects of dexamethasone.
CYP3A4 inhibitors/inducers: May increase/decrease effects of dexamethasone.
CYP3A4 substrates, cyclosporine: Dexamethasone may decrease levels and effects of substrates.
Digoxin: May increase digoxin toxicity caused by hypokalemia.
Diuretics, insulin, oral hypoglycemics, potassium supplements: May decrease the effects of these drugs.
Hepatic enzyme inducers: May decrease the effects of dexamethasone.
Live-virus vaccines: May decrease the patient's antibody response to vaccine, increase vaccine side effects, and potentiate virus replication.
Salicylates: Salicylates may increase the GI adverse effects of corticosteroids.
Thalidomide: May increase risk of DVT.
Warfarin: May alter effects of warfarin.
Herbal
None known.
Food
None known.

DIAGNOSTIC TEST EFFECTS

May increase blood glucose and serum lipid, amylase, and sodium levels. May decrease serum calcium, potassium, and thyroxine levels.

IV INCOMPATIBILITIES

Calcium chloride, calcium gluconate, caspofungin (Cancidas), cefuroxime (Zinacef), chlorpromazine, ciprofloxacin (Cipro), dantrolene, daunorubicin (Cerubidine), diazepam (Valium), diphenhydramine (Benadryl), dobutamine, epirubicin (Ellence), erythromycin lactobionate, esmolol (Brevibloc), fenoldopam (Corlopam), gentamicin, haloperidol (Haldol), hydroxyzine, idarubicin (Idamycin), labetalol, magnesium sulfate, midazolam (Versed), minocycline (Minocin), mitoxantrone (Novantrone), pantoprazole (Protonix), phenytoin, prochlorperazine, promethazine, protamine, quinupristin/dalfopristin (Synercid), rocuronium (Zemuron), sulfamethoxazole-trimethoprim, tobramycin, topotecan (Hycamtin).

SIDE EFFECTS

D

Frequent

Inhalation: Cough, dry mouth, hoarseness, throat irritation.
Intranasal: Burning, mucosal dryness.
Ophthalmic: Blurred vision.
Systemic: Insomnia, facial swelling or cushingoid appearance, moderate abdominal distention, indigestion, increased appetite, nervousness, facial flushing, diaphoresis.

Occasional

Inhalation: Localized fungal infection, such as thrush.
Intranasal: Crusting inside nose, nosebleed, sore throat, ulceration of nasal mucosa.
Ophthalmic: Decreased vision, watering of eyes, eye pain, burning, stinging, redness of eyes, nausea, vomiting.
Systemic: Dizziness, decreased or blurred vision.
Topical: Allergic contact dermatitis, purpura or blood-containing blisters, thinning of skin with easy bruising, telangiectasis or raised dark red spots on skin.

Rare

Inhalation: Increased bronchospasm, esophageal candidiasis.
Intranasal: Nasal and pharyngeal candidiasis, eye pain.
Systemic: General allergic reaction (such as rash and hives); pain, redness, or swelling at injection site; psychologic changes; false sense of well-being; hallucinations; depression.

SERIOUS REACTIONS

- Long-term therapy may cause immunosuppression, Kaposi sarcoma, muscle wasting (especially in the arms and legs), osteoporosis, spontaneous fractures, amenorrhea, cataracts, glaucoma, peptic ulcer disease, and congestive heart failure (CHF).
- The ophthalmic form may cause glaucoma, ocular hypertension, and cataracts.
- May cause adrenal suppression with high doses or extended treatment periods. Taper therapy slowly to avoid adrenal crisis.
- Abrupt withdrawal following long-term therapy may cause severe joint pain, severe headache, anorexia, nausea, fever, rebound inflammation, fatigue, weakness, lethargy, dizziness, and orthostatic hypotension.
- May cause psychiatric disturbances, depression, euphoria, insomnia.
- Myocardial rupture following recent MI.

PRECAUTIONS & CONSIDERATIONS

Caution is warranted with cirrhosis, hepatic impairment, renal impairment, CHF, diabetes mellitus, high thromboembolic risk, hypertension, hyperthyroidism, adrenal insufficiency, myasthenia gravis, ocular herpes simplex, osteoporosis, peptic ulcer disease, respiratory tuberculosis, seizure disorders, ulcerative colitis, and untreated systemic infections. The ophthalmic form should be used cautiously in long-term therapy because prolonged use may result in cataracts or glaucoma. Dexamethasone crosses the placenta and is distributed in breast milk. Prolonged treatment with high dosages may decrease the short-term growth rate and cortisol secretion in children. Elderly patients are at higher risk for developing hypertension or osteoporosis. Severe stress, including serious infection, surgery, or trauma, may require an increase in dexamethasone dosage. Dentists or other physicians should be informed of dexamethasone therapy if taken within the past 12 mo.

Mood swings, ranging from euphoria to depression, may occur. Notify the physician of fever, muscle aches, sore throat, and sudden weight gain or swelling. Blood glucose level, intake and output, BP, serum electrolyte levels, height, and weight should be monitored before and during therapy. Be alert to signs and symptoms of infection caused by reduced immune response, including fever, sore throat, and vague symptoms. In long-term therapy, signs and symptoms of hypocalcemia (such as muscle twitching, cramps, and positive Chvostek's or Trousseau's sign) or hypokalemia (such as ECG changes, nausea and vomiting, irritability, weakness and muscle cramps, and numbness or tingling, especially in the lower extremities) should be assessed.

Administration

Take oral dexamethasone with milk or food. Do not abruptly discontinue the drug or change the dosage or schedule. Expect to taper the drug after chronic use.

Dexamethasone sodium phosphate may be given by IV push or IV infusion. For IV push, give over 1-4 min. For IV infusion, mix with 0.9% NaCl or D5W and infuse over 15-30 min. If administering to a neonate, solution must be preservative free. May give deep IM, preferably in the gluteus maximus.

Shake ophthalmic suspension well before use. For ophthalmic use, to administer the solution or suspension, place a gloved finger on the lower eyelid and pull it out until a pocket is formed between the eye and lower lid. Hold the dropper above the pocket and place the correct number of drops into the pocket. Close the eye gently. Apply digital pressure to the lacrimal sac for 1-2 min to minimize drainage to the nose and throat, thereby reducing the risk of systemic effects. Remove excess around the eye with a tissue.

The intravitreal insert is applied by a physician trained in intravitreal techniques.

Dexchlorpheniramine

dex′klor-fen-eer′a-meen

CATEGORY AND SCHEDULE

Pregnancy Risk Category: B

Classification: Antihistamines, H_1 receptor antagonist, sedating

MECHANISM OF ACTION

A propylamine derivative that competes with histamine for H_1-receptor sites on effector cells in the GI tract, blood vessels, and respiratory tract. Dexchlorpheniramine is the dextro-isomer of chlorpheniramine and is approximately 2 times more active. *Therapeutic Effect:* Prevents allergic response, produces mild bronchodilation, blocks histamine-induced allergic responses.

PHARMACOKINETICS

Route	Onset	Peak	Duration
PO	0.5 h	1-2 h	3-6 h

Well absorbed from the GI tract. Protein binding: 70%. Widely distributed. Metabolized in liver to active metabolite; undergoes extensive first-pass metabolism. Excreted primarily in urine. Not removed by hemodialysis. *Half-life:* 20 h.

AVAILABILITY

Syrup: 2 mg/5 mL.

INDICATIONS AND DOSAGES

▸ **Allergic rhinitis, common cold, angioedema, urticaria, vasomotor rhinitis**

PO

Adults, Elderly, Children 12 yr or older. 2 mg q4-6h.
Children 6-11 yr. 1 mg (oral syrup) q4-6h.
Children 2-5 yr. 0.5 mg q4-6h.

CONTRAINDICATIONS

History of hypersensitivity to antihistamines, newborn or premature infants, third trimester of pregnancy, MAOIs.

INTERACTIONS

Drug

Alcohol, central nervous system (CNS) depressants: May increase CNS depression.
MAOIs: May cause severe hypotension.
Methacholine: May interfere with interpretation of pulmonary function tests after a methacholine bronchial challenge.
Procarbazine: May increase CNS depression.

Herbal

None known.

Food

None known.

DIAGNOSTIC TEST EFFECTS

May interfere with methacholine bronchial challenge test or allergy testing.

SIDE EFFECTS

Frequent

Drowsiness; dizziness; headache; dry mouth, nose, or throat; urinary retention; thickening of bronchial secretions; sedation; hypotension.

Occasional

Epigastric distress, flushing, blurred vision, tinnitus, paresthesia, sweating, chills.

SERIOUS REACTIONS

- Children may experience dominant paradoxical reactions, including restlessness, insomnia, euphoria, nervousness, and tremors.
- Hypersensitivity reaction, such as eczema, pruritus, rash, cardiac disturbances, and photosensitivity, may occur.
- Overdosage may vary from CNS depression, including sedation, apnea, hypotension, cardiovascular collapse, or death, to severe paradoxical reaction, such as hallucinations, tremor, and seizures.

PRECAUTIONS & CONSIDERATIONS

Caution is warranted with asthma, cardiovascular disease, chronic obstructive pulmonary disease (COPD), narrow-angle glaucoma, peptic ulcer disease, prostatic hypertrophy, pyloroduodenal or bladder neck obstruction, thyroid disease, and severe CNS depression or coma. Be aware that timed-release tablets should be avoided in children 5 yr and younger. It is unknown whether dexchlorpheniramine crosses the placenta or is distributed in breast milk. Dexchlorpheniramine should not be used in patients during the third trimester of pregnancy or while breastfeeding. No age-related precautions have been noted in elderly patients, although they may be more sensitive to adverse effects.

Dizziness, drowsiness, and dry mouth are expected side effects of dexchlorpheniramine. Tasks that require mental alertness or motor skills should be avoided until the effects are established. Alcohol should be avoided during therapy.

Storage

Store at room temperature.

Administration

Take without regard to meals.

Dexlansoprazole

dex'lan-soe'pra-zole

Dexilant

Do not confuse Dexilant with Dexedrine.

CATEGORY AND SCHEDULE

Pregnancy Risk Category: B

Classification: Gastrointestinal agents, proton pump inhibitors (PPI)

MECHANISM OF ACTION

A proton-pump inhibitor that selectively inhibits the parietal cell membrane enzyme system (hydrogen, potassium adenosine triphosphatase) or proton pump. *Therapeutic Effect:* Suppresses gastric acid secretion.

PHARMACOKINETICS

Formulated as a dual delayed-release capsule that results in two distinct peaks; the first peak occurs in 1-2 h, followed by a second peak within 4-5 h. Protein binding: Roughly 97%. Extensively metabolized in the liver to inactive metabolites. Eliminated in feces and urine. Not removed by hemodialysis. *Half-life:* 1-2 h (plasma); > 24 h at gastric site of action (increased in those with hepatic impairment).

AVAILABILITY

Capsules (Delayed Release): 30 mg, 60 mg.

INDICATIONS AND DOSAGES

▸ **Healing and maintenance of erosive esophagitis**

PO

Adults, Elderly. 60 mg/day for up to 8 wks. If healing does not occur within 8 wks, may give for additional 8 wks. Maintenance: 30 mg/day for up to 6 mo.

▸ **Symptomatic nonerosive gastroesophageal reflux (GERD)**

PO

Adults, Elderly. 30 mg/day for up to 4 weeks; repeat courses may be given.

▸ **Dosage adjustment in hepatic impairment**

Adults. No adjustment needed if impairment mild. If Child-Pugh class B or C, maximum is 30 mg/day PO. (No studies in patients with class C cirrhosis are available.)

CONTRAINDICATIONS

Hypersensitivity to dexlansoprazole, lansoprazole, or any product components.

INTERACTIONS

Drug

Ampicillin, digoxin, iron salts, ketoconazole: May interfere with the absorption of ampicillin, digoxin, iron salts, and ketoconazole.

Sucralfate: May delay the absorption of lansoprazole.

Atazanavir: Do not give PPI with atazanavir because levels of atazanavir will be decreased and

effectiveness against HIV will be diminished.
Tacrolimus: May increase tacrolimus concentrations.
Warfarin: Monitor INR as anticoagulant effect may be increased.
Herbal and Food
None known.

DIAGNOSTIC TEST EFFECTS
May increase AST (SGOT), ALT (SGPT), serum alkaline phosphatase, bilirubin, creatinine, glucose and potassium levels. May reduce platelet, RBC, and WBC counts.

SIDE EFFECTS
More common (≥ 2%)
Diarrhea, abdominal pain, nausea, vomiting, flatulence, mild upper respiratory infection.
Infrequent (< 2%)
Altered taste, headache, rash, dizziness, myalgia/arthralgia, bronchospasm.

SERIOUS REACTIONS
- Hepatomegaly (rare).
- Serious hypersensitivity/dermatologic reactions (rare), such as angioedema, anaphylaxis, Stevens-Johnson syndrome.
- Neutropenia or thrombocytopenia.

PRECAUTIONS & CONSIDERATIONS
Caution is warranted in impaired hepatic function. It is unknown whether dexlansoprazole is distributed in human breast milk; caution is warranted in pregnancy and lactation. Safety and efficacy of dexlansoprazole have not been established in children. No age-related precautions have been noted in the elderly.

Laboratory values, including CBC and blood chemistry, should be obtained before therapy. Monitor for gastric symptom improvement.
Storage
Store at room temperature.
Administration
May take without regard to meals. Do not chew or crush delayed-release capsules; swallow whole. May open capsules and sprinkle granules on 1 tbsp of applesauce; swallow immediately.

Dexmedetomidine Hydrochloride
decks-meh-deh-tome′ih-deen
★ 🍁 Precedex
Do not confuse Precedex with Peridex or Percocet.

CATEGORY AND SCHEDULE
Pregnancy Risk Category: C

Classification: Central-acting adrenergic agonists, sedatives

MECHANISM OF ACTION
A selective centrally acting α_2-adrenergic agonist. *Therapeutic Effect:* Produces analgesic, hypnotic, and sedative effects.

PHARMACOKINETICS
Protein binding 94%. Metabolized in liver. Excreted primarily in urine. *Half-life:* 6 min, terminal 2 h. Onset of action is rapid.

AVAILABILITY
Injection: 100 mcg/mL.

INDICATIONS AND DOSAGES
▸ **Sedation before, during, and after intubation and mechanical ventilation while in the intensive care unit (ICU)**
IV

Adults. Loading dose of 1 mcg/kg over 10 min followed by maintenance infusion of 0.2-0.7 mcg/kg/h.
Elderly. May require decreased dosage. No guidelines available.

▸ **Procedural sedation**

IV

Adults. Load 1 mcg/kg (or 0.5 mcg/kg if procedure less invasive) over 10 min followed by infusion of 0.6 mcg/kg/h. Titrate within range of 0.2-1 mcg/kg/h. If patient receiving awake fiberoptic intubation, give maintenance of 0.7 mcg/kg/h until endotracheal tube is secured.
Elderly. Load 0.5 mcg/kg over 10 min then titrate to desired level of sedation. Usual infusion rates lower than those of adults

▸ **Patients with hepatic impairment:** For all indications, consider dosage reduction.

CONTRAINDICATIONS

None known.

INTERACTIONS

Drug

Anesthetics, opioids, other sedative-hypnotics: May enhance the effects of dexmedetomidine.
CYP2D6 substrates: Dexmedetomidine may increase levels/effects of substrates.

Herbal

None known.

Food

None known.

DIAGNOSTIC TEST EFFECTS

May increase serum potassium, alkaline phosphatase, AST (SGOT), and ALT (SGPT) levels.

IV INCOMPATIBILITIES

Do not mix dexmedetomidine with amphotericin, blood, serum, or plasma.

Additional incompatibilities include diazepam (Valium), pantoprazole (Protonix), phenytoin.

IV COMPATIBILITIES

0.9% NaCl, D5W, 20% mannitol, alfentanil, amikacin, aminophylline, amiodarone, ampicillin, ampicillin-sulbactam (Unasyn), atracurium, atropine, azithromycin (Zithromax), aztreonam (Azactam), bretylium, bumetanide, butorphanol, calcium gluconate, cefazolin, cefepime (Maxipime), cefoperazone sodium, cefotaxime, cefotetan, cefoxitin, ceftazidime (Fortaz), ceftizomine, ceftriaxone (Rocephin), cefuroxime, chlorpromazine, cimetidine, ciprofloxacin (Cipro), cisatracurium, clindamycin (Cleocin), dexamethasone sodium phosphate, digoxin, diltiazem, diphenhydramine, dobutamine, dolasetron, dopamine, doxycycline, droperidol, enalaprilat, ephedrine, epinephrine, erythromycin, esmolol, etomidate, famotidine, fenoldopam, fentanyl, fluconazole (Diflucan), furosemide (Lasix), gatifloxacin, gentamicin, glycopyrrolate, granisetron (Kytril), haloperidol, heparin, hydrocortisone sodium succinate, hydromorphone (Dilaudid), hydroxyzine, inamrinone, isoproterenol, ketorolac, labetalol, lactated Ringer's, levofloxacin (Levaquin), lidocaine, linezolid (Zyvox), lorazepam, magnesium sulfate, meperidine, methylprednisolone sodium succinate, metoclopramide, metronidazole, midazolam, milrinone, mivacurium, morphine, nalbuphine (Nubain), nitroglycerin, norepinephrine, ofloxacin, ondansetron (Zofran), pancuronium, phenylephrine, piperacillin/tazobactam (Zosyn), potassium chloride, procainamide, prochloperazine, promethazine, propofol, ranitidine, rapacuronium, remifentanil, rocuronium, sodium bicarbonate, sodium nitroprusside, succinylcholine, sufentanil, sulfamethoxazole-trimethoprim, theophylline, thiopental, ticarcillin-clavulanate (Timentin), tobramycin, vancomycin, vecuronium, verapamil, and a plasma substitute.

SIDE EFFECTS

Frequent

Hypotension (30%), hypertension (16%), nausea (11%). When infused for more than 6 h, nervousness, agitation, and headaches may occur for up to 48 h.

Occasional (2%-5%)

Pain, fever, vomiting, dry mouth, oliguria, thirst.

SERIOUS REACTIONS

- Bradycardia, hypotension, and sinus arrest may occur with too-rapid IV infusion.
- Atrial fibrillation, tachycardia, arrhythmia, hypoxia, anemia, hemorrhage, and pleural effusion have occurred.

PRECAUTIONS & CONSIDERATIONS

! Use only in intensive care setting. Caution is warranted with CHF, advanced heart block, hypovolemia, chronic hypertension, ventricular dysfunction, diabetes hepatic or renal impairment, and those on a continuous cardiac monitor and pulse oximeter. Be aware that dexmedetomidine will provide relaxation and sedation before, during, and after insertion of the endotracheal tube, and during mechanical ventilation. Comfort measures, such as mouth care and repositioning, should be provided. Transient hypertension may occur initially and may require reduction in infusion rate.

Before dexmedetomidine use, baseline vital signs, ECG, and liver function tests should be obtained. ECG for atrial fibrillation, BP for hypotension and level of sedation, pulse rate for bradycardia, and respiratory rate and rhythm should be monitored during therapy. Monitor for weakness, confusion, excessive sweating, abdominal pain, salt cravings, dizziness.

Storage

Store vials at room temperature. Infusions in NS are stable for up to 24 h at room temperature.

Administration

! Do not infuse the drug for longer than 24 h.

For IV use, dilute 2 mL of dexmedetomidine with 48 mL of 0.9% NaCl. (Final concentration: 4 mcg/mL.) Administer the drug as a maintenance infusion using a controlled infusion device, as prescribed. Titrate dose to desired clinical effect for individual patient. The rate of maintenance infusion should be adjusted to achieve desired level of sedation. Dexmedetomidine has been continuously infused in mechanically ventilated patients before, during, and after extubation. It is not necessary to discontinue dexmedetomidine before extubation provided the infusion does not exceed 24 h.

Dexmethylphenidate

dex-meth-ill-fen′i-date

★ Focalin, Focalin XR

CATEGORY AND SCHEDULE

Pregnancy Risk Category: C

Controlled Substance Schedule: II

Classification: Stimulants, central nervous system (CNS)

MECHANISM OF ACTION

A CNS stimulant that blocks the reuptake of norepinephrine and dopamine into presynaptic neurons, increasing the release of these neurotransmitters into the synaptic cleft. *Therapeutic Effect:* Decreases motor restlessness and fatigue; increases motor activity, mental alertness, and attention span; elevates mood.

PHARMACOKINETICS

Readily absorbed from the GI tract. Plasma concentrations increase rapidly. Time to peak: 1-1.5 h (tablet); 1.5 h and 6.5 h (extended-release capsule). Metabolized in the liver. Excreted as metabolites in urine. *Half-life:* 2.2 h. Duration of action: 4-5 h (tablet), 12 h (extended-release capsule).

AVAILABILITY

Tablets: 2.5 mg, 5 mg, 10 mg.
Capsules (Extended Release): 5 mg, 10 mg, 15 mg, 20 mg, 30 mg, 40 mg.

INDICATIONS AND DOSAGES

▸ **Attention-deficit-hyperactivity disorder (ADHD)**

PO

Adults. Patients new to dexmethylphenidate or methylphenidate. *Tablets:* 2.5 mg twice a day (5 mg/day). May adjust dosage in 2.5- to 5-mg increments. Maximum: 40 mg/day. *Capsule:* 10 mg daily. May adjust dose in 10-mg increments at weekly intervals. Maximum dose: 40 mg/day.
Children 6 yr and older. Patients new to dexmethylphenidate or methylphenidate. *Tablets:* 2.5 mg twice a day (5 mg/day). May adjust dosage in 2.5- to 5-mg increments. Maximum dose: 30 mg/day. *Capsule:* 5 mg daily. May adjust dose in 5-mg increments at weekly intervals. Maximum dose: 30 mg/day.
Patients currently taking methylphenidate. Half the methylphenidate dosage.
Patients changing from dexmethylphenidate immediate-release tablets to dexmethylphenidate extended release. Convert at same daily dose. Capsules are given once daily.

CONTRAINDICATIONS

Hypersensitivity to drug or methylphenidate. Diagnosis or family history of Tourette syndrome; glaucoma; history of marked agitation, anxiety, or tension; motor tics; use within 14 days of MAOIs.

INTERACTIONS

Drug

Amitriptyline, phenobarbital, phenytoin, primidone, anticonvulsants: Dosage of these drugs may need to be decreased.
Antihypertensives: Decreased effect of antihypertensives may occur.
Clonidine: Severe toxic reactions occur with methylphenidate.
MAOIs, linezolid: May increase the effects of dexmethylphenidate such as severe hypertensive episodes. MAOIs are contraindicated.
Other CNS stimulants: May have an additive effect.
Warfarin: May inhibit the metabolism of warfarin. Monitor INR.

Herbal

None known.

Food

None known.

DIAGNOSTIC TEST EFFECTS

None known.

SIDE EFFECTS

Frequent

Headache, abdominal pain, nausea, anorexia, fever, restlessness.

D

Occasional
Tachycardia, arrhythmias, palpitations, insomnia, twitching.
Rare
Blurred vision, rash, arthralgia, insomnia.

SERIOUS REACTIONS

- Withdrawal after prolonged therapy may unmask symptoms of the underlying disorder.
- CNS stimulant use associated with serious cardiovascular events and sudden death in patients with cardiac abnormalities or serious heart problems.
- Dexmethylphenidate may lower the seizure threshold in those with a history of seizures.
- Overdose produces excessive sympathomimetic effects, including vomiting, tremor, hyperreflexia, seizures, confusion, hallucinations, and diaphoresis.
- Prolonged administration to children may delay growth.

PRECAUTIONS & CONSIDERATIONS

Caution is warranted with cardiovascular disease, structural cardiac abnormalities, or other cardiac problems, psychosis, seizure disorders, hypertension, and history of substance abuse. It is unknown whether dexmethylphenidate is excreted in breast milk; avoid breastfeeding. Children are more prone to develop abdominal pain, insomnia, anorexia, and weight loss. Long-term dexmethylphenidate use may inhibit growth in children. In psychotic children, dexmethylphenidate use may exacerbate behavior disturbances and abnormal thoughts. No age-related precautions have been noted in elderly patients.

Tasks that require mental alertness and motor skills should be avoided until response to the drug is established. CBC, WBC count with differential, and platelets should be monitored. Baseline height and weight should be obtained at the beginning and periodically throughout therapy.

Storage
Store at room temperature; keep tightly closed.

Administration
Take dexmethylphenidate without regard to food. Take the last dose of the day several hours before bedtime to prevent insomnia.

Do not crush or chew extended-release capsule. Capsules may be opened and sprinkled over a spoonful of cool applesauce. Capsules given once daily in the morning.

Dextran

dex′tran

★ Gentran

Do not confuse with Genprine.

CATEGORY AND SCHEDULE

Pregnancy Risk Category: C

Classification: Plasma expanders

MECHANISM OF ACTION

A branched polysaccharide that produces plasma volume expansion as a result of high colloidal osmotic effect. Draws interstitial fluid into the intravascular space. May also increase blood flow in microcirculation. *Therapeutic Effect:* Increases central venous pressure, cardiac output, stroke volume, BP, urine output, capillary perfusion, and pulse pressure. Decreases heart rate, peripheral resistance, and blood viscosity. Corrects hypovolemia.

AVAILABILITY

Injection (High Molecular Weight [Gentran]): 6% dextran 70 in 500 mL 0.9% NaCl.
Injection (Low Molecular Weight [Gentran LMD]): 10% dextran 40 in 500 mL D5W, 10% dextran 40 in 500 mL 0.9% NaCl.

INDICATIONS AND DOSAGES

▸ **Volume expansion, shock**

IV

Adults, Elderly (Dextran 40 or 70). 500-1000 mL at a rate of 20-40 mL/min. Maximum dose: 20 mL/kg for first 24 h and 10 mL/kg thereafter.

Children (Dextran 40 or 70). Total dose not to exceed 20 mL/kg on day 1 and 10 mL/kg/day thereafter.

▸ **Prevention of venous thrombosis/ pulmonary embolism**

IV (DEXTRAN 40)

Adults. 50-100 g on day of surgery, then 50 g every 2-3 days as needed based on risk, up to 2 wks.

CONTRAINDICATIONS

Hypervolemia, renal failure with severe oliguria or anuria, severe bleeding disorders, severe cardiac decompensation, severe thrombocytopenia.

INTERACTIONS

Drug
None known.
Herbal
None known.
Food
None known.

DIAGNOSTIC TEST EFFECTS

Prolongs bleeding time and depresses platelet count. Decreases clotting factors V, VIII, and IX. May falsely elevate glucose assays.

IV INCOMPATIBILITIES

Do not add medications to dextran solution.

SIDE EFFECTS

Occasional
Mild hypersensitivity reaction, including urticaria, nasal congestion, wheezing.

SERIOUS REACTIONS

- Severe or fatal anaphylaxis, manifested by marked hypotension and cardiac or respiratory arrest, may occur early during IV infusion, generally in those not previously exposed to IV dextran.
- Renal failure has occurred.

PRECAUTIONS & CONSIDERATIONS

Caution is warranted with chronic hepatic disease and extreme dehydration and in patients with active hemorrhage. Observe for bleeding, and monitor hematocrit to keep above 30%. Fluid overload can occur; use with caution in patients with hypovolemia. Be aware of signs and symptoms of fluid overload, such as peripheral or pulmonary edema, and impending congestive heart failure. Women may experience a heavier menstrual flow than usual. An electric razor and soft toothbrush should be used to prevent bleeding during dextran therapy. Do not take any medications, including OTC drugs (especially aspirin), without physician approval.

Notify the physician of bleeding from the surgical site, chest pain, dyspnea, black or red stool, coffee-ground emesis, dark or red urine, or red-speckled mucus from cough. Urine output, vital signs, and laboratory values, such as bleeding time, platelet count, and clotting factors, should be monitored. Central venous pressure

(CVP) should also be assessed to detect blood volume overexpansion.

Storage

Store at room temperature. Use only clear solutions, and discard partially used containers.

Administration

! Therapy should not continue longer than 5 days.

Give by IV infusion only. Monitor closely during first 15 min of infusion for anaphylactic reaction. Monitor vital signs every 5 min. Monitor urine flow rate during administration. Discontinue dextran 40 and give an osmotic diuretic, as prescribed, if oliguria or anuria occurs to minimize vascular overloading. If dextran is given by rapid injection, monitor CVP. Immediately discontinue the drug and notify the physician if CVP rises precipitously. Monitor BP diligently during infusion. Stop the infusion immediately if marked hypotension occurs, a sign of imminent anaphylactic reaction. If evidence of blood volume overexpansion occurs, discontinue the drug until blood volume is adjusted by diuresis.

Dextroamphetamine

dex-troe-am-fet′a-meen

★ Procentra, Dexedrine Spansule

Do not confuse dextroamphetamine with dextromethorphan, or Dexedrine with Dextran or Excedrin.

CATEGORY AND SCHEDULE

Pregnancy Risk Category: C

Controlled Substance Schedule: II

Classification: Adrenergic agonists, amphetamines, stimulants

MECHANISM OF ACTION

An amphetamine that enhances the action of dopamine and norepinephrine by blocking their reuptake from synapses; also inhibits monoamine oxidase and facilitates the release of catecholamines. *Therapeutic Effect:* Increases motor activity and mental alertness; decreases motor restlessness, drowsiness, and fatigue; suppresses appetite.

AVAILABILITY

Capsules, Sustained Release (Dexedrine Spansule): 5 mg, 10 mg, 15 mg.

Tablets: 5 mg, 10 mg.

Oral Solution (Procentra): 1 mg/mL.

INDICATIONS AND DOSAGES

▸ **Narcolepsy**

PO

Adults, Children older than 12 yr. Initially, 10 mg/day. Increase by 10 mg/day at weekly intervals until therapeutic response is achieved. Maximum: 60 mg/day.

Children 6-12 yr. Initially, 5 mg/day. Increase by 5 mg/day at weekly intervals until therapeutic response is achieved. Maximum dose: 60 mg/day.

▸ **Attention-deficit-hyperactivity disorder (ADHD)**

PO

Adults: Initially, 5 mg once or twice daily. Titrate at weekly intervals. Usual maximum: 60 mg/day.

Children 6 yr and older. Initially, 5 mg once or twice a day. Increase by 5 mg/day at weekly intervals until therapeutic response is achieved. Maximum: 40 mg/day. Usual dose: 5-20 mg/day.

Children 3-5 yr. Initially, 2.5 mg/day. Increase by 2.5 mg/day at weekly intervals until therapeutic response is achieved. Maximum dose: 40 mg/day. Usual range

0.1-0.5 mg/kg/day. Do not use Spansule.

▸ **Appetite suppressant**

PO

Adults, Children older than 12 yr. 5-30 mg daily in divided doses of 5-10 mg each, given 30-60 min before meals; or 1 extended-release capsule in the morning. Usually no longer than 3-6 wks.

CONTRAINDICATIONS

Advanced arteriosclerosis, agitated states, glaucoma, history of drug abuse, hypersensitivity to sympathomimetic amines, hyperthyroidism, moderate to severe hypertension, symptomatic cardiovascular disease, use within 14 days of MAOIs.

INTERACTIONS

Drug

Antihypertensives: May decrease efficacy of antihypertensives.
Antipsychotics: Efficacy of antipsychotics may be decreased.
β-Blockers: May increase the risk of bradycardia, heart block, and hypertension.
Digoxin: May increase the risk of arrhythmias.
MAOIs, linezolid: May prolong and intensify the effects of dextroamphetamine, including severe hypertensive episodes.
Meperidine: May increase the risk of hypotension, respiratory depression, seizures, and vascular collapse.
Other CNS stimulants: May increase the effects of dextroamphetamine.
SSRIs: May increase risk of serotonin syndrome.
Thyroid hormones: May increase the effects of either drug.
Tricyclic antidepressants: May increase cardiovascular effects.

Herbal

None known.

Food

None known.

DIAGNOSTIC TEST EFFECTS

May increase plasma corticosteroid concentrations.

SIDE EFFECTS

Frequent

Irregular pulse, increased motor activity, talkativeness, nervousness, mild euphoria, insomnia.

Occasional

Headache, chills, dry mouth, GI distress, worsening depression in patients who are clinically depressed, tachycardia, palpitations, chest pain, dizziness, decreased appetite.

SERIOUS REACTIONS

- CNS stimulant use associated with serious cardiovascular events and sudden death in patients with cardiac abnormalities or serious heart problems.
- Overdose may produce skin pallor or flushing, arrhythmias, and psychosis.
- Abrupt withdrawal after prolonged use of high doses may produce lethargy lasting for weeks.
- Prolonged administration to children with ADHD may inhibit growth.

PRECAUTIONS & CONSIDERATIONS

Caution is warranted in debilitated and elderly patients; in those with hypertension, psychiatric disorders, seizure disorder, and Tourette syndrome; and in those who are tartrazine sensitive. Safety and efficacy have not been established in children. Distributed in breast milk; breastfeeding should be avoided. Mental status, BP, and weight should be assessed. Tasks that require mental alertness or motor skills should be avoided until response to the drug has been established. Notify the physician if decreased appetite, dizziness, dry mouth, or pronounced nervousness occurs.

Administration

Take the last dose of the day several hours before bedtime to prevent insomnia. Tolerance to the drug's appetite-suppressant and mood-elevating effects usually occurs within a few weeks. Dexedrine Spansule is not for initial therapy; patients should be established on regular-release formulations first. Spansule is usually administered once daily.

Dextromethorphan

dex-troe-meth-or′fan

★ Buckley's DM Cough, Buckley's Mixture Suspension, Delsym 12-Hour, Robitussin Honey/Cough, Robitussin Maximum Strength, Silphen-DM, Vicks Formula 44

CATEGORY AND SCHEDULE

Pregnancy Risk Category: C
OTC

Classification: Antitussive, nonnarcotic

MECHANISM OF ACTION

A chemical relative of morphine without the narcotic properties that acts on the cough center in the medulla oblongata by elevating the threshold for coughing. *Therapeutic Effect:* Suppresses cough.

PHARMACOKINETICS

Rapidly absorbed from the GI tract. Distributed into cerebrospinal fluid (CSF). Extensively and poorly metabolized in liver to dextrorphan (active metabolite). Excreted unchanged in urine. *Half-life:* 1.4-3.9 h (parent compound), 3.4-5.6 h (dextrorphan). Onset of action: 15-30 min.

AVAILABILITY

Suspension (Extended Release): 30 mg/5 mL (Delsym).
Syrup: 10 mg/5 mL (Robitussin Honey Cough, Silphen-DM), 12.5 mg/5 mL (Buckley's DM), 15 mg/5 mL (Robitussin Maximum Strength Cough), 30 mg/15 mL (Vicks Formula 44).

INDICATIONS AND DOSAGES

▸ **Cough**

PO

Adults, Elderly, Children 12 yr and older. 10-20 mg q4h or 30 mg q6-8h or extended release 60 mg twice a day. Maximum: 120 mg/day.
Children 6-12 yr. 5-10 mg q4h or 15 mg q6-8h or extended release 30 mg twice a day. Maximum: 60 mg/day.
Children 4-5 yr. 2.5-7.5 mg q4-8h or extended release 15 mg twice a day. Maximum: 30 mg/day.

CONTRAINDICATIONS

Coadministration with monoamine oxidase inhibitors (MAOIs), hypersensitivity to dextromethorphan or its components.

INTERACTIONS

Drug

Other cough/cold products: Read ingredients carefully to avoid duplication and potential overdose.
MAOIs, phenelzine, SSRIs, sibutramine: May increase the risk of serotonin syndrome. MAOIs are contraindicated.
Haloperidol, quinidine, CYP2D6 inhibitors: May increase adverse effects associated with dextromethorphan.

Herbal
None known.
Food
None known.

DIAGNOSTIC TEST EFFECTS
None known.

SIDE EFFECTS
Rare
Abdominal discomfort, constipation, dizziness, drowsiness, GI upset, nausea.

SERIOUS REACTIONS
• Overdosage may result in muscle spasticity, increase or decrease in BP, blurred vision, blue fingernails and lips, nausea, vomiting, hallucinations, and respiratory depression.

PRECAUTIONS & CONSIDERATIONS
Dextromethorphan has become a drug of abuse. Be aware that dextromethorphan should not be used for chronic and persistent cough accompanying a disease state or cough associated with excessive secretions. It is unknown whether dextromethorphan crosses the placenta or is distributed in breast milk. Be aware that dextromethorphan is not recommended for use in children younger than 4 yr of age. No age-related precautions have been noted in elderly patients. If fever, rash, headache, or sore throat persists, notify the physician.
Storage
Store syrup, suspension, liquid at room temperature.
Administration
Give dextromethorphan without regard to meals.
Shake oral suspension well before use.

Diazepam
dye-az′e-pam
Diastat, Diazepam Intensol, Valium
Apo-Diazepam, Diazemuls, Diastat, Vivol, Valium
Do not confuse diazepam with diazoxide or Ditropan, or Valium with Valcyte.

CATEGORY AND SCHEDULE
Pregnancy Risk Category: D
Controlled Substance Schedule: IV

Classification: Anxiolytics, benzodiazepines, relaxants, skeletal muscle

MECHANISM OF ACTION
A benzodiazepine that depresses all levels of the central nervous system (CNS) by enhancing the action of γ-aminobutyric acid, a major inhibitory neurotransmitter in the brain. *Therapeutic Effect:* Produces anxiolytic effect, elevates the seizure threshold, produces skeletal muscle relaxation.

PHARMACOKINETICS

Route	Onset	Peak	Duration
PO	30 min	1-2 h	2-3 h
IV	1-5 min	15 min	15-60 min
IM	15 min	30-90 min	30-90 min

Well absorbed from the GI tract. Widely distributed. Protein binding: 98%. Metabolized in the liver to active metabolite. Excreted in urine. Minimally removed by hemodialysis. *Half-life:* 20-70 h (increased in patients with hepatic dysfunction and in elderly patients).

AVAILABILITY
Oral Concentrate (Diazepam Intensol): 5 mg/mL.
Oral Solution: 5 mg/5 mL.

Tablets: 2 mg, 5 mg, 10 mg.
Injection: 5 mg/mL.
Rectal Gel (Diastat): 2.5 mg, 5 mg, 20 mg; or Accudial delivery system, 10 mg, 20 mg.

D

INDICATIONS AND DOSAGES

▸ **Anxiety, skeletal muscle relaxation**
PO
Adults. 2-10 mg 2-4 times a day.
Elderly. 2.5 mg twice a day.
Children. 0.12-0.8 mg/kg/day in divided doses q6-8h.
IV, IM
Adults. 2-10 mg repeated in 3-4 h.
Children. 0.04-0.3 mg/kg/dose q2-4h. *Maximum:* 0.6 mg/kg in an 8-h period.

▸ **Preanesthesia**
IV
Adults, Elderly. 5-15 mg 5-10 min before procedure.
Children. 0.2-0.3 mg/kg. Maximum: 10 mg.

▸ **Alcohol withdrawal**
PO
Adults, Elderly. 10 mg 3-4 times during first 24 h, then reduced to 5-10 mg 3-4 times a day as needed.
IV, IM
Adults, Elderly. Initially, 10 mg, followed by 5-10 mg q3-4h as needed.

▸ **Status epilepticus**
IV
Adults, Elderly. 5-10 mg q10-15 min up to 30 mg/8 h.
Children 5 yr and older. 0.05-0.3 mg/kg/dose q15-30 min. Maximum: 10 mg/dose.
Children 1 mo to 5 yr. 0.05-0.3 mg/kg/dose q15-30 min. Maximum: 5 mg/dose.

▸ **Control of increased seizure activity in patients with refractory epilepsy who are on stable regimens of anticonvulsants**
RECTAL GEL
Adults, Elderly, Children 12 yr and older. 0.2 mg/kg; may be repeated in 4-12 h. Round dose up to nearest dosage form for adults and down for elderly.
Children 6-11 yr. 0.3 mg/kg; may be repeated in 4-12 h.
Children 2-5 yr. 0.5 mg/kg; may be repeated in 4-12 h.

▸ **Dose in hepatic dysfunction (cirrhosis)**
Consider reduced dosage, but no specific recommendations are available.

OFF-LABEL USES

Treatment of panic disorder, tremors, benzodiazepine withdrawal, insomnia.

CONTRAINDICATIONS

Angle-closure glaucoma, coma, children younger than 6 mo, pregnancy.

INTERACTIONS

Drug
Alcohol, other CNS depressants: May increase CNS depression.
CYP2C19, CYP3A4 inhibitors: May increase levels/effects of diazepam.
CYP2C19, CYP3A4 inducers: May decrease levels/effects of diazepam.
Herbal
Kava kava, valerian: May increase CNS depression.
Food
Grapefruit juice: May increase sedative effect by increasing diazepam levels.

DIAGNOSTIC TEST EFFECTS

May elevate serum LDH, alkaline phosphatase, bilirubin, AST (SGOT), and ALT (SGPT) levels. May produce abnormal renal function test results. Therapeutic serum drug level is 0.5-2 mcg/mL; toxic serum drug level is > 3 mcg/mL.

IV INCOMPATIBILITIES

Acyclovir (Zovirax), alfentanil (Alfenta), amikacin (Amikar), aminophylline, amphotericin B cholesteryl (Amphotec), amphotericin B liposomal (AmBisome), ampicillin, ampicillin/sulbactam (Unasyn), ascorbic acid, atracurium (Tracrium), atropine, azathioprine, aztreonam (Azactam), benztropine (Cogentin), bivalirudin (Angiomax), bretylium, bumetanide (Bumex), buprenorphine (Buprenex), butorphanol (Stadol), calcium chloride, calcium gluconate, carboplatin, caspofungin (Cancidas), cefazolin, cefepime (Maxipime), cefotaxime (Claforan), cefotetan (Cefotan), cefoxitin (Mefoxin), ceftazidime (Ceptaz, Fortaz, Tazicef, Tazidime), ceftizoxime (Cefizox), ceftriaxone (Rocephin), cefuroxime (Zinacef), chloramphenicol, chlorpromazine, cimetidine (Tagamet), cisplatin, clindamycin (Cleocin), cyanocobalamin, cyclophosphamide (Cytoxan), cyclosporine (Sandimmune), dactinomycin (Cosmegen), dantrolene, dexamethasone sodium phosphate, dexmedetomidine (Precedex), digoxin (Lanoxin), diltiazem (Cardizem), diphenhydramine (Benadryl), dopamine (Intropin), doripenem (Doribax), doxorubicin (Adriamycin), enalaprilat, ephedrine, epinephrine, epirubicin (Ellence), epoetin alfa (Procrit), ertapenem (Invanz), erythromycin lactobionate, esmolol (Brevibloc), etoposide phosphate (Etopophos), famotidine (Pepcid), fenoldopam (Corlopam), fluconazole (Diflucan), fludarabine (Fludara), fluorouracil, folic acid, foscarnet (Foscavir), furosemide (Lasix), ganciclovir, gemcitabine (Gemzar), gentamicin, granisetron (Kytril), haloperidol (Haldol), heparin, hetastarch, hydralazine, hydrocortisone sodium succinate (Solu-Cortef), hydroxyzine, imipenem/cilastatin (Primaxin), insulin (regular, Humulin R, Novolin R), isoproterenol (Isuprel), ketorolac, labetalol, lactated Ringer's, lansoprazole (Prevacid), levofloxacin (Levaquin), lidocaine, linezolid (Zyvox), magnesium sulfate, mannitol, meperidine (Demerol), meropenem (Merrem IV), methicillin, methotrexate, methylprednisolone sodium succinate, metoclopramide (Reglan), metoprolol (Lopressor), metronidazole (Flagyl), midazolam (Versed), milrinone (Primacor), minocycline (Minocin), mitoxantrone (Novantrone), multiple vitamins injection, nalbuphine (Nubain), naloxone (Narcan), nitroglycerin, nitroprusside sodium (Nitropress), norepinephrine (Levophed), oxacillin, oxaliplatin (Eloxatin), oxytocin (Pitocin), paclitaxel (Taxol), palonosetron (Aloxi), pancuronium, pemetrexed (Alimta), pencillin G potassium, penicillin G sodium, pentobarbital, phenobarbital, phenytoin, piperacillin, potassium chloride, procainamide, prochloperazine, promethazine propofol (Diprivan), propranolol, quinupristin/dalfopristin (Synercid), ranitidine (Zantac), rocuronium (Zemuron), sodium acetate, sodium bicarbonate, streptokinase, succinylcholine, sulfamethoxazole/trimethoprim, tacrolimus (Prograf), theophylline, ticarcillin (Ticar), ticarcillin/clavulanate (Timentin), tigecycline (Tygacil), tirofibran (Aggrastat), tobramycin, vancomycin, vasopressin, vecuronium (Norcuron), verapamil, vincristine (Vincasar), vinorelbine (Navelbine), vitamin B complex with C, voriconazole (Vfend).

D

IV COMPATIBILITIES

Daptomycin (Cubicin), docetaxel (Taxotere), methadone, piperacillin/tazobactam (Zosyn), teniposide (Vumon).

SIDE EFFECTS

Frequent
Pain with IM injection, somnolence, fatigue, ataxia.
Occasional
Slurred speech, confusion, depression, orthostatic hypotension, headache, hypoactivity, constipation, nausea, blurred vision.
Rare
Paradoxical CNS reactions, such as hyperactivity or nervousness in children and excitement or restlessness in elderly or debilitated patients (generally noted during first 2 wks of therapy, particularly in presence of uncontrolled pain).

SERIOUS REACTIONS

- IV administration may produce pain, swelling, thrombophlebitis, and carpal tunnel syndrome.
- Abrupt or too-rapid withdrawal may result in pronounced restlessness, irritability, insomnia, hand tremor, abdominal or muscle cramps, diaphoresis, vomiting, and seizures.
- Anterograde amnesia may occur.
- Abrupt withdrawal in patients with epilepsy may produce an increase in the frequency or severity of seizures.
- Overdose results in somnolence, confusion, diminished reflexes, and coma.

PRECAUTIONS & CONSIDERATIONS

Caution is warranted in patients with hypoalbuminemia, hepatic and renal impairment, impaired gag reflex, respiratory depression, uncontrolled pain, history of drug abuse, depression, and in those who are taking other CNS depressants. Diazepam crosses the placenta and is distributed in breast milk. Diazepam may increase the risk of fetal abnormalities if administered during the first trimester of pregnancy. Chronic diazepam use during pregnancy may produce withdrawal symptoms in the patient and CNS depression in the neonate. For children and elderly patients, expect to administer a reduced dose initially and to increase dosage gradually to prevent ataxia and excessive sedation. Females should use effective contraception during therapy and notify the physician immediately if they become or suspect they are pregnant.

Drowsiness and dizziness may occur. Change positions slowly from recumbent to sitting before standing to prevent dizziness. Alcohol, caffeine, and tasks that require mental alertness or motor skills should also be avoided. Autonomic responses, such as cold, clammy hands and diaphoresis, and motor responses, such as agitation, trembling, and tension, should be assessed. Seizure frequency and intensity should be assessed. BP, pulse rate, and respiratory rate, rhythm, and depth should be obtained immediately before giving diazepam. The duration, location, onset, and type of pain should be recorded, and immobility, stiffness, and swelling should be assessed in those being treated for musculoskeletal spasm.

Storage

Store unopened vials at room temperature.

Administration

Take oral diazepam without regard to food. Crush tablets as needed, but do not crush or break capsules. Dilute the oral concentrate with juice, water, or a carbonated beverage or mix it with a semisolid food, such as applesauce or pudding.

For IV use, administer IV push into the tubing of a free-flowing IV solution as close to the vein insertion point as possible. Be aware of solution incompatibilities, which are many. Administer directly into a large vein to reduce the risk of phlebitis and thrombosis. Do not use small veins, such as those of the wrist or dorsum of the hand. Administer IV at a rate not exceeding 5 mg/min (adults). For children, give over a 3-min period because a too-rapid IV may result in hypotension and respiratory depression. Monitor respirations every 5-15 min for 2 h. Stay recumbent for up to 3 h after parenteral administration to reduce the drug's hypotensive effect.

For IM use, inject the IM dose deep into the deltoid muscle. IM injection may be painful.

! For rectal use, do not administer the rectal gel more often than once every 5 days or 5 times a month. See specialized instructions for use. If using the Accudial dose form, a pharmacist must dial in the dose and lock the rectal syringe prior to dispensing. It is ready when the "Green Ready Band" is clearly visible.

D

Diclofenac

dye-kloe′fen-ak

Cataflam, Flector, Solaraze, Voltaren Emulgel, Voltaren Ophthalmic, Voltaren Rapid, Zipsor

Novo-Difenac, Voltaren

Do not confuse diclofenac with Diflucan or Duphalac, or Voltaren with Verelan.

CATEGORY AND SCHEDULE

Pregnancy Risk Category: B (topical), C (oral, transdermal; D if used in third trimester or near delivery), C (ophthalmic solution)

Classification: Analgesics, nonnarcotic, nonsteroidal anti-inflammatory drugs, ophthalmics

MECHANISM OF ACTION

An NSAID that inhibits prostaglandin synthesis, reducing the intensity of pain. Also constricts the iris sphincter. May inhibit angiogenesis (the formation of blood vessels) by inhibiting substance P or blocking the angiogenic effects of prostaglandin E. *Therapeutic Effect:* Produces analgesic and anti-inflammatory effects. Prevents miosis during cataract surgery. May reduce angiogenesis in inflamed tissue.

PHARMACOKINETICS

Route	Onset	Peak	Duration
PO	30 min	2-3 h	Up to 8 h

Completely absorbed from the GI tract; penetrates cornea after ophthalmic administration (may

D

be systemically absorbed). Topical absorption 6%-10%. Protein binding: > 99%. Widely distributed. Metabolized in the liver. Primarily excreted in urine. Minimally removed by hemodialysis. *Half-life:* 1.2-2 h, patch 12 h. Diclofenac potassium more rapid onset than diclofenac sodium.

AVAILABILITY

Topical Gel (Solaraze): 3%.
Topical Gel (Voltaren): 1%.
Topical Patch (Flector): 1.3%.
Tablets (Cataflam): 50 mg.
Tablets (Enteric-Coated, Delayed-Release Diclofenac Sodium): 25 mg, 50 mg, 75 mg.
Tablets (Extended Release [Voltaren XR]): 100 mg.
Ophthalmic Solution (Voltaren Ophthalmic): 0.1%.
Capsules (Liquid-Filled, Zipsor): 25 mg.

INDICATIONS AND DOSAGES

▸ **Osteoarthritis**

PO (CATAFLAM, DICLOFENAC DELAYED RELEASE)
Adults, Elderly. 50 mg 2-3 times a day or delayed release 75 mg twice a day.
PO (VOLTAREN XR)
Adults, Elderly. 100 mg/day as a single dose.
TOPICAL GEL (VOLTAREN GEL)
Adults. Apply 4 g to knee, ankle, foot 4 times a day (maximum 16 g/joint daily). Apply 2 g to elbow, hand, wrist 4 times a day (maximum 8 g/joint a day). Maximum 32 g/day total for all joints.

▸ **Rheumatoid arthritis**

PO (CATAFLAM, DICLOFENAC DELAYED RELEASE)
Adults, Elderly. 50 mg 2-4 times a day or delayed release 75 mg twice a day. Maximum: 225 mg/day.
PO (VOLTAREN XR)
Adults, Elderly. 100 mg once a day. Maximum: 100 mg twice a day.

▸ **Ankylosing spondylitis**

PO (DICLOFENAC DELAYED RELEASE)
Adults, Elderly. 100-125 mg/day in 4-5 divided doses.

▸ **Analgesia, primary dysmenorrhea**

PO (CATAFLAM)
Adults, Elderly. 50 mg 3 times a day.

▸ **Usual pediatric dosage**

PO
Children. 2-3 mg/kg/day in 2-4 divided doses.

▸ **Actinic keratoses**

TOPICAL GEL (SOLARAZE)
Adults, Adolescents. Apply twice a day to lesion for 60-90 days.

▸ **Cataract surgery**

OPHTHALMIC
Adults, Elderly. Apply 1 drop to eye 4 times a day commencing 24 h after cataract surgery. Continue for 2 wks afterward.

▸ **Pain, relief of photophobia in patients undergoing corneal refractive surgery**

OPHTHALMIC
Adults, Elderly. Apply 1 drop to affected eye 1 h before surgery, within 15 min after surgery, then 4 times a day for 3 days.

▸ **Acute pain from sprains, contusions**

TOPICAL PATCH
Adults. Apply patch twice a day to the affected area.

OFF-LABEL USES

Treatment of vascular headaches (oral).

CONTRAINDICATIONS

Hypersensitivity to aspirin, diclofenac, and other NSAIDs; perioperative use with CABG.

INTERACTIONS

Drug

Acetylcholine, carbachol: May decrease the effects of these drugs (with ophthalmic diclofenac).

Antihypertensives, diuretics: May decrease the effects of these drugs.

Aspirin, other salicylates: May increase the risk of GI side effects such as bleeding. NSAID use may negate cardioprotective effect.

Bone marrow depressants: May increase the risk of hematologic reactions.

Cyclosporine: Diclofenac may increase risk for nephrotoxicity.

Epinephrine, other antiglaucoma medications: May decrease the antiglaucoma effect of these drugs.

Heparin, oral anticoagulants, thrombolytics: May increase the effects of these drugs.

Lithium: May increase the blood concentration and risk of toxicity of lithium.

Methotrexate: May increase the risk of methotrexate toxicity.

Probenecid: May increase diclofenac blood concentration.

Herbal

Supplements with antiplatelet or anticoagulant effects (e.g., feverfew, garlic, ginger, ginkgo biloba, ginseng, red clover, sweet clover, white willow): May increase effects on platelets or risk of bleeding.

Food

Alcohol: May increase dizziness; may increase risk of G1 bleeding.

DIAGNOSTIC TEST EFFECTS

May increase BUN level; urine protein level; and serum LDH, potassium, alkaline phosphatase, creatinine, AST (SGOT), and ALT (SGPT) levels. May decrease serum uric acid level.

SIDE EFFECTS

Frequent (4%-9%)

PO: Headache, abdominal cramps, constipation, diarrhea, nausea, dyspepsia.

Ophthalmic (6%-30%): Lacrimation, keratitis, increased intraocular pressure, burning or stinging on instillation, ocular discomfort.

Topical: Pruritus, rash, dry skin, pain, numbness.

Occasional (1%-3%)

PO: Flatulence, dizziness, epigastric pain.

Ophthalmic (5%-10%): Ocular itching or tearing, corneal changes, blurred/ abnormal vision, eyelid swelling.

Rare (< 1%)

PO: Rash, peripheral edema or fluid retention, visual disturbances, vomiting, drowsiness.

SERIOUS REACTIONS

- Overdose may result in acute renal failure.
- Rare reactions with long-term use include peptic ulcer disease, GI bleeding, gastritis, a severe hepatic reaction (jaundice), nephrotoxicity (hematuria, dysuria, proteinuria), and a severe hypersensitivity reaction (bronchospasm or angioedema) or serious skin reactions, such as Stevens-Johnson syndrome.

PRECAUTIONS & CONSIDERATIONS

Caution is warranted with hepatic or renal impairment, a predisposition to fluid retention, and history of GI tract disease such as active peptic ulcer disease, chronic inflammation of GI tract, GI bleeding or ulceration. Use the lowest effective dose for the shortest time. Anaphylactoid reactions have occurred in patients with aspirin triad hypersensitivity. Do not use in patients with aspirin-sensitive asthma. Cardiovascular event risk may be increased with duration of use or preexisting cardiovascular risk factors or disease. Use caution with fluid retention, heart failure, or hypertension. Use the lowest effective dose for the shortest time. Risk of myocardial infarction and stroke may be increased following coronary artery bypass graft surgery. Do not administer within 4-6 half-lives before surgical procedures. Diclofenac crosses the placenta; it is unknown whether the drug is distributed in breast milk. Notify the physician of pregnancy. Diclofenac should not be used during the last trimester of pregnancy because it may cause adverse effects in the fetus, such as premature closure of the ductus arteriosus. The safety and efficacy of diclofenac have not been established in children. In elderly patients, GI bleeding or ulceration is more likely to cause serious complications, and age-related renal impairment may necessitate dose reduction.

Notify the physician of persistent headache, black stools, changes in vision, pruritus, rash, or weight gain. Pattern of daily bowel activity and stool consistency should be assessed. Therapeutic response, such as decreased pain, stiffness, swelling, tenderness, improved grip strength, and increased joint mobility, should be evaluated.

Storage

Store at controlled room temperature. Protect gels from heat and avoid freezing. Keep patches in sealed pouch until time of use.

Administration

Do not crush or break enteric-coated tablets. Take diclofenac with food, milk, or antacids if GI distress occurs.

For ophthalmic use, place a finger on the lower eyelid and pull it out until a pocket is formed between the eye and lower lid. Hold the dropper above the pocket, and place the prescribed number of drops in the pocket. Gently close the eye, and apply digital pressure to the lacrimal sac for 1-2 min to minimize drainage into the nose and throat, reducing the risk of systemic effects. Remove excess with a tissue. Do not use Hydrogel soft contact lenses during ophthalmic therapy.

Topical gels: Follow prescribed use. For external use only; avoid eyes and mucous membranes. Voltaren gel has dose card to measure dosage. Wash hands after application.

Topical patch: Remove liner before adhering to normal intact skin. Patch should be applied to affected area. Apply only 1 patch at a time.

Dicloxacillin

dye-klox′a-sill-in

Do not confuse dicloxacillin with dicyclomine.

CATEGORY AND SCHEDULE

Pregnancy Risk Category: B

Classification: Antibiotics, antistaphylococcal penicillins, penicillinase-resistant penicillins

MECHANISM OF ACTION

A penicillin that acts as a bactericidal in susceptible microorganisms. *Therapeutic Effect:* Inhibits bacterial cell wall synthesis.

PHARMACOKINETICS

Absorption 35%-76% from the GI tract. Rate and extent reduced by food. Distributed throughout body, including CSF (low). Protein binding: 96%. Partially metabolized in liver. Primarily excreted in feces and urine. Not removed by hemodialysis. *Half-life:* 0.7 h.

AVAILABILITY
Capsules: 250 mg, 500 mg.

INDICATIONS AND DOSAGES
▸ **Infections due to susceptible penicillinase-producing staphylococci**

PO

Adults, Elderly, Children weighing 40 kg. 125-250 mg q6h.

Children weighing < 40 kg. 25-50 mg/kg/day divided q6h.

CONTRAINDICATIONS
Hypersensitivity to any penicillin.

INTERACTIONS
Drug

Oral contraceptives: May decrease the effects of oral contraceptives.

Probenecid: May increase blood concentration and risk for dicloxacillin toxicity.

Warfarin: May decrease effects of warfarin.

DIAGNOSTIC TEST EFFECTS
May cause positive Coombs' test.

SIDE EFFECTS
Frequent

GI disturbances (mild diarrhea, nausea, or vomiting), headache.

Occasional

Generalized rash, urticaria.

SERIOUS REACTIONS
- Altered bacterial balance may result in potentially fatal superinfections and antibiotic-associated colitis as evidenced by abdominal cramps, watery or severe diarrhea, and fever.
- Severe hypersensitivity reactions, including anaphylaxis and acute interstitial nephritis, occur rarely. Immediate reactions occur within 20 min to 48 h and include anaphylaxis, pruritus, urticaria, hypotension, laryngospasm. Delayed allergic reactions occur after 48 h and include serum sickness-like symptoms.
- Neurotoxic reactions may occur with large intravenous doses, especially in patients with renal dysfunction.

PRECAUTIONS & CONSIDERATIONS
Be aware that dicloxacillin crosses the placenta and is distributed in breast milk in low concentrations. Be aware that dicloxacillin use should be avoided in neonates due to immature elimination processes. No age-related precautions have been noted for elderly patients. History of allergies, especially to cephalosporins or penicillins, should be determined before giving the drug. If diarrhea, rash, or symptoms occur during treatment, notify the physician.

Storage

Store at room temperature.

Administration

Best to take on empty stomach 1 h before or 2 h after meals. Continue dicloxacillin for the full length of treatment.

Dicyclomine
dye-sye′kloe-meen

★ Bentyl

🍁 Bentylol, Formulex, Protylol

Do not confuse dicyclomine with doxycycline or dyclomine, or Bentyl with Aventyl or Benadryl.

CATEGORY AND SCHEDULE
Pregnancy Risk Category: B

Classification: Anticholinergics, gastrointestinals

D

MECHANISM OF ACTION
A GI antispasmodic and anticholinergic agent that directly acts as a relaxant on smooth muscle. *Therapeutic Effect:* Reduces tone and motility of GI tract.

PHARMACOKINETICS

Route	Onset	Peak	Duration
PO	1-2 h	N/A	4 h

Readily absorbed from the GI tract. Widely distributed. Metabolized in the liver. *Half-life:* 9-10 h.

AVAILABILITY
Capsules: 10 mg.
Tablets: 20 mg.
Syrup, Solution: 10 mg/5 mL.
Injection: 10 mg/mL.

INDICATIONS AND DOSAGES
▸ Functional disturbances of GI motility
PO
Adults. 20 mg 4 times a day, then increase up to 40 mg 4 times/day.
Children older than 2 yr. 10 mg 3-4 times a day.
Children 6 mo to 2 yr. 5 mg 3-4 times a day.
Elderly. 10-20 mg 4 times a day. May increase up to 40 mg 4 times/day.
IM
Adults. 20 mg 4 times a day for 1-2 days, switch to PO as soon as possible.

CONTRAINDICATIONS
Bladder neck obstruction, myasthenia gravis in patients not treated with neostigmine, narrow-angle glaucoma, obstructive disease of the GI tract, paralytic ileus, severe ulcerative colitis, tachycardia, unstable cardiovascular status in acute hemorrhage, reflux esophagitis, breastfeeding, infants < 6 mo.

INTERACTIONS
Drug
Antacids: May decrease the absorption of dicyclomine.
Antidiarrheals: Additive effects and may increase risk for toxic megacolon.
Digoxin: May increase absorption of digoxin.
Ketoconazole: May decrease the absorption of ketoconazole.
Other anticholinergics: May increase the effects of dicyclomine.
Potassium chloride: May increase the severity of GI lesions with the wax matrix formulation of potassium chloride.
Herbal
None known.
Food
None known.

DIAGNOSTIC TEST EFFECTS
None known.

SIDE EFFECTS
Frequent
Dry mouth (sometimes severe), dizziness, constipation, blurred vision, nausea, diminished sweating ability.
Occasional
Photophobia; urinary hesitancy; somnolence (with high dosage); agitation, excitement, confusion, or somnolence noted in elderly patients (even with low dosages); transient light-headedness (with IM route), irritation at injection site (with IM route).
Rare
Confusion, hypersensitivity reaction, increased intraocular pressure, vomiting, unusual fatigue.

SERIOUS REACTIONS
• Overdose may produce temporary paralysis of ciliary muscle; pupillary dilation; tachycardia; palpitations;

hot, dry, or flushed skin; absence of bowel sounds; hyperthermia; increased respiratory rate; ECG abnormalities; nausea; vomiting; rash over face or upper trunk; central nervous system (CNS) stimulation.

• Psychosis (marked by agitation, restlessness, rambling speech, visual hallucinations, paranoid behavior, and delusions, followed by depression).

PRECAUTIONS & CONSIDERATIONS

Extreme caution should be used with autonomic neuropathy, diarrhea, known or suspected GI infections, and mild to moderate ulcerative colitis. Caution is also warranted with congestive heart failure, chronic obstructive pulmonary disease, coronary artery disease, or hiatal hernia associated with reflux esophagitis, gastric ulcer, hyperthyroidism, hypertension, hepatic or renal disease, tachyarrhythmias, prostatic hypertrophy, and in elderly patients. It is unknown whether dicyclomine crosses the placenta. Dicyclomine is excreted in breast milk and is contraindicated during lactation. Infants and young children are more susceptible to the drug's toxic effects. Dicyclomine use in elderly patients may cause agitation, confusion, somnolence, or excitement. Avoid hot baths, saunas, and becoming overheated while exercising in hot weather because this may cause heatstroke. Tasks that require mental alertness or motor skills should also be avoided until response to the drug has been established. Antacids or antidiarrheals should not be taken within 1 h of taking dicyclomine because they will decrease dicyclomine's effectiveness.

BP, body temperature, pattern of daily bowel activity and stool consistency, and hydration status should be monitored. The patient should void before taking the drug to reduce the risk of urine retention.

Storage

Store capsules, tablets, syrup, and parenteral form at room temperature. Do not freeze.

Administration

Dicyclomine may be given without regard to meals.

The injection normally appears colorless. Do not administer IV or subcutaneously. Inject IM deep into large muscle mass. Do not give for longer than 2 days, as prescribed.

Didanosine (ddI)

dye-dan'o-seen

★ Videx, Videx-EC 🍁 Videx-EC

CATEGORY AND SCHEDULE

Pregnancy Risk Category: B

Classification: Antiretrovirals, nucleoside reverse transcriptase inhibitors

MECHANISM OF ACTION

A purine nucleoside analogue that is intracellularly converted into a triphosphate, which interferes with RNA-directed DNA polymerase (reverse transcriptase). *Therapeutic Effect:* Inhibits replication of retroviruses, including HIV.

PHARMACOKINETICS

Variably absorbed from the GI tract. Protein binding: < 5%. Rapidly metabolized intracellularly to active form. Primarily excreted in urine. Partially (20%) removed by hemodialysis. *Half-life:* 1.5 h; metabolite: 8-24 h.

D

AVAILABILITY

Capsules (Delayed Release): 125 mg, 200 mg, 250 mg, 400 mg.
Pediatric Powder for Oral Solution: 10 mg/mL.

INDICATIONS AND DOSAGES

▸ **HIV infection (in combination with other antiretrovirals)**
PO
DELAYED-RELEASE CAPSULES
Adults, Children 13 yr and older, weighing 60 kg or more. 400 mg once a day.
Adults, Children 13 yr and older, weighing < 60 kg. 250 mg once a day.
PEDIATRIC POWDER FOR ORAL SOLUTION
Adults, Children 13 yr and older weighing 60 kg or more. 250 mg q12h.
Adults, Children 13 yr and older weighing < 60 kg. 167 mg q12h.
Children 2 wks to 8 mo. 100 mg/m^2 twice daily.
Children > 8 mo. 120 mg/m^2 twice daily.

▸ **Dosage in renal impairment**
For adults or adolescents weighing 60 kg or more.

CrCl (mL/min)	Powder for Oral Solution	Delayed-Release Capsule
30-59	100 mg twice daily	200 mg daily
10-29	167 mg daily	125 mg daily
< 10	100 mg daily	125 mg daily

For adults or adolescents weighing < 60 kg:

CrCl (mL/min)	Powder for Oral Solution	Delayed-Release Capsule
30-59	100 mg twice daily	125 mg daily
10-29	100 mg daily	125 mg daily
< 10	100 mg daily	Do not use capsule

CONTRAINDICATIONS

Hypersensitivity to didanosine or any of its components. Use of allopurinol or ribavirin with didanosine is contraindicated.

INTERACTIONS

Drug
Allopurinol: May increase didanosine concentration. Contraindicated.
Atazanavir: Levels of both drugs may be decreased.
Dapsone, fluoroquinolones, itraconazole, ketoconazole, tetracyclines: May decrease absorption of these drugs.
Delavirdine, indinavir: Levels of these agents may be decreased. Administer 1 h before didanosine.
Medications producing pancreatitis or peripheral neuropathy: May increase the risk of pancreatitis or peripheral neuropathy.
Methadone: Decreased didanosine levels may occur.
Stavudine: May increase the risk of fatal lactic acidosis in pregnancy.
Tenofovir, ribavirin: Increased levels of didanosine and toxicity including pancreatitis, hyperglycemia, lactic acidosis, and peripheral neuropathy. Ribavirin is contraindicated.
Herbal
None known.
Food
All foods: Decreases absorption of didanosine.

DIAGNOSTIC TEST EFFECTS

May increase serum alkaline phosphatase, amylase, bilirubin, lipase, triglyceride, AST (SGOT), ALT (SGPT), and uric acid levels. May decrease serum potassium levels.

SIDE EFFECTS

Frequent

Adults (> 10%): Diarrhea, neuropathy, chills, and fever.

Children (> 25%): Chills, fever, decreased appetite, pain, malaise, nausea, vomiting, diarrhea, abdominal pain, headache, nervousness, cough, rhinitis, dyspnea, asthenia, rash, pruritus.

Occasional

Adults (2%-9%)

Rash, pruritus, headache, abdominal pain, nausea, vomiting, pneumonia, myopathy, decreased appetite, dry mouth, dyspnea.

Children (10%-25%)

Failure to thrive, weight loss, stomatitis, oral thrush, ecchymosis, arthritis, myalgia, insomnia, epistaxis, pharyngitis.

SERIOUS REACTIONS

- Pneumonia and opportunistic infections occur occasionally.
- Peripheral neuropathy, potentially fatal pancreatitis, lactic acidosis, severe hepatomegaly with steatosis, retinal changes, and optic neuritis are the major toxic effects.
- Myocardial infarction.

PRECAUTIONS & CONSIDERATIONS

Extreme caution should be used in patients with history of pancreatitis. Caution is warranted with alcoholism, elevated triglycerides, and renal or liver dysfunction, T-cell counts < 100 cells/mm^3, and phenylketonuria and sodium-restricted diets because didanosine contains phenylalanine and sodium. Myocardial infarction risk may be greatest in patients with recent use and those with existing risk factors for heart disease. Be aware that didanosine should be used during pregnancy only if clearly needed and that breastfeeding should be discontinued. Pregnancy increases risk for fatal lactic acidosis. Be aware that didanosine is well tolerated in children older than 3 mo. Elderly patients are at higher risk for pancreatitis. In elderly patients, age-related renal impairment may require dosage adjustment. Didanosine is not a cure for HIV infection, nor does it reduce risk of transmission to others. Avoid alcohol.

! Contact the physician if abdominal pain, elevated serum amylase or triglycerides, nausea, and vomiting occur, because these symptoms may indicate pancreatitis. Assess for signs and symptoms of peripheral neuropathy, including burning feet, "restless legs syndrome" (unable to find comfortable position for legs and feet), and lack of coordination, and for signs and symptoms of opportunistic infections, including cough or other respiratory symptoms, fever, or oral mucosa changes. Assess for nausea, abdominal pain, vomiting, and weight loss as well as visual or hearing difficulty. Expect to obtain baseline values for complete blood count (CBC), renal and liver function tests, vital signs, and weight.

Storage

Store at room temperature. Pediatric powder for oral solution, following reconstitution as directed, is stable for 30 days refrigerated.

Administration

Take oral didanosine 1 h before or 2 h after meals because food decreases the rate and extent of didanosine absorption.

Add 100 mL or 200 mL water to 2 or 4 g of the unbuffered pediatric powder, respectively, to provide a concentration of 20 mg/mL. Immediately mix with an equal amount of an antacid to provide a concentration of 10 mg/mL. Shake thoroughly before removing each dose. Recommended antacid: Maximum strength Mylanta. Keep in mind antacids decrease absorption of some medications and may need to separate administration times.

Swallow enteric-coated capsules whole; take them on an empty stomach.

Diethylpropion

die-ethyl-prop′ion

★ Radtue

CATEGORY AND SCHEDULE

Pregnancy Risk Category: B
Controlled Substance Schedule: IV

Classification: Anorexiants, stimulants, central nervous system

MECHANISM OF ACTION

A sympathomimetic amine that stimulates the release of norepinephrine and dopamine. *Therapeutic Effect:* Decreases appetite.

PHARMACOKINETICS

Rapidly absorbed from the GI tract. Widely distributed. Metabolized in liver to active metabolite and undergoes extensive first-pass metabolism. Excreted in urine. Unknown whether removed by hemodialysis. *Half-life:* 4-6 h.

AVAILABILITY

Tablets: 25 mg.
Tablets (Extended Release): 75 mg.

INDICATIONS AND DOSAGES

▸ **Obesity**

PO

Adults. 25 mg 3 times/day before meals *or* Extended Release: 75 mg at midmorning.

CONTRAINDICATIONS

Agitated states, use of MAOIs within 14 days, glaucoma, history of drug abuse, hyperthyroidism, advanced arteriosclerosis or severe cardiovascular disease, severe hypertension, pulmonary hypertension, glaucoma, history of drug abuse, other anorectic agents, and hypersensitivity to sympathomimetic amines. Do not use with sibutramine.

INTERACTIONS

Drug

Anorectic agents, sympathomimetics: May increase the risk of cardiac effects of diethylpropion.
Anesthetics: May increase the risk of arrhythmias.
Antidiabetic agents, insulin: May alter blood glucose concentrations.
Guanethidine: May decrease the effects of guanethidine.
MAOIs, linezolid: May increase the risk of hypertensive crisis. MAOI use is contraindicated.
Phenothiazines: May decrease the effects of diethylpropion.
Tricyclic antidepressants: May increase the cardiac and CNS effects of diethylpropion.

Sibutramine: Contraindicated due to risk of increased heart rate and BP.
Herbal
None known.
Food
None known.

DIAGNOSTIC TEST EFFECTS

(+) Urine screen for amphetamines.

SIDE EFFECTS

Frequent
Elevated blood pressure, nervousness, insomnia.
Occasional
Dizziness, drowsiness, tremor, headache, nausea, stomach pain, fever, rash.
Rare
Blurred vision.

SERIOUS REACTIONS

- Overdose may produce agitation, tachycardia, palpitations, cardiac irregularities, chest pain, psychotic episode, seizures, and coma.
- Hypersensitivity reactions, psychosis, cerebrovascular accident, seizures, and blood dyscrasias occur rarely.
- Primary pulmonary hypertension and valvular heart disease have been associated with anorexients.

PRECAUTIONS & CONSIDERATIONS

Caution is required in patients with diabetes, epilepsy, Tourette syndrome, hypertension, and cardiovascular disease. Diethylpropion crosses the placenta and is distributed in breast milk. No age-related precautions have been noted in elderly patients. Safety and efficacy have not been evaluated in pediatric patients. Alcohol should be avoided during therapy. Should not be used if other anorexients used within the past year.

Storage
Store at room temperature.
Administration
Generally, do not take in the afternoon or evening because the drug can cause insomnia. Do not crush or break sustained-release capsules. Take immediate-release tablets 1 h before meals. Expect to reassess weight loss after 4 wks to determine risk/benefit of continued use.

Diflorasone

die-flor'a-sone
★ Apexicon, Apexicon-E

CATEGORY AND SCHEDULE

Pregnancy Risk Category: C

Classification: Corticosteroids, topical; dermatologics, high-potency

MECHANISM OF ACTION

A high-potency, fluorinated corticosteroid that decreases inflammation by suppression of migration of polymorphonuclear leukocytes and reversal of increased capillary permeability. The exact mechanism of the anti-inflammatory process is unclear. *Therapeutic Effect:* Decreases or prevents tissue response to the inflammatory process.

PHARMACOKINETICS

Poor absorption; occlusive dressings increase absorption. Metabolized in liver. Primarily excreted in urine.

AVAILABILITY

Cream: 0.05%.
Ointment: 0.05%.

INDICATIONS AND DOSAGES

▸ **Corticosteroid-responsive dermatoses**

TOPICAL

Adults, Elderly. Cream: Apply sparingly 2-4 times/day. Ointment: Apply sparingly 1-3 times/day. Maximum: 50 grams/wk topically.

CONTRAINDICATIONS

History of hypersensitivity to diflorasone or other corticosteroids.

INTERACTIONS

Drug

None known.

Herbal

None known.

Food

None known.

DIAGNOSTIC TEST EFFECTS

None known.

SIDE EFFECTS

Rare

Itching, redness, dryness, irritation, burning at site of application, hypertrichosis, folliculitis, maceration, atrophy, secondary skin infection.

SERIOUS REACTIONS

- Overdosage symptoms include moon face, central obesity, hypertension, diabetes, hyperlipidemia, peptic ulcer, increased susceptibility to infection, electrolyte and fluid imbalance, psychosis, and hallucinations.
- The serious reactions of long-term therapy and the addition of occlusive dressings are reversible hypothalamic-pituitary-adrenal (HPA) axis suppression, manifestations of Cushing syndrome, hyperglycemia, and glucosuria.
- Kaposi sarcoma has been reported with prolonged treatment with corticosteroids.

PRECAUTIONS & CONSIDERATIONS

Caution should be used over large surface areas, with prolonged use, addition of occlusive dressings, and uncontrolled infections. Skin irritation should be reported. HPA axis suppression should be evaluated by ACTH stimulation test, AM plasma cortisol test, or urinary free cortisol test. It is unknown whether diflorasone diacetate crosses the placenta or is distributed in breast milk. Children may absorb larger amounts and may be more susceptible to toxicity. Safety and efficacy of diflorasone diacetate have not been established in children or in elderly patients.

Storage

Store at room temperature.

Administration

Diflorasone diacetate ointments are recommended for dry, scaly lesions; creams are recommended for moist lesions. Gently cleanse area before application. Use occlusive dressings only as directed. Apply a thin film over affected area and rub into area gently and thoroughly. Wash hands after application. In general, avoid face, groin, and axillae.

Diflunisal

dye-floo′ni-sal

★ Dolobid 🍁 Apo-Diflunisal

Do not confuse diflunisal with Dicarbosil, or Dolobid with Slo-Bid.

CATEGORY AND SCHEDULE

Pregnancy Risk Category: C (D if used in third trimester or near delivery)

Classification: Analgesics, anti-inflammatory agents, salicylates

MECHANISM OF ACTION
A nonsteroidal anti-inflammatory and difluorophenyl derivative of salicylic acid that inhibits prostaglandin synthesis, reducing inflammatory response and intensity of pain stimulus reaching sensory nerve endings. *Therapeutic Effect:* Produces analgesic and anti-inflammatory effect.

PHARMACOKINETICS

Route	Onset	Peak	Duration
PO	1 h	2-3 h	8-12 h

Completely absorbed from the GI tract. Widely distributed. Protein binding: > 99%. Metabolized in liver. Unlike other salicylates, not metabolized to salicylic acid. Primarily excreted in urine as metabolites. Not removed by hemodialysis. *Half-life:* 8-12 h.

AVAILABILITY
Tablets: 500 mg.

INDICATIONS AND DOSAGES
▸ **Mild to moderate pain**

PO

Adults, Elderly. Initially, 0.5-1 g, then 250-500 mg q8-12h. Maximum: 1.5 g/day.

▸ **Rheumatoid arthritis, osteoarthritis**

PO

Adults, Elderly. 0.5-1 g/day in 2 divided doses. Maximum: 1.5 g/day.

OFF-LABEL USES
Treatment of psoriatic arthritis, migraine, vascular headache.

CONTRAINDICATIONS
Active GI bleeding, hypersensitivity to aspirin or NSAIDs, perioperative use with coronary artery bypass graft.

INTERACTIONS
Drug

Antihypertensives, diuretics: May decrease the effects of these drugs.
Aspirin, antiplatelets, salicylates: May increase the risk of GI bleeding and side effects. NSAID may diminish cardioprotective effect of ASA.
Bisphosphonates, corticosteroids: Increased risk of GI ulceration.
Bone marrow depressants: May increase the risk of hematologic reactions.
Cyclosporine, pemetrexed: May increase levels and effects of cyclosporine, pemetrexed.
Heparin, oral anticoagulants, thrombolytics: May increase the effects of these drugs.
Lithium: May increase the blood concentration and risk of toxicity of lithium.
Methotrexate: May increase the risk of toxicity of methotrexate.
Probenecid: May increase diflunisal blood concentration.

Herbal

Supplements with antiplatelet or anticoagulant effects e.g., feverfew, garlic, ginger, ginkgo biloba, ginseng, red clover, sweet clover, white willow, etc.: May increase effects on platelets or risk of bleeding.

Food

Alcohol: May increase dizziness; may increase risk of GI bleeding.

DIAGNOSTIC TEST EFFECTS
May increase serum AST (SGOT) and ALT (SGPT) levels. May decrease serum uric acid levels.

SIDE EFFECTS
Side effects are less common with short-term treatment.

Occasional (0%-3%)

Nausea, dyspepsia (heartburn, indigestion, epigastric pain), diarrhea, headache, rash.

D

Rare (1%-3%)
Vomiting, constipation, flatulence, dizziness, somnolence, insomnia, fatigue, tinnitus.

SERIOUS REACTIONS

- Overdosage may produce drowsiness, vomiting, nausea, diarrhea, hyperventilation, tachycardia, diaphoresis, stupor, and coma.
- Peptic ulcer, GI bleeding, gastritis, and severe hepatic reaction, including cholestasis, jaundice occur rarely.
- Nephrotoxicity, including dysuria, hematuria, proteinuria, and nephrotic syndrome, and severe hypersensitivity reaction, marked by bronchospasm and angioedema, or serious skin rashes, like Stevens-Johnson syndrome, occur rarely.

PRECAUTIONS & CONSIDERATIONS

Caution is warranted with hepatic or renal impairment, a predisposition to fluid retention, and a history of GI tract disease such as active peptic ulcer disease, chronic inflammation of GI tract, GI bleeding or ulceration. Use the lowest effective dose for the shortest duration. Anaphylactoid reactions have occurred in patients with aspirin triad hypersensitivity. Do not use in patients with aspirin-sensitive asthma. Cardiovascular event risk may be increased with duration of use or preexisting cardiovascular risk factors or disease. Use caution with fluid retention, heart failure, or hypertension. Use the lowest effective dose for the shortest duration. Risk of myocardial infarction and stroke may be increased following coronary artery bypass graft surgery. Do not administer within 4-6 half-lives before surgical procedures.

Caution is also warranted in patients with factor VII or factor IX deficiencies, platelet and bleeding disorders, and vitamin K deficiency. Be aware that diflunisal crosses the placenta and is distributed in breast milk. Avoid diflunisal use during the last trimester of pregnancy, since the drug may adversely affect the fetal cardiovascular system, causing premature closure of the ductus arteriosus. Be aware that the safety and efficacy of this drug have not been established in children. Reye syndrome is possible with diflunisal. In elderly patients, GI bleeding or ulceration is more likely to cause serious adverse effects. In elderly patients, age-related renal impairment may require a lower dose.

Notify the physician if GI distress, headache, or rash occurs. Baseline laboratory tests, including PT, aPTT, renal and liver function studies, and CBC, should be obtained. Skin for rash, pattern of daily bowel activity and stool consistency, and therapeutic response should be assessed.

Storage
Store at room temperature.

Administration
Take diflunisal with meals, milk, or water. Do not crush or break film-coated tablets.

Digoxin

di-jox'in

Lanoxin Toloxin

Do not confuse digoxin with Desoxyn or doxepin, or Lanoxin with Levsinex or Lonox.

CATEGORY AND SCHEDULE

Pregnancy Risk Category: C

Classification: Antiarrhythmics, cardiac glycosides, inotropes

MECHANISM OF ACTION

A cardiac glycoside that increases the influx of calcium from extracellular to intracellular cytoplasm.

Therapeutic Effect: Potentiates the activity of the contractile cardiac muscle fibers and increases the force of myocardial contraction. Slows the heart rate by decreasing conduction through the SA and AV nodes.

PHARMACOKINETICS

Route	Onset	Peak	Duration
PO	0.5-2 h	2-8 h	3-4 days
IV	5-30 min	1-4 h	3-4 days

Readily absorbed from the GI tract. Widely distributed. Protein binding: 30%. Partially metabolized in the liver. Primarily excreted in urine. Minimally removed by hemodialysis. *Half-life (adults):* 36-48 h (increased with impaired renal function and in elderly patients).

AVAILABILITY

Elixir: 50 mcg/mL.
Tablets (Lanoxin): 125 mcg, 250 mcg.
Injection (Lanoxin): 250 mcg/mL, 100 mcg/mL.

INDICATIONS AND DOSAGES

▸ **Rapid loading dose for the management and treatment of CHF; control of ventricular rate in patients with atrial fibrillation; treatment and prevention of recurrent paroxysmal atrial tachycardia**

PO

Adults, Elderly. Initially, 0.5-0.75 mg, additional doses of 0.125-0.375 mg at 6- to 8-h intervals. Range: 0.75-1.25 mg.
Children older than 10 yr. 10-15 mcg/kg.
Children 5-10 yr. 20-35 mcg/kg.
Children 2-5 yr. 30-40 mcg/kg.
Children 1-24 mo. 35-60 mcg/kg.
Neonate, full-term. 25-35 mcg/kg.
Neonate, premature. 20-30 mcg/kg.
One-half of loading dose given initially, followed by equal portions of the remaining dose at 4- to 8-h intervals.

IV

Adults, Elderly. Initially, 0.25-0.5 mg, usually followed by additional doses of 0.125-0.25 mg at 6- to 8-h intervals for 2-3 doses, then switch to maintenance dosing.
Children older than 10 yr. 8-12 mcg/kg.
Children 5-10 yr. 15-30 mcg/kg.
Children 2-5 yr. 25-35 mcg/kg.
Children 1-24 mo. 30-50 mcg/kg.
Neonates, full-term. 20-30 mcg/kg.
Neonates, premature. 15-25 mcg/kg.
One-half of loading dose given initially, followed by equal portions of the remaining dose at 4- to 8-h intervals.

▸ **Maintenance dosage for CHF; control of ventricular rate in patients with atrial fibrillation; treatment and prevention of recurrent paroxysmal atrial tachycardia**

PO, IV

Adults, Elderly. 0.125-0.375 mg/day.
Children. If giving IV, dose is roughly 25%-35% loading dose (20%-30% for premature neonates) divided every 12 h in children < 10 yr.
General guidelines as follows for PO children's maintenance dose per day (Note: If child < 10 yr, usually divide daily dose into 2 doses):
Children > 10 yr. 3-5 mcg/kg/day.
Children 5-10 yr. 7-10 mcg/kg/day. Doses as low as 5 mcg/kg/day recommended.
Children 2-5 yr. 10-15 mcg/kg/day. Doses as low as 7.5 mcg/kg/day recommended.
Children < 2 yr. 10-15 mcg/kg/day.
Full-term neonates. 6-10 mcg/kg/day.
Preterm neonates. 5-7.5 mcg/kg/day.

▸ **Dosage in renal impairment**
Dosage adjustment is based on creatinine clearance. Total digitalizing dose: Decrease by 50% in end-stage renal disease.

Creatinine Clearance	Adult Dosage
10-50 mL/min	25%-75% usual or every 36 h
Less than 10 mL/min	10%-25% usual or every 48 h

CONTRAINDICATIONS
Hypersensitivity to digoxin or other digitalis preparations, ventricular fibrillation, ventricular tachycardia unrelated to congestive heart failure.

INTERACTIONS
Drug
Amiodarone: May increase digoxin blood concentration and risk of toxicity; may have an additive effect on the SA and AV nodes. Reduce digoxin dose by 50% when initiating amiodarone.
Amphotericin, glucocorticoids, potassium-depleting diuretics: May increase risk of toxicity due to hypokalemia.
Antiarrhythmics, parenteral calcium, sympathomimetics: May increase risk of arrhythmias.
Antidiarrheals, cholestyramine, colestipol, sucralfate: May decrease absorption of digoxin.
β-Blockers: May have additive effect on heart rate.
Carvedilol, diltiazem, fluoxetine, quinidine, verapamil: May increase digoxin blood concentration. Reduce dose 25%-50% when initiating quinidine. Reduce digoxin dose with others.
Cyclosporine, itraconazole: May increase digoxin levels.
Parenteral magnesium: May cause cardiac conduction changes and heart block.
Herbal
Siberian ginseng: May increase serum digoxin levels.
Licorice: Hypokalemic effects may increase digoxin toxicity.
Food
None known.

DIAGNOSTIC TEST EFFECTS
Prolongs PR interval of ECG. Clinical status, not serum levels, guide treatment. Roughly ⅔ of adults considered adequately digitalized (without toxicity) have serum digoxin concentrations 0.8-2 ng/mL. However, many have clinical benefits at levels below this "therapeutic" range. About ⅔ of patients with toxicity have serum digoxin concentrations > 2 ng/mL, but ⅓ will have clinical toxicity within the "normal" range. Values < 2 ng/mL do not rule out digoxin toxicity.

IV INCOMPATIBILITIES
Amiodarone, all forms of amphotericin B, caspofungin (Cancidas), dantrolene, diazepam (Valium), doxorubicin (Adriamycin), fluconazole (Diflucan), foscarnet (Foscavir), lansoprazole (Prevacid), minocycline (Minocin), mitoxantrone (Novantrone), paclitaxel (Taxol), phenytoin, propofol (Diprivan), quinupristin/dalfopristin (Synercid), sulfamethoxazole/trimethoprim.

SIDE EFFECTS
Most side effects occur at doses greater than needed for therapeutic effect. However, there is a very narrow margin of safety between a

therapeutic and a toxic result. Long-term therapy may produce mammary gland enlargement in women, but this is reversible when the drug is withdrawn.

Occasional (< 10%)

Dizziness, headache, mental disturbances, diarrhea, nausea, rash.

SERIOUS REACTIONS

- The most common early manifestations of digoxin toxicity are GI disturbances (anorexia, nausea, vomiting) and neurologic abnormalities (fatigue, headache, depression, weakness, drowsiness, confusion, nightmares). In children, the early signs are cardiac arrhythmias, including sinus bradycardia.
- Facial pain, personality change, and ocular disturbances (photophobia, light flashes, halos around bright objects, yellow or green color perception) may be noted.
- Proarrhythmic effects occur with digoxin.

PRECAUTIONS & CONSIDERATIONS

Caution is warranted in patients who have had an acute myocardial infarction (i.e., within 6 mo), advanced cardiac disease, heart failure, cor pulmonale, hypokalemia, hypomagnesemia, hypothyroidism, impaired hepatic or renal function, incomplete AV block, sinus nodal disease, or pulmonary disease. Digoxin crosses the placenta and is distributed in breast milk. Premature infants are more susceptible to toxicity. Keep in mind that infants and children experience signs of overdose differently than adults do. The first sign of overdose in children is usually an arrhythmia, such as bradycardia, followed by nausea, vomiting, diarrhea, anorexia, and CNS disturbances. In elderly patients, age-related hepatic or renal function impairment may require dosage adjustment. Also, there is an increased risk of loss of appetite in this age group. Withhold or reduce dose 1-2 days before elective electrical cardioversion.

Notify the physician if decreased appetite, diarrhea, nausea, visual changes, or vomiting occurs. Apical pulse should be assessed for 60 seconds or 30 seconds if the person is receiving maintenance therapy. If the pulse rate is 60 beats/min or lower in adults or 70 beats/min or lower in children, withhold the drug and contact the physician. Blood samples for digoxin level should be obtained 6-8 h after digoxin administration or just before administration of the next digoxin dose. Be aware that signs and symptoms of digoxin toxicity are GI disturbances and neurologic abnormalities.

Storage

Store at room temperature.

Administration

! Avoid giving digoxin by the IM route, because the drug may cause severe local irritation and is erratically absorbed (IV preferred). Only if no other route is possible, give deep into the muscle followed by massage. Give no more than 2 mL at any one site. Expect to adjust the digoxin dosage in elderly patients and in those with renal dysfunction. Know that larger digoxin doses are often required for adequate control of ventricular rate with atrial fibrillation or flutter. Administer digoxin loading dosage in several doses at 4- to 8-h intervals, as prescribed.

May take oral digoxin without regard to meals. Crush tablets if necessary. Do not increase or skip digoxin doses. Carefully measure oral solution to ensure accurate dosage.

For IV use, give undiluted or dilute with at least a fourfold volume of sterile water for injection, NS, or D5W, because using less than this amount may cause a precipitate to form. Use immediately. Give IV slowly over at least 5 min. If tuberculin syringes are used to measure very small doses, be aware of the problem of inadvertent overadministration of digoxin. The syringe should not be flushed after its contents are expelled into an indwelling vascular catheter.

Digoxin Immune Fab

di-jox'in im'myoon-fab

★ Digibind, DigiFab

Do not confuse digoxin with Desoxyn or doxepin.

CATEGORY AND SCHEDULE

Pregnancy Risk Category: C

Classification: Antidotes

MECHANISM OF ACTION

An antidote that binds molecularly to digoxin in the extracellular space and the complex is excreted by kidneys. *Therapeutic Effect:* Makes digoxin unavailable for binding at its site of action on cells in the body.

PHARMACOKINETICS

Route	Onset	Peak	Duration
IV	30 min	N/A	3-4 days

Widely distributed into extracellular space. Excreted in urine. *Half-life:* 15-20 h.

AVAILABILITY

Powder for Injection (Digibind): 38-mg vial.
Powder for Injection (DigiFab): 40-mg vial.

INDICATIONS AND DOSAGES

▸ **Potentially life-threatening digoxin overdose**

IV

Adults, Elderly, Children. Dosage varies according to amount of digoxin to be neutralized. Refer to manufacturer's dosing calculation guidelines. In general, 20 vials are adequate to treat most life-threatening ACUTE ingestions. Monitor for volume overload in children. Consider up to 10 vials, observing patient's response, and following with an additional 10 vials if indicated. Most cases of toxicity were reversed with 10 vials in clinical trials. For toxicity from CHRONIC use, 6 vials are usually adequate to reverse most cases of toxicity.

CONTRAINDICATIONS

None known.

INTERACTIONS

Drug
None known.
Herbal
None known.
Food
None known.

DIAGNOSTIC TEST EFFECTS

May cause a decline in serum potassium level as toxicity is reversed; monitor serum potassium frequently. Serum digoxin concentration may increase precipitously and persist for up to 1 wk until Fab/digoxin complex is eliminated from the body.

IV INCOMPATIBILITIES
None known.

SIDE EFFECTS
Allergic reaction, phlebitis.

SERIOUS REACTIONS
- Hyperkalemia may occur as a result of digitalis toxicity. Signs and symptoms of hyperkalemia include diarrhea, paresthesia of extremities, heaviness of legs, decreased BP, cold skin, grayish pallor, hypotension, mental confusion, irritability, flaccid paralysis, tented T waves, widening QRS interval, and ST depression.
- Hypokalemia may develop rapidly when the effect of digitalis is reversed. Signs and symptoms of hypokalemia include muscle cramping, nausea, vomiting, hypoactive bowel sounds, abdominal distention, difficulty breathing, and orthostatic hypotension.
- Low cardiac output and congestive heart failure exacerbations may occur rarely when digoxin level is reduced.

PRECAUTIONS & CONSIDERATIONS
Use with caution if a history of allergy to sheep proteins or mannitol, or to other components of the products. Caution is warranted with impaired cardiac and renal function. Be aware of signs and symptoms of digoxin toxicity, including anorexia, nausea, and vomiting, as well as visual changes. It is unknown whether digoxin immune Fab crosses the placenta or is distributed in breast milk. No age-related precautions have been noted in children. In elderly patients, age-related renal impairment may require cautious use.

BP, ECG, serum potassium level, and temperature should be monitored during and after drug administration. Changes from the initial assessment should be assessed. Hypokalemia may result in cardiac arrhythmias, changes in mental status, muscle cramps, muscle strength changes, or tremor. Hyperkalemia may result in cold and clammy skin, confusion, and diarrhea. Signs and symptoms of an arrhythmia (such as palpitations) or heart failure (such as dyspnea and edema) should also be assessed if the digoxin level falls below the therapeutic level.

Storage

Refrigerate vials. After reconstitution, use the solution immediately. If it is not used immediately, store the solution in the refrigerator for up to 4 h.

Administration

Serum digoxin level should be obtained before administering the drug. If the serum digoxin level was drawn < 6 h before the last digoxin dose, the serum digoxin level may be unreliable. Impaired renal function may require more than 1 wk before serum digoxin assay is reliable; however, this fact does not alter recommendations for acute treatment. Monitor for prolonged toxicity.

Reconstitute each 38-mg vial with 4 mL sterile water for injection to provide a concentration of 9.5 mg/mL. Reconstitute each 40-mg vial with 4 mL of sterile water for injection to provide a concentration of 10 mg/mL. The reconstituted product (total dosage) may be diluted with 0.9% NaCl to a convenient volume. Infuse over 30 min. It is recommended that the solution be infused through a 0.22-μm filter. If cardiac arrest is imminent, may give drug by IV push. In children, may need to watch for fluid overload, depending on the number of vials to be given.

D

Dihydroergotamine

dye-hye-droe-er-got′a-meen

D.H.E. 45, Migranal

CATEGORY AND SCHEDULE

Pregnancy Risk Category: X

Classification: Ergot alkaloids and derivatives

MECHANISM OF ACTION

An ergotamine derivative, α-adrenergic blocker that directly stimulates vascular smooth muscle. May also have antagonist effects on serotonin. *Therapeutic Effect:* Peripheral and cerebral vasoconstriction.

PHARMACOKINETICS

Slow, incomplete absorption from the GI tract; rate of absorption of intranasal varies. Protein binding: > 90%. Undergoes extensive first-pass metabolism in liver. Metabolized to active metabolite. Eliminated in feces via biliary system. *Half-life:* 7-9 h.

AVAILABILITY

Injection: 1 mg/mL (D.H.E. 45).
Nasal Spray: 4 mg/mL (0.5 mg/spray) (Migranal).

INDICATIONS AND DOSAGES

▸ Migraine headaches, cluster headaches

IM/SUBCUTANEOUS/IV

Adults, Elderly. 1 mg at onset of headache; repeat hourly if needed for up to 3 total doses. Usual maximum for IV use: 2 mg/24 h. Maximum: 3 mg/day; 6 mg/wk.

INTRANASAL

Adults, Elderly. 1 spray (0.5 mg) into each nostril; repeat in 15 min, up to 4 sprays. Maximum: 6 sprays/day; 8 sprays/wk.

OFF-LABEL USES

Orthostatic hypotension.

CONTRAINDICATIONS

Previous hypersensitivity to ergot alkaloids, coronary artery disease, angina, hypertension, impaired liver or renal function, malnutrition, peripheral vascular diseases, such as thromboangiitis obliterans, syphilitic arteritis, severe arteriosclerosis, thrombophlebitis, coronary artery vasospasm/Prinzmetal angina, hemiplegic or basilar migraine, Raynaud disease, sepsis, severe pruritus (biliary disease), high-dose aspirin therapy, potent CYP3A4 inhibitors, within 24 h of serotonin agonists, within 2 wks of MAOIs, pregnancy, breastfeeding.

INTERACTIONS

Drug

β-Blockers: May increase the risk of vasospasm.

Potent CYP3A4 inhibitors (e.g., ritonavir, nelfinavir, indinavir, erythromycin, clarithromycin, troleandomycin, ketoconazole, itraconazole): Increase toxicity of dihydroergotamine. Contraindicated.

Ergot alkaloids, systemic vasoconstrictors: May increase pressor effect.

Less potent CYP3A4 inhibitors (e.g., saquinavir, nefazodone, fluconazole, fluoxetine, other azole antifungals): May increase risk of ergotism.

MAOIs, serotonin agonists, ("triptans"), sibutramine: May increase risk of serotonin syndrome. Contraindicated.

Nicotine: Nicotine may provoke vasoconstriction.

Nitroglycerin: May decrease the effect of nitroglycerin.

Herbal

None known.

Food
None known.

DIAGNOSTIC TEST EFFECTS
None known.

SIDE EFFECTS
Frequent (> 25%)
Nasal spray: Rhinitis.
Occasional
Nasal spray: Nausea, cough, dizziness, altered taste, throat and nose irritation.
Rare
Muscle pain, fatigue, diarrhea, upper respiratory infection, dyspepsia.

SERIOUS REACTIONS
- Prolonged administration or excessive dosage may produce ergotamine poisoning manifested as nausea, vomiting, weakness of legs, pain in limb muscles, numbness and tingling of fingers or toes, precordial pain, tachycardia or bradycardia, and hypertension or hypotension.
- Coronary artery vasospasm, myocardial ischemia, myocardial infarction, ventricular tachycardia, ventricular fibrillation, cerebrovascular hemorrhage, stroke.
- Localized edema and itching due to vasoconstriction of peripheral arteries and arterioles may occur.
- Feet or hands will become cold, pale, and numb.
- Muscle pain may occur when walking and later, even at rest.
- Gangrene may occur.
- Pleural and retroperitoneal fibrosis have occurred with prolonged daily use.
- Occasionally confusion, depression, drowsiness, and seizures appear.

PRECAUTIONS & CONSIDERATIONS
Dihydroergotamine use is contraindicated in pregnancy because it produces uterine stimulant action, resulting in possible fetal death or retarded fetal growth, and it increases vasoconstriction of placental vascular bed. It is distributed in breast milk and may prohibit lactation.

Dihydroergotamine use may produce diarrhea or vomiting in the neonate. It may be used safely in children older than 6 yr, but use only when the patient is unresponsive to other medication. In elderly patients, age-related occlusive peripheral vascular disease increases the risk of peripheral vasoconstriction. In elderly patients, age-related renal impairment may require caution.

Irregular heartbeat, nausea, numbness or tingling of the fingers and toes, pain or weakness of the extremities, and vomiting should be reported.

Storage
Store at room temperature below 77° F. Protect from light. Do not refrigerate or freeze. Do not refrigerate or freeze injection or nasal spray.

Administration
Injection may be given subcutaneously, IM, or IV.

Before intranasal administration, nasal spray must be primed (pumped 4 times). Use no more than 4 sprays (2 mg) for a single administration; do not use > 6 sprays in a 24-h period or 8 sprays in a week. Inhale deeply through the nose while spraying or immediately after spraying to allow the drug to be absorbed through the skin in the nose. Do not tilt the head back or inhale through the nose. Initiate treatment at the first sign of symptom of an attack. Nasal spray may be administered at any time during a migraine attack. Once spray is prepared, use within 8 h. Discard unused solution.

Diltiazem

dil-tye′a-zem

★ Cardizem, Cardizem CD, Cardizem LA, Cartia XT, Dilacor XR, Diltia XT, Taztia XT, Tiazac

🍁 Cardizem CD, Nu-Diltiaz, Tiazac, Tiazac XC

Do not confuse Cardizem with Cardene or Cardene SR, or Tiazac with Ziac.

CATEGORY AND SCHEDULE

Pregnancy Risk Category: C

Classification: Antiarrhythmics, class IV, antianginals, antihypertensives, calcium channel blockers

MECHANISM OF ACTION

An antianginal, antihypertensive, and antiarrhythmic agent that inhibits calcium movement across cardiac and vascular smooth-muscle cell membranes. This action causes the dilation of coronary arteries, peripheral arteries, and arterioles. *Therapeutic Effect:* Decreases BP, heart rate, and myocardial contractility; slows SA and AV conduction; and decreases total peripheral vascular resistance by vasodilation.

PHARMACOKINETICS

Route	Onset	Peak	Duration
PO	0.5-1 h	2-3 h	N/A
PO (extended release)	2-3 h		10-18 h N/A
IV	3 min		15 min N/A

Well absorbed from the GI tract. Protein binding: 70%-80%. Undergoes first-pass metabolism in the liver to active metabolite. Primarily excreted in urine. Not removed by hemodialysis. *Half-life* (immediate-release tablet): 3-4.5 h. *Half-life* (extended-release tablet): 6-9 h. *Half-life* (extended-release capsules): 5-10 h.

AVAILABILITY

Capsules (Sustained Release [Diltiazem Sustained Release]): 60 mg, 90 mg, 120 mg.
Capsules (Extended Release [Cardizem CD]): 120 mg, 180 mg, 240 mg, 300 mg, 360 mg.
Capsules (Extended Release [Cartia XT]): 120 mg, 180 mg, 240 mg, 300 mg.
Capsules (Extended Release [Dilacor XR]): 120 mg, 180 mg, 240 mg.
Capsules (Extended Release [Diltia XT]): 120 mg, 180 mg, 240 mg.
Capsules (Extended Release [Taztia XT]): 120 mg, 180 mg, 240 mg, 300 mg, 360 mg.
Capsules (Extended Release [Tiazac]): 120 mg, 180 mg, 240 mg, 300 mg, 360 mg, 420 mg.
Tablets (Cardizem): 30 mg, 60 mg, 90 mg, 120 mg.
Tablets (Extended Release [Cardizem LA]): 120 mg, 180 mg, 240 mg, 300 mg, 360 mg, 420 mg.
Injection (Solution): 5 mg/mL.
Injection (Powder): 100 mg.

INDICATIONS AND DOSAGES

▸ **Angina related to coronary artery spasm (Prinzmetal variant), chronic stable angina (effort-associated)**

PO

Adults, Elderly. Initially, 30 mg 4 times a day. Increase up to 180-360 mg/day in 3-4 divided doses at 1- to 2-day intervals.

Adults, Elderly (Cardizem LA). Initially, 180 mg/day. May increase at intervals of 7-14 days up to 360 mg/day.
Adults, Elderly (Cardizem CD, Cartia XT, Dilacor XR, Diltia XT, Tiazac). Initially, 120-180 mg/day; titrate over 7-14 days. Range: Up to 480 mg/day.

▸ **Essential hypertension**

PO
Adults, Elderly. (Cardizem CD, Cartia XT, Dilacor XR, Diltia XT): Initially, 180-240 mg once a day. May increase at 2-wk intervals. Maintenance 240-360 mg/day. Maximum: 480 mg once a day (Cardizem CD, Cartia XT, Dilacor XR). Maximum: 540 mg once a day (Diltia XT).
(Cardizem LA): Initially, 180-240 mg once a day. May increase at 2-wk intervals. Maintenance: 120-540 mg/day. (Taztia XT, Tiazac): Initially, 120-240 mg once a day. May increase at 2-wk intervals. Maximum: 540 mg once a day.

▸ **Temporary control of rapid ventricular rate in atrial fibrillation or flutter, rapid conversion of paroxysmal supraventricular tachycardia to normal sinus rhythm**

IV BOLUS
Adults, Elderly. Initially, 0.25 mg/kg actual body weight over 2 min. May repeat in 15 min at dose of 0.35 mg/kg actual body weight. Subsequent doses individualized.
IV INFUSION
Adults, Elderly. After initial bolus injection, may begin infusion at 5-10 mg/h; may increase by 5 mg/h up to a maximum of 15 mg/h. Infusion duration should not exceed 24 h.

OFF-LABEL USES

Migraine prophylaxis, diabetic nephropathy, unstable angina, dilated cardiomyopathy.

CONTRAINDICATIONS

Acute myocardial infarction, pulmonary congestion, severe hypotension (< 90 mm Hg, systolic), sick sinus syndrome, second- or third-degree AV block (except in the presence of a pacemaker), IV administration within hour of IV β-blockers, ventricular tachycardia, hypersensitivity.

INTERACTIONS

Drug
α-Blockers: Increased hypotensive effect.
Aprepitant/fosaprepitant: May increase levels of each drug.
β-Blockers: May have additive effect.
Carbamazepine: May decrease levels of diltiazem. May increase levels of carbamazepine.
Cyclosporine: Levels of each drug may be increased.
CYP3A4 inhibitors/inducers: May increase or decrease levels and effects of diltiazem, respectively.
CYP3A4 substrates, HMG-CoA reductase inhibitors: Diltiazem may increase levels of substrates.
Digoxin: May increase serum digoxin concentration.
Procainamide, quinidine: May increase risk of QT-interval prolongation.
Herbal
St. John's wort: May decrease levels of diltiazem.
Food
None known.

DIAGNOSTIC TEST EFFECTS

PR interval may be increased.

IV INCOMPATIBILITIES

Acetazolamide (Diamox), acyclovir (Zovirax), allopurinol (Aloprim), aminophylline, amphotericin B liposomal (AmBisome), ampicillin, ampicillin/sulbactam (Unasyn), cefepime (Maxipime), chloramphenicol, dantrolene, diazepam (Valium), fluorouracil, furosemide (Lasix), ganciclovir (Cytovene), heparin, insulin, ketorolac, lansoprazole (Prevacid), methotrexate, micafungin (Micardis), nafcillin, pantoprazole (Protonix), pentobarbital, phenobarbital, phenytoin (Dilantin), piperacillin/tazobactam (Zosyn), rifampin (Rifadin), sodium bicarbonate, thiopental.

D

IV COMPATIBILITIES

Albumin, alfentanil (Alfenta), amifostine (Ethyol), amikacin (Amikar), amiodarone, argatroban, atenolol, atracurium (Tracrium), aztreonam (Azactam), bivalirudin (Angiomax), bretylium, bumetanide (Bumex), buprenorphine (Buprenex), busulfan (Busulfex), butorphanol (Stadol), calcium chloride, calcium gluconate, carboplatin, caspofungin (Cancidas), cefazolin (Ancef), cefotaxime (Claforan), cefotetan (Cefotan), cefoxitin (Mefoxin), ceftazidime (Ceptaz, Fortaz, Tazicef, Tazidime), ceftizoxime (Cefizox), ceftriaxone (Rocephin), cefuroxime (Zinacef), chlorpromazine, cimetidine (Tagamet), ciprofloxacin (Cipro), cisatracurium (Nimbex), cisplatin, clindamycin (Cleocin), cyclophosphamide (Cytoxan), cyclosporine (Sandimmune), dactinomycin (Cosmegen), daptomycin (Cubicin), dexamethasone sodium phosphate, dexmedetomidine (Precedex), digoxin (Lanoxin), diphenhydramine (Benadryl), dobutamine (Dobutrex), docetaxel (Taxotere), dopamine (Intropin), doripenem (Doribax), doxorubicin (Adriamycin), doxycycline, droperidol, enalaprilat, ephedrine, epinephrine, epirubicin (Ellence), ertapenem (Invanz), erythromycin lactobionate, esmolol (Brevibloc), etoposide phosphate (Etopophos), famotidine (Pepcid), fenoldopam (Corlopam), fentanyl (Sublimaze), fluconazole (Diflucan), fludarabine (Fludara), foscarnet (Foscavir), fosphenytoin (Cerbyx), gemcitabine (Gemzar), granisetron (Kytril), haloperidol (Haldol), gentamicin (Garamycin), hydromorphone (Dilaudid), hydroxyzine, imipenem/cilastatin (Primaxin), isoproterenol (Isuprel), labetalol, levofloxacin (Levaquin), lidocaine, linezolid (Zyvox), lorazepam (Ativan), magnesium sulfate, mannitol, melphalan (Alkeran), meperidine (Demerol), meropenem (Merrem), metoclopramide (Reglan), metoprolol (Lopressor), metronidazole (Flagyl), midazolam (Versed), milrinone (Primacor), minocycline (Minocin), mitoxantrone (Novantrone), morphine, multivitamins, nalbuphine (Nubain), naloxone (Narcan), nesiritide (Natrecor), nicardipine (Cardene), nitroglycerin, nitroprusside sodium (Nitropress), norepinephrine (Levophed), ondansetron (Zofran), oxacillin, oxaliplatin (Eloxatin), oxytocin (Pitocin), paclitaxel (Taxol), palonosetron (Aloxi), pancuronium, pemetrexed (Alimta), penicillin G potassium, piperacillin, potassium chloride, potassium phosphate, prochlorperazine, promethazine, propranolol, quinupristin/dalfopristin (Synercid), ranitidine (Zantac), remifentanil (Ultiva), sodium acetate, succinylcholine, sufentanil (Sufenta), sulfamethoxazole/trimethoprim, tacrolimus (Prograf), teniposide (Vumon), theophylline, thiotepa (Thioplex), ticarcillin (Ticar), ticarcillin/clavulanate

(Timentin), tigecycline (Tygacil), tirofibran (Aggrastat), tobramycin, vancomycin, vasopressin, vecuronium (Norcuron), verapamil, vincristine (Vincasar), vinorelbine (Navelbine), voriconazole (Vfend), zidovudine (Retrovir).

SIDE EFFECTS

Frequent (1%-5%)
Peripheral edema, dizziness, light-headedness, headache, pain, bradycardia, asthenia (loss of strength, weakness), dyspepsia.
Occasional (2%-5%)
Nausea, constipation, flushing, ECG changes, injection site reactions (burning, itching).
Rare (< 2%)
Rash, micturition disorder (polyuria, nocturia, dysuria, frequency of urination), abdominal discomfort, somnolence.

SERIOUS REACTIONS

- Abrupt withdrawal may increase frequency or duration of angina.
- Congestive heart failure (CHF) and second- and third-degree AV block and sinus bradycardia occur rarely.
- Overdose produces nausea, somnolence, confusion, slurred speech, and profound bradycardia.

PRECAUTIONS & CONSIDERATIONS

Caution is warranted in patients with CHF, hypertrophic obstructive cardiomyopathy, and impaired hepatic or renal function. It is unclear whether diltiazem crosses the placenta. It should be used during pregnancy only if the benefit to the mother outweighs the risk to the fetus. Diltiazem is distributed in breast milk. No age-related precautions have been noted in children. In elderly patients, age-related renal impairment may require cautious use. Tasks that require alertness and motor skills should also be avoided.

Dizziness or light-headedness may occur. Rise slowly from a lying to a sitting position and wait momentarily before standing to avoid diltiazem's hypotensive effect. Notify the physician of constipation, irregular heartbeat, nausea, pronounced dizziness, or shortness of breath. The onset, type (sharp, dull, or squeezing), radiation, location, intensity, and duration of anginal pain and its precipitating factors, such as exertion and emotional stress, should be documented before therapy. Pulse, BP, and renal and hepatic function test results should be monitored before and during therapy. Skin should be assessed for flushing and peripheral edema, especially behind the medial malleolus.

Storage
Store oral products at room temperature.

Refrigerate single-use solution for injection (may store at room temperature 1 mo). Store powder for reconstitution at room temperature. After dilution, solution is stable for 24 h.

Administration
Take oral immediate-release diltiazem before meals and at bedtime. Taztia XT and Tiazac capsules may be opened and sprinkled on applesauce. Do not crush or open other sustained-release capsules. In general administer at the same time each day for extended-release dosage forms. Dilacor XR or Diltia XT should be given on an empty stomach. Other extended-release capsules are taken without regard to food.

IV bolus given over 2 min. Add 125 mg to 100 mL D5W or 0.9% NaCl to provide an IV infusion concentration of 1 mg/mL. The maximum concentration is 5 mg/mL. Infuse per dilution or rate chart provided by manufacturer.

Dimenhydrinate

dye-men-hye′dri-nate

★ Dramamine, Driminate, Wal-Dram 🍁 Dinate, Gravol, Nausetrol

CATEGORY AND SCHEDULE

Pregnancy Risk Category: B

Classification: Anticholinergics, antiemetics/antivertigo

OTC, Rx

MECHANISM OF ACTION

An antihistamine and anticholinergic that competes for H_1 receptor sites on effector cells of the GI tract, blood vessels, and respiratory tract. The anticholinergic action diminishes vestibular stimulation and depresses labyrinthine function. *Therapeutic Effect:* Prevents symptoms of motion sickness.

AVAILABILITY

Tablets, Chewable: 50 mg.
Tablets: 50 mg.
Injection: 50 mg/mL.

INDICATIONS AND DOSAGES

▸ **Motion sickness**

PO

Adults, Elderly, Children older than 12 yr. 50-100 mg q4-6h. Maximum: 400 mg/day.
Children 6-12 yr. 25-50 mg q6-8h. Maximum: 150 mg/day.
Children 2-5 yr. 12.5-25 mg q6-8h. Maximum: 75 mg/day.

IM/IV

Adults. 50 mg as needed every 4 h. Maximum: 300 mg/day.
Children. 1.25 mg/kg or 37.5 mg/m2 4 times daily. Maximum 300 mg a day. Do not use in neonates.

CONTRAINDICATIONS

Hypersensitivity to dimenhydrinate. Do not use in neonates because injectable product contains benzyl alcohol.

INTERACTIONS

Drug

Alcohol, other central nervous system (CNS) depressants: May increase CNS depression.
Aminoglycosides: Masks signs and symptoms of ototoxicity associated with aminoglycosides.
Other anticholinergics: Increases anticholinergic effect.

DIAGNOSTIC TEST EFFECTS

None known.

SIDE EFFECTS

Frequent

Dry mouth, drowsiness.

Occasional

Hypotension, palpitations, tacycardia, headache, somnolence, dizziness, paradoxical stimulation (especially in children), anorexia, constipation, dysuria, blurred vision, tinnitus, wheezing, chest tightness.

Rare

Photosensitivity, rash, urticaria.

SERIOUS REACTIONS

- None significant.

PRECAUTIONS & CONSIDERATIONS

Caution is warranted in patients with asthma, bladder neck obstruction, cardiovascular disease, history of seizures, angle-closure glaucoma, thyroid dysfunction, and benign prostatic hyperplasia. Alcohol, tasks that require mental alertness or motor skills, and excessive exposure to sunlight should be avoided. Skin should not come in contact with the oral concentrate and syrup because it can cause contact dermatitis. Should not be used in children younger than 2 yr. Elderly patients are more susceptible to side effects.

Drowsiness, dizziness, and dry mouth may occur. BP should be monitored. Be alert for paradoxical reactions, especially in children, and signs and symptoms of motion sickness.

Storage
Store at room temperature. Protect from moisture and light.

Administration
Take without regard to meals. Chewable tablets may be chewed or swallowed whole with or without water. For motion sickness, take dimenhydrinate 1-2 h before the activity that may cause motion sickness.

IM: Inject into large muscle mass.
IV: Dilute dose in 10 mL of 0.9% NaCl, give by slow IV push over 2 min.

Dimercaprol

dye-mer-kap′role
BAL in Oil

CATEGORY AND SCHEDULE

Pregnancy Risk Category: C

Classification: Antidotes, chelators

MECHANISM OF ACTION

A chelating agent that contains two sulfhydryl groups that form a stable, nontoxic chelate 5-membered heterocyclic ring with heavy metals. *Therapeutic Effect:* Prevents the metal from combining with sulfhydryl groups on physiologic proteins and keeps them inactive until they can be excreted.

PHARMACOKINETICS

Time to peak after IM administration occurs in 30-60 min. Widely distributed to all tissues, including the brain and, mainly, intracellular space. Rapidly metabolized by the liver to inactive metabolites. Excreted in the urine and bile. Removed by hemodialysis. *Half-life:* 4 h.

AVAILABILITY

Injection, Oil: 100 mg/mL (BAL in Oil).

INDICATIONS AND DOSAGES

▸ **Poisoning, arsenic (mild)**
IM
Adults, Elderly, Children. 2.5 mg/kg 4 times/day for 2 days, 2 times on day 3, then once daily for 10 days or recovery.

▸ **Poisoning, arsenic (severe)**
IM
Adults, Elderly, Children. 3 mg/kg q4h for 2 days, 4 times on day 3, then twice daily for 10 days or until recovery.

▸ **Poisoning, gold (mild)**
IM
Adults, Elderly, Children. 2.5 mg/kg 4 times/day for 2 days, 2 times on day 3, then once daily for 10 days or until recovery.

▸ **Poisoning, gold (severe)**
IM
Adults, Elderly, Children. 3 mg/kg q4h for 2 days, 4 times on day 3, then twice daily for 10 days or until recovery.

▸ **Poisoning, lead (mild)**
IM
Adults, Elderly, Children. Initially, 4 mg/kg, then 3 mg/kg q4h for 2-7 days in combination with

edetate calcium disodium injection beginning with second dose at different injection sites.

▸ **Poisoning, lead (severe)**

IM

Adults, Elderly, Children. 4 mg/kg q4h usually for 5 days. In combination with edetate calcium disodium injection beginning with second dose at different injection sites. A second 5-day course may be used in severe poisoning. Wait at least 5-7 days before administering a third course, if needed.

▸ **Poisoning, mercury**

IM

Adults, Elderly, Children. 5 mg/kg for 1 day, followed by 2.5 mg/kg 1 or 2 times/day for 10 days.

▸ **Dosage in renal impairment**

Quantitative dosage recommendations are not available. The manufacturer states the drug should be discontinued or used with extreme caution if acute renal insufficiency occurs during treatment.

OFF-LABEL USES

Antimony poisoning, bismuth poisoning, silver poisoning, vanadium poisoning.

CONTRAINDICATIONS

Hepatic insufficiency (unless due to arsenic poisoning); use in iron, cadmium, or selenium poisoning; hypersensitivity to dimercaprol or any component of the formulations, such as peanut oil.

INTERACTIONS

Drug

Gold compounds: Compromise anti-inflammatory effect by chelating gold.

Iron, cadmium, selenium, uranium: May increase risk of toxicity, especially to the kidneys.

DIAGNOSTIC TEST EFFECTS

Iodine (^{131}I) thyroidal uptake values may be decreased. May result in false-positive reaction with nitroprusside test. May increase ALT and AST values.

IV INCOMPATIBILITIES

Edetate calcium disodium.

SIDE EFFECTS

Frequent

Hypertension, dose-related tachycardia, headache. Injection site reactions occur in 30% of children.

Occasional

Nausea, vomiting.

Rare

Burning eyes, lips, mouth, throat, and penis; nervousness; pain at injection site; salivation; fever; dysuria.

SERIOUS REACTIONS

- Abscess formation at injection site, blepharospasm, convulsions, thrombocytopenia, and transient neutropenia occur rarely.
- Fever may occur and persist in children.

PRECAUTIONS & CONSIDERATIONS

Caution is warranted with hypotension because of dose-related increase in blood pressure and heart rate; renal impairment including oliguria; and glucose 6-phosphate dehydrogenase (G6PD) deficiency. Contains peanut oil. Ensure alkalinization of urine to protect the kidney. Caution is also necessary with people receiving iron supplementation. Avoid use until 24 h after last dose of dimercaprol.

Be aware that dimercaprol is effective for acute poisoning by mercury salts if therapy is initiated within 1-2 h after ingestion. Dimercaprol is not effective for chronic mercury poisoning. Serum alkaline phosphatase concentration, blood urea nitrogen (BUN) concentration, serum calcium, creatinine, electrolyte concentrations, hemoglobin (especially in mercury toxicity), and phosphorus concentrations should be monitored.

Storage

Store ampules at room temperature.

Administration

Be careful not to mix with edetate calcium disodium. Administer at different sites.

Administer deep IM injection only. Adjust dose if receiving dialysis.

The injection is painful and causes a sterile abscess in some patients.

Dinoprostone (PGE_2)

dye-noe-prost'one

Cervidil, Prepidil Gel, Prostin E2

Do not confuse Cervidil or Prepidil with bepridil, or Prostin with Prostigmin.

CATEGORY AND SCHEDULE

Pregnancy Risk Category: C

Classification: Oxytocics, prostaglandins, abortifacents (suppositories)

MECHANISM OF ACTION

A prostaglandin that directly acts on the myometrium, causing softening and dilation effect of the cervix. *Therapeutic Effect:* Stimulates myometrial contractions in gravid uterus, promotes cervical ripening.

PHARMACOKINETICS

Undergoes rapid enzymatic deactivation, primarily in maternal lungs. Protein binding: 73%. Primarily excreted in urine. *Half-life:* < 5 min. Onset of action (vaginal suppository): Within 10 min. Duration (vaginal insert): 12 h. Duration (vaginal suppository): 2-3 h.

AVAILABILITY

Vaginal Gel (Prepidil): 0.5 mg.
Vaginal Inserts (Cervidil): 10 mg.
Vaginal Suppositories (Prostin E2): 20 mg.

INDICATIONS AND DOSAGES

▸ Incomplete miscarriage, hydatidiform mole, or intrauterine fetal death, or for second-trimester pregnancy termination

INTRAVAGINAL

Adults. 20 mg (one suppository) high into vagina. May repeat at 3- to 5-h intervals until abortion occurs. Do not administer for > 2 days.

▸ Ripening of unfavorable cervix

INTRACERVICAL

Adults. Initially, 0.5 mg (2.5 mL) (Prepidil); if no cervical or uterine response, may repeat 0.5-mg dose in 6 h. Maximum: 1.5 mg (7.5 mL) for a 24-h period. Alternatively 10 mg (Cervidil) over 12-h period; remove upon onset of active labor or 12 h after insertion.

CONTRAINDICATIONS

Suppository: Active cardiac, hepatic, pulmonary, or renal disease; acute pelvic inflammatory disease; hypersensitivity to dinoprostone or other prostaglandins.

Gel, insert: Fetal malpresentation/distress; hypersensitivity to dinoprostone or other prostaglandins; significant cephalopelvic disproportion; more than 6 previous term pregnancies; unexplained vaginal bleeding; obstetrical emergencies.

D

INTERACTIONS

Drug

Oxytocics: May cause uterine hypertonus, possibly resulting in uterine rupture or cervical laceration. Wait 6-12 h after dinoprostone gel administration or at least 30 min after removal of vaginal insert before initiating oxytocin.

DIAGNOSTIC TEST EFFECTS

None known.

SIDE EFFECTS

Frequent

Vomiting (66%), temperature elevations (50%), diarrhea (40%), nausea (33%).

Occasional

Headache (10%), chills or shivering (10%), transient diastolic BP decrease (10%), hives, bradycardia, increased uterine pain accompanying abortion, peripheral vasoconstriction.

Rare

Flushing, vulvar edema.

SERIOUS REACTIONS

- Overdose may cause uterine hypertonicity with spasm and tetanic contraction, leading to cervical laceration or perforation, and uterine rupture or hemorrhage.
- Uterine hyperstimulation with or without fetal distress.

PRECAUTIONS & CONSIDERATIONS

Do not exceed recommended doses. Suppository: Caution is warranted in patients with anemia, cardiovascular disease, cervicitis, compromised or scarred uterus, diabetes mellitus, epilepsy, hepatic disease, history of asthma, hypertension or hypotension, infected endocervical lesions or acute vaginitis, jaundice, renal disease, and uterine fibroids. Notify the physician if chills, fever, foul-smelling or increased vaginal discharge, or uterine cramps or pain occurs.

Gel, vaginal insert: Caution is warranted with ruptured membranes, nonsingle pregnancy, glaucoma, asthma, nonvertex pregnancy, renal and hepatic impairment.

The character of the cervix, including dilation and effacement, fetal status, including heart rate as well as uterine activity, including the onset of uterine contractions, should be monitored in those receiving the vaginal gel. Bishop score should be monitored before and after therapy.

Uterine tone and duration, frequency, and strength of contractions should be checked if receiving the suppository form. Vital signs should be monitored every 15 min until stable and then hourly until abortion is complete. Expect to give medications to relieve GI adverse effects, if indicated, or abdominal cramps in those receiving the suppository form.

Storage

Refrigerate gel; bring to room temperature just before use to avoid forcing warming process. Keep suppository frozen (< 4° F [15.6° C]); bring to room temperature just before use. Remove foil wrapper after suppository reaches room temperature. Vaginal insert should be stored in freezer.

Administration

Use gel with caution when handling to prevent skin contact. Wash hands thoroughly with soap and water following administration. Assemble dosing apparatus as described in manufacturer's insert. Place the person in the dorsal position, and use a speculum to visualize the cervix. Introduce gel into cervical canal just below level of internal os. After administration, remain in the supine position for at least 15-30 min to minimize leakage of the drug from the cervical canal.

Administer suppository only in a hospital setting, with emergency equipment available. Avoid skin contact because of risk of absorption. Insert high in the vagina. Remain supine for 10 min after administration.

Diphenhydramine

dye-fen-hye'dra-meen

★ Altaryl, Banophen, Benadryl, Ben-Tann, Diphedryl, Diphenhist, Dytan, ElixSure, Genahist, Nytol, Pediacare Nighttime, Q-Dryl, Quenalin, Siladryl, Silphen, Sominex 🍁 Allerdryl, Hydramine Nytol

Do not confuse diphenhydramine with dimenhydrinate, or Benadryl with benazepril, Bentyl, or Benylin, or Banophen with Baclophen.

CATEGORY AND SCHEDULE

Pregnancy Risk Category: B
OTC

Classification: Antihistamines, H_1, sedating

MECHANISM OF ACTION

An ethanolamine that competitively blocks the effects of histamine at peripheral H_1 receptor sites. *Therapeutic Effect:* Produces anticholinergic, antipruritic, antitussive, antiemetic, antidyskinetic, and sedative effects.

PHARMACOKINETICS

Route	Onset	Peak	Duration
PO	15-30 min	1-4 h	4-6 h
IV, IM	< 15 min	1-4 h	4-6 h

Well absorbed after PO or parenteral administration. Protein binding: 98%-99%. Widely distributed. Metabolized in the liver. Primarily excreted in urine. *Half-life:* 2-10 h.

AVAILABILITY

Capsules (Banophen, Benadryl, Diphedryl, Diphenhist, Genahist, Q-Dryl): 25 mg, 50 mg (generic).
Capsules (Nytol): 50 mg.
Elixir (Banophen): 12.5 mg/5 mL.
Oral solution (Altaryl, Banophen, Benadryl, Diphenhist, ElixSure, Genahist, Hydramine, Pediacare Nighttime, Q-Dryl, Siladryl): 12.5 mg/5 mL.
Oral Suspension (Ben-Tann, Dytan): 25 mg/5 mL.
Syrup (Quenalin, Silphen): 12.5 mg/5 mL.
Tablets (Banophen, Benadryl, Diphedryl, Diphenhist, Genahist): 25 mg.
Tablets (Nytol, Sominex): 25 mg, 50 mg.
Chewable Tablets: 12.5 mg (Benadryl Allergy), 25 mg (Dytan)
Orally Disintegrating Tablets (Benadryl Fastmelt): 19 mg.
Strips, Oral Dissolving Film (Benadryl Quick Dissolve): 12.5 mg, 25 mg.
Injection: 50 mg/mL.
Cream (Benadryl): 2%.
Topical Gel (Benadryl): 2%.
Topical Solution (Benadryl Stick): 2%.
Spray: 2%.

INDICATIONS AND DOSAGES

▸ **Moderate to severe allergic reaction**

PO, IV, IM

Adults, Elderly. 10-50 mg q4-6h. Maximum: 400 mg/day.
Children. 5 mg/kg/day in divided doses q6-8h. Maximum: 300 mg/day.

D

▸ **Dystonic reaction**
IV, IM
Adults, Elderly. 10-50 mg/single dose. May repeat in 20-30 min if needed.
Children. 0.5-1 mg/kg/dose.

▸ **Motion sickness, minor allergic rhinitis**
PO
Adults, Elderly, Children 12 yr and older. 25-50 mg q4-6h. Maximum: 300 mg/day.
Children 6-11 yr. 12.5-25 mg q4-6h. Maximum: 150 mg/day.
Children 2-5 yr. 6.25 mg q4-6h. Maximum: 37.5 mg/day.

▸ **Antitussive**
PO
Adults, Elderly, Children 12 yr and older. 25 mg q4h. Maximum: 150 mg/day.
Children 6-11 yr. 12.5 mg q4h. Maximum: 75 mg/day.
Children 2-5 yr. 6.25 mg q4h. Maximum: 37.5 mg/day. NOTE: The FDA recommends against use in children < 6 years of age (2008).

▸ **Nighttime sleep aid**
PO
Adults, Elderly. 25-50 mg at bedtime.

▸ **Pruritus**
TOPICAL
Adults, Elderly, Children 2 yr and older. Apply 2% cream or spray 3-4 times a day.

CONTRAINDICATIONS

Acute exacerbation of asthma, use within 14 days of MAOIs, newborn or premature infants, breastfeeding, narrow-angle glaucoma, prostatic hypertrophy, bladder neck obstruction, pyloroduodenal obstruction, stenosing peptic ulcer.

INTERACTIONS

Drug

Alcohol, other central nervous system (CNS) depressants: May increase CNS-depressant effects.
Anticholinergics: May increase anticholinergic effects.
CYP2D6 substrates: Levels of substrates may be increased.
MAOIs: May increase the anticholinergic and CNS-depressant effects of diphenhydramine.

Herbal and Food

None known.

DIAGNOSTIC TEST EFFECTS

May suppress wheal and flare reactions to antigen skin testing unless the drug is discontinued 4 days before testing.

IV INCOMPATIBILITIES

Allopurinol (Aloprim), aminophylline, amphotericin B cholesteryl (Amphotec), ampicillin, azathioprine, cefazolin, cefepime (Maxipime), cefotaxime (Claforan), cefotetan (Cefotan), cefoxitin (Mefoxin), ceftazidime (Ceptaz, Fortaz, Tazicef, Tazidime), ceftriaxone (Rocephin), cefuroxime (Zinacef), chloramphenicol, dantrolene, dexamethasone (Decadron), diazepam (Valium), fluorouracil, foscarnet (Foscavir), furosemide (Lasix), ganciclovir (Cytovene), insulin (regular, Humulin R, Novolin R), ketorolac, lansoprazole (Prevacid), methylprednisolone sodium succinate (Solu-Medrol), metronidazole (Flagyl), milrinone (Primacor), nitroprusside sodium (Nitropress), pantoprazole (Protonix), pentobarbital, phenobarbital, phenytoin, sodium bicarbonate, sulfamethoxazole/trimethoprim.

SIDE EFFECTS

Frequent

Somnolence, dizziness, muscle weakness, hypotension, urine retention, thickening of bronchial secretions, dry mouth, nose, throat,

or lips; in elderly, sedation, dizziness, hypotension.
Occasional
Epigastric distress, flushing, visual or hearing disturbances, paresthesia, diaphoresis, chills. Contact dermatitis may occur with topical application.

SERIOUS REACTIONS

- Hypersensitivity reactions, eczema, pruritus, rash, cardiac disturbances, and photosensitivity may occur.
- Overdose symptoms may vary from CNS depression, including sedation, apnea, hypotension, cardiovascular collapse, and death, to severe paradoxical reactions, such as hallucinations, tremor, and seizures.
- Children and neonates may experience paradoxical reactions, including restlessness, insomnia, euphoria, nervousness, and tremors.
- Overdosage in children may result in hallucinations, seizures, and death.

PRECAUTIONS & CONSIDERATIONS

Caution is warranted in patients with asthma, cardiovascular disease, chronic obstructive pulmonary disease (COPD), hypertension, hyperthyroidism, angle-closure glaucoma, increased intraocular pressure, peptic ulcer disease, benign prostatic hyperplasia, pyloroduodenal or bladder neck obstruction, and seizure disorders. Diphenhydramine crosses the placenta and appears in breast milk. Its use by breastfeeding women may inhibit lactation and produce irritability in breastfeeding infants. Use of the drug during the third trimester of pregnancy increases the risk of seizures in neonates and premature infants. Diphenhydramine is not recommended for neonates or premature infants. The FDA recommends that OTC cough and cold medications not be used in children < 2 yr old. FDA also recommends against use as a sleep aid in children. Elderly patients are at increased risk for developing confusion, dizziness, hyperexcitability, hypotension, and sedation. Avoid drinking alcoholic beverages and performing tasks that require alertness or motor skills until response to the drug is established.

Drowsiness, dizziness, and dry mouth may occur; tolerance usually develops to sedative effects. Respiratory rate, depth, and rhythm; pulse rate and quality; BP; and therapeutic response should be monitored.
Storage
Store at room temperature.
Administration
Take diphenhydramine without regard to food. Crush scored tablets as needed. Do not crush, break, or open capsules or film-coated tablets.

For IM use, inject diphenhydramine deep into a large muscle mass.

For IV use, diphenhydramine may be given undiluted. Administer IV injection no faster than 25 mg/min.

Topical products are for external use only. Avoid mucus membranes. Apply gently to affected area; discontinue use if sensitivity noted.

Diphenoxylate and Atropine

dye-fen-ox′i-late, a′troe-peen
Lomotil, Lonox Lomotil
Do not confuse Lomotil with Lamictal, or Lonox with Lanoxin, Loprox, or Lovenox.

CATEGORY AND SCHEDULE

Pregnancy Risk Category: C

Classification: Antidiarrheals

MECHANISM OF ACTION
A meperidine derivative that acts locally and centrally on gastric mucosa. *Therapeutic Effect:* Reduces intestinal motility.

PHARMACOKINETICS
Well absorbed from the GI tract. Metabolized in the liver to active metabolite. Primarily eliminated in feces. *Half-life:* 2.5 h; metabolite, 12-24 h. Onset: 45-60 min. Duration 3-4 h.

AVAILABILITY
Tablets (Lomotil, Lonox): 2.5 mg/0.025 mg.
Liquid (Lomotil): 2.5 mg/0.025 mg per 5 mL.

INDICATIONS AND DOSAGES
▸ **Diarrhea**
PO
Adults, Elderly. Initially, 5 mg 4 times a day, then reduce dose to 2.5 mg 2-3 times per day. Maximum: 20 mg/day.
Children 2-12 yr. 0.3-0.4 mg/kg/day in 4 divided doses, then reduce dose. Maximum: 10 mg/day. Use liquid form only.

CONTRAINDICATIONS
Hypersensitivity, children younger than 2 yr, obstructive jaundice, narrow-angle glaucoma, diarrhea from pseudomembranous colitis, or enterotoxin-producing bacteria.

INTERACTIONS
Drug
Alcohol, other CNS depressants: May increase CNS-depressant effects.
Anticholinergics: May increase the effects of atropine.
MAOIs: May precipitate hypertensive crisis.
Herbal
None known.
Food
None known.

DIAGNOSTIC TEST EFFECTS
May increase serum amylase level.

SIDE EFFECTS
Frequent
Somnolence, light-headedness, dizziness, nausea.
Occasional
Headache, dry mouth.
Rare
Flushing, tachycardia, urine retention, constipation, paradoxical reaction (marked by restlessness and agitation), blurred vision.

SERIOUS REACTIONS
- Hypersensitivity reactions, including pruritus, gum swelling, urticaria, anaphylaxis.
- Dehydration may aggravate electrolyte imbalance. Correct fluid balance before administering.
- Paralytic ileus and toxic megacolon (marked by constipation, decreased appetite, and stomach pain with nausea or vomiting) occur rarely.
- Severe anticholinergic reaction, manifested by severe lethargy, hypotonic reflexes, and hyperthermia, may result in severe respiratory depression and coma.

PRECAUTIONS & CONSIDERATIONS
Caution is warranted in patients with acute ulcerative colitis, cirrhosis, hepatic or renal disease, and renal impairment. It is unknown whether diphenoxylate crosses the placenta or is distributed in breast milk. Diphenoxylate is not recommended for use in children < 2 yrs because of the increased risk of toxicity, which can lead to respiratory depression. Use extreme caution in young

children. Elderly patients are more susceptible to the anticholinergic effects of diphenoxylate, and they may experience confusion and respiratory depression. Tasks that require mental alertness or motor skills should be avoided until response to the drug has been established. Alcohol and barbiturates should also be avoided during drug therapy.

Notify the physician if abdominal distention, fever, palpitations, or persistent diarrhea occurs. Pattern of daily bowel activity and stool consistency and hydration status should be monitored.

Storage

Store at room temperature; store liquid in original container.

Administration

Take without regard to meals. If GI irritation occurs, give with food. Administer only the liquid form to children 2-12 yr of age using a graduated dropper for accurate measurement.

Dipyridamole

dye-peer-id'a-mole

★ Persantine

🍁 Apo-Dipyridamole, Persantine

Do not confuse dipyridamole with disopyramide, or Persantine with Periactin.

CATEGORY AND SCHEDULE

Pregnancy Risk Category: B

Classification: Platelet inhibitors

MECHANISM OF ACTION

A blood modifier and platelet aggregation inhibitor that inhibits the activity of adenosine deaminase and phosphodiesterase, enzymes causing accumulation of adenosine and cyclic adenosine monophosphate. *Therapeutic Effect:* Inhibits platelet aggregation; may cause coronary vasodilation.

PHARMACOKINETICS

Slowly, variably absorbed from the GI tract. Widely distributed. Protein binding: 91%-99%. Metabolized in the liver. Primarily eliminated via biliary excretion. *Half-life:* 10-15 h.

AVAILABILITY

Tablets: 25 mg, 50 mg, 75 mg.
Injection: 5 mg/mL.

INDICATIONS AND DOSAGES

▸ **Prevention of thromboembolic disorders after cardiac valve replacement**

PO

Adults, Elderly, Children 12 yr and older. 75-100 mg four times/day in combination with other medications.

▸ **Diagnostic aid, coronary artery disease**

IV

Adults, Elderly (based on weight). 0.142 mg/kg/min infused over 4 min; although a maximum has not been determined, doses > 60 mg have been determined to be unnecessary for any patient.

OFF-LABEL USES

Prevention of myocardial reinfarction, treatment of transient ischemic attacks.

CONTRAINDICATIONS

None known.

INTERACTIONS

Drug

Anticoagulants, aspirin, heparin, salicylates, thrombolytics: May increase the risk of bleeding with these drugs.

Adenosine: Effects may be increased.
Caffeine, theophylline: Methylxanthines, through antagonism of adenosine, may cause false-negative results from dipyridamole-thallium 201 stress testing.
Herbal
None known.
Food
None known.

DIAGNOSTIC TEST EFFECTS
None known.

IV INCOMPATIBILITIES
No information available via Y-site administration. Do not mix with other medications.

SIDE EFFECTS
Oral:
Frequent (14%)
Dizziness.
Occasional (2%-6%)
Abdominal distress, headache, rash.
Rare (< 2%)
Diarrhea, vomiting, flushing, pruritus.
Injection:
Frequent (12%-20%)
Angina pectoris exacerbation, dizziness, headache.
Occasional (2%-10%)
Hypotension, ECG changes, nausea, pain, flushing, hypertension.
Rare (< 2%).
Fatigue, paresthesia.

SERIOUS REACTIONS
- Overdose produces peripheral vasodilation, resulting in hypotension.
- Hepatic failure and enzyme elevations have occurred.

PRECAUTIONS & CONSIDERATIONS
Caution is warranted in patients with hypotension, unstable angina, recent myocardial infarction, or hepatic impairment. Dipyridamole is distributed in breast milk. Safety and efficacy of dipyridamole have not been established in children. No age-related precautions have been noted in elderly patients. Avoid alcohol because it increases the risk of stomach bleeding and dizziness, possibly resulting in a fall.

Dizziness may occur. Do not rise suddenly from a lying or sitting position. Notify the physician of unusual bleeding or chest pain. BP for hypotension and skin for erythema and rash should be monitored.
Storage
Store injection and tablets at room temperature.
Administration
Take oral dipyridamole on an empty stomach with full glass of water. Therapeutic response may not be achieved before 2-3 mo of continuous therapy.

For IV use, dilute to at least 1:2 ratio with 0.9% NaCl or D5W for total volume of 20-50 mL because undiluted solution may cause irritation. Infuse over 4 min. Inject thallium within 5 min after dipyridamole infusion has ended, as prescribed.

Disopyramide
dye-soe-peer'a-mide
Norpace, Norpace CR
Rythmodan
Do not confuse disopyramide with desipramine or dipyridamole, or Rythmodan with Rythmol.

CATEGORY AND SCHEDULE
Pregnancy Risk Category: C

Classification: Antiarrhythmics, class IA

D

MECHANISM OF ACTION
An antiarrhythmic that prolongs the refractory period of the cardiac cell by direct effect, decreasing myocardial excitability and conduction velocity. *Therapeutic Effect:* Depresses myocardial contractility. Has anticholinergic and negative inotropic effects.

AVAILABILITY
Capsules (Norpace): 100 mg, 150 mg.
Capsules (Extended Release [Norpace CR]): 100 mg, 150 mg.

INDICATIONS AND DOSAGES
▸ **Suppression and prevention of ventricular ectopy, unifocal or multifocal premature ventricular contractions, paired ventricular contractions (couplets), and episodes of ventricular tachycardia**
PO
! Do not use extended-release capsules for rapid control.
Adults, Elderly weighing 50 kg and more. 150 mg q6h (300 mg ql2h with extended-release capsules).
Adults, Elderly weighing < 50 kg. 100 mg q6h (200 mg q12h with extended-release capsules).
▸ **Rapid control of arrhythmias**
PO
Adults, Elderly weighing 50 kg and more. Initially, 300 mg (immediate release), then 150 mg q6h or 300 mg (controlled release) q12h.
Adults, Elderly weighing < 50 kg. Initially, 200 mg (immediate release), then 100 mg q6h or 200 mg (controlled release) q12h.
▸ **Severe refractory arrhythmias**
NOTE: Patient should be hospitalized during the initial treatment period.
PO
Adults, Elderly. Up to 400 mg q6h.
Children 12-18 yr. 6-15 mg/kg/day in divided doses q6h.
Children 5-12 yr. 10-15 mg/kg/day in divided doses q6h.
Children 1-4 yr. 10-20 mg/kg/day in divided doses q6h.
Children younger than 1 yr. 10-30 mg/kg/day in divided doses q6h.
▸ **Dosage in renal impairment**
With or without loading dose of 150 mg:

Creatinine Clearance (mL/min)	Dosage
≥ 40	100 mg q6h (extended release, 200 mg q12h)
30-39	100 mg q8h
15-29	100 mg q12h
< 15	100 mg q24h

▸ **Dosage in liver impairment**
Adults, Elderly weighing 50 kg and more. 100 mg q6h (200 mg q12h with extended-release capsules).
▸ **Dosage in cardiomyopathy, cardiac decompensation**
Adults, Elderly weighing 50 kg and more. No loading dose; 100 mg q6-8h with gradual dosage adjustments.

OFF-LABEL USES
Prophylaxis and treatment of supraventricular tachycardia (atrial fibrillation, atrial flutter).

CONTRAINDICATIONS
Cardiogenic shock, narrow-angle glaucoma (unless patient is undergoing cholinergic therapy), preexisting second- or third-degree atrioventricular (AV) block, congenital QT syndrome.

INTERACTIONS
Drug
CYP3A4 inducers/inhibitors: May decrease/increase levels and effects of disopyramide.

Other antiarrhythmics, including diltiazem, propranolol, verapamil: May prolong cardiac conduction, decrease cardiac output.
Pimozide: May increase cardiac arrhythmias.
QT-prolonging agents: May increase risk for QT prolongation.
Herbal and Food
None known.

DIAGNOSTIC TEST EFFECTS
May decrease blood glucose levels. May cause ECG changes. May increase serum cholesterol and triglyceride levels. Therapeutic serum level is 2-8 mcg/mL, and the toxic serum level is > 8 mcg/mL.

SIDE EFFECTS
Frequent (> 9%)
Dry mouth (32%), urinary hesitancy, constipation.
Occasional (3%-9%)
Blurred vision; dry eyes, nose, or throat; urinary retention; headache; dizziness; fatigue; nausea.
Rare (< 1%)
Impotence, hypotension, edema, weight gain, shortness of breath, syncope, chest pain, nervousness, diarrhea, vomiting, decreased appetite, rash, itching.

SERIOUS REACTIONS
- May produce or aggravate congestive heart failure (CHF).
- May produce severe hypotension, shortness of breath, chest pain, syncope (especially in patients with primary cardiomyopathy or CHF).
- May cause arrhythmias, monitor for QT prolongation.
- Hepatotoxicity occurs rarely.

PRECAUTIONS & CONSIDERATIONS
Reserve drug use for those with life-threatening ventricular arrhythmias. Caution is warranted in patients with atrial fibrillation or flutter, bundle-branch block, CHF, impaired liver or renal function, myasthenia gravis, prostatic hypertrophy (avoid use), glaucoma (avoid use), sick sinus syndrome (sinus bradycardia alternating with tachycardia), and Wolff-Parkinson-White syndrome. Nasal decongestants or OTC cold preparations, especially those containing stimulants, should be avoided without the physician's approval. Alcohol and salt consumption should also be avoided.Dizziness and light-headedness may occur. Notify the physician if cough or shortness of breath occurs. The patient should urinate before taking this drug to reduce the risk of urine retention. BP; ECG for cardiac changes; blood glucose; liver enzyme and serum alkaline phosphatase, bilirubin, and potassium should be assessed.
Storage
Store at room temperature. A compounded oral suspension is stable for 4 wks refrigerated in an amber glass bottle.
Administration
Dosage must be individualized. Do not chew or break extended-release capsules. For children, the manufacturer provides for an oral suspension that may be compounded from immediate-release capsules. Shake well before each use.

Disulfiram
die-sul'fi-ram
★ Antabuse

CATEGORY AND SCHEDULE
Pregnancy Risk Category: C

Classification: Substance abuse agents, alcohol deterrent

MECHANISM OF ACTION

A thiuram derivative and an irreversible aldehyde dehydrogenase inhibitor. When taken with alcohol, there is an increase in serum acetaldehyde levels. *Therapeutic Effect:* Produces an acute sensitivity to alcohol.

PHARMACOKINETICS

Slowly absorbed from the GI tract. Metabolized in liver. Primarily excreted in urine. Up to 20% of dose remains in body for at least 1 wk. *Half-life:* Unknown.

AVAILABILITY

Tablets: 250 mg, 500 mg

INDICATIONS AND DOSAGES

▸ **Adjunct in management of selected chronic alcoholic patients who want to remain in state of enforced sobriety**

PO

Adults, Elderly. Initially, administer maximum of 500 mg daily given as a single dose for 1-2 wks. Maintenance: 250 mg daily (normal range: 125-500 mg). Do not exceed maximum daily dose of 500 mg.

CONTRAINDICATIONS

Severe heart disease, psychosis, hypersensitivity to disulfiram or any component of the formulation; patients receiving or using ethanol, metronidazole, paraldehyde, or ethanol-containing products.

DRUG INTERACTIONS

Alcohol, alcohol-containing syrups, elixirs, solutions: Increased disulfiram reaction Contraindicated.
Long-acting benzodiazepines: Increased central nervous system (CNS) depression.
Metronidazole (do not use), tricyclic antidepressants: Risk of psychosis.
Phenytoin: Increased phenytoin levels.
Isoniazid: May increase neurotoxicity.
Warfarin: Increased anticoagulant effect. Monitor INR.
CYP2C9 substrates: Disulfiram inhibits metabolism of these drugs.
Food
Alcohol-containing extracts, vinegars, ciders, foods: Increased disulfiram reaction.

DIAGNOSTIC TEST EFFECTS

Increased liver enzymes.

SIDE EFFECTS/ADVERSE REACTIONS

Frequent
Drowsiness.
Occasional
Headache, restlessness, optic neuritis (impaired color perception, altered vision), peripheral neuropathy, metallic or garlic taste, rash.

SERIOUS REACTIONS

- Disulfiram-alcohol reactions to ingestion of alcohol in any form include flushing/throbbing in head and neck, throbbing headache, nausea, copious vomiting, diaphoresis, dyspnea, hyperventilation, tachycardia, hypotension, marked uneasiness, vertigo, blurred vision, confusion, and death.
- Hepatitis and hepatic failure occur rarely.

PRECAUTIONS & CONSIDERATIONS

Never administer to patient in state of alcohol intoxication or without patient's full knowledge. Do not administer until patient has abstained from alcohol for at least 12 h. Fully inform patient of the disulfiram-alcohol reaction. Advise patients to avoid all alcohol-containing products, including mouthwashes, OTC products, and skin products. Use with caution in patients with diabetes mellitus, hypothyroidism, seizure disorders, cerebral damage, chronic or acute nephritis, or hepatic disease. Safety and effectiveness have not been established in children. Unique precautions have not been observed in the elderly. Not known if excreted in breast milk; do not breastfeed.

Storage

Store at room temperature.

Administration

May be taken in the evening if causes sedation. Tablets may be crushed and mixed with water or juice.

Dobutamine

doe-byoo′ta-meen

Do not confuse dobutamine with Dopamine.

CATEGORY AND SCHEDULE

Pregnancy Risk Category: B

Classification: Adrenergic agonists, inotropes

MECHANISM OF ACTION

A direct-acting inotropic agent acting primarily on β_2-adrenergic receptors. *Therapeutic Effect:* Decreases preload and afterload, and enhances myocardial contractility, stroke volume, and cardiac output. Improves renal blood flow and urine output indirectly.

PHARMACOKINETICS

Route	Onset	Peak	Duration
IV	1-2 min	10 min	Length of infusion

Metabolized in the liver and tissues. Primarily excreted in urine. Not removed by hemodialysis. *Half-life:* 2 min.

AVAILABILITY

Injection (Premix with Dextrose): 1000 mg/250 mL, 250 mg/250 mL, 250 mg/500 mL, 500 mg/250 mL, 500 mg/500 mL.

Injection: 12.5-mg/mL vial.

INDICATIONS AND DOSAGES

▸ **Short-term management of cardiac decompensation**

IV INFUSION

Adults, Elderly, Children. 2.5-15 mcg/kg/min. Rarely, drug can be infused at a rate of up to 40 mcg/kg/min to increase cardiac output.

CONTRAINDICATIONS

Idiopathic hypertrophic subaortic stenosis, sulfite sensitivity.

INTERACTIONS

Drug

β-Blockers: May antagonize the effects of dobutamine.

Digoxin: May increase the risk of arrhythmias and enhance the inotropic effect of both drugs.

MAOIs, oxytocics, tricyclic antidepressants: May increase the adverse effects of dobutamine, such as arrhythmias and hypertension. MAOIs are contraindicated.

Herbal and Food

None known.

DIAGNOSTIC TEST EFFECTS

Decreases serum potassium level.

IV INCOMPATIBILITIES

Acyclovir (Zovirax), alteplase (Activase), aminophylline, amphotericin B cholesteryl (Amphotec), amphotericin B liposomal (AmBisome), ampicillin,

ampicillin/sulbactam (Unasyn), azathioprine, cefazolin, cefotetan (Cefotan), cefoxitin (Mefoxin), ceftriaxone (Rocephin), cefuroxime (Zinacef), chloramphenicol, dantrolene, dexamethasone sodium phosphate, ertapenem (Invanz), fluorouracil, folic acid, foscarnet (Foscavir), ganciclovir, hydrocortisone sodium succinate (Solu-Cortef), indomethacin, ketorolac, lansoprazole (Prevacid), methicillin, methotrexate, micafungin (Mycamine), oxacillin, pantoprazole (Protonix), pemetrexed (Alimta), penicillin G potassium, penicillin G sodium, pentobarbital, phenobarbital, phenytoin, piperacillin, piperacillin/tazobactam (Zosyn), sodium bicarbonate, sulfamethoxazole/trimethoprim, ticarcillin (Ticar), ticarcillin/clavulanate (Timentin), warfarin.

IV COMPATIBILITIES

Alfentanil (Alfenta), alprostadil (Prostin VR), amifostine (Ethyol), amikacin (Amikar), amiodarone (Cordarone), anidulafungin (Eraxis), argatroban, ascorbic acid, atracurium (Tracrium), atropine, aztreonam (Azactam), benztropine (Cogentin), bretylium, buprenorphine (Buprenex), butorphanol (Stadol), calcium chloride, carboplatin, caspofungin (Cancidas), chlorpromazine, cimetidine (Tagamet), ciprofloxacin (Cipro), cisatracurium (Nimbex), cisplatin, cladribine (Leustatin), clonidine, cyanocobalamin, cyclophosphamide (Cytoxan), cyclosporine (Sandimmune), dactinomycin (Cosmegen), daptomycin (Cubicin), dexmedetomidine (Precedex), digoxin (Lanoxin), diltiazem (Cardizem), diphenhydramine (Benadryl), docetaxel (Taxotere), doxorubicin (Adriamycin), doxorubicin liposomal (Doxil), enalaprilat, ephedrine, epinephrine, epirubicin (Ellence), erythromycin lactobionate, etoposide phosphate (Etopophos), famotidine (Pepcid), fenoldopam (Corlopam), fentanyl (Sublimaze), fluconazole (Diflucan), fludarabine (Fludara), gemcitabine (Gemzar), gentamicin, granisetron (Kytril), hydromorphone (Dilaudid), hydroxyzine, isoproterenol (Isuprel), labetalol, levofloxacin (Levaquin), lidocaine, linezolid (Zyvox), lorazepam (Ativan), mannitol, meperidine (Demerol), methylprednisolone sodium succinate, metoclopramide (Reglan), metoprolol (Lopressor), milrinone (Primacor), minocycline (Minocin), mitoxantrone (Novantrone), morphine, nafcillin, nalbuphine (Nubain), naloxone (Narcan), nicardipine (Cardene), nitroglycerin, norepinephrine (Levophed), ondansetron (Zofran), oxaliplatin (Eloxatin), oxytocin (Pitocin), paclitaxel (Taxol), palonosetron (Aloxi), pancuronium, potassium chloride, procainamide, prochlorperazine, promethazine, propofol (Diprivan), propranolol, ranitidine (Zantac), remifentanil (Ultiva), rituximab (Rituxan), sodium acetate, streptokinase, succinylcholine, sufentanil (Sufenta), tacrolimus (Prograf), teniposide (Vumon), theophylline, thiotepa (Thioplex), tigecycline (Tygacil), tirofibran (Aggrastat), tobramycin, trastuzumab (Herceptin), vancomycin, vasopressin, vecuronium (Norcuron), verapamil, vincristine (Vincasar), vinorelbine (Navelbine), voriconazole (Vfend), zidovudine (Retrovir).

SIDE EFFECTS

Frequent (> 5%)
Increased heart rate, increased BP.

Occasional (3%-5%)
Pain at injection site, phlebitis.
Rare (1%-3%)
Nausea, headache, anginal pain, shortness of breath, fever.

SERIOUS REACTIONS

- Overdose may produce a marked increase in heart rate (by 30 beats/min or higher), marked increase in BP (by 50 mm Hg or higher), anginal pain, and premature ventricular contractions (PVCs).
- May cause hypotension in some patients. Tachycardia, marked increases in BP, or ventricular ectopy may occur.

PRECAUTIONS & CONSIDERATIONS

Caution is warranted in patients with atrial fibrillation, aortic stenosis, hypovolemia, post-myocardial infarction, and hypertension. Hypovolemia should be corrected with volume expanders. It is unknown whether dobutamine crosses the placenta or is distributed in breast milk; therefore, it is not administered to pregnant women. No age-related precautions have been noted in children or in elderly patients. Start at lower end of dosage range for elderly patients.

Notify the physician of chest pain or palpitations during infusion or pain or burning at the IV site. Cardiac monitoring should be performed continuously to check for arrhythmias. BP, heart rate, urine output, and respiration should be checked before and during treatment. Serum potassium and dobutamine plasma levels should be monitored; keep in mind that dobutamine's therapeutic range is 40-190 ng/mL.

Storage
Store at room temperature because freezing produces crystallization. Pink discoloration of the solution, caused by oxidation, does not indicate loss of potency if the solution is used within the recommended period. Further diluted solution for infusion must be used within 24 h.

Pre-mix infusion stored at room temperature in overwrap until time of use; do not freeze.

Administration
! Dobutamine dosage is determined by the patient's response to the drug. Plan to correct hypovolemia with volume expanders before dobutamine infusion. Expect to administer digoxin to patients with atrial fibrillation before infusion. Administer by IV infusion only.

For IV use, Further dilute the injection concentrate with either D5W or 0.9% NaCl. Usual final concentrations are 2000 mcg/mL or 4000 mcg/mL. Maximum should not exceed 5000 mcg/mL. Infuse into a large vein. Also available in pre-mixed solutions for infusion.

During CPR, may be infused via the intraosseous route if IV is not available. Use infusion pump to control flow rate. Titrate dosage to individual response, as prescribed.

Docosanol

do-cos'ah-nole
Abreva

CATEGORY AND SCHEDULE

Pregnancy Risk Category: B
OTC

Classification: Topical antiviral

MECHANISM OF ACTION

A highly lipophilic, fatty alcohol that prevents fusion of lipid-enveloped viruses with cell membranes, thereby blocking viral replication.

PHARMACOKINETICS

Topical: Negligible absorption.

AVAILABILITY
Cream: 10%.

INDICATIONS AND DOSAGES
▸ **Recurrent herpes labialis**
TOPICAL
Adult, Children older than 12 yr.
Apply a small amount to the affected area on the face or lips or at the first sign of lesion 5 times a day until healed.

CONTRAINDICATIONS
Hypersensitivity.

INTERACTIONS
Drug
None reported.

SIDE EFFECTS
CNS: Headache.
Integument: Site reaction, rash, pruritus, dry skin, acne.

PRECAUTIONS & CONSIDERATIONS
Avoid application into eyes or mouth; for external use only. Not for use in children less than 12 yr of age.
Storage
Store at room temperature. Do not freeze.
Administration
Wash hands before and after use.

Docusate
dok'yoo-sate
Colace, Correctol, Diocto, Doc-Q-Lace, DOK, Kao-Tin, Phillips' Stool Softener, Silace, Sur-Q-Lax

CATEGORY AND SCHEDULE
Pregnancy Risk Category: C
OTC

Classification: Laxatives, stool softeners

MECHANISM OF ACTION
A laxative that decreases surface film tension by mixing liquid and bowel contents. *Therapeutic Effect:* Increases infiltration of liquid to form a softer stool.

PHARMACOKINETICS
Minimal absorption from the GI tract. Acts in small and large intestines. Results usually occur 1-2 days after first dose but may take 3-5 days.

AVAILABILITY
Capsules (Docusate Sodium; Colace, DOK): 50 mg, 100 mg, 250 mg.
Capsules, Liquid Filled (Correctol, Doc-Q-Lace, Phillips'): 100 mg.
Capsules (Docusate Calcium; Sur-Q-Lax): 240 mg.
Capsules, Liquid Filled (Docusate Calcium; Kao-Tin: 240 mg.
Syrup (Colace, Diocto): 50 mg/5 mL, 60 mg/15 mL, 20 mg/5 mL *(Silace).*

INDICATIONS AND DOSAGES
▸ **Stool softener**
PO
Adults, Elderly, Children 12 yr and older. 50-300 mg/day in 1-4 divided doses.
Children 6-11 yr. 40-150 mg/day in 1-4 divided doses.
Children 3-5 yr. 20-60 mg/day in 1-4 divided doses.
Children younger than 3 yr. 10-40 mg/day in 1-4 divided doses.

CONTRAINDICATIONS
Acute abdominal pain, concomitant use of mineral oil, intestinal obstruction, nausea, vomiting, hypersensitivity.

INTERACTIONS
Drug
Mineral oil: May increase the absorption of mineral oil.
Herbal and Food
None known.

DIAGNOSTIC TEST EFFECTS
None known.

SIDE EFFECTS
Occasional
Mild GI cramping, throat irritation (with liquid preparation), diarrhea.
Rare
Rash.

SERIOUS REACTIONS
• None known.

PRECAUTIONS & CONSIDERATIONS
It is unknown whether docusate is distributed in breast milk, considered compatible with breastfeeding. No age-related precautions have been noted in elderly patients.

Notify the physician if unrelieved constipation, dizziness, muscle cramps or pain, rectal bleeding, or weakness occurs. Maintain adequate fluid intake. Monitor pattern of daily bowel activity and stool consistency.
Storage
Store at room temperature. Protect capsules from moisture.
Administration
Drink 6-8 glasses of water a day to aid in stool softening. Take each dose with full glass of water or fruit juice. Administer docusate liquid with infant formula, fruit juice, or milk to mask the bitter taste. To promote defecation, increase fluid intake, exercise, and eat a high-fiber diet.

Dofetilide
doe-fet′ill-ide
★ Tikosyn

CATEGORY AND SCHEDULE
Pregnancy Risk Category: C

Classification: Antiarrhythmics, class III

MECHANISM OF ACTION
A selective potassium channel blocker that prolongs repolarization without affecting conduction velocity by blocking one or more time-dependent potassium currents. Dofetilide has no effect on sodium channels or adrenergic α or β receptors. *Therapeutic Effect:* Terminates reentrant tachyarrhythmias, preventing reinduction.

AVAILABILITY
Capsules: 125 mcg, 250 mcg, 500 mcg.

INDICATIONS AND DOSAGES
▸ Maintain normal sinus rhythm after conversion from atrial fibrillation or flutter
NOTE: Patient must be hospitalized during the initial treatment period.
PO
Adults, Elderly. Individualized using a seven-step dosing algorithm dependent on calculated creatinine clearance and QT-interval measurements. See prescribing information. Usual range: 125-500 mcg twice daily. Maximum: 500 mcg twice daily.
▸ Starting dosage in renal impairment
CrCl > 60 mL/min: 500 mcg twice a day.
CrCl 40-60 mL/min: 250 mcg twice a day.
CrCl 20-39 mL/min: 125 mcg twice a day.
CrCl < 20 mL/min: Do not use.

CONTRAINDICATIONS
Hypersensitivity to dofetilide; concurrent use of drugs that prolong the QT interval; concurrent use of amiodarone, cimetidine, hydrochlorothiazide, megestrol, metformin, prochlorperazine, trimethoprim, or verapamil;

congenital or acquired prolonged QT syndrome; paroxysmal atrial fibrillation; severe renal impairment.

INTERACTIONS

Drug

Amiloride, megestrol, metformin, prochlorperazine, triamterene: May increase plasma levels of dofetilide. Contraindicated.

Bepridil, phenothiazines, tricyclic antidepressants, other QT-interval prolonging agents: May prolong the QT interval.

Cimetidine, verapamil: Increases levels of dofetilide. Contraindicated.

Diuretics, drugs that deplete potassium or magnesium: May increase dofetilide toxicity. Hydrochlorothiazide contraindicated.

Ketoconazole, itraconazole, trimethoprim: Increase plasma concentration of dofetilide. Contraindicated.

Food

Grapefruit juice: Can increase dofetilide plasma levels.

DIAGNOSTIC TEST EFFECTS

None known.

SIDE EFFECTS

Occasional (< 15%)

Headache, chest pain, dizziness, dyspnea, nausea, insomnia, back and abdominal pain, diarrhea, rash.

SERIOUS REACTIONS

- Angioedema, bradycardia, cerebral ischemia, facial paralysis, and serious ventricular arrhythmias or various forms of heart block may be noted.

PRECAUTIONS & CONSIDERATIONS

Continuous cardiac and BP monitoring should be instituted. ECG for ventricular arrhythmias and for prolongation of the QT interval and serum creatinine level for changes should be monitored. Patients must have continuous ECG monitoring for 3 days, and drug should be initiated in hospital setting. Should reserve dofetilide for symptomatic atrial fibrillation/flutter. Avoid in patients with 2nd- or 3rd-degree heart block or sinus sick syndrome. Correct electrolyte imbalances before and during dofetilide therapy. Caution is warranted in hepatic and renal impairment. Safety and efficacy have not been evaluated in children. Notify the physician if dizziness, severe diarrhea, or other adverse effects occur.

Storage

Store at room temperature, tightly closed. Protect from moisture/humidity.

Administration

! Expect patient to be hospitalized for a minimum of 3 days when treatment is instituted. Administer dofetilide at the same times each day without regard to food. Follow dosing instructions diligently. Continuous cardiac monitoring is essential at the initiation of treatment.

If dofetilide needs to be discontinued to allow for dosing of potentially interacting drugs, a 2-day washout period should be followed before starting the other drug.

Dolasetron

doe-lass'eh-tron

★ 🍁 Anzemet

Do not confuse Anzemet with Aldomet.

CATEGORY AND SCHEDULE

Pregnancy Risk Category: B

Classification: Antiemetics, serotonin receptor antagonists

MECHANISM OF ACTION
A 5-HT3 receptor antagonist that acts centrally in the chemoreceptor trigger zone and peripherally at the vagal nerve terminals. *Therapeutic Effect:* Prevents nausea and vomiting.

PHARMACOKINETICS
Readily absorbed from the GI tract after PO administration. Protein binding: 69%-77%. Metabolized in the liver. Primarily excreted in urine. Unknown if removed by hemodialysis. *Half-life:* 5-10 h.

AVAILABILITY
Tablets: 50 mg, 100 mg.
Injection: 20 mg/mL in single-use 0.625-mL amps, 0.625-mL fill-in 2-mL Carpuject and 5-mL vials.

INDICATIONS AND DOSAGES
▸ **Prevention of chemotherapy-induced nausea and vomiting**
PO
Adults. 100 mg within 1 h of chemotherapy.
Children 2-16 yr. 1.8 mg/kg within 1 h of chemotherapy. Maximum: 100 mg.
IV
Adults, Children 2-16 yr. 1.8 mg/kg as a single dose 30 min before chemotherapy. Maximum: 100 mg.
▸ **Treatment (IV) or prevention of postoperative nausea or vomiting (IV/PO)**
PO
Adults. 100 mg within 2 h of surgery.
Children 2-16 yr. 1.2 mg/kg within 2 h of surgery. Maximum: 100 mg.
IV
Adults. 12.5 mg 15 min before cessation of anesthesia or as soon as nausea occurs.
Children 2-16 yr. 0.35 mg/kg 15 min before cessation of anesthesia or as soon as nausea occurs. Maximum: 12.5 mg.

OFF-LABEL USES
Radiation therapy-induced nausea and vomiting.

CONTRAINDICATIONS
Hypersensitivity.

INTERACTIONS
Drug
Agents that cause QTc prolongation: Caution should be used with these agents.

DIAGNOSTIC TEST EFFECTS
May transiently increase AST (SGOT) and ALT (SGPT) levels.

IV INCOMPATIBILITIES
Amphotericin B liposomal (AmBisome), pantoprazole (Protonix).

IV COMPATIBILITIES
Azithromycin (Zithromax), bivalirudin (Angiomax), caspofungin (Cancidas), cefazolin, cefepime (Maxipime), cefotaxime (Claforan), cyclophosphamide (Cytoxan), daptomycin (Cubicin), dexmedetomidine (Precedex), doxorubicin (Adriamycin), epirubicin (Ellence), ertapenem (Invanz), fenoldopam (Corlopam), levofloxacin (Levaquin), linezolid (Zyvox), mannitol, meperidine (Demerol), oxaliplatin (Eloxatin), oxytocin (Pitocin), pemetrexed (Alimta), quinupristin/dalfopristin (Synercid), sodium acetate, tacrolimus (Prograf), tigecycline (Tygacil), tirofibran (Aggrastat), vecuronium (Norcuron), vincristine (Vincasar), voriconazole (Vfend).

SIDE EFFECTS
Frequent (4%-24%)
Headache, diarrhea, fatigue, hypotension.

Occasional (1%-5%)
Fever, dizziness, pruritus, bradycardia, tachycardia, hypertension, dyspepsia.

SERIOUS REACTIONS

- Overdose may produce a combination of central nervous system (CNS) stimulant and depressant effects.
- Changes in ECG intervals, including QT, have occurred within hours after IV administration and rarely lead to heart block or arrhythmia.

PRECAUTIONS & CONSIDERATIONS

Caution is warranted in patients with congenital prolonged QT interval syndrome, hypokalemia, hypomagnesemia, and prolonged cardiac conduction intervals. Caution should also be used with concurrent use of diuretics, because this can cause electrolyte disturbances, antiarrhythmics that may lead to prolonged QT interval, and high doses of anthracyclines. It is unknown whether dolasetron is distributed in breast milk. The safety and efficacy of this drug have not been established in children younger than 2 yr. No age-related precautions have been noted in elderly patients.

Storage
Store at room temperature and protect from light. After dilution, store IV for up to 24 h at room temperature or up to 48 h if refrigerated.

Administration
Do not cut, break, or chew film-coated tablets. For children aged 2-16 yr, the injection form may be mixed in apple or apple-grape juice and given orally, if needed; see children's oral dosage. May be at room temperature for 2 h.

For IV use, may administer undiluted or may dilute the injection in 0.9% NaCl, D5W, dextrose 5% in 0.45% NaCl, lactated Ringer's (LR) solution, D5LR, or 10% mannitol injection to 50 mL. Administer by IV push as rapidly as 100 mg/30 seconds or by intermittent or piggyback IV infusion over 15 min.

Donepezil

dah-nep'eh-zil
★ 🍁 Aricept
Do not confuse Aricept with Aciphex or Ascriptin.

CATEGORY AND SCHEDULE

Pregnancy Risk Category: C

Classification: Cholinesterase inhibitors

MECHANISM OF ACTION

A cholinesterase inhibitor that inhibits the enzyme acetylcholinesterase, thus increasing the concentration of acetylcholine at cholinergic synapses and enhancing cholinergic function in the central nervous system (CNS). *Therapeutic Effect:* Slows the progression of Alzheimer disease.

PHARMACOKINETICS

Well absorbed after PO administration. Protein binding: 96%. Extensively metabolized. Eliminated in urine and feces. *Half-life:* 70 h.

AVAILABILITY

Tablets: 5 mg, 10 mg, 23 mg.
Orally Disintegrating Tablets: 5 mg, 10 mg.

D

INDICATIONS AND DOSAGES

▸ **Alzheimer disease**

PO

Adults, Elderly. 5-10 mg/day as a single dose. If initial dose is 5 mg, do not increase to 10 mg for 4-6 wks. For patients with moderate to severe AD, after patient has received 10 mg/day for at least 3 mo, a dose of 23 mg/day may be initiated, if clinically warranted.

CONTRAINDICATIONS

History of hypersensitivity to donepezil or piperidine derivatives, acute jaundice, active GI bleeding.

INTERACTIONS

Drug

Anticholinergics: May decrease the effect of donepezil.

Cholinergic agonists, neuromuscular blockers, succinylcholine: May increase cholinergic effects.

Ketoconazole, quinidine, CYP3A4 inhibitors: May inhibit the metabolism of donepezil.

NSAIDs: Increase GI irritation. Monitor for GI bleeding.

Paroxetine, CYP2D6 inhibitors: May decrease the metabolism and increase the blood concentration of donepezil.

Herbal

None known.

Food

None known.

DIAGNOSTIC TEST EFFECTS

May increase blood glucose, alkaline phosphatase, and serum creatinine kinase and LDH concentrations. May decrease the serum potassium level.

SIDE EFFECTS

Frequent (8%-19%)

Nausea, diarrhea, headache, insomnia, nonspecific pain, dizziness, infection, anorexia.

Occasional (3%-6%)

Mild muscle cramps, fatigue, vomiting, ecchymosis.

Rare (2%-3%)

Depression, abnormal dreams, weight loss, hypertension, arthritis, somnolence, syncope, frequent urination.

SERIOUS REACTIONS

- Vagotonic effects may include bradycardia, heart block, and syncopal episodes.
- Overdose may result in cholinergic crisis, characterized by severe nausea, increased salivation, diaphoresis, bradycardia, hypotension, flushed skin, abdominal pain, respiratory depression, seizures, and cardiorespiratory collapse. Increasing muscle weakness may result in death if respiratory muscles are involved. The antidote is 1-2 mg IV atropine sulfate with subsequent doses based on therapeutic response.

PRECAUTIONS & CONSIDERATIONS

Caution is warranted with asthma; bladder outflow obstruction; prostatic hypertrophy; chronic obstructive pulmonary disease (COPD); peptic ulcer disease; history of seizures, sick sinus syndrome, or other supraventricular conduction disturbances (bradycardia); and concurrent use of NSAIDs. It is unknown whether donepezil is distributed in breast milk. Donepezil is not prescribed for children. No age-related precautions have been noted in elderly patients. Be aware that donepezil is not a cure for Alzheimer disease but may slow the progression of its symptoms. Safety and efficacy have not been evaluated in children.

Notify the physician if abdominal pain, diarrhea, excessive sweating or salivation, dizziness, or nausea and vomiting occur. Baseline vital signs should be assessed. Cholinergic reactions, such as diaphoresis, dizziness, excessive salivation, facial warmth, abdominal cramps or discomfort, lacrimation, pallor, and urinary urgency, should be monitored.

Storage

Store at room temperature. Keep ODT in package until time of use; gently remove from packaging with dry hands.

Administration

Take donepezil without regard to food. The drug may be given in the morning or evening; however, best results (limited side effects) may be achieved if it is given at bedtime. Allow orally disintegrating tablet to dissolve on tongue. It can be given with or without liquid.

Dopamine

doe′pa-meen

Do not confuse dopamine with dobutamine or Dopram.

CATEGORY AND SCHEDULE

Pregnancy Risk Category: C

Classification: Adrenergic agonists, inotropes

MECHANISM OF ACTION

A sympathomimetic (adrenergic agonist) that stimulates adrenergic receptors. Effects are dose dependent. Low dosages (0.5-2 mcg/kg/min) stimulate dopaminergic receptors, causing renal vasodilation. Low to moderate dosages (2-10 mcg/kg/min) have a positive inotropic effect by direct action and release of norepinephrine. High dosages (> 10 mcg/kg/min) stimulate α-receptors. *Therapeutic Effect:* With low dosages, increases renal blood flow, urine flow, and sodium excretion. With low to moderate dosages, increases myocardial contractility, stroke volume, and cardiac output. With high dosages, increases peripheral resistance, renal vasoconstriction, and systolic and diastolic BP.

PHARMACOKINETICS

Route	Onset	Peak	Duration
IV	1-2 min	N/A	< 10 min

Widely distributed. Does not cross blood-brain barrier. Metabolized in the liver, kidney, and plasma. Primarily excreted in urine. Not removed by hemodialysis. *Half-life:* 2 min.

AVAILABILITY

Injection: 40 mg/mL, 80 mg/mL, 160 mg/mL.

Injection (Premix with Dextrose): 200 mg/250 mL, 400 mg/250 mL, 400 mg/500 mL, 800 mg/250 mL, 800 mg/500 mL.

INDICATIONS AND DOSAGES

▸ **Treatment and prevention of acute hypotension; shock (associated with cardiac decompensation, myocardial infarction, open heart surgery, renal failure, or trauma); treatment of low cardiac output; treatment of congestive heart failure**

IV

Adults, Elderly. 1-5 mcg/kg/min up to 50 mcg/kg/min; titrate to desired response. Increase rate by 1-4 mcg/kg/min at 10- to 30-min intervals.

Children. 1-20 mcg/kg/min. Maximum: 20 mcg/kg/min. Rates > 20 mcg/kg/min in children and infants may result in excessive vasoconstriction.

Neonates. 1-20 mcg/kg/min.

D

CONTRAINDICATIONS

Pheochromocytoma, sulfite sensitivity, uncorrected tachyarrhythmias, ventricular fibrillation.

INTERACTIONS

Drug

β-Blockers: May decrease the effects of dopamine.
Digoxin: May increase the risk of arrhythmias.
Ergot alkaloids: May increase vasoconstriction.
MAOIs: May increase cardiac stimulation and vasopressor effects.
Tricyclic antidepressants, oxytocics: May increase cardiovascular effects.

Herbal and Food

None known.

DIAGNOSTIC TEST EFFECTS

None known.

IV INCOMPATIBILITIES

Acyclovir (Zovirax), amphotericin B cholesteryl (Amphotec), amphotericin B liposomal (AmBisome), ampicillin, azathioprine, cefazolin, cefepime (Maxipime), chloramphenicol, dantrolene, diazepam (Valium), ganciclovir (Cytovene), furosemide (Lasix), indomethacin, lansoprazole (Prevacid), methotrexate, phenytoin, sodium bicarbonate, sulfamethoxazole/trimethoprim.

IV COMPATIBILITIES

Alfentanil (Alfenta), alprostadil (Prostin VR), amifostine (Ethyol), amikacin (Amikar), aminophylline, amiodarone (Cordarone), anidulafungin (Eraxis), argatroban, ascorbic acid, atracurium (Tracrium), atropine, aztreonam (Azactam), benztropine (Cogentin), bivalirudin (Angiomax), bretylium, bumetanide (Bumex), buprenorphine (Buprenex), butorphanol (Stadol), calcium chloride, calcium gluconate, carboplatin, caspofungin (Cancidas), cefotaxime (Claforan), cefotetan (Cefotan), cefoxitin (Mefoxin), ceftazidime (Ceptaz, Fortaz, Tazicef, Tazidime), ceftizoxime (Cefizox), ceftriaxone (Rocephin), cefuroxime (Zinacef), chlorpromazine, cimetidine (Tagamet), ciprofloxacin (Cipro), cisatracurium (Nimbex), cisplatin, clindamycin (Cleocin), clonidine, cyclophosphamide (Cytoxan), cyclosporine (Sandimmune), dactinomycin (Cosmegen), daptomycin (Cubicin), dexamethasone sodium phosphate, dexmedetomidine (Precedex), digoxin (Lanoxin), diltiazem (Cardizem), diphenhydramine (Benadryl), dobutamine (Dobutrex), docetaxel (Taxotere), doripenem (Doribax), doxorubicin (Adriamycin), doxorubicin liposomal (Doxil), droperidol, enalaprilat, ephedrine, epinephrine, epirubicin (Ellence), epoetin alfa (Procrit), ertapenem (Invanz), erythromycin lactobionate, esmolol (Brevibloc), etoposide phosphate (Etopophos), famotidine (Pepcid), fenoldopam (Corlopam), fentanyl (Sublimaze), fluconazole (Diflucan), fludarabine (Fludara), fluorouracil, folic acid, foscarnet (Foscavir), gemcitabine (Gemzar), gentamicin, granisetron (Kytril), heparin, hydrocortisone sodium phosphate, hydrocortisone sodium succinate (Solu-Cortef), hydromorphone (Dilaudid), hydroxyzine, imipenem/cilastatin (Primaxin), isoproterenol (Isuprel), ketorolac, labetalol, levofloxacin (Levaquin), lidocaine, linezolid (Zyvox), lorazepam (Ativan), magnesium sulfate, mannitol, meperidine (Demerol), methicillin, methylprednisolone (Solu-Medrol), metoclopramide (Reglan), metoprolol (Lopressor), micafungin (Mycamine), midazolam (Versed), milrinone (Primacor), minocycline (Minocin), mitoxantrone (Novantrone), morphine, nafcillin, nalbuphine (Nubain), naloxone (Narcan), nicardipine (Cardene), nitroglycerin, nitroprusside sodium (Nitropress), norepinephrine (Levophed), ondansetron (Zofran), oxacillin, oxaliplatin (Eloxatin), oxytocin (Pitocin), paclitaxel (Taxol), palonosetron (Aloxi), pancuronium, pemetrexed (Alimta), penicillin G sodium, pentobarbital, phenobarbital, piperacillin, piperacillin/tazobactam (Zosyn), potassium chloride, procainamide, prochloperazine, promethazine, propofol (Diprivan), propranolol, ranitidine (Zantac), remifentanil (Ultiva), rituximab (Rituxan), sargramostim (Leukine), sodium acetate, streptokinase, succinylcholine, sufentanil (Sufenta), tacrolimus (Prograf), teniposide (Vumon), theophylline, thiotepa (Thioplex), ticarcillin (Ticar), ticarcillin/clavulanate (Timentin), tigecycline (Tygacil), tirofibran (Aggrastat), tobramycin, trastuzumab (Herceptin), vancomycin, vasopressin, vecuronium (Norcuron), verapamil, vincristine (Vincasar), vinorelbine (Navelbine), vitamin B complex with C, voriconazole (Vfend), warfarin, zidovudine (Retrovir).

SIDE EFFECTS

Frequent

Headache, ectopic beats, tachycardia, anginal pain, palpitations, vasoconstriction, hypotension, nausea, vomiting, dyspnea.

Occasional

Piloerection or goose bumps, bradycardia, widening of QRS complex.

SERIOUS REACTIONS

- High doses may produce ventricular arrhythmias, tachycardia.
- Patients with occlusive vascular disease are at high risk for further compromise of circulation to the extremities, which may result in gangrene.
- Tissue necrosis with sloughing may occur with extravasation of IV solution.

PRECAUTIONS & CONSIDERATIONS

Caution is warranted in patients with ischemic heart disease, cardiac arrhythmias, post-myocardial infarction, and occlusive vascular disease. Be aware that dopamine dosage may have to be reduced if MAOIs were taken within the last 2-3 wks. It is unknown whether dopamine crosses the placenta or is distributed in breast milk. Closely monitor children, because gangrene attributable to extravasation has been reported. No age-related precautions have been noted in elderly patients.

Cardiac monitoring should be performed continuously to check for arrhythmias. BP, heart rate, urine output, and respiration should be checked before and during treatment. Notify the physician of chest pain, palpitations, arrhythmias, decreased peripheral circulation (marked by cold, pale, or mottled extremities), decreased urine output, or significant changes in BP or heart rate, or burning at the IV site.

Storage

Unopened vials are stored at room temperature.

Dopamine is stable for 24 h after dilution. Do not use solutions darker than slightly yellow or solutions that have discolored to brown or pink to purple, because

D

these discolorations indicate decomposition of drug.

Store pre-mix bags at room temperature in original overwrap. Do not freeze.

Administration

! Expect to correct blood volume depletion before administering dopamine. Blood volume replacement may occur simultaneously with dopamine infusion.

For IV use, dilute 200-400 mg vial in 250-500 mL 0.9% NaCl, D5W/0.45% NaCl, D5W/lactated Ringer's, or lactated Ringer's. Keep in mind that the concentration is dependent on the dosage and the patient's fluid requirements. Remember that a 200 mg/250 mL solution yields 800 mcg/mL and that a 200 mg/500 mL solution yields 400 mcg/mL. The maximum infusion concentration is 3200 mcg/mL. The drug is available prediluted in 250 or 500 mL of D5W. Administer into large vein, such as the antecubital or subclavian vein, to prevent drug extravasation. Use an infusion pump to control rate of flow. Titrate dosage to the desired hemodynamic values or optimum urine flow, as prescribed. If extravasation occurs, immediately infiltrate the affected tissue with 10-15 mL 0.9% NaCl solution containing 5-10 mg phentolamine mesylate, as ordered.

During CPR, if IV is not available, may be administered by intraosseous infusion.

Doripenem

dor-i-pen′em

Doribax

CATEGORY AND SCHEDULE

Pregnancy Risk Category: B

Classification: Antibiotics, carbapenems

MECHANISM OF ACTION

A carbapenem that penetrates the bacterial cell wall of microorganisms and binds to penicillin-binding proteins, inhibiting cell wall synthesis. Good activity against methicillin-sensitive gram-positive and gram-negative nonbetalactamase-forming bacteria, with good activity against *Pseudomonas* species. *Therapeutic Effect:* Produces bacterial cell death.

PHARMACOKINETICS

Widely distributed into most body fluids and tissues, including bile, gallbladder, peritoneal and retroperitoneal fluid, and urine. Plasma protein binding: 8.1%. Minimally metabolized to an inactive metabolite (doripenem-M1) via dehydropeptidase-I. Primarily excreted unchanged by kidneys into the urine. Removed (52%) by hemodialysis. *Half-life:* 1 h (increased with renal impairment).

AVAILABILITY

Injection Powder for Reconstitution: 500 mg.

INDICATIONS AND DOSAGE

▸ Complicated intra-abdominal infection or complicated UTI (e.g., pyelonephritis)

IV INFUSION

Adults, Elderly. 500 mg every 8 h.

▸ Dosage in renal impairment (adults)

CrCl > 50 mL/min	No change
CrCl 30-50 mL/min	250 mg q8h IV
CrCl 11-29 mL/min	250 mg q12h IV
CrCl < 10 mL/min or ESRD with dialysis	Insufficient data for recommendations

CONTRAINDICATIONS
History of hypersensitivity to doripenem or other carbapenems (imipenem, meropenem, ertapenem) or anaphylaxis to β-lactams.

INTERACTIONS
Drug
Probenecid: Reduces renal excretion by interfering with active tubular secretion of doripenem, increases concentration. Avoid co-use.
Valproic acid: Reduces serum levels of valproic acid. Monitor levels and adjust dose.
Herbal and Food
None known.

DIAGNOSTIC TEST EFFECTS
May increase AST (SGOT) and ALT (SGPT) levels. May decrease platelet count, WBC count, and serum potassium level.

IV INCOMPATIBILITIES
The manufacturer recommends that doripenem not be mixed with or added to solutions containing other drugs. Known Y-site incompatibilities include amphotericin B (conventional and liposomal forms), diazepam (Valium), phenytoin, potassium phosphates, propofol (Diprivan).

SIDE EFFECTS
Frequent (≥ 5%)
Headache, nausea, diarrhea, rash, infused vein complications (phlebitis); anemia.
Occasional (2%-5%)
Pruritus, hepatic enzyme elevation.
Rare (< 2%)
Dizziness, insomnia, oral or vulva or vaginal candidiasis, colitis.

SERIOUS REACTIONS
- Antibiotic-associated colitis [e.g., *Clostridium dificile* associated diarrhea (CDAD)] and other superinfections may occur.
- Anaphylactic reactions have been reported.
- Serious skin rashes, such as Stevens-Johnson syndrome.
- Seizures may occur in those with central nervous system (CNS) disorders (including patients with brain lesions or a history of seizures), bacterial meningitis, or severe renal impairment, but seizures are more rare with doripenem versus other drugs in the carbapenem class.
- Inhalation of the drug has caused pneumonitis; interstitial pneumonitis reported with infusional use very rarely.

PRECAUTIONS & CONSIDERATIONS
Caution is warranted with CNS disorders (particularly with brain lesions or history of seizures), renal impairment or end-stage renal disease, or a hypersensitivity to cephalosporins, penicillins, or other β-lactams. It is not known if doripenem is distributed in breast milk. There are no adequate studies in pregnancy. Be aware that the safety and efficacy have not been established in children. In elderly patients, age-related renal dysfunction may prompt dosage adjustment.

History of allergies, particularly to β-lactams, cephalosporins, and penicillins, should be obtained before beginning drug therapy. Hydration status, nausea, vomiting, skin (for rash), sleep pattern, and mental status should be evaluated. Report any diarrhea, rash, seizures, tremors, or other new symptoms.
Storage
Store vials at room temperature. Constituted vials may be held for up to 1 h prior to further dilution in the infusion bag. Diluted infusion solutions are stable for up to

12 h in 0.9% NaCl or 4 h in D5W at room temperature OR under refrigeration for up to 72 h in 0.9% NaCl or 24 h in D5W. Do not freeze.

Administration

For IV infusion only. For IV use, first dilute 500-mg vial with 10 mL of sterile water for injection or 0.9% NaCl. Gently shake to form an even suspension. Must be diluted further before infusion. Further dilute with 100 mL 0.9% NaCl or D5W for a 500-mg dose. Shake the bag gently until clear. Final concentration is 4.5 mg/mL. For a 250-mg dose, the manufacturer recommends preparing the 500-mg infusion as listed, then removing 55 mL from the 500-mg infusion bag to make the 250-mg dose. Give doses by intermittent IV infusion (piggyback). Do not give IV push. Infuse over 1 h (60 min).

Dornase Alfa

door′nace al′fa

Pulmozyme

CATEGORY AND SCHEDULE

Pregnancy Risk Category: B

Classification: Enzymes, respiratory, recombinant DNA origin

MECHANISM OF ACTION

An enzyme that selectively splits and hydrolyzes DNA in sputum. *Therapeutic Effect:* Reduces sputum viscosity and elasticity.

AVAILABILITY

Inhalation: 2.5-mg ampules for nebulization.

INDICATIONS AND DOSAGES

▸ To improve management of pulmonary function in patients with cystic fibrosis

NEBULIZATION

Adults, Children 3 mo and older. 2.5 mg (1 ampule) once daily by recommended nebulizer. May increase to 2.5 mg twice daily.

CONTRAINDICATIONS

Sensitivity to dornase alfa.

INTERACTIONS

Drug, Herbal, and Food

None known.

DIAGNOSTIC TEST EFFECTS

None known.

SIDE EFFECTS

Frequent (> 10%)

Pharyngitis, fever, rhinitis, dyspnea, chest pain or discomfort, voice changes.

Occasional (3%-10%)

Conjunctivitis, hoarseness, rash.

SERIOUS REACTIONS

- None significant.

PRECAUTIONS & CONSIDERATIONS

Hoarseness, chest pain, and sore throat may occur during dornase alfa therapy. Viscosity of pulmonary secretions should be checked. Drink plenty of fluids. Use in children < 5 yr is limited.

Storage

Refrigerate unopened ampules and protect them from light. Keep in foil pouch until ready to use.

Administration

For nebulization, do not mix any other medications in the nebulizer with dornase alfa.

Doxapram

dox'a-pram

Dopram

Do not confuse doxapram with doxepin or Ultram.

CATEGORY AND SCHEDULE

Pregnancy Risk Category: B

Classification: Analeptics, stimulants, central nervous system (CNS)

MECHANISM OF ACTION

A CNS stimulant that directly stimulates the respiratory center in the medulla or indirectly by effects on the carotid. *Therapeutic Effect:* Increases pulmonary ventilation by increasing resting minute ventilation, tidal volume, respiratory frequency, and inspiratory neuromuscular drive and enhances the ventilatory response to carbon dioxide.

PHARMACOKINETICS

IV onset 20-40, peak 1-2 min, duration 5-12 min. Metabolized in the liver to metabolites, ketodoxapram (active), and desethyldoxapram (inactive). Partially excreted in the urine. Not removed by hemodialysis. *Half-life:* 2.4-9.9 h.

AVAILABILITY

Injection: 20 mg/mL (Dopram).

INDICATIONS AND DOSAGES

▸ **Chronic obstructive pulmonary disease (COPD)**

IV INFUSION

Adults, Elderly, Children older than 12 yr. Initially, 1-2 mg/min. Maximum: 3 g/day for no more than 2 h.

▸ **Drug-induced CNS depression**

IV INJECTION

Adults, Elderly, Children older than 12 yr. Initially, 1-2 mg/kg, repeat after 5 min. May repeat at 1- to 2-h intervals, until sustained consciousness. Maximum: 3 g/day.

IV INFUSION

Adults, Elderly, Children older than 12 yr. Initially, bolus dose of 1-2 mg/kg, repeat after 5 min. If no response, wait 1-2 h and repeat. If stimulation is noted, initiate infusion at 1-3 mg/min. Infusion should not be continued for more than 2 h. Maximum: 3 g/day.

▸ **Respiratory depression following anesthesia**

IV INJECTION

Adults, Elderly, Children older than 12 yr. Initially, 0.5-1 mg/kg. May repeat at 5-min intervals in patients who demonstrate initial response. Maximum: 2 mg/kg.

IV INFUSION

Adults, Elderly, Children older than 12 yr. Initially, 5 mg/min until adequate response or adverse effects are seen. Decrease to 1-3 mg/min. Maximum: 4 mg/kg.

OFF-LABEL USES

Sleep apnea, post-anesthetic shivering.

CONTRAINDICATIONS

Convulsive disorders, cardiovascular impairment, cerebral edema, head injury or cerebrovascular accident, severe hypertension, pulmonary embolism, mechanical ventilation disorders, hypersensitivity to doxapram.

INTERACTIONS

Drug

Cyclopropane, enflurane, halothane: May increase catecholamine release. Delay the

initiation of doxapram therapy for at least 10 min following discontinuation of these anesthetics known to sensitize the myocardium.
CNS-stimulant medications: May increase risk of stimulation to excessive levels, causing nervousness, insomnia, irritability, or possibly cardiac arrhythmias or seizures.
MAOIs, sympathomimetic agents: May increase the pressor effects of these medications or doxapram.
Herbal
None known.
Food
None known.

DIAGNOSTIC TEST EFFECTS
May decrease hemoglobin, hematocrit, or red blood cell counts. May further decrease WBC in the presence of preexisting leukopenia. May increase BUN and albuminuria.

IV INCOMPATIBILITIES
Alkaline solutions, aminophylline, ascorbic acid, cefotaxime (Claforan), cefotetan (Cefotan), cefuroxime (Zinacef), clindamycin (Cleocin), dexamethasone sodium phosphate, diazepam (Valium), digoxin, dobutamine, folic acid, furosemide (Lasix), hydrocortisone sodium succinate (Solu-Cortef), ketamine (Ketalar), methylprednisolone, minocycline (Minocin), sodium bicarbonate, thiopental (Pentothal), ticarcillin (Ticar).

IV COMPATIBILITIES
Amikacin (Amikin), ampicillin, bumetanide (Bumex), caffeine citrate (Cafcit), calcium chloride, calcium gluconate, cefazolin, ceftazidime (Fortaz), chlorpromazine, cimetidine (Tagamet), cisplatin, cyclophosphamide (Cytosar), deslanoside, dopamine, doxycycline (Doxy-100), epinephrine, erythromycin lactobionate, fentanyl (Sublimaze), gentamicin, heparin, insulin (regular, Humulin R, Novolin R), hydroxyzine, isoniazid (Nydrazid), lincomycin (Lincocin), methotrexate, metoclopramide (Reglan), metronidazole (Flagyl), oxacillin, phenobarbital, phytonadione, pyridoxine, ranitidine (Zantac), terbutaline (Brethine), thiamine, tobramycin (Nebcin), vancomycin, vincristine.

SIDE EFFECTS
Occasional
Flushing, sweating, pruritus, disorientation, headache, dizziness, hyperactivity, convulsions, dyspnea, cough, tachypnea, hiccough, rebound hypoventilation, phlebitis, variations in heart rate, arrhythmias, chest pain, nausea, vomiting, diarrhea, stimulation of urinary bladder with spontaneous voiding.

SERIOUS REACTIONS
- Overdosage may produce extensions of the pharmacologic effects of the drug. Excessive pressor effect, skeletal muscle hyperactivity, tachycardia, and enhanced deep tendon reflexes may be early signs of overdosage.
- May cause severe CNS toxicity, including seizures.

PRECAUTIONS & CONSIDERATIONS
Caution is warranted with hypermetabolic states, such as hyperthyroidism and pheochromocytoma as well as arrhythmias, diabetes mellitus, glaucoma, hypertension, impaired renal or liver function, peptic ulcer disease. It is unknown whether doxapram crosses the placenta or is excreted in breast milk, so it is not administered to pregnant women. No age-related precautions have been

noted for the elderly. Safety and efficacy have not been evaluated in children younger than 12 yr. Be aware that doxapram is contraindicated in neonates. Benzyl alcohol may cause gasping syndrome in neonates.

Storage

Store vials at room temperature.

Administration

Doxapram dosage is determined by response to the drug. Discontinue if sudden hypotension or dyspnea develops. The rate of infusion should not be increased in severely ill patients with chronic obstructive pulmonary disease (COPD). Monitor closely during administration and for some time afterward until the patient is fully alert for 30-60 min to ensure that reflexes have been restored and to prevent rebound hypoventilation. Before doxapram administration, ensure adequate airway and oxygenation in postanesthetic or drug-induced respiratory depression. Avoid extravasation or use of a single injection site over an extended period. Local irritation or thrombophlebitis may result. Doxapram is stable and compatible with D5W, D10W, or 0.9% NaCl.

Doxepin

dox'eh-pin

★ 🍁 Novo-Doxepin, Prudoxin, Silenor, Zonalon

Do not confuse doxepin with doxapram, doxazosin, or Doxidan.

CATEGORY AND SCHEDULE

Pregnancy Risk Category: C (B for topical form)

Classification: Antidepressants, tricyclic; dermatologics

MECHANISM OF ACTION

A tricyclic antidepressant, antianxiety agent, antineuralgic agent, antipruritic agent, and antiulcer agent that increases synaptic concentrations of norepinephrine and serotonin. *Therapeutic Effect:* Produces antidepressant and anxiolytic effects.

PHARMACOKINETICS

Rapidly and well absorbed from the GI tract. Protein binding: 80%-85%. Metabolized in the liver to active metabolite. Primarily excreted in urine. Not removed by hemodialysis. *Half-life:* 6-8 h. *Topical:* Absorbed through the skin to levels similar to those of oral administration. Distributed to body tissues. Metabolized to active metabolite. Excreted in urine.

AVAILABILITY

Capsules: 10 mg, 25 mg, 50 mg, 75 mg, 100 mg, 150 mg.
Oral Concentrate: 10 mg/mL.
Cream (Prudoxin, Zonalon): 5%.
Tablets (Silenor): 3 mg, 6 mg.

INDICATIONS AND DOSAGES

▸ **Depression, anxiety**

PO

Adults. 25-150 mg/day at bedtime or in 2-3 divided doses. May increase to 300 mg/day.
Elderly. Initially, 10-25 mg at bedtime. May increase by 10-25 mg/day every 3-7 days. Maximum: 75 mg/day.
Adolescents. Initially, 25-50 mg/day as a single dose or in divided doses. May increase to 100 mg/day.

▸ **Pruritus associated with eczema**

TOPICAL

Adults, Elderly. Apply thin film 4 times a day with at least 3-4 h between applications.

D

▸ **Insomnia with difficulty in sleep maintenance:**
PO (SILENOR):
Adults. 6 mg once daily within 30 min of bedtime; 3 mg PO may be sufficient in some.
Elderly. 3 mg PO once daily within 30 min of bedtime; may increase to 6 mg if clinically indicated.

OFF-LABEL USES

Treatment of neurogenic pain, panic disorder; prevention of vascular headache, pruritus in idiopathic urticaria.

CONTRAINDICATIONS

Angle-closure glaucoma, hypersensitivity to other tricyclic antidepressants, urine retention, acute post-myocardial infarction period.

INTERACTIONS

Drug
Alcohol, other central nervous system (CNS) depressants: May increase CNS and respiratory depression and the hypotensive effects of doxepin.
Anticholinergics: Additive anticholinergic effects may occur.
Antithyroid agents: May increase the risk of agranulocytosis.
Bupropion: May increase doxepin levels.
Cimetidine: May increase doxepin blood concentration and risk of toxicity.
Clonidine, guanadrel: May decrease the effects of these drugs.
CYP1A2 inducers/inhibitors: May decrease/increase levels and effects of doxepin.
CYP2D6 inhibitors: May increase levels and effects of doxepin.
CYP3A4 inducers/inhibitors: May decrease/increase levels and effects of doxepin.
Lithium: Increased risk of neurotoxicity.
MAOIs, linezolid: May increase the risk of seizures, hyperpyrexia, and hypertensive crisis. MAOIs are contraindicated.
Phenothiazines: May increase the anticholinergic and sedative effects of doxepin.
Sympathomimetics: May increase cardiac effects.
QT-prolonging agents: May increase risk of QT prolongation of tricyclics.
Herbal and Food
None known.

DIAGNOSTIC TEST EFFECTS

May alter blood glucose levels and ECG readings. Therapeutic serum drug level is 110-250 ng/mL; toxic serum drug level is > 300 ng/mL.

SIDE EFFECTS

Frequent
Oral: Orthostatic hypotension, somnolence, dry mouth, headache, increased appetite, weight gain, nausea, unusual fatigue, unpleasant taste.
Topical: Drowsiness; edema; increased itching, eczema, burning, or stinging at application site; altered taste; dizziness; somnolence; dry skin; dry mouth; fatigue; headache; thirst.
Occasional
Oral: Blurred vision, confusion, constipation, hallucinations, difficult urination, eye pain, irregular heartbeat, fine muscle tremors, nervousness, impaired sexual function, diarrhea, diaphoresis, heartburn, insomnia.
Topical: Anxiety, skin irritation or cracking, nausea.
Rare
Oral: Allergic reaction, alopecia, tinnitus, breast enlargement.
Topical: Fever, photosensitivity.

SERIOUS REACTIONS

- Overdose may produce confusion; seizures; severe somnolence; fast, slow, or irregular heartbeat; fever; hallucinations; agitation; dyspnea; vomiting; and unusual fatigue or weakness.
- Abrupt withdrawal after prolonged therapy may produce headache, malaise, nausea, vomiting, and vivid dreams.

PRECAUTIONS & CONSIDERATIONS

Antidepressants increase the risk of suicidal ideation in children, adolescents, and young adults with depression and psychiatric disorders. Closely monitor when initiating therapy, especially the first 2 mo.

Caution is warranted with cardiac disease, diabetes mellitus, glaucoma, hiatal hernia, history of seizures, history of urinary obstruction or urine retention, hyperthyroidism, increased intraocular pressure, renal or hepatic disease, benign prostatic hyperplasia, mania, bipolar disorder, and schizophrenia. Doxepin crosses the placenta and is distributed in breast milk. The safety and efficacy of this drug have not been established in children. Lower doxepin dosages are recommended for elderly patients because they are at increased risk for toxicity. Exposure to sunlight or artificial light sources should be avoided.

Drowsiness and dizziness may occur. Change positions slowly from recumbent to sitting, before standing, to prevent dizziness. Alcohol, caffeine, and tasks that require mental alertness or motor skills should also be avoided until drug effects are known. BP, pulse rate, weight, and ECG should also be monitored. Appearance, behavior, level of interest, mood, and speech pattern should be assessed.

Storage

Store at room temperature, protect from light and excessive heat.

Administration

Take doxepin with food or milk if GI distress occurs. Dilute the oral concentrate in 8 oz fruit juice (such as grapefruit, orange, pineapple, or prune), milk, or water. Avoid diluting in carbonated drinks because they are incompatible with doxepin. Maintenance dose for depression may be administered as daily dose at bedtime to reduce daytime sedation and improve sleep. An improvement should occur within 2-5 days of starting therapy, but the maximum therapeutic effect for depression usually takes 2-3 wks to appear.

Topical cream is for external use only; apply to affected area and rub in gently.

Doxercalciferol

dox-er-cal-sif'er-ol

★ Hectorol

CATEGORY AND SCHEDULE

Pregnancy Risk Category: B

Classification: Vitamins/ minerals, vitamin D analogues

MECHANISM OF ACTION

A fat-soluble vitamin that is essential for absorption, utilization of calcium phosphate, and normal calcification of bone. *Therapeutic Effect:* Stimulates calcium and phosphate absorption from small intestine, promotes secretion of calcium from bone to blood, promotes renal tubule phosphate resorption, acts on bone cells to stimulate skeletal growth and on parathyroid gland to suppress hormone synthesis and secretion.

D

PHARMACOKINETICS

Readily absorbed from small intestine. Metabolized in liver. Partially eliminated in urine. Not removed by hemodialysis. *Half-life:* Up to 96 h.

AVAILABILITY

Capsule: 0.5 mcg, 2.5 mcg.
Injection: 2 mcg/mL.

INDICATIONS AND DOSAGES

▸ **Secondary hyperparathyroidism, dialysis patients**

IV

Adults, Elderly. Titrate dose to lower immunoreactive parathyroid hormone (iPTH) to 150-300 pg/mL. Adjust dose at 8-wk intervals to a maximum dose of 18 mcg/wk. Initially, if iPTH level is more than 400 pg/mL, give 4 mcg 3 times/wk after dialysis, administered as a bolus dose.

Dose titration:

The iPTH level decreased by 50% and more than 300 pg/mL: Dose may be increased by 1-2 mcg at 8-wk intervals as needed.

iPTH level 150-300 pg/mL: Maintain the current dose.

iPTH level < 100 pg/mL: Suspend drug for 1 wk and resume at a reduced dose of at least 1 mcg lower.

PO

Adults, Elderly. Dialysis patients: Titrate dose to lower iPTH to 150-300 pg/mL. Adjust dose at 8-wk intervals to a maximum dose of 20 mcg 3 times/wk. Initially, if iPTH is more than 400 pg/mL, give 10 mcg 3 times/wk at dialysis.

Dose titration:

Level decreased by 50% and more than 300 pg/mL: Increase dose to 12.5 mcg 3 times/wk for 8 wks or longer. This titration process may continue at 8-wk intervals. Each increase should be by 2.5 mcg/dose.

iPTH level 150-300 pg/mL: Maintain current dose.

iPTH level < 100 pg/mL: Suspend drug for 1 wk and resume at a reduced dose. Decrease each dose by at least 2.5 mcg.

▸ **Secondary hyperparathyroidism, predialysis patients**

PO

Adults, Elderly. Titrate dose to lower iPTH to 35-70 pg/mL with stage 3 disease or to 70-110 pg/mL with stage 4 disease. Dose may be adjusted at 2-wk intervals with a maximum dose of 3.5 mcg/day. Begin with 1 mcg/day.

Dose titration:

iPTH level more than 70 pg/mL with stage 3 disease or more than 110 pg/mL with stage 4 disease: Increase dose by 0.5 mcg every 2 wks as needed.

iPTH level 35-70 pg/mL with stage 3 disease or 70-110 pg/mL with stage 4 disease: Maintain current dose.

iPTH level is < 35 pg/mL with stage 3 disease or < 70 pg/mL with stage 4 disease: Suspend drug for 1 wk, then resume at a reduced dose of at least 0.5 mcg lower.

CONTRAINDICATIONS

Hypercalcemia, vitamin D toxicity, hypersensitivity to doxercalciferol or other vitamin D analogues.

INTERACTIONS

Drug

Aluminum-containing antacid (long-term use): May increase aluminum concentration and aluminum bone toxicity.

Calcium-containing preparations, thiazide diuretics: May increase the risk of hypercalcemia.

Magnesium-containing antacids: May increase magnesium concentration.

Vitamin D, other supplements: May increase risk of toxicity.
Herbal
None known.
Food
None known.

DIAGNOSTIC TEST EFFECTS

Decreases iPTH levels. May increase serum cholesterol, calcium, magnesium, and phosphate levels. May decrease serum alkaline phosphatase.

SIDE EFFECTS

Occasional
Edema (34%), headache (28%), malaise (28%), dizziness (12%), nausea (24%), vomiting (24%), dyspnea (12%).
Rare (< 10%)
Bradycardia, sleep disorder, pruritus, anorexia, constipation.

SERIOUS REACTIONS

- Excessive vitamin D may cause progressive hypercalcemia, hypercalciuria, hyperphosphatemia, and adynamic bone disease.
- Early signs of overdosage are manifested as weakness, headache, somnolence, nausea, vomiting, dry mouth, constipation, muscle and bone pain, and metallic taste sensation.
- Later signs of overdosage are evidenced by polyuria, polydipsia, anorexia, weight loss, nocturia, photophobia, rhinorrhea, pruritus, disorientation, hallucinations, hyperthermia, hypertension, and cardiac arrhythmias.

PRECAUTIONS & CONSIDERATIONS

Caution is necessary with coronary artery disease, kidney stones, and hepatic impairment. Correct hyperphosphatemia before starting therapy. Mineral oil should be avoided during doxercalciferol use. It is unknown whether doxercalciferol crosses the placenta or is distributed in breast milk. Safety and efficacy have not been established in children. No age-related precautions have been noted in elderly patients.

During titration, iPTH, serum calcium, and serum phosphorus levels should be obtained weekly. If hypercalcemia, hyperphosphatemia, or a serum calcium × phosphorus product > 70 is noted, the drug should be immediately suspended until these parameters are appropriately lowered, then, the drug should be restarted at a lower dose.
Storage
Store at room temperature. Protect from light.
Administration
Individualize dosing based on serum iPTH levels. Injection for IV use only. Give oral doxercalciferol without regard to food. Swallow whole and avoid crushing, chewing, or opening the capsules.

Doxorubicin

dox-oh-roo′bi-sin
(US) Adriamycin, Doxil
(Canada) Adriamycin, Caelyx, Myocet
Do not confuse with daunorubicin, Idamycin, or idarubicin. Do NOT confuse conventional doxorubicin with doxorubicin liposomal (Doxil) due to different indications and dosage regimens.

CATEGORY AND SCHEDULE

Pregnancy Risk Category: D

Classification: Antineoplastics, anthracyclines

D

MECHANISM OF ACTION

An anthracycline antibiotic that inhibits DNA and DNA-dependent RNA synthesis by binding with DNA strands. Liposomal encapsulation increases uptake by tumors, prolongs action, and may decrease toxicity. *Therapeutic Effect:* Prevents cellular division.

PHARMACOKINETICS

Widely distributed. Protein binding: Unknown. Metabolized in liver. Minimal excretion in urine. *Half-life:* 45-55 h.

AVAILABILITY

Injection, Powder for Solution: 10 mg, 20 mg, 50 mg, 150 mg.
Injection, Solution: 2 mg/mL.
Liposomal Injection (Doxil): 2 mg/mL.

INDICATIONS AND DOSAGES

NOTE: Regimens vary with indication for use, and other medications employed. Consult specialized references to confirm protocols.

▸ **Acute lymphocytic leukemia (ALL):**
IV INFUSION
Adults, Children. Conventional doxorubicin. 30 mg/m^2 IV once weekly for 4 wks, or 30 mg/m^2 IV on days 1, 2, and 14 of induction, or 20 mg/m^2 IV on days 15, 16, and 17 as part of a multidrug regimen.

▸ **Acute myelogenous leukemia (AML):**
IV INFUSION
Adults, Children. Conventional doxorubicin. 30 mg/m^2/day IV bolus for 3 days of induction in combination with cytarabine.

▸ **For treatment of small cell lung carcinoma (SCLC):**
IV INFUSION
Adults. Conventional doxorubicin. 40-50 mg/m^2/dose IV once monthly in combination with other antineoplastics.

▸ **Adjuvant treatment in early breast cancer with axillary lymph nodes**
IV INFUSION
Adults. Conventional doxorubicin. 60 mg/m^2 with cyclophosphamide (600 mg/m^2) administered on day 1 of each 21-day cycle for 4 cycles. Give 75% of usual dose for neutropenic fever/infection. Delay next cycle if needed until ANC ≥ 1000 cells/mm^3 and platelet count ≥ 100,000 cells/mm^3 and nonhematologic toxicities resolved.

▸ **AIDS-related Kaposi sarcoma**
IV INFUSION
Adults. Liposomal doxorubicin. 20 mg/m^2 over 30 min q3wk.
Neoplastic conditions (ovarian, breast, prostate, thyroid, gastric, lung cancers; lymphomas).
IV INFUSION
Adults. Conventional doxorubicin. As a single agent, 60-75 mg/m^2 q3wk. In combination with other chemotherapy, 40-60 mg/m^2 q3-4 wk.

▸ **Ovarian cancer progressed despite platinum treatment**
IV INFUSION
Adults. Liposomal doxorubicin. 50 mg/m^2 q 4 wk.

▸ **Dosage in hepatic impairment (both forms of doxorubicin)**
If serum bilirubin 1.2-3 mg/dL, give 50% of usual dose. If serum bilirubin > 3 mg/dL, give 25% of usual dose. If bilirubin is > 5 mg/dL, then dose is held.

CONTRAINDICATIONS

Myelosuppression; previous receipt of complete cumulative doses of doxorubicin, daunorubicin, idarubicin, or other anthracyclines; nursing mothers, hypersensitivity to doxorubicin compounds or daunorubicin.

DRUG INTERACTIONS

Cyclosporine: Increased doxorubicin concentrations and toxicity.

Live vaccines: Increased risk infection by vaccine.

IV INCOMPATIBILITIES

Conventional doxorubicin: Allopurinol, aminophylline, cephalothin, dexamethasone, diazepam, ertapenem (Invanz), etoposide, fluorouracil, fosphenytoin, furosemide, gallium nitrate, heparin, hydrocortisone, lansoprazole (Prevacid IV), magnesium sulfate, meropenem (Merrem), pantoprazole (Protonix), phenytoin, piperacillin sodium/tazobactam, potassium or sodium phosphates, rituximab (Rituxan), TPN, vincristine, voriconazole (VFend).
Liposomal doxorubin: Benzyl alcohol. Doxorubicin liposomal should not be mixed with any other medications.

SIDE EFFECTS

Conventional doxorubicin:
Frequent
Nausea, vomiting, alopecia, mucositis, myelosuppression.
Occasional
Anorexia, diarrhea, hyperpigmentation of nailbeds, phalangeal and dermal creases.
Rare
Fever, chills, urticaria, conjunctivitis, lacrimation.
Liposomal doxorubicin:
Frequent (> 20%)
Asthenia, fatigue, fever, anorexia, nausea, vomiting, stomatitis, diarrhea, constipation, hand and foot syndrome, rash, neutropenia, thrombocytopenia, anemia.

SERIOUS REACTIONS

- Bone marrow depression manifested as hematologic toxicity (principally leukopenia and, to a lesser extent, anemia, thrombocytopenia) may occur.
- Cardiotoxicity noted as either acute, transient abnormal ECG findings or cardiomyopathy manifested as congestive heart failure may occur.
- Acute infusion-related reactions with liposomal doxorubicin.

PRECAUTIONS & CONSIDERATIONS

Probability of cardiac toxicity increases with higher total cumulative dose. Maximum lifetime cumulative dosage of doxorubicin is 550 mg/m^2 IV; 450 mg/m^2 IV in patients who have received previous mediastinal radiation. Risk of cardiotoxicity increased in patients with prior mediastinal irradiation, concurrent cyclophosphamide therapy, concurrent calcium channel blocker therapy, preexisting heart disease, or early or advanced age. Monitor cardiac function. Use with caution in patients with impaired hepatic function. Women of childbearing potential should be advised to avoid becoming pregnant.
Excreted in breast milk; do not breastfeed.

Storage
Store lyophilized powder at room temperature. Protect from light. Store conventional solution in the refrigerator for up to 48 h. Protect from light.

Store liposomal solution in the refrigerator.

Administration
CAUTION: Observe and exercise appropriate precautions for handling, preparing, and administering cytotoxic drugs.
Conventional doxorubicin:
Reconstitute lyophilized powder with NS (nonpreserved) to a concentration of 2 mg/mL. Do not administer IM or SC. Severe local tissue damage will occur with IV extravasation. Slowly administer into tubing of a freely running

IV infusion of NS or D5W into a large vein. Administer over at least 3 to 5 min. Use of a butterfly needle inserted into a large vein is preferred.

! Do not substitute liposomal doxorubicin for conventional doxorubicin on a mg per mg basis. Do not use in-line filter with liposomal formulation. Dilute liposomal doxorubicin with D5W, not to exceed 90 mg/250 mL D5W. Infuse at an initial rate of 1 mg/min to decrease the risk of infusion reactions. Administer over at least 1 hr.

Doxycycline

dox-i-sye′kleen

Adoxa, Alodox, Doryx, Doxy-100, Monodox, Oraxyl, Periostat, Vibramycin Apo-Doxy, Doxycin, Vibra-Tabs

Do not confuse doxycycline with dicyclomine or doxylamine, or Monodox with Monopril.

CATEGORY AND SCHEDULE

Pregnancy Risk Category: D

Classification: Antibiotics, tetracyclines

MECHANISM OF ACTION

A tetracycline antibiotic that inhibits bacterial protein synthesis by binding to ribosomes. *Therapeutic Effect:* Bacteriostatic.

PHARMACOKINETICS

Well absorbed after oral administration. Protein binding: 90%. Widely distributed except in the central nervous system (CNS; poor). Excreted in urine and feces. *Half-life:* 12-15 h.

AVAILABILITY

Capsules (Doxycycline, Monodox): 50 mg, 75 mg, 100 mg.
Capsules (Vibramycin): 100 mg.
Capsules (Adoxa): 150 mg.
Capsules (Oraxyl): 20 mg.
Capsules, Delayed Release: 75 mg, 100 mg.
Capsules, Delayed Release (Oracea): 40 mg.
Oral Suspension (Vibramycin): 50 mg/5 mL, 25 mg/5 mL.
Syrup (Vibramycin): 50 mg/5 mL.
Tablets (Adoxa): 50 mg, 75 mg, 100 mg, 150 mg.
Tablets (Alodox, Periostat): 20 mg.
Tablet, Delayed Release (Doryx): 75 mg, 100 mg.
Injection, Powder for Reconstitution (Doxy-100): 100 mg.

INDICATIONS AND DOSAGES

▸ **Respiratory, skin, and soft-tissue infections; urinary tract infection; pelvic inflammatory disease (PID); brucellosis; trachoma; Rocky Mountain spotted fever; typhus; Q fever; rickettsia; severe acne (Adoxa); smallpox; psittacosis; ornithosis; granuloma inguinale; lymphogranuloma venereum; intestinal amebiasis (adjunctive treatment); prevention of rheumatic fever**

PO

Adults, Elderly, Children older than 8 yr and weighing > 45 kg. Initially, 100 mg q12h, then 100 mg/day as single dose or 50 mg q12h or 100 mg q12h for severe infections.

Children older than 8 yr and weighing < 45 kg. Initially, 4 mg/kg/day, then 2-4 mg/kg/day divided q12-24h. Maximum: 200 mg/day.

IV

Adults, Elderly, Children older than 8 yr and weighing > 45 kg. Initially, 200 mg as 1-2 infusions;

then 100-200 mg/day in 1-2 divided doses.
Children older than 8 yr and < 45 kg. 2-4 mg/kg/day divided q12-24h. Maximum: 200 mg/day.

▸ **Acute gonococcal infections**
PO
Adults. 100 mg twice daily for 7 days.

▸ **Syphilis**
PO, IV
Adults. 200 mg/day in divided doses for 14-28 days.

▸ **Traveler's diarrhea, prophylaxis**
PO
Adults, Elderly. 100 mg/day during a period of risk (up to 14 days) and for 2 days after returning home.

▸ **Periodontitis**
PO
Adults (Periostat, Alodox, Oraxyl). 20 mg twice a day.

▸ **Malaria, prophylaxis**
PO
Adults. 100 mg once a day beginning 1-2 days before travel, during travel, and 4 wks after returning home.
Children over 8 yr. 2 mg/kg once a day beginning 1-2 days before travel, during travel, and 4 wks after returning home.

▸ **Rosacea**
PO (Oracea)
Adults. 40 mg once daily.

OFF-LABEL USES

Treatment of atypical mycobacterial infections, rheumatoid arthritis, gonorrhea, and malaria; prevention of Lyme disease; prevention or treatment of traveler's diarrhea.

CONTRAINDICATIONS

Children 8 yr and younger, hypersensitivity to tetracyclines or sulfites, pregnancy, severe hepatic dysfunction.

INTERACTIONS

Drug

Antacids and supplements containing aluminum, calcium, or magnesium and oral iron preparations; laxatives containing magnesium: Decrease doxycycline absorption; separate administration.
Barbiturates, carbamazepine, phenytoin: May decrease doxycycline blood concentrations.
Cholestyramine, colestipol: May decrease doxycycline absorption; separate administration.
Methotrexate: May increase levels of methotrexate.
Oral contraceptives: May decrease the effects of oral contraceptives.
Warfarin: May increase anticoagulation of warfarin.

Herbal

None known.

Food

None known.

DIAGNOSTIC TEST EFFECTS

May increase serum alkaline phosphatase, amylase, bilirubin, AST (SGOT), and ALT (SGPT) levels. May alter CBC.

IV INCOMPATIBILITIES

Allopurinol (Aloprim), amphotericin B cholesteryl (Amphotec), amphotericin B liposomal (AmBisome), ampicillin, ampicillin/sulbactam (Unasyn), cefazolin, cefotetan (Cefotan), cefoxitin (Mefoxin), ceftazidime (Ceptaz, Fortaz, Tazicef, Tazidime), ceftizoxime (Cefizox), cefuroxime (Zinacef), chloramphenicol, dantrolene, diazepam, erythromycin lactobionate, fluorouracil, folic acid, furosemide (Lasix), ganciclovir (Cytovene), heparin, hydrocortisone sodium succinate (Solu-Cortef), indomethacin, ketorolac, methicillin, methotrexate, methylprednisolone sodium succinate, nafcillin, oxacillin, palonosetron (Aloxi), pemetrexed (Alimta), penicillin G potassium, penicillin G sodium, pentobarbital, phenytoin, piperacillin, piperacillin/tazobactam (Zosyn), sodium bicarbonate, sulfamethoxazole/trimethoprim.

SIDE EFFECTS

Frequent

Anorexia, nausea, vomiting, diarrhea, dysphagia, possibly severe photosensitivity.

Occasional

Rash, urticaria.

SERIOUS REACTIONS

- Superinfection (especially fungal) and benign intracranial hypertension (headache, visual changes) may occur.
- Hepatoxicity, fatty degeneration of the liver, and pancreatitis occur rarely. Autoimmune syndromes have been reported.

PRECAUTIONS & CONSIDERATIONS

Caution should be used in those who cannot avoid sun or ultraviolet exposure, because such exposure, may produce a severe photosensitivity reaction.

History of allergies, especially to tetracyclines or sulfites, should be determined before drug therapy. Caution is warranted in renal impairment. Avoid use in children, because it may cause permanent tooth discoloration, enamel hypoplasia. Pattern of daily bowel activity, stool consistency, food intake and tolerance, renal function, and skin for rash should be assessed. Be alert for signs and symptoms of superinfection, such as anal or genital pruritus, diarrhea, and ulceration or changes of the oral mucosa or tongue. Loss of consciousness should be monitored because of the potential for increased intracranial pressure.

Storage

Store capsules and tablets at room temperature. Store oral suspension for up to 2 wks at room temperature. After reconstitution, the IV piggyback infusion may be stored for up to 12 h at room temperature or up to 72 h if refrigerated. Protect the drug from direct sunlight. Discard it if a precipitate forms.

Administration

Take oral doxycycline with a full glass of fluid. It may also be given with food or milk. An exception is Oracea, which is best taken on an empty stomach 1 h before or 2 h after a meal. Take oral doxycycline 1-2 h before or after antacids that contain aluminum, calcium, or magnesium; laxatives that contain magnesium; or oral iron preparations, because these drugs may impair doxycycline absorption. Shake suspension well before use.

! Do not administer doxycycline IM or subcutaneously. Space doses evenly around the clock. Reconstitute each 100-mg vial with 10 mL of sterile water for injection to yield a concentration of 10 mg/mL. Further dilute each 100 mg with at least 100 mL to concentration of 0.1 mg/mL to 1 mg/mL with D5W, 0.9% NaCl, or lactated Ringer's solution. Give the intermittent IV (piggyback) infusion over 1-4 h. Avoid extravasation.

Dronabinol

droe-nab′i-nol

Marinol

Do not confuse dronabinol with droperidol.

CATEGORY AND SCHEDULE

Pregnancy Risk Category: C

Controlled Substance Schedule: III

Classification: Antiemetics/antivertigo, appetite stimulant

MECHANISM OF ACTION
An antiemetic and appetite stimulant that may act by inhibiting vomiting control mechanisms in the medulla oblongata. *Therapeutic Effect:* Inhibits vomiting and stimulates appetite.

PHARMACOKINETICS
Well absorbed after oral administration. Distributes to adipose tissue. Protein binding > 97%. Metabolized in liver, extensive first-pass effect. *Half-life:* 25-36 h. Primarily excreted in feces. Onset of action: 1 h. Duration of appetite stimulation: 24 h.

AVAILABILITY
Capsules (Gelatin): 2.5 mg, 5 mg, 10 mg.

INDICATIONS AND DOSAGES
▸ **Prevention of chemotherapy-induced nausea and vomiting**

PO

Adults, Children. Initially, 5 mg/m^2 1-3 h before chemotherapy, then q2-4h after chemotherapy for total of 4-6 doses a day. May increase by 2.5 mg/m^2 up to 15 mg/m^2 per dose.

▸ **Appetite stimulant in patients with AIDS or cancer (off-label use)**

PO

Adults. Initially, 2.5 mg twice a day (before lunch and dinner). Range: 2.5-20 mg/day.

CONTRAINDICATIONS
Hypersensitivity to marijuana or any cannabinoid or sesame oil.

INTERACTIONS
Drug

Alcohol, other CNS depressants: May increase CNS depression.

Amphetamines, cocaine, sympathomimetics: Hypertension, tachycardia, cardiotoxicity may occur.

Anticholinergics, antihistamines: Additive tachycardia drowsiness may occur.

Tricyclic antidepressants: Tachycardia, hypertension, or drowsiness may occur.

Herbal and Food

None known.

DIAGNOSTIC TEST EFFECTS
None known.

SIDE EFFECTS
Frequent (3%-24%)

Euphoria, dizziness, paranoid reaction, somnolence, abnormal thinking.

Occasional (1%-3%)

Asthenia, ataxia, confusion, abdominal pain, depersonalization.

Rare (< 1%)

Diarrhea, depression, nightmares, speech difficulties, headache, anxiety, tinnitus, flushed skin.

SERIOUS REACTIONS
- Withdrawal symptoms may occur upon abrupt discontinuation.
- Mild intoxication may produce increased sensory awareness (including taste, smell, and sound), altered time perception, reddened conjunctiva, dry mouth, and tachycardia.
- Moderate intoxication may produce memory impairment and urine retention.
- Severe intoxication may produce lethargy, decreased motor coordination, slurred speech, and orthostatic hypotension.

PRECAUTIONS & CONSIDERATIONS
Caution is warranted in patients with heart disease, hypertension, a history of drug or alcohol abuse, hepatic impairment, seizure

disorder, depression, mania, and schizophrenia. Dependence has been noted. Use with caution in elderly patients because postural hypotension can occur.

Dronabinol use is not recommended for children with AIDS-related anorexia. Alcohol, barbiturates, other CNS depressants, should be avoided. Patients should be specifically warned not to drive, operate machinery, or engage in any hazardous activity until it is established that they are able to tolerate the drug and perform such tasks safely. BP, heart rate, and behavioral and mood reactions should be monitored.

Storage

Keep tightly closed. Store in refrigerator. Protect from freezing.

Administration

Take dronabinol before lunch and dinner to stimulate appetite. Relief from nausea and vomiting generally occurs within 15 min of drug administration. A dose of the drug is usually given 1-3 h prior to chemotherapy.

Dronedarone

Dro-neh′da-rone

Multaq

Do not confuse dronedarone with amiodarone.

CATEGORY AND SCHEDULE

Pregnancy Risk Category: X

Classification: Antiarrhythmics

MECHANISM OF ACTION

A benzofuran derivative of amiodarone with a complex electrophysical profile. Possesses antiarrhythmic properties belonging to all four Vaughan-Williams classes. Like class III agents (e.g., amiodarone), lengthens cardiac action potential and refractory periods by inhibiting the potassium currents. Also inhibits sodium channels and inhibits the slow L-type calcium channels. Exhibits some antiadrenergic properties. Prolongs the PR and QT interval. *Therapeutic Effect:* Suppresses atrial arrhythmias; keeps heart in sinus rhythm longer than without the medication.

PHARMACOKINETICS

Presystemic first-pass metabolism; bioavailability without food is low, about 4%, but improves to 15% when taken with a high-fat meal. Peak plasma concentrations of drug and main active metabolite are reached within 3-6 h. After repeated administration, steady state reached in 4-8 days. A 2-fold increase in dose results in an approximate 2.5- to 3-fold increase with respect to Cmax and AUC of main metabolite and parent drug. Protein binding: > 98%, mainly to albumin. Extensively metabolized in liver, mainly by CYP3 A. There are over 30 uncharacterized inactive metabolites. Mainly excreted in the feces as metabolites, only 6% excreted in urine. *Half-life:* 13-19 h.

AVAILABILITY

Tablets (Multaq): 400 mg.

INDICATIONS AND DOSAGES

▸ **Paroxysmal AFib or AFlutter with recent episode now in sinus rhythm or to be cardioverted, with CV risk factors**

PO

Adults, Elderly. 400 mg twice per day.

D

CONTRAINDICATIONS

QT prolongation, severe hepatic impairment, pregnancy, breastfeeding, NYHA class IV heart failure or NYHA class II- III heart failure with a recent decompensation, 2nd- or 3rd-degree AV block or sick sinus syndrome (except with functioning pacemaker), bradycardia < 50 bpm, concomitant use of strong CYP3 A inhibitors OR concomitant use of drugs/herbals that prolong the QT interval and might increase the risk of torsades de pointes (see Interactions).

INTERACTIONS

Drug

Antiarrhythmics: May increase cardiac effects. Do not give with class I or class III antiarrhythmics due to risk of torsades.

Strong CYP3A inhibitors or QT-prolonging drugs (e.g., azole antifungals, cisapride, cyclosporine, pimozide, fluoroquinolones, macrolides, nefazodone, ranolazine, ritonavir and certain other protease inhibitors, thioridazine, ziprasidone, phenothiazines, tricyclic antidepressants: Contraindicated. Risk of cardiac arrhythmias, including torsades de pointes, may be increased, either due to decreased dronedarone metabolism or due to additive QT prolongation. List may not be complete for all strong CYP3A inhibitors or drugs that prolong the QT interval.

β-Blockers: May increase effect of β-blockers.

CYP2D6 substrates (e.g., fluoxetine and other SSRIs) or CYP3A substrates (e.g., midazolam, alprazolam, triazolam, pimozide, sirolimus, tacrolimus): May increase concentrations of these drugs; monitor for dose adjustment.

CYP3A inducers: Avoid rifampin or other CYP3A inducers such as phenobarbital, carbamazepine, phenytoin, because they decrease dronedarone exposure significantly.

Digoxin: May increase drug concentration and risk of toxicity of digoxin; additive cardiac effects; lower dose of digoxin recommended.

Diuretics: May cause electrolyte imbalances that could increase risk of arrhythmia. Monitor closely.

HMG-CoA reductase inhibitors ("statins"): May increase risk of myopathy/rhabdomyolysis; follow statin labeling recommendations.

Verapamil or diltiazem: Increased dronedarone exposure; monitor closely.

Warfarin: Possible increased anticoagulant effect; closely monitor INR.

Herbal

St. John's wort: Significantly reduces dronedarone concentrations. Avoid.

Food

All foods: Food increases the extent of absorption. Dose with meals.

Grapefruit juice: Increased dronedarone concentrations. Avoid grapefruit juice.

DIAGNOSTIC TEST EFFECTS

Commonly increases serum creatinine roughly 0.1 mg/dL due to a reduction in kidney tubular secretion. May increase AST (SGOT), ALT (SGPT) levels. Prolongs PR and QT interval of ECG.

SIDE EFFECTS

Frequent (≥ 3%)

Diarrhea, nausea, abdominal pain, bradycardia, and asthenia, skin rashes (generalized, macular, maculopapular, erythematous).

D

Occasional (1%-2%)
Headache, dyspepsia, vomiting, pruritus, eczema, allergic dermatitis.
Rare (< 1%)
Decreased libido, dizziness, dysguesia, paresthesias, photosensitivity, fatigue, tremor.

SERIOUS REACTIONS

- May worsen existing arrhythmias or produce new arrhythmias (called proarrhythmias).
- Worsening heart failure.
- Serious allergic reactions/hypersensitivity.
- Hepatic dysfunction or hepatic failure (rare).

PRECAUTIONS & CONSIDERATIONS

Certain patients with heart failure must not be given dronedarone due to a noted increase in mortality (see Contraindications). Patients with stable, mild heart failure should be monitored very closely. Caution is warranted with thyroid disease and hepatic impairment, in patients receiving diuretic therapy or who have a history of potassium or magnesium imbalance. Per animal studies, dronedarone crosses the placenta and adversely affects fetal development. Contraindicated during pregnancy. Effective contraception must be used if the female is of childbearing potential. It readily crosses into breast milk; breastfeeding is contraindicated. Safety and efficacy have not been established in children. Elderly patients may be more sensitive to dronedarone's effects. The drug may cause photosensitivity; wear sunscreen and sun-protective clothing.

ECG, liver enzyme tests, serum electrolytes, and serum creatinine should be obtained at baseline and during therapy. Apical pulse and BP should be assessed immediately before giving. Withhold the medication and notify the physician if the pulse rate is 55 beats/min or lower or the systolic BP is < 90 mm Hg, unless physician has given other parameters. Pulse rate for bradycardia, an irregular rhythm, and quality should be monitored. ECG for changes such as widening of the QRS complex and prolonged PR and QT intervals should be assessed. Signs and symptoms of heart failure should be assessed in patients with potential risk factors, including dyspnea, edema, fatigue.

Storage
Store tablets at room temperature.

Administration
Take with meals; one tablet with morning meal and one with evening meal. Do not take with grapefruit juice.

! Treatment with class I or III antiarrhythmics (e.g., amiodarone, flecainide, propafenone, quinidine, disopyramide, dofetilide, sotalol) or drugs that are strong inhibitors of CYP3A must be stopped before starting this drug.

Droperidol

droe-pear'ih-dall

CATEGORY AND SCHEDULE

Pregnancy Risk Category: C

Classification: Antiemetics

MECHANISM OF ACTION

A general anesthetic and antiemetic agent that antagonizes dopamine neurotransmission at synapses by blocking postsynaptic dopamine receptor sites; partially blocks adrenergic receptor binding sites. *Therapeutic Effect:* Produces tranquilization, antiemetic effect.

D

PHARMACOKINETICS
Onset of action occurs within 3-10 min, peak 30 min. Well absorbed. Metabolized in liver. Excreted in urine and feces. Duration of action: 2-4 h. *Half-life:* 2.3 h.

AVAILABILITY
Injection: 2.5 mg/mL.

INDICATIONS AND DOSAGES
▸ **Prevention of nausea and vomiting with surgery**
IM/IV
Adults, Elderly, Children 12 yr and older. Initially, up to 2.5 mg. Additional doses of 1.25 mg may be given.
Children 2-12 yr. Initially, up to 0.1 mg/kg.

CONTRAINDICATIONS
Known or suspected QT prolongation, hypersensitivity to droperidol or any component of the formulation. Droperidol is not recommended for any use other than for the treatment of perioperative nausea and vomiting in patients for whom other treatments are ineffective or inappropriate.

INTERACTIONS
Drug
Central nervous system (CNS) depressants: May increase CNS-depressant effect.
Class I, IA, or III antiarrhythmics, cisapride, cyclobenzaprine, phenothiazines, pimozide, quinolone antibiotics, tricylic antidepressants: May increase risk of QT prolongation.
Hypotensive agents: May increase hypotension.
Metoclopramide: Increased risk for extrapyramidal symptoms.
Propofol: Increased nausea and vomiting.
Herbal
None known.
Food
None known.

IV INCOMPATIBILITIES
Allopurinol (Aloprim), amphotericin B cholesteryl (Amphotec), amphotericin B liposomal (AmBisome), cefepime (Maxipime), ertapenem (Invanz), fluorouracil, foscarnet (Foscavir), furosemide (Lasix), lansoprazole (Prevacid), leucovorin, nafcillin, pantoprazole (Protonix), pemetrexed (Alimta), piperacillin/tazobactam (Zosyn).

IV COMPATIBILITES
Amifostine (Ethyol), azithromycin (Zithromax), aztreonam (Azactam), bivalirudin (Angiomax), bleomycin (Blenoxane), carboplatin, caspofungin (Cancidas), cisatracurium (Nimbex), cisplatin, cladribine (Leustatin), cyclophosphamide (Cytoxan), cytarabine, dactinomycin (Cosmegen), daptomycin (Cubicin), dexmedetomidine (Precedex), diltiazem (Cardizem), docetaxel (Taxotere), dopamine (Intropin), doxorubicin (Adriamycin), doxorubicin liposomal (Doxil), epirubicin (Ellence), famotidine (Pepcid), fenoldopam (Corlopam), fentanyl (Sublimaze), filgrastim (Neupogen), fluconazole (Diflucan), fludarabine (Fludara), gemcitabine (Gemzar), granisetron (Kytril), hydrocortisone sodium succinate (Solu-Cortef), hydromorphone (Dilaudid), idarubicin (Idamycin), ketamine (Ketalar), levofloxacin (Levaquin), linezolid (Zyvox), lorazepam (Ativan), melphalan (Alkeran), meperidine (Demerol), metoclopramide (Reglan), milrinone (Primacor), mitoxantrone (Novantrone), oxaliplatin (Eloxatin),

oxytocin (Pitocin), paclitaxel (Taxol), palonosetron (Aloxi), potassium chloride, quinupristin/dalfopristin (Synercid), rituximab (Rituxan), sargramostim (Leukine), tacrolimus (Prograf), teniposide (Vumon), thiotepa (Thioplex), tigecycline (Tygacil), tirofibran (Aggrastat), trastuzumab (Herceptin), vasopressin, vecuronium (Norcuron), vinblastine (Velban), vincristine (Vincasar), vinorelbine (Navelbine), vitamin B complex with C, voriconazole (Vfend).

SIDE EFFECTS

Frequent
Mild to moderate hypotension.
Occasional
Tachycardia, postoperative drowsiness, dizziness, chills, shivering.
Rare
Postoperative nightmares, facial sweating, bronchospasm.

SERIOUS REACTIONS

- Extrapyramidal symptoms may appear as akathisia (motor restlessness) and dystonias: torticollis (neck muscle spasm), opisthotonos (rigidity of back muscles), and oculogyric crisis (rolling back of eyes).
- Overdosage includes symptoms of hypotension, tachycardia, hallucinations, and extrapyramidal symptoms.
- Prolonged QT interval (> 10%), torsade de pointes, seizures, neuroleptic malignant syndrome, orthostatic hypotension, and arrhythmias have been reported.

PRECAUTIONS & CONSIDERATIONS

Use with caution in patients with risk factors for QT prolongation, such as congenital risks, uncorrected electrolyte abnormalities, or taking other medications that might prolong the QT interval. All patients should have EKG prior to administration to determine if QT interval is prolonged.

Caution is warranted in patients with impaired hepatic, renal, or cardiac function, bradycardia, seizure disorder, pheochromocytoma, myasthenia gravis, or glaucoma. Droperidol readily crosses the placenta, and it is unknown whether droperidol is distributed in breast milk. Be aware that dystonias are more likely in children. Be aware that elderly patients may be more susceptible to sedative and hypotensive effects. Safety and efficacy have not been established in children < 2 yr of age. Monitor ECG.

Change positions slowly to avoid orthostatic hypotension and avoid tasks that require mental alertness or motor skills.

Storage
Store vials at room temperature. Protect from light.
Administration
Be aware that the person must remain recumbent for 30-60 min in head-low position with legs raised, to minimize hypotensive effect.

For IM administration, inject slow and deep into upper outer quadrant of gluteus maximus.

For IV administration, may give undiluted as IV push at a rate of 10 mg or less over 1 min.

Drotrecogin Alfa

droh-tree-koh′gen al′fa
★ 🍁 Xigris

CATEGORY AND SCHEDULE

Pregnancy Risk Category: C

Classification: Thrombolytics

D

MECHANISM OF ACTION
A recombinant form of human-activated protein C that exerts an antithrombotic effect by inhibiting factors Va and VIIIa and may exert an indirect profibrinolytic effect by inhibiting plasminogen activator inhibitor-1 and limiting the generation of activated thrombin-activatable fibrinolysis-inhibitor. The drug may also exert an anti-inflammatory effect by inhibiting tumor necrosis factor (TNF) production by monocytes, by blocking leukocyte adhesion to selectins, and by limiting thrombin-induced inflammatory responses.
Therapeutic Effect: Produces anti-inflammatory, antithrombotic, and profibrinolytic effects.

PHARMACOKINETICS
Inactivated by endogenous plasma protease inhibitors. Clearance occurs within 2 h of initiating infusion.
Half-life: 1.6 h.

AVAILABILITY
Powder for Infusion: 5 mg, 20 mg.

INDICATIONS AND DOSAGES
▸ **Severe sepsis (Apache II score ≥ 25)**
IV INFUSION
Adults, Elderly. 24 mcg/kg/h for 96 h. Dose is based on actual body weight.

CONTRAINDICATIONS
Active internal bleeding, evidence of cerebral herniation, intracranial neoplasm or mass lesion, presence, of an epidural catheter, recent (within the past 3 mo) hemorrhagic stroke, recent (within the past 2 mo) intracranial or intraspinal surgery or severe head trauma, trauma with an increased risk of life-threatening bleeding.

INTERACTIONS
Drug
Antiplatelets, anticoagulants, thrombolytics: May increase risk for bleeding.
Herbal
None known.
Food
None known.

DIAGNOSTIC TEST EFFECTS
May prolong aPTT.

IV INCOMPATIBILITIES
Do not mix drotrecogin alfa with other medications.

IV COMPATIBILITIES
Lactated Ringer's solution, 0.9% NaCl, and dextrose are the only solutions that can be administered through the same line.

SIDE EFFECTS
Occasional
Bleeding, bruising.

SERIOUS REACTIONS
- Bleeding (intrathoracic, retroperitoneal, GI, genitourinary, intra-abdominal, intracranial) occurs in about 2% of patients.

PRECAUTIONS & CONSIDERATIONS
Caution is warranted in patients with chronic, severe hepatic disease, intracranial aneurysm, platelet count < 30,000/mm^3, INR > 3, or prolonged PT, and in those who have had GI bleeding within the past 6 wks. Caution should be used in those who are using heparin concurrently and in those who have had thrombolytic therapy within the past 3 days or anticoagulant or aspirin therapy within the past 7 days. Caution should also be used when administering other drugs that affect hemostasis. It is unknown whether

D

drotrecogin alfa causes fetal harm or is excreted in breast milk. The safety and efficacy of drotrecogin alfa have not been established in children or in elderly patients.

The following criteria must be met before initiating drotrecogin alfa therapy: age of at least 18 yr; weight < 135 kg; no pregnancy or breastfeeding; 3 or more systemic inflammatory response criteria (fever, heart rate > 90 beats/min, respiratory rate > 20 breaths/min, increased WBC count); and at least 1 sepsis-induced organ or system failure (cardiovascular, hepatic, renal, respiratory, or unexplained metabolic acidosis). Monitor for hemorrhagic complications. Bleeding may occur for up to 28 days after treatment. Notify the physician if signs and symptoms of unusual bleeding occur. Study in pediatric patients was terminated early due to lack of efficacy and increased side effects.

Storage

Store unreconstituted vials at room temperature. Reconstituted vials should be used within 3 hr to prepare infusion. If not used immediately, the infusion may be refrigerated for up to 12 h, but the maximum time limit for use of the IV solution is 24 h from the time of vial dilution.

Administration

! If clinically important bleeding occurs, immediately stop the infusion.

Reconstitute the 5- and 20-mg vials by slowly adding 2.5 mL or 10 mL of sterile water for injection, respectively, to yield a concentration of 2 mg/mL. Swirl the vial gently to mix; do not shake or invert it. Must further dilute, either in infusion bags or in syringe-pump syringes. Add the reconstituted drug to an infusion bag containing 0.9% NaCl, and dilute to a final concentration of 100-200 mcg/mL. Direct the stream to the side of the bag to minimize agitation. Invert the infusion bag to mix the solution. If using syringes, slowly withdraw the reconstituted Xigris solution from the vial(s) into a syringe that will be used in the syringe pump. Into the same syringe, slowly withdraw 0.9% NaCl to obtain the desired final volume. Gently invert and/or rotate to mix. The syringe pump must be primed according to manufacturer's directions before use. Start the infusion within 3 h after reconstitution. Administer the drug through a dedicated IV line or a dedicated lumen of a multilumen central venous catheter at a rate of 24 mcg/kg/h for 96 h. If the infusion is interrupted, restart it at 24 mcg/kg/h, as prescribed. Stop infusion 2 h before invasive procedures. Resume immediately after minimally invasive procedures; delay for 12 h after major invasive procedures or surgery.

Duloxetine

du-lox′uh-teen

★🍁 Cymbalta

CATEGORY AND SCHEDULE

Pregnancy Risk Category: C

Classification: Antidepressants, selective serotonin/norepinephrine (SNRI) reuptake inhibitor

MECHANISM OF ACTION

An antidepressant that appears to inhibit serotonin and norepinephrine reuptake at neuronal presynaptic membranes; is a less potent inhibitor of dopamine reuptake. *Therapeutic Effect:* Relieves depression.

D

PHARMACOKINETICS

Well absorbed from the GI tract. Protein binding: > 90%. Extensively metabolized to active metabolites. Excreted primarily in urine and, to a lesser extent, in feces. *Half-life:* 8-17 h.

AVAILABILITY

Capsules, Delayed Release: 20 mg, 30 mg, 60 mg.

INDICATIONS AND DOSAGES

▸ **Major depressive disorder**

PO

Adults. 20 mg twice a day, increased up to 60 mg/day as a single dose or in 2 divided doses. Maximum: 120 mg/day.

▸ **Diabetic neuropathy**

PO

Adults. 60 mg once daily. Maximum: 120 mg/day.

▸ **Fibromyalgia**

PO

Adults. 30 mg/day, titrated to 60 mg/day after 1 wk. Maximum 120 mg/day.

▸ **Generalized anxiety**

Adults. 60 mg once daily (may start at 30 mg once daily for 1 wk, then titrate). Maximum: 120 mg/day.

▸ **Dosage in renal impairment**

Consider lower starting dosage. If creatinine clearance < 30 mL/min, use is not recommended.

OFF-LABEL USES

Chronic pain syndromes, stress incontinence.

CONTRAINDICATIONS

Uncontrolled angle-closure glaucoma; use within 14 days of MAOIs.

INTERACTIONS

Drug

Alcohol: Increases the risk of hepatic injury.

Buspirone, meperidine, serotonin agonists, SSRIs/SNRIs, sibutramine, tramadol, trazodone: May increase risk of serotonin syndrome.

CYP1A2 inhibitors/inducers: May increase/decrease duloxetine levels and effects. Potent inhibitors of CYP1A2 should be avoided (e.g., cimetidine, ciprofloxacin, fluvoxamine).

Fluoxetine, fluvoxamine, paroxetine, quinidine, quinolone antimicrobials, CYP2D6 inhibitors: May increase duloxetine plasma concentration.

MAOIs, linezolid: May cause serotonin syndrome, characterized by autonomic hyperactivity, coma, diaphoresis, excitement, hyperthermia, and rigidity. MAOIs are contraindicated.

Thioridazine: May produce ventricular arrhythmias.

Warfarin: May increase warfarin concentration; monitor INR.

Herbal

St John's wort: May increase adverse effects.

DIAGNOSTIC TEST EFFECTS

May increase serum bilirubin, AST (SGOT), and ALT (SGPT) levels.

SIDE EFFECTS

Frequent (11%-20%)

Nausea, dry mouth, diarrhea, constipation, insomnia, somnolence, headache.

Occasional (9%-59%)

Dizziness, fatigue, anorexia, diaphoresis/hyperhidrosis, vomiting.

Rare (2%-4%)

Blurred vision, erectile dysfunction, delayed or failed ejaculation, anorgasmia, anxiety, decreased libido, hot flashes, increased BP.

SERIOUS REACTIONS

• Duloxetine use may slightly increase the patient's heart rate or cause orthostatic hypotension.

• Colitis, dysphagia, gastritis, hepatotoxicity, and irritable bowel syndrome occur rarely.
• Activation of mania or hypomania in bipolar patients can occur. Monotherapy is not recommended in these patients.
• SIADH and hyponatremia occur with SSRIs and SNRIs.
• Withdrawal syndrome may occur with abrupt discontinuation. Gradually taper dose.

PRECAUTIONS & CONSIDERATIONS

Antidepressants increase the risk of suicidal ideation in children, adolescents, and young adults with depression and psychiatric disorders. Closely monitor when initiating therapy, especially the first 2 mo.

Caution is warranted with conditions that may slow gastric emptying, hepatic impairment, history of anemia, history of seizures, renal impairment, mania, hypomania, bipolar, and suicidal tendencies. Be aware that duloxetine use in pregnant women may produce neonatal adverse reactions, including constant crying, feeding difficulty, hyperreflexia, and irritability. Be aware that duloxetine is distributed in breast milk. Breastfeeding is not recommended. Be aware that the safety and efficacy of duloxetine have not been established in children. Exercise caution when increasing duloxetine doses in elderly patients.

Drowsiness and dizziness may occur, so avoid alcohol and tasks that require mental alertness or motor skills. Blood chemistry tests to assess hepatic and renal function should be performed before and periodically during therapy.

Storage
Store at room temperature.

Administration
Take without regard to meals. Take with food or milk if GI distress occurs. Do not crush or chew enteric-coated capsules. Do not sprinkle capsule contents on food or mix with liquids. The therapeutic effects will be noted within 1-4 wks. Do not abruptly discontinue duloxetine.

Dutasteride

du-tas'tur-ide
Avodart

CATEGORY AND SCHEDULE

Pregnancy Risk Category: X

Classification: 5-α-Reductase inhibitors, antiandrogens, hormones/hormone modifiers

MECHANISM OF ACTION

An androgen hormone inhibitor that inhibits 5-α reductase, an intracellular enzyme that converts testosterone into dihydrotestosterone (DHT) in the prostate gland, reducing the serum DHT level. *Therapeutic Effect:* Reduces size of the prostate gland and BPH symptoms.

PHARMACOKINETICS

Route	Onset	Peak	Duration
PO	24 h	N/A	3-8 wks

Moderately absorbed after PO administration; can be absorbed through skin. Widely distributed. Protein binding: 99%. Metabolized in the liver. Primarily excreted in feces. *Half-life:* Up to 5 wks.

AVAILABILITY

Capsule: 0.5 mg.

INDICATIONS AND DOSAGES

▸ **Benign prostatic hyperplasia (BPH)**

PO

Adults, Elderly. 0.5 mg once a day.

OFF-LABEL USES

Treatment of hair loss in males.

CONTRAINDICATIONS

Females, physical handling of capsules by those who are or may be pregnant, hypersensitivity to dutasteride or other 5-α reductase inhibitors, children.

INTERACTIONS

Drug

Calcium channel antagonists, cimetidine, CYP3A4 inhibitors: May increase dutasteride concentrations.

Herbal

None known.

Food

None known.

DIAGNOSTIC TEST EFFECTS

Decreases the serum prostate-specific antigen (PSA) level, testosterone increased, TSH increased.

SIDE EFFECTS

Occasional

Gynecomastia, sexual dysfunction (decreased libido, impotence, and decreased volume of ejaculate).

SERIOUS REACTIONS

- Toxicity may be manifested as rash, diarrhea, and abdominal pain.
- Allergic reaction, angioedema, pruritus, rash, urticaria may occur.

PRECAUTIONS & CONSIDERATIONS

Caution is warranted with hepatic impairment, preexisting sexual dysfunction (such as impotence and decreased libido), and obstructive uropathy. The drug has a pregnancy risk category of X and carries the risk of causing anomalies in the male fetus. Pregnant women or women trying to conceive should not consume or handle dutasteride.

Dutasteride may cause impotence and decrease ejaculate volume. Serum PSA determinations should be obtained before and periodically during therapy. A new baseline must be established after 3-6 mo of use. Intake and output and improvement in BPH signs and symptoms should also be monitored. Avoid blood donation during therapy and for 6 mo after last dose. Safety and efficacy have not been established in children; contraindicated.

Storage

Store at room temperature of 77° F or lower. Higher temps may cause capsules to become soft, leak, or stick together.

Administration

Do not break, crush, or open capsules. Take dutasteride without regard to food. Urinary flow may not improve for up to 6 mo after beginning treatment.

Women who are pregnant or are trying to become pregnant should not handle open or broken capsules or capsule contents.

Dyphylline

dye′fi-lin

★ Dylix, Lufyllin

Do not confuse dyphylline with Dilacor.

CATEGORY AND SCHEDULE

Pregnancy Risk Category: C

Classification: Bronchodilators, xanthine derivatives

MECHANISM OF ACTION

A xanthine derivative that acts as a bronchodilator by directly relaxing smooth muscle of the bronchial airway and pulmonary blood vessels similar to theophylline. *Therapeutic Effect:* Relieves bronchospasm, increases vital capacity, produces cardiac and skeletal muscle stimulation.

D

PHARMACOKINETICS

Rapid absorption after PO administration. Protein binding: Unknown. Not metabolized to theophylline in vivo. Excreted in urine. *Half-life:* 2 h.

AVAILABILITY

Elixir: 100 mg/15 mL (Dylix).
Tablet: 200 mg, 400 mg (Lufyllin).

INDICATIONS AND DOSAGES

▸ **Chronic bronchospasm, asthma**

PO

Adults, Elderly. 15 mg/kg up to 4 times/day. Individualize dosage to condition and response; patients may respond to lower dosage.

▸ **Dosage in renal impairment:**

Creatinine Clearance (mL/min)	Dosage Percent
50-80	Administer 75% of dose
10-50	Administer 50% of dose
< 10	Administer 25% of dose

CONTRAINDICATIONS

History of hypersensitivity to dyphylline, related xanthine derivatives, or any component of the formulation.

INTERACTIONS

Drug

Adenosine, benzodiazepines: Effects may be decreased by dyphylline.

β-Blockers, nonselective: May decrease bronchodilator effects of dyphylline.

Cimetidine, ciprofloxacin, erythromycin, norfloxacin, probenecid, zileuton: May increase dyphylline concentrations and risk of toxicity.

Glucocorticoids: May produce hypernatremia.

Phenytoin, primidone, rifampin: May increase dyphylline metabolism.

Smoking: May decrease dyphylline concentrations.

Herbal

Ma huang, ephedra: Increased CNS stimulation.

Food

Caffeine: Increased CNS stimulation.

SIDE EFFECTS

Frequent

Tachycardia, nervousness, restlessness.

Occasional

Heartburn, vomiting, headache, mild diuresis, insomnia, nausea.

SERIOUS REACTIONS

• Ventricular arrhythmias, hypotension, circulatory failure, seizures, hyperglycemia, and syndrome of inappropriate antidiuretic hormone (SIADH) have been reported.

PRECAUTIONS & CONSIDERATIONS

Uncontrolled arrhythmias, hyperthyroidism.

Caution is necessary with congestive heart failure (CHF), hypertension, impaired cardiac or renal function, hyperthyroidism, peptic ulcer disease, and seizure disorder. Be aware that dyphylline is equivalent to 70% theophylline. Dyphylline should not be used to treat status asthmaticus. Serious dosing errors can occur if dyphylline serum levels are monitored by theophylline serum assay. Smoking, charcoal-broiled food, and a high-protein, low-carbohydrate diet may decrease dyphylline level. Caffeine derivatives such as chocolate, coffee, cola, cocoa, and tea should be avoided.

Oxygen depletion may occur and is evident by blue or gray lips, blue or dusky-colored fingernails in light-skinned patients, and gray fingernails in dark-skinned persons.

Storage

Store at room temperature.

Administration

Give oral dyphylline with food to avoid GI distress. Give with plenty of water.

Ecallantide

e-kal′lan-tide

★ 🍁 Kalbitor

CATEGORY AND SCHEDULE

Pregnancy Risk Category: C

Classification: Kallikrein inhibitors

MECHANISM OF ACTION

A potent, selective, reversible inhibitor of kallikrein that blocks the production of kallikrein, a precursor to bradykinin. *Therapeutic Effect:* Reduces edema, improving symptoms based on the site of the hereditary angioedema (HAE) attack.

PHARMACOKINETICS

Time to peak serum concentration 2-3 h; ecallantide is a small protein (7054 Da), and renal elimination via the urine has been demonstrated. *Half-life:* About 2 h.

AVAILABILITY

Injection Solution: 10 mg/mL.

INDICATIONS AND DOSAGES

▸ **Acute attacks of hereditary angioedema (HAE)**

SC

Adults and Children 16 yr and older. 30 mg (given as three 10-mg injections). If attack persists, may give an additional 30-mg dose within a 24-h period.

CONTRAINDICATIONS

Ecallantide hypersensitivity.

INTERACTIONS

Drug, Herbal, Food

None known.

DIAGNOSTIC TEST EFFECTS

Neutralizing antibodies form in roughly 4.7% of patients. aPTT prolongation has been observed with intravenous use.

SIDE EFFECTS

Frequent (≥10%)

Headache, nausea, fatigue, diarrhea, upper respiratory infection.

Occasional (3%-9%)

Injection site reactions, nasopharyngitis, vomiting, pruritus, abdominal pain, pyrexia.

SERIOUS REACTIONS

- Hypersensitivity reactions: Anaphylaxis occurs in 3.9% of patients and is similar in appearance to the disease itself. Pruritus, rash and urticaria may also be present.

PRECAUTIONS & CONSIDERATIONS

Administer in a setting equipped to manage anaphylaxis and hereditary angioedema. Given the similarity in hypersensitivity symptoms and acute HAE symptoms, monitor patients closely for hypersensitivity reactions. There are no data in pregnant women. It is unknown if the drug is excreted in breast milk. The safety and efficacy of ecallantide have not been established in children under 16 yr of age. There are no data in patients with renal or hepatic dysfunction.

Storage

Refrigerate. Do not freeze. Protect from light; store in original carton until administration. The solution should be colorless and clear.

Administration

For subcutaneous use only. Using aseptic technique, withdraw 1 mL (10 mg) from the vial using a large-bore needle. Change the needle on the syringe to a 27 gauge, or other needle suitable for subcutaneous injection. Inject into the skin of the abdomen, thigh, or upper arm. Repeat procedure until all 3 vials (entire dose) administered. Each of the injections may be in the same or in different anatomic locations (abdomen, thigh, upper arm). There is no need for site rotation. Separate each injection by at least 2 inches (5 cm) and keep away from the anatomical site of attack. The same instructions apply to an additional dose administered within 24 h. Different injection sites or the same anatomical location (as used for the first administration) may be used.

Econazole

e-kone'a-zole

CATEGORY AND SCHEDULE

Pregnancy Risk Category: C

Classification: Antifungals, topical azole antifungals

MECHANISM OF ACTION

An imidazole derivative that changes the permeability of the fungal cell wall. *Therapeutic Effect:* Inhibits fungal biosynthesis of triglycerides, phospholipids. Fungistatic.

PHARMACOKINETICS

Penetrates into stratum corneum, but low systemic absorption. Less than 1% of applied dose recovered in urine or feces as metabolites.

AVAILABILITY

Cream: 1%.

INDICATIONS AND DOSAGES

▸ **Treatment of tinea pedis, tinea cruris, tinea corporis, tinea versicolor**

TOPICAL

Adults, Elderly, Children. Apply once daily to affected area for 2-4 wks. Tinea pedis for 1 mo.

▸ **Treatment of cutaneous candidiasis**

TOPICAL

Adults, Elderly, Children. Apply twice daily to affected area for 2 wks.

CONTRAINDICATIONS

Hypersensitivity to econazole.

INTERACTIONS

Drug

None known.

Herbal

None known.

Food

None known.

DIAGNOSTIC TEST EFFECTS

None known.

SIDE EFFECTS

Occasional (1%-10%)

Burning, itching, stinging, redness at application site.

Rare (< 1%)

Contact dermatitis.

SERIOUS REACTIONS

• None known.

PRECAUTIONS & CONSIDERATIONS

Caution should be used during pregnancy. Econazole should be avoided during the first trimester of pregnancy. Use only if clearly needed in the second and third trimesters. It is unknown whether econazole is distributed in breast milk.

Storage

Store at room temperature. Protect from heat and light.

Administration

Apply and rub gently into affected areas. Prolonged therapy over weeks or months may be necessary. Avoid occlusive dressings and wear light clothing for ventilation. Avoid getting in the eyes.

Eculizumab

e'coo-liz'oo-mab

★ 🍁 Soliris

Do not confuse Soliris with Solage or Solaraze.

CATEGORY AND SCHEDULE

Pregnancy Risk Category: C

Classification: Biologic response modifiers, monoclonal antibodies, complement inhibitors

MECHANISM OF ACTION

A monoclonal antibody that specifically and with high affinity binds to the complement protein C5, thereby inhibiting its cleavage to C5a and C5b and preventing the generation of the terminal complement complex C5b-9. *Therapeutic Effect:* Inhibits terminal complement-mediated intravascular hemolysis in PNH patients, lowering need for RBC transfusion and improving fatigue.

PHARMACOKINETICS

Complement activity inhibited for less than 2 wks following single dose. Reduction of hemolysis (as determined by reduction in LDH concentrations) is maintained at least 52 wks. Metabolic fate not well characterized; catabolized in various tissues via diffuse cellular processes. Minimal excretion in urine expected due to large molecular size. Small quantities found in bile. *Half-life:* Approximately 272 h.

AVAILABILITY

Injection Solution: 300 mg (10 mg/mL).

INDICATIONS AND DOSAGES

▸ **Reduction of hemolysis from paroxysmal nocturnal hemoglobinuria (PNH)**

IV INFUSION

Adults. 600 mg every 7 days for 4 wks, then 900 mg for the 5th dose given 7 days later, and then 900 mg every 14 days.

CONTRAINDICATIONS

Patients with unresolved serious *Neisseria meningitidis* infection or who are not currently vaccinated against *N. meningitidis.*

INTERACTIONS

Drug, Herbal, Food

None known.

DIAGNOSTIC TEST EFFECTS

A reduction in LDH should correspond with reduction in hemolysis during treatment.

SIDE EFFECTS

Frequent (≥ 10%)

Headache, rhinitis, sore throat, back pain, nausea, fatigue.

Occasional (2%-9%)

Myalgia, sinusitis, respiratory tract infection, herpes infection, constipation, pain in an extremity, flu-like symptoms.

Rare

Infusion reactions.

SERIOUS REACTIONS

- Serious and potentially life-threatening infections (e.g., sepsis, meningitis); the drug increases the risk of meningococcal infection, which may rapidly become life threatening or fatal if not recognized and treated early.

• As with other protein infusions, potential for anaphylaxis or other hypersensitivity reactions (rare).

PRECAUTIONS & CONSIDERATIONS

Serious meningococcal infections have occurred during treatment. Patients being treated with eculizumab will automatically be enrolled in a registry (Soliris Safety Registry) established to monitor long-term safety of the drug and limit distribution to those patients enrolled in the program with their prescribers. Patients should carry a card stating they are receiving eculizumab treatment. Patients are required to receive a meningococcal vaccination at least 2 wks prior to receiving the first dose, if they have not previously been vaccinated. They must be revaccinated according to current medical guidelines while on therapy. There are no data in pregnant women. It is unknown if the drug is excreted in breast milk. The safety and efficacy of eculizumab have not been established in children under the age of 18 yrs. There are no particular precautions for elderly patients.

Monitor patient for infusion-related reactions. Between treatments, patients should immediately report signs or symptoms of infection, particularly high fever (> 103° F) and photophobia, severe headache, stiff neck, flu-like symptoms, or other severe or unusual symptoms. Patients should receive their treatments within 2 days of their dose due date. If treatments are suddenly discontinued, rebound hemolysis and associated symptoms of the disease may occur; if patients must stop treatments, they should be carefully monitored for at least 8 wks.

Storage

Refrigerate unopened vials and keep in original carton until time of use. Do not freeze; protect from light; do not shake. Infusions are stable for 24 h under refrigeration and at room temperature.

Administration

For IV infusion only. Do not administer as an intravenous push or bolus. Withdraw the required amount for the dose from the vials into a sterile syringe. Transfer the recommended dose to an infusion bag. Dilute to a final infusion concentration of 5 mg/mL by adding the appropriate (equal) amount of 0.9% NaCl, 0.45% NaCl, D5W, or Ringer's injection to the infusion bag. The final admixed infusion volume is 120 mL for 600-mg doses or 180 mL for 900-mg doses. Gently invert the infusion bag to ensure thorough mixing of the product and diluent. Discard any unused portion left in a vial, as the product contains no preservatives. Allow the infusion to come to room temperature before infusion; do not heat.

Administer IV infusion over 35 min. If an adverse reaction occurs during infusion, the infusion may be slowed or stopped at the discretion of the physician. If the infusion is slowed, the total infusion time should not exceed 2 h. Monitor patient for 1 h after every infusion for infusion-related reactions.

Edetate Calcium Disodium (Calcium EDTA)

ed-eh-tate kal-see-um dye-sow-dee-um

★ Calcium Disodium Versenate

Do not confuse with edetate disodium.

Do not use EDTA as abbreviation to avoid potential confusion.

CATEGORY AND SCHEDULE

Pregnancy Risk Category: B

Classification: Antidotes, heavy metal

E

MECHANISM OF ACTION

A chelating agent that reduces the blood concentration of heavy metals, especially lead, forming stable complexes. *Therapeutic Effect:* Allows heavy metal excretion in urine.

PHARMACOKINETICS

Well absorbed after parenteral administration; poorly absorbed from the GI tract. Penetrates to extracellular fluid and slowly diffuses into cerebrospinal fluid (CSF). No metabolism occurs. Excreted in the urine either unchanged or as the metal chelates. *Half-life:* 20-60 min (IV), 1.5 h (IM). Onset for chelation of lead: 1 h.

AVAILABILITY

Injection: 200 mg/mL.

INDICATIONS AND DOSAGES

▸ **Diagnosis of lead poisoning**

IM/IV

Adults, Elderly for 8-h or 24-h mobilization test. 500 mg/m^2 IV over 1 h or IM. Maximum: 1g.

Adults, Eldery for 8-h mobilization test. 50 mg/kg. Maximum: 1g IM as one dose is alternate.

IM/IV

Children for 24-h mobilization test. 500 mg/m^2 as single-dose IV over 1h, or 500 mg/m^2 IM divided into doses at 12-h intervals (maximum: 1 g). NOTE: Mobilization tests should not be performed in symptomatic patients or those with blood levels > 55 mcg/dL as therapy is indicated.

▸ **Symptomatic (without encephalopathy), or asymptomatic lead poisoning with blood lead levels > 70 mcg/dL**

IM/IV

Adults, Elderly, Children. 1-1.5 g/m^2 daily as 8-24 h IV infusion or divided every 12 h or 167 mg/m^2 IM every 4 h for 3-5 days (if blood lead concentration > 70 mcg/dL, calcium edetate usually given with dimercaprol until levels < 50 mcg/dL). Allow at least 2-4 days, up to 2-3 wks, between courses of therapy. Adults should not be given more than 2 courses of therapy.

▸ **Lead poisoning (with encephalopathy) with or without blood lead levels > 70 mcg/dL**

IM

Adults, Elderly, Children. Initially, dimercaprol 4 mg/kg; then give dimercaprol 4 mg/kg and calcium EDTA 250 mg/m^2 IM 4 h later and q4h for 5 days. Can also be given IV 50 mg/kg/day as 24-h continuous infusion or 1-1.5 g/m^2 as 8- to 24-h infusion or divided into 2 doses every 12 h. Allow at least 2 days before considering repeating course. Give dimercaprol for at least first 3 days.

▸ **Asymptomatic lead poisoning in children with blood lead level 45-69 mcg/dL**

IV

1 g/m^2/day IV infusion over 8-24 h is preferred regimen. 25 mg/kg/day for 5 days as an 8- to 24-h infusion or divided into 2 doses every 12 h. May also give dose IM at 8- to 12-h intervals.

CONTRAINDICATIONS

Anuria, severe renal disease, hepatitis, hypersensitivity to EDTA or any component of the formulation.

INTERACTIONS

Drug

Insulin preparations: May bind to zinc components of some insulin preparations increasing active amount of insulin while decreasing duraction of action.

Zinc: May decrease the effects of zinc.

Herbal and Food
None known.

IV INCOMPATIBILITIES
Amphotericin B cholesteryl (Amphotec), hydralazine, dextrose 10%, lactated Ringer's, Ringer's.

IV COMPATIBILITIES
Epinephrine.

SIDE EFFECTS
Frequent
Chills, fever, anorexia, headache, histamine-like reaction (sneezing, stuffy nose, watery eyes), decreased BP, nausea, vomiting, thrombophlebitis, pain at IM injection site.
Rare
Frequent urination, secondary gout (severe pain in feet, knees, elbows).

SERIOUS REACTIONS
• Drug may produce same signs of renal damage as severe acute lead poisoning (proteinuria, microscopic hematuria). Transient anemia/bone marrow depression, hypercalcemia (constipation, drowsiness, dry mouth, metallic taste) occur occasionally.

PRECAUTIONS & CONSIDERATIONS
Edetate calcium disodium is capable of producing toxic effects that can be fatal. Dosage schedules should be followed, and at no time should the recommended daily dose be increased. It is unknown whether EDTA is distributed in breast milk. Lead encephalopathy is usually rare in adults but occurs more often in children. No age-related precautions have been noted in children or elderly patients. Edetate calcium disodium can produce the same renal damage as lead poisoning, such as proteinuria and microscopic hematuria. Discontinue if severe oliguria or anuria occurs. Monitor for cardiac arrhythmias.

Do not confuse with edetate disodium. The FDA recommends that edetate disodium never be given for chelation therapy as fatal hypocalcemia can occur if edetate disodium is used instead of edetate calcium disodium for chelation. Do not use abbreviation EDTA. Only edetate calcium disodium should be used for lead intoxication.

Administration
Be aware that when administering IV, calcium EDTA may be given in 2 divided doses at 12-h intervals or 8- to 24-h infusions; when administered IM and used alone, it may be given in divided doses at 8- to 12-h intervals; when given IM with dimercaprol in divided doses, administer at 4-h intervals.

Be aware that total dose is dependent on severity of lead poisoning, patient response, and tolerance to medication. Consult specific protocols.

For IV administration, add total daily dose to 250-500 mL of 0.9% NaCl or D5W. Preferably infused over 8-12 hr. Avoid rapid infusion.

Patients with lead encephalopathy and cerebral edema may experience a lethal increase in intracranial pressure following IV infusion; the IM route is preferred for these patients. In cases where the IV route is necessary, avoid rapid infusion. The dosage schedule should be followed, and at no time should the recommended daily dose be exceeded. Rapid IV infusion may be lethal due to increased intracranial pressure.

For IM injection, should add lidocaine or prilocaine to injection: 1 mL of 1% procaine hydrochloride or lidocaine 1% to each mL of edetate calcium disodium to minimize pain at injection site. The total daily dose is usually divided into equal doses given 8-12 h apart.

E

Edetate Disodium

ed′eh-tate dye-sow′dee-um

Do not confuse with edetate calcium disodium.

Do not use EDTA as abbreviation to avoid potential confusion.

CATEGORY AND SCHEDULE

Pregnancy Risk Category: C

Classification: Antidotes, chelators

MECHANISM OF ACTION

A chelating agent that forms a soluble chelate with calcium, resulting in rapid decrease in plasma calcium concentrations. *Therapeutic Effect:* Allows calcium to be excreted in urine.

PHARMACOKINETICS

Distributed in extracellular fluid and does not appear in red blood cells. No metabolism occurs. Rapidly excreted in the urine. *Half-life:* 1.4-3 h. Prolonged in renal impairment. Chelation occurs in 24-48 h.

AVAILABILITY

Injection: 150 mg/mL.

INDICATIONS AND DOSAGES

▸ **Digitalis toxicity (ventricular arrhythmia), hypercalcemia**

IV

Adults, Elderly. 50 mg/kg/day over 3 h or more, daily for 5 days, skip 2 days, repeat as needed up to 15 doses. Maximum: 3 g/day.

Children. 40 mg/kg/day over 3 h or more, daily for 5 days, skip 5 days, repeat as needed. Maximum: 70 mg/kg/day.

CONTRAINDICATIONS

Anuria, renal impairment, hypersensitivity to edetate disodium or any component of the formulation.

INTERACTIONS

Drug

Insulin: May increase the effects of some forms of insulin containing zinc.

Herbal

None known.

Food

None known.

SIDE EFFECTS

Frequent

Abdominal cramps or pain, diarrhea, nausea, vomiting, circumoral paresthesia, headache, numbness, postural hypotension.

Rare

Exfoliative dermatitis, toxic skin and mucous membrane reactions, thrombophlebitis (at injection site).

SERIOUS REACTIONS

- Nephrotoxicity may occur with excessive dosages.
- Hypomagnesemia may occur with prolonged use.
- Hypokalemia can occur as potassium excretion may increase.

PRECAUTIONS & CONSIDERATIONS

Caution is warranted in patients with diabetes mellitus, clinical or subclinical hypokalemia, intracranial lesions, seizures, renal impairment, and limited cardiac reserve or incipient congestive heart failure. Be aware that edetate sodium is recommended only when the severity of the clinical condition justifies the aggressive measures associated with this type of therapy. It is unknown whether edetate disodium is distributed in breast milk. No age-related precautions have been noted in children or elderly patients.

Stop edetate sodium immediately and notify physician if frequent or sudden urges to urinate occur.

Do not confuse with edetate calcium disodium. The FDA recommends that edetate disodium never be given for chelation therapy as fatal hypocalcemia can occur if edetate disodium is used instead of edetate calcium disodium for chelation. Do not use abbreviation EDTA. Only edetate calcium disodium should be used for lead intoxication.

Administration

Be aware that edetate disodium is rarely used to treat digitalis-induced ventricular arrhythmias because other, more effective agents are available. It should be used only in emergency situations. It is not for IM use.

Dilute solution for injection with 500 mL of D5W or 0.9% NaCl before IV administration; in pediatric patients, concentration should not exceed 3% (30 mg/mL). Administer by IV infusion only after dilution. Be careful not to exceed recommended dose or rate of administration (over at least 3 h). A precipitous drop in serum calcium concentrations may occur. Calcium replacement suitable for IV administration should be instantly available.

Efavirenz

e-fahv′er-ins

Sustiva

Do not confuse with Survanta. Do not confuse efavirenz with etravirine.

CATEGORY AND SCHEDULE

Pregnancy Risk Category: D

Classification: Antiretroviral, nonnucleoside reverse transcriptase inhibitor

MECHANISM OF ACTION

A nonnucleoside reverse transcriptase inhibitor that inhibits the activity of HIV reverse transcriptase of HIV-1 and the transcription of HIV-1 RNA to DNA. *Therapeutic Effect:* Interrupts HIV replication, slowing the progression of HIV infection.

PHARMACOKINETICS

Rapidly absorbed after PO administration, increased by fatty meals. Protein binding: 99% (primarily albumin). Metabolized to inactive metabolites in the liver via CYP3A4 and CYP2B6. Eliminated in urine and feces. *Half-life:* 40-55 h.

AVAILABILITY

Capsules: 50 mg, 200 mg.
Tablets: 600 mg.

INDICATIONS AND DOSAGES

▸ **HIV infection (in combination with other antiretrovirals)**

PO

Adults, Elderly, Children 3 yr and older weighing 40 kg or more. 600 mg once a day at bedtime.

Children 3 yr and older weighing 32.5 kg to < 40 kg. 400 mg once a day.

Children 3 yr and older weighing 25 kg to < 32.5 kg. 350 mg once a day.

Children 3 yr and older weighing 20 kg to < 25 kg. 300 mg once a day.

Children 3 yr and older weighing 15 kg to < 20 kg. 250 mg once a day.

Children 3 yr and older weighing 10 kg to < 15 kg. 200 mg once a day.

▸ **Dosage adjustment with voriconazole (adults)**

The voriconazole maintenance dose should be increased to 400 mg every 12 h, and the efavirenz dose should be decreased to 300 mg once daily using the capsule formulation (one 200-mg and two 50-mg capsules or six 50-mg capsules).

E

CONTRAINDICATIONS

Efavirenz as monotherapy; hypersensitivity to efavirenz. The following drugs are contraindicated with efavirenz: ergot alkaloids, midazolam, triazolam, bepridil, cisapride, pimozide, and St. John's wort.

INTERACTIONS

Drug

Alcohol, benzodiazepines, psychoactive drugs: May produce additive central nervous system (CNS) effects.

Amprenavir, atazanavir, diltiazem, HMG-CoA reductase inhibitors, indinavir, itraconazole, lopinavir, methadone, saquinavir, sertraline, voriconazole: Decreases the plasma concentrations of these drugs. Some of these medications significantly increase efavirenz concentrations.

Carbamazepine: Levels of carbamazepine and/or efavirenz may decrease.

Clarithromycin: Decreases clarithromycin plasma levels.

CYP2B6, CYP3A4 inducers: May decrease concentration of efavirenz.

CYP2C9, CYP2C19 substrates: May increase concentration of substrates.

CYP3A4 substrates: Concentration of substrates may be altered.

Ergot derivatives, midazolam, triazolam: May cause serious or life-threatening reactions, such as arrhythmias, prolonged sedation, or respiratory depression. Contraindicated.

Nelfinavir, ritonavir, ethinyl estradiol: Increases the plasma concentrations of these drugs.

Phenobarbital, rifabutin, rifampin: Lowers efavirenz plasma concentration.

Warfarin: Alters warfarin plasma concentration.

Herbal

St. John's wort: Decreases efavirenz concentration; contraindicated.

Food

High-fat meals: May increase drug absorption.

DIAGNOSTIC TEST EFFECTS

May produce false-positive urine test results for cannabinoid and increased total cholesterol, AST (SGOT), ALT (SGPT), serum amylase, and serum triglyceride levels.

SIDE EFFECTS

Frequent (52%)

Mild to severe: Dizziness, vivid dreams, insomnia, confusion, impaired concentration, amnesia, agitation, depersonalization, hallucinations, euphoria, somnolence (mild symptoms do not interfere with daily activities; severe symptoms interrupt daily activities). Insomnia is often transient.

Occasional

Mild to moderate: Maculopapular rash (27%); nausea, fatigue, headache, diarrhea, fever, cough (< 26%) (moderate symptoms may interfere with daily activities).

Rare

Fat redistribution syndrome with buffalo hump, asymptomatic amylasemia, visual impairment, convulsions.

SERIOUS REACTIONS

- Convulsions and immune reconstitution syndrome rarely occur. Psychiatric symptoms, including aggressive behavior, paranoid reactions, severe depression, suicidal ideations, and manic reactions, may occur.
- Pancreatitis or hepatic failure.
- Serious skin rashes, including Stevens-Johnson syndrome (rare, but may be more common in children).

PRECAUTIONS & CONSIDERATIONS

Caution is warranted in patients with a history of liver impairment, mental illness, or substance abuse. Breastfeeding is not recommended for mothers with HIV-1 infection. Reports of neural tube defects in infants born to women with first-trimester exposure, includes cases of meningomyelocele and Dandy-Walker syndrome; data indicate drug may cause fetal harm when administered during the first trimester. Pregnancy should be avoided in women receiving efavirenz. Barrier contraception must be used in combination with other methods (e.g., hormonal contraceptives). Use of adequate contraceptive measures for 12 wks after discontinuation of the drug is recommended. The safety and efficacy of efavirenz have not been established in children younger than 3 yr. In children, there may be an increased incidence of rash. No age-related precautions have been noted in elderly patients. Efavirenz is not a cure for HIV infection, nor does it reduce risk of transmission to others. Use in combination with other antiretrovirals; do not use as monotherapy.

Expect to obtain history of all prescription and nonprescription medications before giving the drug because efavirenz interacts with several drugs. Monitor for signs and symptoms of adverse CNS psychological side effects, such as abnormal dreams, dizziness, impaired concentration, insomnia, severe acute depression including suicidal ideation or attempts, and somnolence. Avoid tasks that require mental alertness or motor skills until response to the drug is established.

Storage

Store at room temperature.

Administration

Take on empty stomach at bedtime. Giving drug at bedtime helps attenuate some CNS effects. Administration with food may increase side effects; avoid. Take the medication every day as prescribed. Do not alter the dose or discontinue the medication without first notifying the physician.

Eflornithine

eh-floor′nigh-theen

Vaniqa

CATEGORY AND SCHEDULE

Pregnancy Risk Category: C

Classification: Antiprotozoals, depilatory agents, dermatologics

MECHANISM OF ACTION

A topical that inhibits ornithine decarboxylase cell division and synthetic function in the skin. When given systemically, the drug has antiprotozoal activity. *Therapeutic Effect:* Reduces rate of hair growth. Treats protozoal infection systemically.

PHARMACOKINETICS

Absorption is < 1% from intact skin. Not metabolized. Primarily excreted as unchanged drug in urine. *Half-life:* 8 h.

AVAILABILITY

Cream: 13.9%.

INDICATIONS AND DOSAGES

▸ **For reduction of unwanted facial hair in women**

Topical

Adults, Elderly. Apply a thin layer to affected area of the face and adjacent involved areas under chin; rub in thoroughly. Use twice daily at least 8 h apart. Do not wash area for at least 4 h.

E

OFF-LABEL USES
Outside of U.S., systemic forms used for pneumocystis pneumonia (PCP), African sleeping sickness.

CONTRAINDICATIONS
Hypersensitivity to eflornithine or any component of the formulation.

INTERACTIONS
Drug, Herbal, and Food
None known.

DIAGNOSTIC TEST EFFECTS
May elevate serum transaminases.

SIDE EFFECTS
Frequent (> 10%)
Acne, pseudofolliculitis barbae.
Occasional (2%-10%)
Headache, stinging/burning skin, tingling skin, dry skin, pruritus, erythema, dyspepsia.
Rare (<1%)
Bleeding skin, rash, herpes simplex, folliculitis, rosacea.

SERIOUS REACTIONS
• Bleeding skin, cheilitis, contact dermatitis, herpes simplex, lip swelling, nausea, and weakness have been reported.

PRECAUTIONS & CONSIDERATIONS
It is unknown whether eflornithine is distributed in breast milk. Safety and efficacy of eflornithine have not been established in children. No age-related precautions have been noted in elderly patients.

Transient stinging or burning may occur when applied to broken or abraded skin.

Storage
Store at room temperature; do not freeze.

Administration
Continue to use other hair-removal techniques in conjunction with eflornithine. Apply eflornithine more than 5 min after hair removal. Avoid application on abraded or broken skin. Cosmetics or sunscreen may be applied over treated areas after cream has dried. Therapeutic improvement noted in 4-8 wks. Condition may return to pretreatment levels 8 wks after discontinuing treatment.

Eletriptan
elé-trip'tan
Relpax

CATEGORY AND SCHEDULE
Pregnancy Risk Category: C

Classification: Migraine agents, serotonin agonists

MECHANISM OF ACTION
A serotonin receptor agonist that binds selectively to vascular serotonin 5-HT1B, 5-HT1D, and 5-HT1F receptors, producing a vasoconstrictive effect on cranial blood vessels. *Therapeutic Effect:* Relieves migraine headache.

PHARMACOKINETICS
Well absorbed after PO administration (50% bioavailability), peaks with 1.5 h. Metabolized by the liver to inactive metabolite by CYP3A4. Eliminated in urine (90%). *Half-life:* 4.4 h increased in patients with hepatic impairment and in elderly patients (older than 65 yr).

AVAILABILITY
Tablets: 20 mg, 40 mg.

INDICATIONS AND DOSAGES
▸ **Acute migraine headache with or without aura**

PO
Adults, Elderly. 20-40 mg. If headache improves but then returns, dose may be repeated after 2 h. Maximum: 80 mg/day.

CONTRAINDICATIONS

Hypersensitivity to eletriptan, arrhythmias associated with angina, conduction disorders, coronary artery disease, ischemic heart disease, history of myocardial infarction, cerebrovascular disease, peripheral vascular disease, ischemic bowel disease, hemiplegic or basilar migraine, severe hepatic impairment, uncontrolled hypertension. Eletriptan should not be used within 24 h of another serotonin agonist (triptan) or an ergot-type medication; do not use within 72 h of a potent CYP3A4 inhibitor.

INTERACTIONS

Drug
Clarithromycin, itraconazole, ketoconazole, nefazodone, nelfinavir, ritonavir, CYP3A4 inhibitors: May decrease eletriptan metabolism. Contraindicated within 72 h of eletriptan use. This list is not inclusive of all potent CYP3A4 inhibitors.
Ergotamine-containing medications: May produce a vasospastic reaction. Contraindicated within 24 h of eletriptan use.
Sibutramine: May produce serotonin syndrome (marked by altered level of consciousness, CNS irritability, motor weakness, myoclonus, and shivering).
Serotonin reuptake inhibitors/ serotonin agonists (triptans): May increase risk of serotonin syndrome.
Herbal and Food
None known.

DIAGNOSTIC TEST EFFECTS

None known.

SIDE EFFECTS

Occasional (5%-6%)
Dizziness, somnolence, asthenia, nausea.
Rare (2%-4%)
Paresthesia, headache, dry mouth, warm or hot sensation, dyspepsia, dysphagia.

SERIOUS REACTIONS

- Cardiac reactions (including ischemia, coronary artery vasospasm, and myocardial infarction) and noncardiac vasospasm-related reactions (such as hemorrhage and cerebrovascular accident [CVA]) occur rarely, particularly in patients with hypertension, diabetes, or a strong family history of coronary artery disease; obese patients; smokers; males older than 40 yr; and postmenopausal women.
- Serotonin syndrome has occurred; avoid concomitant use of serotonergic drugs. Increased BP and hypertensive crisis have occurred in patients with and without a history of hypertension.

PRECAUTIONS & CONSIDERATIONS

Caution is warranted in patients with controlled hypertension, mild to moderate hepatic or renal impairment, and a history of CVA. Eletriptan should not be given to patients with risk factors predictive of coronary artery disease unless clinical evaluation demonstrates that the patient is free of cardiovascular disease. Eletriptan is distributed in breast milk, and caution should be exercised in lactating women. Eletriptan effects in pregnancy are unknown and may suppress ovulation. The safety and efficacy of eletriptan have not been established in children. Elderly patients are at increased risk for hypertension. Tasks that require mental alertness or motor skills should be avoided.

Notify the physician immediately if palpitations, pain or tightness in the chest or throat, pain or weakness in the extremities, or sudden or severe abdominal pain occurs.
BP for evidence of uncontrolled hypertension should be assessed before treatment. Migraines and associated symptoms, including nausea and vomiting, photophobia, and phonophobia (sound sensitivity), should be assessed before and during treatment.

Storage

Store at room temperature. Protect from light and moisture.

Administration

Take film-coated tablets whole with fluids; don't crush or break them.

Emedastine

eh-med′ah-steen

Emadine

CATEGORY AND SCHEDULE

Pregnancy Risk Category: B

Classification: Ophthalmic antihistamine

MECHANISM OF ACTION

An ophthalmic H_1 receptor antagonist that inhibits histamine-stimulated vascular permeability in the conjunctiva. *Therapeutic Effect:* Relieves ocular itching associated with allergic conjunctivitis.

PHARMACOKINETICS

Negligible absorption after ophthalmic administration; amounts mostly below detection limits for assay.

AVAILABILITY

Ophthalmic Solution: 0.05%.

INDICATIONS AND DOSAGES

▸ **Allergic conjunctivitis**

OPHTHALMIC

Adults, Elderly, Children 3 yr and older. 1 drop in affected eye(s) up to 4 times daily.

CONTRAINDICATIONS

Hypersensitivity to emedastine or any other component of the formulation.

DRUG INTERACTIONS

Drug

None reported.

Herbal and Food

None known.

SIDE EFFECTS

Frequent

Headache.

Occasional

Abnormal dreams, asthenia (loss of strength, energy), bad taste, blurred vision, burning or stinging, dry eyes, foreign body sensation, tearing.

Rare

- Somnolence and malaise occur rarely.

SERIOUS REACTIONS

None reported.

PRECAUTIONS & CONSIDERATIONS

For topical ophthalmic use only. Safety and effectiveness have not been established in children < 3 yr of age. Not known to what extent it is distributed in breast milk; use with caution.

Storage

Store at room temperature. Do not use more than 30 days after opening.

Administration

Wash hands before use. Tilt head back slightly and gently pull the lower eyelid to form a pouch. Instill the drops and gently close eyes. Do not touch the tip of the dropper to any surface. Wait at least 10 min after use before inserting contact lenses.

Emtricitabine

em-tri-site′uh-been

Emtriva

CATEGORY AND SCHEDULE

Pregnancy Risk Category: B

Classification: Antiretroviral, nucleoside reverse transcriptase inhibitors

MECHANISM OF ACTION

An antiretroviral that inhibits HIV-1 reverse transcriptase by incorporating itself into viral DNA, resulting in chain termination. *Therapeutic Effect:* Interrupts HIV replication, slowing the progression of HIV infection.

PHARMACOKINETICS

Rapidly and extensively absorbed from the GI tract. Bioavailability of capsules 93%, oral solution 75%. Relative bioavailability of oral solution approximately 80% of capsules. Excreted primarily in urine (86%) and, to a lesser extent, in feces (14%); 30% removed by hemodialysis. Unknown whether removed by peritoneal dialysis. *Half-life:* 10 h, children 5-18 h.

AVAILABILITY

Capsules: 200 mg.
Oral Solution: 10 mg/mL.

INDICATIONS AND DOSAGES

▸ **HIV infection (in combination with other antiretrovirals)**

PO

Adults, Elderly. 200-mg capsule or 240-mg (24-mL) oral solution once a day.

Children 3 months to 17 yr. 6 mg/kg (maximum 240 mg) of oral solution once daily.

Infants 0-3 months. 3mg/kg once daily (oral solution).

▸ **Adult dosage in renal impairment**

Dosage and frequency are modified based on creatinine clearance.

Creatinine Clearance (mL/min)	Capsule Dosage	Oral Solution Dosage
30-49	200-mg capsule q24h	120 mg (12 mL) q24h
15-29	200-mg capsule q72h	80 mg (8 mL) q24h
< 15	200-mg capsule q72h	60 mg (6 mL) q24h

▸ **Hemodialysis patients (give after hemodialysis)**

Adults. 200 mg q96h capsule or 60 mg q24h oral solution.

OFF-LABEL USES

Part of non-occupational and occupational postexposure prophylaxis regimen for HIV infection (adults and children), reduction of perinatal transmission from HIV-infected mother to newborn.

CONTRAINDICATIONS

Hypersensitivity.

INTERACTIONS

Drug

Ribavirin, interferons: Risk of hepatic decompensation may be increased.

Herbal and Food

None known.

DIAGNOSTIC TEST EFFECTS

May elevate serum amylase, lipase, ALT (SGPT), AST (SGOT), creatinine kinase, and triglyceride levels. May alter blood glucose levels.

SIDE EFFECTS

Frequent (13%-23%)
Headache, rhinitis, rash, diarrhea, nausea, fever, skin hyperpigmentation (especially children).
Occasional (4%-14%)
Cough, vomiting, abdominal pain, insomnia, abnormal dreams, depression, paresthesia, fatigue, dizziness, peripheral neuropathy, dyspepsia, myalgia.
Rare (2%-3%)
Arthralgia, redistribution of body fat.

SERIOUS REACTIONS

- Lactic acidosis and hepatomegaly with steatosis occur rarely and may be severe. Severe acute exacerbations of hepatitis B may occur.
- Anemia has been reported more commonly in children.

PRECAUTIONS & CONSIDERATIONS

Caution is warranted in patients with impaired liver, and dosage adjustments recommended for renal dysfunction. Be aware that breastfeeding is not recommended. In elderly patients, age-related decreased renal function may require dosage adjustment. Emtricitabine is not a cure for HIV infection, nor does it reduce risk of transmission to others. Emtricitabine is not indicated for hepatitis B. Patients with hepatitis B may have flare-ups on discontinuation, and liver function should be monitored closely.

Expect to obtain baseline laboratory testing, especially liver function tests and triglycerides, before beginning emtricitabine therapy and at periodic intervals during therapy. Assess for any nausea or vomiting and skin for rash and urticaria. Determine pattern of bowel activity and stool consistency.

Storage
Store capsules at room temperature. Store the oral solution in a refrigerator; do not freeze. May keep at room temperature for up to 3 mo; discard any remaining solution after that time.
Administration
Take without regard to food, at approximately the same time daily. Continue emtricitabine therapy for the full length of treatment.

Enalapril

en-al'a-pril
★ 🍁 Vasotec
Do not confuse with Anafranil, Eldepryl, or ramipril.

CATEGORY AND SCHEDULE

Pregnancy Risk Category: D (C if used in first trimester)

Classification: Antihypertensives, angiotensin-converting enzyme inhibitors

MECHANISM OF ACTION

This angiotensin-converting enzyme (ACE) inhibitor suppresses the renin-angiotensin-aldosterone system and prevents conversion of angiotensin I to angiotensin II, a potent vasoconstrictor; it may inhibit angiotensin II at local vascular, renal sites. Decreases plasma angiotensin II, increases plasma renin activity, and decreases aldosterone secretion. *Therapeutic Effect:* In hypertension, reduces peripheral arterial resistance. In congestive heart failure (CHF), increases cardiac output; decreases peripheral vascular resistance, BP, pulmonary capillary wedge pressure, heart size.

PHARMACOKINETICS

Route	Onset	Peak	Duration
PO	1 h	4-6 h	24 h
IV	15 min	1-4 h	6 h

Readily absorbed from the GI tract (not affected by food). Protein binding: 50%-60%. Enalaprilat, the IV form, is rapidly converted to active metabolite. Primarily excreted in urine. Removed by hemodialysis. *Half-life:* 11 h (half-life is increased in those with impaired renal function).

AVAILABILITY

Tablets: 2.5 mg, 5 mg, 10 mg, 20 mg.
Injection: 1.25 mg/mL.

INDICATIONS AND DOSAGES

▸ **Hypertension alone or in combination with other antihypertensives**
PO
Adults, Elderly. Initially, 2.5-5 mg/day. Range: 10-40 mg/day in 1-2 divided doses.
Children > 1 mo. 0.08 mg/kg/day (up to 5 mg) in 1-2 divided doses. Maximum: 0.58 mg/kg/day (not to exceed 40 mg).
IV
Adults, Elderly. 0.625-1.25 mg q6h up to 5 mg q6h.
Children >1 mo. 5-10 mcg/kg/dose q8-24h.

▸ **Adjunctive therapy for congestive heart failure**
PO
Adults, Elderly. Initially, 2.5-5 mg/day. Range: 5-20 mg/day in 2 divided doses. Maximum dose: 40 mg/day in 2 divided doses.

▸ **Adult oral dosage in renal impairment**
Dosage is modified based on creatinine clearance.

Creatinine Clearance (mL/min)	% Usual PO Dose
10-50	75-100
< 10	50

Enalapril should not be used in children with CrCl ≤ 30 mL/min.

OFF-LABEL USES

Treatment of diabetic nephropathy, nondiabetic kidney disease, or renal crisis in scleroderma, left ventricular dysfunction after myocardial infarction, Raynaud phenomenon.

CONTRAINDICATIONS

Hypersensitivity or history of angioedema from previous treatment with ACE inhibitors, idiopathic or hereditary angioedema, bilateral renal artery stenosis.

INTERACTIONS

Drug
Alcohol, antihypertensives, diuretics: May increase the effects of enalapril.
Aspirin: May decrease effectiveness of enalapril.
Lithium: Increased risk of lithium toxicity.
NSAIDs: Renal adverse effects may be increased.
Potassium-sparing diuretics, drospirenone, potassium supplements: Increased risk of hyperkalemia.
Herbal and Food
None known.

DIAGNOSTIC TEST EFFECTS

May increase BUN and serum alkaline phosphatase, serum bilirubin, serum creatinine, serum potassium, SGOT (AST), and SGPT (ALT) levels. May decrease serum sodium levels. May cause positive ANA titer or decreased WBC.

IV INCOMPATIBILITIES

Amphotericin B (Fungizone), caspofungin (Cancidas), cefepime (Maxipime), dantrolene, diazepam (Valium), lansoprazole (Prevacid), nesiritide (Natrecor), phenytoin.

SIDE EFFECTS

Frequent (5%-7%)
Headache, dizziness, hypotension, increased serum creatinine.
Occasional (2%-3%)
Orthostatic hypotension, fatigue, diarrhea, cough, syncope.
Rare (< 2%)
Angina, abdominal pain, vomiting, nausea, rash, asthenia (loss of strength, energy), syncope.

SERIOUS REACTIONS

- Excessive hypotension (first-dose syncope) may occur in patients with CHF and in those who are severely salt or volume depleted.
- Angioedema (swelling of face, lips; especially after first dose).
- Hyperkalemia may occur, especially with concomitant potassium-altering agents.
- Agranulocytosis and neutropenia may be noted in collagen vascular diseases, including scleroderma and systemic lupus erythematosus, and impaired renal function.
- Nephrotic syndrome may be noted in those with history of renal disease.
- Cholestatic jaundice, which may progress to hepatic necrosis.
- Renal dysfunction may occur. Increases in serum creatinine may occur after initiation of therapy. Monitor serum creatinine and discontinue if progressive or severe decline in function.

PRECAUTIONS & CONSIDERATIONS

Caution is warranted with cerebrovascular and coronary insufficiency, hypovolemia, renal impairment, unilateral renal artery stenosis, valvular stenosis, sodium depletion, and those on dialysis or receiving diuretics or anesthesia. Be aware that enalapril crosses the placenta and is distributed in breast milk. Enalapril may cause fetal or neonatal morbidity or mortality and should not be used during pregnancy. Discontinue as soon as pregnancy is detected. Enalapril is not used in neonates or in children with severe renal impairment. Elderly patients may be more susceptible to the hypotensive effects of enalapril.

Dizziness may occur. Be alert to fluctuations in BP. If an excessive reduction in BP occurs, place the person in the supine position with legs elevated. CBC and blood chemistry should be obtained before beginning enalapril therapy, then every 2 wks for the next 3 mo, and periodically thereafter.

Storage
Store tablets and vials at room temperature; compounded oral suspension should be refrigerated and used within 30 days of preparation.

Administration
Tablets: May administer without regard to meals.
IV: May be administered undiluted, or in up to 50 mL of a compatible IV solution (e.g., D5W, 0.9% NaCl). Administer IV over at least 5 min.

The manufacturer allows for the preparation of an oral suspension if needed for children; shake well before each use.

Enfuvirtide

en-few'vir-tide

★ 🍁 Fuzeon

Do not confuse Fuzeon with Furoxone.

CATEGORY AND SCHEDULE

Pregnancy Risk Category: B

Classification: Antivirals, fusion inhibitors

MECHANISM OF ACTION

A fusion inhibitor that interferes with the entry of HIV-1 into $CD4^+$ cells by inhibiting the fusion of vial and cellular membranes. *Therapeutic Effect:* Impairs HIV replication, slowing the progression of HIV infection.

PHARMACOKINETICS

Comparable absorption when injected into subcutaneous tissue of abdomen, arm, or thigh. Protein binding: 92% (mainly albumin). Undergoes catabolism to amino acids. *Half-life:* 3.8 h.

AVAILABILITY

Powder for Injection: 108-mg (approximately 90 mg/mL when reconstituted) single-use vials.

INDICATIONS AND DOSAGES

▸ **HIV infection (in combination with other antiretrovirals)**

SUBCUTANEOUS

Adults, Elderly. 90 mg (1 mL) twice a day.

▸ **Pediatric dosing guidelines**

Children 6-16 yr. 2 mg/kg twice a day. Maximum: 90 mg twice a day.

Weight: kg	Dosage (mg/mL)
11-15.5	27 (0.3) (give BID)
15.6-20	36 (0.4) (give BID)
20.1-24.5	45 (0.5) (give BID)
24.6-29	54 (0.6) (give BID)
29.1-33.5	63 (0.7) (give BID)
33.6-38	72 (0.8) (give BID)
38.1-42.5	81 (0.9) (give BID)
> 42.5	90 (1) (give BID)

CONTRAINDICATIONS

Hypersensitivity to enfuvirtide or any of its components.

INTERACTIONS

None known.

DIAGNOSTIC TEST EFFECTS

May elevate blood glucose and serum amylase, CK, lipase, triglyceride, AST (SGOT), and ALT (SGPT) levels. May decrease blood hemoglobin levels and WBC count.

SIDE EFFECTS

Expected (98%)

Local injection site reactions (pain, discomfort, induration, erythema, nodules, cysts, pruritus, ecchymosis).

Frequent (16%-26%)

Diarrhea, nausea, fatigue.

Occasional (4%-11%)

Insomnia, peripheral neuropathy, depression, cough, decreased appetite or weight loss, sinusitis, anxiety, asthenia, myalgia, cold sores, infections.

Rare (2%-3%)

Constipation, influenza, upper abdominal pain, anorexia, conjunctivitis, infection at injection site, flu-like syndrome.

SERIOUS REACTIONS

- Enfuvirtide use may potentiate bacterial pneumonia.
- Hypersensitivity (rash, fever, chills, rigors, hypotension), thrombocytopenia, neutropenia, and renal insufficiency or failure may occur rarely.

E

PRECAUTIONS & CONSIDERATIONS

Caution is warranted in patients with liver function impairment. Breastfeeding is not recommended because of the possibility of HIV transmission. Be aware that the safety and efficacy of enfuvirtide have not been established in children younger than 6 yr of age. No age-related precautions have been noted in elderly patients. Increased rate of bacterial pneumonia has occurred with enfuvirtide use. Seek medical attention if cough with fever, rapid breathing, or shortness of breath occurs. Enfuvirtide is not a cure for HIV infection, nor does it reduce risk of transmission to others.

Expect to obtain baseline laboratory testing, especially liver function tests and serum triglyceride levels, before beginning enfuvirtide therapy and at periodic intervals during therapy. Assess for hypersensitivity reaction and local injection site reaction, fatigue or nausea, depression, and insomnia.

Storage

Store at room temperature or in a refrigerator. Do not freeze. Refrigerate reconstituted solution; use within 24 h. Bring reconstituted solution to room temperature before injection.

Administration

Reconstitute with 1.1 mL sterile water for injection. Gently tap vial for 10 seconds and then gently roll between the hands to avoid foaming and to ensure that all particles of drug are in contact with the liquid and no drug remains on the vial wall. Allow to stand until the powder goes completely into solution, which could take up to 45 min. Reconstitution time can be reduced by gently rolling the vial between the hands until completely dissolved. Ensure solution is clear, colorless, and without bubbles. Final concentration is 90 mg/mL. Discard unused portion. Administer subcutaneously into the upper abdomen, anterior thigh, or upper arm. Administer each injection at a different site and only where there is no injection site reaction. Continue taking enfuvirtide for the full length of treatment.

Enoxaparin

e-nox-ah-pair′in

★ 🍁 Lovenox

Do not confuse Lovenox with Lotronex.

CATEGORY AND SCHEDULE

Pregnancy Risk Category: B

Classification: Anticoagulants, low-molecular-weight heparins

MECHANISM OF ACTION

A low-molecular-weight heparin that potentiates the action of antithrombin III and inactivates coagulation factor Xa. *Therapeutic Effect:* Produces anticoagulation. Does not significantly influence bleeding time, PT, or aPTT.

PHARMACOKINETICS

Route	Onset	Peak	Duration
Subcutaneous	N/A	3-5 h	12 h

Well absorbed after subcutaneous (SC) administration. Eliminated primarily in urine. Not removed by hemodialysis. *Half-life:* 4.5 h.

AVAILABILITY

Injection: 30 mg/0.3 mL, 40 mg/ 0.4 mL, 60 mg/0.6 mL, 80 mg/0.8 mL, 100 mg/mL, 120 mg/0.8 mL, 150 mg/mL in prefilled syringes. Multidose vial 100 mg/mL (3 mL).

INDICATIONS AND DOSAGES

▸ **Prevention of deep vein thrombosis (DVT) after hip and knee surgery**

SC

Adults, Elderly. 30 mg twice a day, generally for 7-10 days. Initial dose 12-24 h after surgery (if hemostasis established). For hip replacement, initial dose may be given 12 h before surgery. After initial thromboprophylaxis in hip replacement, 40 mg once daily for 3 wks is recommended.

▸ **Prevention of DVT after abdominal surgery**

SC

Adults, Elderly. 40 mg once a day for 7-10 days. Initial dose given 2 h before surgery.

▸ **Prevention of long-term DVT in nonsurgical acute illness**

SC

Adults, Elderly. 40 mg once a day for 6-11 days, up to 14 days in clinical trials.

▸ **Prevention of ischemic complications of unstable angina and non-Q-wave MI (with oral aspirin therapy)**

SC

Adults, Elderly. 1 mg/kg q12h. Should be given for minimum of 2 days and until clinical stabilization, usual duration 2-8 days.

▸ **Treatment of acute ST-segment elevation myocardial infarction**

IV/SC

Adults. Bolus 30 mg IV once followed by 1 mg/kg SC, then 1 mg/kg SC q12h (maximum 100 mg for first two doses, followed by 1 mg/kg dosing for remaining doses).
Elderly > 75 yr. Do not give IV bolus. Start with 0.75 mg/kg SC q12h (maximum 75 mg for the first two doses, followed by 0.75 mg/kg dosing for remaining doses).
Note, all STEMI patients: When administered in conjunction with a thrombolytic, give between 15 min before and 30 min after the start of therapy. All patients should receive aspirin for STEMI and maintained with 75-325 mg once daily unless contraindicated. Treatment duration until hospital discharge. For patients managed with percutaneous coronary intervention (PCI): If the last SC administration was given < 8 h before balloon inflation, no additional dosing is needed. If the SC administration was given more than 8 h before balloon inflation, an IV bolus of 0.3 mg/kg should be administered.

▸ **Acute DVT**

SC

Adults, Elderly. 1 mg/kg q12h or 1.5 mg/kg once daily. Initiate warfarin within 72 h. Continue enoxaparin for minimun of 5 days and until therapeutic INR achieved (INR 2-3).

▸ **Usual pediatric dosage**

SC

Children > 2 mo to 18 yr. 0.5 mg/kg q12h (prophylaxis); 1 mg/kg q12h (treatment).

▸ **Dosage in renal impairment**

Clearance of enoxaparin is decreased when creatinine clearance is < 30 mL/min. Monitor patient and adjust dosage as necessary. Monitoring of anti-factor Xa activity may be warranted. When enoxaparin is used in abdominal, hip, or knee surgery or acute illness, the adult dosage in renal impairment is 30 mg once a day. When used to treat DVT, angina, or non-Q-wave MI, the dosage in renal impairment is 1 mg/kg once a day. Treatment of acute ST-segment elevation MI (< 75 yr of age) dose is 30 mg IV bolus plus 1 mg/kg SC dose followed by 1 mg/kg SC once daily. Treatment of acute ST-segment elevation MI (> 75 yr) is 1 mg/kg SC once daily.

E

IV INCOMPATIBILITIES
Do not mix with other medications.

OFF-LABEL USES
Prevention of DVT following general surgical procedures, acute arterial thrombosis, prevention of thrombosis with hemodialysis, lichen planus, thrombophilia in pregnancy.

CONTRAINDICATIONS
Active major bleeding, concurrent heparin therapy, hypersensitivity to heparin or pork products, hypersensitivity to benzyl alcohol (multidose vial), thrombocytopenia associated with positive in vitro test for antiplatelet antibodies.

INTERACTIONS
Drug
Anticoagulants, platelet inhibitors: May increase bleeding.
Herbal
Supplements with antiplatelet or anticoagulant effects (e.g., feverfew, garlic, ginger, ginkgo biloba, ginseng, red clover, sweet clover, white willow, etc.): May increase effects on platelets or risk of bleeding.
Food
None known.

DIAGNOSTIC TEST EFFECTS
Increases (reversible) LDH, serum alkaline phosphatase, AST (SGOT), ALT (SGPT), and anti-factor Xa levels. May decrease platelet counts.

SIDE EFFECTS
Occasional (1%-4%)
Injection site hematoma, fever, nausea, hemorrhage, peripheral edema.

SERIOUS REACTIONS
- Overdose may lead to bleeding complications ranging from local ecchymoses to major hemorrhage. Antidote: Protamine sulfate (1% solution) equal to the dose of enoxaparin injected. 1 mg protamine sulfate neutralizes 1 mg enoxaparin. A second dose of 0.5 mg protamine sulfate per 1 mg enoxaparin may be given if aPTT tested 2-4 h after first injection remains prolonged.
- Spinal or epidural hematomas resulting in paralysis have occurred. Risk is increased in patients with postoperative indwelling epidural catheters.
- Heparin-induced thrombocytopenia.

PRECAUTIONS & CONSIDERATIONS
Caution is warranted in patients with conditions associated with increased risk of hemorrhage (e.g., bacterial endocarditis, congenital or acquired bleeding disorders, active ulcerative and angiodysplastic GI disease, hemorrhagic stroke, or shortly after brain, spinal, or ophthalmologic surgery, or in patients treated concomitantly with platelet inhibitors), history of recent GI ulceration and hemorrhage, history of heparin-induced thrombocytopenia, impaired renal function, uncontrolled arterial hypertension, thrombocytopenia, indwelling epidural catheters, and in elderly patients. Enoxaparin should be used with caution in pregnant women, particularly during the last trimester and immediately postpartum, because

it increases the risk of maternal hemorrhage. It is unknown whether enoxaparin is excreted in breast milk. Safety and efficacy of enoxaparin have not been established in children. Elderly patients may be more susceptible to bleeding. Women may experience heavier menstrual flow. Other medications, including OTC drugs, should be avoided. An electric razor and soft toothbrush should be used to prevent bleeding during therapy.

Notify the physician of abdominal or back pain, severe headache or neurologic impairment, black or red stool, coffee-ground vomitus, dark or red urine, or red-speckled mucus from cough. CBC and stool for occult blood should be periodically monitored. Be aware of signs of bleeding, including bleeding at injection or surgical sites or from gums, blood in stool, bruising, hematuria, and petechiae.

Storage

Store at room temperature.

Administration

! Do not give IM. Give initial dose as soon as possible after surgery but not more than 24 h after surgery.

The patient should lie down before administering by deep subcutaneous injection. Inject between the left and right anterolateral and left and right posterolateral abdominal wall. Introduce entire length of needle (one-half inch) into skinfold held between thumb and forefinger, holding skinfold during injection. Alternate sites of administration; do not rub injection site after administration.

For IV use: Use the multiple-dose vial and use a graduated syringe to ensure proper dosing.

Give IV bolus through line. Do not mix or give with other drugs. Flush the IV access port with a sufficient amount of compatible IV solution before and after administration. May be safely administered with 0.9% NaCl or D5W.

E

Entacapone

en-tak'a-pone

★ 🍁 Comtan

CATEGORY AND SCHEDULE

Pregnancy Risk Category: C

Classification: Antiparkinsonian agents, COMT inhibitors

MECHANISM OF ACTION

An antiparkinsonian agent that inhibits the enzyme catechol *O*-methyltransferase (COMT), potentiating dopamine activity and increasing the duration of action of levodopa. *Therapeutic Effect:* Decreases signs and symptoms of Parkinson disease.

PHARMACOKINETICS

Rapidly absorbed after PO administration (peak effect 1 h). Protein binding: 98% (primarily albumin). Metabolized in the liver. Primarily eliminated by biliary excretion. Not removed by hemodialysis. *Half-life:* 2.4 h.

AVAILABILITY

Tablets: 200 mg.

INDICATIONS AND DOSAGES

▸ **Adjunctive treatment of Parkinson disease**

PO

Adults, Elderly. 200 mg concomitantly with each dose of carbidopa and levodopa up to a maximum of 8 times a day (1600 mg).

CONTRAINDICATIONS

Hypersensitivity, use within 14 days of nonselective MAOIs.

INTERACTIONS

Drug

Ampicillin, cholestyramine, erythromycin, probenecid: May decrease the excretion of entacapone.
Bitolterol, dobutamine, dopamine, epinephrine, isoetharine, isoproterenol, epinephrine, methyldopa, norepinephrine: May increase the risk of arrhythmias and changes in BP.
Nonselective MAOIs (including phenelzine): May inhibit catecholamine metabolism and increase risk of cardiovascular side effects such as hypertensive crisis. Contraindicated.
Other central nervous system (CNS) depressants: May increase CNS depression.

Herbal

None known.

Food

None known.

DIAGNOSTIC TEST EFFECTS

None known.

SIDE EFFECTS

Frequent (> 10%)

Dyskinesia, hyperkinesia, nausea, dark yellow or orange urine and sweat, diarrhea.

Occasional (3%-9%)

Abdominal pain, vomiting, constipation, hallucinations, dry mouth, fatigue, back pain.

Rare (< 2%)

Anxiety, somnolence, agitation, dyspepsia, flatulence, diaphoresis, asthenia, dyspnea.

SERIOUS REACTIONS

- Rhabdomyolysis and neuroleptic malignant syndrome have occurred rarely.
- Rare reports of loss of impulse control, such as urge to gamble excessively or unusual sexual urges.

PRECAUTIONS & CONSIDERATIONS

Caution is warranted with hepatic or renal impairment, dyskinesia, orthostatic hypotension, and syncope. It is unknown whether entacapone is distributed in breast milk. There are no human pregnancy data. This drug is not indicated for children. No age-related precautions have been noted in elderly patients.

Tasks that require mental alertness or motor skills should be avoided until drug effects are known. Notify the physician if uncontrolled movement of the hands, arms, legs, eyelids, face, mouth, or tongue occurs. Baseline vital signs should be obtained. Relief of symptoms, such as improvement of mask-like facial expression, muscular rigidity, shuffling gait, and resting tremors of the hands and head, should be assessed during treatment. Dyskinesia, diarrhea, and orthostatic hypotension should also be monitored. Do not withdraw abruptly as rapid withdrawal may lead to hyperpyrexia and confusion resembling neuroleptic malignant syndrome.

Storage

Store at room temperature.

Administration

! Always administer entacapone with carbidopa and levodopa.

Take entacapone without regard to food.

Entecavir

en-te'ca-veer

Baraclude

CATEGORY AND SCHEDULE

Pregnancy Risk Category: C

Classification: Antivirals, nucleoside reverse transcriptase inhibitors

MECHANISM OF ACTION

A guanosine nucleoside analogue with activity against HBV polymerase. Drug inhibits all three activities of the HBV polymerase (reverse transcriptase): (1) base priming, (2) reverse transcription of the negative strand from the pregenomic messenger RNA, and (3) synthesis of the positive strand of HBV DNA. NOTE: Unlike other NRTIs, is not recommended as monotherapy in HBV-positive patients coinfected with the HIV virus due to the development of drug resistance. *Therapeutic Effect:* Interrupts HBV replication, slowing the progression of or improving the clinical status of hepatitis infection.

PHARMACOKINETICS

Rapidly and completely absorbed from the GI tract. Administration with food significantly decreases oral absorption. Protein binding: 13%. Widely distributed. Primarily excreted in urine predominantly unchanged and small amounts of glucuronide and sulfate metabolites via glomerular filtration and net tubular secretion. Some removal by hemodialysis. *Terminal Half-life:* 128-149 h (intracellular), 15 h (serum, adults), (increased in impaired renal function).

AVAILABILITY

Oral Solution: 0.05 mg/mL.
Tablets: 0.5 mg, 1 mg.

INDICATIONS AND DOSAGES

▸ **Chronic hepatitis B**

▸ **For nucleoside-treatment-naïve patients**

PO

Adults, Children > 16 yr. 0.5 mg once daily. Optimal duration of therapy unknown.

▸ **For patients with lamivudine resistance**

PO

Adults, Children > 16 yr. 1 mg once daily. Optimal duration of therapy unknown.

▸ **Dosage in renal impairment (adult and adolescent)**

Dosage and frequency are modified based on creatinine clearance. Use once-daily dose options whenever possible. NOTE: For doses less than 0.5 mg, use the oral solution.

CrCl (mL/min)	Naïve Patients	Lamivudine-refractory Patients
≥ 50	Use usual dose	Use usual dose
30-49	0.25 mg QD or 0.5 mg q48h	0.5 mg QD or 1 mg q48h
10-29	0.15 mg QD or 0.5 mg q72h	0.3 mg QD or 1 mg q72h
< 10 (includes hemodialysis or CAPD)*	0.05 mg QD or 0.5 mg every 7 days	0.1 mg QD or 1 mg every 7 days

*If administered on a hemodialysis day, administer after the hemodialysis session.

CONTRAINDICATIONS

Hypersensitivity.

INTERACTIONS

Drug

Metformin: Theoretically, competition for tubular secretion may increase risk of lactic acidosis.

Herbal

None known.

Food

All food: Decrease oral absorption. Take on empty stomach.

DIAGNOSTIC TEST EFFECTS

May increase serum AST (SGOT) and ALT (SGPT). Occasionally see elevated blood glucose, serum creatinine, or serum lipase.

SIDE EFFECTS

Frequent

Headache, fatigue, dizziness, nausea.

Occasional

Diarrhea, dyspepsia/indigestion, vomiting, sleepiness, insomnia.

Rare

Rash, alopecia.

SERIOUS REACTIONS

- Anaphylactoid reactions occur rarely.
- Lactic acidosis.
- Severe hepatomegaly with steatosis.

PRECAUTIONS & CONSIDERATIONS

Lactic acidosis and severe hepatomegaly with steatosis, including fatal cases, have been reported with the use of nucleoside analogues alone or in combination with antiretrovirals; females appear to have a higher risk. Obesity and prolonged nucleoside exposure may be risk factors. Caution is warranted in patients with impaired renal function. Be aware that the drug is likely to cross the placenta, and that there are no adequate dates in pregnant women. It is unknown whether entecavir is distributed in breast milk. Breastfeeding is not recommended in patients coinfected with HIV due to risk of HIV transmission. Be aware that the safety and efficacy of this drug have not been established in children younger than 16 yr. In elderly patients, age-related renal impairment may require dosage adjustment.

Before starting drug therapy, check baseline lab values, especially renal function. Expect to monitor serum liver function tests, BUN, and serum creatinine. Assess for altered sleep patterns, dizziness, headache, nausea, and pattern of daily bowel activity and stool consistency. Avoid activities that require mental acuity if dizziness occurs until the effects of the drug are known. Patients should be advised not to stop taking the drug suddenly, as this can cause a worsening of hepatitis that may be sudden. Treatment with entecavir does not reduce the risk of transmission of HBV to others through sexual contact or blood contamination.

Storage

Store at room temperature in tightly closed container. Protect from moisture and light.

Administration

Take on an empty stomach (2 h before or 2 h after meals) at about the same time each day. If using the oral solution, use the dosing spoon provided. Rinse the spoon with water after each use and allow it to air dry.

Ephedrine

eh-fed′rin

Do not confuse with epinephrine.

CATEGORY AND SCHEDULE

Pregnancy Risk Category: C

Classification: Adrenergic agonists, decongestants, vasopressors.

MECHANISM OF ACTION

An adrenergic agonist that stimulates α-adrenergic receptors causing vasoconstriction and pressor effects; β_1-adrenergic receptors, resulting in cardiac stimulation; and β_2-adrenergic receptors, resulting in bronchial dilation and vasodilation. *Therapeutic Effect:* Increases BP and pulse rate.

PHARMACOKINETICS

Well absorbed after oral, nasal, and parenteral absorption. Metabolized in liver to small extent. Excreted in urine. *Half-life:* 3-6 h. Onset of bronchodilation: 15 min to 1 h. Duration (oral): 3-6 h.

AVAILABILITY

Injection: 50 mg/mL.

INDICATIONS AND DOSAGES

▸ **Asthma**

IM/IV/SQ

Adults. 12.5-25 mg. Maximum dose: 150 mg/day.

Children > 2 yr. 2-3 mg/kg/day or 100 mg/m²/day divided into 4-6 doses/day.

▸ **Hypotension**

IM

Adults. 25-50 mg as a single dose. Maximum: 150 mg/day.

IV

Adults. 5 mg/dose slow IVP as prevention. 10-25 mg/dose slow IVP repeated q5-10 min as treatment. Maximum: 150 mg/day.

Children. 0.2-0.3 mg/kg/dose slow IVP q4-6h.

SUBCUTANEOUS

Adults. 25-50 mg q4-6h. Maximum: 150 mg/day.

Children. 3 mg/kg/day in divided doses q4-6 h.

CONTRAINDICATIONS

Anesthesia with cyclopropane or halothane, diabetes (ephedrine injection), hypersensitivity to ephedrine or other sympathomimetic amines, hypertension or other cardiovascular disorders, myocardial infarction, angina, arrhythmias, obstetrics with maternal blood pressure above 130/80, thyrotoxicosis, angle-closure glaucoma.

INTERACTIONS

Drug

Atropine, MAOIs, oxytocics, tricyclic antidepressants: May increase cardiovascular effects.

α-Adrenergic, β-adrenergic blockers: May blunt ephedrine vasopressor effects.

Caffeine: May increase cardiac stimulation.

Cardiac glycosides, sympathomimetics, theophylline, general anesthetics: May increase toxic cardiac stimulation.

Herbal

Ephedra (ma huang) guarana, kola nut, green tea, bitter orange, yohimbe: May increase central nervous system (CNS) and cardiovascular stimulation and effects.

Food

Excessive amounts of caffeine such as in chocolate, cocoa, coffee, cola, or tea should be avoided.

DIAGNOSTIC TEST EFFECTS

May result in false-positive amphetamine EMIT assay. Lactic acid serum values may be increased.

IV INCOMPATIBILITIES

Dantrolene, diazepam, hydrocortisone sodium succinate (Solu-Cortef), pantoprazole (Protonix), phenobarbital (Luminal), phenytoin, thiopental (Thioplex).

IV COMPATIBILITIES

Chloramphenicol, etomidate (Amidate), fenoldopam (Corlopam), lidocaine, methotrexate, milrinone

(Primacor), nafcillin (Unipen), penicillin G, propofol (Diprivan), tetracycline, tigecycline (Tygacil), vecuronium (Norcuron).

SIDE EFFECTS

Frequent
Hypertension, anxiety, agitation.
Occasional
Nausea, vomiting, palpitations, tremor, chest pain, BP changes, tachycardia, hallucinations, restlessness, diaphoresis, xerostomia.
Nasal: Burning, stinging, runny nose.
Rare
Psychosis, decreased/painful urination, necrosis at injection site from repeated injections.

SERIOUS REACTIONS

- Excessive doses may cause hypertension, intracranial hemorrhage, anginal pain, arrhythmias (including ventricular tachycardia), myocardial infarction, cardiac arrest.
- Stroke, transient ischemic attack, seizures.
- Prolonged or excessive use may result in metabolic acidosis as a result of increased serum lactic acid concentrations.
- Observe for disorientation, weakness, hyperventilation, headache, nausea, vomiting, and diarrhea.

PRECAUTIONS & CONSIDERATIONS

Caution is warranted with angina, coronary artery disease, diabetes, hypoxia (lack of oxygen), heart attack, psychiatric disorders, tachycardia, severe liver or kidney impairment, seizure disorder, thyroid disorders, prostatic hypertrophy, and in elderly patients. Ephedrine crosses the placenta and is distributed in breast milk and breastfeeding should be avoided. Changes in vital signs and proper lung function should be monitored.

Storage
Injectable should be stored at room temperature and protected from light.
Administration
Ampule should be shaken thoroughly. Solution should not be used if it appears discolored or contains a precipitate. A tuberculin syringe for subcutaneous injection into lateral deltoid muscle region should be used and injection site massaged.

For IV use, each 1 mg of 1:1000 solution is diluted with 10 mL 0.9% NaCl to provide 1:10,000 solution, and injected as each 1 mg or fraction thereof over more than 1 min. For infusion, preparation should be further diluted with 250-500 mL D5W. Maximum concentration is 64 mg/250 mL, the recommended rate of IV infusion is 1-10 mcg/min, adjusted to desired response.

Epinastine

ep'i-nas'teen
★ Elestat

CATEGORY AND SCHEDULE

Pregnancy Risk Category: C

Classification: Antihistamines, H_1, ophthalmics

MECHANISM OF ACTION

An ophthalmic H_1 receptor antagonist that inhibits the release of histamine from the mast cell. *Therapeutic Effect:* Prevents pruritus associated with allergic conjunctivitis.

PHARMACOKINETICS

Low systemic exposure. Protein binding: 64%. Less than 10% is metabolized. Excreted primarily in urine and, to a lesser extent, in feces. *Half-life:* 12 h.

AVAILABILITY

Ophthalmic Solution: 0.05% (5 mL).

INDICATIONS AND DOSAGES

▸ **Allergic conjunctivitis**

OPHTHALMIC

Adults, Elderly, Children 3 yr and older. 1 drop in each eye twice a day. Continue treatment until period of exposure (pollen season, exposure to offending allergen) is over.

CONTRAINDICATIONS

Hypersensitivity to epinastine or any of its components.

INTERACTIONS

Drug

None known.

Herbal

None known.

Food

None known.

DIAGNOSTIC TEST EFFECTS

None known.

SIDE EFFECTS

Occasional

Ocular (1%-10%): Burning sensation in the eye, hyperemia, pruritus.

Nonocular (10%): Cold symptoms, upper respiratory tract infection.

Rare (1%-3%)

Headache, rhinitis, sinusitis, increased cough, pharyngitis.

SERIOUS REACTIONS

• None known.

PRECAUTIONS & CONSIDERATIONS

Not to be used to treat contact lens-associated irritation. It is not known whether epinastine is distributed in breast milk. The safety and efficacy of epinastine have not been established in children younger than 3 yr. No age-related precautions have been noted in elderly patients. Therapeutic response should be monitored.

Storage

Store bottle at room temperature.

Administration

For ophthalmic use, place a finger on the lower eyelid, and pull it out until a pocket is formed between the eye and lower lid. Don't let the applicator tip touch any surface. Place the prescribed number of drops in the pocket. Close the affected eye gently. Apply gentle pressure to the lacrimal sac at the inner canthus for 1 min after installation to lessen the risk of systemic absorption. Remove contact lenses before instilling epinastine because the lenses may absorb the drug's preservatives. The lenses may be reinserted 10 min after administration unless the treated eye is red.

Epinephrine

ep-i-nef′rin

★ Adrenalin, Adrenaclick, Bronchial Mist, EpiPen, EpiPen Jr., Primatene Mist, S2, Twinject

🍁 Adrenilin, EpiPen, EpiPen Jr, Anapen, Anapen Jr, S2

Do not confuse epinephrine with ephedrine.

CATEGORY AND SCHEDULE

Pregnancy Risk Category: C

Rx: Injection, topical solution

OTC: Inhalation aerosol

Classification: Adrenergic agonists, bronchodilators, inotropes

MECHANISM OF ACTION

A sympathomimetic, adrenergic agonist that stimulates β-adrenergic receptors, causing vasoconstriction

and pressor effects; β_1-adrenergic receptors, resulting in cardiac stimulation; and β_2-adrenergic receptors, resulting in bronchial dilation and vasodilation.
Therapeutic Effect: Relaxes smooth muscle of the bronchial tree, produces cardiac stimulation, and dilates skeletal muscle vasculature.

E

PHARMACOKINETICS

Route	Onset (min)	Peak (min)	Duration (h)
IM	5-10	20	1-4
Subcutaneous	5-10	20	1-4
Inhalation	1-5	20	1-3

Well absorbed after parenteral administration; minimally absorbed after inhalation. Metabolized in the liver, other tissues, and sympathetic nerve endings. Excreted in urine.

AVAILABILITY

Injection: 0.1 mg/mL, 1 mg/mL.
Injection (EpiPen): 0.3 mg/0.3 mL, 0.15 mg/0.3 mL.
Injection (Twinject): 0.15 mg/0.15 mL and 0.3 mg/0.3 mL
Inhalation, Aerosol (Primatene Mist): 0.22 mg/inhalation.
Inhalation, Solution: 2.25% (racepinephrine).

INDICATIONS AND DOSAGES

▸ **Asystole**
IV
Adults, Elderly. 1 mg q3-5min up to 0.1 mg/kg q3-5min.
Infants, Children. 0.01 mg/kg (0.1 mL/kg of 1:10,000 solution). May repeat q3-5min. Subsequent doses of 0.1 mg/kg (0.1 mL/kg) of a 1:1000 solution q3-5min. Maximum: 1 mg (10 mL).
ENDOTRACHEAL
Adults. 2-2.5 mg via ET, may repeat every 3-5 min.
Children, Infants. 0.1 mg/kg (0.1 mL/kg of 1:1000 solution). May repeat q3-5min. Maximum: 10 mg.

▸ **Bradycardia**
IV INFUSION
Adults, Elderly. 1-10 mcg/min titrated to desired effect.
IV
Infants, Children. 0.01 mg/kg (0.1 mL/kg of 1:10,000 solution) q3-5min. Maximum: 1 mg (10 mL).

▸ **Bronchodilation**
IM, SUBCUTANEOUS
Adults, Elderly. 0.3-0.5 mg (1:1000) q20min to 4 h for 3 doses.
SUBCUTANEOUS
Children. 10 mcg/kg (0.01 mL/kg of 1:1000). Maximum: 0.5 mg every 5 min up to 3 doses.
INHALATION
Adults, Elderly, Children 4 yr and older. 1 inhalation, may repeat in at least 1 min. Give subsequent doses no sooner than 3-4 h.
NEBULIZER
Adults, Elderly, Children 4 yr and older. 1-3 deep inhalations. Give subsequent doses no sooner than 3 h.

▸ **Hypersensitivity reaction**
IM, SUBCUTANEOUS
Adults, Elderly. 0.3-0.5 mg q15-20min.
SUBCUTANEOUS
Children. 0.01 mg/kg q15min for 2 doses, then q4h. Maximum single dose: 0.5 mg.
AUTOINJECTORS
Adults. Twinject (subcutaneous/IM) 0.3 mg. EpiPen (IM) 0.3 mg. May repeat once after 10-20 min.
Children 15-30 kg. Twinject (subcutaneous/IM) 0.15 mg. EpiPen (IM) 0.15 mg.
Children > 30 kg. Twinject (subcutaneous/IM) 0.3 mg. EpiPen (IM) 0.3 mg.

OFF-LABEL USES

Treatment of gingival or pulpal hemorrhage, priapism.

CONTRAINDICATIONS

Cardiac arrhythmias, cerebrovascular insufficiency, hypertension, hyperthyroidism, ischemic heart disease, labor, narrow-angle glaucoma, shock (except anaphylactic).

INTERACTIONS

Drug

β-Blockers: May decrease the effects of β-blockers.

Digoxin, sympathomimetics, halogenated inhalational anesthetics: May increase the risk of arrhythmias and toxicity.

Ergonovine, methergine, oxytocin: May increase vasoconstriction.

MAOIs, tricyclic antidepressants: May increase cardiovascular effects. Contraindicated within 2 wks of MAOI.

Herbal

Ephedra (ma huang), bitter orange, yohimbe: May increase central nervous system (CNS) and cardiovascular stimulation and effects.

Food

None known.

DIAGNOSTIC TEST EFFECTS

May decrease serum potassium level.

IV INCOMPATIBILITIES

Acyclovir (Zovirax), aminophylline, azathioprine, ampicillin, dantrolene, diazepam (Valium), fluorouracil, ganciclovir (Cytovene), indomethacin, micafungin (Mycamine), pantoprazole (Protonix), pentobarbital, phenobarbital, phenytoin, thiopental, sodium bicarbonate, sulfamethoxazole/trimethoprim.

IV COMPATIBILITIES

Alfentanil (Alfenta), amikacin (Amikar), amiodarone, amphotericin B liposomal (AmBisome), anidulafungin (Eraxis), ascorbic acid, atracurium (Tracrium), atropine, aztreonam (Azactam), benztropine (Cogentin), bivalirudin (Angiomax), bretylium, bumetanide (Bumex), bupivacaine, calcium chloride, calcium gluconate, carboplatin, caspofungin (Cancidas), cefazolin, cefotaxime (Claforan), cefotetan (Cefotan), cefoxitin (Mefoxin), ceftazidime (Ceptaz, Fortaz, Tazicef, Tazidime), ceftizoxime (Cefizox), ceftriaxone (Rocephin), cefuroxime (Zinacef), chloramphenicol, chlorpromazine, cimetidine (Tagamet), cisatracurium (Nimbex), cisplatin, clindamycin (Cleocin), clonidine, cyanocobalamin, cyclophosphamide (Cytoxan), cyclosporine (Sandimmune), dactinomycin (Cosmegen), daptomycin (Cubicin), dexamethasone sodium phosphate, dexmedetomidine (Precedex), digoxin (Lanoxin), diltiazem (Cardizem), diphenhydramine (Benadryl), dobutamine (Dobutrex), docetaxel (Taxotere), dopamine (Intropin), doxorubicin (Adriamycin), edetate calcium disodium, enalaprilat, ephedrine, epirubicin (Ellence), epoetin alfa (Procrit), ertapenem (Invanz), erythromycin lactobionate, esmolol (Brevibloc), etoposide phosphate (Etopophos), famotidine (Pepcid), fenoldopam (Corlopam), fentanyl (Sublimaze), fluconazole (Diflucan), fludarabine (Fludara), folic acid, furosemide (Lasix), gemcitabine (Gemzar), gentamicin, granisetron (Kytril), heparin, hydrocortisone sodium succinate (Solu-Cortef), hydromorphone (Dilaudid), hydroxyzine, imipenem/cilastatin (Primaxin), isoproterenol (Isuprel), ketorolac, labetalol, levofloxacin (Levaquin), lidocaine, linezolid (Zyvox), lorazepam (Ativan), magnesium sulfate, mannitol, meperidine (Demerol), methicillin, methotrexate, methylprednisolone sodium succinate, metoclopramide (Reglan), metoprolol (Lopressor), metronidazole (Flagyl), midazolam (Versed), milrinone (Primacor), minocycline (Minocin), mitoxantrone (Novantrone), morphine, multiple vitamins injection, nafcillin, nalbuphine (Nubain), naloxone (Narcan), nicardipine (Cardene), nitroglycerin, nitroprusside sodium (Nitropress), norepinephrine (Levophed), ondansetron (Zofran), oxacillin, oxaliplatin (Eloxatin), oxytocin (Pitocin), paclitaxel (Taxol), pancuronium, pemetrexed (Alimta), penicillin G potassium, penicillin G sodium, phytonadione, potassium chloride, procainamide, prochlorperazine, promethazine, propofol (Diprivan), propranolol, quinupristin/dalfopristin (Synercid), ranitidin (Zantac), remifentanil (Ultiva), streptokinase, succinylcholine, sufentanil (Sufenta), tacrolimus (Prograf), teniposide (Vumon), ticarcillin (Ticar), ticarcillin/clavulanate (Timentin), tigecycline (Tygacil), tirofibran (Aggrastat), tobramycin, vancomycin, vasopressin, vecuronium (Norcuron), verapamil, vincristine (Vincasar), vinorelbine (Navelbine), vitamin B complex with C, voriconazole (Vfend), warfarin.

SIDE EFFECTS

Frequent

Systemic: Tachycardia, palpitations, nervousness, dizziness.
Ophthalmic: Headache, eye irritation, watering of eyes.

Occasional

Systemic: Dizziness, light-headedness, facial flushing, headache, diaphoresis, increased BP, nausea, trembling, insomnia, vomiting, fatigue, urinary retention.
Ophthalmic: Blurred or decreased vision, eye pain.

Rare

Systemic: Chest discomfort or pain, arrhythmias, bronchospasm, dry mouth or throat.

SERIOUS REACTIONS

- Excessive doses may cause acute hypertension or arrhythmias or cerebrovascular hemorrhage.
- Prolonged or excessive use may result in metabolic acidosis as a result of increased serum lactic acid concentrations. Metabolic acidosis may cause disorientation, fatigue, hyperventilation, headache, nausea, vomiting, and diarrhea.

PRECAUTIONS & CONSIDERATIONS

Caution is warranted with angina, diabetes, coronary artery disease, cerebrovascular disease, thyroid disease, seizure disorders, prostatic hypertrophy, hypoxia (lack of oxygen), heart attack, psychiatric disorders, tachycardia, severe liver or kidney impairment, and in elderly patients. Avoid extravasation as tissue necrosis can occur. Epinephrine crosses the placenta and is distributed in breast milk. Changes in vital signs and proper lung function should be monitored.

Storage

Injectable solutions should be stored at room temperature.

Administration

For racepinephrine, vial should be shaken thoroughly. Do not use if brown or cloudy in appearance.
For use in a hand-held rubber bulb nebulizer. Add 0.5 mL (contents of one vial) of solution to nebulizer and administer as directed.

For injection, each 1 mg of 1:1000 solution is diluted with 10 mL 0.9% NaCl to provide 1:10,000 solution, and injected as each 1 mg or fraction thereof over more than 1 min. For continuous IV infusion: Dilute 1 mg epinephrine in 250 or 500 mL of D5W or other compatible IV solution to a concentration of 4 or 2 mcg/mL, respectively. Administer into a large vein, if possible. Concentrated solutions (e.g., 16 to 32 mcg/mL) may be used when administered through a central line. The recommended rate of IV infusion is 1-10 mcg/min, adjusted to desired response.

Eplerenone

e-plear'a-nown

Inspra

CATEGORY AND SCHEDULE

Pregnancy Risk Category: B

Classification: Antihypertensives, selective aldosterone receptor antagonist

MECHANISM OF ACTION

An aldosterone receptor antagonist that binds to the mineralocorticoid receptors in the kidney, heart, blood vessels, and brain, blocking the binding of aldosterone. *Therapeutic Effect:* Reduces BP and promotes sodium, chloride, and water excretion.

PHARMACOKINETICS

Absorption is unaffected by food. Protein binding: 50%. Metabolized by CYP3A4. No active metabolites. Excreted in the urine with a lesser amount eliminated in the feces. Not removed by hemodialysis. *Half-life:* 4-6 h. Onset of full hypertensive effect may take 4 wks.

AVAILABILITY

Tablets: 25 mg, 50 mg.

INDICATIONS AND DOSAGES

▸ Hypertension

PO

Adults, Elderly. 50 mg once a day. If 50 mg once a day produces an inadequate BP response, may increase dosage to 50 mg twice a day (max dose). If patient is concurrently receiving erythromycin, saquinavir, verapamil, or fluconazole, reduce initial dose to 25 mg once a day.

▸ Congestive heart failure following myocardial infarction

PO

Adults, Elderly. Initially, 25 mg once a day. If tolerated, titrate up to 50 mg once a day within 4 wks. If potassium < 5 mEq/L, increase the dose from 25 mg every other day to 25 mg daily or increase dose from 25 to 50 mg daily. No dose adjustment if potassium 5-5.4 mEq/L. If potassium 5.5-5.9 mEq/L, decrease the dose from 50 to 25 mg daily or from 25 mg daily to 25 mg every other day or 25 mg every other day to withhold. If potassium > 6 mEq/L, withhold dose until potassium < 5.5 mEq/L, then give 25 mg every other day.

CONTRAINDICATIONS

ALL patients: Serum K + > 5.5 mEq/L at initiation, CrCl ≤ 30 mL/min, concomitant administration of strong CYP3A4 inhibitors (e.g., ketoconazole, itraconazole, nefazodone, troleandomycin, clarithromycin, ritonavir, and nelfinavir).

For patients being treated for HTN: Type 2 diabetes with microalbuminuria, SCr > 2 mg/dL in males or > 1.8 mg/dL in females, CrCl < 50 mL/min, or concurrent use of potassium supplements or potassium-sparing diuretics (e.g., amiloride, spironolactone, triamterene).

INTERACTIONS

Drug

ACE inhibitors, angiotensin II antagonists, potassium-sparing diuretics, potassium supplements: Increases the risk of hyperkalemia.
CYP3A4 inhibitors such as calcium channel blockers, erythromycin, fluconazole, saquinavir, verapamil: May increase levels and toxicity such as hyperkalemia. Strong inhibitors such as clarithromycin, itraconazole, and ketoconazole should not be used concomitantly.
CYP3A4 inducers: May decrease levels of eplerenone.
NSAIDs: May decrease antihypertensive effect.

Herbal

St. John's wort: Decreases eplerenone effectiveness.

Food

Grapefruit juice: Produces small increase in exposure to eplerenone (25%).

DIAGNOSTIC TEST EFFECTS

May increase serum potassium level, serum creatinine, triglycerides, cholesterol, ALT, and GGT levels. May decrease serum sodium level.

SIDE EFFECTS

Common (≥ 2%)

Patients with CHF: Hyperkalemia and increased serum creatinine.
Patients with HTN: Dizziness, diarrhea, cough, fatigue, and flu-like symptoms.

Rare

Abdominal pain, abnormal vaginal bleeding, gynecomastia.

SERIOUS REACTIONS

- Hyperkalemia may occur, particularly in patients with type 2 diabetes mellitus and microalbuminuria. Monitor closely.
- Rare reports of angioneurotic edema or rash.

PRECAUTIONS & CONSIDERATIONS

Caution is warranted with hyperkalemia and hepatic or renal impairment. Diabetic patients with CHF, post-MI, or proteinuria should be treated with particular caution, due to increased rates of hyperkalemia. It is unknown whether eplerenone crosses the placenta or is distributed in breast milk. The safety and efficacy of eplerenone have not been established in children. No age-related precautions have been noted in elderly patients. Exercising outside during hot weather should be avoided because of the risks of dehydration and hypotension.

Dizziness and light-headedness may occur. Tasks that require mental alertness or motor skills should be avoided. Apical heart rate and BP should be obtained immediately before each dose, in addition to regular monitoring. Be alert to BP fluctuations. If an excessive reduction in BP occurs, place in the supine position with feet slightly elevated, and notify the physician. Pattern of daily bowel activity and stool consistency and potassium and sodium levels should also be monitored.

Storage

Store at room temperature. Protect from moisture.

Administration

Film-coated tablets should not be broken, crushed, or chewed. May give without regard to food.

Epoetin Alfa (Erythropoietin)

eh-poh′ee-tin al′fa

Epogen, Procrit Eprex

Do not confuse Epogen with Neupogen.

CATEGORY AND SCHEDULE

Pregnancy Risk Category: C

Classification: Hematopoietic agents, erythropoiesis-stimulating agents (ESAs)

MECHANISM OF ACTION

A glycoprotein that stimulates division and differentiation of erythroid progenitor cells in bone marrow. *Therapeutic Effect:* Induces erythropoiesis and releases reticulocytes from bone marrow to raise hemoglobin and hematocrit.

PHARMACOKINETICS

Well absorbed after subcutaneous (SC) administration. Following administration, an increase in reticulocyte count occurs within 10 days, and increases in hemoglobin, hematocrit, and RBC count are seen within 2-6 wks. *Half-life:* 4-13 h (chronic renal failure); half-life is shorter in those without renal dysfunction.

AVAILABILITY

Injection, Single-Dose Vials: 2000 units/mL, 3000 units/mL, 4000 units/mL, 10,000 units/mL, 40,000 units/mL.

INDICATIONS AND DOSAGES

▸ Treatment of anemia in chemotherapy patients

IV, SC

Adults, Elderly. 150 units/kg/dose SC 3 times/wk. Maximum: 1200 units/kg/wk. Weekly dosing: 40,000 units SC weekly. Reduce dose by 25% when hemoglobin approaches 12 g/dL or increases by more than 1 g/dL in any 2-wk period. If hemoglobin exceeds 12 g/dL, hold dose until hemoglobin is < 11 g/dL and restart at 25% reduction in previous dose. If hemoglobin does not increase 1 g/dL or more after 4 wks for weekly dosing, increase dose to 60,000 units/wk. If hemoglobin does not increase with 3 times/wk dosing, after 8 wks increase dose to 300 units/kg 3 times/wk.

Children: 600 units/kg IV once per week. Maximum: 40,000 units/dose. If hemoglobin does not increase 1 g/dL or more after 4 wks, increase dose to 900 units/kg IV weekly.

▸ Reduction of allogenic blood transfusions in elective surgery

SC

Adults, Elderly. 300 units/kg/day 10 days before, the day of, and 4 days after surgery. Alternate dose: 600 units/kg once weekly (21, 14, and 7 days before surgery) and the day of surgery.

▸ Chronic renal failure

IV BOLUS, SC

Adults, Elderly. Initially, 50-100 units/kg 3 times a week. Target hemoglobin for patients not on dialysis 10-12 g/dL. Hematocrit range: 30%-36%. Adjust dosage no earlier than 1-mo intervals unless prescribed. Decrease dosage if hemoglobin is approaching 12 g/dL, reduce dose by 25%. If level continues to increase, withhold dose until hemoglobin decreases and restart at 25% reduction. If increase in hemoglobin is < 1 g/dL in 4 wks (with adequate iron stores), increase dose by 25% of previous dose. Maintenance: For patients on dialysis, 75 units/kg 3 times/wk.

Range: 12.5-525 units/kg. For patients not on dialysis, 75-150 units/kg/wk.
Children on Dialysis. Initially, 50 units/kg 3 times/wk. Maintenance: For children on hemodialysis, median dose of 167 units/kg/wk administered in divided doses 2-3 times weekly. For children on peritoneal dialysis, median dose of 76 units/kg/wk in divided doses 2-3 times weekly.

▸ **HIV infection in patients treated with zidovudine (AZT)**

IV, SC
Adults. Initially, 100 units/kg 3 times a week for 8 wks; may increase by 50-100 units/kg 3 times a week. Evaluate response q4-8wk thereafter. Adjust dosage by 50-100 units/kg 3 times/wk. If dosages larger than 300 units/kg 3 times/wk are not eliciting response, it is unlikely patient will respond. Maintenance: Titrate to maintain desired hematocrit; hemoglobin not to exceed 12 g/dL.

OFF-LABEL USES

Prevention of anemia in patients donating blood before elective surgery to reduce autologous transfusion, treatment of anemia in critical illness.

CONTRAINDICATIONS

History of sensitivity to hamster cell–derived products or human albumin, uncontrolled hypertension.

INTERACTIONS

Drug
Heparin: An increase in RBC volume may enhance blood clotting. Heparin dosage may need to be increased.
Herbal
None known.
Food
None known.

DIAGNOSTIC TEST EFFECTS

May increase BUN, serum phosphorus, serum potassium, serum creatinine, serum uric acid, and sodium levels. May decrease bleeding time, iron concentration, and serum ferritin levels.

IV INCOMPATIBILITIES

Do not mix with other medications. Amphotericin B cholesteryl sulfate complex (Amphotec), chlorpromazine, dantrolene, diazepam (Valium), haloperidol (Haldol), inamrinone, midazolam, minocycline (Minocin), phenytoin, prochlorperazine, sulfamethoxazole/trimethoprim, vancomycin.

IV COMPATIBILITIES

Alfentanil (Alfenta), amikacin (Amikar), aminophylline, ascorbic acid, atracurium (Tracrium), atropine, azathioprine, aztreonam (Azactam), benztropine (Cogentin), bretylium, bumetanide (Bumex), buprenorphine (Buprenex), butorphanol (Stadol), calcium chloride, calcium gluconate, cefazolin, cefotaxime (Claforan), cefotetan (Cefotan), cefoxitin (Mefoxin), ceftazidime (Ceptaz, Fortaz, Tazicef, Tazidime), ceftizoxime (Cefizox), ceftriaxone (Rocephin), cefuroxime (Zinacef), chloramphenicol, cimetidine (Tagamet), clindamycin (Cleocin), cyanocobalamin, cyclosporine (Sandimmune), dexamethasone sodium phosphate, digoxin (Lanoxin), diltiazem (Cardizem), diphenhydramine (Benadryl), dobutamine (Dobutrex), dopamine (Intropin), enalaprilat, ephedrine, epinephrine, erythromycin lactobionate, esmolol (Brevibloc), famotidine (Pepcid), fentanyl (Sublimaze), fluconazole (Diflucan), folic acid, furosemide (Lasix), ganciclovir (Cytovene), heparin, hydrocortisone sodium succinate (Solu-Cortef), hydroxyzine, imipenem/cilastatin (Primaxin), insulin (regular, Humulin R, Novolin R), isoproterenol (Isuprel), ketorolac, labetalol, lidocaine, magnesium sulfate, mannitol, meperidine (Demerol), methicillin, methylprednisolone sodium succinate, metoclopramide (Reglan), metoprolol (Lopressor), metronidazole (Flagyl), morphine, multiple vitamins injection, nafcillin, nalbuphine (Nubain), naloxone (Narcan), nitroglycerin, nitroprusside sodium (Nitropress), norepinephrine (Levophed), ondansetron (Zofran), oxacillin, oxytocin (Pitocin), penicillin G potassium, penicillin G sodium, pentobarbital, phenobarbital, phytonadione, potassium chloride, procainamide, promethazine, propranolol, ranitidine (Zantac), sodium bicarbonate, streptokinase, succinylcholine, sufentanil (Sufenta), theophylline, ticarcillin (Ticar), ticarcillin/clavulanate (Timentin), tobramycin, vasopressin, verapamil.

SIDE EFFECTS

▸ **Patients receiving chemotherapy**

Frequent (17%-20%)
Fever, diarrhea, nausea, vomiting, edema.

Occasional (11%-13%)
Asthenia, shortness of breath, paresthesia.

Rare (3%-5%)
Dizziness, trunk pain.

▸ **Patients with chronic renal failure**

Frequent (11%-24%)
Hypertension, headache, nausea, arthralgia.

Occasional (7%-9%)
Fatigue, edema, diarrhea, vomiting, chest pain, skin reactions at administration site, asthenia, dizziness, clotted access.

▸ **Patients with HIV infection treated with AZT**

Frequent (15%-38%)
Fever, fatigue, headache, cough, diarrhea, rash, nausea.

Occasional (9%-14%)
Shortness of breath, asthenia, skin reaction at injection site, dizziness.

SERIOUS REACTIONS

- Hypertensive encephalopathy, thrombosis, cerebrovascular accident, myocardial infarction (MI), and seizures have occurred rarely.
- Epoetin alfa increased the risk for death and serious cerebrovascular events in controlled clinical trials when administered to target a hemoglobin of more than 12 g/dL and in cancer patients receiving chemotherapy. There is increased risk of serious arterial and venous thromboembolic reactions, including MI, stroke, congestive heart failure (CHF), and hemodialysis graft occlusion. To reduce cerebrovascular risks, use the lowest dose of epoetin alfa that will gradually increase the hemoglobin concentration to a level sufficient to avoid the need for RBC transfusion. The hemoglobin concentration should not exceed 12 g/dL; the rate of hemoglobin increase should not exceed 1 g/dL in any 2-wk period.
- Epoetin alfa has shortened time to tumor progression and reduced survival time in solid tumor patients with target hemoglobin > 12 g/dL.
- Hyperkalemia occurs occasionally in patients with chronic renal failure, usually in those who do not conform to medication regimen, dietary guidelines, and frequency of dialysis regimen.

• Cases of pure red cell aplasia and severe anemia, with or without other cytopenias, associated with neutralizing antibodies to erythropoietin, have been reported in patients treated with epoetin alfa. This has been reported predominantly in patients with chronic renal failure (CRF) receiving epoetin alfa by SC administration.

PRECAUTIONS & CONSIDERATIONS

Caution is warranted with a history of seizures and known porphyria (an impairment of erythrocyte formation in bone marrow). It is unknown whether epoetin alfa crosses the placenta or is distributed in breast milk. Safety and efficacy of epoetin alfa have not been established in children 1 mo of age and younger. No age-related precautions have been noted in elderly patients. Avoid potentially hazardous activities during the first 90 days of therapy. There is an increased risk of seizure development in those with chronic renal failure during the first 90 days of therapy.

Notify the physician of severe headache. Hemoglobin and hematocrit should be monitored diligently. The dosage should be reduced if hematocrit level increases more than 4 points in 2 wks. Hemoglobin should not exceed 12 g/dL or increase by 1 g/dL in any 2-wk period. CBC should also be monitored. In addition, BP must be monitored aggressively for an increase because 25% of persons taking epoetin alfa require antihypertensive therapy and dietary restrictions. Keep in mind that most patients need supplemental iron therapy.

Storage

Refrigerate vials. Do not shake. Protect from light.

Administration

! Avoid excessive agitation of vial; do not shake because it can denature medication, rendering it inactive.

IV route is preferred for patients on hemodialysis. For IV use, reconstitution is not necessary. May be given as an IV bolus. To limit adherence to the tubing, inject while blood is still in the IV line, followed by a saline flush.

For SC administration, use 1 dose per vial; do not reenter vial. Discard unused portion. To minimize SC injection site discomfort, may dilute single-use vial dose in a 1:1 ratio with bacteriostatic 0.9% NaCl injection with benzyl alcohol 0.9%.

Epoprostenol (Prostacyclin)

e-poe-pros'ten-ol

Flolan

CATEGORY AND SCHEDULE

Pregnancy Risk Category: B

Classification: Platelet inhibitors, vasodilators

MECHANISM OF ACTION

An antihypertensive that directly dilates pulmonary and systemic arterial vascular beds and inhibits platelet aggregation. *Therapeutic Effect:* Reduces right and left ventricular afterload; increases cardiac output and stroke volume.

AVAILABILITY

Injection, Powder for Reconstitution: 0.5 mg, 1.5 mg.

INDICATIONS AND DOSAGES

▸ **Long-term treatment of New York Heart Association Class III and IV primary pulmonary hypertension and pulmonary hypertension associated with scleroderma spectrum of disease in New York Heart Association Class II and IV who do not respond adequately to conventional therapy**

IV INFUSION

Adults, Elderly. Procedure to determine dose range: Initially, 2 ng/kg/min, increased in increments of 2 ng/kg/min q15min until dose-limiting adverse effects occur.

Increments in dose should be considered if symptoms of pulmonary hypertension persist or recur after improving. The infusion should be increased by 1- to 2-ng/kg/min increments at intervals sufficient to allow assessment of clinical response; these intervals should be at least 15 min. In clinical trials, incremental increases in dose occurred at intervals of 24-48 h or longer. Avoid abrupt withdrawal or sudden large dose reductions.

OFF-LABEL USES

Primary pulmonary arterial hypertension in children.

CONTRAINDICATIONS

Long-term use in patients with CHF (severe ventricular systolic dysfunction) or chronically in patients who develop pulmonary edema during initiation.

INTERACTIONS

Drug

Acetate in dialysis fluids, other vasodilators, antihypertensives, diuretics: May increase hypotensive effect.

Anticoagulants, antiplatelets: May increase the risk of bleeding.

Vasoconstrictors: May decrease effects of epoprostenol.

Herbal

Supplements with antiplatelet or anticoagulant effects (e.g., feverfew, garlic, ginger, ginkgo biloba, ginseng, red clover, sweet clover, white willow, etc.): May increase effects on platelets or risk of bleeding.

Food

None known.

DIAGNOSTIC TEST EFFECTS

None known.

IV INCOMPATIBILITIES

Do not mix epoprostenol with other medications.

IV COMPATIBILITIES

Bivalirudin (Angiomax).

SIDE EFFECTS

Frequent

Acute phase: Flushing (58%), headache (49%), nausea (32%), vomiting (32%), hypotension (16%), anxiety (11%), chest pain (11%), dizziness (8%).

Chronic phase (> 20%): Dyspnea, asthenia, dizziness, headache, chest pain, nausea, vomiting, palpitations, edema, jaw pain, tachycardia, flushing, myalgia, nonspecific muscle pain, diarrhea, anxiety, chills, fever, or flu-like symptoms.

Occasional

Acute phase (2%-5%): Bradycardia, abdominal pain, muscle pain, dyspnea, back pain.

Chronic phase (10%-20%): Rash, depression, hypotension, paresthesia, pallor, syncope, bradycardia, ascites, tachycardia.

Rare

Acute phase: Paresthesia, diaphoresis, dyspepsia, tachycardia.

E

SERIOUS REACTIONS

- Angina, myocardial infarction, and thrombocytopenia occur rarely.
- Abrupt withdrawal, including a large reduction in dosage or interruption in drug delivery, may produce rebound pulmonary hypertension as evidenced by dyspnea, dizziness, and asthenia.
- Sepsis during long-term follow-up.

PRECAUTIONS & CONSIDERATIONS

Interruptions in the IV infusion should be avoided because even a short break in the infusion can result in rebounding pulmonary hypertension. The patient should be closely monitored during initiation of therapy. Use epoprostenol cautiously in elderly patients.

Before beginning therapy, a backup infusion pump and IV infusion sets should be obtained to avoid interruptions in therapy. A central venous catheter must be in place. Vital signs should be monitored before and during therapy. Standing and supine BP should be monitored for several hours after a dosage adjustment. Therapeutic evidence is evidenced by decreased chest pain, dyspnea on exertion, fatigue, pulmonary arterial pressure, pulmonary vascular resistance, and syncope, and improved pulmonary function.

Storage

Store unopened vial at room temperature. Do not freeze. Reconstituted solutions are stable for up to 48 h if refrigerated. Discard if frozen or if reconstituted > 48 h.

Administration

! Infuse epoprostenol continuously through an indwelling central venous catheter. If necessary and on a temporary basis, infuse through a peripheral vein. Use only the diluent provided by the manufacturer.

Follow instructions of manufacturer for dilution to specific concentrations; use only sterile water for injection or 0.9% NaCl. Give as pump infusion only. Adjustments to dose should be done only by physician.

Eprosartan

eh-pro-sar'tan

★ 🍁 Teveten

CATEGORY AND SCHEDULE

Pregnancy Risk Category: C (D if used in second or third trimester)

Classification: Angiotensin II receptor antagonists

MECHANISM OF ACTION

An angiotensin II receptor antagonist that blocks the vasoconstrictor and aldosterone-secreting effects of angiotensin II, inhibiting the binding of angiotensin II to the AT1 receptors. *Therapeutic Effect:* Causes vasodilation, decreases peripheral resistance, and decreases BP.

PHARMACOKINETICS

Rapidly absorbed after PO administration. Protein binding: 98%. Minimally metabolized in liver. Excreted in urine (90%) and biliary system. Minimally removed by hemodialysis. *Half-life:* 5-9 h.

AVAILABILITY

Tablets: 400 mg, 600 mg.

INDICATIONS AND DOSAGES

▸ **Hypertension**

PO

Adults, Elderly. Initially, 600 mg/day (given in 1 or 2 doses). Range: 400-800 mg/day.

CONTRAINDICATIONS

Hypersensitivity to eprosartan.

INTERACTIONS

Drug

Potassium-sparing diuretics, potassium supplements: May increase risk of hyperkalemia.

Herbal

Licorice, ma huang, yohimbine: May decrease the effectiveness of eprosartan.

Food

None known.

DIAGNOSTIC TEST EFFECTS

May increase BUN, serum alkaline phosphatase, serum bilirubin, serum creatinine, potassium, AST (SGOT), and ALT (SGPT) levels. May decrease blood hemoglobin levels.

SIDE EFFECTS

Occasional (2%-8%)

Upper respiratory infection, rhinitis, cough, abdominal pain.

Rare (< 2%)

Muscle pain, fatigue, diarrhea, urinary tract infection, depression, hypertriglyceridemia, hyperkalemia.

SERIOUS REACTIONS

- Overdosage may manifest as hypotension and tachycardia. Bradycardia occurs less often.
- Angioedema is rare.

PRECAUTIONS & CONSIDERATIONS

Caution is warranted with preexisting renal insufficiency, significant aortic and mitral stenosis, hyperaldosteronism, and bilateral or unilateral renal artery stenosis. Salt and volume-depletion should be corrected before starting therapy. Eprosartan has caused fetal or neonatal morbidity or mortality, particularly in 2nd and 3rd trimesters; discontinue as soon as pregnancy is known. Also, because of the potential for adverse effects on the infant, patients taking eprosartan should not breastfeed. Safety and efficacy of eprosartan have not been established in children. No age-related precautions have been noted in elderly patients.

Apical pulse and BP should be assessed immediately before each eprosartan dose and regularly throughout therapy. Be alert to fluctuations in apical pulse and BP. If an excessive reduction in BP occurs, place the person in the supine position with feet slightly elevated and notify the physician. Tasks that require mental alertness or motor skills should be avoided. BUN, serum electrolytes, serum creatinine levels, heart rate for tachycardia, and urinalysis results should be obtained before and during therapy.

Administration

Take eprosartan without regard to food. Do not crush or break tablets.

Eptifibatide

ep-tih-fib'ah-tide

Integrilin

CATEGORY AND SCHEDULE

Pregnancy Risk Category: B

Classification: Platelet inhibitors, glycoprotein IIb/IIIa inhibitors

MECHANISM OF ACTION

A glycoprotein IIb/IIIa inhibitor that rapidly inhibits platelet aggregation by preventing binding of fibrinogen to receptor sites on platelets. *Therapeutic Effect:* Prevents closure of treated coronary arteries. Also prevents acute cardiac ischemic complications.

AVAILABILITY

Injection Solution: 0.75 mg/mL, 2 mg/mL.

INDICATIONS AND DOSAGES

▸ Adjunct to percutaneous coronary intervention (PCI)

IV BOLUS, IV INFUSION

Adults, Elderly. 180 mcg/kg bolus (maximum 22.6 mg) before PCI initiation; then continuous drip of 2 mcg/kg/min and a second 180 mcg/kg bolus (maximum 22.6 mg) 10 min after the first. Maximum: 15 mg/h. Continue until hospital discharge or for up to 18-24 h. Minimum 12 h is recommended. Concurrent aspirin and heparin therapy is recommended.

▸ Acute coronary syndrome

IV BOLUS, IV INFUSION

Adults, Elderly. 180 mcg/kg bolus (max 22.6 mg) then 2 mcg/kg/min until discharge or coronary artery bypass graft, up to 72 h. Maximum: 15 mg/h. Concurrent aspirin and heparin therapy is recommended.

▸ Dosage in renal impairment

Serum creatinine 2-4 mg/dL or CrCl < 50 mL/min: Use 180 mcg/kg bolus (maximum 22.6 mg) and 1 mcg/kg/min infusion (maximum 7.5 mg/h). For PCI, a second bolus dose should be administered (180 mcg/kg, maximum 22.6 mg) 10 min after the first bolus.

CONTRAINDICATIONS

Active internal bleeding within previous 30 days, history of stroke within 30 days, or any history of hemorrhagic stroke, recent (6 wks or less) surgery or trauma, severe uncontrolled hypertension, thrombocytopenia (< 100,000 cells/μL), renal dialysis, administration of another parenteral GP IIb/IIIa inhibitor, hypersensitivity.

INTERACTIONS

Drug

Anticoagulants, heparin: May increase the risk of hemorrhage.

Dextran, drotrecogin alfa, other platelet aggregation inhibitors (such as aspirin), thrombolytic agents: May increase the risk of bleeding.

Herbal

None known.

Food

None known.

DIAGNOSTIC TEST EFFECTS

Increases aPTT, PT, and clotting time. Decreases platelet count.

IV INCOMPATIBILITIES

Administer in separate line; do not add other medications to infusion solution.

Furosemide (Lasix).

IV COMPATIBILITIES

Alteplase (Activase), amiodarone, argatroban, atropine, bivalirudin (Angiomax), daptomycin (Cubicin), dobutamine, ertapenem (Invanz), heparin, lidocaine, meperidine (Demerol), metoprolol (Lopressor), micafungin (Mycamine), midazolam, morphine, nitroglycerin, oxytocin (Pitocin), palonosetron (Aloxi), potassium chloride, teniposide (Vumon), tigecycline (Tygacil), tirofibran (Aggrastat), verapamil, 0.9% NaCl, 0.9% NaCl-D5%W.

SIDE EFFECTS

Occasional (7%)

Hypotension.

SERIOUS REACTIONS

- Minor to major bleeding complications may occur, most commonly at arterial access site for cardiac catheterization.

• Thrombocytopenia, intracranial hemorrhage and stroke, anaphylaxis have occurred rarely.

PRECAUTIONS & CONSIDERATIONS

Caution is warranted in patients with PTCA < 12 h from the onset of symptoms of acute myocardial infarction, prolonged PTCA that is > 70 min, and failed PTCA. Caution should also be used in persons who weigh < 75 kg or are older than 65 yr; have a history of GI disease or GI or genitourinary bleeding; have an AV malformation or aneurysm, intracranial tumors, platelet count < 100,000, renal dysfunction, hemorrhagic retinopathy; or are receiving aspirin, heparin, or thrombolytics. It is unknown whether eptifibatide causes fetal harm or can affect reproduction capacity. It is unknown whether eptifibatide is distributed in breast milk. Safety and efficacy of eptifibatide have not been established in children. In elderly patients, the risk of major bleeding is increased.

Hemoglobin, hematocrit, and platelet count should be obtained before treatment. If platelet count is < 90,000/mm^3, additional platelet counts should be obtained routinely to avoid development of thrombocytopenia. Nasogastric tube and urinary catheter use should be avoided, if possible.

Storage

Store vials in refrigerator. Vials may be stored at room temperature for up to 2 mo.

Administration

Solution normally appears clear and is colorless. Do not shake. Discard unused portions. Also discard if preparation contains any opaque particles. Withdraw bolus dose from 10-mL vial (2 mg/mL); for IV infusion, withdraw from 100-mL vial (0.75 mg/mL). May give IV push and infusion undiluted. Give bolus dose IV push over 1-2 min. Infusion should be given via a controlled infusion pump.

Ergoloid Mesylates

ur'go-loyd mess'ah-lates

🍁 Hydergine

CATEGORY AND SCHEDULE

Pregnancy Risk Category: C

Classification: Ergot alkaloids and derivatives

MECHANISM OF ACTION

There is no specific evidence that clearly establishes the mechanism by which ergoloid mesylates preparations produce mental effects, nor is there conclusive evidence that the drug particularly affects cerebral arteriosclerosis or cerebrovascular insufficiency.

PHARMACOKINETICS

Rapidly, incompletely absorbed from GI tract. Metabolized in liver. Eliminated primarily in feces. *Half-life:* 2-5 h.

AVAILABILITY

Tablets: 1 mg.

INDICATIONS AND DOSAGES

▸ **Age-related decline in mental capacity**

PO

Adults, Elderly. Initially, 1 mg 3 times/day. Range: 1.5-12 mg/day. Usual dose: 1-2 mg 3 times/day.

CONTRAINDICATIONS

Acute or chronic psychosis (regardless of etiology), hypersensitivity to ergoloid mesylates, or any component of the formulation; pregnancy.

INTERACTIONS

Drug

Potent CYP450 3A4 inhibitors: May increase risk of ergotism (nausea, vomiting, vasospastic ischemia).

Frovatriptan, naratriptan, rizatriptan, sumatriptan, zolmitriptan, other serotonergic agents: May prolong vasospastic reactions (ergot derivatives).

Herbal

None known.

Food

Grapefruit juice: May increase risk of ergotism (nausea, vomiting, vasospastic ischemia).

SIDE EFFECTS

Occasional

GI distress, transient nausea, sublingual irritation.

SERIOUS REACTIONS

- Overdose may produce blurred vision, dizziness, syncope, headache, flushed face, nausea, vomiting, decreased appetite, stomach cramps, and stuffy nose.

PRECAUTIONS & CONSIDERATIONS

It is unknown whether ergoloid mesylates cross the placenta or are distributed in breast milk. Most ergot alkaloids are excreted into breast milk and are considered contraindicated during pregnancy because of their oxytocic and uterine stimulant properties. Be aware that the safety and efficacy of ergoloid mesylates have not been established in children. There are no age-related precautions noted in elderly patients.

Clinical improvement is gradual, and results may not be noted for 3-4 wks.

Storage

Store at room temperature.

Administration

Give with food to avoid GI upset.

Ergotamine & Ergotamine-Caffeine

er-got'a-meen

Ergotamine: Ergomar

Ergotamine-Caffeine:

Cafergot, Migergot

CATEGORY AND SCHEDULE

Pregnancy Risk Category: X

Classification: Ergot alkaloids and derivatives

MECHANISM OF ACTION

An ergotamine derivative and α-adrenergic blocker that directly stimulates vascular smooth muscle, resulting in peripheral and cerebral vasoconstriction. May also have antagonist effects on serotonin. *Therapeutic Effect:* Suppresses vascular headaches.

PHARMACOKINETICS

Slowly and incompletely absorbed from the GI tract; rapidly and extensively absorbed after rectal administration. Protein binding: > 90%. Undergoes extensive first-pass metabolism in the liver to active metabolite. Eliminated in feces by the biliary system. *Half-life:* 2 h.

AVAILABILITY

Tablets (Sublingual [Ergomar]): 2 mg.
Tablets (Ergotamine and Caffeine [Cafergot]): 1 mg, with 100 mg caffeine.
Suppositories (Ergotamine and Caffeine [Migergot]): 2 mg, with 100 mg caffeine.

INDICATIONS AND DOSAGES

▸ **Vascular headaches**

PO (CAFERGOT [FIXED COMBINATION OF ERGOTAMINE AND CAFFEINE])

Adults, Elderly. 1-2 tablets at onset of headache, then 1-2 tablets q30min. Maximum: 6 tablets/episode; 10 tablets/wk.

Children. 1 tablet at onset of headache, then 1 tab q30min as needed. Maximum: 3 mg/episode.

SUBLINGUAL (ERGOMAR)

Adults, Elderly. 1 tablet at onset of headache, then 1 tablet q30min as needed. Maximum: 3 tablets/24 h; 5 tablets/wk.

SUBLINGUAL (ERGOMAR)

Children > 10 yr. 1 mg at onset of headache, then 1 mg q30min. Maximum: 3 mg/episode.

RECTAL (MIGERGOT)

Adults, Elderly. 1 suppository at onset of headache; may repeat dose in 1 h. Maximum: 2 suppositories/episode; 5 suppositories/wk.

Children > 10 yr. One-fourth to one-half of suppository; may repeat dose in 1 h. Maximum: 2 mg ergotamine/attack.

CONTRAINDICATIONS

Coronary artery disease, hypertension, impaired hepatic or renal function, malnutrition, peripheral vascular diseases (such as thromboangiitis obliterans, syphilitic arteritis, severe arteriosclerosis, thrombophlebitis, and Raynaud disease), sepsis, severe pruritus, pregnancy.

INTERACTIONS

Drug

β-Blockers: May increase the risk of vasospasm.

CYP3A4 inhibitors: May increase levels and effects of ergotamine. Ketoconazole, itraconazole, protease inhibitors, and macrolide antibiotics are contraindicated.

Ergot alkaloids, systemic vasoconstrictors: May increase pressor effect.

MAOIs, serotonergic agonists, SSRIs: May increase risk of serotonin syndrome. Do not use within 24 h of a serotonin agonist for migraine ("triptan").

Nitroglycerin: May decrease the effects of nitroglycerin.

Herbal

None known.

Food

Caffeine: May increase caffeine levels.

Grapefruit: May increase ergotamine levels.

DIAGNOSTIC TEST EFFECTS

None known.

SIDE EFFECTS

Frequent (6%-10%)

Nausea, vomiting.

Occasional (2%-5%)

Cough, dizziness.

Rare (< 2%)

Myalgia, fatigue, diarrhea, dry mouth, upper respiratory tract infection, dyspepsia, confusion, drowsiness.

SERIOUS REACTIONS

• Prolonged administration or excessive dosage may produce ergotamine poisoning, manifested as nausea and vomiting; paresthesia, muscle pain, or weakness; precordial pain; angina; tachycardia or bradycardia; and hypertension or hypotension. Vasoconstriction of peripheral arteries and arterioles may result in localized edema and pruritus. Muscle pain will occur when walking and later, even at rest. Other rare effects include confusion, depression, drowsiness, seizures, pancreatitis, ischemic colitis, myocardial infarction, and gangrene. Ergotismy can occur at dose < 5 mg but are most likely to occur with > 15 mg/24 h or 40 mg in a few days.

PRECAUTIONS & CONSIDERATIONS

Ergotamine use is contraindicated in pregnancy because it may result in fetal harm and even death. Ergotamine is distributed in breast milk and may inhibit lactation. Ergotamine use may produce diarrhea or vomiting in neonates; it may be used safely in children 10 yr and older but should be used only when patient is unresponsive to other drugs. In elderly patients, age-related occlusive peripheral vascular disease increases the risk of peripheral vasoconstriction; in addition, age-related renal impairment may require cautious use.

Notify the physician immediately if the drug does not relieve the headache or if irregular heartbeat, nausea or vomiting, numbness or tingling of the fingers and toes, or pain or weakness of the extremities occurs. Peripheral circulation, including the temperature, color, and strength of pulses in the extremities, should be assessed.

Storage

Store rectal suppositories in refrigerator. Store tablets at room temperature, protected from light and moisture.

Administration

! Do not exceed daily, per attack, or weekly dosage limits. Patients should not use serotonin agonist (triptans) within 24 h of ergot use.

For sublingual use, place the sublingual tablet under the tongue, let it dissolve, and swallow the saliva. Do not administer it with water.

Tablets may be taken with fluids. For rectal suppository, if too soft, run wrapper under cool water. Remove wrapper; moisten with water before insertion.

Erlotinib

er-low'tih-nib

Tarceva

CATEGORY AND SCHEDULE

Pregnancy Risk Category: D

Classification: Antineoplastics, miscellaneous

MECHANISM OF ACTION

A human epidermal growth factor that inhibits tyrosine kinases (TKs) associated with transmembrane cell surface receptors found on both normal and cancer cells. One such receptor is epidermal growth factor receptor (EGFR). *Therapeutic Effect:* TK activity appears to be vitally important to cell proliferation and survival.

AVAILABILITY

Tablets: 25 mg, 100 mg, 150 mg.

INDICATIONS AND DOSAGES

▸ **Locally advanced or metastatic non–small cell lung carcinoma after failure of first-line therapy**

PO

Adults, Elderly. 150 mg/day.

▸ **Locally advanced, unresectable, or metastatic pancreatic cancer, first-line therapy**

Adults, Elderly. 100 mg/day with gemcitabine.

▸ **Concomitant therapy with strong CYP3A4 inhibitor**

Consider erlotinib dose reduction if adverse reactions occur.

▸ **Concomitant therapy with strong CYP3A4 inducer**
Consider treatments lacking CYP3A4-inducing activity or consider dose > 150 mg.
▸ **Dosage-hepatic impairment**
Expect to interrupt or reduce dose treatment if severe changes in total bilirubin or liver transaminase levels occur.

OFF-LABEL USES
Metastatic renal cell carcinoma.

CONTRAINDICATIONS
Pregnancy.

INTERACTIONS
Drug
CYP3A4 inducers, aminoglutethimide, carbamazepine, nafcillin, nevirapine, phenobarbital, phenytoin, rifampin: May decrease the levels and effects of erlotinib.
CYP3A4 inhibitors, azole antifungals, ciprofloxacin, clarithromycin, diclofenac, doxycycline, erythromycin, imatinib, isoniazid, ketoconazole, nefazodone, nicardipine, propofol, protease inhibitors, quinidine, verapamil: May increase the levels and effects of erlotinib.
Herbal
St. John's wort: May increase metabolism and decrease serum erlotinib concentration. Avoid.
Food
All foods: Give erlotinib at least 1 h before or 2 h after ingestion of food. Bioavailability without food 60%, with food 100%.
Other
Cigarette smoking: Decreases erlotinib exposure. Advise patients to quit smoking.

DIAGNOSTIC TEST EFFECTS
May increase hepatic enzyme levels.

SIDE EFFECTS
Frequent (10%-88%)
Acneiform rash, pruritus, diarrhea, fatigue, pyrexia, anorexia, nausea, edema, constipation, bone pain, anxiety, headache, dry skin, vomiting, mucositis, dry mouth, depression, dizziness, insomnia, erythema, alopecia, dyspepsia, weight loss, abdominal pain, myalgia, arthralgia, rigors, paresthesia, dyspnea, cough, infection.
Occasional (4%-9%)
Keratitis, pneumonitis, deep vein thrombosis.

SERIOUS REACTIONS
- Renal dysfunction.
- Interstitial lung disease has been reported.
- Myocardial infarction, cerebrovascular accident, and microangiopathic hemolytic anemia with thrombocytopenia.

PRECAUTIONS & CONSIDERATIONS
Caution is warranted with dehydration, hepatic or severe renal impairment. Erlotinib may cause fetal harm and should not be used during pregnancy or lactation. Safety and efficacy have not been established in children. No age-related precautions have been noted in elderly patients.
Storage
Store at controlled room temperature.
Administration
CAUTION: Observe and exercise appropriate precautions for handling and administering cytotoxic drugs. Take erlotinib at least 1 h before or 2 h after ingestion of food (on an empty

stomach). Administer at roughly the same time each day.

Ertapenem

er-ta-pen′em

★ 🍁 Invanz

CATEGORY AND SCHEDULE

Pregnancy Risk Category: B

Classification: Antibiotics, carbapenems

MECHANISM OF ACTION

A carbapenem that penetrates the bacterial cell wall of microorganisms and binds to penicillin-binding proteins, inhibiting cell wall synthesis. Not effective against methicillin-resistant *Staphylococcus, Enterococcus* spp., penicillin-resistant strains of *S. pneumoniae*, β-lactamase-positive strains of *H. influenzae*, or most *P. aeruginosa*. *Therapeutic Effect:* Produces bacterial cell death.

PHARMACOKINETICS

Almost completely absorbed after IM administration. Protein binding: 85%-95%. Widely distributed. Primarily excreted in urine with smaller amount eliminated in feces. Removed by hemodialysis. *Half-life:* 4 h.

AVAILABILITY

Injection Powder for Reconstitution: 1 g.

INDICATIONS AND DOSAGES

▸ Intra-abdominal infection

IM, IV

Adults, Elderly, Children 13 yr and older. 1 g/day for 5-14 days.

Children 3 mo to 12 yr. 15 mg/kg twice daily (maximum 1 g/day) for 5-14 days.

▸ Skin and skin-structure infection

IM, IV

Adults, Elderly, Children 13 yr and older. 1 g/day for 7-14 days.

Children 3 mo to 12 yr. 15 mg/kg twice daily (maximum 1 g/day) for 7-14 days.

▸ Community-acquired pneumonia, urinary tract infection (UTI)

IM, IV

Adults, Elderly, Children 13 yr and older. 1 g/day for 10-14 days.

Children 3 mo to 12 yr. 15 mg/kg twice daily (maximum 1 g/day) for 10-14 days.

▸ Pelvic/gynecologic infection

IM, IV

Adults, Elderly, Children 13 yr and older. 1 g/day for 3-10 days.

Children 3 mo to 12 yr. 15 mg/kg twice daily (maximum 1 g/day) for 3-10 days.

▸ Prophylaxis of surgical site infection following colorectal surgery

IV

Adults, Elderly. 1 g given 1 h before surgical incision.

▸ Dosage in renal impairment

For adults and elderly patients with creatinine clearance ≤ 30 mL/min or on hemodialysis, dosage is 500 mg once a day.

CONTRAINDICATIONS

History of hypersensitivity to other carbapenems (imipenem, meropenem) or anaphylaxis to beta-lactams, hypersensitivity to lidocaine or amide-type local anesthetics (IM).

INTERACTIONS

Drug

Probenecid: Reduces renal excretion of ertapenem, increases concentration.

Valproic acid: Reduces serum levels of valproic acid. Monitor levels and adjust dose.

Herbal and Food

None known.

DIAGNOSTIC TEST EFFECTS

May increase serum alkaline phosphatase, AST (SGOT), and ALT (SGPT) levels. May decrease platelet count, blood hematocrit and hemoglobin levels, and serum potassium level.

IV INCOMPATIBILITIES

Do not use diluents or IV solutions containing dextrose.

Allopurinol (Aloprim), amiodarone, amphotericin B cholesteryl sulfate complex (Amphotec), anidulafungin (Eraxis), caspofungin (Cancidas), chlorpromazine, dantrolene, daunorubicin (Cerubidine), diazepam (Valium), dobutamine, doxorubicin (Adriamycin), droperidol, epirubicin (Ellence), hydralazine, hydroxyzine, idarubicin (Idamycin PFS), midazolam, minocycline (Minocin), mitoxantrone (Novantrone), nicardipine (Cardene), ondansetron (Zofran), phenytoin, prochlorperazine, promethazine, quinupristin/dalfopristin (Synercid), topotecan (Hycamtin), verapamil.

IV COMPATIBILITIES

Acyclovir (Zovirax), alfentanil (Alfenta), amifostine (Ethyol), amikacin (Amikar), aminocaproic acid, aminophylline, amphotericin B lipid complex (Abelcet), amphotericin B liposome (AmBisome), argatroban, arsenic trioxide (Trisenox), atenolol, atracurium (Tracrium), azithromycin (Zithromax), aztreonam (Azactam), bivalirudin (Angiomax), bleomycin (Blenoxane), bretylium, bumetanide (Bumex), buprenorphine (Buprenex), busulfan (Bulsulfex), butorphanol (Stadol), calcium chloride, calcium gluconate, carboplatin, carmustine (BiCNU), cimetidine (Tagamet), ciprofloxacin (Cipro), cisatracurium (Nimbex), cisplatin, cyclophosphamide (Cytoxan), cyclosporine (Sandimmune), cytarabine (Tarabine), dacarbazine (DTIC-Dome), dactinomycin (Cosmegen), daptomycin (Cubicin), dexamethasone sodium phosphate, dexrazoxane (Zinecard), digoxin (Lanoxin), diltiazem (Cardizem), diphenhydramine (Benadryl), docetaxel (Taxotere), dopamine, enalaprilat, ephedrine, epinephrine, eptifibatide (Integrilin), erythromycin lactobionate, esmolol (Brevibloc), etoposide (VePesid), etoposide phosphate (Etopophos), famotidine (Pepcid), fenoldopam (Corlopam), fluconazole (Diflucan), fludarabine (Fludara), fluorouracil, foscarnet (Foscavir), fosphenytoin (Cerebyx), furosemide (Lasix), ganciclovir (Cytovene), gemcitabine (Gemzar), gentamicin, granisetron (Kytril), haloperidol lactate (Haldol), heparin, hetastarch in NS, hydrocortisone sodium succinate (Solu-Cortef), hydromorphone (Dilaudid), ifosfamide (Ifex), insulin (regular, Humulin R, Novolin R), irinotecan (Camptosar), isoproterenol (Isuprel), ketorolac, labetalol, leucovorin, levofloxacin (Levaquin), lidocaine, linezolid (Zyvox), lorazepam (Ativan), magnesium sulfate, melphalan (Alkeran), meperidine (Demerol), mesna (Mesnex), methotrexate, methylprednisolone sodium succinate, metoclopramide (Reglan), metronidazole (Flagyl), milrinone (Primacor), mitomycin (Mutamycin), morphine, moxifloxacin (Avelox), nalbuphine (Nubain), naloxone (Narcan), nesiritide (Natrecor), nitroglycerin, nitroprusside sodium (Nitropress), norepinephrine (Levophed), oxaliplatin (Eloxatin), oxytocin (Pitocin), paclitaxel (Taxol), pamidronate (Aredia), pantoprazole (Protonix), pemetrexed (Alimta), pentobarbital, phenobarbital, phenylephrine, potassium acetate, potassium chloride, potassium phosphates, procainamide, propranolol, ranitidine (Zantac), remifentanil (Ultiva), rocuronium (Zemuron), sodium acetate, sodium phosphates, succinylcholine (Anectine, Quelicin), sufentanil (Sufenta), tacrolimus (Prograf), teniposide (Vumon), theophylline, thiotepa (Thioplex), tigecycline (Tygacil), tirofibran (Aggrastat), tobramycin, vancomycin, vasopressin, vecuronium (Norcuron), vinblastine (Velban), vincristine (Vincasar), vinorelbine (Navelbine), voriconazole (Vfend), water for injection, 0.9% NaCl, zidovudine (Retrovir), zolendronic acid (Zometa).

E

SIDE EFFECTS

Frequent (6%-10%)
Diarrhea, nausea, headache, infused vein complications.

Occasional (2%-5%)
Altered mental status, insomnia, rash, abdominal pain, constipation, vomiting, edema, fever.

Rare (< 2%)
Dizziness, cough, oral candidiasis, anxiety, tachycardia, hypertension, hypotension, phlebitis at IV site, extravasation.

SERIOUS REACTIONS

- Antibiotic-associated colitis and other superinfections may occur.
- Anaphylactic reactions have been reported.
- Seizures may occur in those with central nervous system (CNS) disorders (including patients with brain lesions or a history of seizures), bacterial meningitis, or severe renal impairment.

PRECAUTIONS & CONSIDERATIONS

Caution is warranted with CNS disorders (particularly with brain lesions or history of seizures), a hypersensitivity to cephalosporins, penicillins, or other allergens, and impaired renal function. Be aware that ertapenem is distributed in breast milk. Be aware that the safety and efficacy of ertapenem have not been established in children younger than 3 mo. In elderly patients, advanced renal insufficiency and end-stage renal insufficiency may require dosage adjustment.

History of allergies, particularly to β-lactams, cephalosporins, and penicillins, should be obtained before beginning drug therapy. Hydration status, nausea, vomiting, skin for rash, sleep pattern, and mental status should be evaluated. Report any diarrhea, rash, seizures, tremors, or other new symptoms.

Storage
Store vials at room temperature. Solution normally appears colorless to yellow (variation in color does not affect potency). Discard if solution contains precipitate. Reconstituted solution is stable for 6 h at room temperature, 24 h if refrigerated and used within 4 h after removing.

Administration
For IM use, reconstitute with 3.2 mL 1% lidocaine HCl injection (without epinephrine). Shake vial thoroughly. Give deep IM injections slowly to minimize patient discomfort. To further minimize discomfort, administer IM injections into the gluteus maximus instead of the lateral aspect of the thigh. Administer IM within 1 h after preparation.

For IV use, dilute 1-g vial with 10 mL, 0.9% NaCl or bacteriostatic water for injection. Shake well to dissolve. Further dilute with 50 mL 0.9% NaCl to concentration 20 mg/mL or less. Give by intermittent IV infusion (piggyback). Do not give IV push. Infuse over 20-30 min. Dextrose solutions are not compatible with ertapenem.

Erythromycin

er-ith-roe-mye′sin

★ Akne-Mycin, E.E.S., Emcin, Emgel, EryDerm, Erygel, EryPed, Ery-Tab, Erythrocin, My-E, PCE

🍁 AK-Mycin, Diomycin, EES, EryBID, Eryc, Erymycin, Erythrocin, Erythro-S, PCE

Do not confuse with Emct, azithromycin, Ethmozine, or Pedialyte.

CATEGORY AND SCHEDULE

Pregnancy Risk Category: B

Classification: Anti-infectives, macrolides

MECHANISM OF ACTION

A macrolide that reversibly binds to bacterial ribosomes, inhibiting bacterial protein synthesis. *Therapeutic Effect:* Bacteriostatic.

PHARMACOKINETICS

Variably absorbed from the GI tract (depending on dosage form used; better with salt forms than base form). Protein binding: 70%-90%. Widely distributed. Metabolized in the liver by CYP3A4. Primarily eliminated in feces by bile. Not removed by hemodialysis. *Half-life:* 1.4-2 h (increased in impaired renal function).

AVAILABILITY

Topical Gel (Emgel, Erygel): 2%.
Injection Powder for Reconstitution (Erythrocin): 500 mg, 1 g.
Ophthalmic Ointment: 5 mg/g (0.5%).
Topical Ointment (Akne-Mycin): 2%.
Oral Suspension (EryPed, E.E.S): 200 mg/5 mL, 400 mg/5 mL.
Topical Solution (EryDerm): 2%.
Capsule (Delayed Release): 250 mg.
Tablets (Ery-Tab): 250 mg, 333 mg, 500 mg.
Tablets (E.E.S): 400 mg.
Tablets (Erythrocin): 250 mg, 500 mg.
Tablets (PCE): 333 mg, 500 mg.
Topical Medicated Pledget (Emcin Clear, Ery): 2%.

INDICATIONS AND DOSAGES

▸ **Mild to moderate infections of the upper and lower respiratory tract, pharyngitis, skin infections**

PO

Adults, Elderly (base). 250 mg q6h, 500 mg q12h, or 333 mg q8h. Maximum: 4 g/day.

Adults, Elderly (ethylsuccinate). 400-800 mg q6-12h. Maximum: 4 g/day.

Children. 30-50 mg/kg/day in 2-4 divided doses up to 60-100 mg/kg/day for severe infections.

IV

Adults, Elderly, Children. 15-20 mg/kg/day in divided doses q6h or 500-1000 mg q6h. Maximum: 4 g/day.

▸ **Preoperative intestinal antisepsis**

PO

Adults, Elderly. 1 g at 1 PM, 2 PM, and 11 PM on the day before surgery (with neomycin).

Children. 20 mg/kg at 1 PM, 2 PM, and 11 PM on day before surgery (with neomycin).

▸ **Acne vulgaris**

TOPICAL

Adults, Children. Apply thin layer to affected area twice a day.

PO
Adults. 250 mg 4 times daily.
▸ **Gonococcal ophthalmia neonatorum prevention**
OPHTHALMIC
Neonates. 0.5-2 cm to each eye no later than 1 h after delivery.

E

OFF-LABEL USES

Systemic: Chancroid, *Campylobacter enteritis,* gastroparesis, Lyme disease.
Ophthalmic: Treatment of blepharitis, conjunctivitis, keratitis, chlamydial trachoma.

CONTRAINDICATIONS

Administration of fixed-combination product; history of hepatitis due to macrolides; hypersensitivity to macrolides; preexisting hepatic disease (estolate only).

INTERACTIONS

Drug
Buspirone, cyclosporine, felodipine, lovastatin, simvastatin: May increase the blood concentration and toxicity of these drugs.
Carbamazepine: May inhibit the metabolism of carbamazepine.
Chloramphenicol, clindamycin: May decrease the effects of these drugs.
Hepatotoxic medications: May increase the risk of hepatotoxicity.
Theophylline: May increase the risk of theophylline toxicity.
Warfarin: May increase warfarin's effects.
Herbal and Food
None known.

DIAGNOSTIC TEST EFFECTS

May increase serum alkaline phosphatase, bilirubin, AST (SGOT), and ALT (SGPT) levels.

IV INCOMPATIBILITIES

Amphotericin B cholesteryl sulfate complex (Amphotec), amphotericin B liposome (AmBisome), ascorbic acid, aztreonam (Azactam), cefazolin, cefepime (Maxipime), cefoxitin (Mefoxin), chloramphenicol, dantrolene, dexamethasone sodium phosphate, diazepam (Valium), fluconazole (Diflucan), furosemide (Lasix), ganciclovir (Cytovene), indomethacin, ketorolac, linezolid (Zyvox), minocycline (Minocin), nitroprusside sodium (Nitropress), pemetrexed (Alimta), pentobarbital, phenobarbital, phenytoin, rocuronium (Zemuron), sulfamethoxazole/trimethoprim, ticarcillin (Ticar), ticarcillin/clavulanate (Timentin).

IV COMPATIBILITIES

Acyclovir (Zovirax), alfentanil (Alfenta), amikacin (Amikar), aminophylline, amiodarone (Cordarone), anidulafungin (Eraxis), atracurium (Tracrium), atropine, azathioprine, benztropine (Cogentin), bivalirudin (Angiomax), bretylium, bumetanide (Bumex), buprenorphine (Buprenex), butorphanol (Stadol), calcium chloride, calcium gluconate carboplatin, caspofungin (Cancidas), cefotaxime (Claforan), ceftriaxone (Rocephin), cefuroxime (Zinacef), chlorpromazine, cimetidine (Tagemet), cisplatin, cyclophosphamide (Cytoxan), cyclosporine (Sandimmune), dactinomycin (Cosmegen), daptomycin (Cubicin), digoxin (Lanoxin), diltiazem (Cardizem), diphenhydramine (Benadryl), dobutamine (Dobutrex), docetaxel (Taxotere), dopamine (Intropin), doxorubicin (Adriamycin), enalaprilat, ephedrine, epinephrine, epirubicin (Ellence), epoetin alfa (Procrit), ertapenem (Invanz), esmolol (Brevibloc), etoposide phosphate (Etopophos), famotidine (Pepcid), fenoldopam (Corlopam), fentanyl (Sublimaze), fludarabine (Fludara), fluorouracil, folic acid, foscarnet (Foscavir), gemcitabine (Gemzar), gentamicin, granisetron (Kytril), hydrocortisone sodium succinate, hydromorphone (Dilaudid), hydroxyzine, idarubicin (Idamycin), imipenem/cilastatin (Primaxin), insulin (regular, Humulin R, Novolin R), isoproterenol (Isuprel), labetalol, levofloxacin (Levaquin), lidocaine, lorazepam (Ativan), meperidine (Demerol), methicillin, methotrexate, methylprednisolone sodium succinate, metoclopramide (Reglan), metronidazole (Flagyl), midazolam (Versed), milrinone, mitoxantrone (Novantrone), morphine, multivitamins, nafcillin, nalbuphine (Nubain), naloxone (Narcan), nicardipine (Cardene), nitroglycerin, norepinephrine (Levophed), ondansetron (Zofran), oxacillin, oxaliplatin (Eloxatin), oxytocin (Pitocin), paclitaxel (Taxol), palonosetron (Aloxi), perphenazine, piperacillin, piperacillin/tazobactam (Zosyn), procainamide, prochlorperazine, promethazine, propranolol, protamine, pyridoxine, ranitidine, sodium acetate, sodium bicarbonate, streptokinase, succinylcholine, sufentanil (Sufenta), tacrolimus (Prograf), teniposide (Vumon), theophylline, thiotepa (Thioplex), tigecycline (Tygacil), tirofibran (Aggrastat), tobramycin, vancomycin, vasopressin, vecuronium (Norcuron), verapamil, vincristine (Vincasar), vinorelbine (Navelbine), voriconazole (Vfend), zidovudine (Retrovir).

SIDE EFFECTS

Frequent

IV: Abdominal cramping or discomfort, phlebitis or thrombophlebitis.
Topical: Dry skin (50%).

Occasional

Nausea, vomiting, diarrhea, rash, urticaria.

Rare

Ophthalmic: Sensitivity reaction with increased irritation, burning, itching, and inflammation.
Topical: Urticaria.

SERIOUS REACTIONS

- Antibiotic-associated colitis and other superinfections may occur.
- High dosages in patients with renal or hepatic impairment may lead to reversible hearing loss.
- Anaphylaxis and hepatotoxicity occur rarely.
- Ventricular arrhythmias and prolonged QT interval occur rarely with the IV drug form.

PRECAUTIONS & CONSIDERATIONS

Caution is warranted with hepatic dysfunction. Caution should also be used with the combination drug Pediazole (erythromycin and sulfisoxazole) in patients with impaired renal or hepatic function, severe allergies, bronchial asthma, or glucose-6-phosphate dehydrogenase deficiency. Major inhibitor of CYP3A4, which may lead to serious drug interactions. Use with caution in patients with myasthenia gravis (aggravation of disease). Infantile hypertrophic pyloric stenosis has occurred in infants. Determine whether there is a history of hepatitis or allergies to erythromycin or other macrolides before beginning therapy. Erythromycin crosses the placenta and is distributed in breast milk.

Erythromycin estolate may increase liver function test results in pregnant women. Elderly patients may be at increased risk for hearing loss or torsades de pointes at doses > 4 g/day.

WBC should be monitored to determine whether the infection is improving. Diarrhea, GI discomfort, headache, nausea, pattern of daily bowel activity and stool consistency, as well as signs and symptoms of superinfection, including anal or genital pruritus, moderate to severe diarrhea, abdominal cramps, fever, and sore mouth or tongue, should be assessed. Signs of hearing loss should be monitored because high dosages can cause hearing loss with hepatic and renal dysfunction.

Storage

Store capsules and tablets at room temperature. The oral suspension is stable for 14 days at room temperature. Store the parenteral form at room temperature. The initial reconstituted solution in vial is stable for 8 h at room temperature and 2 wks if refrigerated. Diluted IV solutions are stable for 8 h at room temperature and 24 h if refrigerated. Discard the solution if a precipitate forms.

Administration

Administer erythromycin base or stearate 1 h before or 2 h after a meal. Erythromycin estolate and ethylsuccinate may be given without regard to food but are absorbed better when given on an empty stomach. Give tablets or capsules with 8 oz of water. If the patient has difficulty swallowing, sprinkle the capsule contents in a teaspoonful of applesauce and follow with water. Chew or crush chewable tablets.

For IV use, reconstitute each 500-mg vial with 10 mL or each 1-g vial with 20 mL sterile water for injection without a preservative to provide a concentration of 50 mg/mL. Further dilute with 100-250 mL D5W or 0.9% NaCl. Administer intermittent IV infusion (piggyback) over 20-60 min. Administer continuous infusion over 6-24 h. Assess for pain along vein frequently.

For topical use, gently cleanse and dry area before application. Apply thin film. Avoid eyes and mucous membranes.

For ophthalmic use, place a gloved finger on the lower eyelid and pull it out until a pocket is formed between the eye and the lower lid. Place ¼ to ½ inch of ointment into the pocket. Close the eye for 1-2 min and roll the eyeball gently to increase the drug's distribution. Remove excess ointment around the eye with tissue.

Escitalopram

es-sy-tal'oh-pram

Lexapro Cipralex

CATEGORY AND SCHEDULE

Pregnancy Risk Category: C

Classification: Antidepressants, selective serotonin reuptake inhibitors

MECHANISM OF ACTION

A selective serotonin reuptake inhibitor that blocks the uptake of the neurotransmitter serotonin at neuronal presynaptic membranes, increasing its availability at postsynaptic receptor sites. *Therapeutic Effect:* Relieves depression.

PHARMACOKINETICS

Well absorbed after PO administration. Primarily metabolized in the liver.

Primarily excreted in feces, with a lesser amount eliminated in urine. *Half-life:* 35 h, extended with hepatic impairment. Oral solution and tablet bioequivalent.

AVAILABILITY

Oral Solution: 1 mg/mL (240 mL).
Tablets: 5 mg, 10 mg, 20 mg.

INDICATIONS AND DOSAGES

▸ Depression, general anxiety disorder (GAD)

PO
Adults. Initially, 10 mg once a day in the morning or evening. May increase to 20 mg after a minimum of 1 wk.
Elderly. 10 mg/day for depression; up to 20 mg/day for anxiety.
Children 12 yr and older. Initially, 10 mg once a day (indicated for depression only). May increase to 20 mg after a minimum of 3 wks.

▸ Dose adjustment for hepatic impairment

Limit dose to 10 mg/day PO.

OFF-LABEL USES

Trichotillomania, panic disorder.

CONTRAINDICATIONS

Use within 14 days of MAOIs, hypersensitivity to eitalopram or escitalopram; use with pimozide.

INTERACTIONS

Drug
Alcohol, other CNS depressants: May increase CNS depression.
Anticoagulants, antiplatelets, NSAIDs: May increase risk of bleeding.
Antifungals, cimetidine, macrolide antibiotics, CYP3A4 inhibitors: May increase plasma level of escitalopram.
Carbamazepine, CYP2C19 inducers, CYP3A4 inducers: May decrease plasma level of escitalopram.
CYP2C19 inhibitors, delavirdine, fluconazole, gemfibrozil, omeprazole: May increase plasma level of escitalopram.
MAOIs, linezolid, meperidine, selegiline: May cause serotonin syndrome, marked by autonomic hyperactivity, coma, diaphoresis, excitement, hyperthermia, and rigidity, and neuroleptic malignant syndrome. Avoid combination with MAOIs and allow 14-day washout.
Metoprolol: Increases plasma level of metoprolol.
Pimozide: Increases QTc interval significantly; mechanism unknown. Contraindicated.
SSRIs, SNRIs, buspirone, sibutramine, tramadol, triptans: May increase risk for serotonin syndrome.
Herbal
St. John's wort: May increase risk for serotonin syndrome and/or decrease escitalopram plasma level.
Food
None known.

DIAGNOSTIC TEST EFFECTS

May reduce serum sodium level.

SIDE EFFECTS

Frequent (9%-21%)
Nausea, dry mouth, somnolence, insomnia, abnormal ejaculation.
Occasional (4%-8%)
Tremor, diarrhea, diaphoresis, dyspepsia, fatigue, anxiety, decreased libido.
Rare (2%-3%)
Sinusitis, vomiting, constipation, anorexia, sexual dysfunction, menstrual disorder, abdominal pain, agitation.

SERIOUS REACTIONS

- Overdose is manifested as dizziness, drowsiness, tachycardia, somnolence, confusion, and seizures.
- Serotonin syndrome, activation of hypomania/mania, abnormal bleeding, hyponatremia/SIADH.

E

PRECAUTIONS & CONSIDERATIONS

Antidepressants increased the risk of suicidal thinking and behavior (suicidality) in short-term studies in children and adolescents with depression and other psychiatric disorders. Caution is warranted with hepatic or severe renal impairment; those with a history of hypomania, mania, or seizures; and patients concurrently using CNS depressants. Neonates exposed to escitalopram late in the third trimester have developed complications requiring prolonged hospitalization, respiratory support, and tube feeding. Consider tapering escitalopram in the third trimester of pregnancy. Escitalopram is distributed in breast milk. Escitalopram use may increase anticholinergic effects and hyperexcitability in children. Elderly patients are more sensitive to the drug's anticholinergic effects, such as dry mouth, and are more likely to experience confusion, dizziness, hyperexcitability, and sedation.

Alcohol and tasks that require mental alertness or motor skills should be avoided until the effects of the drug are known. CBC and liver and renal function tests should be performed before and periodically during therapy, especially with long-term use. Gradual discontinuation is advised to avoid withdrawal symptoms.

Storage

Store at room temperature.

Administration

! Make sure at least 14 days elapse between the use of MAOIs and escitalopram.

Take escitalopram without regard to food. Do not crush film-coated tablets. Do not abruptly discontinue escitalopram or increase the dosage.

Esmolol

ess'moe-lol

★ 🍁 Brevibloc

CATEGORY AND SCHEDULE

Pregnancy Risk Category: C

Classification: Antiadrenergics, β-blocking; antiarrhythmics, class II

MECHANISM OF ACTION

An antiarrhythmic that selectively blocks β1-adrenergic receptors. *Therapeutic Effect:* Slows sinus heart rate, decreases cardiac output, reducing BP.

AVAILABILITY

Injection: 10 mg/mL (250 mL, 10 mL), 20 mg/mL (5 mL, 100 mL). *Premixed IV Infusion:* 2500 mg/250 mL; 2000 mg/100 mL

INDICATIONS AND DOSAGES

▸ **Supraventricular tachyarrhythmias, including sinus tachycardia or PSVT, or to control ventricular rate in patients with AFib or AFlutter**

IV

Adults, Elderly. Initially, a loading dose of 500 mcg/kg over 1 min, followed by 50 mcg/kg/min for 4 min. If optimum response is not attained in 5 min, give a second loading dose of 500 mcg/kg/min for 1 min, followed by infusion of 100 mcg/kg/min for 4 min. An additional loading dose can be given and infusion increased by 50 mcg/kg/min, up to 200 mcg/kg/min, for 4 min. Once the desired response is attained, cease loading dose and decrease infusion by no more than 25 mcg/kg/min at 10-min intervals. Infusion is usually administered over 24-48 h in most patients. Range: 50-200 mcg/kg/min, with average dose of 100 mcg/kg/min.

▸ **Intraoperative tachycardia or hypertension (immediate control)**

IV

Adults, Elderly. Initially, 80 mg over 30 seconds, then 150 mcg/kg/min infusion up to 300 mcg/kg/min. Titrate to desired heart rate and/or BP.

OFF-LABEL USES

Postoperative hypertension and SVT in children.

CONTRAINDICATIONS

Cardiogenic shock, overt cardiac failure, second- and third-degree heart block, sinus bradycardia, pregnancy (2nd and 3rd trimesters).

INTERACTIONS

Drug

Calcium channel blockers: Effects of verapamil, nifedipine may be potentiated. Diltiazem, felodipine, nicardipine may increase esmolol effects.

Digoxin: Increase in digoxin levels.

Insulin, oral hypoglycemics: May mask symptoms of hypoglycemia and prolong hypoglycemic effect of these drugs.

MAOIs: May cause significant hypertension or bradycardia.

Morphine: Increase in esmolol levels.

Succinylcholine: Prolonged duration of neuromuscular blockade.

Sympathomimetics, xanthines: May mutually inhibit effects.

Herbal

None known.

Food

None known.

DIAGNOSTIC TEST EFFECTS

None known.

IV INCOMPATIBILITIES

Acyclovir (Zovirax), amphotericin B cholesteryl sulfate complex (Amphotec), azathioprine, cefotetan (Cefotan), dantrolene, dexamethasone sodium phosphate, diazepam (Valium), furosemide (Lasix), ganciclovir (Cytovene), indomethacin, ketorolac, lansoprazole (Prevacid), minocycline (Minocin), oxacillin, pantoprazole (Protonix), pentobarbital, phenobarbital.

IV COMPATIBILITIES

Alfentanil (Alfenta), amikacin (Amikar), aminophylline, amiodarone (Cordarone), amphotericin B liposomal (AmBisome), ascorbic acid, atracurium (Tracrium), atropine, aztreonam (Azactam), benztropine (Cogentin), bivalirudin (Angiomax), bretylium, bumetanide (Bumex), buprenorphine (Buprenex), butorphanol (Stadol), calcium chloride, calcium gluconate, carboplatin, caspofungin (Cancidas), cefazolin, cefotaxime (Claforan), cefoxitin (Mefoxin), ceftazidime (Ceptaz, Fortaz, Tazicef, Tazidime), ceftizoxime (Cefizox), ceftriaxone (Rocephin), cefuroxime (Zinacef), chlorpromazine, cimetidine (Tagamet), cisatracurium (Nimbex), cisplatin, clindamycin (Cleocin), cyanocobalamin, cyclophosphamide

(Cytoxan), cyclosporine (Sandimmune), dactinomycin (Cosmegen), daptomycin (Cubicin), dexmedetomidine (Precedex), digoxin (Lanoxin), diltiazem (Cardizem), diphenhydramine (Benadryl), dobutamine (Dobutrex), docetaxel (Taxotere), dopamine (Intropin), doxorubicin (Adriamycin), enalaprilat, ephedrine, epinephrine, epoetin alfa (Procrit), ertapenem (Invanz), erythromycin lactobionate, etoposide phosphate (Etopophos), famotidine (Pepcid), fenoldopam (Corlopam), fentanyl (Sublimaze), fluconazole (Diflucan), fludarabine (Fludara), fluorouracil, folic acid, gemcitabine (Gemzar), gentamicin, granisetron (Kytril), heparin, hydromorphone (Dilaudid), hydroxyzine, imipenem/cilastatin (Primaxin), insulin (regular, Humulin R, Novolin R), isoproterenol (Isuprel), labetalol, levofloxacin (Levaquin), lidocaine, linezolid (Zyvox), lorazepam (Ativan), magnesium sulfate, mannitol, meperidine (Demerol), methicillin, methotrexate, metoclopramide (Reglan), metoprolol (Lopressor), metronidazole (Flagyl), micafungin (Mycamine), midazolam (Versed), mitoxantrone (Novantrone), morphine, multiple vitamins injection, nalbuphine (Nubain), naloxone (Narcan), nicardipine (Cardene), nitroglycerin, nitroprusside sodium (Nitropress), norepinephrine (Levophed), ondansetron (Zofran), oxaliplatin (Eloxatin), oxytocin (Pitocin), paclitaxel (Taxol), palonosetron (Aloxi), pancuronium, pemetrexed (Alimta), penicillin G potassium, penicillin G sodium, phytonadione, potassium chloride, prochloperazine, promethazine, propofol (Diprivan), propranolol, quinupristin/dalfopristin (Synercid), ranitidin (Zantac), remifentanil (Ultiva), sodium bicarbonate, streptokinase, succinylcholine, sufentanil (Sufenta), tacrolimus (Prograf), teniposide (Vumon), theophylline, thiotepa (Thioplex), ticarcillin (Ticar), ticarcillin/clavulanate (Timentin), tigecycline (Tygacil), tirofibran (Aggrastat), tobramycin, vancomycin, vasopressin, vecuronium (Norcuron), verapamil, vincristine (Vincasar), voriconazole (Vfend), warfarin.

SIDE EFFECTS

Esmolol is generally well tolerated, with transient and mild side effects.

Frequent (> 10%)

Hypotension (systolic BP < 90 mm Hg) asymptomatic or symptomatic manifested as dizziness, nausea, diaphoresis, headache, cold extremities, fatigue.

Occasional

Nausea, dizziness, anxiety, drowsiness, flushed skin, vomiting, confusion, pain or inflammation at injection site, fever.

SERIOUS REACTIONS

- Overdose may produce profound hypotension, bradycardia, dizziness, syncope, drowsiness, breathing difficulty, bluish fingernails or palms of hands, and seizures.
- Esmolol administration may potentiate insulin-induced hypoglycemia in diabetic patients.

PRECAUTIONS & CONSIDERATIONS

Caution is warranted in patients with bronchial asthma, conduction disorder (e.g., sinus sick syndrome), bronchitis, congestive heart failure, diabetes, emphysema, history of allergy, myasthenia gravis, depression, peripheral vascular disease, and impaired renal function. Extravasation may cause tissue necrosis. Safety and efficacy have not been evaluated in children.

Notify the physician of cold extremities, dizziness, faintness, or nausea. BP for hypotension, respiratory status for shortness of breath, pattern of daily bowel activity and stool consistency, ECG for arrhythmias, and pulse for quality, rate, and rhythm should be monitored during treatment. If pulse rate is 55 beats/min or lower or systolic BP is < 90 mm Hg, withhold the medication and contact the physician. Signs and symptoms of congestive heart failure, such as decreased urine output, distended neck veins, dyspnea (particularly on exertion or lying down), night cough, peripheral edema, and weight gain, should also be assessed.

Storage

After dilution, solution is stable for 24 h. Store unopened vials at room temperature.

Premixed infusions are stored at room temperature in overwrap until time of use.

Administration

! Give esmolol by IV infusion. Avoid using butterfly needles and very small veins.

For IV administration, use only clear and colorless to light yellow solution. Discard solution if it is discolored or if precipitate forms. For IV infusion, make sure the prescribed amount of esmolol is diluted to provide a concentration of 10 mg/mL or 20 mg/mL. Premixed bags are available. Administer by controlled infusion device, and titrate according to the patient's tolerance and response. Infuse IV loading dose over 1-2 min. Monitor the patient for hypotension (a systolic BP of < 90 mm Hg), especially during the first 30 min of infusion.

Esomeprazole

es-om-eh-pray'zole

Nexium

CATEGORY AND SCHEDULE

Pregnancy Risk Category: B

Classification: Gastrointestinals, proton pump inhibitors

MECHANISM OF ACTION

A proton pump inhibitor that is converted to active metabolites that irreversibly bind to and inhibit hydrogen-potassium adenosine triphosphates, an enzyme on the surface of gastric parietal cells. Inhibits hydrogen ion transport into gastric lumen. *Therapeutic Effect:* Increases gastric pH, reducing gastric acid production.

PHARMACOKINETICS

Well absorbed after oral administration. Protein binding: 97%. Extensively metabolized by the liver by CYP219 and CYP3A4. Primarily excreted in urine. *Half-life:* 1-1.5 h.

AVAILABILITY

Capsules (Delayed Release): 20 mg, 40 mg.

Suspension (Delayed Release): 10 mg/packet, 20 mg/packet, 40 mg/packet.

Injection, Powder for Reconstitution: 20 mg, 40 mg.

INDICATIONS AND DOSAGES

▸ **Erosive esophagitis healing**

PO

Adults, Elderly, Adolescents. 20-40 mg once daily for 4-8 wks.

Children 1-11 yr of age weighing < 20 kg. 10 mg once daily for up to 8 wks.

Children 1-11 yr of age weighing > 20 kg. 10-20 mg once daily for up to 8 wks.

▸ **To maintain healing of erosive esophagitis**

PO

Adults, Elderly. 20 mg/day.

▸ **Gastroesophageal reflux disease**

PO

Adults, Elderly. 20 mg once a day for 4-8 wks.

Adolescents aged 12-17 yr. 20-40 mg once daily for up to 8 wks.

Children aged 1-11 yr. 10 mg once daily for up to 8 wks.

IV

Adults, Elderly. 20-40 mg once daily.

▸ **Duodenal ulcer caused by Helicobacter pylori**

PO

Adults, Elderly. 40 mg (esomeprazole) once a day, with amoxicillin 1000 mg and clarithromycin 500 mg twice a day for 10-14 days.

▸ **Prevention of NSAID-induced gastric ulcer**

PO

Adults, Elderly. 20-40 mg once daily for up to 6 mo.

▸ **Hypersecretory conditions (e.g., Zollinger-Ellison syndrome)**

PO

Adults, Elderly. 40 mg twice daily.

▸ **Dose in hepatic impairment (Child-Pugh Class C)**

PO

Adults, Elderly. Dose should not exceed 20 mg/day.

CONTRAINDICATIONS

Hypersensitivity to other PPIs or esomeprazole.

INTERACTIONS

Drug

Digoxin, iron, ketoconazole, atazanavir, indinavir: May decrease the concentration of digoxin, iron, atazanavir, indinavir, and ketoconazole.

Benzodiazepines (diazepam, midazolam, triazolam): May increase levels of benzodiazepines metabolized by oxidation.

CYP2C19 inducers: May decrease esomeprazole level.

CYP2C19 inhibitors: May increase esomeprazole level.

Methotrexate: May decrease excretion of methotrexate, monitor for side effects.

Herbal

None known.

Food

None known.

DIAGNOSTIC TEST EFFECTS

None known.

IV INCOMPATIBILITIES

Do not administer concomitantly with any other medications through the same IV site and/or tubing. Specific incompatibilities include tacrolimus (Prograf).

IV COMPATIBILITIES

Doripenem (Doribax).

SIDE EFFECTS

Frequent (> 10%)

Headache.

Occasional (2%-9%)

Diarrhea, abdominal pain, flatulence, nausea, hypertension, pain, anxiety, insomnia, local injection site reaction (IV).

Rare (< 2%)

Dizziness, dyspepsia, asthenia or loss of strength, vomiting, constipation, rash, cough, anemia.

SERIOUS REACTIONS

• Pancreatitis, Stevens-Johnson syndrome, toxic epidermal necrolysis, erythema multiforme occur rarely.

PRECAUTIONS & CONSIDERATIONS

It is unknown whether esomeprazole crosses the placenta or is distributed in breast milk. However, omeprazole is distributed in breast milk. Safety and efficacy of esomeprazole have not been established in children < 1 yr. No age-related precautions have been noted in elderly patients. Notify the physician if headache, diarrhea, discomfort, or nausea occurs during esomeprazole therapy.

Storage

Store oral product and unopened IV vials at room temperatue, protected from light. Once IV reconstituted with LR or NaCl, use within 12 h. If infusion in D5W, use within 6 h.

Administration

Take 1 h or more before eating. Do not crush or open capsule; swallow the capsule whole. May open the capsule and mix pellets with 1 tbsp of applesauce; swallow the spoonful without chewing. Mix contents of oral suspension packet with 1 tbsp (15 mL) of water, then leave 2-3 min to thicken. Stir and drink within 30 min. If any material remains after drinking, add more water, stir, and drink immediately.

IV may be given as either IV injection or as IV infusion. NOTE: The IV line should always be flushed with either 0.9% NaCl, lactated Ringer's, or D5W both prior to and after giving the drug. To prepare injection, dilute either 20 mg or 40 mg with 5 mL of 0.9% NaCl and give IV over no less than 3 min. For IV infusion, further dilute vial to a final volume of 50 mL with 0.9% NaCl, lactated Ringer's, or D5W. Infuse over a period of 10-30 min.

Estazolam

es-tay'zoe-lam

CATEGORY AND SCHEDULE

Pregnancy Risk Category: X
Controlled Substance Schedule: IV

Classification: Sedatives/hypnotics, benzodiazepines

MECHANISM OF ACTION

A benzodiazepine that enhances action of gamma aminobutyric acid (GABA) neurotransmission in the central nervous system (CNS). *Therapeutic Effect:* Produces depressant effect at all levels of CNS.

PHARMACOKINETICS

Rapidly absorbed from the GI tract. Onset of action 1 h. Protein binding: 93%. Metabolized in liver extensively. Primarily excreted in urine, minimal in feces. *Half-life:* 10-24 h.

AVAILABILITY

Tablets: 1 mg, 2 mg.

INDICATIONS AND DOSAGES

▸ **Insomnia**

PO

Adults (older than 18 yr). 1-2 mg at bedtime.

Elderly, debilitated, liver disease, low serum albumin. 0.5-1 mg at bedtime.

CONTRAINDICATIONS

Pregnancy, hypersensitivity to other benzodiazepines.

INTERACTIONS

Drug

Alcohol, CNS depressants: May increase CNS and respiratory depression and have hypotensive effects.

Herbal

Kava kava, valerian: May increase CNS depressant effect.

Food

None known.

SIDE EFFECTS

Frequent

Drowsiness, sedation, hypokinesia, rebound insomnia (may occur for 1-2 nights after drug is discontinued), dizziness, confusion, euphoria, abnormal coordination.

Occasional

Weakness, anorexia, diarrhea.

Rare

Paradoxical CNS excitement, restlessness (particularly noted in elderly or debilitated patients).

SERIOUS REACTIONS

- Overdosage results in somnolence, confusion, diminished reflexes, and coma.
- Hypersensitivity reactions, including anaphylaxis and angioedema, have been reported.

PRECAUTIONS & CONSIDERATIONS

Caution should be used with impaired renal or liver function, respiratory disease, decreased gag reflex, or depression. Be aware that estazolam is contraindicated in pregnancy. Estazolam crosses the placenta and is distributed in breast milk. Safety and efficacy of estazolam have not been established in children. Use small initial doses and gradually increase them to avoid excessive sedation or ataxia as evidenced by muscular incoordination in elderly patients. Patients taking benzodiazepines are at risk for falls. Rebound insomnia may occur when drug is discontinued after short-term therapy. Avoid alcohol.

Storage

Store at room temperature.

Administration

Take at bedtime. May be taken without regard to meals.

Estradiol

ess-tra-dye′ole

★ 🍁 Alora, Climara, Delestrogen, Depo-Estradiol, Divigel, Elestrin, Estrace, Estraderm, Estrasorb, EstroGel, Estring, Evamist, Femring, Femtrace, Gynodiol, Menostar, Vagifem, Vivelle-Dot.

Do not confuse Estraderm with Testoderm.

CATEGORY AND SCHEDULE

Pregnancy Risk Category: X

Classification: Estrogens, hormones/hormone modifiers

MECHANISM OF ACTION

An estrogen that increases the synthesis of DNA, RNA, and proteins in target tissues; reduces release of gonadotropin-releasing hormone from the hypothalamus; and reduces follicle-stimulating hormone and luteinizing hormone (LH) release from the pituitary. *Therapeutic Effect:* Promotes normal growth, promotes development of female sex organs, and maintains genitourinary function and vasomotor stability. Prevents accelerated bone loss by inhibiting bone resorption, restoring balance of bone resorption and formation. Inhibits LH and decreases serum testosterone concentration.

PHARMACOKINETICS

Well absorbed from the GI tract. Widely distributed. Protein binding: 50%-80%. Metabolized in the liver. Primarily excreted in urine. *Half-life:* 1-2 h.

AVAILABILITY

Tablets (micronized, Estrace, Femtrace, Gynodiol): 0.5 mg, 1 mg, 1.5 mg, 2 mg.
Tablets (acetate, Femtrace): 0.45 mg, 0.9 mg, 1.8 mg.
Emulsion (Topical [Estrasorb]): 2.5 mg/g (0.25%).
Injection (Cypionate [Depo-Estradiol]): 5 mg/mL.
Injection (Valerate [Delestrogen]): 10 mg/mL, 20 mg/mL, 40 mg/mL.
Topical Gel (Divigel, Elestrin, EstroGel): 0.06%, 0.1%.
Topical Spray (Evamist): 1.53 mg/actuation.
Transdermal System (Alora): twice weekly: 0.025 mg, 0.05 mg, 0.075 mg, 0.1 mg.
Transdermal System (Climara): once weekly: 0.025 mg, 0.0375 mg, 0.05 mg, 0.06 mg, 0.075 mg, 0.1 mg.
Transdermal System (Estraderm): twice weekly: 0.05 mg, 0.1 mg.
Transdermal System (Menostar): once a week: 1 mg estradiol (14 mcg/24 h).
Transdermal System (Vivelle-Dot): twice weekly: 0.025 mg, 0.0375 mg, 0.05 mg, 0.075 mg, 0.1 mg.
Vaginal Cream (Estrace): 0.1 mg/g (0.01%).
Vaginal Ring (Estring): 2 mg.
Vaginal Ring (Femring): 0.05 mg, 0.1 mg.
Vaginal Tablet (Vagifem): 25 mcg.

INDICATIONS AND DOSAGES

▸ **Prostate cancer (palliative)**
IM (VALERATE)
Adults, Elderly. 30 mg or more q1-2 wk.
PO
Adults, Elderly. 10 mg 3 times a day for at least 3 mo.

▸ **Breast cancer (palliative)**
PO
Adults, Elderly. 10 mg 3 times a day for at least 3 mo.

▸ **Osteoporosis prophylaxis in postmenopausal females**
PO
If intact uterus, give 14 days progestin every 6-12 mo.
Adults, Elderly. 0.5 mg/day cyclically (3 wks on, 1 wk off).
TRANSDERMAL (CLIMARA)
Adults, Elderly. Initially, 0.025 mg weekly, adjust dose as needed.
TRANSDERMAL (ALORA, VIVELLE-DOT)
Adults, Elderly. Initially, 0.025 mg patch twice weekly, adjust dose as needed.
TRANSDERMAL (ESTRADERM)
Adults, Elderly. 0.05 mg twice weekly.
TRANSDERMAL (MENOSTAR)
Adults, Elderly. 1 mg weekly.

▸ **Female hypoestrogenism**
PO
Adults, Elderly. 1-2 mg/day, adjust dose as needed.
IM (ESTRADIOL CYPIONATE)
Adults, Elderly. 1.5-2 mg monthly.
IM (ESTRADIOL VALERATE)
Adults, Elderly. 10-20 mg q4wk.
TRANSDERMAL (CLIMARA)
Adults, Elderly. 0.025 mg once weekly.

▸ **Vasomotor symptoms associated with menopause**
PO
Adults, Elderly. 1-2 mg/day cyclically (3 wks on, 1 wk off), adjust dose as needed.
IM (ESTRADIOL CYPIONATE)
Adults, Elderly. 1-5 mg q3-4wk.
IM (ESTRADIOL VALERATE)
Adults, Elderly. 10-20 mg q4wk.
TOPICAL EMULSION (ESTRASORB)

Adults, Elderly. 3.84 g once a day in the morning.
TOPICAL GEL (ESTROGEL)
Adults, Elderly. 1.25 g/day.
TOPICAL GEL (DIVIGEL)
Adults, Elderly. 0.25 g/day. Range 0.25-1 g/day.
TOPICAL GEL (ELESTRIN)
Adults, Elderly. 0.87 g/day.
TOPICAL SPRAY (EVAMIST)
Adults, Elderly. One spray/day. Range 1-3 sprays/day based on response.
TRANSDERMAL (CLIMARA)
Adults, Elderly. 0.025 mg weekly. Adjust dose as needed.
TRANSDERMAL (ALORA, ESTRADERM, VIVELLE-DOT)
Adults, Elderly. 0.05 mg twice a week.
VAGINAL RING (FEMRING)
Adults, Elderly. 0.05 mg once q90 days. May increase to 0.1 mg if needed.

▸ **Vaginal atrophy**
VAGINAL RING (ESTRING)
Adults, Elderly. 2 mg once q90 days.
VAGINAL CREAM (ESTRACE)
Adults, Elderly. 2-4 g/day for 2 wks, then reduce to ½ initial dose for 2 wks, then 1 g 1-3 times a week.
TOPICAL GEL (ESTROGEL)
Adults, Elderly. 1.25 g/day.
TOPICAL GEL (ELESTRIN)
Adults, Elderly. 0.87 g/day.
TRANSDERMAL (CLIMARA)
Adults, Elderly. 0.025 mg once a week.

▸ **Atrophic vaginitis**
VAGINAL TABLET (VAGIFEM)
Adults, Elderly. Initially, 1 tablet/day for 2 wks. Maintenance: 1 tablet twice a week.

OFF-LABEL USES

Treatment of Turner syndrome.

CONTRAINDICATIONS

Abnormal vaginal bleeding, active arterial thrombosis, blood dyscrasias, estrogen-dependent cancer, known or suspected breast cancer, pregnancy, thrombophlebitis or thromboembolic disorders, thyroid dysfunction, severe hepatic dysfunction.

INTERACTIONS

Drug

Aromatase inhibitors: May interfere with effects of aromatase inhibitors.
Bromocriptine: May interfere with the effects of bromocriptine.
Corticosteroids: May increase effects of hydrocortisone and prednisone.
Cyclosporine: May increase blood cyclosporine concentration and the risk of hepatotoxicity and nephrotoxicity.
CYP3A4 inducers/inhibitors: May alter levels of estradiol.
Hepatotoxic medications, cyclosporine: May increase the risk of hepatotoxicity. May increase the level of cyclosporine.
Thyroid medications: May decrease effects of thyroid medications.

Herbal

Saw palmetto: Increases the effects of saw palmetto.
St. John's wort: May decrease effects of estradiol.

Food

None known.

DIAGNOSTIC TEST EFFECTS

May increase blood glucose, HDL, serum calcium, and triglyceride levels. May decrease serum cholesterol levels and LDH concentrations. May affect metapyrone testing and thyroid function tests.

SIDE EFFECTS

Frequent

Anorexia, nausea, swelling of breasts, peripheral edema marked by swollen ankles and feet.

Transdermal: Skin irritation, redness.
Occasional
Vomiting, especially with high doses; headache that may be severe; intolerance to contact lenses; hypertension; glucose intolerance; brown spots on exposed skin.
Vaginal: Local irritation, vaginal discharge, changes in vaginal bleeding, including spotting, and breakthrough or prolonged bleeding.
Rare
Chorea or involuntary movements, hirsutism or abnormal hairiness, loss of scalp hair, depression.

SERIOUS REACTIONS

- Prolonged administration increases the risk of gallbladder disease, thromboembolic disease, and breast, cervical, vaginal, endometrial, and hepatic carcinoma.
- Myocardial infarction, stroke, venous thromboembolism.
- Cholestatic jaundice occurs rarely.
- Retinal vascular thrombosis.

PRECAUTIONS & CONSIDERATIONS

Estrogen therapy should not be used to prevent cardiovascular disease, and other options for osteoporosis should be considered if being used solely for prevention of osteoporosis because it increases the risk of cardiovascular events. Use with caution in patients with cardiovascular disease. Use with caution in patients with history of cholestatic jaundice with past estrogen use or pregnancy. Estrogen therapy should be used for the shortest duration and lowest dose possible. Caution is warranted in patients with diseases exacerbated by fluid retention and with hepatic or renal insufficiency and with gallbladder disease, hypocalcemia, porphyria, or lupus. Should be discontinued at least 4 wks before and for 2 wks following surgical procedures or prolonged immobilizations (risk of thromboembolism). Estradiol is distributed in breast milk and may be harmful to the infant. Estradiol should not be used during breastfeeding. Estradiol should be used cautiously in children whose bone growth is not complete because the drug may accelerate epiphyseal closure. The risk of dementia is increased in postmenopausal women aged > 65 yr.

Avoid smoking because of the increased risk of blood clot formation and myocardial infarction. Limit alcohol and caffeine intake.

Notify the physician of calf or chest pain, depression, numbness or weakness of an extremity, severe abdominal pain, shortness of breath, speech or vision disturbance, sudden headache, unusual bleeding, or vomiting. BP, weight, blood glucose, hepatic enzyme, and serum calcium levels should be monitored.
Storage
Store all products at room temperature; do not freeze. Alcohol-based topical products are flammable; avoid heat and flame exposure. Keep transdermal systems and vaginal ring in sealed pouch until time of use.
Administration
Take oral estradiol at the same time each day.

For IM use, rotate the vial to disperse drug in oil. Give deep IM injection into the gluteus maximus. NOT for intravenous use.

For vaginal use, apply estradiol cream at bedtime for best absorption. To administer, insert the end of the filled applicator into the vagina, directing the applicator slightly toward the sacrum; push the plunger down completely. To prevent topical absorption of the drug, do not allow the cream to contact the skin.

Apply topical gels, lotions, and spray at the same time each day topically as directed for each specific product.

E

Apply vaginal rings high in vagina as directed; they are left in place for 90 days, then removed and replaced.

! Transdermal Climara is administered once weekly; many transdermal forms of estradiol are applied twice weekly. Follow the directions for each specific brand.

To apply the transdermal system, remove the old patch and select a new site. Consider using the buttocks as an alternative application site. Peel off the protective strip on the patch to expose the adhesive surface. Apply to clean, dry, intact skin on the trunk of the body in an area with as little hair as possible. Press in place for at least 10 seconds. Do not apply the patch to breasts or waistline.

Estrogens, Conjugated

ess'troe-jenz

★ Cenestin, Enjuvia, Premarin

🍁 C.E.S., Congest, Premarin

Do not confuse with Primaxin or Remeron.

CATEGORY AND SCHEDULE

Pregnancy Risk Category: X

Classification: Estrogens, hormones/hormone modifiers

MECHANISM OF ACTION

An estrogen that increases the synthesis of DNA, RNA, and various proteins in target tissues; reduces release of gonadotropin-releasing hormone from the hypothalamus; and reduces follicle-stimulating hormone (FSH) and luteinizing hormone (LH) release from the pituitary gland. *Therapeutic Effect:* Promotes normal growth, promotes development of female sex organs, and maintains genitourinary function and vasomotor stability. Prevents accelerated bone loss by inhibiting bone resorption, restoring balance of bone resorption and formation. Inhibits LH and decreases serum concentration of testosterone.

PHARMACOKINETICS

Well absorbed from the GI tract. Widely distributed. Protein binding: 50%-80%. Metabolized in the liver. Primarily excreted in urine. *Half-life (metabolite):* 27 h.

AVAILABILITY

Tablets (Cenestin, Premarin): 0.3 mg, 0.45 mg, 0.625 mg, 0.9 mg, 1.25 mg.
Tablets (Enjuvia): 0.3 mg, 0.45 mg, 0.625 mg, 0.9 mg, 1.25 mg.
Injection: 25 mg.
Vaginal Cream: 0.625 mg/g.

INDICATIONS AND DOSAGES

▸ **Vasomotor symptoms associated with menopause, atrophic vaginitis, kraurosis vulvae**

PO

Adults, Elderly. 0.3-0.625 mg/day cyclically (21 days on, 7 days off) or continuously.

INTRAVAGINAL

Adults, Elderly. 0.5-2 g/day cyclically, such as 21 days on and 7 days off.

▸ **Female hypogonadism**

PO

Adults. 0.3-0.625 mg/day in divided doses for 20 days; then a rest period of 10 days.

▸ **Female castration, primary ovarian failure**
PO
Adults. Initially, 1.25 mg/day cyclically. Adjust dosage, upward or downward, according to severity of symptoms and patient response. For maintenance, adjust dosage to lowest level that will provide effective control.
▸ **Osteoporosis**
PO
Adults, Elderly. 0.3-0.625 mg/day, cyclically, such as 25 days on and 5 days off.
▸ **Breast cancer palliation**
PO
Adults, Elderly. 10 mg 3 times a day for at least 3 mo.
▸ **Prostate cancer (palliative)**
PO
Adults, Elderly. 1.25-2.5 mg 3 times a day.
▸ **Abnormal uterine bleeding**
PO
Adults. 1.25 mg q4h for 24 h, then 1.25 mg/day for 7-10 days.
IV, IM
Adults. 25 mg; may repeat once in 6-12 h.

OFF-LABEL USES

Prevention of estrogen deficiency–induced premenopausal osteoporosis.
Cream: Prevention of nosebleeds.

CONTRAINDICATIONS

Breast cancer (with some exceptions), severe hepatic disease, thrombophlebitis or thromboembolic disorders, undiagnosed vaginal bleeding, active arterial thrombosis, blood dyscrasias, estrogen-dependent cancer, pregnancy, thyroid dysfunction.

INTERACTIONS

Drug
Aromatase inhibitors: May interfere with effects of aromatase inhibitors.
Bromocriptine: May interfere with the effects of bromocriptine.
Corticosteroids: May increase effects of hydrocortisone and prednisone.
Cyclosporine: May increase blood cyclosporine concentration and the risk of hepatotoxicity and nephrotoxicity.
CYP3A4 inducers/inhibitors: May alter levels of estrogens.
Hepatotoxic medications: May increase the risk of hepatotoxicity.
Thyroid medications: May decrease effects of thyroid medications.
Herbal
St. John's wort: May decrease the effects of estrogens.
Food
None known.

DIAGNOSTIC TEST EFFECTS

May increase blood glucose, HDL, serum calcium, and triglyceride levels. May decrease serum cholesterol levels and LDH concentrations. May affect serum metapyrone testing and thyroid function tests.

IV INCOMPATIBILITIES

Pantoprazole.

IV COMPATIBILITIES

Heparin, hydrocortisone sodium succinate, potassium chloride, vitamin B complex with C.

SIDE EFFECTS

Frequent
Vaginal bleeding, such as spotting or breakthrough bleeding; breast pain or tenderness; gynecomastia.
Occasional
Headache, hypertension, intolerance to contact lenses.
High doses: Anorexia, nausea.
Rare
Loss of scalp hair, depression.

SERIOUS REACTIONS

- Prolonged administration may increase the risk of gallbladder disease, thromboembolic disease, and breast, cervical, vaginal, endometrial, and hepatic carcinoma.
- Myocardial infarction, stroke, venous thromboembolism.
- Cholestatic jaundice occurs rarely.
- Retinal vascular thrombosis.

PRECAUTIONS & CONSIDERATIONS

Estrogen therapy should not be used to prevent cardiovascular disease; because of the increased risk of cardiovascular disease, other options for osteoporosis should be considered if it is being used solely for prevention of osteoporosis. Use with caution in patients with cardiovascular disease. Use with caution in patients with a history of cholestatic jaundice with past estrogen use or pregnancy. Estrogen therapy should be used for the shortest duration and lowest dose possible. Caution is warranted in patients with diseases exacerbated by fluid retention, such as asthma, cardiac dysfunction, diabetes mellitus, epilepsy, migraine headaches, heart failure, and renal impairment. Caution is warranted in patients with hepatic and with gallbladder disease, hypocalcemia, porphyria, lupus. Should be discontinued at least 4 wks before and for 2 wks following surgical procedures or prolonged immobilizations (risk of thromboembolism). Conjugated estrogens are distributed in breast milk and may be harmful to the infant. The drug should be discontinued in a pregnant woman. Estrogens should not be used during breastfeeding. Safety and efficacy of conjugated estrogens have not been established in children. Estrogens should be used cautiously in children whose bone growth is not complete because the drug may accelerate epiphyseal closure. The risk of dementia is increased in postmenopausal women aged > 65 yr. Avoid smoking because of the increased risk of blood clot formation and MI. Limit alcohol and caffeine intake.

Notify the physician of weight gain of more than 5 lb in a week, abnormal vaginal bleeding, depression, or signs and symptoms of blood clots. Also, signs and symptoms of thromboembolic or thrombotic disorders, including loss of coordination, numbness or weakness of an extremity, shortness of breath, speech or vision disturbance, sudden severe headache, and pain in the chest, leg, or groin, should be reported immediately. Breast self-examinations should be made monthly. Weight and BP should be monitored.

Storage

Store tablets and vaginal cream at room temperature. Refrigerate injection. The reconstituted solution is stable for 60 days refrigerated. Do not use if solution darkens or precipitate forms.

Administration

Take at the same time each day with food or milk if nausea occurs.

Administer vaginal cream at bedtime to reduce side effects. Use applicator provided and fill to mark corresponding with dose. After use, wash applicator with warm (not hot), soapy water

For IV and IM use, reconstitute with 5 mL sterile water for injection containing benzyl alcohol (provided). Slowly add diluent, shaking gently. Avoid vigorous shaking. For the IV form, give slowly to prevent flushing. (no more than 5 mg/min).

Estrogens, Esterified

ess'troe-jenz

Menest Estragyn

CATEGORY AND SCHEDULE

Pregnancy Risk Category: X

Classification: Estrogens, hormones/hormone modifiers

MECHANISM OF ACTION

A combination of sodium salts of sulfate esters of estrogenic substances (principal component is estrone) that increases synthesis of DNA, RNA, and various proteins in responsive tissues. Reduces release of gonadotropin-releasing hormone, reducing follicle-stimulating hormone (FSH) and luteinizing hormone (LH). *Therapeutic Effect:* Promotes vasomotor stability, maintains genitourinary function, normal growth, development of female sex organs. Prevents accelerated bone loss by inhibiting bone resorption, restoring balance of bone resorption and formation.

PHARMACOKINETICS

Readily absorbed from the GI tract. Widely distributed. Protein binding: 50%-80%. Rapidly metabolized in liver and GI tract to estrone sulfate and conjugated and unconjugated metabolites. Excreted in urine and bile. *Half-life:* Unknown.

AVAILABILITY

Tablets: 0.3 mg, 0.625 mg, 1.25 mg.

INDICATIONS AND DOSAGES

▸ **Vasomotor symptoms associated with menopause, atrophic vaginitis, kraurosis vulvae**

PO

Adults, Elderly. 0.3-1.25 mg/day cyclically.

▸ **Female hypogonadism**

PO

Adults. 2.5-7.5 mg/day in divided doses for 20 days; rest 10 days.

▸ **Female castration, primary ovarian failure**

PO

Adults. Initially, 1.25 mg/day cyclically.

▸ **Breast cancer palliation**

PO

Adults, Elderly. 10 mg 3 times/day for at least 3 mo.

▸ **Prostate cancer**

PO

Adults, Elderly. 1.25-2.5 mg 3 times/day.

▸ **Osteoporosis in postmenopausal women**

PO

Adults, Elderly. 0.3-1.25 mg/day cyclically.

CONTRAINDICATIONS

Breast cancer (with some exceptions), liver disease, thrombophlebitis or thromboembolic disorders, undiagnosed vaginal bleeding, active arterial thrombosis, blood dyscrasias, estrogen-dependent cancer, pregnancy, thyroid dysfunction, severe hepatic dysfunction.

INTERACTIONS

Drug

Aromatase inhibitors: May interfere with effects of aromatase inhibitors.

Bromocriptine: May interfere with effects of bromocriptine.

Corticosteroids: May increase effects of hydrocortisone and prednisone.

Cyclosporine: May increase blood concentration and nephrotoxicity of cyclosporine.

Liver toxic medications: May increase the risk of liver toxicity.
CYP3A4 inducers/inhibitors: May alter levels of estrogens.
Thyoid medications: May decrease effects of thyroid medications.
Herbal
St. John's wort: May decrease levels of esterified estrogens.
Black cohosh, dong quai: May increase estrogenic activity.
Red clover, saw palmetto, ginseng: May increase hormonal effects.

DIAGNOSTIC TEST EFFECTS

May affect metapyrone testing, thyroid function tests. May decrease serum cholesterol levels and LDH concentrations. May increase blood glucose levels, HDL concentrations, serum calcium and triglyceride levels.

SIDE EFFECTS

Frequent
Change in vaginal bleeding, such as spotting or breakthrough bleeding, breast pain or tenderness, gynecomastia.
Occasional
Headache, increased BP, intolerance to contact lenses, nausea.
Rare
Loss of scalp hair, clinical depression.

SERIOUS REACTIONS

- Prolonged administration may increase risk of gallbladder or thromboembolic disease, and breast, cervical, vaginal, endometrial, and liver carcinoma.
- Myocardial infarction, stroke, venous thromboembolism.
- Cholestatic jaundice occurs rarely.
- Retinal vascular thrombosis.

PRECAUTIONS & CONSIDERATIONS

Estrogen therapy should not be used to prevent cardiovascular disease. Other options for osteoporosis should be considered if estrogen therapy is being used solely for prevention of osteoporosis because of the increased risk of cardiovascular events. Use with caution in patients with cardiovascular disease. Use with caution in patients with history of cholestatic jaundice with past estrogen use or pregnancy. Estrogen therapy should be used for the shortest duration and lowest dose possible. Caution is warranted in patients with diseases exacerbated by fluid retention, such as asthma, cardiac dysfunction, diabetes mellitus, epilepsy, migraine headaches, and renal impairment. Caution is warranted with hepatic insufficiency and with gallbladder disease, hypocalcemia, porphyria, or lupus. Should be discontinued at least 4 wks before and for 2 wks following surgical procedures or prolonged immobilizations (risk of thromboembolism). Be aware that esterified estrogen is distributed in breast milk and may be harmful to infants. Esterified estrogen should not be used during breastfeeding or pregnancy. Be aware that the safety and efficacy of this drug have not been established in children. Esterified estrogen should be used cautiously in children whose bone growth is not complete because the drug may accelerate epiphyseal closure. The risk of dementia is increased in postmenopausal women aged > 65 yr. Smoking should be strongly discouraged because of increased risk of blood clot formation and myocardial infarction. Limit alcohol and caffeine intake.

Signs and symptoms of thromboembolic or thrombotic

disorders are evident by loss of coordination; numbness or weakness of an extremity; pain in the chest, leg, or groin; shortness of breath; speech or vision disturbance; or sudden severe headache. Abnormal vaginal bleeding, tenderness, and swelling may be signs and symptoms of blood clots.

Storage
Store at room temperature.

Administration
Administer at the same time each day. Give esterified estrogen with food or milk if the patient experiences nausea.

Estropipate

es-tro-pip'ate

★ 🍁 Ogen

CATEGORY AND SCHEDULE

Pregnancy Risk Category: X

Classification: Estrogens, hormones/hormone modifiers

MECHANISM OF ACTION

An estrogen that increases synthesis of DNA, RNA, and proteins in target tissues; reduces release of gonadotropin-releasing hormone from the hypothalamus; and reduces follicle-stimulating hormone (FSH) and luteinizing hormone (LH) from the pituitary. *Therapeutic Effect:* Promotes normal growth, promotes development of female sex organs, and maintains genitourinary function and vasomotor stability. Prevents accelerated bone loss by inhibiting bone resorption, restoring balance of bone resorption and formation. Inhibits LH and decreases serum testosterone concentration.

AVAILABILITY

Tablets: 0.625 mg (0.75 mg estropipate), 1.25 mg (1.5 mg estropipate), 2.5 mg (3 mg estropipate).

INDICATIONS AND DOSAGES

▸ **Vasomotor symptoms, atrophic vaginitis, kraurosis vulvae**

PO

Adults, Elderly. 0.625-5 mg/day (0.75-6 mg estropipate) cyclically.

▸ **Female hypogonadism, castration, primary ovarian failure**

PO

Adults, Elderly. 1.25-7.5 mg/day (1.5-9 mg estropipate) for 21 days; then off for 8-10 days. Repeat if bleeding does not occur by end of off cycle.

▸ **Prevention of osteoporosis**

PO

Adults, Elderly. 0.625 mg/day (0.75 mg estropipate) (25 days of 31-day cycle).

CONTRAINDICATIONS

Abnormal vaginal bleeding, active arterial thrombosis, blood dyscrasias, estrogen-dependent cancer, known or suspected breast cancer, pregnancy, thrombophlebitis or thromboembolic disorders, thyroid dysfunction, severe liver disease.

INTERACTIONS

Drug

Aromatase inhibitors: May interfere with effects of aromatase inhibitors.

Bromocriptine: May interfere with the effects of bromocriptine.

Corticosteroids: May increase effects of hydrocortisone and prednisone.

Cyclosporine: May increase blood cyclosporine concentration and the risk of hepatotoxicity and nephrotoxicity.

E

CYP3A4 inducers/inhibitors: May alter levels of estropipate.
Hepatotoxic medications: May increase the risk of hepatotoxicity.
Thyroid medications: May decrease effects of thyroid medications.

Herbal
Saw palmetto: Increases the effects of saw palmetto.
St. John's wort: May decrease levels of estropipate.
Food
None known.

DIAGNOSTIC TEST EFFECTS

May increase blood glucose, HDL, serum calcium, and triglyceride levels. May decrease serum cholesterol and LDH concentrations. May affect metapyrone testing and thyroid function tests.

SIDE EFFECTS

Frequent
Anorexia, nausea, swelling of breasts, peripheral edema marked by swollen ankles and feet.
Occasional
Vomiting, especially with high doses; headache that may be severe; intolerance to contact lenses; hypertension; glucose intolerance; brown spots on exposed skin.
Vaginal: Local irritation, vaginal discharge, changes in vaginal bleeding, including spotting, and breakthrough or prolonged bleeding.
Rare
Chorea or involuntary movements, hirsutism or abnormal hairiness, loss of scalp hair, depression.

SERIOUS REACTIONS

- Prolonged administration increases the risk of gallbladder disease; thromboembolic disease; and breast, cervical, vaginal, endometrial, and hepatic carcinoma.
- Myocardial infarction, stroke, venous thromboembolism.
- Retinal vascular thrombosis.
- Cholestatic jaundice occurs rarely.

PRECAUTIONS & CONSIDERATIONS

Estrogen therapy should not be used to prevent cardiovascular disease. Because of the increased risk for cardiovascular events, other options for osteoporosis should be considered if estrogen therapy is being used solely for the prevention of osteoporosis. Use with caution in patients with cardiovascular disease. Use with caution in patients with a history of cholestatic jaundice with past estrogen use or pregnancy. Estrogen therapy should be used for the shortest duration and lowest dose possible. Caution is warranted with diseases exacerbated by fluid retention such as asthma, cardiac dysfunction, diabetes, epilepsy, migraine headaches, and renal insufficiency. Caution is warranted in patients with hepatic insufficiency and with gallbladder disease, hypocalcemia, porphyria, or lupus. Should be discontinued at least 4 wks before and for 2 wks following surgical procedures or prolonged immobilizations (risk of thromboembolism). Estropipate is distributed in breast milk and may be harmful to the infant. Estropipate should not be used during breastfeeding. Estropipate should be used cautiously in children whose bone growth is not complete because the drug may accelerate epiphyseal closure. The risk of dementia is increased in postmenopausal women aged > 65 yr. Limit alcohol and caffeine intake. Avoid smoking because of the increased risk of blood clot formation and myocardial infarction.

Notify the physician of depression or abnormal vaginal bleeding. Signs and symptoms of thromboembolic or thrombotic disorders, including peripheral paresthesia, shortness of breath, speech or vision disturbance, and sudden headache, should be immediately reported. BP, weight, blood glucose, hepatic enzyme, and serum calcium levels should be monitored.

Storage
Store in a tightly-closed container at room temperature.

Administration
Take estropipate at the same time each day. Administration with food may decrease GI upset.

Eszopiclone

es-zoe-pick′lone
★ Lunesta

CATEGORY AND SCHEDULE

Pregnancy Risk Category: C

Classification: Sedatives/hypnotics

MECHANISM OF ACTION

A nonbenzodiazepine that may interact with GABA-receptor complexes at binding domains located close to or allosterically coupled to benzodiazepine receptors. *Therapeutic Effect:* Induces sleep and helps maintain sleep at night.

AVAILABILITY

Tablets (Film-Coated): 1 mg, 2 mg, 3 mg.

INDICATIONS AND DOSAGES

▸ **Insomnia**

PO

Adults. 2 mg immediately before bedtime. Maximum: 3 mg.
Adults using CYP3A4 inhibitors concurrently. 1 mg before bedtime; may be increased to 2 mg if needed.
Elderly (difficulty falling asleep). 1 mg before bedtime. Maximum: 2 mg.
Adults, Elderly (difficulty maintaining sleep). 2 mg before bedtime. Maximum: 3 mg.

▸ **Severe hepatic impairment**

PO

Adults. Initially, 1 mg at bedtime. Maximum: 2 mg.

CONTRAINDICATIONS

None known.

INTERACTIONS

Drug

Alcohol, olanzapine: May lead to decreased psychomotor function.
Aminoglutethimide, carbamazepine, nafcillin, nevirapine, phenobarbital, phenytoin, rifampicin, CYP3A4 inducers: May decrease the blood level and effects of eszopiclone.
Clarithromycin, ketoconazole, nefazodone, nelfinavir, ritonavir, traconazole, troleandomycin, CYP3A4 inhibitors: May increase the blood level and effects of eszopiclone.
CNS depressants: May increase adverse effects.

Herbal

Gotu kola, kava kava, St. John's wort, valerian: May increase CNS depression.

Food

Heavy meals: May reduce onset of eszopiclone action if taken with or immediately after a heavy meal.

DIAGNOSTIC TEST EFFECTS
None known.

SIDE EFFECTS
Frequent (21%-34%)
Unpleasant taste, headache.
Occasional (4%-10%)
Somnolence, dry mouth, dyspepsia, dizziness, nervousness, pain, nausea, rash, pruritus, depression, diarrhea.
Rare (2%-3%)
Hallucinations, anxiety, confusion, abnormal dreams, decreased libido, neuralgia, dysmenorrhea, gynecomastia.

SERIOUS REACTIONS
- Chest pain and peripheral edema occur occasionally.
- Complex, bizarre, and potentially risky behavior, agitation, and "sleep driving" while not fully awake, often with amnesia to the events.

PRECAUTIONS & CONSIDERATIONS
Caution is warranted in patients with clinical depression, drug abuse, hepatic impairment, and compromised respiratory function. Abnormal thinking and behavioral changes may occur, so monitor. Amnesia, CNS depression, and hypersensitivity reactions can occur. Use cautiously in elderly patients and reduce dose.
Safety and efficacy have not been evaluated in children.
Avoid abrupt cessation of therapy to avoid withdrawal symptoms.
Administration
Take immediately before bedtime. Do not take with, or immediately following, a high-fat meal. Do not crush or break tablets. Patients should be able to devote time for a full night's rest.

Etanercept
e-tan′er-cept
Enbrel

CATEGORY AND SCHEDULE
Pregnancy Risk Category: B

Classification: Disease-modifying antirheumatic drugs, immunomodulators, tumor necrosis factor modulators.

MECHANISM OF ACTION
A protein that binds to tumor necrosis factor (TNF), blocking its interaction with cell surface receptors. Elevated levels of TNF, which is involved in inflammatory and immune responses, are found in the synovial fluid of rheumatoid arthritis patients. *Therapeutic Effect:* Relieves the symptoms of rheumatoid arthritis, psoriasis, and other inflammatory conditions.

PHARMACOKINETICS
Well absorbed after subcutaneous administration. *Half-life:* 115 h. Onset of action: 1-3 wks.

AVAILABILITY
Powder for Injection: 25 mg.
Prefilled Syringe: 50 mg/mL.

INDICATIONS AND DOSAGES
▸ **Rheumatoid arthritis, psoriatic arthritis, ankylosing spondylitis**
SUBCUTANEOUS
Adults, Elderly. 25 mg twice weekly given 72-96 h apart or 50 mg as one injection or two 25-mg injections on the same day.
▸ **Juvenile rheumatoid arthritis**
SUBCUTANEOUS
Children 2-17 yr. 0.8 mg/kg/wk. Once-weekly dosing maximum is

50 mg/dose. Alternatively, 0.4 mg/kg (maximum 25 mg dose) twice weekly given 72-96 h apart.

▸ **Plaque psoriasis**

SUBCUTANEOUS

Adults, Elderly. 50 mg twice a week (give 3-4 days apart) for 3 mo. Maintenance: 50-mg/week given as once-weekly 50-mg injection or as a 25-mg injection twice weekly 3-4 days apart.

CONTRAINDICATIONS

Serious active infection or sepsis, hypersensitivity to etanercept, significant hematologic abnormalities, latex hypersensitivity (auto-injection), benzyl alcohol hypersensitivity (diluent for powder for injection).

INTERACTIONS

Drug

Abatacept, anakinara: May increase the risk of infection.

Cyclophosphamide: Increase in risk for noncutaneous solid malignancies when used concurrently, avoid concomitant use.

Live vaccines: Secondary transmission of infection by the live vaccine may occur.

Herbal and Food

None known.

DIAGNOSTIC TEST EFFECTS

None known.

SIDE EFFECTS

Frequent (20%-37%)

Injection site erythema, pruritus, pain, and swelling; abdominal pain (children 19%), upper respiratory infection.

Occasional (4%-19%)

Headache, rhinitis, dizziness, pharyngitis, cough, asthenia, abdominal pain (adults 5%), stomatitis, dyspepsia, vomiting (more common in children than adults), rash, nausea.

Rare (< 3%)

Sinusitis, allergic reaction, lupus-like symptoms.

SERIOUS REACTIONS

- Infections (such as pyelonephritis, cellulitis, osteomyelitis, wound infection, leg ulcer, septic arthritis, diarrhea, bronchitis, and pneumonia) occur in 29%-38% of patients.
- Rare adverse effects include heart failure, hypertension, hypotension, pancreatitis, GI hemorrhage, and dyspnea. The patient also may develop autoimmune antibodies.
- Nervous system problems such as seizures, optic neuritis, weakness of arms or legs (rare).
- Rare reports of malignancies (leukemia, lymphoma, nonmelanoma skin cancer) in patients receiving TNF blockers.

PRECAUTIONS & CONSIDERATIONS

Serious infections (including bacterial sepsis and tuberculosis) leading to hospitalization or death have been observed in patients treated with etanercept. Screen patients for latent tuberculosis infection before beginning etanercept. Patients should be educated about the symptoms of infection and closely monitored for signs and symptoms of infection during and after treatment with the drug. Patients who develop an infection should be evaluated for appropriate antimicrobial treatment and, in patients who develop a serious infection, etanercept should be discontinued. Use with caution in patients with seizure disorders, preexisting neurological conditions, multiple sclerosis, or with preexisting heart failure.

Caution is warranted in patients with history of recurrent infections and illnesses that predispose to infection, such as diabetes mellitus. It is unknown whether etanercept is excreted in breast milk. No age-related precautions have been noted in elderly patients or in children 4 yr and older. Avoid receiving live-virus vaccines during treatment. Discontinue therapy and expect to treat with varicella-zoster immune globulin, as prescribed, if the patient experiences significant exposure to varicella virus during treatment.

Notify the physician of bleeding, bruising, pallor, or persistent fever. CBC and erythrocyte sedimentation rate or C-reactive protein level should be monitored. Signs of a therapeutic response, including improved grip strength, increased joint mobility, reduced joint tenderness, and relief of pain, stiffness, and swelling, should be assessed.

Storage

Refrigerate unopened vials and prefilled syringes. Do not freeze. Protect from light. Once reconstituted, the drug may be stored for up to 14 days in the refrigerator.

Administration

! Do not add other medications to the solution. Do not use a filter during reconstitution or administration. Allow to come to room temperature before administering prefilled syringes or autoinjector syringe.

! If using vials, reconstitute only with 1 mL sterile bacteriostatic water for injection (containing 0.9% benzyl alcohol). Slowly inject the diluent into the vial. Some foaming will occur. To avoid excessive foaming, slowly swirl the contents until the powder is dissolved (< 5 min). The reconstituted solution normally appears clear and colorless. Discard if it contains particles or becomes cloudy or discolored. Withdraw all the solution into the syringe. The final volume should be approximately 1 mL.

Subcutaneously inject into the abdomen, thigh, or upper arm. Rotate injection sites. Administer each new injection at least 1 inch. from an old site, avoiding tender, bruised, hard, or red areas. Injection site reactions generally occur in the first month of treatment and decrease in frequency with continued etanercept therapy.

Ethambutol

e-tham′byoo-tole

Myambutol Etibi

Do not confuse ethambutol or Myambutol with Nembutal.

CATEGORY AND SCHEDULE

Pregnancy Risk Category: C

Classification:

Antimycobacterials

MECHANISM OF ACTION

An isonicotinic acid derivative that interferes with RNA synthesis.

Therapeutic Effect: Suppresses the multiplication of mycobacteria.

PHARMACOKINETICS

Rapidly and well absorbed from the GI tract (80%). Protein binding: 20%-30%. Widely distributed. Metabolized in the liver. Primarily excreted in urine. Removed by hemodialysis. *Half-life:* 3-4 h (increased in impaired renal function).

AVAILABILITY

Tablets: 100 mg, 400 mg.

INDICATIONS AND DOSAGES

▸ **Tuberculosis**

PO

Adults, Elderly, Adolescents 13 yr and older. 15-25 mg/kg/day as a single dose (maximum 1600 mg/dose) or 50 mg/kg 2 times/wk (maximum 4 g/dose). Consult recommended initial dosing and retreatment schedules, because treatment regimens can vary.

Children 6-12 yr (off-label). 20 mg/kg/day as a single dose (maximum 2.5 g/day).

▸ **Dosage in renal impairment**

Dosage interval is modified based on creatinine clearance.

Creatinine Clearance (mL/min)	Dosage Interval
10-50	q24-36h
< 10	q48h

OFF-LABEL USES

Treatment of atypical mycobacterial infections, use in children 6-13 yr.

CONTRAINDICATIONS

Optic neuritis and patients who cannot report visual changes, hypersensitivity to ethambutol.

INTERACTIONS

Drug

Neurotoxic medications: May increase the risk of neurotoxicity.

Aluminum antacids: Decrease absorption of ethambutol, administer 4 h apart.

Herbal and Food

None known.

DIAGNOSTIC TEST EFFECTS

May increase serum uric acid levels, may elevate liver enzyme levels.

SIDE EFFECTS

Occasional

Acute gouty arthritis (chills, pain, swelling of joints with hot skin), confusion, abdominal pain, nausea, vomiting, anorexia, headache.

Rare

Rash, fever, blurred vision, eye pain, red-green color blindness.

SERIOUS REACTIONS

- Optic neuritis and sometimes irreversible blindness (more common with high-dosage or long-term ethambutol therapy), peripheral neuritis, liver toxicities, and an anaphylactoid reaction occur rarely.
- Thrombocytopenia.

PRECAUTIONS & CONSIDERATIONS

Caution is warranted in patients with cataracts, diabetic retinopathy, gout, recurrent ocular inflammatory conditions, and renal dysfunction. Ethambutol use is not recommended for children younger than 13 yr of age. Be aware that ethambutol crosses the placenta and is excreted in breast milk. In elderly patients, age-related renal impairment may require dosage adjustment.

Initial complete blood count (CBC) and renal and liver function test results should be evaluated. Uric acid levels should be monitored and signs and symptoms of gout, including hot, painful, or swollen joints, especially in the ankle, big toe, or knee, should be assessed. Signs and symptoms of peripheral neuritis as evidenced by burning, numbness, or tingling of the extremities should also be assessed. Notify the physician if peripheral neuritis occurs. In addition, notify the physician immediately of any visual problems. Monthly eye exams are advised. Visual effects are generally reversible after ethambutol is discontinued, but in rare cases visual problems may take up to a year to disappear or may become permanent.

Storage

Store at room temperature. Protect from light and moisture.

Administration

Administer daily doses at roughly the same time each day. Give with food to decrease GI upset. Do not skip drug doses and take ethambutol for the full length of therapy, which may be months or years.

Ethionamide

e-thye-on'am-ide

Trecator

Do not confuse with Tricor.

CATEGORY AND SCHEDULE

Pregnancy Risk Category: C

Classification:

Antimycobacterials

MECHANISM OF ACTION

An antitubercular agent that inhibits peptide synthesis. *Therapeutic Effect:* Suppresses mycobacterial multiplication. Bactericidal.

PHARMACOKINETICS

Rapidly absorbed from the GI tract. Widely distributed. Protein binding: 30%. Metabolized in liver. Primarily excreted in urine. Removed by hemodialysis. *Half-life:* 2-3 h (increased with impaired renal function).

AVAILABILITY

Tablets: 250 mg (Trecator).

INDICATIONS AND DOSAGES

▸ **Tuberculosis**

PO

Adults, Elderly. 15-20 mg/kg/day; initiate dose at 250 mg/day for 1-2 days, then 250 mg twice daily for 1-2 days; increase to highest tolerated dose; average adult dose 750 mg/day. Maximum 1000 mg/day in 3-4 divided doses.

Children. 10-20 mg/kg/day in 2 or 3 divided doses or 15 mg/kg once daily. Maximum: 1 g/day.

OFF-LABEL USES

Treatment of atypical mycobacterial infections.

CONTRAINDICATIONS

Severe hepatic impairment, hypersensitivity to ethionamide.

INTERACTIONS

Drug

Cycloserine, isoniazid: May increase the risk of toxicity.

Rifampin: May increase the risk of hepatotoxicity.

Herbal

None known.

Food

Ethanol: Psychotic reaction has occurred. Avoid alcoholic beverages.

DIAGNOSTIC TEST EFFECTS

May increase ALT and AST, may increase TSH.

SIDE EFFECTS

Occasional

Abdominal pain, nausea, vomiting, weakness, postural hypotension, psychiatric disturbances, drowsiness, dizziness, headache, confusion, anorexia, headache, metallic taste, diarrhea, stomatitis, peripheral neuritis, acne, alopecia, photosensitivity, impotence.

Rare

Rash, fever, blurred vision, seizures, hypothyroidism, hypoglycemia, gynecomastia, thrombocytopenia, jaundice, hypersensitivity reaction.

SERIOUS REACTIONS

- Peripheral neuropathy, anorexia, seizures, and joint pain rarely occur.
- Optic neuritis and loss of vision may occur.

PRECAUTIONS & CONSIDERATIONS

Caution is warranted in patients receiving cycloserine or isoniazid, diabetics, patients with thyroid disease, epileptics, and psychiatric illness. Ethionamide crosses the placenta and is excreted in breast milk.

In elderly patients, age-related renal impairment may require dosage adjustment.

Stomach upset, loss of appetite, metallic taste, burning, numbness, tingling of the feet or hands, and pain and swelling of joints should be reported.

Storage

Store at room temperature.

Administration

May take without regard to food. However, administration at mealtimes usually improves GI tolerance. Do not skip drug doses and take for the full length of therapy.

! Expect use with pyridoxine to help decrease neurotoxicity.

Ethosuximide

eth-oh-sux′i-mide

★ 🍁 Zarontin

Do not confuse with Zaroxolyn or Neurontin.

CATEGORY AND SCHEDULE

Pregnancy Risk Category: C

Classification: Anticonvulsants, succinimides

MECHANISM OF ACTION

An anticonvulsant that increases the seizure threshold and suppresses paroxysmal spike-and-wave pattern in absence seizures; depresses nerve transmission in the motor cortex. *Therapeutic Effect:* Produces anticonvulsant activity.

PHARMACOKINETICS

Well absorbed from the GI tract. Metabolized in the liver. Excreted in urine. Removed by hemodialysis. *Half-life:* 50-60 h (in adults); 30 h (in children). Time to peak: 2-4 h (capsule), < 2-4 h (syrup).

AVAILABILITY

Capsule: 250 mg.
Syrup: 250 mg/5 mL.

INDICATIONS AND DOSAGES

▸ **Absence seizures**

PO

Adults, Elderly, Children older than 6 yr. Initially, 250-500 mg/day or 15 mg/kg/day in 2 divided doses. Maintenance: 15-40 mg/kg/day in 2 divided doses. Maximum: 1.5 g/day in 2 divided doses.

Children 3-6 yr. Initially, 250 mg/day in 2 divided doses, increased by 250 mg as needed every 4-7 days. Maintenance: 20-40 mg/kg/day in 2 divided doses. Maximum: 1.5 g/day in 2 divided doses.

CONTRAINDICATIONS

Hypersensitivity to succinimides.

INTERACTIONS

Drug

Alcohol, central nervous system (CNS) depressants: May increase CNS depression.

Carbamazepine, phenobarbital, phenytoin, primidone, valproic acid, CYP3A4 inducers: May

decrease ethosuximide blood concentration.
Azole antifungals, ciprofloxacin, clarithromycin, isoniazid, quinidine, protease inhibitors, verapamil, CYP3A4 inhibitors: May increase ethosuximide blood concentration.
Herbal
Evening primrose oil: May decrease effectiveness of ethosuximide.
Ginkgo: May decrease effectiveness of ethosuximide.
St. John's wort: May decrease ethosuximide blood concentrations.
Food
Ethanol: CNS depression; avoid use.

DIAGNOSTIC TEST EFFECTS

May lower WBC counts, alter other blood parameters. A relationship between ethosuximide toxicity and plasma levels has not been established. Usual serum levels are 40-100 mcg/mL, although levels as high as 150 mcg/mL have been reported without signs of toxicity.

SIDE EFFECTS

Occasional
Dizziness, drowsiness, double vision, headache, ataxia, nausea, diarrhea, vomiting, somnolence, urticaria.
Rare
Agranulocytosis, gum hypertrophy, leukopenia, myopia, swelling of the tongue, systemic lupus erythematosus, vaginal bleeding, inability to concentrate.

SERIOUS REACTIONS

- Abrupt withdrawal may increase seizure frequency.
- Blood dyscrasias, Stevens-Johnson syndrome, systemic lupus erythematosus have been associated with succinimides.
- Overdosage results in nausea, vomiting, and CNS depression including coma with respiratory depression.

PRECAUTIONS & CONSIDERATIONS

Caution should be used with renal or hepatic function impairment. Ethosuximide should be used cautiously when given alone in mixed types of epilepsy. Ethosuximide crosses the placenta; use in pregnancy and during breastfeeding only when clearly needed. Alcohol and tasks that require mental alertness and motor skills should be avoided until response to the drug is established.

Have patients promptly report any easy bruising, fever, joint pain, mouth ulcerations, sore throat, and unusual bleeding.
Storage
Store at room temperature; protect from light. Do not freeze.
Administration
Take with meals to reduce risk of GI distress. Do not abruptly discontinue.

Etidronate

ee-tid′roe-nate
★ Didronel
Do not confuse etidronate with etidocaine or etomidate.

CATEGORY AND SCHEDULE

Pregnancy Risk Category: C

Classification: Bisphosphonates

MECHANISM OF ACTION

A bisphosphonate that decreases mineral release and matrix in bone and inhibits osteocytic osteolysis. *Therapeutic Effect:* Decreases bone resorption.

AVAILABILITY
Tablets: 200 mg, 400 mg.

INDICATIONS AND DOSAGES
▸ Paget disease
PO
Adults, Elderly. Initially, 5-10 mg/kg/day not to exceed 6 mo, or 11-20 mg/kg/day not to exceed 3 mo. Repeat only after drug-free period of at least 90 days.
▸ Heterotopic ossification caused by spinal cord injury
PO
Adult, Elderly. 20 mg/kg/day for 2 wks; then 10 mg/kg/day for 10 wks.
▸ Heterotopic ossification complicating total hip replacement
PO
Adults, Elderly. 20 mg/kg/day for 1 mo before surgery; then 20 mg/kg/day for 3 mo after surgery.
▸ Hypercalcemia associated with malignancy
PO
Adults, Elderly. 20 mg/kg/day for 30 days. If needed, maximum 90 days.

OFF-LABEL USES
Postmenopausal osteoporosis.

CONTRAINDICATIONS
Clinically overt osteomalacia, renal failure (SCr ≥ 5 mg/dL, hypersensitivity to etidronate or other bisphosphonates.

INTERACTIONS
Drug
Antacids containing aluminum, calcium, magnesium; calcium supplements, iron: May decrease the absorption of etidronate. Separate by at least 2 h.
Warfarin: Concurrent use may alter bleeding times.
Herbal
None known.
Food
Foods with calcium: May decrease the absorption of etidronate.

DIAGNOSTIC TEST EFFECTS
May increase serum phosphate.

SIDE EFFECTS
Frequent
Nausea; diarrhea; continuing or more frequent bone pain in patients with Paget disease.
Occasional
Bone fractures, especially of the femur. Metallic, altered taste.
Rare
Hypersensitivity reaction.

SERIOUS REACTIONS
- Nephrotoxicity, including hematuria, dysuria, and proteinuria, has occurred with parenteral route.
- Serious hypersensitivity (rare).
- Osteonecrosis of the jaw.
- Esophageal irritation occurs if not administered as recommended.

PRECAUTIONS & CONSIDERATIONS
Caution is warranted in patients with hyperphosphatemia, impaired renal function, and restricted calcium and vitamin D intake. Patients with Paget disease may be at increased risk for osteomalacia and fracture of long bones when used for periods > 6 mo. Etidronate may cause skeletal malformations in the fetus. It is unknown whether etidronate is excreted in breast milk. Do not give to women who are breastfeeding. Safety and efficacy of etidronate have not been established in children.

Notify the physician of diarrhea. Serum electrolytes, BUN, fluid intake and output should be monitored.
Storage
Store at room temperature.

E

Administration
Take on an empty stomach. Swallow with a full glass of water (6-8 oz). Patients should not lie down after taking to avoid esophageal irritation. If GI discomfort occurs, the dose may be divided. Take etidronate 2 h before antacids, food, or vitamins. The full therapeutic response may take up to 3 mo.

E

Etodolac

e-toe-doe′lak
Taro-Etodolac

CATEGORY AND SCHEDULE

Pregnancy Risk Category: C (D if used in third trimester or near delivery)

Classification: Analgesics, nonsteroidal anti-inflammatory drugs

MECHANISM OF ACTION

An NSAID that produces analgesic and anti-inflammatory effects by inhibiting prostaglandin synthesis. *Therapeutic Effect:* Reduces the inflammatory response and intensity of pain.

PHARMACOKINETICS

Route	Onset	Peak	Duration
PO (analgesic)	30 min	N/A	4-12 h

Well absorbed from the GI tract. Protein binding: > 99%. Widely distributed. Metabolized in the liver. Primarily excreted in urine. Not removed by hemodialysis. *Half-life:* 6-7 h. Onset of analgesia: 2-4 h. Maximum anti-inflammatory: Several days.

AVAILABILITY

Capsules: 200 mg, 300 mg.
Tablets: 400 mg, 500 mg.
Tablets (Extended Release): 400 mg, 500 mg, 600 mg.

INDICATIONS AND DOSAGES

▸ **Osteoarthritis or rheumatoid arthritis**
PO (IMMEDIATE RELEASE)
Adults, Elderly. Initially, 300 mg 2-3 times a day or 400-500 mg twice daily. Maintenance: 600-1200 mg/day.
PO (EXTENDED RELEASE)
Adults, Elderly. Initially, 400 mg once daily. Maximum: 1000 mg once daily.

▸ **Analgesia**
PO (IMMEDIATE RELEASE)
Adults, Elderly. 200-400 mg q6-8h as needed. Maximum: 1200 mg/day.

▸ **Juvenile rheumatoid arthritis**
PO (EXTENDED RELEASE)
Children 6-16 yr. 20-30 kg: 400 mg once daily. 31-45 kg: 600 mg once daily. 46-60 kg: 800 mg once daily. > 60 kg: 1000 mg once daily.

OFF-LABEL USES

Treatment of acute gouty arthritis, vascular headache.

CONTRAINDICATIONS

History of hypersensitivity to aspirin or NSAIDs, within 10-14 days of coronary artery bypass graft (CABG).

INTERACTIONS

Drug
ACE inhibitors, ARBs: May increase risk of renal dysfunction.
Antihypertensives, diuretics: May decrease the effects of these drugs.
Aspirin, antiplatelets, other salicylates, corticosteroids: May increase the risk of GI side effects

such as bleeding. NSAID use may negate cardioprotective effect of ASA.
Bisphosphonates: Increased risk for gastrointestinal ulceration.
Bone marrow depressants: May increase the risk of hematologic reactions.
Cyclosporine: Nephrotoxicity and cyclosporine levels may be increased.
Heparin, oral anticoagulants, thrombolytics: May increase the bleeding effects of these drugs.
Lithium: May increase the blood concentration and risk of toxicity of lithium.
Methotrexate: May increase the risk of methotrexate toxicity.
Pemetrexed: May increase levels and effects of pemetrexed. Avoid etodolac 2-5 days before pemetrexed and 2 days following.
Probenecid: May increase etodolac blood concentration.
Vancomycin: May increase level of vancomyin.
Herbal
Supplements with antiplatelet or anticoagulant effects (e.g., feverfew, garlic, ginger, ginkgo biloba, ginseng, red clover, sweet clover, white willow, etc.): May increase effects on platelets or risk of bleeding.
Food
Alcohol: May increase dizziness, may increase risk of GI bleeding.

DIAGNOSTIC TEST EFFECTS

May increase bleeding time, liver function test results, and serum creatinine level. May decrease serum uric acid level.

SIDE EFFECTS

Occasional (4%-9%)
Dizziness, headache, abdominal pain or cramps, bloated feeling, diarrhea, nausea, indigestion, flatulence, weakness.
Rare (1%-3%)
Constipation, rash, pruritus, visual disturbances, tinnitus, depression, nervousness.

SERIOUS REACTIONS

- Overdose may result in acute renal failure.
- Rare reactions with long-term use include peptic ulcer disease, GI bleeding, gastritis, severe hepatic reactions (jaundice), nephrotoxicity (hematuria, dysuria, proteinuria), and a severe hypersensitivity reaction (bronchospasm, angioedema).
- Hepatic and renal impairment have occurred.

PRECAUTIONS & CONSIDERATIONS

Caution is warranted in patients with hepatic or renal impairment, a predisposition to fluid retention, and history of GI tract disease such as active peptic ulcer disease, chronic inflammation of GI tract, GI bleeding or ulceration. Use the lowest effective dose for the shortest duration of time. Anaphylactoid reactions have occurred in patients with aspirin triad hypersensitivity. Do not use in patients with aspirin-sensitive asthma. Cardiovascular event risk may be increased with duration of use or preexisting cardiovascular risk factors or disease. Use caution in patients with fluid retention, heart failure, or hypertension. Risk of myocardial infarction and stroke may be increased following CABG surgery. Do not administer within 4-6 half-lives before surgical procedures. It is unknown whether etodolac crosses the placenta or is distributed in breast milk. Etodolac should not be used during the last trimester of pregnancy because it may cause adverse effects in the fetus, such as premature closure of the ductus arteriosus. Notify the physician if the patient is pregnant. The safety and efficacy of etodolac have not been established in children < 6 yr of age. In elderly paients, GI bleeding or ulceration is more likely to cause serious complications, and age-related renal impairment may increase the risk of hepatotoxicity or renal toxicity; a decreased dosage is recommended. Tasks that require mental alertness or motor skills should be avoided until response to the drug has been established.

Notify the physician of edema, GI distress, headache, rash, signs of bleeding, or visual disturbances. CBC and blood chemistry studies should be monitored to assess hepatic and renal function. Therapeutic response, such as decreased pain, stiffness, swelling, or tenderness, improved grip strength, and increased joint mobility, should be evaluated.

Storage

Store at room temperature.

Administration

Do not crush, open, or break capsules or extended-release tablets. Take etodolac with food or milk, or antacids if GI distress occurs.

Etoposide, VP-16

e-toe-poe′side

★ Etopophos, Toposar 🍁 VePesid

Do not confuse etoposide with Etopophos.

CATEGORY AND SCHEDULE

Pregnancy Risk Category: D

Classification: Antineoplastics, epipodophyllotoxins

MECHANISM OF ACTION

An epipodophyllotoxin that induces single- and double-stranded breaks in DNA. Cell cycle–dependent and phase-specific; most effective in the S and G_2 phases of cell division. *Therapeutic Effect:* Inhibits or alters DNA synthesis.

PHARMACOKINETICS

Variably absorbed from the GI tract (25%-75%). Rapidly distributed, low concentrations in cerebrospinal fluid (CSF). Protein binding: 97%. Metabolized in the liver. Etoposide phosphate rapidly converted to etoposide in plasma. Primarily excreted in urine. Not removed by hemodialysis. *Half-life:* 3-12 h, children 6-8 h.

AVAILABILITY

Capsules (VePesid): 50 mg.
Injection Solution (Toposar). 20 mg/mL.
Powder for Injection (water-soluble etoposide phosphate [Etopophos]). 100-mg vial.

INDICATIONS AND DOSAGES

▸ **Refractory testicular tumors**

IV

Adults. 50-100 mg/m²/day on days 1-5, or 100 mg/m²/day on days 1, 3, 5 (as combination therapy) every 3-4 wks.

▸ **Acute myelocytic leukemia**

IV

Children. Remission: 150 mg/m²/day for 2-3 days and 2-3 cycles. Intensification or consolidation: 250 mg/m²/day for 3 days courses 2-5.

▸ **Malignant glioma**

IV

Children. 150 mg/m²/day on days 2 and 3 of treatment course.

▸ **Neuroblastoma**

IV

Children. 100 mg/m²/day on days 1-5 of treatment course; repeated q4wk.

▸ **Small cell lung carcinoma**

PO

Adults. Twice the IV dose rounded to nearest 50 mg. Give once a day for doses 400 mg or less or in divided doses for dosages > 400 mg.

IV

Adults. 35 mg/m²/day for 4 consecutive days; up to 50 mg/m²/day for 5 consecutive days (as combination therapy) every 3-4 wks.

▸ **Dosage in renal impairment**

Creatinine clearance 15-50 mL/min. 75% of normal dose.

Creatinine clearance < 15 mL/min. 50% of normal dose.

OFF-LABEL USES

Treatment of acute myelocytic leukemia, AIDS-associated Kaposi sarcoma, Ewing sarcoma, Hodgkin disease, non-Hodgkin lymphoma, platinum-resistant ovarian cancer.

CONTRAINDICATIONS

Hypersensitivity.

INTERACTIONS

Drug

Bone marrow depressants: May increase myelosuppression.

Cyclosporine: High-dose cyclosporine has increased etoposide levels by 80%. Monitor for increased toxic effects of etoposide if cyclosporine is initiated, the dose is increased, or it has been recently discontinued.

Live-virus vaccines: May potentiate virus replication, increase vaccine side effects, and decrease the patient's antibody response to the vaccine.

Herbal and Food

None known.

DIAGNOSTIC TEST EFFECTS

Decreased platelet counts, WBC, RBC.

IV INCOMPATIBILITIES

VePesid: Cefepime (Maxipime), filgrastim (Neupogen), idarubicin (Idamycin), lansoprazole (Prevacid), pantoprazole (Protonix).

Etopophos: Allopurinol (Aloprim), amphotericin B (Fungizone), amphotericin B liposomal (Ambisome), cefepime (Maxipime), chlorpromazine (Thorazine), dantrolene, diazepam (Valium), imipenem/cilastatin (Primaxin), methylprednisolone sodium succinate (Solu-Medrol), mitomycin (Mutamycin), pantoprazole (Protonix), phenytoin, prochlorperazine (Compazine).

SIDE EFFECTS

Frequent (43%-66%)

Mild to moderate nausea and vomiting, alopecia, ovarian failure, amenorrhea.

Occasional (6%-13%)

Diarrhea, anorexia, stomatitis.

Rare (Up to 2%)

Hypotension (with rapid infusion), peripheral neuropathy.

SERIOUS REACTIONS

- Myelosuppression may result in hematologic toxicity, manifested as anemia, leukopenia (occurring 5-7 days after drug administration), thrombocytopenia (occurring 9-16 days after administration), anemia, and, to lesser extent, pancytopenia. Bone marrow recovery occurs by day 20-28.
- Hepatotoxicity occurs occasionally.
- Anaphylactic reaction to IV infusion.

PRECAUTIONS & CONSIDERATIONS

Caution is warranted with myelosuppression or hepatic or renal impairment. Patients with low serum albumin or displaced binding due to elevated bilirubin may be more at risk for toxicity. Because of the risk of fetal harm, pregnant women should not take etoposide, especially during the first trimester. Dose-limiting bone marrow suppression is the most significant toxicity associated with etoposide therapy. Treatment should be withheld for platelets < 50,000/mm^3 or absolute neutrophil count (ANC) < 500/mm^3. Use with caution and reduce dose in patients with hepatic or renal dysfunction. Breastfeeding women also should not take this drug. The safety and efficacy of etoposide have not been established in children. Preparations with polysorbate 80 should be avoided in neonates. Anaphylactic reactions have been reported in children. In elderly patients, age-related renal impairment may require dosage adjustment. Vaccinations and coming in contact with anyone who has recently received a live-virus vaccine should be avoided.

Notify the physician of easy bruising, fever, signs of local infection, sore throat, or unusual bleeding from any site. Hematology test results should be monitored before and frequently during etoposide therapy. WBC counts, hemoglobin and hematocrit levels, pattern of daily bowel activity and stool consistency, signs and symptoms of paresthesia and peripheral neuropathy, signs and symptoms of stomatitis should be assessed. Alopecia may occur and is reversible, but new hair growth may have a different color or texture.

Storage

Refrigerate gelatin capsules. Do not freeze.

Store most etoposide injections at room temperature before dilution. Reconstituted solution is stable at room temperature for up to 96 h at 0.2 mg/mL and 48 h at 0.4 mg/mL. Discard solution if crystallization occurs. Refrigerate Etopophos vials before reconstitution. Protect from light. After reconstitution, Etopophos is stable for up to 24 h at room temperature or refrigerated. Etoposide injection diluted for oral use to 10 mg/mL in NS may be stored at room temperature for 22 days. Mix with apple or orange juice to concentration < 0.4 mg/mL and use within 3 h.

Administration

CAUTION: Observe and exercise appropriate precautions for handling, preparing, and administering cytotoxic drugs.

! Etoposide dosage is individualized based on clinical response and tolerance of the drug's adverse effects. Treatment is repeated at 3- to 4-wk intervals. Administer parenteral etoposide by slow IV infusion.

Etoposide solution concentrate for injection normally is clear and yellow. For IV use, dilute each 100-mg (5-mL) vial with at least 250 mL D5W or 0.9% NaCl to provide a concentration of 0.4 mg/mL (or 500 mL for a concentration of 0.2 mg/mL). Stability is concentration dependent and precipitates may occur > 0.4 mg/mL. Infuse slowly, over 30-60 min. Rapid IV infusion may produce marked hypotension. Monitor for an anaphylactic reaction manifested as back, chest, or throat pain; chills; diaphoresis; dyspnea; fever; lacrimation; and sneezing.

For Etopophos IV, reconstitute each 100 mg of Etopophos with 5-10 mL sterile water for injection, D5W, or 0.9% NaCl to provide a concentration of 20 mg/mL or 10 mg/mL, respectively. Etopophos may be given without further dilution or may be further diluted with 0.9% NaCl or D5W to a concentration as low as 0.1 mg/mL. Administer Etopophos over 5-10 min, as appropriate.

Etravirine

e-tra-vir'een

Intelence

Do not confuse with efavirenz.

CATEGORY AND SCHEDULE

Pregnancy Risk Category: B

Classification: Antiretroviral, nonnucleoside reverse transcriptase inhibitor

MECHANISM OF ACTION

A nonnucleoside reverse transcriptase inhibitor that inhibits the activity of HIV reverse transcriptase of HIV-1 and the transcription of HIV-1 RNA to DNA. *Therapeutic Effect:* Interrupts HIV replication, slowing the progression of HIV infection.

PHARMACOKINETICS

Absolute oral bioavailability unknown; fasting decreases absorption by 50% so the drug should be taken with food. Protein binding: 99.9% (primarily albumin). Metabolized to inactive metabolites in the liver via CYP3A4 and CYP2C9, and CYP2C19. Eliminated primarily (> 93%) in the feces; no unchanged drug found in urine. *Half-life:* 21-61 h.

AVAILABILITY

Tablets: 100 mg.

INDICATIONS AND DOSAGES

▸ **HIV infection (in combination with other antiretrovirals)**

PO

Adults, Elderly. 200 mg (two 100-mg tablets) twice daily following meals.

CONTRAINDICATIONS

Etravirine as monotherapy; hypersensitivity to etravirine.

INTERACTIONS

NOTE: Etravirine is an inducer of CYP3A and inhibitor of CYP2C9, CYP2C19, and P-glycoprotein and may alter the therapeutic effect or adverse reaction profile of the coadministered drug(s). See manufacturer literature for specific recommendations on management.

Drug

Alcohol, benzodiazepines, psychoactive drugs: May produce additive central nervous system (CNS) effects.

Potent CYP3A4 inhibitors: May significantly increase etravirine concentrations.

Clopidogrel: May negate clopidogrel effectiveness.

CYP3A4 substrates: Concentration of substrates may be altered.

Carbamazepine, phenobarbital, rifabutin, rifampin: Lower etravirine plasma concentration.

HMG-CoA reductase inhibitors ("statins"): May increase or decrease some statin concentrations and risk for adverse effects.

Warfarin: Alters warfarin plasma concentration. May increase bleeding risk. Monitor INR

Herbal

St. John's wort: May decrease etravirine concentration. Avoid.

Food

Meals: Increase drug absorption.

DIAGNOSTIC TEST EFFECTS

May increase total cholesterol, AST (SGOT), ALT (SGPT), and serum triglyceride levels. May increase serum amylase, lipase, serum creatinine, or blood glucose. Decreased WBC, platelets, or hemoglobin may occur.

SIDE EFFECTS

Frequent (4%-10%)
Rash, peripheral neuropathy, nausea.
Common
Fatigue, dyspepsia, flatulence, anxiety, sleep disorders, disorientation, nervousness, headache, nightmares, hyperglycemia, vertigo, blurred vision, increased blood pressure.
Rare
Fat redistribution syndrome with buffalo hump.

SERIOUS REACTIONS

- Immune reconstitution syndrome.
- Pancreatitis or hepatic failure.
- Serious skin rashes, including Stevens-Johnson syndrome and erythema multiforme.

PRECAUTIONS & CONSIDERATIONS

Severe, potentially life-threatening, and fatal skin reactions have been reported. These include cases of Stevens-Johnson syndrome, toxic epidermal necrolysis, and erythema multiforme. Hypersensitivity reactions have also been reported and were characterized by rash, constitutional findings, facial swelling, oral lesions, and sometimes organ dysfunction, including hepatic failure. Discontinue immediately if such skin reactions occur. Caution is warranted in patients with a history of liver impairment. Breastfeeding is not recommended for mothers with HIV-1 infection due to the risk of transmission of the virus. There are no adequate data during pregnancy. The safety and efficacy of etravirine have not been established in children. Etravirine is not a cure for HIV infection, nor does it reduce risk of transmission to others.

Expect to obtain history of all prescription and nonprescription medications before giving the drug because etravirine interacts with multiple drugs. Monitor for signs and symptoms of serious skin rashes, liver dysfunction, and adverse CNS side effects. Patients should report skin rashes promptly for evaluation. Avoid tasks that require mental alertness or motor skills until response to the drug is established.
Storage
Store at room temperature in the original bottle. Keep the bottle tightly closed and protect from moisture. Do NOT remove the desiccant pouches.
Administration
Take the doses following a meal. If patient unable to swallow the tablets whole, disperse the tablets in a glass of water. Once dispersed, stir well and drink immediately. Rinse glass with water several times and completely swallow to ensure the entire dose is consumed. Take the medication every day as prescribed. Do not alter the dose or discontinue the medication without first notifying the physician.

Everolimus

e-ve-ro′li-mus
★ 🍁 Afinitor, Zortress
Do not confuse Afinitor with Zortress due to different indications and dosages.

CATEGORY AND SCHEDULE

Pregnancy Risk Category: C (Zortress), D (Afinitor)

Classification: Antineoplastics, immunosuppressants

MECHANISM OF ACTION

An immunosuppressant with antineoplastic activity that inhibits T-lymphocyte proliferation. Prevents activation of the enzyme target of rapamycin (mTOR), a key regulatory kinase in cell-cycle progression. As an inhibitor of mTOR, the drug results in complex formation and inhibition of mTOR kinase activity. Everolimus reduced the activity of cellular protein synthesis and reduced the expression of vascular endothelial growth factor (VEGF). *Therapeutic Effect:* Suppresses the immunologically mediated inflammatory response; prevents kidney organ transplant rejection. Fights cancer by reducing cell proliferation, angiogenesis.

PHARMACOKINETICS

Variably absorbed after PO administration. Protein binding: 74%–97%. Extensively metabolized in the liver. Excreted in feces. Not removed by hemodialysis. *Half-life:* 11.7 h, with a range up to 30 h.

AVAILABILITY

Tablets (Afinitor): 2.5 mg, 5 mg, 10 mg.
Tablets (Zortress): 0.25 mg, 0.5 mg, 0.75 mg.

INDICATIONS AND DOSAGES

▸ Prevention of kidney transplant rejection

PO (ZORTRESS)

Adults. Initially, 0.75 mg every 12 h in combination with basiliximab induction, cyclosporine USP modified, and corticosteroids. Therapeutic drug monitoring of everolimus and cyclosporine is recommended for all patients to guide adjustments. If needed, adjust everolimus dose at 4-5 day intervals.

▸ Zortress -Dosage adjustment for hepatic impairment

For Child-Pugh class B hepatic impairment, reduce daily dose by half and monitor blood concentrations.

▸ Advanced renal cell carcinoma after failure with sunitinib or sorafenib

PO (AFINITOR)

Adults. 10 mg once daily.

▸ Afinitor -If moderate inhibitors of CYP3A4 or P-glycoprotein (PgP) are required

Reduce dose to 2.5 mg once daily; if tolerated, consider increase to 5 mg once daily.

▸ Afinitor -If strong inducers of CYP3A4 are required

Increase dose in 5-mg increments to a max of 20 mg once daily.

▸ Afinitor -Dosage adjustment for hepatic impairment

For Child-Pugh class B hepatic impairment, reduce dose to 5 mg once daily.

▸ Afinitor -Dosage adjustment for side effects

Interruption and/or dose reduction to 5 mg daily may be needed to manage adverse drug reactions.

CONTRAINDICATIONS

Hypersensitivity to everolimus, other rapamycin derivatives, or ingredients in the formulation.

INTERACTIONS

Drug

Aminoglycosides, amphotericin B, cisplatin: May increase the risk of renal dysfunction.

ACE inhibitors: Increased risk for angioedema.

CYP3A4 inhibitors or Pgp inhibitors: May affect everolimus concentrations. Blood concentration monitoring is recommended; consider dose adjustment. Avoid if possible.

Azole antifungals, calcium channel blockers, clarithromycin, diltiazem, erythromycin, protease inhibitors, verapamil: Increase everolimus blood concentration and risk of toxicity.
CYP3A4 inducers (e.g., carbamazepine, efavirenz, nevirapine, phenobarbital, phenytoin, rifampin): Decrease everolimus blood concentration. Blood concentration monitoring is recommended; consider dose adjustment. Avoid if possible.
Digoxin: Inhibits Pgp and may decrease the efflux of everolimus from intestinal cells and increase everolimus blood concentrations.
HMG-CoA reductase inhibitors ("statins"): May increase risk of statin side effects, like myopathy.
Live-virus vaccines: May potentiate virus replication, increase vaccine side effects, and decrease the patient's antibody response to the vaccine. Avoid live-virus vaccines during treatment.
Cyclosporine and other immunosuppressants: May increase the risk of nephrotoxicity, or immunosuppression. Cyclosporine inhibits CYP3A and Pgp and raises everolimus blood concentrations.
Herbal
St. John's wort: May decrease the effects of everolimus.
Food
Grapefruit, grapefruit juice: May alter the effects of the drug. Avoid.

DIAGNOSTIC TEST EFFECTS

May increase blood glucose and serum creatinine levels. May decrease WBC, RBC indices, and platelet counts. Increases cholesterol and triglycerides. May alter serum liver function tests, potassium or magnesium levels. May cause proteinuria. Trough concentrations of everolimus are monitored; recommended everolimus therapeutic range is 3-8 ng/mL.

SIDE EFFECTS

Common
Peripheral edema, constipation, hypertension, nausea, anemia, UTI or other infections, hyperlipidemia, stomatitis, cough, diarrhea, headache.
Occasional
Rash, pruritus, anorexia, asthenia, dyspepsia, abdominal pain, fatigue, dry skin, taste disturbance, dyspnea, epistaxis, dizziness, paresthesia, delayed wound healing, photosensitivity, new-onset hyperglycemia/diabetes, proteinuria, arthralgia. Azoospermia and infertility possible in men.

SERIOUS REACTIONS

- Hypersensitivity.
- Nephrotoxicity or acute renal failure.
- Noninfectious pneumonitis; rarely fatal. Be alert for dyspnea and cough.
- Pericardial and pleural effusions or ascites.
- Kidney arterial or venous thrombosis of transplant graft.
- Increased risk of sepsis; opportunistic infections occur occasionally.
- Possible risk of lymphoma or other malignancy (i.e., non-melanoma skin cancers). Appears related to intensity and duration of use of the immunosuppressant drug.

PRECAUTIONS & CONSIDERATIONS

Caution is warranted in those patients with a listed hypersensitivity to similar medications (e.g., sirolimus).

Caution is warranted in patients with chickenpox, herpes zoster, hepatitis B, and other infection. Use with caution in those with immunosuppression, hypertension, diabetes, actively healing wounds, and hepatic impairment. Patients with rare disorders of galactose intolerance should not use the drug. Everolimus crosses the placenta and may cause fetal harm. The drug is distributed to breast milk; women taking this drug should not breastfeed. This drug may cause infertility or sperm changes in males. Patients should use an effective method of contraception during therapy and for 8 wks after ending treatment. The safety and efficacy of everolimus have not been established in children.

Review all medications, including nonprescription, prior to prescribing to manage drug interactions. Avoid crowds and people with infection. Also avoid exposure to sunlight and artificial light because these may cause a photosensitivity reaction. Notify the physician of change in mental status, chest pain, dizziness, headache, decreased urination, rash, respiratory infection, difficulty breathing, or unusual bleeding or bruising. CBC should be monitored routinely. Liver function test results and serum creatinine and potassium levels should also be assessed regularly.

Storage

Store in the original container at room temperature, protect from light and moisture.

Administration

May take without regard to food. Do not break, chew, or crush Afinitor tablets. Zortress 0.75-mg tablets are scored if a dose needs to be divided. Swallow with a full glass of water. Take doses at about the same time daily. Do not give this drug with grapefruit juice.

Exemestane

ex-uh-mess'tane

★ 🍁 Aromasin

CATEGORY AND SCHEDULE

Pregnancy Risk Category: D

Classification: Aromatase inhibitors, hormones/hormone modifiers

MECHANISM OF ACTION

Inactivates aromatase, the principal enzyme that converts androgens to estrogens in both premenopausal and postmenopausal women, thereby lowering the circulating estrogen level. *Therapeutic Effect:* Inhibits the growth of breast cancers that are stimulated by estrogens.

PHARMACOKINETICS

Rapidly absorbed after PO administration. Protein binding: 90%. Distributed extensively into tissues. Metabolized extensively in the liver; eliminated in urine and feces. *Half-life:* 24 h.

AVAILABILITY

Tablets: 25 mg.

INDICATIONS AND DOSAGES

▸ **Breast cancer, advanced after tamoxifen therapy**

PO

Adults, Elderly. 25 mg once a day after a meal.

If potent CYP3A4 inducer coprescribed, give 50 mg once daily after a meal.

CONTRAINDICATIONS
Hypersensitivity to exemestane.

INTERACTIONS
Drug
CYP3A4 inducers: May decrease levels and effects of exemestane.
Herbal
St. John's wort: May decrease levels and effects of exemestane. Avoid use.
Food
None known.

DIAGNOSTIC TEST EFFECTS
May increase serum alkaline phosphatase, AST (SGOT), ALT (SGPT), creatinine, and bilirubin levels.

SIDE EFFECTS
Frequent (10%-22%)
Fatigue, nausea, depression, hypertension, alopecia, arthralgia, hot flashes, pain, insomnia, anxiety, dyspnea.
Occasional (5%-8%)
Headache, dizziness, vomiting, dermatitis, peripheral edema, abdominal pain, weight gain, anorexia, flu-like symptoms, diaphoresis, constipation, visual disturbances.
Rare (4%)
Diarrhea.

SERIOUS REACTIONS
- Myocardial infarction, angina, and thromboembolism have been reported.

PRECAUTIONS & CONSIDERATIONS
Exemestane is not for use in premenopausal women. Exemestane is indicated only for postmenopausal women. Use with caution in renal or hepatic insufficiency. This drug is not used in children. No age-related precautions have been noted in elderly patients. Should not be used during pregnancy.

Potential side effects, including dizziness, headache, insomnia, depression, may occur. Notify the physician if hot flashes or nausea become unmanageable. Nausea and vomiting may be prevented or treated with an antiemetic. Baseline vital signs, especially BP, should be assessed because exemestane may cause hypertension.
Storage
Store at room temperature.
Administration
Give oral exemestane after a meal.

Exenatide
ex-en'a-tide
★ 🍁 Byetta

CATEGORY AND SCHEDULE
Pregnancy Risk Category: C

Classification: Antidiabetic agents, incretin mimetics

MECHANISM OF ACTION
A synthetic peptide initially derived from the saliva of the Gila monster lizard; some of the peptide sequence overlaps with human glucagon-like peptide-1 (GLP-1). Incretins, such as GLP-1, enhance glucose-dependent insulin secretion and exhibit other antihyperglycemic actions following their release into the circulation from the gut. Exenatide is a GLP-1 receptor agonist that enhances glucose-dependent insulin secretion by the pancreatic β-cell, suppresses inappropriately elevated glucagon secretion, and slows gastric emptying. *Therapeutic Effect:* Lowers blood glucose concentration and also HbA1c over time.

PHARMACOKINETICS

Native GLP-1 has a very short half-life (< 1 min) and is not clinically useful; exenatide has an extended therapeutic profile in comparison. Median plasma concentration occurs 2.1 h after subcutaneous injection. Primarily eliminated by glomerular filtration followed by proteolytic degradation. *Half-life:* 2.4 h (significantly prolonged in severe renal impairment and end-stage renal disease).

AVAILABILITY

Injection (250 mcg/mL): Available in 5-mcg and 10-mcg prefilled pens containing 60 doses each.

INDICATIONS AND DOSAGES

▸ **Type 2 diabetes mellitus**

SC

Adults, Elderly. Initially, 5 mcg twice daily, with dose given 60 min prior to morning and evening meals (or before the 2 main meals of the day with doses at least 6 h apart). Increase to 10 mcg twice daily after 1 mo based on clinical response.

▸ **Dosage in renal impairment**

Use caution in increasing doses for those with mild or moderate renal impairment. Do not use in patients with severe renal impairment (CrCl < 30 mL/min) or end-stage renal disease.

CONTRAINDICATIONS

Hypersensitivity to exenatide or product components. Not for type 1 diabetes mellitus or diabetic ketoacidosis. For patients with a history of pancreatitis, selection of other antidiabetic medications is strongly suggested (see Serious Reactions). Do not use in severe renal impairment or end-stage renal disease.

INTERACTIONS

Drug

β-Blockers: May mask signs of hypoglycemia.

Oral medications (e.g., oral contraceptives, antibiotics): Exenatide slows GI transit times. For oral medications dependent on normal transit times efficacy, such as contraceptives and antibiotics, patients should be advised to take those drugs at least 1 h before exenatide, or at a meal or snack when exenatide is not administered.

Corticosteroids: May increase blood sugar.

Sulfonylureas: May increase risk of hypoglycemia; lower sulfonylurea dose may be needed.

Warfarin: May increase the effects of warfarin, resulting in increased INR. Monitor INR closely.

Herbal

Alfalfa, aloe, bilberry, bitter melon, burdock, celery, damiana, fenugreek, garcinia, garlic, ginger, ginseng (American), gymnema, marshmallow, stinging nettle: May enhance hypoglycemic effects.

Food

Alcohol: Hypoglycemia is more likely to occur if alcohol is ingested. High and chronic alcohol use may increase risk for pancreatitis.

DIAGNOSTIC TEST EFFECTS

Lowers blood sugar. May increase serum creatinine, amylase, or lipase.

SIDE EFFECTS

Frequent

Nausea, hypoglycemia, vomiting, diarrhea, nervousness, dizziness, headache, dyspepsia. Nausea subsides with time.

Occasional

Gastroesophageal reflux (GERD), decreased appetite, asthenia, hyperhidrosis.

Rare
Injection site reaction, abdominal pain, eructation, flatulence, abdominal distention, taste disturbance, pruritus, urticaria, maculopapular rash.

SERIOUS REACTIONS

- Overdose may produce severe hypoglycemia, along with severe GI symptoms and vomiting.
- Pancreatitis, including nonfatal hemorrhagic and necrotizing pancreatitis.
- Rare reports of serious allergic reactions, including angioedema and serious rashes.
- Worsened renal function or acute renal failure.

PRECAUTIONS & CONSIDERATIONS

Caution is warranted in patients with debilitation, impaired renal function, potential risk factors for pancreatitis (hypertriglyceridemia, alcoholism, other), and significant GI disease (e.g., gastroparesis) where slowing of GI transit time may aggravate the condition. Be alert to conditions that alter blood glucose requirements or dietary intake, such as fever, increased activity, stress, or a surgical procedure. There are no data regarding exenatide use during pregnancy. It is unknown whether the drug is distributed in breast milk; caution is recommended. The drug may alter the efficacy of oral hormonal contraceptives and the choice of an additional or alternate contraceptive may be desirable. Safety and efficacy of exenatide have not been established in children. Hypoglycemia may be difficult to recognize in elderly patients. With time, development of antibodies to the drug may present as treatment failure.

Food intake and blood glucose should be monitored before and during therapy. Be aware of signs and symptoms of hypoglycemia (anxiety, cool wet skin, diplopia, dizziness, headache, hunger, numbness in the mouth, tachycardia, tremors), or hyperglycemia (deep rapid breathing, dim vision, fatigue, nausea, polydipsia, polyphagia, polyuria, vomiting); carry candy, sugar packets, or other sugar supplements for immediate response to hypoglycemia.

Consult the physician when glucose demands are altered (such as with fever, heavy physical activity, infection, stress, trauma). Exercise, good personal hygiene (including foot care), not smoking, and weight control are essential parts of therapy.

Storage
Store unopened pens in the original carton in a refrigerator. Do not freeze. Once opened and set up for first use, the pen can be kept at a temperature not to exceed 77° F for up to 30 days. Always protect the pen from light and keep it dry. Do not store the pen with the needle attached, as this will cause leakage from the pen and air bubbles may form in the cartridge.

Administration
For subcutaneous injection only; doses are given anytime within the 60 min prior to the start of a main meal. If using a new pen, make sure you have prepared the pen for routine use. For routine use, wash hands. Check that the right pen is selected. Pull off blue pen cap. The cartridge liquid should be clear, colorless, and free of particles. Attach the needle and dial in the pen dose as the manufacturer directs. Inject the dose SC as directed in the thigh, abdomen, or upper arm; rotate injection sites with each use. After injection, reset

the pen, remove and dispose of the used needle properly, and store the pen for next use by replacing the blue pen cap.

Ezetimibe

eh-zet′eh-mibe

Zetia Ezetrol

Do not confuse Zetia with Zestril.

CATEGORY AND SCHEDULE

Pregnancy Risk Category: C

Classification:

Antihyperlipidemics

MECHANISM OF ACTION

An antihyperlipidemic that inhibits cholesterol absorption in the small intestine, leading to a decrease in the delivery of intestinal cholesterol to the liver. *Therapeutic Effect:* Reduces total serum cholesterol, LDL cholesterol, and triglyceride levels and increases HDL cholesterol concentration.

PHARMACOKINETICS

Variable absorption following oral administration. Protein binding: > 90%. Metabolized in the small intestine and liver. Excreted by the kidneys and bile. *Half-life:* 22 h.

AVAILABILITY

Tablets: 10 mg.

INDICATIONS AND DOSAGES

▸ **Hypercholesterolemia**

PO

Adults, Elderly, Children > 10 yr. Initially, 10 mg once a day, given with or without food. If the patient is also receiving a bile acid sequestrant, give ezetimibe at least 2 h before or at least 4 h after the bile acid sequestrant.

CONTRAINDICATIONS

Hypersensitivity to ezetimibe.

NOTE: If given with an HMG-CoA reductase inhibitor ("statin"), follow statin contraindications (e.g., patients with active hepatic disease or unexplained persistent elevations in serum transaminase levels, moderate or severe hepatic insufficiency, pregnancy, breastfeeding).

INTERACTIONS

Drug

Aluminum and magnesium-containing antacids: Decrease ezetimibe plasma concentration.

Cyclosporine: Increases ezetimibe concentration; cyclosporine level may also increase.

Fenofibrate, gemfibrozil: Increases ezetimibe plasma concentration. Fibrates may increase risk of cholelithiasis.

Cholestyramine: Decreases drug effectiveness. Administer 2 h before or 4 h after bile acid sequestrants.

Herbal and Food

None known.

DIAGNOSTIC TEST EFFECTS

May increase serum alkaline phosphatase, serum bilirubin, AST (SGOT), and ALT (SGPT) levels.

SIDE EFFECTS

Frequent (> 10%)

Upper respiratory tract infection.

Occasional (3%-9%)

Headache, back pain, diarrhea, myalgia, arthralgia, sinusitis, abdominal pain, chest pain.

Rare (2%)

Cough, pharyngitis, fatigue.

SERIOUS REACTIONS

- None known.

E

PRECAUTIONS & CONSIDERATIONS

Caution is warranted in patients with chronic renal failure, diabetes, hypothyroidism, liver function impairment, and obstructive liver disease. It is unknown whether ezetimibe crosses the placenta or is distributed in breast milk. Safety and efficacy of ezetimibe have not been established in children 10 yr of age and younger. This drug is not recommended for use in patients with moderate or severe hepatic impairment.

Notify the physician of any abdominal disturbances and back pain. Pattern of daily bowel activity and stool consistency should be assessed. Serum cholesterol and triglyceride levels should be checked at baseline and periodically thereafter.

Storage

Store at room temperature. Protect from moisture.

Administration

Take ezetimibe without regard to food. Separate administration from that of bile sequestrants.

Factor IX Complex and Factor IX Concentrates

AlphaNine SD, Bebulin VH, BeneFIX, Mononine, Profilnine SD
BeneFIX, Immunine VH

CATEGORY AND SCHEDULE

Pregnancy Risk Category: C

Classification: Antihemophilic agents, blood clotting factors

MECHANISM OF ACTION

A blood modifier that raises the plasma levels of factor IX, restoring hemostasis in patients with factor IX deficiency. *Therapeutic Effect:* Increases blood clotting factor IX to restore hemostasis.

PHARMACOKINETICS

Mean half-time is 22 h (range, 11-36 h). Mean increase in circulating factor IX activity after infusion is 0.67-1.15 units/dL rise per units/kg body weight.

AVAILABILITY

Injection: Number of units is indicated on each vial.
AlphaNine SD: Contains factor IX; contains only low or nontherapeutic levels of factors II, VII, and X.
Mononine: Purified by monoclonal antibody process to isolate factor IX.
BeneFIX: Recombinant human factor IX.
Profilnine SD, Bebulin VH: Contains factor IX; also contains some factors, II, VII, and X and proteins S and C.

INDICATIONS AND DOSAGES

▸ **Bleeding caused by factor IX deficiency (hemophilia B, Christmas disease)**

IV INFUSION

Adults, Elderly, Children. Amount of factor IX required is individualized. Dosage depends on degree of deficiency, level of each factor desired, patient's weight, and severity of bleeding.

OFF-LABEL USES

Emergency reversal of oral anticoagulant effects.

CONTRAINDICATIONS

Sensitivity to mouse protein (Mononine) or hamster protein (BeneFIX).

INTERACTIONS

Drug and Food

Aminocaproic acid: May increase the risk of thrombosis.

Herbal and Food

None known.

DIAGNOSTIC TEST EFFECTS

None known.

IV INCOMPATIBILITIES

Do not mix with other medications.

SIDE EFFECTS

Rare

Mild hypersensitivity reaction marked by fever, chills, change in BP and pulse rate, rash, and urticaria.
Nausea, discomfort at IV site, altered taste, burning sensation in the jaw and skull, allergic rhinitis, light-headedness, headache, dizziness, chest tightness, phlebitis, or cellulitis at IV site. Rapid infusion rate: headache, flushing, changes in BP or pulse rate, transient fever, chills, tingling, urticaria, nausea, and vomiting may occur. Symptoms disappear promptly on discontinuation. Except in the most reactive individuals, the infusion may be resumed at a slower rate. Chills and fever (particularly when large doses are used).

SERIOUS REACTIONS

- There is a high risk of venous thrombosis during the postoperative period.
- Acute hypersensitivity reaction or anaphylactic reaction may occur.
- There is a risk of transmitting viral hepatitis and other viral diseases.
- High doses may be associated with myocardial infarction, disseminated intravascular coagulation, venous thrombosis, and pulmonary embolism.

PRECAUTIONS & CONSIDERATIONS

Caution is warranted with hepatic impairment, recent surgery, and sensitivity to factor IX. OTC medications should be avoided without physician approval. Efficacy and safety in children under age 6 yr have not been evaluated.

Notify the physician of abdominal or back pain, gingival bleeding, black or red stool, coffee-ground emesis, dark or red urine, or red-speckled mucus from cough. Intake and output and vital signs should be monitored. IV site should be assessed for oozing every 5-15 min for 1-2 h after administration.

Factor levels and hematologic and coagulation tests are frequently monitored during and between treatments.

Storage

AlphaNine SD: May also be stored at room temperature not to exceed 30° C (86° F) for up to 1 mo.

BeneFIX: May also be stored at room temperature, not to exceed 25° C (77° F) for up to 6 mo. Reconstituted solution at room temperature should be used within 3 h.

Mononine: May also be stored at room temperature not to exceed 25° C (77° F) for up to 1 mo.

Administration

Gently agitate vial until powder is completely dissolved so that the active components will not be removed when the solution is filtered during administration. Bring diluent and factors to room temperature before combining. Filter before administration. Begin administration within 3 h of reconstitution. Administer by IV infusion. Infuse slowly, no faster than 2 mL/min (Bebulin and Mononine), 10 mL/min (Profilnine and AlphaNine), and over several minutes (BeneFIX). Too rapid an IV infusion may produce a change in BP and pulse rate, headache, flushing, and a tingling sensation.

Famciclovir

fam-si'klo-veer

★ 🍁 Famvir

Do not confuse Famvir with Femhrt.

CATEGORY AND SCHEDULE

Pregnancy Risk Category: B

Classification: Antivirals

MECHANISM OF ACTION

A synthetic nucleoside that inhibits viral DNA synthesis. *Therapeutic Effect:* Suppresses replication of herpes simplex virus and varicella-zoster virus.

PHARMACOKINETICS

Rapidly and extensively absorbed after PO administration. Protein binding: 20%-25%. Rapidly metabolized to penciclovir by enzymes in the GI wall, liver, and plasma. Eliminated unchanged in urine. Removed by hemodialysis. *Half-life:* 2 h.

AVAILABILITY

Tablets: 125 mg, 250 mg, 500 mg.

INDICATIONS AND DOSAGES

▸ **Herpes zoster (shingles)**

PO

Adults. 500 mg q8h for 7 days.
CrCl 40-59 mL/min: Administer 500 mg every 12 h.
CrCl 20-39 mL/min: Administer 500 mg every 24 h.
CrCl < 20 mL/min: Administer 250 mg every 24 h.
Hemodialysis: Administer 250 mg after each dialysis session.

▸ **Recurrent genital herpes**

PO

Adults. 1000 mg twice a day for 1 day within 6 h of symptom onset.
CrCl 40-59 mL/min: Administer 500 mg every 12 h for 1 day.
CrCl 20-39 mL/min: Administer 500 mg as a single dose.
CrCl < 20 mL/min: Administer 250 mg as a single dose.
Hemodialysis: Administer 250 mg as a single dose after dialysis session.

▸ **Suppression of recurrent genital herpes**

PO

Adults. 250 mg twice a day for up to 1 yr.
CrCl 20-39 mL/min: Administer 125 mg every 12 h.
CrCl < 20 mL/min: Administer 125 mg every 24 h.
Hemodialysis: Administer 125 mg after each dialysis session.

▸ **Recurrent herpes labialis (cold sores)**

PO

Adults. 1500 mg as a single dose earliest sign or symptom of a cold sore.
CrCl 40-59 mL/min: Administer 750 mg as a single dose.
CrCl 20-39 mL/min: Administer 500 mg as a single dose.
CrCl < 20 mL/min: Administer 250 mg as a single dose.
Hemodialysis: Administer 250 mg as a single dose after dialysis session.

▸ **Recurrent orolabial or genital herpes simplex infection in patients with HIV infection**

PO

Adults. 500 mg twice a day for 7 days.
CrCl 20-39 mL/min: Administer 500 mg every 24 h.
CrCl < 20 mL/min: Administer 250 mg every 24 h.
Hemodialysis: Administer 250 mg after each dialysis session.

OFF-LABEL USES

Bell's palsy, prophylaxis of postherpetic neuralgia.

CONTRAINDICATIONS

Hypersensitivity to famciclovir or penciclovir.

INTERACTIONS

Drug
Probenecid: May inhibit active tubular secretion and increase levels of penciclovir.
Herbal
None known.
Food
None known.

DIAGNOSTIC TEST EFFECTS

Increases in AST, ALT. Decreases in WBC.

SIDE EFFECTS

Frequent (>10%)
Headache, nausea.
Occasional (2%-10%)
Diarrhea, abdominal pain, dysmenorrhea, fatigue, vomiting, pruritus, flatulence, paresthesia.

F

Rare (< 2%)
Insomnia, migraine.

SERIOUS REACTIONS

- Acute renal failure in patients with underlying renal dysfunction.
- Delirium or disorientation; reported more commonly in elderly patients.
- Rare allergic reactions, including pruritus, erythema multiforme, Stevens-Johnson syndrome, or toxic epidermal necrolysis.
- Rare reports of cholestatic jaundice.

PRECAUTIONS & CONSIDERATIONS

Caution is warranted in patients with renal impairment because acute renal failure may occur with inappropriately high doses. Dose adjustment is recommended for patients with CrCl < 60 mL/min. The safety and efficacy of famciclovir have not been established in children. The efficacy of famciclovir has not been established for initial-episode genital herpes infection, ophthalmic zoster, disseminated zoster, or in immunocompromised patients with herpes zoster. Famciclovir tablets contain lactose. Patients with rare hereditary problems of galactose intolerance, a severe lactase deficiency, or glucose-galactose malabsorption should not take famciclovir tablets. It is unknown whether famciclovir crosses the placenta or is distributed in breast milk. Efficacy and safety have not been established in children. No age-related precautions have been noted in elderly patients.

Storage
Store at room temperature.

Administration
May be taken without regard to meals.

Famotidine

fam-oh'tah-deen
★ Pepcid, Pepcid AC
🍁 Pepcid, Pepcid AC, Peptic Guard, Ulcidine

CATEGORY AND SCHEDULE

Pregnancy Risk Category: B
Rx (10-mg tablets, 20-mg tablets, 40-mg tablets, injection, orally disintegrating tablets, oral suspension)
OTC (10-mg tablets, 20-mg tablets)

Classification: Gastrointestinal agents, antiulcer agents, histamine H_2 receptor antagonist

MECHANISM OF ACTION

An antiulcer agent and gastric acid secretion inhibitor that inhibits histamine action at H_2 receptors of parietal cells. *Therapeutic Effect:* Inhibits gastric acid secretion when fasting, at night, or when stimulated by food, caffeine, or insulin.

PHARMACOKINETICS

Route	Onset	Peak	Duration
PO	1 h	1-4 h	10-12 h
IV	0.5-1 h	0.5-3 h	10-12 h

Rapidly, incompletely absorbed from the GI tract. Protein binding: 15%-20%. Partially metabolized in the liver. Primarily excreted in urine. Not removed by hemodialysis. *Half-life:* 2.5-3.5 h (increased with impaired renal function).

AVAILABILITY

Tablets (OTC): 10 mg, 20 mg.
Chewable tablets (OTC): 10 mg.
Gelcaps (OTC): 10 mg.
Tablets (Rx): 10 mg, 20 mg, 40 mg.

Orally Disintegrating Tablets (Rx): 20 mg, 40 mg.
Oral Suspension (Rx): 40 mg/5 mL.
Injection (Rx): 10 mg/mL (1-mL, 2-mL, 4-mL, 20-mL, 50-mL vials; premixed 20 mg/50 mL).

INDICATIONS AND DOSAGES

▸ **Acute treatment of duodenal and gastric ulcers**
PO
Adults, Elderly, Children 17 yr and older. 40 mg/day at bedtime.
Children 1-16 yr. 0.5 mg/kg/day at bedtime. Maximum: 40 mg/day.

▸ **Duodenal ulcer maintenance**
PO
Adults, Elderly, Children 17 yr and older. 20 mg/day at bedtime.

▸ **Gastroesophageal reflux disease (GERD)**
PO
Adults, Elderly, Children 12 yr and older. 20 mg twice a day (maximum 40 mg BID).
Children aged 1-11 yr. 1 mg/kg/day in 2 divided doses (maximum 40 mg BID).
Children aged 3-12 mo. 0.5 mg/kg/dose twice a day.
Children younger than 3 mo. 0.5 mg/kg/dose once a day.

▸ **Esophagitis**
PO
Adults, Elderly, Children 12 yr and older. 20-40 mg twice a day.

▸ **Hypersecretory conditions**
PO
Adults, Elderly, Children 12 yr and older. Initially, 20 mg q6h. May increase up to 160 mg q6h.

▸ **Acid indigestion, heartburn (OTC)**
PO
Adults, Elderly, Children 12 yr and older. 10-20 mg 15-60 min before eating. Maximum: 2 doses per day.

▸ **Usual parenteral dosage**
IV
Adults, Elderly, Children 12 yr and older. 20 mg q12h.
Children 1-11 yr. 0.25-0.5 mg 1 kg q12h.

▸ **Dosage in renal impairment**
Dosing frequency is modified on the basis of creatinine clearance. May decrease dose by 50% or modify frequency, as follows:

Creatinine Clearance(mL/min)	Dosage Interval
10-50	q36-48h
< 10	q36-48h

OFF-LABEL USES

Urticaria, prevention of paclitaxel hypersensitivity reactions, stress ulcer prophylaxis in critically ill.

CONTRAINDICATIONS

Hypersensitivity to famotidine or other H_2 antagonists.

INTERACTIONS

Drug
Causes decreased oral absorption of following medications: May decrease the absorption of azole antifungals (monitor), atazanavir (boost with ritonovir), cefpodoxime (separate oral doses by 2 h), cefuroxime (separate oral doses by 2 h), dasatinib (avoid), saquinavir (monitor), gefitinib (monitor), cefditoren (avoid use), some modified release dosage forms may be altered as well.
Cyclosporine: Histamine H_2 antagonists may increase the serum concentration of cyclosporine (monitor).
Herbal and Food
None known.

DIAGNOSTIC TEST EFFECTS

May rarely cause decreases in WBC counts.

F

IV INCOMPATIBILITIES

Amphotericin B cholesteryl sulfate complex (Amphotec), azathioprine, azithromycin (Zithromax), cefepime (Maxipime), dantrolene, diazepam (Valium), ganciclovir (Cytovene), lansoprazole (Prevacid), minocycline (Minocin), pantoprazole (Protonix), piperacillin/tazobactam (Zosyn), rocuronium (Zemuron), sulfamethoxazole/trimethoprim.

IV COMPATIBILITIES

Acyclovir (Zovirax), alfentanil (Alfenta), allopurinol (Aloprim), amifostine (Ethyol), aminophylline, amiodarone, anakinra (Kineret), anidulafungin (Eraxis), ascorbic acid, atracurium (Tracrium), atropine, aztreonam (Azactam), benztropine (Cogentin), bivalirudin (Angiomax), bretylium, bumetanide (Bumex), buprenorphine (Buprenex), butorphanol (Stadol), calcium chloride, calcium gluconate, carboplatin, caspofungin (Cancidas), cefazolin, cefotaxime (Claforan), ceftazidime (Ceptaz, Fortaz, Tazicef, Tazidime), cefuroxime (Zinacef), chlorpromazine, cisatracurium (Nimbex), cisplatin, cladribine (Leustatin), clindamycin (Cleocin), cyclophosphamide (Cytoxan), cytarabine (Tarabine), dactinomycin (Cosmegen), daptomycin (Cubicin), dexamethasone sodium phosphate, dextran 40, digoxin (Lanoxin), diltiazem (Cardizem), diphenhydramine (Benadryl), dobutamine, docetaxel (Taxotere), dopamine, doripenem (Doribax), doxorubicin (Adriamycin), doxorubicin liposome (Doxil), droperidol (Inapsine), enalaprilat, epinephrine, epirubicin (Ellence), ertapenem (Invanz), erythromycin lactobionate, esmolol (Brevibloc), etoposide (VePesid), fenoldopam (Corlopam), fentanyl citrate (Sublimaze), filgrastim (Neupogen), fluconazole (Diflucan), fludarabine (Fludara), fluorouracil, folic acid, gemcitabine (Gemzar), gentamicin, granisetron (Kytril), heparin, hydrocortisone, hydrocortisone sodium succinate (Solu-Cortef), hydromorphone (Dilaudid), hydroxyzine, imipenem/cilastatin (Primaxin), isoproterenol (Isuprel), ketorolac, labetalol (Trandate), levofloxacin (Levaquin), lidocaine, linezolid (Zyvox), lorazepam (Ativan), magnesium sulfate, mannitol, melphalan (Alkeran), meperidine (Demerol), methotrexate, methylprednisolone sodium succinate (Solu-Medrol), metoclopramide (Reglan), metoprolol (Lopressor), metronidazole (Flagyl), midazolam, milrinone (Primacor), mitoxantrone (Novantrone), morphine, nafcillin, naloxone (Narcan), nicardipine (Cardene), nitroglycerin, norepinephrine (Levophed), ondansetron (Zofran), oxacillin, oxaliplatin (Eloxatin), oxytocin (Pitocin), paclitaxel (Taxol), palonosetron (Aloxi), pemetrexed (Alimta), penicillin G potassium, penicillin G sodium, phenylephrine (Neo-Synephrine), phytonadione, potassium chloride, potassium phosphates, procainamide, promethazine, propofol (Diprivan), propranolol (Inderal), protamine, ranitidine (Zantac), remifentanil (Ultiva), rituximab (Rituxan), sargramostim (Leukine), sodium acetate, sodium nitroprusside (Nitropress), succinylcholine (Anectine, Quelicin), sufentanil (Sufenta), tacrolimus (Prograf), teniposide (Vumon), theophylline, thiamine, thiotepa (Thioplex), ticarcillin (Ticar), ticarcillin/

clavulanate potassium (Timentin), tigecycline (Tygacil), tirofiban (Aggrastat), tobramycin, trastuzumab (Herceptin), vecuronium (Norcuron), verapamil, vincristine (Vincasar), vinorelbine (Navelbine), voriconazole (Vfend).

SIDE EFFECTS

Occasional (2%-10%)
Headache.
Rare (1% or less)
Constipation, diarrhea, dizziness.

SERIOUS REACTIONS

- Rare: agranulocytosis, pancytopenia, leukopenia, thrombocytopenia.

PRECAUTIONS & CONSIDERATIONS

Caution is warranted in patients with moderate to severe renal impairment because CNS adverse reactions may occur. Famotidine crosses the placenta and is distributed in breast milk. No age-related precautions have been noted in elderly patients. RPD and chewable tablets contain aspartame (caution: phenylketonuria).

Storage
Store tablets at controlled room temperature.

Store injection vials in the refrigerator; do not freeze. Store premixed infusion at room temperature. If solution freezes, bring to room temperature; allow sufficient time to solubilize.

Solution is stable for 7 days at room temperature when added to or diluted with most commonly used IV solutions. When added to or diluted with sodium bicarbonate injection, a precipitate may form. Diluted solutions of famotidine injection should be refrigerated and used within 48 h.

Administration
IV push: Dilute no more than 20 mg to total volume 5 or 10 mL and inject over not < 2 min.

IV infusion: Dilute with 50-100 mL of solution and administer over 15-30 min.

Shake oral suspension well prior to each use. For oral use to relieve symptoms, may give without regard to meals. To prevent symptoms, give 60 min before eating food that causes heartburn.

Febuxostat

feb-ux'oh-stat
Uloric

CATEGORY AND SCHEDULE

Pregnancy Risk Category: C

Classification: Antigout agents, antihyperuricemic, xanthine-oxidase inhibitor

MECHANISM OF ACTION

A xanthine oxidase inhibitor that decreases uric acid production by inhibiting xanthine oxidase, an enzyme. *Therapeutic Effect:* Reduces uric acid concentrations in both serum and urine.

PHARMACOKINETICS

Well absorbed from the GI tract. Protein binding: Roughly 99%. Widely distributed. Metabolized in the liver to four active metabolites. Excreted in urine and feces as unchanged drug and metabolites. Removed by hemodialysis. *Half-life:* 5-8 h (febuxostat); metabolites, 12-30 h.

AVAILABILITY

Tablet: 40 mg, 80 mg.

INDICATIONS AND DOSAGES

▸ For chronic management of hyperuricemia due to gout

PO

Adults, Elderly. Initially, 40 mg once daily. Testing for the target serum uric acid level of less than 6 mg/dL may be performed as early as 2 wks after initiating therapy.

After 2 wks may increase to 80 mg once daily if needed to achieve goal. No dose modifications are needed in mild or moderate renal or hepatic impairment. Use caution in patients with CrCl < 30 mL/min.

CONTRAINDICATIONS

History of hypersensitivity to febuxostat, and in patients being treated with azathioprine, mercaptopurine, or theophylline.

INTERACTIONS

Drug

Azathioprine, mercaptopurine: May increase toxicity of azathioprine and mercaptopurine via inhibition of xanthine oxidase. Contraindicated.

Theophylline: May increase toxicity of theophylline via inhibition of xanthine oxidase. Contraindicated.

Herbal

None known.

Food

None known.

DIAGNOSTIC TEST EFFECTS

Expected to lower uric acid level. May increase AST (SGOT) and ALT (SGPT) levels. May alter blood counts. Increased blood glucose, lipids, serum creatinine occasionally reported.

SIDE EFFECTS

Occasional (≥ 1%)

Liver function enzyme increase, nausea, arthralgia, and rash.

Rare (<1%)

Headache, change in appetite, constipation, insomnia, alopecia, urinary disturbances.

SERIOUS REACTIONS

- Severe hypersensitivity is rare.
- Bone marrow depression.
- Hepatic toxicity occurs very rarely.
- Increased rate of thromboembolic events, such as heart attack and stroke; these occur rarely and causality is not established.

PRECAUTIONS & CONSIDERATIONS

No recommended for patients who have asymptomatic hyperuricemia. Caution is warranted with cardiac disease, diabetes mellitus, hypertension, and severely impaired renal or hepatic function. It is unknown whether febuxostat crosses the placenta. It is likely the drug is excreted in breast milk based on animal studies; use with caution in nursing women. No age-related precautions have been noted in elderly patients. Not approved for use in children. The drug should be discontinued if rash or other evidence of allergic reaction appears. Avoid tasks that require mental alertness or motor skills until response to the drug has been established.

Encourage good fluid intake. Gout flares occur in early therapy but treatment can be continued. Monitor CBC, liver function tests, and serum uric acid levels. Signs and symptoms of a therapeutic response, including improved joint range of motion and reduced redness, swelling, and tenderness, should be evaluated.

Storage

Store at room temperature. Protect from light.

Administration

May take with food or antacids. Drink enough fluid daily to maintain good urine output. It may take 1-2 wks for the full therapeutic effect of the drug to be evident.

Felbamate

fel′ba-mate

Felbatol

CATEGORY AND SCHEDULE

Pregnancy Risk Category: C

Classification: Anticonvulsant (carbamate derivative)

MECHANISM OF ACTION

An anticonvulsant, structurally similar to meprobamate, that weakly blocks repetitive, sustained firing of neurons by enhancing the ability of γ-aminobutyric acid (GABA) and antagonizes the strychnine-insensitive glycine recognition site of the *N*-methyl-d-aspartate receptor-ionophore complex. *Therapeutic Effect:* Decreases seizure activity.

PHARMACOKINETICS

Rapidly and almost completely absorbed after PO administration. Protein binding: 22%-25%, primarily to albumin. Partially excreted unchanged in the urine (40%-50% of absorbed dose). Unidentified metabolites and conjugates account for 40% of dose. *Half-life:* 20-23 h.

AVAILABILITY

Tablets: 400 mg, 600 mg.
Oral Suspension: 600 mg/5mL (240 mL and 960 mL).

INDICATIONS AND DOSAGES

Not indicated as first-line antiepileptic treatment.

▸ **Monotherapy or adjunctive therapy in the treatment of partial seizures, with and without generalization**

PO

Adults, Children 14 yr and older. Initially, 1200 mg/day in divided doses 3-4 times a day. Increase the felbamate dosage by 600-mg increments every 2 wks to 2400 mg/day based on clinical response up to 3600 mg/day as clinically indicated. Reduce the dosage of other antiepileptic drugs (AEDs) by one third of their original dosage at initiation of felbamate. At wk 2, increase dose of felbamate to 2400 mg/day and reduce dose of other AEDs by an additional one third of their original dose. At wk 3, increase the felbamate dosage up to 3600 mg/day and continue to reduce the dosage of other AEDs as clinically indicated.

▸ **Adjunctive therapy in the treatment of partial seizures, with and without generalization**

PO

Adults, Children 14 yr and older. Add 1200 mg/day in divided doses 3-4 times a day while reducing present AEDs by 20% in order-control plasma concentrations of concurrent phenytoin, valproic acid, and carbamazepine and its metabolites. Increase dosage by 1200 mg/day increments at weekly intervals to 3600 mg/day. Continuous reduction of the other AEDs may be necessary to control side effects.

▸ **Lennox-Gastaut syndrome**

PO

Children 2-14 yr. Add felbamate at 15 mg/kg/day in divided doses 3-4 times a day while reducing present AEDs by 20% in order-control plasma concentrations of concurrent phenytoin, valproic acid, and carbamazepine and its metabolites. Increase the dosage of felbamate by

15 mg/kg/day increments at weekly intervals to 45 mg/kg/day. Continuous reduction of the other AEDs may be necessary to control side effects.

▸ **Dosage in renal impairment**

Manufacturer recommends reducing usual dosages by 50%.

OFF-LABEL USES

None known.

CONTRAINDICATIONS

History of any blood dyscrasia or hepatic dysfunction, hypersensitivity to felbamate, its ingredients, or known sensitivity to other carbamates.

INTERACTIONS

Drug

Carbamazepine: Concentration of carbamazepine decreased, felbamate concentration decreased. Carbamazepine epoxide metabolite concentration increased.

CYP inducers and inhibitors: May affect felbamate concentrations.

Phenobarbital: Concentration of phenobarbital increased.

Phenytoin: Concentration of phenytoin increased, felbamate decreased (20% reduction in phenytoin dose resulted in phenytoin levels similar to baseline).

Valproate: Concentration of valproate increased.

Herbal and Food

None known.

DIAGNOSTIC TEST EFFECTS

Hemoglobin decreases. AST, ALT, GGT increases. Prothrombin increased or decreased. Be alert to decreased WBC, platelet, or reticulocyte counts.

SIDE EFFECTS

Frequent (> 10%)

Anorexia, vomiting, insomnia, nervousness, nausea, headache, dizziness, somnolence, fatigue, constipation, dyspepsia, fever (children), upper respiratory infection.

Occasional (1%-10%)

Rhinitis, tremor, diplopia, taste perversion, abnormal vision, abnormal gait, abdominal pain, depression, anxiety, ataxia, paresthesia, rash, acne, intramenstrual bleeding, weight decrease, facial edema, myalgia, pharyngitis, chest pain, dry mouth, weight increase, palpitations, tachycardia, psychologic disturbance, aggressive reaction.

Rare (< 1%)

Anaphylactoid reaction, delusion, hallucinations, urinary retention, acute renal failure.

SERIOUS REACTIONS

- Aplastic anemia has been reported during felbamate therapy.
- Hepatic failure resulting in death has been reported. Hepatotoxicity can develop without warning signs; discontinue drug if liver enzymes are ≥ 2 times the upper limit of normal.

PRECAUTIONS & CONSIDERATIONS

Warning of increased risk of aplastic anemia, hepatic failure; safety and efficacy in children with other types of seizures have not been established. Rapid withdrawal of antiepileptic drugs could result in rebound seizures. Should be used with caution in renal dysfunction. Antiepileptic drugs (AEDs) may increase the risk of suicidal thoughts or behavior; monitor for the emergence or worsening of depression, suicidal thoughts, and/or any unusual changes in mood or behavior. Felbamate is likely to cross the placenta and is excreted in breast milk. Do not use during lactation.

Seizure frequency, liver function, and CBC should be regularly monitored.

Storage
Store at room temperature, keep tightly closed.
Administration
Administer without regard to food. Shake suspension well before use.

Felodipine

fell-oh'da-peen
Plendil Renedil
Do not confuse Plendil with Pletal or Prinivil.

CATEGORY AND SCHEDULE

Pregnancy Risk Category: C

Classification: Antihypertensive agents, calcium channel blockers

MECHANISM OF ACTION

An antihypertensive and antianginal agent that inhibits calcium movement across cardiac and vascular smooth-muscle cell membranes. Potent peripheral vasodilator (does not depress SA or AV nodes) (dihydropyridine derivative). *Therapeutic Effect:* Increases myocardial contractility, heart rate, and cardiac output; decreases peripheral vascular resistance and BP.

PHARMACOKINETICS

Route	Onset	Peak	Duration
PO	2-5 h	N/A	24 h

Rapidly, completely absorbed from the GI tract. Protein binding: > 99%. Undergoes first-pass metabolism in the liver (205%). Primarily excreted in urine. Not removed by hemodialysis. *Half-life:* 11-16 h.

AVAILABILITY

Tablets, Extended Release: 2.5 mg, 5 mg, 10 mg.

INDICATIONS AND DOSAGES

▸ **Hypertension**
PO
Adults. Initially, 5 mg/day as single dose. Adjust dosage at no less than 2-wk intervals. Usual range: 2.5-10 mg/day.
Elderly, Patients with impaired hepatic function. Initially, 2.5 mg/day. Adjust dosage at no less than 2-wk intervals. Maintenance: 2.5-10 mg/day.

OFF-LABEL USES

Chronic angina pectoris, pediatric hypertension.

CONTRAIDICATIONS

Hypersensitivity, sick sinus syndrome, second- or third-degree heart block, SBP < 90 mm Hg.

INTERACTIONS

Drug
Amiodarone: May result in bradycardia, atrioventricular block, and/or sinus arrest.
β-Blockers: Increased pharmacodynamic effects.
Carbamazepine, phenobarbital, phenytoin: Decreased felodipine concentration.
CYP inducers and inhibitors: May affect felodipine concentrations.
CYP2C8 substrates: Felodipine may inhibit metabolism of substrates.
Fentanyl: May result in severe hypotension.
Itraconazole (and other azole antifungals), erythromycin, cimetidine, cyclosporine: Increased felodipine concentration.
Nafcillin, rifampin: Decreased felodipine concentration.
NSAIDs: Decreased hypotensive effect or increased risk for GI complications.
Sildenafil, tadalafil, vardenafil: Additive hypotensive effects possible.
Tacrolimus: Concentration increased by felodipine.

Herbal
St. John's wort: May decrease felodipine levels.
Food
Grapefruit juice: Increases felodipine concentration.

SIDE EFFECTS

Frequent (> 10%)
Headache, peripheral edema.
Occasional (1%-10%)
Flushing, respiratory infection, dizziness, light-headedness, palpitations, dyspepsia, asthenia (loss of strength, weakness), constipation, mild gingival hyperplasia.
Rare
Paresthesia, abdominal discomfort, nervousness, muscle cramping, cough, diarrhea.

SERIOUS REACTIONS

- Overdose produces nausea, somnolence, confusion, slurred speech, hypotension, and bradycardia. Contact Poison Control Center if overdose suspected.
- Hypotension, syncope, reflex tachycardia. Arrhythmia, myocardial infarction.

PRECAUTIONS & CONSIDERATIONS

Congestive heart failure, hypotension < 90 mm Hg systolic, hepatic injury/impairment, children, renal disease, elderly patients. It is unknown whether felodipine is distributed in breast milk; there are no adequate data in human pregnancy.
Storage
Store at room temperature; keep tightly closed and protect from light.
Administration
Take without food or give only with a light meal. Swallow whole and do not crush or chew. Generally avoid taking with grapefruit juice to avoid increased maximal concentrations.

Fenofibrate

fee-no-fye′brate
🇺🇸 Antara, Fenoglide, Lipofen, Lofibra, TriCor, Triglide
🇨🇦 Apo-Fenofibrate, Feno-Micro, Fenomax, Lipidil
Do not confuse Tricor with Tracleer.

CATEGORY AND SCHEDULE

Pregnancy Risk Category: C

Classification: Antihyperlipidemics, fibric acid derivatives

MECHANISM OF ACTION

An antihyperlipidemic that enhances synthesis of lipoprotein lipase and reduces triglyceride-rich lipoproteins and VLDLs. *Therapeutic Effect:* Increases VLDL catabolism and reduces total triglyceride levels. Increases HDL levels.

PHARMACOKINETICS

Well absorbed from the GI tract. Micronized and nonmicronized forms are bioequivalent. Absorption increased when given with food. Protein binding: 99%. Rapidly metabolized in the liver to active metabolite. Excreted primarily in urine; lesser amount in feces. Not removed by hemodialysis. *Half-life:* 16-23 h.

AVAILABILITY

Tablets: 40 mg, 48 mg, 50 mg, 54 mg, 107 mg, 120 mg, 145 mg, 160 mg.
Capsules: 50 mg, 150 mg.
Capsules, Micronized Fenofibrate: 43 mg, 67 mg, 130 mg, 134 mg, 200 mg.

INDICATIONS AND DOSAGES

▸ **Hypertriglyceridemia**
PO
Adults, Elderly. Antara (micronized) capsule: Initially, 43-130 mg/day; may increase to 130 mg/day.

Fenoglide (nonmicronized) tablet: Initially, 40-120 mg/day; may increase to 120 mg/day.
Lipofen (nonmicronized) capsule: Initially, 50-150 mg/day; may increase to 150 mg/day.
Lofibra (micronized) capsule: Initially, 67-200 mg/day; may increase to 200 mg/day.
Lofibra (nonmicronized) tablet: Initially, 54-160 mg/day; may increase to 160 mg/day.
TriCor (nonmicronized) tablet: Initially, 48-145 mg/day; may increase to 145 mg/day.
Triglide (nonmicronized) tablet: Initially, 50-160 mg/day; may increase to 160 mg/day.

Dosage in renal impairment
Antara (micronized) capsule: Initially, 43 mg/day.
Fenoglide (nonmicronized) tablet: CrCl 31-80 mL/min initially, 40 mg/day, CrCl < 30 mL/min contraindicated.
Lipofen (nonmicronized) capsule: Initially, 50 mg/day.
Lofibra (micronized) capsule: Initially, 67 mg/day.
Lofibra (nonmicronized) tablet: Initially, 54 mg/day.
TriCor (nonmicronized) tablet: CrCl 31-80 mL/min initially, 48 mg/day, CrCl < 30 mL/min contraindicated.
Triglide (nonmicronized) tablet: CrCl 11-49 mL/min initially, 50 mg/day. CrCl < 10 mL/min contraindicated.

OFF-LABEL USES
Hyperuricemia, gout, metabolic syndrome.

CONTRAINDICATIONS
Gallbladder disease, hypersensitivity to fenofibrate, severe renal or hepatic dysfunction (including primary biliary cirrhosis, unexplained persistent liver function abnormality).

INTERACTIONS
Drug
Bile acid sequestrants: Decrease absorption of fenofibrate (give fenofibrate 1 h before or 4-6 h after).
Cyclosporine: Concomitant use may lead to renal dysfunction.
Ezetimibe: Fenofibrate may increase concentrations.
HMG-CoA reductase inhibitors (atorvastatin, fluvastatin, lovastatin, pravastatin, rosuvastatin, simvastatin): May increase the risk of myopathy and rhabdomyolysis. Extreme caution is warranted if used concomitantly or avoid use. Monitor.
Sulfonylureas: Enhanced hypoglycemic effects.
Warfarin: May increase the anticoagulant effect of warfarin; monitor INR closely and adjust warfarin dose as needed.
Herbal
None known.
Food
None known.

DIAGNOSTIC TEST EFFECTS
Increased AST, ALT, CPK, creatinine, GGT.

SIDE EFFECTS
Occasional (1%-10%)
AST/ALT elevation, respiratory disorder, abdominal pain, back pain, headache, flu symptoms, asthenia, nausea, vomiting, diarrhea, rhinitis, constipation, asthenia.
Rare (< 1%)
Anxiety, acne, anorexia, anemia, edema, arthralgia, insomnia, polyuria, cough, abnormal vision, eye floaters, earache.

SERIOUS REACTIONS

- Fenofibrate may increase excretion of cholesterol into bile, leading to cholelithiasis.
- Hypersensitivity reactions, pancreatitis, hepatitis, thrombocytopenia, and agranulocytosis occur rarely.

PRECAUTIONS & CONSIDERATIONS

Monitor liver function; may lead to pancreatitis or cholelithiasis; can be associated with myositis, myopathy, or rhabdomyolysis; renal function impairment; discontinue use if no response in 2 mo; base dose in elderly on renal function, monitor for adverse effects.

Not recommended for use in pregnancy or lactation due to potential tumorigenicity. Safety and efficacy in children have not been established.

Storage

Store at room temperature. Protect from moisture and light.

Administration

Fenoglide, Lofibra, Lipofen should be administered with meals.
Antara, TriCor may be administered with or without meals.
Triglide may be administered with or without meals.

Fenoprofen

fen-oh-proe′fen

★ Nalfon

Do not confuse Nalfon with Naldecon.

CATEGORY AND SCHEDULE

Pregnancy Risk Category: B (D if used in third trimester or near delivery)

Classification: Analgesics, nonsteroidal anti-inflammatory drugs

MECHANISM OF ACTION

An NSAID that produces analgesic, antipyretic, and anti-inflammatory effects by inhibiting prostaglandin synthesis. *Therapeutic Effect:* Reduces the inflammatory response, fever, and intensity of pain.

AVAILABILITY

Capsules: 200 mg, 400 mg.
Tablets: 600 mg.

INDICATIONS AND DOSAGES

▸ **Mild to moderate pain**

PO

Adults, Elderly. 200 mg q4-6h as needed.

▸ **Rheumatoid arthritis, osteoarthritis**

PO

Adults, Elderly. 400-600 mg 3-4 times a day. Total daily dose should not exceed 3200 mg.

OFF-LABEL USES

Treatment of ankylosing spondylitis, migraine, psoriatic arthritis, tendinitis, vascular headaches.

CONTRAINDICATIONS

Active peptic ulcer disease, chronic inflammation of GI tract, GI bleeding or ulceration, history of hypersensitivity to aspirin or NSAIDs, significant renal impairment; use within 14 days of coronary artery bypass graft (CABG) surgery.

INTERACTIONS

Drug

Antihypertensives, diuretics: May decrease the effects of these drugs.
Aspirin, other salicylates: May increase the risk of GI side effects such as bleeding. NSAID use may negate cardioprotective effect of ASA.
Bile acid sequestrants: May decrease absorption.

Corticosteroids: May increase risk of GI ulceration.
Cyclosporine: May increase nephrotoxicity and serum levels of cyclosporine.
Heparin, oral anticoagulants, antiplatelets, thrombolytics: May increase the effects of these drugs.
Lithium: May increase the blood concentration and risk of toxicity of lithium.
Methotrexate: May increase the risk of methotrexate toxicity and methotrexate levels.
SSRIs, SNRIs: Increased risk of GI bleeding.
Warfarin: Effects on GI bleeding are synergistic; risk of serious GI bleeding higher than users of either drug alone.
Vancomycin: May increase levels of vancomycin.

Herbal

Supplements with antiplatelet or anticoagulant effects (e.g., feverfew, garlic, ginger, ginkgo biloba, ginseng, red clover, sweet clover, white willow): May increase effects on platelets or risk of bleeding.

Food

Alcohol: May increase risk of dizziness or GI irritation/bleeding.

DIAGNOSTIC TEST EFFECTS

May increase bleeding time, BUN and blood glucose levels, and serum protein, alkaline phosphatase, LDH, creatinine, AST (SGOT), and ALT (SGPT) levels.

SIDE EFFECTS

Frequent (3%-10%)
Headache, somnolence, dyspepsia, nausea, vomiting, constipation, dizziness, sweating, pruritus, rash, blurred vision.

Occasional (1%-2%)
Dizziness, nervousness, asthenia, diarrhea, abdominal cramps, flatulence, tinnitus, peripheral edema, tremor, confusion, and fluid retention.

SERIOUS REACTIONS

- Overdose may result in acute hypotension and tachycardia.
- Rare reactions with long-term use include peptic ulcer disease, GI bleeding, gastritis, severe hepatic reaction (jaundice), nephrotoxicity (hematuria, dysuria, proteinuria), and a severe hypersensitivity reaction (bronchospasm, angioedema).
- Hypersensitivity may include serious skin rash such as Stevens-Johnson syndrome.

PRECAUTIONS & CONSIDERATIONS

Caution is warranted with hepatic or renal impairment and history of GI disease. Caution is warranted in patients with a history of active peptic ulcer disease, chronic inflammation of GI tract, GI bleeding, or ulceration. Use the lowest effective dose for the shortest duration of time. Anaphylactoid reactions have occurred in patients with aspirin triad hypersensitivity. Cardiovascular event risk may be increased with duration of use or preexisting cardiovascular risk factors or disease. Use caution in patients with fluid retention, heart failure, or hypertension. Risk of myocardial infarction and stroke may be increased following CABG surgery.

Fenoprofen crosses the placenta and is distributed in breast milk. Fenoprofen should not be used during the last trimester of pregnancy because it may cause adverse effects in the fetus, such as premature closure of the ductus arteriosus. The safety and efficacy of fenoprofen have not been established in children. In elderly patients, GI bleeding or ulceration is more likely to cause serious complications, and age-related renal impairment may increase the risk of hepatotoxicity or renal toxicity; a decreased drug dosage is recommended. Tasks that require mental alertness or motor skills should be avoided until response to the drug has been established.

Baseline bleeding time, BUN and blood glucose levels, creatinine, liver function tests, and urinary protein levels should be obtained at the beginning of therapy. Pattern of daily bowel activity and stool consistency should be assessed. Therapeutic response, such as decreased pain, stiffness, swelling, and tenderness, improved grip strength, and increased joint mobility, should be evaluated.

Storage

Store at room temperature.

Administration

Swallow whole; do not crush, open, or break. Administer with food to decrease GI irritation.

Fentanyl

fen'ta-nil

★ Actiq, Duragesic, Fentora, Onsolis, Sublimaze 🍁 Duragesic

Do not confuse fentanyl with alfentanil, remifentanil, or sufentanil.

CATEGORY AND SCHEDULE

Pregnancy Risk Category: C (D if used for prolonged periods or at high dosages at term)

Controlled Substance Schedule: II

Classification: Analgesics, narcotic; anesthetics, general

MECHANISM OF ACTION

An opioid agonist that binds to opioid receptors in the CNS, reducing stimuli from sensory nerve endings and inhibiting ascending pain pathways. *Therapeutic Effect:* Alters pain reception and increases the pain threshold.

PHARMACOKINETICS

Route	Onset	Peak	Duration
IV	1-2 min	3-5 min	0.5-1 h
IM	7-15 min	20-30 min	1-2 h
Transdermal	6-8 h	24 h	72 h
Transmucosal	5-15 min	20-30 min	1-2 h

Well absorbed after IM or topical administration. Transmucosal form absorbed through the buccal mucosa and GI tract. Protein binding: 80%-85%. Metabolized in the liver by CYP3A4. Primarily eliminated by biliary system. *Half-life:* 2-4 h IV; 17 h transdermal patch; 3.2-5.9 h transmucosal lozenge; 3-12 h buccal tablet.

AVAILABILITY

Injection (Sublimaze): 50 mcg/mL.
Transdermal Patch (Duragesic): 12.5 mcg/h, 25 mcg/h, 50 mcg/h, 75 mcg/h, 100 mcg/h.
Transmucosal Lozenges (Actiq): 200 mcg, 400 mcg, 600 mcg, 800 mcg, 1200 mcg, 1600 mcg.
Transmucosal Buccal Tablets: 100 mcg, 200 mcg, 400 mcg, 600 mcg, 800 mcg.
Transmucosoal Buccal Film (Onsolis): 200 mcg, 400 mcg, 600 mcg, 800 mcg, 1200 mcg.

INDICATIONS AND DOSAGES

▸ **Premedication**

IV, IM

Adults, Elderly, Children 12 yr and older. 50-100 mcg/dose 30-60 min before surgery.

▸ **Adjunct to general anesthesia**
IV
Adults, Elderly, Children 12 yr and older. Low dose: 0.5-2 mcg/kg/dose; moderate dose: 2-20 mcg/kg/dose; high dose: 20-50 mcg/kg.
Children 2-12 yr. Induction and maintenance. 2-3 mcg/kg/dose.

▸ **Adjunct to regional anesthesia**
IV, IM
Adults, Elderly, Children 12 yr and older. 25-100 mcg over 1-2 min.

▸ **Postoperative pain**
IM
Adults, Elderly, Children 12 yr and older. 50-100 mcg every 1-2 h as needed.

▸ **Chronic pain management**
USUAL TRANSDERMAL DOSE
Adults, Elderly, Children 12 yr and older. Use dose conversion chart to convert patients from oral or IV opioids. May increase after 3 days and then every 6 days thereafter. Should not be used in opioid-naïve patients. Upon system removal, 17 h or more are required for a 50% decrease in serum fentanyl concentrations. Effects on respiratory system may persist for longer.

▸ **Breakthrough cancer pain**
USUAL TRANSMUCOSAL DOSE (LOZENGE)
Adults, Children. Initial 200 mcg. May start second unit 15 min after completing first if needed. If more than one lozenge is needed per episode for several episodes, consider prescribing next highest strength.
USUAL TRANSMUCOSAL DOSE (BUCCAL TABLET)
Adults, Children. Initial 100 mcg; redosing can occur 30 min after start of first tablet, if necessary. Dose titration should be done in 100-mcg increments up to 400 mcg. See prescribing information for converting from lozenge.
USUAL TRANSMUCOSAL DOSE (BUCCAL FILM)
Adults: Initial 200 mcg; redosing can occur 2 h after start of first film, if necessary. Dose titration should be done in 200-mcg increments. Maximum is 4 × 200 mcg films or one 1200 mcg film per dose. NMT 4 doses per day are allowed; doses should be separated by at least 2 h. See prescribing information.
USUAL EPIDURAL DOSE
Adults, Elderly. Bolus dose of 100 mcg, followed by continuous infusion of 10 mcg/mL concentration at 4-12 mL/h.

▸ **Continuous analgesia**
IV
Adults, Elderly, Children 1-12 yr. Bolus dose of 1-2 mcg/kg, followed by continuous infusion of 1 mcg/kg/h. Range: 1-5 mcg/kg/h.
Children younger than 1 yr. Bolus dose of 1-2 mcg/kg, followed by continuous infusion of 0.5-1 mcg/kg/h.

▸ **Dosage in renal impairment**
Dosage is modified based on creatinine clearance.

Creatinine Clearance	Dosage
10-50 mL/min	75% of usual dose
< 10 mL/min	50% of usual dose

CONTRAINDICATIONS
Increased intracranial pressure, severe hepatic or renal impairment, severe respiratory depression, severe bronchial asthma, paralytic ileus. Hypersensitivity to fentanyl. Fentanyl lozenge, buccal tablet, and transdermal patch are contraindicated for acute or postoperative pain and opioid nontolerant patients.

INTERACTIONS

Drug

Amiodarone: Profound bradycardia, sinus arrest, and hypotension have occurred with coadministration.

Benzodiazepines, CNS depressants: May increase the risk of hypotension and respiratory depression, sedation.

Buprenorphine: May decrease the effects of fentanyl.

CYP3A4 inhibitors: May increase concentration of fentanyl. CYP3A4 inducers may decrease concentration of fentanyl.

MAOIs: Should not be used.

Ritonavir: Increases fentanyl concentrations.

Herbal

St. John's wort: May decrease fentanyl levels.

Food

None known.

DIAGNOSTIC TEST EFFECTS

May increase serum amylase and lipase concentrations.

IV INCOMPATIBILITIES

Azithromycin (Zithromax), dantrolene, hydroxocobalamin, pantoprazole (Protonix), phenytoin (Dilantin), sulfamethoxazole/trimethoprim.

IV COMPATIBILITIES

Abciximab (Reopro), acyclovir (Zovirax), alfentanil (Alfenta), alprostadil (Prostin VR), amikacin (Amikin), aminophylline, amiodarone, amphotericin B cholesteryl complex (Amphotec), amphotericin B liposome (AmBisome), anidulafungin (Eraxis), argatroban, ascorbic acid, atracurium (Tracrium), atropine, azathioprine, aztreonam (Azactam), benztropine (Cogentin), bivalirudin (Angiomax), bretylium, bumetanide (Bumex), bupivacaine (Marcaine, Sensorcaine), buprenorphine (Buprenex), butorphanol (Stadol), caffeine citrate (Cafcit), calcium chloride, calcium gluconate, carboplatin, caspofungin (Cancidas), cefazolin, cefotaxime (Claforan), cefoxitin (Mefoxin), ceftazidime (Ceptaz, Fortaz, Tazicef, Tazidime), ceftizoxime (Cefizox), cefuroxime (Zinacef), chloramphenicol, chlorpromazine, cimetidine, cisatracurium (Nimbex), cisplatin, clindamycin (Cleocin), clonidine (Duraclon), cyanocobalamin, cyclophosphamide (Cytoxan), cyclosporine (Sandimmune), dactinomycin (Cosmegen), daptomycin (Cubicin), dexamethasone sodium phosphate, digoxin (Lanoxin), diltiazem (Cardizem), diphenhydramine (Benadryl), dobutamine (Dobutrex), docetaxel (Taxotere), dopamine (Intropin), doripenem (Doribax), doxorubicin (Adriamycin), droperidol (Inapsine), emolol (Brevibloc), enalaprilat, ephedrine, epinephrine, epirubicin (Ellence), epoetin alfa (Procrit), erythromycin lactobionate, etomidate (Amidate), etoposide phosphate (Etopophos), famotidine (Pepcid), fenoldopam (Corlopam), fluconazole (Diflucan), fludarabine (Fludara), folic acid, furosemide (Lasix), ganciclovir (Cytovene), gemcitabine (Gemzar), gentamicin, glycopyrrolate, granisetron (Kytril), heparin, hydrocortisone sodium succinate (Solu-Cortef), hydromorphone (Dilaudid), hydroxyzine, imipenem/cliastatin (Primaxin), inamrinone, insulin (regular, Humulin R, Novolin R), isoproterenol (Isuprel), ketamine (Ketalar), ketorolac, labetalol, lansoprazole (Prevacid), levofloxacin (Levaquin), lidocaine, linezolid (Zyvox), lorazepam (Ativan), magnesium sulfate, mannitol, meperidine (Demerol), methicillin, methotrexate, methylprednisolone sodium succinate, metoclopramide (Reglan), metoprolol (Lopressor), metronidazole (Flagyl), midazolam, milrinone (Primacor), minocycline (Minocin), mitoxantron (Novantrone), mivacurium (Mivacron), morphine, nafcillin, nalbuphine (Nubain), naloxone (Narcan), nesiritide (Natrecor), nicardipine (Cardene), nitroglycerin, nitroprusside (Nitropress), norepinephrine (Levophed), ondansetron (Zofran), oxacillin, oxytocin (Pitocin), paclitaxel (Taxol), palonosetron (Aloxi), pancuronium, pemetrexed (Alimta), pencillin G potassium, pencillin G sodium, phenobarbital, phytonadione, piperacillin, piperacillin/tazobactam (Zosyn), potassium chloride, procainamide, promethazine, propofol (Diprivan), propranolol (Inderal), protamine, pyridoxine, quinupristin/dalfopristin (Synercid), ranitidine (Zantac), remifentanil (Ultiva), rituximab (Rituxan), sargramostim (Leukine), scopolamine, sodium acetate, sodium bicarbonate, streptokinase, succinylcholine (Anectine, Quelicin), sufentanil (Sufenta), tacrolimus (Prograf), teniposide (Vumon), theophylline, thiamine, thiotepa (Thioplex), ticarcillin (Ticar), ticarcillin/clavulanate (Timentin), tigecycline (Tygacil), tirofiban (Aggrastat), tobramycin, trastuzumab (Herceptin), vancomyin, vecuronium (Norcuron), verapamil, vincristine (Vincasar), vinorelbine (Navelbine), voriconazole (Vfend).

SIDE EFFECTS

Frequent

IV: Postoperative drowsiness, nausea, vomiting, dizziness.
Transdermal (3%-10%): Headache, pruritus, nausea, vomiting, diaphoresis, dyspnea, confusion, dizziness, somnolence, diarrhea, constipation, decreased appetite.
Lozenge (> 10%): Nausea, dizziness, somnolence, vomiting, constipation.
Buccal tablet (> 10%): Dizziness, nausea, headache, somnolence, asthenia, constipation.

Occasional

IV: Postoperative confusion, blurred vision, chills, hypertension, orthostatic hypotension, constipation, difficulty urinating.
Transdermal (1%-3%): Chest pain, arrhythmias, erythema, pruritus, swelling of skin, syncope, agitation, tingling or burning of skin.
Lozenge (2%-10%): Asthenia, headache, confusion, constipation, dyspnea, anxiety, abnormal gait, nervousness, pruritus, rash, sweating, abnormal vision, vasodilation.
Buccal tablet (2%-10%): Application-site reactions (pain, ulcer, irritation), vomiting, fatigue, confusion, depression, insomnia, abdominal pain, diarrhea, anorexia, weight decreased, arthralgia, back pain.

SERIOUS REACTIONS

- Respiratory depression, apnea, rigidity, and bradycardia are most common serious adverse reactions. If untreated, could lead to respiratory arrest, circulatory depression, or cardiac arrest.
- Overdose or too-rapid IV administration may produce severe respiratory depression and skeletal and thoracic muscle rigidity (which may lead to apnea), laryngospasm, bronchospasm, cold and clammy skin, cyanosis, and coma.
- The patient who uses fentanyl repeatedly may develop a tolerance to the drug's analgesic effect.

F

PRECAUTIONS & CONSIDERATIONS

Caution is warranted with bradycardia; head injuries; altered level of consciousness; hepatic, renal, or respiratory disease; history of drug abuse; and concurrent use of MAOIs within 14 days of fentanyl administration. Fentanyl readily crosses the placenta; it is unknown whether fentanyl is distributed in breast milk. Fentanyl may prolong labor if administered in the latent phase of the first stage of labor or before the cervix has dilated 4-5 cm. Fentanyl may cause respiratory depression in the neonate if it is given to the mother during labor. The transdermal form of fentanyl is not recommended for children younger than 12 yr or children younger than 18 yr and < 50 kg. Neonates and elderly patients are more susceptible to the drug's respiratory depressant effects. Age-related renal impairment may require a dosage adjustment in elderly patients. Abrupt discontinuation after prolonged use may result in withdrawal.

Dizziness and drowsiness may occur, so change positions slowly and avoid alcohol, CNS depressants, and tasks that require mental alertness or motor skills until response to the drug is established. BP, heart rate, respiratory rate, oxygen saturation, pattern of daily bowel activity and stool consistency, and clinical improvement of pain should be monitored.

Storage

Store the parenteral form at room temperature. Keep buccal and transmucosal forms away from moisture and protect from freezing. Transdermal patches should be kept in foil overwrap until time of application.

Administration

! Keep in mind that fentanyl may be combined with a local anesthetic, such as bupivacaine. Discontinue fentanyl slowly after long-term use.

For IV use, make sure resuscitative equipment and an opiate antagonist (naloxone 0.5 mcg/kg) are readily available before administering the drug. For initial anesthesia induction, give a small amount by tuberculin syringe, as prescribed. Give by slow IV push, over 1-2 min. A too-rapid IV infusion increases the risk of severe adverse reactions, such as anaphylaxis, bronchospasm, laryngospasm, peripheral circulatory collapse, cardiac arrest, and skeletal and thoracic muscle rigidity (which may result in apnea).

For transdermal patch use, clean the patch site before application; use only water, because soap and oils may irritate the skin. Allow the skin to dry. Apply the patch to a flat, unirritated, nonhairy (or clip hair; do not shave) area of intact skin on the upper torso, chest, back, flank, or upper arm. Apply immediately after removing from sealed package. Do not cut or alter patch. Press the patch onto the skin firmly and evenly for 30 seconds, ensuring that it comes in full contact with the skin, especially around the edges. Each patch should be worn continuously for 72 h. Rotate application sites. Patients must avoid exposing the patch to excessive heat, because this promotes the release of fentanyl from the patch and increases the absorption of fentanyl through the skin, which can result in fatal overdose. Monitor patients with a fever carefully. Carefully fold used patches so that they adhere to themselves, and discard them in the toilet. Patients should dispose of any patches remaining from a prescription as soon as they are no longer needed. Unused patches should be removed from their pouches, folded so that the adhesive side of the patch adheres to itself, and flushed down the toilet. If the gel from the drug reservoir accidentally contacts the skin of the patient or caregiver, the skin should be washed with copious amounts of water. Do not use soap, alcohol, or other solvents to remove the gel, because they may enhance the drug's ability to penetrate the skin. Keep out of the reach of children. Oral ingestion of gel from patches may cause fatality.

Transmucosal lozenge: Open the blister package with scissors immediately before product use. Place the unit in the patient's mouth between the cheek and lower gum, moving it from one side to the other, using the handle. Instruct the patient to suck, not chew, the lozenge for 15 min for optimal efficacy. If signs of excessive opioid effects appear before the unit is consumed, remove the drug matrix from the patient's mouth immediately and decrease future doses. Fentanyl lozenge contains medicine in an amount that could be fatal to a child. Dispose of units remaining from a prescription as soon as they are no longer needed. Dispose of all units immediately after use. Partially consumed units represent a special risk because they are no longer protected by the child-resistant pouch and yet may contain enough medicine to be fatal to a child. A temporary storage bottle is provided to be used in the event that a partially consumed unit cannot be disposed of promptly.

Transmucosal buccal tablet: Open the blister pack immediately before use. The blister backing should then be peeled back to expose the tablet. Patients should NOT attempt to push the tablet through the blister because to do so may cause damage to the tablet. The tablet should not be stored once it has been removed from the blister package because the tablet's integrity may be compromised and because this increases the risk of accidental exposure to the tablet. Remove the tablet from the blister unit and immediately place the entire fentanyl buccal tablet in the buccal cavity (above a rear molar, between the upper cheek and gum). Patients should not attempt to split the tablet. Do not suck, chew, or swallow tablet because to do so will result in lower plasma concentrations than when taken as directed. The fentanyl buccal tablet should be left between the cheek and gum until it has disintegrated, which usually takes approximately 14-25 min. After 30 min, if remnants from the fentanyl buccal tablet remain, they may be swallowed with a glass of water. Dispose of any remaining tablets immediately. May be fatal to a child.

Transmucosal buccal film: Apply to the inside of the cheek. Wet the affected area with tongue or with water prior to application. Open package with dry hands. Do not cut or tear the film. Using a dry finger on the white side of the film, place 1 film in the mouth with the pink side facing the cheek; hold in place for approximately 5 seconds to adhere. If using more than 1 film per dose, place films separately, using both sides of the mouth as needed; do not overlap. Allow to dissolve over 15 to 30 min. Do not chew or swallow. Do not drink within 5 min after application or eat before the film has fully dissolved.

Ferrous Salts

fer-rous

★ Femiron, Feostat, Ferretts, Ferro-Sequels, Hemocyte, Nephro-Fer, Fergon, Fer-Gen-Sol, Fer-In-Sol, Fer-Iron, Slow-Fe

🍁 Apo-Ferrous Gluconate, Apo-Ferrous Sulfate, Palafer

F

CATEGORY AND SCHEDULE

Pregnancy Risk Category: A
OTC

Classification: Hematinics

MECHANISM OF ACTION

An enzymatic mineral that is an essential component in the formation of hemoglobin, myoglobin, and enzymes. Promotes effective erythropoiesis and transport and utilization of oxygen (O_2). *Therapeutic Effect:* Prevents and treats iron deficiency.

PHARMACOKINETICS

Absorbed in the duodenum and upper jejunum. Ten percent absorbed in patients with normal iron stores; increased to 20%-30% in those with inadequate iron stores. Bound primarily to serum transferrin. Excreted in urine, sweat, and sloughing of intestinal mucosa and by menses. *Half-life:* 6 h.

AVAILABILITY

Ferrous Fumarate

Tablets (Femiron): 63 mg (20 mg elemental iron).
Tablets (Ferretts): 325 mg (106 mg elemental iron).
Tablets (Hemocyte): 324 mg (106 mg elemental iron).
Tablets (Nephro-Fer): 350 mg (115 mg elemental iron).
Tablets (Chewable [Feostat]): 100 mg (33 mg elemental iron).
Tablets (Timed Release [Ferro-Sequels]): 150 mg (50 mg elemental iron).

Ferrous Gluconate

Tablets: 325 mg (36 mg elemental iron).
Tablets (Fergon): 240 mg (27 mg elemental iron).

Ferrous Sulfate

Tablets: 325 mg (65 mg elemental iron).
Tablets, Exsiccated: 200 mg (65 mg elemental iron).
Tablets (Timed Release [Slow FE]): 160 mg (50 mg elemental iron).
Elixir: 220 mg/5 mL (44 mg elemental iron per 5 mL).
Oral Drops (Fer-Gen-Sol, Fer-In-Sol, Fer-Iron): 75 mg/0.6 mL (15 mg/0.6 mL elemental iron).

INDICATIONS AND DOSAGES

▸ **Iron deficiency anemia**

Dosage is expressed in terms of milligrams of elemental iron, degree of anemia, patient weight, and presence of any bleeding. Expect to use periodic hematologic determinations as guide to therapy.

PO

Adults, Elderly. Ferrous fumarate: 60-100 mg twice a day; ferrous gluconate: 60 mg 2-4 times a day; ferrous sulfate: 325 mg 2-4 times a day.

Children. Ferrous fumarate, ferrous gluconate, ferrous sulfate: 3-6 mg/kg/day in 2-3 divided doses.

▸ **Prevention of iron deficiency anemia**

PO

Adults, Elderly. Ferrous fumarate: 60-100 mg/day; ferrous gluconate: 60 mg/day; ferrous sulfate: 325 mg/day.

Children. Ferrous fumarate, ferrous gluconate, ferrous sulfate: 1-2 mg/kg/day, maximum 15 mg/day.

CONTRAINDICATIONS

Hemochromatosis, hemosiderosis, hemolytic anemias, peptic ulcer disease, regional enteritis, ulcerative colitis.

INTERACTIONS

Drug

Ascorbic acid: May increase absorption of iron by > 30%.
Antacids, H_2 antagonists, proton pump inhibitors, calcium supplements, pancreatin, pancrelipase: May decrease the absorption of ferrous fumarate, ferrous gluconate, and ferrous sulfate.
Etidronate, levodopa, levothyroxine, quinolones, tetracyclines: May decrease the absorption of etidronate, levodopa, levothyroxine, quinolones, and tetracyclines.

Herbal

None known.

Food

Eggs, dietary fiber, coffee, milk: Inhibit ferrous fumarate absorption.

DIAGNOSTIC TEST EFFECTS

May increase serum bilirubin level. May decrease serum calcium level. May obscure occult blood in stools.

SIDE EFFECTS

Occasional

Mild, transient nausea.

Rare

Heartburn, anorexia, constipation, diarrhea.

SERIOUS REACTIONS

- Large doses may aggravate existing GI tract disease, such as peptic ulcer disease, regional enteritis, and ulcerative colitis.
- Severe iron poisoning occurs most often in children and is manifested as vomiting, severe abdominal pain, diarrhea, and dehydration, followed by hyperventilation, pallor or cyanosis, and cardiovascular collapse. If accidental overdose occurs, contact the Poison Control Center immediately.

PRECAUTIONS & CONSIDERATIONS

Caution is warranted in patients with bronchial asthma and iron hypersensitivity. Iron crosses the placenta and is distributed in breast milk. No age-related precautions have been noted in children or elderly patients.

Urine may darken in color. Hemoglobin, reticulocyte count, ferritin and serum iron levels, and total iron-binding capacity should be monitored. Daily bowel activity and stool consistency should be assessed. Clinical improvement should also be assessed, and relief of iron deficiency symptoms (fatigue, headache, irritability, pallor, and paresthesia of extremities) should be recorded.

Storage

Store all forms, including tablets, capsules, suspension, and drops, at room temperature and out of reach of children.

Administration

Take between meals with water unless GI discomfort occurs; if so, give with meals. To avoid transient staining of mucous membranes and teeth, place liquid on back of tongue with a dropper or straw. Do not crush the sustained-release form. Avoid simultaneous administration of antacids.

F

Fesoterodine

fes'oh-ter'oh-deen

Toviaz

CATEGORY AND SCHEDULE

Pregnancy Risk Category: C

Classification: Anticholinergics, urinary antispasmodics, urinary incontinence agents

F

MECHANISM OF ACTION

An antispasmodic that exhibits potent antimuscarinic activity by selectively blocking cholinergic muscarinic receptors, particularly in the bladder. Inhibits urinary bladder contraction and decreases detrussor pressure. *Therapeutic Effect:* Decreases urinary frequency, urgency.

PHARMACOKINETICS

Rapidly and well absorbed after PO administration. Protein binding: Only 50%. Once absorbed, rapidly metabolized to an active metabolite. Extensively metabolized in the liver (CYP2D6 and CYP3A4) to inactive metabolites. Metabolites excreted primarily (70%) in urine. Unknown whether removed by hemodialysis. *Half-life*: 7-9 h.

AVAILABILITY

Tablets (Extended Release): 4 mg, 8 mg.

INDICATIONS AND DOSAGES

▸ **Overactive bladder**

PO (EXTENDED RELEASE)

Adults, Elderly. Initially, 4 mg once a day, may increase to 8 mg once a day if needed and tolerated.

▸ **Dosage in severe renal impairment or taking strong inhibitors of CYP3A4**

PO (EXTENDED RELEASE)

Adults, Elderly. Do not exceed 4 mg once a day.

▸ **Severe hepatic impairment**

Do not use.

CONTRAINDICATIONS

Urinary retention, gastric retention, uncontrolled narrow-angle glaucoma, known hypersensitivity to fesoterodine or its ingredients.

INTERACTIONS

Drug

Anticholinergics: May have additive anticholinergic effects.

Clarithromycin, erythromycin, itraconazole, ketoconazole, and other strong inhibitors of CYP3A4 (e.g., ritonavir): May increase fesoterodine concentration. Use lowered fesoterodine dose.

Herbal and Food

None known.

DIAGNOSTIC TEST EFFECTS

None known or expected.

SIDE EFFECTS

Frequent (≥ 4%)

Dry mouth, constipation.

Occasional (1%-4%)

Headache, abdominal pain, dysuria, dyspepsia (heartburn, indigestion, epigastric discomfort), urinary tract infection, urinary retention, dry eyes, nausea, back pain, insomnia.

Rare

Dizziness, fatigue, somnolence, abnormal vision (accommodation problems), rash, dry skin.

SERIOUS REACTIONS

- Overdose can result in severe anticholinergic effects, including abdominal cramps, facial warmth, excessive salivation or lacrimation, diaphoresis, pallor, urinary urgency, blurred vision, and prolonged QT interval.
- Rare reports of hypersensitivity, including angioedema.

PRECAUTIONS & CONSIDERATIONS

Caution is warranted in patients with renal impairment, hepatic impairment, myasthenia gravis, clinically significant bladder outflow obstruction (increases risk of urine retention), GI obstructive disorders such as pyloric stenosis (increases risk of gastric retention and reduces gastric motility), and treated angle-closure glaucoma. It is unknown whether the drug is distributed in breast milk. However, breastfeeding is not recommended. The safety and efficacy of this drug have not been established in children. No age-related precautions have been noted in elderly patients.

Blurred vision, GI upset, constipation, and dry eyes and dry mouth may occur. Notify the physician of a change in vision. Incontinence and residual urine in the bladder should be determined.

Storage

Store at room temperature. Protect from moisture.

Administration

Take fesoterodine without regard to food. Take with liquid and swallowed whole. Do not chew, divide, or crush extended-release tablets.

Fexofenadine

fex-oh-fen′eh-deen

Allegra

CATEGORY AND SCHEDULE

Pregnancy Risk Category: C

Rx and OTC

Classification: Antihistamines, H_1 receptor antagonists, non-sedating

MECHANISM OF ACTION

A piperidine that competes with histamine for H_1 receptor sites on effector cells. *Therapeutic Effect:* Relieves allergic rhinitis symptoms.

PHARMACOKINETICS

Rapidly absorbed after PO administration. Protein binding: 60%-70%. Does not cross the blood-brain barrier. Minimally metabolized. Eliminated in feces and urine. Not removed by hemodialysis. *Half-life:* 14.4 h (increased in renal impairment).

AVAILABILITY

Tablets: 30 mg, 60 mg, 180 mg.
Oral Disintegrating Tablets (ODT): 30 mg.
Oral Suspension: 30 mg/5 mL.

INDICATIONS AND DOSAGES

▸ **Allergic rhinitis, chronic idiopathic urticaria**

PO

Adults, Elderly, Children 12 yr and older. 60 mg twice a day or 180 mg once a day.

Children aged 6-11 yr. 30 mg twice a day.

▸ **Dosage in renal impairment**

Adults, Elderly, and Children 12 yr and older. Dosage is reduced to 60 mg once a day. For children aged 6-11 yr, dosage is reduced to 30 mg once a day.

▸ **Allergic rhinitis, chronic idiopathic urticaria**

PO

Children aged 2-11 yr. Oral suspension 30 mg twice a day. For children with renal dysfunction, dosage is reduced to 30 mg once daily.

▸ **Chronic idiopathic urticaria**

PO

Children aged 6 mo to 2 yr. Oral suspension 15 mg twice a day. For children with renal dysfunction, dosage is reduced to 15 mg once daily.

CONTRAINDICATIONS

Hypersensitivity.

INTERACTIONS

Drug

Antacids: May decrease fexofenadine absorption if given within 15 min of a fexofenadine dose.

Herbal

None known.

Food

Fruit juice.

DIAGNOSTIC TEST EFFECTS

May suppress wheal and flare reactions to antigen skin testing unless drug is discontinued at least 4 days before testing.

SIDE EFFECTS

Rare (< 2%)

Somnolence, headache, fatigue, nausea, vomiting, abdominal distress, dysmenorrhea.

SERIOUS REACTIONS

- Rare serious hypersensitivity reactions.

PRECAUTIONS & CONSIDERATIONS

ODTs contain phenylalanine (phenylketonuria).

Caution is warranted with severe renal impairment. It is unknown whether fexofenadine crosses the placenta or is distributed in breast milk. No age-related precautions have been noted in elderly patients. Avoid drinking alcoholic beverages and performing tasks that require alertness or motor skills until response to the drug is established.

Drowsiness may occur. Respiratory rate, depth, and rhythm; pulse rate and quality; BP; and therapeutic response should be monitored.

Storage

Store at room temperature. ODT should be kept protected from moisture and not removed from blister foil until administration time.

Administration

Take fexofenadine without regard to food. ODTs are designed to disintegrate on the tongue, followed by swallowing with or without water, and should be taken on an empty stomach. Do not chew ODT. Shake oral suspension well before each use.

Filgrastim

fil-gra'stim

★🍁 Neupogen

Do not confuse Neupogen with Epogen or Nutramigen.

CATEGORY AND SCHEDULE

Pregnancy Risk Category: C

Classification: Hematopoietic agents, recombinant DNA origin

MECHANISM OF ACTION

A biologic modifier that stimulates production, maturation, and activation of neutrophils to increase their migration and cytotoxicity. *Therapeutic Effect:* Increases neutrophil count and enhances count recovery. Decreases incidence of infection.

PHARMACOKINETICS

Readily absorbed after subcutaneous (SC) administration. Not removed by hemodialysis. *Half-life:* 3.5 h.

AVAILABILITY

Injection, Single-Dose Vials: 300 mcg/mL, 480 mcg/0.8 mL. *Prefilled Syringes (Single Ject):* 300 mcg, 480 mcg.

INDICATIONS AND DOSAGES

▸ **Myelosuppression from chemotherapy**

IV OR SC INFUSION, SC INJECTION

Adults, Elderly. Initially, 5 mcg/kg/day. May increase by 5 mcg/kg for each chemotherapy cycle based on duration or severity of absolute neutrophil count nadir. Administer daily for up to 2 wks until the ANC has reached 10,000/mm^3 following the expected chemotherapy-induced neutrophil nadir.

▸ **Bone marrow transplant**

IV OR SC INFUSION

Adults, Elderly. 10 mcg/kg/day given as an IV infusion of 4 or 24 h or as a continuous 24-h SC infusion. Adjust dosage daily during period of neutrophil recovery based on neutrophil response.

▸ **Mobilization progenitor cells**

SC INJECTION OR INFUSION

Adults. 10 mcg/kg/day beginning at least 4 days before first leukapheresis and continuing until last leukapheresis.

▸ **Chronic neutropenia, congenital neutropenia**

SC

Adults, Children. 6 mcg/kg/dose twice a day.

▸ **Idiopathic or cyclic neutropenia**

SC

Adults, Children. 5 mcg/kg/dose once a day.

OFF-LABEL USES

Treatment of AIDS-related neutropenia; drug-induced agranulocytosis; febrile neutropenia; myelodysplastic syndrome.

CONTRAINDICATIONS

Hypersensitivity to *Escherichia coli*–derived proteins; use within 24 h before or after cytotoxic chemotherapy.

INTERACTIONS

Drug

Lithium: May increase white blood cell count greater than expected.

Topotecan: May prolong the duration of neutropenia.

Herbal

None known.

Food

None known.

DIAGNOSTIC TEST EFFECTS

Transient increase in neutrophils occurs 1-2 days after initiation. May increase LDH concentrations, leukocyte alkaline phosphatase (LAP) scores, and serum alkaline phosphatase and uric acid levels.

IV INCOMPATIBILITIES

Amphotericin (Fungizone), cefepime (Maxipime), cefotaxime (Claforan), cefoxitin (Mefoxin), ceftizoxime (Cefizox), ceftriaxone (Rocephin), cefuroxime (Zinacef), clindamycin (Cleocin), dactinomycin (Cosmegen), etoposide (VePesid), fluorouracil, furosemide (Lasix), heparin, mannitol, methylprednisolone (Solu-Medrol), metronidazole (Flagyl), mitomycin (Mutamycin), piperacillin, thiotepa (Thioplex), prochlorperazine (Compazine).

SIDE EFFECTS

Frequent

Nausea or vomiting (57%), mild to severe bone pain (22%) that occurs more frequently with high-dose IV form and less frequently with low-dose subcutaneous form; alopecia (18%), diarrhea (14%), fever (12%), fatigue (11%).

Occasional (5%-9%)

Anorexia, dyspnea, headache, cough, rash.

Rare (< 5%)

Psoriasis, hematuria or proteinuria, osteoporosis.

F

SERIOUS REACTIONS

- Long-term administration occasionally produces chronic neutropenia and splenomegaly.
- Splenic rupture, allergic-type reactions, and sickle cell crisis have occurred.
- Alveolar hemorrhage has occurred in healthy patients undergoing peripheral blood progenitor cell mobilization.
- Thrombocytopenia, myocardial infarction, and arrhythmias occur rarely.
- Adult respiratory distress syndrome may occur in patients with sepsis.

PRECAUTIONS & CONSIDERATIONS

Caution is warranted in patients with gout, malignancy with myeloid characteristics (because of the potential for granulocyte-colony-stimulating factor to act as a growth factor), preexisting cardiac conditions, and psoriasis. It is unknown whether filgrastim crosses the placenta or is distributed in breast milk. No age-related precautions have been noted in children or elderly patients. Avoid situations that might present risk for contracting an infectious disease, such as influenza.

Notify the physician of chest pain, chills, fever, palpitations, or severe bone pain. BP should be monitored for a transient decrease. Also, body temperature, hematocrit, CBC, and hepatic enzyme and serum uric acid levels should be assessed. CBC should be obtained before the start of filgrastim therapy and twice weekly thereafter. Those with preexisting cardiac conditions should be closely watched. Be alert for adult respiratory distress syndrome in those with sepsis. Abdominal exams should include palpation for splenomegaly.

Storage

Refrigerate vials for IV use. Filgrastim is stable for up to 24 h at room temperature, provided vial contents are clear and contain no particulate matter. The drug remains stable if accidentally exposed to freezing temperature. Store vials for SC use in refrigerator, but remove before use and allow to warm to room temperature.

Administration

! May be given by subcutaneous injection or short IV infusion (15-30 min) or by continuous IV infusion. Begin filgrastim therapy at least 24 h after last dose of chemotherapy; discontinue at least 24 h before next dose of chemotherapy. Begin therapy at least 24 h after bone marrow infusion.

For IV administration, use single-dose vial. Do not reenter vial. Do not shake. Dilute with 10-50 mL D5W to a concentration of 15 mcg/mL or higher. For a concentration from 5 to 14 mcg/mL, add 2 mL of 5% albumin to each 50 mL D5W to provide a final concentration of 2 mg/mL. Do not dilute to a final concentration of < 5 mcg/mL. For intermittent infusion (piggyback), infuse over 15-30 min. For continuous infusion, give single dose over 4-24 h. In all situations, flush IV line with D5W before and after administration.

Finasteride

feen-as'ter-ide

Propecia, Proscar

Do not confuse Proscar with Posicor, ProSom, Prozac, or Psorcon.

CATEGORY AND SCHEDULE

Pregnancy Risk Category: X

Classification: 5-α-Reductase inhibitors, antiandrogens, hormones/hormone modifiers

MECHANISM OF ACTION

An androgen hormone inhibitor that inhibits 5-α-reductase, an intracellular enzyme that converts testosterone into dihydrotestosterone (DHT) in the prostate gland, resulting in a decreased serum DHT level.
Therapeutic Effect: Reduces size of the prostate gland, decreases BPH symptoms, increases hair growth.

PHARMACOKINETICS

Route	Onset	Peak	Duration
PO	24 h	2-6 h	5-7 days

Rapidly absorbed from the GI tract. Protein binding: 90%. Widely distributed. Metabolized in the liver. *Half-life:* 6-8 h. Onset of clinical effect: 3-6 mo of continued therapy.

AVAILABILITY

Tablets (Propecia): 1 mg.
Tablets (Proscar): 5 mg.

INDICATIONS AND DOSAGES

▸ **Benign prostatic hyperplasia (BPH)**

PO

Adults, Elderly. 5 mg once a day (for a minimum of 6 mo).

▸ **Male-pattern hair loss**

PO

Adults. 1 mg/day (for a minimum of 3 mo).

OFF-LABEL USES

Adjuvant monotherapy after radical prostatectomy in treatment of prostate cancer, female hirsutism, prophylaxis of prostate cancer.

CONTRAINDICATIONS

Hypersensitivity, exposure to the patient's semen or handling of finasteride tablets, or ingestion by those who are or may become pregnant.

INTERACTIONS

Drug

Androgens: Oppose finasteride.

Herbal

Saw palmetto: Effects may be additive on prostate tissue, but unstudied.

Food

None known.

DIAGNOSTIC TEST EFFECTS

Decreases (falsely) the serum prostate-specific antigen (PSA) level, even in patients with prostate cancer. After 6 mo of use, the PSA value should be doubled for comparison with normal levels in untreated men.

SIDE EFFECTS

Rare (1%-4%)

Gynecomastia, sexual dysfunction (impotence, decreased libido, decreased volume of ejaculate, ejaculation disorder), postural hypotension, weakness, dizziness.

SERIOUS REACTIONS

- Male breast neoplasia has been reported. High-grade prostate cancer has been reported.

PRECAUTIONS & CONSIDERATIONS

Caution is warranted in patients with hepatic impairment. Finasteride is not indicated for use in children. The efficacy of this drug has not been established in elderly patients. It is unknown whether finasteride is excreted in breast milk, and it should not be taken by pregnant or lactating women.

Finasteride may cause impotence and decrease ejaculate volume. Be aware that urinary flow might not improve, even if the prostate gland shrinks. Serum PSA determinations should be obtained before and periodically during therapy. Intake and output should also be monitored.

Storage
Store at room temperature tightly closed and protect from light and moisture.
Administration
Do not break or crush film-coated tablets. Take finasteride without regard to food. Full therapeutic effect may take up to 6 mo.

Women should not handle crushed or broken finasteride tablets when they are pregnant or may potentially be pregnant because of possible exposure to finasteride and the subsequent potential risk to a male fetus. Tablets are coated and this will normally prevent contact with the active ingredient, provided that the tablets are not broken or crushed.

F

Flavocoxid

fla-vo-cox′id
★ Limbrel
Do not confuse Limbrel with Limbitrol.

CATEGORY AND SCHEDULE

Pregnancy Risk Category: Not classified.

Classification: Medical food, oral nutritional supplements

MECHANISM OF ACTION

An oral nutritional supplement that inhibits prostaglandin synthesis and arachidonic acid metabolism, reducing the production of leukotrienes. Also acts through an antioxidant mechanism. *Therapeutic Effect:* Produces anti-inflammatory and analgesic effects and increases mobility in osteoarthritis.

PHARMACOKINETICS

Undergoes hydrolysis at the gut mucosal border. Food decreases absorption. Little hepatic metabolism.

AVAILABILITY

Capsules: 250 mg, 500 mg.

INDICATIONS AND DOSAGES

▸ **Osteoarthritis**
PO
Adults 18 yr and older, Elderly. 250- or 500-mg capsule q12h.

CONTRAINDICATIONS

Hypersensitivity to flavocoxid and any component of flavocoxid.

INTERACTIONS

Drug
None known.
Herbal
None known.
Food
All foods: Decrease the absorption of flavocoxid.

DIAGNOSTIC TEST EFFECTS

None known.

SIDE EFFECTS

Rare (≥ 2%)
Increase in varicose veins, psoriasis, mild hypertension, fluid accumulation in knee, reduced flexibility.

SERIOUS REACTIONS

- GI bleeding, perforation, and ulceration occur rarely in patients currently or previously treated with NSAIDs or COX-2 inhibitors or with previous history of GI ulceration or bleeding.

PRECAUTIONS & CONSIDERATIONS

Not recommended for patients with a history of peptic ulcer. It is unknown whether flavocoxid crosses the placenta or is distributed in breast milk. Flavocoxid use is not recommended during pregnancy. The safety and efficacy of flavocoxid have not been established in children younger than 18 yr. No age-related precautions have been noted in elderly patients.

Therapeutic response, including improved grip strength, increased joint mobility, reduced joint tenderness, and relief of pain, stiffness, and swelling, should be assessed.

Storage

Store at room temperature protected from light and moisture.

Administration

Do not take flavocoxid within 1 h of eating because food decreases the supplement's absorption. However, if GI discomfort occurs, may take with food.

Flavoxate

fla-vox′ate

CATEGORY AND SCHEDULE

Pregnancy Risk Category: B

Classification: Antispasmodic

MECHANISM OF ACTION

An anticholinergic that relaxes detrusor and other smooth muscles by cholinergic blockade, counteracting muscle spasm in the urinary tract. *Therapeutic Effect:* Produces anticholinergic, local anesthetic, and analgesic effects, relieving urinary symptoms.

AVAILABILITY

Tablets: 100 mg.

INDICATIONS AND DOSAGES

▸ **To relieve symptoms of nocturia, incontinence, suprapubic pain, dysuria, frequency and urgency associated with urologic conditions (symptomatic only)**

PO

Adults, Elderly, Children > 12 yr. 100-200 mg 3-4 times a day.

CONTRAINDICATIONS

Duodenal or pyloric obstruction, GI hemorrhage or obstruction, ileus, lower urinary tract obstruction.

INTERACTIONS

Drug

Anticholinergic agents: May have additive effects.

Herbal

None known.

Food

None known.

DIAGNOSTIC TEST EFFECTS

None known.

SIDE EFFECTS

Frequent

Somnolence, dry mouth and throat.

Occasional

Constipation, difficult urination, blurred vision, dizziness, headache, increased light sensitivity, nausea, vomiting, abdominal pain.

Rare

Confusion (primarily in elderly), hypersensitivity, increased intraocular pressure, leukopenia.

SERIOUS REACTIONS

- Overdose may produce anticholinergic effects, including unsteadiness, severe dizziness, somnolence, fever, facial flushing, dyspnea, nervousness, and irritability.

PRECAUTIONS & CONSIDERATIONS

Caution is warranted in patients with glaucoma. Avoid tasks that require mental alertness and motor skills until response to the drug is established. Use with caution in pregnancy or lactation. Not approved for children < 12 yr of age. Symptomatic relief should be assessed. Notify the physician of symptoms of flavoxate overdose, including unsteadiness, severe dizziness, drowsiness, fever, flushed face, shortness of breath, nervousness, and irritability.

Storage

Store at room temperature.

Administration

May administer with food if GI upset occurs.

F

Flecainide

fle'kah-nide

Tambocor

CATEGORY AND SCHEDULE

Pregnancy Risk Category: C

Classification: Antiarrhythmics, class IC

MECHANISM OF ACTION

An antiarrhythmic that slows atrial, AV, His-Purkinje, and intraventricular conduction. Decreases excitability, conduction velocity, and automaticity. *Therapeutic Effect:* Controls atrial, supraventricular, and ventricular arrhythmias.

AVAILABILITY

Tablets: 50 mg, 100 mg, 150 mg.

INDICATIONS AND DOSAGES

▸ Life-threatening ventricular arrhythmias, sustained ventricular tachycardia

PO

Adults, Elderly. Initially, 100 mg q12h, increased by 100 mg (50 mg twice a day) every 4 days until effective dose or maximum of 400 mg/day is attained. If CrCl 35 mL/min or less, initiate with 100 mg once daily or 50 mg twice daily.

▸ Paroxysmal supraventricular tachycardia (PSVT), paroxysmal atrial fibrillation (PAF)

PO

Adults, Elderly. Initially, 50 mg q12h, increased by 100 mg (50 mg twice a day) every 4 days until effective dose or maximum of 300 mg/day is attained.

CONTRAINDICATIONS

Cardiogenic shock, preexisting second- or third-degree AV block, right bundle-branch block (without presence of a pacemaker), recent MI, and known hypersensitivity to the drug.

INTERACTIONS

Drug

Amiodarone: Decrease the usual flecainide dosage by 50%.

Antipsychotic agents, azoles, fluoroquinolones, macrolides, tricyclic antidepressants: May increase risk of cardiotoxicity, QT prolongation.

β-Blockers: May increase negative inotropic effects.

Bupropion, cinacalcet, quinidine, protease inhibitors: May increase flecainide concentrations.

Cimetidine: May increase flecainide concentrations.

Digoxin: May increase blood concentration of digoxin.

Other antiarrhythmics: May have additive effects.

Urinary acidifiers: May increase the excretion of flecainide.

Urinary alkalinizers: May decrease the excretion of flecainide.

Herbal

Black cohosh, gingko, ginseng: May increase flecainide concentrations.

Ephedra: May increase risk of cardiotoxicity.

Food

None known.

DIAGNOSTIC TEST EFFECTS

May prolong QTc interval of ECG. Trough plasma levels are generally targeted between 0.2 and 1 mcg/mL.

SIDE EFFECTS
Frequent (10%-19%)
Dizziness, dyspnea, headache.
Occasional (4%-9%)
Nausea, fatigue, palpitations, chest pain, asthenia (loss of strength, energy), tremor, constipation.

SERIOUS REACTIONS
• Flecainide may worsen existing arrhythmias or produce new ones.
• Congestive heart failure (CHF) may occur, or existing CHF may worsen.
• Overdose may increase QRS duration, prolong QT interval, cause conduction disturbances, reduce myocardial contractility, and cause hypotension.
• Very rare reports of serious hypersensitivity, cholestatic jaundice with hepatic failure, or blood dyscrasias.

PRECAUTIONS & CONSIDERATIONS
Only to be used for refractory, life-threatening ventricular arrhythmias. Caution is warranted with CHF, recent MI, impaired myocardial function, second- and third-degree AV block (with pacemaker), and sick sinus syndrome. Nasal decongestant or OTC cold preparations should be avoided without physician approval.

The side effects of flecainide therapy usually disappear with continued use or decreased dosage. Tasks that require mental alertness or motor skills should be avoided. Continuous cardiac monitoring should be given. ECG measurements, including QRS duration and QT interval, should be performed before and periodically during therapy. Pulmonary status, weight gain, intake and output, and dyspnea should be monitored in those with CHF.

Storage
Store at room temperature. Keep tightly closed. Protect from light.

Administration
Crush scored tablets as needed. May take without regard to food.

Fluconazole
floo-con′a-zole
Diflucan, Diflucan, Apo-Fluconazole
Do not confuse Diflucan with diclofenac.

CATEGORY AND SCHEDULE
Pregnancy Risk Category: C

Classification: Antifungals

MECHANISM OF ACTION
A fungistatic antifungal that interferes with cytochrome P-450, an enzyme necessary for ergosterol formation. *Therapeutic Effect:* Directly damages fungal membrane, altering its function.

PHARMACOKINETICS
Well absorbed from GI tract. Widely distributed, including to cerebrospinal fluid. Protein binding: 11%. Partially metabolized in the liver. Excreted unchanged, primarily in urine. Partially removed by hemodialysis. *Half-life:* 20-30 h (increased in impaired renal function).

AVAILABILITY
Tablets: 50 mg, 100 mg, 150 mg, 200 mg.
Powder for Oral Suspension: 10 mg/mL, 40 mg/mL.
Injection: 2 mg/mL (in 100- or 200-mL containers).

INDICATIONS AND DOSAGES
▸ **Oropharyngeal candidiasis**
PO, IV
Adults, Elderly. 200 mg once, then 100 mg/day for at least 14 days.

Children. 6 mg/kg/day once, then 3 mg/kg/day.

▸ **Esophageal candidiasis**

PO, IV

Adults, Elderly. 200 mg once, then 100 mg/day (up to 400 mg/day) for 21 days and at least 14 days following resolution of symptoms.

Children. 6 mg/kg/day once, then 3 mg/kg/day (up to 12 mg/kg/day) for 21 days and at least 14 days following resolution of symptoms.

▸ **Vaginal candidiasis**

PO

Adults. 150 mg once.

▸ **Prevention of candidiasis in patients undergoing bone marrow transplantation**

PO

Adults. 400 mg/day.

▸ **Systemic candidiasis**

PO, IV

Adults, Elderly. 400 mg once, then 200 mg/day (up to 400 mg/day) for at least 28 days and at least 14 days following resolution of symptoms.

Children. 6-12 mg/kg/day.

▸ **Cryptococcal meningitis**

PO, IV

Adults, Elderly. 400 mg once, then 200 mg/day (up to 800 mg/day) for 10-12 wks after cerebrospinal fluid becomes negative (200 mg/day for suppression of relapse in patients with AIDS).

Children. 12 mg/kg/day once, then 6-12 mg/kg/day (6 mg/kg/day for suppression of relapse in patients with AIDS).

▸ **Onychomycosis**

PO

Adults. 150 mg/wk.

▸ **Dosage in renal impairment (adults)**

After a loading dose of 400 mg, the daily dosage is based on creatinine clearance:

Creatinine Clearance	% of Recommended Dose
> 50 mL/min	100
21-50 mL/min	50
11-20 mL/min	25
Dialysis	Dose after dialysis

OFF-LABEL USES

Treatment of coccidioidomycosis, cryptococcosis, fungal pneumonia, onychomycosis.

CONTRAINDICATIONS

Hypersensitivity to fluconazole or other azole antifungal agents. Coadministration of terfenadine is contraindicated in patients receiving ≥ 400 mg/day of fluconazole. Coadministration of drugs known to prolong the QT interval and also metabolized by CYP3A4 (e.g., cisapride, astemizole, pimozide, and quinidine) is contraindicated.

INTERACTIONS

Drug

Cyclosporine: High fluconazole doses increase cyclosporine blood concentration.

Oral antidiabetics: May increase blood concentration and effects of oral antidiabetics.

Phenytoin, warfarin: May decrease the metabolism of these drugs.

Rifampin: May increase fluconazole metabolism.

Systemic coadministration with QT-prolonging drugs metabolized by CYP3A4 (e.g., cisapride, pimozide, quinidine, dofetilide, astemizole, terfenadine): Contraindicated. Do not use.

Theophylline: May increase theophylline concentrations.

Warfarin: Anticoagulant effect of warfarin may be increased. Monitor INR.

Herbal

None known.

Food
None known.

DIAGNOSTIC TEST EFFECTS
May increase serum alkaline phosphatase, serum bilirubin, SGOT (AST), and SGPT (ALT) levels.

IV INCOMPATIBILITIES
Amphotericin B (Fungizone), amphotericin B complex (Abelcet, AmBisome, Amphotec), ampicillin (Polycillin), calcium gluconate, cefotaxime (Claforan), ceftazidime (Fortaz), ceftriaxone (Rocephin), cefuroxime (Zinacef), chloramphenicol (Chloromycetin), clindamycin (Cleocin), co-trimoxazole (Bactrim), dantrolene (Dantrium), diazepam (Valium), digoxin (Lanoxin), erythromycin (Erythrocin), furosemide (Lasix), haloperidol (Haldol), hydroxyzine (Vistaril), imipenem and cilastatin (Primaxin), pantoprazole (Protonix), sulfamethoxazole and trimethoprim.

IV COMPATIBILITIES
Acyclovir, aldesleukin, alfentanil, allopurinol, amifostine, amikacin, aminophylline, amiodarone, ascorbic acid, atracurium, atropine, azathioprine, aztreonam, benztropine, bivalirudin, bretylium, bumetanide, buprenorphine, butorphanol, calcium chloride, carboplatin, cefamandole, cefazolin, cefepime, cefmetazole, cefonicid, cefoperazone, cefotetan, cefoxitin, ceftizoxime, cephalothin, chlorpromazine, cimetidine, cisatracurium, cisplatin, cyanocobalamin, cyclophosphamide, cyclosporine, dactinomycin, daptomycin, dexamethasone, diltiazem (Cardizem), dimenhydrinate, diphenhydramine, dobutamine (Dobutrex), docetaxel, dopamine (Intropin), doripenem, doxacurium, doxycycline, droperidol, drotecogin alfa, enalaprilat, ephedrine sulfate, epinephrine, epirubicin, epoetin alfa, ertapenem, erythromycin lactobionate, esmolol, etoposide, famotidine, fenoldopam, fentanyl, filgrastim, fludarabine, fluorouracil, folic acid, foscarnet, furosemide, gallium nitrate, ganciclovir, gatifloxacin, gemcitabine, gentamicin, glycopyrrolate, granisetron, heparin, hetastarch 6% (Hextend), hydrocortisone sodium phosphate, hydrocortisone sodium succinate, hydromorphone, hydroxyzine, immune globulin, inamrinone lactate, indomethacin, insulin-regular, isoproterenol, ketorolac, labetolol, lactated Ringer's, lansoprazole, leucovorin, levofloxacin, lidocaine, linezolid, lorazepam (Ativan), magnesium sulfate, mannitol, meclorethamine, melphalan, meperidine, meropenem, metaraminol, methicillin, methoxamine, methyldopate, methylprednisolone, metoclopramide, metoprolol tartrate, metronidazole, mezlocillin, miconazole, midazolam (Versed), milrinone, minocycline, mitoxantrone, morphine sulfate, moxalactam, multiple vitamins, nafcillin, nalbuphine, naloxone, netilmicin, nitroglycerin, nitroprusside sodium, norepinephrine, ondansetron, oxacillin, paclitaxel, palonosetron, pancronium, pantoprazole, papaverine, pemetrexed, penicillin G potassium, penicillin G sodium, pentamidine, pentazocine, pentobarbital, phentolamine, phenylephrine, phytanadione, piperacillin and tazobactam, polymixin B, potassium chloride, procainamide, prochlorperazine, promethazine, propofol (Diprivan), propranolol, protamine sulfate, pyridoxine, quinidine, quinupristin and dalfopristin, ranitidine,

remifentanil, ritodrine, rituximab, sargramostim, sodium acetate, sodium bicarbonate, streptokinase, succinylcholine, sufentanil, tacrolimus, teniposide, theophylline, thiotepa, ticarcillin, ticarcillin and clavulanate, tigecycline, tirofiban, tobramycin, tolazoline, trastuzumab, trimetaphan, urokinase, vancomycin, vasopressin, vecuronium, verapamil, vincristine, vinorelbine, voriconazole, zidovudine.

SIDE EFFECTS

Occasional (1%-4%)

Hypersensitivity reaction (including chills, fever, pruritus, and rash), dizziness, drowsiness, dyspepsia, headache, constipation, diarrhea, nausea, vomiting, abdominal pain, taste perversion.

SERIOUS REACTIONS

• Exfoliative skin disorders, serious hepatic effects, QT prolongation, torsade de pointes, seizures, and blood dyscrasias (such as eosinophilia, thrombocytopenia, anemia, and leukopenia) have been reported rarely.

PRECAUTIONS & CONSIDERATIONS

Caution is warranted in patients with liver or renal impairment; hypersensitivity to other triazoles, such as itraconazole or terconazole; or hypersensitivity to imidazoles, such as butoconazole and ketoconazole. Be aware that it is unknown whether fluconazole is excreted in breast milk. No age-related precautions have been noted in children. In elderly patients, age-related renal impairment may require dosage adjustment.

Expect to monitor the complete blood count (CBC), liver and renal function test results, platelet count, and serum potassium levels. Report any itching or rash promptly. Monitor the temperature daily. Assess the daily pattern of bowel activity and stool consistency. Evaluate for dizziness and provide assistance as needed; do not drive or use machinery until response to the drug is established. If dark urine, pale stool, rash with or without itching, or yellow skin or eyes occur, notify the physician. Patients with oropharyngeal infections should be taught good oral hygiene. Administer with caution in patients with proarrhythmic conditions.

Storage

Store at room temperature.

Administration

Give oral fluconazole without regard to meals. Be aware that PO and IV therapy are equally effective. Shake oral suspension well before each use.

For IV administration, do not remove from outer wrap until ready to use. Squeeze inner bag to check for leaks. Do not use parenteral form if the solution is cloudy, a precipitate forms, the seal is not intact, or it is discolored. Do not add another medication to the solution. Do not exceed maximum flow rate of 200 mg/h.

Flucytosine

floo-sye′toe-seen

★ Ancobon

CATEGORY AND SCHEDULE

Pregnancy Risk Category: C

Classification: Antifungals

MECHANISM OF ACTION
An antifungal that penetrates fungal cells and is converted to fluorouracil, which competes with uracil interfering with fungal RNA and protein synthesis. *Therapeutic Effect:* Damages fungal membrane.

PHARMACOKINETICS
Well absorbed from GI tract. Widely distributed, including cerebrospinal fluid. Protein binding: 2%-4%. Metabolized in liver. Partially removed by hemodialysis. *Half-life:* 3-8 h (half-life is increased with impaired renal function).

AVAILABILITY
Capsule: 250 mg, 500 mg.

INDICATIONS AND DOSAGES
▸ Fungal infections, candidiasis, cryptococcosis
PO
Adults, Elderly, Children. 50-150 mg/kg/day in equally divided doses q6h.
▸ Dosage in renal function impairment
Based on creatinine clearance:

Creatinine Clearance (mL/min)	Dosage Interval
20-40	q12h
10-20	q24h
0-10	q24-48h

CONTRAINDICATIONS
Hypersensitivity to flucytosine.

INTERACTIONS
Drug
Amphotericin B: May increase the effects of flucytosine.
Cytarabine: May decrease flucytosine efficacy.
Zidovudine: May increase the risk of hematologic toxicity.
Herbal
None known.
Food
None known.

DIAGNOSTIC TEST EFFECTS
Measurement of serum creatinine should be determined by the Jaffe reaction or other modern laboratory methods, as the drug does not interfere with these methods. Most automated equipment makes use of non-interfering assays. Therapeutic blood serum level is 25-100 mcg/mL. Prolonged serum levels over this range may result in hematologic changes or hepatitis. Drug may cause decreased WBC, platelets, or increased liver function tests.

SIDE EFFECTS
Occasional
Pruritus, rash, photosensitivity, dizziness, drowsiness, headache, diarrhea, nausea, vomiting, abdominal pain, increased liver enzymes, jaundice, increased BUN and creatinine, weakness, hearing loss.

SERIOUS REACTIONS
- Hepatic dysfunction and severe bone marrow suppression occur rarely.

PRECAUTIONS & CONSIDERATIONS
Caution is warranted in patients with liver or renal impairment, hematologic disease, or bone marrow suppression. Monotherapy should be avoided. There are no adequate data in pregnant women. It is unknown whether flucytosine is excreted in breast milk. No age-related precautions have been noted in children. In elderly patients, age-related renal impairment may require dosage adjustment.

F

Be alert to bone marrow suppressive symptoms. Unexplained fever, sore throat, rash or hives, trouble breathing, yellow skin or eyes, persistent chest pain, or bloody urine should be reported.

Blood concentrations, renal and hepatic function, and hematologic status should be monitored routinely.

Because of resistance, this medication should be used in combination with amphotericin B for treatment of systemic candidiasis and cryptococcosis.

Storage

Store at room temperature.

Administration

To avoid GI upset, take a few capsules at a time over 15 min with food until full dose is taken. Flucytosine doses should be spaced evenly around the clock to promote less variation in peak and trough blood serum levels.

Fludrocortisone

floo-droe-kor'ti-sone

Florinef

CATEGORY AND SCHEDULE

Pregnancy Risk Category: C

Classification: Corticosteroid, mineralocorticoid

MECHANISM OF ACTION

A mineralocorticoid that acts at distal tubules. *Therapeutic Effect:* Increases potassium and hydrogen ion excretion. Replaces sodium loss and raises blood pressure (with low dosages). Inhibits endogenous adrenal cortical secretion, thymic activity, and secretion of corticotropin by pituitary gland (with higher dosages).

PHARMACOKINETICS

Well absorbed from the GI tract. Protein binding: 42%. Widely distributed. Metabolized in the liver and kidney. Primarily excreted in urine. *Half-life:* 3.5 h.

AVAILABILITY

Tablets: 0.1 mg.

INDICATIONS AND DOSAGES

▸ **Addison disease**

PO

Adults, Elderly. 0.05-0.1 mg/day. Range: 0.1 mg 3 times a week to 0.2 mg/day. Administration with cortisone or hydrocortisone preferred.

▸ **Salt-losing adrenogenital syndrome**

PO

Adults, Elderly. 0.1-0.2 mg/day.

▸ **Usual pediatric dosage**

Children. 0.05-0.1 mg/day.

OFF-LABEL USES

Diagnosis of acidosis in renal tubular disorders, idiopathic orthostatic hypotension, congenital hypoaldosteronism, postoperative cerebral salt wasting syndrome.

CONTRAINDICATIONS

Systemic fungal infection, hypersensitivity to fludrocortisone.

INTERACTIONS

Drug

Antidiabetic agents (oral agents and insulin): Antidiabetic effect may be decreased. Monitor for signs of hyperglycemia; adjust dose if necessary.

Digoxin: May increase the risk of digoxin toxicity caused by hypokalemia.

Hepatic enzyme inducers (such as phenytoin): May increase the metabolism of fludrocortisone.

Hypokalemia-causing medications: May increase the effects of fludrocortisone.
Sodium-containing medications: May increase BP, incidence of edema, and serum sodium level.
Herbal and Food
None known.

DIAGNOSTIC TEST EFFECTS

May increase serum sodium level. May decrease hematocrit and serum potassium level.

SIDE EFFECTS

Frequent
Increased appetite, exaggerated sense of well-being, abdominal distention, weight gain, insomnia, mood swings.
High dosages, prolonged therapy, too-rapid withdrawal: Increased susceptibility to infection with masked signs and symptoms, delayed wound healing, hypokalemia, hypocalcemia, GI distress, diarrhea or constipation, hypertension.
Occasional
Headache, dizziness, menstrual difficulty or amenorrhea, gastric ulcer development.
Rare
Hypersensitivity reaction.

SERIOUS REACTIONS

- Long-term therapy may cause muscle wasting (especially in the arms and legs), osteoporosis, spontaneous fractures, amenorrhea, cataracts, glaucoma, peptic ulcer disease, and congestive heart failure.
- Abruptly withdrawing the drug after long-term therapy may cause anorexia, nausea, fever, headache, joint pain, rebound inflammation, fatigue, weakness, lethargy, dizziness, and orthostatic hypotension.

PRECAUTIONS & CONSIDERATIONS

Due to sodium retention, caution is warranted with edema, hypertension, and impaired renal function. It is unknown whether fludrocortisone crosses the placenta or is distributed in breast milk. Fludrocortisone use in children may suppress growth and inhibit endogenous steroid production. Effects of fludrocortisone use in elderly patients are unknown.

Mood swings, ranging from euphoria to depression, may occur. Notify the physician of fever, muscle aches, sore throat, and sudden weight gain or swelling. Blood glucose level, serum renin, BP, serum electrolyte levels, height, and weight should be monitored before and during therapy. Be alert to signs and symptoms of infection caused by reduced immune response, including fever, sore throat, and vague symptoms.
Storage
Store at room temperature; protect from light and excessive heat.
Administration
Take fludrocortisone with food or milk. Taper the dosage slowly if fludrocortisone is to be discontinued. Expect to lower dosage if transient hypertension develops.

Flumazenil

flew-maz′ah-nil
★ Romazicon 🍁 Anexate

CATEGORY AND SCHEDULE

Pregnancy Risk Category: C

Classification: Antidotes

MECHANISM OF ACTION

An antidote that antagonizes the effect of benzodiazepines on the γ-aminobutyric acid receptor complex in the CNS. *Therapeutic Effect:* Reverses sedative effect of benzodiazepines.

PHARMACOKINETICS

Route	Onset	Peak	Duration
IV	1-2 min	6-10 min	< 1 h

F

Duration and degree of benzodiazepine reversal depend on dosage and plasma concentration. Protein binding: 50%. Metabolized by the liver; excreted in urine.

AVAILABILITY

Injection: 0.1 mg/mL.

INDICATIONS AND DOSAGES

▸ **Reversal of conscious sedation or general anesthesia**

IV

Adults, Elderly. Initially, 0.2 mg (2 mL) over 15 seconds; may repeat dose in 45 seconds; then at 60-second intervals. Maximum: 1-mg (10-mL) total dose.

Children. Initially, 0.01 mg/kg; may repeat in 45 seconds, then at 60-second intervals. Maximum: 0.2-mg single dose; 0.05-mg/kg or 1-mg cumulative dose.

▸ **Benzodiazepine overdose**

IV

Adults, Elderly. Initially, 0.2 mg (2 mL) over 30 seconds; if desired level of consciousness is not achieved after 30 seconds, 0.3 mg (3 mL) may be given over 30 seconds. Further doses of 0.5 mg (5 mL) may be administered over 30 seconds at 60-second intervals. Maximum: 3 mg (30 mL) total dose. If resedation occurs, may repeat regimen in 20 min.

Children. Initially, 0.01 mg/kg; may repeat in 45 seconds, then at 60-second intervals. Maximum: 0.2-mg single dose; 1-mg cumulative dose.

CONTRAINDICATIONS

Anticholinergic signs (such as mydriasis, dry mucosa, and hypoperistalsis), arrhythmias, cardiovascular collapse, history of hypersensitivity to benzodiazepines, patients with signs of serious cyclic antidepressant overdose (such as motor abnormalities), patients who have been given a benzodiazepine for control of a potentially life-threatening condition (such as control of status epilepticus or increased intracranial pressure).

INTERACTIONS

Drug

Tricyclic antidepressants: May produce seizures and arrhythmias as flumazenil reverses the sedative effects of tricyclic antidepressants.

Herbal and Food

None known.

DIAGNOSTIC TEST EFFECTS

None known.

IV INCOMPATIBILITIES

No information available for Y-site administration.

IV COMPATIBILITIES

Heparin.

SIDE EFFECTS

Frequent (4%-11%)

Agitation, anxiety, dry mouth, dyspnea, insomnia, palpitations, tremors, headache, blurred vision, dizziness, ataxia, nausea, vomiting, pain at injection site, diaphoresis.

Occasional (1%-3%)

Fatigue, flushing, auditory disturbances, thrombophlebitis, rash.

Rare (< 1%)

Urticaria, pruritus, hallucinations.

SERIOUS REACTIONS

- Toxic effects, such as seizures and arrhythmias, of other drugs taken in overdose, especially tricyclic antidepressants; may emerge with reversal of sedative effect of benzodiazepines.
- Flumazenil may provoke a panic attack in those with a history of panic disorder.

PRECAUTIONS & CONSIDERATIONS

Caution is warranted with head injury, impaired hepatic function, alcoholism, or drug dependency. Be aware that it is unknown whether flumazenil crosses the placenta or is distributed in breast milk. It is not recommended during labor and delivery. Be aware that flumazenil is not approved for infants or neonates. Be aware that benzodiazepine-induced sedation tends to be deeper and more prolonged, requiring careful monitoring in elderly patients. Be aware that flumazenil may wear off before effects of benzodiazepines. Repeat dosing may be necessary. Obtain arterial blood gases before and at 30-min intervals during IV administration. Prepare to intervene in reestablishing airway, assisting ventilation. Tasks that require alertness or motor skills, ingestion of alcohol, or taking of nonprescription drugs should be avoided until at least 18-24 h after discharge.

Storage

Store parenteral form at room temperature. Discard after 24 h once medication is drawn into syringe, is mixed with any solutions, or if particulate or discoloration is noted.

Administration

Be aware that flumazenil is compatible with D5W, lactated Ringer's, or 0.9% NaCl. Be aware that if resedation occurs, dose should be repeated at 20-min intervals. Maximum: 1 mg (given as 0.2 mg/min) at any one time, 3 mg in any 1 h. Administer through freely running IV infusion into large vein (local injection produces pain, inflammation at injection site). For reversing conscious sedation or general anesthesia, administer over 15 seconds. For benzodiazepine overdose, administer over 30 seconds. Take care to avoid extravasation. Observe patient for at least 2 h for signs of resedation and hypoventilation.

Flunisolide

floo-niss'oh-lide

★ AeroBid, Aerobid-M

🍁 Rhinaler

Do not confuse flunisolide with fluocinonide, or Nasalide with Nasalcrom.

CATEGORY AND SCHEDULE

Pregnancy Risk Category: C

Classification: Corticosteroids, inhalation

MECHANISM OF ACTION

An adrenocorticosteroid that controls the rate of protein synthesis, depresses migration of polymorphonuclear leukocytes, reverses capillary permeability, and stabilizes lysosomal membranes. *Therapeutic Effect:* Prevents or controls inflammation.

PHARMACOKINETICS

After oral inhalation of 1 mg, total systemic availability was 40%. Swallowed flunisolide is rapidly and extensively converted to the 6β-OH metabolite and to water-soluble conjugates via first pass through the liver. Therefore, there is low systemic activity. Inhaled flunisolide absorbed through the bronchial tree is converted to the same metabolites. Does not accumulate with repeat inhalations. Intranasal doses act locally with little systemic absorption. *Half-life:* 1.8 h.

AVAILABILITY

Aerosol (AeroBid, Aerobid-M). 250 mcg/activation.
Nasal Spray 25 mcg/spray.

INDICATIONS AND DOSAGES

▸ Long-term control of bronchial asthma, assists in reducing or discontinuing oral corticosteroid therapy

INHALATION

Adults, Elderly. 2 inhalations twice a day, morning and evening. Maximum: 4 inhalations twice a day.
Children 6-15 yr. 2 inhalations twice a day.

▸ Relief of symptoms of perennial and seasonal rhinitis

INTRANASAL

Adults, Elderly. Initially, 2 sprays each nostril twice a day, may increase at 4- to 7-day intervals to 2 sprays 3 times a day. Maximum: 8 sprays in each nostril daily.
Children aged 6-14 yr. Initially, 1 spray 3 times a day or 2 sprays twice a day. Maximum: 4 sprays in each nostril daily. Maintenance: 1 spray into each nostril each day.

OFF-LABEL USES

To prevent recurrence of nasal polyps after surgery, bronchopulmonary dysplasia of newborns, sinusitis.

CONTRAINDICATIONS

Hypersensitivity to any of the products' ingredients, persistently positive sputum cultures for *Candida albicans,* primary treatment of status asthmaticus, systemic fungal infections, untreated local infection (nasal).

INTERACTIONS

Drug
None significant.
Herbal and Food
None known.

DIAGNOSTIC TEST EFFECTS

None known.

SIDE EFFECTS

Frequent
Inhalation (10%-25%): Unpleasant taste, nausea, vomiting, sore throat, diarrhea, upset stomach, cold symptoms, nasal congestion.
Occasional
Inhalation (3%-9%): Dizziness, irritability, nervousness, tremors, abdominal pain, heartburn, oropharynx candidiasis, edema.
Nasal: Mild nasopharyngeal irritation or dryness, rebound congestion, bronchial asthma, rhinorrhea, altered taste.

SERIOUS REACTIONS

- An acute hypersensitivity reaction, marked by urticaria, angioedema, and severe bronchospasm, occurs rarely.
- A transfer from systemic to local steroid therapy may unmask previously suppressed bronchial asthma condition or may precipitate systemic signs of steroid withdrawal.
- Nasal septal perforation with prolonged or inappropriate use of nasal spray.

PRECAUTIONS & CONSIDERATIONS

If patient transferred from systemic steroid, be alert to signs of adrenal insufficiency. Use with caution if tuberculosis, fungal, bacterial, or systemic viral infections are present. Although systemic effects have been minimal with recommended doses, the potential for HPA axis suppression increases with excessive dosages. Use nasal form with caution in patients who have experienced recent nasal septal ulcers, recurrent epistaxis, or nasal surgery or trauma. Use with caution during pregnancy and lactation. Safety and efficacy not established for children under 6 yr of age.

Drink plenty of fluids to decrease the thickness of lung secretions. Pulse rate and quality, ABG levels, and respiratory rate, depth, rhythm, and type should be monitored. Notify the physician of nasal irritation or if symptoms, such as sneezing, fail to improve.

Storage

Store inhalers and nasal spray at controlled room temperature. Keep inhalation canisters away from excessive heat (may combust).

Administration

Expect to see improvement of the symptoms within a few days and relief of symptoms within 2 wks. Prepare to discontinue the drug after 3 wks if significant improvement does not occur. Do not abruptly discontinue or change the dosage schedule. The dosage must be tapered gradually under medical supervision.

For inhalation, first shake the container well. Exhale completely and place the mouthpiece between the lips. Inhale and hold breath for as long as possible before exhaling. Allow 1 min between inhalations to promote deeper bronchial penetration. Avoid spraying in the eyes. Rinse mouth with water immediately after inhalation to prevent mouth and throat dryness and oral candidiasis. If using a bronchodilator inhaler concomitantly with a steroid inhaler, use the bronchodilator several minutes before using the corticosteroid to help the steroid penetrate into the bronchial tree.

Clear nasal passages prior to intranasal use. Prime the unit before first use. Pump the activator (using care not to spray toward others) 7 or 8 times until a fine spray appears. Reprime the unit if not used in 5 days by pumping the activator once or twice. Tilt head slightly forward. Insert spray tip up into the nostril, pointing toward inflamed nasal turbinates, away from the nasal septum. Spray the drug into the nostril while holding the other nostril closed, and at the same time inhale through the nose.

Fluocinolone Acetonide

floo-oh-sin'oh-lone a-seat'oh-nide

★ Capex, Derma-Smoothe/FS, Synalar, Tri-Luma 🍁 Capex, Dermotic, Derma-Smoothe/FS, Fluoderm, Synalar

CATEGORY AND SCHEDULE

Pregnancy Risk Category: C

Classification: Corticosteriods, topical, dermatologics

MECHANISM OF ACTION

A fluorinated topical corticosteroid that controls the rate of protein synthesis; depresses migration of polymorphonuclear leukocytes and fibroblasts; reduces capillary permeability; prevents or controls inflammation. *Therapeutic Effect:* Decreases tissue response to inflammatory process.

PHARMACOKINETICS

Use of occlusive dressings may increase percutaneous absorption. Protein binding: More than 90%.

Excreted in urine. *Half-life:* Unknown.

AVAILABILITY

Cream: 0.01%, 0.025% (Synalar, Tri-Luma).
Oil: 0.01% (Derma-Smoothe/FS).
Ointment: 0.025% (Synalar).
Shampoo: 0.01% (Capex, FS).
Solution: 0.01% (Synalar).

INDICATIONS AND DOSAGES

▸ Corticosteroid-responsive dermatoses

TOPICAL

Adults, Elderly. Apply 3-4 times/day.
Children 2 yr and older. Apply 2 times/day.

▸ Scalp psoriasis

TOPICAL OIL

Adults, Elderly. Apply to damp or wet hair and leave on overnight or for at least 4 h. Remove by washing hair with shampoo.

▸ Seborrheic dermatitis, scalp

SHAMPOO

Adults, Elderly. Apply 1 oz once daily. Allow to remain on scalp for at least 5 min.

CONTRAINDICATIONS

Hypersensitivity to fluocinolone, other corticosteroids, or any components of specific products. For example, Derma-Smoothe/FS contains peanut oil and those with peanut allergy may experience hypersensitivity.

INTERACTIONS

Drug, Herbal, and Food

None known.

DIAGNOSTIC TEST EFFECTS

None known.

SIDE EFFECTS

Occasional

Burning, dryness, itching, stinging.

Rare

Allergic contact dermatitis, purpura or blood-containing blisters, thinning of skin with easy bruising, telangiectasis or raised dark red spots on skin.

SERIOUS REACTIONS

- When taken in excessive quantities, systemic hypercorticism and adrenal suppression may occur.

PRECAUTIONS & CONSIDERATIONS

It is unknown whether fluocinolone crosses the placenta and is distributed in breast milk. Be aware that the safety and efficacy of fluocinolone have not been established in children younger than 2 yr. Be aware that children may absorb larger amounts of topical corticosteroids, which should be used sparingly. No age-related precautions have been noted in elderly patients. HPA axis suppression should be monitored by urinary free cortisol tests and an ACTH stimulation test.

Storage

Store at room temperature. Shampoo is stable for 3 mo after mixing by pharmacist.

Administration

Gently cleanse area before topical application. Use occlusive dressings only as ordered. Apply sparingly, and rub into area thoroughly. When using topical oil preparation on scalp, massage through dampened hair and scalp. Cover with shower cap. Leave on overnight or for at least 4 h. Remove by washing hair with shampoo. When using shampoo preparation, first shake well. Apply to wet hair, massage for 1 min, and allow to remain on scalp for 5 min. Rinse thoroughly.

Fluorescein

flure′e-seen

AK-Fluor, Fluorescite, Fluor-I-Strip-AT, Ful-Glo BioGlo, Diofluor, Flourets

Do not confuse with fluoride.

CATEGORY AND SCHEDULE

Pregnancy Risk Category: X (parenteral), C (topical)

Classification: Diagnostics, nonradioactive, ophthalmic

MECHANISM OF ACTION

An indicator dye used as a diagnostic agent with a low molecular weight, high water solubility, and fluorescence that penetrates any break in epithelial barrier to permit rapid penetration. Emits light at a wavelength of 520-530 nm (green-yellow) when exposed to light in the blue wavelength (465-490 nm). *Therapeutic Effect:* Diagnosis of corneal and conjunctival abnormalities.

PHARMACOKINETICS

Rapidly absorbed. Protein binding: 85%. Widely distributed. Metabolized in liver to an active metabolite, fluorescein monoglucuronide. Primarily excreted in urine. *Half-life:* 24 min (parent compound), 4 h (metabolite).

AVAILABILITY

Injection, Solution: 10% (AK-Fluor, Fluorescite).

Strip, Ophthalmic: 0.6 mg (Ful-Glo), 1 mg (Fluor-I-Strip-AT, Ful-Glo).

INDICATIONS AND DOSAGES

▸ Retinal angiography

INJECTION

Adults, Elderly. Inject contents (500 mg) of ampule or vial of 10% solution rapidly into the antecubital vein. If laser ophthalmoscope used, a reduced dose of 200 mg may be appropriate.

Children. 7.7 mg/kg (actual body weight) not to exceed 500 mg.

▸ Applanation tonometry

OPHTHALMIC STRIPS

Adults, Elderly. Place strip, which has been moistened with a drop of sterile water, at the fornix in the lower cul-de-sac close to the punctum. Patient should close lid tightly over strip until desired amount of staining is observed or retract upper lid and touch tip of strip to the bulbar conjunctiva on the temporal side until adequate staining is achieved.

CONTRAINDICATIONS

Concomitant soft contact lens use (ophthalmic strips), hypersensitivity to fluorescein or any component of the formulation.

INTERACTIONS

Drug, Herbal, and Food

None known.

IV COMPATIBILITIES

Do not mix or dilute with other solutions on drugs.

DIAGNOSTIC TEST EFFECTS

May interfere with digoxin assay results.

SIDE EFFECTS

Occasional

Ophthalmic: Burning sensation in the eye.

Injection: Stinging, bronchospasm, generalized hives and itching, hypersensitivity, headache, gastrointestinal distress, nausea, strong taste, vomiting, hypotension, syncope.

Rare
Injection: Anaphylaxis, basilar artery ischemia, cardiac arrest, severe shock, convulsions, thrombophlebitis at injection site.

SERIOUS REACTIONS

- Anaphylactic reactions have occurred, leading to laryngeal edema, bronchospasm, shock, and even death.

PRECAUTIONS & CONSIDERATIONS

Injection preparation should be used cautiously with bronchial asthma or history of allergy. It is unknown whether fluorescein crosses the placenta or is distributed in breast milk. Safety and efficacy have not been established in children. No age-related precautions have been noted in elderly patients. Blockages or leakage should be assessed on map location for possible treatment. Normal values will appear normal in size. Skin and urine may temporarily turn yellow. Abnormal results can mean diabetic or other retinopathy, macular degeneration, cancer, tumors, circulatory problems, inflammation or edema, microaneurysms, or swelling of the optic disc.

Storage
Store at room temperature. Do not freeze.

Administration
Allow a few seconds for staining when using ophthalmic preparation. Wash out excess with sterile water or irrigating solution. Blink several times after application of strip.

For fluorescein injection, inject rapidly into antecubital vein (5-10 seconds). Take care to avoid extravasation. Flush IV cannula with saline flush before and after use to prevent physical incompatability with other drugs.

Fluoride, Sodium

Epiflur, Fluorabon, Fluor-A-Day, Fluoritab, Flura-Loz, Ludent, Luride NaFrinse, Prevident, ReNaf

Fluor-A-Day

Do not confuse with Fludara.

CATEGORY AND SCHEDULE

Pregnancy Risk Category: B (topical gels/rinses), C (oral)

Classification: Dental preparations, minerals

MECHANISM OF ACTION

A trace element that increases tooth resistance to acid dissolution. *Therapeutic Effect:* Promotes remineralization of decalcified enamel, inhibits dental plaque bacteria, increases resistance to development of caries, maintains bone strength.

AVAILABILITY

Oral Solution Drops: 0.25 mg/mL, 0.5 mg/mL.
Tablets (Chewable): 0.25 mg, 0.5 mg, 1 mg.
NOTE: Many topical fluoride agents exist OTC as dental rinses, toothpastes, and gels (e.g., Prevident).

INDICATIONS AND DOSAGES

▸ Dietary supplement for prevention of dental caries in children

Fluoride Level in Water (ppm)	Age	Oral Dosage (mg/day)*
< 0.3	6 mo to 2 yr	0.25
	3-5 yr	0.5
	6-16 yr	1
0.3-0.6	Younger than 2 yr	None
	3-5 yr	0.25
	6-16 yr	0.5

ppm, Parts per million.
*Expressed as fluoride ion.

CONTRAINDICATIONS
Arthralgia, GI ulceration, severe renal insufficiency (CrCl < 20 mL/min), areas where fluoride level in water exceeds 0.6 ppm.

INTERACTIONS
Drug
Aluminum hydroxide, calcium: May decrease the absorption of fluoride.
Herbal
None known.
Food
Dairy products: May decrease fluoride's absorption. Do not eat or drink dairy products within 1 h of fluoride adminsitration.

DIAGNOSTIC TEST EFFECTS
May increase serum alkaline phosphatase and AST (SGOT) levels.

SIDE EFFECTS
Rare
Oral mucous membrane ulceration.

SERIOUS REACTIONS
- Hypocalcemia, tetany, bone pain (especially in ankles and feet), electrolyte disturbances, and arrhythmias occur rarely.
- Fluoride use may cause skeletal fluorosis, osteomalacia, and osteosclerosis.

PRECAUTIONS & CONSIDERATIONS
Take care to avoid overdosage. Use in infants < 6 mo is not recommended by current American Dental Association and American Academy of Pediatrics guidelines. Use with caution in pregnancy and lactation. Heavy exposure to fluoride during in utero development may result in skeletal fluorosis, which becomes evident in childhood.

Storage
Store at room temperature, protected from humidity. Keep solutions tightly closed.
Administration
Chewable tablets should be chewed before swallowing. Oral drops can be given directly in mouth or mixed with cereal or fruit juice.

Administration at bedtime after brushing teeth is recommended for tablets.

There are many topical forms of fluoride for dental use. Always supervise young children. Avoid ingestion of any of these products.

Fluorouracil, 5-FU
flure-oh-yoor′ah-sill
Adrucil, Carac, Efudex, Fluoroplex Efudex, Fluoroplex
Do not confuse Efudex with Efidac.

CATEGORY AND SCHEDULE
Pregnancy Risk Category: D

Classification: Antineoplastic, antimetabolite

MECHANISM OF ACTION
An antimetabolite that blocks formation of thymidylic acid. Cell-cycle–specific for S phase of cell division. *Therapeutic Effect:* Inhibits DNA and RNA synthesis. Topical form destroys rapidly proliferating cells.

PHARMACOKINETICS
Widely distributed. Crosses the blood-brain barrier. Rapidly metabolized in tissues to active metabolite, which is localized intracellularly. Primarily excreted by lungs as carbon dioxide. Removed by hemodialysis. *Half-life:* 20 h.

F

AVAILABILITY

Cream: 0.5%, 1%, 5%.
Solution, Topical: 2%, 5%.
Injection: 50 mg/mL.

INDICATIONS AND DOSAGES

▸ **Carcinoma of breast, colon, pancreas, rectum, and stomach; in combination with levamisole after surgical resection in patients with Duke's stage C colon cancer**

IV

Adults, Elderly. Initially, 12 mg/kg/day for 4-5 days. Maximum: 800 mg/day. Followed by 6 mg/kg every other day for 4 doses. Maintenance: Repeat initial dose every 30 days; or 10-15 mg/kg/wk as a single dose not to exceed 1 g/wk.

! NOTE: After adult IV doses given, lower dosages are recommended for debilitated patients.

▸ **Multiple actinic or solar keratoses**

TOPICAL 0.5% CREAM

Adults, Elderly. Apply once a day.

TOPICAL 1% & 5% CREAM, 2% SOLUTION

Adults, Elderly. Apply twice a day.

▸ **Basal cell carcinoma**

TOPICAL 5% SOLUTION

Adult, Elderly. Apply twice a day.

CONTRAINDICATIONS

Myelosuppression, poor nutritional status, potentially serious infections, hypersensitivity to fluorouracil or product ingredients, dihydropyrmidine dehydrogenase enzyme deficiency.

INTERACTIONS

Drug

Leucovorin, levoleucovorin, metronidazole, tinidazole: Increased 5-FU toxicity.

Phenytoin: Altered phenytoin concentrations (mostly lowered) have been reported.

Warfarin: Increased risk of bleeding.

Live vaccines: Defer vaccination due to potential virus replication, adverse reactions to the virus, immunosuppression.

Herbal

None reported.

Food

None reported.

IV INCOMPATIBILITIES

Aldesleukin, amiodarone, buprenorphine, calcium chloride, caspofungin (Cancidas), ciprofloxacin (Cipro), cisplatin, cytarabine, diazepam, doxorubicin, droperidol, epirubicin, filgrastim, gallium nitrate, haloperidol, idarubicin, lansoprazole (Prevacid IV), leucovorin, levofloxacin (Levaquin), levoleucovorin, lorazepam, methotrexate, metoclopramide, midazolam, morphine, nicardipine, ondansetron, phenytoin, quinupristin-dalfopristin (Synercid), topotecan, TPN, vancomycin, vinorelbine.

SIDE EFFECTS

Occasional

Parenteral: Anorexia, diarrhea, minimal alopecia, fever, dry skin, skin fissures, scaling, erythema. Topical: Pain, pruritus, hyperpigmentation, irritation, inflammation, and burning at application site; photosensitivity.

Rare

Nausea, vomiting, anemia, esophagitis, proctitis, GI ulcer, confusion, headache, lacrimation, visual disturbances, angina, allergic reactions.

SERIOUS REACTIONS

• The earliest sign of toxicity, which may occur 4-8 days after beginning therapy, is stomatitis (as evidenced by dry mouth, burning sensation, mucosal erythema, and ulceration at inner margin of lips).

• Hematologic toxicity may be manifested as leukopenia (generally within 9-14 days after drug administration, but possibly as late as the 25th day), thrombocytopenia (within 7-17 days after administration), pancytopenia, or agranulocytosis.
• The most common dermatologic toxicity is a pruritic rash on the extremities or, less frequently, the trunk. Delayed serious hypersensitivity reactions may also occur.

PRECAUTIONS & CONSIDERATIONS

Patients should be hospitalized during the initial course of IV fluorouracil therapy. Use with caution in patients with a history of high-dose pelvic irradiation or previous use of alkylating agents, metastatic bone marrow involvement, or impaired hepatic or renal function. Discontinue therapy in patients developing stomatitis, leukopenia, intractable vomiting, diarrhea, GI ulceration or bleeding, thrombocytopenia, or hemorrhage from any site. Severe toxicity (abdominal pain, bloody diarrhea, neutropenia, neurotoxicity, chills, fever or vomiting) while receiving topical or systemic fluorouracil may occur in those with dipyrimidine dehydrogenase (DPD) deficiency; deficiency results in prolonged fluorouracil clearance. It is not known if fluorouracil is excreted in breast milk; avoid use. Safety and effectiveness of topical fluorouracil have not been established in children. No age-related precautions have been observed in the elderly. Avoid application of topical fluorouracil to mucous membranes. Use with occlusive dressings cautiously; may increase penetration and incidence of inflammatory reactions in adjacent healthy skin. Avoid prolonged exposure to sunlight.

Storage
Injectable, topical cream and solution should be stored at room temperature. Protect from light and freezing. Infusions have extended stability once prepared, but refer to specialized resources for details as stability is concentration dependent.

Administration
CAUTION: Observe and exercise appropriate precautions for handling and administering cytotoxic drugs.

Fluorouracil injection should be administered IV, either by slow IV push or IV infusion. Use care to avoid extravasation. No dilution is required. However, the drug is often administered as an IV infusion and diluted in 0.9% NaCl or D5W (usual max concentrations 10 mg/mL dilutions). Protect from light.

Cleanse the affected area and wait 10 min before applying topical fluorouracil. Apply with fingertips and wash hands as soon as finish application. A moisturizer/sunscreen may be applied 2 h after fluorouracil.

Fluoxetine

floo-ox′e-teen

★ Prozac, Prozac Weekly, Sarafem, Selfemra

🍁 Prozac

Do not confuse fluoxetine with fluvastatin; Prozac with Prilosec, Proscar, or ProSom; or Sarafem with Serophene.

CATEGORY AND SCHEDULE

Pregnancy Risk Category: C

Classification: Antidepressants, selective serotonin reuptake inhibitors

F

MECHANISM OF ACTION

A psychotherapeutic agent that selectively inhibits serotonin uptake in the CNS, enhancing serotonergic function. *Therapeutic Effect:* Relieves depression; reduces obsessive-compulsive and bulimic behavior.

PHARMACOKINETICS

Well absorbed from the GI tract. Crosses the blood-brain barrier. Protein binding: 94%. Metabolized in the liver to active metabolite. Primarily excreted in urine. Not removed by hemodialysis. *Half-life:* 2-3 days; metabolite 7-9 days.

AVAILABILITY

Capsules (Prozac): 10 mg, 20 mg, 40 mg.
Capsules (Sarafem, Selfemra): 10 mg, 20 mg.
Capsules (Enteric Coated [Prozac Weekly]): 90 mg.
Oral Solution (Prozac): 20 mg/5 mL.
Tablets: 10 mg, 20 mg, 40 mg.
Tablets (Sarafem): 10 mg, 15 mg, 20 mg.

INDICATIONS AND DOSAGES

▸ Depression, obsessive-compulsive disorder

PO

Adults and Elderly. Initially, 20 mg each morning. If therapeutic improvement does not occur after 2 wks, gradually increase to maximum of 80 mg/day in 2 equally divided doses in morning and at noon. Prozac Weekly: 90 mg/wk, begin 7 days after last dose of 20 mg.

Children aged 8 yr and older for depression, 7 yr and older for OCD. Initially, 10-20 mg/day. Begin with 10 mg/day in lower weight or younger children. Usual dosage is 20 mg/day. Do not exceed 60 mg/day for OCD.

▸ Panic disorder

PO

Adults, Elderly. Initially, 10 mg/day. May increase to 20 mg/day after 1 wk. Maximum: 60 mg/day.

▸ Bulimia nervosa

PO

Adults. 60 mg each morning. May need to titrate up from lower dosage.

▸ Premenstrual dysphoric disorder

PO

Adults. 20 mg/day continuously, or 20 mg/day starting 14 days before the anticipated start of menstruation and continue through the first full day of menses.

OFF-LABEL USES

Treatment of hot flashes, fibromyalgia, posttraumatic stress disorder.

CONTRAINDICATIONS

Use within 14 days of MAOIs, also contraindicated with thioridazine. Hypersensitivity.

INTERACTIONS

NOTE: Of the SSRI-type drugs, fluoxetine inhibits multiple CYP isozymes significantly (particularly CYP 2D6, 2C19, 3A4 (weak), 2C9, and 2C10. Increased serum concentrations and toxicity of concomitant medications may occur.

Drug

Alcohol, other CNS depressants: May increase CNS depression.
Highly protein-bound medications (including oral anticoagulants): May increase adverse effects.
MAOIs: May produce serotonin syndrome and neuroleptic malignant syndrome. Contraindicated.
Phenytoin: May increase phenytoin blood concentration and risk of toxicity.
Platelet inhibitors: May increase risk of bleeding.

Ritonavir: Fluoxetine dose reduction may be necessary.
Serotonergic agents: Increased risk of serotonin syndrome.
Thioridazine: Increased thioridazine concentrations. Contraindicated with fluoxetine.
Herbal
St. John's wort: May increase fluoxetine's pharmacologic effects and risk of toxicity.
Food
None known.

DIAGNOSTIC TEST EFFECTS

May increase liver enzymes. May cause lowered serum sodium; may cause platelet dysfunction.

SIDE EFFECTS

Frequent (>10%)
Headache, asthenia, insomnia, anxiety, nervousness, somnolence, nausea, diarrhea, decreased appetite.
Occasional (2%-9%)
Dizziness, tremor, fatigue, vomiting, constipation, dry mouth, abdominal pain, nasal congestion, diaphoresis, rash.
Rare (< 2%)
Flushed skin, light-headedness, impaired concentration, platelet dysfunction with or without bleeding.

SERIOUS REACTIONS

• Overdose may produce seizures, nausea, vomiting, agitation, and restlessness (serotonin syndrome). As a result of long half-life, effects may be prolonged.
• SIADH and hyponatremia have been reported rarely, most commonly in elderly patients.

PRECAUTIONS & CONSIDERATIONS

Caution is warranted in patients with hepatic and renal impairment and in those with a history of hypomania, mania, and seizures. Fluoxetine is distributed in breast milk and should be used with caution in pregnancy because adverse neonatal outcomes have been reported, including drug withdrawal syndromes. Antidepressants have been reported to increase the risk of suicidal thinking and behavior in children, adolescents, and young adults (18-24 yr of age) with major depressive disorder (MDD) and other psychiatric disorders. Patients should be closely monitored for clinical worsening, suicidality, or unusual changes in behavior, particularly during the initial 1-2 mo of therapy or following dosage adjustments. Elderly patients are more sensitive to the drug's effects, such as dry mouth.

Drowsiness and dizziness may occur, so avoid alcohol and tasks that require mental alertness or motor skills until the drug effects are known. CBC and liver and renal function tests should be performed before and periodically during long-term therapy. Assess pattern of daily bowel activity and stool consistency, skin for rash, and blood glucose level.
Storage
Store all products at room temperature.
Administration
! Make sure that at least 14 days elapse between the use of MAOIs and fluoxetine.

Take fluoxetine with food or milk if GI distress occurs. Avoid administration at night. The therapeutic effects of fluoxetine will be noted within 1 to 4 wks. Do not abruptly discontinue fluoxetine. Divided doses can be given at morning and noon.

Prozac Weekly: Swallow whole; do not crush or chew.

Fluoxymesterone

floo-ox-ih-mes′te-rone

★ Androxy

CATEGORY AND SCHEDULE

Pregnancy Risk Category: X

Controlled Substance Schedule: III

Classification: Androgens, hormones/hormone modifiers

MECHANISM OF ACTION

An androgen that suppresses gonadotropin-releasing hormone, LH, and FSH. *Therapeutic Effect:* Stimulates spermatogenesis, development of male secondary sex characteristics, and sexual maturation at puberty. Stimulates production of red blood cells (RBCs).

PHARMACOKINETICS

Rapidly absorbed from the GI tract. Protein binding: 98%. Metabolized in liver. Excreted in urine. *Half-life:* 9.2 h.

AVAILABILITY

Tablets: 10 mg.

INDICATIONS AND DOSAGES

Dosage must be strictly individualized; suggested dose for androgens varies, depending on the age, sex, and diagnosis of the patient. Dosage is adjusted according to the patient's response and the appearance of adverse reactions.

▸ **Males (hypogonadism)**

PO

Adults. 5-20 mg/day.

▸ **Males (delayed puberty)**

PO

Adults. 2.5-10 mg/day for 4-6 mo. Maximum: 20 mg/day.

▸ **Females (inoperable breast cancer)**

PO

Adults. 10-40 mg/day in divided doses for 1-3 mo.

CONTRAINDICATIONS

Serious cardiac, renal, or hepatic dysfunction, men with carcinomas of the breast or prostate, hypersensitivity to fluoxymesterone or any component of the formulation including tartrazine, known or suspected pregnancy, breastfeeding.

INTERACTIONS

Drug

Cyclosporine: May increase the risk of cyclosporine toxicity.

Hepatotoxic medications: May increase the risk of hepatotoxicity.

Oral anticoagulants: May increase the effect of these drugs.

Herbal

Chaparral, comfrey, eucalyptus, germander, Jin Bu Huan, kava kava, pennyroyal, skullcap, valerian: May increase the risk of liver damage.

Food

None known.

DIAGNOSTIC TEST EFFECTS

May decrease levels of thyroxine-binding globulin, total T4 serum levels, and resin uptake of T3 and T4. May increase alkaline phosphatase, SGOT (AST), bilirubin, calcium, potassium, sodium, hemoglobin, hematocrit, LDL. May decrease HDL.

SIDE EFFECTS

Frequent

Females: Amenorrhea, virilism (e.g., acne, decreased breast size, enlarged clitoris, male pattern baldness), deepening voice.

Males: Urinary tract infection, breast soreness, gynecomastia, priapism, virilism (e.g., acne, early pubic hair growth).

Occasional
Edema, nausea, vomiting, mild acne, diarrhea, stomach pain.
Males: Impotence, testicular atrophy.

SERIOUS REACTIONS

- Peliosis hepatitis (liver, spleen replaced with blood-filled cysts), hepatic neoplasms, and hepatocellular carcinoma have been associated with prolonged high dosage.

PRECAUTIONS & CONSIDERATIONS

Caution is warranted with impaired renal or liver function, benign prostate hypertrophy, hypercalcemia (may be aggravated in patients with metastatic breast cancer), history of myocardial infarction, and diabetes mellitus. This drug should not be used to enhance athletic performance. Fluoxymesterone use is contraindicated during pregnancy lactation. Safety and efficacy of fluoxymesterone have not been established in children, so use with caution. Fluoxymesterone use in elderly patients may increase the risk of hyperplasia or stimulate growth of occult prostate carcinoma.
Acne, nausea, pedal edema, or vomiting should be reported to the physician. In particular, female patients should report deepening of voice, hoarseness, and menstrual irregularities; male patients should report difficulty urinating, frequent erections, and gynecomastia.
Patients should be monitored for hypercalcemia.

Storage
Store at room temperature.

Administration
Give with food to minimize GI upset. May cut scored tablet to adjust dosage.

Fluphenazine

floo-fen′a-zeen
Modecate
Do not confuse decanoate injection with other injectable forms of the drug.

CATEGORY AND SCHEDULE

Pregnancy Risk Category: C

Classification: Antipsychotics, phenothiazines

MECHANISM OF ACTION

A phenothiazine that antagonizes dopamine neurotransmission at synapses by blocking postsynaptic dopaminergic receptors in the brain. *Therapeutic Effect:* Decreases psychotic behavior. Also produces weak anticholinergic, sedative, and antiemetic effects and strong extrapyramidal effects.

PHARMACOKINETICS

Erratic and variable absorption from the GI tract. Widely distributed. Metabolized in liver. Primarily excreted in urine. *Half-life:* 163-232 h.

AVAILABILITY

Elixir: 2.5 mg/5 mL.
Tablets: 1 mg, 2.5 mg, 5 mg, 10 mg.
Injection: 2.5 mg/mL.
Injection Suspension (Decanoate): 25 mg/mL.

INDICATIONS AND DOSAGES

▸ **Psychosis**

PO
Adults, Elderly. 0.5-10 mg/day in divided doses q6-8h. Doses above 20 mg/day are rarely needed.
IM
Adults, Elderly. Initially, 1.25-2.5 mg IM q6-8h. Usual effective dose:

1.5-10 mg/day in divided doses q6-8h or 12.5 mg (decanoate) q3wks.

CONTRAINDICATIONS

Severe CNS depression, comatose states, severe depression, subcortical brain damage, presence of blood dyscrasias or liver damage, hypersensitivity to fluphenazine or any component of the formulation including tartrazine.

INTERACTIONS

Drug

Alcohol, other CNS depressants: May increase hypotensive and CNS and respiratory depressant effects.
Antithyroid agents: May increase the risk of agranulocytosis.
Extrapyramidal symptom-producing medications: May increase extrapyramidal symptoms.
Hypotension-producing medications: May increase hypotension.
Levodopa: May decrease the effects of this drug.
Lithium: May decrease the absorption of fluphenazine and produce adverse neurologic effects.
MAOIs, tricyclic antidepressants: May increase anticholinergic and sedative effects.

Herbal and Food

None known.

DIAGNOSTIC TEST EFFECTS

Causes elevated prolactin levels. May produce false-positive pregnancy and phenylketonuria test results. May cause ECG changes, including Q- and T-wave disturbances.

SIDE EFFECTS

Frequent

Hypotension, dizziness, and syncope (occur frequently after first injection, occasionally after subsequent injections, and rarely with oral doses).

Occasional

Somnolence (during early therapy), dry mouth, blurred vision, lethargy, constipation or diarrhea, nasal congestion, peripheral edema, urine retention. Elevates prolactin levels.

Rare

Ocular changes, altered skin pigmentation (with prolonged use of high doses).

SERIOUS REACTIONS

- Extrapyramidal symptoms appear to be related to high dosages and are divided into three categories: akathisia (inability to sit still, tapping of feet), parkinsonian symptoms (such as hypersalivation, mask-like facial expression, shuffling gait, and tremors), and acute dystonias (such as torticollis, opisthotonos, and oculogyric crisis).
- Tardive dyskinesia, manifested as tongue protrusion, puffing of the cheeks, and chewing or puckering of the mouth, occurs rarely but may be irreversible.
- Abrupt withdrawal after long-term therapy may precipitate dizziness, gastritis, nausea and vomiting, and tremors.
- Blood dyscrasias, particularly agranulocytosis and mild leukopenia, may occur.
- Fluphenazine use may lower the seizure threshold.
- Neuroleptic Malignant Syndrome (NMS).

PRECAUTIONS & CONSIDERATIONS

Caution is warranted with Parkinson disease and seizures. Drowsiness may occur, so tasks that require mental alertness or motor skills should be avoided. Exposure to light and sunlight should also be avoided. Signs of tardive dyskinesia such as fine tongue movement and therapeutic response should be monitored. BP for hypotension, WBC for blood dyscrasias, and therapeutic response should be assessed during therapy. This medication is known to cross the placenta, and it is unknown if it appears in breast milk.

Storage

Store at room temperature and protect from light.

Administration

May take with food to decrease GI effects. Do not take antacids within 1 h.

For IM use, administer deep injection in large muscle mass, keep patient recumbent for 30 min after injection to minimize hypotension.

Administer decanoate injection deep IM into gluteal area.

Flurandrenolide

flure-an-dren′oh-lide

★ Cordran, Cordran SP

CATEGORY AND SCHEDULE

Pregnancy Risk Category: C

Classification: Corticosteroids, topical, dermatologics

MECHANISM OF ACTION

A fluorinated corticosteroid that decreases inflammation by suppression of the migration of polymorphonuclear leukocytes and reversal of increased capillary permeability. *Therapeutic Effect:* Decreases tissue response to inflammatory process. The amount of corticosteroid absorbed from the skin depends on the intrinsic properties of the drug, the vehicle used, the duration of exposure, the skin surface area, and the condition of the skin.

PHARMACOKINETICS

Repeated applications may lead to percutaneous absorption. Absorption is about 36% from scrotal area, 7% from forehead, 4% from scalp, and 1% from forearm. Metabolized in liver. Excreted in urine. *Half-life:* Unknown.

AVAILABILITY

Cream: 0.025%, 0.05% (Cordran SP).
Lotion: 0.05% (Cordran).
Ointment: 0.025%, 0.05% (Cordran).
Tape, Topical: 4 mcg/cm^2 (Cordran).

INDICATIONS AND DOSAGES

▸ Anti-inflammatory, immunosuppressant, corticosteroid replacement therapy

TOPICAL

Adults, Elderly. Apply 2-3 times/day.
Children. Apply 1-2 times/day, once daily if tape used.

CONTRAINDICATIONS

Hypersensitivity to flurandrenolide or any component of the formulation; viral, fungal, or tubercular skin lesions.

INTERACTIONS

Drug

None known.

Herbal

None known.

Food

None known.

DIAGNOSTIC TEST EFFECTS

None known.

SIDE EFFECTS

Occasional

Itching, dry skin, folliculitis.

Rare

Intracranial hemorrhage, acne, striae, miliaria, allergic contact dermatitis, telangiectasis, or raised dark red spots on the skin.

SERIOUS REACTIONS

- When taken in excessive quantities, systemic hypercorticism and adrenal suppression may occur.

PRECAUTIONS & CONSIDERATIONS

Caution should be exercised when used over large areas of body, in denuded areas, for prolonged periods, with occlusive dressings, and in small children. It is unknown whether flurandrenolide crosses the placenta or is distributed in breast milk. Be aware that the safety and efficacy of flurandrenolide have not been established in children. Therefore, use the smallest dose necessary to achieve optimal results. Be aware that children are at an increased risk of systemic toxicity and side effects.

No age-related precautions have been noted in elderly patients. Urinary free cortisol test and ACTH stimulation test should be obtained for suspected HPA axis suppression.

Storage

Store at room temperature.

Administration

Avoid contact with eyes. Gently cleanse area before application. Use occlusive dressings only as ordered. Apply sparingly and rub into area thoroughly. Children using flurandrenolide tape should use it only once a day.

Flurazepam

flure-az′e-pam

Dalmane SomPam, Somnol

Do not confuse with Dialume.

CATEGORY AND SCHEDULE

Pregnancy Risk Category: X

Controlled Substance Schedule: IV

Classification: Benzodiazepines, sedatives/hypnotics

MECHANISM OF ACTION

A benzodiazepine that enhances the action of inhibitory neurotransmitter γ-aminobutyric acid (GABA). *Therapeutic Effect:* Produces hypnotic effect due to central nervous system (CNS) depression.

PHARMACOKINETICS

Route	Onset	Peak	Duration
PO	15-20 min	3-6 h	7-8 h

Well absorbed from the GI tract. Protein binding: 97%. Crosses the blood-brain barrier. Widely distributed. Metabolized in liver to active metabolite. Primarily excreted in urine. Not removed by hemodialysis. *Half-life:* 2.3 h; metabolite: 40-114 h.

AVAILABILITY

Capsules: 15 mg, 30 mg.

INDICATIONS AND DOSAGES

▸ **Insomnia**

PO

Adults. 15-30 mg at bedtime.

Elderly, debilitated, liver disease, low serum albumin, Children 15 yr and older. 15 mg at bedtime.

CONTRAINDICATIONS

Acute alcohol intoxication, acute angle-closure glaucoma, pregnancy or breastfeeding, sleep apnea.

INTERACTIONS

Drug

Alcohol, CNS depressants: May increase CNS depression.

Digoxin: Increased digoxin serum levels and toxicity may increase.

Herbal

Dong quai, kava kava, magnolia, passionflower, skullcap, valerian: May increase CNS depression.

St. John's wort: Decreased efficacy of flurazepam.

Food
None known.

DIAGNOSTIC TEST EFFECTS

None known.

SIDE EFFECTS

Frequent
Drowsiness, dizziness, ataxia, sedation.

Morning drowsiness may occur initially.

Occasional
GI disturbances, nervousness, blurred vision, dry mouth, headache, confusion, skin rash, irritability, slurred speech.

Rare
Paradoxical CNS excitement or restlessness, particularly noted in elderly or debilitated patients.

SERIOUS REACTIONS

- Abrupt or too-rapid withdrawal after long-term use may result in pronounced restlessness and irritability, insomnia, hand tremors, abdominal or muscle cramps, vomiting, diaphoresis, and seizures.
- Overdose results in somnolence, confusion, diminished reflexes, and coma.

PRECAUTIONS & CONSIDERATIONS

Caution is warranted with impaired liver or renal function. Flurazepam crosses the placenta and may be distributed in breast milk. Chronic flurazepam ingestion during pregnancy may produce withdrawal symptoms and CNS depression in neonates. The safety and efficacy of flurazepam have not been established in children younger than 15 yr of age. Use small initial doses with gradual dose increases to avoid ataxia or excessive sedation in elderly patients. Avoid smoking, because it reduces the drug's effectiveness. Flurazepam may be habit-forming. Assess BP, pulse, and respirations immediately before beginning flurazepam administration. Disturbed sleep 1-2 nights after discontinuing the drug may occur.

Storage
Store at room temperature and protect from light.

Administration
Take flurazepam without regard to meals. If desired, empty capsules and mix with food. Take before bedtime. Do not abruptly withdraw the medication after long-term use.

Flurbiprofen

flure-bi′-proe-fen

Ansaid, Ocufen

Do not confuse Ocufen with Ocuflox.

CATEGORY AND SCHEDULE

Pregnancy Risk Category: B (D if used in third trimester or near delivery; C for ophthalmic solution)

Classification: Nonsteroidal anti-inflammatory, ophthalmic anti-inflammatory

MECHANISM OF ACTION

A phenylalkanoic acid that produces analgesic and anti-inflammatory effect by inhibiting prostaglandin synthesis. Also relaxes the iris sphincter. *Therapeutic Effect:* Reduces the inflammatory response and intensity of pain. Prevents or decreases miosis during cataract surgery.

PHARMACOKINETICS

Well absorbed from the GI tract; ophthalmic solution penetrates cornea after administration, and may be systemically absorbed. Protein binding: 99%. Widely distributed. Metabolized in the liver. Primarily excreted in urine. *Half-life:* 3-4 h.

AVAILABILITY

Tablets: 50 mg, 100 mg.
Ophthalmic Solution: 0.03%.

INDICATIONS AND DOSAGES

▸ Rheumatoid arthritis, osteoarthritis
PO
Adults, Elderly. 200–300 mg/day in 2-4 divided doses. Maximum: 100 mg/dose or 300 mg/day.
▸ Dysmenorrhea, pain
PO
Adults. 50 mg 4 times a day.
▸ Intraoperative miosis
OPHTHALMIC
Adults, Elderly, Children. Apply 1 drop q30min starting 2 h before surgery for total of 4 doses.

CONTRAINDICATIONS

Active peptic ulcer, chronic inflammation of GI tract, GI bleeding or ulceration, history of hypersensitivity to aspirin or NSAIDs; treatment of perioperative pain following CABG surgery.

DRUG INTERACTIONS

Aspirin, alcohol, corticosteroids: GI ulceration, bleeding. NSAID use may negate cardioprotective effect of ASA.
Salicylates: Decreased action.
Oral anticoagulants, oral antidiabetics, lithium, methotrexate: Risk of increased effects.
Diuretics: Decreased effects.
SSRIs, SNRIs: Increased risk GI bleeding.
Herbal
Herbs with antiplatelet effects (e.g., ginkgo, white willow): Increased risk of bleeding.
Food
Alcohol: May increase dizziness or risk of GI bleeding.

SIDE EFFECTS

Occasional
PO: Headache, abdominal pain, diarrhea, indigestion, nausea, fluid retention.
Ophthalmic: Burning or stinging on instillation, keratitis, elevated intraocular pressure.
Rare
PO: Blurred vision, flushed skin, dizziness, somnolence, nervousness, insomnia, unusual fatigue, constipation, decreased appetite, vomiting, confusion.

SERIOUS REACTIONS

- Overdose may result in acute renal failure.
- Rare reactions with long-term use include peptic ulcer disease, GI bleeding, gastritis, severe hepatic reaction (jaundice), nephrotoxicity (hematuria, dysuria, proteinuria), a severe hypersensitivity reaction (angioedema, bronchospasm), and cardiac arrhythmias.

PRECAUTIONS & CONSIDERATIONS

Use with caution in patients with CHF, hypertension, fluid retention, dehydration, history of GI disease (bleeding or ulcers), coagulation disorders, asthma, hepatic impairment, or renal impairment. Flurbiprofen should not be used in the third trimester of pregnancy as it may lead to premature closure of the ductus arteriosis. Flurbiprofen is excreted in breast milk; use in nursing mothers is not recommended. Safety and effectiveness have not been established in children. The elderly are at increased risk of adverse effects, particularly GI effects and renal toxicity.

Anaphylactoid reactions have occurred in patients with aspirin triad hypersensitivity. Do not use in patients with aspirin-sensitive asthma. Cardiovascular event risk may be increased with duration of use or preexisting cardiovascular risk factors or disease. Use caution in patients with fluid retention, heart failure, or hypertension. Use the lowest effective dose for the shortest duration. Risk of myocardial infarction and stroke may be increased following CABG surgery. Do not administer within 4-6 half-lives before surgical procedures.

Notify the physician of edema, GI distress, headache, rash, signs of bleeding, or visual disturbances. CBC and blood chemistry studies should be monitored to assess hepatic and renal function. Therapeutic response, such as decreased pain, stiffness, swelling or tenderness, improved grip strength, and increased joint mobility, should be evaluated.

Storage
Store at room temperature.

Administration
May be taken with food, milk, or antacid to reduce GI effects.

Flutamide

floo'ta-mide

🍁 Euflex

Do not confuse flutamide with Flumadine.

CATEGORY AND SCHEDULE

Pregnancy Risk Category: D

Classification: Antineoplastics, antiandrogens, hormones/hormone modifiers

MECHANISM OF ACTION

An antiandrogen hormone that inhibits androgen uptake and prevents androgen from binding to androgen receptors in target tissue. Used in conjunction with leuprolide to inhibit the stimulant effects of flutamide on serum testosterone levels. *Therapeutic Effect:* Suppresses testicular androgen production and decreases the growth of prostate carcinoma.

PHARMACOKINETICS

Completely absorbed from the GI tract. Protein binding: 94%-96%. Metabolized in the liver to active metabolite. Primarily excreted in urine. Not removed by hemodialysis. *Half-life:* 6 h (increased in elderly patients).

AVAILABILITY

Capsules: 125 mg.

INDICATIONS AND DOSAGES

▸ **Prostatic carcinoma (in combination with leuprolide)**

PO

Adults, Elderly. 250 mg q8h.

CONTRAINDICATIONS

Severe hepatic impairment, pregnancy, hypersensitivity to the drug.

INTERACTIONS

Drug
Warfarin: May increase risk of bleeding.

Herbal
Chaparral, comfrey, eucalyptus, germander, Jin Bu Huan, kava kava, pennyroyal, skullcap, valerian: May increase risk of hepatotoxicity.

Food
None known.

DIAGNOSTIC TEST EFFECTS

May increase blood glucose level and serum estradiol, testosterone, bilirubin, creatinine, AST (SGOT), and ALT (SGPT) levels.

SIDE EFFECTS

Frequent

Hot flashes (50%); decreased libido, diarrhea (24%); generalized pain (23%); asthenia (17%); constipation (12%); nausea, nocturia (11%).

Occasional (6%-8%)

Dizziness, paresthesia, insomnia, impotence, peripheral edema, gynecomastia.

Rare (4%-5%)

Rash, diaphoresis, hypertension, hematuria, vomiting, urinary incontinence, headache, flu-like symptoms, photosensitivity.

SERIOUS REACTIONS

- Hepatoxicity, including hepatic encephalopathy, and hemolytic anemia may be noted.

PRECAUTIONS & CONSIDERATIONS

Flutamide is not used in pregnant women or in children. No age-related precautions have been noted in elderly patients.

Clinical progression and drug therapy may be evaluated by PSA levels.

Overexposure to the sun or ultraviolet light should be avoided and protective clothing should be worn outdoors until tolerance of ultraviolet light is determined.

Urine may become amber or yellow-green during flutamide therapy. Liver function test results should be obtained before beginning drug therapy and periodically thereafter. If initial ALT result exceeds upper normal limits, use of the drug is not recommended.

Storage

Store at room temperature.

Administration

Take oral flutamide without regard to food. Do not abruptly discontinue the drug.

Fluticasone

flu-tic'a-zone

Cutivate, Flonase, Flovent Diskus, Flovent HFA, Veramyst

CATEGORY AND SCHEDULE

Pregnancy Risk Category: C

Classification: Corticosteroids, inhalation, topical

MECHANISM OF ACTION

A corticosteroid that controls the rate of protein synthesis, depresses migration of polymorphonuclear leukocytes, reverses capillary permeability, and stabilizes lysosomal membranes. *Therapeutic Effect:* Prevents or controls inflammation and asthma.

PHARMACOKINETICS

Inhalation/intranasal: Protein binding: 91%. Undergoes extensive first-pass metabolism in liver. Excreted in urine. *Half-life:* 3-7.8 h. Topical: Amount absorbed depends on affected area and skin condition (absorption increased with fever, hydration, inflamed or denuded skin).

AVAILABILITY

Aerosol for Oral Inhalation (Flovent HFA): 44 mcg/inhalation, 110 mcg/inhalation, 220 mcg/inhalation.
Powder for Oral Inhalation (Flovent Diskus): 50 mcg, 100 mcg, 250 mcg.

Intranasal Spray (Flonase):
50 mcg/spray.
Intranasal Spray (Veramyst):
27.5 mcg/spray.
Topical Cream & Lotion (Cutivate):
0.05%.
Topical Ointment (Cutivate):
0.005%.

INDICATIONS AND DOSAGES

▸ **Allergic rhinitis**

INTRANASAL

Adults, Elderly, and Children 12 yr and older. Initially, 2 sprays in each nostril once daily for a few days. Maintenance: Some patients can reduce to 1 spray in each nostril once daily.

Children 2 to 11 yr. Initially, 1 spray in each nostril once daily. Maximum: 2 sprays/nostril once daily for a short time, then decrease to 1 spray/nostril per day.

▸ **Relief of inflammation and pruritus associated with steroid-responsive disorders, such as contact dermatitis and eczema**

TOPICAL

Adults, Elderly, Children older than 3 mo. Apply sparingly to affected area once or twice a day.

▸ **Maintenance treatment for asthma for those previously treated with bronchodilators**

INHALATION POWDER (FLOVENT DISKUS)

Adults, Elderly, Children 12 yr and older. Initially, 100 mcg q12h. Maximum: 500 mcg twice daily.

INHALATION (ORAL, FLOVENT HFA)

Adults, Elderly, Children 12 yr and older. Initially, 88 mcg twice a day. Maximum: 440 mcg twice a day.

▸ **Maintenance treatment for asthma for those previously treated with inhaled steroids**

INHALATION POWDER (FLOVENT DISKUS)

Adults, Elderly, Children 12 yr and older. Initially, 100-250 mcg q12h. Maximum: 500 mcg q12h.

INHALATION, ORAL (FLOVENT HFA)

Adults, Elderly, Children 12 yr and older. 88-220 mcg twice a day. Maximum: 440 mcg twice a day.

▸ **Maintenance treatment for asthma for those previously treated with oral steroids**

INHALATION POWDER (FLOVENT DISKUS)

Adults, Elderly, Children 12 yr and older. 500-1000 mcg twice a day.

INHALATION (ORAL, FLOVENT HFA)

Adults, Elderly, Children 12 yr and older. 440-880 mcg twice a day.

CONTRAINDICATIONS

Primary treatment of status asthmaticus or other acute asthma episodes (inhalation); severe allergies to milk proteins (inhalation); untreated localized infection of nasal mucosa; hypersensitivity to the drug or components of the various formulations.

INTERACTIONS

Drug

Ketoconazole, protease inhibitors: May increase plasma fluticasone concentrations following nasal or inhalational administration of fluticasone.

Herbal and Food

None known.

DIAGNOSTIC TEST EFFECTS

None known.

SIDE EFFECTS

Frequent

Inhalation: Throat irritation, hoarseness, dry mouth, cough, temporary wheezing, oropharyngeal candidiasis (particularly if the mouth

is not rinsed with water after each administration).
Intranasal: Mild nasopharyngeal irritation; nasal burning, stinging, or dryness; rebound congestion; rhinorrhea; loss of taste.
Occasional
Inhalation: Oral candidiasis.
Intranasal: Nasal and pharyngeal candidiasis, headache.
Topical: Skin burning, pruritus.

SERIOUS REACTIONS

- Anaphylaxis, hypersensitivity reactions, and glaucoma occur rarely.
- Nasal septal perforation with prolonged innappropriate use.

PRECAUTIONS & CONSIDERATIONS

Caution is warranted with active or quiescent tuberculosis, ocular herpes simplex infection, and untreated systemic infections (including fungal, bacterial, or viral). It is unknown whether fluticasone crosses the placenta or is distributed in breast milk. The safety and efficacy of fluticasone have not been established in children younger than 2-4 yr, depending on product. Children may experience growth suppression with prolonged or high doses. No age-related precautions have been noted in elderly patients. Drink plenty of fluids to decrease the thickness of lung secretions. Pulse rate and quality, ABG levels, and respiratory rate, depth, rhythm, and type should be monitored. Notify the physician of nasal irritation or if symptoms, such as sneezing, fail to improve.
Storage
Store products at room temperature. Aerosol canisters should not be punctured and should not be used or stored near heat or open flame. Do not freeze or refrigerate.
Administration
For inhalation, first shake the container well. Exhale completely and place the mouthpiece between the lips. Inhale and hold the breath for as long as possible before exhaling. Allow 1 min between inhalations to promote deeper bronchial penetration. Rinse mouth with water immediately after inhalation to prevent mouth and throat dryness and oral candidiasis.

Clear the nasal passages before using nasal spray. Prime nasal spray units before first use by shaking the contents well and releasing 6 sprays into the air away from the face. If unit has not been used for more than 30 days or if the cap has been left off the bottle for 5 days or longer, reprime until fine mist appears. Shake the nasal spray well before each use. Tilt head slightly forward. Insert spray tip up into the nostril, pointing toward the inflamed nasal turbinates, away from nasal septum. Spray the drug into the nostril while holding the other nostril closed, and at the same time inhale through the nose.

For topical fluticasone, rub a thin film gently on the affected area. Use the drug only on the prescribed area and for no longer than prescribed. Keep the preparation away from the eyes.

Fluvastatin

floo′va-sta-tin
★ ✚ Lescol, Lescol XL
Do not confuse fluvastatin with fluoxetine.

CATEGORY AND SCHEDULE

Pregnancy Risk Category: X

Classification: Antihyperlipidemics, HMG-CoA reductase inhibitors

MECHANISM OF ACTION
An antihyperlipidemic that inhibits HMG-CoA reductase, the enzyme that catalyzes the early step in cholesterol synthesis. *Therapeutic Effect:* Decreases LDL cholesterol, VLDL, and triglyceride levels. Slightly increases HDL cholesterol concentration.

PHARMACOKINETICS
Well absorbed from the GI tract and is unaffected by food. Does not cross the blood-brain barrier. Protein binding: > 98%. Primarily eliminated in feces. *Half-life:* 1.2 h.

AVAILABILITY
Capsules (Lescol): 20 mg, 40 mg.
Tablets (Extended Release [Lescol XL]): 80 mg.

INDICATIONS AND DOSAGES
▸ **Hyperlipoproteinemia**
PO
Adults, Elderly. Initially, 20 mg/day (capsule) in the evening. May increase up to 40 mg/day. Maintenance: 20-40 mg/day in a single dose or divided doses. Patients requiring more than a 25% decrease in LDL cholesterol: 40-mg capsule 1-2 times a day or 80-mg extended-release tablet once a day.
Children 9 yr of age and older. Initially, 20 mg/day in the evening. May increase slowly at 6-wk intervals to up to 40 mg/day, either as 40 mg twice per day or extended-release 80 mg once daily.
▸ **Dosage in renal impairment**
Generally recommend not to exceed 40 mg/day.

CONTRAINDICATIONS
Active hepatic disease, unexplained increased serum transaminase levels, pregnancy, breastfeeding, hypersensitivity to the drug.

INTERACTIONS
Drug
Cyclosporine, fibrates, phenytoin, fluconazole, immunosuppressants, niacin: Increases the risk of acute renal failure and rhabdomyolysis with these drugs.
Bile acid sequestrant: Administer statin 2 h apart to avoid interaction.
Glyburide: At higher fluvastatin doses may see increased hypoglycemic effect.
Warfarin: Interactions not expected, but increased INRs reported with other "statins"; monitor INR.
Herbal and Food
Red yeast rice: May increase risk of myopathy due to "statin"-like components. Avoid.

DIAGNOSTIC TEST EFFECTS
May increase serum CK and transaminase concentrations.

SIDE EFFECTS
Frequent (5%-8%)
Headache, dyspepsia, back pain, myalgia, arthralgia, diarrhea, abdominal cramping, rhinitis.
Occasional (2%-4%)
Nausea, vomiting, insomnia, constipation, flatulence, rash, pruritus, fatigue, cough, dizziness.

SERIOUS REACTIONS
- Myositis (inflammation of voluntary muscle) with or without increased CK and muscle weakness occur rarely. These conditions may progress to frank rhabdomyolysis and renal impairment.

PRECAUTIONS & CONSIDERATIONS
Use fluvastatin cautiously in those who are receiving anticoagulant therapy, have a history of liver disease, or consume substantial amounts of alcohol. Caution is also warranted with hypotension, major

surgery, severe acute infection, renal failure secondary to rhabdomyolysis, uncontrolled seizures, and severe electrolyte, endocrine, and metabolic disorders. Expect to discontinue or withhold fluvastatin if these conditions appear. Fluvastatin use is contraindicated in pregnancy because the suppression of cholesterol biosynthesis may cause fetal toxicity. It is unknown whether fluvastatin is distributed in breast milk; therefore, it is contraindicated during lactation. Safety and efficacy of fluvastatin have not been established in children under 9 yr of age. No age-related precautions have been noted in elderly patients.

Notify the physician of any muscle pain and weakness, especially if accompanied by fever or malaise. Pattern of daily bowel activity and stool consistency should be assessed. Serum lipid cholesterol and triglyceride levels and hepatic function should be checked at baseline and periodically during treatment. Therapy with lipid-altering agents should be used in addition to a diet restricted in saturated fat and cholesterol.

Storage

Store products at room temperature, tightly closed. Protect from light.

Administration

Take fluvastatin without regard to food.

Fluvoxamine

floo-vox'a-meen

Luvox CR

CATEGORY AND SCHEDULE

Pregnancy Risk Category: C

Classification: Antidepressants, serotonin selective reuptake inhibitors

MECHANISM OF ACTION

An antidepressant and antiobsessive agent that selectively inhibits neuronal reuptake of serotonin. *Therapeutic Effect:* Relieves anxiety and symptoms of obsessive-compulsive disorder.

AVAILABILITY

Tablets: 25 mg, 50 mg, 100 mg.
Extended-Release Capsule: 100 mg,150 mg.

INDICATIONS AND DOSAGES

▸ **Obsessive-compulsive disorder**

PO

Adults. 50 mg at bedtime; may increase by 50 mg every 4-7 days. Dosages > 100 mg/day given in 2 divided doses. Maximum: 300 mg/day. Also may give as extended release, with target dose given once daily at bedtime. Maximum: 300 mg/day.

Children 8-17 yr. 25 mg at bedtime; may increase by 25 mg every 4-7 days. Dosages > 50 mg/day given in 2 divided doses. Maximum: 200 mg/day.

▸ **Social anxiety disorder**

PO (EXTENDED RELEASE)

Adults. 100 mg po at bedtime. Titrate at 50-mg increments weekly as needed. Maximum: 300 mg/day.

OFF-LABEL USES

Treatment of depression, panic disorder, anxiety disorders in children.

CONTRAINDICATIONS

Coadministration of alosetron, tizanidine, thioridazine, or pimozide, and use within 14 days of MAOIs contraindicated, hypersensitivity to fluvoxamine or any of the excipients.

INTERACTIONS

Drug

Benzodiazepines, carbamazepine, clozapine, theophylline: May increase the blood concentration and risk of toxicity of these drugs.

Lithium, tryptophan: May enhance fluvoxamine's serotonergic effects.
MAOIs: May produce excess serious reactions, including hyperthermia, rigidity, and myoclonus. Contraindicated.
Tricyclic antidepressants: May increase the fluvoxamine blood concentration.
Warfarin: May increase the effects of warfarin.
Herbal
St. John's wort: May increase fluvoxamine's pharmacologic effects and risk of toxicity.
Food
None known.

DIAGNOSTIC TEST EFFECTS
None known.

SIDE EFFECTS
Frequent
Nausea (40%); headache, somnolence, insomnia (21%-22%).
Occasional (8%-14%)
Nervousness, dizziness, diarrhea, dry mouth, asthenia, weakness, dyspepsia, constipation, abnormal ejaculation.
Rare (3%-6%)
Anorexia, anxiety, tremor, vomiting, flatulence, urinary frequency, sexual dysfunction, altered taste.

SERIOUS REACTIONS
- Overdose may produce seizures, nausea, vomiting, and extreme agitation and restlessness.

PRECAUTIONS & CONSIDERATIONS
Caution is warranted in patients with hepatic and renal impairment and in those with a history of hypomania, mania, and seizures. The drug is distributed in breast milk and should generally not be used during lactation or in pregnancy because adverse neonatal outcomes have been reported, including drug withdrawal syndromes. Antidepressants have been reported to increase the risk of suicidal thinking and behavior in children, adolescents, and young adults (18-24 yr of age) with major depressive disorder (MDD) and other psychiatric disorders. Patients should be closely monitored for clinical worsening, suicidality, or unusual changes in behavior, particularly during the initial 1-2 mo of therapy or following dosage adjustments.

Dizziness, somnolence, and dry mouth may occur. Alcohol and tasks that require mental alertness or motor skills should be avoided. CBC and blood chemistry tests should be performed before and periodically during therapy, especially with long-term use.

Storage
Store at room temperature. Keep tightly closed. Protect from humidity and avoid exposure to temperatures above 86° F.
Administration
Do not abruptly discontinue the drug. Fluvoxamine's maximum therapeutic response may require 4 wks or more to appear.

Extended release given with or without food as a single daily dose at bedtime. Do not crush or chew extended-release capsules.

Folic Acid
foe'lik a'sed

CATEGORY AND SCHEDULE
Pregnancy Risk Category: A
OTC (0.4-mg and 0.8-mg tablets only); Rx only (1-mg tablets and injection)

Classification: Vitamins, B vitamins, water soluble

MECHANISM OF ACTION

A coenzyme that stimulates production of platelets, RBCs, and WBCs. *Therapeutic Effect:* Essential for nucleoprotein synthesis and maintenance of normal erythropoiesis.

PHARMACOKINETICS

PO form almost completely absorbed from the GI tract (upper duodenum). Protein binding: High. Metabolized in the liver and plasma to active form. Excreted in urine. Removed by hemodialysis.

AVAILABILITY

Tablets: 0.4 mg, 0.8 mg, 1 mg.
Injection: 5 mg/mL.

INDICATIONS AND DOSAGES

▸ **Vitamin B_9 deficiency**

PO, IV, IM, Subcutaneous

Adults, Elderly, Children 12 yr and older. Initially, 1 mg/day. Maintenance: 0.5 mg/day.
Children 1-11 yr. Initially 1 mg/day. Maintenance: 0.1-0.4 mg/day.
Infants. 50 mcg/day.

▸ **Dietary supplement**

PO, IV, IM, SUBCUTANEOUS

Adults, Elderly, Children 4 yr and older. 0.4 mg/day.
Children 1 to less than 4 yr. 0.3 mg/day.
Children younger than 1 yr. 0.1 mg/day.
Pregnant women. 0.8 mg/day.

CONTRAINDICATIONS

Previous folic acid hypersensitivity. Administration of folic acid monotherapy is improper for pernicious anemia and other megaloblastic anemias in which vitamin B_{12} is deficient.

INTERACTIONS

Drug

Analgesics, carbamazepine, estrogens: May increase folic acid requirements.
Antacids, cholestyramine: May decrease the absorption of folic acid.
Hydantoin anticonvulsants: May decrease the effects of these drugs (rare).
Methotrexate, triamterene, trimethoprim: May antagonize the effects of folic acid.

Herbal and Food

None known.

DIAGNOSTIC TEST EFFECTS

May decrease vitamin B_{12} concentration.

IV INCOMPATIBILITIES

Amikacin, calcium chloride, diazepam, dobutamine, doxycycline, gentamicin, haloperidol, hydralazine, inamrinone, methyldopate, morphine, nafcillin, nalbuphine, norepinephrine, phenytoin, promethazine, protamine, tobramycin, verapamil.

SIDE EFFECTS

No adverse effects commonly reported at usual doses. At high doses (15 mg/day or more) patients may report insomnia, bad taste, nausea, irritability, or other similar effects.

SERIOUS REACTIONS

- Allergic hypersensitivity occurs rarely.

PRECAUTIONS & CONSIDERATIONS

Use with extreme caution in patients with undiagnosed anemia. Folic acid corrects the hematologic manifestations of pernicious anemia, while the neurologic complications progress, potentially causing irreversible central nervous system effects. Doses above 0.4 mg/day should be avoided until the diagnosis of pernicious anemia is ruled out. Folic acid is distributed in breast milk. No age-related precautions have been noted in children or elderly patients. Eating foods rich in folic acid, including fruits, vegetables, and organ meats, is encouraged.

Therapeutic improvement, including improved sense of well-being and relief from iron deficiency symptoms, such as fatigue, headache, pallor, dyspnea, and sore tongue, should be assessed. Be aware that persons with alcoholism, decreased hematopoiesis, or deficiency of vitamin B_6, B_{12}, C, or E and those using antimetabolic drugs may develop a resistance to treatment.

Storage

Store at room temperature protected from light. Folic acid injection mixed in D5W, 0.9% NaCl, or TPN is stable for 24 h at room temperature.

Administration

May give orally without regard to food.

Folic acid injection may be given IV, IM, or subcutaneously. For IV use, may give IV directly at a rate of 5 mg over at least 1 min. For infusion, may add dose to any large-volume or piggyback solution containing D5W or saline, or a mixure thereof. May be added to TPN solution.

Fomepizole

foe-mep'i-zoll

Antizol

CATEGORY AND SCHEDULE

Pregnancy Risk Category: C

Classification: Antidotes

MECHANISM OF ACTION

An alcohol dehydrogenase inhibitor that inhibits the enzyme that catalyzes the metabolism of ethanol, ethylene glycol, and methanol to their toxic metabolites. *Therapeutic Effect:* Inhibits conversion of ethylene glycol and methanol into toxic metabolites.

PHARMACOKINETICS

Protein binding: Low. Rapidly distributes to total body water after IV infusion. Extensively metabolized by the liver. Minimal excretion in the urine. Removed by hemodialysis. *Half-life:* 5 h.

AVAILABILITY

Solution for Injection: 1 g/mL (Antizol).

INDICATIONS AND DOSAGES

▸ Ethylene glycol or methanol intoxication

IV infusion

Adults, Elderly. 15 mg/kg as loading dose, followed by 10 mg/kg q12h for 4 doses, then 15 mg/kg q12h until ethylene glycol or methanol concentrations are below 20 mg/dL. All doses should be administered as a slow IV infusion over 30 min.

▸ Dosage in renal impairment

During hemodialysis: 15 mg/kg as a loading dose, followed by 10 mg/kg q4h for 4 doses, then 15 mg/kg q4h until ethylene glycol or methanol concentrations are below 20 mg/dL.

After hemodialysis: If the time between the last dose and end of hemodialysis is < 1 h, do not give dose. If the time between is 1-3 h, give 50% of next scheduled dose. If time is > 3 h, give next scheduled dose.

OFF-LABEL USES

Butoxyethanol intoxication, diethylene glycol intoxication, ethanol sensitivity.

CONTRAINDICATIONS

Hypersensitivity to fomepizole or other pyrazoles.

F

INTERACTIONS

Drug

Alcohol: May reduce elimination of both drugs.

Herbal and Food

None known.

DIAGNOSTIC TEST EFFECTS

None known.

IV INCOMPATIBILITIES

Data not available.

SIDE EFFECTS

Frequent

Hypertriglyceridemia, headache, nausea, dizziness.

Occasional

Abnormal sense of smell, nystagmus, visual disturbances, ringing in ears, agitation, seizures, anorexia, heartburn, anxiety, vertigo, light-headedness, altered sense of awareness.

Rare

Anuria, disseminated intravascular coagulopathy.

SERIOUS REACTIONS

- Mild allergic reactions including rash and eosinophilia occur rarely.
- Overdose may cause nausea, dizziness, and vertigo.

PRECAUTIONS & CONSIDERATIONS

Caution is warranted in patients with liver disease or renal impairment. Dialysis should be considered in addition to fomepizole in cases of renal failure. If < 6 h has passed since the last dose, do not give dose. If more than 6 h has passed since the last dose, give the next scheduled dose. It is unknown whether fomepizole crosses the placenta or is distributed in breast milk. Safety and efficacy of fomepizole have not been established in children. Age-related renal impairment may require dosage adjustment in elderly patients.

Monitor for signs or symptoms of allergic reactions during administration. This medication is given to treat antifreeze or windshield wiper fluid ingestion. If not treated, these poisons will cause kidney damage, eye damage, seizures, coma, and possibly death.

Storage

Do not freeze. Store unopened vial at room temperature. Fomepizole solidifies at temperatures less than 77° F. If solid in the vial, the solution should be liquefied by running the vial under warm water or by holding in the hand.

Solidification does not affect the efficacy, safety, or stability of the solution. Once mixed for infusion, the infusion solution should be used within 24 h.

Administration

Dilute in at least 100 mL of 0.9% NaCl or D5W. Administer fomepizole as a slow IV infusion over 30 min. Do not give undiluted or by bolus injection.

Fondaparinux

fawn-da-pear'ih-nux

Arixtra

CATEGORY AND SCHEDULE

Pregnancy Risk Category: B

Classification: Anticoagulants, factor Xa inhibitors

MECHANISM OF ACTION

A factor Xa inhibitor and pentasaccharide that selectively binds to antithrombin and increases its affinity for factor Xa, thereby inhibiting factor Xa and stopping the blood coagulation cascade.

Therapeutic Effect: Indirectly prevents formation of thrombin and subsequently the fibrin clot.

PHARMACOKINETICS

Well absorbed after subcutaneous administration. Undergoes minimal, if any, metabolism. Highly bound to antithrombin III. Distributed mainly in blood and to a minor extent in extravascular fluid. Excreted unchanged in urine. Removed by hemodialysis. *Half-life:* 17-21 h (prolonged in patients with impaired renal function).

AVAILABILITY

Injection, Prefilled Syringes: 2.5 mg/0.5 mL, 5 mg/0.4 mL, 7.5 mg/0.6 mL, 10 mg/0.8 mL.

INDICATIONS AND DOSAGES

▸ **Prevention of venous thromboembolism**

SUBCUTANEOUS

Adults 50 kg or greater. 2.5 mg once a day for 5-9 days after surgery. Initial dose should be given 6-8 h after surgery. Only approved for patients weighing 50 kg or more.

Adults less than 50 kg: Contraindicated for this indication.

▸ **Treatment of pulmonary embolism or DVT in conjunction with warfarin**

Adults. 5 mg SC once daily; if < 50 kg, 50-100 kg 7.5 mg SC once daily; if > 100 kg, 10 mg SC once daily. Usual duration 5-9 days; continue until warfarin treatment achieves INR 2-3.

▸ **Dosage in renal impairment**

Adults. Use cautiously in those with CrCl 30-50 mL/min: CrCl < 30 mL/min: Contraindicated.

CONTRAINDICATIONS

Active major bleeding, bacterial endocarditis, severe renal impairment (with creatinine clearance < 30 mL/min), thrombocytopenia associated with antiplatelet antibody formation in the presence of fondaparinux.

INTERACTIONS

Drug

Anticoagulants, platelet inhibitors, thrombolytics: May increase risk of bleeding.

Herbal

Ginger, gingko: May increase risk of bleeding.

Food

None known.

DIAGNOSTIC TEST EFFECTS

Increases reversible serum creatinine, AST (SGOT), and ALT (SGPT) levels. May decrease hemoglobin, hematocrit, and platelet count.

NOTE: The anti-factor Xa activity of the drug can be measured by anti-Xa assay using appropriate calibrator (fondaparinux); it cannot be compared with activities of heparin or low-molecular-weight heparins.

SIDE EFFECTS

Occasional (14%)

Fever.

Rare (1%-4%)

Injection site hematoma, nausea, peripheral edema.

SERIOUS REACTIONS

- Accidental overdose may lead to bleeding complications ranging from local ecchymoses to major hemorrhage.
- Thrombocytopenia occurs rarely.

PRECAUTIONS & CONSIDERATIONS

The needle guard of prefilled syringe contains natural latex rubber; use caution in those with latex sensitivity. Caution is warranted in patients with conditions associated with increased risk of hemorrhage, such as concurrent use of antiplatelet

F

agents, GI ulceration, hemophilia, history of cerebrovascular accident, severe uncontrolled hypertension, history of heparin-induced thrombocytopenia, impaired renal function, indwelling epidural catheter or neuraxial anesthesia, and in elderly patients. Fondaparinux should be used with caution in pregnant women, particularly during the last trimester and immediately postpartum, because it increases the risk of maternal hemorrhage. It is unknown whether fondaparinux is excreted in breast milk. Safety and efficacy of fondaparinux have not been established in children. In elderly patients, age-related decreased renal function may increase the risk of bleeding. Women may experience heavier menstrual flow. Other medications, including OTC drugs, should be avoided. An electric razor and soft toothbrush should be used to prevent bleeding during therapy.

Notify the physician of bleeding from surgical site, chest pain, dyspnea, severe or sudden headache, swelling in the feet or hands, unusual back pain, bruising, weakness, black or red stool, coffee-ground vomitus, dark or red urine, or red-speckled mucus from cough. Monitor for neurologic impairment; promptly report any changes in neurologic status. CBC, BUN and creatinine levels, BP, pulse, and stool of occult blood should be monitored. Be aware of signs of bleeding, including bleeding at injection or surgical sites or from gums, blood in stool, bruising, hematuria, and petechiae.

Storage

Store at room temperature. Do not freeze. The parenteral form normally appears clear and colorless; discard if discoloration or particulate matter is noted.

Administration

For subcutaneous use only. Do not expel the air bubble from the prefilled syringe before injection to avoid expelling drug. Pinch a fold of the patient's skin at the injection site between the thumb and forefinger. Introduce the entire length of subcutaneous needle into the skinfold. Inject into fatty tissue between the left and right anterolateral or the left and right posterolateral abdominal wall. Rotate injection sites.

Formoterol

for-moe'ter-ol

★ Foradil Aerolizer, Perforomist

🍁 Foradil, Oxeze Turbuhaler

CATEGORY AND SCHEDULE

Pregnancy Risk Category: C

Classification: Adrenergic agonists, bronchodilators, long-acting β-agonist

MECHANISM OF ACTION

A long-acting bronchodilator that stimulates β_2-adrenergic receptors in the lungs, resulting in relaxation of bronchial smooth muscle. Also inhibits release of mediators from various cells in the lungs, including mast cells, with little effect on heart rate. *Therapeutic Effect:* Relieves bronchospasm, reduces airway resistance. Improves bronchodilation, nighttime asthma control, and peak flow rates.

PHARMACOKINETICS

Route	Onset	Peak	Duration
Inhalation	1-3 min	0.5-1 h	12 h

Absorbed from bronchi after inhalation. Metabolized in the

liver. Primarily excreted in urine. Unknown if removed by hemodialysis. *Half-life:* 10 h.

AVAILABILITY

Inhalation Powder in Capsules: 12 mcg.
Nebulizer Solution: 20 mcg/2 mL.

INDICATIONS AND DOSAGES

▸ **Asthma, chronic obstructive pulmonary disease (COPD), exercise-induced bronchospasm**
INHALATION
Adults, Elderly, Children 5 yr and older. 12 mcg q12h.
NEBULIZER INHALATION (COPD)
Adults, Elderly. 20 mcg nebulized twice daily, morning and evening.
▸ **Exercise-induced bronchospasm**
INHALATION
Adults, Elderly, Children 5 yr and older. 12 mcg at least 15 min before exercise. Do not repeat for another 12 h.

CONTRAINDICATIONS

Status asthmaticus. Formoterol should always be administered in conjunction with an inhaled corticosteroid; use without corticosteroid treatment is contraindicated.

INTERACTIONS

Drug
β-Blockers: May antagonize formoterol's bronchodilating effects.
Diuretics, steroids, xanthine derivatives: May increase the risk of hypokalemia.
Drugs that can prolong QT interval (including erythromycin, quinidine, and thioridazine), MAOIs, tricyclic antidepressants: May potentiate cardiovascular effects.
Herbal and Food
None known.

DIAGNOSTIC TEST EFFECTS

May decrease serum potassium level. May increase blood glucose level.

SIDE EFFECTS

Occasional
Tremor, muscle cramps, tachycardia, insomnia, headache, irritability, irritation of mouth or throat.

SERIOUS REACTIONS

• Excessive sympathomimetic stimulation may produce palpitations, extrasystole, and chest pain.

PRECAUTIONS & CONSIDERATIONS

Caution is warranted in patients with cardiovascular disease, hypertension, a seizure disorder, and thyrotoxicosis. It is unknown whether formoterol crosses the placenta or is distributed in breast milk. The safety and efficacy of formoterol have not been established in children younger than 5 yr. The nebulizer solution is approved only in adults. Elderly patients may be more prone to tachycardia and tremor because of increased sensitivity to sympathomimetics. Drink plenty of fluids to decrease the thickness of lung secretions. Avoid excessive use of caffeinated products, such as chocolate, cocoa, cola, coffee, and tea. Monotherapy with formoterol may increase risk of asthma-related events, such as hospitalization or mortality.

Pulse rate and quality, ECG, respiratory rate, depth, rhythm, and type, ABG, and serum potassium levels should be monitored. Keep a log of measurements of peak flow readings.

Storage
Before dispensing, store nebulizer solution in refrigerator. After dispensing, may be stored at room temperature for up to 3 mo. The nebulizer solution should remain in

the foil pouch until just prior to use. Formoterol capsules for inhalation are kept at room temperature, protected from heat and moisture, in original packaging.

Administration

Keep capsules in individual blister packs until immediately before use. Do not swallow the capsules. Do not use with a spacer. Pull off the aerolizer inhaler cover, twisting the mouthpiece in the direction of the arrow to open. Place the capsule in the chamber and twist the mouthpiece closed. Press both buttons on the side of the aerolizer only once. This action punctures the capsule. Exhale completely, then place mouth on the mouthpiece and close the lips. Inhale quickly and deeply through the mouth, which causes the capsule to spin and dispense the drug. Hold breath for as long as possible before exhaling slowly. Check the capsule to make sure all the powder is gone. If not, inhale again to receive the rest of the dose. Rinse mouth with water immediately after inhalation to prevent mouth and throat dryness. Never swallow capsules orally. Never wash the aerolizer inhaler.

The nebulizer solution should be administered using a standard jet nebulizer connected to an air compressor. Do not mix with any other drugs.

Fosamprenavir

fos'am-pren-a-veer

★ Lexiva 🍁 Telzir

CATEGORY AND SCHEDULE

Pregnancy Risk Category: C

Classification: Antivirals, protease inhibitors

MECHANISM OF ACTION

An antiretroviral that is rapidly converted to amprenavir, which inhibits HIV-1 protease by binding to the enzyme's active site, thus preventing the processing of viral precursors and resulting in the formation of immature, noninfectious viral particles. *Therapeutic Effect:* Impairs HIV replication and proliferation.

PHARMACOKINETICS

Rapidly absorbed after PO administration. Protein binding: 90%. Metabolized in the liver. Excreted in urine and feces. *Half-life:* 7.7 h.

AVAILABILITY

Tablets: 700 mg (equivalent to 600 mg amprenavir).
Oral Suspension: 50 mg/mL (equivalent to 43 mg/mL amprenavir).

INDICATIONS AND DOSAGES

▸ **HIV infection in patients who have not had previous protease inhibitor therapy**

PO

Adults, Elderly. 700 mg given with ritonavir (100 mg) twice daily OR 1400 mg once daily (without ritonavir) OR 1400 mg with ritonavir (100 or 200 mg) once daily.
Children 6 yr and older. Oral suspension 30 mg/kg twice daily (maximum 1400 mg twice daily) OR 18 mg/kg (not to exceed 700 mg) plus ritonavir (3 mg/kg, maximum 100 mg/dose) given twice daily. Those ≥ 39 kg may receive tablets; those at least 47 kg may receive adult dose regimen.
Children 2 to 5 yr. Oral suspension 300 mg/kg twice daily (not to exceed 1400 mg twice daily).

▸ **HIV infection in patients who have had previous protease inhibitor therapy**
PO
Adults, Elderly. 700 mg twice daily plus ritonavir 100 mg twice daily.
Children 6 yr and older. Oral suspension 18 mg/kg (maximum 700 mg) plus ritonavir (3 mg/kg, maximum 100 mg) given twice daily. Those ≥ 39 kg may receive tablets; those at least 47 kg may receive adult regimen.

▸ **Concurrent therapy with efavirenz**
PO
Adults, Elderly. In patients receiving fosamprenavir plus once-daily ritonavir with efavirenz, an additional 100 mg/day ritonavir (300 mg total/day) should be given.

▸ **Dosage in hepatic impairment**
Consult prescribing information. Dosages must be adjusted in moderate and severe hepatic impairment.

CONTRAINDICATIONS

Clinically significant hypersensitivity to fosamprenavir OR amprenavir. Contraindicated when coadministered with drugs highly dependent on CYP3A4 metabolism when elevated concentrations are associated with serious and/or life-threatening events (see drug interactions and prescribing information). Also see ritonavir contraindications.

INTERACTIONS

Drug
NOTE: *The following drugs are CONTRAINDICATED with fosamprenavir*:
Alfuzosin: Increased alfuzosin levels and severe hypotension.
Cisapride, pimozide: Risk of life-threatening cardiac arrhythmias.
Delavirdine: May cause loss of virologic response to delavirdine, with possible resistance emergence.
Flecainide and propafenone: If used with ritonavir, significant increases in cardiac drug levels and toxicity.
Ergotamine and other ergot alkaloids: May cause ergot toxicity.
HMG-CoA reductase inhibitors (statins) (lovastatin and simvastatin): Increased risk of myopathy.
Midazolam, triazolam: Risk for over sedation and prolonged sedation.
PDE5 inhibitors (e.g., sildenafil for pulm HTN): May increase risk for priapism, hypotension.
Rifampin: Decreases fosamprenavir blood concentration and reduces antiviral activity.
OTHER IMPORTANT INTERACTIONS:
Antacids, didanosine: May decrease the absorption of fosamprenavir.
Carbamazepine, phenobarbital, phenytoin: May decrease the fosamprenavir blood concentration.
Amiodarone, cyclosporine, and other immunosuppressants, warfarin: May increase blood levels of many medicatons; carefully monitor drugs with narrow therapeutic index.
Herbal
St. John's wort: May decrease the fosamprenavir blood concentration. Contraindicated.
Food
None known.

DIAGNOSTIC TEST EFFECTS

May increase serum lipase, triglyceride, AST (SGOT), and ALT (SGPT) levels. May increase blood sugar or decrease WBC count.

SIDE EFFECTS

Frequent
Nausea, rash, diarrhea.

Occasional
Headache, vomiting, fatigue, depression, fat redistribution syndrome/buffalo hump, hyperglycemia, hyperlipidemia.
Rare
Pruritus, abdominal pain, perioral paresthesia.

F

SERIOUS REACTIONS

- Severe and possibly life-threatening dermatologic reactions occur rarely.
- Other potentially serious reactions include acute hemolytic anemia, new-onset diabetes, nephrolithiasis, immune reconstitution syndrome.
- Hepatitis or reactivation of hepatitis B or C.
- Increased risk of bleeding noted in patients with hemophilia.

PRECAUTIONS & CONSIDERATIONS

Fosamprenavir contains a sulfonamide moiety; use with caution in those allergic to sulfonamide-class drugs. Extreme caution should be used with liver impairment. Caution is also warranted in patients with diabetes mellitus, impaired renal function, and in elderly patients. Breastfeeding is not recommended in this population because of the possibility of HIV transmission. Use with caution during pregnancy. Fosamprenavir is not a cure for HIV infection, nor does it reduce risk of transmission to others.

Obtain baseline lab values, including blood glucose, serum lipase, SGPT (ALT), SGOT (AST), and serum triglyceride levels. Find out which other drugs the person is taking. Report any side effects, including rash or diarrhea.
Storage
Tablets are stored at room temperature tightly closed. Suspension may be at room temperature or refrigerated; do not freeze. Refrigeration may help palatability of oral suspension.
Administration
Do not chew, crush, or break film-coated tablets. May take without regard to food. Shake oral suspension well before each use.

Fosaprepitant

fos′a-pre′pi-tant
Emend IV
Do not confuse fosaprepitant with aprepitant.

CATEGORY AND SCHEDULE

Pregnancy Risk Category: B

Classification: Antiemetics, substance P antagonists

MECHANISM OF ACTION

A selective human substance P and neurokinin-1 (NK1) receptor antagonist that inhibits chemotherapy-induced nausea and vomiting by crossing the blood brain barrier to act centrally to occupy receptors in the chemoreceptor trigger zone. *Therapeutic Effect:* Prevents the acute and delayed phases of chemotherapy-induced emesis, including vomiting caused by high-dose cisplatin.

PHARMACOKINETICS

A prodrug that is rapidly converted to aprepitant after administration (within 30 min). The mean aprepitant plasma concentration 24 h after an infusion of fosaprepitant 115 mg IV is similar to that seen with aprepitant 125 mg PO. Plasma protein binding: 95%. Crosses the blood-brain barrier. Aprepitant is extensively metabolized in the liver to weakly active metabolites and is not excreted renally. *Half-life:* 9-13 h.

AVAILABILITY

Powder for Injection: 115-mg vial.
NOTE: See aprepitant monograph for oral form.

INDICATIONS AND DOSAGES

▸ **Prevention of chemotherapy-induced nausea and vomiting**
IV INFUSION
Adults, Elderly. 115 mg given 30 min prior to chemotherapy as an alternative to the first dose of oral aprepitant on day 1 of the aprepitant-CINV regimen (see aprepitant monograph). Given as part of regimens that include a steroid and a 5-HT3 antagonist.

CONTRAINDICATIONS

Hypersensitivity to fosaprepitant, aprepitant, or polysorbate 80. Concurrent use of pimozide (Orap), cisapride (Propulsid) is contraindicated due to risk of cardiac arrhythmias.

INTERACTIONS

Drug
Alprazolam, docetaxel, etoposide, ifosfamide, imatinib, irinotecan, midazolam, paclitaxel, triazolam, vinblastine, vincristine, vinorelbine: May increase the plasma concentrations of these drugs that are substrates for CYP3A4.
Antifungals, clarithromycin, diltiazem, nefazodone, nelfinavir, ritonavir: Increase aprepitant plasma concentration; diltiazem concentration may increase.
Carbamazepine, phenytoin, rifampin: Decrease aprepitant plasma concentration.
Contraceptives: May decrease the effectiveness of estrogen or progestin contraceptives. Alternative or backup methods of contraception should be used during treatment and for 1 mo following the last dose.
Corticosteroids: Increase levels of systemic corticosteroids. If the patient is also receiving a steroid, expect to reduce the IV steroid dose by 25% and the oral dose by 50%.
Paroxetine: May decrease the effectiveness of either drug.
Warfarin: Fosaprepitant is an inducer of isoenzyme CYP2C9, an enzyme involved in warfarin metabolism. May decrease the effectiveness of warfarin. Monitor INR.
Herbal
St. John's wort: May decrease aprepitant levels.
Food
None.

IV INCOMPATIBILITIES

Do not dilute or infuse with any solutions containing divalent cations (e.g., calcium or magnesium), including lactated Ringer's or Hartmann's solution, calcium chloride, calcium gluconate, TPN, magnesium sulfate.

DIAGNOSTIC TEST EFFECTS

May increase BUN level and serum creatinine, AST (SGOT), and ALT (SGPT) levels. May produce proteinuria.

SIDE EFFECTS

Extrapolated from data with oral aprepitant.
Frequent (≥ 10%)
Fatigue, nausea, hiccups, diarrhea, constipation, anorexia.
Occasional (4%-9%)
Headache, vomiting, dizziness, dehydration, heartburn or epigastric discomfort, infusion site reactions, tinnitus.
Rare (≤ 3%)
Abdominal pain, gastritis, insomnia, hyperpyrexia.

SERIOUS REACTIONS

- Neutropenia and mucous membrane disorders occur rarely.

PRECAUTIONS & CONSIDERATIONS

Chronic use of this drug is not recommended. Use caution in hepatic impairment; there are no data in patients with severe hepatic impairment. It is unknown whether fosaprepitant crosses the placenta or is distributed in breast milk. The safety and efficacy of fosaprepitant have not been established in children. No age-related precautions have been noted in elderly patients.

Nausea and vomiting should be relieved shortly after drug administration. Notify the physician if headache or persistent vomiting occurs. Pattern of daily bowel activity and stool consistency should be assessed.

Storage

Store vials under refrigeration in original package. Do not freeze. The IV infusion, once prepared, is stable for 24 h at ambient room temperature.

Administration

As prescribed, fosaprepitant is given with corticosteroids and a serotonin (5-HT3) antagonist when given prior to chemotherapy.

Fosaprepitant is for intravenous infusion only. To prepare the IV infusion: Dilute vial with 5 mL of 0.9% NaCl (NS), directing toward the wall of the vial to prevent foaming. Swirl the vial gently. Prepare an infusion bag filled with 110 mL of NS. Withdraw the dose from the vial and transfer to the infusion bag. The total volume will be 115 mL, with a final concentration of 1 mg/1 mL. Gently invert the bag 2 to 3 times. Infuse IV over 15 minutes.

Foscarnet

foss-car′net

CATEGORY AND SCHEDULE

Pregnancy Risk Category: C

Classification: Antivirals

MECHANISM OF ACTION

An antiviral that selectively inhibits binding sites on virus-specific DNA polymerase and reverse transcriptase. *Therapeutic Effect:* Inhibits replication of herpes virus.

PHARMACOKINETICS

Sequestered into bone and cartilage. Protein binding: 14%-17%. Primarily excreted unchanged in urine. Removed by hemodialysis. *Half-life:* 3.3-6.8 h (increased in impaired renal function).

AVAILABILITY

Injection: 24 mg/mL.

INDICATIONS AND DOSAGES

▸ **Cytomegalovirus (CMV) retinitis**

IV

Adults, Elderly. Initially, 60 mg/kg q8h or 100 mg/kg q12h for 2-3 wks. Maintenance: 90-120 mg/kg/day as a single IV infusion.

▸ **Herpes infection**

IV

Adults. 40 mg/kg q8-12h for 2-3 wks or until healed.

▸ **Dosage in renal impairment**

Dosages are individualized based on creatinine clearance. Refer to the dosing guide provided by the manufacturer.

CONTRAINDICATIONS

None known.

INTERACTIONS

Drug

Nephrotoxic medications: May increase the risk of nephrotoxicity.

Pentamidine (IV): May cause reversible hypocalcemia, hypomagnesemia, and nephrotoxicity.

Zidovudine (AZT): May increase the risk of anemia.

Herbal and Food

None known.

DIAGNOSTIC TEST EFFECTS

May increase serum alkaline phosphatase, bilirubin, creatinine, AST (SGOT), and ALT (SGPT) levels. May decrease serum magnesium and potassium levels. May alter serum calcium and phosphate concentrations.

IV INCOMPATIBILITIES

Acyclovir (Zovirax), amphotericin B (Fungizone), co-trimoxazole (Bactrim), diazepam (Valium), digoxin (Lanoxin), diphenhydramine (Benadryl), dobutamine (Dobutrex), droperidol (Inapsine), ganciclovir (Cytovene), haloperidol (Haldol), leucovorin, midazolam (Versed), pentamidine (Pentam IV), prochlorperazine (Compazine), vancomycin (Vancocin). Also incompatible with any divalent cations, such as calcium or magnesium.

IV COMPATIBILITIES

Dopamine (Intropin), heparin, hydromorphone (Dilaudid), lorazepam (Ativan), morphine, potassium chloride.

SIDE EFFECTS

Frequent

Fever (65%); nausea (47%); vomiting, diarrhea (30%).

Occasional (≥ 5%)

Anorexia, pain and inflammation at injection site, fever, rigors, malaise, headache, paresthesia, dizziness, rash, diaphoresis, abdominal pain.

Rare (1%-5%)

Back or chest pain, edema, flushing, pruritus, constipation, dry mouth.

SERIOUS REACTIONS

- Nephrotoxicity occurs to some extent in most patients.
- Seizures and serum mineral or electrolyte imbalances may be life threatening.

PRECAUTIONS & CONSIDERATIONS

Caution is warranted in patients with altered serum calcium or other serum electrolyte levels, a history of renal impairment, or cardiac or neurologic abnormalities. Be aware that it is unknown whether foscarnet is distributed in breast milk. Be aware that the safety and efficacy of foscarnet have not been established in children. In elderly patients, age-related renal impairment may require dosage adjustment.

The severity of renal impairment is reduced by ensuring sufficient fluid intake to promote diuresis before and during dosing. Frequent monitoring of renal parameters, such as serum creatinine, is essential. Signs and symptoms of anemia, such as bleeding, superinfections, and tremors, should be assessed. Institute safety measures for potential seizures. Report numbness in the extremities, paresthesias, or perioral tingling, during or after infusion, as this may indicate electrolyte abnormalities.

Storage

Store parenteral vials at room temperature. After dilution, foscarnet is stable for 24 h at room temperature. Do not use if foscarnet solution is discolored or contains particulate material.

F

Administration
Use the standard 24 mg/mL solution without diluting it when a central venous catheter is used for infusion; the 24 mg/mL solution must be diluted to 12 mg/mL when giving the drug through a peripheral vein catheter. Use only D5W or 0.9% NaCl injection for dilution. Because foscarnet dosage is calculated on body weight, remove the unneeded quantity before the start of infusion to avoid overdosage. Use an IV infusion pump to administer foscarnet and prevent accidental overdose. Use aseptic technique and administer the solution within 24 h of the first entry into the sealed bottle.

! Do not give foscarnet as an IV injection or by rapid infusion because these routes increase the drug's toxicity. Administer foscarnet by IV infusion at a rate not faster than 1 h for doses up to 60 mg/kg and 2 h for doses > 60 mg/kg. To minimize the risk of phlebitis and toxicity, use central venous lines or veins with an adequate blood flow to permit rapid dilution and dissemination of foscarnet. Administer hydration fluid with each dose.

Fosfomycin

foss-fo-mye′sin

★ 🍁 Monurol

Do not confuse Monurol with Monopril.

CATEGORY AND SCHEDULE

Pregnancy Risk Category: B

Classification: Antibiotics, miscellaneous, antiseptics, urinary tract

MECHANISM OF ACTION

An antibiotic that prevents bacterial cell wall formation by inhibiting the synthesis of peptidoglycan. *Therapeutic Effect:* Bactericidal.

AVAILABILITY

Powder for Oral Solution: 3 g.

INDICATIONS AND DOSAGES

▸ **Uncomplicated urinary tract infection in females**

PO

Females. 3 g mixed in 4 oz water as a single dose.

▸ **Uncomplicated urinary tract infection in males**

Males. 3 g/day for 2-3 days.

CONTRAINDICATIONS

Known hypersensitivity to fosfomycin.

INTERACTIONS

Drug

Metoclopramide: Lowers serum concentration and urinary excretion of fosfomycin.

Herbal and Food

None known.

DIAGNOSTIC TEST EFFECTS

May increase blood eosinophil count and serum alkaline phosphatase, bilirubin, AST (SGOT), and ALT (SGPT) levels. May alter platelet and WBC counts. May decrease blood hematocrit and hemoglobin levels.

SIDE EFFECTS

Occasional (3%-9%)

Diarrhea, nausea, headache, back pain.

Rare (< 2%)

Dysmenorrhea, pharyngitis, abdominal pain, rash.

SERIOUS REACTIONS

• Rare reports of serious hypersensitivity such as angioedema or hepatic reactions.

PRECAUTIONS & CONSIDERATIONS

Symptoms should improve 2-3 days after the dose of fosfomycin. Use with caution during pregnancy and lactation. Safety and efficacy not established in children under 12 yr.

Storage

Store sachets at room temperature.

Administration

Take fosfomycin without regard to food. Always mix with 3-4 oz of water before consuming. Do not use with hot water. Duration of treatment is always a single dose.

Fosinopril

fo-sin′o-pril

★ 🍁 Monopril

Do not confuse Monopril with Monurol.

CATEGORY AND SCHEDULE

Pregnancy Risk Category: C (D if used in second or third trimester)

Classification:

Antihypertensives, angiotensin-converting enzyme inhibitors

MECHANISM OF ACTION

An ACE inhibitor that suppresses the renin-angiotensin-aldosterone system and prevents conversion of angiotensin I to angiotensin II, a potent vasoconstrictor; may also inhibit angiotensin II at local vascular and renal sites. Decreases plasma angiotensin II, increases plasma renin activity, and decreases aldosterone secretion. *Therapeutic Effect:* Reduces peripheral arterial resistance, pulmonary capillary wedge pressure; improves cardiac output, exercise tolerance.

PHARMACOKINETICS

Route	Onset	Peak	Duration
PO	1 h	2-6 h	24 h

Slowly absorbed from the GI tract. Protein binding: 97%-98%. Metabolized in the liver and GI mucosa to active metabolite. Primarily excreted in urine. Minimal removal by hemodialysis. *Half-life:* 11.5 h.

AVAILABILITY

Tablets: 10 mg, 20 mg, 40 mg.

INDICATIONS AND DOSAGES

▸ **Hypertension (monotherapy)**

PO

Adults, Elderly. Initially, 10 mg/day. Maintenance: 20-40 mg/day. Maximum: 80 mg/day.

▸ **Hypertension (with diuretic)**

PO

Adults, Elderly. Initially, 10 mg/day titrated to patient's needs.

▸ **Heart failure**

PO

Adults, Elderly. Initially, 10 mg once daily. Use 5 mg initially if patient has hypovolemia or moderate to severe renal impairment or is vigorously treated with diuretics. Maintenance: 20-40 mg/day. Target dose: 40 mg/day if tolerated.

OFF-LABEL USES

Treatment of diabetic and nondiabetic nephropathy, post-myocardial infarction, left ventricular dysfunction, renal crisis in scleroderma.

CONTRAINDICATIONS

Hypersensitivity or history of angioedema from previous treatment with ACE inhibitors, idiopathic or hereditary angioedema, bilateral renal artery stenosis.

F

INTERACTIONS

Drug

Alcohol, antihypertensives, diuretics: May increase the effects of fosinopril.

Lithium: May increase lithium blood concentration and risk of lithium toxicity.

NSAIDs: May decrease the effects of fosinopril.

Potassium-sparing diuretics, drospirenone, eplerenone, potassium supplements: May cause hyperkalemia.

Herbal and Food

None known.

DIAGNOSTIC TEST EFFECTS

May increase BUN, serum alkaline phosphatase, serum bilirubin, serum creatinine, serum potassium, AST (SGOT), and ALT (SGPT) levels. May decrease serum sodium levels. May cause positive antinuclear antibody titer.

SIDE EFFECTS

Frequent (9%-12%)

Dizziness, cough.

Occasional (2%-4%)

Hypotension, nausea, vomiting, upper respiratory tract infection, hyperkalemia.

SERIOUS REACTIONS

- Excessive hypotension (first-dose syncope) may occur in patients with congestive heart failure and in those who are severely salt and volume depleted.
- Angioedema (swelling of face and lips) occurs rarely.
- Agranulocytosis and neutropenia may be noted in those with collagen vascular disease, including scleroderma and systemic lupus erythematosus, and impaired renal function.
- Nephrotic syndrome may be noted in those with history of renal disease.

PRECAUTIONS & CONSIDERATIONS

Caution is warranted with cerebrovascular and coronary insufficiency, hypovolemia, renal impairment, sodium depletion, and those on dialysis or receiving diuretics. Fosinopril crosses the placenta, is distributed in breast milk, and may cause fetal or neonatal morbidity or mortality. Safety and efficacy of fosinopril have not been established in children. Neonates and infants may be at increased risk for neurologic abnormalities and oliguria. Elderly patients may be more sensitive to the hypotensive effects of fosinopril.

Dizziness may occur. BP should be obtained immediately before giving each fosinopril dose, in addition to regular monitoring. Be alert to fluctuations in BP. If an excessive reduction in BP occurs, place the person in the supine position with legs elevated. CBC and blood chemistry should be obtained before beginning fosinopril therapy, then every 2 wks for the next 3 mo, and periodically thereafter in patients with autoimmune disease or renal impairment, and in those who are taking drugs that affect immune response or leukocyte count. BUN, serum creatinine, and serum potassium should also be monitored in those who are receiving a diuretic. Crackles and wheezes should be assessed in persons with congestive heart failure.

Storage

Store at room temperature.

Administration

Take fosinopril without regard to food. Crush tablets if necessary.

Fosphenytoin

fos-fen′i-toyn

Cerebyx

Do not confuse Cerebyx with Celebrex or Celexa.

CATEGORY AND SCHEDULE

Pregnancy Risk Category: D

Classification: Anticonvulsants, hydantoins

MECHANISM OF ACTION

A hydantoin anticonvulsant that stabilizes neuronal membranes by decreasing sodium and calcium ion influx into the neurons. Also decreases post-tetanic potentiation and repetitive discharge. *Therapeutic Effect:* Decreases seizure activity.

PHARMACOKINETICS

Completely absorbed after IM administration. Protein binding: 95%-99%. Rapidly and completely hydrolyzed to phenytoin after IM or IV administration. Time of complete conversion to phenytoin: 4 h after IM injection; 2 h after IV infusion. *Half-life:* 8-15 min (for conversion to phenytoin).

AVAILABILITY

Injection: 75 mg/mL (equivalent to 50 mg/mL phenytoin).

INDICATIONS AND DOSAGES

▸ **Status epilepticus**

IV

Adults. Loading dose: 15-20 mg phenytoin equivalent (PE)/kg infused at rate of 100-150 mg PE/min.

▸ **Nonemergent seizures**

IV, IM

Adults. Loading dose: 10-20 mg PE/kg. Maintenance: 4-6 mg PE/kg/day.

▸ **Short-term substitution for oral phenytoin**

IM, IV

Adults. May substitute for oral phenytoin at same total daily dose of phenytoin equivalent (PE).

CONTRAINDICATIONS

Adams-Stokes syndrome, hypersensitivity to fosphenytoin or phenytoin, second- or third-degree AV block, severe bradycardia, sinoatrial block.

INTERACTIONS

Drug

NOTE: Like phenytoin, fosphenytoin induces the metabolism of many important drugs.

Alcohol, other CNS depressants: May increase CNS depression.

Amiodarone, anticoagulants, cimetidine, disulfiram, fluoxetine, isoniazid, sulfonamides: May increase fosphenytoin blood concentration, effects, and risk of toxicity.

Antiretroviral protease inhibitors: May decrease PI blood concentrations, leading to loss of antiviral effect.

Fluconazole, ketoconazole, miconazole: May increase fosphenytoin blood concentration.

Glucocorticoids: May decrease the effects of glucocorticoids.

Lidocaine, propranolol: May increase cardiac depressant effects.

Valproic acid: May increase the blood concentration and decrease the metabolism of fosphenytoin.

Theophylline and other xanthines: May increase the metabolism of xanthines.

Warfarin: May alter effects of warfarin; monitor INR.

Herbal and Food

None known.

DIAGNOSTIC TEST EFFECTS

May increase blood glucose, serum GGT, and serum alkaline phosphatase levels.

IV INCOMPATIBILITIES

Caspofungin, doxorubicin, epirubicin, idarubicin, midazolam (Versed), quinupristin-dalfopristin.

IV COMPATIBILITIES

Lorazepam (Ativan), phenobarbital, potassium chloride.

SIDE EFFECTS

Frequent

Dizziness, paresthesia, tinnitus, pruritus, headache, somnolence.

Occasional

Morbilliform rash.

SERIOUS REACTIONS

- An elevated fosphenytoin blood concentration may produce ataxia, nystagmus, diplopia, lethargy, slurred speech, nausea, vomiting, and hypotension. As the drug level increases, extreme lethargy may progress to coma.
- Hypersensitivity can manifest as serious skin reactions (e.g., Stevens-Johnson syndrome) that can be life threatening.

PRECAUTIONS & CONSIDERATIONS

Caution is warranted with hypoalbuminemia, hypotension, hepatic and renal disease, porphyria, and severe myocardial insufficiency. Fosphenytoin use during pregnancy may increase the risk of congenital malformations in the fetus. It is unknown whether fosphenytoin is excreted in breast milk. The safety of this drug has not been established in children. A lower fosphenytoin dosage is recommended for elderly patients.

Drowsiness and dizziness may occur, so alcohol and tasks that require mental alertness or motor skills should be avoided. Assess history of the seizure disorder, including the duration, frequency, and intensity of seizures. BP, ECG, and cardiac and respiratory function should be monitored during and for 10-20 min after infusion. Blood level of fosphenytoin should be assessed 2 h after IV infusion or 4 h after IM injection.

Storage

Refrigerate unopened vials. Do not store the drug at room temperature for longer than 48 h; discard vials that contain particulate matter. After dilution, the solution is stable for 8 h at room temperature or 24 h if refrigerated.

Administration

! Always confirm dosage and injection amount before administration to avoid overdose.

! Know that 150 mg fosphenytoin yields 100 mg phenytoin and that the dose, concentration solution, and infusion rate of fosphenytoin are expressed in terms of phenytoin equivalents (PEs).

For IV use, dilute the drug in D5W or 0.9% NaCl to a concentration of 1.5-25 mg PE/mL. Administer at < 150 mg PE/min to decrease the risk of hypotension and arrhythmias. May also be given IM.

As with all anticonvulsants, therapy is tapered when discontinued, rather than abruptly discontinued.

Fospropofol

fos-pro-poe′fall

Lusedra

CATEGORY AND SCHEDULE

Pregnancy Risk Category: B

Controlled Substance Schedule: IV

Classification: Anesthetics, general

MECHANISM OF ACTION

Fospropofol's action is due to the conversion to propofol, a rapidly acting general anesthetic that appears to depress NMDA-mediated excitatory neurotransmission. It also has agonistic activity at the GABA-A receptor. *Therapeutic Effect:* Produces sedation, anesthesia, and amnesia.

PHARMACOKINETICS

Following IV injection, fospropofol is metabolized by alkaline phosphatases to propofol, the active drug, and formaldehyde. The conversion time results in differences in onset of activity from propofol.

Route	Onset	Peak	Duration
IV	1-20 min	4-13 min	5-15 min after onset

Rapidly and extensively distributed once propofol liberated. Protein binding: 98%. Propofol is metabolized in the liver. Excreted primarily in urine. *Terminal half-life:* 48-60 min.

AVAILABILITY

Injection Solution: 1050 mg/30 mL.

INDICATIONS AND DOSAGES

▸ Anesthesia

IV

(NOTE: The manufacturer provides weight-based dose tables for easy conversions)

Adults, American Society of Anesthesiologists (ASA) I and II patients (dose is weight based).

> 90 kg: 577.5 mg IV bolus; then supplemental doses up to 140 mg IV/dose to achieve desired level of sedation; give no more frequently than every 4 min; lower doses may be used for lighter sedation if desired.

61-89 kg: 6.5 mg/kg (maximum 577.5 mg) IV bolus; then as needed, give supplemental doses up to 1.6 mg/kg/dose (maximum 140 mg/dose) IV to achieve desired level of sedation; give no more frequently than every 4 min; lower doses may be used for lighter sedation if desired.

≤ 60 kg: 385 mg IV bolus; then as needed, give supplemental doses up to 1.2 mg/kg/dose (maximum of 105 mg IV/dose) to achieve desired level of sedation; give no more frequently than every 4 min; lower doses may be used for lighter sedation if desired.

Elderly, Debilitated, Hypovolemic, OR ASA III or IV Adult patients (dose is weight based). Use 75% of the standard dosing regimen based on weight.

CONTRAINDICATIONS

None.

INTERACTIONS

Drug

Alcohol, narcotics, sedative hypnotics, antipsychotics, skeletal muscle relaxants, general anesthetics, other CNS depressants: May increase hypotensive and CNS and respiratory depressant effects of fospropofol.

Herbal

None known.

Food

None known.

DIAGNOSTIC TEST EFFECTS

None known.

IV INCOMPATIBILITIES

Do NOT mix with other drugs prior to administration; NOT compatible with midazolam or meperidine and has not been evaluated with other medications.

SIDE EFFECTS

Frequent (> 20%)
Paresthesia, pruritus. Involuntary muscle movements, apnea (common during induction; lasts longer than 60 seconds).
Occasional
Hypotension, nausea, vomiting, twitching, headache, dizziness, fever, abdominal cramps, coldness, cough, hiccups, facial flushing.
Rare
Agitation, confusion.

SERIOUS REACTIONS

- Overdose may result in extreme somnolence, respiratory depression, and circulatory depression; metabolites such as formate may contribute to the toxicities.
- Nonsustained ventricular tachycardia has been reported.
- Hypotension may require supportive measures.

PRECAUTIONS & CONSIDERATIONS

Caution is warranted in patients with cardiovascular disease, hepatic disease, renal disease, severe respiratory disorder, or history of epilepsy. Use with caution in debilitated patients. Consider the risk for hypotension and resultant decreased perfusion in patients with impaired cerebral circulation and monitor closely. Propofol (active component of fospropofol) crosses the placenta and fospropofol is not recommended for obstetric use. Propofol (active component of fospropofol) is distributed in breast milk and fospropofol is not recommended for breastfeeding women. The safety and efficacy of fospropofol have not been established in children. Lower fospropofol dosages are recommended for elderly or debilitated patients.

Drug should be administered only by qualified personnel trained in anesthesia; resuscitative equipment should be available. Use supplemental oxygen. Frequent monitoring of ECG is recommended. Physician should be notified if patient's respirations are < 10/min and also for possible CNS changes or cardiac or respiratory dysfunction. Vital signs should be obtained before fospropofol administration. ABG levels, BP, heart and respiratory rates, oxygen saturation, depth of sedation should be monitored. Overdosage is treated by discontinuing the drug, using artificial ventilation, volume replacement, vasopressor agents, or other supportive measures.
Storage
Store fospropofol at room temperature.
Administration
! Do not give fospropofol through the same IV line as blood or plasma. Prepare immediately before use. Draw medication from vial into a sterile syringe after opening. Discard any unused vials and medication at the end of the procedure.
! Do not mix with other drugs prior to administration. Administer via intravenous (IV) bolus into a freely flowing peripheral IV line of D5W; D5W-0.2% NaCl; D5W-0.45% NaCl; D5LR; LR; 0.45% NaCl; 0.9%NaCl; or D5W-0.45% NaCl with 20 mEq KCl solutions only; do not mix with other fluids. Flush IV line with normal saline before and after administration. Fospropofol does not require filtration prior to use.

Frovatriptan

fro-va-trip'tan
★ 🍁 Frova

CATEGORY AND SCHEDULE

Pregnancy Risk Category: C

Classification: Serotonin receptor agonists, antimigraine agents

MECHANISM OF ACTION

A serotonin receptor agonist that binds selectively to vascular receptors, producing a vasoconstrictive effect on cranial blood vessels. *Therapeutic Effect:* Relieves migraine headache.

PHARMACOKINETICS

Well absorbed after PO administration. Metabolized by the liver to inactive metabolite. Eliminated in urine. *Half-life:* 26 h (increased in hepatic impairment).

AVAILABILITY

Tablets: 2.5 mg.

INDICATIONS AND DOSAGES

▸ Acute Migraine Attack

PO

Adults, Elderly. Initially 2.5 mg. If headache improves but then returns, dose may be repeated after 2 h. Maximum: 7.5 mg/day.

CONTRAINDICATIONS

Basilar or hemiplegic migraine, cerebrovascular or peripheral vascular disease, coronary artery disease, ischemic heart disease (including angina pectoris, history of myocardial infarction, silent ischemia, and Prinzmetal angina), uncontrolled hypertension, use within 24 h of ergotamine-containing preparations or another serotonin receptor agonist.

INTERACTIONS

Drug

Ergotamine-containing medications: May produce a vasospastic reaction. Do not use triptan within 24 h of ergot drug.

SSRIs, SNRIs: May produce serotonin syndrome.

Herbal and Food

St. John's wort: Additive serotonin effects.

SIDE EFFECTS

Occasional

Dizziness, paresthesia, fatigue, flushing.

Rare

Hot or cold sensation, dry mouth, dyspepsia.

SERIOUS REACTIONS

- Cardiac reactions (including ischemia, coronary artery vasospasm, and MI), and noncardiac vasospasm-related reactions (such as hemorrhage and CVA), occur rarely, particularly in patients with hypertension, diabetes, or a strong family history of coronary artery disease; obese patients; smokers; males older than 40 yr; and postmenopausal women.

PRECAUTIONS & CONSIDERATIONS

Avoid use in patients with risk factors for heart disease unless receive a satisfactory cardiovascular evaluation. Reassess cardiovascular status periodically in all patients receiving frovatriptan. It is unknown if frovatriptan is excreted in breast milk. Safety and effectiveness have not been established in children. No age-related precautions have been identified in the elderly; however, frovatriptan concentrations are increased 1.5 to 2 times in the elderly compared with younger adults.

Storage

Store at room temperature.

Administration

Swallow tablets with liquid.

Fulvestrant

full'veh-strant

★ Faslodex

Do not confuse Faslodex with Fosamax.

CATEGORY AND SCHEDULE

Pregnancy Risk Category: D

Classification: Antineoplastics, antiestrogens, hormones/hormone modifiers

F

MECHANISM OF ACTION

An estrogen antagonist that competes with endogenous estrogen at estrogen receptor binding sites. *Therapeutic Effect:* Inhibits tumor growth.

PHARMACOKINETICS

Extensively and rapidly distributed after IM administration. Protein binding: 99%. Metabolized in the liver. Eliminated by hepatobiliary route; excreted in feces. *Half-life:* 40 days in postmenopausal women. Peak serum levels occur in 7-9 days.

AVAILABILITY

Prefilled Syringe: 250 mg/5 mL syringe.

INDICATIONS AND DOSAGES

▸ **Hormone-receptor positive breast cancer**

IM

Adults, Elderly. 500 mg, given as two 5-mL injections, 1 in each buttock, on days 1, 15, 29, and once monthly thereafter.

▸ **Patients with hepatic impairment**

With moderate (Child-Pugh class B) impairment, reduce to 250 mg IM on days 1, 15, 29, and once monthly thereafter. Not studied in severe hepatic impairment (Child-Pugh class C).

CONTRAINDICATIONS

Known or suspected pregnancy, intravenous use, breastfeeding.

INTERACTIONS

Drug, Herbal, and Food

None known.

DIAGNOSTIC TEST EFFECTS

None known.

SIDE EFFECTS

Frequent (13%-26%)

Nausea, hot flashes, pharyngitis, asthenia, vomiting, vasodilation, headache.

Occasional (5%-12%)

Injection site pain, constipation, diarrhea, abdominal pain, anorexia, dizziness, insomnia, paresthesia, bone or back pain, depression, anxiety, peripheral edema, rash, diaphoresis, fever.

Rare (1%-2%)

Vertigo, weight gain.

SERIOUS REACTIONS

- Urinary tract infections, vaginitis, anemia, thromboembolic phenomena, and leukopenia occur rarely.

PRECAUTIONS & CONSIDERATIONS

Due to the IM route of administration, fulvestrant should be used with caution in those receiving anticoagulant therapy and in those with bleeding diathesis, estrogen receptor-negative breast cancer, hepatic disease or reduced hepatic flow, and thrombocytopenia. Do not administer fulvestrant to pregnant women. It is unknown whether fulvestrant is excreted in breast milk. Fulvestrant is not for use in children. No age-related precautions have been noted in elderly patients.

Notify the physician if weakness, hot flashes, or nausea becomes unmanageable. An estrogen receptor assay test should be performed before therapy, and a computed tomography scan should be performed before and periodically thereafter during and following fulvestrant therapy. Blood chemistry and lipid levels should also be monitored.

Storage

Store unopened syringes in original packaging in the refrigerator. Do not freeze. Protect from light.

Administration

For IM use only; do not give intravenously. Prior to beginning therapy, pregnancy must be excluded. For a 500-mg dose, 2 syringes must be administered. Follow the manufacturer's directions for use of the SafetyGlide needle. Inject IM deeply into the buttock. Administer over 1-2 min. The second syringe should be administered in the opposite buttock. Rotate injection sites.

Furosemide

fur-oh'se-mide

Lasix

Do not confuse Lasix with Lidex, Luvox, or Luxiq, or furosemide with torsemide.

CATEGORY AND SCHEDULE

Pregnancy Risk Category: C (D if used in pregnancy-induced hypertension)

Classification: Diuretics, loop

MECHANISM OF ACTION

A loop diuretic that enhances excretion of sodium, chloride, and potassium by direct action at the ascending limb of the loop of Henle. *Therapeutic Effect:* Produces diuresis and lowers BP.

PHARMACOKINETICS

Route	Onset (min)	Peak	Duration (h)
PO	30-60	1-2 h	6-8
IV	5	20-60 min	2
IM	30	N/A	N/A

Well absorbed from the GI tract. Protein binding: 91%-97%. Partially metabolized in the liver. Primarily excreted in urine (nonrenal clearance increases in severe renal impairment). Not removed by hemodialysis. *Half-life:* 30-90 min (increased in renal or hepatic impairment, and in neonates).

AVAILABILITY

Oral Solution: 10 mg/mL.
Tablets: 20 mg, 40 mg, 80 mg.
Injection: 10 mg/mL.

INDICATIONS AND DOSAGES

▸ Edema, hypertension

PO

Adults, Elderly. Initially, 20-80 mg/dose; may increase by 20-40 mg/dose q6-8h. May titrate up to 600 mg/day in severe edematous states.
Children. 1-6 mg/kg/day in divided doses q6-12h.

IV, IM

Adults, Elderly. 20-40 mg/dose; may increase by 20 mg/dose q1-2h. Once desired dosage confirmed, give once or twice daily to maintain effect. Maximum: 80 mg/dose. Usual initial dose for pulmonary edema is 40 mg.
Children. 1-2 mg/kg/dose q6-12h. Maximum: 6 mg/kg/day.
Neonates. 1-2 mg/kg/dose q12-24h. Maximum: 1 mg/kg/day if premature.

IV INFUSION

Adults, Elderly. Bolus of 0.1 mg/kg, followed by infusion of 0.1 mg/kg/h; may double q2h. Maximum: 0.4 mg/kg/h.

Children. 0.05 mg/kg/h; titrate to desired effect.

OFF-LABEL USES

Hypercalcemia.

CONTRAINDICATIONS

Anuria, hepatic coma, severe electrolyte depletion, hypersensitivity to furosemide.

INTERACTIONS

Drug

Amphotericin B, nephrotoxic and ototoxic medications: May increase the risk of nephrotoxicity and ototoxicity.

Lithium: May increase the risk of lithium toxicity.

Other hypokalemia-causing medications: May increase the risk of hypokalemia.

Herbal and Food

None known.

DIAGNOSTIC TEST EFFECTS

May increase blood glucose, BUN, and serum uric acid levels. May decrease serum calcium, chloride, magnesium, potassium, and sodium levels.

IV INCOMPATIBILITIES

Cimetidine, ciprofloxacin (Cipro), diltiazem (Cardizem), dobutamine (Dobutrex), dopamine (Intropin), doxorubicin (Adriamycin), droperidol (Inapsine), esmolol (Brevibloc), famotidine (Pepcid), filgrastim (Neupogen), fluconazole (Diflucan), gemcitabine (Gemzar), gentamicin (Garamycin), idarubicin (Idamycin), inamrinone, labetalol (Trandate), meperidine (Demerol), metoclopramide (Reglan), midazolam (Versed), milrinone (Primacor), nicardipine (Cardene), ondansetron (Zofran), quinidine, thiopental (Pentothal), vecuronium (Norcuron), vinblastine (Velban), vincristine (Oncovin), vinorelbine (Navelbine).

IV COMPATIBILITIES

Aminophylline, bumetanide (Bumex), calcium gluconate, heparin, hydromorphone (Dilaudid), lidocaine, nitroglycerin, potassium chloride, propofol (Diprivan).

SIDE EFFECTS

Expected

Increased urinary frequency and urine volume.

Frequent

Nausea, dyspepsia, abdominal cramps, diarrhea or constipation, electrolyte disturbances.

Occasional

Dizziness, light-headedness, headache, blurred vision, paresthesia, photosensitivity, rash, fatigue, bladder spasm, restlessness, diaphoresis.

Rare

Flank pain.

SERIOUS REACTIONS

- Vigorous diuresis may lead to profound water loss and electrolyte depletion, resulting in hypokalemia, hyponatremia, and dehydration.
- Sudden volume depletion may result in increased risk of thrombosis, circulatory collapse, and sudden death.
- Acute hypotensive episodes may occur, sometimes several days after beginning therapy.
- Ototoxicity—manifested as deafness, vertigo, or tinnitus—may occur, especially in patients with severe renal impairment.
- Furosemide use can exacerbate diabetes mellitus, systemic lupus erythematosus, gout, and pancreatitis.
- Blood dyscrasias have been reported.

PRECAUTIONS & CONSIDERATIONS

Caution is warranted in patients with hepatic cirrhosis. Furosemide crosses the placenta and is distributed in breast milk. Neonates may require an increased dosage interval because the drug's half-life is increased in this age group. Elderly patients may be more sensitive to the drug's electrolyte and hypotensive effects and are at increased risk for circulatory collapse and thromboembolic effects. Age-related renal impairment may require a dosage adjustment in elderly patients. Consuming foods high in potassium, such as apricots; bananas; legumes; meat; orange juice; raisins; whole grains, including cereals; and white and sweet potatoes, is encouraged. Avoid prolonged exposure to sunlight.

An increase in the frequency and volume of urination and hearing abnormalities, such as a sense of fullness or ringing in the ears, may occur. BP, vital signs, electrolytes, intake and output, and weight should be monitored before and during treatment. Be aware of signs of electrolyte disturbances such as hypokalemia or hyponatremia. Hypokalemia may cause arrhythmias, altered mental status, muscle cramps, asthenia, and tremor. Hyponatremia may result in cold and clammy skin, confusion, and thirst.

Storage

Store all products at room temperature and protected from light (amber containers).

Administration

Take furosemide with food to avoid GI upset, preferably with breakfast to help prevent nocturia.

The solution for injection normally appears clear and colorless. Discard yellow solutions. Furosemide is compatible with D5W, 0.9% NaCl, and lactated Ringer's solution, but it may also be given undiluted. Administer each 20-40 mg or less by IV push over 1-2 min. Do not exceed an infusion administration rate of 4 mg/min in adults or 0.5 mg/kg/min in children.

After IM use, monitor for temporary pain at the injection site.

Gabapentin

ga'ba-pen-tin

Neurontin

Do not confuse Neurontin with Noroxin.

CATEGORY AND SCHEDULE

Pregnancy Risk Category: C

Classification: Anticonvulsants, GABA analog

MECHANISM OF ACTION

An anticonvulsant and antineuralgic agent whose exact mechanism is unknown. May increase the synthesis or accumulation of γ-aminobutyric acid by binding to as-yet-undefined receptor sites in brain tissue. *Therapeutic Effect:* Reduces seizure activity and neuropathic pain.

PHARMACOKINETICS

Well absorbed from the GI tract (not affected by food). Protein binding: < 5%. Widely distributed. Crosses the blood-brain barrier. Primarily excreted unchanged in urine. Removed by hemodialysis. *Half-life:* 5-7 h (increased in patients with impaired renal function and in elderly patients).

AVAILABILITY

Capsules: 100 mg, 300 mg, 400 mg.
Oral Solution: 250 mg/5 mL.
Tablets: 100 mg, 300 mg, 400 mg, 600 mg, 800 mg.

INDICATIONS AND DOSAGES

▸ **Adjunctive therapy for seizure control**

PO

Adults, Elderly, Children 12 yr and older. Initially, 300 mg 3 times a day. May titrate dosage. Range: 900-1800 mg/day in 3 divided doses. Maximum: 3600 mg/day.

Children 3-12 yr. Initially, 10-15 mg/kg/day in 3 divided doses. May titrate up to 25-35 mg/kg/day (for children 5-12 yr) and 40 mg/kg/day (for children 3-4 yr) Maximum: 50 mg/kg/day.

▸ **Postherpetic neuralgia**

PO

Adults, Elderly. 300 mg on day 1, 300 mg twice a day on day 2, and 300 mg 3 times a day on day 3. Titrate up to 1800 mg/day.

▸ **Dosage in renal impairment**

Adults, Children 12 yr and older. Dosage and frequency are modified based on creatinine clearance: An example is given below. See manufacturer prescribing information for full table.

CrCl (mL/min)	Dosage
60 or higher	400 mg q8h
30-59	300 mg q12h
16-29	300 mg daily
< 16	300 mg every other day
Hemodialysis	200-300 mg after each 4-h hemodialysis session

OFF-LABEL USES

Treatment of essential tremor, hot flashes, diabetic neuropathy.

CONTRAINDICATIONS

Hypersensitivity to gabapentin.

INTERACTIONS

Drug

Antacids: May decrease gabapentin absorption; separate administration by 2 h.
Hydrocodone: Gabapentin may decrease hydrocodone concentrations.
Cimetidine: Appears to slightly reduce gabapentin renal excretion
Naproxen: Increases oral absorption of gabapentin by roughly 15%.

Morphine: May increase plasma concentrations of gabapentin.
Herbal
Evening primrose oil, ginkgo: May decrease anticonvulsant effectiveness.
Food
None known.

DIAGNOSTIC TEST EFFECTS

May decrease serum WBC count.

SIDE EFFECTS

Frequent (10%-19%)
Fatigue, somnolence, dizziness, ataxia.
Occasional (3%-8%)
Nystagmus, tremor, diplopia, rhinitis, weight gain.
Rare (< 2%)
Nervousness, dysarthria, memory loss, dyspepsia, pharyngitis, myalgia, emotional lability, aggression or hostility.

SERIOUS REACTIONS

- Abrupt withdrawal may increase seizure frequency.
- Overdosage may result in diplopia, slurred speech, drowsiness, lethargy, and diarrhea.
- Children < 12 yr old with epilepsy may experience behavioral problems; hostility or aggressive behavior; concentration problems; hyperkinesia (restlessness and hyperactivity).

PRECAUTIONS & CONSIDERATIONS

Caution is warranted in patients with renal impairment. It is unknown whether gabapentin is distributed in breast milk. There are no adequate and well-controlled studies in pregnant women; use only if the benefit justifies the potential fetal risk. The safety and efficacy have not been established in children < 3 yr. In elderly patients, age-related renal impairment may require dosage adjustment. Alcohol and tasks requiring mental alertness or motor skills should be avoided. Antiepileptic drugs (AEDs), including gabapentin, increase the risk of suicidal thoughts or behavior. Monitor for the emergence or worsening of depression, suicidal thoughts, or any unusual changes in mood or behavior.

Seizure disorder or nerve pain, including the onset, duration, frequency, and intensity, should be assessed before and during treatment. Weight, renal function, and behavior should also be monitored.

Storage
Store capsules and tablets at room temperature. Store oral solution in refrigerator. Do not freeze.

Administration
! The interval between drug doses should not exceed 12 h.

Gabapentin may be taken with food to reduce GI upset. If the scored 600- or 800-mg tablet is divided to administer a half-tablet, the unused half-tablet should be used with the next dose. Half-tablets not used within several days of breaking should be discarded. If gabapentin treatment will be discontinued or another anticonvulsant added to the treatment regimen, expect to make the changes gradually over at least 1 wk to prevent loss of seizure control.

Galantamine

ga-lan'ta-mene
Razadyne Reminyl, Reminyl ER
Do not confuse Razadyne with Rozerem or Reyataz.

CATEGORY AND SCHEDULE

Pregnancy Risk Category: B

Classification: Cholinesterase inhibitors

MECHANISM OF ACTION

A cholinesterase inhibitor that inhibits the enzyme acetylcholinesterase, thus increasing the concentration of acetylcholine at cholinergic synapses and enhancing cholinergic function in the CNS. *Therapeutic Effect:* Slows the progression of Alzheimer disease.

PHARMACOKINETICS

Rapidly absorbed from the GI tract. Protein binding: 18%. Distributed to blood cells; binds to plasma proteins, mainly albumin. Metabolized in the liver. Excreted in urine.
Half-life: 7 h.

AVAILABILITY

Capsule (Extended Release): 8 mg, 16 mg, 24 mg.
Oral Solution: 4 mg/mL.
Tablets (Immediate Release): 4 mg, 8 mg, 12 mg.

INDICATIONS AND DOSAGES

▸ Alzheimer disease

PO

Adults, Elderly. Initially, 4 mg twice a day (8 mg/day) of the immediate-release tablets or 8 mg once daily of the extended-release capsules. After a minimum of 4 wks (if well tolerated), may increase to 8 mg twice a day (16 mg/day) of the immediate-release tablets or 16 mg once daily of the extended-release capsules. After another 4 wks, may increase to 12 mg twice daily (24 mg/day) of the immediate-release tablets or 24 mg once daily of the extended-release capsules. Range: 16-24 mg/day in 2 divided doses for the immediate-release tablets or once daily for the extended-release capsules.

▸ Dosage in renal or hepatic impairment

For moderate impairment, maximum dosage is 16 mg/day. Drug is not recommended for patients with severe impairment (CrCl < 9 mL/min or Child-Pugh class C).

CONTRAINDICATIONS

Hypersensitivity, severe hepatic or renal impairment.

INTERACTIONS

Drug

Anticholinergics: May oppose effects of galantamine.
Bethanechol, succinylcholine: May interfere with the effects of these drugs.
Cimetidine, erythromycin, ketoconazole, paroxetine: May increase the galantamine blood concentration.

Herbal and Food

None known.

DIAGNOSTIC TEST EFFECTS

None known.

SIDE EFFECTS

Frequent (5%-17%)
Nausea, vomiting, diarrhea, anorexia, weight loss.
Occasional (4%-9%)
Abdominal pain, insomnia, depression, headache, dizziness, fatigue, rhinitis.
Rare (< 3%)
Tremors, constipation, confusion, cough, anxiety, urinary incontinence.

SERIOUS REACTIONS

- Overdose may cause cholinergic crisis, characterized by increased salivation, lacrimation, severe nausea and vomiting, bradycardia, respiratory depression, hypotension, and increased muscle weakness. Treatment usually consists of supportive measures and an anticholinergic such as atropine.
- Heart block, bradycardia.

PRECAUTIONS & CONSIDERATIONS

Caution is warranted in patients with asthma, bladder outflow obstruction, chronic obstructive pulmonary disease (COPD), significant GI disease, including peptic ulcer disease, a history of seizures, moderate hepatic or renal impairment, supraventricular conduction disturbances, and concurrent use of NSAIDs. It is unknown whether galantamine crosses the placenta or is distributed in breast milk. Galantamine is not prescribed for children. Be aware that galantamine is not a cure for Alzheimer disease, but it might slow the progression of its symptoms.

Notify the physician if the patient experiences excessive sweating, tearing, or salivation, depression, dizziness, excessive fatigue, muscle weakness, insomnia, weight loss, or persistent GI disturbances. Liver and renal function test results should be assessed, and periodically monitor pulse rate and quality.

Storage

Store at room temperature tightly closed. Do not freeze oral solution.

Administration

! If galantamine therapy is interrupted for several days or longer, reinstitute therapy as prescribed.

Take immediate-release galantamine with morning and evening meals, and take the extended-release capsule with morning meals.

Ganciclovir

gan-sy′clo-ver

★ Zirgan, Vitrasert 🍁 Cytovene

Do not confuse Cytovene with Cytosar.

CATEGORY AND SCHEDULE

Pregnancy Risk Category: C

Classification: Antivirals, nucleoside analogue

MECHANISM OF ACTION

This synthetic nucleoside competes with viral DNA polymerase and is incorporated into growing viral DNA chains. *Therapeutic Effect:* Interferes with synthesis and replication of viral DNA.

PHARMACOKINETICS

Widely distributed. Protein binding: 1-2%. Undergoes minimal metabolism. Excreted unchanged primarily in urine. Removed by hemodialysis. *Half-life:* 2.5-3.6 h (increased in patients with impaired renal function).

AVAILABILITY

Capsules: 250 mg, 500 mg.
Powder for Injection (Cytovene): 500 mg.
Implant (Vitrasert): 4.5 mg.
Ophthalmic Gel (Zirgan): 0.15%.

INDICATIONS AND DOSAGES

▸ **Cytomegalovirus (CMV) retinitis**

IV

Adults, Children 3 mo and older. 10 mg/kg/day in divided doses q12h for 14-21 days, then 5 mg/kg/day as a single daily dose 7 days/wk or 6 mg/kg/day as a single daily dose 5 days/wk.

G

▸ **Prevention of CMV disease in transplant patients**
IV
Adults, Children. 10 mg/kg/day in divided doses q12h for 7-14 days, then 5 mg/kg/day as a single daily dose 7 days/wk or 6 mg/kg/day as a single daily dose 5 days/wk.
ORAL
Adults. 1000 mg 3 times daily; continue for 14 wks.

▸ **Other CMV infections**
IV
Adults. Initially, 10 mg/kg/day in divided doses q12h for 14-21 days, then 5 mg/kg/day as a single daily dose 7 days/wk or 6 mg/kg/day as a single daily dose 5 days/wk. Maintenance: 1000 mg orally 3 times a day or 500 mg q3h (6 times a day) after IV regimen.
Children. Initially, 10 mg/kg/day in divided doses q12h for 14-21 days, then 5 mg/kg/day as a single daily dose 7 days/wk or 6 mg/kg/day as a single daily dose 5 days/wk. Maintenance: 30 mg/kg/dose q8h. PO.

▸ **Intravitreal implant**
Adults. 1 implant q6-9mo plus oral ganciclovir (1-1.5 g 3 times daily).
Children 9 yr and older. 1 implant q6-9mo plus oral ganciclovir (30 mg/dose q8h).

▸ **Actue herpes simplex keratitis (dendritic keratitis)**
OPHTHALMIC GEL
Adults, Children 2 yr and older. 1 drop in the affected eye(s) 5 times per day (q3h while awake) until corneal ulcer heals, and then 1 drop in the affected eye(s) 3 times per day for 7 days.

▸ **Adult dosage in renal impairment**
Dosage and frequency are modified based on CrCl.

CrCl (mL/min)	IV Induction Dosage	IV Maintenance Dosage	Oral
50-69	2.5 mg/kg q12h	2.5 mg/kg q24h	1500 mg/day
25-49 daily	2.5 mg/kg q24h	1.25 mg/kg q24h	1000 mg/day
10-24	1.25 mg/kg q24h	0.625 mg/kg q24h	500 mg/day
< 10	1.25 mg/kg 3 times/wk	0.625 mg/kg 3 times/wk	500 mg 3 times/wk

CrCl, Creatinine clearance.

OFF-LABEL USES

Treatment of other CMV infections, such as gastroenteritis, hepatitis, and pneumonitis.

CONTRAINDICATIONS

Absolute neutrophil count < 500/mm^3, platelet count < 25,000/mm^3, hypersensitivity to acyclovir or ganciclovir, immunocompetent patients, patients with congenital or neonatal CMV disease.

INTERACTIONS

Drug

Bone marrow depressants: May increase bone marrow depression.
Didanosine: May increase ganciclovir levels.
Imipenem and cilastatin: May increase the risk of seizures.
Nephrotoxic agents: May cause added risk of nephrotoxicity.
Probenecid: May decrease the clearance of ganciclovir.
Zidovudine (AZT): May increase the risk of hepatotoxicity.

Herbal and Food

None known.

DIAGNOSTIC TEST EFFECTS

May increase serum alkaline phosphatase, bilirubin, AST (SGOT), and ALT (SGPT) levels.

IV INCOMPATIBILITIES

Aldesleukin (Proleukin), amifostine (Ethyol), amikacin (Amikin), aminophylline, amphotericin B colloidal (Amphotec), ampicillin (Polycillin), ampicillin and sulbactam (Unasyn), amsacrine (Amsa P-D), ascorbic acid, atracurium (Tracrium), azathioprine (Imuran), aztreonam (Azactam), benztropine (Cogentin), bumetanide (Bumex), buprenorphine (Buprenex), butorphanol (Stadol), calcium chloride, cefamandole (Mandol), cefazolin (Ancef), cefepime (Maxipime), cefmetazole (Zefazone), cefonicid (Monocid), cefoperazone (Cefobid), cefotaxime (Claforan), cefotetan (Cefotan), cefoxitin (Mefixitin), ceftazidime (Fortaz), ceftizoxime (Cefizox), ceftriaxone (Rocephin), cefuroxime (Zinacef), cephalothin (Keflin), cephapirin (Cefadyl), chloramphenicol (Chloromycetin), chlorpromazine (Thorazine), cimetidine (Tagamet), cisatracurium (Nimbex), clindamycin (Cleocin), cytarabine (ARA-C), dantrolene (Dantrium), diazepam (Valium), diazoxide (Proglycem), diltiazem (Cardizem), diphenhydramine (Benadryl), dobutamine (Dobutrex), dopamine (Intropin), doxorubicin (Adriamycin), doxycycline (Vibramycin), ephedrine, epinephrine, epirubicin (Ellence), erythromycin lactobionate (Erythrocin), esmolol (BreviBloc), famotidine (Pepcid), fenoldopam (Corlopam), fludarabine (Fludara), foscarnet (Foscavir), gemcitabine (Gemzar), gentamicin (Garamycin), haloperidol (Haldol), hydralazine (Apresoline), hydrocortisone sodium succinate (Solu-Cortef), inamrinone (Inocor), isoproterenol (Isuprel), ketorolac (Toradol), levofloxacin (Levofloxacin), lidocaine, magnesium sulfate, meperidine (Demerol), metaraminol (Aramine), methicillin (Staphcillin), methoxamine (Vasoxyl), methyldopate (Aldomet), methylprednisolone (Solu-Medrol), metoclopramide (Reglan), metronidazole (Flagyl), mezlocillin (Mezlin), midazolam (Versed), minocycline (Minocin), morphine sulfate (Avinza, Kadian, Robinul), moxalactam (Moxam), multiple vitamins, nalbuphine (Nubain), netilmicin (Netromycin), norepinephrine (Levophed), ondansetron (Zofran), oxacillin (Bactocil), palonosetron (Aloxi), papaverine, penicillin G potassium (Pfizerpen), penicillin G sodium, pentamidine (Pentam), pentazocine (Talwin), phentolamine (Regitine), phenylephrine, phenytoin (Dilantin), piperacillin (Piperacil), piperacillin and tazobactam (Zosyn), procainamide (Pronestyl), prochlorperazine (Compazine), promethazine (Phenergan), pyridoxine, quinidine, quinupristin and dalfopristin (Synercid), sargramostim (Leukine), sodium bicarbonate, streptokinase (Streptase), succinylcholine (Anectine), sulfamethoxazole and trimethoprim (Bactrim), tacrolimus (Prograf), theophylline (Theodur), thiamine, ticarcillin (Ticar), ticarcillin and clavulanate (Timentin), tobramycin (Nebcin), tolazoline (Tolazolin), urokinase (Abbokinase), vancomycin (Vancocin), verapamil (Calan), vinorelbine (Navelbine).

SIDE EFFECTS

Frequent

Diarrhea (41%), fever (40%), nausea (25%), abdominal pain (17%), vomiting (13%).

Occasional (6%-11%)

Diaphoresis, infection, paresthesia, flatulence, pruritus.

Rare (2%-4%)

Headache, stomatitis, dyspepsia, phlebitis.

G

SERIOUS REACTIONS

- Hematologic toxicity occurs commonly: Leukopenia, thrombocytopenia, anemia.
- Intraocular insertion occasionally results in visual acuity loss, vitreous hemorrhage, and retinal detachment.
- GI hemorrhage occurs rarely.
- Aspermatogenesis.

PRECAUTIONS & CONSIDERATIONS

Caution should be used in pediatric patients. The long-term safety of this drug has not been determined because of the potential for long-term adverse reproductive and carcinogenic effects. Caution is warranted with impaired renal function, neutropenia, and thrombocytopenia. Be aware that ganciclovir should not be used during pregnancy and that breastfeeding should be discontinued during ganciclovir use. Breastfeeding may be resumed no sooner than 72 h after the last dose of ganciclovir. Be aware that effective contraception should be used during ganciclovir therapy. Ganciclovir may temporarily or permanently inhibit sperm production in males and suppress fertility in females. Barrier contraception should be used during ganciclovir administration and for 90 days after therapy because of mutagenic potential. Be aware that the safety and efficacy of ganciclovir have not been established in children younger than 12 yr of age. In elderly patients, age-related renal impairment may require dosage adjustment.

Specimens (blood, feces, throat culture, urine) should be obtained for culture and sensitivity testing, as ordered, before giving the drug. Keep in mind that test results are needed to support the differential diagnosis and rule out retinal infection as the result of hematogenous dissemination. Intake and output should be monitored as well as adequate hydration (minimum 1500 mL/24 h). Hematology reports for decreased platelets, neutropenia, and thrombocytopenia should be evaluated. Altered vision, complications, and therapeutic improvement should be assessed.

Storage

Store products at room temperature. Do not refrigerate. Reconstituted solution in vial is stable for 12 h at room temperature. After dilution, refrigerate and use within 24 h. Discard the solution if precipitate forms or discoloration occurs.

Administration

CAUTION: Due to pontential mutagenicity, the manufacturer recommends preparation, administration, and handling in a manner similar to cytotoxic drugs. Give ganciclovir orally with food. Do not open or crush the capsules.

Reconstitute 500-mg vial with 10 mL sterile water for injection to provide a concentration of 50 mg/mL; do not use bacteriostatic water, which contains parabens and is therefore incompatible with ganciclovir. Further dilute with 100 mL D5W, 0.9% NaCl, lactated Ringer's, or any combination thereof, to provide a concentration of 5 mg/mL. Do not give by IV push or rapid IV infusion because these routes increase the risk of ganciclovir toxicity. Administer only by IV infusion over 1 h. Protect from infiltration because the high pH of this drug causes severe tissue irritation. Use large veins to permit rapid dilution and dissemination of ganciclovir and to minimize the risk of phlebitis. Keep in mind that central venous ports tunneled under subcutaneous tissue may reduce catheter-associated infection.

For the ophthalmic gel, wash hands before and after use. Tilt the head back slightly and pull the lower eyelid down to form a pouch. Squeeze the prescribed number of drops. Close eyes to spread drops. Patients should not wear contact lenses during treatment.

Gatifloxacin

gah-tee-floks'a-sin

Zymar, Zymaxid Zymar

CATEGORY AND SCHEDULE

Pregnancy Risk Category: C

Classification: Antibiotics, quinolones, ophthalmic

MECHANISM OF ACTION

A fluoroquinolone that inhibits two enzymes, topoisomerase II and IV, in susceptible microorganisms. *Therapeutic Effect:* Interferes with bacterial DNA replication. Prevents or delays resistance emergence. Bactericidal.

AVAILABILITY

Ophthalmic Solution (Zymar): 0.3%.
Ophthalmic Solution (Zymaxid): 0.5%.

INDICATIONS AND DOSAGES

▸ **Bacterial conjunctivitis (Zymar)**

Adults, Elderly, Children 1 yr and older. 1 drop q2h while awake for 2 days, then 1 drop up to 4 times/day for days 3-7.

▸ **Bacterial conjunctivitis (Zymaxid)**

Adults, Elderly, Children 1 yr and older. On day 1, instill 1 drop to affected eye(s) q2h while awake, up to 8 times daily. On days 2-7, instill 1 drop 2-4 times per day while awake.

CONTRAINDICATIONS

Hypersensitivity to quinolones.

INTERACTIONS

Drug
None known.
Herbal
None known.
Food
None known.

DIAGNOSTIC TEST EFFECTS

None known.

SIDE EFFECTS

Occasional (5%-10%)
Ophthalmic: Conjunctival irritation, increased tearing, corneal inflammation.
Rare (0.1%-3%)
Ophthalmic: Corneal swelling, dry eye, eye pain, eyelid swelling, headache, red eye, reduced visual acuity, altered taste.

SERIOUS REACTIONS

- Conjunctival hemorrhage has been reported.
- May cause severe hypersensitivity (rare).

PRECAUTIONS & CONSIDERATIONS

Patients should be advised to avoid contact lens use while they have signs and symptoms of bacterial conjunctivitis. It is unknown if gatifloxacin is distributed in breast milk. The safety and efficacy of gatifloxacin have not been established in children < 1 yr. History of hypersensitivity to gatifloxacin and other quinolones should be determined before therapy.

Storage

Store at room temperature; do not freeze.

Administration

Tilt head backward and look up. Gently pull the lower eyelid down until a pocket is formed. Hold the dropper above the pocket, and without touching the eyelid or conjunctival sac, place drops into the center of the pocket. Close the eye, and then apply gentle digital pressure to the lacrimal sac at the inner canthus. Remove excess solution around the eye with a tissue.

Gefitinib

ge-fi'tye-nib

Iressa

CATEGORY AND SCHEDULE

Pregnancy Risk Category: D

Classification: Antineoplastic; epidermal growth factor receptor inhibitor

MECHANISM OF ACTION

Blocks the signaling pathway that binds to the epidermal growth factor receptor (EGFR) on the surface of normal and cancer cells. EGFR activates the enzyme tyrosine kinase, which sends signals instructing the cells to grow. *Therapeutic Effect:* Inhibits the growth of cancer cells.

PHARMACOKINETICS

Slowly absorbed and extensively distributed throughout the body. Protein binding: 90%. Undergoes extensive metabolism in the liver. Excreted in the feces. *Half-life:* 48 h.

AVAILABILITY

Tablets: 250 mg.

INDICATIONS AND DOSAGES

▸ **Non–small cell lung carcinoma (only in those patients showing benefit from current or past use)**

PO

Adults, Elderly. 250 mg/day; may increase to 500 mg/day for patients receiving drugs that may decrease gefitinib blood concentrations (CYP3A4 inducers), such as rifampin and phenytoin.

CONTRAINDICATIONS

Severe hypersensitivity to the drug.

INTERACTIONS

Drug

CYP3A4 inducers (e.g., rifamycins, phenytoin): Reduce gefitinib concentrations. Dosage adjustment and careful monitoring recommended.

Erythromycin, fluconazole, itraconazole, ketoconazole, and CYP3A4 inhibitors: May increase gefitinib blood concentration and toxicity.

H_2 antagonists (e.g., cimetidine, ranitidine): Decrease absorption of gefitinib.

Vinorelbine: Increased risk of neutropenia.

Warfarin: Increases the risk of bleeding.

Herbal

St. John's wort: May reduce gefitinib concentrations. Avoid.

Food

None known.

DIAGNOSTIC TEST EFFECTS

May increase serum alkaline phosphatase, bilirubin, AST (SGOT), and ALT (SGPT) levels.

SIDE EFFECTS

Frequent (25%-48%)
Diarrhea, rash, acne.
Occasional (8%-13%)
Dry skin, nausea, vomiting, pruritus.
Rare (2%-7%)
Anorexia, asthenia, weight loss, peripheral edema, eye pain.

SERIOUS REACTIONS

- Pancreatitis and ocular hemorrhage occur rarely.
- Hypersensitivity reaction produces angioedema and urticaria.
- Interstitial lung disease has been reported and if it occurs, requires discontinuation of the drug.

PRECAUTIONS & CONSIDERATIONS

Distribution of this drug is limited under a risk management plan called the Iressa Access Program.

Caution is warranted in patients with hepatic impairment and severe renal impairment. Gefitinib may cause fetal harm and result in termination of pregnancy. Pregnant or breastfeeding women should not receive this drug. Pregnancy should be avoided during therapy, and contraceptive methods should be used during treatment and for up to 12 mo afterward. The safety and efficacy of gefitinib have not been established in children. No age-related precautions have been noted in elderly patients. Vaccinations without the physician's approval and crowds and people with known infections should be avoided.

Notify the physician of anorexia, nausea, vomiting, persistent or severe diarrhea, and signs and symptoms of infection, including fever and flu-like symptoms. Periodic liver function monitoring is advised.

Adequate hydration should be maintained. Bowel sounds for hyperactivity and pattern of daily bowel activity and stool consistency should be assessed. Antidiarrheals and antiemetics may help prevent and treat diarrhea, nausea, and vomiting. For those who cannot tolerate diarrhea, expect to interrupt gefitinib therapy for up to 14 days. If dyspnea, cough, or other pulmonary symptoms occur, interrupt therapy until cause is determined.

Storage
Store at room temperature.
Administration
Take gefitinib without regard to food. For patients who have difficulty swallowing, the tablets may be dropped in a half glass of noncarbonated drinking water and stirred to dissolve (approximately 10 min); then drink the liquid immediately. Rinse the glass with half a glass of water and drink that as well. The liquid may also be given via nasogastric tube.

Gemcitabine

gem-site'a-been
Gemzar

CATEGORY AND SCHEDULE

Pregnancy Risk Category: D

Classification: Antineoplastics, antimetabolites, pyrimidine analogues

MECHANISM OF ACTION

An antineoplastic agent chemically related to cytarabine. Gemcitabine undergoes intracellular conversion to gemcitabine monophosphate via the enzyme deoxycytidine kinase.

Gemcitabine monophosphate is subsequently converted to gemcitabine triphosphate (deoxydifluorocytidine triphosphate, dFdCTP) and gemcitabine diphosphate (deoxydifluorocytidine diphosphate). Gemcitabine triphosphate competes with deoxycytadine triphosphate (dCTP) for incorporation into DNA strands. After insertion of the gemcitabine analogue into DNA, an additional base pair is added before DNA polymerase is stopped. The "masked termination" inhibits both DNA replication and repair. Cell cycle–specific for S phase of cell division. *Therapeutic Effect:* Potent antineoplastic activity; blocks cancer cell replication, particularly in solid tumors.

PHARMACOKINETICS

Metabolized by cytidine deaminase to the inactive metabolite, 2', 2'-difluorodeoxyuridine (dFdU). Protein binding: Less than 10%. Primarily excreted in urine, with 92%-98% recovery as inactive metabolite and < 10% as active drug. *Half-life:* 40-50 min following 30-min infusion (increased in females and elderly).

AVAILABILITY

Injection Powder for Solution: 200-mg, 1-g vials.

INDICATIONS AND DOSAGES

▸ For metastatic breast cancer with paclitaxel

IV INFUSION

Adults, Elderly. 1250 mg/m^2 on days 1 and 8 of a 21-day cycle in combination with paclitaxel (175 mg/m^2 given on day 1 prior to gemcitabine).

▸ For ovarian cancer that has relapsed at least 6 mo after platinum-based treatment

IV INFUSION

Adults, Elderly. 1000 mg/m^2 on days 1 and 8 of a 21-day cycle in combination with carboplatin (AUC4; given on day 1 after gemcitabine infusion).

▸ For non–small cell lung carcinoma along with cisplatin

IV INFUSION

Adults, Elderly. 1000 mg/m^2 on days 1, 8, and 15 of a 28-day cycle OR 1250 mg/m^2 on days 1 and 8 of a 21-day cycle. Cisplatin (100 mg/m^2 IV) is given following the gemcitabine infusion on day 1 of either regimen.

▸ For pancreatic cancer as a single agent

IV INFUSION

Adults, Elderly. 1000 mg/m^2 once weekly for up to 7 wks, followed by 1 wk of rest.

▸ Dosage modifications

NOTE: Expect to modify the dose regimen as needed based on the cancer type and toxicities that present. See prescribing information for detailed information.

CONTRAINDICATIONS

Hypersensitivity to gemcitabine.

INTERACTIONS

Drug

Paclitaxel: May increase gemcitabine concentrations and risk of toxicity; monitor closely.
Warfarin: May increase anticoagulant effect; monitor INR.
Live vaccines: Defer vaccination due to potential virus replication, adverse reactions to the virus, immunosuppression.
Radiation: Drug has radiosensitizing activity.

Herbal
None known.
Food
None known.

DIAGNOSTIC TEST EFFECTS

May increase AST (SGOT) and ALT (SGPT) levels. May decrease blood hematocrit, hemoglobin level, and WBC and platelet count. May cause proteinuria or hematuria.

IV INCOMPATIBILITIES

Acyclovir, amphotericin B (Abelcet, AmBisome), cefepime (Maxipime), cefotaxime, daptomycin, diazepam, furosemide, ganciclovir (Cytovene), imipenem-cilastatin (Primaxin IV), irinotecan, lansoprazole (Prevacid), methotrexate, methylprednisolone sodium succinate (Solu-Medrol), nafcillin, pantoprazole (Protonix), pemetrexed, phenytoin, piperacillin-tazobactam (Zosyn), prochlorperazine, thiopental.

SIDE EFFECTS

Expected
Leukopenia, neutropenia, thrombocytopenia, anemia.
Frequent (> 5%)
Nausea, vomiting, dyspnea, fever, infections, mild hematuria or proteinuria, alopecia, rash.
Occasional (≤ 5%)
Stomatitis, somnolence, paresthesias.

SERIOUS REACTIONS

• Serious reactions may include myelosuppression (evidenced by neutropenia, thrombocytopenia, and anemia); myelosuppression is the most frequent adverse drug event and often requires dose adjustment.
• Severe pulmonary events/toxicity.
• Serious hepatotoxicity, including liver failure and death, has been reported very rarely.
• Hemolytic uremic syndrome (HUS) reported rarely.
• Anaphylactoid reactions are rare.

PRECAUTIONS & CONSIDERATIONS

CAUTION: Prolongation of the infusion time beyond 60 min and more frequent than weekly dosing have been shown to increase toxicity. Myelosuppression is the main side effect. Use cautiously in patients with a history of pulmonary disease or renal or hepatic impairment, and in those receiving radiation treatments. Caution is also warranted in elderly patients. Avoid use in pregnant women. It is unknown whether gemcitabine is distributed in breast milk. Safety and efficacy of the drug have not been established in children.

Monitor for signs of infection or bleeding. Monitor for hematologic toxicity with a CBC, including differential and platelet count prior to each dose or on day 8 of combination therapy and prior to the next cycle. Expect dosage modifications if hematologic toxicity occurs. Monitor renal function and hepatic enzymes, as well as respiratory status, closely.

Storage
Unopened vials are stored at room temperature. Reconstituted infusions are stable at room temperature for 24 h. Do not refrigerate as this will cause crystallization.

Administration
CAUTION: Observe and exercise usual cautions for handling and preparing solutions of cytotoxic drugs.

For intravenous administration as an IV infusion. To reconstitute, add

5 mL of 0.9% NaCl to the 200-mg vial or 25 mL to the 1-g vial. Do not use any other diluents. Shake to dissolve. Final vial concentration will be 38 mg/mL. The appropriate dose of drug may be administered as prepared or further diluted with 0.9% NaCl injection to concentrations as low as 0.1 mg/mL. Infuse IV over 30 min. Longer infusion times increase toxicity.

G

Gemfibrozil

gem-fi′broe-zil

Lopid

Do not confuse with Lorabid or Levbid.

CATEGORY AND SCHEDULE

Pregnancy Risk Category: C

Classification: Antihyperlipidemics, fibric acid derivatives

MECHANISM OF ACTION

A fibric acid derivative that inhibits lipolysis of fat in adipose tissue, decreases liver uptake of free fatty acids, and reduces hepatic triglyceride production. Inhibits synthesis of VLDL carrier apolipoprotein B. *Therapeutic Effect:* Lowers serum cholesterol and triglycerides (decreases VLDL, LDL; increases HDL).

PHARMACOKINETICS

Well absorbed from the GI tract. Protein binding: 99%. Metabolized in liver. Primarily excreted in urine. Not removed by hemodialysis. *Half-life:* 1.5 h.

AVAILABILITY

Tablets: 600 mg.

INDICATIONS AND DOSAGES

▸ **Hyperlipidemia, hypertriglyceridemia**

PO

Adults, Elderly. 1200 mg/day in 2 divided doses 30 min before breakfast and dinner.

CONTRAINDICATIONS

Hypersensitivity, liver dysfunction (including primary biliary cirrhosis), preexisting gallbladder disease, severe renal dysfunction, administration with cerivastatin or with repaglinide.

INTERACTIONS

Drug

Bile acid sequestrants: Reduce gemfibrozil absorption; administer 2 h or more apart.

Cyclosporine: May potentiate renal problems.

HMG-CoA reductase inhibitors, especially cerivastatin, lovastatin: May increase risk of rhabdomyolysis, leading to acute renal failure.

Pioglitazone, repaglinide: May increase the effect of these drugs. Use with repaglinide contraindicated due to risk of severe hypoglycemia.

Warfarin: May increase effects of warfarin; reduce anticoagulant dose and closely monitor INR.

Herbal

None known.

Food

None known.

DIAGNOSTIC TEST EFFECTS

May increase serum alkaline phosphatase, serum bilirubin, serum creatinine kinase, serum LDH concentrations, and SGOT (AST) and SGPT (ALT) levels. May decrease blood hemoglobin and hematocrit levels, leukocyte counts, and serum potassium levels.

SIDE EFFECTS

Frequent (20%)
Dyspepsia.
Occasional (2%-10%)
Abdominal pain, diarrhea, nausea, vomiting, fatigue.
Rare (< 2%)
Constipation, acute appendicitis, vertigo, headache, rash, pruritus, altered taste.

SERIOUS REACTIONS

- Cholelithiasis, cholecystitis, acute appendicitis, and pancreatitis occur rarely.
- Rhabdomyolysis when administered with a "statin" is rare.

PRECAUTIONS & CONSIDERATIONS

Caution is warranted in patients with diabetes mellitus, gallbladder disease, receiving estrogen or anticoagulant therapy, and with hypothyroidism. Be aware that it is unknown whether gemfibrozil crosses the placenta or is distributed in breast milk. Animal studies show some tumorigenic potential. Be aware that gemfibrozil use is not recommended in children. In elderly patients, age-related renal impairment may require dosage adjustment.

Notify the physician of any abdominal pain, diarrhea, dizziness, nausea, or vomiting. Pattern of daily bowel activity and stool consistency should be assessed. Serum LDL, VLDL, triglyceride, and cholesterol levels should be checked at baseline and periodically during treatment. Hematology and liver function test results should also be assessed. Blood glucose should be monitored in those with diabetes mellitus.

Be aware of the increased risk of developing rhabdomyolysis when coadministered with a statin. Lovastatin should be limited to a maximum of 20 mg/day if given concomitantly with gemfibrozil.

Storage
Store at room temperature. Protect from light and humidity.
Administration
Take gemfibrozil 30 min before morning and evening meals.

Gemifloxacin

gem-ih-flocks'ah-sin
★ Factive

CATEGORY AND SCHEDULE

Pregnancy Risk Category: C

Classification: Antibiotics, quinolones

MECHANISM OF ACTION

A fluoroquinolone that inhibits the enzyme DNA gyrase in susceptible microorganisms, interfering with bacterial cell replication and repair. *Therapeutic Effect:* Bactericidal.

PHARMACOKINETICS

Rapidly and well absorbed from the GI tract. Protein binding: 70%. Widely distributed. Penetrates well into lung tissue and fluid. Undergoes limited metabolism in the liver. Primarily excreted in feces; lesser amount eliminated in urine. Partially removed by hemodialysis. *Half-life:* 4-12 h.

AVAILABILITY

Tablets: 320 mg.

INDICATIONS AND DOSAGES

▸ **Acute bacterial exacerbation of chronic bronchitis**

PO

Adults, Elderly. 320 mg once a day for 5 days.

▸ **Community-acquired pneumonia**

PO

Adults, Elderly. 320 mg once a day for 7 days.

▸ **Dosage in renal impairment**

Dosage and frequency are modified based on creatinine clearance.

Creatinine Clearance (mL/min)	Dosage
> 40	320 mg once a day
≤ 40	160 mg once a day

CONTRAINDICATIONS

Hypersensitivity to gemifloxacin or to other fluoroquinolones.

INTERACTIONS

Drug

Aluminum and magnesium-containing antacids, bismuth subsalicylate, didanosine, iron preparations and other metals, sucralfate, zinc preparations: May decrease the absorption of gemifloxacin. Avoid administration within 3 h before or 2 h after gemifloxacin.

Antipsychotics, class 1A and class III antiarrhythmics, erythromycin, tricyclic antidepressants, pimozide, thioridazine: May increase the risk of prolonged QTc interval and life-threatening arrhythmias.

Corticosteroids: May increase risk of tendon rupture, especially in elderly patients.

Cyclosporine: Increases the risk of nephrotoxicity.

Probenecid: Increases gemifloxacin serum concentration.

Warfarin: May increase the effect of warfarin.

Herbal and Food

None known.

DIAGNOSTIC TEST EFFECTS

May increase BUN and serum alkaline phosphatase, bilirubin, LDH, creatinine, AST (SGOT), and ALT (SGPT) levels.

SIDE EFFECTS

Occasional (2%-4%)

Diarrhea, rash, nausea.

Rare (≤ 1%)

Headache, abdominal pain, dizziness, tremor, nervousness.

SERIOUS REACTIONS

- Antibiotic-associated colitis may result from altered bacterial balance.
- Hypersensitivity reactions, including photosensitivity (as evidenced by rash, pruritus, blisters, edema, and burning skin), have occurred in patients receiving fluoroquinolones. With gemifloxacin, serious rashes occur more frequently in women under 40 and women of any age receiving hormone replacement therapy.
- Tendon ruptures and peripheral neuropathy have been reported.
- Convulsions (rare).
- QT interval prolongation and risk of proarrhythmia.

PRECAUTIONS & CONSIDERATIONS

Caution is warranted in patients with acute myocardial ischemia or impaired hepatic or renal function. Use with caution in patients with cardiac arrhythmias; should not be used unmonitored in patients with known QT prolongation.

Conditions that might increase the risk of proarrythmia include electrolyte imabalances and use of drugs that prolong the QT interval. Fluoroquinolones increase the risk of tendonitis and tendon rupture, which may be seen more often in the elderly, in those taking corticosteroids, and in patients with organ transplants. There are no adequate data regarding the use of gemifloxacin in pregnancy or breastfeeding. The safety and efficacy of gemifloxacin have not been established in children 18 yr of age and younger. Age-related renal impairment may require a dosage adjustment in elderly patients.

Dizziness, headache, nausea, signs of infection, and skin for rash should be evaluated. Pattern of daily bowel activity and stool consistency should be assessed. Liver function and white blood cell (WBC) count should be monitored. QT interval should be checked for prolongation. History of hypersensitivity to gemifloxacin and other quinolones should be determined before therapy.

Fluoroquinolone use has been associated with hypoglycemia in patients with and without diabetes. Patients with diabetes should be monitored frequently while taking gemifloxacin. Excessive exposure to sunlight and UV light should be avoided due to potential photosensitivity.

Storage

Store at room temperature and protect from light.

Administration

Take gemifloxacin without regard to food. Do not crush or break tablets. Take 2 h before giving antacids, buffered tablets or solutions, ferrous sulfate, or multivitamins with minerals. Drink plenty of fluids.

Gentamicin

jen-ta-mye′sin

★ Garamycin, Gentasol, Gentak

🍁 Diogent, Garamycin, Gentak

CATEGORY AND SCHEDULE

Pregnancy Risk Category: C

Classification: Anti-infectives, ophthalmic, topical, antibiotics, aminoglycosides, dermatologics

MECHANISM OF ACTION

An aminoglycoside antibiotic that irreversibly binds to the protein of bacterial ribosomes. *Therapeutic Effect:* Interferes with protein synthesis of susceptible microorganisms. Bactericidal.

PHARMACOKINETICS

Rapid, complete absorption after IM administration. Protein binding: < 30%. Widely distributed (does not cross the blood-brain barrier, low concentrations in CSF). Excreted unchanged in urine. Removed by hemodialysis. *Half-life:* 2-4 h (increased in impaired renal function and neonates; decreased in cystic fibrosis and burn or febrile patients).

AVAILABILITY

Injection: 10 mg/mL, 40 mg/mL.
Ophthalmic Solution (Gentasol): 0.3%.
Ophthalmic Ointment (Gentak): 0.3%.
Cream: 0.1%.
Ointment: 0.1%.

INDICATIONS AND DOSAGES

▸ **Acute pelvic, bone, intra-abdominal, joint, respiratory tract, burn wound, postoperative, and skin or skin-structure infections; complicated urinary tract infection; septicemia; meningitis**

IV, IM

Adults, Elderly. Usual dosage, 3-6 mg/kg/day in divided doses q8h or 4-7 mg/kg once a day.

Children 5-12 yr. Usual dosage 2-2.5 mg/kg/dose q8h.

Children younger than 5 yr. Usual dosage, 2.5 mg/kg/dose q8h.

Neonates. Usual dosage 2.5-3.5 mg/kg/dose q8-12h.

▸ **Intrathecal (preservative-free injection only)**

Adults. 4-8 mg/day.

Children 3 mo to 12 yr. 1-2 mg/day.

Neonates. 1 mg/day.

▸ **Superficial eye infections**

OPHTHALMIC OINTMENT

Adults, Elderly. Usual dosage, apply thin strip to conjunctiva 2-3 times a day.

OPHTHALMIC SOLUTION

Adults, Elderly, Children. Usual dosage, 1-2 drops q2-4h up to 2 drops/h.

▸ **Superficial skin infections**

TOPICAL

Adults, Elderly. Usual dosage, apply 3-4 times/day.

▸ **Dosage in renal impairment (adults)**

For traditional dosing regimens.

Creatinine clearance 40-60 mL/min. Dosage interval q12h.

Creatinine clearance 20-40 mL/min. Dosage interval q24h.

Creatinine clearance < 20 mL/min. Monitor levels to determine dosage interval.

▸ **Hemodialysis**

IV, IM

Adults, Elderly. 1-1.7 mg/kg after dialysis.

Children. 1-1.7 mg/kg/dose after dialysis.

CONTRAINDICATIONS

Hypersensitivity to gentamicin, other aminoglycosides (cross-sensitivity), or their components. Injection contains sodium metabisulfite, a sulfite that may cause anaphylactic symptoms in certain susceptible people (seen more commonly in those with asthma).

INTERACTIONS

Drug

Nephrotoxic medications, other aminoglycosides, ototoxic medications: May increase the risk of nephrotoxicity or ototoxicity.

Neuromuscular blockers and botulinum toxins: May increase neuromuscular blockade.

Herbal

None known.

Food

None known.

DIAGNOSTIC TEST EFFECTS

May increase serum creatinine, serum bilirubin, BUN, serum LDH, SGOT (AST), and SGPT (ALT) levels. May decrease serum calcium, magnesium, potassium, and sodium concentrations. In traditional dose regimens, the therapeutic peak serum level is 6-10 mcg/mL and trough is 0.5-2 mcg/mL. For all regimens, toxic trough level is > 2 mcg/mL.

IV INCOMPATIBILITIES

Allopurinol (Aloprim), amphotericin B complex (Abelcet, AmBisome, Amphotec), ampicillin (Polycillin), cefamandole (Mandol), cefepime (Maxipime), cefotaxime (Claforan), cefotetan (Cefotan), cefuroxime (Ancef), clindamycin (Cleocin), cytarabine (Cytosar), dopamine

(Intropin), filgrastim (Neupogen), furosemide (Lasix), heparin, hetastarch (Hespan), idarubicin (Idamycin), indomethacin (Indocin), nafcillin (Unipen), phenytoin (Dilantin), propofol (Diprivan), ticarcillin (Ticar), warfarin (Coumadin).

IV COMPATIBILITIES

Acyclovir (Zovirax), alatrofloxacin (Trovan), amifostine (Ethyol), amiodarone (Cordarone), amsacrine (AMSA), atracurium (Tracrium), aztreonam (Azactam), bleomycin (Blenoxane), cefoxitin (Mefixitin), cimetidine (Tagamet), ciprofloxacin (Cipro), cisatracurium (Nimbex), clarithromycin (Biaxin), cyclophosphamide (Cytoxan), diltiazem (Cardizem), enalaprilat (Vasotec), esmolol (BreviBloc), etoposide (VePesid), famotidine (Pepcid), fluconazole (Diflucan), fludarabine (Fludara), foscarnet (Foscavir), gatifloxacin (Tequin), gemcitabine (Gemzar), granisetron (Kytril), hydromorphone (Dilaudid), insulin, labetolol (Normodyne, Trandate), levofloxacin (Levaquin), lidocaine (Xylocaine), linezolid (Zyvox), lorazepam (Ativan), magnesium sulfate, melphalan (Alkeran), meperidine (Demerol), meropenem (Merrem), metronidazole (Flagyl), midazolam (Versed), morphine, multivitamins, ondansetron (Zofran), paclitaxel (Taxol), pancuronium (Pavulon), perphenazine (Trilafon), ranitidine (Zantac), remifentanil (Ultiva), sargramostim (Leukine), tacrolimus (Prograf), teniposide (Vumon), theophylline (Theodur), thiotepa (Thioplex), tolazone (Tolazolin), vecuronium (Norcuron), verapamil (Calan), vinorelbine (Navelbine), vitamin B complex with C, zidovudine (Retrovir).

SIDE EFFECTS

Occasional

IM: Pain, induration.
IV: Phlebitis, thrombophlebitis, hypersensitivity reactions (fever, pruritus, rash, urticaria).
Ophthalmic: Burning, tearing, itching, blurred vision.
Topical: Redness, itching.

Rare

Alopecia, hypertension, weakness.

SERIOUS REACTIONS

- Nephrotoxicity (as evidenced by increased BUN and serum creatinine levels and decreased creatinine clearance) may be reversible if the drug is stopped at the first sign of symptoms.
- Irreversible ototoxicity (manifested as tinnitus, dizziness, ringing or roaring in the ears, and diminished hearing) and neurotoxicity (as evidenced by headache, dizziness, lethargy, tremor, and visual disturbances) occur occasionally. The risk of these effects increases with higher dosages or prolonged therapy and when the solution is applied directly to the mucosa.
- Superinfections, particularly with fungal infections, may result from bacterial imbalance no matter which administration route is used.
- Ophthalmic application may cause paresthesia of conjunctiva or mydriasis.

PRECAUTIONS & CONSIDERATIONS

! Cumulative gentamicin effects may occur with concurrent systemic administration and topical application to large areas. Caution is warranted with neuromuscular disorders (because of the potential for respiratory depression), prior hearing loss, renal impairment, and vertigo and in elderly and neonatal patients because of age-related renal insufficiency or immaturity. Gentamicin readily crosses the placenta; it is unknown whether it is distributed in breast milk.

Before giving gentamicin, determine whether the patient has a history of allergies, especially to aminoglycosides, sulfites, and parabens (for topical and ophthalmic forms). Expect to correct dehydration before beginning parenteral therapy. Establish baseline hearing acuity before starting therapy. Intake and output should be monitored. Drink fluids to maintain adequate hydration. Monitor urinalysis results for casts, RBCs, WBCs, and decreased specific gravity. Be alert for ototoxic and neurotoxic side effects. If giving ophthalmic gentamicin, monitor the patient's eye for burning, itching, redness, and tearing. If giving topical gentamicin, monitor for itching and redness. Be alert for signs and symptoms of superinfection, particularly changes in the oral mucosa, diarrhea, and genital or anal pruritus. Monitor peak and trough serum drug levels.

Storage

Store ophthalmic preparations, topicals, and solution vials for injection at room temperature. The solution normally appears clear or slightly yellow. Intermittent IV infusion or IV piggyback solution is stable for 24 h at room temperature. Discard the IV solution if a precipitate forms.

Administration

! Space parenteral doses evenly around the clock. Gentamicin dosage is based on ideal body weight. As ordered, monitor peak and trough serum drug levels periodically to maintain the desired serum concentrations and to minimize the risk of toxicity.

For IV administration, dilute with 50-200 mL of D5W or 0.9% NaCl. The amount of diluent for infants and children depends on individual needs. Infuse over 30-60 min for adults and older children. Infuse over 60-120 min for infants and young children.

Administer the IM injection slowly and deep in the gluteus maximus rather than the lateral aspect of the thigh to minimize injection site pain.

For intrathecal administration, use only 2 mg/mL of the intrathecal preparation without preservative. Mix with 10% of the estimated cerebrospinal fluid volume or preservative-free 0.9% NaCl. Use the intrathecal form immediately after preparation. Discard any unused portion. Give over 3-5 min.

For ophthalmic use, place a gloved finger on the lower eyelid and pull it out until a pocket is formed between the eye and lower lid. Hold the dropper above the pocket, and place the correct number of drops (or ¼ to ½ inch of ointment) into the pocket. Close the eye gently. After administering ophthalmic solution, apply digital pressure to the lacrimal sac for 1-2 min to minimize drainage into the nose and throat, thereby reducing the risk of systemic effects. After applying ophthalmic ointment, close eye for 1-2 min. Roll the eyeball to increase the drug's contact with the eye. Use tissue to remove excess solution or ointment around the eye.

Glatiramer

gla-teer'a-mer

Copaxone

Do not confuse Copaxone with Compazine.

CATEGORY AND SCHEDULE

Pregnancy Risk Category: B

Classification:

Immunosuppressives

MECHANISM OF ACTION

An immunosuppressive whose exact mechanism is unknown. May act by modifying immune processes thought to be responsible for the pathogenesis of multiple sclerosis (MS). *Therapeutic Effect:* Slows progression of MS.

PHARMACOKINETICS

Substantial fraction of glatiramer is hydrolyzed locally. Some fraction of injected material enters the lymphatic circulation, reaching regional lymph nodes; some may enter systemic circulation intact.

AVAILABILITY

Injection: 20 mg/mL in prefilled syringes.

INDICATIONS AND DOSAGES

▸ **MS**

SUBCUTANEOUS

Adults, Elderly. 20 mg once a day.

CONTRAINDICATIONS

Hypersensitivity to glatiramer or mannitol.

INTERACTIONS

Drug

None known.

Herbal

None known.

Food

None known.

DIAGNOSTIC TEST EFFECTS

None known.

SIDE EFFECTS

Expected (40%-73%)

Pain, erythema, inflammation, or pruritus at injection site; asthenia.

Frequent (18%-27%)

Arthralgia, vasodilation, anxiety, hypertonia, nausea, transient chest pain, dyspnea, flu-like symptoms, rash, pruritus.

Occasional (10%-17%)

Palpitations, back pain, diaphoresis, rhinitis, diarrhea, urinary urgency.

Rare (6%-8%)

Anorexia, fever, neck pain, peripheral edema, ear pain, facial edema, vertigo, vomiting.

SERIOUS REACTIONS

- Infection is a common effect.
- Lymphadenopathy occurs occasionally.
- Hypertension may occur.
- Transient eosinophilia may occur.

PRECAUTIONS & CONSIDERATIONS

Caution is warranted with an immediate post-injection reaction, including anxiety, chest pain, dyspnea, flushing, palpitations, and urticaria. This reaction is usually transient and self-limiting. Pregnancy should be avoided during therapy. It is unknown whether glatiramer is distributed in breast milk. The safety and efficacy of glatiramer have not been established in children. No information is available on glatiramer use in elderly patients.

Notify the physician of rash, weakness, difficulty breathing or swallowing, or itching or swelling of the legs. Vital signs, including temperature, should be obtained at baseline.

Storage

Refrigerate syringes. Do not freeze.

Administration

For subcutaneous use only. Bring syringe to room temperature before injecting. To avoid loss of medicine, do not expel or attempt to expel the air bubble from the syringe before use. Each day, pick a different injection site. Do not inject in the same area more than once a week.

Administer as subcutaneous injection in the upper arms, abdomen, thighs, or hips.

G

Glimepiride

gly-mep′er-ide

Amaryl

Do not confuse glimepiride with glipizide or glyburide.

CATEGORY AND SCHEDULE

Pregnancy Risk Category: C

Classification: Antidiabetic agents, sulfonylureas, second generation

MECHANISM OF ACTION

A second-generation sulfonylurea that promotes release of insulin from β cells of the pancreas and increases insulin sensitivity at peripheral sites. *Therapeutic Effect:* Lowers blood glucose concentration.

PHARMACOKINETICS

Route	Onset	Peak	Duration
PO	N/A	2-3 h	24 h

Completely absorbed from the GI tract. Protein binding: > 99%. Metabolized in the liver. Excreted in urine and eliminated in feces. *Half-life:* 5-9.2 h.

AVAILABILITY

Tablets: 1 mg, 2 mg, 4 mg.

INDICATIONS AND DOSAGES

▸ **Type 2 diabetes mellitus**

PO

Adults, Elderly. Initially, 1-2 mg once a day, with breakfast or first main meal. Maintenance: 1-4 mg once a day. After dose of 2 mg/day is reached, dosage should be increased in increments of up to 2 mg q1-2wk, based on blood glucose response. Maximum: 8 mg/day.

▸ **Dosage in renal impairment**

PO

Adults. Initially, 1 mg once a day. Titrate with care.

CONTRAINDICATIONS

Hypersensitivity, type 1 diabetes or diabetic ketoacidosis (with or without coma) as these conditions require insulin.

INTERACTIONS

Drug

β-Blockers: May increase the hypoglycemic effect of glimepiride and mask signs of hypoglycemia.

Cimetidine, ciprofloxacin, fluconazole, MAOIs, quinidine, ranitidine, tricyclic antidepressant agents, large doses of salicylates: May increase the effects of glimepiride.

Corticosteroids, lithium, thiazide diuretics: May decrease the effects of glimepiride.

Inhibitors of CYP2C9: May increase glimepiride blood concentrations and risk of hypoglycemia.

Cyclosporine: Sulfonylureas may increase cyclosporine levels.

Oral anticoagulants: May increase the effects of oral anticoagulants.

Herbal
Alfalfa, aloe, bilberry, bitter melon, burdock, celery, damiana, fenugreek, garcinia, garlic, ginger, ginseng (American), gymnema, marshmallow, stinging nettle: May enhance the hypoglycemic effects of glimepiride.
Food
Alcohol: Hypoglycemia is more likely to occur if alcohol is ingested.

DIAGNOSTIC TEST EFFECTS

May increase BUN and LDH concentrations and serum alkaline phosphatase, creatinine, and AST (SGOT) levels.

SIDE EFFECTS

Frequent
Altered taste sensation, dizziness, somnolence, weight gain, constipation, diarrhea, heartburn, nausea, vomiting, stomach fullness, headache.
Occasional
Increased sensitivity of skin to sunlight, peeling of skin, itching, rash.

SERIOUS REACTIONS

- Overdose or insufficient food intake may produce hypoglycemia, especially with increased glucose demands.
- GI hemorrhage, cholestatic hepatic jaundice, leukopenia, thrombocytopenia, pancytopenia, agranulocytosis, and aplastic or hemolytic anemia occur rarely.

PRECAUTIONS & CONSIDERATIONS

Use with caution in patients with pervious sulfonamide or sulfonylurea allergies.

Caution is warranted in patients with adrenal insufficiency, debilitation, hepatic disease, impaired renal or hepatic function, intestinal obstruction, malnutrition, pituitary insufficiency, prolonged vomiting, severe diarrhea, uncontrolled hyperthyroidism, and stress situations (including severe infection, trauma, surgery). Be alert to conditions that alter blood glucose requirements, such as fever, increased activity, stress, or a surgical procedure. Glimepiride use is not recommended during pregnancy. It is unknown whether glimepiride is distributed in breast milk. Safety and efficacy of glimepiride have not been established in children. Hypoglycemia may be difficult to recognize in elderly patients. Also, age-related renal impairment may increase sensitivity to glucose-lowering effect. Wear sunscreen and protective eyewear to prevent the effects of light sensitivity.

Food intake and blood glucose should be monitored before and during therapy. Be aware of signs and symptoms of hypoglycemia (anxiety, cool wet skin, diplopia, dizziness, headache, hunger, numbness in the mouth, tachycardia, tremors), or hyperglycemia (deep rapid breathing, dim vision, fatigue, nausea, polydipsia, polyphagia, polyuria, vomiting); carry candy, sugar packets, or other sugar supplements for immediate response to hypoglycemia. Consult the physician when glucose demands are altered (such as with fever, heavy physical activity, infection, stress, trauma). Exercise, good personal hygiene (including foot care), not smoking, and weight control are essential parts of therapy.
Storage
Store at room temperature.
Administration
Take glimepiride with breakfast or the first main meal.

Glipizide

glip'i-zide

★ Glucotrol, Glucotrol XL

Do not confuse glipizide with glimepiride or glyburide.

CATEGORY AND SCHEDULE

Pregnancy Risk Category: C

Classification: Antidiabetic agents, sulfonylureas, second generation

MECHANISM OF ACTION

A second-generation sulfonylurea that promotes the release of insulin from β cells of the pancreas and increases insulin sensitivity at peripheral sites. *Therapeutic Effect:* Lowers blood glucose concentration.

PHARMACOKINETICS

Route	Onset	Peak	Duration
PO	15-30 min	2-3 h	12-24 h
Extended release	2-3 h	6-12 h	24 h

Well absorbed from the GI tract. Protein binding: 99%. Metabolized in the liver. Excreted in urine. *Half-life:* 2-4 h.

AVAILABILITY

Tablets (Glucotrol): 5 mg, 10 mg.
Tablets (Extended Release [Glucotrol XL]): 2.5 mg, 5 mg, 10 mg.

INDICATIONS AND DOSAGES

▸ **Type 2 diabetes mellitus**

PO

Adults. Initially, 5 mg/day or 2.5 mg in elderly patients. Adjust dosage in 2.5- to 5-mg increments at intervals of several days. Maximum single dose: 15 mg. Maximum dose: 40 mg/day (rarely needed). Maintenance (extended-release tablet): Usually 5-20 mg once daily.

Patients with hepatic impairment: Begin at 2.5 mg once daily; titrate cautiously.

CONTRAINDICATIONS

Hypersensitivity, type 1 diabetes or diabetic ketoacidosis (with or without coma) as these conditions require insulin.

INTERACTIONS

Drug

β-Blockers: May increase the hypoglycemic effect of glipizide and mask signs of hypoglycemia.

Cimetidine, ciprofloxacin, fluconazole, MAOIs, quinidine, ranitidine, large doses of salicylates: May increase the effects of glipizide.

Corticosteroids, lithium, thiazide diuretics: May decrease the effects of glipizide.

Cyclosporine: Sulfonylureas may increase cyclosporine levels.

Oral anticoagulants: May increase the effects of oral anticoagulants.

Herbal

Alfalfa, aloe, bilberry, bitter melon, burdock, celery, damiana, fenugreek, garcinia, garlic, ginger, ginseng (American), gymnema, marshmallow, stinging nettle: May enhance the hypoglycemic effects of glipizide.

Food

Alcohol: Hypoglycemia is more likely to occur if alcohol is ingested.

DIAGNOSTIC TEST EFFECTS

May increase BUN and LDH concentrations and serum alkaline phosphatase, creatinine, and AST (SGOT) levels.

SIDE EFFECTS

Frequent

Feeling nervous, diarrhea, and gas are most common. Altered taste sensation, dizziness, somnolence, weight gain, constipation, heartburn, nausea, vomiting, stomach fullness, headache.

Occasional

Increased sensitivity of skin to sunlight, peeling of skin, itching, rash.

SERIOUS REACTIONS

- Overdose or insufficient food intake may produce hypoglycemia, especially with increased glucose demands.
- GI hemorrhage, cholestatic hepatic jaundice, leukopenia, thrombocytopenia, pancytopenia, agranulocytosis, and aplastic or hemolytic anemia occur rarely.

PRECAUTIONS & CONSIDERATIONS

Caution is warranted with adrenal or pituitary insufficiency, hypoglycemic reactions, and impaired hepatic or renal function. Be alert to conditions that alter blood glucose requirements, such as fever, increased activity, stress, or a surgical procedure. Insulin is the drug of choice during pregnancy. Glipizide given within 1 mo of delivery may produce neonatal hypoglycemia. Glipizide crosses the placenta and is minimally distributed in breast milk. Safety and efficacy of glipizide have not been established in children. Hypoglycemia may be difficult to recognize in elderly patients. Also, age-related renal impairment may increase sensitivity to the glucose-lowering effect. Wear sunscreen and protective eyewear to prevent the effects of light sensitivity.

Food intake and blood glucose should be monitored before and during therapy. Be aware of signs and symptoms of hypoglycemia (anxiety, cool wet skin, diplopia, dizziness, headache, hunger, numbness in mouth, tachycardia, tremors) or hyperglycemia (deep rapid breathing, dim vision, fatigue, nausea, polydipsia, polyphagia, polyuria, vomiting); carry candy, sugar packets, or other sugar supplements for immediate response to hypoglycemia. Consult the physician when glucose demands are altered (such as with fever, heavy physical activity, infection, stress, trauma). Exercise, good personal hygiene (including foot care), not smoking, and weight control are essential parts of therapy.

Storage

Store at room temperature. Protect from moisture.

Administration

Take glipizide 30 min before a meal; the extended-release tablets should be taken with breakfast. Do not cut, crush, or chew extended-release tablets. The tablet shell may be noted in a bowel movement and is not cause for concern.

Glucagon Hydrochloride

gloo′ka-gon

★ 🍁 Glucagen Hypokit; Glucagen; Glucagon Diagnostic Kit; Glucagon Emergency Kit

Do not confuse glucagon with Glaucon.

CATEGORY AND SCHEDULE

Pregnancy Risk Category: B

Classification: Antihypoglycemics, hormones/hormone modifiers

MECHANISM OF ACTION
A glucose-elevating agent that promotes hepatic glycogenolysis, gluconeogenesis. Stimulates the production of cyclic adenosine monophosphate (cAMP), which results in increased plasma glucose concentration, smooth muscle relaxation, and an inotropic myocardial effect. *Therapeutic Effect:* Increases plasma glucose level and relaxes GI tract.

G

AVAILABILITY
Powder for Injection: 1 mg.

INDICATIONS AND DOSAGES
▸ **Hypoglycemia**

IV, IM, SUBCUTANEOUS

Adults, Elderly, Children weighing more than 20 kg. 1 mg. May give 1 or 2 additional doses if response is delayed.

Children weighing 20 kg or less. 0.5 mg or, alternatively, 0.02-0.03 mg/kg. Maximum: 1 mg.

▸ **Diagnostic aid**

IV, IM

Adults, Elderly. 0.25-2 mg 10 min before procedure. Use 1-2 mg if given IM.

OFF-LABEL USES
Treatment of esophageal obstruction by solid food (food impaction), toxicity associated with β-blockers or calcium channel blockers.

CONTRAINDICATIONS
Hypersensitivity to glucagon or beef or pork proteins, known pheochromocytoma or insulinoma.

INTERACTIONS
Drug

Anticoagulants: May increase the effects of these drugs.

Herbal and Food

None known.

DIAGNOSTIC TEST EFFECTS
May decrease serum potassium level.

IV INCOMPATIBILITIES
Do not mix glucagon with any other medications.

SIDE EFFECTS
Occasional

Nausea, vomiting.

Rare

Allergic reaction, such as urticaria, respiratory distress, and hypotension.

SERIOUS REACTIONS
- Overdose may produce persistent nausea and vomiting and hypokalemia, marked by severe weakness, decreased appetite, irregular heartbeat, and muscle cramps.
- Serious allergic reactions are rare.

PRECAUTIONS & CONSIDERATIONS
Caution is warranted in patients with a history suggestive of insulinoma or pheochromocytoma. Be aware of how to recognize symptoms of hypoglycemia, including anxiety, increased sweating, difficulty concentrating, headache, hunger, nausea, nervousness, pale and cool skin, shakiness, unusual fatigue, weakness, and unconsciousness. Treat early signs of hypoglycemia with a simple sugar first, such as hard candy, honey, orange juice, sugar cubes, or table sugar dissolved in water or juice, followed by a protein source, such as cheese and crackers, half a sandwich, or a glass of milk.

Storage

Store vials and kits at room temperature. Do not freeze. After reconstitution, use immediately and discard unused portion. Do not store for later use. Do not use glucagon solution unless it is clear.

Administration

! Place the patient on his or her side to avoid aspiration because glucagon (as well as hypoglycemia) may produce nausea and vomiting.

! If patient fails to respond in 15 min, get emergency assistance.

Administer IV dextrose if the patient fails to respond to glucagon.

May give glucagon intravenously, IM, or subcutaneously. Reconstitute the powder with the diluent supplied by the manufacturer. To provide 1 mg glucagon/mL, reconstitute the 1-mg vial with 1 mL diluent. Rate of IV administration is 1 mg/min, and glucagon is compatible with dextrose solutions. The patient will usually awaken in 5-20 min. If the patient fails to respond after 1 or 2 additional doses, give IV dextrose as prescribed. When the patient awakens, give oral carbohydrates to restore hepatic glycogen stores and prevent secondary hypoglycemia.

Glyburide

glye'byoor-ide

🇺🇸 DiaBeta, Glynase 🇨🇦 DiaBeta, Euglucon, Mylan-Glybe

Do not confuse glyburide with glimepiride or glipizide.

CATEGORY AND SCHEDULE

Pregnancy Risk Category: C

Classification: Antidiabetic agents, sulfonylureas, second generation

MECHANISM OF ACTION

A second-generation sulfonylurea that promotes the release of insulin from β cells of the pancreas and increases insulin sensitivity at peripheral sites. *Therapeutic Effect:* Lowers blood glucose concentration.

PHARMACOKINETICS

Route	Onset	Peak	Duration
PO	0.25-1 h	1-2 h	12-24 h

Well absorbed from the GI tract. Protein binding: 99%. Metabolized in the liver to weakly active metabolite. Primarily excreted in urine. Not removed by hemodialysis. *Half-life:* 1.4-1.8 h.

AVAILABILITY

Tablets (DiaBeta): 1.25 mg, 2.5 mg, 5 mg.

Tablets (Glynase): 1.5 mg, 3 mg, 6 mg.

INDICATIONS AND DOSAGES

▸ **Diabetes mellitus Type 2**

PO

Adults. Initially 2.5-5 mg. May increase by 2.5 mg/day at weekly intervals. Maintenance: 1.25-20 mg/day. Maximum: 20 mg/day.

Elderly. Initially, 1.25-2.5 mg/day. May increase by 1.25-2.5 mg/day at 1- to 3-wk intervals.

PO (MICRONIZED TABLETS [GLYNASE])

Adults, Elderly. Initially, 0.75-3 mg/day. May increase by 1.5 mg/day at weekly intervals. Maintenance: 0.75-12 mg/day as a single dose or in divided doses.

▸ **Dosage in renal impairment**

Glyburide is not recommended in patients with creatinine clearance < 50 mL/min.

CONTRAINDICATIONS

Hypersensitivity, type 1 diabetes or diabetic ketoacidosis (with or without coma) as these conditions

G

require insulin. Concurrent use of bosentan.

INTERACTIONS

Drug

β-Blockers: May increase the hypoglycemic effect of glyburide and mask signs of hypoglycemia.
Bosentan: May increase the risk of hepatotoxicity. Manufacturer of bosentan considers co-use contraindicated.
Cimetidine, ciprofloxacin, fluconazole, MAOIs, quinidine, ranitidine, tricyclic antidepressant agents, large doses of salicylates: May increase the effects of glyburide.
Corticosteroids, lithium, thiazide diuretics: May decrease the effects of glyburide.
Oral anticoagulants: May increase the effects of oral anticoagulants.

Herbal

Alfalfa, aloe, bilberry, bitter melon, burdock, celery, damiana, fenugreek, garcinia, garlic, ginger, ginseng (American), gymnema, marshmallow, stinging nettle: May increase the risk of hypoglycemia.

Food

Alcohol: Hypoglycemia is more likely to occur if alcohol is ingested.

DIAGNOSTIC TEST EFFECTS

May increase BUN and LDH concentrations and serum alkaline phosphatase, creatinine, and AST (SGOT) levels.

SIDE EFFECTS

Frequent

Altered taste sensation, dizziness, somnolence, weight gain, constipation, diarrhea, heartburn, nausea, vomiting, stomach fullness, headache.

Occasional

Increased sensitivity of skin to sunlight, peeling of skin, itching, rash.

SERIOUS REACTIONS

- Overdose or insufficient food intake may produce hypoglycemia, especially in patients with increased glucose demands.
- Cholestatic jaundice, leukopenia, thrombocytopenia, pancytopenia, agranulocytosis, and aplastic or hemolytic anemia occur rarely.

PRECAUTIONS & CONSIDERATIONS

Caution is warranted in patients with adrenal or pituitary insufficiency, hypoglycemic reactions, sulfonamide hypersensitivity, and impaired hepatic or renal function. Be alert to conditions that alter blood glucose requirements, such as fever, increased activity, stress, or a surgical procedure. Insulin is the drug of choice during pregnancy. Glyburide crosses the placenta and is distributed in breast milk. Glyburide use within 2 wks of delivery may produce neonatal hypoglycemia. Safety and efficacy of glyburide have not been established in children. Hypoglycemia may be difficult to recognize in elderly patients. Also, age-related renal impairment may increase sensitivity to the glucose-lowering effect. Wear sunscreen and protective eyewear to prevent the effects of light sensitivity.

Food intake and blood glucose should be monitored before and during therapy. Be aware of signs and symptoms of hypoglycemia (anxiety, cool wet skin, diplopia, dizziness, headache, hunger, numbness in the mouth, tachycardia, tremors) or hyperglycemia (deep rapid breathing, dim vision, fatigue, nausea, polydipsia, polyphagia, polyuria, vomiting); carry candy, sugar packets, or other sugar supplements for immediate response to hypoglycemia. Consult the physician when glucose demands are altered (such as with fever, heavy physical activity, infection, stress, trauma). Exercise, good personal hygiene (including foot care), not smoking, and weight control are essential parts of therapy.

Storage

Store at room temperature in a tightly closed container.

Administration

Daily doses of glyburide are administered with breakfast or the first main meal. If taking more than 1 dose per day, give with breakfast and dinner.

Glycerin

gli′ser-in

★ Advanced Eye Relief Dry Eye Environmental Lubricant Eye Drops, Fleet Babylax, Fleet Liquid Glycerin Suppositories for Adults and Children, Fleet Glycerin Suppositories for Adults, Fleet Glycerin Suppositories for Children, Fleet Maximum-Strength Glycerin Suppositories, Glyrol, Osmoglyn, Sani-Supp

CATEGORY AND SCHEDULE

Pregnancy Risk Category: B
OTC (suppositories)

Classification: Osmotic diuretic, antiglaucoma, laxative

MECHANISM OF ACTION

An osmotic dehydrating agent that increases osmotic pressure and draws fluid into the colon and stimulates evacuation of inspissated feces. Lowers both intraocular and intracranial pressure by osmotic dehydrating effects. Increases blood flow to ischemic areas, decreases serum free fatty acids, and increases synthesis of glycerides in the brain. *Therapeutic Effect:* Aids in fecal evacuation.

PHARMACOKINETICS

Well absorbed after PO administration but poorly absorbed after rectal administration. Widely distributed to extracellular space. Rapidly metabolized in liver. Primarily excreted in urine. *Half-life:* 30-45 min.

AVAILABILITY

Ophthalmic Solution: 1% (Advanced Eye Relief Dry Eye Environmental Lubricant Eye Drops).
Oral Solution: 50% (Osmoglyn).
Rectal Solution: 2.3 g (Fleet Babylax), 5.6 g (Fleet Liquid Glycerin Suppositories).
Suppositories: 1 g (Fleet Glycerin Suppositories for Children), 2 g (Fleet Glycerin Suppositories), 3 g (Fleet Maximum-Strength Glycerin Suppositories), 82.5% (Sani-Supp).

INDICATIONS AND DOSAGES

▸ Constipation

RECTAL

Adults, Elderly, Children 6 yr and older. 3 g/day.
Children younger than 6 yr. 1-1.5 g/day.

▸ Dry, irritated eyes

OPHTHALMIC

Adults, Elderly, Children. 1 or 2 drops as needed.

▸ Reduction of intraocular pressure

PO

Adults, Elderly. 1-1.5 g/kg. Maximum reduction in IOP occurs in 1 h and lasts approximately 5 h. May give twice to 4 times a day.

CONTRAINDICATIONS

Hypersensitivity to any component in the preparation, well-established anuria, severe dehydration, frank or impending acute pulmonary edema, severe cardiac decompensation.

INTERACTIONS

Drug

PO medications: Oral glycerin may decrease transit time of concurrently administered oral medication, decreasing absorption.

Herbal

Licorice: May increase risk of hypokalemia.

Food

None known.

DIAGNOSTIC TEST EFFECTS

None known.

SIDE EFFECTS

Frequent

Oral: Nausea, headache, vomiting.
Rectal: Some degree of abdominal discomfort, nausea, mild cramps, headache, vomiting.

Occasional

Oral: Diarrhea, dizziness, dry mouth or increased thirst.
Ophthalmic: Pain and irritation may occur upon instillation.
Rectal: Faintness, weakness, abdominal pain, bloating.

SERIOUS REACTIONS

• Laxative abuse includes symptoms of abdominal pain, weakness, fatigue, thirst, vomiting, edema, bone pain, fluid and electrolyte imbalance, hypoalbuminemia, and syndromes that mimic colitis.

PRECAUTIONS & CONSIDERATIONS

Caution is warranted in patients with diabetes mellitus because product orally will increase blood sugar and osmotic load. Hemolytic anemia; altered hydration; cardiac, renal, or hepatic disease. It is unknown whether glycerin crosses the placenta or is excreted in breast milk. No age-related precautions have been noted in children. Be aware that glycerin may increase the risk of dehydration in elderly patients because it reduces the water in the body. Unrelieved constipation, dizziness, muscle cramps or pain, rectal bleeding, confusion, irregular heartbeat, and weakness should be reported.

Storage

Discard ophthalmic preparation 6 mo after dropper is first placed in drug solution. Store at room temperature away from damp places like the bathroom or near the kitchen sink as well as heat and direct light because it may cause the medicine to break down. Refrigerate suppositories.

Administration

Instill ophthalmic drops of solution in each lower conjunctival sac. Close eye gently to help spread the solution to all areas of the conjunctiva. Gently wipe away excess solution from the eyelids and surrounding skin with tissue.

Mix oral glycerin unflavored 50% oral solution with orange juice. Pour solution over crushed ice and drink through a straw to improve palatability. Have patient drink over 5-10 min to reduce vomiting risk. May administer doses at 5-h intervals for the reduction of intraocular pressure. Tell the patient to lie down after oral solution to minimize risk of developing headache.

If rectal suppository is too soft, chill for 30 min in refrigerator or run cold water over foil wrapper.

Remove wrapper and moisten suppository with cold water before inserting well into rectum. Lie on the left side. Insert suppository high in rectum and retain for 15 min. If administering liquid glycerin rectally, gently insert stem with steady pressure at tip pointing toward the navel and squeeze unit until almost all the liquid has been delivered. A small amount of liquid will remain. Withdraw unit.

Increase fluid intake, exercise, and eat a high-fiber diet to promote defecation. Warn the patient to notify the physician if he or she experiences unrelieved constipation, dizziness, muscle cramps or pain, rectal bleeding, confusion, irregular heartbeat, and weakness.

Glycopyrrolate

glye-koe-pye′roe-late

★ Cuvposa, Robinul, Robinul Forte

Do not confuse Robinul with Reminyl.

CATEGORY AND SCHEDULE

Pregnancy Risk Category: B

Classification: Anticholinergics, gastrointestinals

MECHANISM OF ACTION

A quaternary anticholinergic that inhibits the action of acetylcholine at postganglionic parasympathetic sites in smooth muscle, secretory glands, and the central nervous system (CNS). *Therapeutic Effect:* Reduces salivation and excessive secretions of respiratory tract; reduces gastric secretions and acidity.

PHARMACOKINETICS

Poorly and irregularly absorbed from GI tract after oral administration. Metabolized in the liver. Primarily excreted in urine. *Half-life:* 1.7 h.

AVAILABILITY

Injection: 0.2 mg/mL.
Tablets: 1 mg, 2 mg.
Oral Solution: 1 mg/5 mL.

INDICATIONS AND DOSAGES

▸ **Preoperative inhibition of salivation and excessive respiratory tract secretions**

IM

Adults, Elderly. 4 mcg/kg 30-60 min before procedure.
Children 2 yr and older. 4 mcg/kg.
Children younger than 2 yr. 4-9 mcg/kg. Do not use in neonates (< 1 mo).

▸ **To block the effects of anticholinesterase agents**

IV

Adults, Elderly, Children. 0.2 mg for each 1 mg neostigmine or 5 mg pyridostigmine.

▸ **Peptic ulcer disease, adjunct**

IV, IM

Adults, Elderly. 0.1 mg IV or IM 3-4 times a day.

PO

Adults, Elderly. 1-2 mg 2-3 times a day. Maximum: 8 mg/day.

▸ **For severe drooling in children with cerebral palsy**

PO

Children 3 to 16 yr. Initially, 0.02mg/kg 3 times per day and titrate by 0.02 mg/kg q 5-7 days as needed and tolerated. Maximum: 0.1 mg/kg 3 times daily, and not to exceed 1.5-3 mg per dose.

CONTRAINDICATIONS

Acute hemorrhage, myasthenia gravis, narrow-angle glaucoma, obstructive uropathy, paralytic ileus, tachycardia, ulcerative colitis, obstructive diseases of the GI tract, neonates. With chronic use, do not use sold oral dosage forms of potassium chloride.

INTERACTIONS

Drug

Antacids, antidiarrheals: May decrease the absorption of glycopyrrolate. Do not take within 1 h of taking oral glycopyrrolate.
Digoxin tablets: Can increase digoxin serum levels. Monitor patients closely.
Atenolol or metformin: May increase serum levels of atenolol or metformin.
Haloperidol or levodopa: May decrease serum levels of haloperidol or levodopa.
Ketoconazole: May decrease the absorption of ketoconazole.
Other anticholinergics: May increase the effects of glycopyrrolate.
Potassium chloride: May increase the severity of GI lesions with the wax matrix formulation of potassium chloride.
Pramlinitide: May increase anticholinergic effects.

Herbal

None known.

Food

None known.

DIAGNOSTIC TEST EFFECTS

May decrease serum uric acid levels.

IV INCOMPATIBILITIES

Chloramphenicol, dexamethasone sodium phosphate (Decadron), diazepam (Valium), dimenhydrinate (Dramamine), methohexital (Brevital), methylprednisolone sodium succinate (Solu-Medrol), pentazocine (Talwin), pentobarbital (Nembutal), secobarbital (Seconal), sodium bicarbonate, thiopental (Pentothal).

IV COMPATIBILITIES

Atropine, buprenorphine (Buprenex), butorphanol (Stadol), chlorpromazine (Thorazine), cimetidine (Tagamet), codeine, diphenhydramine (Benadryl), droperidol (Inapsine), hydromorphone (Dilaudid), hydroxyzine (Vistaril), levorphanol (Levo-Dromoran), lidocaine, meperidine (Demerol), midazolam (Versed), morphine, nalbuphine (Nubain), neostigmine, ondansetron (Zofran), oxymorphone (Opana), physostigmine, procaine (Pronestyl), prochlorperazine (Compazine), promazine (Sparine), promethazine (Phenergan), propofol (Diprivan), pyridostigmine (Mestinon), ranitidine (Zantac), scopolamine, triflupromazine (Vesprin), trimethobenzamide (Tigan).

SIDE EFFECTS

Frequent

Dry mouth, decreased sweating, constipation.

Occasional

Blurred vision, gastric bloating, urinary hesitancy, somnolence (with high dosage), headache, intolerance to light, loss of taste, nervousness, flushing, insomnia, impotence, mental confusion or excitement (particularly in the elderly and children), temporary light-headedness (with parenteral form), local irritation (with parenteral form).

Rare

Dizziness, faintness.

SERIOUS REACTIONS

- Overdose may produce temporary paralysis of the ciliary muscle; pupillary dilation; tachycardia; palpitations; hot, dry, or flushed skin; absence of bowel sounds; hyperthermia; increased respiratory rate; ECG abnormalities; nausea; vomiting; rash over face or upper trunk; CNS stimulation; and psychosis (marked by agitation, restlessness, rambling speech, visual hallucinations, paranoid behavior, and delusions, followed by depression).

PRECAUTIONS & CONSIDERATIONS

Caution is warranted with congestive heart failure, diarrhea, fever, GI infections, hepatic or renal disease, prostatic hypertrophy, hypertension, ulcerative colitis, hypothyroidism, and reflux esophagitis. Avoid hot baths, saunas, and becoming overheated while exercising in hot weather because they may cause heatstroke. Tasks that require mental alertness or motor skills should also be avoided until response to the drug has been established.

Dry mouth may occur. BP, body temperature, heart rate, pattern of daily bowel activity and stool consistency, and urine output should be monitored. The patient should void before receiving the drug to reduce the risk of urine retention.

Storage

Store tablets and unopened injection vials at room temperature.

Administration

For direct injection, administer undiluted through the tubing of a free-flowing compatible IV solution, over 1-2 min.

For IM use, administer undiluted or diluted with D5W, $D_{10}W$, or 0.9% NaCl.

Take oral tablets 30-60 min before meals. Oral solution is given 1 h before or 2 h after meals.

Gold Sodium Thiomalate

gold so′dee-um thye-oh-mah′late

★ 🍁 Myochrysine

CATEGORY AND SCHEDULE

Pregnancy Risk Category: C

Classification: Disease-modifying antirheumatic drugs, gold compounds

MECHANISM OF ACTION

A gold compound whose mechanism of action is unknown. May decrease prostaglandin synthesis or alter cellular mechanisms by inhibiting sulfhydryl systems. *Therapeutic Effect:* Decreases synovial inflammation, retards cartilage and bone destruction, suppresses or prevents—but does not cure—arthritis and synovitis.

AVAILABILITY

Injection: 50 mg/mL.

INDICATIONS AND DOSAGES

▸ **Rheumatoid arthritis**

IM

Adults, Elderly. Initially, 10 mg, followed by 25 mg for second dose, then 25-50 mg/wk until improvement noted. Maintenance: 25-50 mg q2wk for 2-20 wks; if stable, may increase intervals to q3-4wk. Maximum: 100 mg/dose. Continued until the cumulative dose reaches 1 g unless toxicity occurs; if no improvement, discontinue use.

▸ **JRA (JIA)**

Children. Initially, 10 mg, then 1 mg/kg/wk up to a maximum single dose of 50 mg. Maintenance: 1 mg/kg/dose q2-4wk.

▸ **Dosage in renal impairment**
Dosage is modified based on creatinine clearance.

CrCL (mL/min)	Dosage
50-80	50% of usual dose
< 50	Not recommended

OFF-LABEL USES

Treatment of psoriatic arthritis.

CONTRAINDICATIONS

Colitis; concurrent use of antimalarials, immunosuppressive agents, penicillamine, or phenylbutazone; congestive heart failure; exfoliative dermatitis; history of blood dyscrasias; severe hepatic or renal impairment; systemic lupus erythematosus, hypersensitivity to the drug or benzyl alcohol.

INTERACTIONS

Drug
ACE inhibitors: May increase toxic effects of gold sodium thiomalate.
Bone marrow depressants, hepatotoxic and nephrotoxic medications: May increase the risk of toxicity.
Penicillamine: May increase the risk of adverse hematologic or renal effects.
Herbal and Food
None known.

DIAGNOSTIC TEST EFFECTS

May decrease hemoglobin level, hematocrit, and WBC and platelet counts. May increase urine protein level. May alter liver function test results.

SIDE EFFECTS

Frequent
Pruritic dermatitis, stomatitis, diarrhea, abdominal pain, nausea.
Occasional
Vomiting, anorexia, flatulence, dyspepsia, conjunctivitis, photosensitivity.
Rare
Constipation, urticaria, rash.

SERIOUS REACTIONS

• Signs and symptoms of gold toxicity include decreased hemoglobin level, decreased granulocyte count (< 150,000/mm^3), proteinuria, hematuria, blood dyscrasias (anemia, leukopenia [WBC < 4000 mm^3], thrombocytopenia, and eosinophilia), glomerulonephritis, nephrotic syndrome, and cholestatic jaundice.

PRECAUTIONS & CONSIDERATIONS

Avoid exposure to sunlight, which may turn skin gray or blue. Oral hygiene should be diligently maintained to help prevent stomatitis. Gold appears in breast milk; discontinue breastfeeding during treatment. Gold therapy is avoided during pregnancy.

Pattern of daily bowel activity and stool consistency, urine for hematuria and proteinuria, CBC (particularly hemoglobin level, hematocrit, and WBC and platelet counts), renal and liver function tests (especially BUN level and serum alkaline phosphatase, creatinine, AST [SGOT], and ALT [SGPT] levels), skin for rash, and oral mucous membranes for stomatitis should be monitored. Analyze urine for protein and sediment changes. Therapeutic response, including improved grip strength, increased joint mobility, reduced joint tenderness, and relief of pain, stiffness, and swelling, should also be assessed.

Storage
Store at room temperature. Protect from light. Solution should be clear

or pale yellow. Vials are for multiple dose use.

Administration

! Give gold sodium thiomalate IM only, as prescribed.

Full therapeutic effect may take 6 mo or longer to appear.

Inject intragluteally with patient lying down; intragluteally keep recumbent for 10 min after injection.

Golimumab

goe-lim′u-mab

Simponi

CATEGORY AND SCHEDULE

Pregnancy Risk Category: B

Classification: Immunomodulators, disease-modifying antirheumatic drugs (DMARDs), TNF modulators

MECHANISM OF ACTION

A monoclonal antibody that neutralizes the biological activity of tumor necrosis factor (TNF)-α by binding to it and blocking its interaction with cell surface TNF receptors, decreasing inflammation and immune responses. *Therapeutic Effect:* Reduces inflammation, swelling, and joint destruction for those with psoriatic arthritis, rheumatoid arthritis, or ankylosing spondylitis, improving symptoms.

PHARMACOKINETICS

Time to steady state reached at roughly 12 wks of treatment. *Half-life:* Approximately 14 days.

AVAILABILITY

Injection: 50 mg/0.5 mL in an autoinjector or prefilled syringes.

INDICATIONS AND DOSAGES

▸ Moderate to severe rheumatoid arthritis (RA), psoriatic arthritis, or active ankylosing spondylitis

SC

Adults: 50 mg SC given once every month. Treatment is given with methotrexate for RA.

CONTRAINDICATIONS

None. Withhold in any patient with a clinically important, active, serious infection, especially active TB.

INTERACTIONS

Drug

Other biologics for arthritis (e.g., rituximab, etc.) and traditional immunosuppressives: There may be an increased risk of serious infections with combined use. Abetacept co-therapy not recommended. Methotrexate is given with golimumab for the treatment of RA.

Narrow therapeutic index drugs metabolized via CYP450 enzymes (e.g., theophylline, cyclosporine, warfarin): Golimumab may alter CYP enzyme activity and thus reduce clearance and increase levels; monitor closely.

Vaccines, live: Avoid use. Altered immune response and increased risk of secondary transmission of infection from vaccine.

DIAGNOSTIC TEST EFFECTS

May increase liver enzymes or decrease various blood cell components.

SIDE EFFECTS

Frequent (≥5%)

Nasopharyngitis, mild upper respiratory infections (bronchitis, sinusitis, pharyngitis, rhinitis).

Occasional (1%-5%)
Increased liver enzymes, hypertension, dizziness, injection site erythema, pyrexia, oral herpes, paresthesia.
Rare (< 1%)
Headache, fatigue. See Serious Reactions.

SERIOUS REACTIONS

- Rare reactions include serious hypersensitivity reactions, risk for malignancies (e.g., lymphomas and nonmelanoma skin malignancy), new or worsening heart failure, hepatitis, lupus-like syndromes, neurologic events (demyelinating disorders), and serious infections (such as pneumonia, tuberculosis, reactivation of hepatitis B).
- Post-market reports of pancytopenia, leukopenia, neutropenia, aplastic anemia, and thrombocytopenia in patients receiving similar TNF blockers.

PRECAUTIONS & CONSIDERATIONS

Serious infections, sepsis, tuberculosis, and opportunistic infections have occurred during therapy. Patients should be screened for active or recent infection, tuberculosis risk factors, and latent tuberculosis infection before initiating therapy. Closely monitor patients for the development of infection during therapy. Caution is warranted with neurologic disease, history of sensitivity to monoclonal antibodies, preexisting or recent onset of CNS disturbances, those with heart failure or cardiac disease, or a history of malignancy. There are no adequate data in pregnant women; animal studies do not show teratogenic effects. It is unknown if the drug is excreted in breast milk. The safety and efficacy of golimumab have not been established in children. Cautious use in the elderly is necessary because they may be at increased risk for serious infection and malignancy. Avoid receiving live vaccines during treatment. The needle cover on the product contains latex and may cause sensitivity in those with latex allergy.
Storage
Refrigerate. Do not freeze. Protect from light; store in original carton until administration. Do not shake.
Administration
For subcutaneous use only; rotate injection sites. The solution should be colorless to slightly yellow and may contain a few small translucent/white particles. Do not use if discolored, cloudy. Do not shake. Allow the autoinjector or prefilled syringe to come to room temperature (roughly 30 min) before use. Injection sites include the front middle thigh, abdominal region, and the outer area of upper arm. Do not inject within 2 inches of the navel. Do not administer where skin is tender, bruised, red, or hard. Do not rub injection site. Discard any unused portion.

Goserelin

go'seh-rel-in
★ 🍁 Zoladex, Zoladex LA

CATEGORY AND SCHEDULE

Pregnancy Risk Category: D (advanced breast cancer), X (endometriosis, endometrial thinning)

Classification: Hormones/hormone modifiers, gonadotropin-releasing hormone analogues

MECHANISM OF ACTION
A gonadotropin-releasing hormone analogue and antineoplastic agent that stimulates the release of luteinizing hormone (LH) and follicle-stimulating hormone (FSH) from the anterior pituitary gland. *Therapeutic Effect:* In females, reduces estrogen levels, produces a reduction in ovarian size and function, a reduction in uterine and mammary gland size, and regression of sex-hormone-responsive tumors. In men, it produces decreased testosterone levels, pharmacologic castration, and decreases the growth of abnormal prostate tissue.

AVAILABILITY
Implant: 3.6 mg (monthly).
Implant: 10.8 mg (every 3 mo).

INDICATIONS AND DOSAGES
▸ **Prostatic cancer**
IMPLANT
Adult males. 3.6 mg every 28 days or 10.8 mg q12wk subcutaneously into upper abdominal wall.
▸ **Breast cancer, endometriosis**
IMPLANT
Adult females. 3.6 mg every 28 days subcutaneously into upper abdominal wall. Do not use 10.8-mg implant in females.

OFF-LABEL USES
Uterine fibroids, endometrial thinning before ablation procedure.

CONTRAINDICATIONS
Pregnancy; hypersensitivity to goserelin products, luteinizing hormone-releasing hormone (LHRH), or LHRH analogues; breastfeeding.

INTERACTIONS
Drug, Herbal, and Food
None known.

DIAGNOSTIC TEST EFFECTS
In men, causes transient increases in serum levels of testosterone at treatment initiation. May increase blood sugar, liver enzymes, or blood lipids.

SIDE EFFECTS
Frequent
Headache (60%), hot flashes (55%), depression (54%), diaphoresis (45%), sexual dysfunction (21%), decreased erection (18%), lower urinary tract symptoms (13%).
Occasional (5%-10%)
Pain, lethargy, dizziness, insomnia, anorexia, nausea, rash, upper respiratory tract infection, hirsutism, abdominal pain.
Rare
Pruritus.

SERIOUS REACTIONS
- Arrhythmias, congestive heart failure, and hypertension occur rarely.
- Ureteral obstruction and spinal cord compression have been observed. An immediate orchiectomy may be necessary if these conditions occur.
- Deep vein thrombosis has been reported.
- Decreased bone mineral density/osteoporosis with long-term use/fractures.

PRECAUTIONS & CONSIDERATIONS
In men at particular risk of developing ureteral obstruction or spinal cord compression, monitor closely. Use with caution in patients with existing diabetes mellitus.

Goserelin crosses the placenta and may cause fetal harm. Women who are or may be pregnant should not use this drug. Pregnancy status should be determined before beginning therapy. Women should use nonhormonal contraceptive measures during therapy. It is unknown whether goserelin is excreted in breast milk. The safety and efficacy of goserelin have not been established in children. No age-related precautions have been noted in elderly patients.

Women should notify the physician if regular menstruation persists or if they become pregnant. Breakthrough bleeding may occur if a goserelin dose is missed. Signs and symptoms of worsening of prostatic cancer, especially in the first month, should be monitored. Decreased bone mineral density secondary to this medication may be irreversible. Caution should be used if other risk factors are present.

Storage

Store at room temperature in original packaging and do not remove from foil pouch until time of use.

Administration

! Confirm implant dosage against patient prescription before insertion.

Inspect for damage before opening. If the package is damaged, do not use the syringe. Remove the sterile syringe from the package immediately before use. Check that implant is visible in the translucent chamber. Place patient in a comfortable position with the upper part of the body slightly raised. Prepare area of the anterior abdominal wall below the navel with alcohol. Grasp the safety tab and pull away from the syringe and discard. Remove needle cover. Do not remove air bubbles as this may displace the implant.

Using aseptic technique, pinch up the skin area for subcutaneous implant. With the bevel of the needle up, insert at a 30-45° angle to the skin in one continuous motion until the protective sleeve touches the skin; take care not to penetrate muscle.

! If the needle penetrates a large vessel, blood will be seen instantly in the syringe chamber. If a vessel is penetrated, withdraw the needle and inject with a new syringe at a different site.

To administer the implant and activate the protective sleeve, grasp the barrel at the finger grip and depress plunger until it cannot depress any further. When the sleeve "clicks," it will automatically begin to slide to cover the needle. Withdraw the needle and allow protective sleeve to cover it. Dispose of in an approved receptacle.

In case of the need to surgically remove the implant, it may be localized by ultrasound.

Granisetron

gra-ni'se-tron

★ Kytril, Sancuso 🍁 Kytril

CATEGORY AND SCHEDULE

Pregnancy Risk Category: B

Classification: Antiemetics/antivertigo, serotonin receptor antagonists

MECHANISM OF ACTION

A 5-HT_3 receptor antagonist that acts centrally in the chemoreceptor trigger zone or peripherally at the vagal nerve terminals. *Therapeutic Effect:* Prevents nausea and vomiting.

PHARMACOKINETICS

Route	Onset	Peak	Duration
IV	1-3 min	N/A	24 h

Rapidly and widely distributed to tissues. Protein binding: 65%. Metabolized in the liver to active metabolite. Eliminated in urine and feces. *Half-life:* 10-12 h (increased in the elderly).

AVAILABILITY

Oral Solution: 1 mg/5 mL.
Tablets: 1 mg.
Injection: 1 mg/mL, 0.1 mg/mL.
Transdermal patch: 3.1 mg/24 h

INDICATIONS AND DOSAGES

▸ **Prevention of chemotherapy-induced nausea and vomiting**

PO

Adults, Elderly, Children 2 yr and older. 2 mg once a day up to 1 h before chemotherapy or 1 mg twice a day, with first dose 1 h before chemotherapy.

TRANSDERMAL PATCH

Adults. Apply a single patch 24 h before chemotherapy. May apply up to a maximum of 48 h before chemotherapy as appropriate. Remove 24 h after completion of chemotherapy. Each patch can be worn for up to 7 days depending on the duration of chemo regimen.

IV

Adults, Elderly, Children 2 yr and older. 10 mcg/kg/dose (or 1 mg/dose) within 30 min of chemotherapy.

▸ **Prevention of radiation-induced nausea and vomiting**

PO

Adults, Elderly. 2 mg once a day given 1 h before radiation therapy.

▸ **Postoperative nausea or vomiting**

IV

Adults, Elderly. 1 mg as a single postoperative dose.

CONTRAINDICATIONS

Hypersensitivity to drug or similar agents. (Use caution.)

Hypersensitivity to benzyl alcohol (IV form).

INTERACTIONS

Drug

Apomorphine: May cause significant hypotension.

Hepatic enzyme inducers: May decrease the effects of granisetron.

Ketoconazole and strong CYP3A inhibitors: May reduce granisetron metabolism.

Qtc-prolonging drugs: Use with caution due to potential additive effects on QT interval.

Herbal

St. John's wort: May decrease levels of granisetron.

Food

None known.

DIAGNOSTIC TEST EFFECTS

May increase AST (SGOT) and ALT (SGPT) levels.

IV INCOMPATIBILITIES

Amphotericin B (Fungizone), diazepam, lansoprazole, phenytoin.

IV COMPATIBILITIES

Acyclovir (Zovirax), allopurinol (Aloprim), amifostine (Ethyol), amikacin (Amikin), aminophylline, amphotericin B cholesteryl sulfate complex (Amphotec), ampicillin (Polycillin), ampicillin and sulbactam (Unasyn), amsacrine (Amsa), aztreonam (Azactam), bleomycin (Blenoxane), bumetanide (Bumex), buprenorphine (Buprenex), butorphanol (Stadol), calcium gluconate, carboplatin (Paraplatin), carmustine (BiCNU), cefazolin (Ancef), cefepime (Maxipime), cefoperazone (Cefobid), cefotaxime (Claforan), cefotetan (Cefotan), cefoxitin (Mefixitin), ceftazidime (Fortaz), ceftizoxime (Cefizox), ceftriaxone

(Rocephin), cefuroxime (Zinacef), chlorpromazine (Thorazine), cimetidine (Tagamet), ciprofloxacin (Cipro), cisplatin (Platinol), cladribine (Leustatin), clindamycin (Cleocin), co-trimoxazole (Bactrim), cyclophosphamide (Cytoxan), cytarabine (Ara-C), dacarbazine (DTIC-Dome), dactinomycin (Cosmegen), daunorubicin (Cerubidine), dexamethasone (Decadron), diphenhydramine (Benadryl), docetaxel (Taxotere), dopamine (Intropin), doxorubicin (Adriamycin), doxycycline (Vibramycin), droperidol (Inapsine), enalaprilat (Vasotec), etoposide (VePesid), famotidine (Pepcid), filgrastim (Neupogen), floxuridine (FUDR), fluconazole (Diflucan), fludarabine (Fludara), fluorouracil (Efurix), furosemide (Lasix), ganciclovir (Cytovene), gatifloxacin (Tequin), gemcitabine (Gemzar), gentamicin (Garamycin), haloperidol (Haldol), heparin, hydrocortisone sodium phosphate, hydrocortisone sodium succinate (Solu-Cortef), hydromorphone (Dilaudid), hydroxyzine (Vistaril), idarubicin (Idamycin), ifosfamide (Ifex), imipenem and cilastatin (Primaxin), leucovorin, linezolid (Zyvox), lorazepam (Ativan), magnesium, mechlorethamine (Mustargen), melphalan (Alkeran), meperidine (Demerol), mesna (Mesnex), methotrexate, methylprednisolone sodium succinate (Solu-Medrol), metoclopramide (Reglan), metronidazole (Flagyl), minocycline (Minocin), mitomycin (Mutamycin), mitoxantrone (Novantrone), morphine (Avinza, Kadian, Roxanol), nalbuphine (Nubain), netilmicin (Netromycin), ofloxacin (Floxin), paclitaxel (Taxol), piperacillin (Piperacil), piperacillin and tazobactam (Zosyn), plicamycin (Mithracin), potassium, prochlorperazine (Compazine), promethazine (Phenergan), propofol (Diprivan), ranitidine (Zantac), sargramostim (Leukine), sodium bicarbonate, streptozocin (Zanosar), teniposide (Vumon), thiotepa (Thioplex), ticarcillin (Ticar), ticarcillin and clavulanate (Timentin), tobramycin (Nebcin), topotecan (Hycamtin), vancomycin (Vancocin), vinblastine (Velban), vincristine (Oncovin), vinorelbine (Navelbine), zidovudine (Retrovir).

SIDE EFFECTS

Frequent (14%-21%)
Headache, constipation, asthenia.
Occasional (6%-8%)
Diarrhea, abdominal pain.
Rare (< 2%)
Altered taste, hypersensitivity reaction.

SERIOUS REACTIONS

• Serious hypersensitivity and anaphylaxis are rare.

PRECAUTIONS & CONSIDERATIONS

Should be used with caution in patients with preexisting arrhythmias or cardiac conduction disorders. Patients with cardiac disease, on cardiotoxic chemotherapy, with electrolyte abnormalities, and/or on QT-prolonging medications are particularly at risk. It is unknown whether granisetron is distributed in breast milk. The safety and efficacy of granisetron have not been established in children younger than 2 yr. No age-related precautions have been noted in elderly patients.

Notify the physician if headache occurs. The pattern of daily bowel activity and stool consistency should be assessed.

Storage
Keep the bottle of oral solution tightly closed. Protect the bottle from light and store it in an upright position. Store vials for IV use at room temperature; the solution normally appears clear and colorless. After dilution, the solution for injection is stable for at least 24 h at room temperature. Keep patch in sealed pouch until time of use.

Administration
! Administer only on days of chemotherapy, as prescribed. Administer oral granisetron within 1 h and the IV form within 30 min before starting chemotherapy.

For IV use, administer granisetron undiluted or dilute it with 20-50 mL 0.9% NaCl or D5W. Do not mix it with other medications. Administer the undiluted drug by IV push over 30 seconds. For IV piggyback, infuse over 5-20 min, depending on the volume of diluent used.

For transdermal patch use, apply to clean, dry, intact healthy skin on the upper outer arm a minimum of 24 h before chemotherapy. Do not place on skin that is red, irritated, or damaged. The patch should not be cut into pieces.

Griseofulvin

griz-ee-oh-full′vin
★ Grifulvin V, Gris-PEG

CATEGORY AND SCHEDULE

Pregnancy Risk Category: X

Classification: Antifungals

MECHANISM OF ACTION

An antifungal that inhibits fungal cell mitosis by disrupting mitotic spindle structure. *Therapeutic Effect:* Fungistatic.

AVAILABILITY

Oral Suspension (Grifulvin V): 125 mg/5 mL.
Tablets (Microsize [Grifulvin V]): 500 mg.
Tablets (Ultramicrosize [Gris-PEG]): 125 mg, 250 mg.

INDICATIONS AND DOSAGES

▸ Tinea capitis, tinea corporis, tinea cruris, tinea pedis, tinea unguium

MICROSIZE TABLETS, ORAL SUSPENSION
Adults. Usually, 500 mg once daily or in 2 divided doses.
Children 2 yr and older. Usual dosage, 10-20 mg/kg/day in 1 dose or 2 divided doses.
ULTRAMICROSIZE TABLETS.
Adults. Usual dosage, 300-750 mg/day as a single dose or in divided doses.
Children 2 yr and older. 5-10 mg/kg/day.

CONTRAINDICATIONS

Hepatocellular failure, porphyria, pregnancy, hypersensitivity.

INTERACTIONS

Drug
Barbiturates: May decrease the effects of griseofulvin.
Cyclosporine: Cyclosporine levels may be decreased.
Oral contraceptives, warfarin: May decrease the effects of these drugs.
Herbal
None known.
Food
Alcohol: May cause disulfiram-like reaction.

DIAGNOSTIC TEST EFFECTS

None known.

SIDE EFFECTS

Occasional
Hypersensitivity reaction (including pruritus, rash, and

urticaria), headache, nausea, diarrhea, excessive thirst, flatulence, oral thrush, dizziness, insomnia.
Rare
Paresthesia of hands or feet, proteinuria, photosensitivity reaction.

SERIOUS REACTIONS

- Granulocytopenia occurs rarely.
- Hepatotoxicity.

PRECAUTIONS & CONSIDERATIONS

Because griseofulvin is produced by a species of *Penicillium,* patients with penicillin allergy might have cross-sensitivity; however, patients with penicillin allergy have received griseofulvin without adverse effects. Determine any history of allergies, especially to griseofulvin and penicillins, before giving the drug. Caution is warranted in those who are exposed to sun or ultraviolet light because photosensitivity may develop. Avoid alcohol and exposure to sunlight. Maintain good hygiene to help prevent superinfection. Separate personal items that come in direct contact with affected areas. Do not give to a pregnant woman; considered teratogenic.There are no data of use during lactation; avoid use during lactation.

Monitor the granulocyte count as appropriate. If granulocytopenia develops, notify the physician and expect to discontinue the drug. If headache occurs, establish and document the headache's location, onset, and type. Assess for dizziness. Evaluate skin for rash and therapeutic response to the drug. Assess daily pattern of bowel activity and stool consistency.
Storage
Store at room temperature; protect from light.
Administration
The duration of treatment depends on the site of infection. Take oral griseofulvin with foods high in fat, such as milk or ice cream, to reduce GI upset and assist in drug absorption. Shake oral suspension well before each use. Keep affected areas dry and wear light clothing for ventilation.

Guaifenesin

gwye-fen′e-sin
★ Allfen, Altarussin, Bidex, Diabetic Tussin Mucus Relief, Ganidin NR, Guiatuss, Liquibid, Mucinex, Mucinex Childrens, Mucinex Junior, Organidin NR, Q-Tussin, Robafen, Robitussin, Scott-Tussin, Situssin SA, XPECT
🍁 Robitussin Chest Congestion, Balminil, Benylin Chest Congestion, Vicks DayQuil Mucus Control
Do not confuse guaifenesin with guanfacine.

CATEGORY AND SCHEDULE

Pregnancy Risk Category: C
OTC

Classification: Expectorants

MECHANISM OF ACTION

An expectorant that stimulates respiratory tract secretions by decreasing the adhesiveness and viscosity of phlegm. *Therapeutic Effect:* Promotes removal of viscous mucus.

PHARMACOKINETICS

Well absorbed from the GI tract. Metabolized in the liver. Excreted in urine.

AVAILABILITY

Granules (Mucinex Childrens, Mucinex Junior): 50 mg/packet, 100 mg/packet.
Tablets: 200 mg, 400 mg.
Tablets, Extended Release (Mucinex): 600 mg, 1200 mg.
Syrup: 100 mg/5 mL.

INDICATIONS AND DOSAGES

▸ **Expectorant**

PO

Adults, Elderly, Children older than 12 yr. 200-400 mg q4h.
Children 6-12 yr. 100-200 mg q4h. Maximum: 1.2 g/day.
Children 2-5 yr. 50-100 mg q4h.
Children younger than 2 yr. 12 mg/kg/day in 6 divided doses.

PO (EXTENDED RELEASE)

Adults, Elderly, Children older than 12 yr. 600-1200 mg q12h. Maximum: 2.4 g/day.

CONTRAINDICATIONS

None known.

INTERACTIONS

Drug
None known.
Herbal
None known.
Food
None known.

DIAGNOSTIC TEST EFFECTS

None known.

SIDE EFFECTS

Rare
Dizziness, headache, rash, diarrhea, nausea, vomiting, abdominal pain.

SERIOUS REACTIONS

- Overdose may produce nausea and vomiting.

PRECAUTIONS & CONSIDERATIONS

It is unknown whether guaifenesin crosses the placenta or is distributed in breast milk. Be alert to liquid formulas that may contain alcohol. No age-related precautions have been noted in children or in elderly patients. Use guaifenesin cautiously in children younger than 2 yr with a persistent cough. Avoid tasks that require mental alertness or motor skills until response to the drug has been established. Fluid intake and environmental humidity should be increased to lower the viscosity of secretions.

Notify the physician of cough that persists or is accompanied by fever, rash, headache, or sore throat. Clinical improvement should be assessed.

Storage
Store syrup, liquid, and tablets at room temperature.

Administration
Take guaifenesin without regard to food. Do not crush or break extended-release tablets. Take extended release at 12-h intervals, as prescribed. Granules may be sprinkled on soft food and then swallowed without chewing or crushing. Do not take for chronic cough.

Maintain adequate fluid intake to aid expectoration.

Guanabenz

gwan'a-benz
Do not confuse with guanfacine.

CATEGORY AND SCHEDULE

Pregnancy Risk Category: C

Classification:
Antihypertensives, central-acting adrenergic agents

MECHANISM OF ACTION
An α-adrenergic agonist that stimulates α_2-adrenergic receptors within the CNS, inhibiting sympatheic nervous system outflow. Inhibits sympathetic cardioaccelerator and vasoconstrictor center to heart, kidneys, peripheral vasculature. *Therapeutic Effect:* Decreases systolic, diastolic BP. Chronic use decreases peripheral vascular resistance.

G

PHARMACOKINETICS
Well absorbed from GI tract. Widely distributed. Protein binding: 90%. Metabolized in liver. Excreted in urine and feces. Not removed by hemodialysis. *Half-life:* 6 h.

AVAILABILITY
Tablets: 4 mg, 8 mg.

INDICATIONS AND DOSAGES
▸ **Hypertension**

PO

Adults. Initially, 4 mg 2 times/day. Increase by 4-8 mg at 1- to 2-wk intervals. Usual effective range is 8-32 mg/day.

Elderly. Initially, 4 mg/day. May increase q1-2wk. Maintenance: 8-16 mg/day. Maximum: 32 mg/day.

CONTRAINDICATIONS
History of hypersensitivity to guanabenz or any component of the formulation.

INTERACTIONS
Drug

β-Blockers, hypotensive-producing medications: May increase antihypertensive effect.

Nitroprusside: May cause additive hypotension.

Noncardioselective β-blockers: May exacerbate rebound hypertension.

Tricyclic antidepressant agents: May decrease effects of guanabenz.

Herbal

Licorice, yohimbine: May decrease guanabenz effectiveness.

Food

None known.

DIAGNOSTIC TEST EFFECTS
May decrease cholesterol, total triglyceride concentrations.

SIDE EFFECTS
Frequent

Drowsiness, dry mouth, dizziness.

Occasional

Weakness, headache, nausea, decreased sexual ability.

Rare

Ataxia, sleep disturbances, rash, itching, diarrhea, constipation, altered taste, muscle aches.

SERIOUS REACTIONS
- Abrupt withdrawal may result in rebound hypertension manifested as nervousness, agitation, anxiety, insomnia, hand tingling, tremor, flushing, and sweating.
- Overdosage produces hypotension, somnolence, lethargy, irritability, bradycardia, and miosis (pupillary constriction).

PRECAUTIONS & CONSIDERATIONS
Caution is warranted in patients with severe coronary insufficiency, recent myocardial infarction, cerebrovascular disease, severe hepatic or renal impairment. It is unknown whether guanabenz crosses the placenta or is distributed in breast milk. Safety and efficacy of guanabenz have not been established in children. No age-related precautions have been noted in elderly patients. Diabetic patients should be educated that this medication may mask symptoms of hypoglycemia.

Side effects such as dry mouth, drowsiness, dizziness, headache, decreased sexual ability, and GI upset may occur during the first 2 wks of therapy but generally diminish during continued therapy. If increased or decreased heartbeat or swollen ankles or feet occur, notify the physician. Avoid alcohol, and caution should be used driving or operating machinery until tolerance to medication is established.

Storage

Store at room temperature and protect from light.

Administration

Give with or without food.

Avoid skipping doses or abruptly discontinuing drug because it may produce severe rebound hypertension.

Guanfacine

gwan′fa-seen

★ Intuniv, Tenex

Do not confuse with guanabenz.

CATEGORY AND SCHEDULE

Pregnancy Risk Category: B

Classification: Antihypertensives, central-acting adrenergic agents

MECHANISM OF ACTION

An α-adrenergic agonist that stimulates α_2-adrenergic receptors within CNS, inhibiting sympathetic nervous system outflow to heart, kidneys, peripheral vasculature. Mechanism in ADHD is not clear. *Therapeutic Effect:* Decreases systolic, diastolic BP and peripheral vascular resistance in HTN; in ADHD, improves hyperactivity and impulsiveness and improves attention span.

PHARMACOKINETICS

Well absorbed from GI tract. Widely distributed. Protein binding: 71%. Metabolized in liver. Excreted in urine and feces. Not removed by hemodialysis. *Half-life:* 17 h.

AVAILABILITY

Tablets: 1 mg, 2 mg.

Tablets, Extended Release (Intuniv): 1 mg, 2 mg, 3 mg, 4 mg.

INDICATIONS AND DOSAGES

▸ **Hypertension**

PO

Adults, Elderly. Initially, 1 mg/day. Increase by 1 mg/day at intervals of 3-4 wks up to 3 mg/day in single or divided doses.

▸ **Attention-deficit hyperactivity disorder (ADHD)**

PO (Extended Release, Intuniv).

Children 6 yr and older. Initially, 1 mg once daily and adjust by no more than 1 mg/wk. Dose range 1-4 mg/day. Alternatively, consider weight-based dosing. Starting doses of 0.05-0.08 mg/kg once daily. Doses up to 0.12 mg/kg once daily may provide benefit. Maximum: 4 mg/day.

▸ **Dosage in hepatic or renal impairment (all patients)**

Drug is equally cleared by hepatic and renal routes; dose adjustments may be needed in either hepatic or renal impairment, but specific recommendations not available.

CONTRAINDICATIONS

History of hypersensitivity to guanfacine or any component of the formulation.

INTERACTIONS

Drug

β-Blockers, hypotensive-producing medications: May increase antihypertensive effect.

Bupropion: May increase risk of seizure activity.

Nitroprusside: May have additive hypotensive effects.
Noncardioselective β-blockers: May exacerbate rebound hypertension when guanfacine is withdrawn.
Tricyclic antidepressant agents: May decrease the hypotensive effects of guanfacine.
Valproic acid/divalproex: Drug can increase valproic acid concentrations.
CYP3A inhibitors: May increase guanfacine concentrations.
Drugs with sedative properties: Increase risk of sedation.
Herbal
Licorice, yohimbine: May decrease guanfacine effectiveness.
Ma huang: May increase BP.
Food
Alcohol: Manufacturer recommends avoidance.
High-fat foods: Increase risk of side effects from extended-release tablets.

DIAGNOSTIC TEST EFFECTS

May increase growth hormone concentration. May decrease urinary catecholamine and VMA excretion.

SIDE EFFECTS

Frequent
Somnolence sedation, lowered blood pressure, abdominal pain, dizziness, dry mouth, and constipation.
Occasional
Fatigue, headache, asthenia (loss of strength, energy).
Rare
Excessive hypotension, syncope, bradycardia (see Serious Reactions).

SERIOUS REACTIONS

- Overdosage may produce difficult breathing, dizziness, faintness, severe drowsiness, bradycardia.

PRECAUTIONS & CONSIDERATIONS

Caution should be used with impaired renal function. Guanfacine crosses the placenta, and it is unknown if it is distributed in breast milk. Be aware that guanfacine is not recommended in treatment of acute hypertension associated with preeclampsia. Safety and efficacy of guanfacine have not been established in children under 6 yr of age. There are no age-related precautions noted in the elderly. Diabetic patients should be educated that this medication may mask symptoms of hypoglycemia.

Therapeutic effect may take 1 wk and peak effect should be noted in 1-3 mo. Avoid alcohol, and caution should be used driving or operating machinery until the effects of the drug are known.

Storage
Store at room temperature and protect from light.
Administration
Give immediate-release tablets at bedtime. For extended-release tablets, do not cut, crush, or chew. Swallow dose whole once daily with water, milk, or liquid and do NOT administer with high-fat foods as this will increase drug exposure.

! NOTE: Do not substitute immediate-release tablets for the extended-release tablets on a mg-mg basis; they are NOT equivalent.

Avoid skipping doses or abruptly discontinuing drug, which may produce severe rebound hypertension. When discontinuing, taper the dose by no more than 1 mg every 3-7 days.

Halcinonide

hal-sin'o-nide

★ Halog

CATEGORY AND SCHEDULE

Pregnancy Risk Category: C

Classification: Corticosteroids, topical, dermatologics, anti-inflammatory

MECHANISM OF ACTION

A topical high-potency corticosteroid that inhibits accumulation of inflammatory cells, phagocytosis, lysosomal enzyme release, and synthesis or release of mediators of inflammation. *Therapeutic Effect*: Decreases or prevents tissue response to inflammatory process.

PHARMACOKINETICS

Repeated application results in a cumulative depot effect in the skin, which may lead to a prolonged duration of action and increased systemic absorption. Large variation in absorption among sites. Protein binding: Varies. Metabolized in liver. Primarily excreted in urine.

AVAILABILITY

Cream: 0.1% (Halog).
Ointment: 0.1% (Halog).

INDICATIONS AND DOSAGES

▸ **Corticosteroid-responsive dermatoses**

Topical

Adults, Elderly, Children. Apply sparingly 1-3 times/day.

CONTRAINDICATIONS

History of hypersensitivity to halcinonide or other corticosteroids; viral, fungal, or tubercular skin lesions.

INTERACTIONS

Drug

None known.

Herbal

None known.

Food

None known.

DIAGNOSTIC TEST EFFECTS

None known.

SIDE EFFECTS

Occasional

Itching, redness, irritation, burning at site of application, dryness, folliculitis, acneiform eruptions, hypopigmentation.

Rare

Allergic contact dermatitis, maceration of the skin, secondary infection, skin atrophy.

SERIOUS REACTIONS

- The serious reactions of long-term therapy and the addition of occlusive dressings are reversible hypothalamic-pituitary-adrenal (HPA) axis suppression, manifestations of Cushing syndrome, hyperglycemia, and glucosuria.

PRECAUTIONS & CONSIDERATIONS

Caution should be used over large surface areas and with prolonged use. It is unknown whether halcinonide is excreted in breast milk. Drugs of this class should not be used extensively on pregnant patients, in large amounts, or for prolonged periods of time. Notify physician if irritation occurs. Absorption is more likely with occlusive dressings or extensive application in young children.

Storage

Store at room temperature and away from excessive heat. Do not freeze.

Administration

Gently cleanse area before application preferably after bath or shower for best absorption. Use occlusive dressings only as directed. Apply sparingly. Rub into area gently and thoroughly. Avoid contact with eyes.

Halobetasol

hal-oh-be′ta-sol

★ 🍁 Ultravate

CATEGORY AND SCHEDULE

Pregnancy Risk Category: C

Classification: Corticosteroids, topical, dermatologics

MECHANISM OF ACTION

A very-high-potency corticosteroid that inhibits accumulation of inflammatory cells at inflammation sites, phagocytosis, lysosomal enzyme release, and synthesis or release of mediators of inflammation. *Therapeutic Effect:* Decreases or prevents tissue response to inflammatory process.

PHARMACOKINETICS

Variation in absorption among individuals and sites: scrotum 36%, forehead 7%, scalp 4%, forearm 1%.

AVAILABILITY

Cream: 0.05% (Ultravate).
Ointment: 0.05% (Ultravate).

INDICATIONS AND DOSAGES

▸ **Dermatoses, corticosteroid-responsive**

Topical

Adults, Elderly, Children 12 yr and older. Apply 1-2 times/day. Maximum: 50 g/wk for no more than 2 wks.

CONTRAINDICATIONS

Hypersensitivity to halobetasol or other corticosteroids; viral, fungal, or tubercular skin lesions.

INTERACTIONS

Drug
None known.
Herbal
None known.
Food
None known.

DIAGNOSTIC TEST EFFECTS

None known.

SIDE EFFECTS

Frequent
Burning, stinging, pruritus.
Rare
Cushing syndrome, hyperglycemia, glucosuria, HPA axis suppression.

SERIOUS REACTIONS

• Overdosage can occur from topically applied halobetasol absorbed in sufficient amounts to produce systemic effects producing reversible hypothalamic-pituitary-adrenal (HPA) axis suppression, manifestations of Cushing syndrome, hyperglycemia, and glucosuria in some patients.

PRECAUTIONS & CONSIDERATIONS

Occlusive dressings should be avoided. It is unknown whether halobetasol crosses the placenta or is distributed in the breast milk. Drugs of this class should not be used extensively on pregnant patients, in large amounts, or for prolonged periods of time. Safety and efficacy have not been established in children less than 12 yr of age. No age-related precautions have been noted in elderly patients.

Storage
Store at room temperature and away from excessive heat.

Administration
Avoid the use of occlusive dressings unless otherwise directed by a physician. Apply sparingly to the skin or scalp and rub into area thoroughly. Administer for no longer than 2 wks. Only small areas should be treated at one time. Discontinue treatment when control is achieved. Do not apply on face, groin, or axillae. Avoid contact with eyes.

Haloperidol

ha-loe-per'idole
★ Haldol, Haldol Decanoate
🍁 Apo-Haloperidol
Do not confuse Haldol with Halcion, Halog, or Stadol.

CATEGORY AND SCHEDULE
Pregnancy Risk Category: C

Classification: Antipsychotics, butyrophenone

MECHANISM OF ACTION
An antipsychotic, antiemetic, and antidyskinetic agent that competitively blocks postsynaptic dopamine receptors, interrupts nerve impulse movement, and increases turnover of dopamine in the brain. Has strong extrapyramidal and antiemetic effects, weak anticholinergic and sedative effects. *Therapeutic Effect:* Produces tranquilizing effect.

PHARMACOKINETICS
Readily absorbed from the GI tract. Protein binding: 92%. Extensively metabolized in the liver. Primarily excreted in urine. Not removed by hemodialysis. *Half-life:* 12-37 h PO; 10-19 h IV; 17-25 h IM.

AVAILABILITY
Oral Concentrate: 2 mg/mL.
Tablets: 0.5 mg, 1 mg, 2 mg, 5 mg, 10 mg, 20 mg.
Injection (Lactate): 5 mg/mL.
Injection (Decanoate): 50 mg/mL, 100 mg/mL.

INDICATIONS AND DOSAGES
▸ **Treatment of psychotic disorders**
PO
Adults, Children 12 yr and older. Initially, 0.5-5 mg 2-3 times/day. Dosage gradually adjusted as needed.
Elderly. 0.5-2 mg 2-3 times/day. Dosage gradually adjusted as needed.
Children 3-12 yr or weighing 15-40 kg. Initially, 0.05 mg/kg/day in 2-3 divided doses. May increase by 0.5-mg increments at 5- to 7-day intervals. Maximum: 0.15 mg/kg/day in divided doses.
IM (LACTATE)
Adults, Elderly, Children 12 yr and older. Initially, 2-5 mg. May repeat at 1-h intervals as needed. Convert to oral treatment as soon as possible.
IM (DECANOATE)
Adults, Elderly, Children 12 yr and older. Initially, 10-15 times previous daily oral dose up to maximum initial dose of 100 mg. Injections are given once every 28 days. Maximum: 300 mg/mo.
▸ **Treatment of nonpsychotic disorders, Tourette syndrome**
PO
Children 3-12 yr or weighing 15-40 kg. Initially, 0.05 mg/kg/day in 2-3 divided doses. May increase by 0.5 mg at 5- to 7-day intervals. Maximum: 0.075 mg/kg/day.

OFF-LABEL USES
Treatment of nausea or vomiting associated with cancer chemotherapy, used IV off-label for agitation in hospitalized patients.

H

CONTRAINDICATIONS

Angle-closure glaucoma, severe central nervous system (CNS) depression, Parkinson disease, coma, hypersensitivity.

INTERACTIONS

Drug

Alcohol, other CNS depressants: May increase CNS depression.
Amphetamines, selected β-blockers, dextromethorphan, fluoxetine, lidocaine, mirtazapine, nefazodone, paroxetine, risperidone, ritonavir, thioridazine, tricyclic antidepressants, venlafaxine, and other CYP2D6 substrates: May increase the levels of haloperidol.
Antihypertensives: May cause additive hypotension.
Azole antifungals, clarithromycin, diclofenac, doxycycline, erythromycin, imatinib, isoniazid, nefazodone, nicardipine, propofol, protease inhibitors, quinidine, telithromycin, verapamil, and other CYP3A4 inhibitors: May increase the effects of haloperidol.
Carbamazepine, nafcillin, nevirapine, phenobarbital, phenytoin, rifamycins, and other CYP3A4 inducers: May decrease the effects of haloperidol.
Chlorpromazine, delavirdine, fluoxetine, miconazole, paroxetine, pergolide, quinidine, quinine, ritonavir, ropinirole, and other CYP2D6 inhibitors: May increase the levels of haloperidol.
Epinephrine: May block α-adrenergic effects.
Extrapyramidal symptom-producing medications: May increase extrapyramidal symptoms.
Lithium: May increase neurologic toxicity.
QT-prolonging medications: May increase the risk of QT prolongation.
SSRIs: May increase the risk of extrapyramidal symptoms.
Tricyclic antidepressants: May cause increased toxicity.

Herbal

Valerian, St. John's wort, kava kava, gotu kola: May increase CNS depression.

Food

Alcohol: May increase CNS depression.

DIAGNOSTIC TEST EFFECTS

May decrease WBC or increase LFTs. Therapeutic serum drug level is 0.2-1 mcg/mL; toxic serum drug level is > 1 mcg/mL.

IV INCOMPATIBILITIES

Allopurinol (Aloprim), amphotericin B complex (Abelcet, AmBisome, Amphotec), cefepime (Maxipime), calcium chloride, most cephalosporins, clindamycin (Cleocin), diazepam (Valium), digoxin (Lanoxin), diphenhydramine (Benadryl), epoetin alfa (Epogen, Procrit), fluconazole (Diflucan), foscarnet (Foscavir), furosemide, heparin, hydroxyzine (Vistaril), imipenem-cilastatin (Primaxin), ketorolac (Toradol), lansoprazole (Prevacid), magnesium sulfate, methylprednisolone (Solu-Medrol), nitroprusside (Nipride), pantoprazole (Protonix), phenobarbital, phenytoin, piperacillin and tazobactam (Zosyn), potassium chloride, sodium bicarbonate, vancomycin.

IV COMPATIBILITIES

Amifostine (Ethyol), amsacrine (Amsa), aztreonam (Azactam), cimetidine (Tagamet), cisatracurium (Nimbex), cladribine (Leustatin), dobutamine (Dobutrex), docetaxel (Taxotere), dopamine (Intropin), doxorubicin (Rubex), etoposide (VePesid), famotidine (Pepcid), fentanyl (Sublimaze), filgrastim (Neupogen), fludarabine (Fludara), gatifloxacin (Tequin), gemcitabine (Gemzar), granisetron (Kytril), hydromorphone (Dilaudid), lidocaine, linezolid (Zyvox), lorazepam (Ativan), midazolam (Versed), morphine, nitroglycerin, norepinephrine (Levophed), ondansetron (Zofran), paclitaxel (Taxol), phenylephrine, propofol (Diprivan), remifentanil (Ultiva), sufentanil (Sufenta), tacrolimus (Prograf), teniposide (Vumon), theophylline (Theodur), thiotepa (Thioplex), vinorelbine (Navelbine).

SIDE EFFECTS

Frequent

Blurred vision, constipation, orthostatic hypotension, dry mouth, swelling or soreness of female breasts, peripheral edema.

Occasional

Allergic reaction, difficulty urinating, decreased thirst, dizziness, decreased sexual function, drowsiness, nausea, vomiting, photosensitivity, lethargy.

SERIOUS REACTIONS

- Extrapyramidal symptoms appear to be dose related and typically occur in the first few days of therapy. Marked drowsiness and lethargy, excessive salivation, and fixed stare occur frequently. Less common reactions include severe akathisia (motor restlessness) and acute dystonias (such as torticollis, opisthotonos, and oculogyric crisis).
- Tardive dyskinesia (tongue protrusion, puffing of the cheeks, chewing or puckering of the mouth) may occur during long-term therapy or after discontinuing the drug and may be irreversible. Elderly women have a greater risk of developing this reaction.
- Rare reports of agranulocytosis or liver dysfunction with jaundice.
- Rare QT prolongation and torsades de pointes; high doses and IV use may result in higher risk.

PRECAUTIONS & CONSIDERATIONS

Caution is warranted in patients with cardiovascular disease, hepatic or renal dysfunction, a history of seizures, and with concurrent use with medications that may prolong the QT interval. Haloperidol crosses the placenta and is distributed in breast milk. Children are more susceptible to dystonias. Haloperidol use is not recommended for children younger than 3 yr. A decreased dosage is recommended for elderly patients, who are more susceptible to extrapyramidal and anticholinergic effects, orthostatic hypotension, and sedation. Elderly patients with dementia-related psychosis have a significantly higher incidence of cerebrovascular adverse events (e.g., stroke, TIA) and increased risk of mortality. Exposure to sunlight and any conditions that may cause dehydration or overheating should be avoided because they may increase the risk of heatstroke.

Drowsiness may occur but generally subsides with continued therapy. Alcohol and tasks that require mental alertness or motor skills should be avoided. Notify the physician if muscle stiffness occurs. Fine tongue movement, mask-like facial expression, rigidity, and tremor should be assessed if they occur.

Storage

Store vials, tablets, and oral solution at room temperature. Protect them from freezing and light. Discard the solution if it becomes discolored or contains precipitate. Do not refrigerate the decanoate injection.

Administration

! Only haloperidol lactate is given IV.

Widely accepted practice but not FDA approved: Off-label, haloperidol may be given undiluted by IV push. Flush with at least 2 mL 0.9% NaCl before and after administration. To dilute, add the drug to 30-50 mL of most solutions; D5W is preferred. Give IV push at 5 mg/min. Infuse IV piggyback over 30 min. For IV infusion, administer up to 25 mg/h, titrating dosage to patient response.

Prepare haloperidol decanoate IM injection using a 21-gauge needle. Do not exceed 3 mL per IM injection site. Slowly inject the drug deep into the upper outer quadrant of the gluteus maximus. Keep recumbent (head low and legs raised) for 30-60 min after administration to minimize hypotensive effects.

Take oral haloperidol without regard to food. Crush scored tablets as needed. Full therapeutic effect may take up to 6 wks to appear. Do not abruptly discontinue the drug after long-term use.

Heparin

hep'a-rin

Hep-Lock, Hep-Lock U/P

Hepalean, Hepalean-Lok

Do not confuse heparin with Hespan.

CATEGORY AND SCHEDULE

Pregnancy Risk Category: C

Classification: Anticoagulants

MECHANISM OF ACTION

A blood modifier that interferes with blood coagulation by blocking the conversion of prothrombin to thrombin and fibrinogen to fibrin. *Therapeutic Effect:* Prevents further extension of existing thrombi or new clot formation. Has no effect on existing clots.

PHARMACOKINETICS

Well absorbed following subcutaneous administration. Protein binding: Very high. Metabolized in the liver. Removed from the circulation via uptake by the reticuloendothelial system. Primarily excreted in urine. Not removed by hemodialysis. *Half-life:* 1-6 h.

AVAILABILITY

Injection: 10 units/mL, 100 units/mL, 1000 units/mL, 2500 units/mL, 5000 units/mL, 7500 units/mL, 10,000 units/mL, 20,000 units/mL.

Pre-mixed IV infusion: 25,000 units/500 mL infusion.

INDICATIONS AND DOSAGES

▸ **Line flushing**

IV

Adults, Elderly, Children. 100 units q6-8h.

Infants weighing < 10 kg. 10 units q6-8h. Caution: Always verify strength of solution before giving heparin flush to infants.

▸ **Treatment of venous thrombosis, pulmonary embolism, peripheral arterial embolism, atrial fibrillation with embolism**

INTERMITTENT IV

Adults, Elderly. Initially, 10,000 units, then 50-70 units/kg (5000-10,000 units) q4-6h, adjust to aPTT.

Children 1 yr and older. Initially, 50-100 units/kg, then 50-100 units q4h, adjust to aPTT.

IV INFUSION

Adults, Elderly. Loading dose: 80 units/kg, then 18 units/kg/h, with adjustments based on aPTT. Range: 10-30 units/kg/h.

Children 1 yr and older. Loading dose: 75 units/kg, then 20 units/kg/h with adjustments based on aPTT.

Children younger than 1 yr. Loading dose: 75 units/kg, then 28 units/kg/h, adjust to aPTT.

▸ **Prevention of venous thrombosis, pulmonary embolism, peripheral arterial embolism, atrial fibrillation with embolism**

SUBCUTANEOUS

Adult, Elderly. 5000 units q8-12h.

CONTRAINDICATIONS

Intracranial hemorrhage, severe hypotension, severe thrombocytopenia, subacute bacterial endocarditis, uncontrolled bleeding, history of heparin-induced thrombocytopenia (HIT).

INTERACTIONS

Drug

Antithyroid medications, cefoperazone, cefotetan, valproic acid: May cause hypoprothrombinemia.

Other anticoagulants, platelet aggregation inhibitors, thrombolytics: May increase the risk of bleeding.

Probenecid: May increase the effects of heparin.

Herbal

Cat's claw, dong quai, evening primrose, feverfew, red clover, horse chestnut, garlic, green tea, ginseng, ginkgo: May have an additive effect.

Food

None known.

DIAGNOSTIC TEST EFFECTS

May increase AST (SGOT) and ALT (SGPT) levels. May decrease serum cholesterol and triglyceride levels. Increases aPTT, may decrease platelets.

IV INCOMPATIBILITIES

Alatrofloxacin (Trovan), alteplase (Activase), amikacin (Amikin), amiodarone (Cordarone), amphotericin B complex (Abelcet, AmBisome, Amphotec), amsacrine (Amsa), atracurium (Tracrium), chlorpromazine (Thorazine), ciprofloxacin (Cipro), clarithromycin (Biaxin), cytarabine (Cytosar), dacarbazine (DTIC), daunorubicin (Cerubidine), diazepam (Valium), dobutamine (Dobutrex), doxorubicin (Adriamycin), doxycycline (Vibramycin), droperidol (Inapsine), erythromycin (Erythrocin), filgrastim (Neupogen), gatifloxacin (Tequin), gentamicin (Garamycin), haloperidol (Haldol), idarubicin (Idamycin), isosorbide dinitrate, kanamycin (Kantrex), labetalol (Trandate), levofloxacin (Levaquin), levorphanol (Levo-Dromoran), meperidine (Demerol), morphine (Avinza, Kadian, Roxanol), nicardipine (Cardene), phenytoin (Dilantin), promethazine (Phenergan), quinidine, tobramycin (Nebcin), vancomycin (Vancocin), warfarin (Coumadin).

IV COMPATIBILITIES

Acyclovir (Zovirax), aldesleukin (Proleukin), allopurinol (Alloprim), amifostine (Ethyol), aminophylline, ampicillin (Polycillin), ampicillin/sulbactam (Unasyn), ascorbic acid, atropine, aztreonam (Azactam), betamethasone sodium phosphate (Celestone), bleomycin (Blenoxane), calcium gluconate, cefamandole (Mandol), cefazolin (Ancef), cefepime (Maxipime), cefoperazone (Cefobid), cefotaxime (Claforan), cefotetan (Cefotan), cefoxitin (Mefixitin), ceftazidime (Fortaz), ceftriaxone (Rocephin), chloramphenicol (Chloromycetin), chlordiazepoxide (Librium), cimetidine (Tagamet), cisplatin (Platinol-AQ), cladribine (Leustatin), clindamycin (Cleocin), cyanocobalamin, cyclophosphamide (Cytoxan), cytarabine (Cytosar), dexamethasone sodium phosphate (Decadron), digoxin (Lanoxin), diltiazem (Cardizem), diphenhydramine (Benadryl), docetaxel (Taxotere), dopamine (Intropin), doxorubicin (Rubex), edrophonium (Tensilon), enalapril (Vasotec), epinephrine, erythromycin lactobionate (Erythrocin), esmolol (BreviBloc), estrogens (conjugated), ethacrynate (Edecrin), etoposide (VePesid), famotidine (Pepcid), fentanyl (Sublimaze), fluconazole (Diflucan), fludarabine (Fludara), fluorouracil (Efurix), foscarnet (Foscavir), furosemide (Lasix), gemcitabine (Gemzar), granisetron (Kytril), hydralazine (Apresoline), hydrocortisone sodium succinate (Solu-Cortef), hydromorphone (Dilaudid), insulin, isoproterenol (Isuprel), leucovorin, lidocaine, linezolid (Zyvox), lorazepam (Ativan), magnesium sulfate, methotrexate, methylprednisolone (Solu-Medrol), metoclopramide (Reglan), metronidazole (Flagyl), midazolam (Versed), milrinone (Primacor), minocycline (Minocin), mitomycin (Mutamycin), nafcillin (Unipen), neostigmine, nitroglycerin, norepinephrine (Levophed), ondansetron (Zofran), oxacillin (Bactocil), oxytocin (Pitocin), paclitaxel (Taxol), pancuronium (Pavulon), penicillin G potassium (Pfizerpen), pentazocine (Talwin), phytonadione, piperacillin (Piperacil), piperacillin/tazobactam (Zosyn), potassium chloride, procainamide (Pronestyl), propofol (Diprivan), propranolol (Inderal), pyridostigmine (Mestinon), ranitidine (Zantac), remifentanil (Ultiva), sargramostim (Leukine), scopolamine, sodium bicarbonate, sodium nitroprusside (Nitropress), streptokinase (Streptase), succinylcholine (Anectine), tacrolimus (Prograf), theophylline (Theodur), thiopental (Pentothal), thiotepa (Thioplex), ticarcillin (Ticar), ticarcillin/clavulanate potassium (Timentin), tirofiban (Aggrastat), trimethaphan camsylate (Arfonad), trimethobenzamide (Tigan), trimethoprim/sulfamethoxazole (Bactrim), vecuronium (Norcuron), vinblastine (Velban), vincristine (Oncovin), zidovudine (Retrovir).

SIDE EFFECTS

Occasional

Itching, burning (particularly on soles of feet) caused by vasospastic reaction.

Rare

Pain, cyanosis of extremity 6-10 days after initial therapy lasting 4-6 h; hypersensitivity reaction, including chills, fever, pruritus, urticaria, asthma, rhinitis, lacrimation, and headache.

SERIOUS REACTIONS

- Bleeding complications ranging from local ecchymoses to major hemorrhage occur more frequently in high-dose therapy, in intermittent IV infusion, and in women 60 yr of age and older.
- Antidote: Protamine sulfate 1-1.5 mg, IV, for every 100 units heparin subcutaneous within 30 min of overdose, 0.5-0.75 mg for every 100 units heparin subcutaneous if within 30-60 min of overdose, 0.25-0.375 mg for every 100 units heparin subcutaneous if 2 h have elapsed since overdose, 25-50 mg if heparin was given by IV infusion.
- Immune-mediated heparin-induced thrombocytopenia (HIT) and resulting risk of thrombosis.

PRECAUTIONS & CONSIDERATIONS

Caution should be used during menstruation in persons receiving IM injections and in those with peptic ulcer disease, recent invasive or surgical procedures, and severe hepatic or renal disease. Heparin should be used with caution in pregnant women, particularly during the last trimester and immediately postpartum, because it increases the risk of maternal hemorrhage. Heparin does not cross the placenta and is not distributed in breast milk. The benzyl alcohol preservative may cause gasping syndrome in infants. NOTE: Extreme caution should be used during the preparation, dispensing, and administration of heparin flushes, heparin-containing fluids, and therapeutic doses of heparin for children and infants. Fatal hemorrhages have occurred in pediatric patients (including neonates) due to medication errors. Elderly patients are more susceptible to hemorrhage, and age-related decreased renal function may increase the risk of bleeding. Other medications, including OTC drugs, should be avoided. An electric razor and soft toothbrush should be used to prevent bleeding during therapy.

Notify the physician of bleeding from surgical site, chest pain, dyspnea, severe or sudden headache, swelling in the feet or hands, unusual back pain, bruising, weakness, black or red stool, coffee-ground vomitus, dark or red urine, or red-speckled mucus from cough. CBC, BUN and creatinine levels, BP, pulse, potassium, and stool for occult blood should be monitored. Be aware of signs of bleeding, including bleeding at injection or surgical sites or from gums, blood in stool, bruising, hematuria, and petechiae.

Storage

Store at room temperature.

Administration

! Do not give by IM injection because it may cause pain, hematoma, ulceration, and erythema. The subcutaneous route is used for low-dose therapy.

! Always confirm the choice of correct heparin vial or solution before administration. Fatal medication errors may occur with incorrect selections.

For subcutaneous use, after withdrawing heparin from the vial, change the needle before injection to prevent leakage along the needle track. Inject the heparin dose above the iliac crest or in the abdominal fat layer. Do not inject within 2 inches of umbilicus or scar tissue.

For IV use, dilute IV infusion in isotonic sterile saline, D5W, or lactated Ringer's solution. Invert IV bag at least 6 times to ensure mixing and to prevent pooling of the medication. Use constant-rate IV infusion pump.

Hepatitis B Immune Globulin (Human)

hep-ah-tie′tis B ih-mewn′ glah′byew-lin

HepaGam B, HyperHEP B, Nabi-HB

CATEGORY AND SCHEDULE

Pregnancy Risk Category: C

Classification: Immune globulins

MECHANISM OF ACTION

An immune globulin of inactivated hepatitis B virus that provides passive immunity against hepatitis B virus.

AVAILABILITY

Injection: 1-mL, 5-mL vials.

INDICATIONS AND DOSAGES

▸ **Prevention of hepatitis B infection**

IM

Adults, Elderly. Usual 0.06 mL/kg. Repeat 28-30 days after exposure.

▸ **Perinatal exposure of infants born to HBsAg-positive mothers**

Infants. 0.5 mL IM after stable at birth, preferably within 12 h of birth.

▸ **For prevention of hepatitis B infection recurrence after liver transplantation in HBsAg-positive liver transplant patients:**

IV INFUSION (HEPAGAM B ONLY)

Adults. 20,000 IU concurrent with grafting of the transplanted liver, then 20,000 IU/day on days 1 to 7 postoperatively, then 20,000 IU q2wk starting on day 14 postoperatively, then 20,000 IU every month starting at month 4 postoperatively. The target serum antiHBs concentration is > 500 IU/L. Regularly monitor the serum antiHBs and HBsAg. If the serum antiHBs concentration is < 500 IU/L the first week, increase the dose to 10,000 IU q6h until target antiHBs concentration attained.

CONTRAINDICATIONS

Allergies to gamma globulin or thimerosal, IgA deficiency, IM injection in patients with coagulation disorders or thrombocytopenia.

INTERACTIONS

Drug

Live-virus vaccines: May decrease immune response.

Herbal and Food

None known.

DIAGNOSTIC TEST EFFECTS

None known.

SIDE EFFECTS

Frequent

Headache (26%), injection site pain (12%).

Occasional (5%)

Malaise, nausea, myalgia.

SERIOUS REACTIONS

- Agents derived from human plasma carry a very rare risk of transmission of certain infectious agents.

PRECAUTIONS & CONSIDERATIONS

Caution is warranted in patients with coagulation disorders; thrombocytopenia; IgA deficiency; and allergies to gamma globulin, eggs, chicken, or thimerosal. Notify the physician of any side effects, including headache or injection site pain. Baseline and periodic liver function studies and hepatitis B antibody levels should be obtained. Live vaccine administration should be deferred for 3 mo after immune globulin.

Storage

Refrigerate this drug; do not freeze it. Use within 6 h of opening.

Administration

HyperHEP B and Nabi-HB are for IM use only. In adults, administer by IM injection only in the gluteal or deltoid area. Complete full course of immunization.

For infants, administer IM in the anterolateral muscles of the thigh.

HepaGam B (ONLY) may be administered via IV infusion for prophylaxis following liver transplant. Calculate the volume needed for each 20,000 IU or 10,000 IU dose by using the measured potency of the HepaGam B lot. The potency is stamped on the vial label. Aseptically prepare the dose. Administer at 2 mL/min through a separate IV line using an IV infusion pump. Decrease the infusion rate to 1 mL/min or less if the patient has infusion-related discomfort.

Hetastarch

het'ah-starch

Hespan, Hextend, Voluven

Hextend

CATEGORY AND SCHEDULE

Pregnancy Risk Category: C

Classification: Plasma expanders

MECHANISM OF ACTION

A plasma volume expander that exerts osmotic pull on tissue fluids. *Therapeutic Effect:* Reduces hemoconcentration and blood viscosity; increases circulating blood volume.

PHARMACOKINETICS

Smaller molecules: < 50,000 molecular weight, rapidly excreted by kidneys; larger molecules: 50,000 molecular weight and greater, slowly degraded to smaller-sized molecules, then excreted. Not removed by hemodialysis. *Half-life:* 17 days.

AVAILABILITY

Injection: 6 g/100 mL 0.9% NaCl (500-mL infusion container).

INDICATIONS AND DOSAGES

▸ **Plasma volume expansion**

IV

Adults, Elderly. 500-1000 mL/day up to 1500 mL/day (20 mg/kg) at a rate up to 20 mL/kg/h in hemorrhagic shock and at a slower rate in burns and septic shock.

Children. Limited clinical data for the Voluven product are available. A mean dose of 16 ± 9 mL/kg was given. Adapt dose to the individual patient colloid needs, taking into account the disease state, as well as the hemodynamic and hydration status. Use in newborns should be carefully evaluated, given the limited numbers of infants studied.

▸ **Leukapheresis**

IV

Adults, Elderly. 250-700 mL infused at a constant rate, usually 1:8 to venous whole blood.

CONTRAINDICATIONS

Known hypersensitivity to hydroxyethyl cellulose, pre-existing coagulation or bleeding disorders, CHF or pulmonary edema where volume overload is a potential problem; do not use in renal disease with oliguria or anuria not related to hypovolemia.

INTERACTIONS

Drug

None significant.

Herbal and Food

None known.

DIAGNOSTIC TEST EFFECTS

May prolong bleeding, and clotting times, PTT, and PT. May decrease Hct concentration. May elevate indirect bilirubin levels and serum amylase.

IV INCOMPATIBILITIES

Amikacin (Amikin), amphotericin B (Fungizone), ampicillin (Polycillin), cefamandole (Mandol), cefazolin (Ancef, Kefzol), cefoperazone (Cefobid), cefotaxime (Claforan), cefoxitin (Mefoxin), diazepam (Valium), gentamicin (Garamycin), ranitidine (Zantac), sodium bicarbonate, theophylline (Theodur), tobramycin (Nebcin).

IV COMPATIBILITIES

Alatrofloxacin (Trovan), alfentanil (Alfenta), aminophylline, amiodarone (Cordarone), ampicillin (Polycillin), ampicillin-sulbactam (Unasyn), atracurium

(Tracrium), azithromycin (Zithromax), bumetanide (Bumex), butorphanol (Stadol), calcium gluconate, cefepime (Maxipime), cefotaxime (Claforan), cefotetan (Cefotan), ceftazidime (Fortaz), ceftizoxime (Cefizox), ceftriaxone (Rocephin), cefuroxime (Zinacef), chlorpromazine (Thorazine), cimetidine (Tagamet), ciprofloxacin (Cipro), cisatracurium (Nimbex), clindamycin (Cleocin), dexamethasone (Decadron), digoxin (Lanoxin), diltiazem (Cardizem), diphenhydramine (Benadryl), dobutamine (Dobutrex), dolasetron (Anzemet), dopamine (Intropin), doxycycline (Vibramycin), droperidol (Inapsine), enalaprilat (Vasotec), ephedrine, epinephrine, erythromycin (Erythrocin), esmolol (BreviBloc), famotidine (Pepcid), fentanyl (Sublimaze), fluconazole (Diflucan), furosemide (Lasix), granisetron (Kytril), haloperidol (Haldol), heparin, hydrocortisone (Solu-Cortef), hydromorphone (Dilaudid), hydroxyzine (Vistaril), inamrinone (Inocor), isoproterenol (Isuprel), ketorolac (Toradol), labetalol (Normodyne, Trandate), levofloxacin (Levaquin), lidocaine (Xylocaine), lorazepam (Ativan), magnesium, mannitol, meperidine (Demerol), methylprednisolone (Solu-Medrol), metoclopramide (Reglan), metronidazole (Flagyl), midazolam (Versed), milrinone (Primacor), mivacurium (Mivacron), morphine (Avinza, Kadian, Roxanol), nalbuphine (Nubain), nitroglycerin (Nitrobid), norepinephrine (Levophed), ofloxacin (Floxin), ondansetron (Zofran), pancuronium (Pavulon), phenylephrine, piperacillin (Piperacil), piperacillin-tazobactam (Zosyn), potassium chloride, procainamide (Pronestyl), prochlorperazine (Compazine), promethazine (Phenergan), rocuronium (Zemuron), sodium nitroprusside (Nitropress), succinylcholine (Anectine), sufentanil (Sufenta), thiopental (Pentothal), ticarcillin (Ticar), ticarcillin-clavulanate (Timentin), tobramycin (Nebcin), trimethoprim-sulfamethoxazole (Bactrim), vancomycin (Vancocin), vecuronium (Norcuron), verapamil (Calan).

SIDE EFFECTS

Rare

Allergic reaction resulting in vomiting, mild temperature elevation, chills, itching, submaxillary and parotid gland enlargement, peripheral edema of lower extremities, mild flu-like symptoms, headache, muscle aches.

SERIOUS REACTIONS

- Fluid overload may occur marked by increased BP and distended neck veins. Neurologic changes that may occur include headache, weakness, blurred vision, behavioral changes, incoordination, and isolated muscle twitching. Pulmonary edema may also occur, manifested by rapid breathing, crackles, wheezing, and coughing.
- Anaphylactic reaction, including periorbital edema, urticaria, and wheezing, may occur.

PRECAUTIONS & CONSIDERATIONS

Use with caution in those with corn hypersensitivity as they may also be allergic to hetastarch. Caution is warranted with congestive heart failure, hepatic disease, pulmonary edema, sodium-restricted diets, thrombocytopenia, and in elderly patients or children. An electric razor and soft toothbrush should be used to prevent bleeding during therapy.

Notify the physician of bleeding, wheezing, itching, rash, black or red stool, coffee-ground emesis. Urine output, vital signs, and laboratory tests, including coagulation studies and CBC, should be monitored. Central venous pressure (CVP) should also be monitored to detect blood volume overexpansion. Be aware of signs and symptoms of fluid overload, such as peripheral or pulmonary edema, and impending congestive heart failure.

Storage

Store solution at room temperature. Solution normally appears clear, pale yellow to amber. Do not use if discolored a deep turbid brown or if precipitate forms.

Administration

Administer only by IV infusion. Do not add drugs to the IV infusion. If administration is by pressure infusion, all air should be withdrawn or expelled from the bag through the medication port prior to infusion. Additionally, take care to turn off infusion pump before the bag runs dry to avoid air embolism. In acute hemorrhagic shock, administer at a rate approaching 1.2 g/kg/h (20 mL/kg/h), as prescribed. Expect to use slower rates in burns and septic shock. Monitor CVP when giving by rapid infusion. If CVP rises precipitously, immediately discontinue the drug, as prescribed, to prevent blood volume overexpansion.

Hyaluronan

★ Euflexxa, Hyalgan, Orthovisc, Supartz, Synvisc Injection

CATEGORY AND SCHEDULE

Pregnancy Risk Category: NR

Classification: Hyaluronic acid derivatives

MECHANISM OF ACTION

A natural complex sugar of the glycosaminoglycan family that enhances viscoelastic properties of synovial fluid. *Therapeutic Effect:* Produces lubrication for knee joint and relieves pain and increases mobility.

PHARMACOKINETICS

Not known.

AVAILABILITY

Prefilled Syringe: 8 mg/1 mL (Synvisc), 10 mg/1 mL (Euflexxa, Hyalgan, Supartz), 15 mg/1 mL (Orthovisc).

INDICATIONS AND DOSAGES

▸ Knee osteoarthritis

PO

Adults, Elderly. Euflexxa: inject 20 mg into one knee weekly for 3 wks; *Hyalgan:* inject 20 mg into one knee weekly for 3-5 wks; *Orthovisc:* inject 30 mg into one knee weekly for 3 or 4 wks; *Supartz:* inject 25 mg into one knee weekly for 5 wks; *Synvisc:* inject 16 mg into one knee weekly for 3 wks.

OFF-LABEL USES

Treatment of psoriatic arthritis.

CONTRAINDICATIONS

Allergies to avian or avian-derived products (including eggs, feathers, or poultry), skin disease or infection in area of injection site, hypersensitivity to hyaluronate preparations or any one of its components, including preservatives.

INTERACTIONS

Drug

Anticoagulants or antiplatelet agents: May increase the risk of injection site bleeding.

Herbal
None known.
Food
None known.

DIAGNOSTIC TEST EFFECTS
None known.

SIDE EFFECTS
Occasional
Arthralgia, back pain, pain at injection site.
Rare
Joint stiffness, swelling.

SERIOUS REACTIONS
- Transient increases in inflammation in the injected knee following hyaluronan injection have been reported in some patients with OA.
- Rare allergic reactions.

PRECAUTIONS & CONSIDERATIONS
Be aware that the safety and effectiveness of hyaluronan have not been established in joints other than the knee. Be aware that use of disinfectants containing quartenary ammonium salts for skin preparation as hyaluronic acid can precipitate in their presence. Safety and efficacy of this drug have not been tested in pregnant, nursing women, or children. No age-related precautions have been noted in elderly patients. Strenuous activity or weight-bearing activities should be avoided within 48 h following injection.
Storage
Store syringes at room temperature. Do not freeze.
Administration
Be aware that the prefilled syringe is for single use only. Discard syringe after administering. Remove the protective rubber cap on the tip of the syringe, and attach small-gauge needle (18-21 gauge) to the tip. Inject full contents of syringe into one knee. If treatment is bilateral, use a separate syringe for each knee.

Hydralazine
hye-dral'a-zeen
(Canada) Apresoline, Nu-Hydral, Novo-Hylazin
Do not confuse hydralazine with hydroxyzine.

CATEGORY AND SCHEDULE
Pregnancy Risk Category: C

Classification: Vasodilators, antihypertensive

MECHANISM OF ACTION
An antihypertensive with direct vasodilating effects on arterioles. *Therapeutic Effect:* Decreases BP and systemic resistance.

PHARMACOKINETICS

Route	Onset (min)	Peak	Duration
PO	20-30	N/A	2-4 h
IV	5-20	N/A	2-6 h

Well absorbed from the GI tract. Widely distributed. Protein binding: 85%-90%. Metabolized in the liver to active metabolite. Primarily excreted in urine. Not removed by hemodialysis. *Half-life:* 3-7 h (increased with impaired renal function).

AVAILABILITY
Tablets: 10 mg, 25 mg, 50 mg, 100 mg.
Injection: 20 mg/mL.

INDICATIONS AND DOSAGES
▸ **Moderate to severe hypertension**
PO
Adults. Initially, 10 mg 4 times a day. May increase by 10-25 mg/dose q2-5 days. Maximum: 300 mg/day.
Children. Initially, 0.75-1 mg/kg/day in 2-4 divided doses, not to exceed

25 mg/dose. May increase over 3-4 wks. Maximum: 7.5 mg/kg/day (5 mg/kg/day in infants).
IV, IM
Adults, Elderly. Initially, 10-20 mg/dose q4-6h. Maximum: 20 mg per dose IV, 50 mg IM.
Children. Initially, 0.1-0.2 mg/kg/dose (maximum 20 mg) q4-6h, as needed, up to 1.7-3.5 mg/kg/day in divided doses q4-6h.

▸ **Dosage in renal impairment**
Dosage interval is based on creatinine clearance.

CrCl (mL/min)	Dosage Interval
10-50	q8h
< 10	q8-24h

OFF-LABEL USES
Treatment of congestive heart failure, hypertension secondary to eclampsia and preeclampsia, primary pulmonary hypertension.

CONTRAINDICATIONS
Hypersensitivity to hydralazine; coronary artery disease; mitral valvular rheumatic heart disease.

INTERACTIONS
Drug
Diuretics, other antihypertensives: May increase hypotensive effect.
Herbal
Licorice, ma huang, yohimbine: May decrease the effectiveness of hydralazine.
Food
None known.

DIAGNOSTIC TEST EFFECTS
May produce positive direct Coombs' test.

IV INCOMPATIBILITIES
Do not add hydralazine to any IV solutions. Aminophylline, ampicillin (Polycillin), chlorothiazide (Diuril), edetate calcium disodium, ethacrynate (Edecrin), furosemide (Lasix), hydrocortisone sodium succinate (Solu-Cortef), methohexital (Brevital), nitroglycerin (Nitrobid), phenobarbital, verapamil (Calan).

SIDE EFFECTS
Frequent
Headache, palpitations, tachycardia (generally disappears in 7-10 days).
Occasional
GI disturbance (nausea, vomiting, diarrhea), paresthesia, fluid retention, peripheral edema, dizziness, flushed face, nasal congestion.

SERIOUS REACTIONS
- High dosage may produce lupus erythematosus-like reaction, including fever, facial rash, muscle and joint aches, and splenomegaly.
- Severe orthostatic hypotension, skin flushing, severe headache, myocardial ischemia, and cardiac arrhythmias may develop.
- Peripheral neuritis (paresthesia, numbness, and tingling). Published evidence suggests an antipyridoxine effect. Pyridoxine should be added to regimen if symptoms develop.
- Profound shock may occur with severe overdosage.

PRECAUTIONS & CONSIDERATIONS
Hydralazine may produce a clinical picture simulating systemic lupus erythematosus, including glomerulonephritis. In such patients hydralazine should usually be discontinued. Caution is warranted with cerebrovascular disease, pulmonary hypertension, and impaired renal function. Hydralazine crosses the placenta; it is unknown whether

it is distributed in breast milk. Hematomas, leukopenia, petechial bleeding, and thrombocytopenia have occurred in newborns; these conditions resolve within 1-3 wks. No age-related precautions have been noted in children. Elderly patients are more sensitive to the drug's hypotensive effects. In elderly patients, age-related renal impairment may require dosage adjustment.

Dizziness and light-headedness may occur. Rise slowly from a lying to a sitting position, and permit legs to dangle from the bed momentarily before standing to reduce the hypotensive effect of hydralazine. Those receiving high doses of hydralazine should notify the physician if fever (lupus-like reaction) or joint and muscle aches occur. Also, notify the physician if headache, palpitations, tachycardia, or peripheral edema of the hands and feet occurs. BP and pulse should be obtained immediately before each hydralazine dose, in addition to regular BP monitoring. Be alert for BP fluctuations. Daily bowel activity and stool consistency should also be monitored.

Storage

Store drug at room temperature. Use injection immediately after the vial is opened. Injection may discolor upon contact with metal; discolored solutions should be discarded.

Administration

Hydralazine is best given with food or regularly spaced meals. Crush tablets if necessary.

For IV use, give undiluted. Do not add to infusion solutions. Give single dose IV at a rate not to exceed 10 mg/min. Hydralazine injection may also be given IM if needed.

Hydrochlorothiazide

hye-droe-klor-oh-thye′a-zide

★ Ezide, Microzide

🍁 Apo-Hydro, Nu-Hydro, Novo-Hydrazide, Urozide

CATEGORY AND SCHEDULE

Pregnancy Risk Category: B (D if used in pregnancy-induced hypertension)

Classification: Diuretics, thiazide and derivatives

MECHANISM OF ACTION

A sulfonamide derivative that acts as a thiazide diuretic, and antihypertensive. As a diuretic, blocks reabsorption of water, sodium, and potassium at the cortical diluting segment of the distal tubule. As an antihypertensive, reduces plasma, extracellular fluid volume, and peripheral vascular resistance by direct effect on blood vessels. *Therapeutic Effect:* Promotes diuresis; reduces BP.

PHARMACOKINETICS

Route	Onset	Peak	Duration
PO (diuretic)	2 h	4-6 h	6-12 h

Variably absorbed from the GI tract. Primarily excreted unchanged in urine. Not removed by hemodialysis. *Half-life:* 5.6-14.8 h.

AVAILABILITY

*Capsules (Microzide):*12.5 mg.
Oral Solution: 50 mg/5 mL.
Tablets: 12.5 mg, 25 mg, 50 mg,

INDICATIONS AND DOSAGES

▸ **Edema, hypertension**

PO

Adults. 12.5-100 mg/day, given in 1-2 divided doses. Maximum: 200 mg/day.

▸ **Usual pediatric dosage**

PO

Children 6 mo to 12 yr. 1-2 mg/kg/day once daily or in 2 divided doses. Maximum for aged 2-12 yr: 100 mg/day. Maximum for up to 2 yr: 12.5-37.5 mg/day.

Infants younger than 6 mo. 2-3 mg/kg/day in 2 divided doses.

OFF-LABEL USES

Treatment of diabetes insipidus, prevention of calcium-containing renal calculi.

CONTRAINDICATIONS

Anuria, history of hypersensitivity to thiazide diuretics or other sulfonamide derivatives.

INTERACTIONS

Drug

β-Blockers: May increase hyperglycemic effects in type 2 diabetics.

Cholestyramine, colestipol: May decrease the absorption and effects of hydrochlorothiazide.

Cyclosporine: Concurrent use with hydrochlorothiazide may increase the risk of gout or renal toxicity.

Digoxin: May increase the risk of digoxin toxicity associated with hydrochlorothiazide-induced hypokalemia.

Lithium: May increase the risk of lithium toxicity.

Neuromuscular blocking agents: May prolong blockade.

Herbal

Ephedra, ginseng, ginkgo biloba, ma huang, yohimbine: May increase BP.

Garlic: May have additive hypotensive effects.

Licorice: May increase risk of hypokalemia and reduce the effectiveness of hydrochlorothiazide.

Food

None known.

DIAGNOSTIC TEST EFFECTS

May increase blood glucose and serum cholesterol, LDL, bilirubin, calcium, creatinine, uric acid, and triglyceride levels. May decrease urinary calcium levels and serum magnesium, potassium, and sodium levels.

SIDE EFFECTS

Expected

Increase in urinary frequency and urine volume.

Frequent

Potassium depletion.

Occasional

Orthostatic hypotension, headache, GI disturbances, photosensitivity.

SERIOUS REACTIONS

• Vigorous diuresis may lead to profound water and electrolyte depletion, resulting in hypokalemia, hyponatremia, and dehydration.
• Acute hypotensive episodes may occur.
• Hyperglycemia may occur during prolonged therapy.
• Pancreatitis, blood dyscrasias, pulmonary edema, allergic pneumonitis, and dermatologic reactions occur rarely.
• Overdose can lead to lethargy and coma without changes in electrolytes or hydration.

PRECAUTIONS & CONSIDERATIONS

Caution is warranted in patients with diabetes mellitus, gout, thyroid disorders, hepatic impairment, severe renal disease, and in elderly patients and debilitated patients. Hydrochlorothiazide crosses the placenta, and a small amount is distributed in breast milk. Breastfeeding is not recommended.

No age-related precautions have been noted in children, except that jaundiced infants may be at risk for hyperbilirubinemia. Elderly patients may be more sensitive to the drug's electrolyte and hypotensive effects. Age-related renal impairment may require cautious use in elderly patients. Consuming foods high in potassium such as apricots, bananas, legumes, meat, orange juice, raisins, whole grains, including cereals, and white and sweet potatoes, is encouraged. Avoid prolonged exposure to sunlight and ultraviolet rays because a photosensitivity reaction may occur.

Dizziness or light-headedness may occur, so change positions slowly and let legs dangle momentarily before standing. An increase in the frequency and volume of urination may also occur. BP, vital signs, electrolytes, intake and output, and weight should be monitored before and during treatment. Be aware of signs of electrolyte disturbances such as hypokalemia or hyponatremia. Hypokalemia may cause arrhythmias, altered mental status, muscle cramps, asthenia, and tremor. Hyponatremia may result in cold and clammy skin, confusion, and thirst.

Storage

Store at room temperature and protect from light, moisture, and do not freeze.

Administration

Take hydrochlorothiazide with food or milk if GI upset occurs, preferably with breakfast to help prevent nocturia. Tablets may be crushed and mixed with fluid, if necessary.

Hydrocodone

hye-droe-koe′done

★ Hydrocodone and acetaminophen. Co-Gesic, Dolorex Forte, Duocet, Hycet, Hydrocet, Lorcet, Lorcet Plus, Lortab, Margesic H, Maxidone, Norco, Polygesic, Stagesic, Vicodin, Vicodin ES, Vicodin HP, Xodol, Zydone hydrocodone and chlorpheniramine (Tussionex, Tussicaps); hydrocodone and guaifenesin (Codiclear DH, Kwelcof, Vitussin, Xpect-HC); hydrocodone and homatropine (Hydromet, Mycodone, Tussigon); hydrocodone and ibuprofen (Reprexain, Vicoprofen); hydrocodone and pseudoephedrine (P-V Tussin)

CATEGORY AND SCHEDULE

Pregnancy Risk Category: C (D if used for prolonged periods, high dosages at term)

Controlled Substance Schedule: III

Classification: Antitussive, narcotic analgesic, opiate derivative, phenathrene derivative

MECHANISM OF ACTION

Hydrocodone blocks pain perception in the cerebral cortex by binding to specific opiate receptors (μ and κ). This binding results in a decreased synaptic chemical transmission throughout the central nervous system (CNS), thus inhibiting the flow of pain sensations into the higher centers.

Therapeutic Effect: Alters perception of pain and produces analgesic effect. Reduces coughing.

PHARMACOKINETICS

Well absorbed. Metabolized in liver. Excreted in urine. *Half-life:* 3.3-3.4 h.

AVAILABILITY

NOTE: Other products may exist on the market; the following listing includes the more common brands available.

Hydrocodone and Acetaminophen

Acetaminophen/Hydrocodone Capsule (5/500): *Dolorex Forte, Polygesic, Margesic H, Stagesic.*
Acetaminophen/Hydrocodone Tablet (5/300): *Xodol 5/300.*
Acetaminophen/Hydrocodone Tablet (5/325): *Norco 5/325.*
Acetaminophen/Hydrocodone Tablet (5/400): *Zydone 5/400.*
Acetaminophen/Hydrocodone Tablet (5/500): *Vicodin, Lortab 5/500, Co-Gesic, Duocet.*
Acetaminophen/Hydrocodone Tablet (7.5/300): *Xodol 7.5/300.*
Acetaminophen/Hydrocodone Tablet (7.5/325): *Norco 7.5/325.*
Acetaminophen/Hydrocodone Tablet (7.5/400): *Zydone 7.5/400.*
Acetaminophen/Hydrocodone Tablet (7.5/500): *Lortab 7.5/500.*
Acetaminophen/Hydrocodone Tablet (7.5/650): *Lorcet Plus.*
Acetaminophen/Hydrocodone Tablet (7.5/750): *Vicodin ES.*
Acetaminophen/Hydrocodone Tablet (10/300): *Xodol 10/300.*
Acetaminophen/Hydrocodone Tablet (10/325): *Norco 10/325.*
Acetaminophen/Hydrocodone Tablet (10/400): *Zydone 10/400.*
Acetaminophen/Hydrocodone Tablet (10/500): *Lortab 10/500.*
Acetaminophen/Hydrocodone Tablet (10/650): *Lorcet.*
Acetaminophen/Hydrocodone Tablet (10/660): *Vicodin HP.*
Acetaminophen/Hydrocodone Tablet (10/750): *Maxidone.*

Hydrocodone and Chlorpheniramine

Oral Suspension, Extended Release: Hydrocodone polistirex 10 mg and chlorpheniramine polistirex 8 mg/5 mL (Tussionex).
Capsules, Extended Release: Hydrocodone polistirex 10 mg and chlorpheniramine polistirex 8 mg per capsule OR hydrocodone polistirex 5 mg and chlorpheniramine polistirex 4 mg per capsule (Tussicaps).

Hydrocodone and Guaifenesin

Liquid: Hydrocodone bitartrate 5 mg and guaifenesin 100 mg/5 mL (Codiclear DH, Kwelcof, Vitussin).
Tablets: Hydrocodone bitartrate 5 mg and guaifenesin 600 mg (Xpect-HC).

Hydrocodone and Homatropine

Syrup: Hydrocodone bitartrate 5 mg and homatropine methylbromide 1.5 mg/5 mL (Hydromet, Mycodone).
Tablets: Hydrocodone bitartrate 5 mg and homatropine methylbromide 1.5 mg (Tussigon).

Hydrocodone and Ibuprofen

Tablets: Hydrocodone bitartrate 5 mg and ibuprofen 200 mg (Reprexain), hydrocodone bitartrate 7.5 mg and ibuprofen 200 mg (Vicoprofen).

Hydrocodone and Pseudoephedrine

Tablets: Hydrocodone bitartrate 5 mg and pseudoephedrine 60 mg (P-V Tussin).

INDICATIONS AND DOSAGES

NOTE: Due to the many available product combinations and dosage forms, dose recommendations may vary from product to product. The most common dosages are listed here. Check prescribing information for the specific product chosen.

▸ **Hydrocodone and acetaminophen**

Analgesia

PO (DOSAGE GIVEN AS HYDROCODONE)
Adults, Children older than 13 yr or > 50 kg. 2.5-10 mg q4-6h. Maximum: 60 mg/day hydrocodone. Maximum dose of acetaminophen: 4 g/day.

Elderly. 2.5-5 mg hydrocodone q4-6h. Titrate dose to appropriate analgesic effect. Maximum: 4 g/day acetaminophen.
Children 2-13 yr or < 50 kg. 0.135 mg/kg/dose hydrocodone q4-6h. Maximum: 6 doses/day of hydrocodone or maximum recommended dose of acetaminophen. See weight-based dosage chart in manufacturer's prescribing information for liquid dosage forms.

▸ **Hydrocodone and chlorpheniramine**
Adults, Elderly, Children 12 yr and older. 5 mL q12h. Maximum: 10 mL/24h.
Children 6-12 yr. 2.5 mL q12h. Maximum: 5 mL/24h.

▸ **Hydrocodone and guaifenesin**
Adults, Elderly, Children 12 yr and older. 5 mL q4h. Maximum: 30 mL/24h.
Children 2-12 yr. 2.5 mL q4h.
Children < 2 yr. 0.3 mg/kg/day (hydrocodone) in 4 divided doses.

▸ **Hydrocodone and homatropine**
Adults, Elderly. 10 mg (hydrocodone) q4-6h. A single dose should not exceed 15 mg and not more frequently than q4h.
Children. 0.6 mg/kg/day (hydrocodone) in 3-4 divided doses. Do not administer more frequently than q4h.

▸ **Hydrocodone and ibuprofen**
Adults. 7.5-15 mg (hydrocodone) q4-6h as needed for pain. Maximum: 5 tablets/day.

▸ **Hydrocodone and pseudoephedrine**
Adults, Elderly. 1 tablet q4-6h as needed, up to 4 doses/day.

CONTRAINDICATIONS

Central nervous system (CNS) depression, severe respiratory depression, hypersensitivity to hydrocodone or to any component of the formulation.

INTERACTIONS

Drug

Alcohol, CNS depressants: May increase hypotension and CNS or respiratory depression.
CYP2D6 inhibitors (e.g., chlorpromazine): May decrease the effects of hydrocodone.
Hepatotoxic medications (e.g., phenytoin), liver enzyme inducers (e.g., cimetidine): May increase the risk of hepatotoxicity associated with acetaminophen with prolonged high dose or single toxic dose.
MAOIs, tricyclic antidepressants: May increase effects of MAOIs and TCAs and hydrocodone.
Warfarin: May increase the risk of bleeding with regular use.

Herbal

Valerian, St. John's wort, SAMe, kava kava: May increase sedative effects.

Food

None known.

DIAGNOSTIC TEST EFFECTS

None known.

SIDE EFFECTS

Frequent

Dizziness, sedation, drowsiness, bradycardia.

Occasional

Anxiety, dysphoria, euphoria, fear, lethargy, light-headedness, malaise, mental clouding, mental impairment, mood changes, physiologic dependence, sedation, somnolence, constipation, bradycardia, heartburn, nausea, vomiting.

Rare

Hypersensitivity reaction, rash.

SERIOUS REACTIONS

• Cardiac arrest, circulatory collapse, coma, hypotension, hypoglycemic coma, ureteral spasm, urinary retention, vesical sphincter

spasm, agranulocytosis, bleeding time prolonged, hemolytic anemia, iron deficiency anemia, occult blood loss thrombocytopenia, hepatic necrosis, hepatits, skeletal muscle rigidity, renal toxicity, and renal tubular necrosis have been reported.
• Hearing impairment or loss has been reported with chronic overdose.
• Acute airway obstruction, apnea, dyspnea, and respiratory depression occur rarely and are usually dose related.

PRECAUTIONS & CONSIDERATIONS

Caution is warranted with hypersensitivity reactions to other phenanthrene derivative opioid agonists (morphine, hydrocodone, hydromorphone, levorphanol, oxycodone, oxymorphone). Be aware that tablets with metabisulfite may cause allergic reactions. Information is not available for hydrocodone during pregnancy. The manufacturers recommend discontinuing the medication or to discontinue nursing during therapy. Be aware that hydrocodone should be used cautiously in children and elderly patients.

Drug dependence or tolerance may occur with prolonged use of high dosages. Avoid alcohol and tasks that require mental alertness or motor skills. Change positions slowly to avoid orthostatic hypotension. Be aware that ambulatory persons and those not in severe pain may experience dizziness, hypotension, nausea, and vomiting more frequently than patients in the supine position or with severe pain. Be aware to expect to reduce the initial dosage in those with concurrent central nervous system (CNS) depressants, elderly, and debilitated.

Storage
Store at room temperature.

Administration
Take without regard to meals. Shake any oral liquid or suspension well before use to avoid improper dosing.

Extended-release products should not be crushed or chewed. Do not exceed maximum dosages for any given product or combination. NOTE: Maximum acetaminophen PO dosage 4000 mg/day in adults and 75 mg/kg/day in children.

H

Hydrocortisone

hye-dro-kor′ti-sone

★ A-HydroCort, Anusol-HC, Caldecort, Cortaid, Cortef, Cortizone-5, Cortizone-10, Hytone, Locoid, Nupercainal Hydrocortisone Cream, Preparation-H, Hydrocortisone, Protocort, Solu-Cortef, Westcort

🍁 A-HydroCort, Anusol-HC, Cortef, Solu-Cortef

CATEGORY AND SCHEDULE

Pregnancy Risk Category: C (D if used in first trimester)
OTC (hydrocortisone 0.5% and 1% cream, gel, and ointment)

Classification: Corticosteroids, topical, dermatologics, anti-inflammatory

MECHANISM OF ACTION

An adrenocortical steroid that inhibits the accumulation of inflammatory cells at inflammation sites, phagocytosis, lysosomal enzyme release, and synthesis and release of mediators of inflammation. *Therapeutic Effect:* Prevents or suppresses cell-mediated immune reactions. Decreases or prevents tissue response to inflammatory process.

PHARMACOKINETICS

Route	Onset	Peak	Duration
IV	N/A	4-6 h	8-12 h

Well absorbed after IM administration. Widely distributed. Metabolized in the liver. *Half-life:* Plasma, 1.5-2 h; biologic, 8-12 h.

AVAILABILITY

Tablet (Cortef): 5 mg, 10 mg, 20 mg.
Cream (Rectal [Nupercainal Hydrocortisone Cream, Cortizone-10, Preparation-H Hydrocortisone]): 1%.
Cream (Topical [Cortizone-5]): 0.5%.
Cream (Topical [Caldecort, Cortizone-10]): 1%.
Cream (Topical [Hytone]): 2.5%.
Ointment (Topical [Locoid]): 0.1%.
Ointment (Topical [Westcort]): 0.2%.
Ointment (Topical [Cortizone-5]): 0.5%.
Ointment (Topical [Anusol-HC, Cortaid, Cortizone-10]): 1%.
Ointment (Topical [Hytone]): 2.5%.
Suppositories (Anusol-HC): 25 mg.
Suppositories (Emcort, Protocort): 30 mg.
Injection (A-HydroCort, Solu-Cortef): 100 mg, 250 mg, 500 mg, 1 g.

INDICATIONS AND DOSAGES

▸ **Acute adrenal insufficiency**
IV
Adults, Elderly. 100 mg IV bolus; then 300 mg/day in divided doses q8h.
Children. 1-2 mg/kg IV bolus; then 150-250 mg/day in divided doses q6-8h.
Infants. 1-2 mg/kg/dose IV bolus; then 25-150 mg/day in divided doses q6-8h.

▸ **Anti-inflammation, immunosuppression**
IV, IM
Adults, Elderly. 15-240 mg q12h.
Children. 1-5 mg/kg/day in divided doses q12h.

▸ **Physiologic replacement**
PO
Children. 0.5-0.75 mg/kg/day in divided doses q8h.
IM
Children. 0.25-0.35 mg/kg/day as a single dose.

▸ **Corticosteroid Responsive Dermatoses**
TOPICAL
Adults, Children. Apply topical product of choice to the affected area as a thin film 2 or 3 times daily depending on the severity of the condition.

▸ **Status asthmaticus**
IV
Adults, Elderly. 100-500 mg q6h.
Children. 2 mg/kg/dose q6h.

▸ **Shock**
IV
Adults, Elderly, Children 12 yr and older. 100-500 mg q6h.

▸ **Adjunctive treatment of ulcerative colitis**
RECTAL (RETENTION ENEMA)
Adults, Elderly. 100 mg at bedtime for 21 nights or until clinical and proctologic remission occurs (may require 2-3 mo of therapy).
RECTAL SUPPOSITORIES
Adults. Suppository 2-3 times/day. Usually for 2 wks.
RECTAL (CORTIFOAM)
Adults, Elderly. 1 applicator 1-2 times a day for 2-3 wks, then every second day until therapy ends.

▸ **Hemorrhoidal irritation**
TOPICAL
Adults, Elderly. Apply sparingly 2-4 times a day.

CONTRAINDICATIONS

Fungal, tuberculosis, or viral skin lesions; serious infections.

INTERACTIONS

Drug

Amphotericin: May increase hypokalemia.

Cyclosporine: May increase the effects of cyclosporine.

Digoxin: May increase the risk of digoxin toxicity caused by hypokalemia.

Diuretics, insulin, oral hypoglycemics, potassium supplements: May decrease the effects of these drugs.

Hepatic enzyme inducers: May decrease the effects of hydrocortisone.

Live-virus vaccines: May decrease the patient's antibody response to vaccine, increase vaccine side effects, and potentiate virus replication.

Herbal

Cat's claw, echinacea: Avoid use because of its immunostimulant properties.

St. John's wort: May decrease hydrocortisone levels.

Food

Calcium: May interfere with calcium absorption.

DIAGNOSTIC TEST EFFECTS

May increase blood glucose and serum lipid, amylase, and sodium levels. May decrease serum calcium, potassium, and thyroxine levels.

IV INCOMPATIBILITIES

Bleomycin (Blenoxane), ciprofloxacin (Cipro), diazepam (Valium), doxapram (Dopram), ephedrine, hydralazine (Apresoline), idarubicin (Idamycin), midazolam (Versed), nafcillin (Unipen), pentobarbital (Nembutal), phenobarbital, phenytoin (Dilantin), prochlorperazine (Compazine), promethazine (Phenergan), sargramostim (Leukine).

IV COMPATIBILITIES

Acyclovir (Zovirax), allopurinol (Alloprim), amikacin (Amikin), amifostine (Ethyol), aminophylline, amphotericin, ampicillin (Polycillin), amsacrine (Amsa), atracurium (Tracrium), atropine, aztreonam (Azactam), betamethasone sodium phosphate (Celestone), calcium gluconate, cefepime (Maxipime), chloramphenicol (Chloromycetin), chlordiazepoxide (Librium), chlorpromazine (Thorazine), cisatracurium (Nimbex), cladribine (Leustatin), clindamycin (Cleocin), corticotropin, cyanocobalamin, cytarabine (Cytosar), daunorubicin (Cerubidine), dexamethasone sodium phosphate (Decadron), digoxin (Lanoxin), diltiazem (Cardizem), diphenhydramine (Benadryl), docetaxel (Taxotere), dopamine (Intropin), doxorubicin (Rubex), droperidol (Inapsine), edrophonium (Tensilon), enalaprilat (Vasotec), epinephrine, erythromycin (Erythrocin), esmolol (BreviBloc), estrogens (conjugated), ethacrynate sodium (edecrin), etoposide (VePesid), famotidine (Pepcid), fentanyl (Sublimaze), filgrastim (Neupogen), fludarabine (Fludara), fluorouracil (Efurix), foscarnet (Foscavir), furosemide (Lasix), gatifloxacin (Tequin), gemcitabine (Gemzar), granisetron (Kytril), heparin, inamrinone (Inocor), insulin, isoproterenol (Isuprel), kanamycin (Kantrex), lidocaine, linezolid (Zyvox), lorazepam (Ativan), magnesium sulfate, meperidine (Demerol), metronidazole (Flagyl), metoclopramide (Reglan), methoxamine (Vasoxyl), methylergonovine (Methergine), minocycline (Minocin), mitomycin (Mutamycin), mitoxantrone (Novantrone), morphine, neostigmine, norepinephrine (Levophed), ondansetron (Zofran), oxacillin (Floxin), oxytocin (Pitocin), paclitaxel (Taxol), pancuronium (Pavulon), penicillin G potassium (Pfizerpen), pentazocine (Talwin), phytonadione, piperacillin/tazobactam (Zosyn), potassium chloride, procainamide (Pronestyl), propofol (Diprivan), propranolol (Inderal), pyridostigmine, remifentanil (Ultiva), scopolamine, sodium bicarbonate, succinylcholine (Anectine), tacrolimus (Prograf), teniposide (Vumon), theophylline (Theodur), thiopental (Pentothal), thiotepa (Thioplex), trimethaphan camsylate (Arfonad), trimethobenzamide (Tigan), vancomycin (Vancocin), vecuronium (Norcuron), verapamil (Calan), vinorelbine (Navelbine).

SIDE EFFECTS

Frequent

Insomnia, heartburn, nervousness, abdominal distention, diaphoresis, acne, mood swings, increased appetite, facial flushing, delayed wound healing, increased susceptibility to infection, diarrhea, or constipation.

Occasional

Headache, edema, change in skin color, frequent urination.
Topical: Itching, redness, irritation.

Rare

Tachycardia, allergic reaction (such as rash and hives), psychologic changes, hallucinations, depression.
Topical: Allergic contact dermatitis, purpura.
Systemic: Absorption more likely with use of occlusive dressings or extensive application in young children.

SERIOUS REACTIONS

- Long-term therapy may cause hypocalcemia, hypokalemia, muscle wasting (especially in arms and legs), osteoporosis, spontaneous fractures, amenorrhea, cataracts, glaucoma, peptic ulcer disease, and congestive heart failure.
- Abruptly withdrawing the drug after long-term therapy may cause anorexia, nausea, fever, headache, sudden severe joint pain, rebound inflammation, fatigue, weakness, lethargy, dizziness, and orthostatic hypotension.
- Chronic corticosteroids raise risk of immunosuppression and resultant increased risk for infection.
- Long-term use may increase intraocular pressure or produce cataracts.

PRECAUTIONS & CONSIDERATIONS

Caution is warranted in patients with cirrhosis, congestive heart failure, diabetes mellitus, hypertension, hyperthyroidism, osteoporosis, peptic ulcer disease, seizure disorders, thromboembolic tendencies, thrombophlebitis, and ulcerative colitis. Hydrocortisone crosses the placenta and is distributed in breast milk. Persons taking hydrocortisone should not breastfeed. Prolonged hydrocortisone use during the first trimester of pregnancy may produce cleft palate in the neonate. Prolonged treatment or high dosages may decrease the cortisol secretion and short-term growth rate in children. Elderly patients may be more susceptible to developing hypertension or osteoporosis. Dentist and other physicians should be informed of hydrocortisone therapy if taken within the past 12 mo. Consult with the physician before taking aspirin or other medications. Avoid alcohol, and limit caffeine intake. Hydrocortisone should not be overused for symptomatic relief.

Mood swings, ranging from euphoria to depression, may occur.

Notify the physician of fever, muscle aches, sore throat, and sudden weight gain or swelling. Blood glucose level, intake and output, BP, serum electrolyte levels, height, and weight should be monitored before and during therapy. Be alert to signs and symptoms of infection caused by reduced immune response, including fever, sore throat, and vague symptoms. In long-term therapy, signs and symptoms of hypocalcemia or hypokalemia (such as ECG changes, weakness and muscle cramps, and numbness or tingling, especially in the lower extremities) should be assessed.

Storage

Store at room temperature. After reconstitution, store hydrocortisone sodium succinate solution at room temperature and use within 72 h.

Administration

For IV administration, use immediately if further diluted with D5W, 0.9% NaCl, or other compatible diluent. For hydrocortisone sodium succinate IV push, dilute to 50 mg/mL; for intermittent infusion, dilute to 1 mg/mL. Administer hydrocortisone sodium succinate solution IV push over 3-5 min. Give intermittent infusion over 20-30 min.

For topical use, gently cleanse area before applying drug; apply topical hydrocortisone valerate after bath or shower for best absorption. Apply sparingly, and rub into area thoroughly. Use occlusive dressings only as ordered.

For rectal use of suppository, moisten the suppository with cold water before inserting it well into the rectum.

For rectal enema use, shake homogeneous suspension well. Lie on the left side with left leg extended and right leg flexed. Gently insert applicator tip into rectum, pointed slightly toward umbilicus, and slowly instill medication.

Hydrocortisone therapy should not be abruptly discontinued. Taper slowly to avoid disease flare or withdrawal symptoms.

Hydromorphone

hye-droe-mor′fone

Dilaudid, Dilaudid HP, Exalgo

Dilaudid, Dilaudid XP, Hydromorph Contin, Jurnista

Do not confuse with morphine or Dilantin.

CATEGORY AND SCHEDULE

Pregnancy Risk Category: C (D if used for prolonged periods or at high dosages at term)

Controlled Substance Schedule: II

Classification: Analgesics, narcotic

MECHANISM OF ACTION

An opioid agonist that binds to opioid receptors in the CNS, reducing the intensity of pain stimuli from sensory nerve endings. *Therapeutic Effect:* Alters the perception of and emotional response to pain; suppresses cough reflex.

PHARMACOKINETICS

Route	Onset (min)	Peak (min)	Duration (h)
PO	30	90-120	4
IV	10-15	15-30	2-3
IM	15	30-60	4-5
Subcutaneous	15	30-90	4
Rectal	15-30	N/A	N/A

Well absorbed from the GI tract after IM administration. Widely distributed. Metabolized in the liver. Excreted in urine. *Half-life:* 1-3 h.

AVAILABILITY

Liquid (Dilaudid): 5 mg/5 mL.
Tablets (Dilaudid): 2 mg, 4 mg, 8 mg.
Injection (Dilaudid): 1 mg/mL, 2 mg/mL, 4 mg/mL.
Injection (Dilaudid HP): 10 mg/mL.
Suppository (Dilaudid): 3 mg.
Extended-Release Tablets (Exalgo): 8 mg, 12 mg, 16 mg.

H

INDICATIONS AND DOSAGES

▸ **Analgesia**

PO (IMMEDIATE-RELEASE)

Adults, Elderly, Children weighing 50 kg and more. 2-4 mg q3-4h. Usual Single Dose Range: 2-8 mg/dose.
Children older than 6 mo and weighing < 50 kg. 0.03-0.08 mg/kg/dose q3-4h.

IV

Adults, Elderly, Children weighing more than 50 kg. 0.2-0.6 mg q2-3h.
Children weighing 50 kg or less. 0.015 mg/kg/dose q3-6h as needed.

RECTAL

Adults, Elderly. 3 mg q6-8h.

▸ **Patient-controlled analgesia (PCA)**

IV

Adults, Elderly. 0.05-0.5 mg at 5-15 min lockout. Maximum (4-h): 4-6 mg.

EPIDURAL

Adults, Elderly. Bolus dose of 1-1.5 mg at rate of 0.04-0.4 mg/h. Demand dose of 0.15 mg at 30-min lockout.

▸ **For moderate to severe pain in opioid-tolerant patients:**

PO (conversion from immediate release hydromorphone to extended-release tablets—EXALGO)
Adults. May be converted to Exalgo by giving the total daily immediate-release oral hydromorphone dose once daily. If necessary, titrate q3-4days until adequate pain relief with tolerable side effects has been achieved.

PO (conversion from other oral opioid analgesics to EXALGO)
Adults. For conversion from other opioids to Exalgo, utilize relative potency information, understanding that conversion ratios are approximate. In general, initiate hydromorphone extended-release tablets at 50% of the calculated total daily equivalent; give the dose q24h. Titrate not more often than q3-4 days.

PO (conversion from transdermal fentanyl patch to EXALGO)
Adults. Initiate Exalgo 18 h after removal of a transdermal fentanyl patch. For each 25-mcg/h dose of transdermal fentanyl, the equianalgesic dose of Exalgo is roughly 12 mg q24h. An appropriate starting dose is 50% of the calculated Exalgo dose; give every 24h. Titrate patients to adequate pain relief with dose increases not more often than q3-4days.

CONTRAINDICATIONS

Respiratory depression in the absence of resuscitative equipment, status asthmatics, depressed ventilatory function, obstetric anesthesia, severe CNS depression, pregnancy.

INTERACTIONS

Drug

Alcohol, other CNS depressants: May increase CNS or respiratory depression and hypotension.
MAOIs: May produce a severe, sometimes fatal, reaction; plan to administer one quarter of the usual hydromorphone dose. When possible, MAOI therapy should generally be discontinued 14 days prior to use.
Selective serotonin reuptake inhibitors (SSRIs): May cause additive serotonergic symptoms leading to serotonin syndrome.

Herbal
Gotu kola, kava kava, St. John's wort, valerian: May cause additive sedative effects.
Food
None known.

DIAGNOSTIC TEST EFFECTS

May increase serum amylase and lipase concentrations.

IV INCOMPATIBILITIES

Amphotericin B complex (Abelcet, AmBisome, Amphotec), ampicillin (Polycillin), cefazolin (Ancef, Kefzol), diazepam (Valium), hyaluronidase (Wydase), minocycline (Minocin), phenobarbital, phenytoin (Dilantin), sargramostim (Leukine), sodium bicarbonate, tetracycline (Sumycin), thiopental (Pentothal).

IV COMPATIBILITIES

Acyclovir (Zovirax), albuterol (Ventolin), allopurinol (Alloprim), amifostine (Ethyol), amikacin (Amikin), amsacrine (Amsa), atropine, aztreonam (Azactam), bupivacaine (Marcaine), cefamandole (Mandol), cefepime (Maxipime), cefoperazone (Cefobid), cefotaxime (Claforan), cefoxitin (Mefixitin), ceftazidime (Fortaz), ceftizoxime (Cefizox), cefuroxime (Zinacef), chloramphenicol (Chloromycetin), chlorpromazine (Thorazine), cimetidine (Tagamet), cisatracurium (Nimbex), cisplatin (Platinol-AQ), cladribine (Leustatin), clindamycin (Cleocin), cyclophosphamide (Cytoxan), cytarabine (Cytosar), diltiazem (Cardizem), dimenhydrinate (Dramamine), diphenhydramine (Benadryl), dobutamine (Dobutrex), docetaxel (Taxotere), dopamine (Intropin), doxorubicin (Rubex), doxycycline (Vibramycin), epinephrine, erythromycin lactobionate (Erythrocin), etoposide (VePesid), famotidine (Pepcid), fentanyl (Sublimaze), filgrastim (Neupogen), fludarabine (Fludara), fluorouracil (Efurix), foscarnet (Foscavir), furosemide (Lasix), gatifloxacin (Tequin), gemcitabine (Gemzar), gentamicin (Garamycin), glycopyrrolate (Robinul), granisetron (Kytril), haloperidol (Haldol), heparin, hydroxyzine (Vistaril), kanamycin (Kantrex), labetalol (Normodyne, Trandate), linezolid (Zyvox), lorazepam (Ativan), magnesium sulfate, melphalan (Alkeran), methotrexate, metoclopramide (Reglan), metronidazole (Flagyl), midazolam (Versed), milrinone (Primacor), morphine, nafcillin (Unipen), nicardipine (Cardene), nitroglycerin (Nitrobid), norepinephrine (Levophed), ondansetron (Zofran), oxacillin (Bactocil), paclitaxel (Taxol), penicillin G potassium (Pfizerpen), pentazocine (Talwin), pentobarbital (Nembutal), piperacillin (Piperacil), piperacillin/tazobactam (Zosyn), prochlorperazine (Compazine), promethazine (Phenergan), propofol (Diprivan), ranitidine (Zantac), remifentanil (Ultiva), tacrolimus (Prograf), teniposide (Vumon), thiotepa (Thioplex), ticarcillin (Ticar), tobramycin (Nebcin), trimethobenzamide (Tigan), trimethoprim/sulfamethoxazole (Bactrim), vancomycin (Vancocin), vecuronium (Norcuron), verapamil (Calan), vinorelbine (Navelbine).

SIDE EFFECTS

Frequent
Somnolence, dizziness, hypotension (including orthostatic hypotension), decreased appetite.
Occasional
Confusion, diaphoresis, facial flushing, urine retention, constipation,

dry mouth, nausea, vomiting, headache, pain at injection site.

Rare

Allergic reaction, depression.

SERIOUS REACTIONS

- Overdose results in respiratory depression, skeletal muscle flaccidity, cold or clammy skin, cyanosis, and extreme somnolence progressing to seizures, stupor, and coma.
- The patient who uses hydromorphone repeatedly may develop a tolerance to the drug's analgesic effect as well as physical dependence.
- This drug may have a prolonged duration of action and cumulative effect in patients with hepatic or renal impairment.

PRECAUTIONS & CONSIDERATIONS

Extreme caution should be used in patients with acute alcoholism, anoxia, CNS depression, hypercapnia, respiratory depression or dysfunction, seizures, shock, and untreated myxedema. Caution is also warranted in patients with acute abdominal conditions, Addison disease, COPD, hypotension, hypothyroidism, hepatic impairment, increased intracranial pressure, benign prostatic hyperplasia, and urethral stricture. Hydromorphone readily crosses the placenta; it is unknown whether it is distributed in breast milk. Regular use of opioids during pregnancy may produce withdrawal symptoms in the neonate, including diarrhea, excessive crying, fever, hyperactive reflexes, irritability, seizures, sneezing, tremors, vomiting, and yawning. Hydromorphone use may prolong labor if administered in the latent phase of the first stage of labor or before cervical dilation of 4-5 cm. The neonate may develop respiratory depression if the mother receives hydromorphone during labor. Children younger than 2 yr may be more susceptible to respiratory depression. Elderly patients may be more susceptible to respiratory depression and paradoxical excitement. In elderly patients, age-related benign prostatic hyperplasia, obstruction, or renal impairment may increase the risk of urine retention; a dosage adjustment is recommended.

Dizziness and drowsiness may occur, so change positions slowly and avoid alcohol, CNS depressants, and tasks that require mental alertness or motor skills until response to the drug is established. Vital signs, pattern of daily bowel activity and stool consistency, and clinical improvement of pain should be monitored. The drug should be held and the physician should be notified if the respiratory rate is 12 breaths/min or less in an adult or 20 breaths/min or less in a child.

Storage

Store tablets, oral solution, vials at room temperature; protect from light. A slight yellow discoloration of the parenteral form does not indicate a loss of potency. Refrigerate suppositories.

Administration

! Ambulatory patients and those not in severe pain may be more prone to dizziness, hypotension, nausea, and vomiting than patients in the supine position and those in severe pain.

Take oral hydromorphone without regard to food. Crush immediate-release tablets as needed. Measure oral liquid carefully using calibrated oral syringe.

For extended-release product (e.g., Exalgo), discontinue all other extended-release opioids when beginning. Administer only once every 24 h with or without food. Do not crush, break, dissolve, or chew the tablets. If the tablets are not swallowed intact, a fatal dose of hydromorphone may be delivered.

! Be aware that a high concentration injection (10 mg/mL) should be used only in patients currently receiving high doses of another opioid agonist for severe, chronic pain caused by cancer or those who have developed a tolerance to high doses of other opioids.

For IV use, hydromorphone may be given undiluted as IV push over 2-5 min, or it may be further diluted with 5 mL sterile water for injection or 0.9% NaCl. Be aware that rapid IV administration increases the risk of a severe anaphylactic reaction, marked by apnea, cardiac arrest, and circulatory collapse.

For IM and subcutaneous administration, use a short 25- to 30-gauge needle for subcutaneous injection. Administer the drug slowly; rotate injection sites. Know that those with circulatory impairment are at increased risk for overdose because of delayed absorption of repeated injections.

For rectal use, unwrap, then moisten the suppository with cold water before inserting it well into the rectum.

Hydroquinone

hye-droe-kwin′one

Alphaquin HP, Alustra, Claripel, Eldopaque, Eldopaque Forte, Eldoquin, EpiQuin Micro, Esoterica Regular, Glyquin, Lustra, Lustra-AF, Melanex, Melpaque HP, Melquin-3, Melquin HP, NeoStrata AHA, Nuquin HP, NeoStrata HQ, Palmer's Skin Success Fade Cream, Solaquin, Solaquin Forte

Esoterica, Lustra, NeoStrata HQ, Palmer's Skin Success Fade Cream

CATEGORY AND SCHEDULE

Pregnancy Risk Category: C

Classification: Depigmenting agents, dermatologics

MECHANISM OF ACTION

A depigmenting agent that suppresses melanocyte metabolic processes of the skin. Inhibits the enzymatic oxidation of tyrosine to DOPA (3,4-dihydroxyphenylalanine). Sun exposure reverses this effect and causes repigmentation. *Therapeutic Effect:* Lighten hyperpigmented areas.

PHARMACOKINETICS

Onset and duration of depigmentation vary among individuals. About 35% is absorbed.

AVAILABILITY

Cream: 2% (Eldopaque, Esoterica Regular, Palmer's Skin Success Fade Cream), 4% (Alphaquin HP, Alustra, EpiQuin Micro, Lustra, Melquin HP, Nuquin HP).
Cream, with Sunscreen: 2% (Solaquin), 4% (Claripel, Glyquin, Solaquin, Solaquin Forte, Lustra-AF, Melpaque HP).
Gel: 2% (NeoStrata AHA).
Gel, with Sunscreen: 4% (Nuquin HP, Solaquin Forte)
Solution, Topical: 3% (Melanex, Melquin-3)

INDICATIONS AND DOSAGES

▸ **Hyperpigmentation, melanin**

TOPICAL

Adults, Elderly, Children 12 yr and older. Apply twice daily.

OFF-LABEL USES

None known.

CONTRAINDICATIONS

Hypersensitivity to hydroquinone, sulfites, or any other component of its formulation.

INTERACTIONS

Drug
None known.
Herbal
None known.

H

Food
None known.

DIAGNOSTIC TEST EFFECTS
None known.

SIDE EFFECTS
Occasional
Burning, itching, stinging, erythema, such as localized contact dermatitis.
Rare
Conjunctival changes, fingernail staining.

H

SERIOUS REACTIONS
• Gradual blue-black darkening of skin has been reported.
• Occasional cutaneous hypersensitivity (localized contact dermatitis) may occur.

PRECAUTIONS & CONSIDERATIONS
Some products contain sulfites that may cause sensitivity in sensitive individuals. It is unknown whether hydroquinone crosses the placenta or is distributed in breast milk. Caution should be used in pregnant women. Therapeutic effect may take several weeks. Be aware that safety and efficacy of hydroquinone have not been established in children younger than 12 yr. No age-related precautions have been noted in elderly patients. Sun exposure should be avoided. Protective sunscreen or clothing to cover the skin should be used if sun is unavoidable.
Storage
Store at room temperature. Keep tightly closed.
Administration
Hydroquinone is for external use only. It is recommended to try a test response in a small area of skin and monitor for irritation or blistering over 24 h before using on a larger skin surface. Gently cleanse the area before application. Limit to small areas of the body at one time. Apply sparingly on skin spots and rub into area thoroughly. Avoid contact with eyes.

Hydroxychloroquine
hye-drox-ee-klor′oh-kwin
★ Plaquenil
🍁 Apo-Hydroxyquine, Plaquenil
Do not confuse hydroxychloroquine with hydrocortisone or hydroxyzine.

CATEGORY AND SCHEDULE
Pregnancy Risk Category: C

Classification: Antiprotozoals, disease-modifying antirheumatic drugs, antimalarial

MECHANISM OF ACTION
An antimalarial and antirheumatic that concentrates in parasite acid vesicles, increasing the pH of the vesicles and interfering with parasite protein synthesis. Antirheumatic action may involve suppressing formation of antigens responsible for hypersensitivity reactions. *Therapeutic Effect:* Inhibits parasite growth anti-inflammatory actions.

PHARMACOKINETICS
PO: Peak 1-2 h. *Half-life:* 3-5 days; metabolized in liver; excreted in urine, feces, breast milk; crosses placenta.

AVAILABILITY
Tablets: 200 mg (155 mg base).

INDICATIONS AND DOSAGES
▸ **Treatment of acute attack of malaria (dosage in mg base)**
PO

Dose	Times	Adults (mg)	Children (mg/kg)
Initial	Day 1	620	10
Second	6 h later	310	5
Third	Day 2	310	5
Fourth	Day 3	310	5

▸ **Suppression of malaria**
PO
Adults. 400 mg (310 mg base) weekly on same day each week, beginning 2 wks before entering an endemic area and continuing for 4-6 wks after leaving the area. If therapy is not begun before exposure, administer a loading dose of 800 mg (620 mg base), then begin the usual suppressive dose.
Children. 5 mg base/kg/wk, beginning 2 wks before entering an endemic area and continuing for 4-6 wks after leaving the area. If therapy is not begun before exposure, administer a loading dose of 10 mg base/kg in 2 equally divided doses 6 h apart, followed by the usual dosage regimen.

▸ **Rheumatoid arthritis**
PO
Adults. Initially, 400-600 mg (310-465 mg base) daily for 5-10 days; gradually increased to optimum response level. Maintenance (usually within 4-12 wks): Dosage decreased by 50% and then continued at maintenance dose of 200-400 mg/day. Maximum effect may not be seen for several months. If symptoms not improved in 6 months, discontinue.

▸ **Lupus erythematosus**
PO
Adults. Initially, 400 mg once or twice a day for several weeks or months. Maintenance: 200-400 mg/day.

OFF-LABEL USES
Sarcoidosis.

CONTRAINDICATIONS
Long-term therapy for children, hypersensitivity to 4-aminoquinolines, retinal or visual field changes attributable to 4-aminoquinolines.

INTERACTIONS
Drug
Aurothioglucose: May increase the risk of blood dyscrasias.
Cimetidine: May increase levels of hydroxychloroquine.
Digoxin: May increase serum digoxin concentrations.
Penicillamine: May increase blood penicillamine concentration and the risk of hematologic, renal, or severe skin reactions.
Herbal
None known.
Food
None known.

DIAGNOSTIC TEST EFFECTS
None known.

SIDE EFFECTS
Frequent
Mild, transient headache; anorexia; nausea; vomiting.
Occasional
Visual disturbances, nervousness, fatigue, pruritus (especially of palms, soles, and scalp), irritability, personality changes, diarrhea.
Rare
Stomatitis, dermatitis, impaired hearing.

SERIOUS REACTIONS
- Ocular toxicity, especially retinopathy, may occur and may progress even after drug is discontinued.
- Prolonged therapy may result in peripheral neuritis, neuromyopathy, hypotension, ECG changes, agranulocytosis, aplastic anemia, thrombocytopenia, seizures, and psychosis.

H

• Overdosage may result in headache, vomiting, visual disturbances, drowsiness, seizures, and hypokalemia followed by cardiovascular collapse and death.

PRECAUTIONS & CONSIDERATIONS

Caution is warranted in patients with glucose-6-phosphate dehydrogenase deficiency, hepatic disease, and alcoholism. May precipitate attacks of porphyria. Use of hydroxychloroquine for psoriasis may precipitate a severe attack of psoriasis. Children are especially susceptible to hydroxychloroquine's effects.

Avoid in pregnancy unless essential for malaria treatment; the drug may affect the fetal retina. Use caution with use during breastfeeding.

Report decreased hearing, tinnitus, visual difficulties, muscle weakness, or any other new symptoms. Visual disturbances, impaired hearing, and GI distress should be monitored. Liver function should be assessed. The skin should be checked for pruritus.

Storage

Store at room temperature.

Administration

! Be aware that 200 mg hydroxychloroquine equals 155 mg of base. Take with food or milk to limit GI effects.

Hydroxyzine

hye-drox'i-zeen

Vistaril Apo-Hydroxyzin, Atarax, Novo-Hydroxyzin

Do not confuse hydroxyzine with hydralazine or hydroxyurea.

CATEGORY AND SCHEDULE

Pregnancy Risk Category: X, first trimester

Classification: Antihistamines, H_1 antagonists, anxiolytics, sedatives/hypnotics, antivertigo

MECHANISM OF ACTION

A piperazine derivative that competes with histamine for receptor sites in the GI tract, blood vessels, and respiratory tract. May exert CNS depressant activity in subcortical areas. Diminishes vestibular stimulation and depresses labyrinthine function. *Therapeutic Effect:* Produces anxiolytic, anticholinergic, antihistaminic, and analgesic effects; relaxes skeletal muscle; controls nausea and vomiting.

PHARMACOKINETICS

Route	Onset	Peak	Duration
PO	15-30 min	N/A	4-6 h

Well absorbed from the GI tract and after parenteral administration. Metabolized in the liver. Primarily excreted in urine. Not removed by hemodialysis. *Half-life:* 20-25 h (increased in elderly patients).

AVAILABILITY

Capsules (Vistaril): 25 mg, 50 mg, 100 mg.
Oral Suspension: 25 mg/5 mL.
Syrup: 10 mg/5 mL.
Tablets (ANX): 10 mg, 25 mg, 50 mg.
Injection (Vistaril): 25 mg/mL, 50 mg/mL.

INDICATIONS AND DOSAGES

▸ **Anxiety**

PO

Adults, Elderly. 25-100 mg 4 times a day. Maximum: 400 mg/day.

▸ **Nausea and vomiting**

IM

Adults, Elderly. 25-100 mg/dose q4-6h.

▸ **Pruritus**

PO

Adults, Elderly. 25 mg 3-4 times a day.

▸ **Preoperative sedation**
PO
Adults, Elderly. 50-100 mg.
IM
Adults, Elderly. 25-100 mg.
▸ **Usual pediatric dosage**
PO
Children. 2 mg/kg/day in divided doses q6-8h.
IM
Children. 0.5-1 mg/kg/dose q4-6h.

CONTRAINDICATIONS

Early pregnancy, hypersensitivity to hydroxyzine or certirizine, intravenous administration.

INTERACTIONS

Drug
Alcohol, other CNS depressants: May increase CNS depressant effects.
MAOIs: May increase anticholinergic and CNS depressant effects.
Herbal
Gotu kola, kava kava, St. John's wort, valerian: May cause additive CNS depressant effects.
Food
None known.

DIAGNOSTIC TEST EFFECTS

May cause false-positive urine 17-hydroxycorticosteroid determinations.

SIDE EFFECTS

Side effects are generally mild and transient.
Frequent
Somnolence, dry mouth, marked discomfort with IM injection.
Occasional
Dizziness, ataxia, asthenia, slurred speech, headache, agitation, increased anxiety.
Rare
Paradoxical CNS reactions, such as hyperactivity or nervousness in children and excitement or restlessness in elderly or debilitated patients (generally noted during first 2 wks of therapy, particularly in presence of uncontrolled pain).

SERIOUS REACTIONS

- A hypersensitivity reaction, including wheezing, dyspnea, and chest tightness, may occur.
- Inadvertent IV administration can cause hemolysis, hypotension, cardiac or respiratory instability, or severe localized injection reactions.

PRECAUTIONS & CONSIDERATIONS

Caution is warranted in patients with asthma, bladder neck obstruction, COPD, angle-closure glaucoma, and benign prostatic hyperplasia. It is unknown whether hydroxyzine crosses the placenta or is distributed in breast milk. Hydroxyzine use is not recommended for neonates or premature infants because they are at increased risk for anticholinergic effects. Children may experience paradoxical excitement. Elderly patients are at increased risk for confusion, dizziness, sedation, hypotension, and hyperexcitability. Be aware of dehydration, which can occur with severe vomiting.

Drowsiness and dizziness may occur. Change positions slowly from recumbent to sitting before standing to prevent dizziness. Alcohol, caffeine, and tasks that require mental alertness or motor skills should also be avoided. Autonomic responses, such as cold, clammy hands and diaphoresis, and motor responses, such as agitation, trembling, and tension, should be assessed. CBC and blood chemistry tests should be performed periodically in long-term therapy. Breath sounds, electrolyte levels, and CNS reactions should also be assessed.

Storage
Store at room temperature; protect from light.
Administration
Crush scored tablets as needed, but do not crush or break capsules. Shake the oral suspension well before each use.
! Do not give hydroxyzine by the subcutaneous, intra-arterial, or IV route because doing so can cause significant tissue damage, thrombosis, and gangrene; IV administration may cause hemolysis.
The IM form may be given undiluted. Inject the drug deep into the gluteus maximus or midlateral thigh in adults and the midlateral thigh in children. Use the Z-track technique of injection to prevent subcutaneous infiltration. IM injection may cause marked discomfort.

Hyoscyamine

hye-oh-sye′a-meen
★ Anaspaz, Colytrol Pediatric Drops, Colidrops Pediatric Drops, Cystospaz, Cystospaz-M, HyoMax, HyoMax-DT, HyoMax-FT, HyoMax-SL, HyoMax SR, Hyosyne, Levbid, Levsin, Levsin SL, Medispaz, NuLev, Spacol, Spacol T/S, Spasdel, Symax FasTabs, Symax DuoTabs, Symax SL
Do not confuse Anaspaz with Anaprox.

CATEGORY AND SCHEDULE

Pregnancy Risk Category: C

Classification: Anticholinergics, gastrointestinals, urinary antispasmodic

MECHANISM OF ACTION

A GI antispasmodic and anticholinergic agent that inhibits the action of acetylcholine at post-ganglionic (muscarinic) receptor sites. *Therapeutic Effect:* Decreases secretions (bronchial, salivary, sweat gland) and gastric juices and reduces motility of GI and urinary tract.

AVAILABILITY

Tablets (Anaspaz, HyoMax, Levsin, Medispaz, Spasdel): 0.125 mg, 0.15 mg.
Tablets (Oral Disintegrating [HyoMax-FT, NuLev, Symax FasTabs]): 0.125 mg.
Tablets (Sublingual [HyoMax-SL, Levsin SL, Symax SL]): 0.125 mg.
Tablets (Extended Release [HyoMax-SR, Levbid, Symax SR]): 0.375 mg.
Capsules (Extended Release [Cystospaz-M]): 0.375 mg.
Elixir (Hyosyne, Spasdel, Spacol): 0.125 mg/5 mL.
Oral Solution Drops (Hyosyne, Colidrops): 0.125 mg/5 mL.
Oral Solution Drops (Colytrol): 0.03 mg/mL.
Injection (Levsin): 0.5 mg/mL.

INDICATIONS AND DOSAGES

▸ **GI tract disorders**
PO or SL
Adults, Elderly, Children 12 yr and older. 0.125-0.25 mg q4h as needed. Extended release: 0.375-0.75 mg PO q12h. Maximum: 1.5 mg/day.
Children 2-11 yr. 0.0625-0.125 mg q4h as needed. Maximum: 0.75 mg/day.
IM, IV
Adults, Elderly, Children 12 yr and older. 0.25-0.5 mg q4h for 1-4 doses.
▸ **Hypermotility of lower urinary tract**
PO, SUBLINGUAL
Adults, Elderly. 0.15-0.3 mg 4 times a day; or extended release 0.375 mg PO q12h.

▸ **Infant colic**
PO
Infants. Individualized drops dosed q4h as needed. See manufacturer-provided weight-based dosing.

CONTRAINDICATIONS

GI or genitourinary obstruction, myasthenia gravis, narrow-angle glaucoma, paralytic ileus, severe ulcerative colitis, intestinal atony of elderly or debilitated patients, toxic megacolon complicating ulcerative colitis, unstable cardiovascular status in acute hemorrhage, myocardial ischemia.

INTERACTIONS

Drug
Antacids, antidiarrheals: May decrease the absorption of hyoscyamine.
Haloperidol, phenothiazines, tricyclic antidepressants: May have additive adverse effects.
Ketoconazole: May decrease the absorption of this drug.
Other anticholinergics: May increase the effects of hyoscyamine.
Potassium chloride: May increase the severity of GI lesions with the matrix formulation of potassium chloride.
Herbal
None known.
Food
None known.

DIAGNOSTIC TEST EFFECTS

None known.

SIDE EFFECTS

Frequent
Dry mouth (sometimes severe), decreased sweating, constipation.
Occasional
Blurred vision, bloated feeling, urinary hesitancy, somnolence (with high dosage), headache, intolerance to light, loss of taste, nervousness, flushing, insomnia, impotence, mental confusion or excitement (particularly in elderly patients and children) temporary light-headedness (with parenteral form), local irritation (with parenteral form).
Rare
Dizziness, faintness.

SERIOUS REACTIONS

• Overdose may produce temporary paralysis of ciliary muscle; pupillary dilation; tachycardia; palpitations; hot, dry, or flushed skin; absence of bowel sounds; hyperthermia; increased respiratory rate; ECG abnormalities; nausea; vomiting; rash over face or upper trunk; CNS stimulation; and psychosis (marked by agitation, restlessness, rambling speech, visual hallucinations, paranoid behavior, and delusions, followed by depression).

PRECAUTIONS & CONSIDERATIONS

Carefully evaluate GI symptoms prior to use. For example, diarrhea may be an early sign of incomplete intestinal obstruction. Caution is warranted with cardiac arrhythmias, congestive heart failure, chronic lung disease, hyperthyroidism, neuropathy, and prostatic hyperplasia. Avoid hot baths, saunas, and becoming overheated while exercising in hot weather. Tasks that require mental alertness or motor skills should also be avoided until response to the drug has been established.

Dry mouth may occur, so good oral hygiene should be maintained. Notify the physician of constipation, difficulty urinating, eye pain, or rash. Pattern of daily bowel activity, stool consistency, and urine output should be monitored. The patient should void before receiving the drug to reduce the risk of urine retention.

Storage
Store at room temperature. Protect from moisture. Keep ODT forms in package until time of use.

Administration
Give oral hyoscyamine without regard to meals. The sublingual tablets may be taken sublingually, orally, or chewed. Extended-release capsule should be swallowed whole. Orally disintegrating tablets may be placed on tongue; dissolve. May be taken with or without water.

For parenteral use, hyoscyamine may be given undiluted. May be administered IM, intravenously, or subcutaneously. If given IV, inject slowly.

Ibandronate

eye-band′droh-nate

★ Boniva

CATEGORY AND SCHEDULE

Pregnancy Risk Category: C

Classification: Bisphosphonates

MECHANISM OF ACTION

A bisphosphonate that binds to bone hydroxyapatite (part of the mineral matrix of bone) and inhibits osteoclast activity. *Therapeutic Effect:* Reduces rate of bone turnover and bone resorption, resulting in a net gain in bone mass.

PHARMACOKINETICS

Absorbed in the upper GI tract. Extent of absorption impaired by food or beverages (other than plain water). Rapidly binds to bone. Unabsorbed portion is eliminated in urine. Protein binding: 90%. *Half-life:* 10-60 h.

AVAILABILITY

Tablets: 2.5 mg, 150 mg.
Injection: 3 mg/3 mL.

INDICATIONS AND DOSAGES

▸ **Osteoporosis**

PO

Adults, Elderly. 2.5 mg daily or 150 mg once a month.

IV

Adults, Elderly. 3 mg every 3 mo.

CONTRAINDICATIONS

Known hypersensitivity to ibandronate or product components (cross-sensitivity may occur with other bisphosphonates), abnormalities of the esophagus such as stricture or achalasia (oral use), inability to stand or sit upright for at least 60 min (for oral use), uncorrected hypocalcemia, severe renal impairment (e.g., SCr > 2.3 mg/dL or CrCl < 30 ml/min).

INTERACTIONS

Drug

Antacids containing aluminum, calcium, magnesium; vitamin D: Decrease the absorption of ibandronate.

Herbal

None known.

Food

Beverages other than plain water, dietary supplements, food: Interfere with the absorption of ibandronate.

DIAGNOSTIC TEST EFFECTS

May decrease serum alkaline phosphatase level. May increase blood cholesterol level.
May cause transient decrease in serum calcium (IV).

SIDE EFFECTS

Frequent (6%-13%)

Back pain; dyspepsia, including epigastric distress and heartburn; peripheral discomfort; diarrhea; headache; myalgia.

Occasional (3%-4%)

Dizziness, arthralgia, asthenia.

Rare (2% or less)

Vomiting, hypersensitivity reaction.

SERIOUS REACTIONS

- Upper respiratory tract infection occurs occasionally.
- Overdose causes hypocalcemia, hypophosphatemia, and significant GI disturbances.
- Osteonecrosis of the jaw.
- Infrequent reports of severe and occasionally incapacitating bone, joint, and/or muscle pain.
- Increased risk of fractures in thigh bone (rare).

PRECAUTIONS & CONSIDERATIONS

Caution is warranted with GI diseases, including duodenitis, dysphagia, esophagitis, gastritis, ulcers, and mild to moderate renal impairment. Bone, joint, and muscle pain have been reported with ibandronate therapy. Osteonecrosis of the jaw has also been reported with ibandronate therapy and has been associated more commonly in cancer patients and in those with preexisting dental disease. Ibandronate may have teratogenic effects. It is unknown whether ibandronate is excreted in breast milk. Breastfeeding is not recommended for women taking ibandronate. The safety and efficacy of ibandronate have not been established in children. No age-related precautions have been noted in elderly patients. Consider beginning weight-bearing exercises, reduce alcohol consumption, and stop cigarette smoking.

Hypocalcemia and vitamin D deficiencies, if present, should be corrected before beginning ibandronate therapy. BUN, creatinine levels, and serum electrolytes, especially calcium and serum alkaline phosphatase levels, should be monitored during therapy.

Storage

Store tablets at room temperature. Store unopened injection at room temperature in carton until time of use.

Administration

Expect patients to receive calcium and vitamin D during bisphosphonate treatment. Take ibandronate on an empty stomach with 6-8 oz of plain water 60 min before the first food or beverage of the day; give with plain water only. Avoid taking ibandronate with coffee, mineral water, and orange juice because they significantly reduce the absorption of the drug. Stay in an upright position while standing or sitting; do not lie down for 60 min after drug administration. Do not chew or suck the tablet because of the potential for oropharyngeal ulceration. Give once-monthly dose on the same date of the month. Give injection IV only over 15-30 seconds. Do not mix with calcium-containing solutions or any other drugs. Do not administer paravenously or intra-arterially because this may cause tissue damage. Do not give injection more often than every 3 mo.

Ibuprofen

eye-byoo'pro-fen

★ Advil, Advil Children's, Advil Infants' Drops, Advil Junior Strength, Advil Liquigels, Advil Migraine, Midol Cramps and Body Aches, Motrin, Motrin IB, Motrin Infants' Drops, Motrin Junior Strength

CATEGORY AND SCHEDULE

Pregnancy Risk Category: B (D if used in third trimester or near delivery)

Many products are OTC; tablets > 200 mg/tablet are Rx only.

Classification: Analgesics, antipyretics, nonsteroidal anti-inflammatory drug (NSAID)

MECHANISM OF ACTION

An NSAID that inhibits prostaglandin synthesis. Also produces vasodilation by acting centrally on the heat-regulating center of the hypothalamus. *Therapeutic Effect:* Produces analgesic and anti-inflammatory effects and decreases fever.

PHARMACOKINETICS

Route	Onset	Peak	Duration
PO (analgesic)	0.5 h	N/A	4-6 h
PO (antirheumatic)	2 days	1-2 wks	NA

Rapidly absorbed from the GI tract. Protein binding: > 90%. Metabolized in the liver. Primarily excreted in urine. Not removed by hemodialysis. *Half-life:* 2-4 h.

AVAILABILITY

Caplets (Advil, Motrin IB): 100 mg, 200 mg.
Capsules (Advil, Advil Migraine): 200 mg.
Gelcaps (Advil, Motrin IB): 200 mg.
Tablets (Advil, Motrin IB): 200 mg.
Tablets (Rx only): 400 mg, 600 mg, 800 mg.
Tablets (Chewable [Children's Advil, Children's Motrin]): 50 mg.
Tablets (Chewable [Junior Advil, Junior Strength Motrin]): 100 mg.
Oral Suspension (Children's Advil, Children's Motrin): 100 mg/5 mL.
Oral Drops (Infant Advil, Infant Motrin): 40 mg/mL.

INDICATIONS AND DOSAGES

▸ **Acute or chronic rheumatoid arthritis, osteoarthritis, migraine pain, gouty arthritis**

PO

Adults, Elderly. 300-800 mg 3-4 times a day. Maximum: 3.2 g/day.

▸ **Mild to moderate pain, primary dysmenorrhea**

PO

Adults, Elderly. 200-400 mg q4-6h as needed. Maximum: 1.6 g/day.

▸ **Fever, minor aches or pain**

PO

Adults, Elderly. 200-400 mg q4-6h. Maximum: 1.6 g/day.

Children, Infants 6 mo and older. 5-10 mg/kg/dose q6-8h. Maximum: 40 mg/kg/day. OTC: 7.5 mg/kg/dose q6-8h. Maximum: 30 mg/kg/day.

▸ **Juvenile arthritis**

PO

Children. 30-40 mg/kg/day in 3-4 divided doses. Maximum: 400 mg/day in children weighing < 20 kg, 600 mg/day in children weighing 20-30 kg, 800 mg/day in children weighing > 30-40 kg.

OFF-LABEL USES

Treatment of psoriatic arthritis, vascular headaches.

CONTRAINDICATIONS

Active peptic ulcer, chronic inflammation of GI tract, GI bleeding disorders or ulceration, history of hypersensitivity to aspirin or NSAIDs, use within 14 days of coronary artery bypass graft surgery.

INTERACTIONS

Drug

Antihypertensives, diuretics: May decrease the effects of these drugs.
Aspirin, other salicylates: May increase the risk of GI side effects such as bleeding. NSAID use may negate cardioprotective effect of ASA.
Bile acid sequestrants: May decrease the absorption of NSAIDs. Separate administration by at least 2 h.
Corticosteroids: May increase risk of GI ulceration.
Heparin, oral anticoagulants, thrombolytics: May increase the effects of these drugs.
Lithium: May increase the blood concentration and risk of toxicity of lithium.
Methotrexate: May increase the risk of methotrexate toxicity.
Probenecid: May increase the ibuprofen blood concentration.

Herbal
Feverfew: May decrease the effects of feverfew.
Alfalfa, anise, bilberry, bladderwrack, bromelain, cat's claw, celery, chamomile, coleus, cordyceps, dong quai, evening primrose, fenugreek, feverfew, garlic, ginger, ginkgo biloba, ginseng (American, Panax, Siberian), grapeseed, green tea, guggul, horse chestnut seed, horseradish, licorice, prickly ash, red clover, reishi, SAMe (S-adenosylmethionine), sweet clover, turmeric, white willow: May increase the risk of bleeding.
Food
Alcohol: Dizziness and may increase the risk of GI bleeding.

DIAGNOSTIC TEST EFFECTS

May prolong bleeding time. May alter blood glucose level. May increase BUN level, and serum creatinine, potassium, AST (SGOT), and ALT (SGPT) levels. May decrease blood hemoglobin and hematocrit.

SIDE EFFECTS

Occasional (3%-9%)
Nausea with or without vomiting, dyspepsia, dizziness, rash.
Rare (< 3%)
Diarrhea or constipation, flatulence, abdominal cramps or pain, pruritus.

SERIOUS REACTIONS

- Acute overdose may result in metabolic acidosis.
- Rare reactions with long-term use include peptic ulcer disease, GI bleeding, gastritis, a severe hepatic reaction (cholestasis, jaundice), nephrotoxicity (dysuria, hematuria, proteinuria, nephrotic syndrome), and a severe hypersensitivity reaction (particularly in patients with systemic lupus erythematosus or other collagen diseases).

PRECAUTIONS & CONSIDERATIONS

Caution is warranted with dehydration, GI disease (such as GI bleeding or ulcers), hepatic or renal impairment, and concurrent anticoagulant use. Cardiovascular event risk may be increased with duration of use or preexisting cardiovascular risk factors or disease. Use caution in patients with fluid retention, heart failure, or hypertension. The lowest effective dose should be used for the shortest duration of time possible. It is unknown whether ibuprofen crosses the placenta or is distributed in breast milk. Ibuprofen should not be used during the third trimester of pregnancy because it may cause adverse effects in the fetus, such as premature closure of the ductus arteriosus. The safety and efficacy of this drug have not been established in children younger than 6 mo. In elderly patients, GI bleeding or ulceration is more likely to cause serious complications, and age-related renal impairment may increase the risk of hepatotoxicity or renal toxicity; a reduced dosage is recommended. Risk of mycardial infarction and stroke may be increased following CABG surgery. Do not administer within 4-6 half-lives before surgical procedures. Increases the risk of GI bleeding. Because the drug may cause dizziness, do not perform tasks requiring mental concentration until the effects of the drug are known.

Monitor CBC and blood chemistries to assess hepatic and renal function with chronic therapeutic use. Be alert for skin rash or dark stools, or other signs of potential bleeding. Therapeutic response, such as decreased pain, stiffness, swelling, and tenderness, improved grip strength, and increased joint mobility, should be evaluated.

Storage

Store at room temperature; protect liquid-filled capsules and chewable tablets from high humidity/moisture.

Administration

Do not crush or break enteric-coated tablets. Take ibuprofen with food, milk, or antacids. Chewable tablets should be chewed well and swallowed with water or liquid.

Shake suspensions well before each use, including infant drops. Take care to measure accurate dosage.

Ibutilide

eye-byoo'ti-lide

★ 🍁 Corvert

CATEGORY AND SCHEDULE

Pregnancy Risk Category: C

Classification: Antiarrhythmics, class III

MECHANISM OF ACTION

An antiarrhythmic that prolongs both atrial and ventricular action potential duration and increases the atrial and ventricular refractory period. Activates slow, inward current (mostly of sodium); produces mild slowing of sinus node rate and AV conduction; and causes dose-related prolongation of QT interval. *Therapeutic Effect:* Converts atrial arrhythmias to sinus rhythm.

PHARMACOKINETICS

After IV administration, highly distributed, rapidly cleared. Protein binding: 40%. Primarily excreted in urine as metabolite. *Half-life:* 2-12 h (average: 6 h).

AVAILABILITY

Injection: 0.1 mg/mL solution.

INDICATIONS AND DOSAGES

▸ **Rapid conversion of atrial fibrillation or flutter of recent onset to normal sinus rhythm**

IV INFUSION

Adults, Elderly weighing 60 kg or more. One vial (1 mg) given over 10 min. If arrhythmia does not stop within 10 min after the end of initial infusion, a second 1-mg/10-min infusion may be given.

Adults, elderly weighing < 60 kg. 0.01 mg/kg given over 10 min. If arrhythmia does not stop within 10 min after end of initial infusion, a second 0.01-mg/kg, 10-min infusion may be given.

CONTRAINDICATIONS

QTc interval > 440 msec, hypersensitivity.

INTERACTIONS

Drug

Class IA antiarrhythmics (disopyramide, moricizine, procainamide, quinidine), class III antiarrhythmics (amiodarone, bretylium, sotalol): Do not give ibutilide with these drugs or give these drugs within 4 h after infusing ibutilide.

Digoxin: Signs of digoxin toxicity may be masked with coadministration.

H_1 receptor antagonists, phenothiazines, tricyclic and tetracyclic antidepressants: May prolong QT interval.

Herbal

None known.

Food

None known.

DIAGNOSTIC TEST EFFECTS

None known.

IV INCOMPATIBILITIES

No information is available for Y-site administration.

SIDE EFFECTS

Ibutilide is generally well tolerated.

Occasional

Ventricular extrasystoles (5.1%), ventricular tachycardia (4.9%), headache (3.6%), hypotension, orthostatic hypotension (2%).

Rare

Bundle-branch block, AV block, bradycardia, hypertension.

SERIOUS REACTIONS

- Sustained polymorphic ventricular tachycardia, occasionally with QT prolongation (torsades de pointes) occurs rarely.
- Overdose results in central nervous system (CNS) toxicity, including CNS depression, rapid gasping breathing, and seizures.
- Expect prolongation of repolarization.
- Existing arrhythmias may worsen or new arrhythmias may develop.

PRECAUTIONS & CONSIDERATIONS

Caution is warranted with abnormal hepatic function or heart block. Avoid coadministration with other medications that may prolong the QT interval. Because ibutilide is embryocidal and teratogenic in animals, breastfeeding is not recommended during ibutilide therapy. Safety and efficacy of ibutilide have not been established in children. No age-related precautions have been noted in elderly patients.

Notify the physician if palpitations or other adverse reactions occur. BP and ECG should be continuously monitored during therapy. Serum electrolyte levels, especially magnesium and potassium, should be monitored, and arrhythmias requiring overdrive cardiac pacing, electrical cardioversion, or defibrillation should be surveyed. Patients with atrial fibrillation lasting more than 3 days should be given an anticoagulant for at least 2 wks before ibutilide therapy is started. Proarrhythmias may develop.

Storage

Store unopened vials at room temperature in carton. Admixtures with diluent are stable at room temperature for up to 24 h or up to 48 h if refrigerated.

Administration

Have advanced cardiac life-support equipment, medications, and trained personnel on hand during and after ibutilide administration. Ibutilide is compatible with D5W and 0.9% NaCl. It is also compatible with polyvinyl chloride plastic and polyolefin bag. Give undiluted or may dilute in 50 mL 0.9% NaCl or dextrose 5%. Give IV over 10 min.

Iloperidone

eye'low-per'i-done

Fanapt

Do not confuse iloperidone with risperidone or ixabepilone, or Fanapt with Fansidar or Fanatrex.

CATEGORY AND SCHEDULE

Pregnancy Risk Category: C

Classification: Antipsychotics, atypical

MECHANISM OF ACTION

A benzisoxazole derivative that antagonizes dopamine and serotonin receptors; also has α-adrenergic blocking properties. *Therapeutic Effect:* Suppresses psychotic behavior.

PHARMACOKINETICS

Oral form is well absorbed from the GI tract; unaffected by food. Protein binding: 95%. Steady-state levels attained in 3-4 days. Extensively metabolized in the liver to 2 metabolites (P88 and P95) by CYP2D6 (predominantly) and CYP3A4. Poor metabolizers of CYP2D6 or administration with potent CYP2D6 inhibitors greatly increases iloperidone exposure. Drug and metabolites excreted primarily in urine and feces. *Half-life:* For iloperidone, P88 and P95 are 18, 26, and 23 h, respectively (increased in poor metabolizers).

AVAILABILITY

Tablets (Fanapt): 1 mg, 2 mg, 4 mg, 6 mg, 8 mg, 10 mg, 12 mg.

INDICATIONS AND DOSAGES

▸ **Schizophrenia**

PO

Adults. Must be titrated slowly to avoid orthostatic hypotension. Initially, give 1 mg twice daily. May increase to 2 mg twice daily, 4 mg twice daily, 6 mg twice daily, 8 mg twice daily, 10 mg twice daily, and 12 mg twice daily on days 2, 3, 4, 5, 6, and 7, respectively. Effective range is 6-12 mg twice daily. Control of symptoms may be delayed during the first 1-2 wks of treatment due to the titration schedule needed. Maximum: 12 mg twice daily (24 mg/day). NOTE: Whenever treatment is interrupted for more than 3 days, return to the titration schedule.

▸ **Dosage adjustment if a poor metabolizer of CYP2D6**

Reduce dose by 50%.

▸ **Dosage adjustment with CYP2D6 inhibitors**

Reduce dose by 50% when given with strong CYP2D6 inhibitors such as fluoxetine or paroxetine. When the CYP2D6 inhibitor is withdrawn, increase dose.

▸ **Dosage adjustment with CYP3A4 inhibitors**

Reduce dose by 50% when given with strong CYP3A4 inhibitors such as ketoconazole or clarithromycin. When the CYP3A4 inhibitor is withdrawn, increase dose.

▸ **Hepatic impairment of any degree**

Use of this drug is not recommended.

CONTRAINDICATIONS

Hypersensitivity to the drug.

INTERACTIONS

Drug

Alcohol, other CNS depressants: May increase central nervous system (CNS) depression.

Drugs that prolong the QT interval: Do not use in combination with such drugs including class 1A (e.g., quinidine, procainamide) or class III (e.g., amiodarone, sotalol) antiarrhythmics, chlorpromazine, thioridazine, gatifloxacin, moxifloxacin, pentamidine, levomethadyl, methadone.

Strong CYP2D6 inhibitors (e.g., fluoxetine, paroxetine): May increase the levels/effects of iloperidone. Reduce dose by 50%.

Strong CYP3A4 inhibitors (e.g., ketoconazole, clarithromycin, erythromycin): May increase the levels/effects of iloperidone. Reduce dose by 50%.

I

Dopamine agonists, levodopa: May antagonize the effects of these drugs.
Herbal
Kava kava, valerian: May increase CNS depression.
Food
Ethanol: Avoid; may increase CNS depression.

DIAGNOSTIC TEST EFFECTS

Elevates prolactin levels. Infrequently causes hyperglycemia, decreased hemoglobin or hematocrit, decreased potassium. May rarely cause changes in neutrophil counts. May rarely cause ECG changes.

SIDE EFFECTS

Frequent (> 10%)
Dizziness, somnolence, tachycardia, dry mouth, nausea, extrapyramidal symptoms.
Occasional (5%-10%)
Fatigue, nasal congestion, orthostatic hypotension, diarrhea, and weight increase. Hyperprolactinemia may affect fertility.
Less Frequent (< 5%)
Blurry vision, abdominal pain, arthralgia, muscle stiffness, nasopharyngitis, cough, upper respiratory infection, hypotension, dyspnea, rash, ejaculation disturbance, extrapyramidal symptoms, tremor, lethargy.

SERIOUS REACTIONS

- Hypersensitivity may include pruritus and urticaria, or more serious reactions.
- Esophageal dysmotility and risk of aspiration.
- Tardive dyskinesia (characterized by tongue protrusion and chewing, puffing, or puckering of the mouth) and neuroleptic malignant syndrome (marked by hyperpyrexia, muscle rigidity, change in mental status, irregular pulse or BP, tachycardia, diaphoresis, cardiac arrhythmias, rhabdomyolysis, and acute renal failure).
- Potential for QTc prolongation and resultant arrhythmia (rare).
- Priapism.
- Seizures, especially in those with altered seizure thresholds.

PRECAUTIONS & CONSIDERATIONS

Avoid use in patients with congenital/hereditary or preexisting QT prolongation or in those with hepatic impairment. Caution is warranted with cardiovascular (hypotension, heart failure, recent MI) or cerebrovascular diseases (because it may induce hypotension or QTc prolongation); correct any electrolyte imbalances prior to administration and do not give with other medications known to cause QT prolongation. Also use with caution in patients with history of seizures or conditions that may lower the seizure threshold (such as Alzheimer disease), and Parkinson disease (because of potential for exacerbation of movement disorders). Use with caution in patients with diabetes or with risk factors for diabetes due to risk for hyperglycemia or weight gain. It is unknown whether iloperidone crosses the placenta; there are no adequate data during pregnancy and use should generally be avoided. Because this drug is likely to be distributed in breast milk, females should avoid breastfeeding. Elderly patients are more susceptible to orthostatic hypotension and may require lower dosages. Elderly patients with dementia-related psychosis treated with antipsychotic drugs are at an increased risk of death; iloperidone has not been approved for dementia-related psychosis. Most deaths appear to be either CV (e.g., heart failure, sudden death) or infectious (e.g., pneumonia) in nature. The safety and efficacy of iloperidone have not been established in children or adolescents.

Drowsiness and dizziness may occur but generally improve with continued therapy. CNS depressants and alcohol should be avoided. Disruption of temperature regulation may occur and patients should use caution with exercise, exposure to extreme heat, or dehydration. Monitor for extrapyramidal symptoms and tardive dyskinesia. BP, pulse rate, weight, CBC, and therapeutic response should also be monitored. Dehydration and hypovolemia should be corrected before beginning therapy.

Storage

Store at room temperature. Protect from light and moisture.

Administration

Take iloperidone without regard to food.

Iloprost

eye'low-prost

★ Ventavis

CATEGORY AND SCHEDULE

Pregnancy Risk Category: C

Classification: Respiratory agents, pulmonary antihypertensive, prostaglandins

MECHANISM OF ACTION

A prostaglandin that dilates systemic and pulmonary arterial vascular beds, alters pulmonary vascular resistance, and suppresses vascular smooth muscle proliferation. *Therapeutic Effect:* Improves symptoms and exercise tolerance in patients with pulmonary hypertension; delays deterioration of condition.

AVAILABILITY

Solution for Oral Inhalation: 10 mcg/mL or 20 mcg/mL ampules.

INDICATIONS AND DOSAGES

▸ **Pulmonary hypertension in patients with New York Heart Association (NYHA) class III or IV symptoms**

ORAL INHALATION

Adults. Initially, 2.5 mcg/dose; if tolerated, increased to 5 mcg/dose. Administer 6-9 times a day at intervals of 2 h or longer while patient is awake. Maintenance: 5 mcg/dose. Maximum daily dose: 45 mcg (5 mcg given 9 times/day).

CONTRAINDICATIONS

None known. Do not initiate if systolic BP < 85 mmHg.

INTERACTIONS

Drug

Antihypertensives, other vasodilators: May increase the hypotensive effects of iloprost.

Herbal

None known.

Food

None known.

DIAGNOSTIC TEST EFFECTS

May increase serum alkaline phosphatase and GGT levels.

SIDE EFFECTS

Frequent (27%-39%)

Increased cough, headache, flushing.

Occasional (11%-13%)

Flu-like symptoms, nausea, lockjaw, jaw pain, hypotension.

Rare (2%-8%)

Insomnia, syncope, palpitations, vomiting, back pain, muscle cramps.

SERIOUS REACTIONS

- Hemoptysis and pneumonia occur occasionally.
- Congestive heart failure, renal failure, dyspnea, and chest pain occur rarely.

PRECAUTIONS & CONSIDERATIONS

Caution is warranted with renal and hepatic impairment and in those who are concurrently taking medications that may increase the risk of syncope. Discontinue therapy immediately if pulmonary edema occurs.

Storage
Store at room temperature up to 86° F or store in refrigerator; do not freeze.

Administration
Iloprost is administered by inhalation only, using the Prodose ADD or the I-neb AAD systems. Transfer the entire contents of the ampule into the medication chamber. Ampule size used (e.g., 1 or 2 mL) is system dependent. After use, discard any unused portion from the system's medication chamber.

! Do not give doses more frequently than every 2 h, even though the clinical effect of the medication may not last the full 2 h.

Imatinib

im'a-tin-ib

Gleevec

CATEGORY AND SCHEDULE

Pregnancy Risk Category: D

Classification: Antineoplastics, signal transduction inhibitors

MECHANISM OF ACTION

Inhibits Bcr-Abl tyrosine kinase, an enzyme created by the Philadelphia chromosome abnormality found in patients with chronic myeloid leukemia (CML). *Therapeutic Effect:* Suppresses tumor growth during the three stages of CML: blast crisis, accelerated phase, and chronic phase.

PHARMACOKINETICS

Well absorbed after PO administration. Binds to plasma proteins, particularly albumin. Metabolized in the liver. Eliminated mainly in the feces as metabolites. *Half-life:* 18 h.

AVAILABILITY

Tablets: 100 mg, 400 mg.

INDICATIONS AND DOSAGES

▸ **Philadelphia chromosome positive (Ph+) CML**

PO

Adults, Elderly. 400 mg/day for patients in chronic-phase CML; 600 mg/day for patients in accelerated phase or blast crisis. May increase dosage from 400 to 600 mg/day for patients in chronic phase or from 600 to 800 mg (given as 300-400 mg twice a day) for patients in accelerated phase or blast crisis in the absence of a severe drug reaction or severe neutropenia or thrombocytopenia in the following circumstances: progression of the disease, failure to achieve a satisfactory hematologic response after 3 mo or more of treatment, or loss of a previously achieved hematologic response.

Children 2 yr and older. Newly diagnosed CML: 340 mg/m^2/day (maximum: 600 mg). Chronic phase: 260 mg/m^2 a day as a single daily dose or in 2 divided doses.

▸ **Ph+ acute lymphocytic leukemia (ALL)**

PO

Adults. 600 mg once daily.

▸ Kit (CD117) positive unresectable of metastatic gastrointestinal stromal tumors (GIST)
PO
Adults. 400-600 mg once daily. Up to 400 mg twice daily may be considered in patients with disease progression at a lower dose.
▸ Kit-positive GIST after complete gross resection
PO
Adults. 400 mg once daily.
▸ Myelodysplastic syndrome (MDS)/ myeloproliferative disease (MPD) with PDGFR (platelet-derived growth factor receptor) gene rearrangement
PO
Adults. 400 mg once daily.
▸ Hypereosinophilic syndrome (HES) or chronic eosinophilic leukemia (CEL) positive for FIPL1L1-PDGFR α fusion kinase OR for HES or CEL that are negative or unknown
PO
Adults. 400 mg PO once daily (if negative for marker). If positive for FIP1L1-PDGFR α fusion kinase, initially 100 mg/day and increase up to 400 mg if inadequate response.
▸ Aggressive systemic mastocytosis (ASM) without D816V c-Kit mutation or status unknown
PO
Adults. 400 mg once daily.
▸ Unresectable, recurrent, and/or metastatic dermatofibrosarcoma protuberans (DFSP)
PO
Adults. 400 mg twice daily.
▸ Dosage modifications (all indications) if taking strong CYP3A inducer
Increase imatinib dose by at least 50% and monitor clinical response closely.
▸ Dosage adjustments
Dosage adjustments are recommended for hepatic dysfunction and hematologic toxicity. See manufacturer's information.

CONTRAINDICATIONS

Known hypersensitivity to imatinib.

INTERACTIONS

Drug
Carbamazepine, dexamethasone, phenobarbital, phenytoin, rifampin: Decrease imatinib concentration. Increase imatinib dose as directed.
Clarithromycin, erythromycin, itraconazole, ketoconazole: Increase imatinib plasma concentration.
Cyclosporine, pimozide: May alter the therapeutic effects of these drugs.
Dihydropyridine calcium channel blockers, simvastatin, triazolobenzodiazepines: May increase the blood concentration of these drugs.
Digoxin: Imatinib may decrease the absorption of digoxin.
HMG-CoA reductase inhibitors: Imatinib may inhibit the metabolism of HMG-CoA reductase inhibitors.
Lansoprazole: May increase dermatological side effects of imatinib.
Live-virus vaccines: May potentiate viral replication, and decrease the patient's antibody response to the vaccine.
Warfarin: Reduces the effect of warfarin. Use heparin or low-molecular-weight heparin instead during treatment.
Herbal
St. John's wort: Decreases imatinib concentration. Avoid.
Food
Grapefruit juice: Increases imatinib concentration. Avoid.

DIAGNOSTIC TEST EFFECTS

May increase serum bilirubin, AST (SGOT), and ALT (SGPT) levels. May decrease platelet count, WBC count, and serum potassium level.

SIDE EFFECTS

Frequent (24%-68%)
Nausea, diarrhea, vomiting, headache, fluid retention (periorbital, lower extremities), rash, musculoskeletal pain, muscle cramps, arthralgia.

Occasional (10%-23%)
Abdominal pain, cough, myalgia, fatigue, fever, anorexia, dyspepsia, constipation, night sweats, pruritus.

Rare (< 10%)
Nasopharyngitis, petechiae, asthenia, epistaxis, infection.

SERIOUS REACTIONS

- Severe fluid retention (manifested as pleural effusion, pericardial effusion, pulmonary edema, and ascites) and hepatotoxicity occur rarely.
- Neutropenia and thrombocytopenia are expected responses to the drug; bleeding may occur.
- Respiratory toxicity, manifested as dyspnea and pneumonia, may occur.
- Stevens-Johnson syndrome and other bullous skin reactions.
- In HES and cardiac involvement, cases of cardiogenic shock/left ventricular dysfunction have been reported.

PRECAUTIONS & CONSIDERATIONS

Caution is warranted in patients with hepatic and renal impairment and in patients with congestive heart failure or pulmonary disease. Because imatinib may cause severe teratogenic effects, women should avoid becoming pregnant and avoid breastfeeding while taking this drug. The safety and efficacy of imatinib have not been established in children. Elderly patients are at increased risk for fluid retention. Vaccinations without the physician's approval, crowds, and contact with people with known infections should be avoided.

Notify the physician of rapid weight gain, fluid retention, nausea, and vomiting. Antiemetics should be ordered to control nausea and vomiting. Pattern of daily bowel activity and stool consistency should be monitored. CBC for evidence of neutropenia and thrombocytopenia and liver function test results for evidence of hepatotoxicity should be assessed. Neutropenia and thrombocytopenia usually last 2-4 wks.

Storage
Store at room temperature. Protect from moisture.

Administration
Give oral imatinib with a meal and a large glass of water. Do not crush or chew. For patients unable to swallow the tablets, the tablets may be dispersed in a glass of water or apple juice. Use approximately 50 mL of liquid for the 100-mg tablet and 200 mL for a 400-mg tablet. Place tablets in the appropriate volume and stir. The suspension should be administered immediately after complete disintegration.

Imiglucerase

im-i-gloo'ser-ase

★🍁 Cerezyme

Do not confuse Cerezyme with Cerebyx or Ceredase.

CATEGORY AND SCHEDULE

Pregnancy Risk Category: C

Classification: Enzymes, metabolic, recombinant DNA origin

MECHANISM OF ACTION

An enzyme analogue of the enzyme β-glucocerebrosidase, which catalyzes hydrolysis of the glycolipid glucocerebroside to glucose and ceramide. *Therapeutic Effect:* Minimizes conditions associated with Gaucher disease, such as anemia and bone disease.

AVAILABILITY

Powder for Injection: 212 units (equivalent to a reconstituted withdrawal dose of 200 units), 424 units (equivalent to a reconstituted withdrawal dose of 400 units).

INDICATIONS AND DOSAGES

▸ **Gaucher disease**

IV

Adults, Elderly, Children. Initially, 2.5 units/kg infused over 1-2 h 3 times a week up to 60 units/kg/wk. Maintenance: Progressive reduction in dosage while monitoring patient response.

CONTRAINDICATIONS

None known. If serious hypersensitivity occurs, reevaluate continued treatment.

INTERACTIONS

None known.

DIAGNOSTIC TEST EFFECTS

None known.

IV INCOMPATIBILITIES

Do not mix imiglucerase with any solution other than 0.9% NaCl.

SIDE EFFECTS

Frequent (3%)

Headache.

Occasional (< 3% to 1%)

Nausea, abdominal discomfort, dizziness, pruritus, rash, small decrease in BP, urinary frequency.

SERIOUS REACTIONS

- Serious hypersensitivity is rare.

PRECAUTIONS & CONSIDERATIONS

CBC, platelet count, and liver function test results should be monitored. Notify the physician of headache.

Storage

Refrigerate vials. The reconstituted solution is stable for 24 h if refrigerated or 12 h at room temperature.

Administration

For IV use, reconstitute the 200-unit vial with 5.1 mL sterile water (or the 400-unit vial with 10.2 mL) to provide a concentration of 40 units/mL. Further dilute with 100-200 mL 0.9% NaCl. Infuse the solution over 1-2 h.

Imipenem-Cilastatin

i-me-pen′em sye′la-stat′in

Primaxin, Primaxin IM

CATEGORY AND SCHEDULE

Pregnancy Risk Category: C

Classification: Antibiotics, carbapenems

MECHANISM OF ACTION

A fixed-combination carbapenem. Imipenem penetrates the bacterial cell membrane and binds to penicillin-binding proteins, inhibiting cell wall synthesis. Cilastatin competitively inhibits the enzyme dehydropeptidase, preventing renal metabolism of imipenem. *Therapeutic Effect:* Produces bacterial cell death.

PHARMACOKINETICS

Readily absorbed after IM administration. Protein binding: 13%-21%.Widely distributed. Metabolized in the kidneys. Primarily excreted in urine. Removed by hemodialysis. *Half-life:* 1 h (increased in impaired renal function).

AVAILABILITY

IV Injection: 250 mg, 500 mg.
IM Injection: 500 mg, powder for suspension.

INDICATIONS AND DOSAGES

▸ **Serious respiratory tract, skin and skin-structure, gynecologic, bone, joint, intra-abdominal, nosocomial, and polymicrobic infections; UTIs; endocarditis; septicemia**

IV

Adults, Elderly. 2-4 g/day in divided doses q6h.

▸ **Mild to moderate respiratory tract, skin and skin-structure, gynecologic, bone, joint, intra-abdominal, and polymicrobic infections; urinary tract infection; endocarditis; septicemia**

IV

Adults, Elderly. 1-2 g/day in divided doses q6-8h.

Children 4 mo to 12 yr. 60-100 mg/kg/day in divided doses q6h. Maximum: 4 g/day.

Children 1-3 mo. 100 mg/kg/day in divided doses q6h.

Children younger than 1 mo. 20-25 mg/kg/dose q8-24h.

IM (ONLY FOR SKIN, LOWER RESPIRATORY SYSTEM, OR ABDOMINAL INFECTIONS)

Adults, Elderly. 500-750 mg q12h.

▸ **Dosage in renal impairment**

Dosage and frequency must be based on creatinine clearance, patient weight, and the severity of the infection. The manufacturer provides detailed and specific tables for dosage adjustments. See prescribing information. Do not give to children with impaired renal function.

CONTRAINDICATIONS

All dosage forms: Hypersensitivity to primaxin or serious previous hypersensitivity with other β-lactams, such as penicillins or cephalosporins. For IM dosage form (since diluted with lidocaine): Hypersensitivity to amide anesthetics or severe shock or heart block.

INTERACTIONS

Drug

Cyclosporine: May increase neurotoxicity of imipenem; may cause increased levels of cyclosporine.
Ganciclovir: May increase risk of seizures.
Valproic acid: May decrease levels of valproic acid.

Herbal and Food

None known.

DIAGNOSTIC TEST EFFECTS

May increase BUN level and serum alkaline phosphatase, bilirubin, creatinine, LDH, AST (SGOT), and ALT (SGPT) levels. May decrease blood hematocrit and hemoglobin levels.

IV INCOMPATIBILITIES

Allopurinol (Aloprim), amphotericin B complex (Abelcet, AmBisome, Amphotec), azithromycin (Zithromax), ceftriazone (Rocephin), diazepam, drotrecogin alfa (Xigris), etoposide (VesPesid), fluconazole (Diflucan), gemcitabine (Gemzar), haloperidol, inamrinone, lansoprazole (Prevacid), lorazepam (Ativan), mannitol, meperidine (Demerol), methyldopate, midazolam (Versed), phenytoin, quinupristin-dalfopristin (Synercid), sagramostim (Leukine), sodium bicarbonate.

IV COMPATIBILITIES

Acyclovir (Valtrex), amifostine (Ethyol), aztreonam (Azactam), cefepime (Maxipime), cisatracurium

(Nimbex), diltiazem (Cardizem), docetaxel (Taxotere), famotidine (Pepcid), fludarabine (Fludara), foscarnet (Foscavir), granisetron (Kytril), idarubicin (Idamycin), insulin, linezolid (Zyvox), melphalan (Alkeran), methotrexate, ondansetron (Zofran), propofol (Diprivan), remifentanil (Ultiva), tacrolimus (Prograf), teniposide (Vumon), thiotepa (Thioplex), vinorelbine (Navelbine), zidovudine (Retrovir).

SIDE EFFECTS

Occasional (2%-3%)
Diarrhea, nausea, vomiting, pruritus, urticaria.
Rare (1%-2%)
Rash.

SERIOUS REACTIONS

- Antibiotic-associated colitis and other superinfections may occur.
- Anaphylactic reactions have been reported, serious skin reactions.
- Seizures, especially with high doses in presence of renal insufficiency.

PRECAUTIONS & CONSIDERATIONS

Caution is warranted with a history of seizures, renal impairment, and sensitivity to penicillins. Superinfection may occur with prolonged use. Be aware that imipenem crosses the placenta and is distributed in amniotic fluid, breast milk, and cord blood. This drug may be used safely in children younger than 12 yr, but the IM form should not be used. Do not give to children with renal impairment. In elderly patients, age-related renal function impairment may require dosage adjustment. Notify the physician if severe diarrhea occurs, but avoid taking antidiarrheals.

Notify the physician of the onset of troublesome or serious adverse reactions, including infusion site pain, redness, or swelling, nausea or vomiting, or skin rash or itching. History of allergies, particularly to β-lactams, cephalosporins, and penicillins, should be determined before beginning drug therapy.

Storage
IM suspension will be light tan once reconstituted. IV solution normally appears colorless to yellow; discard if solution turns brown. IV infusion (piggyback) is stable for 4 h at room temperature, 24 h if refrigerated. Discard if precipitate forms.

Administration
For IM use, prepare primaxin IM with 1% lidocaine without epinephrine, as prescribed; 500-mg vial with 2 mL, 750-mg vial with 3 mL lidocaine HCl. Administer suspension within 1 h of preparation. Do not mix the suspension with any other medications. Give deep IM injections slowly into a large muscle to minimize patient discomfort. To further minimize discomfort, administer IM injections into the gluteus maximus instead of the lateral aspect of the thigh. Be sure to aspirate with the syringe before injecting the drug to decrease risk of injection into a blood vessel.

For IV use, dilute each 250- or 500-mg vial with 100 mL D5W or 0.9% NaCl. Give by intermittent IV infusion (piggyback). Do not give IV push. Infuse over 20-30 min (1-g dose longer than 40-60 min). Observe the patient during the first 30 min of the infusion for possible hypersensitivity reaction. Infusions can be slowed if patient complains of nausea. Doses > 500 mg in children should be given over 40-60 min.

Imipramine

ih-mih'prah-meen

Tofranil, Tofranil-PM

Apo-Imipramine, Impril

Do not confuse imipramine with desipramine.

CATEGORY AND SCHEDULE

Pregnancy Risk Category: D

Classification: Antidepressants, tricyclic

MECHANISM OF ACTION

A tricyclic antidepressant agent that blocks the reuptake of neurotransmitters, such as norepinephrine and serotonin, at presynaptic membranes, increasing their concentration at postsynaptic receptor sites. *Therapeutic Effect:* Relieves depression and controls nocturnal enuresis.

AVAILABILITY

Tablets: 10 mg, 25 mg, 50 mg.
Capsules: 75 mg, 100 mg, 125 mg, 150 mg.

INDICATIONS AND DOSAGES

▸ **Depression**

PO

Adults. Initially, 75-100 mg/day. May gradually increase to 300 mg/day for hospitalized patients, or 200 mg/day for outpatients; then reduce dosage to effective maintenance level, 50-150 mg/day.

Elderly, Adolescents. Initially, 30-40 mg/day at bedtime. May increase by 10-25 mg every 3-7 days. Range: 50-100 mg/day.

Children older than 6 yr. 1.5 mg/kg/day. May increase by 1 mg/kg every 3-4 days. Maximum: 2.5 mg/kg/day.

▸ **Enuresis**

PO

Children older than 6 yr. Initially, 10-25 mg at bedtime. May increase by 25 mg/day. Maximum: 50 mg if under 12 yr, 75 mg if over 12 yr; do not exceed 2.5 mg/kg/day.

OFF-LABEL USES

Treatment of attention-deficit hyperactivity disorder, cataplexy associated with narcolepsy, neurogenic pain, panic disorder.

CONTRAINDICATIONS

Acute recovery period after myocardial infarction, use within 14 days of MAOIs, pregnancy, hypersensitivity.

INTERACTIONS

Drug

Alcohol, other central nervous system (CNS) depressants: May increase the hypotensive effects and CNS and respiratory depression caused by imipramine.

Anticholinergic agents: May have additive adverse effects.

β-Agonists: May increase risk of arrhythmias.

Bile acid sequestrants: May bind to and decrease levels of tricyclic antidepressants.

Carbamazepine: May increase carbamazepine levels.

CYPZD6 inhibitors (e.g., SSRIs, quinidine, and cimetidine): May increase imipramine blood concentration and risk of toxicity.

Clonidine, guanadrel: May decrease the effects of these drugs.

Linezolid: Serotonin syndrome may occur. Avoid this combination.

MAOIs: May increase the risk of neuroleptic malignant syndrome, hyperpyrexia, hypertensive crisis, and seizures. Contraindicated.

Methylphenidate: May inhibit imipramine metabolism.

Phenothiazines: May increase the anticholinergic and sedative effects of imipramine.
Phenytoin: May decrease the imipramine blood concentration.
Sympathomimetics: May increase the risk of cardiac effects.
Valproic acid: May increase adverse effects.
Herbal
Ginkgo biloba: May decrease seizure threshold.
Kava kava, SAMe, valerian: May increase risk of serotonin syndrome and excessive sedation.
St. John's wort: May increase imipramine's pharmacologic effects and risk of toxicity.
Food
None known.

DIAGNOSTIC TEST EFFECTS

May alter blood glucose levels and ECG readings. Therapeutic serum drug level is 225-300 ng/mL; toxic serum drug level is > 500 ng/mL.

SIDE EFFECTS

Frequent
Somnolence, fatigue, dry mouth, blurred vision, constipation, delayed micturition, orthostatic hypotension, diaphoresis, impaired concentration, increased appetite, urine retention, photosensitivity.
Occasional
GI disturbances (nausea, metallic taste).
Rare
Paradoxical reactions (agitation, restlessness, nightmares, insomnia), extrapyramidal symptoms (particularly fine hand tremor).

SERIOUS REACTIONS

- Overdose may produce seizures; cardiovascular effects, such as severe orthostatic hypotension, dizziness, tachycardia, palpitations, and arrhythmias; and altered temperature regulation, including hyperpyrexia or hypothermia.
- Abrupt discontinuation after prolonged therapy may produce headache, malaise, nausea, vomiting, and vivid dreams.

PRECAUTIONS & CONSIDERATIONS

Caution is warranted with cardiac disease, diabetes mellitus, glaucoma, hiatal hernia, history of seizures, history of urinary obstruction or retention, hyperthyroidism, increased intraocular pressure, benign prostatic hyperplasia, renal or hepatic disease, and schizophrenia. Imipramine is minimally distributed in breast milk. Imipramine use is not recommended for children younger than 6 yr. Antidepressants have been associated with an increased risk of suicidality in adolescents and young adults. Patients should be monitored closely for behavioral changes, such as emotional lability, suicidal thoughts, or other unusual behaviors during treatment. Expect to administer a lower dosage to elderly patients because they are at increased risk for drug toxicity.

Anticholinergic, sedative, and hypotensive effects may occur during early therapy, but tolerance to these effects usually develops. Because dizziness may occur, change positions slowly and avoid alcohol and tasks that require mental alertness or motor skills. Assess pattern of daily bowel activity, bladder for urine retention, BP and pulse rate to detect hypotension and arrhythmias, CBC and blood serum chemistry tests to monitor blood glucose level, and liver and renal function tests.

Storage

Store at room temperature.

Administration

! Make sure at least 14 days elapse between the use of MAOIs and imipramine.

Take imipramine with food or milk if GI distress occurs. Do not crush or break film-coated tablets. To reduce daytime sedation and improve sleep, can administer entire daily dose at bedtime in most patients. Improvement may occur 2-5 days after starting therapy but the full therapeutic effect will likely occur within 2-3 wks. Do not abruptly discontinue imipramine.

Imiquimod

im-ick'wih-mod

Aldara, Zyclara

CATEGORY AND SCHEDULE

Pregnancy Risk Category: C

Classification: Dermatologics, immunomodulators

MECHANISM OF ACTION

An immune response modifier whose mechanism of action is unknown. Induces cytokines such as interferon-alfa; tumor necrosis factor-α; and interleukins 1, 6, and 8, which may result in antiviral actions. Dermatologic antitumor effects may be via upregulation of local α interferon levels and that recruitment of natural killer cells may produce therapeutic response. *Therapeutic Effect:* Reduces genital and perianal warts.

PHARMACOKINETICS

Minimal absorption after topical administration. Minimal excretion in urine and feces.

AVAILABILITY

Cream: 5% (Aldara) 3.75% (Zyclara).

INDICATIONS AND DOSAGES

▸ Condyloma acuminata/genital and perianal warts

TOPICAL

Adults, Elderly, Children 12 yr and older. Apply 3 times/wk before normal sleeping hours; leave on skin 6-10 h. Remove following treatment period. Continue therapy for maximum of 16 wks.

▸ Actinic keratosis

Adults. Apply 5% cream to defined treatment area of face or scalp 2 times/wk (e.g., Monday and Thursday) for 16 wks at bedtime. Leave on skin approximately 8 h before washing.

Adults. Apply 3.75% cream once daily at bedtime to the affected area for two 2-week cycles separated by a 2-week no-treatment period. Up to 2 packets may be applied each time. Leave on skin for approximately 8 h before washing.

▸ Superficial basal cell carcinoma

Adults. Apply 5% cream 5 times/wk before bedtime for a full 6 wks. Leave on skin 8 h, then wash.

CONTRAINDICATIONS

History of hypersensitivity to imiquimod.

INTERACTIONS

None known.

DIAGNOSTIC TEST EFFECTS

None known.

SIDE EFFECTS

Frequent

Local skin reactions: erythema, itching, burning, erosion, excoriation/flaking, fungal infections (women).

Occasional

Pain, induration, ulceration, scabbing, soreness, headache, flu-like symptoms, photosensitivity.

SERIOUS REACTIONS

- If local reactions are intense, continue rest periods from treatment.
- Skin color change (hyperpigmentation or hypopigmentation) may occur. Some changes may be permanent.

PRECAUTIONS & CONSIDERATIONS

Caution should be used with inflammatory conditions of the skin. Safety and efficacy have not been established for basal cell nevus syndrome or xeroderma pigmentosum. It is unknown whether imiquimod crosses the placenta or is distributed in breast milk. Safety and efficacy of imiquimod have not been established in children younger than 12 yr. No age-related precautions have been noted in elderly patients.

If severe local skin reaction occurs, the cream should be removed by washing the treatment area and may be resumed after the reaction has subsided. Avoid exposure to sunlight and sunlamps and follow UV protection guidelines.

Storage

Store at room temperature.

Administration

Wash application site with soap and water 6-10 h after applying. Apply a thin layer to affected area. Avoid contact with eyes, lips, and nostrils. Wash hands after application. Discard any partially used packets.

Immune Globulin IV (IGIV)

im-myoon′glob′yoo-lin

★ Baygam, Carimune NF, Flebogamma, Gamimune N, Gammagard S/D, Gammar-P-IV, Gamunex, Iveegam EN, Polygam S/D, Privigen

🍁 IGIVnex, Gammagard S/D, Gamunex, Privigen

CATEGORY AND SCHEDULE

Pregnancy Risk Category: C

Classification: Immune globulins

MECHANISM OF ACTION

An immune serum that increases antibody titer and antigen-antibody reaction. *Therapeutic Effect:* Provides passive immunity against infection; induces rapid increase in platelet count; produces anti-inflammatory effect.

PHARMACOKINETICS

Evenly distributed between intravascular and extravascular space. *Half-life:* 21-23 days.

AVAILABILITY

Injection Solution (Gamimune N, Gamunex, Privigen): 10%.
Injection Solution (Flebogamma): 5%.
Injection Powder for Reconstitution (Carimune): 1 g, 3 g, 6 g, 12 g.
Injection Powder for Reconstitution (Gammagard S/D, Polygam S/D): 2.5 g, 5 g, 10 g.
Injection Powder for Reconstitution (Gammar-P-IV): 5 g, 10 g.
Injection Powder for Reconstitution (Iveegam EN): 0.5 g, 1 g, 2.5 g, 5 g.

INDICATIONS AND DOSAGES

▸ **Primary immunodeficiency syndrome**

IV

Adults, Elderly, Children. 200-800 mg/kg once monthly.

▸ Idiopathic thrombocytopenic purpura (ITP)
IV
Adults, Elderly, Children. 400-1000 mg/kg/day for 2-5 days.
▸ Kawasaki disease
IV
Adults, Elderly, Children. 2 g/kg as a single dose; 400 mg/kg/day for 4 days has also been used.
▸ Chronic lymphocytic leukemia
IV
Adults, Elderly, Children.
400 mg/kg q3-4wk.
▸ Bone marrow transplant
IV
Adults, Elderly, Children.
400-500 mg/kg/dose every week for 12 wks, then every month.

OFF-LABEL USES
Control and prevention of infections in infants and children with immunosuppression from AIDS or AIDS-related complex; prevention of acute infections in immunosuppressed patients; prevention and treatment of infections in high-risk, preterm, low-birth-weight neonates; treatment of chronic inflammatory demyelinating polyneuropathies and multiple sclerosis.

CONTRAINDICATIONS
Allergies to γ-globulin, thimerosal, or anti-IgA antibodies; isolated IgA deficiency; hyperprolinemia.

INTERACTIONS
Drug
Live-virus vaccines: IVIG contains antibodies that may interfere with proper response to the vaccine.
Herbal and Food
None known.

DIAGNOSTIC TEST EFFECTS
None known.

IV INCOMPATIBILITIES
Administer IGIV by infusion only through separate tubing (dedicated line). Avoid mixing IGIV with other medications or IV infusion fluids.

SIDE EFFECTS
Frequent
Tachycardia, backache, headache, arthralgia, myalgia.
Occasional
Fatigue, wheezing, injection site rash or pain, leg cramps, urticaria, bluish lips and nailbeds, light-headedness.

SERIOUS REACTIONS
- Anaphylactic reactions are rare, but the incidence increases with repeated injections of IGIV. Keep epinephrine readily available.
- Renal dysfunction/failure (especially with sucrose-containing products) as a result of osmotic nephrosis.
- Overdose may produce chest tightness, chills, diaphoresis, dizziness, facial flushing, nausea, vomiting, fever, and hypotension.

PRECAUTIONS & CONSIDERATIONS
Caution is warranted with cardiovascular disease, diabetes mellitus, a history of thrombosis, impaired renal function, sepsis, or volume depletion and concurrent use of nephrotoxic drugs. It is unknown whether IGIV crosses the placenta or is distributed in breast milk. No age-related precautions have been noted in children or elderly patients.

Adequate hydration should be maintained before giving IGIV. Notify the physician if dyspnea, decreased urine output, fluid retention, edema, or sudden weight gain occurs. Vital signs and platelet count should be monitored.
Storage
Refer to individual IV preparations for storage requirements and

information about stability after reconstitution.

Administration

Reconstitute IGIV only as directed by the manufacturer. Discard partially used or turbid preparations. Administer IGIV by infusion only through separate tubing. Avoid mixing IGIV with other medications or IV infusion fluids. The infusion rate varies among products. In general, the initial IV rate should begin slowly. Each rate increase thereafter should be at 15-30 min intervals. Because of the risk of acute renal failure, the FDA recommends a maximum infusion rate of 3 mg sucrose/kg/min (2 mg immune globulin/kg/min). Filtering is not necessary. Control the infusion rate carefully. A too-rapid infusion increases the risk of a precipitous drop in BP and an anaphylactic reaction, marked by chest tightness, chills, diaphoresis, facial flushing, fever, nausea, and vomiting. Monitor BP and vital signs diligently during and immediately after IV administration. Stop the infusion immediately if a suspected anaphylactic reaction occurs or with signs of infusion reaction (fever, chills, nausea, vomiting, shock). Keep epinephrine readily available. A rapid response occurs to therapy lasting 1-3 mo.

Inamrinone Lactate

in-am′ri-nohn

Do not confuse with Amiodarone.

CATEGORY AND SCHEDULE

Pregnancy Risk Category: C

Classification: Inotropes, vasodilators

MECHANISM OF ACTION

A positive inotropic agent that inhibits myocardial cyclic adenosine monophosphate (cAMP) phosphodiesterase activity and directly stimulates cardiac contractility. Peripheral vasodilation reduces both preload and afterload. *Therapeutic Effect:* Reduces preload and afterload; increases cardiac output.

PHARMACOKINETICS

After IV administration, rapidly absorbed from the GI tract. Protein binding: 10%-49%. Partially metabolized in liver. Excreted in urine as both inamrinone and its metabolites. *Half-life:* 3-6 h (half-life increased with congestive heart failure).

AVAILABILITY

Injection: 5 mg/mL.

INDICATIONS AND DOSAGES

▸ **Short-term management of intractable heart failure**

IV INFUSION (CONTINUOUS)

Adults. Initially, 0.75 mg/kg loading dose over 2-3 min followed by a maintenance infusion of 5-10 mcg/kg/min. A repeat bolus dose of 0.75 mg/kg may be given 30 min after the initiation of therapy. Maximum: 10 mg/kg/day.

▸ **Dosage for severe renal impairment**

CrCl < 10 mL/min: Reduce dosage to 50%-75% of the usual dosage.

CONTRAINDICATIONS

Severe aortic or pulmonic valvular disease; hypersensitivity to inamrinone or bisulfites.

INTERACTIONS

Drug

Anagrelide: Additive cAMP effects.

Digitalis: May increase the inotropic effects.

Diuretics: May cause hypovolemia and decrease filling pressure.
Dysopyramide: May cause hypotension.
Herbal and Food
None known.

DIAGNOSTIC TEST EFFECTS

Elevated AST or ALT, decreased platelets.

IV INCOMPATIBILITIES

Furosemide (Lasix), sodium bicarbonate, amphotericin B, ampicillin, aztreonam, calcium gluconate, all cephalosporins, clindamycin, esmolol, imipenem-cilastatin, insulin, levofloxacin, many penicillins, vancomycin.

IV COMPATIBILITIES

Atropine, calcium chloride, cisatracurium (Nimbex), digoxin (Lanoxin), labetalol, lidocaine (Xylocaine), metaraminol (Aramine), nitroprusside (Nitropress), propafenone (Rhythmol), propofol (Diprivan), propranolol (Inderal), remifentanil (Ultiva), verapamil (Calan).

SIDE EFFECTS

Occasional
Arrhythmia, nausea, hypotension, thrombocytopenia.
Rare
Fever, vomiting, abdominal pain, anorexia, chest pain, decreased tear production, hepatotoxicity, and burning at the site of injection, hypersensitivity to inamrinone.

SERIOUS REACTIONS

- Overdose may cause severe hypotension.
- Improved diuresis may cause fluid or electrolyte imbalance.
- If thrombocytopenia is persistent, may require discontinuation of drug.

PRECAUTIONS & CONSIDERATIONS

BP and pulse should be obtained immediately before each inamrinone dose, in addition to regular BP monitoring. Be alert for BP fluctuations. Elderly patients are more sensitive to the drug's hypotensive effects, and age-related renal impairment may require dosage adjustment. Caution should be used in children and elderly patients. Cardiac index, stroke volume, systemic vascular resistance, and pulmonary vascular resistance, BP, heart rate, platelet count, fluid status, and liver and renal function should be monitored.
Storage
Store unopened vial at room temperature. Do not freeze. Protect from light.
Administration
Give IV bolus dose undiluted over 2-3 min. Reconstituted solutions should be used within 24 h. Dosage is based on clinical response. Do not dilute with solutions containing dextrose. Do not administer furosemide in intravenous lines containing inamrinone. Inamrinone is for short-term therapy; use infusions within 24 h of preparation. To make recommended 2.5 mg/mL concentration for infusion, mix inamrinone solution with an equal volume of 0.9% or 0.45% NaCl.

Indapamide

in-dap'a-mide
Lozide
Do not confuse indapamide with iodamide or iopamidol.

CATEGORY AND SCHEDULE

Pregnancy Risk Category: B (D if used in pregnancy-induced hypertension)

Classification: Diuretics, thiazide and derivatives

MECHANISM OF ACTION
A thiazide-like diuretic that blocks the reabsorption of water, sodium, and potassium at the cortical diluting segment of the distal tubule; also reduces plasma and extracellular fluid volume and peripheral vascular resistance by direct effect on blood vessels. *Therapeutic Effect:* Promotes diuresis and reduces BP.

AVAILABILITY
Tablets: 1.25 mg, 2.5 mg.

INDICATIONS AND DOSAGES
▸ **Edema**
PO
Adults. Initially, 2.5 mg/day, may increase to 5 mg/day after 1 wk.
▸ **Hypertension**
PO
Adults, Elderly. Initially, 1.25 mg, may increase to 2.5 mg/day after 4 wks or 5 mg/day after additional 4 wks.

CONTRAINDICATIONS
Hypersensitivity to sulfonamide-derived drugs; anuria; renal decompensation; pregnancy.

INTERACTIONS
Drug
β-Blockers: May increase hyperglycemic effects in type 2 diabetic patients.
Cyclosporine: May increase risk of gout or renal toxicity.
Digoxin: May increase the risk of digoxin toxicity associated with indapamide-induced hypokalemia.
Lithium: May increase the risk of lithium toxicity.
Herbal
Ephedra, ginseng, yohimbe: May cause hypertension.
Food
None known.

DIAGNOSTIC TEST EFFECTS
May increase plasma renin activity. May decrease protein-bound iodine and serum potassium and sodium levels. May increase serum calcium or uric acid.

SIDE EFFECTS
Frequent (≥ 5%)
Fatigue, numbness of extremities, tension, irritability, agitation, headache, dizziness, lightheadedness, insomnia, muscle cramps.
Occasional (< 5%)
Tingling of extremities, urinary frequency, urticaria, rhinorrhea, flushing, weight loss, orthostatic hypotension, depression, blurred vision, nausea, vomiting, diarrhea or constipation, dry mouth, impotence, rash, pruritus.

SERIOUS REACTIONS
- Vigorous diuresis may lead to profound water and electrolyte depletion, resulting in hypokalemia, hyponatremia, and dehydration.
- Acute hypotensive episodes may occur.
- Hyperglycemia may occur during prolonged therapy.
- Pancreatitis, blood dyscrasias, pulmonary edema, allergic pneumonitis, and dermatologic reactions occur rarely.
- Overdose can lead to lethargy and coma without changes in electrolytes or hydration.

PRECAUTIONS & CONSIDERATIONS
Caution is warranted in patients with anuria, diabetes mellitus, a history of hypersensitivity to sulfonamides or thiazide diuretics, hepatic impairment, severe renal disease, thyroid disorders, gout, and in elderly or debilitated patients. Consuming foods high in potassium,

such as apricots, bananas, legumes, meat, orange juice, raisins, whole grains, including cereals, and white and sweet potatoes, is encouraged.

Dizziness or light-headedness may occur, so change positions slowly and let legs dangle momentarily before standing. An increase in the frequency and volume of urination may occur. BP, vital signs, electrolytes, intake and output, and weight should be monitored before and during treatment. Be aware of signs of electrolyte disturbances such as hypokalemia or hyponatremia. Hypokalemia may cause arrhythmias, altered mental status, muscle cramps, asthenia, and tremor. Hyponatremia may result in cold and clammy skin, confusion, and thirst.

Storage

Store at room temperature; avoid excessive heat.

Administration

Take indapamide with food or milk if GI upset occurs, preferably with breakfast to help prevent nocturia. Do not crush or break tablets.

Indinavir

in-din′ah-veer

Crixivan

Do not confuse indinavir with Denavir.

CATEGORY AND SCHEDULE

Pregnancy Risk Category: C

Classification: Antiretrovirals, protease inhibitors

MECHANISM OF ACTION

A protease inhibitor that suppresses HIV protease, an enzyme necessary for splitting viral polyprotein precursors into mature and infectious viral particles. *Therapeutic Effect:* Interrupts HIV replication, slowing the progression of HIV infection.

PHARMACOKINETICS

Rapidly absorbed after PO administration. Protein binding: 60%. Metabolized in the liver. Primarily excreted in urine. Unknown if removed by hemodialysis. *Half-life:* 1.8 h (increased in impaired hepatic function).

AVAILABILITY

Capsules: 100 mg, 200 mg, 400 mg.

INDICATIONS AND DOSAGES

▸ **HIV infection (in combination with other antiretrovirals)**

PO

Adults. 800 mg (two 400-mg capsules) q8h; 400 mg twice daily when used with ritonavir 400 mg twice daily *or* 800 mg twice daily when used with ritonavir 100-200 mg twice daily.

▸ **HIV infection in patients with hepatic insufficiency**

PO

Adults. 600 mg q8h (when used without ritonavir).

OFF-LABEL USES

Prophylaxis following occupational exposure to HIV.

CONTRAINDICATIONS

Hypersensitivity to indinavir; concurrent use of alprazolam, amiodarone, cisapride, triazolam, midazolam, pimozide, ergot alkaloids, atazanavir, alfuzosin, sildenafil, conivaptan, dronedarone, ranolazine, colchicine.

INTERACTIONS

NOTE: Please see detailed manufacturer's information for management of drug interactions. In

some cases, dosage adjustment or an alternate agent is recommended.
Drug
Amiodarone: May increase amiodarone levels. Contraindicated.
Antacids: May decrease absorption of indinavir.
Anticonvulsants, venlafaxine: May decrease levels of indinavir.
Antifungal agents, delavirdine, NNRTIs: May increase levels of indinavir.
Atazanavir: Increases blood bilirubin. Contraindicated.
Calcium channel blockers: Indinavir may increase concentrations of calcium channel blockers.
Conivaptan, dronedarone: Indinavir increases concentrations of these drugs significantly. Contraindicated.
Clarithromycin: May increase levels of clarithromycin.
Cyclosporine, other immunosuppressants: Indinavir may increase concentrations; use with caution and monitor closely.
CYP3A4 inducers: May decrease effects of indinavir.
CYP3A4 inhibitors: May increase effects of indinavir.
CYP3A4 substrates: Levels of CYP3A4 substrates may be increased by indinavir. Contraindicated with cisapride and pimozide.
Didanosine: Separate administration by at least 1 h.
Ergot alkaloids: Effects of ergot alkaloids may be increased. Contraindicated.
Fentanyl: Effects of fentanyl may be increased.
HMG-CoA reductase inhibitors, lidocaine: Indinavir may increase effects. Use not recommended with lovastatin, simvastatin, and rosuvastatin.
Phosphodiesterase-5 inhibitors (e.g., sildenafil, vardenafil, tadalafil): Increases PDE-5 inhibitor levels and risk of hypotension. Contraindicated for use with sildenafil for pulmonary HTN.
Alprazolam, midazolam, triazolam: Increases the risk of arrhythmias and prolonged sedation. Contraindicated.
Ranolazine, cisapride, pimozide: Increases levels of these drugs and risk of QT prolongation. Contraindicated.
Rifamycins: Decrease indinavir concentrations. Avoid.
Herbal
St. John's wort: May decrease indinavir concentration and effect. Avoid.
Food
Grapefruit juice: May decrease indinavir concentration and effect. Avoid.
High-fat, high-calorie, and high-protein meals: May decrease indinavir concentration.

DIAGNOSTIC TEST EFFECTS

May increase serum bilirubin (in 10% of patients), AST (SGOT), and ALT (SGPT) levels, blood glucose, lipids.

SIDE EFFECTS

Frequent
Nausea (12%), abdominal pain (9%), headache (6%), diarrhea (5%).
Occasional
Vomiting, asthenia, fatigue (4%); insomnia; accumulation of fat in waist, abdomen, or back of neck, buffalo hump.
Rare
Abnormal taste sensation, heartburn, symptomatic urinary tract disease, tubulointerstitial nephritis, transient renal dysfunction, hyperglycemia.

SERIOUS REACTIONS

- Nephrolithiasis (flank pain with or without hematuria) occurs in 4% of patients, 24% in children.
- Indinavir should be discontinued if hemolytic anemia develops.
- Hepatitis/liver failure or pancreatitis.
- Serious hypersensitivity reactions have included erythema multiforme or Stevens-Johnson syndrome or anaphylactoid reactions.
- Spontaneous bleeding in patients with hemophilia.

PRECAUTIONS & CONSIDERATIONS

Caution is warranted in patients with renal or liver function impairment. Also use with caution in patients with diabetes mellitus, kidney stones, hemophilia. Be aware that it is unknown whether indinavir is excreted in breast milk. Breastfeeding is not recommended in this population because of the possibility of HIV transmission. Be aware that the safety and efficacy of this drug have not been established in children; children have increased risk of nephrolithiasis. No information on the effects of this drug's use in elderly patients is available.

! Monitor for signs and symptoms of nephrolithiasis as evidenced by flank pain and hematuria, and notify the physician if symptoms occur. If nephrolithiasis occurs, expect therapy to be interrupted for 1-3 days. Establish baseline lab values and monitor renal function before and during therapy; in particular, evaluate the results of the serum creatinine and urinalysis tests. Maintain adequate hydration and drink 48 oz (1.5 L) of liquid over each 24-h period during therapy. Assess the pattern of daily bowel activity and stool consistency. Evaluate for abdominal discomfort or headache.

Storage

Store drug at room temperature, keep it in the original bottle, and protect it from moisture. Keep in mind that indinavir capsules are sensitive to moisture. Leave the desicant in the bottle.

Administration

For optimal drug absorption, take indinavir with water only and without food 1 h before or 2 h after a meal. May take indinavir with coffee, juice, skim milk, tea, or water and with a light meal (e.g., dry toast with jelly). Do not take indinavir with meals high in fat, calories, and protein. If indinavir and didanosine are given concurrently, give the drugs at least 1 h apart on an empty stomach.

Indomethacin

in-doe-meth'a-sin

★ Indocin, Indocin IV, Indocin-SR 🍁 Apo-Indomethacin, Indocid, Novomethacin

Do not confuse Indocin with Imodium or Vicodin.

CATEGORY AND SCHEDULE

Pregnancy Risk Category: B (D if used after 34 wks' gestation, close to delivery, or for longer than 48 h)

Classification: Analgesics, nonnarcotic, nonsteroidal anti-inflammatory drugs, antipyretic

MECHANISM OF ACTION

An NSAID that produces analgesic and anti-inflammatory effects by inhibiting prostaglandin synthesis. Also increases the sensitivity of the premature ductus to the dilating effects of prostaglandins.

Therapeutic Effect: Reduces the inflammatory response and intensity of pain. Closure of the patent ductus arteriosus.

PHARMACOKINETICS

PO: Onset 1-2 h, peak 3 h, duration 4-6 h; 99% plasma-protein binding; metabolized in liver, kidneys; excreted in urine, bile, feces, breast milk; crosses placenta.

AVAILABILITY

Capsules (Indocin): 25 mg, 50 mg.
Capsules (Sustained Release [Indocin-SR]): 75 mg.
Oral Suspension (Indocin): 25 mg/5 mL.
Powder for Injection (Indocin IV): 1 mg.
Suppository: 50 mg.

INDICATIONS AND DOSAGES

▸ **Moderate to severe rheumatoid arthritis, osteoarthritis, ankylosing spondylitis**

PO

Adults, Elderly. Initially, 25 mg 2-3 times a day; increased by 25-50 mg/wk up to 150-200 mg/day. Or 75 mg/day (extended release) up to 75 mg twice a day.
Children. 1-2 mg/kg/day. Maximum: 3 mg/kg/day (or 150-200 mg/day). Do not use extended release.

▸ **Acute gouty arthritis**

PO

Adults, Elderly. 50 mg 3 times a day until pain decreases. For short-term use.

▸ **Acute shoulder pain, bursitis, tendinitis**

PO

Adults, Elderly. 75-150 mg/day in 3-4 divided doses. Usually no more than 7-14 days.

▸ **Usual rectal dosage**

Adults, Elderly. 50 mg 4 times a day. Maximum: 200 mg/day.
Children. Initially, 1.5-2.5 mg/kg/day, increased up to 4 mg/kg/day. Maximum: 150-200 mg/day.

▸ **Patent ductus arteriosus**

IV

Neonates. Initially, 0.2 mg/kg. Subsequent doses are based on age, as follows, and are given at 12-24 h intervals.
Neonates older than 7 days. 0.25 mg/kg for second and third doses.
Neonates 2-7 days. 0.2 mg/kg for second and third doses.
Neonates < 48 h. 0.1 mg/kg for second and third doses.
If ductus arteriosus reopens, a second course may be given (not necessary if ductus closes or significantly reduces within 48 h of first course).

OFF-LABEL USES

Treatment of fever from malignancy, pericarditis, psoriatic arthritis, rheumatic complications associated with Paget disease of bone, vascular headache.

CONTRAINDICATIONS

Active GI bleeding or ulcerations; history of proctitis or recent rectal bleeding, hypersensitivity to aspirin, indomethacin, or other NSAIDs; renal impairment, thrombocytopenia; perioperative pain in the setting of coronary artery bypass graft surgery (use within 14 days of surgery). For IV in neonates: active bleeding, thrombocytopenia, coagulation problems, necrotizing enterocolitis, severe renal dysfunction, if patency ductus arteriosis necessary for blood flow.

INTERACTIONS

Drug

Aminoglycosides: May increase the blood concentration of these drugs in neonates.

Antihypertensives, diuretics: May decrease the effects of these drugs.
Aspirin, other salicylates: May increase the risk of GI side effects such as bleeding.
Bile acid sequestrants: May decrease absorption of NSAIDs.
Bone marrow depressants: May increase the risk of hematologic reactions.
Corticosteroids: May increase risk of GI ulceration.
Heparin, oral anticoagulants, thrombolytics: May increase the effects of these drugs.
Lithium: May increase the blood concentration and risk of toxicity of lithium.
Methotrexate: May increase the risk of methotrexate toxicity.
Probenecid: May increase the indomethacin blood concentration.
Quinolone antibiotics: May increase seizure potential.
Triamterene: May potentiate acute renal failure. Do not give concurrently.

Herbal

Alfalfa, anise, bilberry, bladderwrack, bromelain, cat's claw, celery, chamomile, coleus, cordyceps, dong quai, evening primrose, fenugreek, feverfew, garlic, ginger, ginkgo biloba, ginseng (American, Panax, Siberian), grapeseed, green tea, guggul, horse chestnut seed, horseradish, licorice, prickly ash, red clover, reishi, SAMe (S-adenosylmethionine), sweet clover, turmeric, white willow: May increase the risk of bleeding.
Feverfew: May decrease the effects of feverfew.

Food

None known.

DIAGNOSTIC TEST EFFECTS

May prolong bleeding time. May alter blood glucose level. May increase BUN level, and serum creatinine, potassium, AST (SGOT), and ALT (SGPT) levels. May decrease serum sodium level and platelet count.

IV INCOMPATIBILITIES

Amino acid injection, calcium gluconate, cimetidine (Tagamet), dobutamine (Dobutrex), dopamine (Intropin), gentamicin (Garamycin), levofloxacin (Levaquin), tobramycin (Nebcin).

IV COMPATIBILITIES

Furosemide (Lasix), insulin, potassium, sodium bicarbonate, sodium nitroprusside (Nitropress).

SIDE EFFECTS

Frequent (3%-11%)

Headache, nausea, vomiting, dyspepsia, dizziness.

Occasional (< 3%)

Depression, tinnitus, diaphoresis, somnolence, constipation, diarrhea, bleeding disturbances in patent ductus arteriosus.

Rare

Hypertension, confusion, urticaria, pruritus, rash, blurred vision.

SERIOUS REACTIONS

- Paralytic ileus and ulceration of the esophagus, stomach, duodenum, or small intestine may occur.
- Patients with impaired renal function may develop hyperkalemia and worsening of renal impairment.
- Indomethacin use may aggravate epilepsy, parkinsonism, and depression or other psychiatric disturbances.
- Nephrotoxicity, including dysuria, hematuria, proteinuria, and nephrotic syndrome, occurs rarely.
- Metabolic acidosis or alkalosis, apnea, and bradycardia occur rarely in patients with patent ductus arteriosus.

PRECAUTIONS & CONSIDERATIONS

Caution is warranted in patients with cardiac dysfunction, hypertension, epilepsy, hepatic or renal impairment, and in those receiving anticoagulant therapy concurrently. Use of the lowest effective dose for the shortest duration is recommended. Avoid alcohol and aspirin during therapy because these substances increase the risk of GI bleeding. Tasks that require mental alertness or motor skills should be avoided.

BUN, serum alkaline phosphatase, bilirubin, creatinine, potassium, AST (SGOT), ALT (SGPT) levels, BP, ECG, heart rate, platelet count, serum sodium, blood glucose levels, and urine output should be monitored. Therapeutic response, such as decreased pain, stiffness, swelling, and tenderness, improved grip strength, and increased joint mobility, should be evaluated.

Storage

Store at room temperature below 86° F. Do not freeze. Protect injection from light.

Administration

Take oral indomethacin after meals or with food or antacids. Don't crush extended-release capsules. Shake oral suspension well before each use.

! IV injection is the preferred route for neonates with patent ductus arteriosus. The drug may also be given orally, by nasogastric tube, or rectally. Administer no more than 3 doses at 12- to 24-h intervals.

For IV use, reconstitute by adding only 1 or 2 mL preservative-free sterile water for injection or 0.9% NaCl to the 1-mg vial to provide a concentration of 1 mg or 0.5 mg/mL, respectively. Do not dilute the solution any further. Administer the IV immediately after reconstitution. The solution normally appears clear; discard if it becomes cloudy or contains precipitate; discard any unused portion. Administer the drug over 20-30 min. Restrict fluid intake, as ordered. Take care to avoid extravasation.

For rectal use, if suppository is too soft, refrigerate it for 30 min or run cold water over the foil wrapper. Unwrap. Moisten the suppository with cold water before inserting it into the rectum.

Infliximab

in-flicks'ih-mab

Remicade

Do not confuse Remicade with Reminyl.

CATEGORY AND SCHEDULE

Pregnancy Risk Category: C

Classification: Disease-modifying antirheumatic drugs, gastrointestinals, immunomodulators, monoclonal antibodies, tumor necrosis factor modulators

MECHANISM OF ACTION

A monoclonal antibody that binds to tumor necrosis factor (TNF), inhibiting functional activity of TNF. Reduces infiltration of inflammatory cells. *Therapeutic Effect:* Decreases inflamed areas of the intestine, decreases synovitis and joint erosion.

PHARMACOKINETICS

Route	Onset	Peak	Duration
IV	1-2 wks	N/A	8-48 wks (Crohn disease)
IV	3-7 days	N/A	6-12 wks (rheumatoid arthritis [RA])

Absorbed into the GI tissue; primarily distributed in the vascular compartment. *Half-life:* 9.5 days.

AVAILABILITY

Powder for Injection: 100 mg.

INDICATIONS AND DOSAGES

▸ **Moderate to severe Crohn disease and fistulizing Crohn disease**

IV INFUSION

Adults, Elderly, Children 6 yr and older. Initially, 5 mg/kg followed by additional 5-mg/kg doses at 2 and 6 wks after first infusion. Maintenance: 5 mg/kg q8wk. May increase dose to 10 mg/kg if needed.

▸ **RA**

IV INFUSION

Adults, Elderly. 3 mg/kg; followed by additional doses at 2 and 6 wks after first infusion. Maintenance: 3 mg/kg q8wk. Some receive up to 10 mg/kg per dose.

▸ **Ankylosing spondylitis, prosiatic arthritis, plaque psoriasis, and moderate to severe ulcerative colitis**

IV INFUSION

Adults, Elderly. Initially, 5 mg/kg at wks 0, 2 and 6. Maintenance: 5 mg/kg q6-8wk.

CONTRAINDICATIONS

Sensitivity to infliximab or murine proteins, sepsis, serious active infection, doses > 5 mg/kg in patients with moderate or severe congestive heart failure.

INTERACTIONS

Drug

Abatacept, rilonacept, anakinra: May increase adverse effects such as infection risk.

Immunosuppressants: May reduce frequency of infusion reactions and antibodies to infliximab. May increase risk of serious infection.

Live vaccines: May decrease immune response to vaccine.

Herbal

Echinacea: May decrease effect of infliximab.

Food

None known.

DIAGNOSTIC TEST EFFECTS

None known.

IV INCOMPATIBILITIES

Do not infuse infliximab in the same IV line with other agents.

SIDE EFFECTS

Frequent (10%-22%)

Headache, nausea, fatigue, fever.

Occasional (5%-9%)

Fever or chills during infusion, pharyngitis, vomiting, pain, dizziness, bronchitis, rash, rhinitis, cough, pruritus, sinusitis, myalgia, back pain.

Rare (1%-4%)

Hypotension or hypertension, paresthesia, anxiety, depression, insomnia, diarrhea, urinary tract infection.

SERIOUS REACTIONS

- Hypersensitivity reaction, serum-sickness–like illness, and lupus-like syndrome may occur. Most occur within 2 h of infusion.
- Severe hepatic reactions and reactivation of hepatitis B have been reported with therapy.
- Lymphoma has been reported in adolescents and young adults with Crohn disease.
- New or worsening heart failure.
- Reactivation of latent tuberculosis has occurred; other serious infections.

PRECAUTIONS & CONSIDERATIONS

Caution is warranted in patients with a history of recurrent infections and in patients on concomitant immunosuppresant agents. It is unknown whether infliximab is distributed in breast milk. Safety and efficacy of infliximab have not been established in children for JRA; trials failed to establish effectiveness. Use infliximab cautiously in elderly patients because of a higher rate of infection in this population.

Follow-up tests, such as ESR, C-reactive protein measurement, and urinalysis, should be obtained. Notify the physician of signs of infection, such as fever. Persons with rheumatoid arthritis should report increase in pain, stiffness, or swelling of joints. Persons with Crohn disease should report changes in stool color, consistency, or elimination pattern. Hydration status should be assessed before and during therapy.

Storage

Refrigerate vials.

Administration

Reconstitute each vial with 10 mL sterile water for injection, using 21-gauge or smaller needle. Direct the stream of sterile water to the glass wall of the vial. Swirl the vial gently to dissolve the contents. Do not shake. Allow the solution to stand for 5 min. Because infliximab is a protein, the solution may develop a few translucent particles; do not use if particles are opaque or foreign particles are present. The solution normally appears colorless to light yellow and opalescent; do not use if discolored. Withdraw and waste a volume of 0.9% NaCl from a 250-mL bag that is equal to the volume of reconstituted solution to be injected into the 250-mL bag (approximately 10 mL). Total dose to be infused should equal 250 mL. Slowly add the reconstituted infliximab solution to the 250-mL infusion bag. Gently mix. Infusion concentration should range between 0.4 and 4 mg/mL. Begin infusion within 3 h of reconstitution. Administer IV infusion over 2 h, using set with a low-protein-binding filter.

Insulin

in′sull-in

- *Rapid Acting:* ★ 🍁 Humulin R, Novolin R, Novolog, Humalog, Apidra
- *Intermediate Acting:* ★ 🍁 Humulin N, Novolin N
- *Long Acting:* ★ 🍁 Lantus, Levemir
- *Combinations:* ★ 🍁 NovoLog Mix 70/30, Humalog Mix 50/50, Humalog Mix 75/25, Humulin 70/30, Novolin 70/30.

CATEGORY AND SCHEDULE

Pregnancy Risk Category: B

OTC; some forms are Rx-only, such as insulin analogues

Classification: Antidiabetic agents, insulins and insulin analogues

MECHANISM OF ACTION

Exogenous human insulins facilitate passage of glucose, potassium, and magnesium across the cellular membranes of skeletal and cardiac muscle and adipose tissue. Controls storage and metabolism of carbohydrates, protein, and fats. Promotes conversion of glucose to glycogen in the liver. *Therapeutic Effect:* Controls glucose levels in patients with diabetes or hyperglycemia.

PHARMACOKINETICS

Drug Form/ Analogue	Onset (h)	Peak (h)	Duration (h)*
Regular Insulin	0.5-1	2-5	5-12
Insulin Aspart (Novolog)	0.16-0.33	1-3	3-5
Insulin Glulisine (Apidra)	0.25-0.5	0.75-1	4-5
Insulin Lispro (Humalog)	0.25	0.5-1.5	3-6
Insulin NPH	1-2	6-14	10-24
Insulin Detemir (Levemir)	1.1-2	6-8 (not pronounced)	6-24
Insulin Glargine (Lantus)	1.1	No pronounced peak	11-24 (most 18-24)

*Duration of action may vary from individual to individual.

AVAILABILITY

NOTE: All insulins are available as 100 units/mL concentrations.
Rapid Acting: Humulin R, Novolin R, Novolog, Humalog, Apidra.
Intermediate Acting: Humulin N, Novolin N.
Combinations: NovoLog Mix 70/30, Humalog Mix 50/50, Humalog Mix 75/25, Humulin 70/30, Novolin 70/30.
Long Acting: Lantus, Levemir.

INDICATIONS AND DOSAGES

▸ **Treatment of type 1 (insulin-dependent) OR type 2 diabetes mellitus**

SUBCUTANEOUS

Adults, Elderly, Children. Usually 0.5-1 unit/kg/day in divided doses (usual range 0.1-2.5 units/kg/day). Adjust doses to desired target blood sugar for the patient's individualized goals (NOTE: normal blood sugar is generally 80-110 mg/dL). Note that the dosage range given is quite general; patients with diabetes mellitus type 2 usually receive lower initial doses during initial treatment or if taking oral hypoglycemics. Basal insulins (e.g., insulin glargine, insulin detemir) will have different parameters for daily administration, and are usually initiated at 10 units/day or roughly 0.1-0.2 units/kg/day. Consult individual analog product literature for details of correct dosage, titration, and administration times.

Adolescents (during growth spurt). In general, 0.5-1 unit/kg/day, but may be adjusted to individual patient needs.

▸ **Emergency treatment of diabetic ketoacidosis (DKA) OR hyperosmolar hyperglycemic state of type 2 diabetes mellitus (regular insulin)**

IV INFUSION (REGULAR INSULIN ONLY)

Adults. Initially, 0.15 unit/kg IV bolus, then 0.1 unit/kg/h continuous infusion. Additionally, adequate fluid therapy must be initiated; fluid type and hourly requirements based on estimated patient need and serum osmolality. Blood glucose levels are checked hourly, and the insulin infusion rate is adjusted accordingly. The insulin infusion should cause blood glucose to fall at a rate of about 50 to 75 mg/dL/h; faster blood glucose lowering may cause adverse reactions, like cerebral edema. When blood glucose is 250 mg/dL or less, the insulin infusion rate is usually decreased to 0.05-0.1 unit/kg/h IV and fluid therapy is changed to a dextrose-containing infusion; rates are adjusted to maintain a blood glucose of 150-250 mg/dL until the acidosis is corrected.

OFF-LABEL USES

Widely accepted for use to control blood glucose during hyperalimentation (regular insulin); also for emergency treatment of severe hyperkalemia (regular insulin).

CONTRAINDICATIONS

Hypersensitivity or insulin resistance may require change of type or species' source of insulin.

INTERACTIONS

Drug

β-Adrenergic blockers: May increase the risk of hyperglycemia or hypoglycemia; may mask signs and prolong periods of hypoglycemia.

Glucocorticoids, thiazide diuretics: May increase blood glucose level.

Herbal

Chromium, garlic, gymnema: May increase hypoglycemic effects.

Food

Alcohol: May increase risk of hypoglycemia.

DIAGNOSTIC TEST EFFECTS

Expected to decrease blood glucose levels and also HbA1C over time. May decrease serum potassium concentrations. Rarely causes decrease in serum magnesium and phosphate concentrations.

IV INCOMPATIBILITIES

Regular insulin (ONLY) and the analogs Insulin Lispro and Insulin Glulisine (ONLY) are the only insulins that may be given IV: Consult specialized resources for Y-site and other compatibility.

SIDE EFFECTS

Occasional

Localized redness, swelling, and itching caused by improper injection technique or allergy to cleansing solution or insulin, hypoglycemia.

Infrequent

Hypokalemia; Somogyi effect, including rebound hyperglycemia with chronically excessive insulin dosages: systemic allergic reaction, marked by rash, angioedema, and anaphylaxis; lipoatrophy or depression at injection site from breakdown of adipose tissue (can avoid by using adequate injection site rotation).

Rare

Insulin resistance.

SERIOUS REACTIONS

- Severe hypoglycemia caused by hyperinsulinism may occur with insulin overdose, decrease or delay of food intake, or excessive exercise and in those with unstable diabetes.
- Diabetic ketoacidosis may result from stress, illness, omission of insulin dose, or long-term poor insulin control, even despite insulin therapy.
- Rarely, serious allergic reactions occur.

PRECAUTIONS & CONSIDERATIONS

Dose adjustments may be necessary in renal and hepatic dysfunction. Insulin is the drug of choice for treating diabetes mellitus during pregnancy, but close medical supervision is needed. Insulin needs may change in the postpartum period, so monitor closely after delivery. Insulin is not secreted in breast milk. Breast-feeding may alter maternal insulin requirements. No age-related precautions have been noted in children. Decreased vision and shakiness in elderly patients may lead to inaccurate insulin self-dosing. Be alert to conditions that alter blood glucose requirements, such as fever, increased activity, stress, or a surgical procedure. Food intake and blood glucose should be monitored before and during therapy. Be aware of signs and symptoms of hypoglycemia (anxiety, cool wet skin, diplopia, dizziness, headache, hunger, numbness in mouth, tachycardia, tremors) or hyperglycemia (deep rapid breathing, dim vision, fatigue, nausea, polydipsia, polyphagia, polyuria, vomiting); carry candy, sugar packets, or other sugar supplements for immediate response to hypoglycemia. Consult the physician when glucose demands are altered (such as with fever, heavy physical activity, infection, stress, trauma). Exercise, good personal hygiene (including foot care), not smoking, and weight control are essential parts of therapy.

Storage

Store extra unopened vials or unopened prefilled pens/cartridges in refrigerator; do not freeze.

Store currently used insulin vials at room temperature or refrigerated; avoid extreme temperatures and direct sunlight. Discard open vials after 28 days.

Prefilled pens or pens with cartridges should be stored in the vertical or oblique position to avoid plugging. Once in use and at room temperature, refer to the manufacturer advice for how long the pens/cartridges may be kept in use; recommendations vary depending on the device and insulin brand.

Administration

Know that insulin dosages are highly individualized and monitored. Adjust dosage, as prescribed, to achieve blood glucose goals and HbA1c targets.

! Most insulins and insulin analogues are given subcutaneously only; some may be used in subcutaneous external infusion pumps. For subcutaneous use; warm the drug to room temperature; do not give cold insulin. Roll the drug vial gently between hands; do not shake. Regular insulin normally appears clear. No insulin should have discoloration. Suspensions should be uniform in appearance. Gently roll/rock prefilled pens before use to mix the suspensions/solutions. Be sure to always use an insulin syringe (e.g., U-30, U-50, or U-100) for administration.

Use glucometer to check blood glucose before administration. In health care systems, have a second person double-check the insulin type and dose to be administered.

Administer most insulins approximately 30-60 min before a meal. Insulin lispro should be given 15 min before meals or immediately after a meal. Insulin aspart is given 5-10 min before starting a meal. Insulin glulisine is given 15 min before a meal or within 20 min of starting a meal. Insulin aspart is given immediately before a meal. Once-daily basal insulins, such as Lantus and Levemir, are given at any time of day but are usually initiated once daily at the evening meal or at bedtime.

Always draw either regular insulin, Novolog, Humalog, or Apidra first into the syringe when mixed with NPH. Mixtures must be administered immediately after preparation. NEVER give insulin mixtures intravenously. Lantus and Levemir should NOT be mixed with other insulins.

Give subcutaneous injections in the abdomen, buttocks, thigh, or upper arm. Maintain a careful record of rotated injection sites.

! ONLY regular insulin may be given IV. Novolog or Apidra have also been used in this manner, but use of these analogues is more rare;

use of IV insulin should be limited to monitored clinical settings. May give bolus undiluted. An infusion of regular insulin is prepared by adding 100 units of regular insulin (only) to 100 mL of 0.9% NaCl. ONLY regular insulin may be added to hyperalimentation solutions. Administration rate must be individualized (see dosage). Use with controlled infusion device.

Interferon Alfa-2b

inn-ter-fear′on

★ 🍁 Intron-A

Do not confuse interferon alfa-2b with interferon alfa-2a.

CATEGORY AND SCHEDULE

Pregnancy Risk Category: C

Classification: Immunologic agents, interferons

MECHANISM OF ACTION

A biological response modifier that inhibits viral replication in virus-infected cells, suppresses cell proliferation, increases phagocytic action of macrophages, and augments specific cytotoxicity of lymphocytes for target cells. *Therapeutic Effect:* Prevents rapid growth of malignant cells; inhibits hepatitis virus.

PHARMACOKINETICS

Well absorbed after IM and SC administration. Undergoes proteolytic degradation during reabsorption in kidneys. *Half-life:* 2-3 h.

AVAILABILITY

Injection (Multidose Vial): 6 million units/mL, 10 million units/mL.
Injection (Single-Dose Vial): 10 million units/mL.
Injection (Prefilled Solution): 3 million units/0.2 mL, 5 million units/0.2 mL, 10 million units/0.2 mL.
Injection (Powder for Reconstitution): 10 million units, 18 million units, 50 million units.

INDICATIONS AND DOSAGES

▸ **Hairy cell leukemia**

IM, SC

Adults. 2 million units/m^2 3 times a week. If severe adverse reactions occur, modify dose or temporarily discontinue drug.

▸ **Condyloma acuminatum**

INTRALESIONAL

Adults. 1 million units/lesion 3 times a week for 3 wks. Use only 10-million-unit vial, and reconstitute with no more than 1 mL diluent.

▸ **AIDS-related Kaposi sarcoma**

IM, SC

Adults. 30 million units/m^2 3 times a week. Use only 50-million-unit vials. If severe adverse reactions occur, modify dose or temporarily discontinue drug.

▸ **Chronic hepatitis C**

IM, SC

Adults. 3 million units 3 times a week for up to 6 mo. For patients who tolerate therapy and whose ALT (SGPT) level normalizes within 16 wks, therapy may be extended for up to 18-24 mo.

▸ **Chronic hepatitis B**

IM, SC

Adults. 30-35 million units weekly, either as 5 million units/day or 10 million units 3 times a week.

▸ **Malignant melanoma**

IV

Adults. Initially, 20 million units/m^2 5 times a week for 4 wks. Maintenance: 10 million units IM or subcutaneously 3 times a week for 48 wks.

▸ **Follicular lymphoma**
SC
Adults. 5 million units 3 times a week for up to 18 mo.

OFF-LABEL USES

Treatment of bladder, cervical, or renal carcinoma; chronic myelocytic leukemia; laryngeal papillomatosis; multiple myeloma; mycosis fungoides.

CONTRAINDICATIONS

Decompensated liver disease; autoimmune hepatitis interactions, hypersensitivity to interferon alfa-2b, *E.coli* proteins, albumin.

Drug
Bone marrow depressants: May increase myelosuppression.
Ribavirin: May increase risk of hemolytic anemia.
Theophylline: May increase levels of theophylline.
Zidovudine: May increase levels of zidovudine.
Herbal and Food
None known.

DIAGNOSTIC TEST EFFECTS

May increase PT, aPTT, and serum LDH, alkaline phosphatase, AST (SGOT), and ALT (SGPT) levels. May decrease blood hemoglobin level, hematocrit, and leukocyte and platelet counts.

IV INCOMPATIBILITIES

No information available. Do not mix with other medications for Y-site administration.

SIDE EFFECTS

Frequent
Flu-like symptoms, rash (only in patients with hairy cell leukemia, Kaposi sarcoma).
Patients with Kaposi sarcoma: All previously mentioned side effects plus depression, dyspepsia, dry mouth or thirst, alopecia, rigors.
Occasional
Dizziness, pruritus, dry skin, dermatitis, altered taste.
Rare
Confusion, leg cramps, back pain, gingivitis, flushing, tremor, nervousness, eye pain.

SERIOUS REACTIONS

- Hypersensitivity reactions occur rarely.
- May cause severe psychiatric adverse events in patients with or without previous psychiatric symptoms.
- Severe and even life-threatening side effects occur in 0.1% or greater of patients; these include thyroid, visual, auditory, renal, and cardiac impairment, and pulmonary interstitial fibrosis or serious infection.

PRECAUTIONS & CONSIDERATIONS

Caution is warranted in patients with cardiac diseases or abnormalities, compromised CNS function, hepatic or renal impairment, myelosuppression, and seizure disorders. Interferon alfa-2b should not be used by pregnant or breastfeeding women. Effective contraceptive measures should be used during therapy, and the physician should be notified if the woman is or might be pregnant. The safety and efficacy of interferon alfa-2b have not been established in children. Elderly patients are more prone to cardiotoxicity and neurotoxicity. Age-related renal impairment may require cautious use of interferon alfa-2b in elderly patients. Avoid receiving immunizations without the physician's approval and coming in contact with people who have recently received a live-virus vaccine because interferon alfa-2b lowers the body's resistance. Also, avoid tasks that require mental alertness or motor skills until response to the drug has been established.

Flu-like symptoms may occur but may be minimized by taking the drug at bedtime and tend to diminish with continued therapy. Urinalysis, CBC, platelet count, BUN level, serum alkaline phosphatase, creatinine, AST (SGOT), and ALT (SGPT) levels should be obtained before and routinely during therapy.

Storage

Refrigerate unopened vials and multidose pens; however, the drug remains stable for 7 days at room temperature.

Administration

! Dosage is individualized based on clinical response and tolerance of the drug's adverse effects. When used in combination therapy, consult specific protocols for optimum dosage and sequence of drug administration, as prescribed. Remember that side effects are dose related. The drug's therapeutic effect may take 1-3 mo to appear.

! For most uses, give the drug in the evening with acetaminophen, which alleviates side effects.

For IV use, prepare the solution immediately before use. Reconstitute with the diluent provided by the manufacturer. Withdraw the desired dose and further dilute with 100 mL 0.9% NaCl to provide final concentration at least 10 million units/100 mL. Administer the drug over 20 min.

Do not administer interferon alfa-2b by IM injection if platelet count is < 50,000/m^3; instead give it subcutaneously.

For hairy cell leukemia, reconstitute as follows: Add 1 mL bacteriostatic water for injection to each 3-million-unit vial to provide a concentration of 3 million units/mL, or add 1 mL to each 5-million-unit vial, 2 mL to each 10-million-unit vial, or 5 mL to each 25-million-unit vial to provide a concentration of 5 million units/mL.

For condylomata acuminata, (intralesional use), reconstitute each 10-million-unit vial with 1 mL bacteriostatic water for injection to provide a concentration of 10 million units/mL. Use a tuberculin syringe with a 25- or 26-gauge needle.

For AIDS-related Kaposi sarcoma, reconstitute each 50-million-unit vial with 1 mL bacteriostatic water for injection to provide a concentration of 50 million units/mL. Agitate the vial gently and withdraw the solution with a sterile syringe.

For hepatitis indications, multidose pens are available for ease of chronic treatment. See specialized literature for appropriate use.

Interferon Alfa-n3

in-ter-fear′on

★ Alferon N

CATEGORY AND SCHEDULE

Pregnancy Risk Category: C

Classification: Immunologic agents; interferons

MECHANISM OF ACTION

A biological response modifier that inhibits viral replication in virus-infected cells, suppresses cell proliferation, increases phagocytic action of macrophages, and augments the specific cytotoxicity of lymphocytes for target cells.

Therapeutic Effect: Inhibits viral growth in condylomata acuminatum.

PHARMACOKINETICS

Plasma levels below detectable limits.

AVAILABILITY

Injection: 5 million international units/mL.

INDICATIONS AND DOSAGES

▸ **Condyloma acuminatum**

INTRALESIONAL

Adults. 0.05 mL (250,000 international units) per wart twice a week up to 8 wks. Maximum dose/treatment session: 0.5 mL (2.5 million international units). Do not repeat for 3 mo after initial 8-wk course unless warts enlarge or new warts appear.

CONTRAINDICATIONS

Previous history of anaphylactic reaction to egg protein, murine proteins, or neomycin (trace).

INTERACTIONS

Drug

ACE inhibitors: May increase risk of granulocytopenia.

Bone marrow depressants: May increase myelosuppression.

Prednisone: May decrease effects of interferon.

Theophylline: May increase levels of theophylline.

Warfarin: May increase anticoagulant effects.

Zidovudine: May increase levels of zidovudine.

Herbal and Food

None known.

DIAGNOSTIC TEST EFFECTS

May increase serum LDH, alkaline phosphatase, AST (SGOT), and ALT (SGPT) levels. May decrease blood hemoglobin level, hematocrit, and leukocyte and platelet counts.

SIDE EFFECTS

Frequent

Flu-like symptoms.

Occasional

Dizziness, pruritus, dry skin, dermatitis, altered taste.

Rare

Confusion, leg cramps, back pain, gingivitis, flushing, tremor, nervousness, eye pain.

SERIOUS REACTIONS

- Hypersensitivity reaction occurs rarely.
- Severe and even life-threatening side effects occur in 0.1% or greater of patients; these include thyroid, visual, auditory, renal, psychatric, and cardiac impairment, and pulmonary interstitial fibrosis or serious infection.

PRECAUTIONS & CONSIDERATIONS

Caution is warranted with diabetes mellitus and ketoacidosis, hemophilia, pulmonary embolism, seizure disorders, severe myelosuppression, severe pulmonary disease, thrombophlebitis, uncontrolled congestive heart failure, and unstable angina.

Flu-like symptoms may occur but may be minimized by taking the drug at bedtime and tend to diminish with continued therapy. Diagnostic tests, such as CBC, should be obtained before and routinely during therapy.

Storage

Refrigerate vials. Do not freeze or shake them.

Administration

Using a 30-gauge needle, inject 0.05 mL into the base of each wart. Used intralesionally only.

Interferon Alfacon-1

in-ter-fear′on

Infergen

CATEGORY AND SCHEDULE

Pregnancy Risk Category: C

Classification: Immunologic agents; biologic response modifier, interferons

MECHANISM OF ACTION

A biological response modifier that stimulates the immune system. *Therapeutic Effect:* Inhibits hepatitis C virus.

AVAILABILITY

Injection: 15 mcg/0.5 mL, 9 mcg/0.3 mL.

INDICATIONS AND DOSAGES

▸ **Chronic hepatitis C**

SC

Adults. 9 mcg 3 times a week for 24 wks. May increase to 15 mcg 3 times a week in patients who tolerate but fail to respond to 9-mcg dose, for up to 48 wks.

CONTRAINDICATIONS

History of autoimmune hepatitis or hepatic decompensation, hypersensitivity to any drug or component of the product.

SIDE EFFECTS

Frequent (> 50%)

Headache, fatigue, fever, depression.

SERIOUS REACTIONS

- Bone marrow suppression (rare).
- Cardiac effects, hypertension.
- Hypersensitivity.
- Psychiatric disturbances.

PRECAUTIONS & CONSIDERATIONS

Caution is warranted in patients with a history of autoimmune disease, cardiac disease, depression, endocrine disorders, hepatic disorders, myelosuppression, and renal dysfunction. May cause severe psychiatric adverse events in patients with or without previous psychiatric symptoms. Notify the physician of side effects, including headache or injection site pain, as soon as possible. Serum alkaline phosphatase, AST (SGOT), ALT (SGPT), hepatitis C virus (HCV) antibody, and HCV-RNA levels should be obtained before and during therapy.

Storage

Refrigerate unopened vials; do not freeze. Warm to room temperature before administration.

Administration

! Make sure at least 48 h elapse between doses of interferon alfacon-1.

Administer as SC injection. Sometimes, doses are reduced in 1.5 or 3 mcg increments to help tolerance. The lowest effective dose is 7.5 mcg (0.25 mL).

Interferon Beta-1a

in-ter-fear′on

Avonex, Rebif

Do not confuse interferon beta-1a with interferon beta-1b or Avonex with Avelox.

CATEGORY AND SCHEDULE

Pregnancy Risk Category: C

Classification: Immunologic agents; biologic response modifier, interferons

MECHANISM OF ACTION

A biological response modifier that interacts with specific cell receptors found on the surface of human cells. *Therapeutic Effect:* Produces antiviral and immunoregulatory effects.

PHARMACOKINETICS

Peak serum levels attained 3-15 h after IM administration. Biological markers increase within 12 h and remain elevated for 4 days. *Half-life:* 10 h (Avonex); 69 h (Rebif).

AVAILABILITY

Injection Solution (Prefilled Syringe [Avonex]): 30 mcg/0.5 mL.
Injection Solution (Prefilled Syringe [Rebif]): 22 mcg/0.5 mL, 44 mcg/0.5 mL.
Rebif Titration Pack (Prefilled Syringes): 8.8 mcg/0.2 mL and 22 mcg/0.5 mL.

INDICATIONS AND DOSAGES

▸ **Relapsing-remitting multiple sclerosis**

IM (AVONEX)
Adults. 30 mcg once weekly.
SC (REBIF)
Adults. Initially 8.8 mcg 3 times a week; may increase to 44 mcg 3 times a week over 4-6 wks.

OFF-LABEL USES

Treatment of AIDS, AIDS-related Kaposi sarcoma, malignant melanoma, renal cell carcinoma.

CONTRAINDICATIONS

Hypersensitivity to albumin or interferon.

INTERACTIONS

Drug

Hepatotoxic agents: May increase risk of hepatotoxicity.
Theophylline: May increase levels of theophylline.
Warfarin: May increase anticoagulant effects.
Telbivudine: May increase neuropathy.
Zidovudine: May increase effects of zidovudine.

Herbal

None known.

Food

Ethanol: Limit or avoid because may increase risk of hepatic adverse effects.

DIAGNOSTIC TEST EFFECTS

May increase blood glucose and BUN levels and serum alkaline phosphatase, bilirubin, calcium, AST (SGOT), and ALT (SGPT) levels. May decrease blood hemoglobin level and neutrophil, platelet, and WBC counts.

SIDE EFFECTS

Frequent

Headache (67%), flu-like symptoms (61%), myalgia (34%), upper respiratory tract infection (31%), generalized pain (24%), asthenia, chills (21%), sinusitis (18%), infection (11%).

Occasional

Abdominal pain, arthralgia (9%), chest pain, dyspnea (6%), malaise, syncope (4%).

Rare

Injection site reaction, hypersensitivity reaction (3%).

SERIOUS REACTIONS

- Anemia occurs in 8% of patients.
- Severe and even life-threatening side effects occur in 0.1% or greater of patients; these include thyroid, visual, auditory, renal, psychiatric, and cardiac impairment, and pulmonary interstitial fibrosis or serious infection.

PRECAUTIONS & CONSIDERATIONS

Caution is warranted with chronic, progressive multiple sclerosis and in children younger than 18 yr. May cause severe psychiatric adverse events in patients with or without previous psychiatric symptoms. Interferon beta-1a may cause spontaneous abortion. It is unknown whether interferon beta-1a is distributed in breast milk. Interferon beta-1a should be used cautiously in children because its safety and efficacy have not been established in this age group. No information is available on the use of interferon beta-1a in elderly patients.

Notify the physician of flu-like symptoms, headache, or muscle pain or weakness. CBC and serum alkaline phosphatase, AST (SGOT), and ALT (SGPT) levels should be obtained before and during therapy.

Storage

Refrigerate Avonex prefilled syringes; warm to room temperature before use. Use Avonex prefilled syringe within 12 h after removal from refrigerator. Refrigerate Rebif prefilled syringes; if refrigeration is unavailable, the drug may be stored at room temperature, away from heat and light up to 30 days.

Administration

For IM use (Avonex powder for injection), reconstitute 30 mcg MicroPin (6.6-million-unit) vial with 1.1 mL of the diluent, provided by the manufacturer. Discard it if it becomes discolored or contains a precipitate.

! Gently swirl, do not shake the vial, to dissolve the drug.

For IM use (Avonex prefilled syringes), allow the drug to warm to room temperature prior to use. Administer on the same day each week.

For subcutaneous use (Rebif prefilled syringes), administer the drug at the same time of day 3 days each week. Separate doses by at least 48 h.

Interferon Beta-1b

in-ter-fear′on

★ 🍁 Betaseron, Extavia

Do not confuse interferon beta-1b with interferon beta-1a.

CATEGORY AND SCHEDULE

Pregnancy Risk Category: C

Classification: Immunologic agents; biologic response modifier, interferons

MECHANISM OF ACTION

A biological response modifier that interacts with specific cell receptors found on the surface of human cells. *Therapeutic Effect:* Produces antiviral and immunoregulatory effects.

PHARMACOKINETICS

Half-life: 8 min-4.3 h.

AVAILABILITY

Powder for Injection: 0.3 mg (9.6 million units).

INDICATIONS AND DOSAGES

▸ **Relapsing-remitting multiple sclerosis**

SC

Adults. Target dose is 0.25 mg (8 million units) every other day. Start with 62.5 mcg SC every other day and increase to 125 mcg every other day after 2 wks, etc.

CONTRAINDICATIONS

Hypersensitivity to albumin or interferon.

INTERACTIONS

Drug

Theophylline: May increase levels of theophylline.

Herbal and Food

None known.

DIAGNOSTIC TEST EFFECTS

May increase blood glucose and BUN levels and serum alkaline phosphatase, bilirubin, calcium, AST (SGOT), and ALT (SGPT) levels. May decrease blood hemoglobin level and neutrophil, platelet, and WBC counts.

SIDE EFFECTS

Frequent

Injection site reaction (85%), headache (84%), flu-like symptoms (76%), fever (59%), asthenia (49%), myalgia (44%), sinusitis (36%), diarrhea, dizziness (35%), mental status changes (29%), constipation (24%), diaphoresis (23%), vomiting (21%).

Occasional

Malaise (15%), somnolence (6%), alopecia (4%).

SERIOUS REACTIONS

- Seizures occur rarely.
- May cause severe psychiatric adverse events in patients with or without previous psychiatric symptoms.
- Injection site necrosis.
- Rare serious hypersensitivity.
- Severe and even life-threatening side effects occur in 0.1% or greater of patients; these include thyroid, visual, auditory, renal, and cardiac impairment, and pulmonary interstitial fibrosis or serious infection.

PRECAUTIONS & CONSIDERATIONS

Caution is warranted with chronic, progressive multiple sclerosis and in children younger than 18 yr. Pregnancy should be avoided. It is unknown whether interferon beta-1b is distributed in breast milk. The safety and efficacy of interferon beta-1b have not been established in children. No information is available on the use of interferon beta-1b in elderly patients. Sunscreen and protective clothing should be worn when exposed to sunlight or ultraviolet light until the extent of photosensitivity has been determined.

Notify the physician of flu-like symptoms, headache, or muscle pain or weakness. CBC and serum alkaline phosphatase, AST (SGOT), and ALT (SGPT) levels should be obtained before and during therapy. Pattern of daily bowel activity and stool consistency and food intake should be monitored.

Storage

Store vials at room temperature. After reconstitution, the solution is stable for 3 h if refrigerated. Use the solution within 3 h of reconstitution.

Administration

! Gently swirl do not shake the vial to dissolve the drug.

For subcutaneous injection, reconstitute the 0.3-mg (9.6-million-unit) vial with 1.2 mL of the diluent supplied by the manufacturer to provide a concentration of 0.25 mg/mL (8 million units/mL). Using a 27-gauge needle, inject the appropriate dose of the solution subcutaneously into the abdomen, arms, hips, or thighs. Discard the solution if it becomes discolored or contains a precipitate. Discard any unused portion because the solution contains no preservative.

Interferon Gamma-1b

in-ter-fear'on

Actimmune

CATEGORY AND SCHEDULE

Pregnancy Risk Category: C

Classification: Immunologic agents; biologic response modifier, interferons

MECHANISM OF ACTION

A biological response modifier that induces the activation of macrophages in blood monocytes to phagocytes, which is necessary in the body's cellular immune response to intracellular and extracellular pathogens. Enhances phagocytic function and antimicrobial activity of monocytes. *Therapeutic Effect:* Decreases signs and symptoms of serious infections in chronic granulomatous disease.

PHARMACOKINETICS

Slowly absorbed after subcutaneous administration.

AVAILABILITY

Injection: 100 mcg (2 million units).

INDICATIONS AND DOSAGES

▸ **Chronic granulomatous disease; severe, malignant osteopetrosis**

SC

Adults, Children older than 1 yr. 50 mcg/m^2 (1.5 million units/m^2) in patients with body surface area (BSA) > 0.5 m^2; 1.5 mcg/kg/dose in patients with BSA 0.5 m^2 or less. Give 3 times a week.

CONTRAINDICATIONS

Hypersensitivity to *Escherichia coli*–derived products, mannitol, ortho drug.

INTERACTIONS

Drug

Bone marrow depressants: May increase myelosuppression.

Theophylline: May increase levels of theophylline.

Herbal and Food

None known.

DIAGNOSTIC TEST EFFECTS

May elevate AST or ALT.

SIDE EFFECTS

Frequent

Fever (52%); headache (33%); rash (17%); chills, fatigue, diarrhea (14%).

Occasional (10%-13%)

Vomiting, nausea.

Rare (3%-6%)

Weight loss, myalgia, anorexia.

SERIOUS REACTIONS

- Interferon gamma-1b may exacerbate preexisting central nervous system (CNS) disturbances, including decreased mental status, seizures, gait disturbance, and dizziness.
- Neutropenia or thrombocytopenia.
- Severe and even life-threatening side effects occur in 0.1% or greater of patients; these include thyroid, visual, auditory, renal, and cardiac impairment, and pulmonary interstitial fibrosis or serious infection.

PRECAUTIONS & CONSIDERATIONS

Caution is warranted with compromised CNS function, myelosuppression, preexisting cardiac disorders (including arrhythmias, congestive heart failure, and myocardial ischemia), and seizure disorders. It is unknown whether interferon gamma-1b crosses the placenta or is distributed in breast milk. The safety and efficacy of interferon gamma-1b have not been established in children younger than 1 yr. Children are more likely to experience flu-like symptoms. No information is available on the use of interferon gamma-1b in elderly patients. Avoid performing tasks that require mental alertness or motor skills until response to the drug has been established.

Notify the physician of flu-like symptoms or rash. CBC, urinalysis, BUN level and serum alkaline phosphatase, creatinine, AST (SGOT), and ALT (SGPT) levels should be obtained before and every 3 mo during therapy.

Storage

Refrigerate unopened vials; do not freeze them. Discard vials kept at room temperature for longer than 12 h.

Administration

! Avoid excessive agitation of the vial; do not shake it.

Vials come in single doses; discard any unused portion. The solution normally appears clear and colorless. Do not use it if it becomes discolored or contains a precipitate. Administer the drug subcutaneously 3 times a week. Rotate injection sites.

Interleukin-2 (Aldesleukin)

in′ter-lu′kin-2 (al-des-loo′kin)

IL-2, Proleukin

Do not confuse interleukin-2 with interferons.

CATEGORY AND SCHEDULE

Pregnancy Risk Category: C

Classification: Antineoplastics, biological response modifiers, interleukins

MECHANISM OF ACTION

A biological response modifier that acts like human recombinant interleukin-2, promoting proliferation, differentiation, and recruitment of T and B cells, lymphokine-activated and natural cells, and thymocytes. *Therapeutic Effect:* Enhances cytolytic activity in lymphocytes.

PHARMACOKINETICS

Primarily distributed into plasma, lymphocytes, lungs, liver, kidney, and spleen. Metabolized to amino acids in the cells lining the kidneys. *Half-life:* 85 min.

AVAILABILITY

Powder for Injection: 22 million units (1.3 mg).

INDICATIONS AND DOSAGES

▸ **Metastatic melanoma, metastatic renal cell carcinoma**

IV

Adults. 600,000 units/kg q8h for 14 doses, followed by 9 days of rest, then another 14 doses for a total of 28 doses per course. Course may be repeated after rest period of at least 7 wks from date of hospital discharge.

OFF-LABEL USES

Treatment of non-Hodgkin lymphoma, acute myelogenous leukemia.

CONTRAINDICATIONS

Hypersensitivity to the drug or mannitol, abnormal pulmonary function or thallium stress test results, bowel ischemia or perforation, coma or toxic psychosis lasting longer than 48 h, GI bleeding requiring surgery, intubation lasting more than 72 h, organ allografts, pericardial tamponade, renal dysfunction requiring dialysis for longer than 72 h, repetitive or difficult-to-control seizures. Retreatment in those who experience any of the following toxicities: angina, MI, recurrent chest pain with EKG changes, sustained ventricular tachycardia, uncontrolled or unresponsive cardiac rhythm disturbances.

INTERACTIONS

Drug

Antihypertensives: May increase hypotensive effect.

Cardiotoxic, hepatotoxic, myelotoxic, or nephrotoxic medications: May increase the risk of toxicity.

Glucocorticoids: May decrease the effects of interleukin.

Herbal

None known.

Food

None known.

DIAGNOSTIC TEST EFFECTS

May increase BUN and serum alkaline phosphatase, bilirubin, creatinine, AST (SGOT), and ALT (SGPT) levels. May decrease serum calcium, magnesium, phosphorus, potassium, and sodium levels.

IV INCOMPATIBILITIES

Ganciclovir (Cytovene), lorazepam (Ativan), pentamidine (Pentam), prochlorperazine (Compazine), promethazine (Phenergan).

IV COMPATIBILITIES

Amikacin (Amikin), amphotericin B (Abelcet, AmBisome, Amphotec), calcium gluconate, co-trimoxazole (Bactrim), diphenhydramine (Benadryl), dopamine (Intropin), fat emulsion 10%, fluconazole (Diflucan), foscarnet (Foscavir), gentamicin (Garamycin), heparin, lorazepam (Ativan), magnesium, metoclopramide (Reglan), morphine (Avinza, Kadian, Roxanol), ondansetron (Zofran), piperacillin (Piperacil), potassium, ranitidine (Zantac), thiethylperazine, ticarcillin (Ticar), tobramycin (Nebcin).

SIDE EFFECTS

Side effects are generally self-limiting and reversible within 2-3 days after discontinuing therapy.

Frequent (48%-89%)

Fever, chills, nausea, vomiting, hypotension, diarrhea, oliguria or anuria, mental status changes, irritability, confusion, depression, sinus tachycardia, pain (abdominal, chest, back), fatigue, dyspnea, pruritus.

Occasional (17%-47%)

Edema, erythema, rash, stomatitis, anorexia, weight gain, infection (urinary tract infection, injection site, catheter tip), dizziness.

Rare (4%-15%)

Dry skin, sensory disorders (vision, speech, taste), dermatitis, headache, arthralgia, myalgia, weight loss, hematuria, conjunctivitis, proteinuria.

SERIOUS REACTIONS

- Anemia, thrombocytopenia, and leukopenia occur commonly.
- GI bleeding and pulmonary edema occur occasionally.
- Capillary leak syndrome results in hypotension (systolic pressure < 90 mm Hg or a 20 mm Hg drop from baseline systolic pressure), extravasation of plasma proteins and fluid into extravascular space, and loss of vascular tone. It may result in cardiac arrhythmias, angina, myocardial infarction, and respiratory insufficiency.
- Other rare reactions include fatal malignant hyperthermia, cardiac arrest, cerebrovascular

accident, pulmonary emboli, bowel perforation, gangrene, and severe depression leading to suicide.

PRECAUTIONS & CONSIDERATIONS

Extreme caution should be used with a history of cardiac or pulmonary disease, even if they have normal thallium stress and pulmonary function test results. Also use the drug cautiously with fixed requirements for large volumes of fluid (such as those with hypercalcemia) or a history of seizures. Interleukin use should be avoided in patients of either sex who do not practice effective contraception. The safety and efficacy of interleukin have not been established in children. Elderly patients may require cautious use of the drug because of age-related renal impairment. They are also less able to tolerate drug-related toxicities.

Notify the physician of difficulty urinating, black tarry stools, pinpoint red spots on the skin, bruising, fever, signs of local infection, sore throat, or unusual bleeding from any site. Treat persons with bacterial infection and those with indwelling central lines with antibiotic therapy before beginning interleukin therapy. A negative CT scan must be obtained before beginning therapy. Immediately report any symptoms of depression or suicidal ideation. CBC, electrolytes, liver and renal function, amylase concentration, BP, mental status, intake and output, extravascular fluid accumulation, platelet count, pulse oximetry values, and weight should be assessed.

Storage

Refrigerate unopened vials; do not freeze. The reconstituted solution is stable for 48 h at room temperature or refrigerated (refrigerated is preferred).

Administration

! Withhold the drug in patients who exhibit moderate to severe lethargy or somnolence because continued administration may result in coma. Restrict interleukin therapy to patients with normal cardiac and pulmonary function as determined by thallium stress testing and pulmonary function testing. Dosage is individualized based on clinical response and tolerance of the drug's adverse effects.

For IV use, reconstitute the 22-million-unit vial with 1.2 mL sterile water for injection to provide a concentration of 18 million units/mL. Do not use bacteriostatic water for injection or 0.9% NaCl. During reconstitution, direct the diluent at the side of the vial. Swirl the contents gently to avoid foaming; do not shake. Further dilute the appropriate dose in 50 mL D5W and infuse over 15 min. Do not use an in-line filter. Warm the solution to room temperature before infusion. Closely monitor the patient for a drop in mean arterial BP, a sign of capillary leak syndrome. Continued treatment may result in edema, pleural effusion, mental status changes, and significant hypotension (systolic pressure < 90 mm Hg or a 20 mm Hg drop from baseline systolic pressure).

Iodoquinol

eye-oh-do-kwin′ole

★ Yodoxin 🍁 Diodoquin

CATEGORY AND SCHEDULE

Pregnancy Risk Category: C

Classification: Antiprotozoals, amebicide

MECHANISM OF ACTION
An antibacterial, antifungal, and antitrichomonal agent that works in the intestinal lumen by an unknown mechanism. *Therapeutic Effect:* Amebicidal.

PHARMACOKINETICS
Partially and irregularly absorbed from the GI tract. Metabolized in liver. Primarily excreted in feces.

AVAILABILITY
Tablets: 210 mg, 650 mg (Yodoxin).

INDICATIONS AND DOSAGES
▸ **Intestinal amebiasis**
PO
Adults, Elderly. 630 mg OR 650 mg 3 times a day for 20 days.
Children. 30-40 mg/kg in 3 divided doses for 20 days. Maximum: 650 mg/dose.

OFF-LABEL USES
Active treatment of infectious diarrhea due to travel, pulmonary aspergillosis.

CONTRAINDICATIONS
Hepatic impairment, hypersensitivity to iodine and 8-hydroxyquinolones.

INTERACTIONS
Drug, Herbal, and Food
None known.

DIAGNOSTIC TEST EFFECTS
May result in false-positive ferric chloride test for phenylketonuria. May increase protein-bound serum iodine concentrations reflecting a decrease in I^{131} uptake.

SIDE EFFECTS
Occasional
Fever, chills, headache, nausea, vomiting, diarrhea, cramps, urticaria, pruritus.

SERIOUS REACTIONS
- Optic neuritis, atrophy, and peripheral neuropathy have been reported with high dosages and long-term use.

PRECAUTIONS & CONSIDERATIONS
This drug is not intended for long-term use. Caution should be used in patients with thyroid disease and neurologic disorders. It is unknown whether iodoquinol is distributed in breast milk. No age-related precautions have been noted in children. Age-related renal impairment may limit the use of iodoquinol in elderly patients.

Nausea, diarrhea, or GI upset may occur. Be aware that iodoquinol may temporarily stain skin, hair, and clothing a yellow-brown color.

Storage
Store at room temperature.

Administration
Give after meals. May crush tablets and mix with applesauce. Avoid long-term use.

Ipratropium
eye-pra-troep′ee-um
★ Atrovent HFA, Atrovent Nasal 🍁 Apo-Ipravent, Gen-Ipratropium, Novo-Impramide, Ratio-Ipratropium
Do not confuse Atrovent with Alupent.

CATEGORY AND SCHEDULE
Pregnancy Risk Category: B

Classification: Anticholinergics, bronchodilators

MECHANISM OF ACTION
An anticholinergic that blocks the action of acetylcholine at parasympathetic sites in bronchial smooth muscle. *Therapeutic*

Effect: Causes bronchodilation and inhibits nasal secretions.

PHARMACOKINETICS

Route	Onset	Peak	Duration
Inhalation	1-3 min	1-2 h	4-6 h

Minimal systemic absorption after inhalation. Metabolized in the liver (systemic absorption). Primarily eliminated in feces. *Half-life:* 1.5-4 h.

AVAILABILITY

Oral Inhalation: 17 mcg/actuation.
Nebulizer Solution for Inhalation: 0.02%.
Nasal Spray: 0.03%, 0.06%.

INDICATIONS AND DOSAGES

▸ **Bronchospasm, acute treatment, adjunctive**
INHALATION
Adults, Elderly, Children. 2 puffs q6h initially.
NEBULIZATION
Adults, Elderly, Children 12 yr and older. 500 mcg q30min for 3 doses, then q2-4h as needed.
Children younger than 12 yr. 250 mcg q20min for 3 doses, then q2-4h as needed.

▸ **Bronchospasm, maintenance treatment, associated with COPD**
INHALATION
Adults, Elderly. 2 puffs q6h.
NEBULIZATION
Adults, Elderly. 500 mcg q6-8h.

▸ **Rhinorrhea, common cold**
INTRANASAL
Adults, Children older than 12 yr. 2 sprays per nostril of (0.06%) solution 3-4 times a day for up to 4 days.

▸ **Rhinorrhea, allergic or nonallergic perennial**
Adults, Children 6 yr and older. 2 sprays per nostril of (0.03%) solution 2-3 times a day. Usually used for up to 4 days.

CONTRAINDICATIONS

Hypersensitivity to ipratropium bromide or other product components; hypersensitivity to atropine or its derivatives.

INTERACTIONS

Drug
Anticholinergic agents: May increase risk of adverse events.
Cromolyn inhalation solution: Avoid mixing these drugs because they form a precipitate.
Herbal and Food
None known.

DIAGNOSTIC TEST EFFECTS

None known.

SIDE EFFECTS

Frequent
Inhalation (3%-6%): Cough, dry mouth, headache, nausea.
Nasal: Dry nose and mouth, headache, nasal irritation.
Occasional
Inhalation (2%): Dizziness, transient increased bronchospasm.
Rare (< 1%)
Inhalation: Hypotension, insomnia, metallic or unpleasant taste, palpitations, urine retention.
Nasal: Diarrhea or constipation, dry throat, abdominal pain, stuffy nose.

SERIOUS REACTIONS

- Worsening of angle-closure glaucoma, acute eye pain, and hypotension occur rarely.
- Paradoxical acute bronchospasm that can be life threatening; usually reported with first use of a new canister.
- Rare reports of serious hypersensitivity reactions, including anaphylaxis.

PRECAUTIONS & CONSIDERATIONS

Caution is warranted in patients with bladder neck obstruction, angle-closure glaucoma, and benign prostatic hyperplasia. It is unknown whether ipratropium is distributed in breast milk. No age-related precautions have been noted in children or elderly patients. Drink plenty of fluids to decrease the thickness of lung secretions. Avoid excessive use of caffeinated products, such as chocolate, cocoa, cola, coffee, and tea.

Pulse rate and quality, respiratory rate, depth, rhythm and type, ABG levels, and serum potassium levels should be monitored. Lips and fingernails should be examined for hypoxemia. Clinical improvement should also be evaluated.

Storage

Store products at room temperature. Keep nebulizer solution protected from light in packet until time of use. Do not expose HFA to high temperatures or flame, as the contents are under pressure and may burst.

Administration

Shake the HFA container well. If a new canister, first do 3 "test sprays" away from the face and others before first use. Exhale completely through mouth; then place the mouthpiece into the mouth and close lips, holding the inhaler upright. Inhale deeply through the mouth while fully depressing the top of the canister. Hold breath for as long as possible before exhaling slowly. Wait 2 min before inhaling the second dose to allow for deeper bronchial penetration. Rinse mouth with water immediately after inhalation to prevent mouth and throat dryness. Do not take more than 2 inhalations at a time because excessive use decreases the drug's effectiveness or may produce paradoxical bronchoconstriction.

Nebulizer solution: Use in nebulizer as directed; may mix with albuterol if will be used within 1 h. Do not mix with cromolyn sodium as the two are not compatible.

Nasal spray: Before using first time, prime unit with 7 sprays; if unit not used for 24 h, prime with 2 sprays, away from body. Blow nose gently to clear before use. Close one nostril, bend head slightly forward, insert nasal tip into open nostril. Point to back and outer wall of nose. Spray and sniff deeply. Repeat then repeat with other nostril (2 sprays per nostril).

Irbesartan

erb'ba-sar-tan

Avapro

CATEGORY AND SCHEDULE

Pregnancy Risk Category: C (D if used in second or third trimester)

Classification: Antihypertensives, angiotensin receptor antagonists

MECHANISM OF ACTION

An angiotensin II receptor, type AT_1, antagonist that blocks the vasoconstrictor and aldosterone-secreting effects of angiotensin II, inhibiting the binding of angiotensin II to the AT_1 receptors. *Therapeutic Effect:* Causes vasodilation, decreases peripheral resistance, and decreases BP.

PHARMACOKINETICS

Rapidly and completely absorbed after PO administration. Protein binding: 90%. Undergoes hepatic metabolism to inactive metabolite. Recovered primarily in feces and, to a lesser extent, in urine. Not removed by hemodialysis. *Half-life:* 11-15 h.

AVAILABILITY

Tablets: 75 mg, 150 mg, 300 mg.

INDICATIONS AND DOSAGES

▸ **Hypertension alone or in combination with other antihypertensives**

PO

Adults, Elderly. Initially, 150 mg/day. May increase to 300 mg/day.

Use lower (75 mg/day) initial dose if volume-depleted.

▸ **Diabetic nephropathy**

PO

Adults, Elderly. Titrate to target dose of 300 mg/day.

OFF-LABEL USES

Treatment of heart failure.

CONTRAINDICATIONS

Hypersensitivity to irbesartan.

INTERACTIONS

Drug

CYP2C9 substrates: May increase levels of CYP2C9 substrates.

Hydrochlorothiazide: Further reduces BP.

NSAIDs: May decrease efficacy of irbesartan.

Salt substitutes, drospirenone, eplerenone, and potassium sparing diuretics: May increase risk of hyperkalemia.

Herbal

Ephedra, ginseng, yohimbe: May increase blood pressure.

Food

None known.

DIAGNOSTIC TEST EFFECTS

May slightly increase BUN and serum creatinine levels. May decrease blood hemoglobin level. Rarely increases serum potassium.

SIDE EFFECTS

Occasional (3%-9%)

Upper respiratory tract infection, fatigue, diarrhea, cough.

Rare (1%-2%)

Heartburn, dizziness, headache, nausea, rash, hyperkalemia.

SERIOUS REACTIONS

- Overdosage may manifest as hypotension and tachycardia. Bradycardia occurs less often.
- Rare serious hypersensitivity reactions.

PRECAUTIONS & CONSIDERATIONS

Caution is warranted in patients with congestive heart failure, coronary artery disease, mild to moderate hepatic dysfunction, sodium and water depletion, renal dysfunction and unilateral renal artery stenosis. It is unknown whether irbesartan is distributed in breast milk. Irbesartan may cause fetal or neonatal morbidity or mortality. Discontinue as soon as pregnancy is detected. Safety and efficacy of irbesartan have not been established in children. The drug has not been effective at lowering BP in children 6-16 yr of age. In clinical studies, irbesartan did not effectively lower blood pressure in hypertensive children. No age-related precautions have been noted in elderly patients.

Apical pulse and BP should be assessed immediately before each irbesartan dose and regularly throughout therapy. Be alert to fluctuations in apical pulse and BP. If an excessive reduction in BP occurs, place the person in the supine position with feet slightly elevated, and notify the physician. Tasks that require mental alertness or motor skills should be avoided until the drug's effects are known. BUN, serum electrolytes, serum creatinine levels, heart rate for tachycardia, and urinalysis results should be obtained before and during therapy. Maintain adequate hydration; exercising outside during hot weather should be avoided to decrease the risk of dehydration and hypotension.

Storage

Store at room temperature.

Administration

Irbesartan may be given concurrently with other antihypertensives; if BP is not controlled by irbesartan alone, a diuretic may also be prescribed.

Take irbesartan without regard to meals.

Irinotecan

eye-ri-noe-tee′kan

Camptosar

CATEGORY AND SCHEDULE

Pregnancy Risk Category: D

Classification: Antineoplastics, topoisomerase inhibitors

MECHANISM OF ACTION

A DNA topoisomerase inhibitor that inhibits the action of topoisomerase I, an enzyme that allows DNA replication by producing reversible single-strand breaks in DNA that relieve torsional strain. Irinotecan prevents religation of the DNA strand, resulting in damage to double-strand DNA and cell death. *Therapeutic Effect:* Kills cancer cells.

PHARMACOKINETICS

Metabolized to active metabolite in the liver after IV administration. Protein binding: 95% (metabolite). Excreted in urine and eliminated by biliary route. *Half-life:* 6 h; metabolite 10 h.

AVAILABILITY

Injection: 20 mg/mL.

INDICATIONS AND DOSAGES

▸ **For advanced colorectal cancer:**

First-line in combination with 5-FU and leucovorin

IV INFUSION (with bolus 5-FU/leucovorin)

Adults. 125 mg/m^2 IV over 90 min, then leucovorin (20 mg/m^2 IV), and then 5-FU (500 mg/m^2 IV) on days 1, 8, 15, and 22. The next course begins on day 43 or when toxicity has recovered.

IV INFUSION (with infusional 5-FU/leucovorin)

Adults. 180 mg/m^2 IV over 90 mins, then leucovorin (200 mg/m^2 IV), then 5-FU (400 mg/m^2 IV bolus, then 600 mg/m^2 IV infusion for 22 hours). Irinotecan is given days 1, 15, and 29, while leucovorin and 5-FU are given days 1, 2, 15, 16, 29, and 30. The next course begins on day 43 or when toxicity has recovered.

Single-agent for metastatic colorectal cancer

IV INFUSION (WEEKLY DOSAGE)

Adults. 125 mg/m^2 IV over 90 min once weekly for 4 wks, then 2 wks of rest; subsequent cycles given every 6 wks.

IV INFUSION (ONCE-EVERY-3-WK DOSAGE)

Adults. 350 mg/m^2 by IV infusion over 90 min, administered once every 3 wks.

Dosage adjustments

NOTE: A reduction in the starting dose of irinotecan by at least 1 dose level should be considered for patients known to be homozygous for the UGT1A1*28 allele. Expect to adjust dosage based on disease

I

type, concomitant treatments, and worst presenting grade of hematologic or nonhematologic toxicity. Dosage is adjusted in 25-50 mg/m^2 increments to as low as 50 mg/m^2 (see prescribing information). Prior to each course, the granulocyte count should be ≥ 1500, the platelet count ≥ 100,000, and treatment-related diarrhea should be fully resolved.

OFF-LABEL USES

Small cell lung cancer, non–small cell lung carcinoma, malignant gliomas, breast and gynecologic cancers; pancreatic and GI cancers.

CONTRAINDICATIONS

Known hypersensitivity to irinotecan; do not use ketoconazole, St. John's wort, or atazanavir with irinotecan.

INTERACTIONS

Drug

Anticonvulsants: May decrease effects of irinotecan.
Atazanavir: May increase levels of irinotecan. Contraindicated.
Bevacizumab: May increase adverse effects of irinotecan.
CYP2B6 inducers: May decrease levels of irinotecan.
CYP2B6 inhibitors: May increase levels of irinotecan.
CYP3A4 inducers: May decrease levels of irinotecan.
CYP3A4 inhibitors: May increase levels of irinotecan.
Diuretics: May increase the risk of dehydration from vomiting and diarrhea.
Ketoconazole: Increases levels of irinotecan and the active metabolite. Contraindicated.
Laxatives: May increase the severity of diarrhea.
Live-virus vaccines: May potentiate virus replication, increase vaccine side effects, and decrease the patient's antibody response to the vaccine.
Other bone marrow depressants: May increase the risk of myelosuppression.
Prochlorperazine: May increase akathisia.

Herbal

St. John's wort: Decreases therapeutic effect of irinotecan. Contraindicated.

Food

None known.

DIAGNOSTIC TEST EFFECTS

May increase serum alkaline phosphatase and AST (SGOT) levels.

IV INCOMPATIBILITIES

Acyclovir, allopurinol, amphotericin B (all formulas), cefepime (Maxipime), cefotaxime, ceftriaxone (Rocephin), diazepam, epirubicin, 5-fluorouracil, fosphenytoin, furosemide, gemcitabine (Gemzar), methylprednisolone sodium succinate (Solu-Medrol), nafcillin, nitroprusside, pemetrexed, phenytoin, piperacillin-tazobactam (Zosyn), trastuzumab.

SIDE EFFECTS

Expected

Nausea (64%), alopecia (49%), vomiting (45%), diarrhea (32%).

Frequent

Constipation, fatigue (29%); fever (28%); asthenia (25%); skeletal pain (23%); abdominal pain, dyspnea (22%).

Occasional

Anorexia (19%); headache, stomatitis (18%); rash (16%).

SERIOUS REACTIONS

• Myelosuppression characterized as neutropenia occurs in 97% of patients; severe neutropenia, a neutrophil count < 50/mm^3, occurs in 78% of patients. Can be prolonged, life-threatening. Start treatment with loperamide at the first sign of diarrhea.

- Thrombocytopenia, anemia, and sepsis are common reactions.
- Severe diarrhea may occur early or late in therapy. Can be prolonged, life-threatening. Start treatment with loperamide at the first sign of diarrhea.

PRECAUTIONS & CONSIDERATIONS

Caution is warranted in those who have previously received abdominal or pelvic irradiation, patients with renal dysfunction, and elderly patients. Because of the risk of fetal harm, pregnant women should not take irinotecan, especially in the first trimester. Breastfeeding is not recommended for patients taking this drug. The safety and efficacy of irinotecan have not been established in children. Elderly patients are at increased risk for diarrhea. Use the drug cautiously in patients older than 65 yr. Vaccinations and coming in contact with crowds, people with known infections, and anyone who has recently received a live-virus vaccine should be avoided.

Notify the physician if diarrhea, rash, or inflammation at the infusion site occurs. Hemoglobin levels, CBC, serum electrolytes, and hydration status should be monitored. Hair loss may occur and is reversible, but new hair may have a different color or texture.

Storage

Store vials at room temperature, and protect them from light. If the solution is reconstituted in D5W, it remains stable for up to 24 h at room temperature or 48 h if refrigerated. However, because the drug contains no preservative, it should be used within 6 h if kept at room temperature or within 24 h if refrigerated. Do not refrigerate the solution if it is diluted with 0.9% NaCl.

Administration

CAUTION: Observe and exercise usual cautions for handling, administering, and preparing solutions of cytotoxic drugs.

Premedication with antiemetic agents is recommended, including dexamethasone plus a serotonin 5-HT$_3$ blocker, given at least 30 min before administration.

Dilute the drug in D5W (the preferred diluent) or 0.9% NaCl to a concentration of 0.12-2.8 mg/mL. Infusion volume is usually 250- 500 mL. Administer all doses by IV infusion over 90 min. Assess the patient for signs and symptoms of extravasation. If extravasation occurs, flush the site with sterile water and apply ice.

Iron Dextran

eye'ern dex'tran

★ Dexferrum, Infed 🍁 Dexiron, Infufer

CATEGORY AND SCHEDULE

Pregnancy Risk Category: C

Classification: Hematinics, minerals

MECHANISM OF ACTION

A trace element and essential component in the formation of hemoglobin. Necessary for effective erythropoiesis and transport and utilization of oxygen. Serves as cofactor of several essential enzymes. *Therapeutic Effect:* Replenishes hemoglobin and depleted iron stores.

PHARMACOKINETICS

Readily absorbed after IM administration. Most absorption occurs within 72 h; remainder within 3-4 wks. Bound to protein to form hemosiderin, ferritin, or transferrin. No physiologic system of elimination. Small amounts lost daily in shedding of skin, hair, and nails and in feces, urine, and perspiration. *Half-life:* 5-20 h.

AVAILABILITY

Injection: 50 mg/mL.

INDICATIONS AND DOSAGES

▸ **Iron deficiency anemia (no blood loss)**

IV, IM

Adults, Elderly. DOSE (mL) = 0.0442 (desired Hb - observed Hb) × LBW + (0.26 × LBW)

(Lean body weight for males = 50 kg + 2.3 kg for each inch over 5 ft. Lean body weight for females = 45.5 kg + 2.3 kg for each inch over 5 ft). Maximum: 100 mg/day.

▸ **Iron replacement secondary to blood loss**

IM, IV

Adults, Elderly. Replacement iron (mg) = blood loss (mL) times hematocrit.

▸ **Maximum daily dosage**

Adults weighing more than 50 kg. 100 mg.

Children weighing 10-50 kg. 100 mg.

Children weighing 5-9 kg. 50 mg.

Infants weighing < 5 kg. 25 mg.

CONTRAINDICATIONS

Hypersensitivity to the product. All anemias except iron deficiency anemia, including pernicious, aplastic, normocytic, and refractory; hemochromatosis; hemolytic anemia.

INTERACTIONS

Drug

Chloramphenicol: May decrease effect of iron dextran.

Herbal and Food

None known.

DIAGNOSTIC TEST EFFECTS

None known.

IV INCOMPATIBILITIES

No information available via Y-site administration. Do not dilute with dextrose injection or mix with parenteral nutrition for infusion.

SIDE EFFECTS

Frequent

Allergic reaction (such as rash and itching), backache, myalgia, chills, dizziness, headache, fever, nausea, vomiting, flushed skin, pain or redness at injection site, brown discoloration of skin, metallic taste.

SERIOUS REACTIONS

- Anaphylaxis has occurred during the first few minutes after injection, causing death rarely. Use test dose prior to therapeutic dosage.
- Leukocytosis and lymphadenopathy occur rarely.

PRECAUTIONS & CONSIDERATIONS

Extreme caution should be used with serious hepatic impairment. Caution is warranted with bronchial asthma, a history of allergies, and rheumatoid arthritis. Iron dextran may cross the placenta in some form, and trace amounts of the drug are distributed in breast milk. No age-related precautions have been noted in children and elderly patients. Avoid taking oral iron while receiving iron injections.

Stools may become black during iron therapy, but this side effect is harmless unless accompanied by abdominal cramping, pain, or red streaking or sticky consistency of stool. Notify the physician of abdominal cramping or pain, back pain, fever, headache, or red streaking or sticky consistency of stool. Be alert for acute exacerbation of joint pain and swelling in persons with rheumatoid arthritis and iron deficiency anemia.

Storage

Store at room temperature.

Administration

! Plan to discontinue oral iron before administering iron dextran because excessive iron intake may produce excessive iron storage (hemosiderosis). Know that a test dose is generally given before the full dose; stay with the patient for several minutes after injection of the test dose because of the potential for anaphylactic reaction.

! Before giving a therapeutic dose, it is customary to give a test dose of 25 mg (adults). The patient is usually observed for 1 h before commencing therapeutic treatment.

For IV use, may give undiluted or dilute in 0.9% NaCl for infusion. Do not exceed an administration rate of 50 mg/min (1 mL/min). A too-rapid IV rate may produce flushing, chest pain, shock, hypotension, and tachycardia. The patient should stay recumbent for 30-45 min after IV administration to minimize orthostatic hypotension.

For IM use, draw up medication with one needle; use new needle for injection to minimize skin staining. Use Z-tract technique by displacing subcutaneous tissue lateral to injection site before inserting needle to minimize skin staining. Administer deep into upper outer quadrant of buttock only.

Iron Sucrose

eye′ern su′crose

Venofer

CATEGORY AND SCHEDULE

Pregnancy Risk Category: B

Classification: Hematinics, minerals

MECHANISM OF ACTION

A trace element that is an essential component in the formation of hemoglobin. It is necessary for effective erythropoiesis and oxygen transport capacity of blood, and transport and utilization of oxygen, and it serves as cofactor of several essential enzymes. *Therapeutic Effect:* Replenishes body iron stores in patients on long-term hemodialysis who have iron deficiency anemia and are receiving erythropoietin.

AVAILABILITY

Injection: 20 mg/mL or 100 mg elemental iron in 5-mL single-dose vial.

INDICATIONS AND DOSAGES

▸ Iron deficiency anemia in patients on chronic hemodialysis

Dosage is expressed in terms of milligrams of elemental iron.

IV

Adults, Elderly. 100 mg elemental iron, delivered during dialysis; administer 1-3 times a wk to total dose of 1000 mg (10 doses). Give no more than 3 times weekly.

NOTE: Other dose regimens are approved for patients receiving peritoneal dialysis and who are nondialysis dependent. See manufacturer's literature.

CONTRAINDICATIONS

Hypersensitivity to iron sucrose; all anemias except iron deficiency anemia, including pernicious, aplastic, normocytic, and refractory anemia; evidence of iron overload.

INTERACTIONS

Drug

Dimercaprol: May increase nephrotoxicity.
Oral iron preparations: Iron sucrose may decrease absorption of oral agents.

Herbal and Food

None known.

DIAGNOSTIC TEST EFFECTS

Increases hemoglobin and hematocrit, serum ferritin level, and serum transferrin saturation.

IV INCOMPATIBILITIES

Do not mix with other medications or add to parenteral nutrition solution for IV infusion.

SIDE EFFECTS

Frequent (23%-36%)

Hypotension, leg cramps, diarrhea.

SERIOUS REACTIONS

- Too-rapid IV administration may produce severe hypotension, headache, vomiting, nausea, dizziness, paresthesia, abdominal and muscle pain, edema, and cardiovascular collapse.
- Hypersensitivity reaction occurs rarely.

PRECAUTIONS & CONSIDERATIONS

Caution is warranted in patients with cardiac dysfunction, bronchial asthma, history of allergies, and hepatic or renal impairment. Notify the physician of leg cramps or diarrhea. Initially, hematocrit, hemoglobin, serum ferritin, and serum transferrin levels should be obtained monthly, then every 2-3 mo as determined by the physician. Iron levels should be obtained 48 h after iron sucrose administration. Monitor closely for hypotension.

Storage

Store unopened vials at room temperature.

Administration

! Administer directly into dialysis line during hemodialysis, as prescribed.

Can be given as undiluted, slow IV injection. However, IV infusion is preferred to avoid hypotension. For IV infusion, dilute each vial in maximum of 100 mL 0.9% NaCl immediately before infusion. For IV injection, administer into the dialysis line at a rate of 1 mL, or 20 mg iron, undiluted solution per minute. Allow 5 min per vial; do not exceed 1 vial per injection. For IV infusion, administer into dialysis line at a rate of 100 mg iron over at least 15 min. Expect to monitor the results of treatment.

Isocarboxazid

eye-soe-kar-box'a-zid

★ Marplan

CATEGORY AND SCHEDULE

Pregnancy Risk Category: C

Classification: Antidepressants, monoamine oxidase inhibitors

MECHANISM OF ACTION

An antidepressant that inhibits the MAO enzyme system at central nervous system (CNS) storage sites. The reduced MAO activity causes an increased concentration in epinephrine, norepinephrine, serotonin, and dopamine at neuron receptor sites. *Therapeutic Effect:* Produces antidepressant effect.

PHARMACOKINETICS

PO: Good absorption; maximum MAO inhibition 5-10 days, duration up to 2 wks; metabolized by liver; excreted by kidneys.

AVAILABILITY

Tablets: 10 mg (Marplan).

INDICATIONS AND DOSAGES

▸ Depression refractory to other antidepressants or electroconvulsive therapy

PO

Adults, Elderly. Initially, 10 mg 3 times/day. May increase to 60 mg/day.

OFF-LABEL USES

Treatment of panic disorder.

CONTRAINDICATIONS

Cardiovascular disease (CVD), cerebrovascular disease, liver impairment, pheochromocytoma.
NOTE: Many drugs are contraindicated for use within 14 days of MAOI use.

INTERACTIONS

Drug

Alcohol, CNS depressants: May increase CNS depressant effects.
Bupropion: May increase neurotoxic effects.
Buspirone: May increase BP.
Caffeine-containing medications: May increase cardiac arrhythmias and hypertension.
Carbamazepine, cyclobenzaprine, maprotiline, other MAOIs: May precipitate hypertensive crises.
CNS depressants: May increase adverse effects.
CNS stimulants: Isocarboxazid may increase hypertensive effects.
COMT inhibitors: May increase adverse effects of isocarboxacid.
Dextromethorphan, trazodone, SSRIs, tricyclic antidepressants: May cause serotonin syndrome. Contraindicated.
Insulin, oral hypoglycemics: May increase effects of insulin and oral hypoglycemics.
Linezolid: Additive MAOI actions. Contraindicated.
Lithium: May increase adverse effects of lithium.
Meperidine, other opioid analgesics: May produce coma, convulsions, death, diaphoresis, immediate excitation, rigidity, severe hypertension or hypotension, severe respiratory distress, or vascular collapse. Meperidine is contraindicated.
Methylphenidate: May increase the CNS stimulant effects of methylphenidate.
Sympathomimetics: May increase the cardiac stimulant and vasopressor effects of isocarboxazid. Contraindicated.
Tramadol: May increase risk of seizures.
Tyramine: May cause severe, sudden hypertension.

Herbal

None known.

Food

Foods high in tyramine: May cause hypertensive crisis.

DIAGNOSTIC TEST EFFECTS

None known.

SIDE EFFECTS

Frequent (> 10%)

Postural hypotension, drowsiness, decreased sexual ability, weakness, trembling, visual disturbances.

Occasional (1%-10%)
Tachycardia, peripheral edema, nervousness, chills, diarrhea, anorexia, constipation, xerostomia.
Rare (< 1%)
Hepatitis, leukopenia, parkinsonian syndrome.

SERIOUS REACTIONS

- Hypertensive crisis, marked by severe hypertension, occipital headache radiating frontally, neck stiffness or soreness, nausea, vomiting, sweating, fever or chilliness, clammy skin, dilated pupils, palpitations, tachycardia or bradycardia, and constricting chest pain.

PRECAUTIONS & CONSIDERATIONS

Caution is warranted in patients with asthma, bronchitis, bipolar disorder, cardiac arrhythmias, cardiovascular disease, diabetes mellitus, epilepsy, headaches, hepatic function impairment, hypertension, hyperthyroidism, Parkinson disease, renal function impairment, schizophrenia, and those with suicidal tendencies. Foods that require bacteria or molds for their preparation or preservation or containing tyramine, including avocados, bananas, beer, broad beans, cheese, figs, meat tenderizers, papaya, raisins, sour cream, soy sauce, wine, yeast extracts, yogurt, or excessive amounts of caffeine, such as chocolate, coffee, and tea, should be avoided. It is unknown whether isocarboxazid crosses the placenta or is distributed in breast milk. Safety and efficacy have not been established in children or elderly patients.

Blurred vision, drowsiness, increased sweating, decreased sexual ability, and dizziness may be experienced while taking isocarboxazid. Headache, neck soreness or stiffness should be reported.

Storage
Store at room temperature.

Administration
Use the lowest effective dose. Take with or without meals.

! Food and drug interactions with isocarboxazid can be serious (see Interactions). Consider patient's intake of foods/beverages containing large amounts of tyramine, tryptophan, and/or caffeine.

Isoniazid (INH)

eye-soe-nye'a-zid
★ INH, Nydrazid 🍁 Isotamine

CATEGORY AND SCHEDULE

Pregnancy Risk Category: C

Classification: Antimycobacterials; antitubercular

MECHANISM OF ACTION

An isonicotinic acid derivative that inhibits mycolic acid synthesis and causes disruption of the bacterial cell wall and loss of acid-fast properties in susceptible mycobacteria. Active only during bacterial cell division. *Therapeutic Effect:* Bactericidal against actively growing intracellular and extracellular susceptible mycobacteria.

PHARMACOKINETICS

Readily absorbed from the GI tract. Protein binding: 10%-15%. Widely distributed (including to the cerebrospinal fluid). Metabolized in the liver. Primarily excreted in urine. Removed by hemodialysis. *Half-life:* 0.5-5 h.

AVAILABILITY

Tablets: 100 mg, 300 mg.
Syrup: 50 mg/5 mL.
Injection: 100 mg/mL.

INDICATIONS AND DOSAGES

▸ **Tuberculosis (in combination with one or more antituberculars)**

PO, IM

Adults, Elderly. 5 mg/kg/day as a single dose. Maximum: 300 mg/day.
Children. 10-15 mg/kg/day as a single dose. Maximum: 300 mg/day.

▸ **Prevention of tuberculosis**

PO, IM

Adults, Elderly. 300 mg/day as a single dose.
Children. 10 mg/kg/day as a single dose. Maximum: 300 mg/day.

CONTRAINDICATIONS

Acute hepatic disease, history of hypersensitivity reactions or hepatic injury with previous isoniazid therapy.

INTERACTIONS

Drug

Acetaminophen: May potentiate adverse effects of acetaminophen.
Alcohol: May increase isoniazid metabolism and the risk of hepatotoxicity.
Antacids: May decrease absorption of isoniazid.
Benzodiazepines: May decrease metabolism of benzodiazepines.
Carbamazepine, phenytoin, valproic acid: May increase the concentrations of these drugs.
Corticosteroids: May decrease concentrations of isoniazid.
CYP2C19 substrates: May increase levels of CYP2C19 substrates.
CYP2E1 substrates: May decrease levels of CYP2E1 substrates.
CYP3A4 substrates: May increase levels of CYP3A4 substrates.
Disulfiram: May increase central nervous system (CNS) effects.
Dronedarone, ranolazine: INH significantly increases levels of these drugs; avoid.
Hepatotoxic medications: May increase the risk of hepatotoxicity.
MAOIs: INH has some MAO-inhibiting activity; actions may be additive. Avoid co-use.
Theophylline: May increase theophylline levels.

Herbal

None known.

Food

All foods: Significantly reduce INH bioavailability.
Tyramine-containing foods: May cause a hypertensive crisis.

DIAGNOSTIC TEST EFFECTS

May increase serum bilirubin, AST (SGOT), and ALT (SGPT) levels.

SIDE EFFECTS

Frequent

Nausea, vomiting, diarrhea, abdominal pain.

Rare

Pain at injection site, hypersensitivity reaction.

SERIOUS REACTIONS

• Rare reactions include neurotoxicity (as evidenced by ataxia and paresthesia), optic neuritis, and hepatotoxicity.

PRECAUTIONS & CONSIDERATIONS

Because there is a higher frequency of isoniazid-associated hepatitis among certain patient groups, including those over 35 yr, daily users of alcohol, those with chronic hepatic disease, injectable drug abusers, and women belonging to minority groups, particularly in the post-partum period, LFTs should be obtained prior to and monthly during therapy, or more frequently as needed. If any of the values exceed 3 times the upper limit of normal (ULN), temporarily discontinue.

Be aware that prophylactic use of isoniazid is usually postponed until after childbirth. Be aware that isoniazid crosses the placenta. The small concentrations of isoniazid in breast milk do not produce toxicity in the nursing neonate; therefore, breastfeeding should not be discouraged. Pyridoxine supplementation in the nursing infant may be advised. No age-related precautions have been noted in children. Elderly patients are more susceptible to developing hepatitis. Avoid consuming alcohol during treatment and taking any other medications without first notifying the physician, including antacids. Avoid foods containing tyramine, including aged cheeses, sauerkraut, smoked fish, and tuna, because these foods may cause a reaction such as headache, a hot or clammy feeling, light-headedness, pounding heartbeat, and red or itching skin.

! Determine whether the patient has any history of hypersensitivity reactions or liver injury from isoniazid as well as sensitivity to nicotinic acid before starting drug therapy. Monitor the patient's liver function test results, and assess the patient for signs and symptoms of hepatitis as evidenced by anorexia, dark urine, fatigue, jaundice, nausea, vomiting, and weakness. If hepatitis is suspected, withhold the drug and notify the physician promptly. In addition, assess for burning, numbness, and tingling of the extremities. People at risk for neuropathy, such as alcoholics, those with chronic liver disease, diabetics, elderly patients, and malnourished individuals, may receive pyridoxine prophylactically.

Storage

Store vials and tablets at room temperature; protect from light. Injection may crystallize at low temperatures. Warm the vial to room temperature before use to redissolve the crystals.

Administration

Give 1 h before or 2 h after meals. Do not give with food. Administer at least 1 h before antacids, especially those containing aluminum. Do not skip doses and continue taking isoniazid for the full length of therapy (6-24 mo).

INH injection is for intramuscular (IM) use only and is used in those unable to take oral therapy.

Isoproterenol

eye-soe-proe-ter′e-nole

★ Isuprel

CATEGORY AND SCHEDULE

Pregnancy Risk Category: C

Classification: Adrenergic agonists, β-agonists, bronchodilators, inotropes

MECHANISM OF ACTION

A sympathomimetic (adrenergic agonist) that stimulates β_1-adrenergic receptors. *Therapeutic Effect:* Increases myocardial contractility, stroke volume, cardiac output.

PHARMACOKINETICS

Readily absorbed. Metabolized in liver. Primarily excreted in urine. *Half-life:* 2.5-5 min.

AVAILABILITY

Injection: 0.02 mg/mL, 0.2 mg/mL (Isuprel).

INDICATIONS AND DOSAGES

▸ Arrhythmias

IV BOLUS

Adults, Elderly. Initially, 0.02-0.06 mg (1-3 mL of diluted solution). Subsequent dose range: 0.01-0.2 mg (0.5-10 mL of diluted solution).

IV INFUSION

Adults, Elderly. Initially, 5 mcg/min (1.25 mL/min of diluted solution). Subsequent dose range: 2-20 mcg/min.

Children. Initially, 0.1 mcg/kg per min. Range: 0.1-1 mcg/kg/min.

▸ Shock and hypoperfusion

IV INFUSION

Adults, Elderly. Rate of 0.5-5 mcg/min (0.25-2.5 mL of 1:500,000 dilution); rate of infusion based on clinical response (heart rate, central venous pressure, systemic BP, urine flow measurements).

CONTRAINDICATIONS

Tachycardia resulting from digitalis toxicity, preexisting arrhythmias, angina, precordial distress, hypersensitivity to isoproterenol, other sympathomimetic amines, or any component of the formulation.

INTERACTIONS

Drug

β-Blockers: May antagonize the effects of isoproterenol.

Digoxin: May increase the risk of arrhythmias.

General anesthetics: May increase risk of arrhythmias.

Tricyclic antidepressants: May increase cardiovascular effects.

Sympathomimetic agents: May increase adverse effects.

Herbal

Ephedra, ma huang, yohimbe: May increase CNS stimulation.

Food

None known.

DIAGNOSTIC TEST EFFECTS

Decreases serum potassium levels.

IV INCOMPATIBILITIES

Aminophylline, furosemide (Lasix), sodium bicarbonate.

IV COMPATIBILITIES

Amiodarone (Cordarone), atracurium (Tracrium), bretylium (Bretylol), calcium chloride, cimetidine (Tagamet), cisatracurium (Nimbex), dobutamine (Dobutrex), famotidine (Pepcid), heparin, hydrocortisone sodium succinate (Solu-Cortef), inamrinone (Inocor), levofloxacin (Levaquin), magnesium sulfate, milrinone (Primacor), pancuronium (Panvulon), potassium chloride, propofol (Diprivan), ranitidine (Zantac), remifentanil (Ultiva), succinylcholine (Anectine), tacrolimus (Prograf), vecuronium (Norcuron), verapamil (Calan), vitamin B complex with C.

SIDE EFFECTS

Frequent

Palpitations, tachycardia, restlessness, nervousness, tremor, insomnia, anxiety.

Occasional

Increased sweating, headache, nausea, flushed skin, dizziness, coughing.

SERIOUS REACTIONS

- Excessive sympathomimetic stimulation may cause palpitations, extrasystoles, tachycardia, chest pain, slight increase in BP followed by a substantial decrease, chills, sweating, and blanching of skin.
- Ventricular arrhythmias may occur if heart rate is above 130 beats/min.
- Parotid gland swelling may occur with prolonged use.

PRECAUTIONS & CONSIDERATIONS

Caution is warranted with hypersensitivity to sulfite, elderly or debilitated, hypertension, cardiovascular disease, impaired renal function, hyperthyroidism, diabetes mellitus, prostatic hypertrophy, seizure disorder, glaucoma. It is unknown whether isoproterenol crosses the placenta or is distributed in breast milk, so it is not administered to pregnant women. Safety and efficacy have not been established in children. Be aware that elderly patients may exhibit decreased therapeutic response (decreased heart rate, peripheral vascular response).

If chest pain or palpitations occur, notify the physician.

Storage

Store solution at room temperature. Do not use if the solution is pink to brown, contains a precipitate, or appears cloudy. Stability of parenteral admixture at room temperature or at refrigeration is 24 h.

Administration

Reconstitutite for IV push by diluting 0.2 mg (1 mL) of 1:5000 solution to a volume of 10 mL 0.9% NaCl or D5W. Give IV push at rate of 1 mL/min.

For IV infusion, dilute 0.2-2 mg (1-10 mL) of 1:5000 solution in 500 mL D5W to provide a solution of 0.4-4 mcg/mL. Rate of IV infusion determined by the person's heart rate, central venous pressure, systemic BP, and urine flow measurements. Use microdrip (60 drops/mL) or infusion pump to administer drug.

Regulate by ECG monitoring. If ECG changes occur, heart rate exceeds 110 beats/min, or premature beats occur, consider reducing rate of infusion or temporarily stopping infusion.

Isosorbide Dinitrate/Mononitrate

Dilatrate SR, Isordil Titradose, IsoChron, IsoDitrate, Imdur, Monoket Apo-ISMN, Imdur, ISDN, Novo-Sorbide, PMS-ISMN, Pro-ISMN

Do not confuse Isordil with Isuprel or Plendil, or Imdur with Inderal or K-Dur.

CATEGORY AND SCHEDULE

Pregnancy Risk Category: C

Classification: Vasodilators; nitrate antianginal

MECHANISM OF ACTION

A nitrate that stimulates intracellular cyclic guanosine monophosphate. *Therapeutic Effect:* Relaxes vascular smooth muscle of both arterial and venous vasculature. Decreases preload and afterload.

PHARMACOKINETICS

Dinitrate poorly absorbed and metabolized in the liver to its active metabolite isosorbide mononitrate. Mononitrate well absorbed after PO administration. Excreted in urine and feces. *Half-life:* Dinitrate, 1-4 h; mononitrate, 4 h.

AVAILABILITY

Isosorbide Dinitrate (ISDN) Capsules, Sustained Release (Dilatrate SR): 40 mg.
Tablets (Isordil Titradose): 5 mg, 10 mg, 20 mg, 30 mg, 40 mg.
Tablets, Extended Release (IsoChron, IsoDitrate): 40 mg.
Tablets, Sublingual: 2.5 mg, 5 mg.
Isosorbide Mononitrate Tablets (Monoket): 10 mg, 20 mg.
Tablets, Extended Release (Imdur): 30 mg, 60 mg, 120 mg.

INDICATIONS AND DOSAGES

▸ **Angina**

PO (ISOSORBIDE DINITRATE)
Adults, Elderly. 5-40 mg 4 times a day. Sustained release: 40 mg q8-12h.

PO (ISOSORBIDE MONONITRATE)
Adults, Elderly. 5-10 mg twice a day given 7 h apart. Sustained release: Initially, 30-60 mg/day in morning as a single dose. May increase dose at 3-day intervals. Usually up to 120 mg/day. Maximum: 240 mg/day.

OFF-LABEL USES

Congestive heart failure, dysphagia, relief of esophageal spasm with gastroesophageal reflux.

CONTRAINDICATIONS

Closed-angle glaucoma, GI hypermotility or malabsorption (extended-release tablets), head trauma, hypersensitivity to nitrates, increased intracranial pressure, orthostatic hypotension, severe anemia (extended-release tablets).

INTERACTIONS

Drug

Antihypertensives, vasodilators: May increase risk of orthostatic hypotension.
CYP3A4 inducers: May decrease levels of isosorbide.
CYP3A4 inhibitors: May increase levels of isosorbide.
Sildenafil, tadalafil, vardenafil: May significantly decrease blood pressure. Concurrent use is contraindicated.

Herbal

None known.

Food

Alcohol: May increase risk of orthostatic hypotension.

DIAGNOSTIC TEST EFFECTS

May increase urine catecholamine and urine vanillylmandelic acid levels.

SIDE EFFECTS

Frequent

Burning and tingling at the oral point of dissolution (sublingual), headache (possibly severe) occurs mostly in early therapy, diminishes rapidly in intensity, and usually disappears during continued treatment, transient flushing of face and neck, dizziness (especially if the patient is standing immobile or is in a warm environment), weakness, orthostatic hypotension, nausea, vomiting, restlessness.

Occasional

GI upset, blurred vision, dry mouth.

SERIOUS REACTIONS

- Blurred vision or dry mouth may occur (drug should be discontinued).
- Isosorbide administration may cause severe orthostatic hypotension manifested by fainting, pulselessness, cold or clammy skin, and diaphoresis.
- Tolerance may occur with repeated, prolonged therapy but may not occur with the extended-release form. Minor tolerance may be seen with intermittent use of sublingual tablets.
- High dosage tends to produce severe headache.

PRECAUTIONS & CONSIDERATIONS

Caution is warranted with acute MI, blood volume depletion from therapy, glaucoma (contraindicated in closed-angle glaucoma), hepatic or renal disease, and systolic BP < 90 mm Hg. It is unknown if isosorbide crosses the placenta or is distributed in breast milk. The safety and efficacy of isosorbide have not been established in children. Elderly patients may be more sensitive to the drug's hypotensive effects. In elderly patients, age-related decreased renal function may require cautious use. Alcohol should be avoided because it intensifies the drug's hypotensive effect. If alcohol is ingested soon after taking nitrates, an acute hypotensive episode marked by pallor, vertigo, and a drop in BP may occur.

Dizziness, light-headedness, and headache may occur. Notify the physician of facial or neck flushing. The onset, type (sharp, dull, or squeezing), radiation, location, intensity, and duration of anginal pain and its precipitating factors, such as exertion and emotional stress, should be recorded before therapy begins.

Storage

Store at room temperature. Protect from moisture and light.

Administration

Best if taken on an empty stomach; however, take oral isosorbide with meals if the headache occurs. Oral tablets, except the extended-release form, may be crushed. Do not crush or break the extended-release form. Do not crush the chewable form before administering.

For sublingual use, do not crush or chew tablets. Dissolve tablets under tongue without swallowing. Isosorbide should be taken at the first sign or symptom of angina. If angina is not relieved within 5 min, dissolve a second tablet under the tongue and then repeat the dosage 5 min later if there is no relief. Do not take more than 3 tablets within 15-30 min.

Isotretinoin

eye-soe-tret′i-noyn

Amnesteem, Claravis, Sotret

Accutane, Clarus

CATEGORY AND SCHEDULE

Pregnancy Risk Category: X

Classification: Retinoids; dermatologic agents, acne therapies

MECHANISM OF ACTION

Reduces the size of sebaceous glands and inhibits their activity. *Therapeutic Effect:* Decreases sebum production; produces antikeratinizing and anti-inflammatory effects.

PHARMACOKINETICS

Metabolized in the liver; major metabolite active. Eliminated in urine and feces. *Half-life:* 21 h; metabolite, 21-24 h.

AVAILABILITY

Capsules: 10 mg, 20 mg, 30 mg, 40 mg.

INDICATIONS AND DOSAGES

▸ **Recalcitrant cystic acne that is unresponsive to conventional acne therapies**

PO

Adults, Children 12 yr of age and older. Initially, 0.5-1 mg/kg/day, divided into 2 doses for 15-20 wks. May repeat after at least 2 mo off therapy. Severe acne may require 2 mg/kg/day.

OFF-LABEL USES

Treatment of gram-negative folliculitis, severe keratinization disorders, severe rosacea.

CONTRAINDICATIONS

Hypersensitivity to isotretinoin or parabens (component of capsules); pregnancy.

INTERACTIONS

Drug

Carbamazepine: May decrease levels of carbamazepine.

Etretinate, tretinoin, vitamin A: May increase toxic effects.

Methotrexate: May increase risk of hepatotoxicity. Avoid.

Oral contraceptives: May decrease efficacy of oral contraceptives.

Tetracycline: May increase the risk of pseudotumor cerebri.
Tigecycline: May cause pseudotumor cerebri.
Warfarin: Retinoids may decrease effect; monitor INR.
Herbal
Dong quai, St John's wort: May cause photosensitization.
Food
Milk: May increase bioavailability of isotretinoin.

DIAGNOSTIC TEST EFFECTS

May increase serum alkaline phosphatase, total cholesterol, LDH, triglyceride, ALT (SGPT), and AST (SGOT) levels; urine uric acid level; erythrocyte sedimentation rate; and fasting blood glucose level. May decrease HDL level. May decrease hemoglobin and hematocrit.

SIDE EFFECTS

Frequent (20%-90%)
Cheilitis (inflammation of lips), dry skin and mucous membranes, skin fragility, pruritus, epistaxis, dry nose and mouth, conjunctivitis, hypertriglyceridemia, nausea, vomiting, abdominal pain.
Occasional (5%-16%)
Musculoskeletal symptoms (including bone pain, arthralgia, generalized myalgia), photosensitivity.
Rare
Decreased night vision, depression.

SERIOUS REACTIONS

- Inflammatory bowel disease and pseudotumor cerebri (benign intracranial hypertension) have been associated with isotretinoin therapy.
- Hearing impairment may occur and may continue after isotretinoin is discontinued.
- Teratogen.

PRECAUTIONS & CONSIDERATIONS

Caution should be used in patients with renal or hepatic dysfunction. Depression, psychosis, aggressive behavior, and suicide have been reported with this medication. Be aware that isotretinoin is contraindicated in pregnancy. Patients, prescribers, wholesalers, and dispensing pharmacists must register with the iPledge program. There is an extremely high risk of major deformities in infants if pregnancy occurs while taking any amount of isotretinoin, even for short periods. The person must be capable of understanding and carrying out instructions and of complying with mandatory contraception (2 forms). Be aware that excretion in breast milk is unknown; due to potential for serious adverse effects, it is not recommended during nursing. No age-related precautions have been noted in children or elderly patients.

Women must have 2 negative serum pregnancy tests within 2 wks before starting therapy; therapy will begin on the second or third day of the next normal menstrual period. Effective contraception (using 2 reliable forms of contraception simultaneously) must be used for at least 1 mo before, during, and for at least 1 mo after therapy. Give both oral and written warnings, with the patient acknowledging in writing that she understands the warnings and consents to treatment. Prescriptions may be written for only 30 days and pregnancy testing and counseling should be repeated monthly. Med Guides are given with each refill. Blood donation must be avoided during treatment and for 1 mo following completion because the donated blood might be given to a pregnant woman and expose a fetus.

Patients may have decreased tolerance to contact lenses during and after therapy. Patients should be cautioned about driving at night due to potential decreases in night vision and should use caution with UV exposure due to photosensitivity. Notify the physician immediately if abdominal pain, severe diarrhea, rectal bleeding (possible inflammatory bowel disease), or headache, nausea and vomiting, visual disturbances (possible pseudotumor cerebri) occur.

Storage

Store at room temperature and protect from light.

Administration

Give isotretinoin with food and a full glass of liquid to reduce esophogeal irritation. Failure to take with food will significantly decrease absorption. Do not crush or open capsules. Patients not responding to treatment should be asked about adherence to administration with meals prior to increasing dosage.

Isradipine

is-rad′ih-peen

★ DynaCirc CR

Do not confuse DynaCirc with Dynabac or Dynacin.

CATEGORY AND SCHEDULE

Pregnancy Risk Category: C

Classification: Calcium channel blockers

MECHANISM OF ACTION

An antihypertensive that inhibits calcium movement across cardiac and vascular smooth-muscle cell membranes. Potent peripheral vasodilator that does not depress SA or AV nodes. *Therapeutic Effect:* Produces relaxation of coronary vascular smooth muscle and coronary vasodilation. Increases myocardial oxygen delivery to those with vasospastic angina.

PHARMACOKINETICS

Route	Onset	Peak	Duration
PO	2-3 h	2-4 wks (with multiple doses)	NA
		8-16 h (with single dose)	
PO (controlled release)	2 h	8-10 h	NA

Well absorbed from the GI tract. Protein binding: 95%. Metabolized in the liver (undergoes first-pass effect). Primarily excreted in urine. Not removed by hemodialysis. *Half-life:* 8 h.

AVAILABILITY

Capsules: 2.5 mg, 5 mg.
Tablets (Controlled Release [DynaCirc CR]): 5 mg, 10 mg.

INDICATIONS AND DOSAGES

▸ **Hypertension**

PO (IMMEDIATE RELEASE)

Adults, Elderly. Initially, 2.5 mg twice a day. May increase by 2.5 mg at 2- to 4-wk intervals. Range: 5-20 mg/day in divided doses twice daily.

PO (EXTENDED RELEASE)

Initially, 5 mg once daily. Usual dose 5-10 mg/day. Maximum: 20 mg/day.

OFF-LABEL USES

Treatment of chronic angina pectoris, Raynaud phenomenon.

CONTRAINDICATIONS

Hypersensitivity.

INTERACTIONS

Drug

β-Blockers: May have additive effect.

Strong CYP3A inhibitors: May increase isradipine levels.

Fentanyl anesthesia: Severe hypotension has been reported; may have additive effects.

Herbal

Melatonin: Reported to reduce hypotensive effects of some calcium channel blockers.

St. John's wort: May reduce isradipine concentrations.

Food

Grapefruit, grapefruit juice: May increase the absorption of isradipine. Avoid.

DIAGNOSTIC TEST EFFECTS

None known.

SIDE EFFECTS

Frequent (4%-7%)

Peripheral edema, palpitations (higher frequency in female patients).

Occasional (3%)

Facial flushing, cough.

Rare (1%-2%)

Angina, tachycardia, rash, pruritus.

SERIOUS REACTIONS

- Overdose produces nausea, drowsiness, confusion, and slurred speech, dizziness, syncope.
- Congestive heart failure occurs rarely.

PRECAUTIONS & CONSIDERATIONS

Caution is warranted in patients with edema, hepatic disease, severe left ventricular dysfunction, sick sinus syndrome, and in those concurrently receiving β-blockers or digoxin. It is unknown whether isradipine crosses the placenta or is distributed in breast milk. The safety and efficacy of isradipine have not been established in children. In elderly patients, age-related renal impairment may require cautious use. Grapefruit juice, which may increase isradipine blood concentration, should be avoided. Tasks that require alertness and motor skills should also be avoided.

Avoid using sodium-containing products, such as IV saline fluids, for patients with a dietary salt restriction. Patients should be assessed for stress-induced angina episodes, which may occur during isradipine therapy.

Notify the physician if irregular heartbeat, nausea, pronounced dizziness, or shortness of breath occurs. Rise slowly from a lying to a sitting position and wait momentarily before standing to avoid isradipine's hypotensive effect. Apical pulse and BP should be assessed immediately before beginning isradipine administration. If the systolic BP is < 90 mm Hg, withhold the medication and contact the physician. Liver function tests should also be performed before and during therapy. Skin should be assessed for flushing and peripheral edema, especially behind the medial malleolus and the sacral area. Blood dyscrasias may occur in patients on chronic isradipine therapy, which may include signs of infection, bleeding, and poor healing.

Storage

Store at controlled room temperature. Protect from moisture and light.

Administration

Do not crush, open, or break extended-release tablets. Do not abruptly discontinue isradipine. Compliance is essential to control hypertension. May take without regard to food. Do not administer with grapefruit juice.

Itraconazole

it-ra-con'a-zol

Sporanox

Do not confuse Sporanox with Suprax.

CATEGORY AND SCHEDULE

Pregnancy Risk Category: C

Classification: Systemic triazole antifungal

MECHANISM OF ACTION

A fungistatic antifungal that inhibits the synthesis of ergosterol, a vital component of fungal cell formation. *Therapeutic Effect:* Damages the fungal cell membrane, altering its function.

PHARMACOKINETICS

Moderately absorbed from the GI tract. Absorption is increased if the drug is taken with food. Protein binding: 99%. Widely distributed, primarily in the fatty tissue, liver, and kidneys. Metabolized in the liver to active metabolite. Primarily excreted in urine. Not removed by hemodialysis. *Half-life:* 21 h; metabolite, 12 h.

AVAILABILITY

Capsules: 100 mg.
Oral Solution: 10 mg/mL.
Injection: 10 mg/mL (25-mL ampule).

INDICATIONS AND DOSAGES

▸ **Blastomycosis, histoplasmosis, and aspergillosis**

PO

Adults, Elderly. Initially, 200 mg once a day. Maximum: 400 mg/day in 2 divided doses.

IV INFUSION

Adults, Elderly. 200 mg twice a day for 4 doses, then 200 mg once a day.

▸ **Life-threatening fungal infections**

PO

Adults, Elderly. 600 mg/day in 3 divided doses for 3-4 days, then 200-400 mg/day in 2 divided doses.

IV

Adults, Elderly. 200 mg twice a day for 4 doses, then 200 mg once a day.

▸ **Esophageal candidiasis**

PO (ORAL SOLUTION ONLY)

Adults, Elderly. Swish 10 mL in mouth for several seconds, then swallow. Maximum: 200 mg/day.

▸ **Oropharyngeal candidiasis**

PO (ORAL SOLUTION ONLY)

Adults, Elderly. Vigorously swish 10 mL in the mouth for several seconds and then swallow (20 mL total daily dose) once a day. Usually given 1-2 wks.

▸ **Onychomycosis of toenails**

PO

Adults. 200 mg once daily for 12 wks.

▸ **Onychomycosis of fingernails**

PO

Adults. Give 200 mg twice daily for 1 wk; rest for 3 wks; then give 200 mg twice daily for 1 wk.

▸ **Dosage in renal impairment**

Do not use itraconazole IV if CrCl < 30 mL/min.

OFF-LABEL USES

Suppression of histoplasmosis; treatment of disseminated sporotrichosis, fungal pneumonia and septicemia, or ringworm of the hand.

CONTRAINDICATIONS

Hypersensitivity to itraconazole, fluconazole, ketoconazole, or miconazole. Do not use itraconazole for treatment of onychomycosis if patient has CHF.

Coadministration with cisapride, pimozide, quinidine, dofetilide, levomethadyl, lovastatin, simvastatin, and ergot alkaloids is contraindicated.

INTERACTIONS

Drug

Antacids, didanosine, H_2 antagonists: May decrease itraconazole absorption; take itraconazole 2 h before taking antacids, didanosine, or H_2 antagonists.

Buspirone, cyclosporine, digoxin, midazolam, triazolam, allopurinol, felodipine: May increase blood concentration of these drugs.

Carbamazepine, phenobarbital: May increase metabolism of itraconazole.

Cyclosporine, protease inhibitors, nisoldipine, haloperidol, carbamazepine, erythromycin, clarithromycin, azithromycin, alfentanil, corticosteroids, zolpidem: May increase plasma level of these drugs.

HMG-CoA reductase inhibitors (statins): May increase side effects and plasma levels of statins; either avoid using itraconazole with statins or lower their dosages when using itraconazole to limit the risk of rhabdomyolysis. Lovastatin and simvastatin are contraindicated.

Oral anticoagulants, warfarin: May inhibit warfarin metabolism; may increase the effect of oral anticoagulants generally.

Oral antidiabetic agents: May increase the risk of hypoglycemia developing.

Phenytoin, rifampin: May decrease itraconazole blood concentration.

Herbal

None known.

Food

Cola products: May increase plasma levels of itraconazole.

Grapefruit juice: May decrease itraconazole absorption. Avoid.

DIAGNOSTIC TEST EFFECTS

May increase serum LDH, serum alkaline phosphatase, serum bilirubin, SGOT (AST), and SGPT (ALT) levels. May decrease serum potassium level.

IV INCOMPATIBILITIES

! Dilution compatibilities of itraconazole with any solution other than 0.9% NaCl are unknown. Don't mix with D5W or lactated Ringer's solution. Do not administer any medication in same bag or through same IV line as itraconazole.

SIDE EFFECTS

Frequent (9%-11%)

Nausea, rash.

Occasional (3%-5%)

Vomiting, headache, diarrhea, hypertension, peripheral edema, fatigue, fever.

Rare (2% or less)

Abdominal pain, dizziness, anorexia, pruritus.

SERIOUS REACTIONS

- Hepatitis (as evidenced by anorexia, abdominal pain, unusual fatigue or weakness, jaundiced skin or sclera, and dark urine) occurs rarely.
- May cause new or worsened heart failure.

PRECAUTIONS & CONSIDERATIONS

Caution is warranted in patients with achlorhydria, hepatitis, HIV infection, hypochlorhydria, or impaired liver function, or patients with heart failure or risk factors for cardiac compromise. Be aware that itraconazole is distributed in breast milk. Be aware that the safety and efficacy of itraconazole have not been established in children. In elderly patients, age-related renal impairment may require dosage adjustment. Carefully assess potential serious drug interactions.

Obtain the baseline temperature, check the liver function test results, as appropriate, and determine whether there is a history of allergies before giving the drug. Assess for signs and symptoms of liver dysfunction. Report any anorexia, dark urine, nausea, pale stool, unusual fatigue, yellow skin, or vomiting to the physician. Development of hepatic problems may require drug discontinuation. Therapy will continue for at least 3 mo and until lab tests and overall condition indicate that the infection is controlled. Be aware that itraconazole has a tendency to create GI side effects; telling the patient to remain in semisupine position while reclining will reduce these effects.

Storage

Store oral formulations and solutions for injection at room temperature. Do not freeze.

Administration

! Doses larger than 200 mg should be given in 2 divided doses. Give capsules with food to increase absorption. Give solution on an empty stomach. Do not give either with grapefruit juice.

For IV administration, use only components provided by the manufacturer. Do not dilute with any other diluent. Add full contents of amp (250 mg/10 mL) to infusion bag provided (50 mL 0.9% NaCl) and mix gently.

! Then withdraw 15 mL of the solution from the bag before administering to patient; otherwise, patient will receive overdosage. Do not give as an IV bolus; slowly infuse over 60 min using the extension line and infusion set provided. After administration, flush infusion set with 15-20 mL 0.9% NaCl and discard entire infusion line.

Ivermectin (Systemic)

eye-ver-mek'tin

★ Stromectol

CATEGORY AND SCHEDULE

Pregnancy Risk Category: C

Classification: Antihelmintics, systemic

MECHANISM OF ACTION

Selectively binds to chloride ion channels in invertebrate nerve/muscle cells, increasing permeability to chloride ions. In general, the following organisms are susceptible to ivermectin: *Onchocerca volvulus,* pediculosis capitis, *Strongyloides stercoralis, Sarcoptes scabiei,* and *Wuchereria bancrofti. Therapeutic Effects:* Causes paralysis/death of parasites.

PHARMACOKINETICS

Does not readily cross the blood-brain barrier. Metabolized in the liver. Excreted in the feces. *Half-life:* 4 h. Well absorbed with plasma concentrations proportional to the dose.

AVAILABILITY

Tablets: 3 mg.

INDICATIONS AND DOSAGES

▸ **Strongyloidiasis**

PO

Adults, Elderly, Children weighing < 3 lb. 200 mcg/kg as a single dose.

▸ **Onchocerciasis (river blindness)**

PO

Adults, Elderly, Children weighing more than 33 lb. 150 mcg/kg as a single dose at 3-12-mo intervals (12 mo is most common).

▸ **Scabies (off-label)**

PO

Adults. 200 mcg/kg as a single dose and repeat 2 wks later.

▸ **Norwegian scabies (crusted scabies infection), superinfected scabies, or resistant scabies (off-label)**

PO

Adults. 200 mcg/kg with repeated treatments or combined with a topical scabicide.

▸ **Pediculosis (resistant cases) (off-label)**

PO

Adults. A regimen of 2 doses of 200 mcg/kg with each dose separated by 10 days.

OFF-LABEL USES

Cutaneous larva migrans, filariasis, pediculosis, scabies, *Wuchereria bancrofti* (Bancroft's filariasis).

CONTRAINDICATIONS

Hypersensitivity to ivermectin or to any one of its components. Should not be used in women who are pregnant, in infants or children under 33 lb.

INTERACTIONS

Drug

Carbamazepine: May decrease the concentration of ivermectin.

Corticosteroids: May have a synergistic effect with ivermectin reducing inflammation caused by river blindness infestation.

CYP3A4 inducers: Decrease the levels of ivermectin.

CYP3A4 inhibitors: Increase the levels of ivermectin.

Warfarin: Reports of increased INR.

Herbal

None known.

Food

None known.

DIAGNOSTIC TEST EFFECTS

May increase SGOT (AST), SGPT (ALT), alkaline phosphatase, BUN, eosinophil count.

May decrease WBC.

SIDE EFFECTS

Occasional

Abdominal pain, anorexia, arthralgia, constipation, diarrhea, dizziness, drowsiness, edema, fatigue, fever, lymphadenopathy, maculopapular or unspecified rash, nausea, vomiting, orthostatic hypotension, pruritus, Stevens-Johnson syndrome, toxic epidermal necrolysis, tremor, urticaria, vertigo, visual impairment, weakness.

Less Common

Eye or eyelid irritation, pain, redness, swelling, headache, swelling of the face, arms, feet, or legs.

Rare

Orthostatic hypotension, loss of appetite, shaking or trembling, sleepiness.

SERIOUS REACTIONS

- Worsening of Mazzotti reactions (e.g., arthralgia, synovitis, lymph node enlargement and tenderness, pruritus, edema, papular and pustular urticarial rash, and fever.
- Seizures (rare).
- Severe allergic reactions are possible, including anaphylaxis or serious skin rashes.
- Hepatitis (rare).

• Cardiovascular reactions, such as orthostatic hypotension and ECG changes (rare).

PRECAUTIONS & CONSIDERATIONS

Caution is warranted in patients with bronchial asthma. Treating *Loa loa* infection with ivermectin may result in encephalopathy. It is unknown whether ivermectin crosses the placenta and should be avoided during pregnancy. Ivermectin is distributed into breast milk; however, it is not reported to cause problems in nursing babies. Safety and efficacy have not been established in children under 33 lb or in elderly patients.

Light-headedness may occur. Tasks that require mental alertness or motor skills should be avoided. Joint or muscle pain; fever; pain and tender glands in neck, armpits, or groin; skin rash; or rapid heartbeat may also occur (primarily during onchocerciasis therapy).

Follow-up medical examination schedules should be adhered to; additional treatment may be required in intervals of 3-12 mo.

Storage

Store at room temperature below 86° F.

Administration

Take as a single dose with a full glass of water on an empty stomach 1 h before breakfast.

Ixabepilone

ix'ab-ep'i-lone

★ 🍁 Ixempra

CATEGORY AND SCHEDULE

Pregnancy Risk Category: D

Classification: Antineoplastics, epothilones

MECHANISM OF ACTION

Ixabepilone is unique chemical class agent, an epothilone, and a microtubule stabilizing agent with activity similar to taxanes. Ixabepilone directly binds to β-tubulin subunits on microtubules and promotes tubulin polymerization and microtubule stabilization via inhibition of depolymerization. The action leads to microtubule bundles. The damage to spindle formation causes G2/M phase cell-cycle arrest, which results in cell death. In addition to direct antitumor activity, ixabepilone inhibits angiogenesis. *Therapeutic Effect:* Arrests cell cycle, promotes apoptosis.

PHARMACOKINETICS

After IV infusion, ixabepilone exhibits linear kinetics. Protein binding: 67%-77%. Extensively distributes to extravascular spaces. Metabolized in the liver by CYP3A4. Over 30 metabolites identified. Excreted in feces (65%) and urine over a period of 7 days. *Half-life:* 52 h.

AVAILABILITY

Powder for Injection: 15 mg, 45 mg; supplied with diluent that includes polyoxyethylated castor oil and dehydrated alcohol.

INDICATIONS AND DOSAGES

▸ **Metastatic breast cancer**

NOTE: Ixabepilone doses for patients with BSA > 2.2 m^2 should be calculated based on 2.2 m^2.

▸ **With capecitabine**

IV INFUSION

Adults. 40 mg/m^2 IV over 3 h, given q3wk in combination with capecitabine (2000 mg/m^2/day PO in divided doses on days 1-14 of 21-day cycle).

▸ Breast cancer resistant to, intolerant of, or progressing despite anthracycline, taxane, or capecitabine
IV INFUSION
Adults. 40 mg/m^2 IV over 3 h, given q3wk.
▸ Dosage with a strong CYP3A4 inhibitor
Reduce to 20 mg/m^2 IV over 3 h, given q3wk. If the strong inhibitor is discontinued, allow a washout period of approximately 1 wk before adjusting to the normal dosage.
▸ Dosage adjustments for neuropathy, neutropenia, or hepatic dysfunction
! Expect reductions dependent on degree of toxicity and the use of other agents (see manufacturer information). In combination with capecitabine do NOT give if AST or ALT > 2.5 times the upper limit of normal (ULN) or bilirubin > 1 times ULN due to an increased risk of toxicity and neutropenia-related death.

CONTRAINDICATIONS

Hypersensitivity to ixabepilone or to any drugs formulated with Cremophor® EL (e.g., polyoxyethylated castor oil); baseline neutrophil count < 1500 cells/mm^3 or a platelet count < 100,000 cells/mm^3. Patients with AST or ALT > 2.5 times the upper limit of normal (ULN) or bilirubin > 1 times ULN must NOT be treated with ixabepilone in combination with capecitabine due to the risk of toxicity and neutropenia-related mortality.

INTERACTIONS

Drug
Potent CYP3A4 inhibitors (e.g., ketoconazole): Increases ixabepilone levels. Try to avoid if possible. If alternative treatment cannot be chosen, a lower dose should be considered; monitor closely. Use caution when using mild or moderate inhibitors (e.g., erythromycin, fluconazole, or verapamil).
Potent CYP3A4 inducers (e.g., rifampin, phenytoin, carbamazepine, rifabutin, phenobarbital): Decreases ixabepilone levels significantly. Avoid. Choose alternate agent if possible. If must be given a strong CYP3A4 inducer, a gradual dose adjustment to 60 mg/m^2 over 4 h may be considered with caution.
Live-virus vaccines: Contraindicated due to viral replication, adverse reactions to the virus, and the immunocompromised status of the patient. May also decrease the patient's antibody response to the vaccine.
Herbal
St. John's wort: May decrease ixabepilone plasma concentrations unpredictably. Avoid.
Food
None known.

DIAGNOSTIC TEST EFFECTS

May increase bilirubin, AST (SGOT), and ALT (SGPT) levels. May decrease WBC, RBC, platelet count, and hemoglobin levels.

IV INCOMPATIBILITIES

Do not infuse or mix with any other medications. Only dilute for infusion in the solutions indicated.

SIDE EFFECTS

Frequent (> 20%)
Peripheral sensory neuropathy, fatigue/asthenia, myalgia/arthralgia, alopecia, nausea, vomiting, stomatitis/mucositis, diarrhea, and musculoskeletal

pain. More than 40% experience neutropenia, leukopenia, anemia, and thrombocytopenia. In combination with capecitabine: also hand-foot syndrome, anorexia, abdominal pain, nail disorders, and constipation.

Occasional (< 20%)

Headache, dizziness, insomnia, edema, myalgia, hot flushes, pruritus.

SERIOUS REACTIONS

- Severe hypersensitivity reactions related to infusion occur in 1% of patients. To help reduce the risk, must premedicate all patients before treatment (see Administration).
- Dose-limiting reactions include myelosuppression (evidenced mostly by neutropenia) and peripheral neuropathy (burning sensation, hyperesthesia, hypoesthesia, paresthesia, discomfort, or neuropathic pain).
- Risk for serious and opportunistic infections.

PRECAUTIONS & CONSIDERATIONS

Must adjust dose in liver dysfunction; do not give to patients in combination with capecitabine if liver dysfunction meets stated parameters. Use with caution in patients with significant renal impairment, anemia, cardiac disease, angina, or arrhythmia. Avoid use in pregnant women due to the risk of fetal harm; screen for pregnancy prior to use. Women should avoid becoming pregnant during treatment. It is unknown whether ixabepilone is distributed in breast milk. Safety and efficacy have not been established in children.

Must premedicate all patients before treatment. Closely monitor for signs of infusion reaction and hypersensitivity. Monitor CBC. Monitor for signs of infection. Monitor for symptoms of neuropathy, primarily sensory.

Storage

Store unopened vials and diluent in the original kit under refrigeration and protected from light; do not freeze. Once reconstituted, may be stored in the vial (not a syringe) for a maximum of 1 h at room temperature and light prior to dilution for infusion. Once diluted for infusion, the final solution must be used within 6 h of preparation.

Administration

CAUTION: Observe and exercise usual cautions for handling, administering, and preparing solutions of cytotoxic drugs.

! Hypersensitivity reactions are common. Must premedicate ALL patients with an H_1 antagonist (e.g., diphenhydramine 50 mg PO or equivalent) and an H_2 antagonist (e.g., ranitidine 150-300 mg PO or equivalent) 1 h before each treatment. Patients who experience a hypersensitivity reaction will also require premedication with corticosteroids (e.g., dexamethasone 20 mg IV 30 min or orally 60 min before infusion).

Ixabepilone is for intravenous (IV) infusion only. Remove the kit from the refrigerator and allow to stand at room temperature for approximately 30 min. When first removed from the refrigerator, a white precipitate may be observed in the diluent, but this will dissolve as it warms.

To allow for withdrawal losses, the vial labeled as 15 mg for injection contains 16 mg of ixabepilone and the vial labeled as 45 mg contains 47 mg of ixabepilone. The vial must be constituted with supplied diluent. The 15-mg vial is constituted with 8 mL of diluent and for the 45-mg vial use 23.5 mL of diluent. Gently swirl and invert the vial until the powder in the drug is completely dissolved. The vial concentration will be 2 mg/mL.

Before infusion, the drug MUST be further diluted to a final ixabepilone concentration of 0.2-0.6 mg/mL. For most doses, a 250-mL bag of fluid is sufficient. The infusion must be prepared in a DEHP [di-(2-ethylhexyl) phthalate] free bag.

The following infusion fluids are compatible: lactated Ringer's injection; or 0.9% NaCl; or PLASMA-LYTE A Injection pH 7.4®. (NOTE: When using 250 mL or 500 mL 0.9% NaCl to prepare, the pH must be adjusted to a pH between 6 and 9 by adding 2 mEq of sodium bicarbonate injection, prior to the addition of the ixabepilone dose.) Thoroughly mix the infusion bag by manual rotation.

The IV infusion solution must be administered over 3 h through an appropriate in-line filter (0.2 to 1.2 micron). DEHP-free infusion containers and administration sets must be used.

Ketamine Hydrochloride

kee'ta-meen high-droh-klor'ide

Ketalar

CATEGORY AND SCHEDULE

Pregnancy Risk Category: B

Classification: Anesthetics, general

MECHANISM OF ACTION

A rapidly acting general anesthetic that selectively blocks afferent impulses and interacts with central nervous system (CNS) transmitter systems. *Therapeutic Effect:* Produces an anesthetic state characterized by profound analgesia and normal pharyngeal-laryngeal reflexes.

PHARMACOKINETICS

Route	Onset	Peak	Duration
IM (anesthetic)	3-4 min	N/A	12-25 min
IM (analgesic)	30 min	N/A	15-30 min
IV (anesthetic)	30 seconds	N/A	5-10 min
IV (analgesic)	10-15 min	N/A	NA

Rapidly distributed. Metabolized in the liver. Primarily excreted in urine. *Half-life:* Distribution: 10-15 min, elimination: 2-3 h.

AVAILABILITY

Injection: 10 mg/mL, 50 mg/mL, 100 mg/mL.

INDICATIONS AND DOSAGES

▸ **Sole anesthetic for short diagnostic and surgical procedures that do not require skeletal muscle relaxation, induction of anesthesia before administering other general anesthetics, supplement to low-potency agents**

IM

Adults, Elderly. 3-8 mg/kg.

Children. 3-7 mg/kg.

IV

Adults, Elderly. 1-4.5 mg/kg.

Children. 0.5-2 mg/kg.

CONTRAINDICATIONS

Known hypersensitivity, aneurysms, angina, congestive heart failure, elevated intracranial pressure, hypertension, thyrotoxicosis.

INTERACTIONS

Drug

All CNS depressants and nondepolarizing muscle relaxants: May increase the risk of hypotension and prolonged respiratory depression.

Herbal and Food

None known.

DIAGNOSTIC TEST EFFECTS

May increase intraocular pressure.

IV INCOMPATIBILITIES

No information available for Y-site administration.

IV COMPATIBILITIES

Bupivacaine (Marcaine), fentanyl (Sublimaze), lidocaine, morphine, propofol (Diprivan).

SIDE EFFECTS

Frequent

Increased BP and pulse rate; emergence reaction (marked by dream-like state, delirium, hallucinations, and vivid imagery; and occasionally accompanied by confusion, excitement, and irrational behavior; lasts from few hours to 24 h after ketamine administration).

Occasional
Pain at injection site.
Rare
Rash.

SERIOUS REACTIONS

- Continuous or repeated intermittent infusion may result in extreme somnolence and circulatory or respiratory depression.
- Too-rapid IV administration of ketamine may produce severe hypotension, respiratory depression, and irregular muscle movements.
- Psychiatric effects: hallucinations, emergence delirium.

PRECAUTIONS & CONSIDERATIONS

Caution is warranted with intoxication, chronic alcoholism, a full stomach, gastroesophageal reflux disease, and hepatic impairment. Ketamine is not recommended for pregnant or breastfeeding women. No age-related precautions have been noted in children or in elderly patients. Avoid tasks requiring mental alertness or motor skills until 24 h after anesthesia has been discontinued.

Patients must be continuously monitored and facilities for maintenance of patent airway, ventilatory support, oxygen supplementation, and circulatory resuscitation should be immediately available.

Strict aseptic techniques must be followed in handling ketamine HCl.

Vital signs should be monitored before and every 3-5 min during and after ketamine administration until the patient has recovered. A barbiturate or hypnotic should be administered in an emergence reaction. Verbal, tactile, and visual stimulation should be minimized during the recovery period. Advise the patient to avoid performing tasks requiring mental alertness or motor skills for 24 h after anesthesia has been discontinued. A responsible person must drive patient home after recovery.

Storage
Store unopened vials at room temperature. Protect from light.
Administration
Give ketamine by IV push over 60 seconds when it is used to induce anesthesia. Dilute the 100 mg/mL vial of ketamine with an equal volume of sterile water for injection, D5W, or 0.9% NaCl. For a maintenance IV infusion, dilute the 50-mg/mL vial (10 mL) or 100-mg/mL vial (5 mL) of ketamine with 250-500 mL D5W or 0.9% NaCl to provide a concentration of 1-2 mg/mL. Administer maintenance dose by IV push slowly at a rate of 0.5 mg/kg/min over 60 seconds. A too-rapid IV administration may result in severe hypotension and respiratory depression.

For IM administration, use the 10-mg/mL vial of ketamine. Do not dilute the 10-mg/mL vial.

Ketoconazole

kee-toe-koe′na-zole
Extina, Kuric, Nizoral, Nizoral A-D, Xolegal Ketoderm, Nizoral, Nu-Ketocon
Do not confuse Nizoral with Nasarel.

CATEGORY AND SCHEDULE

Pregnancy Risk Category: C
OTC (1% shampoo only)

Classification: Imidazole antifungal

K

MECHANISM OF ACTION

A fungistatic antifungal that inhibits the synthesis of ergosterol, a vital component of fungal cell formation. *Therapeutic Effect:* Damages the fungal cell membrane, altering its function.

PHARMACOKINETICS

PO: Peak serum concentrations achieved in 1-2 h; highly protein bound. Metabolized in liver, excreted in bile, feces. Requires acidic pH for absorption; distributed poorly to cerebrospinal fluid (CSF). *Half-life:* 2 h; terminal half-life: 8 h.

K

AVAILABILITY

Tablets (Nizoral): 200 mg.
Cream (Kuric): 2%.
Shampoo (Nizoral AD): 1%.
Topical Foam (Extina): 2%.
Shampoo (Nizoral): 2%.
Topical Gel (Xolegel): 2%.

INDICATIONS AND DOSAGES

▸ **Systemic fungal infections such as histoplasmosis, blastomycosis, candididasis, chronic mucocutaneous candidiasis, coccidioidomycosis, paracoccidioidomycosis, chromomycosis, onychomycosis, oral thrush, candiduria**

PO

Adults, Elderly. 200-400 mg/day. Maximum: 800 mg/day in 2 divided doses.

Children over 2 yr. 3.3-6.6 mg/kg/day.

▸ **Dermatologic conditions such as seborrheic dermatitis, tinea corporsis, tinea capitis, tinea manus, tinea cruris, tinea pedis**

TOPICAL

Adults, Elderly. Apply to affected area 1-2 times a day for 2-4 wks.

SHAMPOO

Adults, Elderly, Children ≥ 12 yr. Use twice weekly for 4 wks, allowing at least 3 days between shampooing. Use intermittently to maintain control.

OFF-LABEL USES

Systemic: Treatment of fungal pneumonia.

CONTRAINDICATIONS

Hypersensitivity, lactation, fungal meningitis.

Systemic coadministration with cisapride, pimozide, quinidine, dofetilide, lovastatin, simvastatin, ergot alkaloids, terfenadine, astemizole, and triazolam is contraindicated.

INTERACTIONS

NOTE: Ketoconazole (oral) is a potent inhibitor of CYP3A4 and is contraindicated with a variety of medications. Review manufacturer contraindications carefully for drug interactions.

Drug

Alcohol, acetaminophen (high-dose, long-term use); carbamazepine, sulfonamides, and other hepatotoxic medications: May increase hepatotoxicity of ketoconazole.

Antacids, anticholinergics, didanosine, H_2 antagonists, proton-pump inhibitors (omeprazole): May decrease ketoconazole absorption; take 2 h after ketoconazole dose.

Benzodiazepines (midazolam, triazolam), warfarin: May inhibit metabolism of these drugs.

Cyclosporine, HMG-CoA reductase inhibitors (statins): May increase blood concentration and risk of hepatotoxicity of these drugs. Contraindicated with lovastatin and simvastatin.

Buspirone, carbamazepine, corticosteroids, haloperidol, indinavir, nisoldipine, ritonavir, saquinavir, tricyclic antidepressants, zolpidem: May increase levels of these drugs.
Isoniazid, rifampin: May decrease blood concentration of ketoconazole.
Tacrolimus: May cause leukocytic disorders.
Systemic coadministration with cisapride, pimozide, quinidine, dofetilide, lovastatin, simvastatin, ergot alkaloids, terfenadine, astemizole, and triazolam: Contraindicated; do not use.
Herbal
Echinacea: May have additive hepatotoxic effects.
Food
None known.

DIAGNOSTIC TEST EFFECTS

May increase serum alkaline phosphatase, serum bilirubin, SGOT (AST), and SGPT (ALT) levels. May decrease serum corticosteroid and testosterone concentrations.

SIDE EFFECTS

Occasional (3%-10%)
Nausea, vomiting.
Rare (< 2%)
Abdominal pain, diarrhea, headache, dizziness, photophobia, pruritus.
Topical: itching, burning, irritation.

SERIOUS REACTIONS

- Hematologic toxicity (as evidenced by thrombocytopenia, hemolytic anemia, and leukopenia) occurs occasionally.
- Hepatotoxicity may occur within 1 wk to several months after starting therapy.
- Anaphylaxis occurs rarely.

PRECAUTIONS & CONSIDERATIONS

Caution is warranted with liver impairment. Use with care in lactation, pregnancy, children, elderly with renal impairment.

Confirm that a culture or histologic test was done for accurate diagnosis; therapy may begin before results are known.

Expect to monitor liver function test results. Be alert for signs and symptoms of hepatotoxicity, including anorexia, dark urine, fatigue, nausea, pale stools, and vomiting, that are unrelieved by giving the medication with food. Monitor complete blood count (CBC) for evidence of hematologic toxicity. Assess the daily pattern of bowel activity and stool consistency. Assess for dizziness, provide assistance as needed, and institute safety precautions. Evaluate skin for itching, rash, and urticaria.

Prolonged therapy over weeks or months is usually necessary. Do not miss a dose, and continue therapy for as long as directed. Avoid alcohol to avoid potential liver toxicity. Avoid tasks that require mental alertness or motor skills until response to the drug is established.

If dark urine, increased irritation in topical use, onset of other new symptoms, pale stool, or yellow skin or eyes develop, notify the physician.

In dermatologic treatment, separate personal items that come in direct contact with the affected area.

Storage
Store products at room temperature. Foam and gels are flammable; keep away from excessive heat and away from flame. Do not freeze.
Administration
Give oral ketoconazole with food to minimize GI irritation. Tablets may be crushed. Ketoconazole requires acidity for absorption in the GI

tract; give didanosine, antacids, anticholinergics, H_2 blockers, and proton-pump inhibitors (all) at least 2 h after dosing.

Apply ketoconazole shampoo to wet hair, massage for 1 min, rinse thoroughly, reapply for 3 min, then rinse. Use initially twice weekly for 4 wks with at least 3 days between shampooing. Further shampooing will be based on the response to the initial treatment.

Apply topical ketoconazole sparingly and rub gently into the affected and surrounding area. Avoid drug contact with the eyes, keep the skin clean and dry, and wear light clothing for ventilation.

Ketoprofen

kee-toe-proe′fen

Apo-Keto

CATEGORY AND SCHEDULE

Pregnancy Risk Category: B (D if used in third trimester or near delivery)

Classification: Analgesics, nonsteroidal anti-inflammatory drug

MECHANISM OF ACTION

An NSAID that produces analgesic and anti-inflammatory effects by inhibiting prostaglandin synthesis. *Therapeutic Effect:* Reduces the inflammatory response and intensity of pain.

PHARMACOKINETICS

PO: Peak levels achieved in 2 h. 99% plasma protein binding. Metabolized in liver, excreted in urine and breast milk as metabolites. *Half-life:* 3-3.5 h.

AVAILABILITY

Capsules: 50 mg, 75 mg.
Capsules (Extended Release): 200 mg.

INDICATIONS AND DOSAGES

▸ **Acute or chronic rheumatoid arthritis and osteoarthritis**

PO (IMMEDIATE RELEASE)

Adults. Initially, 75 mg 3 times a day or 50 mg 4 times a day.

Elderly. Initially, 25-50 mg 3-4 times a day. Maintenance: 150-300 mg/day in 3-4 divided doses.

PO (EXTENDED RELEASE)

Adults, Elderly. 200 mg once a day.

▸ **Mild to moderate pain, dysmenorrhea**

PO

Adults, Elderly. 25-50 mg q6-8h. Maximum: 300 mg/day.

▸ **Dosage in renal impairment**

Mild: 150 mg/day maximum.
Severe: 100 mg/day maximum.

OFF-LABEL USES

Treatment of acute gouty arthritis, psoriatic arthritis, ankylosing spondylitis, vascular headache.

CONTRAINDICATIONS

Previous hypersensitivity to ketoprofen; those who have experienced asthma, urticaria, or serious reactions after taking aspirin or other NSAIDs; use within 14 days of CABG surgery.

INTERACTIONS

Drug

Acetaminophen (long-term or chronic use): Increased risk of nephrotoxicity, hepatotoxicity.

Antihypertensives, diuretics: May decrease the effects of these drugs.

Aspirin, other NSAIDs, corticosteroids, alcohol, or other salicylates: May increase the risk of GI side effects such as bleeding.

NSAIDs may negate cardioprotective effect of ASA.
Bone marrow depressants: May increase the risk of hematologic reactions.
Cyclosporine: Possible decreased renal function.
Diuretics: May decrease diuretic effect.
Heparin, oral anticoagulants, thrombolytics, oral antidiabetic agents: May increase the effects of these drugs.
Lithium: May increase the blood concentration and risk of toxicity of lithium.
Methotrexate: May increase the risk of methotrexate toxicity.
Probenecid: May increase the ketoprofen blood concentration.
Tetracycline: Possible increased photosensitivity.
Herbal
Feverfew: May decrease the effects of feverfew.
Ginkgo biloba: May increase the risk of bleeding.
Food
Alcohol: May increase dizziness; may increase risk of GI bleeding.

DIAGNOSTIC TEST EFFECTS

May prolong bleeding time. May increase serum alkaline phosphatase levels and liver function test results. May decrease hematocrit, blood hemoglobin, and serum sodium levels.

SIDE EFFECTS

Frequent (11%)
Dyspepsia.
Occasional (> 3%)
Nausea, diarrhea or constipation, flatulence, abdominal cramps, headache.
Rare (< 2%)
Anorexia, vomiting, visual disturbances, fluid retention.

SERIOUS REACTIONS

- Rare reactions with long-term use include peptic ulcer disease, GI bleeding, gastritis, and severe hepatic reactions (cholestasis, jaundice), nephrotoxicity (dysuria, hematuria, proteinuria, nephrotic syndrome), and severe hypersensitivity reaction (bronchospasm, angioedema).

PRECAUTIONS & CONSIDERATIONS

Caution is warranted with hepatic or renal impairment, and a predisposition to fluid retention. Caution is warranted in patients with a history of GI tract disease such as active peptic ulcer disease, chronic inflammation of GI tract, GI bleeding or ulceration. Use the lowest effective dose for the shortest duration of time. Anaphylactoid reactions have occurred in patients with aspirin triad hypersensitivity. Cardiovascular event risk may be increased with duration of use or preexisting cardiovascular risk factors or disease. Use caution in patients with fluid retention, heart failure, or hypertension. Risk of myocardial infarction and stroke may be increased following CABG surgery. Drug is excreted in breast milk as metabolite; caution is warranted in lactation. It is not known whether drug crosses placenta; use with caution in pregnancy. No age-related precautions are noted except in cases of impaired renal function where dose adjustment may be required or in individuals age 75 or older.

CBC, blood chemistry, and renal and liver function tests should be obtained at the beginning and throughout therapy. Therapeutic response, such as improved grip strength, increased mobility, improved range of motion, and

K

decreased pain, tenderness, stiffness, and swelling, should be assessed.

Because of possible increased photosensitivity attributed to NSAIDs, patients should be advised to wear a sunscreen with SPF 15 during UV exposure.

Storage

Store at room temperature. Protect from light and moisture.

Administration

Take ketoprofen with food, a full glass (8 oz) of water, or milk to minimize GI distress. Do not break, open, or chew extended-release capsules.

K

Ketorolac Tromethamine

kee-tor'oh-lak tro-meth'ay-meen

★ Acular, Acular LS, Acuvail, Sprix 🍁 Acular, Acular-LS, Toradol

Do not confuse Acular with Acthar or Ocular.

CATEGORY AND SCHEDULE

Pregnancy Risk Category: C (D if used in third trimester)

Classification: Analgesics, nonsteroidal anti-inflammatory drugs, ophthalmics

MECHANISM OF ACTION

An NSAID that inhibits prostaglandin synthesis and reduces prostaglandin levels in the aqueous humor and body. *Therapeutic Effect:* Relieves pain stimulus and reduces intraocular inflammation.

PHARMACOKINETICS

Route	Onset	Peak	Duration
PO	30-60 min	1.5-4 h	4-6 h
IV/IM	30 min	1-2 h	4-6 h

Readily absorbed from the GI tract, after IM administration. Protein binding: 99%. Largely metabolized in the liver. Primarily excreted in urine. Not removed by hemodialysis. *Half-life:* 3.8-6.3 h (increased with impaired renal function and in elderly patients).

AVAILABILITY

Tablets: 10 mg.
Injection: 15 mg/mL, 30 mg/mL.
Nasal (Sprix): 15.75 mg/spray.
Ophthalmic Solution (Acular): 0.5%.
Ophthalmic Solution (Acular LS): 0.4%.
Ophthalmic Solution (Acuvail): 0.45% preservative-free.

INDICATIONS AND DOSAGES

▸ **Short-term relief of moderate pain (multiple doses)**

! The combined use of ketorolac injection and tablets, or use of the nasal form, is not to exceed 5 days.

PO

Adults, Elderly. 10 mg q4-6h. Maximum: 40 mg/24 h.

NOTE: Oral route is only used as continuation following IV or IM dosing, if necessary.

IV/IM

Adults younger than 65 yr. 30 mg q6h. Maximum: 120 mg/24 h.

Elderly 65 yr and older, Adults with renal impairment or weighing < 50 kg. 15 mg q6h. Maximum: 60 mg/24 h.

NASAL (Sprix)

Adults < 65 yrs and ≥ 50 kg: 1 spray (15.75 mg/spray) in each nostril q6-8h. Maximum 126 mg/day.

Elderly or renally impaired adults, or adults < 50 kg: 1 spray (15.75 mg) in ONLY one nostril q 6-8 h. Maximum 63 mg/day.

▸ **Short-term relief of moderate pain (single dose)**

IV

Adults younger than 65 yr, Adolescents 17 yr and older weighing more than 50 kg: 30 mg.
Elderly 65 yr and older, Adults with renal impairment or weighing < 50 kg. 15 mg.
Children 2-16 yr. 0.5 mg/kg. Maximum: 15 mg.
IM
Adults younger than 65 yr, Adolescents 17 yr and older, weighing more than 50 kg. 60 mg.
Elderly 65 yr and older, Adults with renal impairment or weighing < 50 kg. 30 mg.
Children 2-16 yr. 1 mg/kg. Maximum: 30 mg.

▸ **Allergic conjunctivitis**
OPHTHALMIC (ACULAR)
Adults, Elderly, Children 3 yr and older. 1 drop 4 times a day.

▸ **Cataract extraction (ACULAR)**
OPHTHALMIC
Adults, Elderly. 1 drop 4 times a day. Begin 24 h after surgery and continue for 2 wks.
OPHTHALMIC (ACUVAIL)
Adults, Elderly. 1 drop to affected eye(s) twice per day beginning 1 day prior to surgery. Continue on the day of surgery and then for 2 weeks.

▸ **Refractive surgery**
OPHTHALMIC (ACULAR LS)
Adults, Elderly. 1 drop 4 times a day for 4 days.

OFF-LABEL USES

Prevention or treatment of ocular inflammation (ophthalmic form).

CONTRAINDICATIONS

Active peptic ulcer disease, chronic inflammation of the GI tract, GI bleeding or ulceration, history of hypersensitivity to aspirin or NSAIDs, use within 14 days of CABG surgery, advanced renal failure, labor and delivery, breastfeeding, cerebrovascular bleeding and other serious bleeding or risk for such bleeding, use with probenecid or pentoxifylline, use with aspirin or other NSAIDs.

INTERACTIONS

Drug
Aspirin, other salicylates, other NSAIDs, alcohol, corticosteroids: May increase the risk of GI side effects such as bleeding. NSAIDs may negate cardioprotective effect of ASA.
β-Blockers, ACE inhibitors, diuretics: May decrease the antihypertensive effects of these.
Bone marrow depressants: May increase the risk of hematologic reactions.
Cyclosporine: Possible decreased renal function.
Heparin, oral anticoagulants, thrombolytics: May increase the effects of these drugs.
Lithium: May increase the blood concentration and risk of toxicity of lithium.
Methotrexate: May increase the risk of methotrexate toxicity.
Other NSAIDs: Contraindicated for concurrent use.
Pentoxifylline: Contraindicated for concurrent use.
Probenecid: May increase ketorolac blood concentration to dangerous levels; contraindicated; do not use.
Herbal
Feverfew: May decrease the effects of feverfew.
Ginkgo biloba: May increase the risk of bleeding.
Food
Alcohol: Increases dizziness; may increase risk of GI bleeding.

DIAGNOSTIC TEST EFFECTS

May prolong bleeding time.
May increase liver function test results.

K

IV INCOMPATIBILITIES

Promethazine (Phenergan).

IV COMPATIBILITIES

Fentanyl (Sublimaze), hydromorphone (Dilaudid), morphine, nalbuphine (Nubain).

SIDE EFFECTS

Frequent (12%-17%)
Headache, nausea, abdominal cramps or pain, dyspepsia.
Occasional (3%-9%)
Diarrhea.
Ophthalmic: Transient stinging and burning.
Rare (1%-3%)
Constipation, vomiting, flatulence, stomatitis, dizziness.
Ophthalmic: Ocular irritation, allergic reactions, superficial ocular infection, keratitis.

SERIOUS REACTIONS

- Rare reactions with long-term use include peptic ulcer disease, GI bleeding, gastritis, severe hepatic reactions (cholestasis, jaundice), nephrotoxicity (glomerular nephritis, interstitial nephritis, nephrotic syndrome), and an acute hypersensitivity reaction (including fever, chills, and joint pain).
- Hemmorrhage.
- Hypersensitivity.

PRECAUTIONS & CONSIDERATIONS

Caution is warranted in patients with a history of GI tract disease such as chronic inflammation of GI tract. Use the lowest effective dose for the shortest duration of time. Anaphylactoid reactions have occurred in patients with aspirin triad hypersensitivity. Cardiovascular event risk may be increased with duration of use or preexisting cardiovascular risk factors or disease. Use caution in patients with fluid retention, heart failure, or hypertension. Risk of myocardial infarction and stroke may be increased following CABG surgery.
Caution is warranted with hepatic or renal impairment. It is unknown whether ketorolac is excreted in breast milk. Ketorolac should not be used during the third trimester of pregnancy because it can cause adverse effects in the fetus, such as premature closure of the ductus arteriosus. Notify the physician if pregnant. The safety and efficacy of ketorolac have not been established in children, for continued use; a single-dose regimen should be adhered to.

GI bleeding or ulceration is more likely to cause serious complications, and age-related renal impairment may increase the risk of hepatotoxicity or renal toxicity; a decreased dosage is recommended. Tasks that require mental alertness or motor skills should also be avoided.

CBC, liver and renal function tests, urine output, BUN level, and creatinine levels should be assessed. Be alert for signs of bleeding, which may also occur with ophthalmic use. Therapeutic response, such as decreased pain, stiffness, swelling, and tenderness; improved grip strength; and increased joint mobility, should be evaluated.

Storage
Store all products at room temperature. Protect from light. Nasal spray should be discarded within 24 h of opening, even if the bottle still contains some medication.

Administration
! Ketorolac should not be administered by any route or combination of routes for more

than 5 days. This drug may be given as a single dose, on a schedule, or on an as-needed basis, as prescribed.

Take oral ketorolac with food, milk, or antacids if GI distress occurs. Oral dosing is preceded by parenteral use. Duration total not to exceed 5 consecutive days.

For IV use, administer ketorolac undiluted by IV push over at least 15 seconds.

For IM use, slowly inject the drug deeply into a large muscle mass.

For ophthalmic use, place a finger on lower eyelid, and pull it out until a pocket is formed between the eye and lower lid. Hold the dropper above the pocket, and place the prescribed number of drops in the pocket. Gently close eye and apply digital pressure to the lacrimal sac for 1-2 min to minimize the risk of systemic effects. Remove excess solution with a tissue.

Prime the nasal spray before first use; remove the cap cover and press pump down evenly and release 5 times. Blow nose gently to clear nostrils. Gently insert the tip into one nostril and point tip away from the center of the nose. Press down evenly on both sides of pump and spray. For patients needing 2 sprays per dose, repeat the nasal spray in the other nostril. Wipe tip and replace cap.

Ketotifen

kee-toe-teh′fen

🇺🇸 Claritin Eye, Zaditor, Zyrtec Itchy Eye

🇨🇦 Claritin Eye, Zaditen, Zaditor, Zyrtec Itchy Eye

CATEGORY AND SCHEDULE

Pregnancy Risk Category: C
OTC

Classification:
Antihistamines, ophthalmics

MECHANISM OF ACTION

An antihistamine that competes with histamine for histamine receptor sites, and stabilizes mast cells. *Therapeutic Effect:* Relieves symptoms associated with allergic conjunctivitis, such as redness, itching, and excessive tearing.

PHARMACOKINETICS

Minimal systemic absorption via application of eyedrops, especially with lacrimal occlusion. Duration of relief approximately 8-12 h.

K

AVAILABILITY

Ophthalmic Solution: 0.025%.

INDICATIONS AND DOSAGES

▸ **Allergic conjunctivitis**

OPHTHALMIC

Adults, Elderly, Children 3 yr or older. 1 drop into affected eye(s) twice a day, doses separated by 8-12 hours.

CONTRAINDICATIONS

History of hypersensitivity.

INTERACTIONS

Drug
None expected.
Herbal
None known.
Food
None known.

DIAGNOSTIC TEST EFFECTS

None.

SIDE EFFECTS

Frequent
Conjunctival hyperemia, headache, rhinitis.
Occasional
Burning or stinging on application, dry eyes, tearing, ocular pain, eyelid disorder, itching.

Rare
Keratitis, conjunctivitis, temporary photophobia, rash, pharyngitis.

SERIOUS REACTIONS

- Allergic reactions are rare.

PRECAUTIONS & CONSIDERATIONS

It is unknown whether ketotifen crosses the placenta or is distributed in breast milk. The safety and efficacy of this drug have not been established in children younger than 3 yr. No age-related precautions have been noted in elderly patients.

Storage
Store at room temperature. Do not freeze. Keep tightly closed when not in use.

Administration
For ophthalmic use only. To prevent contamination, care should be taken not to touch the dropper tip to any surface. Tilt head back and instill the drops in the conjunctival sac of the affected eye. Close the eye gently; then press gently on the lacrimal sac for 1 min. Wait at least 10 min before inserting contact lenses.

Labetalol Hydrochloride

la-bet'a-lole high-droh-klor'ide
Normodyne, Trandate
Trandate
Do not confuse Trandate with tramadol or Trental.

CATEGORY AND SCHEDULE

Pregnancy Risk Category: C

Classification: Antihypertensives, mixed β- and α-blocker

MECHANISM OF ACTION

An antihypertensive that blocks α_1-, β_1-, and β_2- (large doses) adrenergic receptor sites. Large doses increase airway resistance.
Therapeutic Effect: Slows sinus heart rate; decreases peripheral vascular resistance, cardiac output, and BP.

PHARMACOKINETICS

Route	Onset	Peak	Duration (h)
PO	0.5-2 h	2-4 h	8-12 h
IV	2-5 min	5-15 min	2-4 h

Completely absorbed from the GI tract. Protein binding: 50%. Undergoes first-pass metabolism. Metabolized in the liver. Primarily excreted in urine. Not removed by hemodialysis. *Half-life:* PO, 6-8 h; IV, 5.5 h.

AVAILABILITY

Tablets (Normodyne, Trandate): 100 mg, 200 mg, 300 mg.
Injection: 5 mg/mL.

INDICATIONS AND DOSAGES

▸ **Hypertension**

PO

Adults. Initially, 100 mg twice a day adjusted in increments of 100 mg twice a day q2-3 days. Maintenance: 200-400 mg twice a day. Maximum: 2.4 g/day.
Elderly. Initially, 100 mg 1-2 times a day. May increase as needed.

▸ **Severe hypertension, hypertensive emergency**

IV

Adults. Initially, 20 mg. Additional doses of 20-80 mg may be given at 10-min intervals, up to total dose of 300 mg.

IV INFUSION

Adults. Initially, 2 mg/min up to total dose of 300 mg.

PO (AFTER IV THERAPY)

Adults. Initially, 200 mg; then, 200-400 mg in 6-12 h. Increase dose at 1-day intervals to desired level.

OFF-LABEL USES

Control of hypotension during surgery, treatment of chronic angina pectoris, treatment of HTN in children.

CONTRAINDICATIONS

Bronchial asthma, cardiogenic shock, second- or third-degree heart block, severe bradycardia, uncontrolled congestive heart failure, hypersensitivity.

INTERACTIONS

Drug

Cimetidine: May increase plasma level.
Diuretics, other antihypertensives: May increase hypotensive effect.
Hydrocarbon inhalation anesthetics: May increase risk of hypotension or myocardial depression.
Indomethacin, NSAIDs: May decrease hypotensive effect.
Insulin, oral hypoglycemics: May mask symptoms of hypoglycemia and prolong hypoglycemic effect of these drugs.

Lidocaine: May result in decreased metabolism of labetalol.
MAOIs: May produce hypertension.
Sympathomimetics, xanthines: May mutually inhibit effects.
Herbal
None known.
Food
None known.

DIAGNOSTIC TEST EFFECTS
May increase serum antinuclear antibody titer and BUN, serum LDH, lipoprotein, alkaline phosphatase, bilirubin, creatinine, potassium, triglyceride, uric acid, AST (SGOT), and ALT (SGPT) levels.

IV INCOMPATIBILITIES
Amphotericin B complex (Abelcet, AmBisome, Amphotec), ceftriaxone (Rocephin), furosemide (Lasix), heparin, nafcillin (Nafcil), thiopental, sodium bicarbonate solutions.

IV COMPATIBILITIES
Aminophylline, amiodarone (Cordarone), calcium gluconate, diltiazem (Cardizem), dobutamine (Dobutrex), dopamine (Intropin), enalapril (Vasotec), fentanyl (Sublimaze), hydromorphone (Dilaudid), lidocaine, lorazepam (Ativan), magnesium sulfate, midazolam (Versed), milrinone (Primacor), morphine, nitroglycerin, norepinephrine (Levophed), potassium chloride, potassium phosphate, propofol (Diprivan).

SIDE EFFECTS
Frequent
Drowsiness, difficulty sleeping, unusual fatigue or weakness, diminished sexual ability, transient scalp tingling.
Occasional
Dizziness, dyspnea, peripheral edema, depression, anxiety, constipation, diarrhea, nasal congestion, nausea, vomiting, abdominal discomfort.
Rare
Altered taste, dry eyes, increased urination, paresthesia.

SERIOUS REACTIONS
- Labetolol administration may precipitate or aggravate congestive heart failure (CHF) because of decreased myocardial stimulation.
- Abrupt withdrawal may precipitate ischemic heart disease, producing sweating, palpitations, headache, and tremor.
- May mask signs and symptoms of acute hypoglycemia (tachycardia, BP changes) in patients with diabetes.
- Hepatic injury, necrosis (rare).

PRECAUTIONS & CONSIDERATIONS
Caution is warranted in patients with diabetes mellitus, medication-controlled CHF, impaired cardiac or hepatic function, nonallergic bronchospastic disease, including chronic bronchitis and emphysema. Patients with pheochromocytoma may require higher doses or closer monitoring to avoid paradoxical hypertension. Labetalol crosses the placenta and is distributed in small amounts in breast milk. The safety and efficacy of labetalol have not been established in children. In elderly patients, age-related peripheral vascular disease may increase susceptibility to decreased peripheral circulation. Be aware that salt and alcohol intake should be restricted. Nasal decongestants or OTC cold preparations (stimulants) should not be used without physician approval.

Notify the physician of excessive fatigue, headache, prolonged dizziness, shortness of breath, or weight gain. BP for hypotension, respiratory status for shortness of breath, pattern of daily bowel activity and stool consistency, ECG for arrhythmias, and pulse for quality, rate, and rhythm should be monitored during treatment. If pulse rate is 60 beats/min or lower or systolic BP is < 90 mm Hg, withhold the medication and contact the physician. Signs and symptoms of CHF, such as decreased urine output, distended neck veins, dyspnea (particularly on exertion or lying down), night cough, peripheral edema, and weight gain should also be assessed.

Storage

Store at room temperature. After dilution, IV solution is stable for 24 h.

Administration

Labetalol may be taken without regard to meals. Crush tablets if necessary. Do not abruptly discontinue the drug.

! Place the patient in a supine position for IV administration and for 3 h after receiving the medication. Expect a substantial drop in BP if the patient stands within 3 h following drug administration.

The solution for injection normally appears clear and colorless to light yellow; discard the solution if precipitate forms or discoloration occurs. For IV infusion, dilute 200 mg in 160 mL dextrose 5% in water, 0.9% NaCl, lactated Ringer's solution, or any combination of these solutions to provide a concentration of 1 mg/mL. For IV push, give slowly over 2 min at 10-min intervals. For IV infusion, administer at a rate of 2 mg/min (2 mL/min) initially. Adjust the rate according to the patient's BP. Monitor the patient's BP immediately before and every 5-10 min during IV administration. Maximum effect occurs within 5 min of any IV push injection.

Lacosamide

la-koe'sah-mide

Vimpat

CATEGORY AND SCHEDULE

Pregnancy Risk Category: C

Controlled Substance Schedule: V

Classification: Anticonvulsant

MECHANISM OF ACTION

An antiepileptic medication whose precise mechanism remains to be fully elucidated. Selectively enhances slow inactivation of voltage-gated sodium channels, resulting in stabilization of hyperexcitable neuronal membranes and inhibition of repetitive neuronal firing. Drug binds to collapsin response mediator protein-2 (CRMP-2), a phosphoprotein that is mainly expressed in the nervous system and is involved in neuronal differentiation and control of axonal outgrowth. The role of CRMP-2 binding in seizure control is unknown. *Therapeutic Effect:* Reduces seizure activity.

PHARMACOKINETICS

Well absorbed after PO administration; oral bioequivalent to injection (100%). Protein binding is low (15%). Lacosamide is a CYP2C19 substrate; the primary metabolite has no anticonvulsant activity. Parent drug and metabolite primarily excreted in urine. Removed by hemodialysis. *Half-life:* 13 h.

AVAILABILITY

Tablets: 50 mg, 100 mg, 150 mg, 200 mg.

Oral Solution: 10 mg/mL.

Injection Solution: 200 mg/20 mL.

INDICATIONS AND DOSAGES

▸ **Partial seizures (adjunctive treatment)**

PO OR IV INFUSION

Adults, Elderly, Children 17 yr and older. Initially, give 50 mg twice daily (100 mg/day). The dose may be increased, based on clinical response and tolerability, at weekly intervals by 100 mg/day given as 2 divided doses up to a total of 200-400 mg/day.

SWITCHING FROM PO TO IV INFUSION

The initial total daily IV dose should be equivalent to the total PO daily dosage and frequency. At the end of IV treatment, may switch to PO at the equivalent daily dosage and frequency of IV administration.

▸ **Dosage adjustment for renal impairment**

No dose adjustment is necessary in patients with mild to moderate renal impairment. Max of 300 mg/day is recommended if CrCl ≤ 30mL/min and with end-stage renal disease. Following a 4-h hemodialysis treatment, dosage supplementation of up to 50% of a dose should be considered.

▸ **Dosage adjustment for hepatic impairment**

The dose titration should be performed with caution. Max of 300 mg/day is recommended for mild or moderate hepatic impairment. Not recommended in patients with severe hepatic impairment.

CONTRAINDICATIONS

Hypersensitivity.

INTERACTIONS

Drug

Potent inhibitors of CYP2C19 (e.g., fluconazole, isoniazid, fenofibric acid): In theory may increase lacosamide levels.

Potent inducers of CYP2C19 (e.g., rifampin, barbiturates): In theory may decrease lacosamide levels.

Drugs that prolong PR interval (e.g., atazanavir, digoxin, dronedarone, β-blockers, diltiazem, verapamil): May have additive effects on ECG with lacosamide.

Herbal and Food

None known.

DIAGNOSTIC TEST EFFECTS

May prolong PR interval of ECG. May increase serum AST (SGOT) and ALT (SGPT) levels.

IV INCOMPATIBILITIES

No information regarding Y-site administration is available.

SIDE EFFECTS

Frequent

Diplopia, headache, dizziness, nausea.

Occasional

Somnolence, ataxia, impaired memory or concentration, vertigo, gait disturbance, nystagmus. IV administration: injection site pain or discomfort, irritation, erythema, vomiting.

Rare

Pruritus, tinnitus, irritability, paresthesia, confusion, atrial arrhythmia, syncope.

SERIOUS REACTIONS

- Overdose is characterized by bradycardia, hypotension, respiratory depression, and coma.
- Multiorgan hypersensitivity reactions (also known as drug reaction with eosinophilia and systemic symptoms, or DRESS) have been reported with other anticonvulsants and typically present with fever and rash associated with other organ

system involvement, which may include eosinophilia, hepatitis, nephritis, lymphadenopathy, and/or myocarditis.

PRECAUTIONS & CONSIDERATIONS

Antiepileptic drugs (AEDs) increase the risk of suicidal thoughts or behavior in patients taking these drugs for any indication. Monitor for the emergence or worsening of depression, suicidal thoughts, or unusual changes in behavior or mood. Hepatic or renal dysfunction may require dosage adjustment. Use with caution in patients with known conduction problems (e.g., marked first-degree AV block, second-degree or higher AV block, and sick sinus syndrome without pacemaker) or with severe cardiac disease such as myocardial ischemia or heart failure. Obtaining an ECG prior to initiation is recommended in such patients; repeat tests are recommended during treatment. The drug may cause fetal harm; women of childbearing age must use reliable and adequate contraception. Use with caution during lactation. Safety and efficacy not established in children < 17 yr. The oral solution contains a source of phenylalanine and should be used with caution in phenylketonuria.

May cause dizziness or drowsiness; patients should not drive or operate machinery or do other hazardous tasks until effects of drug are known. Monitor hepatic function and for improvements in seizure control.

Storage

Store at all products at controlled room temperature. Do not freeze injection or oral solution. Discard any unused oral solution remaining after 7 wks of first opening the bottle. If mixed as an IV infusion, the solutions are stable for 24 h at room temperature.

Administration

Oral forms may be taken with or without food. A calibrated oral medicine syringe or spoon should be used to measure oral solution.

The injection is for IV infusion only. The injection can be administered IV without further dilution or may be diluted. May dilute in either 0.9% NaCl or D5W, or lactated Ringer's injection. Infuse IV over 30-60 min.

As with many antiepileptic medications, do not abruptly discontinue treatment; slow tapering is recommended to minimize increasing seizure potential.

Lactulose

lak′tyoo-lose

★ Acilac, Constulose, Enulose, Generlac, Kristalose 🍁 Euro-LAC

Do not confuse lactulose with lactose.

CATEGORY AND SCHEDULE

Pregnancy Risk Category: B

Classification: Laxatives, osmotic

MECHANISM OF ACTION

A lactose derivative that retains ammonia in the colon and decreases serum ammonia concentration; also produces an osmotic effect. *Therapeutic Effect:* Promotes increased peristalsis and bowel evacuation; expels ammonia from the colon.

PHARMACOKINETICS

Route	Onset	Peak	Duration
PO	24-48 h	NA	NA
Rectal	30-60 min	NA	NA

Poorly absorbed from the GI tract. Acts in the colon. Primarily excreted in feces.

AVAILABILITY

Syrup: 10 g/15 mL.
Packets: 10 g, 20 g.

INDICATIONS AND DOSAGES

▸ **Constipation**

PO

Adults, Elderly. 15-30 mL (10-20 g lactulose)/day, up to 60 mL (40 g)/day.

▸ **Portal-systemic encephalopathy**

PO

Adults, Elderly. 30-45 mL (20-30 g) 3-4 times a day. Adjust dose q1-2 days to produce 2-3 soft stools a day. Hourly doses of 30-45 mL may be used for rapid laxation initially; then it may be reduced to recommended daily dose levels.

Children. 40-90 mL/day in divided doses to produce 2-3 soft stools/day.

Infants. 2.5-10 mL/day in divided doses to produce 2-3 soft stools/day.

RECTAL (AS RETENTION ENEMA)

Adults, Elderly. 300 mL with 700 mL water or saline solution; patient should retain 30-60 min. Repeat q4-6h. If evacuation occurs too promptly, repeat immediately.

CONTRAINDICATIONS

Lactulose contains galactose (< 0.3 g/10 g), so contraindicated in those who require a low galactose diet.

INTERACTIONS

Drug

Neomycin, other anti-infectives: May interfere with degradation of lactulose and prevent acidification of colonic contents.

Nonabsorbable antacids: May inhibit colonic acidification.

Oral medication: May decrease transit time of concurrently administered oral medications, decreasing lactulose absorption.

Herbal and Food

None known.

DIAGNOSTIC TEST EFFECTS

Lowers serum ammonia.

SIDE EFFECTS

Occasional

Abdominal cramping, flatulence, increased thirst, abdominal discomfort.

Rare

Nausea, vomiting.

SERIOUS REACTIONS

• Diarrhea indicates overdose; adjust dosage downward.

• Long-term use may result in laxative dependence, chronic constipation, and loss of normal bowel function.

• Excessive dosage can lead to diarrhea with potential complications, such as loss of fluids, hypokalemia, and hypernatremia.

PRECAUTIONS & CONSIDERATIONS

Caution is warranted in patients with diabetes mellitus. It is unknown whether lactulose crosses the placenta or is distributed in breast milk. Lactulose for constipation should generally be avoided in children younger than 6 yr of age as the child may develop hyponatremia and dehydration. No age-related precautions have been noted in elderly patients, but extended use (> 6 mo) may increase risk of dehydration and electrolyte imbalance.

Maintain adequate fluid intake. Electrolyte levels and pattern of daily bowel activity and stool consistency should be monitored. Periodic serum ammonia levels should be obtained.

Storage

Store solution at room temperature.

Administration
Oral solution normally appears pale yellow to yellow and viscous in consistency. However, cloudy, darkened solution does not indicate potency loss. Evacuation occurs in 24-48 h of the initial drug dose. To promote defecation, increase fluid intake, exercise, and eat a high-fiber diet. Some patients find liquid more palatable when mixed with fruit juice, water, or milk.

The powder for oral solution (10- or 20-g packet) should be dissolved in at least 4 oz of water.

To prepare retention enema, mix 300 mL lactulose with 700 mL of water or 0.9% NaCl irrigation. Administer solution rectally using a rectal balloon catheter. Enema should be retained for 30-60 min. May be readministered if inadvertently expelled.

Lamivudine (3TC)

la-miv'yoo-deen

★ Epivir, Epivir-HBV,
🍁 Heptovir

Do not confuse lamivudine with lamotrigine.

CATEGORY AND SCHEDULE

Pregnancy Risk Category: C

Classification: Antiretrovirals, nucleoside reverse transcriptase inhibitors

MECHANISM OF ACTION

An antiviral that inhibits HIV reverse transcriptase by viral DNA chain termination. Also inhibits RNA- and DNA-dependent DNA polymerase, an enzyme necessary for HIV replication. *Therapeutic Effect:* Interrupts HIV replication, slowing the progression of HIV infection.

PHARMACOKINETICS

Rapidly and completely absorbed from the GI tract. Protein binding: 36%. Widely distributed (crosses the blood-brain barrier). Primarily excreted unchanged in urine.
Not removed by hemodialysis or peritoneal dialysis. *Half-life:* 11-15 h (intracellular), 2-11 h (serum, adults), 1.7-2 h (serum, children) (increased in impaired renal function).

AVAILABILITY

Oral Solution: (Epivir): 10 mg/mL; (Epivir-HBV): 5 mg/mL.
Tablets: (Epivir): 150 mg, 300 mg; (Epivir-HBV): 100 mg.

INDICATIONS AND DOSAGES

▸ **HIV infection (in combination with other antiretrovirals)**

PO

Adults, Children >16 yr weighing more than 50 kg (100 lb). 150 mg twice a day or 300 mg once a day.
Children 3 mo to ≤ 16 yr. 4 mg/kg twice a day (up to 150 mg/dose).

▸ **Chronic hepatitis B**

PO

Adults, Children 17 yr and older. 100 mg/day.
Children younger than 17 yr. 3 mg/kg/day. Maximum: 100 mg/day.

▸ **Dosage in renal impairment (adult and adolescent ≥ 30 kg)**

Dosage and frequency are modified based on creatinine clearance.

CrCl (mL/min)	HIV Dosage	Hepatitis B Dosage
≥ 50	150 mg twice a day	100 mg once a day
30-49	150 mg once a day	100 mg first dose, then 50 mg once a day

CrCl (mL/min)	HIV Dosage	Hepatitis B Dosage
15-29	150 mg first dose, then 100 mg once a day	100 mg first dose, then 25 mg once a day
5-14	150 mg first dose, then 50 mg once a day	35 mg first dose, then 15 mg once a day
< 5	50 mg first dose, then 25 mg once a day	35 mg first dose, then 10 mg once a day

L

OFF-LABEL USES

Prophylaxis in health care workers at risk of acquiring HIV after occupational exposure.

CONTRAINDICATIONS

Hypersensitivity, history of pancreatitis as a child.

INTERACTIONS

Drug

Co-trimoxazole: Increases lamivudine blood concentration.
Emtricitabine: Due to similarities between the drugs and therapeutic duplication/toxic effects, do not use.
Interferon alfa: Hepatic decompensation may occur; monitor; consider dose reductions of agents.
Ribavirin: Increased risk of hepatotoxicity; monitor closely.
Zalcitabine: May inhibit intracellular phosphorylation when used concomitantly. Avoid co-use since the action cancels effectiveness of both drugs.

Herbal

St. John's wort: May decrease lamivudine blood concentration and effect. Avoid.

Food

None known.

DIAGNOSTIC TEST EFFECTS

May increase serum amylase, AST (SGOT), and ALT (SGPT) levels. May rarely lower platelet, WBC, or RBC counts.

SIDE EFFECTS

Frequent

Headache (35%), nausea (33%), malaise and fatigue (27%), nasal disturbances (20%), diarrhea, cough (18%), musculoskeletal pain, neuropathy (12%), insomnia (11%), anorexia, dizziness, fever, or chills (10%).

Occasional

Depression (9%), myalgia (8%), abdominal cramps (6%), dyspepsia, arthralgia (5%). Alopecia occurs rarely.

SERIOUS REACTIONS

- Pancreatitis, occurs in 13% of pediatric patients.
- Anemia, neutropenia, and thrombocytopenia occur rarely.
- Lactic acidosis.
- Severe hepatomegaly with steatosis.

PRECAUTIONS & CONSIDERATIONS

Caution is warranted in patients with impaired renal function, a history of pancreatitis, and a history of peripheral neuropathy and in young children. Be aware that lamivudine crosses the placenta, and it is unknown whether lamivudine is distributed in breast milk. Breastfeeding is not recommended in this population because of the possibility of HIV transmission. Be aware that the safety and efficacy of this drug have not been established in children younger than 3 mo. In elderly patients, age-related renal impairment may require dosage adjustment. Lamivudine is not a cure for HIV, and the patient may continue to experience illnesses, including opportunistic infections.

Before starting drug therapy, check the baseline lab values, especially renal function. Expect to monitor the serum amylase, BUN, and serum creatinine levels. Assess for altered sleep patterns, cough, dizziness, headache, nausea, and pattern of daily bowel activity and stool consistency. Avoid activities that require mental acuity if dizziness occurs. Modify diet or administer a laxative, if ordered, as needed. Closely monitor children for symptoms of pancreatitis, manifested as clammy skin, hypotension, nausea, severe and steady abdominal pain often radiating to the back, and vomiting accompanying abdominal pain. If pancreatitis occurs in a child, help the child to sit up or flex at the waist to relieve abdominal pain aggravated by movement.

Storage

Store all products at room temperature, tightly closed.

Administration

Give without regard to meals. Take lamivudine for the full length of treatment and evenly space drug doses around the clock.

Lamotrigine

la-moe-trih'jeen

Lamictal, Lamictal CD, Lamictal ODT, Lamictal XR

Do not confuse lamotrigine with lamivudine.

CATEGORY AND SCHEDULE

Pregnancy Risk Category: C

Classification: Anticonvulsant

MECHANISM OF ACTION

An anticonvulsant whose exact mechanism is unknown. May block voltage-sensitive sodium channels, thus stabilizing neuronal membranes and regulating presynaptic transmitter release of excitatory amino acids. *Therapeutic Effect:* Reduces seizure activity.

PHARMACOKINETICS

Rapidly absorbed from the GI tract. Protein binding: 55%. Metabolized primarily by glucuronic acid conjugation. Excreted in the urine. *Half-life:* 13-30 h.

AVAILABILITY

Chewable Tablets (Lamictal CD): 2 mg, 5 mg, 25 mg.
Tablets: 25 mg, 100 mg, 150 mg, 200 mg.
Tablets, Orally Disintegrating (Lamictal ODT): 25 mg, 50 mg, 100 mg, 200 mg.
Extended-Release Tablets Lamictal XR): 25 mg, 50 mg, 100 mg, 200 mg.

INDICATIONS AND DOSAGES

▸ **Seizure control in patients receiving enzyme-inducing antiepileptic drug (EIAEDs) but not valproic acid**

PO

Adults, Elderly, Children 12 yr and older. Recommended as add-on therapy: 50 mg once a day for 2 wks, followed by 100 mg/day in 2 divided doses for 2 wks. Maintenance: Dosage may be increased by 100 mg/day every week, up to 300-500 mg/day in 2 divided doses.

Children aged 2-12 yr. 0.6 mg/kg/day in 2 divided doses for 2 wks, then 1.2 mg/kg/day in 2 divided doses for wks 3 and 4. Maintenance: 5-15 mg/kg/day. Maximum: 400 mg/day.

▸ Seizure control in patients receiving combination therapy of EIAEDs and valproic acid
PO
Adults, Elderly, Children 12 yr and older. 25 mg every other day for 2 wks, followed by 25 mg once a day for 2 wks. Maintenance: Dosage may be increased by 25-50 mg/day q1-2wk, up to 150 mg/day in 2 divided doses.
Children aged 2-12 yr. 0.15 mg/kg/day in 2 divided doses for 2 wks, then 0.3 mg/kg/day in 2 divided doses for wks 3 and 4. Maintenance: 1-5 mg/kg/day in 2 divided doses. Maximum: 200 mg/day.
▸ Conversion to monotherapy in patients receiving EIAEDs
PO
Adults, Elderly, Children 16 yr and older. Add lamotrigine 50 mg/day in divided doses for 2 wks; then titrate to the desired dose while maintaining EIAED at a fixed level until maintenance dosage is achieved. Gradually discontinue other EIAEDs by 20% each week over 4 wks once maintenance dose is achieved.
▸ Conversion to monotherapy in patients receiving valproic acid
PO
Adults, Elderly, Children 16 yr. and older. Titrate lamotrigine to 200 kg/day, maintaining valproic acid dose. Maintain lamotrigine dose and decrease valproic acid to 500 mg/day not to exceed 500 mg/day/wk, then maintain 500 mg/day for 1 wk. Increase lamotrigine to 300 mg/day, and decrease valproic acid to 250 mg/day and maintain for 1 wk. Then discontinue valproic acid and increase lamotrigine by 100 mg/day each week until maintenance dose of 500 mg/day is reached.
▸ Usual dosage extended release for seizure control
PO (EXTENDED RELEASE)
NOTE: Lamictal XR is given once daily. When converting from immediate release the initial dose of Lamictal XR should match the total daily dose of immediate-release lamotrigine. Some patients may have lower plasma levels with Lamictal XR and should be monitored.
▸ Treatment initiation if not currently on lamotrigine
Adults and Children > 12 yr receiving EIAEDs (e.g., carbamazepine, phenobarbital, phenytoin, primidone), WITHOUT valproic acid: 50 mg PO daily during wks 1-2, then 100 mg daily during wks 3-4, then 200 mg daily during wk 5, then 300 mg daily during wk 6, then 400 mg daily during wk 7. After wk 7, the maintenance range is 400-600 mg daily. Dosage increases after wk 7 should not exceed 100 mg/day at weekly intervals.
Adults and Children > 12 yr receiving nonenzyme-inducing AEDs and WITHOUT valproic acid. 25 mg PO daily during wks 1-2, then 50 mg daily during wks 3-4, then 100 mg daily during wk 5, then 150 mg daily during wk 6, then 200 mg daily during wk 7. After wk 7, the maintenance range is 300-400 mg daily. Dosage increases after wk 7 should not exceed 100 mg/day at weekly intervals.
Adults and Children > 12 yr receiving valproic acid: 25 mg PO every other day during wks 1-2, then 25 mg daily during wks 3-4, then 50 mg daily during wk 5, then 100 mg daily during wk 6, then 150 mg daily during wk 7. After wk 7, the maintenance range is 200-250 mg every day. Dosage increases after wk 7 should not exceed 100 mg/day at weekly intervals.
▸ Bipolar disorder in patients receiving EIAEDs without valproic acid.
PO
Adults, Elderly. 50 mg/day for 2 wks, then 100 mg/day for 2 wks, then

200 mg/day for 1 wk, then 300 mg/day for 1 wk. Then increase to usual maintenance dose of 400 mg/day in divided doses.

▸ **Bipolar disorder in patients receiving valproic acid**

PO

Adults, Elderly. 25 mg/day every other day for 2 wks, then 25 mg/day for 2 wks, then 50 mg/day for 1 wk, then 100 mg/day. Usual maintenance dose with valproic acid: 100 mg/day.

▸ **Discontinuation therapy**

Adults, Children older than 16 yr. A dosage reduction of approximately 50% per week over at least 2 wks is recommended.

▸ **General recommendations for patients with hepatic impairment**

For initial dosing, decrease normal initial dose by 25% for moderate to severe impairment; up to 50% if ascites is present. Escalate and adjust to clinical response.

CONTRAINDICATIONS

Previous hypersensitivity or drug-induced rash from lamotrigine.

INTERACTIONS

Drug

Acetaminophen (long-term, high dose): Possible increased excretion of lamotrigine.

Carbamazepine, phenobarbital, phenytoin, primidone: Decrease lamotrigine blood concentration.

Valproic acid: Doubles lamotrigine concentration.

Oral hormonal contraceptives: may increase CNS side effects; may decrease effectiveness of lamotrigine or oral contraceptive. Adjustment of lamotrigine dose will be required in most patients taking estrogen-containing contraceptives.

Herbal and Food

None known.

DIAGNOSTIC TEST EFFECTS

May increase serum AST or ALT. The value of monitoring plasma levels of lamotrigine has not been established.

SIDE EFFECTS

Frequent

Dizziness (38%), diplopia (28%), headache (29%), ataxia (22%), nausea (19%), blurred vision (16%), somnolence, rhinitis (14%).

Occasional (5%-10%)

Rash, phary-ngitis, vomiting, cough, flu-like symptoms, diarrhea, dysmenorrhea, fever, insomnia, dyspepsia.

Rare

Constipation, tremor, anxiety, pruritus, vaginitis, hypersensitivity reaction.

SERIOUS REACTIONS

- Abrupt withdrawal may increase seizure frequency.
- Serious rashes, including Stevens-Johnson syndrome, requiring hospitalization and discontinuation of treatment, have been reported; can be life threatening.
- Rarely, multisystem organ dysfunction, including liver failure.
- Rarely, neutropenia, leukopenia, anemia, thrombocytopenia, pancytopenia, and, rarely, aplastic anemia and pure red cell aplasia.
- Unknown potential for eye effects due to melanin-binding activity.

PRECAUTIONS & CONSIDERATIONS

Caution is warranted in patients with cardiac, hepatic, and renal impairment. AEDs increase the risk of suicidal thoughts or behavior in patients taking these drugs for any indication. Monitor for the emergence or worsening of depression, suicidal thoughts, or unusual behavior or moods. Safety and efficacy not established in

L

children < 2 yr of age; do not use extended release in children under 13 yr. The effects of lamotrigine on pregnancy are not known. The drug is excreted in breast milk and breastfeeding is not recommended. Exposure to sunlight and artificial light should be avoided.

Drowsiness and dizziness may occur, so alcohol and tasks requiring mental alertness or motor skills should be avoided. Notify the physician if fever, rash, or swollen glands occur. If rash suspected to be drug-related, discontinuation of lamotrigine is recommended. Seizure disorder, including the onset, duration, frequency, intensity, and type of seizures, should be assessed before and during treatment. Changes in frequency or characterization of seizures should be reported to the health care provider immediately.

Storage

Store all dosage forms at room temperature; protect chewable tablets and ODT from moisture; keep ODT in foil blister until time of use.

Administration

! If the patient is currently taking valproic acid, expect to reduce the lamotrigine dosage to less than half the normal dosage.

Take lamotrigine without regard to food. Do not discontinue the drug abruptly after long-term therapy. Strict maintenance of drug therapy is essential for seizure control.

Lamotrigine regular tablets should be swallowed whole because of their bitter taste. The chewable-dispersible tablets may be chewed or dissolved in a small amount of liquid (5 mL) in a spoon, then swallowed.

Lamotrigine ODT should be placed on tongue and moved around in the mouth to facilitate disintegration. The tablet may be swallowed with or without water.

Swallow the extended-release tablets whole. Do not chew, crush, or divide.

Lansoprazole

lan-soe′pray-zole

★ Prevacid, Prevacid IV, Prevacid SoluTab 🍁 Previcid FasTab, Prevacid-SRC

Do not confuse Prevacid with Pepcid, Pravachol, or Prevpac.

CATEGORY AND SCHEDULE

Pregnancy Risk Category: B

Classification: Gastrointestinals, proton-pump inhibitors

MECHANISM OF ACTION

A proton-pump inhibitor that selectively inhibits the parietal cell membrane enzyme system (hydrogen-potassium adenosine triphosphatase) or proton pump. *Therapeutic Effect:* Suppresses gastric acid secretion.

PHARMACOKINETICS

Route	Onset	Peak	Duration
PO (15 mg)	2-3 h	NA	8-24 h
PO (30 mg)	1-2 h	NA	longer than 24 h

Rapid and complete absorption (food may decrease absorption) once the drug has left the stomach. Protein binding: 97%. Distributed primarily to gastric parietal cells and converted to two active metabolites. Extensively metabolized in the liver. Eliminated in bile and urine. Not removed by hemodialysis.

Half-life: 1.5 h (increased in elderly patients and in those with hepatic impairment).

AVAILABILITY

Capsules (Delayed-Release [Prevacid]): 15 mg, 30 mg.
Granules for Oral Suspension (Delayed-Release Granules) (Prevacid): 15 mg/pack; 30 mg/pack.
Injection Powder for Reconstitution (Prevacid IV): 30 mg.
Oral Disintegrating Tablets (Prevacid SoluTab): 15 mg, 30 mg.

INDICATIONS AND DOSAGES

▸ **Duodenal ulcer**
PO
Adults, Elderly. 15 mg/day, before eating, preferably in the morning, for up to 4 wks.
▸ **Healed duodenal ulcer, gastroesophageal reflux disease (GERD)**
PO
Adults. 15 mg/day.
▸ **Erosive esophagitis**
PO
Adults, Elderly. 30 mg/day, before eating, for up to 8 wks. If healing does not occur within 8 wks (in 5%-10% of cases), may give for additional 8 wks. Maintenance: 15 mg/day.
IV
Adults, Elderly. 30 mg once a day for up to 7 days. Switch to oral lansoprazole therapy as soon as the patient can tolerate the oral route.
▸ **Gastric ulcer**
PO
Adults. 30 mg/day for up to 8 wks.
▸ **NSAID gastric ulcer**
PO
Adults, Elderly. (Healing): 30 mg/day for up to 8 wks. (Prevention): 15 mg/day for up to 12 wks.
▸ **Usual pediatric dosage**
Children 1-11 yr, weighing more than 30 kg. 30 mg once daily for up to 12 weeks for GERD or erosive esophagitis, active treatment. See adult dosages for children 12 yr and older.
Children 1-11 yr, weighing ≤ 30 kg. 15 mg once daily for up to 12 weeks for GERD or erosive esophagitis active treatment.
▸ ***Helicobacter pylori* infection**
PO
Adults. 30 mg twice a day for 10 days (with amoxicillin and clarithromycin).
▸ **Pathologic hypersecretory conditions (including Zollinger-Ellison syndrome)**
PO
Adults, Elderly. 60 mg/day. Individualize dosage according to patient needs and for as long as clinically indicated. Doses up to 90 mg twice daily have been used.
▸ **Severe hepatic disease**
Consider dosage reduction.

CONTRAINDICATIONS

Hypersensitivity to lansoprazole or any of its components.

INTERACTIONS

Drug
Ampicillin, digoxin, iron salts, ketoconazole: May interfere with the absorption of ampicillin, digoxin, iron salts, and ketoconazole.
Clopidogrel: PPIs with CYP2C19 inhibiting activity reduce conversion of clopidogrel to active metabolite; may result in cardiovascular events due to decreased efficacy. Avoid PPI use when possible.
Sucralfate: May delay the absorption of lansoprazole.
Atazanavir: Do not give PPI with atazanavir because effectiveness against HIV will be diminished.
Herbal and Food
None known.

DIAGNOSTIC TEST EFFECTS

May increase LDH, serum alkaline phosphatase, bilirubin, cholesterol, creatinine, AST (SGOT), ALT (SGPT), triglyceride, and uric acid levels. May produce abnormal albumin/globulin ratio, electrolyte balance, and platelet, RBC, and WBC counts. May increase hemoglobin and hematocrit levels.

IV INCOMPATIBILITIES

Do not administer with other drugs via Y-site.

SIDE EFFECTS

Occasional (2%-3%)
Diarrhea, abdominal pain, rash, pruritus, altered appetite.
Rare (1%)
Nausea, headache.

SERIOUS REATIONS

- Bilirubinemia, eosinophilia, and hyperlipemia occur rarely.
- Serious hypersensitivity-dermatologic reactions (rare).

PRECAUTIONS & CONSIDERATIONS

Caution is warranted in impaired hepatic function. It is unknown whether lansoprazole is distributed in breast milk; caution is warranted in pregancy and lactation. Safety and efficacy of lansoprazole have not been established in infants. No age-related precautions have been noted in elderly patients. Laboratory values, including CBC and blood chemistry, should be obtained before and periodically during therapy. Some gastric disruption, such as loose stool or flatulence, is common, especially early in therapy.
Storage
Store the drug at room temperature. Keep SoluTab in package until time of administration. Use within 15 min of addition to liquid. IV infusion is stable for up to 24 h at room temperature once prepared with NS (12 h in D5W).
Administration
Take lansoprazole capsules while fasting or before meals. Do not chew or crush delayed-release capsules. May open capsules and sprinkle granules on 1 tbsp of applesauce; swallow immediately. May also sprinkle in 2 oz of apple, orange, or tomato juice. Take lansoprazole 30 min before sucralfate because sucralfate may delay lansoprazole absorption.

SoluTab may be placed on tongue and allowed to dissolve without water. May give SoluTab with oral syringe or NG tube. May dissolve in 4 mL water (15 mg) or 10 mL water (30 mg). Shake gently.

Delayed-release oral suspension: Mix packet with 30 mL of water only. Stir well and drink immediately. Oral suspension not for use with nasogastric tube.

For IV use, infuse over 30 min. The IV vial must only be reconstituted with 5 mL of sterile water for injection. Mix gently. Then add dose to either 50 mL of 0.9% NaCl or Dextrose 5% injection. Must use provided in-line filter (1.2 μm) to deliver. Flush administration port before and after administration.

Lanthanum Carbonate

lan-than′um car′bo-nate
★ 🍁 Fosrenol

CATEGORY AND SCHEDULE

Pregnancy Risk Category: C

Classification: Phosphate-binding agents

MECHANISM OF ACTION

A phosphate regulator that dissociates in the acidic environment of the upper GI tract to lanthanum ions, which bind to dietary phosphate released from food during digestion, forming highly insoluble lanthanum phosphate complexes. *Therapeutic Effect:* Reduces phosphate absorption.

PHARMACOKINETICS

Phosphate complexes are eliminated in urine.

AVAILABILITY

Tablets (Chewable): 500 mg, 750 mg, 1000 mg.

INDICATIONS AND DOSAGES

▸ **Reduce serum phosphate in end-stage renal disease**

PO

Adults, Elderly. 1500 mg/day initially in divided doses, taken with or immediately after a meal. Dosage may be titrated q2-3wk based on serum phosphate levels. Most patients require 1500-3000 mg/day.

CONTRAINDICATIONS

None known.

INTERACTIONS

Drug

Antacids: Interact with lanthanum; separate administration by 2 h.

Herbal and Food

None known.

DIAGNOSTIC TEST EFFECTS

During abdominal x-ray studies, drug may show up similar to a radiopaque imaging agent.

SIDE EFFECTS

Frequent

Nausea (11%), vomiting (9%), dialysis graft occlusion (8%), abdominal pain (5%).

SERIOUS REACTIONS

- None known.

PRECAUTIONS & CONSIDERATIONS

Caution is warranted in patients with acute peptic ulcer disease, bowel obstruction, Crohn disease, and ulcerative colitis. Side effects of nausea and vomiting should decrease over time.

Storage

Store at room temperature. Protect from moisture.

Administration

Chew the tablets thoroughly before swallowing. Take the drug with or immediately after a meal. Take lanthanum 2 h before or after antacids.

Latanoprost

la-tan'oh-prost

★ 🍁 Xalatan

CATEGORY AND SCHEDULE

Pregnancy Risk Category: C

Classification: Ophthalmic agents, prostaglandin analogues, antiglaucoma agents

MECHANISM OF ACTION

A synthetic analogue of prostaglandin with ocular hypotensive activity. *Therapeutic Effect:* Reduces intraocular pressure (IOP) by increasing the outflow of aqueous humor.

PHARMACOKINETICS

Absorbed through the cornea and hydrolyzed to the active free acid form. Peak aqueous humor concentrations occur roughly 2 h after administration. Reduction IOP starts approximately 3 h after administration and peaks after 8-12 h. Plasma levels detectable only in first hour of administration. Any absorbed drug metabolized by liver and metabolites excreted primarily by the kidney. *Half-life:* 17 min.

AVAILABILITY

Ophthalmic Solution: 0.005%.

INDICATIONS AND DOSAGES

▸ **Open-angle glaucoma, ocular hypertension**

OPHTHALMIC

Adults, Elderly. 1 drop in affected eye(s) once daily, in the evening.

CONTRAINDICATIONS

Hypersensitivity to latanoprost or any component of the formulation.

L

DIAGNOSTIC TEST EFFECTS

None known.

SIDE EFFECTS

Frequent

Conjunctival hyperemia, growth of eyelashes, temporary blurring of vision after application, increased iris pigmentation, and ocular pruritus.

Occasional

Ocular dryness, visual disturbance, foreign body sensation, eye pain, pigmentation of the periocular skin, blepharitis, cataract, superficial punctate keratitis, eyelid erythema, ocular irritation, and eyelash darkening.

Rare

Intraocular inflammation (iritis).

SERIOUS REACTIONS

- Systemic adverse events, including infections (colds and upper respiratory tract infections), headaches, skin rash/allergic reactions, have been reported.
- Macular retinal edema may occur.

PRECAUTIONS & CONSIDERATIONS

May permanently increase pigmentation in iris and eyelid and produce changes in eye color and changes in eyelashes (color, length, shape). Use with caution in patients with uveitis or risk factors for macular edema. Effects in pregnancy and lactation not known; use with caution and only if clearly needed in women who are pregnant or breastfeeding. Safety and effectiveness have not been established in children. Remove contact lenses to apply; wait 15 min after administration to reinsert.

Storage

Protect from light. Store unopened bottle under refrigeration. Once a bottle is opened for use, it may be stored at room temperature for up to 6 wks.

Administration

If more than 1 topical ophthalmic agent is being used, wait at least 5 min between administration of each. Remove contact lenses prior to use, and wait 15 min after administration before reinsertion.

Tilt the head back slightly and pull the lower eyelid down with the index finger to form a pouch. Instill drop(s) and gently close the eyes for 1-2 min. Do not blink. Do not touch the tip of the dropper to any surface to avoid contamination.

Leflunomide

le-flu′na-mide

★🍁 Arava

CATEGORY AND SCHEDULE

Pregnancy Risk Category: X

Classification: Disease-modifying antirheumatic drugs, immunosuppressives

MECHANISM OF ACTION

An immunomodulatory agent that inhibits dihydroorotate dehydrogenase, the enzyme involved in autoimmune process that leads to rheumatoid arthritis. *Therapeutic Effect:* Reduces signs and symptoms of rheumatoid arthritis and slows structural damage.

PHARMACOKINETICS

Well absorbed after PO administration. Protein binding: > 99%. Metabolized to active metabolite in the GI wall and liver. Excreted through both renal and biliary systems. Not removed by hemodialysis. *Half-life:* 16 days.

AVAILABILITY

Tablets: 10 mg, 20 mg.

INDICATIONS AND DOSAGES

▸ **Rheumatoid arthritis**

PO

Adults, Elderly. Initially, 100 mg/day for 3 days, then 10-20 mg/day. May eliminate loading dose if patient is at risk for hematologic or hepatic toxicity, such as receiving concurrent methotrexate.

CONTRAINDICATIONS

Pregnancy or plans to become pregnant, OR women of childbearing potential who are not using reliable contraception; known hypersensitivity to the drug. Do not use if preexisting acute or chronic liver disease, or serum ALT > 2 × ULN is present.

INTERACTIONS

Drug

Activated charcoal and cholestyramine: Rapidly decrease concentration of leflunomide's active metabolite.

Hepatotoxic medications: May increase risk of liver toxicity.

Rifampin: Increases the blood concentration of leflunomide's active metabolite; use is generally contraindicated.

Tolbutamide: May increase tolbutamide free fraction; monitor blood glucose.

Vaccines, live: Due to potential immunosuppression, avoid vaccination during treatment.

Warfarin: May increase the effects of warfarin.

Herbal and Food

None known.

DIAGNOSTIC TEST EFFECTS

May increase hepatic enzyme levels, especially AST (SGOT) and ALT (SGPT). Monitor ALT levels at least monthly for 6 mo, and thereafter q6-8wk. May decrease WBC and platelet counts.

SIDE EFFECTS

Frequent (10%-20%)

Diarrhea, respiratory tract infection, alopecia, rash, nausea.

SERIOUS REACTIONS

- Transient thrombocytopenia and leukopenia occur rarely.
- Hypersensitivity, including rare cases of Stevens-Johnson syndrome and TEN.
- Severe liver injury, including fatal liver failure.

! NOTE: If any serious toxicity occurs, a drug elimination procedure, using cholestyramine or activated charcoal, must be given because of the long half-life of the drug.

- Risk of malignancy (lymphoproliferative) is increased with some immunosuppressants.

PRECAUTIONS & CONSIDERATIONS

Caution is warranted in patients with immunodeficiency, bone marrow dysplasia, impaired hepatic or renal function. Severe liver injury has been reported. Use caution when the drug is given with other potentially hepatotoxic, or immunosuppressant drugs. Not recommended for patients with severe immunodeficiency; bone marrow suppression; or severe, uncontrolled infections. If infection occurs, may need to hold therapy. Leflunomide may cause fetal harm. Pregnancy must be excluded before the start of treatment. Pregnancy must be avoided during treatment or prior to the completion of the drug elimination procedure. Although it is not known whether leflunomide is excreted in breast milk, the drug is not recommended for breastfeeding women. The safety and efficacy of leflunomide have not been established in children younger than 18 yr. No age-related precautions have been noted in elderly patients, although decreased renal function or hepatic disease may require decreased dosage or total discontinuation of drug.

Liver function test results should be monitored. Symptomatic relief of rheumatoid arthritis, including relief of pain and improved range of motion, grip strength, and mobility, should be assessed.

Storage

Store at room temperature and protect from light.

Administration

Take leflunomide without regard to food. Therapeutic effect may take longer than 8 wks to appear.

Lenalidomide

lin-e-lid'oh-mide

★ 🍁 Revlimid

Do not confuse lenalidomide with leflunomide.

CATEGORY AND SCHEDULE

Pregnancy Risk Category: X

Classification:

Antineoplastics, immunomodulators, tumor necrosis factor modulators

MECHANISM OF ACTION

An analog of thalidomide, lenalidomide is an immunomodulator whose exact mechanism is unknown. Has anti-inflammatory, antineoplastic, and antiangiogenic activity. Lenalidomide inhibits the secretion of pro-inflammatory cytokines and increases the secretion of anti-inflammatory cytokines from peripheral blood mononuclear cells. Lenalidomide inhibits cell proliferation in some but not all cell lines. Effective in inhibiting Namalwa cells (a human B cell lymphoma cell) and multiple myeloma cells, by inducing cell-cycle arrest and apoptosis. Also inhibits cyclooxygenase-2 (COX-2) but not COX-1. *Therapeutic Effect:* Reduces need for RBC transfusion in myelodysplastic syndromes (MDS); induces apoptosis (cell death) of myeloma cells.

PHARMACOKINETICS

Well absorbed orally. Extent of absorption not affected by food, but a higher Cmax attained if taken on an empty stomach. Plasma concentrations are proportional to the dose given. Protein binding: 30%. Unknown if drug passes into semen. Roughly two-thirds of the drug eliminated unchanged through the urine. Partially actively secreted; drug clearance exceeds GFR. Removed by hemodialysis. *Half-life:* 3 h. (prolonged in moderate to severe renal impairment).

AVAILABILITY

Capsules: 5 mg, 10 mg, 15 mg, 25 mg.

INDICATIONS AND DOSAGES

▸ **Multiple myeloma**

PO

Adults. Initially, 25 mg once per day on days 1-21 of each 28-day cycle. (With dexamethasone –e.g., 40 mg/day PO on days 1-4, 9-12, and 17-20 of each 28-day cycle for the first 4 cycles, and then 40 mg/day PO on days 1-4 every 28 days – NOTE: other dexamethasone dosing options are available, this is a representative regimen). Dosing is continued or modified based upon clinical and laboratory findings.

▸ **Myelodysplastic syndromes (MDS)**

PO

Adults. Initially 10 mg once per day. Dosing is continued or modified based upon clinical and laboratory findings.

▸ **Adjustment for renal function**

PO

Adjust starting doses. Continue or modify dosing based upon clinical and laboratory findings.

CrCl 30-59 ml/min: 5 mg q24h (MDS); 10 mg q24h (multiple myeloma).

CrCl < 30 ml/min (no dialysis): 5 mg q48h (MDS); 15 mg q48h (multiple myeloma).

ESRD (requiring hemodialysis): 5 mg given 3 times per week after each dialysis (MDS); 5 mg once per day, given after dialysis on dialysis days (multiple myeloma).

▸ **Adjustment for neutropenia or thrombocytopenia**

Expect to adjust dosing based on WBC and platelet counts; see manufacturer's prescribing information for adjustments.

CONTRAINDICATIONS

Hypersensitivity to lenalidomide; pregnancy (known teratogen).

INTERACTIONS

Drug

Digoxin: May increase digoxin levels. Monitor digoxin clinically and via levels as indicated.

Medications decreasing efficacy of hormonal contraception: Be alert for medications that might interfere with contraceptive efficacy (e.g., antibiotics, anticonvulsants).

Live-virus vaccines: Due to potential immunosuppression, avoid vaccination during treatment.

Herbal

None known.

Food

All food: Decreases peak levels; best taken with water only.

DIAGNOSTIC TEST EFFECTS

Reduces WBC and platelet counts frequently.

SIDE EFFECTS

Frequent

Diarrhea, itching/pruritus, rash, fatigue, reductions in blood counts, peripheral edema, arthralgia, fever, constipation.

Occasional

Nausea, sore throat, headache, dizziness, weakness, dry skin, epistaxis, cough, infection, poor appetite, sleep disturbance, paresthesias, swelling, sedation.

SERIOUS REACTIONS

- Known teratogen.
- Thromboembolic events are common (DVT and PE).
- Neutropenia and thrombocytopenia.
- Serious hypersensitivity, such as Stevens-Johnson syndrome or TEN, have been reported.

PRECAUTIONS & CONSIDERATIONS

! Lenalidomide is an analog of thalidomide. All prescribers, pharmacists, and patients must be registered in RevAssist™ to prescribe, dispense, or receive lenalidomide. As a known tetratogen, 2 forms of contraception must be used 4 wks before, during, and 4 wks following discontinuation of lenalidomide. Lenalidomide is contraindicated in pregnant women.

Women of childbearing age must receive a pregnancy test within 10-14 days and again 24 h before starting treatment and then testing will occur every 2-4 wks; the 2 negative tests results are required prior to use. Males must always use a latex condom during any sexual contact with females of childbearing potential even if they have undergone a successful vasectomy, as the drug may be present in the semen.

Breastfeeding is contraindicated. The drug is not approved for use in children. Patients with renal impairment or the elderly with renal dysfunction may require dosage adjustment (see Indications and Dosages). The elderly may be more at risk for side effects such as embolism and syncope. Caution is warranted with history of thromboembolic events. Prophylactic anticoagulation may be considered. Risk may be greater with concomitant dexamethasone use.

Patients should be instructed to seek medical care if they develop clot symptoms such as shortness of breath, chest pain, or arm or leg swelling. Patients should drink plenty of fluids. Notify the physician if symptoms of clotting, unusual bruising or bleeding, fever, infection, or extreme fatigue limiting daily activities occur. Monitor CBC frequently and monitor for signs of bone marrow suppression.

Storage

Store capsules at room temperature.

Administration

Administer lenalidomide with water only. Do not break, open, crush, or chew the capsules. Bedtime administration may minimize intolerance to neurologic side effects.

Letrozole

le′tro-zole

Femara

Do not confuse Femara with FemHRT.

CATEGORY AND SCHEDULE

Pregnancy Risk Category: D

Classification: Hormones and hormone modifiers, aromatase inhibitors

MECHANISM OF ACTION

Decreases the level of circulating estrogen by inhibiting aromatase, an enzyme that catalyzes the final step in estrogen production. *Therapeutic Effect:* Inhibits the growth of breast cancers that are stimulated by estrogens.

PHARMACOKINETICS

Rapidly and completely absorbed. Metabolized in the liver. Primarily eliminated by the kidneys. Unknown if removed by hemodialysis. *Half-life:* Approximately 2 days.

AVAILABILITY

Tablets: 2.5 mg.

INDICATIONS AND DOSAGES

▸ **Breast cancer, hormone replacement**

PO

Adults, Elderly. 2.5 mg/day. Continue until tumor progression is evident.

▸ **Dosage in severe hepatic impairment**

Give 2.5 mg every other day.

CONTRAINDICATIONS

Hypersensitivity to letrozole or any of its components, pregnancy, premenopausal women.

INTERACTIONS

Drug

Estrogens: Oppose actions of letrozole.

Herbal

None known.

Food

None known.

DIAGNOSTIC TEST EFFECTS

May increase serum calcium, cholesterol, GGT, AST (SGOT), and ALT (SGPT) levels.

SIDE EFFECTS

Frequent (9%-21%)

Musculoskeletal pain (back, arm, leg), nausea, headache, hot flashes.

Occasional (5%-8%)

Constipation, arthralgia, fatigue, vomiting, diarrhea, abdominal pain, cough, rash, anorexia, hypertension, peripheral edema.

Rare (1%-4%)

Asthenia, somnolence, dyspepsia, weight gain, pruritus.

SERIOUS REACTIONS

- May decrease bone mineral density with long-term use.
- Peripheral thrombotic events.

PRECAUTIONS & CONSIDERATIONS

Caution is warranted in patients with hepatic and severe renal impairment. Women who are or may be pregnant should not use this drug. Pregnancy should be determined before beginning therapy. It is unknown whether letrozole is distributed in breast milk. The safety and efficacy of letrozole have not been established in children. No age-related precautions have been noted in elderly patients.

Notify the physician if weakness, hot flashes, or nausea becomes unmanageable. Vital signs, especially BP, should be assessed before therapy begins because letrozole may cause hypertension. CBC, serum electrolyte levels, thyroid function, and liver and renal function tests should be monitored during therapy. Signs of infection or blood dyscrasias should be reported to health care provider immediately.

Storage

Store at a controlled room temperature.

Administration

Take oral letrozole without regard to food.

Leucovorin Calcium (Folinic Acid, Citrovorum Factor)

loo-koe-vor′in kal′see-um

★ Wellcovorin

Do not confuse Wellcovorin with Wellbutrin or Wellferon. Do not confuse folinic acid with folic acid. Do not confuse leucovorin with levoleucovorin; the two drugs have different dosages.

It is recommended always to use leucovorin as the drug name to avoid drug errors.

CATEGORY AND SCHEDULE

Pregnancy Risk Category: C

Classification: Antineoplastic adjunct; antidotes, folate analogue

MECHANISM OF ACTION

An antidote to folic acid antagonists that may limit the antagonists' action on normal cells by competing with them for the same transport processes into the cells. Actively and passively transported across cell membranes and converted to 5-methyltetrahydrofolic acid (5-methyl-THF), the primary circulating form of active reduced folate. Leucovorin and 5-methyl-THF are polyglutamated intracellularly by the enzyme folylpolyglutamate synthetase. Folypolyglutamates are active and participate in biochemical pathways that require reduced folate. *Therapeutic Effect:* Counteracts toxic effects of folic acid antagonists, such as bone marrow toxicities; has little effect on acute renal toxicity of methotrexate.

PHARMACOKINETICS

Readily absorbed from the GI tract. Widely distributed. Small quantities pass into the CSF. Metabolized in the liver and intestinal mucosa to active metabolite. Primarily excreted in urine. *Half-life:* 5.7 h (terminal).

L

AVAILABILITY

Tablets: 5 mg, 10 mg, 15 mg, 25 mg.
Injection: 10 mg/mL.
Powder for Injection: 50 mg, 100 mg, 200 mg, 350 mg, 500 mg.

INDICATIONS AND DOSAGES

▸ **Rescue dosage following high-dose methotrexate therapy**

IV INFUSION OR PO

Adults, Elderly, Children. 10 mg/m^2 IV q6h for 10 doses start 24 h after the beginning of the methotrexate infusion. Serum creatinine and methotrexate levels are determined at least once daily. Rescue administration, hydration, and urinary alkalinization (pH of 7.0 or more) should be continued until the methotrexate level is $< 5 \times 10^{-8}$ M (0.05 micromolar). If there is delayed early elimination of methotrexate or evidence of acute renal injury, doses of 100 mg/m^2 IV q3h may be given until methotrexate level < 1 micromolar; then give 10 mg/m^2 IV q3h until methotrexate level is < 0.05 micromolar.

▸ **Inadvertent folic acid antagonist overdose**

IV INFUSION/IM/PO

Adults, Elderly, Children. Begin as soon as possible after an inadvertent overdosage, preferably within 24 h. As the time interval between overdose and rescue increases, the effectiveness in counteracting toxicity may decrease. Give 10 mg/m^2 IV q6h until the serum methotrexate level is $< 10^{-8}$ M. Serum creatinine and methotrexate levels should be determined daily. If the 24-h serum creatinine has increased 50% over baseline or if the 24-h methotrexate level is $> 5 \times 10^{-6}$ M or the 48-h level is $> 9 \times 10^{-7}$ M, the dose should be increased to 100 mg/m^2 IV q3h until the methotrexate level is $< 10^{-8}$ M. Hydration (3 L/day) and urinary alkalinization with $NaHCO_3$ should be employed concomitantly to maintain the urine pH at 7.0 or greater.

▸ **Megaloblastic anemia secondary to folate deficiency**

IM/IV

Adults, Elderly, Children. 1 mg/day.

▸ **Prevention of hematologic toxicity (for toxoplasmosis) with sulfadiazine**

PO, IV

Adults, Elderly, Children. 10 mg/day.

▸ **Prevention of hematologic toxicity with pyrimethamine**

PO, IV

Adults, Children. 25 mg once weekly. Regimens may vary depending on other medications used.

OTHER USES

Used with 5-FU in standard approved regimens for colorectal cancer.

CONTRAINDICATIONS

Previous allergic reactions attributed to folic acid or leucovorin calcium (folinic acid). NOTE: Not approved for pernicious anemia and megaloblastic anemias secondary to the lack of vitamin B_{12}. Improper use may cause a hematologic remission while neurologic manifestations continue to progress.

INTERACTIONS

Drug

Anticonvulsants: May decrease the effects of anticonvulsants.

Chemotherapeutic agents: May increase the effects and toxicity of these drugs when taken in combination.

Sulfamethoxazole-trimethoprim (SMZ-TMP): Concomitant use for the acute treatment of PCP in patients with HIV infection is associated with treatment failure and morbidity.

Herbal and Food

None known.

DIAGNOSTIC TEST EFFECTS

None known.

IV INCOMPATIBILITIES

Amphotericin B complex (Abelcet, AmBisome, Amphotec), droperidol (Inapsine), foscarnet (Foscavir).

IV COMPATIBILITIES

Cisplatin (Platinol AQ), cyclophosphamide (Cytoxan), doxorubicin (Adriamycin), etoposide (VePesid), filgrastim (Neupogen), 5-fluorouracil, gemcitabine (Gemzar), granisetron (Kytril), heparin, methotrexate, metoclopramide (Reglan), mitomycin (Mutamycin), piperacillin and tazobactam (Zosyn), vinblastine (Velban), vincristine (Oncovin).

SIDE EFFECTS

Frequent

When combined with chemotherapeutic agents: Diarrhea, stomatitis, nausea, vomiting, lethargy or malaise or fatigue, alopecia, anorexia.

Occasional

Urticaria, dermatitis.

SERIOUS REACTIONS

- Excessive dosage may negate chemotherapeutic effects of folic acid antagonists.
- Anaphylaxis occurs rarely.
- Diarrhea may cause rapid clinical deterioration.

PRECAUTIONS & CONSIDERATIONS

Caution is warranted in patients with bronchial asthma and a history of allergies. Caution should also be used with 5-fluorouracil in persons with GI toxicities. It is unknown whether leucovorin crosses the placenta or is distributed in breast milk. Leucovorin use in epileptic children may increase the risk of seizures by counteracting the anticonvulsant effects of barbiturates and hydantoins. Age-related renal impairment may require a dosage adjustment for elderly patients receiving drug for rescue from effects of high-dose methotrexate therapy. Consuming foods with folic acid, including dried beans, meat proteins, and green leafy vegetables, is encouraged in those with folic acid deficiency.

Caution in individuals with severe anemia or those receiving cancer chemotherapy. Report development of infection immediately.

CBC, BUN, and serum creatinine levels (important in leucovorin rescue) should be monitored. Electrolyte levels and liver function test results in those receiving chemotherapeutic agents in combination with leucovorin should be assessed. For treatment of accidental overdosage of folic acid antagonists, leucovorin should be given as soon as possible (preferably within 1 h), as prescribed.

Storage

Store vials for parenteral use at room temperature. Protect from light. Use the solution immediately if reconstituted with sterile water for injection and within 7 days if reconstituted with bacteriostatic water for injection.

Administration

Scored tablets may be crushed.

The injection solution normally appears clear and yellowish. Reconstitute each 50-mg vial with 5 mL sterile water for injection or bacteriostatic water for injection (containing benzyl alcohol) to provide a concentration of 10 mg/mL. Reconstitute doses >10 mg/m^2 with sterile water for injection. Further dilute with D5W or 0.9% NaCl. Do not exceed an infusion rate of 160 mg/min (because of the drug's calcium content).

! Never administer intrathecally. Do not mix in same infusion as 5-FU.

Leuprolide Acetate

loo′proe-lide ass′eh-tayte

[US] Eligard, Lupron, Lupron Depot, Lupron Depot-Ped, Viadur

[CAN] Eligard, Lupron, Lupron Depot, Lupron Depot-Ped

Do not confuse leuprolide or Lupron with Lopurin or Nuprin.

CATEGORY AND SCHEDULE

Pregnancy Risk Category: X

Classification: Antineoplastics, hormones, gonadotropin-releasing hormone analogue

MECHANISM OF ACTION

A gonadotropin-releasing hormone analogue and antineoplastic agent that stimulates the release of luteinizing hormone (LH) and follicle-stimulating hormone (FSH) from the anterior pituitary gland.

Therapeutic Effect: Produces pharmacologic castration and decreases the growth of abnormal prostate tissue in males, causes endometrial tissue to become inactive and atrophic in females, and decreases the rate of pubertal development in children with central precocious puberty.

PHARMACOKINETICS

Rapidly and well absorbed after SC administration. Absorbed slowly after IM administration. Protein binding: 43%-49%. *Half-life:* 3-4 h.

AVAILABILITY

Implant (Viadur): 65 mg.

Injection Depot Formulation (Eligard): 7.5 mg, 22.5 mg, 30 mg.

Injection Depot Formulation (Lupron Depot): 3.75 mg, 7.5 mg, 11.25 mg, 22.5 mg, 30 mg.

Injection Depot Formulation (Lupron Depot-Ped): 7.5 mg, 11.25 mg, 15 mg.

Injection Solution (Lupron): 5 mg/mL.

INDICATIONS AND DOSAGES

▸ **Advanced prostatic carcinoma**

IM

Adults, Elderly. Lupron Depot: 7.5 mg/mo or 22.5 mg every 3 mo or 30 mg every 4 mo.

SC

Adults, Elderly. Eligard: 7.5 mg every month or 22.5 mg every 3 mo or 30 mg every 4 mo. Lupron: 1 mg/day. Viadur: 65 mg implanted every 12 mo.

▸ **Endometriosis**

IM

Adults, Elderly. Lupron Depot: 3.75 mg/mo for up to 6 mo or 11.25 mg every 3 mo for up to 2 doses.

▸ **Uterine leiomyomata**
IM
Adults, Elderly. Lupron Depot: 3.75 mg/mo for up to 3 mo or 11.25 mg as a single injection.
▸ **Precocious puberty**
IM
Children. Lupron Depot-Ped: 0.3 mg/kg/dose every 28 days. Minimum: 7.5 mg. If downregulation is not achieved, titrate upward in 3.75-mg increments q4wk.
SC
Children. Lupron: 20-45 mcg/kg/day. Titrate upward by 10 mcg/kg/day if downregulation is not achieved.

CONTRAINDICATIONS

Pregnancy, breastfeeding, hypersensitivity to drug or GnRH analogues.

INTERACTIONS

Drug, Herbal, and Food
None known.

DIAGNOSTIC TEST EFFECTS

May increase serum prostatic acid phosphatase (PAP) levels. Initially increases, then decreases, serum testosterone concentration.

SIDE EFFECTS

Frequent
Hot flashes (ranging from mild flushing to diaphoresis).
Females: Amenorrhea, spotting.
Occasional
Arrhythmias; palpitations; blurred vision; dizziness; edema; headache; burning, itching, or swelling at injection site; nausea; insomnia; weight gain.
Females: Deepening voice, hirsutism, decreased libido, increased breast tenderness, vaginitis, altered mood.
Males: Constipation, decreased testicle size, gynecomastia, impotence, decreased appetite, angina.
Rare
Males: Thrombophlebitis.

SERIOUS REACTIONS

- Signs and symptoms of metastatic prostatic carcinoma (such as bone pain, dysuria or hematuria, and weakness or paresthesia of the lower extremities) occasionally worsen 1-2 wks after the initial dose but then subside with continued therapy.
- Pulmonary embolism and MI occur rarely.
- Decreased bone density may lead to osteoporosis.

PRECAUTIONS & CONSIDERATIONS

Caution is warranted when administered to children receiving long-term therapy. Leuprolide use is contraindicated in pregnancy because the drug may cause spontaneous abortion. Pregnancy should be determined before therapy. Nonhormonal contraceptives should be used during leuprolide use. No age-related precautions have been noted in elderly patients.

Females should notify the physician if regular menstruation persists or pregnancy occurs. The patient should be assessed for peripheral edema, arrhythmias and palpitations, sleep-pattern changes, and visual difficulties. Serum testosterone and PAP levels should be obtained periodically during leuprolide therapy in men. Be aware that serum testosterone and PAP levels should increase during the first week of therapy. The testosterone level should decrease to baseline level or less within 2 wks, and the PAP level should decrease within 4 wks.

Storage
Refrigerate Lupron vials. Store Lupron Depot at room temperature; do not freeze and protect from

light and heat. Store Eligard in the refrigerator.

Administration

! Because leuprolide may be carcinogenic, mutagenic, or teratogenic, handle it with extreme care during preparation and administration.

For SC (Lupron) use, the injection should appear clear and colorless. Discard the solution if it appears discolored or contains precipitate. Administer the drug undiluted into the abdomen, anterior thigh, or deltoid muscle.

For IM (Lupron Depot) use, reconstitute only with the diluent provided. Follow mixing instructions provided by the manufacturer. Use the reconstituted solution immediately. Do not use needles smaller than 22 gauge; use syringes provided by the manufacturer (0.5-mL low-dose insulin syringes may be used as an alternative).

For IM (Eligard) use, allow drug to warm to room temperature before reconstitution. Follow mixing instructions provided by the manufacturer. Administer the drug within 30 min after reconstitution.

Viadur implant: Implanted SC in inner aspect of upper arm. Removed after 12 mo.

Levalbuterol

lee-val-byoo′ter-ole

Xopenex, Xopenex HFA

Do not confuse Xopenex with Xanax.

CATEGORY AND SCHEDULE

Pregnancy Risk Category: C

Classification: Adrenergic β_2 agonist, bronchodilator

MECHANISM OF ACTION

A sympathomimetic that stimulates β_2-adrenergic receptors in the lungs resulting in relaxation of bronchial smooth muscle. *Therapeutic Effect:* Relieves bronchospasm and reduces airway resistance.

PHARMACOKINETICS

Route	Onset	Peak	Duration
Inhalation	10-17 min	1.5 h	5-6 h

Metabolized in the liver to inactive metabolite. *Half-life:* 3.3-4 h.

AVAILABILITY

Solution for Nebulization: 0.31 mg in 3-mL vials, 0.63 mg in 3-mL vials, 1.25 mg in 3-mL vials. Also available as 1.25 mg/0.5 mL nebulizer solution.

Inhalation (Aerosol [Xopenex HFA]): 45 mcg/actuation.

INDICATIONS AND DOSAGES

▸ Treatment and prevention of bronchospasm

NEBULIZATION

Adults, Elderly, Children 12 yr and older. Initially, 0.63 mg 3 times a day 6-8 h apart. May increase to 1.25 mg 3 times a day with dose monitoring.

Children aged 6-11 yr. Initially 0.31 mg 3 times a day. Maximum: 0.63 mg 3 times a day.

HFA INHALER

Adults, Elderly, Children 12 yr and older. 90 mcg (2 inhalations) q4-6h; in some, 45 mcg (1 inhalation) q4h may be sufficient.

Children aged 4-11 yr. 90 mcg (2 inhalations) q4-6h; in some, 45 mcg (1 inhalation) q4h may be sufficient.

CONTRAINDICATIONS

History of hypersensitivity to sympathomimetics, particularly albuterol or levalbuterol.

INTERACTIONS

Drug

β-Blockers: Antagonize effects of levalbuterol.
Digoxin: May increase the risk of arrhythmias.
Diuretics: Hypokalemia associated with diuretic may worsen with levalbuterol. Monitor potassium levels.
MAOIs, tricyclic antidepressants: May potentiate cardiovascular effects. MAOIs may cause hypertensive crisis.

Herbal

None known.

Food

Caffeine: Limit use of caffeine, increased CNS stimulation.

DIAGNOSTIC TEST EFFECTS

May increase blood glucose level. May decrease serum potassium level.

SIDE EFFECTS

Frequent

Tremor, nervousness, headache, throat dryness and irritation.

Occasional

Cough, bronchial irritation.

Rare

Somnolence, diarrhea, dry mouth, flushing, diaphoresis, anorexia.

SERIOUS REACTIONS

- Excessive sympathomimetic stimulation may produce palpitations, extrasystoles, tachycardia, chest pain, a slight increase in BP followed by a substantial decrease, chills, diaphoresis, and blanching of skin.
- Too-frequent or excessive use may lead to decreased bronchodilating effectiveness and severe, paradoxical bronchoconstriction.

PRECAUTIONS & CONSIDERATIONS

Caution is warranted in patients with cardiovascular disorders (such as arrhythmias), diabetes mellitus, hypertension, and seizures. Levalbuterol crosses the placenta. It is unknown whether the drug is distributed in breast milk. The safety and efficacy of levalbuterol have not been established in children younger than 4 yr. A lower initial dosage is recommended for elderly patients. Drink plenty of fluids to decrease the thickness of lung secretions. Avoid excessive use of caffeinated products, such as chocolate, cocoa, cola, coffee, and tea.

Pulse rate and quality; respiratory rate, depth, rhythm, and type; ECG; ABG levels; and serum potassium levels should be monitored.

Storage

Store at room temperature. For nebulization, use the solution within 2 wks of opening the foil. Do not freeze; protect from light. Store inhaler with the actuator (or mouthpiece) down. Contents under pressure; exposure to heat or flame will cause bursting.

Administration

For nebulization, discard the solution if it is not colorless. Do not dilute the solution. Do not mix levalbuterol with other medications. Administer levalbuterol over 5-15 min.

For HFA inhalation, shake the container well before inhalation. Prime before first use or if inhaler has not been used for 3 days. Wait 2 min before inhaling the second dose to allow for deeper bronchial penetration. Rinse mouth with water immediately after inhalation to prevent mouth and throat dryness. Excessive use may produce paradoxical bronchoconstriction.

Levetiracetam

leva-tir-ass'eh-tam

Keppra, Keppra XR

Do not confuse Keppra with Kaletra.

CATEGORY AND SCHEDULE

Pregnancy Risk Category: C

Classification: Anticonvulsants

MECHANISM OF ACTION

An anticonvulsant that inhibits burst firing without affecting normal neuronal excitability. *Therapeutic Effect:* Prevents seizure activity.

PHARMACOKINETICS

Oral bioavailability is 100%. Onset 1 h, peak plasma levels attained in 20 min to 2 h. < 10% plasma protein bound; limited hepatic metabolism and renal excretion (66%). *Half-life:* 6-8 h.

AVAILABILITY

Extended-Release Tablets: 500 mg, 750 mg.
Liquid: 100 mg/mL.
Tablets: 250 mg, 500 mg, 750 mg, 1000 mg.
Injection: 100 mg/mL.

INDICATIONS AND DOSAGES

▸ Partial-onset seizures, juvenile myoclonic epilepsy, primary generalized tonic-clonic seizures

PO OR IV

Adults, Elderly, children ≥ 16 yr. Initially, 500 mg q12h. May increase by 1000 mg/day q2wk. Maximum: 3000 mg/day. For extended-release tablets, give usual total daily dose once daily.

Children aged 4-16 yr. 10 mg/kg/day in 2 divided doses. May increase at weekly intervals by 10-20 mg/kg. Maximum: 60 mg/kg.

▸ Replacement therapy (switching from PO to IV)

The initial total daily IV dosage is equivalent to the total daily dosage and frequency of immediate-release PO regimen. At the end of the IV treatment period, may switch to immediate-release PO at the equivalent daily dosage and frequency of the IV.

▸ Dosage in renal impairment

Dosage is modified based on creatinine clearance.

Creatinine Clearance (mL/min)	Adult Dosage (mg q12h)
> 80	500-1500
50-80	500-1000
30-50	250-750
< 30 mL/min	250-500
End-stage renal disease using dialysis	500-1000 every 24 h
After dialysis, supplemental dose is recommended	250-500

NOTE: If extended-release, may give total daily dose q24h, as long as dosage 1000 mg/day, or above. If lower doses/day, require the use of immediate-release dose forms.

CONTRAINDICATIONS

Hypersensitivity reaction.

INTERACTIONS

Drug

Probenecid: competes with metabolite for tubular renal clearance.

Herbal

None known.

Food

None significant.

DIAGNOSTIC TEST EFFECTS

Infrequent decreases in blood hemoglobin level, hematocrit, and RBC and WBC counts.

IV COMPATIBILITIES
Lorazepam, diazepam, valproate sodium. There are no data to support compatibility with any other drugs.

SIDE EFFECTS
Frequent (10%-15%)
Somnolence, asthenia, headache, infection.
Occasional (4%-9%)
Dizziness, pharyngitis, pain, depression, nervousness, vertigo, rhinitis, anorexia.
Rare (< 3%)
Amnesia, anxiety, emotional lability, cough, sinusitis, anorexia, diplopia, neutropenia (mild).

SERIOUS REACTIONS
- Psychotic reactions (rare).
- Abnormal liver function, hepatic failure, hepatitis (rare).
- Blood dyscrasias or bone marrow suppression (rare).

PRECAUTIONS & CONSIDERATIONS
Caution is warranted in patients with renal impairment. Drowsiness and dizziness may occur, so alcohol and tasks requiring mental alertness or motor skills should be avoided. AEDs may increase the risk of suicidal thoughts or behavior in patients taking these drugs for any indication. Monitor for the emergence or worsening of depression, suicidal thoughts, or unusual behavior or moods. Safety and efficacy not established in children < 4 yr of age; do not use extended-release in children under 16 yr. The effects of this drug on pregnancy are not known. Levetiracetam is excreted in breast milk, and breastfeeding is not recommended. Seizure disorder, including the onset, duration, frequency, intensity, and type of seizures, should be assessed before and during treatment.

Report symptoms of blood dyscrasias or infection immediately to health care provider.

Storage
Store all oral products and unopened vials at room temperature. Only prepare infusion immediately prior to use; discard any unused portion.

Administration
Take levetiracetam without regard to food. Because of bitter taste, do not cut tablets; administer whole. Do not crush, cut, or chew extended-release tablets.

IV must be diluted before use with 100 mL of 0.9% NaCl or dextrose 5% injection up to 1500 mg/100 mL. Infuse over 15 min.

Do not discontinue the drug abruptly after long-term therapy. Strict maintenance of drug therapy is essential for seizure control.

Levocetirizine
lee′vo-si-tear′a-zeen
Xyzal
Do not confuse levocetirizine with cetirizine, or Xyzal with Xyrem.

CATEGORY AND SCHEDULE
Pregnancy Risk Category: B

Classification: Antihistamines, H_1, low sedating

MECHANISM OF ACTION
The active enantiomer of cetirizine, levocetirizine is a second-generation piperazine that competes with histamine for H_1 receptor sites on effector cells in the GI tract, blood vessels, and respiratory tract. *Therapeutic Effect:* Prevents allergic response, reduces itching.

PHARMACOKINETICS

Route	Onset	Peak	Duration
PO	< 4-8 h	0.5-1 h	24 h

Rapidly and almost completely absorbed from the GI tract (absorption not affected by food). Protein binding: 92%. Not extensively metabolized by the liver. Drug and metabolites primarily excreted in urine (more than 85%). Levocetirizine is excreted both by glomerular filtration and active tubular secretion. *Half-life:* 8-9 h.

AVAILABILITY

Oral Solution: 2.5 mg/5 mL.
Tablets: 5 mg.

L

INDICATIONS AND DOSAGES

▸ Allergic rhinitis, chronic idiopathic urticaria

PO

Adults, Elderly, Children 12 yr and older. 5 mg once daily.
Children 6-11 yr. 2.5 mg once daily.
Children 6 mo to 5 yr. 1.25 mg once daily.

▸ Dosage in renal impairment (adults and children ≥ 12 yr)

CrCl 50-80 mL/min: 2.5 mg once daily.
CrCl 30-50 mL/min: 2.5 mg once every other day.
CrCl 10-30 mL/min): 2.5 mg twice weekly (give once every 3-4 days).
CrCl < 10 mL/min, ESRD and patients undergoing dialysis: Do not use.

CONTRAINDICATIONS

Hypersensitivity to levocetirizine, cetirizine, or hydroxyzine; CrCl < 10 mL/min or end-stage renal disease; any degree of renal impairment in children 11 yr of age and younger.

INTERACTIONS

Drug

Alcohol, other CNS depressants: May increase CNS depression.
Ritonavir: May increase cetirizine concentrations.

Herbal

None known.

Food

None known.

DIAGNOSTIC TEST EFFECTS

May suppress wheal and flare reactions to antigen skin testing, unless drug is discontinued 4 days before testing.

SIDE EFFECTS

Occasional (2%-10%)

Mild sedation, pharyngitis, fatigue, dry mouth. Additionally, pyrexia, cough, and epistaxis in children 6-12 yr of age. In children < 6 yr, pyrexia, diarrhea, vomiting, otitis media, and constipation were reported.

SERIOUS REACTIONS

- Children may experience paradoxical reactions, including restlessness, insomnia, euphoria, nervousness, and tremor.
- Dizziness, sedation, asthenia, and confusion are more likely to occur in elderly patients.

PRECAUTIONS & CONSIDERATIONS

Caution is warranted with renal impairment or with hepatic impairment when renal impairment is also likely. Levocetirizine use is not recommended during the early months of pregnancy. Levocetirizine is likely to be excreted in breast milk. Breastfeeding is not recommended. Elderly patients are more likely to experience dry mouth and urine retention, as well as dizziness, sedation, and confusion.

Avoid drinking alcoholic beverages, and tasks that require alertness or motor skills until response to the drug is established. Drowsiness may occur at dosages > 5 mg/day. Do not exceed recommended doses, especially in children, whose exposure to the drug increases greatly with increasing dose. Therapeutic response should be monitored.

Storage

Store at room temperature.

Administration

Take levocetirizine without regard to food. Administer in the evening.

Levofloxacin

levo-flox'a-sin

Iquix, Levaquin, Quixin

Levaquin

CATEGORY AND SCHEDULE

Pregnancy Risk Category: C

Classification: Fluoroquinolone anti-infectives

MECHANISM OF ACTION

A fluoroquinolone that inhibits the enzyme DNA gyrase in susceptible microorganisms, interfering with bacterial cell replication and repair. *Therapeutic Effect:* Bactericidal.

PHARMACOKINETICS

Well absorbed after both PO and IV administration. Protein binding: 8%-24%. Penetrates rapidly and extensively into leukocytes, epithelial cells, and macrophages. Lung concentrations are 2-5 times higher than those of plasma. Eliminated unchanged in the urine. Partially removed by hemodialysis. *Half-life:* 8 h.

AVAILABILITY

Tablets (Levaquin): 250 mg, 500 mg, 750 mg.
Oral Solution: 25 mg/mL.
Injection (Levaquin): 500-mg/20-mL.
Premixed IV Solution (Levaquin): 250 mg/50 mL, 500 mg/100 mL, 750 mg/150 mL.
Ophthalmic Solution (Quixin): 1.5%.
Ophthalmic Solution (Iquix): 0.5%.

INDICATIONS AND DOSAGES

▸ **Bronchitis**

PO, IV

Adults, Elderly. 500 mg q24h for 7 days.

▸ **Community-acquired pneumonia**

PO, IV

Adults, Elderly. 750 mg/day for 5 days or use 500 mg/day for 7-14 days.

▸ **Pneumonia nosocomial**

PO, IV

Adults, Elderly. 750 mg q24h for 7-14 days.

▸ **Acute maxillary sinusitis**

PO, IV

Adults, Elderly. 500 mg q24h for 10-14 days or use 750 mg/day for 5 days.

▸ **Skin and skin-structure infections**

PO, IV

Adults, Elderly. 500 mg q24h for 7-10 days or if complicated, 750 mg/day for 7-14 days.

▸ **Urinary tract infection, acute pyelonephritis**

PO, IV

Adults, Elderly. 250 mg q24h for 10 days or use 750 mg/day for 5 days.

▸ **Bacterial conjunctivitis**

OPHTHALMIC

Adults, Elderly, Children 1 yr and older. 1-2 drops q2h for 2 days (up to 8 times a day), then 1-2 drops q4h for 5 days.

▸ **Corneal ulcer**

OPHTHALMIC

Adults, Elderly, Children older than 5 yr. Days 1-3: Instill 1-2 drops q30min to 2 h while awake and 4-6 h after retiring. Days 4 through completion: 1-2 drops q1-4h while awake.

▸ **Dosage in renal impairment**

For bronchitis, pneumonia, sinusitis, and skin and skin-structure infections, dosage and frequency are modified based on creatinine clearance.

Creatinine Clearance (mL/min)	Based on 500 mg/ day* Adult Dosage
50-80	No change
20-49	500 mg initially, then 250 mg q24h
10-19	500 mg initially, then 250 mg q48h
Dialysis	500 mg initially, then 250 mg q48h

*See prescribing information for adjustment for higher 750 mg/day dose.

Creatinine Clearance (mL/min)	Based on 250 mg/ day Adult dosage
20	No change
10-19	250 mg initially, then 250 mg q48h

CONTRAINDICATIONS

Hypersensitivity to levofloxacin, other fluoroquinolones, or nalidixic acid.

INTERACTIONS

Drug

Antacids, didanosine, iron preparations, sucralfate, zinc: Decrease levofloxacin absorption. Separate times of administration by at least 2 h.

Antipsychotics, class 1A and class III antiarrhythmics, erythromycin, tricyclic antidepressants: May increase the risk of prolonged QTc interval.

Corticosteroids: May increase risk of tendon rupture, especially in elderly patients.

Cyclosporine: May increase cyclosporine levels; monitor.

NSAIDs: May increase the risk of central nervous system (CNS) stimulation or seizures.

Warfarin: May increase risk of bleeding.

Herbal

None known.

Food

None known.

DIAGNOSTIC TEST EFFECTS

May alter blood glucose levels.

IV INCOMPATIBILITIES

Cefazolin, diazepam, furosemide (Lasix), heparin, insulin, nitroglycerin, phenytoin, propofol (Diprivan).

IV COMPATIBILITIES

Aminophylline, dobutamine, dopamine, fentanyl (Sublimaze), lidocaine, lorazepam (Ativan), morphine.

SIDE EFFECTS

Occasional (1%-3%)

Diarrhea, nausea, abdominal pain, dizziness, drowsiness, headache, light-headedness.

Ophthalmic: Local burning or discomfort, margin crusting, crystals or scales, foreign body sensation, ocular itching, altered taste.

Rare (< 1%)

Flatulence; altered taste; pain; inflammation or swelling in calves, hands, or shoulder; chest pain; difficulty breathing; palpitations; edema; tendon pain; hypoglycemia.

Ophthalmic: Corneal staining, keratitis, allergic reaction, eyelid swelling, tearing, reduced visual acuity.

SERIOUS REACTIONS

- Antibiotic-associated colitis and other superinfections may occur from altered bacterial balance.
- Hypersensitivity reactions, including photosensitivity (as evidenced by rash, pruritus, blisters, edema, and burning skin) have occurred in patients receiving fluoroquinolones.
- Tendon rupture.
- Peripheral neuropathy.
- Seizures (rare).
- Hepatitis or other liver dysfunction (rare).
- QTc prolongation and potential for arrhythmia (rare).

PRECAUTIONS & CONSIDERATIONS

History of hypersensitivity to levofloxacin and other quinolones should be determined before therapy. Caution is warranted with bradycardia, cardiomyopathy, hypokalemia, hypomagnesemia, impaired renal function, seizure disorders, or suspected CNS disorder. Use with caution in patients with cardiac arrhythmias; should not be used unmonitored in patients with known QT prolongation. Conditions that might increase the risk of proarrythmia include electrolyte imbalances and use of drugs that prolong the QT interval. Fluoroquinolones increase the risk of tendinitis and tendon rupture and may be seen more often in the elderly, in those taking corticosteroids, and in patients with organ transplants. There are no adequate data regarding the use of levofloxacin in pregnancy. The drug is likely excreted in breast milk. The safety and efficacy of levofloxacin have not been established in children younger than 18 yr. Age-related renal impairment may require a dosage adjustment in elderly patients.

Chest pain, difficulty breathing, palpitations, edema, tendon pain, as well as hypersensitivity reactions, including photosensitivity, pruritus, skin rash, and urticaria, should be reported immediately. Be alert for signs and symptoms of superinfection, such as moderate to severe diarrhea, new or increased fever, and ulceration or changes in the oral mucosa. Symptomatic relief should be provided for nausea. Blood glucose levels, liver and renal function, and white blood cell (WBC) count should be monitored.

Discontinue treatment if patient experiences pain or inflammation of a tendon; seek medical consultation, rest and refrain from exercise.

Storage

Store at room temperature; protect injection and premixed infusions from light and freezing. Infusions prepared from vials are stable for 72 h at room temperature or for 14 days if refrigerated. Do not remove overwrap from premixed bags until time of use.

Administration

Take levofloxacin tablets without regard to food. Oral solution should be given 1 h before or 2 h after food. Do not take antacids (containing aluminum or magnesium), sucralfate, iron preparations, or multivitamins containing zinc within 2 h of levofloxacin because these drugs significantly reduce levofloxacin absorption.

Injection is for further dilution as an IV infusion only. For infusion using the single-dose vial, withdraw the desired amount (10 mL for 250 mg, 20 mL for 500 mg). Dilute each 10 mL (250 mg) with at least 40 mL 0.9% NaCl or D5W. Give 250-mg or 500-mg IV infusions over 60 min and 750-mg infusions over 90 min.

For ophthalmic use, place a gloved finger on the lower eyelid, and pull it out until a pocket is formed between the eye and lower lid. Hold the dropper above the pocket, and place the correct number of drops into the pocket. Close the eye gently. Apply digital pressure to the lacrimal sac for 1-2 min to minimize drainage of the medication into the patient's nose and throat, reducing the risk of systemic effects.

Levoleucovorin Calcium

lee'vo-loo'koe-vor'in kal'see-um

Fusilev

Do not confuse Fusilev with Fuzeon. Do not confuse levoleucovorin calcium with leucovorin calcium; the two drugs have different dosages.

CATEGORY AND SCHEDULE

Pregnancy Risk Category: C

Classification: Antineoplastic adjunct; antidotes, folate analogue.

MECHANISM OF ACTION

Levoleucovorin is the pharmacologically active isomer of leucovorin. An antidote to folic acid antagonists that may limit the antagonist's action on normal cells by competing with them for the same transport processes into the cells. Does not require reduction by the enzyme dihydrofolate reductase. Levoleucovorin is actively and passively transported across cell membranes and converted to 5-methyltetrahydrofolic acid (5-methyl-THF), the primary circulating form of active reduced folate. Levoleucovorin and 5-methyl-THF are polyglutamated intracellularly by the enzyme folylpolyglutamate synthetase. Folylpolyglutamates are active and participate in biochemical pathways that require reduced folate. *Therapeutic Effect:* Counteracts toxic effects of folic acid antagonists, such as bone marrow toxicities; has little effect on acute renal toxicity of methotrexate.

PHARMACOKINETICS

After rapid IV administration, serum total tetrahydrofolate (total-THF) concentrations reached a mean peak of 1722 ng/mL. Mean peak serum (6S)-5-methyl-5,6,7,8-tetrahydrofolate concentration was 275 ng/mL and the mean time to peak was 0.9 h. Small quantities of the drug penetrate into the CSF. Metabolized in intestinal mucosa and by the liver. Primarily excreted in urine as active folate metabolites. *Half-life:* 5.1-6.8 h.

AVAILABILITY

Powder for Injection: 50 mg (contains mannitol).

INDICATIONS AND DOSAGES

NOTE: Levoleucovorin dosage is 50% of the normal leucovorin dosage in various rescue dosage regimens.

▸ **Rescue dosage following high-dose methotrexate therapy**

IV INFUSION

Adults, Elderly, Children > 6 yrs. 5 mg/m^2 IV q6h for 10 doses; treatment starts 24 h after the beginning of the methotrexate infusion. Serum creatinine and methotrexate levels are determined at least once daily. Rescue administration, hydration, and urinary alkalinization (pH of 7.0 or more) should be continued until the methotrexate level is $< 5 \times 10^{-8}$ M (0.05 micromolar). If there is delayed early elimination of methotrexate or evidence of acute renal injury, doses of 50 mg/m^2 IV q3h may be given until methotrexate level < 1 micromolar; then give 5 mg/m^2 IV q3h until methotrexate level is < 0.05 micromolar.

▸ **Inadvertent folic acid antagonist overdose**

IV INFUSION

Adults, Elderly, Children > 6 yrs. Begin as soon as possible after an inadvertent overdosage, preferably within 24 h. As the time interval between overdose and rescue increases, the effectiveness in counteracting toxicity may decrease. Give 5 mg/m^2 IV q6h until the serum methotrexate level is < 10^{-8} M. Serum creatinine and methotrexate levels should be determined daily. If the 24-h serum creatinine has increased 50% over baseline or if the 24-h methotrexate level is > 5 × 10^{-6} M or the 48-h level is > 9 × 10^{-7} M, the dose should be increased to 50 mg/m^2 IV q3h until the methotrexate level is < 10^{-8} M. Hydration (3 L/day) and urinary alkalinization with $NaHCO_3$ should be employed concomitantly to maintain the urine pH at 7.0 or greater.

OFF-LABEL USES

Used in place of leucovorin (at 50% the leucovorin dosage) in times of drug shortage along with 5-FU in standard regimens for colorectal cancer. May also be used for overdosage or toxicity of various other folate antagonists (e.g., trimethoprim, pyrimethamine).

CONTRAINDICATIONS

Previous allergic reactions attributed to folic acid or leucovorin calcium (folinic acid). NOTE: Not approved for pernicious anemia and megaloblastic anemias secondary to the lack of vitamin B_{12}. Improper use may cause a hematologic remission while neurologic manifestations continue to progress.

INTERACTIONS

Drug

Anticonvulsants: May decrease the anticonvulsant activity.

Chemotherapeutic agents: May increase the effects and toxicity of these drugs when taken in combination. Occurs especially with 5-FU; watch for dehydration, diarrhea.

Sulfamethoxazole-trimethoprim (SMZ-TMP): Concomitant use for the acute treatment of PCP in patients with HIV infection is associated with treatment failure and morbidity.

Herbal and Food

None known.

DIAGNOSTIC TEST EFFECTS

None known.

IV INCOMPATIBILITIES

Due to the risk of precipitation, do not coadminister with other agents in the same admixture.

SIDE EFFECTS

Frequent

Vomiting (38%), stomatitis (38%), and nausea (19%) were most common.

Occasional

Diarrhea, taste perversion, urticaria, dermatitis, dyspnea.

SERIOUS REACTIONS

- Excessive dosage may negate chemotherapeutic effects of folic acid antagonists.
- Anaphylaxis occurs rarely.
- Diarrhea may cause rapid clinical deterioration.

PRECAUTIONS & CONSIDERATIONS

Monitor patients with renal dysfunction or dehydration closely. It is unknown whether levoleucovorin crosses the placenta or is distributed in breast milk. Consuming foods with folic acid, including dried beans, meat proteins, and green leafy vegetables, is encouraged in those with folic acid deficiency. Caution in individuals with severe anemia or those receiving cancer chemotherapy. Report development of infection immediately. Monitor CBC, BUN, and serum creatinine (important in methotrexate rescue). Electrolyte levels and liver function test results in those receiving chemotherapeutic agents should be assessed. For treatment of accidental overdosage of folic acid antagonists, levoleucovorin should be given as soon as possible.

Storage

Store vials at room temperature; protect from light. Initial reconstitution or infusions using 0.9% NaCl may be held at room temperature for not more than 12 h. Infusions in D5W may be held at room temperature for not more than 4 h.

Administration

For intravenous (IV) infusion use only. NEVER administer intrathecally.

Prior to IV use, the 50-mg vial is reconstituted with 5.3 mL of 0.9% NaCl (unpreserved) to yield a concentration of 10 mg/mL. Further dilute to a concentration between 0.5 mg/mL and 5 mg/mL in 0.9% NaCl or D5W. Because of the calcium content, no more than 16 mL (160 mg of levoleucovorin) should be infused IV per minute.

Levorphanol

lee-vor'fa-nole

★ Levo-Dromoran

CATEGORY AND SCHEDULE

Pregnancy Risk Category: C

Controlled Substance Schedule: II

Classification: Analgesics, narcotic

MECHANISM OF ACTION

An opioid agonist that binds at opiate receptor sites in central nervous system (CNS). *Therapeutic Effect:* Reduced intensity of pain stimuli incoming from sensory nerve endings, altering pain perception and emotional response to pain.

PHARMACOKINETICS

Rapidly absorbed after oral administration; onset of effect within 15-30 min after IM administration. Protein binding: 40%-50%. Extensively distributed. Metabolized in liver. Excreted in urine. Steady-state plasma levels attained by third day of dosing. *Half-life:* 11 h.

AVAILABILITY

Tablets: 2 mg.

Injection: 2 mg/mL (Levo-Dromoran).

INDICATIONS AND DOSAGES

▸ **Pain**

PO

Adults, Elderly. 2 mg. May be increased to 3 mg if needed and may increase dose to 3 mg every 6-8 h. Not to exceed 6-12 mg/day.

IM/SC

Adults, Elderly. 1-2 mg as a single dose. May repeat in 6-8 h as needed. Maximum: 3-8 mg/day.

IV

Adults. Up to 1 mg injection in divided doses by slow injection. May repeat in 3-6 h as needed. Maximum: 4-8 mg/day.

▸ **Preoperative**

IM/SC

Adults, Elderly. 1-2 mg as a single dose 60-90 min before surgery. Adjustment may be needed in elderly patients.

▸ **Perioperative**

IM/SC

Adults, Elderly. Dosing based on age, weight, physical status, underlying pathology, and other anesthetic being used during procedure.

CONTRAINDICATIONS

Hypersensitivity to levorphanol or any component of the formulation.

INTERACTIONS

Drug

Alcohol, barbiturates, general anesthetics, hypnotics, other opioids, phenothiazines, sedatives, skeletal muscle relaxants, tranquilizers, tricyclic antidepressants and other central nervous system (CNS) depressants: May increase CNS or respiratory depression, profound sedation and coma, hypotension.

MAOIs: May produce severe, fatal reaction.

Herbal

None known.

Food

None known.

DIAGNOSTIC TEST EFFECTS

May increase serum amylase and lipase levels.

IV INCOMPATIBILITIES

Do not mix with aminophylline, ammonium dichloride, amobarbital, chlorothiazide, dietholamine, heparin, methicillin, nitrofurantoin, novobiocin, pentobarbital, perphenazine, phenobarbital, phenytoin, secobarbital, sodium bicarbonate, sodium iodide, sulfadiazine, sulfisoxazole, thiopental.

SIDE EFFECTS

Effects are dependent on dosage amount, route of administration. Ambulatory patients and those not in severe pain may experience dizziness, nausea, vomiting, or hypotension more frequently than those in supine position or having severe pain.

Frequent

Dizziness, drowsiness, hypotension, nausea, vomiting.

Occasional

Shortness of breath, confusion, decreased urination, stomach cramps, altered vision, constipation, dry mouth, headache, difficult or painful urination.

Rare

Allergic reaction (rash, itching), histamine reaction (decreased BP, increased sweating, flushed face, wheezing).

SERIOUS REACTIONS

- Overdosage results in respiratory depression, skeletal muscle flaccidity, cold clammy skin, cyanosis, extreme somnolence progressing to convulsions, stupor, coma, hypotension, respiratory depression, and death.
- Tolerance to analgesic effect, physical dependence may occur with repeated use.
- Paralytic ileus may occur with prolonged use.

PRECAUTIONS & CONSIDERATIONS

Extreme caution should be used in patients with acute alcoholism, anoxia, CNS depression, hypercapnia, respiratory depression, respiratory dysfunction, seizures, shock, and untreated myxedema. Caution is also warranted with acute abdominal conditions, biliary surgery, Addison disease, chronic obstructive pulmonary disease (COPD), hypothyroidism, impaired renal or liver function, increased intracranial pressure, benign prostatic hypertrophy, and urethral stricture; expect to reduce the initial dosage in these conditions. biliary surgery, Safety and efficacy in children are not established. Unknown if excreted in breast milk; caution warranted in pregnancy and lactation.

Vital signs should be taken before giving medication. If respirations are 12/min or lower (20/min or lower in children), withhold medication and contact the physician. Vital signs should be monitored after administration as well.

Be aware that ambulatory persons and those not in severe pain may experience dizziness, hypotension, nausea, and vomiting more frequently than persons in the supine position or with severe pain. Avoid alcohol and tasks that require mental alertness or motor skills. Change positions slowly to avoid orthostatic hypotension.

Drug has abuse potential. Caution warranted in patients with addictive disorders.

May cause serious or potentially fatal respiratory depression if given in excessive dose, given too frequently, or given in full dose to compromised patients. Discontinuing after chronic use may result in withdrawal syndrome.

Any of the follwing symptoms should be reported immediately to health care providers: dizziness, light-headedness, sleepiness, drowsiness, difficulty urinating, fainting, shallow breathing, excessive sleepiness.

Storage

Store at room temperature.

Administration

Dosage should be individualized based on degree of pain and physical condition of the person. Administration may be IV, IM, or SC. Give by slow IV injection.

Levothyroxine

lee-voe-thye-rox'een

Levothroid, Levoxyl, Synthroid, Tirosint, Unithroid Eltroxin, Euthyrox, Synthroid

Do not confuse levothyroxine with liothyronine.

CATEGORY AND SCHEDULE

Pregnancy Risk Category: A

Classification: Thyroid hormone

MECHANISM OF ACTION

A synthetic isomer of thyroxine (T4) involved in normal metabolism, growth, and development, especially of the CNS in infants. Possesses catabolic and anabolic effects. *Therapeutic Effect:* Increases basal metabolic rate, enhances gluconeogenesis, and stimulates protein synthesis.

PHARMACOKINETICS

Variable, incomplete absorption from the GI tract. Protein binding: 99%. Widely distributed. Deiodinated in peripheral tissues, minimal metabolism in the liver. Eliminated by biliary excretion. *Half-life:* 6-7 days.

AVAILABILITY

Tablets (Levothroid, Levoxyl, Synthroid, Unithroid): 0.025 mg, 0.05 mg, 0.075 mg, 0.088 mg, 0.1 mg, 0.112 mg, 0.125 mg, 0.137 mg, 0.15 mg, 0.175 mg, 0.2 mg, 0.3 mg.
Capsules (Tirosint): 0.013 mg, 0.025 mg, 0.05 mg, 0.075 mg, 0.125 mg, 0.137 mg, 0.150 mg.
Powder for Injection: 200 mcg, 500 mcg.

INDICATIONS AND DOSAGES

▸ **Hypothyroidism (non-emergent)**

PO

Adults, Elderly. Initially, 12.5-50 mcg. May increase by 25-50 mcg/day q2-4wk. Maintenance: 100-200 mcg/day.

▸ **Usual pediatric dose**

NOTE: Dosing is highly individualized and based on body weight and age (see manufacturer dosing). The information below represents common ranges seen at each age.

Children 13 yr and older. 150 mcg/day.

Children aged 6-12 yr. 100-125 mcg/day.

Children aged 1-5 yr. 75-100 mcg/day.

Children 7-11 mo. 50-75 mcg/day.

Children 3-6 mo. 25-50 mcg/day.

Children 3 mo and younger. 10-15 mcg/day.

▸ **Myxedema (usual dose)**

IV

Adults, Elderly. Initially, 300-500 mcg/day for 1 dose, the 100-300 mcg on second day if needed. Then, 75-100 mcg/day until stabilized and PO therapy feasible.

▸ **Thyroid-stimulating hormone suppression in thyroid cancer, nodules, euthyroid**

PO

Adults, Elderly. 2-6 mcg/kg/day for 7-10 days.

▸ **Usual IV maintenance dosage**

IV

Adults, Elderly, Children. Initial dosage approximately half the previously established oral dosage.

CONTRAINDICATIONS

Hypersensitivity to tablet components, such as tartrazine; uncorrected adrenal insufficiency (may cause acute adrenal crisis); myocardial infarction and thyrotoxicosis uncomplicated by hypothyroidism; treatment of obesity.

INTERACTIONS

Drug

Antidiabetic drugs: As thyroid replacement ensues, antidiabetic requirements may change; monitor.

Cholestyramine, colestipol, enteral feedings, antacids, calcium and iron supplements: May decrease the absorption of levothyroxine. Separate times of administration.

Digoxin: May alter digoxin dose requirements as thyroid function corrected due to increased metabolic rate; monitor.

Oral anticoagulants: May alter the effects of oral anticoagulants.

Sympathomimetics: May increase the risk of coronary insufficiency.

Herbal

None known.

Food

Coffee, dairy foods, soybean flour (infant formula), cotton seed meal, walnuts, and dietary fiber: May decrease absorption.

DIAGNOSTIC TEST EFFECTS

None known. Dose is adjusted based on monitoring of TSH response. Changes in TBG levels must be considered when interpreting T4 and T3 values.

IV INCOMPATIBILITIES

Do not use or mix with other IV solutions.

SIDE EFFECTS

Occasional

Reversible hair loss at the start of therapy (in children).

Rare

Dry skin, GI intolerance, rash, hives, pseudotumor cerebri, or severe headache in children.

SERIOUS REACTIONS

- Excessive dosage produces signs and symptoms of hyperthyroidism, including weight loss, palpitations, increased appetite, tremors, nervousness, tachycardia, hypertension, headache, insomnia, and menstrual irregularities.
- Cardiac arrhythmias occur rarely.

PRECAUTIONS & CONSIDERATIONS

Caution is warranted in patients with angina pectoris, hypertension, other cardiovascular disease, and in elderly patients. Levothyroxine does not cross the placenta and is minimally excreted in breast milk. Thyroid euthymia promotes fetal development and proper lactation, so there are usually no particular precautions for pregnancy or lactation. No age-related precautions have been noted in children. Use caution in interpreting thyroid function tests in neonates. Elderly patients may be more sensitive to thyroid effects. Individualized dosages are recommended for this population. Increased nervousness, excitability, sweating, or tachycardia indicates possible uncontrolled hyperthyroidism or overdosage.

Reversible hair loss or increased aggressiveness may occur during the first few months of therapy. Notify the physician of chest pain, edema of feet or ankles, insomnia, nervousness, tremors, weight loss, or a pulse rate of 100 beats/min or more. Weight and vital signs, especially pulse rate and rhythm, should be monitored. Keep in mind that levothyroxine may intensify the signs and symptoms of adrenal insufficiency, diabetes insipidus, diabetes mellitus, and hypopituitarism. Also, know that adrenocortical steroids should be prescribed before thyroid therapy in persons with coexisting hypoadrenalism and hypothyroidism.

Storage

Store tablets and vials at room temperature. Protect tablets from moisture.

Administration

! Do not use different brands of levothyroxine interchangeably, although problems with bioequivalence among manufacturers are minimized with today's manufacturing process; it is better for patients to use same product throughout treatment or be carefully monitored during product switches. Begin therapy with small doses and increase the dosage gradually, as prescribed.

Take oral levothyroxine at same time each day to maintain hormone levels. Take before breakfast or at bedtime on empty stomach and without other medications or foods. Take with plenty of water. Full therapeutic effect of the drug may take 4-6 wks to appear. Crush tablets as needed. Do not crush or cut capsules. Do not discontinue this drug; replacement therapy for hypothyroidism is lifelong.

For IV use, reconstitute 500-mcg vial with 5 mL or 200-mcg vial with 2 mL 0.9% NaCl to provide a concentration of 100 mcg/mL; shake until clear. Use immediately, and discard unused portion. Give each 100 mcg or less over 1 min.

Lidocaine Hydrochloride

lye′doe-kane high-droh-klor′ide

★ Lidoderm Patch, Lidamantle, Lidomar, Solarcaine, Xylocaine, Xylocaine MPF, Xylocaine Jelly, Xylocaine Topical Solution

🍁 Lidodan, Lidodan Jelly, Xylocard

CATEGORY AND SCHEDULE

Pregnancy Risk Category: B

Classification: Antiarrythmics, class IB; local anesthetics, amide local anesthetics

MECHANISM OF ACTION

An amide anesthetic that inhibits the conduction of nerve impulses. *Therapeutic Effect:* Causes temporary loss of feeling and sensation. Also an antiarrhythmic that decreases depolarization, automaticity, excitability of the ventricle during diastole by direct action.

PHARMACOKINETICS

Route	Onset	Peak	Duration
IV	30-90 seconds	NA	10-20 min
Local	2.5 min	NA	30-60 min anesthetic

Completely absorbed after IM administration. Protein binding: 60%-80%. Widely distributed. Metabolized in the liver. Primarily excreted in urine. Minimally removed by hemodialysis. *Half-life:* 1-2 h.

AVAILABILITY

IV Syringes, Prefilled, 10 mL: 10 mg/mL, 20 mg/mL.
IV Infusion: 4 mg/mL, 8 mg/mL.
Injection (Anesthesia): 0.5%, 1%, 1.5%, 2%, 4%.
Ointment: 2.5%, 5%.
Cream: 0.5%.
Gel: 0.5%, 2.5%.
Topical Spray: 0.5%.
Topical Solution: 2%, 4%.
Topical Jelly: 2%.
Dermal Patch (Lidoderm): 5%.
Viscous Oral Solution: 2%

INDICATIONS AND DOSAGES

▸ **Rapid control of acute ventricular arrhythmias after myocardial infarction, cardiac catheterization, cardiac surgery, or digitalis-induced ventricular arrhythmias**

IV

Adults, Elderly. Initially, 50-100 mg (1 mg/kg) IV bolus at rate of 25-50 mg/min. May repeat in 5 min. Give no more than 200-300 mg in 1 h. Maintenance: 20-50 mcg/kg/min (1-4 mg/min) as IV infusion.

Children, Infants. Initially, 0.5-1 mg/kg IV bolus; may repeat but total dose not to exceed 3-5 mg/kg. Maintenance: 10-50 mcg/kg/min as IV infusion.

▸ **Dental or surgical procedures, childbirth**

INFILTRATION OR NERVE BLOCK

Adults. Local anesthetic dosage varies with the procedure, degree of anesthesia, vascularity, duration. Maximum dose: 4.5 mg/kg. Do not repeat within 2 h.

▸ **Local skin disorders (minor burns, insect bites, prickly heat, skin manifestations of chickenpox, abrasions) and local anesthesia of nasal and laryngeal mucous membranes; relief of discomfort of pruritus ani, hemorrhoids, pruritus vulvae**

TOPICAL

Adults, Elderly. Apply to affected areas as needed. Refer to specific directions of product chosen.

▸ **Postherpetic neuralgia**

TOPICAL (DERMAL PATCH)

Adults, Elderly. Apply to intact skin over most painful area (up to 3 patches once for up to 12 h in a 24-h period).

▸ **Oral pain relief**

ORAL MUCOSAL APPLICATION (VISCOUS ORAL SOLUTIONS)

Adults. 15 mL no more than q3h undiluted as needed. For use in the mouth, swish around in the mouth and spit out. For use in the pharynx, gargle and may be swallowed. Maximum: 8 doses/24 h.

Children > 3 yr. Care must be taken to ensure correct dosage based on age and weight. For example, in a child of 5 yr weighing 50 lb, the dose should not exceed 75-100 mg (3.75-5 mL); do not give more often than q3h. Maximum: 8 doses/24 h.

Infants and Children < 3 yr. 1.25 mL of the solution should be accurately measured and applied to the immediate area with a cotton-tipped

L

applicator. Give no sooner than at 3-h intervals. Not more than 4 doses should be given in a 12-h period.

▸ **Typical dosage for urethral anesthesia**

TOPICAL (JELLY)

Adults. Instill 15 mL (male) or 3-5 mL (female) of 2% jelly or solution into the urethra.

CONTRAINDICATIONS

Adams-Stokes syndrome, hypersensitivity to amide-type local anesthetics, septicemia (spinal anesthesia), supraventricular arrhythmias, Wolff-Parkinson-White syndrome.

L

INTERACTIONS

Drug

Anticonvulsants: May increase cardiac depressant effects.

β-Adrenergic blockers: May increase risk of toxicity.

Other antiarrhythmics: May increase cardiac effects.

Herbal

None known.

Food

None known.

DIAGNOSTIC TEST EFFECTS

Therapeutic blood level is 1.5-6 mcg/mL; toxic blood level is > 6 mcg/mL. Monitor ECG.

IV INCOMPATIBILITIES

Amphotericin B complex (Abelcet, AmBisome, Amphotec), caspofungin (Cancidas), diazepam, haloperidol, lansoprazole (Prevacid), milrinone, nesiritide (Natrecor), pantoprazole (Protonix), phenobarbital, phenytoin, thiopental.

IV COMPATIBILITIES

Aminophylline, amiodarone (Cordarone), calcium gluconate, digoxin (Lanoxin), diltiazem (Cardizem), dobutamine (Dobutrex), dopamine (Intropin), enalapril (Vasotec), furosemide (Lasix), heparin, insulin, nitroglycerin, potassium chloride.

SIDE EFFECTS

Central nervous system (CNS) effects are generally dose-related and of short duration.

Occasional

IM: Pain at injection site.

Topical: Burning, stinging, tenderness at application site.

Rare

Generally with high dose: Drowsiness; dizziness; disorientation; light-headedness; tremors; apprehension; euphoria; sensation of heat, cold, or numbness; blurred or double vision; ringing or roaring in ears (tinnitus); nausea.

SERIOUS REACTIONS

- Although serious adverse reactions to lidocaine are uncommon, high dosage by any route may produce cardiovascular depression, bradycardia, hypotension, arrhythmias, heart block, cardiovascular collapse, and cardiac arrest.
- Potential for malignant hyperthermia.
- CNS toxicity may occur, especially with regional anesthesia use, progressing rapidly from mild side effects to tremors, somnolence, seizures, vomiting, and respiratory depression.
- Methemoglobinemia (evidenced by cyanosis) has occurred following topical application of lidocaine for teething discomfort and laryngeal anesthetic spray.

PRECAUTIONS & CONSIDERATIONS

Caution is warranted in patients with atrial fibrillation, bradycardia, heart block, hypovolemia, liver disease, marked hypoxia, and severe respiratory depression. Be aware that lidocaine crosses the placenta and is distributed in breast milk. No age-related precautions have been noted in children. Elderly patients are more sensitive to the adverse effects of lidocaine. Lidocaine dose and rate of infusion should be reduced in elderly patients. In elderly patients, age-related renal impairment may require dosage adjustment. Chewing gum, drinking, or eating for 1 h after oral mucous membrane lidocaine application should be avoided; the swallowing reflex may be impaired, increasing risk of aspiration, and numbness of tongue or buccal mucosa may lead to trauma.

A loss of feeling or sensation will occur, and patients will need protection from trauma until anesthetic wears off. Hypersensitivity to amide anesthetics and lidocaine should be determined before beginning drug therapy. BP, pulse, respirations, ECG, and serum electrolytes should be obtained at baseline and periodically thereafter.

Storage

Store at room temperature.

Administration

! Keep resuscitative equipment and drugs, including O_2, readily available when administering lidocaine by any injectable route.

For IM administration, use 10% (100 mg/mL) and clearly identify the lidocaine preparation. Give injection in deltoid muscle because the blood level will be significantly higher than if the injection is given in gluteus muscle or lateral thigh. For transdermal use, may cut patch to size before removing adhesive backing.

! Use only lidocaine without preservative, clearly marked for IV use.

For IV infusion, prepare solution by adding 1 g to 1 L D5W to provide concentration of 1 mg/mL (0.1%). Know that commercially available preparations of 0.2%, 0.4%, and 0.8% may be used for IV infusion. Be aware that the maximum concentration is 4 g/250 mL. For IV push, use 1% (10 mg/mL) or 2% (20 mg/mL). Administer IV push at rate of 25-50 mg/min. Administer for IV infusion at rate of 1-4 mg/min (1-4 mL) and use a volume control IV set.

For topical use, be aware that this form is not for ophthalmic use. For skin disorders, apply directly to affected area or put on a gauze or bandage, which is then applied to the skin. For mucous membrane use, apply to desired area as per manufacturer's insert. Administer the lowest dosage possible that still provides anesthesia. Dermal patches may be cut to fit area.

Lindane (Gamma Benzene Hexachloride)

lin'dane

Hexit

Do not confuse lindane with lidocaine.

CATEGORY AND SCHEDULE

Pregnancy Risk Category: C

Classification: Anti-infectives, topical, dermatologics, scabicides/pediculicides

MECHANISM OF ACTION

A scabicidal agent that is directly absorbed by parasites and ova through the exoskeleton. *Therapeutic Effect:* Stimulates the nervous system resulting in seizures and death of parasitic arthropods.

PHARMACOKINETICS

May be absorbed systemically. Metabolized in liver. Excreted in the urine and feces. *Half-life:* 17-22 h.

AVAILABILITY

Lotion: 1%.
Shampoo: 1%.

INDICATIONS AND DOSAGES

NOTE: Only to be used in patients who cannot tolerate or have failed first-line treatment with safer medications.

▸ **Treatment of scabies**

TOPICAL

Adults, Elderly, Children weighing 110 lb (50 kg) or more. Apply thin layer. Massage on skin from neck to the toes. Bathe and remove drug after 8-12 h.

▸ **Head lice**

TOPICAL

Adults, Elderly, Children weighing 110 lb (50 kg) or more. Apply about 30 mL of shampoo to dry hair and massage into hair for 4 min. Add small amounts of water to hair until lather forms, then rinse hair thoroughly and comb with a fine-tooth comb to remove nits. Maximum: 60 mL of shampoo.

CONTRAINDICATIONS

Hypersensitivity to lindane or any component of the formulation, uncontrolled seizure disorders, crusted (Norwegian) scabies, acutely inflamed skin or raw, weeping surfaces, or other skin conditions that might increase systemic absorption.

INTERACTIONS

Drug

Drugs known to decrease seizure threshold (antipsychotics, etc.): Use caution due to neurotoxicity of lindane.

Herbal

None known.

Food

None known.

DIAGNOSTIC TEST EFFECTS

None known.

SIDE EFFECTS

Rare (< 1%)

Burning, stinging, cardiac arrhythmia, ataxia, dizziness, headache, restlessness, seizures, pain, alopecia, contact dermatitis, skin and adipose tissue may act as repositories, eczematous eruptions, pruritus, urticaria, nausea, vomiting, aplastic anemia, hepatitis, paresthesias, hematuria, pulmonary edema.

SERIOUS REACTIONS

- Seizures and death or serious reactions due to neurotoxicity; may occur even with proper, single-dose use.

PRECAUTIONS & CONSIDERATIONS

Lindane is second-line choice because of the potential for systemic absorption and CNS side effects, especially in children. Do not use in children < 50 kg. Caution should be used in people taking medications for seizures. Avoid use during pregnancy and when breastfeeding. Avoid using on infants. No age-related precautions have been noted in elderly patients. Clothing and bedding should be washed in hot water or by dry cleaning to remove infestation.

Administration

! Never apply more than 2 oz of lotion! Wait at least 1 h after bathing or showering to apply. Skin should be clean and free of any lotions, creams, or oils before lindane application. Apply a thin layer and massage onto clean, dry skin from the neck to the toes. Wait 8-12 h, then bathe or shower. Avoid contact with eyes or face.

Apply shampoo to clean, dry hair. Wait at least 1 h after washing hair before applying lindane shampoo. Hair should be washed with a shampoo that does not contain conditioner. Hair should be free of any lotions, oils, or creams before lindane application.

Because of the drug's toxicity, no more than 1 treatment should be applied.

Linezolid

li-nee'zoh-lid

★ Zyvox, 🍁 Zyvoxam

Do not confuse Zyvox with Zovirax or Vioxx.

CATEGORY AND SCHEDULE

Pregnancy Risk Category: C

Classification: Antibiotics, oxazolidinone derivative

MECHANISM OF ACTION

An oxazolidinone anti-infective that binds to a site on bacterial 23S ribosomal RNA, preventing the formation of a complex that is essential for bacterial translation. *Therapeutic Effect:* Bacteriostatic against enterococci and staphylococci; bactericidal against streptococci.

PHARMACOKINETICS

Rapidly and extensively absorbed after PO administration. Protein binding: 31%. Metabolized in the liver by oxidation. Excreted in urine. Removed by dialysis. *Half-life:* 4-5.4 h.

AVAILABILITY

Powder for Oral Suspension: 100 mg/5 mL.
Tablets: 400 mg, 600 mg.
Premixed IV Infusion: 2 mg/mL in 100-mL, 200-mL, 300-mL bags.

INDICATIONS AND DOSAGES

▸ **Vancomycin-resistant infections (VRE, VR-MSRA)**
PO, IV
Adults, Elderly, Children ≥ 12 yr. 600 mg q12h for 14-28 days.

▸ **Pneumonia, complicated skin and skin-structure infections**
PO, IV
Adults, Elderly, Children ≥ 12 yr. 600 mg q12h for 10-14 days.

▸ **Uncomplicated skin and skin-structure infections**
PO
Adults, Elderly. 400 mg q12h for 10-14 days.

▸ **Usual pediatric dosage**
Children ≥ 12 yr. 600 mg q12h.
Children aged 5-11 yr. 10 mg/kg/dose q8-12h.

▸ **Usual neonate dosage**
PO, IV
Neonates. 10 mg/kg/dose q8-12h.

CONTRAINDICATIONS

Hypersensitivity to oxazolidinones or any of their components. Use within 14 days of an MAOI, uncontrolled hypertension.

INTERACTIONS

Drug

Adrenergic agents (indirect-acting sympathomimetics) and vasopressors (dopaminergic drugs, phenylephrine, pseudoephedrine, epinephrine): May increase pressor effects.

L

MAOIs: Additive side effects. Contraindicated.
SSRI antidepressants and other serotonergic drugs: Occasional reports of serotonin syndrome with co-use. Avoid use if possible.
Herbal
None known.
Food
Tyramine-containing foods and beverages: Excessive amounts may cause hypertension.

DIAGNOSTIC TEST EFFECTS

May decrease blood hemoglobin, platelet count, WBC count, and ALT (SGPT) levels; monitor platelet counts and CBC in patients at risk for bleeding.

L

IV INCOMPATIBILITIES

Do not mix with other drugs while infusing.

Amphotericin B complex (Abelcet, AmBisome, Amphotec), chlorpromazine (Thorazine), co-trimoxazole (Bactrim), diazepam (Valium), erythromycin (Erythrocin), pantoprazole (Protonix), pentamidine (Pentam IV), phenytoin (Dilantin), thiopental.

SIDE EFFECTS

Occasional (2%-5%)
Diarrhea, nausea, headache.
Rare (< 2%)
Altered taste, vaginal candidiasis, fungal infection, dizziness, tongue discoloration.

SERIOUS REACTIONS

- Thrombocytopenia and myelosuppression occur rarely.
- Antibiotic-associated colitis and other superinfections may result from altered bacterial balance.
- Serotonin syndrome or hypertension with serotonergic or pressor agents (rare).

PRECAUTIONS & CONSIDERATIONS

Caution is warranted in patients with carcinoid syndrome, pheochromocytoma, severe renal or hepatic impairment, uncontrolled hypertension, or untreated hyperthyroidism. It is unknown whether linezolid is distributed in breast milk. The safety and efficacy of linezolid have not been established in children. No age-related precautions have been noted in elderly patients. Avoid excessive amounts of tyramine-containing foods (such as aged cheese and red wine) because these foods may cause severe reactions and increased hypertension, including diaphoresis, neck stiffness, palpitations, and severe headache. May promote overgrowth of nonsusceptible bacterial strains; monitor platelet counts in patients at risk for bleeding.

Mild GI effects may be tolerable, but severe symptoms may indicate the onset of antibiotic-associated colitis. Pattern of daily bowel activity and stool consistency should be monitored. Be alert for signs and symptoms of superinfection, including abdominal pain, moderate to severe diarrhea, severe anal or genital pruritus, fever or fatigue, and severe mouth soreness. CBC should be monitored weekly.
Storage
Use the oral suspension within 21 days of reconstitution. Store the drug at room temperature and protect it from light. A yellow color does not affect potency. Keep infusion bags in overwrap until ready to use. Protect from freezing.
Administration
Take oral linezolid without regard to food. May take with food or milk if GI upset occurs. Space drug doses evenly around the clock, and

continue linezolid therapy for the full course of treatment.

! Do not mix linezolid for IV use with other medications. If the same line is used to administer another drug, flush it with a compatible fluid (D5W, 0.9% NaCl, lactated Ringer's). Infuse the drug over 30-120 min.

Liothyronine T_3

lye-oh-thye'roe-neen

Cytomel, Triostat Cytomel

Do not confuse liothyronine with levothyroxine.

CATEGORY AND SCHEDULE

Pregnancy Risk Category: A

Classification: Thyroid hormone

MECHANISM OF ACTION

A synthetic form of triiodothyronine (T_3), a thyroid hormone involved in normal metabolism, growth, and development, especially of the central nervous system in infants. Possesses catabolic and anabolic effects. *Therapeutic Effect:* Increases basal metabolic rate, enhances gluconeogenesis, and stimulates protein synthesis.

PHARMACOKINETICS

PO: Peak 12-48 h. *Half-life:* 0.6-1.4 days.

AVAILABILITY

Tablets (Cytomel): 5 mcg, 25 mcg, 50 mcg.
Injection (Triostat): 10 mcg/mL.

INDICATIONS AND DOSAGES

▸ **Hypothyroidism**

PO

Adults, Elderly. Initially, 25 mcg/day. May increase in increments of 12.5-25 mcg/day q1-2wk. Maximum: 100 mcg/day.
Children. Initially, 5 mcg/day. May increase by 5 mcg/day q3-4wk. Maintenance: 100 mcg/day (children older than 3 yr); 50 mcg/day (children 1-3 yr); 20 mcg/day (infants).

▸ **Myxedema**

PO

Adults, Elderly. Initially, 5 mcg/day. Increase by 5-10 mcg q1-2wk (after 25 mcg/day has been reached, may increase in 12.5-mcg increments). Maintenance: 50-100 mcg/day.

▸ **Nontoxic goiter**

PO

Adults, Elderly. Initially, 5 mcg/day. Increase by 5-10 mcg/day q1-2wk. When 25 mcg/day has been reached, may increase by 12.5-25 mcg/day q1-2wk. Maintenance: 75 mcg/day.
Children. 5 mcg/day. May increase by 5 mcg q1-2wk. Maintenance: 15-20 mcg/day.

▸ **Congenital hypothyroidism**

PO

Children. Initially, 5 mcg/day. Increase by 5 mcg/day q3-4 days. Maintenance: Full adult dosage (children older than 3 yr); 50 mcg/day (children 1-3 yr); 20 mcg/day (infants).

▸ **T_3 suppression test**

PO

Adults, Elderly. 75-100 mcg/day for 7 days; then repeat ^{131}I thyroid uptake test.

▸ **Myxedema coma, precoma**

IV

Adults, Elderly. Initially, 25-50 mcg (10-20 mcg in patients with cardiovascular disease). Total dose at least 65 mcg/day.

CONTRAINDICATIONS

Hypersensitivity to tablet components; myocardial infarction; thyrotoxicosis uncomplicated by hypothyroidism; uncorrected adrenal

L

insufficiency (may cause acute adrenal crisis); treatment of obesity.

INTERACTIONS

Drug

Antidiabetic drugs: As thyroid replacement ensues, antidiabetic requirements may change; monitor.
Cholestyramine, colestipol, enteral feedings, antacids, calcium and iron supplements: May decrease the absorption of liothyronine.
Digoxin: May alter digoxin dose requirements as thyroid function corrected due to increased metabolic rate; monitor.
Ketamine: May cause tachycardia or hypertension.
Oral anticoagulants: May alter the effects of these drugs.
Sympathomimetics: May increase the risk of coronary insufficiency and the effects of liothyronine.

Herbal

None known.

Food

None known.

DIAGNOSTIC TEST EFFECTS

None known.

SIDE EFFECTS

Occasional

Reversible hair loss at start of therapy (in children).

Rare

Dry skin, GI intolerance, rash, hives, pseudotumor cerebri or severe headache in children.

SERIOUS REACTIONS

- Excessive dosage produces signs and symptoms of hyperthyroidism, including weight loss, palpitations, increased appetite, tremors, nervousness, tachycardia, hypertension, headache, insomnia, and menstrual irregularities.
- Cardiac arrhythmias occur rarely.

PRECAUTIONS & CONSIDERATIONS

Signs of excessive overdose should be reported immediately and include signs and symptoms of hyperthyroidism, including weight loss, palpitations, increased appetite, tremors, nervousness, tachycardia, hypertension, headache, insomnia, and menstrual irregularities.

Caution is warranted in patients with adrenal insufficiency, cardiovascular disease, coronary artery disease, diabetes insipidus, and diabetes mellitus. Liothyronine does not cross the placenta and is minimally excreted in breast milk. Maternal thyroid health is important to pregnancy and to proper lactation. No age-related precautions have been noted in children. Use caution in interpreting thyroid function test results in neonates. Elderly patients may be more sensitive to thyroid effects. Individualized dosages are recommended.

Reversible hair loss or increased aggressiveness may occur during the first few months of therapy. Notify the physician of chest pain, edema of feet or ankles, insomnia, nervousness, tremors, weight loss, or a pulse rate of 100 beats/min or more. Weight and vital signs, especially pulse rate and rhythm, should be monitored. Keep in mind that liothyronine may intensify the signs and symptoms of adrenal insufficiency, diabetes insipidus, diabetes mellitus, and hypopituitarism.

Also, know that adrenocortical steroids should be prescribed before thyroid therapy in persons with coexisting hypoadrenalism and hypothyroidism.

Storage

Store tablets and unopened vials at room temperature.

Administration

! Initial and subsequent dosages are based on the clinical status and response. Do not use different brands of liothyronine interchangeably because of problems with bioequivalence among manufacturers.

Take at the same time each day, preferably in the morning. Do not abruptly discontinue the drug; replacement therapy for hypothyroidism is lifelong.

Administer IV dose over 4 h but no longer than 12 h apart. For intravenous use only; may give without further dilution.

Liraglutide

lir'a-gloo'tide

Victoza

CATEGORY AND SCHEDULE

Pregnancy Risk Category: C

Classification: Antidiabetic agents, incretin mimetics

MECHANISM OF ACTION

A synthetic peptide similar to exenatide; 97% of the peptide sequence of liraglutide overlaps with human glucagon-like peptide-1 (GLP-1). Incretins, such as GLP-1, enhance glucose-dependent insulin secretion and exhibit other antihyperglycemic actions following their release into the circulation from the gut. Liraglutide is a GLP-1 receptor agonist that enhances glucose-dependent insulin secretion by the pancreatic β-cell, suppresses inappropriately elevated glucagon secretion, and slows gastric emptying. *Therapeutic Effect:* Lowers blood glucose concentration and also HbA1C over time.

PHARMACOKINETICS

Native GLP-1 has a very short half-life (< 1 min) and is not clinically useful; liraglutide has an extended therapeutic profile in comparison. Bioavailability following subcutaneous administration is roughly 55%. Maximum plasma concentration occurs 8-12 h after subcutaneous injection. There is no one organ responsible for liraglutide elimination. *Half-life:* 13 h.

AVAILABILITY

Injection (6 mg/mL): Available in prefilled pens that deliver doses of either 0.6 mg, 1.2 mg or 1.8 mg; each containing 60 doses.

INDICATIONS AND DOSAGES

▸ Type 2 diabetes mellitus

SC

Adults, Elderly. Initially, 0.6 mg once per day for 1 wk. The dose can be given at any time of day and without regard to meals. The initial dose is for titration to limit GI side effects and is not effective for glycemic control. After 1 wk, increase the dose to 1.2 mg once per day. Can then increase to 1.8 mg once per day if needed for glycemic control.

▸ Dosage in renal or hepatic impairment

Use usual dose, but use with caution due to lack of clinical data.

CONTRAINDICATIONS

Hypersensitivity to liraglutide or product components. Do not use in patients with a personal or family history of medullary thyroid carcinoma (MTC) or in patients with multiple endocrine neoplasia syndrome type 2 (MEN 2). Not for type 1 diabetes mellitus or diabetic ketoacidosis.

INTERACTIONS

Drug

β-Blockers: May mask signs of hypoglycemia.

Oral medications (e.g., oral contraceptives, antibiotics): Liraglutide may slow GI transit time. For oral medications dependent on normal transit times efficacy, such as contraceptives and antibiotics, it may be best to take those drugs at least 1 h before liraglutide, or at a meal or snack when liraglutide is not administered.

Corticosteroids: May increase blood sugar.

Digoxin: Liraglutide may reduce digoxin concentrations; monitor for clinical effect, etc.

Sulfonylureas: May increase risk of hypoglycemia; lower sulfonylurea dose may be needed.

Warfarin: May increase the effects of warfarin, resulting in increased INR. Monitor INR closely.

Herbal

Alfalfa, aloe, bilberry, bitter melon, burdock, celery, damiana, fenugreek, garcinia, garlic, ginger, ginseng (American), gymnema, marshmallow, stinging nettle: May enhance hypoglycemic effects.

Food

Alcohol: Hypoglycemia is more likely to occur if alcohol is ingested. High and chronic alcohol use may increase risk for pancreatitis.

DIAGNOSTIC TEST EFFECTS

Lowers blood sugar. May increase serum creatinine, amylase, or lipase.

SIDE EFFECTS

Frequent

Headache, nausea, diarrhea and antiliraglutide antibody formation. Nausea subsides with time.

Occasional

Gastroesophageal reflux (GERD), vomiting, constipation, hypoglycemia, nervousness, dizziness, dyspepsia, decreased appetite, asthenia, hyperhidrosis.

Rare

Injection site reaction, abdominal pain, eructation, flatulence, abdominal distention, taste disturbance, pruritus, urticaria, maculopapular rash.

SERIOUS REACTIONS

- Overdose may produce severe hypoglycemia, along with severe GI symptoms and vomiting.
- Pancreatitis, including nonfatal hemorrhagic and necrotizing pancreatitis.
- Rare reports of serious allergic reactions, including angioedema and serious rashes.
- Potential risk of thyroid tumor.

PRECAUTIONS & CONSIDERATIONS

For patients with a history of pancreatitis, selection of other antidiabetic medications is suggested (see Serious Reactions). Caution is warranted in patients with potential risk factors for pancreatitis (hypertriglyceridemia, alcoholism, other) and patients with significant GI disease (e.g., gastroparesis) where slowing of GI transit time may aggravate the condition. Also use with caution in patients with thyroid disease. Liraglutide may cause dose-dependent and treatment-duration-dependent thyroid C-cell tumors (adenomas and/or carcinomas). Be alert to conditions that alter blood glucose requirements or dietary intake, such as fever, increased activity, stress, or a surgical procedure. There are limited data in patients with organ dysfunction.

There are no data regarding liraglutide use during pregnancy. It is unknown whether the drug is distributed in breast milk; discontinuation of breastfeeding is recommended due to the potential tumorigenicity of the drug. Safety and efficacy of liraglutide have not been established in children. Hypoglycemia may be difficult to recognize in elderly patients. With time, development of antibodies to the drug may present as treatment failure.

Food intake and blood glucose should be monitored before and during therapy. Be aware of signs and symptoms of hypoglycemia (anxiety, cool wet skin, diplopia, dizziness, headache, hunger, numbness in the mouth, tachycardia, tremors) or hyperglycemia (deep rapid breathing, dim vision, fatigue, nausea, polydipsia, polyphagia, polyuria, vomiting); carry candy, sugar packets, or other sugar supplements for immediate response to hypoglycemia. Consult the physician when glucose demands are altered (such as with fever, heavy physical activity, infection, stress, trauma). Exercise, good personal hygiene (including foot care), not smoking, and weight control are essential parts of therapy.

Storage

Prior to first use, store pens in a refrigerator. Do not freeze. After initial use, the pen can be stored for 30 days at controlled room temperature or in a refrigerator. Keep the pen cap on when not in use. Protect from heat and sunlight. Always store the pen without an injection needle attached. This will reduce the potential for contamination, infection, and leakage.

Administration

For subcutaneous injection only. Doses are given any time of day and may be given without regard to meals.

If using a new pen, make sure you have prepared the pen for routine use. For routine use, wash hands. Pull off pen cap. The cartridge liquid should be clear, colorless, and free of particles. Attach the needle and dial in the pen dose as the manufacturer directs. Inject the dose SC as directed in the thigh, abdomen, or upper arm; rotate injection sites with each use. After injection, reset the pen, remove and dispose of the used needle properly, and store the pen for next use by replacing the pen cap.

L

Lisdexamfetamine

lis-dex-am-fet′a-meen

★ 🍁 Vyvanse

Do not confuse Vyvanse with Glucovance.

CATEGORY AND SCHEDULE

Pregnancy Risk Category: C

Controlled Substance Schedule: II

Classification: Adrenergic agonists, amphetamines, stimulants

MECHANISM OF ACTION

Lisdexafetamine is a prodrug of dextroamphetamine, an amphetamine that enhances the action of dopamine and norepinephrine by blocking their reuptake from synapses; also inhibits monoamine oxidase. May also modulate serotonergic pathways. Alters motor activity, mental alertness; decreases drowsiness, fatigue. *Therapeutic Effect:* Improves attention span, decreases distractibility, and decreases impulsivity.

PHARMACOKINETICS

Rapidly absorbed from the GI tract. Converted to dextroamphetamine and L-lysine, which is believed to occur by first-pass intestinal and/or hepatic metabolism. Not metabolized by CYP450. Plasma concentrations of unconverted lisdexamfetamine dimesylate are low and are nonquantifiable roughly 8 h after a dose. There is minor inhibition of CYP2D6 by dextroamphetamine. Dextroamphetamine metabolized in liver, and metabolites and drug excreted in urine; a small amount of lisdexamfetamine appears in feces. *Half-life:* Parent drug: < 1 h; dextroamphetamine: roughly 10 h in adults and 6-8 h in children.

AVAILABILITY

Capsules (Vyvanse): 20 mg, 30 mg, 40 mg, 50 mg, 60 mg, 70 mg.

INDICATIONS AND DOSAGES

▸ **Attention-deficit hyperactivity disorder (ADHD)**

PO

Adults, Children 6 yr and older. Initially, 30 mg once daily in the morning. Titrate at weekly intervals in increments of 10-20 mg if needed. Maximum: 70 mg/day given once daily in the morning.

CONTRAINDICATIONS

Advanced arteriosclerosis, agitated states, glaucoma, history of drug abuse, hypersensitivity to sympathomimetic amines, hyperthyroidism, moderate to severe hypertension, symptomatic cardiovascular disease, use during or within 14 days of MAOIs.

INTERACTIONS

Drug

Antihypertensives: May decrease efficacy of antihypertensives.

Antipsychotics: Efficacy of antipsychotics may be decreased.

β-Blockers: May increase the risk of bradycardia, heart block, and hypertension.

GI antacids, sodium bicarbonate, and urinary alkalinizers: Increase amphetamine absorption and decrease urinary elimination, respectively. Avoid concurrent use.

Lithium and neuroleptic medications: Antagonize effect of amphetamines; concurrent use not recommended.

MAOIs, linezolid: May prolong and intensify the effects of amphetamines, including severe hypertensive episodes. Contraindicated with MAOIs.

Meperidine: May increase the risk of hypotension, respiratory depression, seizures, and vascular collapse.

Methenamine and urinary acidifiers: Increase amphetamine elimination.

Other CNS stimulants: May increase the effects of amphetamines. Concurrent use not recommended.

SSRIs: May increase risk of serotonin syndrome.

Thyroid hormones: May increase the effects of either drug.

Tricyclic antidepressants: May increase cardiovascular effects of TCAs.

Dietary Supplements

Melatonin: Potential for additive neurologic and cardiac effects.

Food

None known.

DIAGNOSTIC TEST EFFECTS

May increase plasma corticosteroid concentrations.

SIDE EFFECTS

Frequent (≥ 5%)

Adults: Upper abdominal pain, diarrhea, nausea, fatigue, feeling

jittery, irritability, anorexia, decreased appetite, headaches, anxiety, and insomnia.
Children: Decreased appetite, dizziness, dry mouth, irritability, insomnia, upper abdominal pain, nausea, vomiting, and decreased weight.

Occasional

Tachycardia, palpitations, emotional lability, blurred vision.

Rare

Change in libido, allergic reactions, elevated blood pressure, chest pain, hallucinations or psychosis at normal doses.

SERIOUS REACTIONS

- CNS stimulant use associated with serious cardiovascular events and sudden death in patients with cardiac abnormalities or serious heart problems.
- Hypersensitivity reactions, including angioedema and anaphylaxis. Serious skin reactions, including Stevens-Johnson syndrome and toxic epidermal necrolysis have been reported.
- Overdose may produce skin pallor or flushing, arrhythmias, seizures, and psychosis.
- Abrupt withdrawal after prolonged use of high doses may produce lethargy.
- Prolonged administration to children with ADHD may inhibit growth. Patients who are not growing or gaining weight as expected may need to have their treatment interrupted.

PRECAUTIONS & CONSIDERATIONS

Amphetamines have a high potential for abuse; prolonged administration may lead to dependence. Misuse of amphetamines may cause sudden death and serious cardiovascular adverse events. Even normal prescription use may cause events in susceptible individuals. Stimulant products generally should not be used in those with known serious structural cardiac abnormalities, cardiomyopathy, serious heart rhythm abnormalities, or other serious cardiac problems that may place them at increased vulnerability to the sympathomimetic effects. Caution is warranted in debilitated and elderly patients and in those with hypertension, psychiatric disorders, seizure disorder, and Tourette syndrome (may exacerbate tics), or with a history of substance abuse. Safety and efficacy have not been established in children less than 6 yr of age; children under 3 yr should not receive amphetamine treatment. Avoid in pregnancy; amphetamines may cause premature delivery, low birth weight, or withdrawal symptoms in the neonate. Distributed in breast milk; breastfeeding should be avoided.

Mental status, BP, and weight should be assessed. Tasks that require mental alertness or motor skills should be avoided until response to the drug has been established. Monitor weight and growth status in children during treatment. Notify the physician if decreased appetite, dizziness, dry mouth, or pronounced nervousness occurs, or if there are unusual changes in behavior or moods. Patients who develop symptoms such as exertional chest pain, unexplained syncope, or other symptoms suggestive of cardiac disease during stimulant treatment should undergo a prompt cardiac evaluation.

Storage

Store capsules at room temperature in a tightly closed container.

Administration
Lisdexafetamine should be taken in the morning; giving the daily dose in the afternoon may cause insomnia.

The capsules may be taken with or without food. Take whole, or the capsule may be opened and the entire contents dissolved in a glass of water. The entire dose of solution should be consumed immediately. The dose of a single capsule should not be divided. Where possible, treatment should be interrupted occasionally to determine if there is a recurrence of behavioral symptoms sufficient to require continued treatment.

L

Lisinopril

ly-sin'oh-pril
Prinivil, Zestril Prinivil, Zestril, Apo-Lisinopril
Do not confuse Prinivil with Desyrel, fosinopril, or Plendil; or Zestril with Zostrix.

CATEGORY AND SCHEDULE

Pregnancy Risk Category: C (D if used in second or third trimester)

Classification: Antihypertensives, angiotensin-converting enzyme (ACE) inhibitors

MECHANISM OF ACTION

This ACE inhibitor suppresses the renin-angiotensin-aldosterone system and prevents the conversion of angiotensin I to angiotensin II, a potent vasoconstrictor; may also inhibit angiotensin II at local vascular and renal sites. Decreases plasma angiotensin II, increases plasma renin activity, and decreases aldosterone secretion.
Therapeutic Effect: Reduces peripheral arterial resistance, BP, afterload, pulmonary capillary wedge pressure (preload), pulmonary vascular resistance. In those with heart failure, also decreases heart size, increases cardiac output, and increases exercise tolerance time.

PHARMACOKINETICS

Route	Onset	Peak	Duration
PO	1 h	6 h	24 h

Incompletely absorbed from the GI tract. Protein binding: 25%. Primarily excreted unchanged in urine. Removed by hemodialysis.
Half-life: 12 h (half-life is prolonged in those with impaired renal function).

AVAILABILITY

Tablets (Prinivil, Zestril): 2.5 mg, 5 mg, 10 mg, 20 mg, 30 mg, 40 mg.

INDICATIONS AND DOSAGES

▸ **Hypertension (used alone)**
PO
Adults. Initially, 10 mg/day. May increase by 5-10 mg/day at 1- to 2-wk intervals. Maximum: 40 mg/day.
Elderly. Initially, 2.5-5 mg/day. May increase by 2.5-5 mg/day at 1- to 2-wk intervals. Maximum: 40 mg/day.
Children 6 yr of age or older. Initially, 0.07 mg/kg once daily (up to 5 mg total). Adjust according to BP response. Doses above 0.61 mg/kg (or 40 mg/day) have not been studied.

▸ **Hypertension (used in combination with other hypertensives)**
PO
Adults. Initially, 2.5-5 mg/day titrated to clinical response.

▸ Adjunctive therapy for management of heart failure
PO
Adults, Elderly. Initially, 2.5-5 mg/day. May increase by no more than 10 mg/day at intervals of at least 2 wks. Maintenance: 5-40 mg/day.

▸ Improve survival in patients after myocardial infarction (MI)
PO
Adults, Elderly. Initially, 5 mg, then 5 mg after 24 h, 10 mg after 48 h, then 10 mg/day for 6 wks. For patients with low systolic BP, give 2.5 mg/day for 3 days, then 2.5-5 mg/day.

▸ Dosage in renal impairment (adults)
Titrate to patient's response/tolerance after giving the following initial dose:

CrCl (mL/min)	Initial Dosage
> 30	10 mg once daily
10-30	5 mg once daily
< 10	2.5 mg once daily

OFF-LABEL USES
Treatment of hypertension or renal crises with scleroderma.

CONTRAINDICATIONS
Hypersensitivity, history of angioedema related to ACE inhibitors, hereditary or idiopathic angioedema.

INTERACTIONS
Drug
Alcohol, phenothiazines, diuretics, hypotensive agents: May increase hypotensive effects.
Gold compounds: May cause facial flushing, hypotension.
Lithium: May increase lithium blood concentration and risk of toxicity.
NSAIDs, indomethacin, sympathomimetics: May decrease hypotensive effects.
Potassium-sparing diuretics, drospirenone, eplerenone, potassium supplements: May cause hyperkalemia.
Herbal
None known.
Food
Salt substitutes: Rich in potassium, these should be avoided during treatment.

DIAGNOSTIC TEST EFFECTS
May increase BUN, serum alkaline phosphatase, serum bilirubin, serum creatinine, serum potassium, SGOT (AST), and SGPT (ALT) levels. May decrease serum sodium levels. May cause positive ANA titer.

SIDE EFFECTS
Frequent (5%-12%)
Headache, dizziness, postural hypotension.
Occasional (2%-4%)
Hyperkalemia, chest discomfort, fatigue, rash, abdominal pain, nausea, diarrhea, upper respiratory infection.
Rare (≤ 1%)
Palpitations, tachycardia, peripheral edema, insomnia, paresthesia, confusion, constipation, dry mouth, muscle cramps.

SERIOUS REACTIONS
- Excessive hypotension ("first-dose syncope") may occur in patients with congestive heart failure (CHF) and severe salt and volume depletion.
- Angioedema (swelling of face and lips) occurs rarely.
- Agranulocytosis and neutropenia may be noted in patients with collagen vascular disease, including

scleroderma and systemic lupus erythematosus, and impaired renal function.

• Nephrotic syndrome may be noted in patients with history of renal disease.

PRECAUTIONS & CONSIDERATIONS

Caution is warranted in patients with cerebrovascular and coronary insufficiency, hypovolemia, renal impairment, sodium depletion, and those on dialysis or receiving diuretics. Be aware that lisinopril crosses the placenta and that it is unknown whether lisinopril is distributed in breast milk; caution is warranted in lactation. Lisinopril has caused fetal or neonatal morbidity or mortality. Discontinue use as soon as possible after pregnancy is detected. Be aware that the safety and efficacy of lisinopril have not been established in children less than 6 yr of age. Elderly patients may be more sensitive to the hypotensive effects of lisinopril.

First-dose syncope may occur in patients with congestive heart failure and severe salt and fluid depletion.

Dizziness may occur. BP should be obtained immediately before giving each lisinopril dose, in addition to regular monitoring. Be alert to fluctuations in BP since orthostatic hypotension may occur; avoid rapid postural changes.

CBC and blood chemistry should be obtained before beginning lisinopril therapy, then every 2 wks for the next 3 mo, and periodically thereafter. Lungs should be ausculated for rales. Pattern of daily bowel activity and stool consistency should be assessed.

Storage
Store tablets at room temperature. Compounded suspension stored at or below 77 °F is stable for up to 4 wks; do not freeze.

Administration
Take lisinopril without regard to food. Crush tablets if necessary.

For pediatric patients, the manufacturer allows for the compounding of an oral suspension. Shake well before each use.

Lithium Carbonate/ Lithium Citrate

lith′ee-um kahr′buh-neyt/sit′rayte

★ Lithobid 🍁 Carbolith, Duralith, Lithane, Lithmax

Do not confuse Lithobid with Levbid, Lithostat, or Lithotabs.

CATEGORY AND SCHEDULE

Pregnancy Risk Category: D

Classification: Psychiatric agents; mood stabilizers.

MECHANISM OF ACTION

A psychotherapeutic agent that affects the storage, release, and reuptake of neurotransmitters. Antimanic effect may result from increased norepinephrine reuptake and serotonin receptor sensitivity. *Therapeutic Effect:* Produces antimanic and antidepressant effects.

PHARMACOKINETICS

Rapidly and completely absorbed from the GI tract. Primarily excreted unchanged in urine. Removed by hemodialysis. *Half-life:* 18-24 h (increased in elderly).

AVAILABILITY

Capsules: 150 mg, 300 mg, 600 mg.
Oral Solution: 300 mg/5 mL.

Tablets: 300 mg.
Tablets (Extended Release): 300 mg, 450 mg.

INDICATIONS AND DOSAGES

ALERT

During acute phase, a therapeutic serum lithium concentration of 1-1.4 mEq/L is required. For long-term control, the desired level is 0.5-1.3 mEq/L. Monitor serum drug concentration and clinical response to determine proper dosage.

▸ **Prevention or treatment of acute mania, manic phase of bipolar disorder (manic-depressive illness)**

PO

Adults. 300 mg 3-4 times a day or 450-900 mg slow-release form twice a day. Maximum: 2.4 g/day.
Elderly. 300 mg twice a day. May increase by 300 mg/day q1wk. Maintenance: 900-1200 mg/day.
Children 12 yr and older. 600-1800 mg/day in 3-4 divided doses (2 doses/day for slow release).
Children 6-12 yr. 15-60 mg/kg/day in 3-4 divided doses.

OFF-LABEL USES

Treatment of depression, treatment of SIADH.

CONTRAINDICATIONS

Debilitated patients, severe cardiovascular disease, severe dehydration, severe renal disease, severe sodium depletion, first trimester of pregnancy.

INTERACTIONS

Drug

Aspirin, indomethacin, other NSAIDs, metronidazole, carbamazepine: May increase risk of toxicity developing.
Antithyroid medications, iodinated glycerol, potassium iodide: May increase the effects of these drugs.
Diuretics, NSAIDs: May increase lithium serum concentration and risk of toxicity.
Haloperidol: May increase extrapyramidal symptoms and the risk of neurologic toxicity.
Molindone: May increase the risk of neurotoxicity.
Neuromuscular blocking agents: May increase effects of these drugs.
Phenothiazines: May decrease the absorption of phenothiazines, increase the intracellular concentration and renal excretion of lithium, and increase delirium and extrapyramidal symptoms. Antiemetic effect of some phenothiazines may mask early signs of lithium toxicity.

Herbal

None known.

Food

Caffeine: Excessive caffeine intake may alter lithium concentrations.
Enteral feedings: Physically incompatible; do not mix together.

DIAGNOSTIC TEST EFFECTS

May increase blood glucose, immunoreactive parathyroid hormone, and serum calcium levels. Therapeutic lithium serum level is 0.6-1.2 mEq/L; toxic serum level is > 1.5 mEq/L.

SIDE EFFECTS

! Side effects are dose related and seldom occur at lithium serum levels < 1.5 mEq/L.

Occasional

Fine hand tremor, polydipsia, polyuria, mild nausea.

Rare

Weight gain, bradycardia or tachycardia, acne, rash, muscle twitching, cold and cyanotic extremities, pseudotumor cerebri (eye pain, headache, tinnitus, vision disturbances).

SERIOUS REACTIONS

- A lithium serum concentration of 1.5-2.0 mEq/L may produce vomiting, diarrhea, drowsiness, confusion, incoordination, coarse hand tremor, muscle twitching, and T-wave depression on ECG.
- A lithium serum concentration of 2.0-2.5 mEq/L may result in ataxia, giddiness, tinnitus, blurred vision, clonic movements, and severe hypotension.
- Acute toxicity may be characterized by seizures, oliguria, circulatory failure, coma, and death.

PRECAUTIONS & CONSIDERATIONS

Caution is warranted in patients with thyroid disease, renal impairment, or cardiovascular disease as well as those receiving medications that alter sodium such as diuretics, ACE inhibitors, and NSAIDs. Caution should also be used if there is a risk of suicide. Lithium crosses the placenta and is excreted in breast milk. Children and elderly are more sensitive to an increased drug dosage and have a higher risk for toxicity. Steady salt and fluid intake should be maintained, especially during summer months.

Serum lithium should be monitored every 4-5 days during initial therapy, then every 1-3 mo when stable. Draw lithium serum concentrations 8-12 h after dose. Closely supervise patients during early therapy. Patients with renal impairment need close monitoring and careful dosing.

Storage

Store at room temperature; protect from moisture.

Administration

Take with food or milk if GI distress occurs. Extended-release tablets must be swallowed whole. Do not crush or chew. Drink 2-3 L of water daily.

Lithium solution may be diluted with fruit juice or other flavored beverage. However, do not mix with other liquid medications or with enteral feedings as incompatibilities may form.

Lodoxamide Tromethamine

loe-dox′a-mide troh-meth′aye-meen

★ 🍁 Alomide

CATEGORY AND SCHEDULE

Pregnancy Risk Category: B

Classification: Mast cell stabilizers, ophthalmics

MECHANISM OF ACTION

A mast cell stabilizer that prevents an increase in cutaneous vascular permeability and antigen-stimulated histamine release and that may prevent calcium influx into mast cells. *Therapeutic Effect:* Inhibits sensitivity reaction.

PHARMACOKINETICS

Nondetectable absorption. *Half-life:* 8.5 h.

AVAILABILITY

Ophthalmic Solution: 0.1% (Alomide).

INDICATIONS AND DOSAGES

▸ **Treatment of vernal keratoconjunctivitis, conjunctivitis, keratitis**

OPHTHALMIC

Adults, Elderly, Children 2 yr or older. 1-2 drops 4 times/day, for up to 3 mo.

CONTRAINDICATIONS

Wearing soft contact lenses (product contains benzalkonium chloride) or hypersensitivity to lodoxamide tromethamine or any component of the formulation.

INTERACTIONS

Drug
None known.
Herbal
None known.
Food
None known.

DIAGNOSTIC TEST EFFECTS

None known.

SIDE EFFECTS

Frequent
Transient stinging, burning, instillation discomfort.
Occasional
Ocular itching, blurred vision, dry eye, tearing/discharge/foreign body sensation, headache.
Rare
Scales on lid or lash, ocular swelling, sticky sensation, dizziness, somnolence, nausea, sneezing, dry nose, rash.

SERIOUS REACTIONS

- None reported.

PRECAUTIONS & CONSIDERATIONS

Be aware that lodoxamide tromethamine is for ophthalmic use only. Not for injection. It is unknown whether lodoxamide tromethamine crosses the placenta or is distributed in breast milk. Be aware that the safety and efficacy of lodoxamide tromethamine have not been established in children younger than 2 yr. No age-related precautions have been noted in elderly patients. Continuous use for longer than 2 wks could result in dry mouth.
Storage
Store at room temperature.
Administration
Tilt the patient's head back; place solution in conjunctival sac. Close eyes, then press gently on the lacrimal sac for 1 min. Do not wear soft contact lenses during therapy. Therapy may last up to 3 mo.

Loperamide

loe-per'a-mide
★ Imodium A-D, Immodium A-D EZ Chews 🍁 Diarr-Eze, Imodium
Do not confuse Imodium with Indocin or Ionamin.

CATEGORY AND SCHEDULE

Pregnancy Risk Category: C
OTC liquid, tablets

Classification: Antidiarrheals, opioids

MECHANISM OF ACTION

An antidiarrheal that directly affects the intestinal wall muscles. *Therapeutic Effect:* Slows intestinal motility and prolongs transit time of intestinal contents by reducing fecal volume, diminishing loss of fluid and electrolytes, and increasing viscosity and bulk of stool.

PHARMACOKINETICS

Poorly absorbed from the GI tract. Protein binding: 97%. Metabolized in the liver. Eliminated in feces and excreted in urine. Not removed by hemodialysis. *Half-life:* 9.1-14.4 h.

AVAILABILITY

Capsules: 2 mg.
Liquid: 1 mg/5 mL or 1 mg/7.5 mL, both OTC.
Tablets: 2 mg (OTC).
Chewable Tablets: 2 mg (OTC).

INDICATIONS AND DOSAGES

▸ **Acute diarrhea**
PO (CAPSULES)

Adults, Elderly. Initially, 4 mg; then 2 mg after each unformed stool. Maximum: 16 mg/day.
Children aged 9-12 yr, weighing more than 30 kg. Initially, 2 mg 3 times a day for 24 h. Maintenance: 0.1 mg/kg given only after loose stool. Maximum: 6 mg/day.
Children aged 6-8 yr, weighing 20-30 kg. Initially, 2 mg twice a day for 24 h. Maintenance: 0.1 mg/kg given only after loose stool. Maximum: 4 mg/day.
Children aged 2-5 yr, weighing 13-20 kg. Initially, 1 mg 3 times/day for 24 h. Maintenance: 0.1 mg/kg only after loose stool.

▸ **Chronic diarrhea**
PO
Adults, Elderly. Initially, 4 mg; then 2 mg after each unformed stool until diarrhea is controlled.
Children. 0.08-0.24 mg/kg/day in 2-3 divided doses. Maximum: 2 mg/dose.

▸ **Traveler's diarrhea (to reduce bowel movement frequency and enable travel while awaiting antibiotics)**
PO
Adults, Elderly. Initially, 4 mg; then 2 mg after each loose bowel movement (LBM). Maximum: 8 mg/day for 2 days.
Children 9-11 yr. Initially, 2 mg; then 1 mg after each LBM. Maximum: 6 mg/day for 2 days.
Children 6-8 yr. Initially, 1 mg; then 1 mg after each LBM. Maximum: 4 mg/day for 2 days.

CONTRAINDICATIONS

Hypersensitivity, acute ulcerative colitis (may produce toxic megacolon), diarrhea associated with pseudomembranous enterocolitis from broad-spectrum antibiotics or with organisms that invade intestinal mucosa (such as *Escherichia coli,* shigella, and salmonella), patients who must avoid constipation, patients with undiagnosed abdominal pain in absence of diarrhea, those with dysentery.

INTERACTIONS

Drug
Opioid (narcotic) analgesics: May increase the risk of constipation.
Herbal
None known.
Food
None known.

DIAGNOSTIC TEST EFFECTS

None known.

SIDE EFFECTS

Rare
Dry mouth, somnolence, abdominal discomfort, allergic reaction (such as rash and itching).

SERIOUS REACTIONS

• Toxicity results in constipation, GI irritation, including nausea and vomiting, and central nervous system (CNS) depression. Activated charcoal is used to treat loperamide toxicity.

PRECAUTIONS & CONSIDERATIONS

Caution is warranted in patients with fluid and electrolyte depletion and hepatic impairment. It is unknown whether loperamide crosses the placenta or is distributed in breast milk. Loperamide use is not recommended in children younger than 6 yr. Infants younger than 3 mo are more susceptible to CNS effects. Loperamide use in elderly patients may mask dehydration and electrolyte depletion. Tasks that require mental alertness or motor skills should be avoided until response to the drug has been established. Alcohol should also be avoided during drug therapy.

Dry mouth may occur. Notify the physician if abdominal distention and pain, diarrhea that does not stop within 3 days, or fever occurs. Pattern of daily bowel activity and stool consistency and hydration status should be monitored.

Storage

Store at room temperature.

Administration

Do not give if bloody diarrhea is present or temperature is > 101° F. When administering the oral liquid to children, use the accompanying plastic dropper to measure the liquid.

Lopinavir/Ritonavir

lop-in'a-veer/rit-on'a-veer

Kaletra

Do not confuse Kaletra with Keppra.

CATEGORY AND SCHEDULE

Pregnancy Risk Category: C

Classification: Antiretrovirals, protease inhibitors

MECHANISM OF ACTION

A protease inhibitor combination drug in which lopinavir inhibits the activity of the enzyme protease late in the HIV replication process and ritonavir increases plasma levels of lopinavir. *Therapeutic Effect:* Formation of immature, noninfectious viral particles.

PHARMACOKINETICS

Readily absorbed after PO administration (absorption increased when taken with food). Protein binding: 98%-99%. Metabolized in the liver. Eliminated primarily in feces. Not removed by hemodialysis. *Half-life:* 5-6 h.

AVAILABILITY

Oral Solution: 80 mg/mL lopinavir/20 mg/mL ritonavir.
Tablets: 100 mg lopinavir/25 mg ritonavir; 200 mg lopinavir/50 mg ritonavir.

INDICATIONS AND DOSAGES

▸ **HIV infection (monotherapy)**

PO

Adults. 400 mg lopinavir/100 mg ritonavir or 5 mL twice a day. Increase to (500 mg lopinavir/125 mg ritonavir) 6.5 mL when taken with efavirenz or nevirapine.

Children aged 6 mo to 12 yr. General: Dose based on lopinavir component of combination:

Children weighing more than 40 kg who are not taking amprenavir, efavirenz, or nevirapine. PO adult dose.

Children weighing 15-40 kg who are not taking efavirenz or nevirapine. 10 mg/kg twice a day.

Children weighing 7-14 kg who are not taking amprenavir, efavirenz, nelfinavir, or nevirapine. 12 mg/kg twice a day.

▸ **HIV infection concomitant therapy with amprenavir, efavirenz, nelfinavir, or nevirapine**

Adults. 400 mg lopinavir/100 mg ritonavir or 5 mL twice a day. Increase to (500 mg lopinavir/125 mg ritonavir) 6.5 mL when taken with efavirenz or nevirapine.

Children aged 6 mo to 12 yr. General: Dose based on lopinavir component of combination:

Children weighing 15-40 kg who are taking efavirenz or nevirapine.

11 mg/kg twice a day.
Children weighing 7-14 kg who are taking amprenavir, efavirenz, or nevirapine. 13 mg/kg twice a day.
Children weighing more than 45 kg who are taking amprenavir, efavirenz, or nevirapine. PO adult dose.

▸ **HIV infection in therapy-naïve patients**
PO
Adults. 400/100 mg twice daily or 800/200 mg once daily. Once daily only for those without resistance mutations.

▸ **HIV infection in therapy-experienced patients**
PO
Adults. 400/100 mg twice daily.

▸ **HIV infection concomitant therapy with amprenavir, efavirenz, nelfinavir, nevirapine**
PO
Adults. A dose increase in lopinavir/ritonavir to 500/125 mg 2 times a day with food is recommended when combined.

CONTRAINDICATIONS

Coadministration with drugs that are highly dependent on CYP3A4 for clearance and for which elevated plasma levels are associated with serious and or life-threatening reactions (astemizole, cisapride, conivaptan, dihydroergotamine, ergonovine, ergotamine, methylergonovine, midazolam, pimozide, ranolazine, sulfasalazine, terfenadine, triazolam).

Hypersensitivity to lopinavir or ritonavir or any of its components; breastfeeding.

INTERACTIONS

! NOTE: Many medications are contraindicated with, or must be used cautiously with, protease inhibitors like ritonavir. Check manufacturer's recommendations for drug interaction management.

Drug

Abacavir, amprenavir, atovaquone, lamotrigine, methadone, oral contraceptives, phenytoin, zidovudine: May reduce serum levels of these drugs, decreasing efficacy.

Antiarrhythmic agents (amiodarone, bepridil, lidocaine systemic, quinidine), antifungal agents (itraconazole, ketoconazole), atorvastatin, buspirone, calcium channel blockers (amiodipine, diltiazem, felodipine, nicardipine, nifedepine), cetirizine, clarithromycin, cyclosporine, dihydropyridine, fexofenadine, fluticasone, phosphodiesterase type 5 inhibitors (sildenafil, tadalafil, vardenafil), protease inhibitors (amprenavir, indinavir, nelfinavir, saquinavir), rifabutin, tacrolimus, tenofovir, trazodone: May increase levels of these drugs, increasing adverse pharmacologic and adverse reactions.

Astemizole, cisapride, conivaptan ergot derivatives (dihydroergotamine, ergonovine, ergotamine, methylergonovine), HMG-CoA reductase inhibitors (lovastatin, simvastatin), midazolam, pimozide, ranolazine, rifampin, sulfasalazine, terfenadine, triazolam: Contraindicated due to potentially life-threatening reactions.

Carbamazepine, dexamethasone, NNRTIs (efavirenz, nevirapine), phenobarbital, pheytoin, protease inhibitors (amprenavir, fosamprenavir, nelfinavir), rifampin: May reduce lopinavir concentrations, decreasing efficacy.

Delavirdine, ritonavir: May elevate lopinavir concentrations, increasing efficacy and adverse effects.
Didanosine: Must be given 1 h before or 2 h after lopinavir/ritonavir capsules or oral solution.
Disulfiram, metronidazole: May produce a disulfiram-like reaction when administered with the oral solution, which contains alcohol.
Oral contraceptives: May decrease efficacy; advise patient to use alternative nonhormonal contraception during therapy.
Warfarin: May affect efficacy; monitor INR levels.
Herbal
St. John's wort: May decrease blood concentration and effects of lopinavir and ritonavir. Avoid.
Food
None known.

DIAGNOSTIC TEST EFFECTS

May increase blood glucose, GGT, total cholesterol, total bilirubin, total cholesterol, and serum uric acid (at least 2%), AST (SGOT), ALT (SGPT), and triglyceride levels, INR.

SIDE EFFECTS

Frequent (14%)
Mild to moderate diarrhea.
Occasional (2%-6%)
Nausea, asthenia, abdominal pain, headache, vomiting.
Rare (< 2%)
Insomnia, rash. Redistribution/accumulation of body fat including buffalo hump, hypercholesterolemia, hyperglycemia with insulin resistance or new-onset diabetes mellitus.

SERIOUS REACTIONS

- Anemia, leukopenia, lymphadenopathy, deep vein thrombosis, Cushing syndrome, and hemorrhagic colitis occur rarely.
- Pancreatitis and hepatotoxicity occur rarely.

PRECAUTIONS & CONSIDERATIONS

! Lopinavir/ritonavir oral solution contains alcohol and should not be given to those receiving metronidazole because this combination may cause a disulfiram-type reaction. Caution is warranted with hepatitis B or C or impaired liver function and pancreatitis where fatalities have been reported. Be aware that it is unknown whether lopinavir/ritonavir is excreted in breast milk. Breastfeeding is not recommended in this population because of the possibility of HIV transmission. Be aware that the safety and efficacy of lopinavir/ritonavir have not been established in children younger than 6 mo. In elderly patients, age-related cardiac function, renal, or liver impairment requires caution. Lopinavir/ritonavir is not a cure for HIV infection, nor does it reduce risk of transmission to others.

Alcohol-related toxicity may occur because of the 42.5% alcohol content of the oral solution; caution warranted in using this product or any other alcohol-containing product or beverage.

Women should be advised to use another nonhormonal-based contraceptive while taking this medication.

Expect to establish baseline values for CBC, renal and liver function tests, and weight. Assess for nausea and vomiting, pattern of daily bowel activity and stool consistency, and signs and symptoms of pancreatitis as evidenced by abdominal pain, nausea, and vomiting. Eat small, frequent meals to offset nausea or vomiting. Evaluate for signs and symptoms of opportunistic infections as evidenced by cough, onset of fever, oral mucosal changes, or other respiratory symptoms. Check the weight at least twice a week.

Storage

Refrigerate until dispensed, and avoid exposure to excessive heat. If stored at room temperature, use within 2 mo.

Administration

Tablets may be taken without regard to food. Oral solution should be given with food to improve absorption. The oral solution is highly concentrated and the dosage ordered should be double-checked to the weight and age of the patient to avoid overdosage. Do not administer lopinavir/ritonavir as a once-daily regimen in combination with amprenavir, efavirenz, nelfinavir, or nevirapine; once-daily administration of lopinavir/ritonavir is not recommended in therapy-experienced patients.

L

Loratadine

loer-at'ah-deen

★ Alavert, Claritin, Claritin Children's, Claritin Liqui-Gels, Claritin RediTabs, Dimetapp, Tavist ND 🍁 Claritin, Claritin Kids

CATEGORY AND SCHEDULE

Pregnancy Risk Category: B

Classification: OTC

Antihistamines, H_1 histamine antagonist, nonsedating

MECHANISM OF ACTION

A long-acting antihistamine that competes with histamine for H_1 receptor sites on effector cells. *Therapeutic Effect:* Prevents allergic responses mediated by histamine, such as rhinitis, urticaria, and pruritus.

PHARMACOKINETICS

Route	Onset	Peak	Duration
PO	1-3 h	8-12 h	Longer than 24 h

Rapidly and almost completely absorbed from the GI tract. Protein binding, 97%; metabolite, 73%-77%. Distributed mainly to the liver, lungs, GI tract, and bile. Metabolized in the liver to active metabolite; undergoes extensive first-pass metabolism. Eliminated in urine and feces. Not removed by hemodialysis. *Half-life:* 8.4 h; metabolite, 28 h (increased in elderly and hepatic impairment).

AVAILABILITY

Syrup (Claritin): 5 mg/5 mL.
Tablets (Alavert, Claritin, Tavist ND): 10 mg.
Tablets (Rapid Disintegrating [Alavert, Claritin RediTabs]): 10 mg.
Chewable Tablets (Claritin Children's): 5 mg
Liquid-Filled Capsule (Claritin Liqui-Gels): 10 mg.

INDICATIONS AND DOSAGES

▸ **Allergic rhinitis, urticaria**

PO

Adults, Elderly, Children 6 yr and older. 10 mg once a day.
Children 2-5 yr. 5 mg once a day.

▸ **Dosage in hepatic impairment**

For adults, elderly, and children 6 yr and older, dosage is reduced to 10 mg every other day. Children 2-5 yr, reduce to 5 mg every other day.

CONTRAINDICATIONS

Hypersensitivity to loratadine or its ingredients.

INTERACTIONS

Drug

All central nervous system (CNS) depressants, alcohol: May increase CNS depressive effects.

Anticholinergics, antihistamines, antiparkinsonian drugs: May increase anticholinergic effects.
Clarithromycin, erythromycin, fluconazole, ketoconazole: May increase the loratadine blood concentration.
Conscious sedation drugs: May cause synergistic sedative activity.
Herbal
None known.
Food
All foods: Delay the absorption of loratadine.

DIAGNOSTIC TEST EFFECTS

May suppress wheal and flare reactions to antigen skin testing unless the drug is discontinued 4 days before testing.

SIDE EFFECTS

Frequent (8%-12%)
Headache, fatigue, somnolence.
Occasional (3%)
Dry mouth, nose, or throat.
Rare
Photosensitivity.

SERIOUS REACTIONS

- None known.

PRECAUTIONS & CONSIDERATIONS

Caution should be used in breastfeeding women, children, and those with hepatic impairment. Loratadine is excreted in breast milk. Children and elderly patients are more sensitive to the drug's anticholinergic effects, such as dry mouth, nose, and throat. Avoid exposure to sunlight, drinking alcoholic beverages, and tasks that require alertness or motor skills until response to the drug is established.

Drowsiness and dry mouth may occur. Respiratory rate, depth, and rhythm; pulse rate and quality; BP; and therapeutic response should be monitored.

Storage
Store at room temperature. Protect RediTabs or ODT form from moisture; keep in foil until time of use. Once package open, use within 6 mo.
Administration
May take oral forms without regard to food. For ODT or RediTabs: Place on tongue; allow to dissolve and then swallow. May be administered with or without water. Chewable tablets are chewed thoroughly then swallowed with water.

Lorazepam

lor-a'ze-pam
★ Ativan, Lorazepam Intensol
🍁 Apo-Lorazepam, Ativan, Novolorazepam, Nu-Loraz
Do not confuse lorazepam with alprazolam.

CATEGORY AND SCHEDULE

Pregnancy Risk Category: D
Controlled Substance Schedule: IV

Classification: Anxiolytics, benzodiazepines

MECHANISM OF ACTION

A benzodiazepine that enhances the action of the inhibitory neurotransmitter γ-aminobutyric acid in the CNS, affecting memory, as well as motor, sensory, and cognitive function. *Therapeutic Effect:* Produces anxiolytic, anticonvulsant, sedative, muscle relaxant, and antiemetic effects.

PHARMACOKINETICS

Route	Onset (min)	Peak	Duration (h)
PO	60	NA	8-12
IV	15-30	NA	8-12
IM	30-60	NA	8-12

Well absorbed after PO and IM administration. Protein binding: 85%. Widely distributed. Metabolized in the liver. Primarily excreted in urine. Not removed by hemodialysis. *Half-life:* 10-20 h.

AVAILABILITY

Tablets (Ativan): 0.5 mg, 1 mg, 2 mg.
Injection (Ativan): 2 mg/mL, 4 mg/mL.
Oral Solution (Lorazepam Intensol): 2 mg/mL.

INDICATIONS AND DOSAGES

▸ **Anxiety**

PO

Adults. 1-10 mg/day in 2-3 divided doses. Average: 2-6 mg/day.
Elderly. Initially, 1-2 mg/day. May increase gradually. Range: 0.5-4 mg.

IV

Adults, Elderly. 0.044 mg/kg or 2 mg single dose, whichever is smaller. Repeat doses may be given every 6-8 h as needed.

IV INFUSION

Adults, Elderly. 0.01-0.1 mg/kg/h.

PO, IV

Children. 0.05 mg/kg/dose q4-8h. Range: 0.02-0.1 mg/kg. Maximum: 2 mg/dose.

▸ **Insomnia due to anxiety**

PO

Adults. 2-4 mg at bedtime.
Elderly. 0.5-1 mg at bedtime.

▸ **Preoperative sedation**

IV

Adults, Elderly. 0.044 mg/kg 15-20 min before surgery. Maximum total dose: 2 mg.

IM

Adults, Elderly. 0.05 mg/kg 2 h before procedure. Maximum total dose: 4 mg.

▸ **Status epilepticus**

IV

Adults, Elderly. 4 mg over 2-5 min. May repeat in 10-15 min. Maximum: 8 mg in 12-h period.
Children. 0.1 mg/kg over 2-5 min. May give second dose of 0.05 mg/kg in 15-20 min. Maximum: 4 mg.
Neonates. 0.05 mg/kg. May repeat in 10-15 min.

OFF-LABEL USES

Treatment of alcohol withdrawal, panic disorders, skeletal muscle spasms, chemotherapy-induced nausea or vomiting, tension headache, tremors; adjunctive treatment before endoscopic procedures (diminishes patient recall).

CONTRAINDICATIONS

Angle-closure glaucoma; pre-existing CNS depression. Known sensitivity to benzodiazepines or injection vehicle (polyethylene glycol, propylene glycol, and benzyl alcohol), patients with sleep apnea or other severe respiratory insufficiency, except in those mechanically ventilated. The use of the injection intra-arterially is contraindicated because it may produce arteriospasm resulting in gangrene, which may require amputation.

INTERACTIONS

Drug

Alcohol, other CNS depressants, probenecid: May increase CNS depression.
Opioid analgesics: Increases CNS effects; reduce dosage by a third in elderly patients.
Scopolamine: Possible increased sedation, hallucination.

Herbal

Kava kava, valerian: May increase CNS depression.

Food

None known.

DIAGNOSTIC TEST EFFECTS

None known. Therapeutic serum drug level is 50-240 mg/mL; toxic serum drug level is unknown.

IV INCOMPATIBILITIES

Aldesleukin (Proleukin), ampicillin, aztreonam (Azactam), idarubicin (Idamycin), ondansetron (Zofran), pantoprazole, sufentanil (Sufenta).

IV COMPATIBILITIES

Bumetanide (Bumex), cefepime (Maxipime), diltiazem (Cardizem), dobutamine (Dobutrex), dopamine (Intropin), heparin, labetalol (Normodyne, Trandate), milrinone (Primacor), norepinephrine (Levophed), piperacillin and tazobactam (Zosyn), potassium, propofol (Diprivan).

SIDE EFFECTS

Frequent
Somnolence (initially in the morning), ataxia, confusion.
Occasional
Blurred vision, slurred speech, hypotension, headache.
Rare
Paradoxical CNS restlessness or excitement in elderly or debilitated.

SERIOUS REACTIONS

- Abrupt or too-rapid withdrawal may result in pronounced restlessness, irritability, insomnia, hand tremor, abdominal or muscle cramps, diaphoresis, vomiting, and seizures.
- Overdose results in somnolence, confusion, diminished reflexes, and coma.

PRECAUTIONS & CONSIDERATIONS

Caution is warranted in patients with pulmonary, hepatic, and renal impairment and in those using other CNS depressants concurrently. Lorazepam may cross the placenta and be distributed in breast milk. Lorazepam may increase the risk of fetal abnormalities if administered during the first trimester of pregnancy. Women on long-term therapy should use effective contraception during therapy and notify the physician immediately if they become or might be pregnant. Chronic lorazepam use during pregnancy may produce withdrawal symptoms in the patient and CNS depression in the neonate. The safety and efficacy of this drug have not been established in children younger than 12 yr. In elderly patients, expect to give small doses initially and to increase dosage gradually to avoid ataxia and excessive sedation.

Lorazepam may be abused by those with addictive propensities; psychologic and physical dependence may occur with chronic administration.

Elderly persons are more prone to orthostatic hypotension and anticholinergic and sedative effects; it may be advisable to reduce their dosages.

Drowsiness and dizziness may occur. Change positions slowly from recumbent, to sitting, before standing to prevent dizziness or orthostatic hypotension from developing. Alcohol, caffeine, and tasks that require mental alertness or motor skills should also be avoided. BP, heart rate, respiratory rate, CBC with differential, and hepatic and renal function should be monitored.

Storage
Oral forms should be stored at room temperature; protect oral solution from light. Refrigerate—do not freeze—parenteral form.

Administration
Take oral lorazepam with food. Crush tablets as needed.

Do not use the solution for injection if it appears discolored or contains a precipitate. Dilute with an equal volume of sterile water for injection, 0.9% NaCl, or D5W. To dilute a prefilled syringe, remove air from a half-filled syringe, aspirate an equal volume of diluent, pull the plunger back slightly to allow for mixing, and gently invert the syringe several times—do not shake vigorously. Give by IV push into the tubing of a free-flowing IV infusion of 0.9% NaCl or D5W at a rate not exceeding 2 mg/min. Keep recumbent after parenteral administration to reduce the drug's hypotensive effect.

For IM use, inject the drug deep into a large muscle mass, such as the gluteus maximus.

Losartan

lo-sar'tan

Cozaar

Do not confuse Cozaar with Zocor.

CATEGORY AND SCHEDULE

Pregnancy Risk Category: C (D if used in second or third trimesters)

Classification: Antihypertensives, angiotensin II receptor antagonists

MECHANISM OF ACTION

An angiotensin II receptor, type AT_1, antagonist that blocks vasoconstrictor and aldosterone-secreting effects of angiotensin II, inhibiting the binding of angiotensin II to the AT_1 receptors. *Therapeutic Effect:* Causes vasodilation, decreases peripheral resistance, and decreases BP.

PHARMACOKINETICS

Route	Onset	Peak	Duration
PO	N/A	6 h	24 h

Well absorbed after PO administration. Protein binding: 98%. Undergoes first-pass metabolism in the liver to active metabolites. Excreted in urine and via the biliary system. Not removed by hemodialysis. *Half-life:* 2 h, metabolite: 6-9 h.

AVAILABILITY

Tablets: 25 mg, 50 mg, 100 mg.

INDICATIONS AND DOSAGES

▸ **Hypertension**

PO

Adults, Elderly. Initially, 50 mg once a day. Maximum: May be given once or twice a day, with total daily doses ranging from 25 to 100 mg.

Children 6 yr of age and older. Initially, 0.7 mg/kg once daily (up to 50 mg total). Adjust according to BP response. Doses > 1.4 mg/kg (or > 100 mg) daily have not been studied.

▸ **Diabetic nephropathy**

PO

Adults, Elderly. Initially, 50 mg/day. May increase to 100 mg/day based on BP response.

▸ **Stroke prophylaxis**

PO

Adults, Elderly. 50 mg/day. Maximum: 100 mg/day.

▸ **Hypertension in patients with impaired hepatic function**

PO

Adults, Elderly. Initially, 25 mg/day.

CONTRAINDICATIONS

Hypersensitivity, second or third trimester of pregnancy.

INTERACTIONS

Drug

Cimetidine: May increase the effects of losartan.

Fluconazole, ketoconazole, troleandomycin: Suspected increase in antihypertensive effects; monitor BP if used concurrently.

General anesthetics: May increase risk of hypotensive episode.

Lithium: May increase lithium blood concentration and risk of lithium toxicity.
Other hypotensive drugs and sedatives: May increase hypotensive effects.
Phenobarbital, rifampin: May decrease hypotensive effects of losartan.
Herbal
None known.
Food
Grapefruit juice: May alter the absorption of losartan.

DIAGNOSTIC TEST EFFECTS

May increase BUN, serum alkaline phosphatase, serum bilirubin, serum creatinine, serum potassium, AST (SGOT), and ALT (SGPT) levels. May decrease blood hemoglobin and hematocrit levels.

SIDE EFFECTS

Frequent (8%)
Upper respiratory tract infection.
Occasional (2%-4%)
Dizziness, diarrhea, cough, hyperkalemia.
Rare (≤ 1%)
Insomnia, dyspepsia, heartburn, back and leg pain, muscle cramps, myalgia, nasal congestion, sinusitis.

SERIOUS REACTIONS

- Overdosage may manifest as hypotension and tachycardia. Bradycardia occurs less often.
- Angioedema (rare).

PRECAUTIONS & CONSIDERATIONS

Caution is warranted in patients with hepatic and renal impairment and renal arterial stenosis. Losartan has caused fetal or neonatal morbidity or mortality and may adversely affect the breastfed infant. Patients should not breastfeed while taking losartan. Safety and efficacy of losartan have not been established in children. No age-related precautions have been noted in elderly patients.

Apical pulse and BP should be assessed immediately before each losartan dose and regularly throughout therapy. Be alert to fluctuations in apical pulse and BP. If an excessive reduction in BP occurs, place the person in the supine position with feet slightly elevated and notify the physician. BUN, serum electrolytes, serum creatinine levels, heart rate, urinalysis, and pattern of daily bowel activity and stool consistency should be assessed. Maintain adequate hydration; exercising outside during hot weather should be avoided to decrease the risk of dehydration and hypotension.

Storage
Store tablets at room temperature. Compounded suspension is stable under refrigeration for up to 4 wks.
Administration
Take losartan without regard to food. Do not crush or break tablets.

For pediatric patients, the manufacturer allows for the compounding of an oral suspension. Shake well before each use.

Lovastatin

lo'va-sta-tin
★ 🍁 Altoprev, Mevacor
Do not confuse with Leustatin, Livostin, or Mivacron.

CATEGORY AND SCHEDULE

Pregnancy Risk Category: X

Classification:
Antihyperlipidemics, HMG-CoA reductase inhibitors

MECHANISM OF ACTION

An antihyperlipidemic that inhibits HMG-CoA reductase, the enzyme that catalyzes the early step in cholesterol synthesis. *Therapeutic Effect:* Decreases LDL cholesterol, VLDL cholesterol, plasma triglycerides; increases HDL cholesterol.

PHARMACOKINETICS

Route	Onset	Peak	Duration
PO	3 days	4-6 wks	NA

Incompletely absorbed from the GI tract (increased on empty stomach). Protein binding: 95%. Hydrolyzed in the liver to active metabolite. Primarily eliminated in feces. Not removed by hemodialysis. *Half-life:* 1.1-1.7 h.

AVAILABILITY

Tablets (Mevacor): 10 mg, 20 mg, 40 mg.
Tablets (Extended Release [Altoprev]): 20 mg, 40 mg, 60 mg.

INDICATIONS AND DOSAGES

▸ Hyperlipoproteinemia, primary prevention of coronary artery disease

PO

Adults, Elderly. Initially, 20 mg/day with evening meal. Increase at 4-wk intervals up to maximum of 80 mg/day. Maintenance: 20-80 mg/day in single or divided doses.
Children 10-17 yr. 10-40 mg/day with evening meal.

PO (EXTENDED RELEASE)

Adults, Elderly. Initially, 20 mg/day. May increase at 4-wk intervals up to 60 mg/day.

▸ Heterozygous familial hypercholesterolemia

PO

Children aged 10-17 yr. Initially, 10 mg/day. May increase to 20 mg/day after 8 wks and 40 mg/day after 16 wks if needed.

CONTRAINDICATIONS

Hypersensitivity, active liver disease, pregnancy, unexplained elevated liver function tests, lactation, rhabdomyolysis. See Drug Interactions for contraindicated drugs.

INTERACTIONS

Drug

Amiodarone, verapamil: Do not exceed lovastatin 40 mg/day.
Cyclosporine, gemfibrozil, other fibrates, danazol, niacin: Increases the risk of acute renal failure, myalgia, and rhabdomyolysis. Do not exceed lovastatin 20 mg/day.
Erythromycin, itraconazole, clarithromycin, HIV protease inhibitors, ergot alkaloids, nefazodone, ketoconazole: Contraindicated.

Herbal

None known.

Food

Grapefruit juice: Large amounts of grapefruit juice may increase risk of side effects, such as myalgia and weakness. Avoid.

DIAGNOSTIC TEST EFFECTS

May increase serum creatinine kinase and serum transaminase concentrations.

SIDE EFFECTS

Generally well tolerated. Side effects usually mild and transient.

Frequent (5%-9%)

Headache, flatulence, diarrhea, abdominal pain or cramps, rash and pruritus.

Occasional (3%-4%)

Nausea, vomiting, constipation, dyspepsia.

Rare (1%-2%)
Dizziness, heartburn, myalgia, blurred vision, eye irritation.

SERIOUS REACTIONS

- There is a potential for cataract development.
- Hepatotoxicity or rhabdomyolysis.

PRECAUTIONS & CONSIDERATIONS

Caution is warranted in patients with history of heavy or chronic alcohol use, renal impairment, and those who use cyclosporine, fibrates, and niacin. Be aware that lovastatin use is contraindicated in pregnancy because the suppression of cholesterol biosynthesis may cause fetal toxicity and in lactation because it is unknown whether lovastatin is distributed in breast milk. Be aware that the safety and efficacy of lovastatin have not been established in children younger than 10 yr. No age-related precautions have been noted in elderly patients.

Notify the physician of changes in the color of stool or urine, muscle weakness, myalgia, severe gastric upset, rash, unusual bruising, vision changes, or yellowing of eyes or skin. Pattern of daily bowel activity and stool consistency should be assessed. Serum cholesterol and triglyceride levels and hepatic function should be checked at baseline and periodically during treatment.

Be aware that diet is an important part of treatment.

Storage
Lovastatin should be kept at room temperature in a container with low light exposure.

Administration
Take lovastatin immediate-release tablets with the evening meal for best effectiveness. Administer extended-release tablets in the evening at bedtime, preferably without food (to increase absorption); do not crush or chew. Do not administer lovastatin with grapefruit juice.

Loxapine

lox′a-peen

★ Loxitane 🍁 Apo-Loxapine, Loxapac, Xylac

CATEGORY AND SCHEDULE

Pregnancy Risk Category: C

Classification: Antipsychotics

MECHANISM OF ACTION

A dibenzodiazepine derivative that interferes with the binding of dopamine at postsynaptic receptor sites in the brain. Strong anticholinergic effects. *Therapeutic Effect:* Suppresses locomotor activity, produces tranquilization.

PHARMACOKINETICS

Onset of action occurs within 1 h. Metabolized to active metabolites 8-hydroxyloxapine, 7-hydroxyloxapine, and 8-hydroxyamoxapine. Excreted in urine. *Half-life:* 4 h.

AVAILABILITY

Capsules: 5 mg, 10 mg, 25 mg, 50 mg (Loxitane).

INDICATIONS AND DOSAGES

▸ **Psychotic disorders**

PO

Adults. 10 mg 2 times/day. Increase dosage rapidly during first week to 50 mg, if needed. Usual therapeutic, maintenance range: 60-100 mg daily in 2-4 divided doses. Maximum: 250 mg/day.

CONTRAINDICATIONS

Severe central nervous system (CNS) depression, comatose states, hypersensitivity to loxapine or any component of the formulation.

INTERACTIONS

Drug

Alcohol, all CNS depressants: May increase CNS depressant effects.
Antacids, antidiarrheals: May decrease absorption of loxapine.
Anticholinergics: May increase effects of both drugs.
Extrapyramidal symptom (EPS)-producing medications: May increase risk of EPS.
Sympathomimetics, carbamazepine: May decrease effect of these drugs.

Herbal

None known.

Food

None known.

DIAGNOSTIC TEST EFFECTS

None known.

SIDE EFFECTS

Frequent

Blurred vision, confusion, drowsiness, dry mouth, dizziness, light-headedness.

Occasional

Allergic reaction (rash, itching), decreased urination, constipation, decreased sexual ability, enlarged breasts, headache, photosensitivity, nausea, vomiting, insomnia, weight gain.

SERIOUS REACTIONS

- Extrapyramidal symptoms frequently noted are akathisia (motor restlessness, anxiety). Less frequently noted are akinesia (rigidity, tremor, salivation, mask-like facial expression, reduced voluntary movements). Infrequently noted dystonias: torticollis (neck muscle spasm), opisthotonos (rigidity of back muscles), and oculogyric crisis (rolling back of eyes). Tardive dyskinesia (protrusion of tongue, puffing of cheeks, chewing/puckering of mouth) occurs rarely but may be irreversible. Risk is greater in elderly women.
- Seizures.

PRECAUTIONS & CONSIDERATIONS

Extreme caution should be used in patients with a history of seizures. Caution is also warranted with cardiovascular disease, glaucoma, prostatic hypertrophy, and urinary retention. It is unknown whether loxapine crosses the placenta or is distributed in breast milk. Safety and efficacy of loxapine have not been established in children under the age of 16 yr. Elderly patients are more susceptible to anticholinergic effects and sedation, increased risk for extrapyramidal effects, and orthostatic hypotension. A decreased dosage is recommended in elderly patients. Avoid alcohol and tasks that require mental alertness or motor skills.

Assess for presence of extrapyramidal motor symptoms, such as tardive dyskinesia and akathisia.

Storage

Store at room temperature.

Administration

Give loxapine with food or a full glass of water or milk to decrease GI irritation. The full therapeutic effect may take up to 6 wks. Do not abruptly discontinue loxapine.

Lubiprostone

loo-bee-pros′tone

Amitiza

CATEGORY AND SCHEDULE

Pregnancy Risk Category: C

Classification: Gastrointestinal agents, GI regulators, laxatives

MECHANISM OF ACTION

A bicyclic fatty acid, prostaglandin E1 (PGE 1) derivative. Increases intestinal fluid secretion by activating specific ClC-2 chloride channels in the luminal cells of the intestinal epithelium. *Therapeutic Effect:* Alters stool consistency and promotes regular bowel movements, without altering serum electrolyte concentrations or producing tolerance.

PHARMACOKINETICS

Minimal absorption following oral administration. Plasma concentrations below the level of quantification, and pharmacokinetic parameters cannot be calculated. Plasma levels of the only known active metabolite are also very low. Minimal distribution occurs beyond the GI tissues.

AVAILABILITY

Capsules, Gelatin (Amitiza): 8 mcg, 24 mcg.

INDICATIONS AND DOSAGES

▸ **Treatment of idiopathic chronic constipation**

PO

Adults, Elderly. 24 mcg twice per day. If intolerance occurs, may reduce to 24 mcg once daily.

▸ **Treatment of irritable bowel syndrome (IBS), constipation-predominant**

PO

Adult, Elderly females. 8 mcg twice per day. If intolerance occurs, may reduce to once daily. Not proved effective in males.

CONTRAINDICATIONS

Hypersensitivity, known or suspected mechanical GI obstruction.

INTERACTIONS

Drug

None known.

Herbal and Food

None.

DIAGNOSTIC TEST EFFECTS

Rare reports of increased AST or ALT.

SIDE EFFECTS

Frequent

Nausea, mild abdominal discomfort, flatulence, loose stools.

Occasional

Diarrhea, headache, dizziness, dyspepsia, dry mouth.

Rare

Fecal incontinence, mild cramps, defecation urgency, frequent bowel movements, hyperhidrosis, anxiety, cold sweat, constipation, cough, dysgeusia, eructation, decreased appetite, myalgia.

SERIOUS REACTIONS

- Chest tightness and dyspnea.
- Severe watery diarrhea (stop drug).
- Allergic-type reactions (including rash, swelling, and throat tightness).

PRECAUTIONS & CONSIDERATIONS

If severe diarrhea occurs, it can lead to fluid and electrolyte imbalance. Do not use in patients with diarrhea-predominant IBS. There are no adequate data in human pregnancy, and there are no data for use during breastfeeding. Lubiprostone is a prostaglandin derivative and is generally not recommended for use in pregnancy due to its chemical classification. Not approved for use in children.

Increasing fluid intake, exercising, and eating a high-fiber diet should be instituted to promote defecation. Notify the physician if dyspnea within an hour of the dosage, unrelieved constipation, dizziness, severe diarrhea, or rectal bleeding weakness occurs. Hydration status, daily bowel activity, and stool consistency should be assessed.

Storage

Store at room temperature; protect from excessive heat.

Administration

Swallow capsules whole with water. Do not cut, crush, or chew. Administer doses in the morning and evening as prescribed. May give with food to reduce nausea. If excessive loose stools occur, a reduction in dose to once daily may alleviate their occurrence.

Mafenide

ma'fe-nide

★ Sulfamylon

CATEGORY AND SCHEDULE

Pregnancy Risk Category: C

Classification: Anti-infectives, topical, dermatologics, sulfonamides

MECHANISM OF ACTION

A topical anti-infective that decreases number of bacteria in avascular tissue of second- and third-degree burns. *Therapeutic Effect:* Bacteriostatic. Promotes spontaneous healing of deep partial-thickness burns.

PHARMACOKINETICS

Absorbed through devascularized areas into systemic circulation following topical administration. Excreted in the form of its metabolite rho-carboxybenzenesulfonamide.

AVAILABILITY

Cream: 85 mg base/g (Sulfamylon).
Powder for Topical Solution: 5%.

INDICATIONS AND DOSAGES

▸ **Burns**

TOPICAL (CREAM)

Adults, Elderly, Children. Apply 1-2 times/day.

CONTRAINDICATIONS

Hypersensitivity to mafenide or sulfonamides or any other component of the formulation.

INTERACTIONS

Drug

None known.

Herbal

None known.

Food

None known.

DIAGNOSTIC TEST EFFECTS

None known.

SIDE EFFECTS

Difficult to distinguish side effects and effects of severe burn.

Frequent

Pain, burning upon application.

Occasional

Allergic reaction (usually 10-14 days after initiation): itching, rash, facial edema, swelling; unexplained syndrome of marked hyperventilation with respiratory alkalosis.

Rare

Delay in eschar separation, excoriation of new skin.

SERIOUS REACTIONS

• Hemolytic anemia, porphyria, bone marrow depression, superinfections (especially with fungi), metabolic acidosis occur rarely.

PRECAUTIONS & CONSIDERATIONS

Caution is warranted with impaired renal function because of the risk of metabolic acidosis. Be aware that cross-sensitivity to sulfonamides is not certain. It is unknown whether mafenide crosses the placenta or is distributed in breast milk. Be aware that mafenide is not recommended in newborn infants because sulfonamides may cause kernicterus. No age-related precautions have been noted in elderly patients.

Signs and symptoms of metabolic acidosis should be monitored.

Storage

Store cream at room temperature.

Administration

Mafenide is for external use only. Apply cream with gloved hands. Burned area should be kept covered with mafenide at all times. Apply to thickness of around 16 mm. For details of preparation and use of topical solution for burns, see manufacturer literature. Dressings may be moistened every 6-8 h as necessary.

Magnesium Hydroxide, Aluminum Hydroxide, Simethicone

mag-nee'zee-um hi-drox'ide, ah-loo'mih-num hi-drox'ide, sye-meth'i-cone

★ Almacone, Maalox, Maalox Max, Maalox Multi-Symptom Suspension, Mag-Al Plus, Mintox Plus, Mylanta, Mylanta Maximum Strength, Rulox

CATEGORY AND SCHEDULE

Pregnancy Risk Category: C

Classification: Gastrointestinal agents, antacid-antigas combination

MECHANISM OF ACTION

An antacid combination that reduces gastric acid. Simethicone disperses gas pockets within the GI tract. *Therapeutic Effect:* Neutralizes acid and increases gastric pH; alleviates GI symptoms and eliminates gas.

PHARMACOKINETICS

In GI tract, antacids react with hydrochloric acid to form chloride salts and water, neutralizing the acid. Roughly 15%-30% of the magnesium chloride formed is available for oral absorption. Most aluminum chloride formed combines with dietary elements in the intestine and is excreted primarily via the feces. Any magnesium systemically absorbed is utilized in the body or excreted by the kidneys. Simethicone is not systemically absorbed. Magnesium may accumulate with chronic use in severe renal impairment.

AVAILABILITY

Chewable Tablets: 200 mg aluminum hydroxide, 200 mg magnesium hydroxide, and 25 mg simethicone per tablet.
Suspension, Regular Strength: 200 mg aluminum hydroxide, 200 mg magnesium hydroxide, and 20 mg simethicone/5 mL.
Suspension, Maximum Strength: 400 mg aluminum hydroxide, 400 mg magnesium hydroxide, and 40 mg simethicone/5 mL.

INDICATIONS AND DOSAGES

▸ **Antacid (with flatulence)**

PO

Adults, Elderly, Children 12 yr of age or older. 10-20 mL or 2-4 chewable tablets 4-6 times/day.

CONTRAINDICATIONS

Not recommended for those with severe renal impairment; hypermagnesemia.

INTERACTIONS

Drug

Bisphosphonates, ketoconazole, quinolones, tetracyclines: Antacids may decrease absorption of these medications; separate times of administration.
Methenamine: May decrease effects of methenamine.

Herbal

None known.

Food

None known.

DIAGNOSTIC TEST EFFECTS

May increase serum gastrin levels and gastric pH.

SIDE EFFECTS

Frequent

Chalky taste, mild constipation, stomach cramps, diarrhea.

Occasional

Nausea, vomiting.

Rare

Hypermagnesemia, hypophosphatemia, osteomalacia.

SERIOUS REACTIONS

- Prolonged constipation may result in intestinal obstruction.
- Excessive or chronic use may produce hypophosphatemia.
- Prolonged use may produce urinary calculi.

PRECAUTIONS & CONSIDERATIONS

Use caution in using magnesium- and aluminum-containing antacids in patients with mild to moderate renal impairment. Caution is warranted with Alzheimer disease, chronic diarrhea, cirrhosis, constipation, dehydration, edema, fecal impaction, fluid restrictions, gastric outlet obstruction, undiagnosed GI or rectal bleeding, heart failure, low sodium diets, symptoms of appendicitis, and in elderly patients. Do not use in children 6 yr or younger without physician approval. Elderly patients may be at increased risk of constipation and fecal impaction.

Storage

Store at room temperature.

Administration

Administer 1-3 h after meals for best antacid effect. Expect the dosage to be individualized based on the neutralizing capacity of the antacid. For chewable tablets, thoroughly chew before swallowing and then drink a glass of water or milk. If administering a suspension, shake well before use.

Magnesium Salts

mag-nee′zee-um salts

Magnesium Citrate

★ Magnesium Hydroxide Phillips Milk of Magnesia, Phillips′ Concentrated Milk of Magnesia, Ex-Lax Milk of Magnesia

★ Magnesium Chloride Mag-64, Slow-Mag

★ Magnesium Gluconate Mag-G, Magtrate, Magonate

★ Magnesium Oxide Uro-Mag, MagOx 400, Phillips′ Cramp Free Caplets

Magnesium Sulfate

Do not confuse magnesium sulfate with manganese sulfate or morphine sulfate.

To avoid prescription confusion, never abbreviate formulas chemically.

CATEGORY AND SCHEDULE

Pregnancy Risk Category: A (parenteral use)

Magnesium citrate, hydroxide, and oxide (OTC).

Most other forms are Rx only.

Classification: Nutritional supplements, electrolytes, minerals, laxatives, antacids

MECHANISM OF ACTION

Magnesium citrate: A hyperosmotic saline laxative that acts by osmotically drawing water into the intestinal lumen; the intestine responds with increased peristalsis and release of cholecystokinin. *Therapeutic Effect:* Produces bowel evacuation and laxative effect.

M

Magnesium hydroxide: Also known as milk of magnesia, is used PO primarily as a laxative. As a relatively nonabsorbable cation, magnesium hydroxide is considered a saline laxative. It is also used as an antacid, primarily in combination products with aluminum hydroxide (see separate monograph).

Magnesium sulfate, oxide, gluconate, and chloride: Primarily used as electrolyte and mineral replacement. This electrolyte is found primarily in intracellular fluids and is essential for enzyme activity, nerve conduction, and muscle contraction. Stabilizes cardiac muscle and conduction. Magnesium sulfate can act as an anticonvulsant; it blocks neuromuscular transmission and the amount of acetylcholine released at the motor endplate. *Therapeutic Effect:* Maintains and restores magnesium levels. Stabilizes nerve conduction and electronic activity.

PHARMACOKINETICS

Oral dosage forms have roughly 15%-30% absorption. IM injection onsets within about an hour; IV effect is immediate. Widely distributed. Approximately one-half of the total body magnesium is in soft tissue; most of the remaining is in bone. Less than 1% of the total body magnesium is present the blood. Crosses the placenta and is excreted into breast milk. Not metabolized. Elimination occurs renally. Approximately 12 mEq of magnesium is excreted in the urine daily and some is reabsorbed in the thick ascending limb of the loop of Henle.

AVAILABILITY

Magnesium citrate
Oral Solution (Citrate of Magnesia): 291 mg/5 mL (also available in low-sodium formula).

Magnesium hydroxide
Oral Liquid (Milk of Magnesia, various): 400 mg/5 mL, 800 mg/5 mL.
Chewable Tablets (Phillips' Milk of Magnesia): 311 mg.

Magnesium chloride
Delayed-Release Tablets (Mag-64): 64 mg.
Enteric-Coated Tablets with added calcium (Slow-Mag): 143 mg.

Magnesium gluconate
Oral Solution (Magonate): 100 mg/5 mL.
Tablets (Mag-G, Magtrate): 500 mg.

Magnesium oxide
Tablets (MagOx 400): 400 mg.
Capsules (Uro-Mag): 140 mg.
Caplets for Constipation (Phillips' Cramp Free Laxative Caplets): 500 mg.

Magnesium sulfate
Premix IVPB Infusion Solution: 1 g/100 mL, 2 g/100 mL.
Injection: 50% (4 mEq/mL or 5 g/10 mL).
Topical Powder for Soaks (Epsom Salts)

INDICATIONS AND DOSAGES

▸ **Dietary supplement (magnesium oxide)**

PO

Adults, Elderly. 400-800 mg PO per day in 1-2 divided doses, dose adjusted depending on patient status. Doses may be given up to 3 times per day for short-term use if deficiency is present.

▸ **Dietary supplement (magnesium chloride)**

PO

Adults, Elderly. 64-429 mg/day in 1-4 divided doses; dose adjusted depending on patient status.

▸ **Dietary supplement (magnesium gluconate)**

PO

Adults, Elderly. 500 mg given 1-3 times per day; dose adjusted depending on patient status.

M

▸ **Acute hypomagnesemia (usual dosages, magnesium sulfate)**
IV, IM
Adults, Elderly. 1 g IM q6h for up to 4 doses; or, 1-2 g IVPB for one dose. Recheck magnesium levels to determine need for additional treatment.
Children. 25-50 mg/kg/dose q4-6h for 3-4 doses. Maximum: 2 g/dose.
▸ **Preeclampsia/eclampsia (magnesium sulfate)**
IV INFUSION
Adult females. Initially, 4-5 g bolus, diluted, then 1-2 g/h given by IV continuous infusion; rate adjustments guided by magnesium levels, urine output, patellar reflexes, contractions, and patient status. Alternatively, up to 10-14 g may be needed in severe cases initially; the dose may be given as two 4- or 5-g injections IM into each buttock if needed.
▸ **Hyperalimentation (magnesium sulfate)**
NOTE: Exact daily requirements must be determined individually.
TPN
Adults, Elderly. Maintenance dose 8-24 mEq (1-3 g) daily.
Infants. 2-10 mEq (0.25-1.25 mEq) daily.
▸ **ACLS protocol use (magnesium sulfate)**
IV
Adults, Elderly. For pulseless cardiac arrest, 1-2 g (diluted in 10 mL D5W or NS) IV over 5-20 min. Alternatively, if a pulse is present, 1-2 g (in 50-100 mL compatible solution), infused slowly over 5-60 min.
▸ **Cathartic or bowel preparation (magnesium citrate)**
PO
Adults, Elderly, Children 12 yr and older. 120-300 mL.
Children 6-11 yr. 100-200 mL.
Children < 6 yr. 0.5 mL/kg up to maximum of 200 mL.

▸ **Constipation**
PO (MOM suspension or concentrate)
Adults, Elderly, Children older than 11 yr. 30-60 mL/day (or 10-20 mL concentrated MOM) once daily as needed.
Children 6-11 yr. 7.5-15 mL/day (or 3.75-7.5 mL concentrated MOM) once daily as needed.
Children 2-5 yr. 2.5-7.5 mL/day (or 1.25-3.75 mL concentrated MOM) once daily as needed.
▸ **Constipation**
PO (magnesium hydroxide chewable tablets)
Adults, Elderly, Children older than 11 yr. 8 tablets at bedtime or given in divided doses throughout the day.
Children 6-11 yr. 4 tablets at bedtime or given in divided doses throughout the day.
Children 3-5 yr. 2 tablets at bedtime or given in divided doses throughout the day.
▸ **Constipation**
PO (magnesium oxide caplets)
Adults, Elderly, Children older than 11 yr: 2-4 caplets daily at bedtime or individually taken throughout the day.

CONTRAINDICATIONS

Antacid/laxative: Appendicitis, ileus or intestinal obstruction, severe renal impairment, undiagnosed rectal bleeding.
Systemic: Renal failure, toxemia of pregnancy during 2 h preceding delivery.

INTERACTIONS

Drug
▸ **ANTACID/LAXATIVE**
Ketoconazole, bisphosphonates, fluoroquinolones, tetracyclines: May decrease the absorption of these drugs; separate times of oral administration.

M

Methenamine: May decrease the effects of methenamine.
Nitrofurantoin: May decrease absorption.

▸ **SYSTEMIC (ELECTROLYTE REPLACEMENT)**

Calcium: May reverse the effects of magnesium (used to treat magnesium toxicity).
Digoxin: May cause changes in cardiac conduction if magnesium is excessive or depleted.
Fluoroquinolones, tetracyclines: May form nonabsorbable complex; separate times of oral administration.
Cisplatin, aminoglycosides, amphotericin B, loop diuretics: May deplete magnesium.

Herbal
None known.

Food
Alcohol: Excessive use may deplete magnesium.

DIAGNOSTIC TEST EFFECTS

Antacid: Increases gastric pH.
Systemic: Normal magnesium serum concentrations are 1.4-2 mEq/L in adults and children, and 1.5-2.3 mEq/L in infants. As an anticonvulsant for eclampsia, effective concentrations reported to be 2.5-7.5 mEq/L.

IV INCOMPATIBILITIES

Amphotericin B complex (Abelcet, AmBisome, Amphotec), anidulafungin (Eraxis), cefepime (Maxipime), ceftriaxone (Rocephin), cefuroxime, ciprofloxacin (Cipro), dexamethasone sodium phosphate, diazepam, doxorubicin, drotrecogin alfa (Xigris), epirubicin, haloperidol, inamrinone, lansoprazole (Prevacid), levofloxacin (Levaquin), methylprednisolone sodium succinate, phenytoin, phytonadione.

SIDE EFFECTS

Frequent
Antacid: Chalky taste, laxative effect.

Occasional
Antacid/laxative: Nausea, cramping, diarrhea, increased thirst, flatulence.
Systemic (dietary supplement, electrolyte replacement): Reduced respiratory rate, decreased reflexes, flushing, hypotension, decreased heart rate.

SERIOUS REACTIONS

- Magnesium as an antacid or laxative has no known serious reactions with routine recommended use, as long as renal function is normal.
- Systemic use of magnesium may produce prolonged PR interval and widening of QRS interval.
- Magnesium toxicity may cause loss of deep tendon reflexes, heart block, respiratory paralysis, and cardiac arrest. Hypocalcemia with tetany may occur with large doses. The antidote for toxicity is 10-20 mL 10% calcium chloride or gluconate (5-10 mEq of calcium).

PRECAUTIONS & CONSIDERATIONS

Magnesium antacids/laxatives should be used cautiously in those with renal impairment and in those with chronic diarrhea, GI disease, and undiagnosed GI and rectal bleeding. Use cautiously in those with diabetes mellitus and in those on a low-salt diet because some magnesium supplements contain sugar or sodium. Due to sodium content, use magnesium citrate with caution if congestive heart failure is present. Occasional use of magnesium hydroxide for constipation is generally considered compatible for pregnancy and lactation.

When magnesium is given for systemic use, it should be used cautiously in severe renal impairment. Parenteral magnesium readily crosses the placenta and is distributed in breast milk. Continuous IV infusion of magnesium increases the risk of magnesium toxicity in the neonate and should not be administered IV during the 2 h preceding delivery. Magnesium should be used cautiously in children younger than 6 yr. Elderly patients are at increased risk for developing magnesium deficiency because of decreased magnesium absorption, other medications they may be taking, and poor diet.

Adequate hydration should be maintained. Notify the physician if signs and symptoms of hypermagnesemia occur, including confusion, hypotension, cramping, dizziness, irregular heartbeat, light-headedness, or unusual fatigue or weakness. ECG, BUN, serum creatinine, and magnesium levels should be monitored in those receiving parenteral or chronic oral therapy. Patellar reflexes monitored to assess for CNS depression. Know that suppressed reflexes may indicate impending respiratory arrest. Patellar reflexes should be present, and respiratory rate should be > 16 breaths/min before each parenteral dose. Report any unrelieved constipation, rectal bleeding, symptoms of electrolyte imbalance, particularly muscle cramps, pain, weakness, and dizziness, immediately.

Storage

May refrigerate magnesium citrate prior to use; do not freeze. Store oral supplements at room temperature protected from moisture. If oral suspension appears nonmiscible, discard. Store parenteral injection vials at room temperature. Once diluted, IVPB and infusions are stable for 24 h at room temperature. Premixed bags should be kept in overwraps until time of use. Do not freeze injection or premixed bags.

Administration

When using magnesium hydroxide suspension, shake well before use. Chew the chewable tablets thoroughly before swallowing. Follow oral laxative with a full glass of water. Take at least 2 h before or 2 h after other medications. Do not take for longer than 1-2 wks, unless directed by the physician.

Magnesium citrate liquid may be chilled before serving for palatability. Follow with clear liquids as physician instructs, especially for bowel preparation. A lower sodium formula is available for those patients who should have lower sodium intake.

For IV use, magnesium sulfate injection solution must be diluted. Dilute for IVPB in an appropriate volume of D5W or 0.9% NaCl. Normally, a 1-2 g IVPB is diluted in 100 mL of fluid and is infused over 1 h. For emergency use, do not exceed infusion rate of 150 mg/min and the concentration should not exceed 20% (200 mg/mL). Do not mix with other IV drugs unless compatibility is established.

For IM use in children, dilute to a maximum of 20% concentration. Adults may receive the 50% solution undiluted for IM use. Inject deep into a large muscle mass, as prescribed.

Mannitol
man′i-tall
Osmitrol

CATEGORY AND SCHEDULE
Pregnancy Risk Category: C

Classification: Diuretics, osmotic

MECHANISM OF ACTION
An osmotic diuretic, antiglaucoma, and antihemolytic agent that elevates osmotic pressure of the glomerular filtrate, inhibiting tubular reabsorption of water and electrolytes, resulting in increased flow of water into interstitial fluid and plasma. *Therapeutic Effect:* Produces diuresis; reduces intraocular pressure (IOP); reduces intracranial pressure (ICP) and cerebral edema.

PHARMACOKINETICS

Route	Onset (min)	Peak	Duration (h)
IV (diuresis)	1-3h	N/A	2-8
IV (reduced ICP)	15-30	N/A	3-8
IV (reduced IOP)	N/A	30-60 min	4-8

Remains in extracellular fluid. Primarily excreted in urine. Removed by hemodialysis. *Half-life:* 45-100 min.

AVAILABILITY
Injection: 5%, 10%, 15%, 20%, 25%.

INDICATIONS AND DOSAGES
▸ **Prevention and treatment of oliguric phase of acute renal failure, to promote urinary excretion of toxic substances (such as aspirin, barbiturates, bromides, and imipramine); to reduce increased ICP due to cerebral edema or edema of injured spinal cord; to reduce increased IOP due to acute glaucoma**
IV
Adults, Elderly, Children. Initially, 0.2-1 g/kg, then 0.25-0.5 g/kg q4-6h.

CONTRAINDICATIONS
Severe dehydration, active intracranial bleeding (except during craniotomy), severe pulmonary edema and congestion, severe renal disease (well established anuria), progressive renal damage or dysfunction after receiving mannitol, including increasing oliguria and azotemia, progressive heart failure. Hypersensitivity to mannitol.

INTERACTIONS
Drug
Digoxin: May increase the risk of digoxin toxicity associated with mannitol-induced hypokalemia.
Lithium: Increases urinary excretion of lithium.
Herbal
None known.
Food
None known.

DIAGNOSTIC TEST EFFECTS
May decrease serum phosphate, potassium, and sodium levels.

IV INCOMPATIBILITIES
Cefepime (Maxipime), diazepam, doxorubicin liposomal (Doxil), filgrastim (Neupogen), imipenemcilastatin (Primaxin), meropenem (Merrem), phenytoin, whole blood for transfusion.

IV COMPATIBILITIES
Cisplatin (Platinol), ondansetron (Zofran), propofol (Diprivan).

SIDE EFFECTS

Frequent

Dry mouth, thirst.

Occasional

Blurred vision, increased urinary frequency and urine volume, headache, arm pain, backache, nausea, vomiting, urticaria, dizziness, hypotension or hypertension, tachycardia, fever, angina-like chest pain.

SERIOUS REACTIONS

- Fluid and electrolyte imbalance may occur from rapid administration of large doses or inadequate urine output resulting in overexpansion of extracellular fluid.
- Circulatory overload may produce pulmonary edema and congestive heart failure.
- Excessive diuresis may produce hypokalemia and hyponatremia.
- Fluid loss in excess of electrolyte excretion may produce hypernatremia and hyperkalemia.

PRECAUTIONS & CONSIDERATIONS

It is unknown whether mannitol crosses the placenta or is distributed in breast milk. The safety and efficacy of mannitol have not been established in children younger than 12 yr. Age-related renal impairment may require cautious use in elderly patients.

Dry mouth and an increase in the frequency and volume of urination may occur. BP, BUN, liver function test results, electrolytes, and urine output should be assessed before and during treatment. Weight should be monitored daily. Be aware of signs of electrolyte disturbances such as hypokalemia or hyponatremia. Hypokalemia may cause arrhythmias, altered mental status, muscle cramps, asthenia, and tremor. Hyponatremia may result in cold and clammy skin, confusion, and thirst.

May increase cerebral blood flow and worsen intracranial hypertension in chldren who develop generalized cerebral hyperemia 24-48 h post injury.

Storage

Store the drug at room temperature. Do not use if container is damaged or solution is not clear. Do not use if crystals are visible; brief storage in a warmer (< 40° C) may help redispense crystals.

Administration

! Assess the IV site for patency before administering each dose. Pain and thrombosis are noted with extravasation. With suspected renal insufficiency or marked oliguria, a test dose should be given. The test dose is 12.5 g for adults (200 mg/kg for children) over 3-5 min to produce a urine flow of at least 30-50 mL/h (1 mL/kg/h for children) over 2-3 h.

If the solution crystallizes, warm the bottle in hot water and shake it vigorously at intervals. Do not use the solution if crystals remain after the warming procedure. Cool the solution to body temperature before administration. Use an in-line filter (< 5 μm) for drug concentrations > 20%. The test dose for oliguria is IV push over 3-5 min. The test dose for cerebral edema or elevated ICP is IV over 20-30 min. Maximum concentration is 25%. Do not add potassium chloride or sodium chloride to mannitol with a concentration of 20% or greater. Do not add mannitol to whole blood for transfusion conjointly. If it is necessary to coadminister whole blood, use at least 20 mEq NaCl added to each liter of mannitol solution to prevent pseudoagglutination.

Do not put into PVC bags for administration.

Maraviroc

mah-rav'i-rock

Selzentry Celsentri

CATEGORY AND SCHEDULE

Pregnancy Risk Category: B

Classification: Antiretrovirals, fusion inhibitors

MECHANISM OF ACTION

A fusion inhibitor that is a CCR5 coreceptor antagonist that interferes with the entry of HIV-1 into CD4+ cells by inhibiting the fusion of viral and cellular membranes. Maraviroc is only effective at reducing viral load in patients with CCR5-tropic HIV strains. *Therapeutic Effect:* Impairs HIV replication, slowing the progression of HIV infection.

PHARMACOKINETICS

Efficacy not affected by food. The drug is a substrate for the efflux transporter P-glycoprotein (Pgp). Protein binding: 76% with moderate affinity for albumin and α-1 acid glycoprotein. Metabolized in liver to inactive metabolites; CYP3A is the major enzyme for metabolism. Maraviroc was the major component present in urine (8% dose) and feces (25% dose); the remainder was excreted as metabolites. *Half-life:* 14-18 h.

AVAILABILITY

Table (Selzentry): 150 mg, 300 mg.

INDICATIONS AND DOSAGES

▸ **CCR5-tropic HIV infection (in combination with other antiretrovirals)**

▸ **With CYP3A inhibitors with or without a CYP3A inducer (e.g., most protease inhibitors, delavirdine, and other strong CYP3A inhibitors)**

PO

Adults, Elderly, Children 16 yr and older. 150 mg twice daily.

▸ **With CYP3A inducers (e.g., efavirenz, rifampin, etravirine, others) with NO strong CYP3A inhibitor**

PO

Adults, Elderly, Children 16 yr and older. 600 mg twice daily.

IF regimen does NOT include ANY CYP3A inducers or inhibitors (e.g., regimens with tipranavir/ritonavir, nevirapine, raltegravir, NRTIs, and enfuvirtide)

PO

Adults, Elderly, Children 16 yr and older. 300 mg twice daily.

▸ **Dosage in Renal impairment**

CrCl ≥30 mL/min: Use usual dosage based on other medications.

CrCl < 30 mL/min: Use not recommended in a patient taking a CYP3A inducer or inhibitor or any such combinations. IF the regimen does NOT include ANY CYP3A inducers or inhibitors, no dosage adjustment is needed; however, if postural hypotension occurs, reduce to 150 mg PO twice daily.

CONTRAINDICATIONS

Hypersensitivity to maraviroc. Do NOT use in severe renal impairment or ESRD (i.e., CrCl < 30 mL/min) if taking potent CYP3A inhibitors or inducers.

INTERACTIONS

Drug

CYP3A inhibitors (including most protease inhibitors [except tipranavir/ritonavir] and delavirdine, ketoconazole, itraconazole, clarithromycin,

nefazodone): Increases the concentration of maraviroc. Decrease maraviroc dosage.
CYP3A inducers (e.g., efavirenz, rifampin, etravirine, carbamazepine, phenobarbital, and phenytoin): Decreases the concentration of maraviroc. Increase maraviroc dosage.
Herbal
St. John's wort: Decreases the concentration of maraviroc. Avoid.
Food
None known. High-fat food decreases absorption some but does not affect final efficacy.

DIAGNOSTIC TEST EFFECTS

May elevate AST (SGOT) and ALT (SGPT) levels. May decrease blood hemoglobin levels and WBC count.

SIDE EFFECTS

Frequent (> 8%)
Upper respiratory tract infections, cough, pyrexia, rash, and dizziness.
Occasional (3%-7%)
Asthenia, arthralgia, insomnia, anxiety, constipation, myalgia, paresthesias, peripheral neuropathy, cold sores, sinus and other infections.
Rare (2% or less)
Change in appetite, conjunctivitis, urinary symptoms, flu-like syndrome. Lowered blood counts, altered fat distribution. Postural hypotension with increased levels of maraviroc.

SERIOUS REACTIONS

- Hepatotoxicity has been reported, which may be preceded by evidence of a systemic allergic reaction (e.g., pruritic rash, eosinophilia, or elevated IgE). Stevens-Johnson syndrome has been reported.
- More cardiovascular events, including myocardial ischemia and/or infarction, were observed in treatment-experienced subjects who received this drug, but more data are needed to assess any risk.
- Because of effects on immune cells, potential risk for infection or increased rate of malignancy. Immune reconstitution syndrome has been reported. Risk currently not proven or known.

PRECAUTIONS & CONSIDERATIONS

Caution is warranted in patients with liver function impairment and in those coinfected with hepatitis B. In patients with renal impairment, carefully screen for drug interactions. Use with caution in patients at increased risk of cardiovascular events or diabetes or at risk of postural hypotension. There are no adequate data in human pregnancy. Breastfeeding is not recommended in this patient population because of the possibility of HIV transmission. Be aware that the safety and efficacy of maraviroc have not been established in children younger than 16 yr of age. No age-related precautions have been noted in elderly patients.

Maraviroc is not a cure for HIV infection, nor does it reduce risk of transmission to others. Expect to obtain baseline laboratory testing, especially CBC, liver function, and renal function, before beginning maraviroc therapy and at periodic intervals. Assess for hypersensitivity reaction, fatigue or nausea, myalgia, paresthesia or neuropathy, and insomnia.
Storage
Store at room temperature. Shelf life is only 1 yr.
Administration
Maraviroc may be taken without regard to food or meals.

Mebendazole

meh-ben'dah-zole

🍁 Vermox

CATEGORY AND SCHEDULE

Pregnancy Risk Category: C

Classification: Antihelmintics, carbamate

MECHANISM OF ACTION

A synthetic benzimidazole derivative that degrades parasite cytoplasmic microtubules and irreversibly blocks glucose uptake in helminthes and larvae. *Therapeutic Effect:* Vermicidal. Depletes glycogen, decreases ATP, causes helminth death.

PHARMACOKINETICS

Poorly absorbed from GI tract (absorption increases with food). Metabolized in liver. Primarily eliminated in feces. *Half-life:* 2.5-9 h (half life increased with impaired renal function).

AVAILABILITY

Tablets, Chewable: 100 mg.

INDICATIONS AND DOSAGES

▸ **Trichuriasis, ascariasis, hookworm**

PO

Adults, Elderly, Children older than 2 yr. 1 tablet in morning and at bedtime for 3 days. For resistant infections (i.e., helminth ova continuing to appear in feces 3-4 wks after initial course), a 2nd course is recommended.

▸ **Enterobiasis (Pinworm)**

PO

Adults, Elderly, Children older than 2 yr. 1 tablet one time.

OFF-LABEL USES

Ancylostoma duodenale or *Necator americanus, trichinosis, visceral larva migrans.*

CONTRAINDICATIONS

Hypersensitivity to mebendazole or any component of the formulation.

INTERACTIONS

Drug

Carbamazepine: May decrease concentrations of mebendazole.

Cimetidine: May increase mebendazole levels.

Herbal

None known.

Food

None known.

DIAGNOSTIC TEST EFFECTS

May increase SGOT (AST), SGPT (ALT), alkaline phosphatase, BUN. May decrease hemoglobin.

SIDE EFFECTS

Occasional

Nausea, vomiting, headache, dizziness, transient abdominal pain, diarrhea with massive infection and expulsion of helminthes.

Rare

Fever.

SERIOUS REACTIONS

- High dosage may produce reversible myelosuppression (granulocytopenia, leukopenia, neutropenia).
- Higher-than-recommended dosages may produce hepatitis.

PRECAUTIONS & CONSIDERATIONS

Be aware that mebendazole is ineffective in hydatid disease. Use with caution in known liver dysfunction and monitor closely. It is unknown whether mebendazole crosses the placenta or is distributed in breast milk; caution is warranted in lactation. Safety and efficacy have not been established in children 2 yr and younger. No age-related precautions have been noted in elderly patients.

Avoid walking barefoot (larval entry into system). Change and launder underclothing, pajamas, bedding, towels, and washcloths daily. Because of the high transmission of pinworm infections, all family members should be treated simultaneously; the infected person should sleep alone and shower frequently.

Storage

Store at room temperature protected from light and moisture.

Administration

For high dosages, take with food. Tablets may be crushed, swallowed, or mixed with food. Take and continue iron supplements as long as ordered (may be 6 mo after treatment) for anemia associated with whipworm and hookworm.

Meclizine Hydrochloride

mek'li-zeen high-droh-klor'ide

★ Antivert, Bonine, Dramamine Less Drowsy 🍁 Bonamine

Do not confuse Antivert with Axert.

CATEGORY AND SCHEDULE

Pregnancy Risk Category: B

OTC, Rx

Classification: Antihistamines, sedating, H_1 antagonists, antivertigo agents

MECHANISM OF ACTION

An anticholinergic that reduces labyrinthine excitability and diminishes vestibular stimulation of the labyrinth, affecting the chemoreceptor trigger zone.

Therapeutic Effect: Reduces nausea, vomiting, and vertigo.

PHARMACOKINETICS

Route	Onset	Peak	Duration
PO	30-60 min	N/A	12-24 h

Well absorbed from the GI tract. Widely distributed. Metabolized in the liver. Primarily excreted in urine. *Half-life:* 6 h.

AVAILABILITY

Tablets (Antivert): 12.5 mg, 25 mg, 50 mg.

Tablets, Chewable (Bonine): 25 mg.

Tablets (Dramamine Less Drowsy): 25 mg.

INDICATIONS AND DOSAGES

▸ **Motion sickness**

PO

Adults, Elderly, Children 12 yr and older. 25-50 mg 1 h before travel. May repeat every 24 h.

▸ **Vertigo**

PO

Adults, Elderly, Children 12 yr and older. 25-100 mg/day in divided doses, as needed.

CONTRAINDICATIONS

Hypersensitivity.

INTERACTIONS

Drug

Alcohol, CNS depressants: May increase CNS depressant effect.

Herbal

None known.

Food

None known.

DIAGNOSTIC TEST EFFECTS

May produce false-negative results in antigen skin testing unless meclizine is discontinued 4 days before testing.

M

SIDE EFFECTS

Frequent
Drowsiness.
Occasional
Blurred vision; dry mouth, nose, or throat.

SERIOUS REACTIONS

- A hypersensitivity reaction, marked by eczema, pruritus, rash, cardiac disturbances, and photosensitivity may occur.
- Overdose may produce CNS depression (manifested as sedation, apnea, cardiovascular collapse, or death) or severe paradoxical reactions (such as hallucinations, tremor, and seizures).
- Children may experience paradoxical reactions, including restlessness, insomnia, euphoria, nervousness, and tremors.
- Elderly patients (older than 60 yr) may have increased risk for agitation, disorientation, dizziness, sedation, hypotension, confusion.

PRECAUTIONS & CONSIDERATIONS

Caution is warranted in patients with asthma, prostate enlargement, angle-closure glaucoma, and obstructive diseases of the GI or genitourinary tract. It is unknown whether meclizine crosses the placenta or is distributed in breast milk. Meclizine use may produce irritability in breastfeeding infants. Safety and efficacy in children under age 12 are not established. Children and elderly patients may be more sensitive to the drug's anticholinergic effects, such as dry mouth. Alcohol and tasks that require mental alertness or motor skills should be avoided until the effects of the drug are known.

Dizziness, drowsiness, and dry mouth may occur. BP, electrolytes, and skin should be assessed.

Storage
Store at room temperature. keep tightly closed and protect from light.
Administration
Take meclizine orally without regard to food. Crush scored tablets if needed. Chewable tablets may be administered with or without water.

Medroxyprogesterone Acetate

me-drox′ee-proe-jess′te-rone ass′e-tayte

★ Depo-Provera, Depo-Provera Contraceptive, Depo-SubQ Provera 104, Provera (Canada) Medroxy, Provera

Do not confuse medroxyprogesterone with hydroxyprogesterone, methylprednisolone, or methyltestosterone.

CATEGORY AND SCHEDULE

Pregnancy Risk Category: X

Classification: Progestogen

MECHANISM OF ACTION

A hormone that transforms endometrium from proliferative to secretory in an estrogen-primed endometrium. Inhibits secretion of pituitary gonadotropins. *Therapeutic Effect:* Prevents follicular maturation and ovulation. Stimulates the growth of mammary alveolar tissue and relaxes uterine smooth muscle. Corrects hormonal imbalance.

PHARMACOKINETICS

Slowly absorbed after IM administration. Protein binding: 90%. Metabolized in the liver. Excreted primarily in urine. *Half-life:* 16 h (oral tablet); 16-43 days (mean, injection suspension).

AVAILABILITY

Tablets (Provera): 2.5 mg, 5 mg, 10 mg.
Injection (Depo-Provera Contraceptive): 150 mg/mL.
Injection (Depo-Provera): 400 mg/mL.
Subcutaneous Injection (Depo-SubQ Provera 104 Contraceptive): 104 mg/0.65 mL.

INDICATIONS AND DOSAGES

▸ **Endometrial hyperplasia**
PO
Adults. 2.5-10 mg/day for 14 days.
▸ **Secondary amenorrhea**
PO
Adults. 5-10 mg/day for 5-10 days, beginning at any time during menstrual cycle or 2.5 mg/day.
▸ **Abnormal uterine bleeding**
PO
Adults. 5-10 mg/day for 5-10 days, beginning on calculated day 16 or day 21 of menstrual cycle.
▸ **Endometrial, renal carcinoma**
IM
Adults, Elderly. Initially, 400-1000 mg; repeat at 1-wk intervals. If improvement occurs and disease is stabilized, begin maintenance with as little as 400 mg/mo.
▸ **Contraception**
IM (DEPO-PROVERA)
Adults. 150 mg q3mo. Do not use for > 2 yr unless necessary.
▸ **Contraception or endometriosis**
SUBCUTANEOUS (DEPO-SUBQ PROVERA 104)
Adults. 104 mg q12-14 wk. Do not use for > 2 yr unless necessary.

CONTRAINDICATIONS

Carcinoma of breast; hormone-dependent neoplasm; history of or active thrombotic disorders, such as cerebral apoplexy, thrombophlebitis, or thromboembolic disorders; hypersensitivity to progestins; known or suspected pregnancy; missed abortion; severe hepatic dysfunction; undiagnosed abnormal genital bleeding; use as pregnancy test.

INTERACTIONS

Drug
Bromocriptine: May interfere with the effects of bromocriptine.
Herbal
None known.
Food
None known.

DIAGNOSTIC TEST EFFECTS

May alter results for serum thyroid and liver function tests, prothrombin time, and metapyrone test.

SIDE EFFECTS

Frequent
Transient menstrual abnormalities (including spotting, change in menstrual flow or cervical secretions, and amenorrhea) at initiation of therapy.
Occasional
Edema, weight change, breast tenderness, nervousness, insomnia, fatigue, dizziness, hot flashes, decreased libido or anorgasmia, acene, rash.
Rare
Alopecia, depression, dermatologic changes, headache, fever, nausea.

SERIOUS REACTIONS

- Thrombophlebitis, pulmonary or cerebral embolism, and retinal thrombosis occur rarely.

M

• Lowered bone mineral density with injectable use > 2 yr; may be nonreversible.

PRECAUTIONS & CONSIDERATIONS

Caution is warranted in patients with conditions aggravated by fluid retention, including asthma, seizures, migraine, cardiac or renal dysfunction, and in those with diabetes mellitus, osteopenia, or history of depression. Medroxyprogesterone should be avoided during pregnancy, especially in the first 4 mo because the drug may cause congenital heart and limb-reduction defects in the neonate. Medroxyprogesterone contraception is compatible with breast-feeding. Safety and efficacy of medroxyprogesterone have not been established in children under the age of 12 yr. No age-related precautions have been noted in elderly patients. Avoid smoking because of the increased risk of blood clot formation and myocardial infarction.

Notify the physician of chest pain, blood-tinged expectorants, hemoptysis, numbness in the arm or leg, severe headache, severe pain or swelling in the calf, severe abdominal pain or tenderness, sudden loss of vision, or unusually heavy vaginal bleeding. BP, weight, blood glucose, hepatic enzyme, and serum calcium levels should be monitored.

Storage

Store all products at room temperature; do not freeze the injection.

Administration

Take oral medroxyprogesterone without regard to meals.

For IM use, shake vial immediately before administering to ensure complete suspension. Inject IM only in upper arm or upper outer aspect of buttock. Rarely, a residual lump, change in skin color, or sterile abscess occurs at injection site.

For use of the subcutaneous injection, shake well immediately before use to ensure complete suspension. Preferred sites of administration are the upper thigh and abdomen.

Mefloquine

me'flow-quine

Lariam

CATEGORY AND SCHEDULE

Pregnancy Risk Category: C

Classification: Antimalarial

MECHANISM OF ACTION

A quinolone-methanol compound structurally similar to quinine that destroys the asexual blood forms of malarial pathogens *Plasmodium falciparum, P. vivax. Therapeutic Effect:* Inhibits parasite growth.

PHARMACOKINETICS

Well absorbed from the GI tract. Protein binding: 98%. Widely distributed, including cerebrospinal fluid (CSF). Metabolized in liver. Primarily excreted in urine. *Half-life:* 21-22 days.

AVAILABILITY

Tablets: 250 mg.

INDICATIONS AND DOSAGES

▸ **Suppression of malaria**

PO

Adults. 250 mg base weekly starting 1-2 wk before travel, continuing weekly during travel and for 4 wks after leaving endemic area.

Children weighing more than 45 kg. 250 mg weekly starting 1-2 wk before travel, continuing weekly

during travel and for 4 wks after leaving the endemic area.
Children weighing 31-45 kg. 187.5 mg (¾ tablet) weekly starting 1-2 wks before travel, continuing weekly during travel, and for 4 wks after leaving the endemic area.
Children weighing 20-30 kg. 125 mg (½ tablet) weekly starting 1-2 wk before travel, continuing weekly during travel, and for 4 wks after leaving the endemic area.
Children weighing 15-19 kg. 62.5 mg (¼ tablet) weekly starting 1 wk before travel, continuing weekly during travel, and for 4 wks after leaving the endemic area.

▸ **Treatment of malaria (if strain not resistant)**

PO
Adults. 1250 mg as a single dose.
Children. 20-25 mg/kg single dose (not to exceed 1250 mg). Splitting the dose into 2 doses taken 6-8 h apart may reduce side effects. Experience in children < 20 kg is limited.

CONTRAINDICATIONS

Cardiac abnormalities; severe psychiatric disorders; epilepsy; history of hypersensitivity to mefloquine; quinine, or quinidine; use with halofantrine.

INTERACTIONS

Drug
Anticonvulsants: May decrease the effect of anticonvulsants.
β-Blockers: May increase bradycardia with β-blockers.
Chloroquine, quinine, quinidine: May increase the risk of toxicity with these drugs (seizures or ECG changes).
Dronedarone: Risk of fatal QT prolongation; do not use.
Halofantrine: Risk of fatal QT prolongation; do not use.
Ketoconazole: Do not use within 15 days of mefloquine as may cause toxicity and QT prolongation.
Medications prolonging the QT interval and/or potently inhibiting CYP3A4: May increase risk of mefloquine toxicity and QT prolongation.
Rifampin: Induces mefloquine metabolism and may cause treatment failure.
Herbal
None known.
Food
None known.

DIAGNOSTIC TEST EFFECTS

None known.

SIDE EFFECTS

Occasional
Mild transient headache, difficulty concentrating, insomnia, lightheadedness, vertigo, diarrhea, nausea, vomiting, visual disturbances, tinnitus, chills, fatigue, myalgia.
Rare
Aggressive behavior, anxiety, bradycardia, depression, hallucinations, hypotension, panic attacks, paranoia, psychosis, syncope, tremor.

SERIOUS REACTIONS

- Prolonged therapy may result in peripheral neuritis, neuromyopathy, hypotension, ECG changes (e.g., QT prolongation), agranulocytosis, aplastic anemia, thrombocytopenia, seizures, and psychosis.
- Overdosage may result in headache, vomiting, visual disturbance, drowsiness, and seizures.
- Acute hypersensitivity.

PRECAUTIONS & CONSIDERATIONS

Caution is warranted in patients with history of depression, epilepsy, liver disease, heart disease, and

M

people who pilot airplanes and operate machines because dizziness and disturbed sense of balance are side effects. It is unknown whether mefloquine crosses the placenta or is excreted in breast milk. Advise female patients to use adequate contraception during the period of prophylaxis or treatment. No age-related precautions have been noted in children or elderly patients.

Any new symptoms of anxiety, confusion, depression, restlessness, tinnitus, and visual difficulties should be reported.

Storage

Store at controlled room temperature in original package until time of use.

Administration

Begin therapy before and continue after trip. Take mefloquine with food and at least 8 oz of water. Tablets may be crushed and mixed with water or sugar water for oral administration. Continue taking mefloquine for the full length of treatment.

! NOTE: Patients with acute *P. vivax* malaria are at high risk of relapse because mefloquine does not eliminate hepatic phase parasites. To avoid relapse after mefloquine treatment, patients should subsequently be treated with an 8-aminoquinoline derivative (e.g., primaquine).

Megestrol Acetate

me-jess′trole ass′ee-tayte

Megace, Megace ES

Apo-Megestrol, Megace OS, Nu-Megestrol

CATEGORY AND SCHEDULE

Pregnancy Risk Category: X (for suspension), D (for tablets)

Classification: Progestin derivative

MECHANISM OF ACTION

A hormone and antineoplastic agent that suppresses the release of luteinizing hormone from the anterior pituitary gland by inhibiting pituitary function. *Therapeutic Effect:* Shrinks tumors. Also increases appetite by an unknown mechanism.

PHARMACOKINETICS

Well absorbed from the GI tract. Metabolized in the liver; excreted in urine.

AVAILABILITY

Tablets: 20 mg, 40 mg.
Suspension: 40 mg/mL, 125 mg/mL.

INDICATIONS AND DOSAGES

▸ Palliative treatment of advanced breast cancer

PO

Adults, Elderly. 160 mg/day in 4 equally divided doses.

▸ Palliative treatment of advanced endometrial carcinoma

PO

Adults, Elderly. 40-320 mg/day in divided doses. Maximum: 800 mg/day in 1-4 divided doses.

▸ Anorexia, cachexia, weight loss

PO (MEGACE)

Adults, Elderly. 400-800 mg/day (equal to 10-20 mL/day).

PO (MEGACE ES)

Adults, Elderly: 625 mg (5 mL) once daily.

OFF-LABEL USES

Appetite stimulant, treatment of hormone-dependent or advanced prostate carcinoma (palliative).

CONTRAINDICATIONS

Hypersensitivity to megestrol acetate or any of its components.

INTERACTIONS

Drug

Antidiabetic agents: Megestrol may alter glucose tolerance. Monitor.

Dofetilide: Megestrol inhibits renal cationic transport and clearance; co-use contraindicated.

Entecavir: Competes with megestrol for renal tubular secretion; monitor.

Warfarin: Megestrol may increase response to warfarin; monitor INR.

Herbal

None known.

Food

None known.

DIAGNOSTIC TEST EFFECTS

May increase blood glucose level.

SIDE EFFECTS

Frequent

Weight gain secondary to increased appetite, hot flashes, sweating, rash, increased blood pressure.

Occasional

Nausea, breakthrough vaginal bleeding, backache, headache, breast tenderness, carpal tunnel syndrome.

Rare

Feeling of coldness.

SERIOUS REACTIONS

- Thrombophlebitis and pulmonary embolism occur rarely.
- New or exacerbation of diabetes mellitus, overt Cushing's syndrome.
- Adrenal insufficiency with megestrol withdrawal after chronic use.

PRECAUTIONS & CONSIDERATIONS

Caution is warranted in patients with a history of thrombophlebitis. Megestrol use should be avoided during pregnancy, if possible, especially in the first 4 mo. Pregnancy should be determined before initiating megestrol therapy. Megestrol has a pregnancy risk category of X in suspension form and D in tablet form. Contraception is imperative during therapy. Breastfeeding is not recommended for patients taking this drug. The safety and efficacy of megestrol have not been established in children. No age-related precautions have been noted in elderly patients.

Notify the physician if calf pain, difficulty breathing, or vaginal bleeding develops.

Patients receiving chemotherapy may require palliative treatment for stomatitis.

Storage

Store suspension and tablets at room temperature; avoid exposure to excessive heat. Do not freeze.

Administration

Tablets and suspensions may be taken without regard to meals. Shake suspension well before using. Note difference in dosage of Megace and Megace ES suspensions.

M

Meloxicam

mel-oks′i-kam

★ Mobic 🍁 Mobicox

CATEGORY AND SCHEDULE

Pregnancy Risk Category: C (D if used in third trimester or near delivery)

Classification: Analgesics, nonsteroidal anti-inflammatory drugs

MECHANISM OF ACTION

An NSAID that produces analgesic and anti-inflammatory effects by inhibiting prostaglandin synthesis. *Therapeutic Effect:* Reduces the inflammatory response and intensity of pain.

PHARMACOKINETICS

Route	Onset	Peak	Duration
PO (analgesic)	30 min	4-5 h	NA

Well absorbed after PO administration. Protein binding: 99%. Metabolized in the liver. Eliminated in urine and feces as inactive metabolites. Not removed by hemodialysis. *Half-life:* 15-20 h.

AVAILABILITY

Tablets: 7.5 mg, 15 mg.
Oral Suspension: 7.5 mg/5 mL.

INDICATIONS AND DOSAGES

▸ **Osteoarthritis, rheumatoid arthritis**

PO

Adults. Initially, 7.5 mg/day. Maximum: 15 mg/day.

▸ **Juvenile rheumatoid arthritis**

PO

Children ≥ 2 yr. 0.125 mg/kg (not to exceed 7.5 mg) once daily.

CONTRAINDICATIONS

Hypersensitivity to meloxicam, other NSAIDs, or aspirin. Use within 14 days of CABG.

INTERACTIONS

Drug

Antihypertensives, diuretics: May decrease the effects of antihypertensives and diuretics.
Aspirin, salicylates, corticosteroids: May increase the risk of GI bleeding and side effects. NSAIDs may negate the cardioprotective effect of ASA.
Cyclosporine: May increase risk of nephrotoxicity.
Heparin, oral anticoagulants, thrombolytics: May increase the effects of heparin, oral anticoagulants, and thrombolytics.
Lithium: May increase the blood concentration and risk of toxicity of lithium.
Methotrexate: May increase the risk of toxicity with methotrexate.

Herbal

Feverfew: May increase the risk of bleeding.
Ginkgo biloba: May increase the risk of bleeding.

Food

Alcohol: May increase risk of dizziness, GI bleeding.

DIAGNOSTIC TEST EFFECTS

May increase serum creatinine, AST (SGOT), and ALT (SGPT) levels.

SIDE EFFECTS

Frequent (7%-9%)

Dyspepsia, headache, diarrhea, nausea.

Occasional (3%-4%)

Dizziness, insomnia, rash, pruritus, flatulence, constipation, vomiting.

Rare (< 2%)

Somnolence, urticaria, photosensitivity, tinnitus.

SERIOUS REACTIONS

- Rare reactions with long-term use include peptic ulcer disease, GI bleeding, gastritis, severe hepatic reaction (jaundice), nephrotoxicity (hematuria, dysuria, proteinuria).
- Severe hypersensitivity reaction (bronchospasm, angioedema).

PRECAUTIONS & CONSIDERATIONS

Caution is warranted in patients with asthma, dehydration, hepatic or renal impairment, a history of GI disorders (such as ulcers), and concurrent anticoagulant use. Cardiovascular event risk may be increased with duration of use or preexisting cardiovascular risk factors or disease. Use caution in patients with fluid retention, heart failure, or hypertension. Risk of myocardial infarction and stroke may be increased following CABG surgery. Do not administer within 4-6 half-lives before surgical procedures. Meloxicam should not be used during pregnancy because it can cause fetal harm. Meloxicam is excreted in breast milk; caution is advisable in lactation. Elderly patients may require dose adjustments due to age-related renal impairment and increased susceptibility to GI toxicity.

Notify the physician if chest pain, difficulty breathing, palpitations, peripheral edema, persistent abdominal cramps or pain, rash, ringing in the ears, severe nausea or vomiting, or unusual bleeding or ecchymosis occurs. CBC, BUN level, and serum alkaline phosphatase, bilirubin, creatinine, AST (SGOT), and ALT (SGPT) levels should be assessed during therapy. Therapeutic response, such as decreased pain, stiffness, swelling, and tenderness, improved grip strength, and increased joint mobility, should be evaluated. Report any indications of infection, bleeding, or poor healing to the health care provider.

Storage

Store at room temperature, tightly closed and protected from moisture.

Administration

Take meloxicam without regard to food.

Memantine Hydrochloride

meh-man′teen high-droh-klor′ide

Namenda Ebixa

CATEGORY AND SCHEDULE

Pregnancy Risk Category: B

Classification: Alzheimer disease agents, NMDA receptor antagonists

MECHANISM OF ACTION

An NMDA receptor antagonist that decreases the effects of glutamate, the principal excitatory neurotransmitter in the brain. Persistent central nervous system (CNS) excitation by glutamate is thought to contribute to the symptoms of Alzheimer disease. *Therapeutic Effect:* May reduce clinical deterioration in moderate to severe Alzheimer disease.

PHARMACOKINETICS

Rapidly and completely absorbed after PO administration. Protein binding: 45%. Undergoes little metabolism; most of the dose is excreted unchanged in urine. *Half-life:* 60-80 h.

AVAILABILITY

Tablets: 5 mg, 10 mg.
Oral Solution: 2 mg/mL.

INDICATIONS AND DOSAGES

▸ **Alzheimer disease**

PO

Adults, Elderly. Initially, 5 mg once a day. May increase dosage at intervals of at least 1 wk in 5-mg increments to 10 mg/day (5 mg twice a day), then 15 mg/day (5 mg and 10 mg as separate doses), and finally 20 mg/day (10 mg twice a day). Target dose: 20 mg/day.

▸ **Dosage in renal impairment (CrCl < 30 mL/min)**

Initially, 5 mg once daily. Target dose is 5 mg twice daily.

CONTRAINDICATIONS

Hypersensitivity to the drug, administration with dofetilide.

INTERACTIONS

Drug

Carbonic anhydrase inhibitors, sodium bicarbonate: May decrease the renal elimination of memantine.

Dofetilide: Competes for renal tubular excretion; contraindicated.
Metformin: Competes for renal tubular excretion and may increase risk of lactic acidosis.
Use with other NDMA antagonists (e.g., dextromethorphan, ketamine, amantadine): Not well studied; use together with caution; may increase risk of side effects.
Herbal
None known.
Food
None known.

DIAGNOSTIC TEST EFFECTS

Increased alkaline phosphatase. Rarely, increased liver function tests. Decreased hemoglobin/hematocrit or decreased WBC noted infrequently.

M

SIDE EFFECTS

Occasional (4%-7%)
Dizziness, headache, confusion, constipation, hypertension, cough.
Rare (2%-3%)
Back pain, nausea, fatigue, anxiety, peripheral edema, arthralgia, insomnia.

SERIOUS REACTIONS

- Atrioventricular block.
- Serious CNS reactions may include aggressive behavior, emotional lability, psychosis or delirium, hallucinations, seizures.
- Rare serious allergic reactions.

PRECAUTIONS & CONSIDERATIONS

Caution is warranted in patients with moderate renal impairment or advanced liver disease. Use with caution in patients with seizure disorders, since not well studied. It is unknown whether memantine crosses the placenta or is distributed in breast milk. Memantine is not used in children. No age-related precautions have been noted in elderly patients. Be aware that memantine is not a cure for Alzheimer disease but may slow the progression of its symptoms.

Adequate fluid intake should be maintained. Renal function and urine pH should be monitored; alkaline urine may lead to an accumulation of the drug and a possible increase in side effects.

Storage
Store all dose forms at room temperature.
Administration
Take memantine without regard to food. Carefully measure the dose using the supplied dosing device. Do not mix the oral solution with any other liquids. Do not abruptly discontinue or adjust the drug dosage. If therapy is interrupted for several days, restart the drug at the lowest dose and increase the dosage at intervals of at least 1 wk to the most recent dose, as prescribed.

Meperidine Hydrochloride

me-per′i-deen high-droh-klor′ide
Demerol Demetrol, Pethidine
Do not confuse Demerol with Demulen or Dymelor.

CATEGORY AND SCHEDULE

Pregnancy Risk Category: C (D if used for prolonged periods or at high dosages at term)
Controlled Substance Schedule: II

Classification: Analgesics, narcotic, opiate agonist, synthetic

MECHANISM OF ACTION

An opioid agonist that binds to opioid receptors in the central nervous system (CNS). *Therapeutic Effect:* Alters the perception of, and emotional response, to pain.

PHARMACOKINETICS

Route	Onset (min)	Peak (min)	Duration (h)
PO	15	60	2-4
IV	< 5	5-7	2-3
IM	10-15	30-50	2-4
Subcutaneous	10-15	30-50	2-4

Variably absorbed from the GI tract; well absorbed after IM administration. Protein binding: 60%-80%. Widely distributed. Metabolized in the liver to active metabolite. Excreted primarily in urine. Not removed by hemodialysis. *Half-life:* 2.4-4 h; metabolite 8-16 h (increased in hepatic impairment and disease).

AVAILABILITY

Syrup: 50 mg/5 mL.
Tablets: 50 mg, 100 mg.
Injection: 10 mg/mL, 25 mg/mL, 50 mg/mL, 75 mg/mL, 100 mg/mL.

INDICATIONS AND DOSAGES

▸ **Analgesia**

PO, IM, SC, IV

Adults, Elderly. 25-150 mg q3-4h.
Children. 1.1-1.5 mg/kg q3-4h. Do not exceed single dose of 100 mg.

▸ **Patient-controlled analgesia (PCA)**

IV

Adults. Loading dose: 50-100 mg. Intermittent bolus: 5-30 mg. Lockout interval: 10-20 min. Continuous infusion: 5-40 mg/h. Maximum (4-h): 200-300 mg.

▸ **Dosage in renal impairment**

Dosage is based on creatinine clearance.

Creatinine Clearance (mL/min)	Dosage
10-50	75% of usual dose
< 10	50% of usual dose

CONTRAINDICATIONS

Hypersensitivity to meperidine; use within 14 days of MAOIs.

INTERACTIONS

Drug

Alcohol, other CNS depressants, alcohol, neuromuscular blocking agents: May increase CNS or respiratory depression and hypotension.
Anticholinergics: Increased anticholinergic effects.
Antihypertensive drugs: May increase risk of hypotension.
MAOIs: May produce a severe, sometimes fatal reaction. Meperidine use is contraindicated.
Ritonavir: Suspected increase in meperidine levels.
Sibutramine: Meperidine use is contraindicated.

Herbal

Valerian: May increase CNS depression.

Food

None known.

DIAGNOSTIC TEST EFFECTS

May increase serum amylase and lipase levels. Therapeutic serum level is 100-550 ng/mL; toxic serum level is > 1000 ng/mL.

IV INCOMPATIBILITIES

Acyclovir, allopurinol (Aloprim), amphotericin B complex (Abelcet, AmBisome, Amphotec), all barbiturates, cefepime (Maxipime), cefoperazone (Cefobid), diazepam, doxorubicin liposomal (Doxil), fospropofol (Lusedra), furosemide (Lasix), heparin, idarubicin (Idamycin), lansoprazole (Prevacid), lorazepam, micafungin (Mycamine), nafcillin (Nafcil), pantoprazole (Protonix), phenytoin, sodium bicarbonate.

IV COMPATIBILITIES

Bumetanide (Bumex), diltiazem (Cardizem), dobutamine (Dobutrex), dopamine (Intropin), insulin, lidocaine, magnesium, oxytocin (Pitocin), potassium, propofol (Diprivan).

SIDE EFFECTS

Frequent
Sedation, hypotension (including orthostatic hypotension), diaphoresis, facial flushing, dizziness, nausea, vomiting, constipation.
Occasional
Confusion, arrhythmias, tremors, urine retention, abdominal pain, dry mouth, headache, irritation at injection site, euphoria, dysphoria.
Rare
Allergic reaction (rash, pruritus), insomnia.

SERIOUS REACTIONS

- Overdose results in respiratory depression, skeletal muscle flaccidity, cold or clammy skin, cyanosis, and extreme somnolence progressing to seizures, stupor, and coma. The antidote is 0.4 mg naloxone.
- CNS toxicity due to accumulation of neurotoxic metabolite; risk of seizures. Many experts do not recommended meperidine use for pain due to potential toxicity.
- The patient who uses meperidine repeatedly may develop a tolerance to the drug's analgesic effect and physical dependence.

PRECAUTIONS & CONSIDERATIONS

Caution is warranted in patients with acute abdominal conditions, cor pulmonale, history of seizures, increased intracranial pressure, hepatic or renal impairment, respiratory abnormalities, supraventricular tachycardia, and in debilitated or elderly patients. Be aware that with renal impairment, meperidine's metabolite may increase and cause seizures, tremors, and twitching. Meperidine crosses the placenta and is distributed in breast milk. Regular use of opiates during pregnancy may produce withdrawal symptoms in the neonate, such as diarrhea, excessive crying, fever, hyperactive reflexes, irritability, seizures, sneezing, tremors, vomiting, and yawning. The neonate may develop respiratory depression if the mother receives meperidine during labor. Children are more prone to develop paradoxical excitement. Children younger than 2 yr and elderly patients are more susceptible to the drug's respiratory depressant effects. In elderly patients, age-related renal impairment may increase the risk of urine retention.

Dizziness and drowsiness may occur, so change positions slowly and avoid alcohol, CNS depressants, and tasks that require mental alertness or motor skills until response to the drug is established. Vital signs, pattern of daily bowel activity and stool consistency, and clinical improvement of pain should be monitored. The drug should be withheld and the physician should be notified if the respiratory rate is 12 breaths/min or less in an adult, or 20 breaths/min or less in a child. Be alert for decreased BP as well as a change in quality and rate of pulse. Psychological and physical dependence may occur with chronic administration; drug has an abuse potential in predisposed individuals.

Storage
Store injection and oral products at room temperature.

Administration
! Be aware that meperidine's side effects are dependent on the dosage and route of administration. Know that ambulatory patients and those

not in severe pain may be more prone to dizziness than those in the supine position and those in severe pain.

Take oral meperidine without regard to food. Dilute the syrup in a half-glass of water to prevent an anesthetic effect on mucous membranes.

! Give meperidine injection by slow IV push or IV infusion.

Meperidine may be given undiluted or may be diluted in D5W, Ringer's solution, lactated Ringer's solution, a dextrose-saline combination (such as 2.5%, 5%, or 10% dextrose and 0.45% or 0.9% NaCl), or Molar (M/6) Sodium Lactate Injection for IV injection or infusion. Place the patient in a recumbent position before administering parenteral meperidine. Administer IV push very slowly, over 2-3 min. Rapid IV administration increases the risk of a severe anaphylactic reaction, marked by apnea, cardiac arrest, and circulatory collapse.

! The IM route is preferred over the SC route because the SC route can produce induration, local irritation, and pain. For IM use, inject the drug slowly.

Meprobamate

me-proe′ba-mate

CATEGORY AND SCHEDULE

Pregnancy Risk Category: D
Controlled Substance Schedule: IV

Classification: Anxiolytics, sedative-hypnotic

MECHANISM OF ACTION

A carbamate derivative that affects the thalamus and limbic system. Appears to inhibit multineuronal spinal reflexes. *Therapeutic Effect:* Anxiolytic and sedative activity.

PHARMACOKINETICS

Slowly absorbed from the GI tract. Protein binding: 0%-30%. Metabolized in liver. Excreted in urine and feces. Moderately dialyzable. *Half-life:* 10 h.

AVAILABILITY

Tablets: 200 mg, 400 mg.

INDICATIONS AND DOSAGES

▸ **Anxiety disorders**

PO

Adults, Children 12 yr and older. 400 mg 3-4 times/day. Maximum: 2400 mg/day.

Children aged 6-12 yr. 100-200 mg 2-3 times/day. Maximum: 600 mg/day.

Elderly. Use lowest effective dose. Maximum: 200 mg 2-3 times/day.

▸ **Dosage in renal impairment**

Creatinine Clearance (mL/min)	Dosage Interval (h)
10-50	Every 9-12 h
< 10	Every 12-18 h

CONTRAINDICATIONS

Acute intermittent porphyria, hypersensitivity to meprobamate or related compounds, such as carisoprodol.

INTERACTIONS

Drug

Alcohol, all central nervous system (CNS) depressants: May increase CNS depression.

Warfarin: Meprobamate has been associated with a decreased anticoagulation response; monitor INR.

Herbal
Gotu kola, kava kava, St. John's wort: May increase CNS depression.
Food
None known.

DIAGNOSTIC TEST EFFECTS

Therapeutic levels range between 6 and 12 mg/mL. Rarely causes decreased WBC, platelets, or changes in LFTs.

SIDE EFFECTS

Frequent
Drowsiness, dizziness.
Occasional
Tachycardia, palpitations, headache, light-headedness, dermatitis, diarrhea, nausea, vomiting, dyspnea, rash, weakness, blurred vision, wheezing.

SERIOUS REACTIONS

- Agranulocytosis, aplastic anemia, leukopenia, anaphylaxis, cardiac arrhythmias, hypotensive crisis, syncope, Stevens-Johnson syndrome, and bullous dermatitis have been reported.
- Overdose may cause CNS depression, ataxia, coma, shock, hypotension, and death.
- Rarely causes seizures in predisposed patients.

PRECAUTIONS & CONSIDERATIONS

Caution is warranted with elderly patients as well as those with liver or renal impairment, those with a history of seizures, and those who use alcohol, psychotropic drugs, or other CNS depressants. Prolonged use of meprobamate may produce dependence. Meprobamate crosses the placenta and is distributed in breast milk. Be aware that the safety and efficacy of meprobamate have not been established in children younger than 6 yr. In elderly patients, there is an increased risk of CNS toxicity, manifested as confusion, hallucinations, mental depression, and sedation. Age-related renal impairment may require a decreased dosage in elderly patients.

Complete blood count (CBC), renal function tests, BUN, serum creatinine, liver function tests should be monitored.

Dizziness and drowsiness are expected side effects with meprobamate. Avoid alcohol and sudden changes in posture to help prevent hypotensive effects. Evaluate the patient's tolerance to stress while on therapy. Psychologic and physical dependence may occur with chronic administration.

Storage
Store at room temperature.
Administration
May give without regard to meals. Give last dose at bedtime. Avoid abrupt discontinuation after prolonged use of meprobamate.

Meropenem

mear-ro-pen'em
★ 🍁 Merrem IV

CATEGORY AND SCHEDULE

Pregnancy Risk Category: B

Classification: Anti-infective, carbapenem

MECHANISM OF ACTION

A carbapenem that binds to penicillin-binding proteins and inhibits bacterial cell wall synthesis. Active against most gram-positive and gram-negative bacteria, including *E. coli, P. aeruginosa,* and methicillin-sensitive *S. aureus*. *Therapeutic Effect:* Produces bacterial cell death in most susceptible organisms.

PHARMACOKINETICS

After IV administration, widely distributed into tissues and body fluids, including cerebrospinal fluid (CSF). Protein binding: 2%. Primarily excreted unchanged in urine. High urinary concentrations maintained for up to 5 h after a dose. Removed by hemodialysis. *Half-life:* 1 h.

AVAILABILITY

Powder for Injection: 500 mg, 1 g.

INDICATIONS AND DOSAGES

▸ **Skin, skin-structure, and intra-abdominal infections**

IV

Adults, Elderly. 0.5-1 g q8h.

Children 3 mo and older. 10-20 mg/kg/dose q8h.

Children younger than 3 mo. 10-20 mg/kg/dose q8-12h.

▸ **Meningitis and concurrent bacteremia**

IV

Adults, Elderly. Children weighing 50 kg or more. 2 g q8h.

Children 3 mo and older weighing < 50 kg. 40 mg/kg q8h. Maximum: 2 g/dose.

▸ **Dosage in renal impairment**

Dosage and frequency are modified based on creatinine clearance.

Creatinine Clearance (mL/min)	Dosage Interval
26-49	Recommended dose q12h
10-25	½ of recommended dose q12h
< 10	½ of recommended dose q24h

OFF-LABEL USES

Lower respiratory tract infections (pneumonia), febrile neutropenia, gynecologic and obstetric infections, sepsis.

CONTRAINDICATIONS

Hypersensitivity to the drug or other carbapenems; use caution in patients with immediate hypersensitivity to other β-lactams.

INTERACTIONS

Drug

Probenecid: Reduces renal excretion of meropenem.

Valproic acid or divalproex: Carbapenems reported to lower valproic acid levels; monitor.

Herbal

None known.

Food

None known.

DIAGNOSTIC TEST EFFECTS

May increase BUN level and serum alkaline phosphatase, bilirubin, creatinine, LDH, AST (SGOT), and ALT (SGPT) levels. May decrease blood hematocrit and hemoglobin levels and serum potassium levels.

IV INCOMPATIBILITIES

According to manufacturer, do not mix with or add to solutions containing other drugs. Acyclovir (Zovirax), amphotericin B (Fungizone), diazepam (Valium), doxycycline (Vibramycin), metronidazole (Flagyl), ondansetron (Zofran), quinupristin-dalfopristin (Synercid).

IV COMPATIBILITIES

Dobutamine (Dobutrex), dopamine (Intropin), heparin, magnesium.

M

SIDE EFFECTS

Frequent (3%-5%)
Diarrhea, nausea, vomiting, headache, inflammation at injection site.
Occasional (2%)
Oral candidiasis, rash, pruritus.
Rare (< 2%)
Constipation, glossitis.

SERIOUS REACTIONS

- Antibiotic-associated colitis and other superinfections may occur.
- Anaphylactic reactions have been reported.
- Seizures may occur in those with CNS disorders (including brain lesions and a history of seizures), bacterial meningitis, or impaired renal function.

M

PRECAUTIONS & CONSIDERATIONS

Caution is warranted in patients with CNS disorders (particularly a history of seizures); hypersensitivity to cephalosporins, penicillins, or other β-lactams; and renal function impairment. Assess penicillin and cephalosporin sensitivity before dosing. Be aware that it is unknown whether meropenem is distributed in breast milk; caution is warranted in lactation. Be aware that the safety and efficacy of meropenem have not been established in children younger than 3 mo. In elderly patients, age-related renal impairment may require dosage adjustment. Notify the physician if severe diarrhea occurs, but avoid taking antidiarrheals.

Notify the physician of the onset of troublesome or serious adverse reactions, including infusion-site pain, redness, or swelling, nausea or vomiting, or skin rash or itching. Electrolytes (especially potassium), intake and output, and renal function test results should be monitored. BP, temperature, and mental status should be monitored. Examine the patient periodically for opportunistic secondary infection. Report any oral soreness, lesions, or bleeding. Drug is to be administered only in a hospital or outpatient institutional setting.

Storage
Store vials at room temperature. After reconstitution with 0.9% NaCl, infusion is stable for 4 h at room temperature, 24 h if refrigerated (with D5W, stable for 1 h at room temperature, 4 h if refrigerated).

Administration
! Space drug doses evenly around the clock.

For IV use, reconstitute each 500 mg with 10 mL sterile water for injection to provide a concentration of 50 mg/mL. Shake to dissolve until clear. May further dilute with 100 mL 0.9% NaCl or D5W. Doses of 500 mg or 1 g may be given by intermittent IV bolus over 3-5 min. If diluted for IV infusion, final concentrations are usually 1-20 mg/mL. Give IV intermittent infusion (piggyback) over 15-30 min.

Mesalamine/5 Aminosalicylic Acid (5-ASA)

mez-al'a-meen
★ Apriso, Asacol, Asacol HD, Canasa, Lialda, Pentasa, Rowasa 🍁 Asacol 800, Mesasal, Mezavant, Pentasa, Salofalk
Do not confuse Asacol with Os-Cal.

CATEGORY AND SCHEDULE

Pregnancy Risk Category: B

Classification: Gastrointestinal anti-inflammatory, 5-aminosalicylate.

MECHANISM OF ACTION

A salicylic acid derivative that locally inhibits arachidonic acid metabolite production, which is increased in patients with chronic inflammatory bowel disease. *Therapeutic Effect:* Blocks prostaglandin production and diminishes inflammation in the colon.

PHARMACOKINETICS

Poorly absorbed from the colon. Moderately absorbed from the GI tract. Metabolized in the liver to active metabolite. Unabsorbed portion eliminated in feces; absorbed portion excreted in urine. Unknown whether removed by hemodialysis. *Half-life:* 0.5-1.5 h; metabolite, 5-10 h.

AVAILABILITY

Tablets (Delayed Release [Asacol]): 400 mg.
Tablets (Delayed Release [Asacol HD]): 800 mg.
Tablets (Delayed Release (Lialda)): 1.2 g.
Capsules (Controlled Release [Pentasa]): 250 mg, 500 mg.
Rectal Suspension (Rowasa): 4 g/60 mL.
Suppositories (Canasa): 1000 mg.
Capsules (Extended Release [Apriso]): 0.375 g.

INDICATIONS AND DOSAGES

▸ **Ulcerative colitis, proctosigmoiditis, proctitis**

PO (ASACOL)
Adults, Elderly. 800 mg (2 × 400 mg tablets) 3 times a day for 6 wks.
PO (ASACOL HD)
Adults, Elderly. 1600 mg (2 × 800 mg) 3 times a day for 6 wks.
PO (LIALDA)
Adults, Elderly. 1.2 g OR 2.4 g once daily for up to 8 wks.
PO (PENTASA)
Adults, Elderly. 1 g 4 times a day for 8 wks.
RECTAL (RETENTION ENEMA)
Adults, Elderly. 60 mL (4 g) at bedtime; retain overnight (about 8 h); treat for 3-6 wks.
RECTAL (SUPPOSITORY)
Adults, Elderly. 1 suppository (500 mg) twice a day, retain 1-3 h; treat for 3-6 wks. Alternatively, 1 suppository (1000 mg) at bedtime.

▸ **Maintenance of remission in ulcerative colitis**

PO (ASACOL)
Adults, Elderly. 800 mg (2 × 400 mg) twice daily or 400 mg 4 times a day.
PO (PENTASA)
Adults, Elderly. 1 g 4 times a day.
PO (APRISO)
Adults. 1.5 g PO once daily.

CONTRAINDICATIONS

Hypersensitivity to drug or other 5-aminosalicylates or salicylates.

INTERACTIONS

Drug

Antacids: Do not administer Apriso capsules with antacids.
Azathioprine, mercaptopurine: May increase side effects of these antineoplastics.

Herbal

None known.

Food

None known.

DIAGNOSTIC TEST EFFECTS

May increase BUN, serum alkaline phosphatase, creatinine, AST (SGOT), and ALT (SGPT) levels.

SIDE EFFECTS

Mesalamine is generally well tolerated, with only mild and transient effects.

M

Frequent (> 6%)
PO: Abdominal cramps or pain, diarrhea, dizziness, headache, nausea, vomiting, rhinitis, unusual fatigue.
Rectal: Abdominal or stomach cramps, flatulence, headache, nausea.
Occasional (2%-6%)
PO: Hair loss, decreased appetite, back or joint pain, flatulence, acne.
Rectal: Hair loss.
Rare (< 2%)
Rectal: Anal irritation.

SERIOUS REACTIONS

- Acute intolerance syndrome may occur in susceptible patients, manifested by cramping, headache, diarrhea, fever, rash, hives, itching, and wheezing. Discontinue drug immediately.
- Hepatitis, pancreatitis, and pericarditis occur rarely with oral use.
- Interstitial nephritis (rare).

M

PRECAUTIONS & CONSIDERATIONS

Caution is warranted in patients with preexisting renal disease and sulfasalazine sensitivity. It is unknown whether mesalamine crosses the placenta or is distributed in breast milk; caution is warranted in lactation. Safety and efficacy of mesalamine have not been established in children. In elderly patients, age-related renal impairment may require cautious use. Avoid tasks that require mental alertness or motor skills until response to the drug has been established.

Be aware that mesalamine use may discolor urine yellow-brown; mesalamine suppositories stain fabrics. Adequate fluid intake should be maintained. Daily bowel activity and stool consistency and skin for rash should be assessed. Mesalamine should be discontinued if cramping, diarrhea, fever, or rash occurs. To avoid the possibility of pseudomembranous colitis developing, medical consultation is warranted before selecting an antibiotic for infection.

Storage
Store rectal suspension, suppositories, and oral forms at room temperature.

Administration
For tablet use, do not break; swallow whole. Take mesalamine without regard to food. Extended- and delayed-release capsules should be swallowed whole.

For rectal use, shake bottle well. Lie on the left side with the lower leg extended, upper leg flexed forward, or assume the knee-chest position. Insert applicator tip into rectum, pointing toward umbilicus. Squeeze bottle steadily until contents are emptied. Retain the enema for as long as tolerable, preferably for a minimum of 8 h.

Metaxalone

me-tax'a-lone
★ 🍁 Skelaxin

CATEGORY AND SCHEDULE

Pregnancy Risk Category: C

Classification: Muscle relaxant

MECHANISM OF ACTION

A central depressant whose exact mechanism is unknown. Many effects due to its central depressant actions. Has no direct effect on muscle contractions, the motor end plate, or the nerve fiber.
Therapeutic Effect: Relieves pain or muscle spasms.

PHARMACOKINETICS

PO route onset 1 h, peak 3 h, duration 4-6 h. Well absorbed from the GI tract. Metabolized in the liver. Excreted primarily in urine. *Half-life:* 9 h.

AVAILABILITY

Tablets: 400 mg, 800 mg (Skelaxin).

INDICATIONS AND DOSAGES

▸ **Muscle relaxant**

PO

Adults, Elderly, Children older than 12 yr. 800 mg 3-4 times/day.

CONTRAINDICATIONS

Significantly impaired renal or hepatic function, history of drug-induced hemolytic anemias or other anemias, history of hypersensitivity to metaxalone.

INTERACTIONS

Drug

Alcohol, central nervous system (CNS) depression-producing medications, tricyclic antidepressants: May increase CNS depression.

Herbal

None known.

Food

None known.

DIAGNOSTIC TEST EFFECTS

May give false-positive Benedict test.

SIDE EFFECTS

Occasional

Drowsiness, headache, lightheadedness, dermatitis, nausea, vomiting, stomach cramps, dyspnea.

SERIOUS REACTIONS

- Overdose may cause CNS depression, coma, shock, and respiratory depression.
- Hemolytic anemia (rare).
- Jaundice.
- Rare reports of anaphylaxis.

PRECAUTIONS & CONSIDERATIONS

Caution should be used in patient with impaired liver or renal function. It is unknown whether metaxalone crosses the placenta or is distributed in breast milk. Safety and efficacy of metaxalone have not been established in children younger than 12 yr. In elderly patients, there is an increased risk of CNS toxicity, manifested as confusion, hallucinations, mental depression, and sedation. Age-related renal impairment may require a decreased dosage in elderly patients. Alcohol as well as tasks that require mental alertness or motor skills should be avoided during therapy.

Storage

Store at room temperature.

Administration

Take metaxalone without regard to food.

Metformin Hydrochloride

met-for′min high-droh-klor′ide

🇺🇸 Fortamet, Glucophage, Glucophage XL, Glumetza, Riomet

🇨🇦 Glucophage, Glucophage XR, Glycon, Glumetza

CATEGORY AND SCHEDULE

Pregnancy Risk Category: B

Classification: Antidiabetic agents, biguanide derivative, oral hypoglycemic

MECHANISM OF ACTION

An antihyperglycemic that decreases hepatic production of glucose. Decreases absorption of glucose and improves insulin sensitivity. *Therapeutic Effect:* Improves glycemic control, stabilizes or decreases body weight, and improves lipid profile.

PHARMACOKINETICS

Slowly, incompletely absorbed after oral administration. Food delays or decreases the extent of absorption. Protein binding: Negligible. Distributed primarily to intestinal mucosa and salivary glands. Primarily excreted unchanged in urine. Removed by hemodialysis. *Half-life:* 3-6 h.

AVAILABILITY

Oral Solution (Riomet): 100 mg/mL.
Tablets (Glucophage): 500 mg, 850 mg, 1000 mg.
Tablets (Extended Release [Glucophage XL]): 500 mg, 750 mg.
Tablets (Extended Release [Fortamet]): 500 mg, 1000 mg.

INDICATIONS AND DOSAGES

▸ **Diabetes mellitus type 2**

PO (500-MG, 1000-MG TABLET)
Adults, Elderly. Initially, 500 mg twice a day, with morning and evening meals. May increase in 500-mg increments every week in divided doses. May give twice a day up to 2000 mg/day (for example, 1000 mg twice a day [with morning and evening meals]). If 2500 mg/day is required, divide dose and give 3 times a day with meals. Maximum: 2500 mg/day.
Children 10-16 yr. Initially, 500 mg twice a day. May increase by 500 mg/day at weekly intervals. Maximum: 2000 mg/day.
PO (850-MG TABLET)
Adults, Elderly. Initially, 850 mg/day, with morning meal. May increase dosage in 850-mg increments every other week, in divided doses. Maintenance: 850 mg twice a day, with morning and evening meals. Maximum: 2550 mg/day (850 mg 3 times a day).
PO (EXTENDED-RELEASE TABLETS)
Adults, Elderly. Initially, 500 mg once a day. May increase by 500 mg/day at weekly intervals. Maximum: 2000 mg once a day.

▸ **Conversion to once-daily extended-release formulation in patients currently taking conventional metformin**

PO (EXTENDED RELEASE)
Adults. May switch to same total daily dose, but give extended release once daily with evening meal. Increase in increments of 500 mg weekly if needed. Maximum for Glucophage XR and Glumetza is 2000 mg/day. Maximum Fortamet is 2500 mg/day.
Elderly, Debilitated Adults: Avoid use if ≥ 80 yr unless normal renal function. Use lower maximum dose.

▸ **Adjunct to insulin therapy**

PO
Adults, Elderly. Initially, 500 mg/day. May increase by 500 mg at 7-day intervals. Maximum: 2500 mg/day (2000 mg/day for extended-release form).

OFF-LABEL USES

Treatment of metabolic complications of AIDS, prediabetes, polycystic ovary syndrome.

CONTRAINDICATIONS

Known hypersensitivity to metformin; renal dysfunction (e.g., as suggested by serum creatinine levels ≥ 1.5 mg/mL [males], ≥ 1.4 mg/mL [females] or abnormal CrCl < 60 mL/min), which may also result from conditions such as cardiovascular collapse (shock), acute MI, and septicemia; acute or chronic metabolic acidosis; diabetic ketoacidosis, with or without coma.

M

Diabetic ketoacidosis should be treated with insulin.

Temporarily discontinue in patients undergoing radiologic studies involving IV iodinated contrast because use may result in acute renal failure.

Contraindicated in use with dofetilide.

INTERACTIONS

Drug

Alcohol, amiloride, cimetidine, digoxin, furosemide, morphine, nifedipine, procainamide, quinidine, quinine, ranitidine, triamterene, trimethoprim, vancomycin: May increase metformin blood concentration.
Dofetilide: Decreases excretion of dofetilide. Contraindicated.
Furosemide, hypoglycemia-causing medications: May require a decrease in metformin dosage.
Iodinated contrast studies: May cause acute renal failure and increased risk of lactic acidosis. Discontinue metformin before such tests and for 48 h after the procedure.
Drugs eliminated by renal tubular secretion (e.g., adefovir, amiloride, cimetidine, entecavir): May decrease metformin excretion.

Herbal

None known.

Food

None known.

DIAGNOSTIC TEST EFFECTS

Rarely causes vitamin B_{12} deficiency and resultant indices of megaloblastic anemia.

SIDE EFFECTS

Occasional (> 3%)

GI disturbances (including diarrhea, nausea, vomiting, abdominal bloating, flatulence, and anorexia) that are transient and resolve spontaneously during therapy. Others include headache, weakness.

Rare (1%-3%)

Unpleasant or metallic taste that resolves spontaneously during therapy.

SERIOUS REACTIONS

- Lactic acidosis occurs rarely but is a fatal complication in 50% of cases. Lactic acidosis is characterized by an increase in blood lactate levels (> 5 mmol/L), a decrease in blood pH, and electrolyte disturbances. Signs and symptoms of lactic acidosis include unexplained hyperventilation, myalgia, malaise, and somnolence, which may advance to cardiovascular collapse (shock), acute CHF, acute MI, and prerenal azotemia.

PRECAUTIONS & CONSIDERATIONS

Caution is warranted in patients with CHF, chronic respiratory difficulty, and uncontrolled hyperthyroidism or hypothyroidism, concurrent use of drugs that affect renal function, conditions that cause hyperglycemia or hypoglycemia or delay food absorption (such as diarrhea, high fever, malnutrition, gastroparesis, and vomiting), and in elderly patients, debilitated, or malnourished with renal impairment. Caution should also be used in those who consume excessive amounts of alcohol; alcohol should be avoided during therapy. Insulin is the drug of choice during pregnancy. Metformin is distributed in breast milk in animals. Safety and efficacy of metformin have not been established in children. In elderly patients, age-related renal impairment or peripheral vascular disease may require dosage adjustment or discontinuation of drug; in general, do not titrate up to adult maximum doses.

Notify the physician of diarrhea, easy bleeding or bruising, change in color of stool or urine, headache, nausea, persistent rash, and vomiting. Hemoglobin and hematocrit, RBC count, and serum creatinine level should be obtained before beginning metformin therapy and annually thereafter. Food intake, blood glucose level, glycosylated hemoglobin, folic acid level, and renal function should also be monitored. Be aware of signs and symptoms of hypoglycemia (anxiety, cool wet skin, diplopia, dizziness, headache, hunger, numbness in mouth, tachycardia, tremors) or hyperglycemia (deep rapid breathing, dim vision, fatigue, nausea, polydipsia, polyphagia, polyuria, vomiting), especially in persons also taking oral sulfonylureas; carry candy, sugar packets, or other sugar supplements for immediate response to hypoglycemia. Consult the physician when glucose demands are altered (such as with fever, heavy physical activity, infection, stress, trauma). Exercise, good personal hygiene (including foot care), not smoking, and weight control are essential parts of therapy.

Notify the physician immediately if any of the following symptoms occur, evidencing lactic acidosis: myalgia, respiratory distress, weakness, diarrhea, malaise, muscle cramps, somnolence. Surgical procedures may warrant stopping metformin therapy or adjustment in dose.

Storage

Store at room temperature.

Administration

! Expect to withhold metformin in patients with conditions that may predispose to lactic acidosis, such as dehydration, hypoperfusion, hypoxemia, and sepsis, radiographic tests using contrast.

Take metformin orally with meals. Do not crush film-coated tablets or extended-release tablets. Once-daily extended-release tablets usually given with evening meal and with a full glass of water. Shake oral suspension well before each use.

Methadone Hydrochloride

meth′a-done high-droh-klor′ide

★ Diskets, Dolophine, Methadone Intensol, Methadose 🍁 Metadol

CATEGORY AND SCHEDULE

Pregnancy Risk Category: C (D if used for prolonged periods or at high dosages at term)

Controlled Substance Schedule: II

For opiate dependence, must comply with Narcotic Addict Treatment Act (NATA) [21USC 823(g)]

Classification: Analgesics, narcotic, opiate agonist, synthetic

MECHANISM OF ACTION

An opioid agonist that binds with opioid receptors in the central nervous system (CNS). *Therapeutic Effect:* Alters the perception of and emotional response to pain; reduces withdrawal symptoms from other opioid drugs.

PHARMACOKINETICS

Route	Peak
Oral	6-8 h
IM	4-5 h
IV	15-30 min

Well absorbed after IM injection. Protein binding: 80%-85%. Metabolized in the liver. Primarily excreted in urine. Not removed by hemodialysis. *Half-life:* 8-59 h.

AVAILABILITY

Oral Concentrate (Methadone Intensol, Methadose): 10 mg/mL.
Oral Solution: 5 mg/5 mL, 10 mg/5 mL.
Tablets (Dolophine, Methadose): 5 mg, 10 mg.
Tablets (Dispersible [Diskets, Methadose]): 40 mg.
Injection (Dolophine): 10 mg/mL.

INDICATIONS AND DOSAGES

▸ Analgesia

PO, IV, IM, SC

Adults. 2.5-10 mg q3-8h as needed up to 5-20 mg q6-8h.

Elderly. 2.5 mg q8-12h.

▸ Detoxification

PO

Adults, Elderly. 15-40 mg/day. For patients preferring a brief course of stabilization followed by medically supervised withdrawal, it is generally recommended that the patient be titrated to a total daily dose of about 40 mg in divided doses to achieve an adequate stabilizing level. Continue stabilization for 2-3 days, after which the dose of methadone should be gradually decreased. The rate at which methadone is decreased is chosen individually. Can decrease daily or at 2-day intervals, but the intake should remain sufficient to keep withdrawal symptoms tolerable. In hospitalized patients, a daily reduction of 20% of the total daily dose may be tolerated. In ambulatory patients, a slower schedule may be needed (e.g., 10% reduction every 10-14 days)

▸ Maintenance treatment of opiate dependence in opiate-tolerant patients

PO

Adults, Elderly. 20-120 mg/day. Dosed initially at 20-40 mg/day if opiate tolerant; reduce initial dose by 50% if little or no tolerance. Additional doses of 10 mg given as needed for distressing symptoms related to abstinence. Daily doses > 120 mg need to be justified in the medical record. Continue maintenance as long as benefit is derived.

CONTRAINDICATIONS

Hypersensitivity to methadone, respiratory depression in absence of monitored setting, acute bronchial asthma, hypercarbia, paralytic ileus.

INTERACTIONS

Drug

Alcohol, narcotics, sedative-hypnotics, skeletal muscle relaxants, benzodiazepines, other CNS depressants: May increase CNS or respiratory depression and hypotension.

Anticholinergics: Increased effects of anticholinergics.

CYP3A4 or CYP2D6 inducers: May decrease methadone effect or precipitate withdrawal.

CYP3A4 or CYP2D6 inhibitors: May increase methadone concentrations.

MAOIs: May produce a severe, sometimes fatal reaction; expect to begin methadone at smaller incremental doses.

Nevirapine, efavirenz, ritonavir: May decrease methadone concentrations.

Medications proloning the QT intervals (e.g., class I and class III antiarrhythmics, others): Possible additive effect on QT interval.

Herbal

Valerian: May increase CNS depression.

M

Food
None known.

DIAGNOSTIC TEST EFFECTS
May increase serum amylase and lipase levels.

SIDE EFFECTS
Frequent
Sedation, decreased BP (including orthostatic hypotension), diaphoresis, facial flushing, constipation, dizziness, nausea, vomiting.
Occasional
Confusion, urine retention, palpitations, abdominal cramps, visual changes, dry mouth, headache, decreased appetite, anxiety, insomnia.
Rare
Allergic reaction (rash, pruritus).

SERIOUS REACTIONS
- Overdose results in respiratory depression, skeletal muscle flaccidity, cold or clammy skin, cyanosis, and extreme somnolence progressing to seizures, stupor, and coma. The antidote is naloxone.
- The patient who uses methadone long-term may develop a tolerance to the drug's analgesic effect and physical dependence.
- Potential for QT prolongation and ECG changes.

PRECAUTIONS & CONSIDERATIONS
! Methadone will accumulate over time. Peak respiratory depressant effects typically occur later, and persist longer, than peak analgesic effects. Thease characteristics can contribute to cases of iatrogenic overdose, particularly during initial dose titration. Dose adjustments should be made cautiously.

Caution is warranted with acute abdominal conditions, cor pulmonale, history of seizures, impaired hepatic or renal function, increased intracranial pressure, respiratory abnormalities, supraventricular tachycardia, and in debilitated or elderly patients. Methadone crosses the placenta and is distributed in breast milk. Regular use of opioids during pregnancy may produce withdrawal symptoms in the neonate, such as diarrhea, excessive crying, fever, hyperactive reflexes, irritability, seizures, sneezing, tremors, vomiting, and yawning. The neonate may develop respiratory depression if the mother receives methadone during labor. Children are more prone to experience paradoxical excitement. Children younger than 2 yr and elderly patients are more susceptible to the drug's respiratory depressant effects. Age-related renal impairment may increase the risk of urine retention in elderly patients.

Dizziness and drowsiness may occur, so change positions slowly and avoid alcohol, CNS depressants, and tasks that require mental alertness or motor skills until response to the drug is established. Vital signs should be monitored for 15-30 min after an IM or SC dose and for 5-10 min after an IV dose. Clinical improvement should be monitored. The drug should be withheld and the physician should be notified if the respiratory rate is 12 breaths/min or less in an adult or 20 breaths/min or less in a child. Psychologic and physical dependence may occur with chronic administration.

Patients in the methadone maintenance program should not receive additional opioids or other controlled substances without a consultation.

Storage
Store all dosage forms at room temperature. Keep dispersible tablets tightly closed.
Administration
Know that oral methadone is one-half as potent as parenteral methadone. Take methadone without regard to food. Dilute the concentrate in 3-4 oz of water or citrus fruit juice to prevent an anesthetic effect on mucous membranes.

Dispersible tablets are placed in 3-4 oz of water, orange juice, citrus Tang, or citrus-flavored Kool-Aid and allowed to disperse (1 min). Drink entire dose after stirring well.

! Be aware that the IM route is preferred over the subcutaneous route because the subcutaneous route may produce induration, local irritation, and pain. Do not use the solution if it appears cloudy or contains a precipitate. Place the patient in the recumbent position before giving parenteral methadone. Inject the drug slowly.

Methazolamide

meth-ah-zole′ah-mide
★ Neptazane
Do not confuse Neptazane with nefazodone.

CATEGORY AND SCHEDULE

Pregnancy Risk Category: C

Classification: Diuretics, anti-glaucoma agents, carbonic anhydrase inhibitors

MECHANISM OF ACTION

A noncompetitive inhibitor of carbonic anhydrase that inhibits the enzyme at the luminal border of cells of the proximal tubule. Increases urine volume and changes to an alkaline pH with subsequent decreases in the excretion of titratable acid and ammonia. *Therapeutic Effect:* Produces a diuretic and antiglaucoma effect.

PHARMACOKINETICS

PO route onset 2-4 h, peak 6-8 h, duration 10-18 h. Well absorbed slowly from the GI tract. Protein binding: 55%. Distributed into the tissues (including CSF). Metabolized slowly from the GI tract. Excreted primarily in urine. Not removed by hemodialysis. *Half-life:* 14 h.

AVAILABILITY

Tablets: 25 mg, 50 mg.

INDICATIONS AND DOSAGES

▸ **Glaucoma**

PO

Adults, Elderly. 50-100 mg/day 2-3 times/day.

OFF-LABEL USES

Prevention of altitude sickness, treatment of essential tremor.

CONTRAINDICATIONS

Hypersensitivity to methazolamide, severe kidney or liver disease, failure of adrenal glands, hyperchloremic acidosis.

INTERACTIONS

Drug
Amphetamines, quinidine, procainamide, methenamine, phenobarbital, salicylates (high doses): May increase the excretion of these drugs.

Aspirin and other salicylates (high doses): May increase the risk for anorexia, tachypnea, lethargy, coma, and death (reported with high dose aspirin treatment).
Corticosteroids (systemic use), diuretics: May cause hypokalemia.
Lithium: May increase the excretion of lithium.
Memantine: May decrease the clearance of memantine.
Steroids: May increase the risk of hypokalemia.
Topiramate: May increase the risk of nephrolithiasis.
Herbal
None known.
Food
None known.

M

DIAGNOSTIC TEST EFFECTS

Monitor complete blood count for blood dyscrasias. May cause decreased serum potassium.

SIDE EFFECTS

Occasional
Paresthesias, hearing dysfunction or tinnitus, fatigue, malaise, loss of appetite, taste alteration, nausea, vomiting, diarrhea, polyuria, drowsiness, confusion, hypokalemia.
Rare
Metabolic acidosis, electrolyte imbalance, transient myopia, urticaria, melena, hematuria, glycosuria, hepatic insufficiency, flaccid paralysis, photosensitivity, convulsions, and rarely crystalluria, renal calculi.

SERIOUS REACTIONS

- Malaise and complaints of tiredness and myalgia are signs of excessive dosing and acidosis in elderly patients.
- Stevens-Johnson syndrome, toxic epidermal necrolysis, fulminant hepatic necrosis, agranulocytosis, aplastic anemia, and other blood dyscrasias have been reported and have caused fatalities.
- Nephrolithiasis.

PRECAUTIONS & CONSIDERATIONS

Caution should be used in patients with allergies to sulfonamides, sulfonylureas, carbonic anhydrase inhibitors, thiazides, and loop diuretics (except ethacrynic acid) because of a risk of cross-reaction. Anorexia, tachypnea, lethargy, coma, and death have been reported with concomitant use of high-dose aspirin and methazolamide. Caution is also warranted with COPD, respiratory acidosis, diabetes mellitus, a history of nephrolithiasis, or mental impairment. It is unknown whether methazolamide crosses the placenta and is excreted in breast milk. Safety and efficacy of this drug have not been established in children. Elderly patients may be at an increased risk for developing hypokalemia.

Hypokalemia may result in cardiac arrhythmias, changes in mental status and muscle strength, muscle cramps, and tremor. In patients with cirrhosis or serious hepatic insufficiency, hepatic coma may be precipitated. Potassium should be assessed before and during treatment. Frequency and volume of urination are expected to increase.
Storage
Store tablets at room temperature.
Administration
Take methazolamide with food to avoid GI upset. Maintain adequate hydration.

Methenamine

Hiprex, Urex Mandelamine

CATEGORY AND SCHEDULE

Pregnancy Risk Category: C

Classification: Anti-infectives, urinary

MECHANISM OF ACTION

A hippuric acid salt that hydrolyzes to formaldehyde and ammonia in acidic urine. *Therapeutic Effect:* Formaldehyde has antibacterial action. Bactericidal.

PHARMACOKINETICS

Readily absorbed from the GI tract. Partially metabolized by hydrolysis (unless protected by enteric coating) and partially by the liver. Primarily excreted in urine. *Half-life:* 3-6 h.

AVAILABILITY

Tablets, as Hippurate: 1 g (Urex, Hiprex).
Tablets, as Mandelate: 500 mg, 1 g.

INDICATIONS AND DOSAGES

▸ **Suppressive therapy for frequently recurring urinary tract infection (UTI)**

PO

Adults, Elderly. 1 g 2 times/day (as hippurate).
Children 6-12 yr. 25-50 mg/kg/day q12h (as hippurate).

OFF-LABEL USES

Hyperhidrosis.

CONTRAINDICATIONS

Moderate to severe renal impairment, hepatic impairment (hippurate salt), tartrazine sensitivity (Hiprex contains tartrazine), hypersensitivity to methenamine or any of its components.

INTERACTIONS

Drug

Acetazolamide, antacids, methazolamide, sodium bicarbonate: May decrease effect secondary to alkalinization of urine.
Dichlorphenamide: May inhibit the action of methenamine to alkalinize the urine.
Sulfonamides: May increase the risk of crystalluria. Avoid.

Herbal

None known.

Food

None known.

DIAGNOSTIC TEST EFFECTS

Formaldehyde, the active form of methenamine, interferes with fluorometric procedures for the determination of urinary catecholamines and vanillylmandelic acid (VMA), causing false high results.

SIDE EFFECTS

Occasional

Rash, nausea, dyspepsia, difficulty urinating.

Rare

Bladder irritation, increased liver enzymes.

SERIOUS REACTIONS

• Crystalluria can occur when there is low urinary output.

PRECAUTIONS & CONSIDERATIONS

Caution should be used in patients with hepatic impairment. It is unknown whether methenamine crosses the placenta or is excreted in breast milk; caution is warranted in lactation. No age-related precautions have been noted in children older than 6 yr of age. Avoid using in elderly patients with age-related renal impairment. Antacids should be avoided. Sun and ultraviolet light should be avoided. If it is not avoidable, sunscreens and protective clothing should be worn. Urine pH should be monitored.

Storage
Store at room temperature.

Administration
Take methenamine with food or milk to reduce GI upset. Usually taken with cranberry juice or ascorbic acid to acidify urine. Maintain adequate hydration. Not to be used as primary treatment of UTI.

Methimazole

meth-im'a-zole
Tapazole

CATEGORY AND SCHEDULE

Pregnancy Risk Category: D

Classification: Thyroid hormone antagonist

MECHANISM OF ACTION

A thiomidazole derivative that inhibits synthesis of thyroid hormone by interfering with the incorporation of iodine into tyrosyl residues. *Therapeutic Effect:* Effectively treats hyperthyroidism by decreasing thyroid hormone levels.

PHARMACOKINETICS

High bioavailability in oral administration (80%-95%). Excreted in breast milk. High transplacental passage. Not bound to plasma proteins. Rapidly metabolized; < 10% eliminated in urine. *Half-life:* 6-13 h.

AVAILABILITY

Tablets: 5 mg, 10 mg.

INDICATIONS AND DOSAGES

▸ **Hyperthyroidism**

PO

Adults, Elderly. Initially, 15-60 mg/day in 3 divided doses. Maintenance: 5-15 mg/day in 3 divided doses. Generally avoid doses > 40 mg/day because of increased risk of blood dyscrasias.
Children. Initially, 0.4 mg/kg/day in 3 divided doses. Maintenance: Half the initial dose, or alternately: 0.5-0.7 mg/kg/day in 3 divided doses initially and half the initial dose for maintenance.

CONTRAINDICATIONS

Hypersensitivity to the drug (including drug-induced agranulocytosis); breastfeeding.

INTERACTIONS

Drug

Anticholinergics and sympathomimetics: May increase cardiovascular side effects in uncontrolled patients.
Amiodarone, iodinated glycerol, iodine, potassium iodide: May decrease response to methimazole.
β-Blockers: May increase effect and toxicity as patient becomes euthyroid.
Central nervous system (CNS) depressants: May have increased response to these drugs in uncontrolled patients.
Digoxin: May increase the blood concentration of digoxin as patient becomes euthyroid.
I^{131}: May decrease thyroid uptake of I^{131}.
Oral anticoagulants: May decrease the effects of oral anticoagulants.
Theophylline: May alter theophylline clearance in hyperthyroid or hypothyroid patients.

Vasoconstrictors: Uncontrolled hypothyroid patients are at higher risk when using methimazole.

Herbal

None known.

Food

None known.

DIAGNOSTIC TEST EFFECTS

May increase LDH, serum alkaline phosphatase, bilirubin, AST (SGOT), and ALT (SGPT) levels and prothrombin time. May decrease prothrombin level and WBC count.

SIDE EFFECTS

Frequent (4%-5%)

Fever, rash, pruritus.

Occasional (1%-3%)

Dizziness, loss of taste, nausea, vomiting, stomach pain, peripheral neuropathy or numbness in fingers, toes, face.

Rare (< 1%)

Swollen lymph nodes or salivary glands.

SERIOUS REACTIONS

- Agranulocytosis as long as 4 mo after therapy, pancytopenia, aplastic anemia, and hepatitis have occurred.

PRECAUTIONS & CONSIDERATIONS

Caution is warranted in patients with concurrent use of other agranulocytosis-inducing drugs, impaired hepatic function, and in persons older than 40 yr. Methimazole is excreted in breast milk and should be avoided during breastfeeding. Methimazole is not the agent of choice in pregnancy because it crosses the placenta. Uncontrolled hyperthyroid patients should not engage in any surgical procedures until blood levels are established.

Notify the physician of illness, unusual bleeding or bruising, sore throat, burning, fever, infection, jaundice, or rash. Weight, pulse, CBC, prothrombin time, thyroid function, and serum hepatic enzymes should be monitored. Overdose is evidenced by nausea, vomiting, epigastric distress, headache, fever, arthralgia, pruritis, edema, pancytopenia, agranulocytosis, exfoliative dermatitis, hepatitis, neuropathies, CNS stimulation, or depression. Drug may cause drowsiness; driving or performing tasks requiring mental alertness should be avoided until the effects of the drug are known.

Storage

Store at room temperature in a light-resistant container.

Administration

Take with food if GI symptoms occur. Space doses evenly around the clock.

Methocarbamol

meth-oh-kar'ba-mole

Robaxin

CATEGORY AND SCHEDULE

Pregnancy Risk Category: C

Classification: Skeletal muscle relaxant

MECHANISM OF ACTION

A carbamate derivative of guaifenesin that causes skeletal muscle relaxation by general central nervous system (CNS) depression. *Therapeutic Effect:* Relieves muscle spasticity.

PHARMACOKINETICS

Rapidly and almost completely absorbed from the GI tract. Protein binding: 46%-50%. Metabolized in liver by dealkylation and hydroxylation. Primarily excreted in urine as metabolites. *Half-life:* 1-2 h.

AVAILABILITY

Injection: 100 mg/mL (Robaxin).
Tablets: 325 mg, 500 mg (Robaxin), 750 mg.

INDICATIONS AND DOSAGES

▸ **Musculoskeletal spasm**

IM/IV

Adults, Children 16 yr and older. 1 g q8h for no more than 3 consecutive days. May repeat course of therapy after a drug-free interval of 48 h.

PO

Adults, Children 16 yr and older. 1.5 g 4 times/day for 2-3 days (up to 8 g/day may be given in severe conditions). Decrease to 4 g/day in 3-6 divided doses.

Elderly. Initially, 500 mg 4 times a day. May gradually increase dosage.

▸ **Tetanus spasm**

IV, FOLLOWED BY NASOGASTRIC ADMINISTRATION OF ORAL TABLETS

Adults. 1-3 g q6h until oral dosing is possible. Injection should be used no more than 3 consecutive days. Oral dosage in tetanus can require up to 24 g/day in divided doses q6h.

Children. 15 mg/kg/dose or 500 mg/m^2/dose q6h as needed. Maximum: 1.8 g/m^2/day for 3 days only.

CONTRAINDICATIONS

Hypersensitivity to methocarbamol or any component of the formulation, renal impairment (injection formulation).

INTERACTIONS

Drug

CNS depressants, including alcohol, narcotics, sedative-hypnotics: May potentiate effects when used with other CNS depressants, including alcohol.

Herbal

Gotu kola, kava kava, St. John's wort: May increase CNS depression.

Food

None known.

DIAGNOSTIC TEST EFFECTS

None known.

SIDE EFFECTS

Frequent

Transient drowsiness, weakness, dizziness, light-headedness, nausea, vomiting.

Occasional

Headache, constipation, anorexia, hypotension, confusion, blurred vision, vertigo, facial flushing, rash.

Rare

Paradoxical CNS excitement and restlessness, slurred speech, tremor, dry mouth, diarrhea, nocturia, impotence, bradycardia, hypotension, syncope.

SERIOUS REACTIONS

• Anaphylactoid reactions, leukopenia, and seizures (IV form) have been reported.
• Methocarbamol overdosage results in cardiac arrhythmias, nausea, vomiting, drowsiness, and coma.

PRECAUTIONS & CONSIDERATIONS

Caution is necessary in patients with oral formulation with renal or hepatic impairment. Due to polyethylene glycol 300, NF in injection, do not use injection in renal impairment. Use injectable formulation cautiously in patients with a history of seizures or hepatic impairment. It is unknown whether methocarbamol crosses the placenta or is distributed in breast milk. Be aware that the safety and efficacy of methocarbamol have not been established in children younger than 16 yr. In elderly patients, there is an increased risk of CNS toxicity, manifested as confusion, hallucinations, mental depression, and sedation.

Age-related renal impairment may necessitate a decreased dosage in elderly patients. Symptoms of overdosage indicated as arrhythmia, nausea, vomiting, drowsiness, and coma should be reported immediately.

Storage

Store tablets and unopened vials at room temperature.

Administration

Maximum of 5 mL can be administered into each gluteal region with IM injection.

! Take care with IV use because pain and sloughing may occur.

IV injection may be administered undiluted as a direct IV bolus at a maximum rate of 3 mL/min. Solution is hypertonic. May dilute 1 g of methocarbamol to no more than 250 mL with 0.9% NaCl or dextrose 5% injection. Do not use for more than 3 consecutive days. Except in tetanus, total parenteral dosage will not exceed 3 vials (30 mL) a day by any route. Administer IV while in recumbent position. Maintain position for 15-30 min following infusion.

Give oral formulation without regard to meals. Tablets may be crushed and mixed with food or liquid if needed. May crush tablets and give by nasogastric (NG) tube if necessary (often necessary in tetanus treatment).

Methotrexate Sodium

meth-oh-trex′ate soe′dee-um

★ Rheumatrex, Trexall,

🍁 Apo-Methotrexate, Metoject

Do not confuse Trexall with Trexan.

CATEGORY AND SCHEDULE

Pregnancy Risk Category: X

Classification: Antineoplastic, disease-modifying antirheumatic drug (DMARD), folic acid antagonist

MECHANISM OF ACTION

An antimetabolite that competes with enzymes necessary to reduce folic acid to tetrahydrofolic acid, a component essential to DNA, RNA, and protein synthesis. This action inhibits DNA, RNA, and protein synthesis. The drug can inhibit replication and function of T and B lymphocytes and can suppress the secretion of interleukin-1, interferon-gamma, and tumor necrosis factor; increase the secretion of interleukin-4; impair the release of histamine from basophils; and decrease chemotaxis of neutrophils. *Therapeutic Effect:* Causes death of cancer cells. In psoriasis, reduces plaque and improves joint symptoms. In inflammatory arthritis, slows progression of joint destruction.

PHARMACOKINETICS

Variably absorbed from the GI tract. Completely absorbed after IM administration. Protein binding: 50%-60%. Widely distributed. Metabolized intracellularly in the liver. Excreted primarily in urine. Removed by hemodialysis but not by peritoneal dialysis. *Half-life:* 8-12 h (large doses, 8-15 h).

AVAILABILITY

Tablets: 2.5 mg, 5 mg, 7.5 mg, 10 mg, 15 mg.
Injection Solution: 25 mg/mL.
Injection, Lyophilized Powder: 1g.

INDICATIONS AND DOSAGES

▸ Head and neck cancer
PO, IV, IM
Adults, Elderly. 25-50 mg/m^2 once weekly.

▸ Choriocarcinoma, chorioadenoma destruens, hydatidiform mole, trophoblastic neoplasms
PO, IM
Adults, Elderly. 15-30 mg/day for 5 days; repeat 3-5 times with 1-2 wks between courses.

▸ Breast cancer
IV
Adults, Elderly. 30-60 mg/m^2 days 1 and 8 q3-4wk.

▸ ALL
PO, IV, IM
Adults, Elderly. Induction: 3.3 mg/m^2/day in combination with other chemotherapeutic agents. Maintenance: 30 mg/m^2/wk PO or IM in divided doses or 2.5 mg/kg IV every 14 days.

▸ Burkitt lymphoma
PO
Adults. 10-25 mg/day for 4-8 days; repeat with 7- to 10-day rest between courses.

▸ Lymphosarcoma
PO
Adults, Elderly. 0.625-2.5 mg/kg/day.

▸ Mycosis fungoides
PO
Adults, Elderly. 5-50 mg once weekly or 15-37.5 mg twice weekly.

▸ Rheumatoid arthritis
PO
Adults, Elderly. 7.5 mg once a wk or 2.5 mg q12h for 3 doses once a wk. Maximum: 20 mg/wk.

▸ Juvenile rheumatoid arthritis
PO
Children. The recommended starting dose is 10 mg/m^2 given once weekly.

▸ Psoriasis
PO
Adults, Elderly. 10-25 mg once a wk or 2.5-5 mg q12h for 3 doses once a wk.
IM
Adults, Elderly. 10-25 mg once a wk.

▸ Antineoplastic dosage for children
PO, IM
Children. 7.5-30 mg/m^2/wk or q2wk.

▸ Dosage in renal impairment
Creatinine clearance 61-80 mL/min. Reduce dose by 25%.
Creatinine clearance 51-60 mL/min. Reduce dose by 33%.
Creatinine clearance 10-50 mL/min. Reduce dose by 50%-70%.

CONTRAINDICATIONS

Contraindicated in nursing mothers and those with hypersensitivity to the drug. In patients with psoriasis or rheumatoid arthritis also contraindicated if pregnant, alcoholic, or have alcoholic liver disease, chronic liver disease, immunodeficiency syndromes, or preexisting blood dyscrasias.

INTERACTIONS

Drug
Amoxicillin, tetracycline, doxycycline: Suspected increase in methotrexate toxicity.
Aspirin, alcohol, NSAIDs: Increased toxicity.
Cyclosporine: Increased levels of both, increased toxicity.

NSAIDs, high-dose IV methotrexate: Possible fatal interactions.
Sulfonamides, co-trimoxazole, trimethoprim: Increased hematologic toxicity.

IV INCOMPATIBILITIES

Amiodarone, amphotericin B, caspofungin (Cancidas), diazepam, diltiazem, dopamine, droperidol, gentamicin, idarubicin, levofloxacin (Levaquin), midazolam, nicardipine, phenytoin, propofol, quinupristin-dalfopristin (Synercid), TPN.

SIDE EFFECTS

Frequent
Nausea, vomiting, stomatitis; burning and erythema at psoriatic site (in patients with psoriasis), photosensitivity.
Occasional
Diarrhea, rash, dermatitis, pruritus, alopecia, dizziness, anorexia, malaise, headache, drowsiness, blurred vision.

SERIOUS REACTIONS

- GI toxicity may produce gingivitis, glossitis, pharyngitis, stomatitis, enteritis, and hematemesis.
- Hepatotoxicity is more likely to occur with frequent small doses than with large intermittent doses.
- Pulmonary toxicity may be characterized by interstitial pneumonitis.
- Hematologic toxicity, which may develop rapidly from marked myelosuppression, may be manifested as leukopenia, thrombocytopenia, anemia, and hemorrhage.
- Dermatologic toxicity may produce a rash, pruritus, urticaria, pigmentation, photosensitivity, petechiae, ecchymosis, and pustules.
- Severe nephrotoxicity may produce azotemia, hematuria, and renal failure.

PRECAUTIONS & CONSIDERATIONS

Methotrexate has been reported to cause fetal death and/or congenital anomalies. Therefore, it is not recommended for women of childbearing potential unless there is clear medical evidence that the benefits can be expected to outweigh the considered risks. Pregnancy should be avoided if either partner is receiving methotrexrate; during and for a minimum of 3 mo after therapy for males, and during and for a least 1 ovulatory cycle after therapy for females. Women on methotrexate should not breastfeed their infants. Use with caution in patients with renal or hepatic impairment, ascites, pleural effusions, debility, peptic ulcer disease, ulcerative colitis, active infection. Baseline assessment should include a complete blood count with differential and platelet counts, hepatic enzymes, renal function tests, and a chest x-ray. Maintain adequate hydration. During therapy of rheumatoid arthritis and psoriasis, monitor CBC at least monthly, renal function and LFTs every 1-2 mo. More frequent monitoring is indicated during antineoplastic therapy.
Storage
Store tablets and injectable at room temperature. Injection solution diluted for administration in D5W or NS is stable for up to 24 h at room temperature.
Administration
CAUTION: Observe usual cautions for handling, preparing, administering, and disposing of parenteral cytotoxic drugs. Formulations containing preservatives must not be used for intrathecal or high-dose therapy.

May be administered IV as slow push, short bolus infusion, or 24- to 42-h continuous infusion. See manufacturer's recommendations for appropriate solutions and volumes.
! For oral use, always check dosage against indication for use. Dosages for ambulatory conditions, such as rheumatoid arthritis, are usually once weekly and do not exceed 20-30 mg/wk maximum in adults. Medication errors that occur can be fatal or cause significant morbidity.

Methscopolamine Bromide

meth-scoe-pol'a-meen bro'myde
★ Pamine, Pamine Forte

CATEGORY AND SCHEDULE

Pregnancy Risk Category: C

Classification: Anticholinergics, gastrointestinals

MECHANISM OF ACTION

A peripheral anticholinergic agent that has limited ability to cross the blood-brain barrier and provides a peripheral blockade of muscarinic receptors. *Therapeutic Effect:* Reduces the volume and the total acid content of gastric secretions, inhibits salivation, and reduces GI motility. The drug has not been shown to be effective at healing peptic ulcers, reducing their recurrence, or preventing complications.

PHARMACOKINETICS

Poorly and unreliably absorbed from the GI tract. Limited ability to cross the blood-brain barrier. Excreted primarily in the urine and the bile. The effects of methscopolamine appear to occur within 1 h and last for 4-6 h. Primarily excreted in urine. *Half-life:* Unknown.

AVAILABILITY

Tablets: 2.5 mg (Pamine), 5 mg (Pamine Forte).

INDICATIONS AND DOSAGES

▸ **Peptic ulcer (historical)**

Adults, Elderly. Initially, 2.5 mg 30 min before meals and 2.5-5 mg at bedtime. Starting dose 12.5 mg/day is most effective. May increase dose by 5 mg every 12 h. Can start with 20 mg/day in 5-mg doses, each half an hour before meals and at bedtime in severe GI distress.

OFF-LABEL USES

Gastrointestinal spasm.

CONTRAINDICATIONS

Reflux esophagitis, glaucoma, obstructed uropathy, obstructed disease of the GI tract (pyloroduodenal stenosis), paralytic ileus, intestinal atony of elderly or debilitated individuals, unstable cardiovascular status in acute hemorrhage, severe ulcerative colitis, toxic megacolon, complicated ulcerative colitis, myasthenia gravis, hypersensitivity to methscopolamine, any component of the formulation, or related drugs.

INTERACTIONS

Drug

Antacids: May decrease absorption of methscopolamine.
Antipsychotic agents: May produce additive anticholinergic effects.
Tricyclic antidepressants, anticholinergics: May produce additive anticholinergic effects.

Herbal

None known.

Food
None known.

DIAGNOSTIC TEST EFFECTS
None known.

SIDE EFFECTS
Occasional
Dry mouth, throat, and nose, urinary hesitancy and/or retention, constipation, tachycardia, palpitations, headache, insomnia, dry skin, urticaria, weakness.

SERIOUS REACTIONS
- Overdosage may vary from central nervous system (CNS) depression, including sedation, apnea, hypotension, cardiovascular collapse, or death to severe paradoxical reaction (such as hallucinations, tremor, and seizures).

PRECAUTIONS & CONSIDERATIONS
Caution is necessary in patients with diarrhea because it may be an early symptom of incomplete intestinal obstruction. Large doses should be used cautiously because methscopolamine may suppress intestinal motility, causing paralytic ileus and precipitate, or aggravate toxic megacolon. Caution is also warranted in patients with autonomic neuropathy, benign prostatic hyperplasia, hyperthyroidism, ulcerative colitis, hepatic or renal dysfunction, arrhythmias, cardiovascular disease, congestive heart failure, hypertension, or in elderly patients. Elderly patients are at an increased risk of developing confusion, dizziness, hyperexcitability, hypotension, and sedation. It is unknown whether methscopolamine crosses the placenta or is excreted in breast milk; caution warranted in lactation. Anticholinergics may suppress lactation. Safety and efficacy have not been established in children.

Expected responses to the drug include dizziness, drowsiness, and dry mouth. Tasks that require mental alertness or motor skills should be avoided until the effects of the drug are known. Report any GI bleeding.

Storage
Store at controlled room temperature.

Administration
Take methscopolamine 30 min before meals and at bedtime.

Methsuximide
meth-sux'i-mide
Celontin
Do not confuse with methoxsalen.

CATEGORY AND SCHEDULE
Pregnancy Risk Category: C

Classification: Anticonvulsants, succinimides

MECHANISM OF ACTION
A succinimide anticonvulsant agent that increases the seizure threshold, suppresses paroxysmal spike-and-wave pattern in absence seizures and depresses nerve transmission in the motor cortex. *Therapeutic Effect:* Controls absence (petit mal) seizures.

PHARMACOKINETICS
Rapidly metabolized in liver to active metabolite, *N*-desmethylmethsuximide. Excreted primarily in urine. Unknown whether it is removed by hemodialysis. *Half-life:* 1.4 h.

AVAILABILITY
Capsules: 300 mg (Celontin).

INDICATIONS AND DOSAGES

▸ **Absence seizures**

PO

Adults, Elderly. Initially, 300 mg/day for the first week. Increase dosage by 300 mg/day at weekly intervals until response is attained. Maintenance: 1200 mg/day divided 2-4 times/day. Do not exceed 1200 mg/day.

Children. Initially, 10-15 mg/kg/day PO given in 3-4 divided doses. Increase weekly up to a maximum of 30 mg/kg/day PO. Maintenance: Mean of 20 mg/kg day for children < 30 kg, and 14 mg/kg/day if > 30 kg.

OFF-LABEL USES

Partial complex (psychomotor) seizures.

M

CONTRAINDICATIONS

Hypersensitivity to succinimides or any component of the formulation.

INTERACTIONS

Drug

Alcohol, benzodiazepines, barbiturates, and other CNS depressants: May cause increased sedative effects.

Anticonvulsants: May increase plasma concentrations of other anticonvulsants.

Cyclosporine: May decrease cyclosporine blood levels by increasing its metabolism.

Haloperidol: May cause change in frequency and pattern of seizures.

Phenothiazines, thioxanthenes, barbiturates: May cause decreased effects of these drugs.

Herbal

Evening primrose oil: May decrease the effects of methsuximide.

Ginkgo biloba: May decrease the effects of methsuximide.

Food

None known.

DIAGNOSTIC TEST EFFECTS

None known.

SIDE EFFECTS

Frequent

Drowsiness, dizziness, nausea, vomiting.

Occasional

Visual abnormalities, such as spots before eyes, difficulty focusing, blurred vision, dry mouth or pharynx, tongue irritation, nervousness, insomnia, headache, constipation or diarrhea, rash, weight loss, proteinuria, edema.

Rare

Systemic lupus-like syndrome.

SERIOUS REACTIONS

- Toxic reactions appear as blood dyscrasias, including aplastic anemia, agranulocytosis, thrombocytopenia, leukopenia, leukocytosis, eosinophilia.
- Dermatologic effects, such as rash, urticaria, pruritus, photosensitivity, Stevens-Johnson syndrome.
- Abrupt withdrawal may precipitate status epilepticus.

PRECAUTIONS & CONSIDERATIONS

Caution is warranted with impaired cardiac, liver, or renal function. Caution should be used in any seizure type. Methsuximide is not first-line therapy. It is unknown if methsuximide crosses the placenta and is distributed in breast milk. Behavioral changes are more likely to occur in children taking methsuximide. Elderly patients are more susceptible to agitation, atrioventricular (AV) block, bradycardia, and confusion. Blood tests should be repeated frequently during first 3 mo of therapy and at monthly intervals thereafter for 2-3 yr. Assess patients for stress tolerance to avoid changes in seizure frequency and frequency of seizure control adjustments being needed.

Drowsiness usually disappears during therapy. Tasks that require mental alertness and motor skills should be avoided.

Storage

Keep at controlled room temperature. Heat of 104° F or higher will melt the drug.

Administration

Take with meals to reduce risk of GI distress. Be aware when replacement by another anticonvulsant is necessary, plan to decrease methsuximide gradually as therapy begins with a low replacement dose. Abrupt withdrawal of the drug may precipitate seizures. Methsuximide must be used in combination with other anticonvulsants in patients with both absence and tonic-clonic seizures.

Methylcellulose

meth-ill-cell'you-los

★ Citrucel

Do not confuse Citrucel with Citracal.

CATEGORY AND SCHEDULE

Pregnancy Risk Category: C

OTC

Classification: Laxatives, bulk-forming

MECHANISM OF ACTION

A bulk-forming laxative that dissolves and expands in water. *Therapeutic Effect:* Provides increased bulk and moisture content in stool, increasing peristalsis and bowel motility.

PHARMACOKINETICS

Route	Onset	Peak	Duration
PO	12-24 h	NA	NA

Acts in small and large intestines. Full effect may not be evident for 2-3 days.

AVAILABILITY

Caplets. 500 mg.

Powder for Oral Solution: Each adult dose contains 2 g; also available sugar-free.

INDICATIONS AND DOSAGES

▸ **Constipation**

PO (POWDER)

Adults, Elderly. 1 tbsp (15 mL) in 8 oz water 1-3 times a day.

Children 6-12 yr. 1 tsp (5 mL) in 4 oz water 3-4 times a day.

PO (CAPLETS)

Adults. 2 caplets up to 6 times/day.

CONTRAINDICATIONS

Abdominal pain, dysphagia, nausea, partial bowel obstruction, symptoms of appendicitis, vomiting, or difficulty swallowing.

INTERACTIONS

Drug

Other oral medications: No specific drug interactions noted; however, it may be advisable to separate fiber administration from that of other oral drugs by 1-2 h.

Herbal

None known.

Food

None known.

DIAGNOSTIC TEST EFFECTS

May increase blood glucose level if taking sugar-containing product.

SIDE EFFECTS

Rare

Some degree of abdominal discomfort, nausea, mild cramps.

SERIOUS REACTIONS

- Esophageal or bowel obstruction may occur if administered with < 250 mL or 1 full glass of liquid.

PRECAUTIONS & CONSIDERATIONS

Methylcellulose can be used safely in pregnancy. Safety and efficacy of methylcellulose have not been established in children younger than 6 yr. No age-related precautions have been noted in elderly patients. Pattern of daily bowel activity and stool consistency should be monitored. Caution is warranted in individuals who have difficulty swallowing, ileostomy, colostomy. Those with diabetes may choose a sugar-free powder, or the caplets, which contain no carbohydrates.

Storage

Store at room temperature, protected from high humidity. Keep tightly closed.

Administration

Powder should not be swallowed in dry form but should be mixed with at least 1 full glass (8 oz) of liquid. For all products, a full glass of water should be taken with each dose; an inadequate amount of fluid may cause choking or swelling in the throat. To promote defecation, increase fluid intake, exercise, and eat a high-fiber diet.

Methyldopa

meth-ill-doe′pa

Aldomet Apo-Methyldopa, Novomedopa

Do not confuse Aldomet with Anzemet.

CATEGORY AND SCHEDULE

Pregnancy Risk Category: B

Classification: Antihypertensives, centrally acting

MECHANISM OF ACTION

An antihypertensive agent that stimulates central inhibitory α-adrenergic receptors, lowers arterial pressure, and reduces plasma renin activity. *Therapeutic Effect:* Reduces BP.

PHARMACOKINETICS

IV form hydrolyzed from methyldopate to methyldopa; onset similar for both PO and IV. Roughly 50% of PO absorbed. Crosses the blood-brain barrier and the placenta, and small amount appears in breast milk. Maximum BP effect at 4-6 h after dose; duration 12-24 h. Eliminated biphasically, 95% during the initial phase (plasma half-life of 2 h) and the rest much more slowly. Unabsorbed drug excreted in the feces. Half-life doubled in renal impairment

AVAILABILITY

Tablets: 250 mg, 500 mg.
Injection: 50 mg/mL.

INDICATIONS AND DOSAGES

▸ **Moderate to severe hypertension**

PO

Adults. Initially, 250 mg 2-3 times a day for 2 days. Adjust dosage at intervals of 2 days (minimum). Maximum: 3 g/day.

Elderly. Initially, 125 mg 1-2 times a day. May increase by 125 mg q2-3 days. Maintenance: 500 mg to 2 g/day in 2-4 divided doses.

Children. Initially, 10 mg/kg/day given in 2-4 divided doses. Maximum: 65 mg/kg/day or 3 g/day, whichever is less.

IV

Adults. 250-1000 mg q6-8h. Maximum: 4 g/day.

Children. Initially, 20-40 mg/kg/day in divided doses q6h. Maximum: 65 mg/kg/day or 3 g/day, whichever is less.

CONTRAINDICATIONS

Hepatic disease, pheochromocytoma, previous liver problems with methyldopa, hypersensitivity, treatment with MAO inhibitors.

INTERACTIONS

Drug

Epinephrine and other sympathomimetics: May increase pressor response.
General anesthetics: May increase hypotensive action of these drugs.
Haloperidol, alcohol and other central nervous system (CNS) depressants: May increase sedative effects of these drugs.
Hypotensive-producing medications, such as antihypertensives and diuretics: May increase the effects of methyldopa.
Indomethacin and other NSAIDs: May decrease effects of methyldopa.
Iron supplements: Decrease oral absorption of methyldopa.
Lithium: May increase the risk of lithium toxicity.
MAOIs: May cause hyperexcitability. Contraindicated.
NSAIDs, tricyclic antidepressants: May decrease the effects of methyldopa.

Herbal

None known.

Food

None known.

IV INCOMPATIBILITIES

Acyclovir, amphotericin B, diazepam, furosemide, imipenem/cilastatin (Primaxin), pentobarbital, phenobarbital, phenytoin, piperacillin/tazobactam (Zosyn).

DIAGNOSTIC TEST EFFECTS

May increase BUN and serum prolactin, alkaline phosphatase, bilirubin, creatinine, potassium, sodium, uric acid, AST (SGOT), and ALT (SGPT) levels. May produce positive Coombs' test and prolong prothrombin time.

SIDE EFFECTS

Frequent

Peripheral edema, somnolence, headache, dry mouth.

Occasional

Mental changes (such as anxiety, depression), decreased sexual function or libido, diarrhea, swelling of breasts, nausea, vomiting, light-headedness, paresthesia, rhinitis.

SERIOUS REACTIONS

- Hepatotoxicity (abnormal liver function test results, jaundice, hepatitis), hemolytic anemia, unexplained fever, and flu-like symptoms may occur. If these conditions appear, discontinue the medication and contact the physician.
- Granulocytopenia.

PRECAUTIONS & CONSIDERATIONS

Caution is warranted in patients with renal impairment. Dizziness, drowsiness, and light-headedness may occur. Tasks requiring mental alertness and motor skills should be avoided. BP, pulse, weight, and liver function tests should be monitored before and during therapy. BP and pulse should be monitored every 30 min until stabilized. Chronic use may cause infection, bleeding, or poor healing, and these symptoms should be reported so medication changes can be considered. Orthostatic hypotension may result with rapid positional changes; caution is warranted.

Storage

Store oral forms and unopened injection at room temperature. Once diluted in D5W for infusion, stable for 24 h at room temperature.

Administration
For IV infusion, add the prescribed dose to 100 mL D5W and infuse over 30-60 min. Alternatively, add the prescribed dose to D5W to make a final concentration of 10 mg/mL and infuse over 30-60 min.

Orally may give without regard to food. Do not give at the same time as iron supplements.

Methylergonovine

meth-ill-er-goe-noe′veen
★ Methergine

CATEGORY AND SCHEDULE

Pregnancy Risk Category: C

Classification: Ergot alkaloids, oxytocics

M

MECHANISM OF ACTION

An ergot alkaloid that stimulates α-adrenergic and serotonin receptors, producing arterial vasoconstriction. Causes vasospasm of coronary arteries and directly stimulates uterine muscle. *Therapeutic Effect:* Increases strength and frequency of uterine contractions. Decreases uterine bleeding.

PHARMACOKINETICS

Route	Onset	Peak	Duration
PO	5-10 min	NA	NA
IV	Immediate	NA	3 h
IM	2-5 min	NA	NA

Rapidly absorbed from the GI tract after IM administration. Distributed rapidly to plasma, extracellular fluid, and tissues. Metabolized in the liver and undergoes first-pass effect. Excreted in urine. *Half-life:* IV (α phase), 2-3 min or less; IV (β phase), 20-30 min or longer.

AVAILABILITY

Tablets: 0.2 mg.
Injection: 0.2 mg/mL.

INDICATIONS AND DOSAGES

▸ **Prevention and treatment of postpartum and postabortion hemorrhage due to atony or involution**

PO

Adults. 0.2 mg 3-4 times a day. Continue for up to 7 days, but 48 h of use is usually sufficient.

IV, IM

Adults. Initially, 0.2 mg. May repeat q2-4h for no more than a total of 0.8 mg/day for no more than 7 days.

OFF-LABEL USES

Treatment of incomplete abortion.

CONTRAINDICATIONS

Hypertension, toxemia, untreated hypocalcemia. Use during pregnancy is contraindicated except following obstetric delivery or abortion. Also, carefully screen for drug interactions.

INTERACTIONS

Drug

Vasoconstrictors, vasopressors: May increase the effects of methylergonovine.

Protease inhibitors, clarithromycin, erythromycin, itraconazole, ketoconazole, and other potent CYP3A4 inhibitors: Increase risk of ergot toxicity. Generally contraindicated.

Less potent CYP3A4 inhibitors (e.g, nefazodone, fluconazole, fluoxetine, fluvoxamine, zileuton): Coadminister with caution as could increase risk of ergot side effects.

Serotonin-receptor agonists ("triptans" for migraine): Do not use within 24 h of ergot alkaloids due to potential for serious coronary or cerebral ischemia.

Tobacco smoking: Increases risk for ergot ischemia; avoid.
Sympathomimetics: May increase effects.
Herbal
None known.
Food
Grapefruit juice: May increase risk of ergot toxicity.

DIAGNOSTIC TEST EFFECTS

May decrease serum prolactin concentration.

IV INCOMPATIBILITIES

No specific information available; compatibility not widely studied.

IV COMPATIBILITIES

Heparin, potassium.

SIDE EFFECTS

Frequent
Nausea, uterine cramping, vomiting.
Occasional
Abdominal pain, diarrhea, dizziness, diaphoresis, tinnitus, bradycardia, chest pain.
Rare
Allergic reaction, such as rash and itching; dyspnea; severe or sudden hypertension.

SERIOUS REACTIONS

- Severe hypertensive episodes may result in cerebrovascular accident, coronary vasospasm and chest pain, serious arrhythmias, and seizures. Hypertensive effects are more frequent with patient susceptibility, rapid IV administration, and concurrent use of regional anesthesia or vasoconstrictors.
- Peripheral ischemia may lead to gangrene.

PRECAUTIONS & CONSIDERATIONS

! Drug is not intended for use in any location other than a hospital setting.
! Methylergonovine should never be used for induction or augmentation of labor.

Caution is warranted in patients with coronary artery disease, hepatic or renal impairment, occlusive peripheral vascular disease, and sepsis. Methylergonovine use is contraindicated during pregnancy. Small amounts of the drug are distributed in breast milk; caution is warranted in lactation, but the drug, in short term (a few days) use, may be given while breastfeeding. Safety and efficacy of methylergonovine use in children or elderly patients are unknown. Avoid smoking because of added effects of vasoconstriction.

Notify the physician of chest pain, increased bleeding, cold or pale feet or hands, cramping, or foul-smelling lochia. Be aware that the drug may diminish circulation. BP, pulse rate, and uterine tone should be monitored every 15 min until stable for 1-2 h.

Storage
Store tablets at room temperature. Refrigerate vials. Protect from light.
Administration
! Methylergonovine should never be used for induction or augmentation of labor.

Administration may be PO, IV, or IM. Initial dose may be given parenterally, followed by an oral regimen.

IM route is the preferred administration. Monitor BP, heart rate, and uterine response prior to and during dosing. Use IV route in life-threatening situations only, as prescribed. Dilute drug with 0.9% NaCl to a volume of 5 mL. Give over at least 1 min, carefully monitoring BP.

M

Methylnaltrexone

meth'ill-nal-trex'own

Relistor

CATEGORY AND SCHEDULE

Pregnancy Risk Category: C

Classification: Gastrointestinal agents, peripheral opioid μ-receptor antagonist

MECHANISM OF ACTION

A unique narcotic antagonist that displaces opioids at opioid-occupied μ-receptor sites in the gastrointestinal tract, without impacting the pain-relieving actions of opioid agonists within the CNS. *Therapeutic Effect:* Reduces opioid-induced constipation.

PHARMACOKINETICS

Following SC use absorbed rapidly, with peak concentrations (Cmax) achieved at approximately 0.5 h. Moderate tissue distribution. Does not cross the blood brain barrier. Protein binding: 11%-15.3%. Minor amounts of metabolites formed. Conversion to methyl-6-naltrexol isomers (5% of total) and methylnaltrexone sulfate (1.3% of total are the primary pathways of metabolism). N-demethylation of methylnaltrexone to produce naltrexone is not significant. The drug is eliminated primarily as the unchanged drug. Approximately 50% is excreted in the urine and somewhat less in feces. *Half-life:* Roughly 8 h.

AVAILABILITY

Injection: 12 mg per 0.6 mL single-use vial (Relistor).

INDICATIONS AND DOSAGES

▸ **Opioid-induced constipation in patients receiving palliative care, when response to laxative therapy has not been sufficient**

SC

Adults, Elderly. The usual dose is given every other day SC, but may be increased to no more frequently than q24h if needed. Dose amount is based on weight as follows; once dose is calculated, round injection volume to the nearest 0.1 mL.

< 38 kg: Give 0.15 mg/kg SC every other day.

38-61 kg: Give 8 mg SC every other day.

62-114 kg: Give 12 mg SC every other day.

115 kg or above: Give 0.15 mg/kg SC every other day.

▸ **Dosage in renal impairment**

CrCl < 30 mL/min: Reduce normal dose by 50%.

CONTRAINDICATIONS

Hypersensitivity; known or suspected mechanical GI obstruction.

INTERACTIONS

Drug, Herbal, and Food

None known.

DIAGNOSTIC TEST EFFECTS

None known.

SIDE EFFECTS

Frequent (> 5%)

Abdominal pain, flatulence, nausea, dizziness, diarrhea, and hyperhidrosis.

SERIOUS REACTIONS

- Rare cases of gastrointestinal (GI) perforation have been reported. Perforations have occurred in the stomach, duodenum, or colon. Any part of the GI tract might be affected.
- Overdosage may produce orthostatic hypotension.

PRECAUTIONS & CONSIDERATIONS

Use with caution in patients with severe renal or hepatic impairment. Also use with caution in patients who may have risk factors for perforation, such as peptic ulcer disease. Has not been studied in patients who have peritoneal catheters in place. Unknown whether crosses placenta or is excreted in breast milk; warrants caution in lactation and in pregnancy. Safety and efficacy are not established in children.

If severe or persistent diarrhea or severe abdominal symptoms occur, advise patients to discontinue therapy and consult their physician.

Storage

Store injection at room temperature and protect from light. Do not freeze. Once drawn into a syringe, the syringe is stable for 24 h at room temperature.

Administration

Methylnaltrexone is for subcutaneous injection only into the upper arm, abdomen, or thigh. Do not administer more than 1 dose in a 24-h period. Most patients have a bowel movement within a few minutes to a few hours after taking a dose; roughly 30% of patients have a bowel movement within 30 min.

Methylphenidate Hydrochloride

meth-ill-fen'i-date high-droh-klor'ide

★ Concerta, Daytrana, Metadate CD, Metadate ER, Methylin Chewable, Methylin Oral Solution, Methylin ER, Ritalin, Ritalin LA, Ritalin SR 🍁 Biphentin, Concerta, Ritalin, Ritalin SR

Do not confuse Ritalin with Rifadin.

CATEGORY AND SCHEDULE

Pregnancy Risk Category: C

Controlled Substance Schedule: II

Classification: Stimulants, central nervous system (CNS)

MECHANISM OF ACTION

A CNS stimulant that blocks the reuptake of norepinephrine and dopamine into presynaptic neurons. *Therapeutic Effect:* The exact mode of action in attention deficit hyperactivity disorder (ADHD) is not know. Decreases motor restlessness and fatigue; increases motor activity, attention span, and mental alertness; produces mild euphoria.

PHARMACOKINETICS

Onset	Peak	Duration
Immediate release	2 h	3-5 h
Sustained release	4-7 h	3-8 h
Extended release	N/A	8-12 h

Slowly and incompletely absorbed from the GI tract. Protein binding: 15%. Metabolized in the liver. Eliminated in urine and in feces by biliary system. Unknown whether it is removed by hemodialysis. *Half-life:* 2-4 h.

AVAILABILITY

Capsules (Extended Release [Metadate CD]): 10 mg, 20 mg, 30 mg.
Capsules (Extended Release [Ritalin LA]): 20 mg, 30 mg, 40 mg.
Tablets (Ritalin): 5 mg, 10 mg, 20 mg.
Tablets (Extended Release [Metadate ER, Methylin ER]): 10 mg, 20 mg.
Tablets (Extended Release [Concerta]): 18 mg, 27 mg, 36 mg, 54 mg.
Tablets (Sustained Release [Ritalin SR]): 20 mg.
Tablets (Chewable [Methylin]): 2.5 mg, 5 mg, 10 mg.
Oral Solution (Methylin): 5 mg/5 mL, 10 mg/5 mL.
Transdermal System (Daytrana 9-h patch): 10 mg, 15 mg, 20 mg, 30 mg.

M

INDICATIONS AND DOSAGES

▸ **Attention-deficit hyperactivity disorder (ADHD)**

PO

Adults, Children 6 yr and older. Immediate release: Initially, 2.5-5 mg before breakfast and lunch. May increase by 5-10 mg/day at weekly intervals. Maximum: 60 mg/day.

TRANSDERMAL (DAYTRANA)

Children 6 yr and older. Initially, 10-mg patch once a day worn for 9 h only; may increase at weekly intervals. Maximum: 30 mg/day. Use the same initial dose even if converting from another dose form.

PO (CONCERTA)

Adults, Children 6 yr and older. Initially, 18 mg once a day; may increase by 18 mg/day at weekly intervals. Maximum: 54-72 mg/day.

PO (METADATE CD)

Adults, Children 6 yr and older. Initially, 20 mg/day. May increase by 20 mg/day at weekly intervals. Maximum: 60 mg/day.

PO (RITALIN LA)

Adults, Children 6 yr and older. Initially, 20 mg/day. May increase by 10 mg/day at weekly intervals. Maximum: 60 mg/day.

Patients changing from methylphenidate multiple daily doses to once-daily extended-release oral forms. Convert at same daily dose and give once daily.

▸ **Narcolepsy**

PO

Adults, Elderly. 10 mg 2-3 times a day. Range: 10-60 mg/day.

OFF-LABEL USES

Treatment of refractory mental depression in adults.

CONTRAINDICATIONS

Hypersensitivity to methylphenidate or dexmethylphenidate or product components. Do not use within 14 days of MAOIs, marked agitation, glaucoma, Tourette or tics, known serious cardiac abnormalities or serious heart rhythmic problems.

INTERACTIONS

Drug

Antihypertensives: Decreased effect of antihypertensives may occur.

Clonidine: Severe toxic reactions occur with methylphenidate.

MAOIs, linezolid: May increase the effects of methylphenidate such as severe hypertensive episodes. MAOIs are contraindicated.

Other CNS stimulants: May have an additive effect.

Phenytoin, phenobarbital: May inhibit the metabolism of these anticonvulsants; monitor.

Tricyclic antidepressants, SSRIs: Dosage of these drugs may need to be decreased.

Warfarin: May inhibit the metabolism of warfarin. Monitor INR.

Herbal

None known.

Food

Caffeine: May be useful to limit caffeinated beverages.

DIAGNOSTIC TEST EFFECTS

None known.

SIDE EFFECTS

Frequent

Anxiety, insomnia, anorexia.

Occasional

Dizziness, drowsiness, headache, nausea, abdominal pain, fever, rash, arthralgia, vomiting.

Rare

Blurred vision, Tourette syndrome (marked by uncontrolled vocal outbursts, repetitive body movements, and tics), palpitations.

SERIOUS REACTIONS

- Withdrawal after prolonged therapy may unmask symptoms of the underlying disorder.
- CNS stimulant use associated with serious cardiovascular events and sudden death in patients with cardiac abnormalities or serious heart problems.
- Methylphenidate may lower the seizure threshold in those with a history of seizures.
- Overdose produces excessive sympathomimetic effects, including vomiting, tremor, hyperreflexia, seizures, confusion, hallucinations, and diaphoresis.
- Prolonged administration to children with ADHD may delay growth.

PRECAUTIONS & CONSIDERATIONS

Caution is warranted in patients with hypertension, seizures, acute stress reaction, emotional instability, and a history of drug dependence. It is unknown whether methylphenidate crosses the placenta or is distributed in breast milk; therefore, caution is warranted in lactation. Children are more prone to develop abdominal pain, anorexia, weight loss, and insomnia. Long-term methylphenidate use may inhibit growth in children. No age-related precautions have been noted in elderly patients.

Tasks that require mental alertness and motor skills should be avoided until response to the drug is established. Notify the physician if fever, anxiety, an increase in hostile or aggressive behavior, palpitations, a rash, vomiting or, for those with a seizure disorder, an increase in the number of seizures, occurs. CBC, WBC count with differential, and platelet should be monitored. Baseline height and weight should be obtained at the beginning and periodically throughout therapy.

Storage

Store all dosage forms at room temperature; keep oral forms tightly closed. Keep transdermal patch in sealed foil wrapper until time of use.

Administration

Take immediate-release methylphenidate 30-45 min before meals (usually before breakfast and lunch). Take the last dose before 6:00 PM to help prevent insomnia. Do not cut, crush, or chew extended-release tablets or capsules. Open the Metadate CD or Ritalin LA or capsule and sprinkle the pellets on applesauce, if desired. Do not chew.

Swallow Concerta whole with liquids; the drug is in a nonabsorbable controlled rate shell. The empty shell matrix may be noted in patient stool but is not cause for alarm. The Daytrana patch is placed on a dry, clean area of the hip and held in place for 30 seconds; apply 2 h before the effect is desired. Do not use on damaged or irritated skin. Do not use patch if it appears damaged after opening. Rotate hips of application daily. Do not cut/trim patch. Do not expose to a heat source as this may cause overdose. Remember to remove patch after no longer than 9 h of wear. Peel off slowly.

Methylprednisolone

meth-il-pred-niss'oh-lone

★ 🍁 Medrol, Depo-Medrol, A-Methapred, Solu-Medrol

Do not confuse methylprednisolone with medroxyprogesterone, or Medrol with Mebaral.

CATEGORY AND SCHEDULE

Pregnancy Risk Category: C

Classification: Glucocorticoid, immediate acting

M

MECHANISM OF ACTION

An adrenocortical steroid that suppresses the migration of polymorphonuclear leukocytes and reverses increased capillary permeability. *Therapeutic Effect:* Decreases inflammation.

PHARMACOKINETICS

Route	Onset	Peak	Duration
PO	NA	1-2 h	30-36 h
IM	NA	4-8 days	1-4 wks

Well absorbed from the GI tract after IM administration. Widely distributed. Metabolized in the liver. Excreted in urine. Removed by hemodialysis. *Half-life:* 3.5 h.

M

AVAILABILITY

Tablets (Medrol): 2 mg, 4 mg, 8 mg, 16 mg, 32 mg.
Injection Powder for Reconstitution (A-Methapred, Solu-Medrol): 40 mg, 125 mg, 500 mg, 1 g.
Injection Suspension (Depo-Medrol): 20 mg/mL, 40 mg/mL, 80 mg/mL.

INDICATIONS AND DOSAGES

▸ **Substitution therapy for deficiency states: acute or chronic adrenal insufficiency, adrenal insufficiency secondary to pituitary insufficiency, and congenital adrenal hyperplasia; nonendocrine disorders: allergic, collagen, hepatic, intestinal tract, ocular, renal, and skin diseases; arthritis, bronchial asthma; cerebral edema; malignancies; rhematoid carditis**

PO

Adults, Elderly. Usual range: 4-60 mg/day, given in 4 divided doses.

IV (METHYLPREDNISOLONE SODIUM SUCCINATE)

Adults, Elderly. Usual range: 40-250 mg q4-6h. Repeat q4-6h for 48-72 h.

▸ **Spinal cord injury**

IV BOLUS AND INFUSION

Adults, Elderly. 30 mg/kg over 15 min. Maintenance dose: 5.4 mg/kg/h for 23 h, to be given within 45 min of bolus dose.

▸ **Usual IM dosage**

IM (METHYLPREDNISOLONE ACETATE)

Adults, Elderly. 10-80 mg. Frequency of repeat doses dependent on condition being treated.

INTRA-ARTICULAR, INTRALESIONAL

Adults, Elderly. 4-40 mg, up to 80 mg q1-5wk.

▸ **Usual pediatric dose**

PO/IM/IV

Pediatric. 0.5-1.7 mg/kg/day or 5-25 mg/m^2/day in 2-4 divided doses.

CONTRAINDICATIONS

Hypersensitivity to product, systemic fungal infections; some injections contain benzyl alcohol and are not for use in neonates.

INTERACTIONS

Drug

Acetaminophen (chronic, high dose): May increase risk of hepatotoxicity.
Alcohol, salicylates, NSAIDs: Possible increase in GI effects.
Amphotericin: May increase hypokalemia.
Barbiturates, rifampin, rifabutin: Possible decreased action.
Digoxin: May increase the risk of digoxin toxicity caused by hypokalemia.
Diuretics, insulin, oral hypoglycemics, potassium supplements: May decrease the effects of these drugs.
Hepatic enzyme inducers: May decrease the effects of methylprednisolone.

Ketoconazole, macrolide antibiotics: Possible increased activity.
Live-virus vaccines: May decrease the patient's antibody response to vaccine, increase vaccine side effects, and potentiate virus replication.
Herbal and Food
None known.

DIAGNOSTIC TEST EFFECTS
May increase blood cholesterol, glucose and serum lipid, amylase, and sodium levels. May decrease serum calcium, potassium, and thyroxine levels.

IV INCOMPATIBILITIES
Ampicillin/sulbactam (Unasyn), calcium chloride or gluconate, caspofungin (Cancidas), cefotaxime, ciprofloxacin (Cipro), diazepam, diltiazem (Cardizem), diphenhydramine, docetaxel (Taxotere), etoposide (VePesid), filgrastim (Neupogen), gemcitabine (Gemzar), haloperidol, hydralazine, ketamine, lansoprazole (Prevacid), magnesium sulfate, paclitaxel (Taxol), pantoprazole (Protonix), phenytoin, potassium chloride, propofol (Diprivan), protamine, quinupristin-dalfopristin (Synercid), thiamine, vecuronium, vinorelbine (Navelbine).

IV COMPATIBILITIES
Dopamine (Intropin), heparin, midazolam (Versed), theophylline.

SIDE EFFECTS
Frequent
Insomnia, heartburn, anxiety, abdominal distention, diaphoresis, acne, mood swings, increased appetite, facial flushing, GI distress, delayed wound healing, increased susceptibility to infection, diarrhea, or constipation.
Occasional
Headache, edema, tachycardia, change in skin color, frequent urination, depression.
Rare
Psychosis, increased blood coagulability, hallucinations.

SERIOUS REACTIONS
- Long-term therapy may cause hypocalcemia, hypokalemia, muscle wasting (especially in arms and legs), osteoporosis, spontaneous fractures, amenorrhea, cataracts, glaucoma, peptic ulcer disease, and congestive heart failure (CHF).
- Abruptly withdrawing the drug after long-term therapy may cause anorexia, nausea, fever, headache, sudden severe myalgia, rebound inflammation, fatigue, weakness, lethargy, dizziness, and orthostatic hypotension.
- Chronic corticosterioids raise risk of immunosuppression and resultant increased risk for infection.
- Long-term use may increase intraocular pressure or produce cataracts.

PRECAUTIONS & CONSIDERATIONS
Caution is warranted with cirrhosis, CHF, diabetes mellitus, hypertension, hypothyroidism, thromboembolic disorders, and ulcerative colitis. Methylprednisolone crosses the placenta and is distributed in breast milk. Women taking methylprednisolone should not breastfeed. Prolonged methylprednisolone use in the first trimester of pregnancy may cause cleft palate in the neonate. Prolonged treatment or high dosages may decrease cortisol secretion and short-term growth rate in children. No age-related precautions have been noted in elderly patients. Severe stress, including serious infection, surgery,

M

or trauma, may require an increase in methylprednisolone dosage. Dentist or another physician should be informed of methylprednisolone therapy if taken within the past 12 mo.

Mood swings, ranging from euphoria to depression, may occur. Notify the physician of fever, muscle aches, sore throat, and sudden weight gain or swelling. Blood glucose level, intake and output, BP, serum electrolyte levels, pattern of daily bowel activity, height, and weight should be monitored before and during therapy. Be alert to signs and symptoms of infection caused by reduced immune response, including fever, sore throat, and vague symptoms. In long-term therapy, signs and symptoms of hypocalcemia (such as muscle twitching, cramps, and positive Chvostek or Trousseau signs) or hypokalemia (such as ECG changes, nausea and vomiting, irritability, weakness and muscle cramps, and numbness or tingling, especially in the lower extremities) should be reported to health care providers immediately.

Storage

Store tablets and vials for injection at room temperature. Use diluted injection within 48 h at room temperature. Infusions and IVPB are stable for 24 h at room temperature.

Administration

! Individualize dosage based on the disease, person, and response.

Take oral methylprednisolone with food or milk. Take single doses before 9:00 AM; give multiple doses at evenly spaced intervals. Do not abruptly discontinue the drug or change the dosage or schedule; the drug must be withdrawn gradually under medical supervision.

ONLY methylprednisolone sodium succinate should be given intravenously (IV). Administer directly into a vein over 2-3 min. Doses ≥ 2 mg/kg or 250 mg usually given as IVPB unless emergent situation. Large doses (≥ 500 mg) given IVPB usually given over 30-60 min. Compatible solutions include D5W and 0.9% NaCl. Large-dose infusions for spinal cord injury are usually prepared in 500 mL 0.9% NaCl.

For IM use, methylprednisolone acetate should not be further diluted. Shake acetate injection suspension well before IM use. Give deep IM injection into gluteus maximus. Methylprednisolone acetate may be given locally as an intra-articular injection.

Methyltestosterone

meth-il-tes-tos′te-rone

★ Android, Methitest, Testred

Do not confuse with methylprednisolone.

CATEGORY AND SCHEDULE

Pregnancy Risk Category: X

Controlled Substance Schedule: III

Classification: Androgens, hormones/hormone modifiers

MECHANISM OF ACTION

A synthetic testosterone derivative with androgen activity that promotes growth and development of male sex organs and maintains secondary sex characteristics in androgen-deficient males. *Therapeutic Effect:* Treats hypogonadism and delayed puberty in males.

PHARMACOKINETICS

Well absorbed from the GI tract. Protein binding: 98%. Metabolized in liver. Primarily excreted in urine. Unknown whether it is removed by hemodialysis. *Half-life:* 10-100 min.

AVAILABILITY

Capsules: 10 mg (Android, Testred).
Tablets: 10 mg (Methitest).

INDICATIONS AND DOSAGES

▸ **Breast cancer, palliative**
PO
Adults, Elderly, Females. 50-200 mg/day.
▸ **Delayed puberty, males**
PO
Adolescents. 5-25 mg/day for 4-6 mo.
BUCCAL
Adolescents. 2.5-12.5 mg/day for 4-6 mo.
▸ **Hypogonadism, males**
PO
Adults. 10-50 mg/day.
BUCCAL
Adults. 5-25 mg/day.

OFF-LABEL USES

Hereditary angioedema.

CONTRAINDICATIONS

Pregnancy, prostatic or breast cancer in males, hypersensitivity to methyltestosterone or any component of its formulation.

INTERACTIONS

Drug
ACTH, corticosteroids: Possible increased edema risk.
Antidiabetic agents, insulin: May alter antidiabetic agent requirements or promote hypoglycemia.
Bupropion: May increase the risk of seizures by decreasing seizure threshold.
Cyclosporine: May increase risk of cyclosporine toxicity.
Liver toxic medications: May increase risk of liver toxicity.
Oral anticoagulants: May increase the effects of oral anticoagulants.
Herbal
None known.
Food
None known.

DIAGNOSTIC TEST EFFECTS

May increase blood hemoglobin and hematocrit, LDL concentrations, serum alkaline phosphatase, bilirubin, calcium, potassium, SGOT (AST) levels, and sodium levels. May decrease HDL concentrations.

SIDE EFFECTS

Frequent
Gynecomastia, acne, amenorrhea or other menstrual irregularities.
Females: Hirsutism, deepening of voice, clitoral enlargement that may not be reversible when drug is discontinued.
Occasional
Edema, nausea, insomnia, oligospermia, priapism, male pattern of baldness, bladder irritability, hypercalcemia in immobilized patients or those with breast cancer, hypercholesterolemia.
Rare
Polycythemia.

SERIOUS REACTIONS

• Cholestatic jaundice, hepatocellular neoplasms, peliosis hepatitis, edema with or without CHF and suppression of clotting factors II, V, VII, and X have been reported.
• Priapism.

PRECAUTIONS & CONSIDERATIONS

Caution is warranted in patients with diabetes, CHF, or preexisting cardiac, liver or renal disease, epilepsy, history of migraine, other conditions that may be aggravated by fluid retention, and hypertension due to the risk of increased BP. Methyltestosterone should not be used during pregnancy or lactation. Safety and efficacy of methyltestosterone have not been

M

established in prepubertal children, so use with caution. Be aware that methyltestosterone use in elderly patients may increase the risk of hyperplasia or stimulate the growth of occult prostate carcinoma. Adequate calories and protein should be consumed.

Acne, nausea, pedal edema, or vomiting may occur. Women should report deepening of voice, hoarseness, and menstrual irregularities. Men should report difficulty urinating, frequent erections, and gynecomastia. Weight should be obtained each day. Weekly weight gains of more than 5 lb should be reported.

Storage

Store at room temperature.

Administration

Give methyltestosterone with meals.

M

Metipranolol Hydrochloride

met-ee-pran′-oh-lol high-droh-klor′ide

☐ OptiPranolol

Do not confuse with metoprolol or propranolol.

CATEGORY AND SCHEDULE

Pregnancy Risk Category: C

Classification: Ophthalmic agents, antiglaucoma agents, β-adrenergic blocker

MECHANISM OF ACTION

An antiglaucoma agent that nonselectively blocks β-adrenergic receptors. Reduces aqueous humor production. *Therapeutic Effect:* Reduces intraocular pressure (IOP).

PHARMACOKINETICS

Route	Onset	Peak	Duration
Eyedrops	0.5-3 h	2-7 h	≥ 24 h

Systemic absorption may occur.

AVAILABILITY

Ophthalmic solution: 0.3%.

INDICATIONS AND DOSAGES

▸ **Glaucoma, ocular hypertension**

OPHTHALMIC

Adults, Elderly. Instill 1 drop 2 times a day.

CONTRAINDICATIONS

Bronchial asthma or chronic obstructive pulmonary disease, cardiogenic shock, overt cardiac failure, second- or third- degree heart atrioventricular block, severe sinus bradycardia, hypersensitivity to metipranolol or any component of the formulation.

DRUG INTERACTIONS

Oral β-blockers: Additive systemic effects.

Calcium channel blockers: Hypotension.

SIDE EFFECTS

Frequent

Eye burning/stinging, hyperemia, blurred vision, headache, fatigue.

Occasional

Sensitivity to light, dizziness.

Rare

Dry eye, conjunctivitis, eye pain, rash.

SERIOUS REACTIONS

- Ophthalmic overdosage may produce bradycardia, hypotension, bronchospasm, and acute cardiac failure.
- Arrhythmias and myocardial infarction have been reported.

PRECAUTIONS & CONSIDERATIONS

Caution in patients with hyperthyroidism, diabetes, cerebrovascular insufficiency, and depression. Safety and efficacy not established in children. No unique precautions in elderly.

Storage

Store at room temperature.

Administration

Tilt the head back slightly and pull the lower eyelid down with the index finger to form a pouch. Instill drop(s) and gently close the eyes for 1-2 min. Do not blink. Use nasolacrimal occlusion to reduce systemic absorption. Do not touch the tip of the dropper to any surface to avoid contamination. Wait several minutes before use of other eyedrops.

Metoclopramide

met′oh-kloe-pra′mide

Reglan, Metozolv ODT

Apo-Metoclop

Do not confuse Reglan with Renagel.

CATEGORY AND SCHEDULE

Pregnancy Risk Category: B

Classification: Gastrointestinal agents, prokinetics, antiemetics

MECHANISM OF ACTION

A dopamine receptor antagonist that stimulates motility of the upper GI tract and decreases reflux into the esophagus. Also raises the threshold of activity in the chemoreceptor trigger zone. *Therapeutic Effect:* Accelerates intestinal transit and gastric emptying; relieves nausea and vomiting.

PHARMACOKINETICS

Route	Onset (min)	Peak	Duration
PO	30-60	NA	NA
IV	1-3	NA	NA
IM	10-15	NA	NA

Well absorbed from the GI tract. Metabolized in the liver. Protein binding: 30%. Primarily excreted in urine. Not removed by hemodialysis. *Half-life:* 4-6 h.

AVAILABILITY

Oral Solution: 5 mg/5 mL.
Tablets: 5 mg, 10 mg.
Injection: 5 mg/mL.
Orally Disintegrating Tablets (ODT): 5 mg, 10 mg.

INDICATIONS AND DOSAGES

▸ Prevention of chemotherapy-induced nausea and vomiting

IV

Adults, Elderly, Children. 1-2 mg/kg 30 min before chemotherapy; repeat q2h for 2 doses, then q3h as needed.

▸ Postoperative nausea and vomiting

IV

Adults, Elderly, Children 15 yr and older. 10 mg; repeat q6-8h as needed.
Children 14 yr and younger. 0.1-0.2 mg/kg/dose; repeat q6-8h as needed.

▸ Diabetic gastroparesis

PO, IV

Adults. 10 mg 30 min before meals and at bedtime for 2-8 wks.

PO

Elderly. Initially, 5 mg 30 min before meals and at bedtime. May increase to 10 mg.

IV

Elderly. 5 mg over 1-2 min. May increase to 10 mg.

▸ Symptomatic gastroesophageal reflux

PO

Adults. 10-15 mg up to 4 times a day or single doses up to 20 mg as needed.
Elderly. Initially, 5 mg 4 times a day. May increase to 10 mg.
Children. 0.4-0.8 mg/kg/day in 4 divided doses.

▸ **To facilitate small bowel intubation (single dose)**

IV

Adults, Elderly. 10 mg as a single dose.
Children 6-14 yr. 2.5-5 mg as a single dose.
Children younger than 6 yr. 0.1 mg/kg as a single dose.

▸ **Dosage in renal impairment**

Initial dosage is modified based on creatinine clearance.

Creatinine Clearance (mL/min)	Initial % of normal dose
< 40 mL/min	50

May be increased or decreased to clinical effect.

OFF-LABEL USES

Prevention of aspiration pneumonia; persistent hiccups, slow gastric emptying, vascular headaches to offset nausea from ergot alkaloids.

CONTRAINDICATIONS

Concurrent use of medications likely to produce extrapyramidal reactions, GI hemorrhage, GI obstruction or perforation, history of seizure disorders, pheochromocytoma, hypersensitivity to metoclopramide.

INTERACTIONS

Drug

Alcohol, other central nervous system (CNS) suppressants: May increase CNS depressant effect.
Anticholinergics, opioids: Decreased GI action.
Digoxin, levodopa: Changes in GI transit time with metoclopramide may alter oral absorption and therapeutic response; monitor.
MAOIs: Use cautiously; may increase risk of hypertension.

Herbal

None known.

Food

None known.

DIAGNOSTIC TEST EFFECTS

May increase serum aldosterone and prolactin concentrations.

IV INCOMPATIBILITIES

Allopurinol (Aloprim), cefepime (Maxipime), diazepam, doxorubicin liposomal (Doxil), furosemide (Lasix), lansoprazole (Prevacid), phenytoin, propofol (Diprivan).

IV COMPATIBILITIES

Dexamethasone, diltiazem (Cardizem), diphenhydramine (Benadryl), fentanyl (Sublimaze), heparin, hydromorphone (Dilaudid), morphine, potassium chloride.

SIDE EFFECTS

Frequent (10%)

Somnolence, restlessness, fatigue, lethargy.

Occasional (3%)

Dizziness, anxiety, headache, insomnia, breast tenderness, altered menstruation, constipation, rash, dry mouth, galactorrhea, gynecomastia.

Rare (< 3%)

Hypotension or hypertension, tachycardia.

SERIOUS REACTIONS

• Extrapyramidal reactions occur most commonly in children and young adults (18-30 yr) receiving large doses (2 mg/kg) during

chemotherapy and are usually limited to akathisia (involuntary limb movement and facial grimacing).
• Neuroleptic malignant syndrome.

PRECAUTIONS & CONSIDERATIONS

Treatment can cause tardive dyskinesia, which is often irreversible. The risk increases with duration of treatment and total cumulative dose. Limit treatment to < 12 wks unless benefits outweigh risks. Caution is warranted in patients with cirrhosis, CHF, and renal impairment. Metoclopramide crosses the placenta and is distributed in breast milk; therefore, caution is warranted in lactation. Children and young adults (aged 18-30 yr) are more susceptible to dystonic reactions at larger doses during chemotherapy, usually evidenced by akathisia of the face and limbs. Elderly patients are more likely to have parkinsonian reactions and dyskinesias after long-term therapy. Alcohol and tasks that require mental alertness or motor skills should be avoided.

Dizziness, drowsiness, and dry mouth may occur. Notify the physician if involuntary eye, facial, or limb movement occurs. BP, heart rate, renal function, skin for rash, and pattern of daily bowel activity and stool consistency should be monitored.

Storage

Store oral dose forms and vials at room temperature. Protect from freezing and light. Protect ODT from moisture; do not remove from package until time of use. After dilution, IV piggyback infusion is stable for 48 h.

Administration

! Metoclopramide may be given by PO and IM routes and by IV push or IV infusion. Doses of 2 mg/kg or more or prolonged therapy may increase the incidence of side effects.

Take oral metoclopramide 30 min before meals and at bedtime. Crush tablets as needed. ODT dose form is taken without liquid. Remove ODT from package with dry hands and place on the tongue. Do not use broken or crumbled tablets. Disintegrates on the tongue in approximately 1 min.

For IV use, dilute doses > 10 mg in 50 mL, 0.9% NaCl (preferred), or dextrose 5%, lactated Ringer's solution. Infuse over 15 min. Give slow IV push of 10 mg over 1-2 min. Too-rapid IV injection may produce intense anxiety or restlessness, followed by drowsiness.

Metolazone

met-tole'a-zone

★ 🍁 Zaroxolyn

Do not confuse metolazone with metaxalone, or Zaroxolyn with Zarontin.

CATEGORY AND SCHEDULE

Pregnancy Risk Category: B (D if used in pregnancy-induced hypertension)

Classification:
Antihypertensives, diuretics, thiazide-like

MECHANISM OF ACTION

An oral quinazoline thiazide-like diuretic and antihypertensive. As a diuretic, blocks reabsorption of sodium, potassium, and chloride at the distal convoluted tubule, increasing renal excretion of sodium and water. As an antihypertensive, reduces plasma and extracellular fluid volume and peripheral vascular resistance. *Therapeutic Effect:* Promotes diuresis and reduces BP.

PHARMACOKINETICS

Route	Onset	Peak	Duration
PO (diuretic)	1 h	2 h	12-24 h

Incompletely absorbed from the GI tract. Protein binding: 95%. Primarily excreted unchanged in urine. Not removed by hemodialysis. *Half-life:* 14 h.

AVAILABILITY

Tablets (Extended Release [Zaroxolyn]): 2.5 mg, 5 mg, 10 mg.

INDICATIONS AND DOSAGES

▸ **Edema**

PO (ZAROXOLYN)

Adults, Elderly. 2.5-20 mg/day.
Children. 0.2-0.4 mg/kg/day in 1-2 divided doses.

▸ **Hypertension**

PO (ZAROXOLYN)

Adults, Elderly. 2.5-5 mg/day.

CONTRAINDICATIONS

Anuria, hepatic coma or precoma. Cross-allergy may occur when given to patients allergic to sulfonamide-derived drugs, thiazides, or quinethazone.

INTERACTIONS

Drug

Cholestyramine, colestipol: May decrease the absorption and effects of metolazone.
Digoxin: May increase the risk of digoxin toxicity when associated with metolazone-induced hypokalemia.
Indomethacin and other NSAIDs: May have decreased hypotensive response.
Lithium: May increase the risk of lithium toxicity.
Tetracyclines: May increase risk of photosensitization.

Herbal

None known.

Food

None known.

DIAGNOSTIC TEST EFFECTS

May increase blood glucose and serum cholesterol, LDL, bilirubin, calcium, creatinine, uric acid, and triglyceride levels. May decrease urinary calcium, and serum magnesium, potassium, and sodium levels.

SIDE EFFECTS

Expected

Increase in urinary frequency and urine volume.

Frequent (9%-10%)

Dizziness, light-headedness, headache.

Occasional (4%-6%)

Muscle cramps and spasm, fatigue, lethargy.

Rare (< 2%)

Asthenia, palpitations, depression, nausea, vomiting, abdominal bloating, constipation, diarrhea, urticaria.

SERIOUS REACTIONS

- Vigorous diuresis may lead to profound water and electrolyte depletion, resulting in hypokalemia, hyponatremia, and dehydration.
- Acute hypotensive episodes may occur.
- Hyperglycemia may occur during prolonged therapy.
- Pancreatitis, paresthesia, blood dyscrasias, pulmonary

edema, allergic pneumonitis, and dermatologic reactions occur rarely.
- Overdose can lead to lethargy and coma without changes in electrolytes or hydration.

PRECAUTIONS & CONSIDERATIONS

Caution is warranted in patients with diabetes, elevated cholesterol and triglyceride levels, gout, hepatic impairment, lupus erythematosus, and severe renal disease. Metolazone crosses the placenta, and a small amount is distributed in breast milk. Breastfeeding is not recommended for patients taking this drug. No age-related precautions have been noted in children. Elderly patients may be more sensitive to the drug's electrolyte and hypotensive effects. Age-related renal impairment may require cautious use in elderly patients. Consuming foods high in potassium, such as apricots, bananas, legumes, meat, orange juice, raisins, whole grains, including cereals, and white and sweet potatoes, is encouraged. Patient should be advised about limiting salt intake and sodium-containing products.

An increase in the frequency and volume of urination may occur. BP, vital signs, electrolytes, intake and output, and weight should be monitored before and during treatment. Be aware of signs of electrolyte disturbances such as hypokalemia or hyponatremia. Hypokalemia may cause arrhythmias, altered mental status, muscle cramps, asthenia, and tremor. Hyponatremia may result in cold and clammy skin, confusion, and thirst. Any of these indicators should be reported immediately. Because of the possible cardiovascular effects, patients should be evaluated for stress tolerance during therapy.

Storage

Store at room temperature protected from light.

Administration

Take metolazone with food or milk if GI upset occurs, preferably with breakfast to help prevent nocturia.

Metoprolol

me-toe'pro-lole

★ Lopressor, Toprol XL

🍁 Apo-Metoprolol, Betaloc, Nu-Metop, Lopressor

Do not confuse metoprolol with metaproterenol or metolazone. Do not confuse Toprol XL with Topamax.

CATEGORY AND SCHEDULE

Pregnancy Risk Category: C (D if used in second or third trimester)

Classification: Antihypertensive, selective β_1-blocker

MECHANISM OF ACTION

An antianginal, antihypertensive, and myocardial infarction (MI) adjunct that selectively blocks β_1-adrenergic receptors; high dosages may block β_2-adrenergic receptors. Decreases oxygen requirements. Large doses increase airway resistance. *Therapeutic Effect:* Slows sinus node heart rate, decreases cardiac output, and reduces BP. Also decreases myocardial ischemia severity.

PHARMACOKINETICS

Route	Onset	Peak	Duration
PO	10-15 min	1h	6 h
PO (extended release)	N/A	6-12 h	24 h
IV	Immediate	20 min	5-8 h

Well absorbed from the GI tract. Protein binding: 12%. Widely distributed. Metabolized in the liver (undergoes significant first-pass metabolism). Primarily excreted in urine. Removed by hemodialysis. *Half-life:* 3-7 h.

AVAILABILITY

Tablets (Lopressor): 25 mg, 50 mg, 100 mg.
Tablets (Extended Release [Toprol XL]): 25 mg, 50 mg, 100 mg, 200 mg.
Injection (Lopressor): 1 mg/mL.

INDICATIONS AND DOSAGES

▸ **Mild to moderate hypertension**
PO
Adults. Initially, 100 mg/day as single or divided dose. Increase at weekly (or longer) intervals. Maintenance: 100-450 mg/day.
Elderly. Initially, 25 mg/day. Range: 25-300 mg/day.
PO (EXTENDED-RELEASE TABLETS)
Adults. 50-100 mg/day as single dose. May increase at least at weekly intervals until optimum BP attained. Maximum: 200 mg/day.

▸ **Chronic, stable angina pectoris**
PO
Adults. Initially, 100 mg/day as single or divided dose. Increase at weekly (or longer) intervals. Maintenance: 100-450 mg/day.
PO (EXTENDED-RELEASE TABLETS)
Adults. Initially, 100 mg/day as single dose. May increase at least at weekly intervals until optimum clinical response achieved. Maximum: 200 mg/day.

▸ **Congestive heart failure (CHF)**
PO (EXTENDED-RELEASE TABLETS)
Adults. Initially, 25 mg/day. May double dose q2wk. Maximum: 200 mg/day.

▸ **Early treatment of MI**
IV
Adults. 5 mg q2min for 3 doses, followed by 50 mg orally q6h for 48 h. Begin oral dose 15 min after last IV dose. Or, in patients who do not tolerate full IV dose, give 25-50 mg orally q6h, 15 min after last IV dose.

▸ **Late treatment and maintenance after an MI**
PO
Adults. Target dose: 100 mg twice a day for at least 3 mo.

OFF-LABEL USES

To increase survival rate in diabetic patients with coronary artery disease (CAD); treatment or prevention of anxiety; cardiac arrhythmias; hypertrophic cardiomyopathy; mitral valve prolapse syndrome; pheochromocytoma; tremors; thyrotoxicosis; vascular headache.

CONTRAINDICATIONS

Cardiogenic shock, MI with a heart rate < 45 beats/min or systolic BP < 100 mm Hg, overt heart failure, second- or third-degree heart block, sinus bradycardia, hypersensitivity to metoprolol and related derivatives (cross-sensitivity between β-blockers can occur), sick sinus syndrome, peripheral arterial circulatory disorders.

INTERACTIONS

Drug

Cimetidine: May increase metoprolol blood concentration.
Didanosine: May decrease effects.
Diphenhydramine: May increase plasma concentrations.
Diuretics, other antihypertensives: May increase hypotensive effect.
Epinephrine, levonordefrin, isoproterenol, other sympathomimetics: May decrease β-blocking, β-adrenergic effects.

Fentanyl derivatives, inhalation anesthetics: Possible increased hypotension and bradycardia.
Indomethacin and other NSAIDs, sympathomimetics: Possible decreased antihypertensive effects.
Insulin, oral hypoglycemics: May mask symptoms of hypoglycemia and prolong hypoglycemic effect of these drugs.
Lidocaine: May slow metabolism of lidocaine.
NSAIDs: May decrease antihypertensive effect.
Sympathomimetics, xanthines: May mutually inhibit effects.
Herbal
None known.
Food
None known.

DIAGNOSTIC TEST EFFECTS

May increase serum antinuclear antibody titer and BUN, serum lipoprotein, serum LDH, serum alkaline phosphatase, serum bilirubin, serum creatinine, serum potassium, serum uric acid, AST (SGOT), ALT (SGPT), and serum triglyceride levels.

IV INCOMPATIBILITIES

Amphotericin B complex (Abelcet, AmBisome, Amphotec), diazepam, lepirudin, pantoprazole, phenytoin.

IV COMPATIBILITIES

Alteplase (Activase), morphine.

SIDE EFFECTS

Metoprolol is generally well tolerated, with transient and mild side effects.
Frequent
Diminished sexual function, drowsiness, insomnia, unusual fatigue or weakness, bradycardia.
Occasional
Anxiety, nervousness, diarrhea, constipation, nausea, vomiting, nasal congestion, abdominal discomfort, dizziness, difficulty breathing, cold hands or feet.
Rare
Altered taste, dry eyes, nightmares, paresthesia, allergic reaction (rash, pruritus).

SERIOUS REACTIONS

- Overdose may produce profound bradycardia, hypotension, and bronchospasm.
- Abrupt withdrawal of metoprolol may result in diaphoresis, palpitations, headache, tremulousness, exacerbation of angina, MI, and ventricular arrhythmias.
- Metoprolol administration may precipitate CHF and MI in patients with heart disease; thyroid storm in those with thyrotoxicosis; and peripheral ischemia in those with existing peripheral vascular disease.
- Hypoglycemia may occur in patients with previously controlled diabetes.

PRECAUTIONS & CONSIDERATIONS

Caution is warranted with bronchospastic disease, diabetes, hyperthyroidism, impaired renal function, inadequate cardiac function, and peripheral vascular disease. Metoprolol crosses the placenta and is distributed in breast milk; therefore, care in lactation is warranted. Metoprolol use should be avoided in pregnant women after the first trimester because it may result in low-birth-weight infants. The drug may also produce apnea, bradycardia, hypoglycemia, or hypothermia during childbirth. The safety and efficacy of metoprolol have not been established in children. In elderly patients, age-related peripheral vascular disease may increase susceptibility to decreased peripheral circulation. Be aware that salt and alcohol intake should be restricted. Nasal decongestants or OTC cold preparations (stimulants) should not be used without physician approval.

Notify the physician of excessive fatigue, headache, prolonged dizziness, shortness of breath, or weight gain. BP for hypotension, respiratory status for shortness of breath, pattern of daily bowel activity and stool consistency, ECG for arrhythmias, and pulse for quality, rate, and rhythm should be monitored during treatment. If pulse rate is 55 beats/min or lower or systolic BP is < 90 mm Hg, withhold the medication and contact the physician. In those receiving metoprolol for treatment of angina, the onset, type (sharp, dull, squeezing), radiation, location, intensity, and duration of anginal pain and its precipitating factors, including exertion and emotional stress, should be recorded. Signs and symptoms of CHF, such as decreased urine output, distended neck veins, dyspnea (particularly on exertion or lying down), night cough, peripheral edema, and weight gain should also be assessed. Do not abruptly discontinue metoprolol; may result in symptoms of diaphoresis, palpitations, headache, tremors, angina, MI, and ventricular arrhythmias.

Storage

Store at room temperature. Protect injection from freezing and light. Once injection opened, use immediately and discard any unused portion.

Administration

Immediate-release tablets are taken with food at regular intervals. May crush tablets if necessary.

Extended-release tablets should not be cut, crushed, or chewed. May take without regard to meals at the same general time each day.

For IV use, give undiluted as necessary. Administer IV injection over 1 min. Monitor the patient's ECG and BP during administration.

Metronidazole Hydrochloride

me-troe-ni'da-zole high-droh-klor'ide

★ Flagyl, Flagyl ER, MetroCream, MetroGel, MetroLotion, Noritate, Nydamax, Vandazol 🍁 Florazole, Florazole ER, NidaGel, Rosasol

CATEGORY AND SCHEDULE

Pregnancy Risk Category: B

Classification: Anti-infectives, nitroimidazoles, amebicides, dermatologic agents

MECHANISM OF ACTION

A nitroimidazole derivative that disrupts bacterial and protozoal DNA, inhibiting nucleic acid synthesis. *Therapeutic Effect:* Produces bactericidal, antiprotozoal, amebicidal, and trichomonacidal effects. Good anaerobic coverage. Produces anti-inflammatory and immunosuppressive effects when applied topically.

PHARMACOKINETICS

Well absorbed from the GI tract; minimally absorbed after topical application. Protein binding: < 20%. Widely distributed; crosses blood-brain barrier. Metabolized in the liver to active metabolite. Primarily excreted in urine; partially eliminated in feces. Removed by hemodialysis. *Half-life:* 8 h (increased in alcoholic hepatic disease and in neonates).

AVAILABILITY

Capsules (Flagyl): 375 mg.
Tablets (Flagyl): 250 mg, 500 mg.
Tablets (Extended Release [Flagyl ER]): 750 mg.
Premixed IV Infusion: 500 mg/100 mL.
Lotion: 0.75%.
Topical Gel (MetroGel): 0.75%.
Topical Cream (MetroCream): 0.75%.
Topical Cream (Noritate): 1%.
Vaginal Gel (MetroGel-Vaginal): 0.75%.

INDICATIONS AND DOSAGES

▸ **Amebiasis**
PO
Adults, Elderly. 500-750 mg q8h for 7-10 days.
Children. 35-50 mg/kg/day in divided doses q8h.

▸ **Trichomoniasis**
PO
Adults, Elderly. 250 mg q8h for 7 days, 375 mg twice daily for 7 days, or 2 g as a single dose.
Children. 15-30 mg/kg/day in divided doses q8h.

▸ **Anaerobic skin and skin-structure infection, CNS, lower respiratory tract, bone, joint, intra-abdominal, gynelogic infections; endocarditis; septicemia**
IV, PO
Adults, Elderly, Children. Loading dose of 15 mg/kg, usually given IV initially. Then, 7.5 mg/kg/dose q6h IV or PO. A common dose in adults is 500 mg q6h. Maximum: 4 g/day.

▸ **Antibiotic-associated pseudomembranous colitis**
PO
Adults, Elderly. 250-500 mg 3-4 times a day for 10-14 days.
Children. 30 mg/kg/day in divided doses q6h for 7-10 days.

▸ **Helicobacter pylori infections**
PO
Adults, Elderly. 250-500 mg 3 times a day (in combination).
Children. 15-20 mg/kg/day in 2 divided doses.

▸ **Bacterial vaginosis**
PO
Adults. 750 mg at bedtime for 7 days.
INTRAVAGINAL
Adults. One full applicator twice a day or once a day at bedtime for 5 days.

▸ **Rosacea**
TOPICAL
Adults. Apply thin layer of lotion or gel to affected area twice a day or cream once a day.

▸ **Dosage in hepatic impairment**
IV OR PO
Reduce dosage or administration frequency. The daily dose may need to be reduced by 50%-60% in severe hapatic disease.

OFF-LABEL USES

Inflammatory bowel disease, pruritus of primary biliary cirrhosis (PBC), pelvic inflammatory disease, dental abscess.

CONTRAINDICATIONS

Hypersensitivity to metronidazole or other nitroimidazole derivatives (also parabens with topical application).

Alcohol and alcohol-containing foods and products.

Do not use during the first trimester of pregnancy for trichomoniasis.

INTERACTIONS

Drug

Alcohol and alcohol-containing products: May cause a

disulfiram-type reaction. Generally, do not ingest during treatment and for 3 days after treatment. Oral medication solutions containing alcohol include amprenavir, ritonavir, sertraline, cough elixirs, and some intravenous products (e.g., paclitaxel).
Bortezomib, possibly other drugs causing neuropathy: Increased risk of peripheral neuropathy.
Busulfan: Decreased busulfan clearance.
Carbamazepine: Increased carbamazepine levels possible; monitor.
Cimetidine: Increased metronidazole concentrations.
5-FU, floxuridine: Possible increased risk of 5-FU toxicity.
Disulfiram: May increase the risk of toxicity.
Lithium: may increase risk of lithium toxicity; monitor.
Mycophenolate, cyclosporine: Alterations in immunosuppressants reported; use with caution.
Phenobarbital: May reduce metronidazole efficacy.
Tacrolimus: Possible increased levels of tacrolimus.
Warfarin: Potentiates anticoagulant effect; monitor INR.

Herbal
None known.

Food
Ethanol: (See Alcohol above).

DIAGNOSTIC TEST EFFECTS

May increase serum LDH, AST (SGOT), and ALT (SGPT) levels. Mild decrease in leukocytes. May interfere with select laboratory assays involving oxidation-reduction of nicotinamide adenine dinucleotide (NADH).

IV INCOMPATIBILITIES

NOTE: The manufacturer recommends against infusing with other medications or infusion solutions. Amphotericin B complex (Abelcet, AmBisome, Amphotec), aztreonam, caspofungin (Cancidas), daptomycin, diazepam, drotrecogen alfa (Xigris), filgrastim (Neupogen), lansoprazole (Prevacid), pantoprazole (Protonix), phenytoin, procainamide, quinupristin/dalfopristin (Synercid).

IV COMPATIBILITIES

Diltiazem (Cardizem), dopamine, heparin, hydromorphone (Dilaudid), lorazepam (Ativan), magnesium sulfate, midazolam (Versed), morphine.

SIDE EFFECTS

Frequent
Systemic: Anorexia, nausea, dry mouth, metallic taste.
Vaginal: Symptomatic cervicitis and vaginitis, abdominal cramps, uterine pain.

Occasional
Systemic: Diarrhea or constipation, vomiting, dizziness, erythematous rash, urticaria, reddish brown urine.
Topical: Transient erythema, mild dryness, burning, irritation, stinging, tearing when applied too close to eyes.
Vaginal: Vaginal, perineal, or vulvar itching; vulvar swelling.

Rare
Mild, transient leukopenia; thrombophlebitis with IV therapy, visual impairment.

SERIOUS REACTIONS

- Oral therapy may result in furry tongue, glossitis, cystitis, dysuria, pancreatitis, and flattening of T waves on ECG readings.
- Peripheral neuropathy, manifested as numbness and tingling in hands or feet, is usually reversible if treatment is stopped immediately after neurologic symptoms appear.
- Seizures occur occasionally.

PRECAUTIONS & CONSIDERATIONS

Caution is warranted with blood dyscrasias, central nervous system (CNS) disorders, severe hepatic dysfunction, predisposition to edema, and in those receiving corticosteroid therapy concurrently. Metronidazole readily crosses the placenta and is distributed in breast milk; caution warranted in lactation. Metronidazole use is contraindicated during the first trimester of pregnancy in women with trichomoniasis. Topical use during pregnancy or breastfeeding is discouraged. No age-related precautions have been noted in children; however, the safety and efficacy of topical administration in those younger than 21 yr have not been established. Age-related hepatic impairment may require a dosage adjustment in elderly patients. Prolonged indwelling catheters should be avoided. Avoid alcohol and alcohol-containing preparations (such as cough syrups and elixirs) during and for at least 3 days post therapy, excessive sunlight, exposure to very hot and cold temperatures, and hot and spicy foods while taking metronidazole. Avoid sexual intercourse, if taking metronidazole for trichomoniasis, until the full treatment is completed.

Urine may become reddish brown during therapy. Skin should be examined for rash and urticaria. Pattern of daily bowel activity and stool consistency should be monitored; document the number and characteristics of stools in those with amebiasis. Be alert for signs and symptoms of superinfection, including abdominal pain, moderate to severe diarrhea, severe anal or genital pruritus, and severe mouth soreness. In addition, be alert for neurologic symptoms such as dizziness and paresthesia. Any of these symptoms should be reported to a health care provider immediately for reevaluation of medical choice. Avoid tasks requiring mental alertness or motor skills until the drug is established. Metronidazole acts on papules, pustules, and erythema but has no effect on ocular problems (conjunctivitis, keratitis, blepharitis), rhinophyma (hypertrophy of nose), or telangiectasia.

Storage

Store all products at room temperature; protect from excessive heat and freezing. Do not remove overwrap of premixed infusion until time of use.

Administration

Regular-release tablets/capsules may be given without regard to meals. Extended-release tablets are taken on an empty stomach, at least 1 h before or 2 h after meals. Do not cut or crush extended-release product.

For topical dermatologic use, apply and rub in a thin film after washing; avoid eye contact.

For vaginal use, use supplied applicators to measure dose and administer. Once-daily dose is given at bedtime.

For IV use, infuse metronidazole over 30-60 min. Do not give as an IV bolus injection.

Metyrosine

me-tye′roe-seen

★ Demser

CATEGORY AND SCHEDULE

Pregnancy Risk Category: C

Classification: Adrenal agents, catecholamine inhibitor

MECHANISM OF ACTION

A tyrosine hydroxylase inhibitor that blocks conversion of tyrosine to dihydroxyphenylalanine, the rate-limiting step in the biosynthetic pathway of catecholamines. *Therapeutic Effect:* Reduces levels of endogenous catecholamines.

PHARMACOKINETICS

Well absorbed from the GI tract. Metabolized in the liver. Excreted primarily in the urine. *Half-life:* 7.2 h.

AVAILABILITY

Capsules: 250 mg (Demser).

INDICATIONS AND DOSAGES

▸ Pheochromocytoma

PO

Adults, Elderly, Children 12 yr and older. Initially, 250 mg 4 times/day. Increase by 250-500 mg/day up to 4 g/day. Maintenance: 2-4 g/day in 4 divided doses.

CONTRAINDICATIONS

Hypertension of unknown etiology, hypersensitivity to metyrosine or any component of the formulation.

INTERACTIONS

Drug

Alcohol and CNS depressants: May increase CNS depressant effects.

Phenothiazines, haloperidol, metoclopramide: May potentiate extrapyramidal symptoms (EPS).

Herbal

None known.

Food

None known.

DIAGNOSTIC TEST EFFECTS

Crystalluria may occur if hydration not adequate. Spurious increases in urinary catecholamines may be observed due to the presence of metabolites of the drug.

SIDE EFFECTS

Frequent

Drowsiness, extrapyramidal symptoms, diarrhea.

Occasional

Galactorrhea, edema of the breasts, nausea, vomiting, dry mouth, impotence, nasal congestion.

Rare

Lower extremity edema, urinary problems, urticaria, anemia, depression, disorientation, crystalluria.

SERIOUS REACTIONS

- Hematologic disorders (including eosinophilia, anemia, thrombocytopenia, and thrombocytosis), increased liver enzymes, peripheral edema, and hypersensitivity reactions such as urticaria and pharyngeal edema have been reported rarely.
- Psychic stimulation when the drug is discontinued.

PRECAUTIONS & CONSIDERATIONS

! Medication may be given in advance of adrenal tumor removal, usually 5-7 days before surgery.

Caution should be used with impaired liver or renal function. It is unknown whether metyrosine is distributed in breast milk; caution in lactation is warranted. Safety and efficacy of metyrosine have not been established in children younger than 12 yr old. Elderly patients with impaired renal function may need dose adjustment. Alcoholic beverages should be avoided during therapy.

Trismus may indicate overdosage and needs to be reported.

Storage
Store at room temperature.
Administration
Take without regard to food.
Maintain adequate fluid intake.

Micafungin

mye'ca-fun'jin
Mycamine

CATEGORY AND SCHEDULE
Pregnancy Risk Category: C

Classification: Antifungal, systemic, echinocandins

MECHANISM OF ACTION

An antifungal that inhibits the synthesis of glucan, a vital component of fungal cell formation, thereby damaging the fungal cell membrane. *Therapeutic Effect:* Fungicidal; active against a variety of *Candida* species.

PHARMACOKINETICS

Distributed in tissue. Protein binding: > 99%. Slowly metabolized in liver to two metabolites. Excreted primarily in feces (72%) and to a lesser extent in the urine. Not removed by hemodialysis. *Half-life:* 13-18 h.

AVAILABILITY

Powder for Injection: 50-mg, 100-mg vials.

INDICATIONS AND DOSAGES

▸ **Invasive candidiasis; candidemia, peritonitis, and abscesses**
IV INFUSION
Adults, Elderly. Give 100 mg daily.
▸ **Esophageal candidiasis**
IV INFUSION
Adults, Elderly. Give 150 mg daily.
▸ **Candida infection prophylaxis following hematopoietic stem cell transplant**
IV INFUSION
Adults, Elderly. Give 50 mg daily.

CONTRAINDICATIONS

Hypersensitivity to micafungin, any component of the product, or other echinocandins.

INTERACTIONS

Drug
Sirolimus, nifedipine, itraconazole: May increase AUC (exposure) of these drugs systemically; monitor for toxicity and need for dosage decrease.
Herbal
None known.
Food
None known.

DIAGNOSTIC TEST EFFECTS

May increase serum alkaline phosphatase, serum creatinine, SGOT (AST), SGPT (ALT). May decrease hemoglobin, hematocrit, platelet count, and serum potassium and magnesium levels.

IV INCOMPATIBILITIES

Do not mix or infuse micafungin with any other medication. Precipitation promptly occurs.

SIDE EFFECTS

Frequent
Diarrhea, nausea, vomiting, pyrexia, hypokalemia, thrombocytopenia, headache, mucosal inflammation, constipation.
Occasional
Phlebitis is more common when given peripherally. Histamine-mediated symptoms, including rash, pruritus, facial swelling, and vasodilatation. Hypomagnesemia, elevated liver enzymes may occur.

M

SERIOUS REACTIONS

- Hypersensitivity reactions (characterized by rash, facial swelling, pruritus, and a sensation of warmth) or anaphylaxis may occur.
- Isolated cases of acute intravascular hemolysis, hemolytic anemia, and hemoglobinuria.
- Isolated cases of hepatic dysfunction, hepatitis, and hepatic failure.
- Isolated cases of acute renal failure.

PRECAUTIONS & CONSIDERATIONS

Caution is warranted for patients with advanced liver function impairment. It is not known if micafungin crosses the placenta or is excreted in human milk; it is possible the drug could cause fetal harm. Be aware that the safety and efficacy of micafungin have not been established in children. There are no special precautions for elderly patients.

Baseline temperature, liver function test results, and history of allergies should be obtained before giving the drug. If increased shortness of breath, itching, facial swelling, or a rash occurs, notify the physician. Report pain, burning, or swelling at the IV infusion site. Monitor for signs of clinical improvement.

Storage

Unopened vials are stored at room temperature. The reconstituted vial solution, before diluted to an infusion solution, may be held at room temperature for 24 h. The final infusion solution can be stored at room temperature for 24 h and must be protected from light. Discard the solution if it contains particulate or is discolored.

Administration

Micafungin is for intravenous infusion only. Aseptically add 5 mL of 0.9% NaCl (without a bacteriostatic agent) to each 50-mg vial or 100-mg vial to obtain a concentration of 10 mg/mL or 20 mg/mL, respectively. Gently swirl (but do not shake) to facilitate dissolution without foaming. The diluted solution should be protected from light. Further dilute with 100 mL of either 0.9% NaCl or D5W for infusion. Administer IV infusion over at least 60 min.

Miconazole

mih-kon'ah-zole

★ Baza Antifungal, Cruex, Desenex, Fungoid, Lotrimin AF Powder and Powder Spray, Micaderm, Micatin, Mitrazol, Monistat-1, Monistat-3, Monistat-7, Neosporin AF, Oravig, Zeasorb AF 🍁 Monistat-1, Monistat-3, Monistat-7, Monistat-Derm, Micatin, Micozole

CATEGORY AND SCHEDULE

Pregnancy Risk Category: C

Topical and vaginal dose forms OTC; buccal tablets Rx only.

Classification: Antifungals, Imidazole

MECHANISM OF ACTION

An imidazole derivative that inhibits synthesis of ergosterol (vital component of fungal cell formation), damaging cell membrane.

Therapeutic Effect: Fungistatic; may be fungicidal, depending on concentration.

PHARMACOKINETICS

Widely distributed in tissues. Metabolized in liver. Primarily excreted in urine. *Half-life:* 24 h.

Topical: No systemic absorption following application to intact skin. Intravaginally: Small amount absorbed systemically. Buccal: Small amount absorbed systemically.

AVAILABILITY

Buccal Tablet: 50 mg (Oravig).
Vaginal Suppository: 100 mg (Monistat-7), 200 mg (Monistat-3), 1200 mg (Monistat-1).
Vaginal Cream: 4% (Monistat-3), 2% (Monistat-7).
Topical Cream: 2% (Baza Antifungal, Micaderm, Neosporin AF).
Topical Powder: 2% (Desenex, Lotrimin AF, Micatin, Mitrazol, Zeasorb AF).
Topical Lotion: 2% (Zeasorb AF).
Topical Ointment: 2%.
Topical Solution: 2% (Fungoid Tincture).
Topical Spray Powder: 2% (Cruex, Desenex, Lotrimin-AF, Neosporin AF).
Topical Spray Solution: 2% (Lotrimin AF, Neosporin AF).
Topical Gel: 2% (Zeasorb AF).

INDICATIONS AND DOSAGES

▸ Vulvovaginal candidiasis

INTRAVAGINALLY

Adults, Elderly. One 200-mg suppository at bedtime for 3 days; one 100-mg suppository or one applicatorful at bedtime for 7 days, or one 1200 mg suppository at bedtime as single dose.

▸ Topical fungal infections, cutaneous candidiasis

TOPICAL

Adults, Elderly, Children 2 yr and older. Apply liberally 2 times/day, morning and evening. Usually for 2-4 wks.

▸ Oral thrush

BUCCAL

Adults, Children 16 yr and older. Apply 50-mg buccal tablet to upper gum region (just above the incisor tooth) once daily for 14 days.

CONTRAINDICATIONS

Hypersensitivity to miconazole or any component of the formulation.
Topically: Children younger than 2 yr old.

INTERACTIONS

Drug

Ergot alkaloids, phenytoin: Although systemic exposure is nominal, could affect clearance of these agents; use caution.
Nonoxynol-9: Vaginal miconazole may inactivate the spermicide, leading to contraceptive failure. Do not use together.
Oral hypoglycemics, warfarin: May increase effects of these drugs, even with nonsystemic use (e.g., vaginal use).

Herbal

None known.

Food

None known.

DIAGNOSTIC TEST EFFECTS

None known.

SIDE EFFECTS

Frequent

Phlebitis, fever, chills, rash, itching, nausea, vomiting.
Buccal use: Diarrhea, headache, nausea, dysgeusia, upper abdominal pain, vomiting.

Occasional

Dizziness, drowsiness, headache, flushed face, abdominal pain, constipation, diarrhea, decreased appetite.

M

Topical: Itching, burning, stinging, erythema, urticaria.
Vaginal: Vulvovaginal burning, itching, irritation, headache, skin rash.

SERIOUS REACTIONS

- Anemia, thrombocytopenia, and liver toxicity occur rarely.

PRECAUTIONS & CONSIDERATIONS

Caution should be used with liver impairment. It is unknown whether miconazole crosses the placenta or is excreted in breast milk; therefore, caution warranted in pregnancy and lactation. No age-related precautions have been noted in children or elderly patients. Medical consultation is necessary before administering antibiotics because of the propensity of antibiotic therapy to evoke a vaginal yeast infection.

Storage
Store at room temperature. Protect buccal tablets from moisture.

Administration
Apply buccal tablet in the morning after brushing the teeth; apply with dry hands. Place rounded surface against upper gum just above the incisor tooth; hold in place for 30 seconds to ensure adhesion. Tablet will gradually dissolve. Alternate sides of the mouth with each application. Do not crush, chew, or swallow. Do not chew gum. If tablet falls off within the first 6 h, reposition the same tablet. If it still does not adhere, a new tablet should be placed.

For intravaginal use, insert high in vagina. Be aware that the base in the vaginal preparation interacts with certain latex products such as contraceptive diaphragm.

For topical administration, wash and dry area before applying medication. Apply a thin layer on affected area. Avoid contact with eyes. Keep areas clean, dry; wear light clothing for ventilation. Separate personal items in contact with affected areas.

Midazolam Hydrochloride

mid-az′zoe-lam high-droh-klor′ide
★ Versed 🍁 Apo-Midazolam
Do not confuse Versed with VePesid.

CATEGORY AND SCHEDULE

Pregnancy Risk Category: D
Controlled Substance Schedule: IV

Classification: Benzodiazepines, preanesthetics, sedatives adjunct

MECHANISM OF ACTION

A benzodiazepine that enhances the action of γ-aminobutyric acid, one of the major inhibitory neurotransmitters in the brain. *Therapeutic Effect:* Produces anxiolytic, hypnotic, anticonvulsant, muscle relaxant, and amnestic effects.

PHARMACOKINETICS

Route	Onset (min)	Peak (min)	Duration
PO	10-20	NA	N/A
IV	1-5	5-7	20-30 min
IM	5-15	15-60	2-6 h

Well absorbed after IM administration. Protein binding: 97%. Metabolized in the liver to active metabolite. Primarily excreted in urine. Not removed by hemodialysis. *Half-life:* 1-5 h.

AVAILABILITY

Syrup: 2 mg/mL.
Injection: 1 mg/mL, 5 mg/mL.

INDICATIONS AND DOSAGES

▸ Preoperative sedation

PO

Children. 0.25-0.5 mg/kg. Maximum: 20 mg.

IV

Children 6-12 yr. 0.025-0.05 mg/kg. Usual maximum: 10 mg.

Children 6 mo to 5 yr. 0.05-0.1 mg/kg. Usual maximum: 6 mg.

IM

Adults, Elderly. 0.07-0.08 mg/kg 30-60 min before surgery.

Children. 0.1-0.15 mg/kg 30-60 min before surgery. Maximum: 10 mg.

▸ Conscious sedation for diagnostic, therapeutic, and endoscopic procedures

IV

Adults, Elderly. 1-2.5 mg over 2 min. Titrate as needed. Maximum total dose: 2.5-5 mg.

▸ Conscious sedation during mechanical ventilation

IV

Adults, Elderly. 0.01-0.05 mg/kg; may repeat q10-15min until adequately sedated. Then continuous infusion at initial rate of 0.02-0.1 mg/kg/h (1-7 mg/h).

Children older than 32 wks. Initially, 1 mcg/kg/min as continuous infusion.

Children 32 wks and younger. Initially, 0.5 mcg/kg/min as continuous infusion.

▸ Status epilepticus

IV

Children older than 2 mo. Loading dose of 0.15 mg/kg followed by continuous infusion of 1 mcg/kg/min. Titrate as needed. Range: 1-18 mcg/kg/min.

CONTRAINDICATIONS

Acute alcohol intoxication, acute angle-closure glaucoma, coma, shock, hypersensitivity to drug, cherries (PO syrup), or other components.

Nelfinavir, ritonavir, indinavir, saquinavir: Contraindicated use.

INTERACTIONS

Drug

Alcohol, other CNS depressants: May increase CNS and respiratory depression and hypotensive effects of midazolam.

Erythromycin, clarithromycin, ketoconazole, itraconazole, fluconazole, miconazole (systemic), diltiazem, fluvoxamine: Likely increased serum levels and prolonged effect of benzodiazepines.

Hypotension-producing medications: May increase hypotensive effects of midazolam.

Protease inhibitors: Increase midazolam concentrations. Generally contraindicated.

Herbal

Kava kava, valerian: May increase CNS depression.

Food

Grapefruit juice: Increases the oral absorption and systemic availability of midazolam.

DIAGNOSTIC TEST EFFECTS

None known.

IV INCOMPATIBILITIES

Albumin, ampicillin and sulbactam (Unasyn), amphotericin B complex (Abelcet, AmBisome, Amphotec), ampicillin (Polycillin), bumetanide (Bumex), co-trimoxazole (Bactrim), dexamethasone (Decadron), fosphenytoin (Cerebyx), furosemide (Lasix), hydrocortisone (Solu-Cortef), methotrexate, nafcillin (Nafcil), sodium bicarbonate, sodium pentothal (Thiopental).

IV COMPATIBILITIES

Amiodarone (Cordarone), calcium gluconate, diltiazem (Cardizem), dobutamine (Dobutrex), dopamine (Intropin), etomidate (Amidate), fentanyl (Sublimaze), heparin, hydromorphone (Dilaudid), insulin, lorazepam (Ativan), milrinone (Primacor), morphine, nitroglycerin, norepinephrine (Levophed), potassium chloride, propofol (Diprivan).

SIDE EFFECTS

Frequent (4%-10%)
Decreased respiratory rate, tenderness at IM or IV injection site, pain during injection, oxygen desaturation, hiccups.
Occasional (2%-3%)
Hypotension, paradoxical CNS reaction.
Rare (< 2%)
Nausea, vomiting, headache, coughing.

SERIOUS REACTIONS

- Inadequate or excessive dosage or improper administration may result in cerebral hypoxia, agitation, involuntary movements, hyperactivity, and combativeness.
- A too-rapid IV rate, excessive doses, or a single large dose increases the risk of respiratory depression or arrest.
- Respiratory depression or apnea may produce hypoxia and cardiac arrest.

PRECAUTIONS & CONSIDERATIONS

Caution is warranted in patients with acute illness, CHF, pulmonary, renal, or hepatic impairment, severe fluid and electrolyte imbalance, and treated angle-closure glaucoma. Midazolam crosses the placenta; it is unknown whether midazolam is distributed in breast milk; caution in lactation is warranted. Women on long-term therapy should use effective contraception during therapy. Notify the physician immediately if she becomes or might be pregnant. Neonates are more likely to experience respiratory depression. In elderly patients, age-related renal impairment may require dosage adjustment.

! Respiratory depression or apnea may produce hypoxia and cardiac arrest. Flumazenil would be reversal agent.

Midazolam produces an amnesic effect. Vital signs should be obtained before and after administering midazolam. Respiratory rate and oxygen saturation should be monitored continuously during parenteral administration to detect apnea and respiratory depression. Sedation should be assessed every 3-5 min.

! All doses of midazolam must be reduced when used in combination with any CNS depressant; serious respiratory and cardiovascular depression, including death, has occurred when midazolam is used in combination with other CNS depressants or is given too rapidly. Medically compromised and elderly patients are at the greatest risk for this effect.

Storage
Store vials at room temperature.

Administration

! Midazolam dosage is individualized based on age, underlying disease, and medications and on the desired effect.

! Oral drug is not for home administration; nor should it be used chronically. Give only if patient is under direct observation of a health care professional.

Midazolam injection may be given undiluted or as an infusion. Ensure that resuscitative supplies, such as endotracheal tubes, suction equipment, and oxygen, are readily available. Administer the drug by slow IV injection in incremental doses. Give each incremental dose over 2 min or more and wait at least 2 min between doses. Reduce the IV rate in patients older than 60 yr, debilitated patients, and those with chronic diseases or impaired pulmonary function. A too-rapid IV rate, excessive doses, or a single large dose increases the risk of respiratory depression or arrest.

For IM use, inject the drug deep into a large muscle mass, such as the gluteus maximus.

! Do NOT inject intrathecally or via epidural.

Midodrine

mid′o-dreen

★ Amatine, ProAmatine

Do not confuse ProAmatine with Amantadine or protamine.

CATEGORY AND SCHEDULE

Pregnancy Risk Category: C

Classification: Vasopressor; orthostatic hypotension adjunct

MECHANISM OF ACTION

A vasopressor that forms the active metabolite desglymidodrine, an α_1-agonist, activating alpha receptors of the arteriolar and venous vasculature. *Therapeutic Effect:* Increases vascular tone and BP.

PHARMACOKINETICS

Peak: 1-2 h. Bioavailability 90%. *Half-life:* 3-4 h.

AVAILABILITY

Tablets: 2.5 mg, 5 mg, 10 mg.

INDICATIONS AND DOSAGES

▸ Orthostatic hypotension

PO

Adults, Elderly. 10 mg 3 times a day. Give during the day when patient is upright, such as upon arising, midday, and late afternoon. Do not give later than 6:00 PM.

▸ Dosage in renal impairment

For adults and elderly patients, give 2.5 mg 3 times a day; increase gradually, as tolerated.

CONTRAINDICATIONS

Acute renal function impairment, persistent hypertension, pheochromocytoma, severe cardiac disease, thyrotoxicosis, urine retention.

INTERACTIONS

Drug

α-Adrenergic agonists: Increased risk of pressor effects.

Digoxin: May have additive bradycardia effects.

Sodium-retaining steroids (such as fludrocortisone): May increase sodium retention.

Vasoconstrictors: May have an additive vasoconstricting effect.

Herbal

None known.

Food

None known.

DIAGNOSTIC TEST EFFECTS

None known.

SIDE EFFECTS

Frequent (7%-20%)

Paresthesia, piloerection, pruritus, dysuria, supine hypertension.

Occasional (< 1%-7%)

Pain, rash, chills, headache, facial flushing, confusion, dry mouth, anxiety.

SERIOUS REACTIONS

- None known.

M

PRECAUTIONS & CONSIDERATIONS

Caution is warranted with a history of vision problems and renal and hepatic impairment. BP and liver and renal function test results should be monitored. OTC medications, such as cough, cold, and diet preparations, should be avoided because they may affect BP.

Administration

Do not take the last dose of the day after the evening meal or < 4 h before bedtime. Do not take the medication while lying down. Caution warranted with position changes due to possible development of orthostatic hypotension.

M

Mifepristone

miff-eh-pris'tone

★ Mifeprex

Do not confuse Mifeprex with Mirapex or mifepristone with misoprostol.

CATEGORY AND SCHEDULE

Pregnancy Risk Category: X

Classification: Abortifacients

MECHANISM OF ACTION

An abortifacient that has antiprogestational activity resulting from competitive interaction with progesterone. Inhibits the activity of endogenous or exogenous progesterone. Also has antiglucocorticoid and weak antiandrogenic activity. *Therapeutic Effect:* Terminates early pregnancy by interrupting progesterone support to the endometrium and sensitizing the uterine muscle to prostaglandins.

PHARMACOKINETICS

Rapidly absorbed; absolute bioavailability (20 mg oral dose) is 90%, 98% protein bound; nonlinear kinetics. Metabolized in liver by CYP450 3A4 hepatic enzymes. Eliminated in feces and urine. *Half-life:* 18 h.

AVAILABILITY

Tablets: 200 mg.

INDICATIONS AND DOSAGES

▸ Termination of pregnancy at ≤ 49 days (7 wks) gestation

PO

Adults. Day 1: 600 mg mifepristone as single dose. Day 3: 400 mcg misoprostol. Day 14: Post-treatment examination.

OFF-LABEL USES

Cushing syndrome, endometriosis, intrauterine fetal death or nonviable early pregnancy, postcoital contraception, refractory hormone-responsive breast cancer.

CONTRAINDICATIONS

Chronic adrenal failure, concurrent long-term steroid or anticoagulant therapy, confirmed or suspected ectopic pregnancy, intrauterine device (IUD) in place, hemorrhagic disorders, inherited porphyria.

INTERACTIONS

Drug

Anticoagulants and chronic corticosteroid therapy: Mifepristone is contraindicated in any patients taking these drugs.

Carbamazepine, phenobarbital, phenytoin, rifampin: May increase the metabolism of mifepristone.

Herbal

St. John's wort: May increase the metabolism of mifepristone.

Food
Grapefruit juice: May inhibit the metabolism of mifepristone.

DIAGNOSTIC TEST EFFECTS
May decrease hemoglobin level and hematocrit and RBC count.

SIDE EFFECTS
Frequent (> 10%)
Headache, dizziness, abdominal pain, nausea, vomiting, diarrhea, fatigue.
Occasional (3%-10%)
Uterine hemorrhage, insomnia, vaginitis, dyspepsia, back pain, fever, viral infections, rigors.
Rare (1%-2%)
Anxiety, syncope, anemia, asthenia, leg pain, sinusitis, leucorrhea.

SERIOUS REACTIONS
- With long-term use or overdose, potential for adrenocortical insufficiency or adrenal failure.
- Remote potential for teratogenesis should pregnancy not be successfully terminated with use.
- Rare reports of allergic reactions, including toxic epidermal necrolysis or serious skin rash.
- Potential for serious systemic bacterial infection following abortion, such as sepsis.
- Prolonged or heavy bleeding following regimen.

PRECAUTIONS & CONSIDERATIONS
Caution is warranted with cardiovascular disease, diabetes, hepatic or renal impairment, hypertension, severe anemia, and in persons older than 35 yr of age or who smoke more than 10 cigarettes a day. Be aware that anticonvulsants, erythromycin, itraconazole, ketoconazole, and rifampin may inhibit the metabolism of mifepristone. Uterine cramping and vaginal bleeding may occur. Hemoglobin level and hematocrit should be monitored. An IUD, if in place, should be removed before therapy begins.

! Sometimes serious or fatal infection and bleeding occur very rapidly following spontaneous, surgical, and medical abortions, including the use of mifepristone. Immediately report sustained fever > 100.4° F, severe abdominal pain, prolonged heavy bleeding, syncope.

! Health care provider must supervise administration of mifepristone. Clinical examination is necessary to confirm complete termination of pregnancy 14 days post treatment. Bleeding for 9-16 days is not unexpected; heavy bleeding must be reported immediately.

Storage
Store tablets in original carton at room temperature.

Administration
! Treatment with mifepristone and misoprostol requires three office visits; only distributed to registered prescribers in the United States.

Complete termination occurs in the majority of patients within 4-24 h after misoprostol.

M

Miglitol
mig-lee'tall
★ Glyset

CATEGORY AND SCHEDULE
Pregnancy Risk Category: B

Classification: Antidiabetic agents, α-glucosidase inhibitors

MECHANISM OF ACTION

An α-glucosidase inhibitor that delays the digestion of ingested carbohydrates into simple sugars such as glucose. *Therapeutic Effect:* Lowers postprandial hyperglycemia.

PHARMACOKINETICS

PO: Peak plasma levels 2-3 h; negligible plasma protein binding, not metabolized, urinary excretion.

AVAILABILITY

Tablets: 25 mg, 50 mg, 100 mg.

INDICATIONS AND DOSAGES

▸ **Diabetes mellitus type 2**

Use as single drug or in combination with insulin or oral hypoglycemics (sulfonylureas, metformin) when diet control is ineffective in controlling blood glucose levels.

PO

Adults, Elderly. Initially, 25 mg 3 times a day with first bite of each main meal. Maintenance: 50 mg 3 times a day. Maximum: 100 mg 3 times a day.

CONTRAINDICATIONS

Colonic ulceration, diabetic ketoacidosis, hypersensitivity to miglitol, inflammatory bowel disease, partial intestinal obstruction. Use in those with severe renal dysfunction (SCr > 2 mg/dL) not recommended.

INTERACTIONS

Drug

Digoxin: May affect bioavailability of oral digoxin, and dose adjustment may be needed.

Herbal

None known.

Food

None known.

DIAGNOSTIC TEST EFFECTS

Transient low serum iron without changes to hemoglobin or hematocrit.

SIDE EFFECTS

Frequent (10%-40%)

Flatulence, loose stools, diarrhea, abdominal pain.

Occasional (5%)

Rash.

SERIOUS REACTIONS

• None reported. Hypoglycemia usually only occurs if other antidiabetic agents are used in the regimen.

PRECAUTIONS & CONSIDERATIONS

Caution is warranted in patients with renal impairment. Adequate studies have not been done in pregnant women. Miglitol is distributed to a very low amount in breast milk; caution warranted in lactation. Safety and efficacy have not been established in children.

Food intake and blood glucose should be monitored before and during therapy. A 1-h postprandial glucose may be helpful in optimizing dosage during initial treatment. Be aware of signs and symptoms of hypoglycemia (anxiety, cool wet skin, diplopia, dizziness, headache, hunger, numbness in mouth, tachycardia, tremors) or hyperglycemia (deep rapid breathing, dim vision, fatigue, nausea, polydipsia, polyphagia, polyuria, vomiting); carry glucose-based supplement for immediate response to hypoglycemia. Consult the physician when glucose demands are altered (such as with fever, heavy physical activity, infection, stress, trauma). Exercise, good personal hygiene (including foot care), not smoking, and weight control are essential parts of therapy. Type 2 diabetic patients may be using insulin concomitantly; if symptomatic hypoglycemia occurs while taking miglitol, use glucose rather than sucrose to reverse hypoglycemic effect owing to interference with sucrose metabolism.

Storage

Store at room temperature.

Administration

Take with the first bite of each main meal. If a meal is skipped, do not give that dose.

Miglustat

mig-lew'stat

★ 🍁 Zavesca

CATEGORY AND SCHEDULE

Pregnancy Risk Category: X

Classification: Metabolic agents, enzyme inhibitor

MECHANISM OF ACTION

A Gaucher disease agent that inhibits the enzyme glucosylceramide synthase, reducing the rate of synthesis of most glycosphingolipids. Allows the residual activity of the deficient enzyme, glucocerebrosidase, to be more effective in degrading lysosomal storage within tissues. *Therapeutic Effect*: Minimizes conditions associated with Gaucher disease, such as anemia and bone disease.

PHARMACOKINETICS

PO: Maximum plasma levels attained in 2-2.5 h; oral bioavailability 97%, no plasma protein binding. Excreted unchanged in the urine. *Half-life:* Approximately 6-7 h.

AVAILABILITY

Capsules: 100 mg.

INDICATIONS AND DOSAGES

▸ Gaucher disease

PO

Adults, Elderly. One 100-mg capsule 3 times a day at regular intervals.

▸ Dosage in renal impairment

Adults. CrCl 50-70 mL/min: Reduce to 100 mg twice a day.

CrCl 30-49 mL/min: 100 mg once a day.

CrCl < 30 mL/min: Not recommended.

CONTRAINDICATIONS

Women who are or may become pregnant, severe renal impairment, hypersensitivity.

INTERACTIONS

Drug

Aspirin, NSAIDs, other salicylates: May decrease platelet aggregation.

Imiglucerase: May decrease the effects of imiglucerase.

Herbal

None known.

Food

None known.

DIAGNOSTIC TEST EFFECTS

None known but should provide pretreatment neurologic evaluation.

SIDE EFFECTS

Expected (65%-89%)

Diarrhea, weight loss.

Frequent (11%-39%)

Hand tremor, flatulence, headache, abdominal pain, nausea.

Occasional (4%-7%)

Paresthesia, anorexia, dyspepsia, leg cramps, vomiting, neuropathy.

M

SERIOUS REACTIONS

- Thrombocytopenia occurs in 7% of patients.
- Overdose produces dizziness and neutropenia.

PRECAUTIONS & CONSIDERATIONS

Caution is warranted in patients with impaired fertility and renal function. Reliable contraceptive methods are necessary during miglustat treatment and for 3 mo afterward. Notify the physician and plan to stop miglustat therapy before trying to conceive. Avoid high-carbohydrate foods during miglustat treatment if diarrhea occurs. Contraindicated in pregnancy; extreme caution is warranted in lactation.

Notify the physician of hand tremor. Adequate hydration should be maintained. Baseline neurologic evaluation should be performed, with follow-up evaluations every 6 mo throughout treatment. Pattern of daily bowel activity and stool consistency and weight should be monitored.

Storage

Store at room temperature.

Administration

Take miglustat without regard to food. Do not open, crush, or break capsules.

Milnacipran

mil-na'sip-ran

Savella

CATEGORY AND SCHEDULE

Pregnancy Risk Category: C

Classification: Antidepressants, selective serotonin/norepinephrine reuptake inhibitor (SNRI)

MECHANISM OF ACTION

An agent related to SNRI antidepressants that inhibits serotonin and norepinephrine reuptake at neuronal presynaptic membranes; is a less potent inhibitor of dopamine reuptake. *Therapeutic Effect:* Relieves fibromyalgia pain through an unknown mechanism.

PHARMACOKINETICS

Well absorbed from the GI tract. Undergoes minimal CYP450 metabolism, with the majority of the dose excreted unchanged in urine (55%), and has a low binding to plasma proteins (13%). *Half-life:* 6-8 h.

AVAILABILITY

Tablets: 12.5 mg, 25 mg, 50 mg, 100 mg.

INDICATIONS AND DOSAGES

▸ Fibromyalgia

PO

Adults, Elderly. Give 12.5 mg once daily on day 1. On days 2-3: give 12.5 mg twice per day. On days 4-7: increase to 25 mg twice per day. After day 7: may give 50 mg twice daily. If needed, maximum is 100 mg twice per day.

▸ Dosage adjustments for renal impairment

CrCl 5-29 mL/min: Reduce maintenance dose to 25 mg PO twice per day. If needed, maximum is 50 mg twice daily.

ESRD: Not recommended.

CONTRAINDICATIONS

Hypersensitivity to drug. Uncontrolled angle-closure glaucoma; use during or within 14 days of MAOIs. Contains FD&C Yellow No. 5

(tartrazine), which may cause allergic-type reactions (including bronchial asthma) in susceptible persons.

INTERACTIONS

Drug

Alcohol: May increase risk of liver dysfunction. Milnacipran may increase the effects of alcohol.

Buspirone, meperidine, serotonin agonists, SSRIs/SNRIs, sibutramine, tramadol, trazodone: May increase risk of serotonin syndrome.

MAOIs, linezolid: May cause serotonin syndrome, characterized by autonomic hyperactivity, coma, diaphoresis, excitement, hyperthermia, and rigidity. MAOIs are contraindicated.

Herbal

St John's wort: May increase risk of serotonin-related adverse effects.

Food

None known.

DIAGNOSTIC TEST EFFECTS

May increase serum bilirubin, AST (SGOT), and ALT (SGPT) levels.

SIDE EFFECTS

Frequent (≥ 10%)

Nausea, constipation, headache, dizziness, hot flash, insomnia.

Occasional (3%-10%)

Vomiting, dry mouth, migraine, fatigue, anorexia, abdominal pain, diaphoresis/hyperhidrosis, anxiety, BP increased, increased heart rate, rash.

Rare (2% or less)

Blurred vision, pruritus, sexual dysfunction, paresthesia, tremor, insomnia, chest discomfort.

SERIOUS REACTIONS

- May slightly increase the patient's heart rate or blood pressure.
- Increased liver enzymes and reports of severe liver injury, including fulminant hepatitis, occur rarely.
- May increase the risk of bleeding events due to platelet dysfunction.
- Activation of mania or hypomania in bipolar patients can occur.
- SIADH and hyponatremia may occur with SSRIs and SNRIs.
- Withdrawal syndrome may occur with abrupt discontinuation. Gradually taper dose.

PRECAUTIONS & CONSIDERATIONS

Antidepressants may increase the risk of suicidal ideation in children, adolescents, and young adults with depression and psychiatric disorders. Closely monitor when initiating therapy, especially the first 2 mo.; monitor for suicidal thoughts, other changes in mood, and for unusual behaviors. Milnacipran is not approved for the treatment of depression. Caution is warranted with conditions that may slow gastric emptying, hepatic impairment, history of anemia, history of seizures, renal impairment, mania, hypomania, bipolar, and suicidal tendencies. The effect of milnacipran on pregnancy or lactation is not known. Breastfeeding is not recommended. Be aware that the safety and efficacy of this drug have not been established in children.

Dizziness may occur, so avoid alcohol and tasks that require mental alertness or motor skills until the effects of the drug are known. Blood chemistry tests to assess hepatic and renal function should be performed before and periodically during therapy. Monitor for improvement in symptoms. Report unusual changes in behavior promptly.

Storage
Store at room temperature.
Administration
Take without regard to meals. Take with food or milk if GI distress occurs. The therapeutic effects (decrease in pain and fibromyalgia scores) will be noted within 1-4 wks. Do not abruptly discontinue the drug.

Milrinone Lactate

mill're-none lack'tayte

CATEGORY AND SCHEDULE

Pregnancy Risk Category: C

Classification: Inotropes

M

MECHANISM OF ACTION

A cardiac inotropic agent that inhibits phosphodiesterase, which increases cyclic adenosine monophosphate and potentiates the delivery of calcium to myocardial contractile systems. *Therapeutic Effect:* Relaxes vascular muscle, causing vasodilation. Increases cardiac output; decreases pulmonary capillary wedge pressure and vascular resistance.

PHARMACOKINETICS

Route	Onset	Peak	Duration
IV	5-15 min	NA	NA

Protein binding: 70%. Primarily excreted unchanged in urine. *Half-life:* 2.4 h.

AVAILABILITY

Injection: 1 mg/mL.
IV Infusion (Premix): 200 mcg/mL.

INDICATIONS AND DOSAGES

▸ **Short-term management of congestive heart failure (CHF)**
IV Infusion
Adults. Initially, 50 mcg/kg over 10 min. Continue with maintenance infusion rate of 0.375-0.75 mcg/kg/min based on hemodynamic and clinical response. Total daily dosage: 0.59-1.13 mg/kg/day.

▸ **Dosage in renal impairment**
The recommended adjusted maintenance infusion rates are as follows; titrate to attain clinical goals.
CrCl > 50 mL/min: No adjustment needed.
CrCl 41-50 mL/min: 0.43 mcg/kg/min.
CrCl 31-40 mL/min: 0.38 mcg/kg/min.
CrCl 21-30 mL/min: 0.33 mcg/kg/min.
CrCl 11-20 mL/min: 0.28 mcg/kg/min.
CrCl 6-10 mL/min: 0.23 mcg/kg/min.
CrCl 5 mL/min or less: 0.20 mcg/kg/min.

CONTRAINDICATIONS

Hypersensitivity.

INTERACTIONS

Drug
Cardiac glycosides: Produces additive inotropic effects.
Herbal
None known.
Food
None known.

DIAGNOSTIC TEST EFFECTS

None known.

IV INCOMPATIBILITIES

Diazepam, esmolol, furosemide (Lasix), imipenem/cilastatin (Primaxin), lansoprazole (Prevacid), lidocaine, ondansetron (Zofran), pantoprazole, (Protonix), phenytoin, procainamide.

IV COMPATIBILITIES

Calcium gluconate, digoxin (Lanoxin), diltiazem (Cardizem), dobutamine (Dobutrex), dopamine (Intropin), heparin, magnesium, midazolam (Versed), nitroglycerin, potassium, propofol (Diprivan).

SIDE EFFECTS

Occasional (1%-3%)
Headache, hypotension.
Rare (< 1%)
Angina, chest pain.

SERIOUS REACTIONS

- Supraventricular and ventricular arrhythmias (12%), nonsustained ventricular tachycardia (2%), and sustained ventricular tachycardia (1%) may occur.

PRECAUTIONS & CONSIDERATIONS

Caution is warranted in patients with atrial fibrillation or flutter, history of ventricular arrhythmias, impaired renal function, and severe obstructive aortic or pulmonic valvular disease. It is unknown whether milrinone crosses the placenta or is distributed in breast milk; therefore, caution is warranted in lactation. The safety and efficacy of milrinone have not been established in children. In elderly patients, age-related renal impairment may require dosage adjustment.

Notify the physician if palpitations or chest pain occurs. Cardiac output, heart rate, BP, renal function, and serum potassium levels should be assessed before beginning treatment and during IV therapy. Breath sounds for crackles and rhonchi and skin for edema should also be assessed. Headache, tremors should be reported immediately; should not use for more than 5 days concurrently.

Storage
Store at room temperature. Do not freeze. Avoid excessive heat. For premix infusion bags, remove overwrap just prior to adminstration.

Administration
For IV infusion, dilute 20-mg (20-mL) vial with 80 mL diluent (0.9% NaCl, D5W) or 10-mg (10-mL) vial with 40 mL diluent to provide concentration of 200 mcg/mL. For a loading-dose IV injection, administer milrinone undiluted slowly over 10 min. Use a controlled-rate infusion device for maintenance infusion. Monitor for arrhythmias and hypotension during IV therapy. If one or both of these conditions occur, reduce or temporarily discontinue infusion until condition stabilizes.

Minocycline Hydrochloride

mi-noe-sye′kleen
high-droh-klor′ide
★ 🍁 Arestin, Dynacin, Minocin, Minocin PAC, Solodyn
Do not confuse Dynacin with Dynabac or Minocin with Mithracin or niacin.

CATEGORY AND SCHEDULE

Pregnancy Risk Category: D

Classification: Tetracycline anti-infective

MECHANISM OF ACTION

A tetracycline antibiotic that inhibits bacterial protein synthesis by binding to ribosomes. *Therapeutic Effects:* Bacteriostatic.

PHARMACOKINETICS

PO: Peak 2-3 h. 55%-88% protein bound; excreted in urine, feces, breast milk; crosses placenta. *Half-life:* 11-17 h.

AVAILABILITY

Capsules (Minocin): 50 mg, 75 mg, 100 mg.
Tablets (Dynacin): 50 mg, 75 mg, 100 mg.
Microspheres for Periodontal Use: 1 mg (Arestin).

Extended-Release Tablets: 45 mg, 55 mg, 65 mg, 80 mg, 90 mg, 105 mg, 115 mg, 135 mg (Solodyn). *Powder for Injection (Minocin):* 100 mg.

INDICATIONS AND DOSAGES

▸ **Mild, moderate, or severe prostate, urinary tract, central nervous system (CNS) infections (excluding meningitis); uncomplicated gonorrhea; brucellosis; skin granulomas; cholera; trachoma; nocardiasis; yaws; syphillis when penicillins are contraindicated**

PO/IV

Adults, Elderly. Initially, 100-200 mg, then 100 mg q12h or 50 mg q6h.

PO/IV

Children older than 8 yr. Initially, 4 mg/kg, then 2 mg/kg q12h.

▸ **Periodontitis**

Adults. 1 unit dose cartridge (1 mg) per periodontal pocket.

▸ **Non-nodular moderate to severe acne vulgaris**

PO

Adults. 200 mg PO for 1 dose, then 100 mg q12h. Alternatively, 100 or 200 mg for 1 dose, then 50 mg q6h.

Children 8 yr and older. Initially 4 mg/kg for 1 dose, then 2 mg/kg q12h (do not exceed adult doses).

PO (EXTENDED-RELEASE TABLETS, SOLODYN)

Adults and Children 12 yr and older. Dose is roughly 1 mg/kg once per day given for 12 wks. Use following conversions for patient weight: 126-135 kg: 135 mg once daily.

103-125 kg: 115 mg once daily.

78-102 kg: 90 mg once daily.

55-77 kg: 65 mg once daily.

45-54 kg: 45 mg once daily.

▸ **Renal impairment dosing**

Do not exceed an adult dose of 200 mg total per day.

CONTRAINDICATIONS

Children younger than 8 yr, hypersensitivity to tetracyclines, last half of pregnancy.

INTERACTIONS

Drug

Carbamazepine, phenytoin: May decrease minocycline blood concentration.

Cholestyramine, colestipol: May decrease minocycline absorption.

Isotretinoin: Contraindicated use.

Oral contraceptives: May decrease the effects of oral contraceptives.

Herbal

St. John's wort: May increase the risk of photosensitivity.

Food

Antacids; milk; other magnesium-, iron-, calcium-, and aluminum-containing products: Decreased anti-infective effect. Separate times of administration.

IV INCOMPATIBILITIES

Do not mix minocycline with any other medications.

DIAGNOSTIC TEST EFFECTS

May increase serum alkaline phosphatase, amylase, bilirubin, AST (SGOT), and ALT (SGPT) levels. May increase eosinophil counts.

SIDE EFFECTS

Frequent

Dizziness, light-headedness, diarrhea, nausea, vomiting, abdominal cramps, possibly severe photosensitivity, drowsiness, vertigo.

Occasional

Altered pigmentation of skin or mucous membranes, rectal or genital pruritus, stomatitis, eosinophilia.

SERIOUS REACTIONS

- Superinfection (especially fungal), anaphylaxis, and benign intracranial hypertension may occur.
- Benign increased intracranial pressure (pseudotumor cerebri).
- Pseudomembranous colitis from *Clostridium difficile* infection may occur during treatment or at any time several mo after therapy is discontinued.
- Tinnitus and hearing loss have been reported during IV use.
- Interstitial nephritis, azotemia, metabolic acidosis, acute renal failure.
- Rare cases of autoimmune syndromes, including a lupus-like syndrome or hepatitis with jaundice, eosinophilia.
- Tooth discoloration and enamel hypoplasia in children.
- Esophageal ulceration from improper administration.

PRECAUTIONS & CONSIDERATIONS

Caution is warranted in patients with renal impairment and in those who cannot avoid sun or ultraviolet exposure because such exposure may produce a severe photosensitivity reaction.

History of allergies, especially to tetracyclines or sulfites, should be determined before drug therapy. Dizziness, drowsiness, and vertigo may occur while taking minocycline. Avoid tasks that require mental alertness or motor skills until response to the drug is established. Pattern of daily bowel activity, stool consistency, food intake and tolerance, renal function, skin for rash should be assessed. Be alert for signs and symptoms of superinfection, such as anal or genital pruritus, diarrhea, sore tongue, fever, fatigue, and ulceration or changes of the oral mucosa or tongue; report symptoms to health care provider immediately. BP and level of consciousness should be monitored because of the potential for increased intracranial pressure. Do not use in patients under 8 yr or in pregnancy because of the likelihood of permanent intrinsic staining in erupted permanent teeth not associated with the calcification stage. Advise patient to report any signs or symptoms associated with frequent loose stools or bloody diarrhea, both of which could indicate pseudomembranous colitis or *C. difficile* infection. Advise patient to maintain compliance with oral contraceptive medications while using an additional nonhormonal form of contraception throughout the duration of therapy.

Storage

Store the drug at room temperature.

Administration

Ingestion of adequate amounts of fluids along with capsule and tablet forms is recommended to reduce the risk of esophageal irritation and ulceration. Do not give oral forms at bedtime. Pellet-filled capsules and extended-release tablets should be swallowed whole.

Microspheres for periodontal use are administered by the periodontist.

Injectable form is rarely used but is given by slow IV infusion only after dilution. Reconstitute vial with 5 mL sterile water for injection and immediately further dilute to 500 mL or 1000 mL with 0.9% NaCl, D5W, D5W/0.9%NaCl, or lactated Ringer's but not with other solutions containing calcium because a precipitate may form, especially in neutral and alkaline solutions. The infusion is acidic and may cause thrombophlebitis. Infuse over a period of 6 h.

M

Minoxidil

min-nox'i-dill

Rogaine, Rogaine Extra Strength, Loniten

Apo-Gain, Minox

Do not confuse Loniten with Lotensin.

CATEGORY AND SCHEDULE

Pregnancy Risk Category: C

OTC (topical solution)

Classification: Antihypertensives, vasodilators

MECHANISM OF ACTION

An antihypertensive and hair growth stimulant that has direct action on vascular smooth muscle, producing vasodilation of arterioles. *Therapeutic Effect:* Decreases peripheral vascular resistance and BP; increases cutaneous blood flow; stimulates hair follicle epithelium and hair follicle growth.

PHARMACOKINETICS

Route	Onset	Peak	Duration
PO	0.5 h	2-8 h	2-5 days

Well absorbed from the GI tract; minimal absorption after topical application. Protein binding: None. Widely distributed. Metabolized in the liver to active metabolite. Primarily excreted in urine. Removed by hemodialysis. *Half-life:* 4.2 h.

AVAILABILITY

Tablets (Loniten): 2.5 mg, 10 mg.

Topical Solution (Rogaine): 2% (20 mg/mL).

Topical Solution (Rogaine Extra Strength): 5% (50 mg/mL).

Topical Foam: 5%

INDICATIONS AND DOSAGES

▸ **Severe symptomatic hypertension, hypertension associated with organ damage; hypertension that has failed to respond to maximal therapeutic dosages of a diuretic or two other antihypertensives**

PO

Adults, Children 12 yr and older. Initially, 5 mg/day. Increase after at least 3-day intervals to 10 mg, then 20 mg, then up to 40 mg/day in 1-2 doses. Maximum: 100 mg/day.

Elderly. Initially, 2.5 mg/day. May increase gradually. Maintenance: 10-40 mg/day. Maximum: 100 mg/day.

Children under 12 yr. Initially, 0.1-0.2 mg/kg (5-mg maximum) daily. Gradually increase at minimum 3-day intervals. Maintenance: 0.25-1 mg/kg/day divided in 1-2 doses. Maximum: 50 mg/day.

▸ **Hair regrowth**

TOPICAL

Adults. 1 mL to affected areas of scalp 2 times a day. Total daily dose not to exceed 2 mL.

CONTRAINDICATIONS

Pheochromocytoma, hypersensitivity.

INTERACTIONS

Drug

Central nervous system (CNS) depressants used in conscious sedation technique: May increase hypotensive effect.

Parenteral antihypertensives: May increase hypotensive effect.

NSAIDs, indomethacin, sympathomimetics: May decrease the hypotensive effects of minoxidil.

Herbal

None known.

Food

None known.

DIAGNOSTIC TEST EFFECTS

May increase plasma renin activity and BUN, serum alkaline phosphatase, serum creatinine, and serum sodium levels. May decrease blood hemoglobin and hematocrit levels and erythrocyte count.

SIDE EFFECTS

Frequent

PO: Edema with concurrent weight gain, hypertrichosis (elongation, thickening, increased pigmentation of fine body hair; develops in 80% of patients within 3-6 wks after beginning therapy).

Occasional

PO: T-wave changes (usually revert to pretreatment state with continued therapy or drug withdrawal).
Topical: Pruritus, rash, dry or flaking skin, erythema.

Rare

PO: Breast tenderness, headache, photosensitivity reaction.
Topical: Allergic reaction, alopecia, burning sensation at scalp, soreness at hair root, headache, visual disturbances.

SERIOUS REACTIONS

• Tachycardia and angina pectoris may occur because of increased oxygen demands associated with increased heart rate and cardiac output.
• Fluid and electrolyte imbalance and CHF may occur, especially if a diuretic is not given concurrently with minoxidil.
• Too rapid reduction in BP may result in syncope, cerebrovascular accident (CVA), myocardial infarction (MI), and ocular or vestibular ischemia.
• Hypersensitivity may occur, usually in form of skin rash; serious rashes include bullous rash and Stevens-Johnson syndrome.
• Pericardial effusion and tamponade may be seen in patients with impaired renal function who are not on dialysis.

PRECAUTIONS & CONSIDERATIONS

Angina may worsen or appear for the first time during treatment; use with caution in patients with recent MI or angina. Also use with caution in patients with fluid retention; may exacerbate CHF or renal impairment. Minoxidil crosses the placenta and is distributed in breast milk; use during pregnancy and lactation is not recommended. No age-related precautions have been noted in children, but dosages must be carefully titrated. Elderly patients are more sensitive to the drug's hypotensive effects. Exposure to sunlight and artificial light sources should be avoided.

BP should be assessed on both arms. Take the patient's pulse for 1 full min immediately before giving the medication. If pulse rate increases 20 beats/min or more over baseline, or systolic or diastolic BP decreases more than 20 mm Hg, withhold minoxidil and contact the physician. Weight and electrolytes should also be monitored during therapy. Report any sudden weight gain over 5 lb, or any dyspnea. Because of the cardiovascular effects of this medication, patients should be assessed for stress tolerance before initiating therapy. Postural changes should be made slowly in consideration of possible orthostatic hypotension developing.

Storage

Store at room temperature away from excessive heat. The topical solutions and foam are flammable and should be kept away from flame.

M

Administration
Take oral minoxidil without regard to food. Can take with food if GI upset occurs. Crush tablets if necessary. Maximum BP response occurs 3-7 days after initiation of minoxidil therapy.

For topical use, shampoo and dry hair before applying medication. Wash hands immediately after application. Avoid getting in the eyes. Treatment must continue on a permanent basis and any cessation of treatment will reverse new hair growth. A response to treatment is usually seen within 4 mo.

Mirtazapine

mir-taz'a-peen

Remeron, Remeron Soltab

Remeron, Remeron RD

Do not confuse Remeron with Premarin.

CATEGORY AND SCHEDULE

Pregnancy Risk Category: C

Classification: Antidepressants, tetracyclic

MECHANISM OF ACTION

A tetracyclic compound that acts as an antagonist at presynaptic α_2-adrenergic receptors, increasing both norepinephrine and serotonin neurotransmission. Has low anticholinergic activity. *Therapeutic Effect:* Relieves depression and produces sedative effects.

PHARMACOKINETICS

Rapidly and completely absorbed after PO administration; absorption not affected by food. Protein binding: 85%. Metabolized in the liver. Primarily excreted in urine. Unknown if removed by hemodialysis. *Half-life:* 20-40 h (longer in males [37 h] than females [26 h]).

AVAILABILITY

Tablets: 7.5 mg, 15 mg, 30 mg, 45 mg.
Tablets (Disintegrating): 15 mg, 30 mg, 45 mg.

INDICATIONS AND DOSAGES

▸ Depression

PO

Adults. Initially, 15 mg at bedtime. May increase by 15 mg/day q1-2wk. Maximum: 45 mg/day.
Elderly. Initially, 7.5 mg at bedtime. May increase by 7.5-15 mg/day q1-2wk. Maximum: 45 mg/day.

OFF-LABEL USES

Essential tremor, intractable pruritus.

CONTRAINDICATIONS

Use within 14 days of MAOIs, hypersensitivity.

INTERACTIONS

Drug

Alcohol, diazepam and other benzodiazepines: May increase impairment of cognition and motor skills.
MAOIs: May increase the risk of neuroleptic malignant syndrome, hypertensive crisis, and severe seizures. Contraindicated.
Opioid analgesics: May impair cognitive or motor performance.

Herbal

None known.

Food

None known.

DIAGNOSTIC TEST EFFECTS

May increase serum cholesterol, triglyceride, AST (SGOT), and ALT (SGPT) levels.

SIDE EFFECTS

Frequent

Somnolence (54%), dry mouth (25%); increased appetite (17%), constipation (13%), weight gain (12%).

Occasional
Asthenia (8%), dizziness (7%), flu-like symptoms (5%), abnormal dreams (4%).
Rare
Abdominal discomfort, vasodilation, paresthesia, acne, dry skin, thirst, arthralgia.

SERIOUS REACTIONS

- Mirtazapine poses a higher risk of seizures than tricyclic antidepressants, especially in those with no previous history of seizures.
- Overdose may produce cardiovascular effects, such as severe orthostatic hypotension, dizziness, tachycardia, palpitations, and arrhythmias.
- Abrupt discontinuation after prolonged therapy may produce headache, malaise, nausea, vomiting, and vivid dreams.
- Agranulocytosis occurs rarely.

PRECAUTIONS & CONSIDERATIONS

Caution is warranted with cardiovascular disorders, GI disorders, angle-closure glaucoma, benign prostatic hyperplasia, hepatic or renal impairment, and urine retention. It is unknown whether mirtazapine is distributed in breast milk; caution is warranted in lactation. Antidepressant drugs increase the risk of suicidal thinking and behavior (suicidality) in children, adolescents, and young adults (ages 18-24) with major depressive disorder (MDD) and other psychiatric disorders. Monitor patients for the emergence of suicidal thoughts, agitation, irritability, or other unusal changes in behavior during therapy. The safety and efficacy of mirtazapine have not been established in children. In elderly patients, age-related renal impairment may require cautious use.

Drowsiness and dizziness may occur, so avoid alcohol and tasks that require mental alertness or motor skills. CBC, serum alkaline phosphatase, bilirubin, AST (SGOT), and ALT (SGPT) levels should be assessed before and periodically during therapy to assess hepatic and renal function in patients on long-term therapy. ECG should also be performed to assess for arrhythmias. Abrupt discontinuation after long-term therapy may produce headache, nausea, malaise, vomiting, and vivid dreams; use caution in surgery with sedation or general anesthesia because of the greater risk of hypotensive episode.
Storage
Store at room temperature. Keep disintegrating tablets in blister pack until time of use.
Administration
! Make sure at least 14 days elapse between the use of MAOIs and mirtazapine.

Take mirtazapine at bedtime without regard to food. Scored tablets may be crushed or broken if needed.

Orally disintegrating tablets may be placed on tongue to dissolve. No water is necessary.

Misoprostol

mis-oh-pros′toll
☒ Cytotec
Do not confuse Cytotec with Cytomel.

CATEGORY AND SCHEDULE

Pregnancy Risk Category: X

Classification: Gastrointestinal agents, prostaglandin analogue, gastric mucosal protectant, abortifacient (when used with mifepristone)

M

MECHANISM OF ACTION
A prostaglandin that inhibits basal, nocturnal gastric acid secretion via direct action on parietal cells. *Therapeutic Effect:* Increases production of protective gastric mucus. Produces uterine contractions and cervical ripening.

PHARMACOKINETICS
Rapidly absorbed from the GI tract. Rapidly converted to active metabolite. Primarily excreted in urine. *Half-life:* 20-40 min.

AVAILABILITY
Tablets: 100 mcg, 200 mcg (Cytotec).

M

INDICATIONS AND DOSAGES
▸ Prevention of NSAID-induced gastric ulcer

PO

Adults. 200 mcg 4 times/day with food (last dose at bedtime). Continue for duration of NSAID therapy. May reduce dosage to 100 mcg if 200-mcg dose is not tolerable.

Elderly. 100-200 mcg 4 times/day with food.

▸ Termination of early pregnancy

PO

See mifepristone monograph for FDA-approved regimen. Only used in combination with mifepristone.

OFF-LABEL USES
Treatment of gastric ulcer; also used in low-dose intravaginal protocols for cervical ripening.

CONTRAINDICATIONS
Pregnancy (produces uterine contractions), hypersensitivity to misoprostol or any component of the formulation.

INTERACTIONS
Drug

Antacids: May decrease misoprostol effectiveness.

NSAIDs: May increase upper GI distress or cause ulceration.

Phenylbutazone: May increase neurosensory effects (headache, dizziness, ataxia).

Herbal

None known.

Food

None known.

DIAGNOSTIC TEST EFFECTS
None known.

SIDE EFFECTS
Frequent

Abdominal pain, diarrhea.

Occasional

Nausea, flatulence, dyspepsia, headache.

Rare

Vomiting, constipation.

SERIOUS REACTIONS
- Overdosage may produce sedation, tremor, convulsions, dyspnea, palpitations, hypotension, and bradycardia.
- Hyperstimulation of uterus and possible uterine rupture (use during labor).

PRECAUTIONS & CONSIDERATIONS
Caution is warranted in patients with renal impairment and women of childbearing age. Females must use an effective contraception method during treatment. Be aware that misoprostol is contraindicated in pregnancy and will produce uterine contractions, uterine bleeding, and expulsion of products of conception. May also be teratogenic in first trimester. Be aware that it is unknown whether misoprostol is distributed in breast

milk; caution is warranted in lactation. Safety and efficacy have not been established in children. No age-related precautions have been noted in elderly patients.

Storage

Store at room temperature in a dry area.

Administration

Take with or after meals to minimize diarrhea. The last dose of the day is taken at bedtime.

Mitotane

mye'toe-tane

★ 🍁 Lysodren

CATEGORY AND SCHEDULE

Pregnancy Risk Category: C

Classification: Antineoplastics, adrenal hormone modifier

MECHANISM OF ACTION

A hormonal agent that inhibits activity of the adrenal cortex. *Therapeutic Effect:* Suppresses functional and nonfunctional adrenocortical neoplasms by direct cytoxic effect.

PHARMACOKINETICS

Adequately absorbed orally (40%). Hepatic metabolism; excreted in urine, bile. *Half-life:* 18-19 days.

AVAILABILITY

Tablets: 500 mg.

INDICATIONS AND DOSAGES

▸ **Adrenocortical carcinomas**

PO

Adults, Elderly. Initially, 2-6 g/day in 3-4 divided doses. Increase by 2-4 g/day every 3-7 days up to 9-10 g/day. Range: 2-16 g/day.

OFF-LABEL USES

Treatment of Cushing syndrome.

CONTRAINDICATIONS

Known hypersensitivity to mitotane.

NOTE: Temporarily discontinue if shock or severe trauma, since adrenal suppression is the drug's prime action, Exogenous steroids should be administered, since the depressed adrenal may not immediately start to secrete steroids in response to the traumatic event.

INTERACTIONS

Drug

All central nervous system (CNS) depressants: May increase CNS depression.

Corticosteroids: Decreased effects; use hydrocortisone instead.

Warfarin: Accelerates warfarin metabolism; monitor INR.

Herbal

None known.

Food

None known.

DIAGNOSTIC TEST EFFECTS

May decrease levels of plasma cortisol, urinary 17-hydroxycorticosteroids, protein-bound iodine, and serum uric acid.

SIDE EFFECTS

Frequent (> 15%)

Anorexia, nausea, vomiting, diarrhea, lethargy, somnolence, adrenocortical insufficiency, dizziness, vertigo, maculopapular rash, hypouricemia.

Occasional (< 15%)

Blurred or double vision, retinopathy, hearing loss, excessive salivation, urine abnormalities (hematuria, cystitis, albuminuria), hypertension, orthostatic hypotension, flushing, wheezing, dyspnea, generalized aching, fever.

SERIOUS REACTIONS

• Brain damage and functional impairment may occur with long-term, high-dosage therapy.
• Adrenal insufficiency may require adrenal steroid replacement.

PRECAUTIONS & CONSIDERATIONS

! Brain damage and functional impairment may occur with long-term, high-dose therapy. Drug may cause adrenal hypofunction; administer hydrocortisone or mineralocorticoid as needed after evaluation and monitoring.

Caution is warranted with impaired hepatic function. Vaccinations and coming in contact with crowds, people with known infections, and anyone who has recently received a live-virus vaccine should be avoided.

Dizziness and drowsiness may occur; tasks that require mental alertness or motor skills should be avoided. Notify the physician if darkening of the skin, diarrhea, depression, loss of appetite, nausea and vomiting, or rash occurs. Adequate hydration should be maintained to prevent urinary side effects. Liver function test results, serum uric acid levels, and urine tests, including urine chemistry and urinalysis, should be assessed. Be aware that neurologic and behavioral assessments are performed periodically on those receiving prolonged therapy (> 2 yr).

Storage

Store at room temperature.

Administration

CAUTION: The manufacturer recommends the following precautions with this cytotoxic drug. To minimize the risk of dermal exposure, always wear impervious gloves when handling. Do not crush the tablets. Perssonnel should avoid exposure to crushed and/or broken tablets. If contact occurs, wash immediately and thoroughly.

Taking with food may improve oral absorption.

Mitoxantrone

mye-toe-zan'trone

★ Novantrone

CATEGORY AND SCHEDULE

Pregnancy Risk Category: D

Classification: Antineoplastics, synthetic anthraquinone

MECHANISM OF ACTION

An anthracenedione that is related to the anthracyclines and that inhibits DNA and RNA synthesis. Active throughout the entire cell cycle. Inhibits B-cell, T-cell, and macrophage proliferation and the secretion of interferon gamma, tumor necrosis factor-α, and interleukin-2. *Therapeutic Effect:* Causes cell death. Slows worsening of neurologic disability and reduces relapse rate in MS.

PHARMACOKINETICS

Protein binding: 78%. Widely distributed. Metabolized in the liver. Primarily eliminated in feces by the biliary system. Not removed by hemodialysis. *Half-life:* 2.3-13 days.

AVAILABILITY

Injection: 2 mg/mL.

INDICATIONS AND DOSAGES

▸ **AML**

IV

Adults, Elderly, Children 2 yr and older. 12 mg/m^2 once a day on days 1-3 is a common first-cycle regimen.

Children younger than 2 yr. 0.4 mg/kg once a day for 3-5 days.

▸ **AML in relapse**

IV

Adults, Elderly, Children older than 2 yr. 12 mg/m^2 once a day for 3-5 days is common regimen.

▸ **Prostate cancer**

IV

Adults, Elderly. 12-14 mg/m^2 every 21 days.

▸ **Multiple sclerosis**

IV

Adults, Elderly. 12 mg/m^2/dose q3mo.

OFF-LABEL USES

Treatment of breast or hepatic carcinoma, ovarian cancer, and various sarcomas, non-Hodgkin lymphoma.

CONTRAINDICATIONS

Baseline left ventricular ejection fraction < 50%, cumulative lifetime mitoxantrone dose of 140 mg/m^2, hypersensitivity.

INTERACTIONS

Drug

Aspirin, other salicylates, NSAIDs: Avoid use.

Antigout medications: May decrease the effects of these drugs.

Bone marrow depressants: May increase myelosuppression.

Live-virus vaccines: May potentiate virus replication, increase vaccine side effects, and decrease the patient's antibody response to the vaccine.

Herbal and Food

None known.

DIAGNOSTIC TEST EFFECTS

May increase serum bilirubin and uric acid, AST (SGOT), and ALT (SGPT) levels.

IV INCOMPATIBILITIES

NOTE: It is recommended that mitoxantrone not be mixed with other drugs.

Amphotericin B, azithromycin, most cephalosporins, clindamycin, dexamethasone, diazepam, digoxin, ertapenem, fosphenytoin, furosemide, heparin, lansoprazole, methylprednisolone, nafcillin, nitroprusside, paclitaxel (Taxol), pantoprazole, phenytoin, pemetrexed, piperacillin/tazobactum (Zosyn), potassium and sodium phosphates, propofol, ticarcillin, TPN, voriconazole.

IV COMPATIBILITIES

Allopurinol (Aloprim), etoposide (VePesid), gemcitabine (Gemzar), granisetron (Kytril), ondansetron (Zofran), potassium chloride.

SIDE EFFECTS

Expected

Temporary discoloration of urine and sclera (blue-green).

Frequent (> 10%)

Nausea, vomiting, diarrhea, cough, headache, stomatitis, abdominal discomfort, fever, alopecia.

Occasional (4%-9%)

Ecchymosis, fungal infection, conjunctivitis, urinary tract infection.

Rare (3%)

Arrhythmias.

SERIOUS REACTIONS

- Myelosuppression may be severe, resulting in GI bleeding, hematologic toxicity, sepsis, and pneumonia.
- Renal failure, seizures, and jaundice may occur.
- Extravasation can cause serious pain, discoloration, skin necrosis.
- Cardiac arrhythmias, ECG changes, heart failure. Decreased ejection fraction may be permanent.
- Anaphylaxis (rare).

PRECAUTIONS & CONSIDERATIONS

Caution is warranted with impaired hepatobiliary function and preexisting myelosuppression and in those who have previously been treated with cardiotoxic medications. Patients with hepatic impairment have higher mitoxantrone exposure because of reduced clearance. Mitoxantrone use should be avoided during pregnancy, especially during the first trimester, because it can cause fetal harm. Contraceptive measures should be used. Breastfeeding also is not recommended. The safety and efficacy of mitoxantrone have not been established in children. No age-related precautions have been noted in elderly patients. Vaccinations and coming in contact with crowds and people with known infections should be avoided.

Urine will appear blue or green and sclera may have a blue tint for 24 h after mitoxantrone administration. Notify the physician if fever, signs of local infection, unusual bleeding from any site, bluish skin, burning or erythema of oral mucosa, difficulty swallowing, oral ulcerations, or sore throat occurs. Adequate hydration should be maintained to protect against renal impairment. Hematologic status and liver, renal, and pulmonary function test.

Storage

Store vials at room temperature. Do not freeze.

Administration

! CAUTION: Observe and exercise appropriate precautions for handling, preparing, and administering cytotoxic drugs.

! Must be diluted before use. Dilute with at least 50 mL D5W or 0.9% NaCl. Do not administer by subcutaneous, IM, intrathecal, or intra-arterial injection. Do not give IV push over < 3 min. Give IV bolus over at least 3 min or intermittent IV infusion over 15-60 min into the tubing of a freely running IV infusion of 0.9% NaCl or dextrose 5% injection. Administer IV infusion of 0.02-0.5 mg/mL in D5W or 0.9% NaCl.

Take care to avoid extravasation. While not a vesicant, significant irritation may occur. If extravasation occurs, the infusion should be stopped and completed via another vein, preferably in another limb. Use of a larger vein is preferable.

M

Modafinil

mode-ah-feen'awl

★ Provigil 🍁 Alertec

CATEGORY AND SCHEDULE

Pregnancy Risk Category: C
Controlled Substance Schedule: IV

Classification: Central nervous system (CNS) stimulants

MECHANISM OF ACTION

An α_1-agonist that may bind to dopamine reuptake carrier sites, increasing α activity and decreasing Θ, T, and β brain wave activity. *Therapeutic Effect:* Reduces the number of sleep episodes and total daytime sleep.

PHARMACOKINETICS

Well absorbed. Protein binding: 60%. Widely distributed. Metabolized in the liver. Excreted by the kidneys. Unknown if removed by hemodialysis. *Half-life:* 8-10 h.

AVAILABILITY

Tablets: 100 mg, 200 mg.

INDICATIONS AND DOSAGES

▸ **Narcolepsy, other sleep disorders**

PO

Adults, Elderly, Adolescents 16 yr and older. 200-400 mg/day.

▸ **Dosage in hepatic impairment**

Reduce normal dosage by 50% in those with moderate to severe liver disease.

CONTRAINDICATIONS

Hypersensitivity to modafinil or armodafinil.

INTERACTIONS

Drug

Antifungals, erythromycins, other CYP450 isoenzyme inhibitors: Could result in increased modafinil concentrations.

Cyclosporine, hormonal contraceptives, theophylline: May decrease plasma concentrations of these drugs.

Diazepam, phenytoin, propranolol, tricyclic antidepressants, warfarin; and other CYPC19 and CYP2C9 substrates: May increase plasma concentrations of these drugs.

Other CNS stimulants: May increase CNS stimulation.

Herbal

None known.

Food

None known.

DIAGNOSTIC TEST EFFECTS

May increase gamma glutamyltransferase (GGT) and alkaline phosphatase.

SIDE EFFECTS

Frequent

Headache, nausea, nervousness, rhinitis, diarrhea, back pain, anxiety, insomnia, dizziness, and dyspepsia.

Occasional

Anorexia, dry mouth or skin, muscle stiffness, polydipsia, paraesthesia, tremor, vomiting.

SERIOUS REACTIONS

- Mania, delusions, hallucinations, suicidal ideation and aggression, some resulting in hospitalization.
- Serious rash, including Stevens-Johnson syndrome, TEN, and eosinophilia.
- Serious hypersensitivity with angioedema (rare).
- Chest pain, palpitations, dyspnea, and transient ischemic T-wave changes reported in assoication with certain cardiac problems.

M

PRECAUTIONS & CONSIDERATIONS

Caution is warranted in patients with hepatic impairment or a history of clinically significant mitral valve prolapse, left ventricular hypertrophy, and seizures. Nonhormonal contraceptive methods should be used during modafinil therapy and 1 mo afterward because modafinil decreases the effectiveness of hormonal contraceptives. It is unknown whether modafinil is excreted in breast milk; caution warranted in lactation. Use caution when giving modafinil to pregnant women. The safety and efficacy of this drug have not been established in children younger than 16 yr. Age-related hepatic or renal impairment may require decreased dosage in elderly patients.

Dizziness may occur, so tasks that require mental alertness and motor skills should be avoided until response to the drug is established. Sleep pattern should be assessed throughout therapy. Should only be used in patients with a diagnosis of narcolepsy, obstructive sleep apnea-hypopnea syndrome, or shift-work sleep disorder.

Storage

Store at room temperature.

Administration

Take modafinil without regard to food. If treating narcolepsy, dose is taken as single dose in the morning. In patients with shift-work sleep disorder, the drug is taken 1 h before the start of the work shift.

Moexipril Hydrochloride

moe-ex′a-prile high-droh-klor′ide

★ Univasc

CATEGORY AND SCHEDULE

Pregnancy Risk Category: C (D if used in second or third trimesters)

Classification: Antihypertensives, angiotensin-converting enzyme (ACE) inhibitors

MECHANISM OF ACTION

An ACE inhibitor that suppresses the renin-angiotensin-aldosterone system and prevents conversion of angiotensin I to angiotensin II, a potent vasoconstrictor; may also inhibit angiotensin II at local vascular and renal sites. *Therapeutic Effect:* Reduces peripheral arterial resistance and lowers BP.

PHARMACOKINETICS

Route	Onset	Peak	Duration
PO	1 h	3-6 h	24 h

Incompletely absorbed from the GI tract. Food decreases drug absorption. Rapidly converted to active metabolite. Protein binding: 50%. Primarily recovered in feces, partially excreted in urine. Unknown whether removed by dialysis.

Half-life: 1 h, metabolite 2-9 h.

AVAILABILITY

Tablets: 7.5 mg, 15 mg.

INDICATIONS AND DOSAGES

▸ **Hypertension**

PO

Adults, Elderly. For patients not receiving diuretics, initial dose is 7.5 mg once a day 1 h before meals. Adjust according to BP effect. Maintenance: 7.5-30 mg a day in 1-2 divided doses 1 h before meals.

▸ **Hypertension in patients with impaired renal function**

PO

Adults, Elderly. 3.75 mg once a day in patients with creatinine clearance of 40 mL/min or less. Maximum: May titrate up to 15 mg/day.

CONTRAINDICATIONS

Hypersensitivity to moexipril, history of angioedema related to ACE inhibitors, hereditary angioedema.

INTERACTIONS

Drug

Alcohol, antihypertensives, diuretics: May increase the effects of moexipril.

Lithium: Increased risk of lithium toxicity.

NSAIDs, salicylates: Renal adverse effects may be increased. May decrease effectiveness of moexipril.

Potassium-sparing diuretics, drospirenone, eplerenone, potassium supplements: Increased risk of hyperkalemia.

Herbal

None known.

Food
All food: Decreases absorption by up to 50%. Administer on empty stomatch.

DIAGNOSTIC TEST EFFECTS

May increase BUN, serum alkaline phosphatase, serum bilirubin, serum creatinine, serum potassium, AST (SGOT), and ALT (SGPT) levels. May decrease serum sodium levels. May cause positive serum antinuclear antibody titer.

SIDE EFFECTS

Occasional
Cough, headache (6%); dizziness (4%); fatigue (3%); hyperkalemia.
Rare
Flushing, rash, myalgia, nausea, vomiting.

SERIOUS REACTIONS

- Excessive hypotension (first-dose syncope) may occur in patients with CHF and in those who are severely salt or volume depleted.
- Angioedema (swelling of face and lips) occurs rarely.
- Agranulocytosis and neutropenia may be noted in those with collagen vascular disease, including scleroderma and SLE, and impaired renal function.
- Nephrotic syndrome may be noted in those with history of renal disease.

PRECAUTIONS & CONSIDERATIONS

Caution is warranted with angina, aortic stenosis, cerebrovascular disease, cerebrovascular and coronary insufficiency, hypovolemia, ischemic heart disease, renal impairment, severe CHF, sodium depletion, and those on dialysis and/or receiving diuretics. Moexipril crosses the placenta and it is unknown whether it is distributed in breast milk; caution is warranted in lactation and pregnancy. Moexipril has caused fetal or neonatal morbidity or mortality. Safety and efficacy of moexipril have not been established in children. In elderly patients, age-related renal impairment may require cautious use of moexipril.

Dizziness may occur. Notify the physician if chest pain, cough, difficulty breathing, fever, sore throat, or swelling of the eyes, face, feet, hands, lips, or tongue occurs. BP should be obtained immediately before giving each moexipril dose, in addition to regular monitoring. Be alert to fluctuations in BP. If an excessive reduction in BP occurs, place the patient in the supine position with legs elevated. CBC and blood chemistry should be obtained before beginning moexipril therapy, then every 2 wks for the next 3 mo, and periodically thereafter. BUN, serum creatinine, serum potassium, renal function, and white blood cell count (WBC) should also be monitored. Lungs should be auscultated for rales. Heart rate should be assessed for irregularities.

Storage
Store at room temperature.
Administration
Take moexipril 1 h before meals. Crush tablets if necessary.

M

Mometasone Furoate

mo-met′a-sone fur′oh-ate
★ Asmanex Twisthaler, Elocon, Nasonex 🍁 Nasonex

CATEGORY AND SCHEDULE

Pregnancy Risk Category: C

Classification: Respiratory agents, dermatologics, synthetic corticosteroids

MECHANISM OF ACTION
A medium-potency adrenocorticosteroid that inhibits the release of inflammatory cells, preventing early activation of the allergic reaction. *Therapeutic Effect:* Decreases response to seasonal and perennial rhinitis, stabilizes asthma, reduces inflammatory skin response.

PHARMACOKINETICS
Undetectable in plasma. Protein binding: 98%-99%. The swallowed portion undergoes extensive metabolism. Excreted primarily through bile and, to a lesser extent, urine. *Half-life:* 5.8 h (nasal).

AVAILABILITY
Nasal Spray: 50 mcg/spray.
Topical Cream: 0.1%.
Topical Ointment: 0.1%.
Topical Lotion: 0.1%.
Oral Inhalation: 110 mcg/actuation, 220 mcg/actuation (Asmanex Twisthaler).

INDICATIONS AND DOSAGES
▸ **Allergic rhinitis**
NASAL SPRAY
Adults, Elderly, Children 12 yr and older. 2 sprays in each nostril once a day.
Children 2-11 yr. 1 spray in each nostril once a day.
▸ **Asthma**
INHALATION
Adults, Elderly, Children 12 yr and older. Initially inhale 220 mcg (1 puff) once a day. Maximum: 880 mcg once a day.
Children 4-11 yr. Initially, 110 mcg once daily.
▸ **Corticosteroid-responsive dermatoses**
TOPICAL
Adults, Elderly, Children 12 yr and older. Apply cream, lotion, or ointment to affected area once a day.
▸ **Nasal polyp**
NASAL SPRAY
Adults, Elderly. 2 sprays in each nostril 2 times/day.

CONTRAINDICATIONS
Hypersensitivity to any corticosteroid, persistently positive sputum cultures for *Candida albicans,* systemic fungal infections, untreated localized infection involving nasal mucosa.

INTERACTIONS
Drug
Ketoconazole (potent inhibitor of CYP3A4): May increase plasma levels of mometasone.
Herbal
None known.
Food
None known.

DIAGNOSTIC TEST EFFECTS
None known.

SIDE EFFECTS
Occasional
Nasal irritation, stinging, sore throat, headache.
Rare
Nasal or pharyngeal candidiasis, sinus infection, HPA axis suppression.

SERIOUS REACTIONS
• An acute hypersensitivity reaction, including urticaria, angioedema, and severe bronchospasm, occurs rarely.
• Transfer from systemic to local steroid therapy may unmask previously suppressed bronchial asthma condition.
• Nasal septum perforation with prolonged improper use of nasal spray.
• Adrenal insufficiency.

PRECAUTIONS & CONSIDERATIONS

Caution is warranted with adrenal insufficiency, cirrhosis, diabetes mellitus, glaucoma, hypothyroidism, osteoporosis, tuberculosis, and untreated infection. It is unknown whether mometasone crosses the placenta or is distributed in breast milk; caution warranted in lactation and pregnancy. In children, prolonged treatment and high dosages may decrease cortisol secretion and short-term growth rate. Some young children do not generate sufficient inspiratory flow to use the dry powder inhaler. No age-related precautions have been noted in elderly patients.

Pulse rate and quality, ABG levels, and respiratory rate, depth, rhythm, and type should be monitored. Symptoms should start to improve within 2 days of the first dose, but the drug's maximum benefit may take up to 2 wks to appear. Notify the physician if symptoms fail to improve.

Storage

Store at room temperature in a dry place protected from light. Discard the Twisthaler 45 days after opening the foil pouch or when dose counter reads "00," whichever is first.

Administration

For inhalation, see instructions for use of the Twisthaler. Exhale completely and place the mouthpiece between the lips. Inhale and hold breath for as long as possible before exhaling. Allow 1 min between inhalations to promote deeper bronchial penetration. Rinse mouth with water immediately after inhalation to prevent mouth and throat dryness and oral candidiasis. Once-daily inhalation doses are administered in the evening.

Clear the nasal passages before using mometasone. Prime nasal unit before first use by pumping the activator 10 times or until a fine spary appears, away from others. If the unit has not been used for 1 wk, reprime by pumping until a fine spray appears. Tilt head slightly forward. Insert spray tip up into the nostril, pointing toward the inflamed nasal turbinates, away from nasal septum. Spray the drug into the nostril while holding the other nostril closed, and at the same time inhale through the nose.

Montelukast

mon-te'loo-kast

★ 🍁 Singulair

CATEGORY AND SCHEDULE

Pregnancy Risk Category: B

Classification: Respiratory agents, anti-inflammatory agents, leukotriene receptor antagonists

MECHANISM OF ACTION

An antiasthmatic that binds to cysteinyl leukotriene receptors, inhibiting the effects of leukotrienes on bronchial smooth muscle. *Therapeutic Effect:* Decreases bronchoconstriction, vascular permeability, mucosal edema, and mucus production.

PHARMACOKINETICS

Route	Onset	Peak	Duration
PO	NA	N/A	24 h
PO (chewable)	NA	N/A	24 h

Rapidly absorbed from the GI tract. Protein binding: 99%. Extensively metabolized in the liver. Excreted almost exclusively in feces. *Half-life:* 2.7-5.5 h (slightly longer in elderly patients).

AVAILABILITY

Oral Granules: 4 mg/packet.
Tablets: 10 mg.
Tablets (Chewable): 4 mg, 5 mg.

INDICATIONS AND DOSAGES

▸ **Bronchial asthma and seasonal and perennial allergic rhinitis**
PO
Adults, Elderly, Adolescents older than 14 yr. One 10-mg tablet a day, taken in the evening.
Children 6-14 yr. One 5-mg chewable tablet a day, taken in the evening.
Children 2-5 yr. One 4-mg chewable tablet a day, taken in the evening, or 1 packet of 4-mg oral granules.
Children, Infants age 6-23 mo. 1 packet 4-mg oral granules daily, in the evening.

▸ **For the prevention of exercise-induced bronchospasm:**
PO
Adults, Children 15 yr and older. 10 mg PO for 1 dose 2 h or more before exercise. Do not take additional doses within 24 h. If already on for another indication, do not take additional dose for exercise. Rescue medications (e.g., β agonists) should be available.

CONTRAINDICATIONS

Hypersensitivity.
Not for acute asthma attacks.

INTERACTIONS

Drug
CYP2C8 substrates (cerivastatin, repaglinide, rosiglitazone, ploglitazone, paclitaxel): Montelukast inhibits CYP2C8 and may raise concentrations and side effect risks of these drugs.
Phenobarbital, rifampin: May decrease montelukast's duration of action.
Herbal
None known.
Food
None known.

DIAGNOSTIC TEST EFFECTS

May increase AST (SGOT) and ALT (SGPT) levels.

SIDE EFFECTS

Adults, adolescents older than 14 yr.
Frequent (18%)
Headache.
Occasional (4%)
Influenza.
Rare (2%-3%)
Abdominal pain, cough, dyspepsia, dizziness, fatigue, dental pain.
Children 6-14 yr: Diarrhea, laryngitis, pharyngitis, nausea, otitis media, sinusitis, viral infection.

SERIOUS REACTIONS

- Systemic eosinophilia, Churg-Strauss syndrome, vasculitis.
- Rare cases of eosinophilic infiltration of the liver (hypersensivity hepatitis), cholestatic hepatitis, liver injury, pancreatitis.
- Reports post-market of agitation, aggressive behavior, confusion (disorientation), hallucinations, seizures, tremor, mood disorders, suicidal ideation.

PRECAUTIONS & CONSIDERATIONS

Caution is warranted in patients with hepatic impairment and in those who are tapering systemic corticosteroid dosage during montelukast therapy. Use montelukast during pregnancy only if necessary. It is unknown whether montelukast is excreted in breast milk. No age-related precautions have been noted in children older than 6 yr or in elderly patients. Parents of children with phenylketonuria should be informed that montelukast chewable tablets contain phenylalanine, a component of aspartame. Be aware montelukast is not intended to treat acute asthma attacks. Drink plenty of fluids to decrease the thickness of lung secretions. Avoid aspirin and NSAIDs while taking montelukast.

Pulse rate and quality, as well as respiratory depth, rate, rhythm, and type, should be monitored. Fingernails and lips should also be assessed for a blue or dusky color in light-skinned patients and a gray color in dark-skinned patients, which may be signs of hypoxemia.

Report any neuropsychiatric events, such as changes in mood, behavior, or sleep, promptly.

Storage

Store all products at room temperature. Granules and chewable tablets should be kept in original containers and protected from light and moisture.

Administration

Take montelukast tablets in the evening without regard to food. Do not abruptly substitute montelukast for inhaled or oral corticosteroids. Take montelukast as prescribed, even during symptom-free periods and exacerbations. Do not alter the dosage or abruptly discontinue other asthma medications.

Chewable tablets should be chewed thoroughly before swallowing. For oral granules, may administer directly in mouth; dissolved in 1 tsp (5 mL) of cold or room-temperature formula or breast milk or mixed with a spoonful of cold food such as applesauce, carrots, rice, or ice cream.

Morphine

mor'feen

Astramorph, Avinza, DepoDur, Duramorph, Infumorph, Kadian, MS Contin, Oramorph SR

Doloral, Kadian, M-Eslon, MS Contin, MS IR, Statex

Do not confuse morphine with hydromorphone.

CATEGORY AND SCHEDULE

Pregnancy Risk Category: C (D if used for prolonged periods or at high dosages at term)

Controlled Substance Schedule: II

Classification: Analgesics, opiate agonists

MECHANISM OF ACTION

An opioid agonist that binds with opioid receptors in the central nervous system (CNS). *Therapeutic Effect:* Alters the perception of and emotional response to pain; produces generalized CNS depression.

PHARMACOKINETICS

Route	Onset	Peak (h)	Duration (h)
Oral solution	NA	1	3-5
Tablets	NA	1	3-5
Tablets (ER)	NA	3-4	8-12
IV	Rapid	0.3	3-5
IM	5-30 min	0.5-1	3-5
Epidural	NA	1	12-20
Subcutaneous	NA	1.1-5	3-5
Rectal	NA	0.5-1	3-7

Variably absorbed from the GI tract. Readily absorbed after IM or SC administration. Protein binding: 20%-35%. Widely distributed. Metabolized in the liver. Primarily excreted in urine. Removed by hemodialysis. *Half-life:* 2-3 h (increased in patients with hepatic disease).

AVAILABILITY

ORAL PRODUCTS
Oral Solution: 10 mg/5 mL, 20 mg/5 mL.
Concentrated Oral Solution: 100 mg/5 mL.
Tablets, Immediate Release: 15 mg, 30 mg.
Capsules (Extended Release [Kadian]): 10 mg, 20 mg, 30 mg, 50 mg, 60 mg, 80 mg, 100 mg
Capules (Biphasic Extended Release [Avinza]): 30 mg, 45 mg, 60 mg, 75 mg, 90 mg, 120 mg.
Tablets (Extended Release) [MS Contin, Oramorph SR]): 15 mg, 30 mg, 60 mg, 100 mg, 200 mg.
RECTAL
Suppository: 5 mg, 10 mg, 20 mg, 30 mg.
INJECTABLE PRODUCTS
Solution for Injection: 0.5 mg/mL, 1 mg/mL, 2 mg/mL, 4 mg/mL, 5 mg/mL, 8 mg/mL, 10 mg/mL, 15 mg/mL, 25 mg/mL, 50 mg/mL.
Solution for Injection (Preservative Free): 0.5 mg/mL, 1 mg/mL, 10 mg/mL, 25 mg/mL, 50 mg/mL.
Epidural and Intrathecal via Infusion Device (Infumorph PF): 10 mg/mL, 25 mg/mL.
Epidural, Intrathecal, IV Infusion Device (Astramorph PF, Duramorph PF): 0.5 mg/mL, 1 mg/mL, 4 mg/mL.
IV Infusion (via Patient-Controlled Analgesia [PCA]): 1 mg/mL, 5 mg/mL.
Liposomal Extended-Release Suspension (DepoDur, Epidural use only): 10 mg/mL, 15 mg/1.5mL.

M

INDICATIONS AND DOSAGES

ALERT
! Dosage should be titrated to desired effect.
! Always double-check selected product and strength against medication order, appropriateness of route, and age and opiate tolerance of the patient.

▸ **Analgesia**
PO (PROMPT RELEASE)
Adults, Elderly. 10-30 mg q3-4h as needed.
Children. 0.15-0.3 mg/kg q3-4h as needed.
PO (EXTENDED RELEASE [AVINZA])
Adults, Elderly. Dosage requirement should be established using prompt-release formulations and is based on total daily dose (one-half the dose is given q12h or one-third the dose is given q8h).
PO (EXTENDED RELEASE [KADIAN])
Adults, Elderly. Dosage requirement should be established using prompt-release formulations and is based on total daily dose. Dose is given once a day or divided and given q12h.
PO (EXTENDED RELEASE [MS CONTIN, ORAMORPH SR]
Adults, Elderly. Dosage requirement should be established using prompt-release formulations and is based on total daily dose. The total daily dose requirement is divided and given q8h or q12h.
Children. 0.3-0.6 mg/kg/dose q12h.
IM
Adults, Elderly. 5-10 mg q3-4h as needed.
Children. 0.1 mg/kg q3-4 h as needed.
IV
Adults, Elderly. 2.5-10 mg q3-4h as needed. NOTE: Repeated doses (e.g., 1-2 mg) may be given more

frequently (e.g., every hour) if needed.
Children. 0.05-0.1 mg/kg q3-4h as needed.
IV CONTINUOUS INFUSION
Adults, Elderly. 0.8-10 mg/h. Range: Up to 80 mg/h.
EPIDURAL (BUT NOT DEPODUR)
Adults, Elderly. Initially, 1-6 mg bolus, infusion rate: 0.1-0.2 mg/h. Maximum: 10 mg/24 h.
INTRATHECAL (UNPRESERVED, E.G., DURAMORPH)
Adults, Elderly. One tenth of the epidural dose: 0.2-1 mg/dose.
EPIDURAL (DEPO-DUR ONLY)
Adults, Elderly, 15-mg single dose. Some patients may benefit from 20 mg, but increased side effect risk.Usually given 30 min before surgery.

▸ **Patient-controlled analgesia PCA**
IV
Adults, Elderly. Loading dose: 5-10 mg. Intermittent bolus: 0.5-3 mg. Lockout interval: 5-12 min. Continuous infusion: 1-10 mg/h. 4-h limit: 20-30 mg.

CONTRAINDICATIONS

Hypersensitivity, acute or severe asthma, GI obstruction, severe hepatic or renal impairment, severe respiratory depression, asthma, severe liver or renal impairment.

INTERACTIONS

Drug
Alcohol, other CNS depressants: May increase CNS or respiratory depression and hypotension.
! Alcohol may result in the rapid release and absorption of a potentially fatal dose of morphine from extended-release products.
Anticholinergics: May increase anticholinergic effects.
MAOIs: May produce a severe, sometimes fatal reaction; expect to administer one-quarter of usual morphine dose.
Herbal
None known.
Food
None known.

DIAGNOSTIC TEST EFFECTS

May increase serum amylase and lipase levels.

IV INCOMPATIBILITIES

Amphotericin B complex (Abelcet, AmBisome, Amphotec), cefepime (Maxipime), doxorubicin liposomal (Doxil), thiopental.

IV COMPATIBILITIES

Amiodarone (Cordarone), bumetanide (Bumex), bupivacaine (Marcaine, Sensorcaine), diltiazem (Cardizem), dobutamine (Dobutrex), dopamine (Intropin), heparin, lidocaine, lorazepam (Ativan), magnesium, midazolam (Versed), milrinone (Primacor), nitroglycerin, potassium, propofol (Diprivan).

SIDE EFFECTS

Frequent
Sedation, decreased BP (including orthostatic hypotension), diaphoresis, facial flushing, constipation, dizziness, somnolence, nausea, vomiting.
Occasional
Allergic reaction (rash, pruritus), dyspnea, confusion, palpitations, tremors, urine retention, abdominal cramps, vision changes, dry mouth, headache, decreased appetite, pain or burning at injection site.
Rare
Paralytic ileus.

SERIOUS REACTIONS

- Overdose results in respiratory depression, skeletal muscle flaccidity, cold or clammy skin, cyanosis, and extreme somnolence progressing to seizures, stupor, and coma.
- The patient who uses morphine repeatedly may develop a tolerance to the drug's analgesic effect and physical dependence.
- The drug may have a prolonged duration of action and cumulative effect in those with hepatic and renal impairment.

PRECAUTIONS & CONSIDERATIONS

Extreme caution should be used with chronic obstructive pulmonary disease (COPD), cor pulmonale, head injury, hypoxia, hypercapnia, increased intracranial pressure, preexisting respiratory depression, and severe hypotension. Caution is also warranted with Addison disease, alcoholism, biliary tract disease, CNS depression, hypothyroidism, pancreatitis, benign prostatic hyperplasia, seizure disorders, toxic psychosis, urethral stricture, and in elderly or debilitated patients. Morphine crosses the placenta and is distributed in breast milk; caution in pregnancy and lactation is warranted. Regular use of opioids during pregnancy may produce withdrawal symptoms in the neonate, such as diarrhea, excessive crying, fever, hyperactive reflexes, irritability, seizures, sneezing, tremors, vomiting, and yawning. Morphine may prolong labor if administered in the latent phase of the first stage of labor or before the cervix is dilated 4-5 cm. The neonate may develop respiratory depression if the mother receives morphine during labor. Children and elderly patients are more prone to experience paradoxical excitement. Children younger than 2 yr and elderly patients are more susceptible to the drug's respiratory depressant effects. Most extended-release products are not appropriate for children. Age-related renal impairment may increase the risk of urine retention in elderly patients.

Dizziness and drowsiness may occur, so change positions slowly and avoid alcohol, CNS depressants, and tasks that require mental alertness or motor skills until response to the drug is established. Pattern of daily bowel activity and clinical improvement should be monitored. Vital signs should be monitored for 5-10 min after IV administration and 15-30 min after IM or SC injection. Be alert for bradycardia and hypotension. The drug should be held and the physician should be notified if the respiratory rate is 12 breaths/min or less in an adult or 20 breaths/min or less in a child. When using scheduled or extended-release dosages, monitor breakthrough pain and need for additional medications.

Storage

Store oral dose forms at room temperature protected from light and moisture. Unopened DepoDur epidural suspension is refrigerated; stable for 30 days once removed from refrigerator. Other injections stored at room temperature. Do not freeze injections. Do not heat sterilize.

Administration

! Expect to reduce morphine dosage for debilitated and elderly patients and those using CNS depressants concurrently. Titrate dosage to desired effect, as prescribed. Morphine's side effects are dependent on the dosage and route of administration.

Ambulatory patients and those not in severe pain are more prone to experience dizziness, nausea, and vomiting than those in the supine position and those in severe pain.

For oral use, mix the liquid form with fruit juice to improve the taste. Do not crush, open, or break extended-release capsules. Kadian (extended-release capsules) contents may be sprinkled on applesauce just before administration or may be flushed down a gastrostomy tube; do not crush or chew during administration.

Morphine may be given undiluted as IV push. For IV injection, 2.5-15 mg morphine may be diluted in 4-5 mL sterile water for injection. For continuous IV infusion, dilute to a concentration of 0.1-1 mg/mL in D5W and administer through a controlled infusion device. Place the patient in the recumbent position before giving parenteral morphine. Always administer IV morphine very slowly because rapid IV administration increases the risk of a severe anaphylactic reaction, marked by apnea, cardiac arrest, and circulatory collapse.

For IM and SC administration, inject the drug slowly; rotate injection sites. Know that patients with circulatory impairment are at increased risk for overdose because of delayed absorption of repeated injections.

For rectal use, if the suppository is too soft, refrigerate it for 30 min or run cold water over the foil wrapper. Remove the foil wrapper; remove and moisten the suppository with cold water before inserting it well into the rectum.

Intrathecal: Only select injections are preservative free and suitable for intrathecal use. Pay close attention to dose limits.

Moxifloxacin Hydrochloride

moks-i-floks'a-sin high-droh-klor'ide

Avelox, Avelox IV, Vigamox

Do not confuse Avelox with Avonex or moxifloxacin with minoxidil.

CATEGORY AND SCHEDULE

Pregnancy Risk Category: C

Classification: Fluoroquinolone anti-infective, ophthalmics, systemic

MECHANISM OF ACTION

A fluoroquinolone that inhibits two enzymes, topoisomerase II and IV, in susceptible microorganisms. *Therapeutic Effect:* Interferes with bacterial DNA replication. Prevents or delays emergence of resistant organisms. Bactericidal.

PHARMACOKINETICS

Well absorbed from the GI tract after PO administration. Protein binding: 50%. Widely distributed throughout body with tissue concentration often exceeding plasma concentration. Metabolized in liver. Primarily excreted in urine with a lesser amount in feces. *Half-life:* 10.7-13.3 h.

AVAILABILITY

Tablets (Avelox): 400 mg.
Injection (Avelox IV): 400 mg.
Ophthalmic Solution (Vigamox): 0.5%.

INDICATIONS AND DOSAGES

▸ **Acute bacterial sinusitis, community-acquired pneumonia, complicated intra-abdominal infection**

IV/PO

Adults, Elderly. 400 mg q24h for 10 days (sinusitis); 7-14 days (pneumonia or intra-abdominal infusion).

▸ Acute bacterial exacerbation of chronic bronchitis.
IV/PO
Adults, Elderly. 400 mg q24h for 5 days.
▸ Skin and skin-structure infection
IV/PO
Adults, Elderly. 400 mg once a day for 7 days (uncomplicated), up to 21 days if complicated.
▸ Topical treatment of bacterial conjunctivitis caused by susceptible strains of bacteria
OPHTHALMIC
Adults, Elderly, Children older than 1 yr. 1 drop 3 times/day for 7 days.

CONTRAINDICATIONS

Hypersensitivity to quinolones.

M

INTERACTIONS

Drug
Antacids, didanosine chewable, buffered tablets or pediatric powder for oral solution, iron preparations, sucralfate, zinc preparations: May decrease moxifloxacin absorption.
Medications prolonging the QT interval (e.g., class 1a and class III antiarrhythmics, erythromycin, tricyclic antidepressants): Possible risk of QT interval elongation.
NSAIDs: Increased risk of central nervous system (CNS) stimulation and seizures.
Herbal and Food
None known.

DIAGNOSTIC TEST EFFECTS

May increase blood sugar. Rare reports of changes in CBC or LFTs.

IV INCOMPATIBILITIES

Do not add or infuse other drugs simultaneously through the same IV line. Flush line before and after use if same IV line is used with other medications.

SIDE EFFECTS

Frequent (6%-8%)
Nausea, diarrhea.
Occasional (2%-3%)
Dizziness, headache, abdominal pain, vomiting.
Ophthalmic (1%-6%): conjunctival irritation, reduced visual acuity, dry eye, keratitis, eye pain, ocular itching, swelling of tissue around cornea, eye discharge, fever, cough, pharyngitis, rash, rhinitis.
Rare (1%)
Change in sense of taste, dyspepsia (heartburn, indigestion), photosensitivity.

SERIOUS REACTIONS

- Pseudomembranous colitis as evidenced by fever, severe abdominal cramps or pain, and severe watery diarrhea may occur.
- Superinfection manifested as anal or genital pruritus, moderate to severe diarrhea, and stomatitis may occur.
- Tendonopathy and tendon rupture.
- QT prolongation.
- Seizures (rare).
- Serious hypersensitivity reaction.

PRECAUTIONS & CONSIDERATIONS

Caution is warranted in patients with cerebral arthrosclerosis, CNS disorders, liver or renal impairment, diabetes mellitus, seizures, those with a prolonged QT interval, uncorrected hypokalemia, and those receiving medications that might prolong the QT interval. Be aware that moxifloxacin may be distributed in breast milk and is generally not recommended for use in pregnancy. Be aware that the safety and efficacy of moxifloxacin have not been established in children. No age-related precautions have been noted in elderly patients.

Avoid exposure to sunlight and ultraviolet light, and wear sunscreen and protective clothing if photosensitivity develops.

Abdominal pain, altered sense of taste, dyspepsia (heartburn, indigestion), headache, vomiting, and signs and symptoms of infections should be assessed. Pattern of daily bowel activity, stool consistency, and WBC count should be monitored. History of hypersensitivity to moxifloxacin and other quinolones should be determined before therapy.

Storage
Store at room temperature. Do not refrigerate. Remove overwrap of premix IV infusion just prior to administration.

Administration
Take oral moxifloxacin without regard to meals. Take 4 h before or 8 h after antacids, didanosine chewable, buffered tablets or pediatric powder for oral solution, iron preparations, multivitamins with minerals, or sucralfate. Take full course of therapy.

For ophthalmic use, tilt the head back, and look up. With a gloved finger, gently pull the lower eyelid down until a pocket is formed. Place drops into the center of the pocket. Close the eye gently, and apply gentle finger pressure to the lacrimal sac at the inner canthus. Remove excess solution around the eye with a tissue.

! Infuse IV over 60 min or longer. IV formulation is available in ready-to-use containers. Give by IV infusion only. Avoid rapid or bolus IV infusion.

Mupirocin

mew-peer'oh-sin

★Bactroban, Centany 🍁 Bactroban

Do not confuse Bactroban with Bactrim or Bacitracin

CATEGORY AND SCHEDULE

Pregnancy Risk Category: B

Classification: Topical anti-infective

MECHANISM OF ACTION

An antibacterial agent that inhibits bacterial protein, RNA synthesis. Less effective on DNA synthesis. Effective against most gram-positive aerobic bacteria, including MRSA. *Therapeutic Effect:* Prevents bacterial growth and replication. Bacteriostatic. Nasal: Eradicates nasal colonization of MRSA.

PHARMACOKINETICS

Metabolized in skin to inactive metabolite. Transported to skin surface; removed by normal skin desquamation.

AVAILABILITY

Ointment: 2% (Bactroban, Centany).
Nasal Ointment: 2% (Bactroban).
Cream: 2% (Bactroban).

INDICATIONS AND DOSAGES

▸ **Impetigo, infected traumatic skin lesions**

TOPICAL

Adults, Elderly, Children. Apply 3 times/day (may cover w/gauze).

▸ **Nasal colonization of resistant *Staphylococcus aureus***

INTRANASAL

Adults, Elderly, Children 12 yr and older. Apply 2 times/day for 5 days.

OFF-LABEL USES

Treatment of infected eczema, folliculitis, minor bacterial skin infections.

CONTRAINDICATIONS

Hypersensitivity to mupirocin or any component of the formulation.

INTERACTIONS

Drug
None known.
Herbal
None known.
Food
None known.

DIAGNOSTIC TEST EFFECTS

None known.

M

SIDE EFFECTS

Frequent
Nasal: Headache, rhinitis, upper respiratory congestion, pharyngitis, altered taste.
Occasional
Nasal: Burning, stinging, cough.
Topical: Pain, burning, stinging, itching.
Rare
Nasal: Pruritis, diarrhea, dry mouth, epistaxis, nausea, rash.
Topical: Rash, nausea, dry skin, contact dermatitis.

SERIOUS REACTIONS

• Superinfection may result in bacterial or fungal infections, especially with prolonged or repeated therapy.

PRECAUTIONS & CONSIDERATIONS

Caution should be used in patients with impaired renal function. It is unknown whether mupirocin crosses the placenta or is distributed in breast milk. Use with caution. Safety and efficacy of nasal preparation have not been established in children younger than 12 yr. No age-related precautions have been noted in children or elderly patients. Isolation precautions will be in effect for those with highly communicable conditions or resistant organisms.
Storage
Store at room temperature.
Administration
Gown and gloves are to be worn until 24 h after therapy is effective. Disease is spread by direct contact with moist discharges. Apply small amount to affected areas. Cover affected areas with gauze dressing if desired.

Apply nasally inside the nose. After application, close the nostrils by pressing together and releasing the sides of the nose repetitively for approximately 1 min. This will spread the ointment throughout the nares. Discard single-use tubes immediately after use.

Mycophenolate

my-co-fen′o-late
★ 🍁 CellCept, Myfortic

CATEGORY AND SCHEDULE

Pregnancy Risk Category: D

Classification:
Immunosuppressives

MECHANISM OF ACTION

An immunologic agent that suppresses the immunologically mediated inflammatory response by inhibiting inosine monophosphate dehydrogenase, an enzyme that deprives lymphocytes of nucleotides necessary for DNA and RNA synthesis, thus inhibiting the proliferation of T and B lymphocytes. *Therapeutic Effect:* Prevents transplant rejection.

PHARMACOKINETICS

Rapidly and extensively absorbed after PO administration (food decreases drug plasma concentration but does not affect absorption). Protein binding: 97%. Completely hydrolyzed to active metabolite mycophenolic acid. Primarily excreted in urine. Not removed by hemodialysis. *Half-life:* 17.9 h.

AVAILABILITY

Mycophenolate Mofetil (CellCept)
Capsules: 250 mg.
Oral Suspension: 200 mg/mL.
Tablets: 500 mg.
Injection: 500 mg.
Mycophenolate Sodium (Myfortic)
Tablets, Extended Release: 180 mg, 360 mg.

INDICATIONS AND DOSAGES

MYCOPHENOLATE MOFETIL (CellCept)

▸ **Prevention of renal transplant rejection**
PO, IV
Adults, Elderly. 1 g twice a day.

▸ **Prevention of heart transplant rejection**
PO, IV
Adults, Elderly. 1.5 g twice a day.

▸ **Prevention of liver transplant rejection**
PO
Adults, Elderly. 1.5 g twice a day.
IV
Adults, Elderly. 1 g twice a day.

▸ **Usual pediatric dosage**
PO
Children. 600 mg/m^2/dose twice a day. Maximum: 1 g/dose.

MYCOPHENOLATE SODIUM (Myfortic)

▸ **Prevention of renal transplant rejection**
PO
Adults, Elderly. 720 mg twice a day in combination with corticosteroids and cyclosporine.

▸ **Usual pediatric dosage**
PO
Children. 400 mg/m^2/dose twice a day. Maximum: 720 mg/dose.

OFF-LABEL USES

Treatment of transplantation rejection, graft-versus-host disease, uveitis, myasthenia gravis.

CONTRAINDICATIONS

Hypersensitivity to mycophenolic acid.

INTERACTIONS

Drug

Acyclovir, ganciclovir: May increase plasma concentrations of both drugs in patients with renal impairment.
Antacids (aluminum and magnesium-containing), cholestyramine: May decrease the absorption of mycophenolate.
Hormonal contraceptives: Mycophenolate can reduce effectiveness; use 2 adequate forms of contraception.
Live-virus vaccines: May potentiate virus replication, increase vaccine side effects, and decrease the patient's antibody response to the vaccine.
Other immunosuppressants: May increase the risk of infection or lymphomas. Azathioprine use not recommended due to bone marrow suppression.
Probenecid: May increase mycophenolate plasma concentration.
Norfloxacin, metronidazole, rifampin: Lower mycophenolate concentrations. Avoid co-use.

Herbal
Echinacea: May decrease the effects of mycophenolate.
Food
All foods: May decrease mycophenolate plasma concentration.

DIAGNOSTIC TEST EFFECTS

Lowered WBC, red cell counts. May increase serum cholesterol, alkaline phosphatase, creatinine, AST (SGOT), and ALT (SGPT) levels. May increase or decrease blood glucose as well as serum lipid, calcium, potassium, phosphate, and uric acid levels.

IV INCOMPATIBILITIES

Mycophenolate is compatible only with D5W. Do not infuse it concurrently with other drugs or IV solutions.

SIDE EFFECTS

Frequent (20%-37%)
Urinary tract infection, hypertension, peripheral edema, diarrhea, constipation, fever, headache, nausea.
Occasional (10%-18%)
Dyspepsia; dyspnea; cough; hematuria; asthenia; vomiting; edema; tremors; abdominal, chest, or back pain; oral candidiasis; acne.
Rare (6%-9%)
Insomnia, respiratory tract infection, rash, dizziness. Phlebitis with intravenous use.

SERIOUS REACTIONS

- Significant anemia, leukopenia, thrombocytopenia, neutropenia, and leukocytosis may occur, particularly in those undergoing renal transplant rejection.
- Sepsis and infection occur occasionally.
- GI tract hemorrhage occurs rarely.
- Patients receiving mycophenolate have an increased risk of developing neoplasms.

PRECAUTIONS & CONSIDERATIONS

Caution is warranted with active serious digestive disease, neutropenia, and renal impairment. Women who might become pregnant should use effective contraception before, during, and for 6 wks after discontinuing mycophenolate therapy, even if there is a history of infertility. Two forms of contraception should be used concurrently (e.g., hormonal and nonhormonal) unless patient will remain abstinent. Pregnancy test should be attained 1 wk before starting treatment. It is unknown whether mycophenolate crosses the placenta or is distributed in breast milk. Women taking this drug should avoid breastfeeding. The safety and efficacy of mycophenolate have not been established in children. Age-related renal impairment may require a dosage adjustment in elderly patients.

Notify the physician of abdominal pain, fever, sore throat, or unusual bleeding or bruising. CBC should be obtained weekly during the first month of therapy, twice monthly during the second and third month, then monthly for the rest of the first year. The dosage should be reduced or discontinued if a rapid fall in WBC count occurs.

Storage
Store tablets at room temperature in tightly closed container. Store the reconstituted suspension in the refrigerator or at room temperature. It remains stable for 60 days after reconstitution. Store vials at room temperature. Do not freeze.

Administration
Give oral mycophenolate mofetil on an empty stomach. Do not open

or crush capsules. Avoid inhaling the powder in capsules, and keep the powder away from the skin and mucous membranes. If contact occurs, wash thoroughly with soap and water, and rinse the eyes profusely with plain water.

The suspension can be administered orally or by nasogastric tube (minimum size: 8 French). Shake well before each use.

Mycophenolate sodium delayed-release tablets and mycophenolate mofetil are not interchangeable because the rate of absorption is not equivalent. Take on an empty stomach 1 h before or 2 h after food. Do not crush, chew, or cut. Swallow whole to maintain the integrity of the enteric coating.

For IV use, reconstitute each 500-mg vial with 14 mL D5W. Gently agitate the vial. For a 1-g dose, further dilute with 140 mL D5W; for a 1.5-g dose, further dilute with 210 mL D5W to provide a concentration of 6 mg/mL. Infuse the drug over at least 2 h.

Nabumetone

na-byu′me-tone

CATEGORY AND SCHEDULE

Pregnancy Risk Category: C (D if used in third trimester or near delivery)

Classification: Analgesics, nonsteroidal anti-inflammatory drugs (NSAIDs)

MECHANISM OF ACTION

An NSAID that produces analgesic and anti-inflammatory effects by inhibiting prostaglandin synthesis. *Therapeutic Effect:* Reduces the inflammatory response and intensity of pain.

PHARMACOKINETICS

Readily absorbed from the GI tract. Protein binding: 99%. Widely distributed. Metabolized in the liver to active metabolite. Excreted primarily in urine. Not removed by hemodialysis. *Half-life:* 22-30 h.

AVAILABILITY

Tablets: 500 mg, 750 mg.

INDICATIONS AND DOSAGES

▸ **Acute or chronic rheumatoid and osteoarthritis**

PO

Adults, Elderly. Initially, 1000 mg as a single dose or in 2 divided doses. May increase up to 2000 mg/day as a single or in 2 divided doses. If patient < 50 kg, usual maximum is 1000 mg/day.

▸ **Dosage in renal impairment**

CrCl ≥ 50 mL/min: No adjustment.
CrCl 30-49 mL/min: Initially 750 mg/day; maximum 1500 mg/day
CrCl 10-30 mL/min: Initially 500 mg/day; maximum 1000 mg/day

CONTRAINDICATIONS

History of hypersensitivity to aspirin or NSAIDs; use within 14 days of coronary artery bypass graft surgery.

INTERACTIONS

Drug

Antihypertensives, diuretics: May decrease the effects of these drugs.
Aspirin, other salicylates, corticosteroids: May increase the risk of GI side effects such as bleeding. NSAIDs may negate the cardioprotective effect of ASA.
Bone marrow depressants: May increase the risk of hematologic reactions.
Cyclosporine: May decrease renal function.
Heparin, oral anticoagulants, thrombolytics: May increase the effects of these drugs.
Lithium: May increase the blood concentration and risk of toxicity of lithium.
Methotrexate: May increase the risk of methotrexate toxicity.
Probenecid: May increase the nabumetone blood concentration.

Herbal

Feverfew: May decrease the effects of feverfew.
Ginkgo biloba: May increase the risk of bleeding.

Food

Alcohol: May increase dizziness or increase risk of GI bleeding.

DIAGNOSTIC TEST EFFECTS

May increase BUN level; urine protein levels; and serum LDH, alkaline phosphatase, creatinine, potassium, AST (SGOT), and ALT (SGPT) levels. May decrease serum uric acid level.

SIDE EFFECTS

Frequent (12%-14%)

Diarrhea, abdominal cramps or pain, dyspepsia.

Occasional (4%-9%)
Nausea, constipation, flatulence, dizziness, headache.
Rare (1%-3%)
Vomiting, stomatitis, confusion.

SERIOUS REACTIONS

- Overdose may result in acute hypotension and tachycardia.
- Rare reactions with long-term use include peptic ulcer disease, GI bleeding, gastritis, nephrotoxicity (dysuria, cystitis, hematuria, proteinuria, nephrotic syndrome), severe hepatic reactions (cholestasis, jaundice), and severe hypersensitivity reactions (bronchospasm, angioedema).

PRECAUTIONS & CONSIDERATIONS

Caution is warranted in patients with hepatic or renal impairment, peptic ulcer disease, and in those using anticoagulants. Nabumetone is distributed in low concentrations in breast milk; caution is warranted in lactation. Nabumetone should not be used during the last trimester of pregnancy because it can cause adverse effects in the fetus, such as premature closing of the ductus arteriosus. The safety and efficacy of this drug have not been established in children. In elderly patients, GI bleeding or ulceration is more likely to cause serious complications, and age-related renal impairment may require a reduced drug dosage.

Cardiovascular event risk may be increased with duration of use or preexisting cardiovascular risk factors. Use caution in patients with fluid retention, heart failure, or hypertension. Use lowest effective dose. Risk of myocardial infarction and stroke may be increased following CABG surgery. Do not administer within 4-6 half-lives before surgical procedures. Because the drug may cause dizziness, do not perform tasks requiring mental concentration until the effects of the drug are known.

Blood chemistry studies, renal and liver function studies, and pattern of daily bowel activity and stool consistency should be assessed before and during therapy. Therapeutic response, such as decreased pain, stiffness, swelling, and increased joint mobility, should be evaluated.
Storage
Store at room temperature.
Administration
Swallow tablets whole. Take nabumetone with food, milk, or antacids if GI distress occurs.

N

Nadolol

nay-doe'lole
Corgard Apo-Nadol
Do not confuse Corgard with Coreg.

CATEGORY AND SCHEDULE

Pregnancy Risk Category: C (D if used in second or third trimester)

Classification: Antihypertensives, antianginal agents, β-adrenergic blockers, nonselective

MECHANISM OF ACTION

A nonselective β-blocker that blocks β_1- and β_2-adrenergic receptors. Large doses increase airway resistance. *Therapeutic Effect:* Slows sinus heart rate, decreases cardiac output and BP. Decreases myocardial ischemia severity by decreasing oxygen requirements.

PHARMACOKINETICS

PO: Onset variable, peak 3-4 h, duration 17-24 h. Not metabolized; excreted unchanged in urine, bile, and breast milk. *Half-life:* 16-24 h.

AVAILABILITY

Tablets: 20 mg, 40 mg, 80 mg.

INDICATIONS AND DOSAGES

▸ **Mild to moderate hypertension or angina**

PO

Adults, Elderly. Initially, 40 mg/day. May increase by 40-80 mg at intervals of 3-7 days. Maximum: 240 mg/day for angina, 320 mg/day for hypertension.

▸ **Dosage in renal impairment**

Dosage is modified based on creatinine clearance.

N

Creatinine Clearance (mL/min)	Dosage Interval
31-50	24-36 h
10-30	24-48 h
< 10	40-60 h

OFF-LABEL USES

Treatment of atrial fibrillation hypertrophic cardiomyopathy, pheochromocytoma, essential tremor, thyrotoxicosis, vascular headache prophylaxis.

CONTRAINDICATIONS

Bronchial asthma, cardiogenic shock, second- or third-degree heart block, sinus bradycardia, overt cardiac failure.

INTERACTIONS

Drug

Cimetidine: May increase nadolol blood concentration.

Diuretics, other antihypertensives: May increase hypotensive effect.

Fentanyl, hydrocarbon inhalation anesthetics: May increase hypotension, myocardial depression.

Indomethacin, other NSAIDs: May decrease hypotensive effects.

Insulin, oral hypoglycemics: May mask symptoms of hypoglycemia and prolong the hypoglycemic effect of insulin and oral hypoglycemics.

Lidocaine: Slows metabolism of nadolol.

NSAIDs: May decrease antihypertensive effect.

Sympathomimetics (epinephrine, norepinephrine, isoproterenol), xanthines: May mutually inhibit effects.

Herbal

None known.

Food

None known.

DIAGNOSTIC TEST EFFECTS

May increase serum antinuclear antibody titer and BUN, serum LDH, serum lipoprotein, serum alkaline phosphatase, serum bilirubin, serum creatinine, serum potassium, serum uric acid, AST (SGOT), ALT (SGPT), and serum triglyceride levels.

SIDE EFFECTS

Nadolol is generally well tolerated, with transient and mild side effects.

Frequent

Diminished sexual ability, drowsiness, unusual fatigue or weakness.

Occasional

Bradycardia, difficulty breathing, depression, cold hands or feet, diarrhea, constipation, anxiety, nasal congestion, nausea, vomiting.

Rare

Altered taste, dry eyes, itching.

SERIOUS REACTIONS

- Overdose may produce profound bradycardia and hypotension.

• Abrupt withdrawal of nadolol may result in diaphoresis, palpitations, headache, tremulousness, exacerbation of angina, MI, and ventricular arrhythmias.
• May precipitate CHF and MI in patients with cardiac disease; thyroid storm in those with thyrotoxicosis; and peripheral ischemia in those with existing peripheral vascular disease.
• Hypoglycemia may occur in patients with previously controlled diabetes.
• Bronchospasm, allergic reactions, or decreased blood counts occur rarely.

PRECAUTIONS & CONSIDERATIONS

Caution is warranted in patients with diabetes mellitus, hyperthyroidism, chronic bronchitis or asthma, impaired hepatic and renal function, and inadequate cardiac function. Nasal decongestants or OTC cold preparations (stimulants) should not be used without physician approval. Tasks that require mental alertness or motor skills should be avoided until drug effects are known. Use caution with postural changes.

Notify the physician of confusion, depression, difficulty breathing, dizziness, fever, rash, slow pulse, sore throat, swelling of arms and legs, or unusual bleeding or bruising. BP for hypotension; respiratory status; pattern of daily bowel activity and stool consistency; and pulse for quality, rate, and rhythm should be monitored. If pulse rate is < 55 beats/min or systolic BP ≤ 90 mm Hg, withhold the medication and contact the physician. In those receiving nadolol for treatment of angina, the onset, type (sharp, dull, squeezing), radiation, location, intensity, and duration of anginal pain and its precipitating factors, including exertion and emotional stress, should be recorded. Signs and symptoms of CHF, such as decreased urine output, distended neck veins, dyspnea (particularly on exertion or lying down), night cough, peripheral edema, and weight gain should also be assessed.

Storage

Store at room temperature.

Administration

Take nadolol without regard to meals. Tablets may be crushed.

Nafcillin Sodium

naph-sil′in

CATEGORY AND SCHEDULE

Pregnancy Risk Category: B

Classification: Antibiotics, antistaphylococcal penicillins, penicillinase-resistant penicillins

MECHANISM OF ACTION

A penicillin that acts as a bactericidal in susceptible penicillinase-producing staphlococcal microorganisms. *Therapeutic Effect:* Inhibits bacterial cell wall synthesis. Bactericidal.

PHARMACOKINETICS

Protein binding: 87%-90%. Widely distributed in bile, pleural, amniotic, synovial fluids. Metabolized in liver. Excreted 30% unchanged primarily in urine. High cerebrospinal fluid penetration with inflamed meninges. Equally cleared by liver and kidney; hemodialysis does not increase rate of clearance. *Half-life:* 0.5-1 h (half-life increased in neonates).

AVAILABILITY

Powder for Injection: 1 g, 2 g (as base).
Premixed IVPB Infusion: 1 g/50 mL, 2 g/100 mL.

INDICATIONS AND DOSAGES

▸ **Methicillin-sensitive staphylococcal infections (bacteremia, endocarditis, meningitis, skin and tissue, pneumonia, bone and joint infections)**

IV

Adults, Elderly. 500 mg q4h or 1-2 g q4h (severe infection), infused over 30-60 min. May give IM if needed.

OFF-LABEL USES

Surgical prophylaxis.

CONTRAINDICATIONS

Hypersensitivity (anaphylactic) to any penicillin or to any component of the formulations.

INTERACTIONS

Drug

Cyclosporine: potential for subtherapeutic cyclosporine levels. In organ transplant patients, monitor cyclosporine levels.

Probenecid: May increase nafcillin blood concentration and risk for nafcillin toxicity.

Warfarin: Nafcillin in high dosages may decrease the effects of warfarin. Monitor INR

Herbal

None known.

Food

None known.

DIAGNOSTIC TEST EFFECTS

May cause positive Coombs' test. May cause false-positive test for urine protein when sulfosalicylic acid test is used.

IV INCOMPATIBILITIES

Caspofungin (Cancidas), diltiazem, droperidol (Inapsine), fentanyl, hydralazine, inamrinone, insulin, labetalol, meperidine, midazolam (Versed), nalbuphine (Nubain), nesiritide, phenytoin, protamine sulfate, succinylcholine, vancomycin, vecuronium, verapamil.

SIDE EFFECTS

Frequent

Mild hypersensitivity reaction (fever, rash, pruritus); GI effects (nausea, vomiting, diarrhea).

Occasional

Phlebitis, thrombophlebitis (more common in elderly).

Rare

Extravasation with IV administration. Increased serum sodium with high IV doses.

SERIOUS REACTIONS

- Superinfections, antibiotic-associated colitis may result from altered bacterial balance.
- Hematologic effects (especially involving platelets, WBCs), severe hypersensitivity reactions, and anaphylaxis occur rarely.
- Thrombophlebitis.
- Neurotoxic reactions (rare).
- Interstitial nephritis (rare).

PRECAUTIONS & CONSIDERATIONS

Caution should be used in patients with antibiotic-associated colitis or a history of allergies, especially to cephalosporins or other beta-lactams. Nafcillin crosses the placenta and is distributed in breast milk in low concentrations, warranting caution in lactation. Not approved for IV use in neonates or children. Delayed excretion may occur in neonates or infants.

Report itching, rash, hives, difficulty breathing, diarrhea, loose foul-smelling stools, and injection site reactions for medical assessment immediately.

Storage

Reconstituted parenteral solution is stable for 3 days at room temperature and 7 days when refrigerated or 12 wks when frozen. Premixed IVPB are delivered frozen. The thawed premixed IVPB is stable for 21 days under refrigeration or 72 h at room temperature. Do not refreeze.

Administration

Be certain to space doses evenly around the clock.

Stop infusion if patient complains of pain. Because of potential for hypersensitivity or anaphylaxis, start the initial dose at a few drops per minute and increase slowly to the ordered rate; stay with the patient for the first 10-15 min, then check every 10 min. Doses are diluted in 50-100 mL of either 0.9% NaCl or dextrose 5% injection. Infuse over 30-60 min.

For IM use, reconstitute with sterile water for injection (unpreserved for neonates), 0.9% NaCl. Add 3.4 mL to the 1-g vial or 6.6 mL to the 2-g vial. Final concentration is 250 mg\mL. After withdrawing required dose, administer by deep intragluteal injection immediately after reconstitution.

Naftifine

naf'ti-feen

★ 🍁 Naftin

Do not confuse naftifine with nafcillin or nafarelin.

CATEGORY AND SCHEDULE

Pregnancy Risk Category: B

Classification: Antifungals, topical, dermatologics

MECHANISM OF ACTION

An antifungal that selectively inhibits the enzyme squalene epoxidase in a dose-dependent manner, which results in the primary sterol, ergosterol, within the fungal membrane not being synthesized. *Therapeutic Effect:* Results in fungal cell death. Fungistatic and fungicidal.

PHARMACOKINETICS

Minimal systemic absorption. Metabolized in the liver. Excreted in the urine as well as the feces and bile. *Half-life:* 48-72 h.

AVAILABILITY

Gel: 1% (Naftin).
Cream: 1% (Naftin).

INDICATIONS AND DOSAGES

▸ **Tinea pedis, tinea cruris, tinea corporis**

TOPICAL

Adults, Elderly, Children 12 yr and older. Apply cream 1 time a day for 4 wks or until signs and symptoms significantly improve. Apply gel 2 times a day for 4 wks or until signs and symptoms significantly improve.

OFF-LABEL USES

Trichomycosis.

CONTRAINDICATIONS

Hypersensitivity to naftifine or any of its components.

INTERACTIONS

Drug

None known.

Herbal

None known.

Food

None known.

DIAGNOSTIC TEST EFFECTS

None known.

SIDE EFFECTS

Frequent

Burning, stinging.

Occasional

Erythema, itching, dryness, irritation.

SERIOUS REACTIONS

• Excessive irritation may indicate hypersensitivity reaction.

PRECAUTIONS & CONSIDERATIONS

Occlusive dressings should be avoided. It is unknown whether naftifine is distributed in breast milk, warranting caution in lactation. Safety and efficacy of naftifine have not been established in children. Use in pregnancy only after determination that benefits outweigh possible risks. No age-related precautions have been noted in elderly patients.

Storage

Store at room temperature. Gel contains a large percentage of alcohol and may be flammable. Avoid heat and flame.

Administration

Naftifine is for external use only. Topical therapy should not exceed 4 wks without clinical reevaluation. Avoid getting the topical form in contact with the eyes, mouth, nose, or other mucous membranes. Wash hands after application.

N

Nalbuphine Hydrochloride

nal′byoo-feen high-droh-klor′ide

Nubain

Do not confuse Nubain with Navane.

CATEGORY AND SCHEDULE

Pregnancy Risk Category: B (D if used for prolonged periods or at high dosages at term)

Classification: Analgesic, mixed opiate agonist-antagonist

MECHANISM OF ACTION

A narcotic agonist-antagonist that binds with opioid receptors in the central nervous system (CNS). Analgesic potency equivalent to that of morphine on a milligram basis; primarily a κ agonist/partial μ antagonist. May displace opioid agonists and competitively inhibit their action; may precipitate withdrawal symptoms. *Therapeutic Effect:* Alters the perception of and emotional response to pain.

PHARMACOKINETICS

Route	Onset (min)	Peak (min)	Duration (h)
IV	2-3	30	3-6
IM	< 15	60	3-6
SC	< 15	NA	3-6

Well absorbed after IM or SC administration. Protein binding: 50%. Metabolized in the liver. Eliminated primarily in feces by biliary secretion. Crosses the placenta. *Half-life:* 3.5-5 h.

AVAILABILITY

Injection: 10 mg/mL, 20 mg/mL.

INDICATIONS AND DOSAGES

▸ **Analgesia (moderate to severe pain, obstetric)**

IV, IM, SC

Adults, Elderly. 10 mg q3-6h as needed. Do not exceed maximum single dose of 20 mg or daily dose of 160 mg. For patients receiving long-term narcotic analgesics of similar duration of action, give 25% of usual dose.

Children. 0.1 mg/kg q3-6h as needed.

▸ **Supplement to anesthesia**

IV

Adults, Elderly. Induction: 0.3-3 mg/kg over 10-15 min. Maintenance: 0.25-0.5 mg/kg as needed.

CONTRAINDICATIONS

Hypersensitivity to nalbuphine.

INTERACTIONS

Drug

Alcohol, other CNS depressants, barbiturates: May increase CNS or respiratory depression and hypotension.

Buprenorphine: May decrease the effects of nalbuphine.

MAOIs: May produce a severe, reaction; plan to administer 25% of the usual nalbuphine dose.

Herbal

None known.

Food

None known.

DIAGNOSTIC TEST EFFECTS

May increase serum amylase and lipase levels.

May interfere with enzymatic methods to detect opioids.

IV INCOMPATIBILITIES

Physically incompatible with nafcillin and keterolac (Toradol). Also incompatible with amphotericin B complex (Abelcet, AmBisome, Amphotec), anidulafungin (Eraxis), cefepime (Maxipime), diazepam, furosemide (Lasix), hydrocortisone (Solu-Cortef), imipenem/cilastatin (Primaxin), indomethacin, methotrexate, methylprednisolone (Solu-Medrol), oxacillin, pantoprazole (Protonix), pentobarbital, phenobarbital, piperacillin and tazobactam (Zosyn), sargramostim (Leukine), sodium bicarbonate, TPN.

IV COMPATIBILITIES

Diphenhydramine (Benadryl), droperidol (Inapsine), glycopyrrolate (Robinul), hydroxyzine (Vistaril), lidocaine, midazolam (Versed), propofol (Diprivan).

SIDE EFFECTS

Frequent (35%)

Sedation.

Occasional (3%-9%)

Diaphoresis, cold and clammy skin, nausea, vomiting, dizziness, vertigo, dry mouth, headache.

Rare (< 1%)

Restlessness, emotional lability, paresthesia, flushing, paradoxical reaction.

SERIOUS REACTIONS

- Abrupt withdrawal after prolonged use may produce symptoms of narcotic withdrawal, such as abdominal cramping, rhinorrhea, lacrimation, anxiety, fever, and piloerection (goose bumps).
- Overdose results in severe respiratory depression, skeletal muscle flaccidity, cyanosis, and extreme somnolence progressing to seizures, stupor, and coma.
- Repeated use may result in drug tolerance and physical dependence.

PRECAUTIONS & CONSIDERATIONS

Caution is warranted in pregnancy and in patients who are opioid dependent or have head trauma, increased intracranial pressure, hepatic or renal impairment, recent MI, respiratory depression, and those about to undergo biliary tract surgery. Nalbuphine readily crosses the placenta and is distributed in breast milk, but the amount is low; use caution. Children may experience paradoxical excitement; not approved for children < 18 yr. Children younger than 2 yr and elderly patients are more likely to develop respiratory depression. In elderly patients, age-related renal impairment may increase the risk of urine retention. Overdose is

N

evidenced by respiratory depression, hypoxemia, sedation.

Low abuse potential but withdrawal symptoms on discontinuation after long-term use; can be abused by patients with narcotic abuse potential. Ensure naloxone, oxygen, resuscitation, and intubation equipment are available if needed.

Dizziness and drowsiness may occur, so change positions slowly and avoid alcohol, CNS depressants, and tasks that require mental alertness or motor skills until response to the drug is established. BP, pulse rate and quality, respirations, pattern of daily bowel activity and stool consistency, and clinical improvement of pain should be monitored.

Storage

Store at room temperature. Do not administer if particulate matter is present or solution is discolored.

Administration

For IV use, nalbuphine may be given undiluted. For IV push, administer each 10 mg over 3-5 min.

For IM use, rotate IM injection sites, inject into a large muscle mass.

Naloxone Hydrochloride

nal-oks′one high-droh-klor′ide

★ Narcan

Do not confuse naloxone with naltrexone, or Narcan with Norcuron.

CATEGORY AND SCHEDULE

Pregnancy Risk Category: B

Classification: Antidotes, narcotic antagonist

MECHANISM OF ACTION

A narcotic antagonist that displaces opioids at opioid-occupied receptor sites in the central nervous system (CNS). *Therapeutic Effect:* Reverses opioid-induced sleep or sedation, increases respiratory rate, raises BP to normal range.

PHARMACOKINETICS

Route	Onset (min)	Peak	Duration (min)
IV	1-2	NA	20-60
IM	2-5	NA	*
SC	2-5	NA	20-60

*IM produces a more prolonged duration than IV.

Well absorbed after IM or SC administration. Metabolized in the liver. Excreted primarily in urine. *Half-life:* 60-100 min.

AVAILABILITY

Injection: 0.4 mg/mL, 1 mg/mL.

INDICATIONS AND DOSAGES

▸ **Opioid toxicity**

IV, IM, SC

Adults, Elderly. 0.4-2 mg q2-3min as needed. May repeat q20-60min. If no response after a cumulative dose of 10 mg; question diagnosis of opioid toxicity.

▸ **Opioid toxicity in children**

! Initially, American Academy of Pediatrics recommends 0.1 mg/kg for infants and children < 5 yr and weighing < 20 kg and if the child is ≥ 5 yr, giving an initial dose of 2 mg.

Children 5 yr and older and weighing ≥ 22 kg. 2 mg/dose; if no response, may repeat q2-3 min. May need to repeat q20-60 min.

Children and Infants younger than 5 yr and weighing < 22 kg. 0.1 mg/kg; if no response, repeat q 2-3 min. May need to repeat q20-60 min.

▸ **Postanesthesia narcotic reversal**
IV
Adults. 0.1-0.2 mg; may repeat q2-3 min.
Children. 0.01 mg/kg; may repeat q2-3 min.

CONTRAINDICATIONS
Hypersensitivity to naloxone.

INTERACTIONS
Drug
Butorphanol, nalbuphine, opioid agonist analgesics, pentazocine: Reverses the analgesic and adverse effects of these drugs and may precipitate withdrawal symptoms.
Herbal
None known.
Food
None known.

DIAGNOSTIC TEST EFFECTS
None known.

IV INCOMPATIBILITIES
Amphotericin B complex (Abelcet, AmBisome, Amphotec), diazepam, lansoprazole (Prevacid), pantoprazole (Protonix), phenytoin.

IV COMPATIBILITIES
Heparin, ondansetron (Zofran), propofol (Diprivan).

SIDE EFFECTS
None known; little or no pharmacologic effect in absence of narcotics.

SERIOUS REACTIONS
- Too-rapid reversal of narcotic-induced respiratory depression may result in nausea, vomiting, tremors, increased BP, and tachycardia.
- Excessive dosage in postoperative patients may produce significant excitement, tremors, and reversal of analgesia.
- Patients with cardiovascular disease may experience hypotension or hypertension, ventricular tachycardia and fibrillation, and pulmonary edema.

PRECAUTIONS & CONSIDERATIONS
! Drug is intended for acute use only. Risk of seizures; be aware of this possibility. Buprenorphine-mediated depression may not be completely reversed.

Caution is warranted in patients with chronic cardiovascular or pulmonary disease, postoperative patients (to avoid cardiovascular complications), and those suspected of having opioid dependence. It is unknown whether naloxone crosses the placenta or is distributed in breast milk. No age-related precautions have been noted in children or elderly patients.

Notify the physician of pain or increased sedation. Vital signs, especially respiratory rate and rhythm, should be monitored. Serious cardiovascular events have been associated with opioid reversal in postoperative patients; doses should be carefully titrated to reduce these events.

Storage
Store the parenteral form at room temperature and protect it from light. The reconstituted solution remains stable in D5W or 0.9% NaCl at 4 mcg/mL for 24 h; discard any unused solution.

Administration
For continuous IV infusion, dilute each 2 mg of naloxone with 500 mL D5W or 0.9% NaCl to provide a concentration of 4 mcg/mL.

Naloxone may also be administered undiluted. Give each 0.4 mg as IV push over 15 seconds. Use the 0.4-mg/mL and 1-mg/mL vials for adults. The 0.4 mg/mL preparation can also be accurately dosed for children and infants using appropriately sized syringes (e.g., 1 mL).

For IM use, inject naloxone in a large muscle mass.

Naltrexone

nal-trex′one

★ ReVia, Vivitrol 🍁 ReVia

CATEGORY AND SCHEDULE

Pregnancy Risk Category: C

Classification: Substance abuse deterrent, narcotic antagonist

MECHANISM OF ACTION

A narcotic antagonist that displaces opioids at opioid-occupied receptor sites in the central nervous system (CNS). *Therapeutic Effect:* Blocks physical effects of opioid analgesics; decreases craving for alcohol and relapse rate in alcoholism.

PHARMACOKINETICS

Rapidly and nearly completely absorbed from GI tract. Peak 2 h followed by second peak 2-3 days later. Extensive first pass effect after oral administration. Low plasma protein binding (20%). Eliminated through urine; undergoes enterohepatic recirculation. *Half-life:* 5-10 days.

AVAILABILITY

Tablets: 50 mg. (ReVia).
Injection for Suspension: 380 mg/vial (Vivitrol).

INDICATIONS AND DOSAGES

▸ **Naloxone challenge test to determine whether patient is opioid dependent (prior to ReVia)**

! Expect to perform the naloxone challenge test if there is any question that the patient is opioid dependent. Do not administer naltrexone until the naloxone challenge test is negative.

IV NALOXONE

Adults, Elderly. Draw 2 mL (0.8 mg) of naloxone into syringe. Inject 0.5 mL (0.2 mg); while needle is still in the vein, observe the patient for 30 seconds for withdrawal signs or symptoms. If no evidence of withdrawal, inject remaining 1.5 mL (0.6 mg); observe patient for additional 20 min for withdrawal signs or symptoms.

SC NALOXONE

Adults, Elderly. Inject 2 mL (0.8 mg) of naloxone; observe patient for 45 min for withdrawal signs or symptoms.

▸ **Treatment of opioid dependence in patients who have been opioid free for at least 7-10 days**

PO (REVIA)

Adults, Elderly. Initially, 25 mg. Observe patient for 1 h. If no withdrawal signs or symptoms appear, give another 25 mg. If a total of 50 mg does not elicit withdrawal, give 50-150 mg/day. Other common regimens are 100 mg every other day or 150 mg every 3 days.

▸ **Adjunctive treatment of alcohol dependence**

PO OR IM

Adults, Elderly. 50 mg once a day for 12 wks (ReVia) or 380 mg IM every 4 wks (Vivitrol).

CONTRAINDICATIONS

Acute opioid withdrawal, failed naloxone challenge test, history of hypersensitivity to naltrexone, opioid dependence (e.g., currently receiving opioid maintenance or opiates for analgesia), positive urine screen for opioids; acute hepatitis or liver failure. Do not use Vivitrol for opioid withdrawal.

INTERACTIONS

Drug

Disulfiram: May increase hepatotoxicity.

Opioid-containing products (including analgesics, antidiarrheals, and antitussives): Blocks the therapeutic effects of these drugs. The concurrent use of any opioid, including methadone, is contraindicated.

Thioridazine: May produce lethargy and somnolence.

Herbal

None known.

Food

None known.

DIAGNOSTIC TEST EFFECTS

May increase AST (SGOT) and ALT (SGPT) levels, bilirubin.

SIDE EFFECTS

Frequent

Insomnia, anxiety, nervousness, headache, low energy, abdominal cramps, nausea, vomiting, arthralgia, myalgia.

Occasional

Dizziness, nervousness, fatigue, insomnia, vomiting, anxiety, suicidal ideation. Irritability, increased energy, anorexia, diarrhea or constipation, rash, chills, increased thirst.

SERIOUS REACTIONS

- Signs and symptoms of opioid withdrawal include stuffy or runny nose, tearing, yawning, diaphoresis, tremor, vomiting, piloerection, feeling of temperature change, bone pain, arthralgia, myalgia, abdominal cramps, and feeling of skin crawling.
- Accidental naltrexone overdose produces withdrawal symptoms within 5 min of ingestion that may last for up to 48 h. Symptoms include confusion, visual hallucinations, somnolence, and significant vomiting and diarrhea.
- Hepatocellular injury may occur with large doses. The margin of separation between the apparently safe dose of naltrexone and the dose causing hepatic injury appears to be only five-fold or less.

PRECAUTIONS & CONSIDERATIONS

Caution is warranted in patients with active hepatic disease. Before treatment, baseline laboratory tests, including creatinine clearance, serum bilirubin, AST (SGOT), and ALT (SGPT) levels, should be obtained. Liver function should be monitored throughout therapy.

Unknown whether excreted in breast milk; warrants caution in lactation. Safety and efficacy in children are not established. Taking opioids while on naltrexone may lead to fatal overdose or coma. Not safe for use in rapid opioid withdrawal procedures.

Be aware that opioid-containing drugs used during naltrexone therapy will have no effect. Any attempt to overcome naltrexone's prolonged 24- to 72-h blockade of opioid effects by taking large amounts of opioids may result in coma, serious injury, or death. Notify the physician if abdominal pain lasts longer than 3 days or if dark urine, white stools, or yellowing of the whites of the eyes occurs. Overdose is evidenced by abdominal pain, dizziness, nausea, and somnolence.

Storage

Store the tablets at room temperature and protect from light.

Injection should be stored in the refrigerator. If removed from refrigerator, injection vial is stable for 7 days at room temperature until mixed.

Administration
Take oral naltrexone with antacids, after meals, or with food to avoid adverse GI effects.

Injection is for intramuscular use only. Remove injection from refrigerator roughly 45 min before giving. Use only diluent provided to reconstitute; 3.4 mL of the supplied diluent will be added to the vial. Vigorously shake to obtain a uniform suspension. After reconstitution the IM suspension will be milky white without clumps. Measure 4 mL of the dose as directed and use immediately. Give IM injection deep into gluteal muscle. Do NOT administer intravenously.

N

Naphazoline

naf-az′oh-leen

★ AK-Con, All Clear, Clear Eyes Redness Relief, Napha Forte

🍁 Abalon, AK-Con, Refresh Redness Relief, Vaphcon Forte

CATEGORY AND SCHEDULE

Pregnancy Risk Category: C
OTC

Classification: Ophthalmic agents, vasoconstrictor

MECHANISM OF ACTION

A sympathomimetic that directly acts on α-adrenergic receptors in conjunctival arterioles. *Therapeutic Effect:* Causes vasoconstriction, resulting in decreased eye redness.

PHARMACOKINETICS

Instillation: Duration 2-3 h.

AVAILABILITY

Ophthalmic Solution: 0.012%, 0.1%.

INDICATIONS AND DOSAGES

▸ **Control of hyperemia in patients with superficial corneal vascularity; relief of congestion and inflammation; for use during ocular diagnostic procedures**

OPHTHALMIC

Adults, Elderly, Children older than 6 yr. 1-2 drops in affected eye up to 4 times per day, for up to 72 h.

CONTRAINDICATIONS

Angle-closure glaucoma, before peripheral iridectomy, patients with a narrow angle who do not have glaucoma.

INTERACTIONS

Drug

Maprotiline, MAOIs, tricyclic antidepressants: May increase pressor effects.

Herbal

None known.

Food

None known.

DIAGNOSTIC TEST EFFECTS

None known.

SIDE EFFECTS

Occasional

Ophthalmic: Blurred vision, dilated pupils, increased eye irritation.

SERIOUS REACTIONS

• If systemically absorbed, the patient may experience tachycardia, palpitations, headache, insomnia, light-headedness, nausea, nervousness, and tremor.

• Overdose in patients older than 60 yr may produce hallucinations, CNS depression, and seizures.

PRECAUTIONS & CONSIDERATIONS

Caution is warranted in patients with diabetes, heart disease (including coronary artery disease), hypertension, and hyperthyroidism.

Storage

Store in a tightly closed container. Do not freeze.

Administration

Avoid touching bottle tip to any surface so contamination does not occur. Do not use while contact lenses are in place. Discontinue the drug and contact the physician if acute eye redness or eye pain, floating spots, vision changes, headache, dizziness, insomnia, irregular heartbeat, tremor, or weakness occurs.

Naproxen/Naproxen Sodium

na-prox'en

★ Naproxen (EC-Naprosyn, Naprelan, Naprosyn)

Naproxen Sodium (Aleve, Anaprox, Anaprox DS, Midol Extended-Relief, Pamprin All Day)

Do not confuse Aleve with Alesse, Anaspaz.

CATEGORY AND SCHEDULE

Pregnancy Risk Category: B (D if used in third trimester or near delivery)

OTC (220-mg gelcaps, 220-mg tablets)

Classification: Analgesics, nonsteroidal anti-inflammatory drugs (NSAIDs)

MECHANISM OF ACTION

An NSAID that produces analgesic and anti-inflammatory effects by inhibiting prostaglandin synthesis. *Therapeutic Effect:* Reduces the inflammatory response and intensity of pain.

PHARMACOKINETICS

Route	Onset	Peak	Duration
PO	< 1 h	NA	≤ 7 h
PO (antirheumatic)	< 14 day	2-4 wks	NA

Completely absorbed from the GI tract. Protein binding: 99%. Metabolized in the liver. Primarily excreted in urine. Not removed by hemodialysis. *Half-life:* 13 h.

AVAILABILITY

Gelcaps (Aleve): 220 mg naproxen sodium (equivalent to 200 mg naproxen) (OTC).

Oral Suspension (Naprosyn): 125 mg/5 mL naproxen.

Tablets (Aleve): 220 mg naproxen (OTC).

Tablets (Anaprox): 275 mg naproxen sodium (equivalent to 250 mg naproxen).

Tablets (Anaprox DS): 550 mg naproxen sodium (equivalent to 500 mg naproxen).

Tablets (Controlled Release [EC-Naprosyn]): 375 mg naproxen, 500 mg naproxen.

Tablets (Controlled Release [Naprelan]): 550 mg naproxen sodium (equivalent to 500 mg naproxen).

INDICATIONS AND DOSAGES

▸ **Rheumatoid arthritis, osteoarthritis, ankylosing spondylitis**

PO

Adults, Elderly. 250-500 mg naproxen (275-550 mg naproxen sodium) twice a day or 250 mg naproxen (275 mg naproxen sodium) in morning and 500 mg naproxen (550 mg naproxen sodium) in evening. Naprelan: 750-1000 mg once a day.

▸ **Acute gouty arthritis**

PO

Adults, Elderly. Initially, 750 mg naproxen (825 mg naproxen sodium), then 250 mg naproxen (275 mg naproxen sodium) q8h until attack subsides. Naprelan: Initially, 1000-1500 mg, then 1000 mg once a day until attack subsides.

▸ **Mild to moderate pain, dysmenorrhea, bursitis, tendinitis**

PO

Adults, Elderly. Initially, 500 mg naproxen (550 mg naproxen sodium), then 250 mg naparoxen (275 mg naproxen sodium) q6-8h as needed. Maximum: 1.25 g/day naproxen (1.375 g/day naproxen sodium). Naprelan: 1000 mg once a day.

▸ **Juvenile rheumatoid arthritis**

PO (NAPROXEN ONLY)

Children. 10-15 mg/kg/day in 2 divided doses. Maximum: 1000 mg/day.

OFF-LABEL USES

Treatment of vascular headaches.

CONTRAINDICATIONS

Hypersensitivity to aspirin, naproxen, or other NSAIDs; use within 14 days of coronary artery bypass graft surgery.

INTERACTIONS

Drug

Antihypertensives, diuretics: May decrease the effects of these drugs.

Aspirin, other salicylates, corticosteroids: May increase the risk of GI side effects such as bleeding. NSAID's may negate cardioprotective effects of ASA.

Bone marrow depressants: May increase the risk of hematologic reactions.

Cyclosporine: Possible risk of decreased renal function.

Heparin, oral anticoagulants, thrombolytics: May increase the effects of these drugs.

Lithium: May increase the blood concentration and risk of toxicity of lithium.

Methotrexate: May increase the risk of methotrexate toxicity.

Probenecid: May increase the naproxen blood concentration.

Tetracyclines: May increase risk of photosensitization.

Herbal

Feverfew: May decrease the effects of feverfew.

Ginkgo biloba: May increase the risk of bleeding.

Food

Alcohol: May increase the risk of side effects such as dizziness or GI bleeding.

DIAGNOSTIC TEST EFFECTS

May prolong bleeding time and alter blood glucose level. May increase serum hepatic function test results. May decrease serum sodium and uric acid levels.

SIDE EFFECTS

Frequent (4%-9%)

Nausea, constipation, abdominal cramps or pain, heartburn, dizziness, headache, somnolence.

Occasional (1%-3%)

Stomatitis, diarrhea, indigestion, fluid retention.

Rare (< 1%)

Vomiting, confusion.

SERIOUS REACTIONS

- Rare reactions with long-term use include peptic ulcer disease, GI bleeding, gastritis, severe hepatic reactions (cholestasis, jaundice), nephrotoxicity (dysuria, hematuria, proteinuria, nephrotic syndrome).
- Severe hypersensitivity reaction (fever, chills, bronchospasm).

PRECAUTIONS & CONSIDERATIONS

Caution is warranted in patients with cardiac disease, hypertension, GI disease, impaired hepatic or renal function, and those using anticoagulants concurrently. Naproxen crosses the placenta and is distributed in breast milk, warranting caution in lactation. Naproxen should not be used during the third trimester of pregnancy because it may cause adverse effects in the fetus, such as premature closing of the ductus arteriosus. The safety and efficacy of naproxen have not been established in children younger than 2 yr. Children older than 2 yr are at an increased risk for developing a rash during naproxen therapy. In elderly patients, GI bleeding or ulceration is more likely to cause serious complications, and age-related renal impairment may increase the risk of hepatotoxicity and renal toxicity; a reduced dosage is recommended. Cardiovascular event risk may be increased with duration of use or preexisting cardiovascular risk factors or disease. Use caution in patients with fluid retention, heart failure, or hypertension. Use lowest effective dose. Risk of myocardial infarction and stroke may be increased following CABG surgery. Do not administer within 4-6 half-lives before surgical procedures. Because the drug may cause dizziness, do not perform tasks requiring mental concentration or motor skills until the effects of the drug are known.

Notify the physician if black or tarry stools, persistent headache, rash, visual disturbances, or weight gain occurs. CBC (particularly hemoglobin, hematocrit, and platelet count), BUN level, serum alkaline phosphatase, bilirubin, creatinine, AST (SGOT), and ALT (SGPT) levels to assess hepatic and renal function, and pattern of daily bowel activity and stool consistency should be assessed during therapy. Therapeutic response, such as decreased pain, stiffness, swelling, and tenderness; improved grip strength; and increased joint mobility, should be evaluated.

Administration

! Each 275- or 550-mg tablet of naproxen sodium equals 250 or 500 mg of naproxen, respectively.

Swallow enteric-coated tablets whole; scored tablets may be broken or crushed. Take naproxen with food, milk, or antacids if GI distress occurs. Shake oral suspension well before each use.

Naratriptan

nare-a-trip′tan

★ 🍁 Amerge

Do not confuse Amerge with Amaryl.

CATEGORY AND SCHEDULE

Pregnancy Risk Category: C

Classification: Migraine agents, serotonin agonists

MECHANISM OF ACTION

A serotonin receptor agonist that binds selectively to vascular receptors, producing a vasoconstrictive effect on cranial blood vessels. *Therapeutic Effect:* Relieves migraine headache.

PHARMACOKINETICS

Well absorbed after PO administration. Protein binding: 28%-31%. Metabolized by the liver to inactive metabolite. Eliminated primarily in urine and, to a lesser extent, in feces.

Half-life: 6 h (increased in hepatic or renal impairment).

AVAILABILITY

Tablets: 1 mg, 2.5 mg.

INDICATIONS AND DOSAGES

▸ **Acute migraine attack**

PO

Adults. 1 mg or 2.5 mg. If headache improves but then returns, dose may be repeated after 4 h. Maximum: 5 mg/24 h.

▸ **Dosage in mild to moderate renal or hepatic impairment**

A lower starting dose is recommended. Do not exceed 2.5 mg/24 h.

CONTRAINDICATIONS

Basilar or hemiplegic migraine, cerebrovascular or peripheral vascular disease, coronary artery disease, ischemic heart disease (including angina pectoris, history of myocardial infarction [MI], silent ischemia, and Prinzmetal angina), severe hepatic impairment—(Child-Pugh grade C), severe renal impairment (serum creatinine < 15 mL/min), uncontrolled hypertension, use within 24 h of ergotamine-containing preparations or another serotonin receptor agonist, use within 14 days of MAOIs.

INTERACTIONS

Drug

5 HT1 agonists: Do not use within 24 h.

Ergotamine-containing medications: May produce a vasospastic reaction. Contraindicated within 24 h.

Fluoxetine, fluvoxamine, paroxetine, sertraline: May produce hyperreflexia, incoordination, and weakness (serotonin syndrome).

MAOIs: Contraindicated within 14 days.

Oral contraceptives: Decrease naratriptan clearance and volume of distribution.

Herbal

None known.

Food

None known.

DIAGNOSTIC TEST EFFECTS

None known.

SIDE EFFECTS

Occasional (5%)

Nausea.

Rare (2%)

Paresthesia; dizziness; fatigue; somnolence; jaw, neck, or throat pressure.

SERIOUS REACTIONS

- Corneal opacities and other ocular defects may occur.
- Cardiac reactions (including ischemia, coronary artery vasospasm, and MI) and noncardiac vasospasm-related reactions (such as hemorrhage or cerebrovascular accident) occur rarely, particularly in patients with hypertension, diabetes, or a strong family history of coronary artery disease; obese patients; smokers; men older than 40 yr; and postmenopausal women.

PRECAUTIONS & CONSIDERATIONS

Caution is warranted with mild to moderate hepatic or renal impairment and cardiovascular risk factors. It is unknown whether naratriptan is excreted in breast milk, warranting caution in lactation. The safety and efficacy of naratriptan have not been established in children. Naratriptan is not recommended for elderly patients. Tasks that require mental alertness or motor skills should be avoided.

Notify the physician immediately if anxiety, chest pain, palpitations, or tightness in the throat occurs. Migraines and associated symptoms, including nausea and vomiting, photophobia, and phonophobia (sound sensitivity), should be assessed before and during treatment.

Storage

Store at room temperature.

Administration

Take naratriptan without regard to food. Swallow tablets whole; do not crush them.

Natalizumab

nat-ah-lih′zoo-mab

★ 🍁 Tysabri

CATEGORY AND SCHEDULE

Pregnancy Risk Category: C

Classification: Neurologic agents, immunologic agents, monoclonal antibodies

MECHANISM OF ACTION

A monoclonal antibody that binds to the surface of leukocytes, inhibiting their adhesion to the vascular endothelial cells of the GI tract and preventing them from migrating across the endothelium into inflamed parenchymal tissue. *Therapeutic Effect:* Decreases clinical exacerbations of multiple sclerosis and decreases GI inflammation.

PHARMACOKINETICS

Half-life: 11 days.

AVAILABILITY

Injection Solution: 300 mg/15 mL.

INDICATIONS AND DOSAGES

▸ **Relapses of multiple sclerosis**

IV INFUSION

Adults, Elderly. 300 mg infused over 1 h every 4 wks.

▸ **Crohn's disease**

IV INFUSION

Adults, Elderly. 300 mg infused over 1 h every 4 wks.

CONTRAINDICATIONS

Multifocal leukoencephalopathy, hypersensitivity to product or murine proteins.

INTERACTIONS

Drug

Antineoplastic, corticosteroid, immunosuppressant, immodulating agents: May cause increase in infection. Not typically used together.

Herbal

None known.

Food

None known.

DIAGNOSTIC TEST EFFECTS

Increases basophil, eosinophil, lymphocyte, monocyte, and RBC counts. May alter liver function test results.

IV INCOMPATIBILITIES

Do not mix natalizumab with any other medication or with any diluent other than 0.9% NaCl.

SIDE EFFECTS

Frequent (15%-35%)

Headache, fatigue, depression, arthralgia.

Occasional (5%-10%)

Abdominal discomfort, rash, urinary frequency or urgency, menstrual irregularities, dysmenorrhea, dermatitis.

Rare (2%-4%)

Pruritus, chest discomfort, local bleeding, rigors, tremor, syncope.

SERIOUS REACTIONS

- Potential increased risk of infection.
- Progressive multifocal leukoencephalopathy.
- Hypersensitivity.
- Hepatotoxicity.

PRECAUTIONS & CONSIDERATIONS

! Increased risk of progressive multifocal leukoencephalopathy that can lead to death or disability. Patients receiving natalizumab must be enrolled and meet conditions of special distribution and registration program (TOUCH program).

Caution is warranted in patients with chronic progressive multiple sclerosis. It is unknown whether natalizumab crosses the placenta or is distributed in breast milk, warranting caution in lactation. The safety and efficacy of natalizumab have not been established in children younger than 18 yr. No age-related precautions have been noted for elderly patients.

Notify the physician of arthralgia, rash, depression, menstrual irregularities, or urinary changes. CBC and liver function test results should be monitored.

Storage

Protect natalizumab vials from light. Do not freeze them. After reconstitution, the solution is stable for 8 h if refrigerated.

Administration

To reconstitute, withdraw 15 mL (300 mg) natalizumab from the vial and inject it into 100 mL 0.9% NaCl. Invert the bag to mix the solution completely. Do not shake it. Inspect the solution for particles. Discard it if it contains particles or becomes discolored. Infuse natalizumab over 1 h. Following the infusion, flush the IV line with 0.9% NaCl. Observe patient for 1 h after infusion.

Natamycin

na-ta-mye′sin

★ Natacyn

Do not confuse with naproxen.

CATEGORY AND SCHEDULE

Pregnancy Risk Category: C

Classification: Antifungals, ophthalmics

MECHANISM OF ACTION

A polyene antifungal agent that increases cell membrane permeability in susceptible fungi. *Therapeutic Effect:* Fungicidal.

PHARMACOKINETICS

Minimal systemic absorption. Adheres to cornea and is retained in conjunctival fornices.

AVAILABILITY

Ophthalmic Suspension: 5% (Natacyn).

INDICATIONS AND DOSAGES

▸ **Fungal keratitis, ophthalmic fungal infections**

OPHTHALMIC

Adults, Elderly. Instill 1 drop in conjunctival sac every 1-2 h. After 3-4 days, reduce to 1 drop 6-8 times daily. Usual course of therapy is 2-3 wks or until the fungal infection is resolved. If limited to blepharitis or conjunctivitis, application 4-6 times/day may be sufficient.

CONTRAINDICATIONS

Hypersensitivity to natamycin or any component of the formulation.

INTERACTIONS

Drug

Topical corticosteroids: May increase risk of toxicity. Concomitant use is contraindicated.

Herbal

None known.

Food

None known.

DIAGNOSTIC TEST EFFECTS

None known.

SIDE EFFECTS

Occasional (3%-10%)

Blurred vision, eye irritation, eye pain, photophobia.

SERIOUS REACTIONS

- Vomiting and diarrhea have occurred with large doses in the treatment of systemic mycoses.

PRECAUTIONS & CONSIDERATIONS

If symptoms do not improve within 7-10 days, or become worse, notify the physician. It is unknown whether natamycin is excreted in breast milk, warranting caution in lactation. Safety and efficacy of natamycin have not been established in children. No age-related precautions have been noted in elderly patients.

Storage

May be stored in refrigerator or at room temperature. Do not freeze. Avoid exposure to light and excessive heat.

Administration

Shake ophthalmic suspension before using. Do not touch dropper to eye. Remove contact lenses and do not wear during treatment. Gently clean eye of any exudate before instilling medication. Form a slight pouch and instill; close the eye and allow the medication to cover the eye before reopening. Wipe away gently any extra medication.

Nateglinide

na-teg'lin-ide

★ 🍁 Starlix

CATEGORY AND SCHEDULE

Pregnancy Risk Category: C

Classification: Antidiabetic agents, meglitinide

MECHANISM OF ACTION

An antihyperglycemic that stimulates the release of insulin from β-cells of the pancreas by depolarizing β-cells, leading to an opening of calcium channels. Resulting calcium influx induces insulin secretion. *Therapeutic Effect:* Lowers blood glucose concentration.

PHARMACOKINETICS

PO: Rapid absorption; peak plasma levels in 1 h; bioavailability 73%. Plasma protein binding 98%, hepatic metabolism by CYP450 A29 isoenzyme (70%) and CYP450 3A4 isoenzyme (30%); excretion in urine and feces.

AVAILABILITY

Tablets: 60 mg, 120 mg.

INDICATIONS AND DOSAGES

▸ **Diabetes mellitus Type 2**

PO

Adult, Elderly. 120 mg 3 times a day before meals. Initially, 60 mg/dose may be given in patients close to goal HbA1C. May be used with metformin or a thiaolidinedione.

CONTRAINDICATIONS

Diabetic ketoacidosis, type 1 diabetes mellitus, hypersensitivity.

N

INTERACTIONS

Drug

β-Blockers, MAOIs, NSAIDs, salicylates: May increase hypoglycemic effect of nateglinide.
Corticosteroids, thiazide diuretics, thyroid medication, sympathomimetics: May decrease hypoglycemic effect of nateglinide.

Herbal

None known.

Food

Liquid meal: Peak plasma levels may be significantly reduced if administered 10 min before a liquid meal.

DIAGNOSTIC TEST EFFECTS

None known.

SIDE EFFECTS

Frequent (10%)
Upper respiratory tract infection.
Occasional (3%-4%)
Back pain, flu symptoms, dizziness, arthropathy, diarrhea.
Rare (2%)
Bronchitis, cough.

SERIOUS REACTIONS

• Hypoglycemia occurs in < 2% of patients.

PRECAUTIONS & CONSIDERATIONS

Use with caution in hepatic or renal impairment. No adequate, well-controlled studies exist in pregnant women. Caution should be exercised when nateglinide is used during pregnancy. It is unknown whether nateglinide is distributed into breast milk. The manufacturer recommends that patients do not breastfeed. The safety and efficacy of nateglinide have not been established in children.

Food intake and blood glucose should be monitored before and during therapy. Be aware of signs and symptoms of hypoglycemia (anxiety, cool wet skin, diplopia, dizziness, headache, hunger, numbness in mouth, tachycardia, tremors) or hyperglycemia (deep rapid breathing, dim vision, fatigue, nausea, polydipsia, polyphagia, polyuria, vomiting); carry candy, sugar packets, or other sugar supplements for immediate response to hypoglycemia. Consult the physician when glucose demands are altered (such as with fever, heavy physical activity, infection, stress, trauma). Exercise, good personal hygiene (including foot care), not smoking, and weight control are essential parts of therapy.

Storage

Store at room temperature, tightly closed.

Administration

Ideally, take within 15 min of a meal; however, may take immediately to as long as 30 min before a meal. Allow at least 1 wk to elapse to assess the response to the drug before new dose adjustment is made.

Nebivolol

na-biv′oh-lol

Bystolic

Do not confuse nebivolol with atenolol or timolol, or Bystolic with bisoprolol.

CATEGORY AND SCHEDULE

Pregnancy Risk Category: C

Classification: Antihypertensive agents, β-blocking

MECHANISM OF ACTION

A β_1-adrenergic blocker that is primarily selective until doses are greater than 10 mg/day, at which some activation of β_2-receptors occurs. Acts as an antihypertensive agent by blocking β_1-adrenergic receptors in vascular tissue and decreasing vascular resistance. *Therapeutic Effect:* Slows sinus node heart rate, decreasing cardiac contractility and BP.

PHARMACOKINETICS

Exact bioavailability has not been determined. Protein binding: 98%. Liver metabolism. Nebivolol is metabolized by a number of routes, including glucuronidation and hydroxylation by CYP2D6. Metabolites contribute to activity. Excreted in urine and feces; 38% of the dose was recovered in urine and 44% in feces in extensive metabolizers. *Half-life:* 12-19 h (increased in severely impaired renal or hepatic function).

AVAILABILITY

Tablets: 2.5 mg, 5 mg, 10 mg, 20 mg.

INDICATIONS AND DOSAGES

▸ Hypertension

PO

Adults. Elderly. Start with 5 mg once daily, as monotherapy or in combination with other agents. The dose can be increased at 2-wk intervals as needed and tolerated up to 40 mg/day.

▸ Dosage in hepatic or renal impairment

For Child-Pugh class A or B or CrCl < 30 mL/min. 2.5 mg once daily initially, titrate carefully to desired clinical effect.

CONTRAINDICATIONS

Severe bradycardia, heart block greater than 1st degree, cardiogenic shock, decompensated CHF, sick sinus syndrome (unless a permanent pacemaker is in place), severe hepatic impairment (Child-Pugh class C), hypersensitive to any component of product.

INTERACTIO

Drug

Cimetidine: May i blood concentration.

Diuretics, other antihy May increase hypotensive calcium channel blockers w additive cardiac conduction ef Discontinue β-blocker several da before a clonidine taper.

CYP2D6 inhibitors (e.g., quinidine, propafenone, fluoxetine, paroxetine): May significantly increase nebivolol exposure.

Insulin, oral hypoglycemics: May mask symptoms of hypoglycemia and prolong hypoglycemic effect of insulin and oral hypoglycemics.

NSAIDs: May decrease antihypertensive effects.

Sympathomimetics: May inhibit blood pressure lowering.

Herbal

None known.

Food

None known.

DIAGNOSTIC TEST EFFECTS

Increase in BUN, uric acid, triglycerides and a decrease in HDL cholesterol and platelet count.

SIDE EFFECTS

Nebivolol is generally well tolerated, with mild and transient side effects.

Frequent

Headache, fatigue, diarrhea, nausea, dizziness.

Occasional

Cold extremities, insomnia, chest pain, bradycardia, hypotension, dyspnea, rash, peripheral edema.

Rare

Urinary frequency, impotence or decreased libido, mental depression. Asthenia, hyperuricemia, hyperlipidemia. Arthralgia, myalgia, confusion (especially in the elderly).

...IONS

...ay produce profound ...a and hypotension.

...t withdrawal may result in ...ioresis, palpitations, headache, ...d tremors.

- May precipitate CHF or MI in patients with cardiac disease; thyroid storm in those with thyrotoxicosis; and peripheral ischemia in those with existing peripheral vascular disease.
- Hypoglycemia may occur in patients with previously controlled diabetes.
- Thrombocytopenia, manifested as unusual bruising or bleeding, occurs rarely.
- Rare hypersensitivity, including anaphylaxis, allergic vasculitis, or angioedema.

PRECAUTIONS & CONSIDERATIONS

Caution is warranted with bronchospastic disease, diabetes, hyperthyroidism, impaired renal or hepatic function, inadequate cardiac function, and peripheral vascular disease. Nebivolol likely crosses the placenta and is likely distributed in breast milk. Use should be avoided in pregnant women after the first trimester because it may result in low-birth-weight infants. The drug may also produce apnea, bradycardia, hypoglycemia, and hypothermia. This drug is not yet approved for use in children. Use cautiously in elderly patients, who may have age-related peripheral vascular disease and impaired renal function.

Be aware that salt and alcohol intake should be restricted. Nasal decongestants or OTC cold preparations (stimulants) should not be used without physician approval. Orthostatic hypotension may occur, so rise slowly from a lying to sitting position and dangle the legs from the bed momentarily before standing. Notify the physician of confusion, depression, dizziness, rash, or unusual bruising or bleeding. BP for hypotension; respiratory status for shortness of breath; and pulse for quality, rate, and rhythm should be monitored during treatment. If pulse rate is < 55 beats/min or systolic BP is < 90 mm Hg, withhold the medication and contact the physician. Signs and symptoms of CHF, such as decreased urine output, distended neck veins, dyspnea (particularly on exertion or lying down), night cough, peripheral edema, and weight gain should also be assessed.

Storage

Store at room temperature.

Administration

Take oral nebivolol without regard to meals. Crush tablets if necessary. Do not abruptly discontinue the drug. Compliance is essential to control hypertension.

Nedocromil Sodium

ned-oh-crow'mil so'dee-um

Alocril

CATEGORY AND SCHEDULE

Pregnancy Risk Category: B

Classification: Ophthalmics, anti-inflammatory agents, mast cell stabilizers

MECHANISM OF ACTION

A mast cell stabilizer that prevents the activation and release of inflammatory mediators, such as histamine, leukotrienes, mast cells, eosinophils, and monocytes. *Therapeutic Effect:* Reduces ocular symptoms of allergies.

PHARMACOKINETICS

Low systemic absorption.

AVAILABILITY
Ophthalmic Solution (Alocril): 2%.

INDICATIONS AND DOSAGES
▸ Allergic conjunctivitis

OPHTHALMIC

Adults, Elderly, Children 3 yr and older. 1-2 drops in each eye twice a day.

CONTRAINDICATIONS
Hypersensitivity to nedocromil.

INTERACTIONS
Drug

None known.

Herbal

None known.

Food

None known.

DIAGNOSTIC TEST EFFECTS
None known.

SIDE EFFECTS
Frequent

Temporary ocular burning, irritation, stinging, unpleasant taste, and nasal congestion.

Rare

Asthma, conjunctivitis, eye redness, photophobia, and rhinitis.

SERIOUS REACTIONS
• None known.

PRECAUTIONS & CONSIDERATIONS
Users of contact lenses should refrain from wearing lenses while exhibiting the signs and symptoms of allergic conjunctivitis. Use with caution in pregnancy and lactation. There are no specific precautions for children over 3 yr of age or the elderly.

Storage

May refrigerate or keep at room temperature. Protect the drug from direct exposure to light.

Administration

Prior to ophthalmic administration, wash hands. Tilt head back slightly, look up, and pull lower eyelid down to form a pouch. Squeeze drop(s) into pouch then close eye gently. Do not touch bottle tip to any surface.

Nefazodone
neh-faz′oh-doan

CATEGORY AND SCHEDULE
Pregnancy Risk Category: C

Classification: Antidepressants, miscellaneous

MECHANISM OF ACTION
Exact mechanism is unknown. Appears to inhibit neuronal uptake of serotonin and norepinephrine and to antagonize α_1-adrenergic receptors. *Therapeutic Effect:* Relieves depression.

PHARMACOKINETICS
Rapidly and completely absorbed from the GI tract; food delays absorption. Protein binding: 99%. Widely distributed in body tissues, including the central nervous system (CNS). Extensively metabolized via the liver to active metabolites. Excreted in urine and eliminated in feces. Unknown whether removed by hemodialysis. *Half-life:* 2-4 h.

AVAILABILITY
Tablets: 50 mg, 100 mg, 150 mg, 200 mg, 250 mg.

INDICATIONS AND DOSAGES
▸ Depression, prevention of relapse in acute depressive episode

PO

Adults. Initially, 200 mg/day in 2 divided doses. Gradually increase

N

by 100-200 mg/day at intervals of at least 1 wk. Range: 300-600 mg/day. *Elderly.* Initially, 100 mg/day in 2 divided doses. Subsequent dosage titration based on clinical response. Range: 200-400 mg/day.

CONTRAINDICATIONS

Do not use within 14 days of MAOIs, previous history of liver problems from nefazodone, or hypersensitivity to nefazodone or trazodone. Coadministration of terfenadine, cisapride, astemizole, pimozide, carbamazepine or triazolam is contraindicated.

INTERACTIONS

NOTE: Because nefazodone is a potent CYP3A4 inhibitor, many prescription medications contraindicate its use. Check prescribing information for other medications carefully before using nefazodone.

N

Drug

Alprazolam: May increase the blood concentration and risk of toxicity of alprazolam.

Carbamazepine: Reduces nefazodone concentrations significantly.

Substrates of CYP3A4: May risk interaction with drugs metabolized with CYP3A4. Important examples of substrates include ergot alkaloids, antiarrhythmic drugs, statins, and protease inhibitors.

MAOIs: May produce severe reactions if used concurrently with or within 14 days of MAOI discontinuation.

Triazolam: Increases triazolam concentration by 75%. Try to avoid, or greatly reduce triazolam dose.

Herbal

St. John's wort: May increase the risk of adverse effects. Avoid.

Food

None known.

DIAGNOSTIC TEST EFFECTS

May increase LFTs.

SIDE EFFECTS

Frequent

Headache (36%); dry mouth, somnolence (25%); nausea (22%); dizziness (17%); constipation (14%); insomnia, asthenia, light-headedness (10%).

Occasional

Dyspepsia, blurred vision (9%); diarrhea, infection (8%); confusion, abnormal vision (7%); pharyngitis (6%); increased appetite (5%); orthostatic hypotension, flushing, feeling of warmth (4%); peripheral edema, cough, flu-like symptoms (3%).

SERIOUS REACTIONS

- Serious reactions, such as hyperthermia, rigidity, myoclonus, extreme agitation, delirium, and coma, will occur due to MAOI interaction.
- Hepatotoxicity.

PRECAUTIONS & CONSIDERATIONS

Caution is warranted in patients with cerebrovascular or cardiovascular disease, recent myocardial infarction, dehydration, hypovolemia, cirrhosis, a history of hypomania or mania, and a history of seizures. It is unknown whether nefazodone crosses the placenta or is distributed in breast milk, warranting caution in lactation. Antidepressants have been reported to increase the risk of suicidal thinking and behavior in children, adolescents, and young adults (18-24 yr of age) with major depressive disorder (MDD) and other psychiatric disorders. Patients should be closely monitored for clinical worsening, suicidality, or unusual changes in behavior, particularly during the initial 1-2 mo of therapy or following dosage adjustments.

The safety and efficacy of this drug have not been established in children. Elderly and debilitated patients are more susceptible to side effects. Lower dosages are recommended for elderly patients, although no age-related precautions have been noted for this age group.

Drowsiness, dizziness, and light-headedness may occur, so avoid alcohol and tasks that require mental alertness or motor skills. BP and pulse rate should be assessed during therapy. Caution is warranted in postural changes because of possible orthostatic hypotension developing.

Patients who develop evidence of hepatocellular injury such as increased serum AST or serum ALT levels ≥ 3 times the upper limit of normal (ULN) should be withdrawn from the drug.

Storage

Store at room temperature.

Administration

! Allow at least 14 days to elapse before switching the patient from an MAOI to nefazodone and at least 7 days to elapse before switching the patient from nefazodone to an MAOI.

Take nefazodone without regard to food.

Nelarabine

nel-are′a-been

Arranon Atriance

Do not confuse nelarabine with cladribine or fludarabine.

CATEGORY AND SCHEDULE

Pregnancy Risk Category: D

Classification: Antineoplastic, antimetabolite, purine analogue

MECHANISM OF ACTION

A prodrug for ARA-G (deoxyguanosine analogue 9-β-D arabinofuranosylguanine), which acts as an intracellular cytotoxic agent and inhibits DNA synthesis. Once inside the cell, ARA-G is mono-phosphorylated and converted to ARA-GTP. Accumulation of ARA-GTP in leukemic blasts allows for incorporation into DNA. Incorporation into DNA halts DNA synthesis and causes apoptosis. Also inhibits RNA synthesis. More toxic to T-lymphoblasts than other blast cells. *Therapeutic Effect:* Leads to tumor cell death.

PHARMACOKINETICS

After IV administration, both nelarabine and ARA-G are rapidly distributed to body tissues. Protein binding: < 25%. The principal route of metabolism for nelarabine is hepatic O-demethylation by adenosine deaminase to form ARA-G, which undergoes hydrolysis to form guanine. In addition, some nelarabine is hydrolyzed to form methylguanine, which is O-demethylated to form guanine. Guanine is N-deaminated to form xanthine, which is further oxidized to yield uric acid. Nelarabine and ARA-G are partially eliminated by the kidneys. *Half-life:* Nelarabine, 18 min; ARA-G, 3.2 h (in adults, slightly shorter in children).

AVAILABILITY

Injection Solution: 250 mg/50 mL (5 mg/mL).

INDICATIONS AND DOSAGES

▸ **T-cell lymphocytic leukemia or T-cell lymphoma**

IV INFUSION

Adults, Elderly. 1500 mg/m^2 over 2 h on days 1, 3, and 5. Cycle is repeated every 21 days.

N

Children. 650 mg/m^2 administered over 1 h daily for 5 consecutive days. Cycle is repeated every 21 days.

▸ Dosage for toxicities

Expect dosage to be discontinued for significant neurotoxicity and delayed for significant hematologic toxicity.

▸ Dosage in renal cell impairment

Give if CrCl < 50 mL/min only when benefits outweigh risks due to lack of data.

CONTRAINDICATIONS

Hypersensitivity.

INTERACTIONS

Drug

Pentostatin: Coadministration is not recommended due to similar actions.

Vaccines, live virus: Avoid use. Altered immune response and increased risk of secondary transmission of infection from vaccine.

Herbal

None known.

Food

None known.

IV INCOMPATIBILITIES

Do not mix with or infuse with other medications.

DIAGNOSTIC TEST EFFECTS

May elevate serum uric acid, serum creatinine. Decreased RBC, WBC, and platelet counts. Electrolyte disturbances may occur.

SIDE EFFECTS

Frequent (> 20%)

Anemia, thrombocytopenia, neutropenia, nausea, diarrhea, vomiting, constipation, fatigue, pyrexia, cough, and dyspnea.

Common (> 10%)

Somnolence, dizziness, weakness, peripheral neuropathy, hypoesthesia, headache, and paresthesia.

Rare

Blurred vision.

SERIOUS REACTIONS

- Dose-limiting toxicity is neurotoxicity. Serious neurotoxicity may cause seizures, paralysis, and coma.
- Bone marrow depression is manifested as hematologic toxicity (principally leukopenia, anemia, thrombocytopenia).
- Hyperkalemia, hyperphosphatemia, hyperuricemia, hypocalcemia, and decreased urine output may be indicative of tumor lysis syndrome (TLS). Appropriate measures must be taken to prevent severe electrolyte imbalances and renal toxicity.

PRECAUTIONS & CONSIDERATIONS

Use with caution and closely monitor patients with hepatic or renal dysfunction. Fetal harm can occur if given to a pregnant woman. Adequate contraception is recommended during treatment. Breastfeeding is not recommended since it is not known if nelarabine is excreted in breast milk. The elderly may be more susceptible to drug toxicities and age-related organ dysfunction.

Monitor CBC with differential and platelet count and renal function before each dose. Patients should avoid those recently vaccinated with live-virus vaccines or crowds. Any of the following symptoms should be reported immediately: rash, hives, difficulty breathing, fever, chills; these symptoms can be indicators of possible infection: bleeding or unusual bruising, mouth sores, dark urine, yellowing of skin or eyes, pain, redness, swelling at injection site; persistent nausea, vomiting, diarrhea, appetite loss, or worsening general body weakness. Maintain adequate hydration during therapy to avoid developing hyperuricemia and urate precipitation.

Storage

Store unopened vials at controlled room temperature. Once transferred to appropriate infusion container, the drug is stable for 8 h at room temperature.

Administration

CAUTION: Observe and exercise usual cautions for handling, preparing, and administering cytotoxic drugs.

Administer nelarabine by IV infusion only. The solution is given undiluted. The appropriate dose is transferred into PVC infusion bags or glass containers and administered as a 2-h infusion in adult patients and as a 1-h infusion in pediatric patients. Appropriate measures (e.g., hydration, urine alkalinization, and prophylaxis with allopurinol) must be taken to prevent hyperuricemia.

Nelfinavir

nel-fin′eh-veer

★ 🍁 Viracept

CATEGORY AND SCHEDULE

Pregnancy Risk Category: B

Classification: Antiretrovirals, protease inhibitors

MECHANISM OF ACTION

Inhibits the activity of HIV-1 protease, the enzyme necessary for the formation of infectious HIV. *Therapeutic Effect:* Formation of immature noninfectious viral particles rather than HIV replication.

PHARMACOKINETICS

Well absorbed after PO administration (absorption increased with food). Protein binding: 98%. Metabolized in the liver. Highly bound to plasma proteins. Eliminated primarily in feces. Unknown if removed by hemodialysis. *Half-life:* 3.5-5 h.

AVAILABILITY

Powder for Oral Suspension: 50 mg/g.

Tablets: 250 mg, 625 mg.

INDICATIONS AND DOSAGES

▸ HIV infection

PO

Adults and Children > 13 yrs. 750 mg (three 250-mg tablets) 3 times a day or 1250 mg twice a day in combination with other antiretroviral agents.

Children aged 2-13 yr. 25-35 mg/kg/dose 3 times a day or 45-55 mg/kg/dose twice daily. Maximum: 750 mg q8h.

CONTRAINDICATIONS

Hypersensitivity; coadministration with amiodarone, quinidine, ergot alkaloids, pimozide, triazolam, midazolam, rifampin, St. John's wort, and proton-pump inhibitors; moderate or severe liver dysfunction.

INTERACTIONS

NOTE: Please see detailed manufacturer's information for management of drug interactions. In some cases, dosage adjustment or an alternate agent is recommended.

Drug

Alcohol, psychoactive drugs: May produce additive central nervous system (CNS) effects.

Alprazolam, midazolam, triazolam: Increases the risk of prolonged sedation. Contraindicated.

Amiodarone: May increase amiodarone levels. Contraindicated.

Anticonvulsants, rifabutin, rifampin: Decrease nelfinavir plasma concentration.
Bosentan, Colchicine: Increases the levels of these drugs. Adjust dose.
Cyclosporine, other immunosuppressants: May increase blood concentrations; use with caution and monitor closely.
Ergot alkaloids: Effects of ergot alkaloids may be increased. Contraindicated.
Erythromycin, ketoconazole: May increase plasma levels.
Fentanyl: May increase plasma concentrations of fentanyl.
HMG-CoA reductase inhibitors: Increases statin concentrations. Use not recommended with lovastatin, simvastatin, and rosuvastatin.
Indinavir, saquinavir: Increases plasma concentration of these drugs.
Oral contraceptives: Decreases the efficacy of the O.C.
Phosphodiesterase-5 inhibitors (e.g., sildenafil, vardenafil, tadalafil): Increases PDE-5 inhibitor blood levels and risk of hypotension. Contraindicated for use with sildenafil for pulmonary HTN.
Ritonavir: Increases nelfinavir plasma concentration.

Herbal

St. John's wort: May decrease plasma concentration and effects of nelfinavir. Avoid, as nelfinavir will become ineffective.

Food

All foods: Increase nelfinavir plasma concentration. Take with food.

DIAGNOSTIC TEST EFFECTS

May decrease hemoglobin values and neutrophil and WBC counts. May increase serum CK, AST (SGOT), and ALT (SGPT) levels. Increased lipids, blood glucose.

SIDE EFFECTS

Frequent

Diarrhea (> 20%), nausea, rash, gas.

Occasional

Asthenia, fatigue; insomnia; accumulation of fat in waist, abdomen, or back of neck (buffalo hump, lipodystrophy).

Rare

Abnormal taste sensation, hyperglycemia, new-onset diabetes, sexual dysfunction.

SERIOUS REACTIONS

- Jaundice, bilirubinemia, rare cases of hepatitis/liver failure or pancreatitis.
- Serious hypersensitivity reactions have included erythema multiforme or Stevens-Johnson syndrome or anaphylactoid reactions.
- Spontaneous bleeding in patients with hemophilia.

PRECAUTIONS & CONSIDERATIONS

Caution is warranted with mild liver function impairment. It is unknown whether nelfinavir is excreted in breast milk. Breastfeeding is not recommended because of the possibility of HIV transmission. Use caution in pregnancy; adherence to contraception should be advised, including the use of non-hormonal methods. No age-related precautions have been noted in children older than 2 yr. Nelfinavir is not a cure for HIV infection, nor does it reduce the risk of transmitting HIV to others.

Monitor the patient for signs and symptoms of opportunistic infections as evidenced by chills, cough, fever, and myalgia. Expect to check to establish an accurate baseline before beginning drug therapy. Assess the pattern of daily bowel activity and stool consistency.

Storage
Store drug at room temperature, keep it in the original container, and protect it from moisture.
Administration
Take with food, a light meal, or snack. Mix oral powder with a small amount of dietary supplement, formula, milk, soy formula, soy milk, or dairy food such as pudding or ice cream. The entire contents must be consumed to receive a full dose. Do not mix with acidic food, such as apple juice, applesauce, or orange juice, or with water. Take the medication every day as prescribed, and evenly space drug doses around the clock.

Neomycin Sulfate
nee-oh-mye′sin sull′fate
★ Neo-Fradin

CATEGORY AND SCHEDULE
Pregnancy Risk Category: D
OTC (topical ointment 0.5% only)

Classification: Antibiotics, aminoglycosides

MECHANISM OF ACTION
An aminoglycoside antibiotic that binds to bacterial 30S ribosomal subunits. *Therapeutic Effect:* Interferes with bacterial protein synthesis; bactericidal.

PHARMACOKINETICS
Poorly absorbed from the GI tract. Rapidly distributed to tissues. Removed by dialysis. 97% eliminated through feces.

AVAILABILITY
Tablets: 500 mg.
Oral Solution: 125 mg/5 mL (Neo-Fradin).
Ointment: 0.5%.

INDICATIONS AND DOSAGES
▸ **Preoperative bowel antisepsis prophylaxis**
PO
Adults, Elderly. 1 g neomycin plus 1 g erythromycin on day prior to surgery at 1:00 PM, 2:00 PM, and 11:00 PM.
▸ **Hepatic encephalopathy**
PO
Adults, Elderly. 4-12 g/day in divided doses q4-6h.
▸ **Diarrhea caused by *Escherichia coli***
PO
Adults, Elderly. 3 g/day in divided doses q6h.
▸ **Minor skin infections**
IRRIGATION, TOPICAL
Adults, Elderly, Children. Usual dosage, apply to affected area 1-3 times/day.

CONTRAINDICATIONS
Hypersensitivity to neomycin, other aminoglycosides (cross-sensitivity), or their components; patients with intestinal stricture, any inflammatory or ulcerative GI disease.

INTERACTIONS
Drug
Anticoagulants: May increase anticoagulant effect and lower vitamin K availability.
Digoxin, fluorouracil, methotrexate, penicillin V, vitamin B_{12}: May inhibit absorption of these drugs.
Nephrotoxic medications, other aminoglycosides, ototoxic, neurotoxic or nephrotoxic medications: May increase

N

nephrotoxicity and ototoxicity if significant systemic absorption occurs.
Potent diuretics (ethacrynic acid, furosemide): May increase neomycin toxicity.
Herbal
None known.
Food
None known.

DIAGNOSTIC TEST EFFECTS
May increase serum creatitine.

SIDE EFFECTS
Frequent
Systemic: Nausea, vomiting, diarrhea, irritation of mouth or rectal area.
Topical: Itching, redness, swelling, rash.
Rare
Systemic: Malabsorption syndrome, neuromuscular blockade (difficulty breathing, drowsiness, weakness).

SERIOUS REACTIONS
• Nephrotoxicity (as evidenced by increased BUN and serum creatinine levels and decreased creatinine clearance) may be reversible if the drug is stopped at the first sign of nephrotoxic symptoms.
• Irreversible ototoxicity (manifested as tinnitus, dizziness, and impaired hearing) and neurotoxicity (as evidenced by headache, dizziness, lethargy, tremor, and visual disturbances) occur occasionally.
• Severe respiratory depression and anaphylaxis occur rarely.
• Superinfections, particularly fungal infections, may occur.

PRECAUTIONS & CONSIDERATIONS
! Systemic absorption may occur after oral administration, increasing the risk of toxicity.

Caution is warranted in elderly patients, infants, and other patients with renal insufficiency, as well as those with neuromuscular disorders, hearing loss, or vertigo. Aminoglycosides can cause fetal harm when administered to a pregnant woman. Use caution in systemic use in lactation.

Expect to correct dehydration before beginning neomycin therapy. Establish the patient's baseline hearing acuity before beginning therapy. Signs and symptoms of hypersensitivity reaction should be monitored. With topical application, symptoms may include a rash, redness, or itching. If dizziness, impaired hearing, or ringing in the ears occurs, notify the physician. Report diarrhea with blood or pus, hearing loss, tinnitus, vestibular symptoms, muscle twitch, numbness, skin tingling, loose or foul-smelling stools.
Storage
Store at controlled room temperature.
Administration
Continue taking neomycin for the full course of treatment, and space doses evenly around the clock.

Neostigmine
nee-oh-stig′meen
★ 🍁 Prostigmin
Do not confuse neostigmine with physostigmine.

CATEGORY AND SCHEDULE
Pregnancy Risk Category: C

Classification: Cholinesterase inhibitors

MECHANISM OF ACTION

A cholinergic that prevents destruction of acetylcholine by inhibiting the enzyme acetylcholinesterase, thus enhancing impulse transmission across the myoneural junction. *Therapeutic Effect:* Improves intestinal and skeletal muscle tone; stimulates salivary and sweat gland secretions.

PHARMACOKINETICS

PO: Onset 45-75 min, duration 2.5-4 h.
IM/SC: Onset 10-30 min, duration 2.5-4 h.
IV: Onset 4-8 min, duration 2-4 h.
Metabolized in the liver, excreted in urine.

AVAILABILITY

Tablets: 15 mg.
Injection: 0.5 mg/mL, 1 mg/mL.

INDICATIONS AND DOSAGES

▸ **Myasthenia gravis**

PO

Adults, Elderly. Initially, 15-30 mg 3-4 times a day. Increase as necessary. Maintenance: 150 mg/day (range of 15-375 mg).

Children. 2 mg/kg/day divided q3-4hr.

IV, IM, SC

Adults. 0.5-2.5 mg as needed q1-3h. Usual maximum: 10 mg/24h.

Children. 0.01-0.04 mg/kg q2-4h.

▸ **Diagnosis of myasthenia gravis**

IM

Adults, Elderly. 0.022 mg/kg. If cholinergic reaction occurs, discontinue tests and administer 0.4-0.6 mg or more atropine sulfate intravenously.

Children. 0.025-0.04 mg/kg preceded by atropine sulfate 0.011 mg/kg subcutaneously.

▸ **Prevention of postoperative urinary retention**

IM, SC

Adults, Elderly. 0.25 mg q4-6h for 2-3 days.

▸ **Postoperative abdominal distention and urine retention**

IM, SC

Adults, Elderly. 0.5-1 mg. Catheterize patient if voiding does not occur within 1 h. After voiding, administer 0.5 mg q3h for 5 injections.

▸ **Reversal of neuromuscular blockade (with atropine)**

IV

Adults, Elderly. 0.5-2.5 mg given slowly.

Children. 0.025-0.08 mg/kg/dose.

Infants. 0.025-0.1 mg/kg/dose.

CONTRAINDICATIONS

GI or genitourinary obstruction, peritonitis, hypersensitivity.

INTERACTIONS

Drug

Anticholinergics: Reverse or prevent the effects of neostigmine; may be contraindicated.

Cholinesterase inhibitors: May increase the risk of toxicity.

Ester-type local anesthetics: May increase risk of toxicity.

Hydrocarbon inhalation anesthetics, corticosteroids: Decreased action.

Neuromuscular blockers: Antagonizes the effects of these drugs.

Procainamide, quinidine: May antagonize the action of neostigmine.

Succinylcholine: May increase activity of succinylcholine.

Herbal

None known.

Food

None known.

DIAGNOSTIC TEST EFFECTS

None known.

IV INCOMPATIBILITIES
None known.

IV COMPATIBILITIES
Glycopyrrolate (Robinul), heparin, ondansetron (Zofran), potassium chloride, thiopental (Pentothal).

SIDE EFFECTS
Frequent
Muscarinic effects (diarrhea, diaphoresis, increased salivation, nausea, vomiting, abdominal cramps or pain).
Occasional
Muscarinic effects (urinary urgency or frequency, increased bronchial secretions, miosis, lacrimation).

SERIOUS REACTIONS
- Overdose produces a cholinergic crisis manifested as abdominal discomfort or cramps, nausea, vomiting, diarrhea, flushing, facial warmth, excessive salivation, diaphoresis, lacrimation, pallor, bradycardia or tachycardia, hypotension, bronchospasm, urinary urgency, blurred vision, miosis, and fasciculation (involuntary muscular contractions visible under the skin).

N

PRECAUTIONS & CONSIDERATIONS
Caution is warranted with arrhythmias, asthma, bradycardia, epilepsy, hyperthyroidism, peptic ulcer disease, and recent coronary occlusion.

Notify the physician of diarrhea, difficulty breathing, increased salivation, irregular heartbeat, muscle weakness, nausea and vomiting, severe abdominal pain, or increased sweating. Vital signs, muscle strength, and fluid intake and output should be monitored. Therapeutic response to the drug, including decreased fatigue, improved chewing and swallowing, and increased muscle strength, should also be assessed.
Storage
Store at room temperature, protect from light.
Administration
! Discontinue all anticholinesterase therapy at least 8 h before testing. Plan to give 0.01 mg/kg atropine sulfate IV simultaneously with neostigmine, or IM 30 min before administering neostigmine, to prevent adverse effects. Give IV at a rate of 0.5 mg over 1 min.

Expect to give larger doses when the patient is most tired. Adminster orally with food or milk to minimize GI irritation.

Nepafenac
neh-pa-fen′ak
Nevanac
Do not confuse nepafenac with bromfenac or diclofenac.

CATEGORY AND SCHEDULE
Pregnancy Risk Category: C (D in late pregnancy)

Classification: Nonsteroidal anti-inflammatory drugs, ophthalmic

MECHANISM OF ACTION
An NSAID prodrug that is rapidly converted to amfenac in the cornea and ocular tissues. The prodrug structure allows nepafenac to rapidly penetrate the cornea and reach its target sites, while minimizing surface accumulation and reducing ocular surface complications. Inhibits prostaglandin synthesis, reducing the intensity of pain and inflammation. In animal eyes, prostaglandins have been shown to produce disruption of

the blood-aqueous humor barrier, vasodilatation, increased vascular permeability, leukocytosis, and increased intraocular pressure. *Therapeutic Effect:* Produces analgesic and anti-inflammatory effects in the eye.

PHARMACOKINETICS

Two to 3 h after bilateral ophthalmic administration, given 3 times daily, low but quantifiable plasma concentrations of nepafenac and amfenac were observed in the majority of subjects. No other data available.

AVAILABILITY

Ophthalmic Suspension (Nevanac): 0.1%.

INDICATIONS AND DOSAGES

▸ Relief of ocular pain and inflammation in patients who have had cataract extraction

OPHTHALMIC

Adults, Elderly, and Children 10 yr of age and older. Apply 1 drop to affected eye(s) 3 times daily beginning 24 h before surgery, then continue on the day of surgery and for 2 wks.

CONTRAINDICATIONS

Hypersensitivity to nepafenac, to other NSAIDs, or any formulation ingredient.

INTERACTIONS

Drug
None known.
Herbal
None known.
Food
None known.

DIAGNOSTIC TEST EFFECTS

None known.

SIDE EFFECTS

Frequent (5%-10%)
Capsular opacity, decreased visual acuity, foreign body sensation, increased intraocular pressure, and sticky sensation.
Occasional (1%-5%)
Conjunctival edema, corneal edema, dry eye, lid margin crusting, ocular discomfort, ocular hyperemia, ocular pain, ocular pruritus, photophobia, tearing, and vitreous detachment. Some effects are probably the result of the surgical procedure.

SERIOUS REACTIONS

- Rare hypersensitivity reactions.
- Corneal adverse events such as thinning, erosion, or perforation.

PRECAUTIONS & CONSIDERATIONS

Use with caution in those with sulfite sensitivity, or previous allergic reactions to other NSAIDS; cross-reactivity may occur. There have been reports that ocularly applied NSAIDs may cause increased bleeding of ocular tissues following ocular surgery. Topical NSAIDS may slow or delay healing, or may cause keratitis. Use with caution in patients with known bleeding tendencies or who are on medications affecting bleeding times. Patients with complicated ocular surgeries, corneal denervation, corneal epithelial defects, diabetes mellitus, dry eye syndrome, or repeat ocular surgeries may be at increased risk for corneal adverse events that may become sight threatening. Use more than 24 h prior to surgery or use beyond 14 days postsurgery may increase patient risk for the occurrence and severity of corneal adverse events. Patients should not wear contact lenses during treatment. The safety and efficacy of nepafenac have not been established in children < 10 yr.

N

Use during pregnancy or lactation only if clearly needed; avoid use in late pregnancy due to potential effect on ductus arteriosis. No particular precautions needed in elderly patients.

Therapeutic response, such as decreased pain, surgical healing, and inflammation, should be assessed.

Storage

Store at controlled room temperature.

Administration

Shake well before each use. Take care to avoid contamination; do not allow dropper tip to touch any surface. Wash hands before use. Place index finger on the lower eyelid and pull gently until a pouch is formed. Place the prescribed number of drops in the pouch. Gently close the eye, and apply digital pressure to the lacrimal sac for 1-2 min to minimize the risk of systemic effects. Blot excess solution with a tissue.

N

Nesiritide

neh-sir′i-tide

Natrecor

CATEGORY AND SCHEDULE

Pregnancy Risk Category: C

Classification: Cardiovascular agents, inotropes, brain natriuretic peptide; endogenous hormone

MECHANISM OF ACTION

A brain natriuretic peptide that facilitates cardiovascular homeostasis and fluid status through counterregulation of the renin-angiotensin-aldosterone system, stimulating cyclic guanosine monophosphate, thereby leading to smooth muscle cell relaxation. *Therapeutic Effect:* Promotes vasodilation, natriuresis, and diuresis, correcting congestive heart failure (CHF).

PHARMACOKINETICS

Route	Onset	Peak	Duration
IV	15-30 min	1-2 h	4 h

Excreted primarily in the heart by the left ventricle. Metabolized by the natriuretic neutral endopeptidase enzymes on the vascular luminal surface. *Half-life:* 18-23 min.

AVAILABILITY

Injection Powder for Reconstitution: 1.5 mg vial.

INDICATIONS AND DOSAGES

▸ Treatment of acutely decompensated CHF in patients with dyspnea at rest or with minimal activity

IV INFUSION

Adults, Elderly. 2 mcg/kg bolus, followed by a continuous IV infusion of 0.01 mcg/kg/min. May be incrementally increased q3h to a maximum of 0.03 mcg/kg/min.

CONTRAINDICATIONS

Cardiogenic shock, systolic BP < 90 mm Hg, low cardiac filling pressures, hypersensitivity to nesiritide or product components, such as *E. coli*–derived proteins.

INTERACTIONS

Drug

ACE inhibitors, IV nitroglycerin, milrinone, nitroprusside: May increase risk of hypotension.

Herbal

None known.

Food

None known.

DIAGNOSTIC TEST EFFECTS

May see elevation in serum creatinine.

IV INCOMPATIBILITIES

Manufacturer states not to mix or infuse with any other medications. Ampicillin, ampicillin-sulbactam (Unasyn), bumetanide (Bumex), cefepime (Maxipime), diazepam, enalapril (Vasotec), ethacrynic acid (Edecrin), furosemide, (Lasix), heparin, hydralazine (Apresoline), insulin, labetalol, micafungin (Mycamine), pantoprazole, (Protonix), phenytoin, piperacillin-tazobactam (Zosyn), sodium metabisulfite.

SIDE EFFECTS

Frequent (11%)
Hypotension.
Occasional (3%-8%)
Headache, nausea, bradycardia, azotemia.
Rare (≤ 1%)
Confusion, paresthesia, somnolence, tremor.

SERIOUS REACTIONS

- Ventricular arrhythmias, including ventricular tachycardia, atrial fibrillation, AV node conduction abnormalities, and angina pectoris occur rarely.
- Hypotension requiring medical intervention.
- Hypersensitivity (rare).

PRECAUTIONS & CONSIDERATIONS

! Drug is intended for acute use in hospitals or emergency rooms.

Caution is warranted in patients with atrial conduction defects, constrictive pericarditis, hypotension, hepatic impairment, pericardial tamponade, renal impairment, restrictive or obstructive cardiomyopathy, significant valvular stenosis, suspected low cardiac filling pressures, and ventricular conduction defects. It is unknown whether nesiritide crosses the placenta or is distributed in breast milk, warranting caution in lactation. The safety and efficacy of nesiritide have not been established in children. No age-related precautions have been noted for elderly patients.

BP should be obtained immediately before each nesiritide dose, in addition to regular monitoring. Be alert to BP fluctuations. Place the patient in the supine position with legs elevated unless an excessive reduction in BP occurs. Intake and output records should be maintained. Notify the physician of chest pain, palpitations, cardiac arrhythmias, decreased urine output, or severe decrease in BP or heart rate.

Storage
Store vial at room temperature. Once reconstituted, store at room temperature or refrigerate; use within 24 h.

Administration
! Do not mix with other injections or infusions. Do not give IM.

Reconstitute one 1.5-mg vial with 5 mL D5W, 0.9% NaCl, 0.2% NaCl, or any combination thereof. Swirl or rock gently, and add to 250-mL bag D5W, 0.9% NaCl, 0.2% NaCl, or any combination thereof yielding a solution of 6 mcg/mL. Give initially as an IV bolus over approximately 60 seconds, followed by continuous IV infusion. The bolus dose is drawn from the infusion bag. Titrate infusion rate up no more frequently than every 3 h.

The catheter must be flushed with a compatible solution between

IV administration of nesiritide and other drugs.

Nevirapine

neh-veer'a-peen

Viramune

CATEGORY AND SCHEDULE

Pregnancy Risk Category: B

Classification: Antiretrovirals, nonnucleoside reverse transcriptase inhibitors (NNRTI)

MECHANISM OF ACTION

A nonnucleoside reverse transcriptase inhibitor that binds directly to HIV-1 reverse transcriptase, thus changing the shape of this enzyme and blocking RNA- and DNA-dependent polymerase activity. *Therapeutic Effect:* Interferes with HIV replication, slowing the progression of HIV infection.

PHARMACOKINETICS

Readily absorbed after PO administration. Protein binding: 60%. Widely distributed. Extensively metabolized in the liver. Excreted primarily in urine. *Half-life:* 45 h (single dose), 25-30 h (multiple doses).

AVAILABILITY

Tablets: 200 mg.
Oral Suspension: 50 mg/5 mL.

INDICATIONS AND DOSAGES

▸ HIV infection

PO

Adults. 200 mg once a day for 14 days (to reduce the risk of rash). Maintenance: 200 mg twice a day in combination with nucleoside analogues.

Children 15 days old and older. 150 mg/m² once daily for 14 days, followed by 150 mg/m² twice daily. Do not exceed 400 mg/day.

OFF-LABEL USES

To reduce the risk of transmitting HIV from infected mother to newborn.

CONTRAINDICATIONS

Hypersensitivity, moderate to severe hepatic impairment.

INTERACTIONS

Drug

Clarithromycin: May decrease activity of clarithromycin.
Efavirenz, methadone: May decrease concentrations of these drugs.
Fluconazone: May increase concentration of nevirapine.
Ketoconazole: Contraindicated; nevirapine negates ketoconazole effectiveness.
Oral contraceptives: May reduce effectiveness of oral contraception.
Rifampin, Rifabutin: May decrease nevirapine levels. Avoid.
Warfarin and other related anticoagualants: May increase INR.

Herbal

St. John's wort: May decrease blood concentration and effects of nevirapine. Avoid.

Food

None known.

DIAGNOSTIC TEST EFFECTS

May significantly increase serum bilirubin, GGT, AST (SGOT), and ALT (SGPT) levels. May significantly decrease hemoglobin level and neutrophil and platelet counts.

SIDE EFFECTS

Frequent (3%-8%)
Rash, fever, headache, nausea, fatigue, myalgia, granulocytopenia (more common in children).
Occasional (1%-3%)
Stomatitis (burning, erythema, or ulceration of the oral mucosa; dysphagia).
Rare (< 1%)
Paresthesia, abdominal pain.

SERIOUS REACTIONS

• Hepatitis and rash may become severe and life threatening. Severe life-threatening and sometimes fatal fulminant and cholestatic hepatic necrosis/failure.

PRECAUTIONS & CONSIDERATIONS

Caution is warranted in elderly patients, infants, and other patients with renal insufficiency or immaturity as well as those with neuromuscular disorders, hearing loss, or vertigo.
! 14-day dosing regimen must be strictly followed, with 18 mo of patient monitoring for skin and hepatic issues.

Drug is excreted in breast milk; breastfeeding is contraindicated. Nevirapine interferes with oral contraceptives; advise patient to remain compliant with oral regimen while adding another nonhormonal form of contraception for the duration of therapy.
Storage
Store at room temperature.
Administration
Continue taking nevirapine for the full course of treatment. May take without regard to food.

The suspension should be shaken gently before each use.

Niacin (Vitamin B_3; Nicotinic Acid)

nye′a-sin
★ 🍁 Niacor, Niaspan, Slo-Niacin
Do not confuse niacin, Niacor, or Niaspan with minocin, Nitro-Bid or nicotine.

CATEGORY AND SCHEDULE

Pregnancy Risk Category: A (C if used at dosages above the recommended daily allowance)

Classification: Vitamins, water soluble; B vitamins

MECHANISM OF ACTION

Nicotinic acid form is an antihyperlipidemic, water-soluble vitamin that is a component of two coenzymes needed for tissue respiration, lipid metabolism, and glycogenolysis. *Therapeutic Effect:* Reduces total, LDL, and VLDL cholesterol levels and triglyceride levels; increases HDL cholesterol concentration.
NOTE: Niacinamide, another form of vitamin B_3, is not effective as an antilipemic and is only used as a dietary supplement.

PHARMACOKINETICS

Widely distributed. Metabolized in the liver. Primarily excreted in urine. *Half-life:* 45 min.

AVAILABILITY

Capsules (Timed Release): 250 mg, 500 mg.
Tablets (Niacor): 50 mg, 100 mg, 250 mg, 500 mg.
Tablets (Timed Release [Slo-Niacin]): 250 mg, 500 mg, 750 mg.
Tablets (Timed Release [Niaspan]): 500 mg, 750 mg, 1000 mg.

N

INDICATIONS AND DOSAGES

▸ Hyperlipidemia

PO (IMMEDIATE RELEASE, NICOTINIC ACID ONLY)

Adults, Elderly. Initially, 50-100 mg twice a day for 7 days. Increase gradually by doubling dose weekly up to 1-1.5 g/day in 2-3 doses. Maximum: 3 g/day.

Children. Initially, 100-250 mg/day (maximum 10 mg/kg/day) in 3 divided doses. May increase by 100 mg/wk or 250 mg q2-3wk. Maximum: 2250 mg/day.

PO (TIMED RELEASE)

Adults, Elderly. Initially, 250 mg OR, 500 mg/day at bedtime for 1 wk; then increase to 500 mg twice a day. Maintenance: 2 g/day.

▸ Nutritional supplement

PO (IMMEDIATE RELEASE)

Adults, Elderly. 10-20 mg/day. Maximum: 100 mg/day.

▸ Pellagra

PO (IMMEDIATE RELEASE)

Adults, Elderly. 50-100 mg 3-4 times a day. Maximum: 500 mg/day.

Children. 50-100 mg 3 times a day.

CONTRAINDICATIONS

Active peptic ulcer disease, arterial hemorrhage, significant hepatic dysfunction, hypersensitivity to niacin or any formulation components.

INTERACTIONS

Drug

Antidiabetic agents, insulin: Niacin use may alter glycemic control. Monitor for needed adjustments.

Lovastatin, pravastatin, simvastatin, and other HMG-CoA reductase inhibitors: May increase the risk of myalgia and rhabdomyolysis.

Warfarin: Occasional reports of increased INR; monitor.

Herbal

None known.

Food

Alcohol and hot drinks: May increase risk of niacin side effects, such as flushing.

DIAGNOSTIC TEST EFFECTS

May increase serum uric acid, AST, ALT, and blood glucose levels. May increase PT. May decrease platelets or serum phosphorus level.

SIDE EFFECTS

Frequent

Flushing (especially of the face and neck) occurring within 20 min of drug administration and lasting for 30-60 min, GI upset, pruritus. Flushing will decrease with continued therapy.

Occasional

Dizziness, hypotension, headache, blurred vision, burning or tingling of skin, flatulence, nausea, vomiting, diarrhea.

Rare

Hyperglycemia, glycosuria, rash, hyperpigmentation, dry skin.

SERIOUS REACTIONS

- Arrhythmias occur rarely.
- Hepatic toxicity, necrosis (rare, but more common with sustained-release dosage forms).

PRECAUTIONS & CONSIDERATIONS

Caution is warranted with diabetes mellitus, gallbladder disease, gout, and a history of hepatic disease or jaundice. Niacin is not recommended for use during pregnancy. Niacin is distributed in breast milk and is not recommended during lactation. No age-related precautions have been noted in children or elderly patients. Niacin use is not recommended for children younger than 2 yr.

Be aware that itching, flushing of the skin, sensation of warmth, and tingling may occur. Notify the physician of dark urine, dizziness, loss of appetite, nausea, vomiting, weakness, yellowing of the skin, blurred vision, headache, or complaints of myalgia. Pattern of daily bowel activity and stool consistency should be assessed. Blood glucose level, serum cholesterol and triglyceride levels, and hepatic function test results should be checked at baseline and periodically during treatment.

Storage
Store at room temperature.

Administration
Avoid administration with alcohol or hot liquids to reduce incidence of flushing. Pretreatment with aspirin or NSAIDs can minimize skin flushing (if patient not allergic). Administration with food can lessen GI distress and pruritus.

Niaspan tablets should be taken at bedtime, after a low-fat snack. Extended-release products should not be broken, crushed, or chewed, but should be swallowed whole.

Nicardipine Hydrochloride

nye-card'i-peen high-droh-klor'ide

★ Cardene SR, Cardene IV

Do not confuse nicardipine with nifedipine, Cardene with codeine, or Cardene SR with Cardizem SR or codeine.

CATEGORY AND SCHEDULE

Pregnancy Risk Category: C

Classification: Antihypertensives, antianginals, calcium channel blockers (dihydropyridine group)

MECHANISM OF ACTION

An antianginal and antihypertensive agent that inhibits calcium ion movement across cell membranes, depressing contraction of cardiac and vascular smooth muscle. *Therapeutic Effect:* Increases heart rate and cardiac output. Decreases systemic vascular resistance and BP.

PHARMACOKINETICS

Route	Onset	Peak	Duration
PO	0.5-2h	1-2 h	8 h

Rapidly, completely absorbed from the GI tract. Protein binding: 95%. Undergoes first-pass metabolism in the liver. Primarily excreted in urine. Not removed by hemodialysis. *Half-life:* 2-4 h.

AVAILABILITY

Capsules: 20 mg, 30 mg.
Capsules, (Sustained Release [Cardene SR]): 30 mg, 45 mg, 60 mg.
Injection (Cardene IV): 2.5 mg/mL.
Premixed Infusion Bags: 20 mg/ 200 mL, 40 mg/200 mL.

INDICATIONS AND DOSAGES

▸ **Chronic stable (effort-associated) angina**

PO

Adults, Elderly. Initially, 20 mg 3 times a day. Range: 20-40 mg 3 times a day.

▸ **Essential hypertension**

PO

Adults, Elderly. Initially, 20 mg 3 times a day. Range: 20-40 mg 3 times a day.

PO (SUSTAINED RELEASE)

Adults, Elderly. Initially, 30 mg twice a day. Range: 30-60 mg twice a day.

▸ **Short-term treatment of hypertension when oral therapy is not feasible or desirable (substitute for oral nicardipine)**

IV INFUSION

Adults, Elderly. 0.5 mg/h (for patient receiving 20 mg PO q8h); 1.2 mg/h (for patient receiving 30 mg PO q8h); 2.2 mg/h (for patient receiving 40 mg PO q8h).

N

▸ **Patients not already receiving nicardipine**
IV INFUSION
Adults, Elderly (gradual BP decrease). Initially, 5 mg/h. May increase by 2.5 mg/h q15min. After BP goal is achieved, decrease rate to 3 mg/h.
Adults, Elderly (rapid BP decrease). Initially, 5 mg/h. May increase by 2.5 mg/h q5min. Maximum: 15 mg/h until desired BP is attained. After BP goal is achieved, decrease rate to 3 mg/h.
▸ **Changing from IV to oral antihypertensive therapy**
Adults, Elderly. A 50% offset of action occurs roughly 30 min after infusion is discontinued. Initiate other antihypertensives upon discontinuation of the infusion. If PO nicardipine is to be used, administer the first dose 1 h prior to weaning infusion off.
▸ **Dosage in hepatic impairment**
PO
For adults and elderly patients, initially give 20 mg twice a day; then titrate to response.
▸ **Dosage in renal impairment**
PO
For adults and elderly patients, initially give 20 mg q8h (30 mg twice a day sustained-release capsules); then titrate to response.

OFF-LABEL USES
Diabetic nephropathy, hypertensive urgency, postoperative hypertension.

CONTRAINDICATIONS
Atrial fibrillation or flutter associated with accessory conduction pathways, cardiogenic shock, congestive heart failure (CHF), second- or third-degree heart block, severe hypotension, sinus bradycardia, ventricular tachycardia, advanced aortic stenosis.

INTERACTIONS
Drug
β-Blockers: May have additive effect.
Carbamazepine: May increase effect of carbamazepine.
Digoxin: May have additive heart effects, monitor digoxin levels.
Erythromycin, ketoconazole, cimetidine, other CYP3A4 inhibitors: May increase plasma levels requiring patient monitoring.
Hypokalemia-producing agents (such as furosemide and certain other diuretics): May increase risk of arrhythmias.
Cyclosporine: May increase cyclosporine levels.
Indomethacin, possibly other NSAIDs, phenobarbital: May decrease effect of nicardipine.
Parenteral and inhalational general anesthetics or other drugs with hypotensive effects: May increase effects of these drugs.
Herbal
St. John's wort: May decrease effect of nicardipine.
Food
Grapefruit, grapefruit juice: May alter absorption of nicardipine and increase serum concentrations.

DIAGNOSTIC TEST EFFECTS
None known.

IV INCOMPATIBILITIES
Ampicillin, ampicillin-sulbactam (Unasyn), cefepime (Maxipime), ertapenem (Invanz), furosemide (Lasix), heparin, lansoprazole (Prevacid IV), micafungin (Mycamine), pantoprazole (Protonix), thiopental (Pentothal), tigecycline (Tygacil).

IV COMPATIBILITIES
Diltiazem (Cardizem), dobutamine (Dobutrex), dopamine (Intropin), epinephrine, hydromorphone (Dilaudid), labetalol (Trandate),

lorazepam (Ativan), midazolam (Versed), milrinone (Primacor), morphine, nitroglycerin, norepinephrine (Levophed).

SIDE EFFECTS

Frequent (7%-10%)
Headache, facial flushing, peripheral edema, light-headedness, dizziness.
Occasional (3%-6%)
Asthenia (loss of strength, energy), palpitations, angina, tachycardia.
Rare (< 2%)
Nausea, abdominal cramps, dyspepsia, dry mouth, rash.

SERIOUS REACTIONS

• Overdose produces confusion, slurred speech, somnolence, marked hypotension, and bradycardia.

PRECAUTIONS & CONSIDERATIONS

Caution is warranted in patients with cardiomyopathy, edema, hepatic or renal impairment, severe left ventricular dysfunction, sick sinus syndrome, and in those concurrently receiving β-blockers or digoxin. It is unclear whether nicardipine crosses the placenta. It should be administered only when the benefit to the mother exceeds the risk to the fetus. It is unknown whether nicardipine is distributed in breast milk, warranting caution in lactation. The safety and efficacy of nicardipine have not been established in children. In elderly patients, age-related renal impairment may require cautious use. Alcohol and caffeine should be limited while taking nicardipine. Patient should be advised to remain compliant with dietary sodium restrictions.

Notify the physician if anginal pain is not relieved by the medication and if constipation, dizziness, irregular heartbeat, nausea, shortness of breath, swelling, or symptoms of hypotension such as light-headedness occur. BP for hypotension, skin for dermatitis, facial flushing and rash, liver function test results, ECG and pulse for tachycardia should be assessed. The onset, type (sharp, dull, or squeezing), radiation, location, intensity, and duration of anginal pain and its precipitating factors, such as exertion and emotional stress, should be recorded. Sublingual nitroglycerin therapy may be used for relief of anginal pain. Caution with postural changes to prevent orthostatic hypotension from developing.

Storage
Store at room temperature. Store diluted IV solution for up to 24 h at room temperature.

Administration
Do not crush, open, or break sustained-release capsules. Take oral nicardipine without regard to food.

For IV use, dilute each 25-mg vial with 250 mL D5W, 0.9% NaCl, 0.45% NaCl, or any combination thereof to provide a concentration of 0.1 mg/mL. Maximum concentration is 0.4 mg/mL. Give by slow IV infusion. Change IV site every 12 h if drug is administered by a peripheral rather than a central venous catheter line.

Nicotine

nik′o-teen
★ Commit, NicoDerm CQ, Nicorette, Nicotrol, Nicotrol NS
🍁 Habitrol
Do not confuse NicoDerm with Nitroderm.

CATEGORY AND SCHEDULE

Pregnancy Risk Category: C (chewing gum), all other forms: D

Classification: Smoking deterrent

N

MECHANISM OF ACTION

A cholinergic-receptor agonist binds to acetylcholine receptors, producing both stimulating and depressant effects on the peripheral and central nervous systems. *Therapeutic Effect:* Provides a source of nicotine during nicotine withdrawal and reduces withdrawal symptoms.

PHARMACOKINETICS

Absorbed slowly after transdermal administration. Protein binding: 5%. Metabolized in the liver. Excreted primarily in urine. *Half-life:* 4 h.

AVAILABILITY

Chewing Gum (Nicorette, OTC): 2 mg, 4 mg.
Lozenge (Commit): 2 mg, 4 mg.
Transdermal Patch (NicoDerm CQ, Nicotrol): 7 mg, 14 mg, 21 mg.
Nasal Spray (Nicotrol NS): 0.5 mg/spray.
Inhalation (Nicotrol Inhaler): 10 mg cartridge.

INDICATIONS AND DOSAGES

▸ **Smoking cessation aid to relieve nicotine withdrawal symptoms**

PO (CHEWING GUM)

Adults, Elderly. Usually, 10-12 pieces/day. Maximum: 30 pieces/day.

PO (LOZENGE)

! For those who smoke the first cigarette within 30 min of waking, administer the 4-mg lozenge; otherwise, administer the 2-mg lozenge.

Adults, Elderly. One 4-mg or 2-mg lozenge q1-2h for the first 6 wks; one lozenge q2-4h for wks 7-9; and one lozenge q4-8h for wks 10-12. Maximum: 1 lozenge at a time, 5 lozenges/6 h, 20 lozenges/day.

TRANSDERMAL

Adults, Elderly who smoke 10 cigarettes or more per day. Follow the guidelines below:
Step 1: 21 mg/day for 4-6 wks.
Step 2: 14 mg/day for 2 wks.
Step 3: 7 mg/day for 2 wks.

Adults, Elderly who smoke < 10 cigarettes per day. Follow the guidelines below:
Step 1: 14 mg/day for 6 wks.
Step 2: 7 mg/day for 2 wks.

Patients weighing < 100 lb, patients with a history of cardiovascular disease. Initially, 14 mg/day for 4-6 wks, then 7 mg/day for 2-4 wks.

NASAL

Adults, Elderly. 1-2 doses/h (1 dose = 2 sprays [1 in each nostril] = 1 mg). Maximum: 5 doses (5 mg)/h; 40 doses (40 mg)/day.

INHALER (NICOTROL)

Adults, Elderly. Puff on nicotine cartridge mouthpiece for about 20 min as needed.

CONTRAINDICATIONS

Immediate post-myocardial infarction (MI) period, lifethreatening arrhythmias, severe or worsening angina, uncontrolled hypertension. Patients with such cardiac disease should be under physician care rather than self-use. Patients who continue to smoke, chew tobacco, use snuff are not candidates.

INTERACTIONS

Drug

Acetaminophen, caffeine, oxazepam, pentazocine, theophylline, β-adrenergic blockers, insulin, warfarin, tricyclic antidepressants, antipsychotics: Increased effects of these drugs as smoking ceases. Expect a need to decrease dose as smoking ceases.

Bupropion: Use of nicotine with bupropion for smoking cessation may elevate blood pressure. Monitor BP.

Cimetidine: May reduce nicotine clearance.

Ergot alkaloids: Increases risk of vasconstriction.
Use of more than 1 nicotine product: Do not use 2 nicotine-contanining products at one time.
Herbal
None known.
Food
Coffee, colas, acidic beverages: May interfere with nicotine gum; do not drink these while gum in mouth.

DIAGNOSTIC TEST EFFECTS

None known.

SIDE EFFECTS

Frequent
All forms: Hiccups, nausea.
Gum: Mouth or throat soreness, nausea, hiccups.
Transdermal: Erythema, pruritus, or burning at application site.
Occasional
All forms: Eructation, GI upset, dry mouth, insomnia, diaphoresis, irritability.
Gum: Hiccups, hoarseness.
Inhaler: Mouth or throat irritation, cough.
Rare
All forms: Dizziness, myalgia, arthralgia.

SERIOUS REACTIONS

• Overdose produces palpitations, tachyarrhythmias, seizures, depression, confusion, diaphoresis, hypotension, rapid or weak pulse, and dyspnea. Lethal dose for adults is 40-60 mg. Death results from respiratory paralysis. NOTE: In children, toxic doses are much smaller.

PRECAUTIONS & CONSIDERATIONS

Caution is warranted in patients with eczematous dermatitis, esophagitis, hyperthyroidism, insulin-dependent diabetes mellitus, oral or pharyngeal inflammation, peptic ulcer disease, pheochromocytoma, or severe renal impairment. Nicotine passes freely into breast milk, and smoking and nicotine are associated with a decrease in fetal breathing movements during pregenancy. The use of nicotine is not recommended for breastfeeding women. Nicotine use is not recommended for children. In elderly patients, an age-related decrease in cardiac function may require cautious use.

Notify the physician of itching or a persistent rash during treatment with the transdermal patch. Vital signs, including BP and pulse rate, should be obtained before and during treatment.

Storage
Store all products at room temperature. Keep gum and patches in overwraps until time of use to prevent loss of potency.

Administration
! Expect to individualize nicotine dosage and to administer the drug when the patient plans to stop smoking.

Chew 1 piece of gum slowly and intermittently for 30 min when there is an urge to smoke. Chew until the distinctive peppery nicotine taste or slight tingling in mouth occurs. Then, park in the cheek. When the tingling is almost gone, after approximately 1 min, repeat the chewing procedure to allow constant, slow buccal absorption. Do not chew too rapidly because this may cause nausea and throat irritation. Do not swallow the gum.

For transdermal use, apply the patch as soon as it has been removed from the protective pouch. Use only an intact pouch. Do not cut the patch. Apply the patch only once daily to a hairless, clean, dry area on the upper body or outer arm. Rotate application sites; do not use the same site for 7 days or the same patch for longer than 24 h. Wash hands with water alone after applying the patch because soap may increase nicotine absorption. To discard a used patch, fold it in half with the sticky sides together, place it in the pouch of the new patch, and discard it in a receptacle that is not accessible to children or pets. Do not smoke while wearing the patch.

To avoid possible burns, remove patch if the patient will go to MRI (magentic resonance imaging) procedures. If insomnia occurs, patients may remove the daily patch at bedtime each day.

To use the inhaler, insert the cartridge into mouthpiece and puff vigorously for 20 min.

N

Nifedipine

nye-fed'i-peen

★ Adalat CC, Afeditab CR, Nifediac CC, Nifedical XL, Procardia, Procardia XL

Do not confuse nifedipine with nicardipine or nimodipine.

CATEGORY AND SCHEDULE

Pregnancy Risk Category: C

Classification: Antihypertensives, anti-anginals, calcium channel blockers (dihydropyridine group)

MECHANISM OF ACTION

An antianginal and antihypertensive agent that inhibits calcium ion movement across cell membranes, depressing contraction of cardiac and vascular smooth muscle. *Therapeutic Effect:* Increases heart rate and cardiac output. Decreases systemic vascular resistance and BP.

PHARMACOKINETICS

Route	Onset	Peak	Duration
Sublingual	1-5 min	NA	N/A
PO	20-30 min	NA	4-8 h
PO (extended release)	2 h	NA	24 h

Rapidly, completely absorbed from the GI tract. Protein binding: 92%-98%. Undergoes first-pass metabolism in the liver. Excreted primarily in urine. Not removed by hemodialysis. *Half-life:* 2-5 h.

AVAILABILITY

Capsules (Procardia): 10 mg.
Tablets (Extended Release [Adalat CC, Afeditab CR, Nifediac CC): 30 mg, 60 mg, 90 mg.
Tablets (Extended Release, Osmotic Release, Procardia XL, Nifedical XL]): 30 mg, 60 mg, 90 mg.

INDICATIONS AND DOSAGES

▸ **Prinzmetal variant angina, chronic stable (effort-associated) angina**

PO

Adults, Elderly. Initially, 10 mg 3 times a day. Increase at 7- to 14-day intervals. Maintenance: 10 mg 3 times a day up to 30 mg 4 times a day.

PO (EXTENDED RELEASE)

Adults, Elderly. Initially, 30-60 mg/day. Maintenance: Up to 90 mg/day.

▸ **Essential hypertension**
PO (EXTENDED RELEASE)
Adults, Elderly. Initially, 30-60 mg/day. Maintenance: Up to 120 mg/day.

OFF-LABEL USES

Premature labor, intractable hiccups, diabetic nephropathy migraine prophylaxis.

CONTRAINDICATIONS

Hypersensitivity, advanced aortic stenosis, severe hypotension. Use of potent CYP3A4 inducers.

INTERACTIONS

Drug
β-Blockers: May have additive effect.
Carbamazepine: May increase effects of carbamazepine.
Digoxin: May increase digoxin blood concentration.
Hypokalemia-producing agents (such as furosemide and certain other diuretics): May increase risk of arrhythmias.
Indomethacin, other NSAIDs, phenobarbital: May decrease effect of these drugs.
Inhibitors of CYP3A4 isoenzymes: May increase effects of nifedipine.
Parenteral and inhalational general anesthetics or other drugs with hypotensive actions: May increase these effects.
Potent CYP3A4 inducers (e.g., rifampin, barbiturates): Decrease effects of nifedipine significantly; contraindicated.
Herbal
None known.
Food
Grapefruit, grapefruit juice: May increase nifedipine plasma concentration. Avoid.

DIAGNOSTIC TEST EFFECTS

Rare, usually transient, but occasionaly significant elevations of enzymes such as alkaline phosphatase, CPK, LDH, SGOT, and SGPT have been noted. Serum creatinine or BUN may also increase rarely. May cause positive ANA and direct Coombs' test.

SIDE EFFECTS

Frequent (11%-30%)
Peripheral edema, headache, flushed skin, dizziness.
Occasional (6%-12%)
Nausea, shakiness, muscle cramps and pain, somnolence, palpitations, nasal congestion, cough, dyspnea, wheezing.
Rare (3%-5%)
Hypotension, rash, pruritus, urticaria, constipation, abdominal discomfort, flatulence, sexual difficulties.

SERIOUS REACTIONS

- Nifedipine may precipitate CHF and myocardial infarction (MI) in patients with cardiac disease and peripheral ischemia.
- Overdose produces nausea, somnolence, confusion, and slurred speech; excessive hypotension, EKG changes may occur, including heart block.
- When given via the sublingual method for rapid control of hypertension, may cause profound hypotension, acute MI, or death. Do not use nifedipine for this purpose.

PRECAUTIONS & CONSIDERATIONS

Caution is warranted in patients with impaired hepatic and renal function. Caution is advised in patients with cardiac conduction problems, heart failure, or existing edema. It is unclear whether nifedipine crosses the placenta. It should be administered only when the benefit to the mother outweighs the risk to the fetus. An insignificant amount of nifedipine is distributed in breast milk. The safety and efficacy of nifedipine have not been established in children. In elderly patients, age-related renal impairment may require cautious use. Alcohol and tasks that require alertness and motor skills should also be avoided until the effects of the drug are known. Patients should be advised to remain compliant with dietary sodium restrictions.

Dizziness or light-headedness may occur. Notify the physician if irregular heartbeat, prolonged dizziness, nausea, or shortness of breath occurs. BP and liver function should be monitored. Skin should be assessed for flushing and peripheral edema, especially behind the medial malleolus and the sacral area. The onset, type (sharp, dull, or squeezing), radiation, location, intensity, and duration of anginal pain and its precipitating factors, such as exertion and emotional stress, should be recorded. Be aware that concurrent administration of sublingual nitroglycerin therapy may be used for relief of anginal pain. Overdose produces nausea, somnolence, confusion, and slurred speech.

Storage

Store at room temperature. Protect from moisture.

Administration

Do not crush or break extended-release tablets. Take oral nifedipine without regard to meals.

! Never give the contents of the immediate-release capsules sublingually.

Avoid coadministration with grapefruit juice.

Nilotinib

ni-loe'ti-nib

★ Tasigna

CATEGORY AND SCHEDULE

Pregnancy Risk Category: D

Classification: Antineoplastic, signal transduction inhibitors

MECHANISM OF ACTION

Highly specific; inhibits BCR-ABL tyrosine kinase, an enzyme created by the Philadelphia chromosome abnormality found in select leukemia cell lines. Also inhibits C-KIT and platelet derived growth factor. *Therapeutic Effect:* Suppresses tumor growth during the three stages of chronic myeloid leukemia (CML): blast crisis, accelerated phase, and chronic phase.

PHARMACOKINETICS

Absorption is greatly increased by food; must take on an empty stomach. Total gastrectomy decreases absorption significantly (53%). Protein binding: 98%. Metabolized in liver, primarily by CYP3A4 to inactive metabolites. Primarily eliminated in feces (93%, 69% as unchanged); minimal excretion in urine (4%, 0.1% unchanged). *Half-life:* 17 h.

AVAILABILITY

Capsules (Hard Gelatin): 150 mg, 200 mg.

INDICATIONS AND DOSAGES

▸ **Chronic phase or accelerated phase Philadelphia chromosome-positive CML, (Ph+ CML), resistant or intolerant to prior therapy, including imatinib**

PO

Adults. 400 mg twice a day (morning and evening).

▸ **Newly diagnosed Ph+ CML**

PO

Adults. 300 mg twice a day.

▸ **Dosage for hepatic impairment**

Patients are given a lower starting dosage initially, then slowly titrated to the full dosage if tolerated. See manufacturer's recommendations based on disease state and hepatic status.

▸ **Dosage adjustment for toxicities**

Expect temporary discontinuation or a reduction in dosage in patients with myelosuppression grade 3 or higher. Withhold therapy if QTc prolongation occurs. Elevated hepatic enzymes, lipase, amylase, or bilirubin may require a dose reduction. See manufacturer's information for recommendations.

CONTRAINDICATIONS

Hypersensitivity to nilotinib or its components. Do not use in patients with hypokalemia, hypomagnesemia, or long QT syndrome.

INTERACTIONS

NOTE: Nilotinib inhibits p-glycoprotein, CYP3A4, CYP2C8, CYP2C9, CYP2D6, and UGT1A1, increasing the concentrations of drugs eliminated by these enzymes. The drug may induce CYP2B6, CYP2C8, and CYP2C9 and decrease the concentrations of drugs that are eliminated by these enzymes.

Drug

H_2 antagonists, proton-pump inhibitors: Decreased nilotinib absorption. Avoid if possible.

Anticoagulants, NSAIDs: Increased risk of bleeding.

Strong CYP3A4 inhibitors (e.g., clarithromycin, erythromycin, ketoconazole, nefazodone, protease inhibitors, voriconazole): May increase the levels and adverse effects of nilotinib. Avoid use when possible. Should treatment with any of these agents be required, interrupt nilotinib treatment or continue dose reduction.

CYP3A4 substrates (midazolam, triazolam): Increased plasma concentrations of these drugs roughly 30% with increased risk of CNS depression.

CYP3A4 inducers (e.g., dexamethasone, phenytoin, carbamazepine, rifampin, rifabutin, rifapentine, phenobarbital): Decreased nilotinib activity and levels. Avoid. Increasing nilotinib dose may not ensure efficacy.

QTc-prolonging medications (e.g., antiarrhythmics: amiodarone, disopyramide, procainamide, quinidine, and sotalol) and other drugs that may prolong QT interval (e.g., cisapride, chloroquine, clarithromycin, haloperidol, methadone, moxifloxacin, pimozide, thioridazine, and others): Avoid co-use. Should treatment with any of these agents be required, interrupt nilotinib treatment.

Herbal

St. John's wort: Decrease nilotinib levels. Avoid.

Food

All food: Increased nilotinib exposure and side effects; must take on empty stomach.

Grapefruit juice: May increase nilotinib levels and adverse effects. Do NOT drink grapefruit juice while taking nilotinib.

DIAGNOSTIC TEST EFFECTS

Elevations in bilirubin, AST/ALT, and alkaline phosphatase. Decreased WBC and platelets. Lowered phosphate, potassium, calcium, and sodium blood concentrations. QTc prolongation on EKG. May elevate serum lipase or amylase.

SIDE EFFECTS

Frequent

Neutropenia, thrombocytopenia, anemia. Also, rash, pruritus, headache, nausea, fatigue, myalgia, nasopharyngitis, constipation, diarrhea, abdominal pain, vomiting, arthralgia, pyrexia, upper urinary tract infection, back pain, cough, and asthenia.

Occasional

Electrolyte imbalances, arthralgia, febrile neutropenia, vertigo, angina, peripheral edema, dyspnea, epistaxis, prolonged QT interval, elevated hepatic enzymes, insomnia, dizziness, hypoesthesia, paresthesia.

Less Common

Hypersensitivity, tumor lysis syndrome, eye hemorrhage, periorbital edema, eye pruritus, conjunctivitis, dry eye, night sweats, eczema, dry skin.

SERIOUS REACTIONS

- Nilotinib may cause severe bone marrow suppression (thrombocytopenia, neutropenia, anemia).
- Hepatitis, jaundice.
- Pancreatitis.
- Fluid retention may cause pulmonary edema.
- QT prolongation, torsades de pointes and other arrhythmias, sudden death.

PRECAUTIONS & CONSIDERATIONS

Use with caution in patients with impaired hepatic function, cardiovascular disease (uncontrolled or significant cardiovascular disease, including recent myocardial infarction, congestive heart failure, unstable angina, or clinically significant bradycardia), pulmonary disease, history of pancreatitis, and patients potentially at risk for QT prolongation. Correct electrolyte imbalance prior to initiating treatment, and carefully monitor serum electrolytes. Safety and effectiveness have not been established in children. Fluid retention may occur more often in the elderly. Women of childbearing potential should be advised to use adequate contraception as the drug may cause fetal harm. Breast milk excretion unknown; do not breastfeed.

Storage

Store at room temperature. Keep in original blister pack until time of use.

Administration

Must take on an empty stomach; do not consume food 2 h before or 1 h after taking a dose. Capsules should be swallowed whole, not crushed or cut. Do not give with grapefruit juice.

Nilutamide

nih-lute′ah-myd

★ Nilandron 🍁 Anandron

CATEGORY AND SCHEDULE

Pregnancy Risk Category: C

Classification: Hormone modifier, anti-androgen, antineoplastic

MECHANISM OF ACTION

An antiandrogen hormone and antineoplastic agent that competitively inhibits androgen action by binding to androgen receptors in target tissue.
Therapeutic Effect: Decreases growth of abnormal prostate tissue.

PHARMACOKINETICS

Consistently well absorbed. Undergoes distribution phase. Moderate protein binding, includes α-1-glycoprotein. Extensively liver metabolized to 5 metabolites; one shows partial activity of the parent drug. Roughly 62% of dose is eliminated in the urine; less than 2% is excreted unchanged. Minor elimination in feces. *Half-Life:*38-59 h (parent drug).

AVAILABILITY

Tablets: 150 mg.

INDICATIONS AND DOSAGES

▸ **Metastatic prostate cancer**

PO

Adults, Elderly. 300 mg once a day for 30 days, then 150 mg once a day. Begin on day of, or day after, surgical castration.

CONTRAINDICATIONS

Severe hepatic impairment, severe respiratory insufficiency, hypersensitivity.

INTERACTIONS

Drug

Warfarin, phenytoin, theophylline, other drugs metabolized by CYP450 with narrow therapeutic margin: Nilutamide may cause delayed elimination and increases the levels of these drugs.

Herbal

None known.

Food

Alcohol: Intolerance to alcohol (facial flushes, malaise, hypotension) may occur. Avoid.

DIAGNOSTIC TEST EFFECTS

May increase serum bilirubin, creatinine, AST (SGOT), and ALT (SGPT) levels.

SIDE EFFECTS

Frequent (> 10%)

Hot flashes, delay in recovering vision after bright illumination (such as sun, television, bright lights), decreased libido, diminished sexual function, mild nausea, gynecomastia, alcohol intolerance.

Occasional (< 10%)

Constipation, hypertension, dizziness, dyspnea, urinary tract infection.

SERIOUS REACTIONS

- Interstitial pneumonitis occurs rarely.
- Hepatitis, severe liver injury.

PRECAUTIONS & CONSIDERATIONS

Caution is warranted in patients with hepatitis and markedly increased serum hepatic function test results. Avoid driving at night. Tinted glasses are recommended to help decrease the visual effect of bright headlights and streetlights.

Notify the physician if signs of hepatotoxicity occur, such as abdominal pain, dark urine, fatigue, and jaundice. A baseline chest radiogram and liver function tests should be obtained before therapy and periodically during long-term therapy.

Be alert for exertional dyspnea, worsening shortness of breath, cough, chest pain, and fever. Get a baseline chest x-ray before treating. Most cases of lung problems occur in the first 3 mo of treatment. X-rays may show intersitial or alveolo-interstitial changes, and PFTs reveal a restrictive pattern if symptoms occur, discontinue the drug and evaluate.

Storage

Store at room temperature protected from light. Keep in foil blister packaging until time of use.

Administration

Take oral nilutamide with or without food.

Nimodipine

nye-mode'i-peen

Nimotop

Do not confuse nimodipine with nifedipine.

CATEGORY AND SCHEDULE

Pregnancy Risk Category: C

Classification: Neurologic agents, selective calcium channel blockers (dihydropyridine group)

MECHANISM OF ACTION

A cerebral vasospasm agent that inhibits movement of calcium ions across vascular smooth-muscle cell membranes. More specific to the CNS than other drugs in the class. *Therapeutic Effect:* Produces favorable effect on severity of neurologic deficits due to cerebral vasospasm. Exerts greatest effect on cerebral arteries; may prevent cerebral spasm.

PHARMACOKINETICS

Rapidly absorbed from the GI tract. Protein binding: 95%. Metabolized in the liver. Excreted in urine; eliminated in feces. Not removed by hemodialysis. *Half-life:* terminal, 3 h.

AVAILABILITY

Capsules: 30 mg.

INDICATIONS AND DOSAGES

▸ **Improvement in neurologic deficits after subarachnoid hemorrhage from ruptured congenital aneurysms**

PO

Adults, Elderly. 60 mg q4h for 21 days. Begin within 96 h of subarachnoid hemorrhage.

▸ **Dosage in hepatic impairment (cirrhosis)**

PO

Adults. 30 mg q4h for 21 days; closely monitor BP and heart rate.

CONTRAINDICATIONS

Hypersensitivity.

INTERACTIONS

Drug

Anesthetics, other antihypertensive medications: May increase risk of hypotension.

β-Blockers: May prolong SA and AV conduction, which may lead to severe hypotension, bradycardia, and cardiac failure.

Cimetidine: Increases nimodipine concentrations.

Erythromycin, itraconazole, ketoconazole, protease inhibitors: May inhibit the metabolism of nimodipine.

Indomethacin and possibly other NSAIDs: May antagonize antihypertensive effect.

Rifabutin, rifampin: May increase the metabolism of nimodipine.

Sympathomimetics: May reduce antihypertensive effects.

Herbal

Garlic: May increase antihypertensive effect.

Ginseng, yohimbe: May worsen hypertension.

Food
Grapefruit juice: May increase nimodipine blood concentration and risk of toxicity. Avoid.

DIAGNOSTIC TEST EFFECTS
None known.

SIDE EFFECTS
Occasional (2%-6%)
Hypotension, peripheral edema, diarrhea, headache.
Rare (< 2%)
Allergic reaction (rash, hives), tachycardia, flushing of skin.

SERIOUS REACTIONS
• Overdose produces nausea, weakness, dizziness, confusion, slurred speech, hypotension, and cardiac effects similar to other CCBs.

PRECAUTIONS & CONSIDERATIONS
Caution is warranted in patients with impaired hepatic and renal function. It is unknown whether nimodipine crosses the placenta or is distributed in breast milk; caution is warranted in lactation. The safety and efficacy of nimodipine have not been established in children. Elderly patients may also experience greater hypotensive response and constipation.

Notify the physician if constipation, dizziness, irregular heartbeat, nausea, shortness of breath, or swelling occurs. Liver function, neurologic response, BP, and heart rate should be assessed before and during therapy. If the pulse rate is 60 beats/min or lower or systolic BP is < 90 mm Hg, withhold the medication and contact the physician.
Storage
Keep at room temperature in original foil packaging until time of use; protect from light and do not freeze.

Administration
If unable to swallow, place a hole in both ends of a capsule with an 18-gauge needle to extract contents into a syringe. Empty contents of syringe into a nasogastric (NG) tube; flush tube with 30 mL normal saline. Avoid coadministration with grapefruit juice.
! Do not administer contents of capsules IV. Fatal medication errors have occurred.

Nisoldipine
nye′soul-dih-peen
★ Sular
Do not confuse nisoldipine with nicardipine.

CATEGORY AND SCHEDULE
Pregnancy Risk Category: C

Classification: Antihypertensives, calcium channel antagonist (dihydropyridine group)

MECHANISM OF ACTION
A calcium channel blocker that inhibits calcium ion movement across cell membrane, depressing contraction of cardiac and vascular smooth muscle. *Therapeutic Effect:* Increases heart rate and cardiac output. Decreases systemic vascular resistance and BP.

PHARMACOKINETICS
Poor absorption from the GI tract. Food increases bioavailability. Protein binding: > 99%. Metabolism occurs in the gut wall. Primarily excreted in urine. Not removed by hemodialysis. *Half-life:* 7-12 h.

AVAILABILITY
Tablets (Extended Release): 8.5 mg, 17 mg, 25.5 mg, 34 mg (Sular).

INDICATIONS AND DOSAGES

▸ Hypertension

PO

Adults. Initially, 17 mg once daily; then increase by 8.5 mg/wk or longer intervals until therapeutic BP response is attained. In the elderly or in those with impaired liver function, start 8.5 mg once daily. Increase by 8.5 mg/wk to therapeutic response. Maintenance: 17-34 mg once daily.

OFF-LABEL USES

Stable angina pectoris.

CONTRAINDICATIONS

Sick sinus syndrome/second- or third degree AV block (except in presence of pacemaker), hypersensitivity to nisoldipine or any component of the formulation.

N

INTERACTIONS

Drug

Amiodarone: May increase risk of bradycardia, atrioventricular block, or sinus arrest.
β-Blockers: May have additive effect.
Delavirdine, ketoconazole, voriconazole: May increase serum nisoldipine concentrations.
Digoxin: May increase digoxin blood concentration.
Epirubicin: May increase risk of heart failure.
Fentanyl: May increase risk of severe hypotension.
NSAIDs, oral anticoagulants: May increase risk of gastrointestinal hemorrhage and/or antagonism of hypotensive effect.
Phenytoin, fosphenytoin: May decrease nisoldipine concentrations.
Quinidine: May increase risk of quinidine toxicity.
Quinupristin/dalfopristin, saquinavir: May increase risk of nisoldipine toxicity.
Rifampin: May decrease nisoldipine efficacy.

Herbal

Licorice, ma huang, peppermint oil, yohimbine: May decrease effectiveness of nisoldipine.
St. John's wort: May decrease bioavailability of nisoldipine.

Food

Grapefruit and grapefruit juice, or high-fat meal: May increase nisoldipine plasma concentration. Avoid.

DIAGNOSTIC TEST EFFECTS

None known.

SIDE EFFECTS

Frequent

Giddiness, dizziness, lightheadedness, peripheral edema, headache, flushing, weakness, nausea.

Occasional

Transient hypotension, heartburn, muscle cramps, nasal congestion, cough, wheezing, sore throat, palpitations, nervousness, mood changes.

Rare

Increase in frequency, intensity, duration of anginal attack during initial therapy.

SERIOUS REACTIONS

- May precipitate CHF and myocardial infarction (MI) in patients with cardiac disease and peripheral ischemia.
- Overdose produces nausea, drowsiness, confusion, and slurred speech.

PRECAUTIONS & CONSIDERATIONS

Caution is warranted in patients with impaired liver or renal function, aortic stenosis, or cirrhosis. It is unknown whether nisoldipine crosses the placenta or is distributed in breast milk, warranting caution in lactation. Safety and efficacy of nisoldipine have not been established in children. Age-related renal impairment may require cautious use in elderly patients.

Rise slowly from lying to sitting position and permit legs to dangle from bed momentarily before standing to reduce hypotensive effect. Contact physician if irregular heartbeat, shortness of breath, pronounced dizziness, or nausea occurs.

Storage

Store at room temperature. Protect from light and moisture.

Administration

Swallow capsule whole. Do not chew, divide, or crush. Take at the same time each day to ensure minimal fluctuation of serum levels.

Do not administer with grapefruit juice. Take on an empty stomach 1 h before on 2 h after a meal.

Nitazoxanide

nigh-tazz-oks′ah-nide

★ Alinia

CATEGORY AND SCHEDULE

Pregnancy Risk Category: B

Classification: Antiprotozoals

MECHANISM OF ACTION

An antiparasitic that interferes with the body's reaction to pyruvate ferredoxin oxidoreductase, an enzyme essential for anaerobic energy metabolism. *Therapeutic Effect:* Produces antiprotozoal activity, reducing or terminating diarrheal episodes.

PHARMACOKINETICS

Rapidly hydrolyzed to an active metabolite. Protein binding: 99%. Excreted in the urine, bile, and feces. *Half-life:* 2-4 h.

AVAILABILITY

Powder for Oral Suspension: 100 mg/5 mL.

Tablet: 500 mg.

INDICATIONS AND DOSAGES

▸ **Infectious diarrhea due to *Giardia lamblia* or *Cryptosporidium parvum***

PO

Adults, Children aged 12 yr and older. 500 mg q12h for 3 days.

Children 4-11 yr. 200 mg (10 mL) q12h for 3 days.

Children aged 12-47 mo. 100 mg (5 mL) q12h for 3 days.

OFF-LABEL USES

Alternative agent for *C dificile*–associated diarrhea.

CONTRAINDICATIONS

History of sensitivity to the drug.

INTERACTIONS

Drug

Warfarin: Potential for displacement from protein-binding sites and increase in effect. Monitor INR.

Herbal

None known.

Food

None known.

DIAGNOSTIC TEST EFFECTS

May increase serum creatinine and ALT (SGPT) levels.

SIDE EFFECTS

Occasional (8%)

Abdominal pain.

Rare (1%-2%)

Diarrhea, vomiting, headache.

SERIOUS REACTIONS

- None known.

PRECAUTIONS & CONSIDERATIONS

Caution is warranted with biliary or hepatic disease, GI disorders, and renal impairment. The oral suspension contains sucrose and caution is warranted if patient has diabetes mellitus. There are no adequate data in pregnancy. It is unknown if nitazoxanide is distributed in breast milk, warranting cautious use in lactation. The safety and efficacy of nitazoxanide have not been established in children less than 1 yr of age. Nitazoxanide is not indicated for use in elderly patients.

Pattern of daily bowel activity and stool consistency, electrolytes, and hydration status should be monitored. Patients should be cautioned to maintain hydration and electrolyte levels following recovery.

Storage

Store unreconstituted powder at room temperature. Reconstituted solution is stable for 7 days at room temperature.

Administration

Take with food. Shake oral suspension well before each use.

Nitrofurantoin

nye-troe-fyoor′an-toyn

★ Furadantin, Macrobid, Macrodantin 🍁 Macrobid

CATEGORY AND SCHEDULE

Pregnancy Risk Category: B

Classification: Antibiotics, nitrofurans, urinary anti-infectives.

MECHANISM OF ACTION

An antibacterial urinary tract infection (UTI) agent that inhibits the synthesis of bacterial DNA, RNA, proteins, and cell walls by altering or inactivating ribosomal proteins. *Therapeutic Effect:* Bacteriostatic (bactericidal at high concentrations).

PHARMACOKINETICS

Microcrystalline form rapidly and completely absorbed; macrocrystalline form more slowly absorbed. Food increases absorption. Protein binding: 60%-90%. Primarily concentrated in urine and kidneys. Metabolized in most body tissues. Primarily excreted in urine. Removed by hemodialysis. *Half-life:* 20-60 min.

AVAILABILITY

Capsules (Macrobid [Macrocrystalline]): 100 mg.
Capsules (Macrodantin [Macrocrystalline]): 25 mg, 50 mg, 100 mg.
Oral Suspension (Furadantin [Microcrystalline]): 25 mg/5 mL.

INDICATIONS AND DOSAGES

▸ **Urinary tract infections (UTIs)**

PO

Adults, Elderly, Children older than 12 yr. (Furadantin, Macrodantin): 50-100 mg q6h with food for 7 days and 3 days thereafter until sterile urine is obtained. Maximum: 400mg/day or roughly 7 mg/g/day. (Macrobid): 100 mg 2 times/day.

Children older than 1 mo and younger than 12 yr. (Furadantin, Macrodantin): 5-7 mg/kg/day in divided doses q6h with food for 7 days and 3 days thereafter until sterile urine is obtained. Maximum: 400 mg/day.

▸ **Long-term prevention of UTIs**

PO (Furadantin, Macrodantin, NOT Macrobid):

Adults, Elderly. 50-100 mg at bedtime.
Children. 1-2 mg/kg/day as a single dose or in 2 divided doses not to exceed maximum: 100 mg/day.

OFF-LABEL USES

Prevention of bacterial UTIs.

CONTRAINDICATIONS

Hypersensitivity, including previous history of cholestatic jaundice/hepatic dysfunction associated with nitrofurantoin. Anuria, oliguria, substantial renal impairment (creatinine clearance < 60 mL/min); infants younger than 1 mo old because of the risk of hemolytic anemia.

INTERACTIONS

Drug

Antacids containing magnesium salts: May decrease absorption and anti-infective activity of nitrofurantoin.
Anticholinergic drugs: May increase absorption of nitrofurantoin.
Probenecid: May increase blood concentration and toxicity of nitrofurantoin.
Zalcitabine: May increase the risk of neurotoxicity.

Herbal

None known.

Food

None known.

DIAGNOSTIC TEST EFFECTS

Urinary creatine elevation and false positive glucose determination with Benedict reagent.

SIDE EFFECTS

Frequent

Anorexia, nausea, vomiting, dark urine.

Occasional

Abdominal pain, diarrhea, rash, pruritus, urticaria, hypertension, headache, dizziness, drowsiness.

Rare

Photosensitivity, transient alopecia, asthmatic exacerbation in those with history of asthma.

SERIOUS REACTIONS

- Hepatotoxicity, peripheral neuropathy (may be irreversible), Stevens-Johnson syndrome, and anaphylaxis occur rarely.
- Hemolytic anemia.
- Intersitial pneumonitis or pulmonary fibrosis.
- Pseudomembranous colitis and other superinfections.

PRECAUTIONS & CONSIDERATIONS

Caution is warranted with debilitated patients (greater risk of peripheral neuropathy) and in patients with anemia, diabetes mellitus, electrolyte imbalance, glucose-6-phosphate dehydrogenase (G6PD) deficiency (greater risk of hemolytic anemia), renal impairment, or vitamin B deficiency. Nitrofurantoin readily crosses the placenta and is distributed in breast milk. Nitrofurantoin use is contraindicated at term and during breastfeeding if the infant is suspected of having G6PD deficiency. No age-related precautions have been noted in children older than 1 mo. Elderly patients are more likely to develop acute pneumonitis and peripheral neuropathy and may require a dosage adjustment because of age-related renal impairment. Avoid sun and ultraviolet light.

Urine may turn dark yellow, orange, or brown. Hair loss may occur but is only temporary.
Notify the physician if chest pain, cough, difficult breathing, fever, or numbness and tingling occur. Intake and output, renal function, bowel activity, skin for rash, and breathing should be monitored. Overdosage is manifested by vomiting.

Storage
Store at room temperature.
Administration
Take nitrofurantoin with food or milk to enhance absorption and reduce GI upset.

Shake suspension well before each use.

Nitroglycerin

nye-troe-gli'ser-in
★ Minitran, Nitro-Bid, Nitro-Dur, Nitrolingual, NitroMist Nitrostat, Nitro-Time 🍁 Nitroject, Transderm-Nitro, Trinipatch
Do not confuse nitroglycerin with nitroprusside; Nitro-Bid with Nicobid; Nitro-Dur with Nicoderm; Nitrostat with Hyperstat, Nilstat.

CATEGORY AND SCHEDULE

Pregnancy Risk Category: C

Classification: Antianginals, vasodilators

N

MECHANISM OF ACTION

A nitrate that decreases myocardial oxygen demand. Reduces left ventricular preload and afterload. *Therapeutic Effect:* Dilates coronary arteries and improves collateral blood flow to ischemic areas within myocardium. IV form produces peripheral vasodilation.

PHARMACOKINETICS

Route	Onset (min)	Peak (min)	Duration
Sublingual	1-3	4-8	30-60 min
Translingual spray	2	4-10	30-60 min
Buccal tablet	2-5	4-10	2 hr
PO (extended release)	20-45	45-120	4-8 h
Topical	15-60	30-120	2-12 h
Transdermal patch	40-60	60-180	18-24 h
IV	Immed-iate	1-2	3-5 min

Well absorbed after PO, sublingual, and topical administration. Undergoes extensive first-pass metabolism. Metabolized in the liver and by enzymes in the bloodstream. Primarily excreted in urine. Not removed by hemodialysis. *Half-life:* 1-4 min.

AVAILABILITY

Capsules (Extended Release [Nitro-Time]): 2.5 mg, 6.5 mg, 9 mg.
Tablets (Sublingual [Nitrostat]): 0.3 mg, 0.4 mg, 0.6 mg.
Spray (Translingual [Nitrolingual, NitroMist]): 0.4 mg/spray.
IV Infusion Solution: 0.1 mg/mL, 0.2 mg/mL, 0.4 mg/mL.
Topical Ointment (Nitro-Bid): 2%.
Transdermal Patch (Minitran): 0.1 mg/h, 0.2 mg/h, 0.3 mg/h, 0.4 mg/h.
Transdermal Patch (NitroDur): 0.1 mg/h, 0.2 mg/h, 0.3 mg/h, 0.4 mg/h, 0.6 mg/h, 0.8 mg/h.
Solution for Injection: 50 mg/10 mL.
Topical Ointment (Nitro-Bid): 2%; 1 inch = 15 mg.

INDICATIONS AND DOSAGES

▸ **Acute relief of angina pectoris, acute prophylaxis**
LINGUAL SPRAY
Adults, Elderly. 1 spray onto or under tongue q3-5min until relief is noted (no more than 3 sprays in 15-min period).
SUBLINGUAL
Adults, Elderly. 0.4 mg or 0.6 mg q5min until relief is noted (no more

than 3 doses in 15-min period). Use prophylactically 5-10 min before activities that may cause an acute attack.

▸ **Long-term prophylaxis of angina**
PO (EXTENDED RELEASE)
Adults, Elderly. 2.5-9 mg q8-12h.
TOPICAL
Adults, Elderly. Initially, ½ inch q8h. Increase by ½ inch with each application. Range: 1-2 inches q8h up to 4-5 inches q4h.
TRANSDERMAL PATCH
Adults, Elderly. Initially, 0.2-0.4 mg/h. Maintenance: 0.4-0.8 mg/h. Consider patch on for 12-14 h, patch off for 10-12 h (prevents tolerance).

▸ **Congestive heart failure (CHF) associated with acute myocardial infarction (MI)**
IV
Adults, Elderly. Initially, 5 mcg/min via infusion pump. Increase in 5-mcg/min increments at 3- to 5-min intervals until BP response is noted or until dosage reaches 20 mcg/min; then increase as needed by 10 mcg/min. Dosage may be further titrated according to clinical, therapeutic response up to 200 mcg/min.
Children. Initially, 0.25-0.5 mcg/kg/min; titrate by 0.5-1 mcg/kg/min, at 3-to 5-min intervals, up to 20 mcg/kg/min.

CONTRAINDICATIONS

Allergic reactions to organic nitrates are extremely rare but do occur; contraindicated if allergic. Allergy to adhesives (transdermal). Also contraindicated in pericardial tamponade, restrictive cardiomyopathy, constrictive pericarditis, increased intracranial pressure, or where cardiac output is dependent upon venous return. Contraindicated with phosphodiesterase (PDE-5) inhibitors (e.g., sildenafil, vardenafil, tadalafil).

INTERACTIONS

Drug
Alcohol, opioids, benzodiazepines, phenthiazines, other drugs used in conscious sedation techniques: May increase hypotensive effects.
Other antihypertensives, vasodilators: May increase risk of orthostatic hypotension.
Sildenafil, tadalafil, vardenafil: Concurrent use of these drugs produces significant hypotension. Contraindicated.
Herbal
None known.
Food
Alcohol: May increase risk of orthostatic hypotension.

DIAGNOSTIC TEST EFFECTS

May increase blood methemoglobin, urine catecholamine, and urine vanillylmandelic acid concentrations.

IV INCOMPATIBILITIES

Alteplase (Activase) diazepam, lansoprazole (Prevacid IV), levofloxacin (Levaquin), phenytoin. Do not administer with blood products.

IV COMPATIBILITIES

Amiodarone (Cordarone), diltiazem (Cardizem), dobutamine (Dobutrex), dopamine (Intropin), epinephrine, famotidine (Pepcid), fentanyl (Sublimaze), furosemide (Lasix), heparin, hydromorphone (Dilaudid), insulin, labetalol (Trandate), lidocaine, lorazepam (Ativan), midazolam (Versed), milrinone (Primacor), morphine, nicardipine (Cardene), nitroprusside (Nipride), norepinephrine (Levophed), propofol (Diprivan).

SIDE EFFECTS

Frequent

Headache (possibly severe; occurs mostly in early therapy, diminishes rapidly in intensity, and usually disappears during continued treatment), transient flushing of face and neck, dizziness (especially if patient is standing immobile or is in a warm environment), weakness, orthostatic hypotension, syncope.
Sublingual: Burning, tingling sensation at oral point of dissolution.
Ointment: Erythema, pruritus.

Occasional

GI upset.
Transdermal: Contact dermatitis.

SERIOUS REACTIONS

- Nitroglycerin should be discontinued if blurred vision or dry mouth occurs; evaluate for overdosage (IV). Rarely, methemoglobinemia occurs.
- Severe orthostatic hypotension may occur, manifested by fainting, pulselessness, cold or clammy skin, and diaphoresis.
- Tolerance may occur with repeated, prolonged therapy; minor tolerance may occur with intermittent use of sublingual tablets.
- High doses of nitroglycerin tend to produce severe headache.

PRECAUTIONS & CONSIDERATIONS

Caution is warranted with acute MI, blood volume depletion from therapy, glaucoma (contraindicated in closed-angle glaucoma), hepatic or renal disease, and systolic BP < 90 mm Hg. It is unknown whether nitroglycerin crosses the placenta or is distributed in breast milk, warranting caution in lactation. The safety and efficacy of nitroglycerin have not been established in children. Elderly patients are more susceptible to the hypotensive effects of nitroglycerin. In elderly patients, age-related renal impairment may require cautious use. Alcohol should be avoided because it intensifies the drug's hypotensive effect. If alcohol is ingested soon after taking nitrates, an acute hypotensive episode marked by pallor, vertigo, and a drop in BP may occur.

Dizziness, light-headedness, and headache may occur. Rise slowly from a lying to a sitting position and dangle legs momentarily before standing to avoid the drug's hypotensive effect. Notify the physician of facial or neck flushing. The onset, type (sharp, dull, or squeezing), radiation, location, intensity, and duration of anginal pain and its precipitating factors, such as exertion and emotional stress, should be recorded before therapy begins. Apical pulse and BP should be determined before administration and periodically after the dose has been given. ECG should be closely monitored during IV administration.

Storage

Keep sublingual tablets in their original container.

Lingual sprays should be stored upright; flammable and under pressure: keep away from heat and flame. Store injection vials and premixed infusion at room temperature, away from heat. Protect from freezing. Prepared infusions stable for up to 48 h at room temperature.

Administration

! The defibrillator must not be discharged through a paddle electrode overlying a nitroglycerin system because to do so may cause burns to the patient or damage the paddle via arching. Do not give nitrates if the patient has recently taken Cialis, Levitra, or Viagra.

Swallow extended-release capsules whole; capsules should not be chewed or crushed. Take nitroglycerin, preferably on an empty stomach; take the medication with meals if headache occurs during therapy.

Prime lingual spray prior to first use. Do not shake aerosol canister before lingual spraying. Use the translingual spray only when sitting down. Spray under the tongue and avoid inhaling or swallowing lingual spray.

For sublingual use, dissolve under the tongue and avoid swallowing. Administer while seated. To lessen the burning sensation under the tongue, place the tablet in the buccal pouch. Take sublingual tablets at the first sign of angina. If anginal pain is not relieved within 5 min of the first dose, seek emergency assistance and dissolve a second tablet under the tongue. If the second dose does not relieve anginal pain within 5 min, dissolve a third tablet under the tongue.

For topical use, spread a thin layer on clean, dry, hairless skin of the upper arm or body, not below the knee or elbow, using the applicator or dose-measuring papers. Do not use fingers; do not rub or massage into skin.

! Transdermal patch should be removed before cardioversion or defibrillation because the electrical current may cause arching, which can burn the person and damage the paddles. Also, remove prior to any MRI procedure to avoid burns.

For transdermal use, apply patch on clean, dry, hairless skin of the upper arm or body, not below the knee or elbow.

The IV form is available in ready-to-use infusions. To use, dilute vials in 250 or 500 mL D5W or 0.9% NaCl to a maximum concentration of 250 mg/250 mL. Use microdrop or infusion pump.

Nitroprusside

nye-troe-pruss′ide

★ Nitropress 🍁 Nipride

Do not confuse nitroprusside with nitroglycerin.

CATEGORY AND SCHEDULE

Pregnancy Risk Category: C

Classification: Antihypertensive agents, vasodilators

MECHANISM OF ACTION

A potent vasodilator used to treat emergent hypertensive conditions; acts directly on arterial and venous smooth muscle. Decreases peripheral vascular resistance, preload and afterload; improves cardiac output. *Therapeutic Effect:* Dilates coronary arteries, decreases oxygen consumption, and relieves persistent chest pain.

PHARMACOKINETICS

Route	Onset	Peak	Duration
IV	1-2 min	Dependent on infusion rate	Dissipates rapidly after stopping IV, 1-10 min

Reacts with hemoglobin in erythrocytes, producing cyanmethemoglobin, and cyanide ions. Excreted primarily in urine. *Half-life:* < 10 min.

AVAILABILITY

Injection: 25 mg/mL.

INDICATIONS AND DOSAGES

▸ **Immediate reduction of BP in hypertensive crisis; to produce controlled hypotension in surgical procedures to reduce bleeding; treatment of acute congestive heart failure (CHF)**

IV

Adults, Elderly, Children. Initially, 0.3 mcg/kg/min. Range: 0.5-10 mcg/kg/min. Do not exceed 10 mcg/kg/min (risk of precipitous drop in BP). Maximal rate for short-term use. To maintain the thiocyanate concentration below 1 mmole/L, the rate of a prolonged infusion (i.e., > 72 h), should not exceed 3 mcg/kg/min and 1 mcg/kg/min in anuric patients.

OFF-LABEL USES

Control of paroxysmal hypertension before and during surgery for pheochromocytoma, peripheral vasospasm caused by ergot alkaloid overdose, treatment adjunct with dopamine for acute myocardial infarction (MI), valvular regurgitation.

CONTRAINDICATIONS

Compensatory hypertension (atrioventricular [AV] shunt or coarctation of aorta), inadequate cerebral circulation, moribund patients (ASA Class 5E), congenital Leber's optic atrophy, tobacco amblyopia, acute CHF with reduced peripheral vascular resistance, pre-existing cyanide toxicity.

INTERACTIONS

Drug

Antihypertensives, ganglionic blockers, volatile anesthetics: May increase hypotensive effect.

Dobutamine: May increase cardiac output and decrease pulmonary wedge pressure.

Herbal

None known.

Food

None known.

DIAGNOSTIC TEST EFFECTS

None known.

IV INCOMPATIBILITIES

Acylovir, caspofungin (Cancidas), ceftazidime (Fortaz), cisatracurium (Nimbex) diazepam, drotrecogin alfa (Xigris), erythromycin, hydralazine, hydroxyzine, levofloxacin (Levaquin), phenytoin, promethazine, quinupristin/dalfopristin (Synercid), voriconazole.

IV COMPATIBILITIES

Diltiazem (Cardizem), dobutamine (Dobutrex), dopamine (Intropin), enalapril (Vasotec), heparin, insulin, labetalol (Normodyne, Trandate), lidocaine, midazolam (Versed), milrinone (Primacor), nitroglycerin, propofol (Diprivan).

SIDE EFFECTS

Occasional

Flushing of skin, increased intracranial pressure, rash, pain or redness at injection site.

SERIOUS REACTIONS

- A too-rapid IV infusion rate reduces BP too quickly.
- Nausea, vomiting, diaphoresis, apprehension, headache, restlessness, muscle twitching, dizziness, palpitations, retrosternal pain, and abdominal pain may occur. Symptoms disappear rapidly if rate of administration is slowed or drug is temporarily discontinued.
- Overdose produces metabolic acidosis and cyanide toxicity (rare).

PRECAUTIONS & CONSIDERATIONS

Caution is warranted in patients with hyponatremia, hypothyroidism, severe hepatic or renal impairment, and in elderly patients. It is unknown whether nitroprusside crosses the placenta or is distributed in breast milk, warranting caution in lactation. The safety and efficacy of nitroprusside have not been established in children. Elderly patients are more sensitive to the drug's hypotensive effect. In elderly patients, age-related renal impairment may require cautious use. Be aware of signs and symptoms of metabolic acidosis, including disorientation, headache, hyperventilation, nausea, vomiting, and weakness. Alcohol should be avoided because it intensifies the drug's hypotensive effect. If alcohol is ingested soon after taking, an acute hypotensive episode marked by pallor, vertigo, and a drop in BP may occur.

Notify the physician of pain, redness, or swelling at the IV insertion, dizziness, headache, nausea, palpitations, or other unusual signs or symptoms. Desired BP levels should be determined with the physician before treatment; it is normally maintained at about 30% to 40% below pretreatment levels. BP and ECG should be monitored before and during treatment. Acid-base balance, electrolyte levels, intake and output, and laboratory results should also be assessed. Nitroprusside should be discontinued if the therapeutic response is not achieved within 10 min after IV infusion at 10 mcg/kg/min is initiated.

! Report symptoms of rare cyanide toxicity from drug metabolism evidenced by venous hyperoxemia with bright red venous blood, lactic acidosis, air hunger, confusion.

Storage

Protect solution from light. Use only freshly prepared solution. Once the solution has been prepared, it must be used within 24 h. Discard unused portion. Protect infusion from light with opaque wrapper.

Administration

Inspect IV solution, which normally appears faint brown. A color change from brown to blue, green, or dark red indicates drug deterioration. Use only freshly prepared solution. Further dilute with 250-500 mL D5W to provide a concentration of 200 mcg/mL to 50 mcg/mL, respectively, up to a maximum concentration of 200 mg/250 mL. Wrap infusion bottle in aluminum foil immediately after mixing to protect from light. Give by IV infusion only using infusion rate chart provided by manufacturer or facility protocol. Administer using IV infusion pump and lock in the rate. The rate of infusion should be monitored frequently. Be alert for extravasation, which produces severe pain and sloughing.

N

Nizatidine

ni-za'ti-deen

★ 🍁 Axid, Axid AR

CATEGORY AND SCHEDULE

Pregnancy Risk Category: B

OTC capsules: 75 mg

Classification: Antihistamines, H_2 receptor antagonist

MECHANISM OF ACTION

An antiulcer agent and gastric acid secretion inhibitor that inhibits histamine action at H_2 receptors of parietal cells. *Therapeutic Effect:* Inhibits basal and nocturnal gastric acid secretion.

PHARMACOKINETICS

Rapidly, well absorbed from the GI tract. Protein binding: 35%. Metabolized in the liver. Excreted primarily in urine. Not removed by hemodialysis. *Half-life:* 1-2 h (increased with impaired renal function).

AVAILABILITY

Capsules: 150 mg, 300 mg.
Oral Solution: 15 mg/mL.
Tables (OTC): 75 mg.

INDICATIONS AND DOSAGES

▸ **Active duodenal ulcer**
PO
Adults, Elderly. 300 mg at bedtime or 150 mg twice a day.
▸ **Prevention of duodenal ulcer recurrence**
PO
Adults, Elderly. 150 mg at bedtime.
▸ **Gastroesophageal reflux disease (GERD)**
PO
Adults, Elderly. 150 mg twice a day.
▸ **Active benign gastric ulcer**
PO
Adults, Elderly. 150 mg twice a day or 300 mg at bedtime.
▸ **Dyspepsia**
PO (OTC)
Adults, Elderly. 75 mg 30-60 min before meals; no more than 2 tablets a day.
▸ **Dosage in renal impairment**
Dosage adjustment is based on creatinine clearance.

Creatinine Clearance (mL/min)	Active Ulcer Disease	Maintenance Therapy
20-50	150 mg every bedtime	150 mg every other day
< 20	150 mg every other day	150 mg every 3 days

OFF-LABEL USES

Gastric hypersecretory conditions, stress-ulcer prophylaxis, pediatric use.

CONTRAINDICATIONS

Hypersensitivity to nizatidine or other H_2 antagonists.

INTERACTIONS

Drug
Antacids: May decrease the absorption of nizatidine.
Aspirin: May increase serum salicylate levels with high doses of aspirin.
Atazanavir, itraconazole, ketoconazole: Nizatidine may decrease absorption.
Herbal
None known.
Food
None known.

DIAGNOSTIC TEST EFFECTS

May increase serum alkaline phosphatase, AST (SGOT), and ALT (SGPT) levels. May cause false-positive tests for urobilinogen with Multistix®.

SIDE EFFECTS

Occasional (2%)
Somnolence, fatigue, headache.
Rare (1%)
Diaphoresis, rash.

SERIOUS REACTIONS

• Asymptomatic ventricular tachycardia, hyperuricemia not associated with gout, and nephrolithiasis occur rarely.

PRECAUTIONS & CONSIDERATIONS

Caution is warranted in patients with impaired hepatic or renal function. Nizatidine crosses the placenta and is distributed in breast milk, warranting caution in pregnancy and lactation. The safety and efficacy of nizatidine have not been established in children younger than 16 yr of age. No age-related precautions have been noted in elderly patients. Tasks that require mental alertness or motor skills should be avoided until response to the drug has been established. Also, avoid alcohol, aspirin, and coffee, all of which may cause GI distress, during nizatidine therapy.

Notify the physician if acid indigestion, gastric distress, or heartburn occurs after 2 wks of continuous nizatidine therapy. Blood chemistry laboratory test results, including BUN, serum alkaline phosphatase, bilirubin, creatinine, AST (SGOT), and ALT (SGPT) levels, to assess hepatic and renal function should be obtained before and during therapy.

Storage

Store at room temperature. Keep tighly closed.

Administration

Take nizatidine without regard to meals. Take right before eating for heartburn prevention. Do not administer within 1 h of magnesium- or aluminum-containing antacids because it can decrease the absorption of nizatidine.

Norepinephrine Bitartrate

nor-ep-i-nef'rin bye-tar'trayte

Levophed

Do not confuse Levophed with Levid or Levbid. Do not confuse norepinephrine with epinephrine, phenylephrine, or Neosynephrine.

CATEGORY AND SCHEDULE

Pregnancy Risk Category: C

Classification: Adrenergic agonists, vasopressors, intropes.

MECHANISM OF ACTION

A sympathomimetic that stimulates β_1-adrenergic receptors and α-adrenergic receptors, increasing peripheral resistance. Enhances contractile myocardial force, increases cardiac output. Constricts resistance and capacitance vessels. *Therapeutic Effect:* Increases systemic BP and coronary blood flow.

PHARMACOKINETICS

Route	Onset	Peak	Duration
IV	Rapid	1-2 min	NA

Localized in sympathetic tissue. Metabolized by MAO and COMT. Primarily excreted in urine.

AVAILABILITY

Injection: 1-mg/mL.

INDICATIONS AND DOSAGES

▸ **Acute hypotension unresponsive to fluid volume replacement**

IV

Adults, Elderly. Initially, administer at 0.5-1 mcg/min. Adjust rate of flow to establish and maintain desired BP. Average maintenance dose: 2-4 mcg/min. Usual maximum 8-12 mcg/min. In cardiac arrest, dose may reach 30 mcg/min.

Children. Initially, 0.05-0.1 mcg/kg/min; titrate to desired effect. Maximum: 1-2 mcg/kg/min.

CONTRAINDICATIONS

Hypovolemic states (unless as an emergency measure), mesenteric or peripheral vascular thrombosis, profound hypoxia.

INTERACTIONS

Drug

β-Blockers: May have mutually inhibitory effects.

N

Digoxin: May increase risk of arrhythmias.
Ergonovine, oxytocin: May increase vasoconstriction.
Halogenated hydrocarbon anesthetics: May increase risk of arrhythmias.
Maprotiline, tricyclic antidepressants, oxytocin, guanethidine: Increased risk of severe hypotension.
Methyldopa: May decrease the effects of methyldopa.
Herbal
None known.
Food
None known.

DIAGNOSTIC TEST EFFECTS
None known.

IV INCOMPATIBILITIES
Aminophylline, amphotericin B, diazepam, drotrecogin alfa (Xigris), regular insulin, pantoprazole (Protonix), phenobarbital, phenytoin, sodium bicarbonate, thiopental.

IV COMPATIBILITIES
Amiodarone (Cordarone), calcium gluconate, diltiazem (Cardizem), dobutamine (Dobutrex), dopamine (Intropin), epinephrine, esmolol (Brevibloc), fentanyl (Sublimaze), heparin, hydromorphone (Dilaudid), labetalol (Trandate), lorazepam (Ativan), magnesium, midazolam (Versed), milrinone (Primacor), morphine, nicardipine (Cardene), nitroglycerin, potassium chloride, propofol (Diprivan).

SIDE EFFECTS
Occasional (3%-5%)
Anxiety, bradycardia, palpitations.
Rare (1%-2%)
Nausea, anginal pain, shortness of breath, fever.

SERIOUS REACTIONS
- Extravasation may produce tissue necrosis and sloughing.
- Overdose is manifested as severe hypertension with violent headache (which may be the first clinical sign of overdose), arrhythmias, photophobia, retrosternal or pharyngeal pain, pallor, excessive sweating, and vomiting.
- Prolonged therapy may result in plasma volume depletion. Hypotension may recur if plasma volume is not restored.

PRECAUTIONS & CONSIDERATIONS
! This drug is used in acute settings in hospitals or emergencies for selected hypotensive episodes.

Caution is warranted in patients with hypertension, hypothyroidism, severe cardiac disease, and concurrent MAOI therapy. Norepinephrine readily crosses the placenta and may produce fetal anoxia as a result of constriction of uterine blood vessels and uterine contraction. Use in pregnancy is contraindicated unless the benefits of therapy clearly outweigh potential risks to the mother and fetus. No age-related precautions have been noted in children or elderly patients.

BP and ECG should be monitored continuously. Be alert to precipitous drops in BP. Intake and output should be assessed hourly or as ordered. If urine output is < 30 mL/h, the infusion should be stopped unless the systolic BP falls below 80 mm Hg. Prolonged therapy may result in plasma volume depleting, causing hypotension to persist or not return to normal levels.
Storage
Store at room temperature. IV infusion is stable for 24 h at room temperature.
Administration
! Expect to restore blood and fluid volume before administering norepinephrine.

Do not use if solution is brown or contains precipitate. Add 4 mL (4 mg) to 1 L of D5W for a 4-mcg/mL solution. A common concentration is 4 mg/250mL for a concentration of 16 mcg/mL. Maximum concentration: 32 mcg/mL. Administer infusion through a central venous catheter, if available, to avoid extravasation. Closely monitor the infusion flow rate with a microdrip or infusion pump. Monitor the BP every 2 min during the infusion until desired therapeutic response is achieved, then every 5 min during the remainder of the infusion. Never leave unattended during the infusion. Be alert to any complaint of headache. Plan to maintain BP at 80-100 mm Hg in previously normotensive patients. Reduce the infusion gradually, as prescribed. Avoid abrupt withdrawal. Check the peripherally inserted catheter IV site frequently for signs of extravasation, including blanching, coldness, hardness, and pallor to the extremity. If extravasation occurs, expect to infiltrate the affected area with 10-15 mL sterile saline containing 5-10 mg phentolamine. Know that phentolamine does not alter the pressor effects of norepinephrine.

For prevention of extravasation effects, phentolamine may be added to the norepinephrine infusion.

Norethindrone

nor-eth'in-drone

★ Aygestin, Camila, Errin, Heather, Jolivette, Micronor, Nora-BE, Nor-QD 🍁 Micronor, Norlutate

CATEGORY AND SCHEDULE

Pregnancy Risk Category: X

Classification: Hormonal agent, progesterone derivative, progestin-only contraceptive

MECHANISM OF ACTION

A synthetic progestin that is used as a single agent or in combination with estrogens for the treatment of gynecological disorders. It inhibits secretion of pituitary gonadotropin (LH), which prevents follicular maturation and ovulation. *Therapeutic Effect:* Transforms endometrium from proliferative to secretory in an estrogen-primed endometrium, promotes mammary gland development, relaxes uterine smooth muscle.

PHARMACOKINETICS

Rapidly absorbed from the GI tract. Widely distributed. Protein binding: 61%. Metabolized in liver. Excreted in urine and feces. *Half-life:* 4-13 h.

AVAILABILITY

Contraceptive Tablets: 0.35 mg (Camila, Errin, Jolivette, Micronor, Nora-BE, Nor-QD).
Tablets, as Norethindrone Acetate: 5 mg (Aygestin).

INDICATIONS AND DOSAGES

▸ **Contraception**

PO

Adults. 1 tablet/day (0.35 mg/day).

▸ **Amenorrhea and abnormal uterine bleeding**

PO (NORETHINDRONE ACETATE)

Adults. 2.5-10 mg per day, given cyclically for 5-10 days.

▸ **Endometriosis**

PO (NORETHINDRONE ACETATE)

Adults. 5 mg/day for 14 days, increase at increments of 2.5 mg/day every 2 wks up to 15 mg/day continue for 6-9 mo or until breakthrough bleeding demands temporary discontinuation.

CONTRAINDICATIONS

Acute liver disease, benign or malignant liver tumors,

N

hypersensitivity to norethindrone or any component of the formulation, known or suspected carcinoma of the breast, known or suspected pregnancy, undiagnosed abnormal genital bleeding.

INTERACTIONS

Drug

Antibiotics such as the penicillins and erythromycin, barbiturates: May decrease effectiveness of norethindrone.

Amprenavir, nelfinavir, nevirapine, ritonavir: May decrease norethindrone concentrations.

Aprepitant: May decrease the effects of both drugs.

Atorvastatin, rosuvastatin: May increase concentrations of norethindrone.

Benzodiazepines: May increase risk of benzodiazepine toxicity.

Cyclosporine: May increase risk of cyclosporine toxicity.

CYP3A4 inducers (carbamazepine, phenobarbital, phenytoin, rifampin, rifabutin): May decrease the levels and/or effects of norethindrone.

Corticosteroids: May prolong the effects of cortisones.

Fluconazole: May increase risk of adverse effects of norethindrone.

Griseofulvin, modafinil, primidone: May decrease effectiveness of norethindrone.

Lamotrigine: May increase or decrease plasma lamotrigine concentrations.

Selegiline: May increase the risk of adverse effects of selegiline.

Theophylline: May increase the risk of theophylline toxicity.

Thiazolidinediones: May decrease the effects of norethindrone.

Warfarin: May increase or decrease anticoagulant effects.

Zolmitriptan: May increase risk of adverse effects of zolmitriptan.

Herbal

Licorice: May increase risk of fluid retention and elevated blood pressure.

Red clover: May alter effectiveness of norethindrone or increase side effects.

St. John's wort: May decrease plasma concentrations of norethindrone.

Vitamin C (at high doses, more than 1 g/day): May increase adverse effects of norethindrone.

Food

Caffeine: May increase CNS stimulation.

DIAGNOSTIC TEST EFFECTS

May increase LDL concentrations and serum alkaline phosphatase levels. May decrease glucose tolerance and HDL concentrations. May cause abnormal thyroid, metapyrone, liver, and endocrine function tests.

SIDE EFFECTS

Occasional

Breast tenderness, dizziness, headache, breakthrough bleeding, amenorrhea, menstrual irregularity, nausea, weakness.

Rare

Mental depression, fever, insomnia, rash, acne, increased breast tenderness, weight gain/loss, changes in cervical erosion and secretions, cholestatic jaundice.

SERIOUS REACTIONS

• Thrombophlebitis, cerebrovascular disorders, retinal thrombosis, cholestatic jaundice, and pulmonary embolism occur rarely.

PRECAUTIONS & CONSIDERATIONS

Caution is warranted in patients with conditions aggravated by fluid retention, delayed follicular atresia or ovarian cysts, asthma, cardiac dysfunction, epilepsy, migraine headache, renal insufficiency, diabetes mellitus, thromboembolism, or a history of mental depression. Norethindrone may be harmful to fetus and is contraindicated in pregnancy. Patient's pregnancy status should be assessed before beginning therapy. If pregnancy is suspected, notify physician immediately. Norethindrone contraception is compatible during breastfeeding. Safety and efficacy of this drug have not been established in children. No age-related precautions have been noted in elderly patients. Avoid smoking while taking norethindrone.

Menstrual spotting may occur between periods. Pain, redness, swelling, or warmth in the calf; chest pain; migraine headache; peripheral paresthesia; sudden decrease in vision; and sudden shortness of breath should be reported immediately. Patient should be advised to use an additional nonhormonal form of birth control during therapy if antibiotics or anti-infectives are prescribed while remaining compliant with the oral contraceptive therapy schedule.

Storage

Store at room temperature; protect from moisture.

Administration

For oral contraception to be effective, take norethindrone at the same time each day. Do not take a break between packs. Do not skip doses.

When used for HRT during menopause, or for other hormonal purposes, take at roughly same time daily; may take with food.

Norfloxacin

nor-flox'a-sin

★ Noroxin 🍁 Apo-Norflox

CATEGORY AND SCHEDULE

Pregnancy Risk Category: C

Classification: Fluoroquinolone anti-infective

MECHANISM OF ACTION

A quinolone that inhibits DNA gyrase in susceptible microorganisms, interfering with bacterial cell replication and repair. *Therapeutic Effect:* Bactericidal.

PHARMACOKINETICS

PO: Peak 1 h, steady state in 2 days. Excreted in urine as active drug and metabolites. *Half-life:* 3-4 h.

AVAILABILITY

Tablets: 400 mg.

INDICATIONS AND DOSAGES

▸ **Urinary tract infections (UTIs)**

PO

Adults, Elderly. 400 mg twice a day for 3-21 days.

▸ **Prostatitis**

PO

Adults. 400 mg twice a day for 4-6 wks.

▸ **Uncomplicated gonococcal infections**

CDC no longer recommends use due to resistant organisms.

PO

Adults. 800 mg as a single dose.

N

▸ **Dosage in renal impairment**
Dosage and frequency are modified based on creatinine clearance.

Creatinine Clearance (mL/min)	Adult Dosage (mg)
≥ 30	400 twice a day
< 30	400 once a day

CONTRAINDICATIONS

Children younger than 18 yr because of risk arthropathy (systemic use). Hypersensitivity to norfloxacin, other quinolones, or their components.

INTERACTIONS

Drug

Antacids, sucralfate, iron supplements, multivitamins with minerals, zinc, didanozine: May decrease norfloxacin absorption.
Cyclosporine: May increase cyclosporine concentrations.
Oral anticoagulants: May increase effects of oral anticoagulants.
Theophylline: Decreases clearance and may increase blood concentration and risk of toxicity of theophylline.

Herbal

None known.

Food

Dairy products: May decrease norfloxacin absorption.

DIAGNOSTIC TEST EFFECTS

May increase BUN level and serum alkaline phosphatase, bilirubin, creatinine, LDH, AST (SGOT), and ALT (SGPT) levels.

SIDE EFFECTS

Burning or discomfort. Other reactions were conjunctival hypermia, chemosis, corneal deposits, photophobia, and a bitter taste following installations.

Frequent

Nausea, headache, dizziness.

Rare

Vomiting, diarrhea, dry mouth, bitter taste, nervousness, drowsiness, insomnia, photosensitivity, tinnitus, crystalluria, rash, fever, seizures.

SERIOUS REACTIONS

- Superinfection, anaphylaxis, Stevens-Johnson syndrome, and arthropathy occur rarely.
- Hypersensitivity reactions, including photosensitivity (as evidenced by rash, pruritus, blisters, edema, and burning skin), have occurred.
- Tendonitis and tendon rupture.
- Hypoglycemia.

PRECAUTIONS & CONSIDERATIONS

Caution is warranted in patients with impaired renal function and a predisposition to seizures. Use with caution in patients with cardiac arrhythmias or risks for QT prolongation. The drug should be used in pregnancy only if clearly needed. The drug is expected to be excreted in breast milk, and use during lactation is not recommended. Safety and effectiveness have not been established in children.

Use appropriate precautions to avoid UV exposure due to potential photosensitivity. Dizziness, headache, nausea, signs of infection, and vaginitis should be evaluated. Patients should be cautioned to watch for pain, swelling, or tenderness in any tendon or ligament in the shoulder, hand, or Achilles tendon, and report any of these symptoms for evaluation by a health care practitioner.

Storage
Store at room temperature.
Administration
Take norfloxacin with 8 oz of water 1 h before or 2 h after a meal and consume several glasses of water between meals. Do not take antacids, divalent cations, dairy products, or didanosine within 2 h of norfloxacin.

Nortriptyline Hydrochloride

nor-trip'ti-leen high-droh-klor'ide
Pamelor Aventyl, Norventyl
Do not confuse nortriptyline with amitriptyline.
Do not confuse Pamelor with Panlor DC.

CATEGORY AND SCHEDULE

Pregnancy Risk Category: D

Classification: Antidepressants, tricyclic

MECHANISM OF ACTION

A tricyclic antidepressant that blocks reuptake of the neurotransmitters norepinephrine and serotonin at neuronal presynaptic membranes, increasing their availability at postsynaptic receptor sites. *Therapeutic Effect:* Relieves depression.

PHARMACOKINETICS

Well absorbed from the GI tract. Protein binding: 86%-95%. Metabolized in the liver. Primarily excreted in the urine. *Half-life:* 17.6 h.

AVAILABILITY

Capsules: 10 mg, 25 mg.
Capsules (Pamelor): 10 mg, 25 mg, 50 mg, 75 mg.
Oral Solution: 10 mg/5 mL.

INDICATIONS AND DOSAGES

▸ Depression

PO
Adults. Initially 25-50 mg/day. Usual dose is 75-100 mg/day in 1-4 divided doses. Reduce dosage gradually to effective maintenance level. Maximum: 150 mg/day.
Elderly. Initially, 10-25 mg at bedtime. May increase by 25 mg every 3-7 days. Maximum: 150 mg/day.
Children 12 yr and older. 30-50 mg/day in 3-4 divided doses.

▸ Enuresis (off-label)

PO
Children 12 yr and older. 25-35 mg/day.
Children aged 8-11 yr. 10-20 mg/day.
Children aged 6-7 yr. 10 mg/day.

OFF-LABEL USES

Treatment of neurogenic pain, panic disorder; prevention of migraine headache, enuresis.

CONTRAINDICATIONS

Acute recovery period after myocardial infarction (MI), use within 14 days of MAOIs, hypersensitivity to drug or other dibenzazepines.

INTERACTIONS

Drug
Alcohol, other central nervous system (CNS) depressants, barbiturates, benzodiazepines: May increase CNS and respiratory depression and the hypotensive effects of nortriptyline.
Antihistamines, phenothiazines, muscarinic blockers: May increase anticholinergic effects.

N

Antithyroid agents: May increase the risk of agranulocytosis.
Cimetidine: May increase the blood concentration and risk of toxicity of nortriptyline.
Clonidine, guanadrel, guanethidine: May decrease the effects of these drugs.
MAOIs: May increase the risk of neuroleptic malignant syndrome, seizures, hyperpyrexia, and hypertensive crisis.
Agents that prolong the OT interval: May increase risk of cardiac arrhythmias.
Phenothiazines: May increase the anticholinergic and sedative effects of nortriptyline.
Sympathomimetics, epinephrine, levonordefrin: May increase the risk of cardiac effects.

Herbal

St. John's wort: Avoid concurrent use with St. John's wort.

Food

None known.

DIAGNOSTIC TEST EFFECTS

May alter blood glucose level and ECG readings. The therapeutic range is 50-150 mg/mL.

SIDE EFFECTS

Frequent

Somnolence, fatigue, dry mouth, blurred vision, constipation, delayed micturition, orthostatic hypotension, diaphoresis, impaired concentration, increased appetite, urine retention.

Occasional

GI disturbances (nausea, GI distress, metallic taste), photosensitivity.

Rare

Paradoxical reactions (agitation, restlessness, nightmares, insomnia), extrapyramidal symptoms (particularly fine hand tremor).

SERIOUS REACTIONS

- Overdose may produce seizures; cardiovascular effects, such as severe orthostatic hypotension, dizziness, tachycardia, palpitations, and arrhythmias; and altered temperature regulation, such as hyperpyrexia or hypothermia.
- Abrupt discontinuation after prolonged therapy may produce headache, malaise, nausea, vomiting, and vivid dreams.

PRECAUTIONS & CONSIDERATIONS

Caution is warranted in patients with cardiac disease, diabetes mellitus, glaucoma, hiatal hernia, history of seizures, history of urinary obstruction or urine retention, hyperthyroidism, increased IOP, prostatic hypertrophy, hepatic or renal disease, and schizophrenia. Children are more sensitive to an acute overdose and are at increased risk for toxicity. Safety and effectiveness of nortriptyline have not been established in children. Antidepressants have been associated with an increased risk of suicidal thinking and behavior in children, adolescents, and young adults with major depressive disorder and other psychiatric disorders. Be alert to suicidal thoughts, irritability, hostility, and other unusual changes in behavior in any patient, especially during early antidepressant treatment and when the dose is adjusted. Elderly patients are more sensitive to the drug's anticholinergic effects. Sunscreens and protective clothing should be worn because the drug may cause photosensitivity to sunlight.

Anticholinergic, sedative, and hypotensive effects may occur, but tolerance usually develops. Because dizziness may occur, change positions slowly, avoid alcohol and tasks that require alertness or motor skills.

Pattern of daily bowel activity and stool consistency, bladder for urine retention, BP and pulse rate, and ECG should be assessed during therapy.

Storage

Store at room temperature.

Administration

! Make sure at least 14 days elapse between the use of MAOIs and nortriptyline.

Take nortriptyline with food or milk if GI distress occurs. Nortriptyline's therapeutic effect may be noted in 2-3 wks.

Nystatin

nye-stat′in

★ Bio-Statin, Pediaderm-AF, Pedi-Dri 🍁 Nyaderm

Do not confuse nystatin or Bio-Statin with HMG-CoA reductase inhibitors ("statins").

CATEGORY AND SCHEDULE

Pregnancy Risk Category: B (vaginal); C (PO, topical)

Classification: Antifungals, polyene type

MECHANISM OF ACTION

A fungistatic antifungal that binds to sterols in the fungal cell membrane. *Therapeutic Effect:* Increases fungal cell-membrane permeability, allowing loss of potassium and other cellular components.

PHARMACOKINETICS

PO: Poorly absorbed from the GI tract. Eliminated unchanged in feces. Topical: Not absorbed systemically from intact skin.

AVAILABILITY

Oral Suspension: 100,000 units/mL.
Capsules (Bio-Statin): 100,000 units, 500,000 units.
Tablets: 500,000 units.
Vaginal Tablets: 100,000 units.
Cream (Pediaderm-AF): 100,000 units/g.
Ointment: 100,000 units/g.
Topical Powder (Pedi-Dri): 100,000 units/g.

INDICATIONS AND DOSAGES

▸ **Intestinal infections**

PO

Adults, Elderly. 500,000-1,000,000 units q8h.

▸ **Oral candidiasis**

PO

Adults, Elderly, Children. 400,000-600,000 units swished and swallowed 4 times/day.

Infants. 200,000 units 4 times/day.

▸ **Vaginal infections**

VAGINAL

Adults, Elderly, Adolescents. 1 tablet/day vaginally at bedtime for 14 days.

▸ **Cutaneous candidal infections**

TOPICAL

Adults, Elderly, Children. Apply 2-4 times/day.

OFF-LABEL USES

Prophylaxis of oropharyngeal candidiasis.

CONTRAINDICATIONS

Hypersensitivity to nystatin or any components in formulation.

INTERACTIONS

Drug, Herbal, and Food

None known.

DIAGNOSTIC TEST EFFECTS

None known.

SIDE EFFECTS

Occasional

PO: Diarrhea, nausea.

N

Topical: Skin irritation.
Vaginal: Vaginal irritation.

SERIOUS REACTIONS

- High dosages of oral form may produce nausea, vomiting, diarrhea, and GI distress.

PRECAUTIONS & CONSIDERATIONS

It is unknown whether nystatin is distributed in breast milk, warranting caution in lactation. During pregnancy, no particular cautions are noted with vaginal tablets other than that manual insertion is desirable over use of applicator. No age-related precautions have been noted for suspension or topical use in children. Lozenges are not recommended for use in children 5 yr old or younger. Topical nystatin is commonly used in neonates/infants in the diaper area. No age-related precautions have been noted in elderly patients.

Confirm that cultures or histologic tests were done for accurate diagnosis before giving the drug. Assess for increased irritation with topical application or increased vaginal discharge with vaginal application. Separate personal items that come in contact with affected areas. Notify the physician if diarrhea, nausea, stomach pain, or vomiting develops.

Storage

Oral, topical, and vaginal products are stored at room temperature. Protect from high heat and freezing.

Administration

Shake suspension well before administration. Place and hold the suspension in the mouth or swish throughout the mouth as long as possible before swallowing. In infants, place half of dose in each cheek/side of mouth.

Use nystatin cream or powder sparingly on erythematous areas. Rub the topical creams or ointments well into affected areas, keep affected areas clean and dry, and wear light clothing for ventilation. Avoid contact with eyes.

Insert the vaginal form high into the vagina at bedtime. Vaginal use should be continued during menses. Consider using condoms during therapy and sexual intercourse.

Octreotide

ok-tree'oh-tide

Sandostatin, Sandostatin LAR

Do not confuse octreotide with OctreoScan, or Sandostatin with Sandimmune or Sandoglobulin.

CATEGORY AND SCHEDULE

Pregnancy Risk Category: B

Classification: Gastrointestinal agents, secretory inhibitor, growth hormone suppressant

MECHANISM OF ACTION

Potent inhibitor of growth hormone, glucagon, and insulin. Blunts LH response to GnRH, decreases splanchnic blood flow, and inhibits secretion of serotonin, gastrin, vasoactive intestinal peptide, secretin, motilin, pancreatic polypeptide, and TSH. *Therapeutic Effect:* Reduces acromegaly; reduces diarrhea due to intestinal carcinoid tumors; helps control bleeding varices.

PHARMACOKINETICS

Route	Onset	Peak	Duration
SC	NA	NA	Up to 12 h

Rapidly and completely absorbed from injection site. Excreted in urine. Removed by hemodialysis. *Half-life:* 1.5 h.

AVAILABILITY

Injection (Sandostatin): 50 mcg/mL, 100 mcg/mL, 200 mcg/mL, 500 mcg/mL, 1 mg/mL.
Suspension for Depot Injection (Sandostatin LAR): 10-mg, 20-mg, 30-mg vials.

INDICATIONS AND DOSAGES

▸ **Carcinoid tumors**

IV, SC (SANDOSTATIN)
Adults, Elderly. 100-600 mcg/day in 2-4 divided doses.
IM (SANDOSTATIN LAR)
Adults, Elderly. 20 mg q4wk.

▸ **VIPomas**

IV, SC (SANDOSTATIN)
Adults, Elderly. 200-300 mcg/day in 2-4 divided doses. Titrate to response.
IM (SANDOSTATIN LAR)
Adults, Elderly. 20 mg q4wk.

▸ **Esophageal varices (Off-label use)**

IV (SANDOSTATIN)
Adults, Elderly. Bolus of 25-50 mcg followed by IV infusion of 25-50 mcg/h.

▸ **Acromegaly**

IV, SC (SANDOSTATIN)
NOTE: GH and IGF-I levels guide titration.
Adults, Elderly. 50 mcg 3 times a day. Increase as needed. Maximum: 500 mcg 3 times a day.
IM (SANDOSTATIN LAR)
Adults, Elderly. 20 mg q4wk for 3 mo. Maximum: 40 mg q4wk.

OFF-LABEL USES

Treatment of AIDS-associated secretory diarrhea, chemotherapy-induced diarrhea, insulinomas, small-bowel fistulas, control of bleeding esophageal varices.

CONTRAINDICATIONS

Sensitivity to the drug or product components.

IV INCOMPATIBILITIES

Not compatible in TPN. Other incompatibilities include diazepam, micafungin, pantoprazole, phenytoin.

INTERACTIONS

Drug

Bromocriptine: May decrease bromocriptine clearance.
Cyclosporine: May lower cyclosporine concentrations, which could increase risk of rejection. Monitor.

Insulin, oral antidiabetics: May alter glucose concentrations.
Vitamin B_{12}: May reduce vitamin B_{12} levels.
Herbal
None known.
Food
None known.

DIAGNOSTIC TEST EFFECTS

May decrease serum thyroxine (T_4) concentration. May increase or decrease blood glucose. Depressed vitamin B_{12} levels and abnormal Schilling tests.

SIDE EFFECTS

Frequent (6%-10%, 30%-35% in acromegaly patients)
Diarrhea, nausea, abdominal discomfort, headache, injection site pain.
Occasional (1%-5%)
Vomiting, flatulence, constipation, alopecia, facial flushing, pruritus, dizziness, fatigue, arrhythmias, ecchymosis, blurred vision.
Rare (< 1%)
Depression, diminished libido, vertigo, palpitations, dyspnea.

SERIOUS REACTIONS

- Severe symptomatic hypoglycemia in patients with diabetes.
- Rare cases of ECG changes, such as QT prolongation, bradycardia.
- Patients using octreotide may develop cholelithiasis or, with prolonged high dosages, hypothyroidism.
- GI bleeding, hepatitis, pancreatitis, and seizures occur rarely.

PRECAUTIONS & CONSIDERATIONS

Caution is warranted in patients with insulin-dependent diabetes and renal failure. It is unknown whether octreotide is excreted in breast milk; therefore, caution is warranted in lactation. The children's dosage has not been established. No age-related precautions have been noted in elderly patients.

Notify the physician of unusual signs or symptoms, such as palpitations or unusual bleeding. Blood glucose levels, BP, pulse rate, respiratory rate, weight, growth hormone, pattern of daily bowel activity and stool consistency, fecal fat, fluid and electrolyte balance, and thyroid function test results should be monitored. Be alert for decreased urine output and peripheral edema, especially of the ankles. Take care in making abrupt postural changes because of the possible risk of orthostatic hypotension developing. Any signs of infection should be reported immediately.

Storage
Store injection solution and depot suspension under refrigeration and protect from light. At room temperature, the injection solution is stable for 14 days if protected from light. If solution is diluted as an IV infusion, stable for 24 h at room temperature.

Administration
! Sandostatin administration may be IV or SC. Sandostatin LAR administration may be only IM.

Do not use solution if it becomes discolored or contains particulates.

Inject Sandostatin LAR depot in a large muscle mass at 4-wk intervals. Avoid deltoid injections.

Sandostatin injection solution is usually administered as an SC injection. Avoid multiple injections at the same site within a week. If injection solution is given IV, it may be diluted in 50-200 mL 0.9% NaCl or D5W and infused over 15-30 min or administered by IV push over 3-5 min. Continuous infusions often given over 24 h.

Ofatumumab

oh'fa-tue'moo-mab

Arzerra.

Do not confuse with omalizumab.

CATEGORY AND SCHEDULE

Pregnancy Risk Category: C

Classification: Antineoplastics, monoclonal antibodies

MECHANISM OF ACTION

Binds to CD20 antigen on B lymphocyte cells and produces complement-dependent cell lysis and antibody-dependent cell-mediated cytotoxicity. *Therapeutic Effect:* Produces cytotoxicity, reducing tumor size.

PHARMACOKINETICS

Due to the depletion of B cells, the clearance of ofatumumab decreased substantially after subsequent infusions compared to the first infusion. *Half-life:* Mean of 14 days between first and 12th doses (range 2.3 days to 61 days).

AVAILABILITY

Solution for Injection: 100 mg/5 mL.

INDICATIONS AND DOSAGES

▸ B-cell chronic lymphocytic leukemia in patients failing alemtuzumab and fludarabine

IV INFUSION

Adults, Elderly. 300 mg via IV infusion for the first dose. Then, 1 wk later, give 2000 mg via IV infusion once weekly for 7 doses; then 4 wks later, give 2000 mg via IV infusion once q4wk for 4 doses. The course is 12 total doses given over 24 wks.

CONTRAINDICATIONS

None.

INTERACTIONS

Drug

Live-virus vaccines: May potentiate viral replication, increase side effects, and decrease the patient's antibody response to the vaccine.

Other immunosuppressants or chemotherapy agents: May enhance adverse effect or toxicity profile; specific data are not available.

Herbal

None known.

Food

None known.

DIAGNOSTIC TEST EFFECTS

May decrease platelet count and WBC count.

IV INCOMPATIBILITIES

Do not mix ofatumumab with any other medications.

SIDE EFFECTS

Frequent (≥ 10%)

Neutropenia, pneumonia, pyrexia, cough, diarrhea, anemia, fatigue, dyspnea, rash, nausea, bronchitis and other upper respiratory tract infections, infections in other sites.

Occasional (< 10%)

Nasopharyngitis, herpes zoster, sepsis, anemia, insomnia, headache, increased BP, tachycardia, hyperhidrosis, urticaria, back pain, muscle cramps, peripheral edema, dizziness, chills.

SERIOUS REACTIONS

- Prolonged and severe thrombocytopenia.
- Serious infections; hepatitis B reactivation, including fulminant hepatitis and death, occurs with other drugs directed against CD20.
- Serious infusion reactions manifesting as bronchospasm, dyspnea, laryngeal edema, pulmonary edema, flushing, hypertension, hypotension, syncope, cardiac ischemia/infarction, back

pain, abdominal pain, pyrexia, rash, urticaria, and angioedema. More common with first 2 infusions.
• Progressive multifocal leukoencephalopathy (PML); discontinue drug if suspected.
• Obstruction of the small intestine.

PRECAUTIONS & CONSIDERATIONS

Use with caution in those with known exposure to hepatitis B or with cardiac disease. Based on animal data, ofatumumab has the potential to cause depletion of B-lymphocytes in the fetus. Effective contraception is recommended for women of childbearing potential; use should be avoided in pregnancy. Discontinue breastfeeding during treatment. The safety and efficacy of ofatumumab have not been established in children. Avoid contact with anyone who has recently received a live-virus vaccine or who has an active infection. Crowds should also be avoided.

Infusion-related reactions, including chills, fever, hypotension, and rigors, should be monitored. Signs and symptoms of hematologic toxicity, including excessive fatigue or weakness, ecchymosis, fever, signs of local infection, sore throat, or unusual bleeding from any site, should be assessed. CBC should be monitored frequently during and after therapy to assess for anemia, neutropenia, and thrombocytopenia.

Storage

Refrigerate unopened injection vial. Do not freeze. Protect from light. Start the infusion within 12 h after preparation; use within 24 h. Discard the solution if it becomes discolored or contains particulate matter.

Administration

! Expect to pretreat with 1000 mg orally of acetaminophen, along with an antihistamine and a corticosteroid. Pretreatment is given 30 min to 2 h before each infusion to minimize infusion-related side effects.

Do not give by IV push or bolus. To prepare the IV infusion, withdraw the needed amount from the vial into a syringe. Inject the dose after removing an equal volume of saline from the 1000 mL 0.9% NaCl infusion bag. Gently invert the bag to mix the contents; do not shake it. The final infusion concentration of the 300 mg initial dose is 0.3 mg/mL. The final concentration for the subsequent 2000 mg infusions will be 2 mg/mL.

Administer using an infusion pump with the in-line filter supplied with product, and polyvinyl chloride (PVC) administration sets. Flush the intravenous line with 0.9% NaCl before and after each dose. The infusion must be titrated during the first dose, second dose, and subsequent doses. See manufacturer's specific instructions. Maximum rate for the first two treatments is 200 mL/h after titration. Other treatments can be given up to 400 mL/h if tolerated after titration.

Ofloxacin

o-flox′a-sin

★ Floxin, Floxin Otic, Ocuflox

🍁 Ocuflox

Do not confuse Floxin with Flexeril or Flexon, or Ocuflox with Ocufen.

CATEGORY AND SCHEDULE

Pregnancy Risk Category: C

Classification: Anti-infectives, fluoroquinolones

MECHANISM OF ACTION

A fluoroquinolone antibiotic that inhibits DNA gyrase in susceptible microorganisms, interfering with bacterial cell replication and repair. *Therapeutic Effect*: Bactericidal.

PHARMACOKINETICS

Rapidly and well absorbed from the GI tract. Protein binding: 20%-25%. Widely distributed (including to the cerebrospinal fluid [CSF]). Metabolized in the liver. Primarily excreted in urine. Removed by hemodialysis. *Half-life:* 4.7-7 h (increased in impaired renal function, cirrhosis, and elderly patients).

AVAILABILITY

Tablets (Floxin): 200 mg, 300 mg, 400 mg.
Ophthalmic Solution (Ocuflox): 0.3%.
Otic Solution (Floxin): 0.3%.

INDICATIONS AND DOSAGES

▸ **Uncomplicated urinary tract infection (UTI)**
PO
Adults, Elderly. 200 mg q12h for 3-7 days.
Complicated urinary tract infection (UTIs)
PO
Adults, Elderly. 200 mg q12h for 10 days.
▸ **Pelvic inflammatory disease (PID)**
PO
Adults, Elderly. 400 mg q12h for 10-14 days.
▸ **Lower respiratory tract, skin, and skin-structure infections**
PO
Adults, Elderly. 400 mg q12h for 10 days.
▸ **Prostatitis, sexually transmitted diseases (cervicitis, urethritis)**
PO
Adults, Elderly. 300 mg q12h for 7 days or for 6 wks for prostatitis.
▸ **Acute, uncomplicated gonorrhea**
NOTE: Due to increased prevalence of quinolone-resistance, CDC no longer recommends.
PO
Adults, Elderly. 400 mg 1 time.
▸ **Bacterial conjunctivitis**
OPHTHALMIC
Adults, Elderly, Children ≥ 1 yr. 1-2 drops q2-4h for 2 days, then 4 times a day for 5 days.
▸ **Corneal ulcers, bacterial**
OPHTHALMIC
Adults. 1-2 drops q30min while awake for 2 days, then q60min while awake for 5-7 days, then 4 times a day.
▸ **Acute otitis media with typanostomy tubes**
OTIC
Children aged 1-12 yr. 5 drops into the affected ear 2 times/day for 10 days.
▸ **Otitis externa**
OTIC
Adults, Elderly, Children 12 yr and older. 10 drops into the affected ear once a day for 7 days.
Children aged 6 mo to 11 yr. 5 drops into the affected ear once a day for 7 days.
▸ **Dosage in hepatic impairment (adults)**
Do not exceed 400 mg/day.
▸ **Dosage in renal impairment (adults)**
After a normal initial dose, systemic dosage and frequency are based on creatinine clearance.

Creatinine Clearance (mL/min)	Adjusted Dose	Dosage Interval (h)
> 50	None	q12
20-50	None	q24
< 20	1/2	q24

CONTRAINDICATIONS

Hypersensitivity to any quinolones.

INTERACTIONS

Drug
Antacids, sucralfate: May decrease absorption and effects of ofloxacin.

Caffeine: May increase the effects of caffeine.
Class IA (quinidine, procainamide), or Class III (amiodarone, sotalol) antiarrhythmic agents: May have additive effects on QT interval.
Corticosteroids: May increase risk of tendon rupture.
Oral antidiabetic agents: May potentiate hypoglycemic actions.
Warfarin: May potentiate anticoagulant effect; monitor INR.
Theophylline: May increase theophylline blood concentration and risk of toxicity.
Herbal
None known.
Food
Caffeine: See above; may limit caffeinated beverages.

DIAGNOSTIC TEST EFFECTS

None known.

SIDE EFFECTS

Frequent (7%-10%)
Nausea, headache, insomnia.
Occasional (3%-5%)
Abdominal pain, diarrhea, vomiting, dry mouth, flatulence, dizziness, fatigue, drowsiness, rash, pruritus, fever.
Rare (< 1%)
Constipation, paresthesia.

SERIOUS REACTIONS

- Antibiotic-associated colitis and other superinfections may occur from altered bacterial balance.
- Hypersensitivity reactions, including photosensitivity (as evidenced by rash, pruritus, blisters, edema, and burning skin), have occurred.
- Arthropathy (swelling, pain, and clubbing of fingers and toes, degeneration of stress-bearing portion of a joint) may occur if the systemic drug is given to children (rare).
- Tendonitis or tendon rupture.
- Rare reports of QT prolongation, arrhythmia, torsade de pointes.
- Hypoglycemia (rare).

PRECAUTIONS & CONSIDERATIONS

Caution is warranted in patients with central nervous system (CNS) disorders, QT prolongation or electrolyte imbalance, diabetes, renal impairment, or seizures. Ofloxacin may mask or delay symptoms of syphilis. Ofloxacin is distributed in breast milk. If possible, pregnant or breastfeeding women should avoid taking the drug because of the risk of arthropathy in the fetus or infant. The safety and efficacy of systemic ofloxacin have not been established in children. Age-related renal impairment may require a dosage adjustment for oral and parenteral forms. Avoid exposure to sunlight and ultraviolet light and wear sunscreen and protective clothing if photosensitivity develops.

Care is important in high sun exposure situations as a result of increased photosensitivity.

Dizziness, drowsiness, headache, and insomnia may occur while taking ofloxacin. Avoid tasks requiring mental alertness or motor skills until response to ofloxacin is established. Maintain hydration. Signs and symptoms of infection, mental status, WBC count, skin for rash, pattern of daily bowel activity and stool consistency should be monitored. Be alert for signs of superinfection, such as anal or genital pruritus, fever, stomatitis, and vaginitis, which should be reported immediately to the health care provider.

Caution is warranted in individuals who are physically active, exercise, and are generally mobile; ruptures of the tendons in the hand, shoulder, and Achilles tendon have been reported with fluoroquinolone use; such injury may require surgical repair and extended disability. Patients experiencing pain or inflammation in a tendon should be advised to rest and refrain from exercise until the situation can be medically evaluated.

Storage

Store at room temperature.

Administration

May take tablets without regard to food. Take antacids containing aluminum or magnesium or products containing iron or zinc within 2 h before or after taking ofloxacin.

For ophthalmic use, tilt the head back and place the solution in the conjunctival sac. Close the eye; then press gently on the lacrimal sac for 1 min. Do not use ophthalmic solutions for injection. To avoid contamination, do not touch tip of dropper to any other surface.

For otic use, lie down with the head turned so that the affected ear is upright. Warm solution in hands for 1-2 min. Instill drops toward the canal wall, not directly on the eardrum. Pull the auricle down and back in children and up and back in adults. Maintain position for 5 min per ear treated to ensure penetration into ear.

Olanzapine

oh-lan'za-peen

Zyprexa, Zyprexa Intramuscular, Zyprexa Relprevv, Zyprexa Zydis

Do not confuse olanzapine with olsalazine, or Zyprexa with Zyrtec or Zyvox.

CATEGORY AND SCHEDULE

Pregnancy Risk Category: C

Classification: Antipsychotics, atypical

MECHANISM OF ACTION

A dibenzapine derivative that antagonizes α_1-adrenergic, dopamine, histamine, muscarinic, and serotonin receptors. Produces anticholinergic, histaminic, and central nervous system (CNS) depressant effects. *Therapeutic Effect*: Diminishes manifestations of psychotic symptoms, stabilizes moods.

PHARMACOKINETICS

Well absorbed after PO administration. Protein binding: 93%. Extensively distributed throughout the body. Undergoes extensive first-pass metabolism in the liver. Excreted primarily in urine and, to a lesser extent, in feces. Not removed by dialysis. *Half-life:* 21-54 h. Extended release injection half life: 30 days.

AVAILABILITY

Tablets (Zyprexa): 2.5 mg, 5 mg, 7.5 mg, 10 mg, 15 mg, 20 mg.
Tablets (Orally Disintegrating [Zyprexa Zydis]): 5 mg, 10 mg, 15 mg, 20 mg.
Injection powder for solution (Zyprexa Intramuscular): 10 mg.

O

Powder for Suspension for IM Use (Zyprexa Relprevv): 210 mg, 300 mg, and 405 mg vials.

INDICATIONS AND DOSAGES

▸ Schizophrenia

PO

Adults. Initially, 5-10 mg once daily. Target dose: 10 mg/day within several days. If further adjustments are indicated, may increase by 5-10 mg/day at 7-day intervals. Range: 10-20 mg/day.
Children 13 yr and older. Initially, 2.5 mg/day. Titrate as necessary, up to 20 mg/day.

IM (ZYPREXA RELPREVV ONLY)

Adults. 150 mg, 210 mg, or 300 mg every 2 wks OR may give 300 mg or 405 mg every 4 wks. Manufacturer information gives titration for PO or IM depot conversion.

▸ Bipolar mania

PO

Adults. Initially, 10-15 mg/day (monotherapy) or 10 mg/day (with lithium or valproate). May increase by 5 mg/day at intervals of at least 24 h. Maximum: 20 mg/day.
Children 13 yr and older. Initially, 2.5 mg/day. Titrate as necessary up to 20 mg/day.

▸ Dosage for elderly or debilitated patients and those predisposed to hypotensive reactions

PO

The initial dosage for these patients is 5 mg/day, then titrate with caution according to indication.

▸ Control of agitation in schizophrenic or bipolar patients

IM (ZYPREXA INJECTION SOLUTION)

Adults, Elderly. 2.5-10 mg. May repeat 2 h after first dose and 4 h after 2nd dose. Maximum: 30 mg/day. Use lower doses (5-7.5 mg) if at risk for hypotension or if debilitated.

O

OFF-LABEL USES

Behavioral disturbance secondary to dementia, adjunct for refractory depression along with conventional antidepressants.

CONTRAINDICATIONS

Hypersensitivity.

INTERACTIONS

Drug

Alcohol, other CNS depressants, diazepam: May increase CNS depressant effects.
Anticholinergic agents: May increase anticholinergic effects.
Antihypertensives: May increase the hypotensive effects of these drugs.
Carbamazepine: Increases olanzapine clearance.
Ciprofloxacin, fluvoxamine: May increase the olanzapine blood concentration.
Dopamine agonists, levodopa: May antagonize the effects of these drugs.
Imipramine, theophylline: May inhibit the metabolism of these drugs.

Herbal

None known.

Food

None known.

DIAGNOSTIC TEST EFFECTS

May significantly increase serum GGT, prolactin, AST (SGOT), and ALT (SGPT) levels, cholesterol or triglycerides, blood sugar.

SIDE EFFECTS

Frequent

Somnolence (26%), agitation (23%), insomnia (20%), headache (17%), nervousness (16%), hostility (15%), dizziness (11%), rhinitis (10%), weight gain.

Occasional

Anxiety, constipation (9%); nonaggressive atypical behavior (8%); dry mouth (7%); weight gain (6%); orthostatic hypotension, fever, arthralgia, restlessness, cough, pharyngitis, visual changes (dim vision) (5%), extrapyramidal symptoms, fatigue.

Rare

Tachycardia; back, chest, abdominal, or extremity pain; tremor.

SERIOUS REACTIONS

- Rare reactions include seizures and neuroleptic malignant syndrome, a potentially fatal syndrome characterized by hyperpyrexia, muscle rigidity, irregular pulse or BP, tachycardia, diaphoresis, and cardiac arrhythmias.
- Extrapyramidal symptoms and dysphagia may also occur.
- Overdose (300 mg) produces drowsiness and slurred speech.
- Development of hyperglycemia/diabetes.
- QT prolongation (rare).
- Zyprexa Relprevv: May cause delirium/sedation syndrome after injection.

PRECAUTIONS & CONSIDERATIONS

Caution is warranted with hypersensitivity, hepatic impairment, cerebrovascular disease, cardiovascular disease (such as conduction abnormalities, heart failure, or history of myocardial infarction [MI] or ischemia), history of seizures or conditions that lower the seizure threshold (such as Alzheimer disease), and conditions predisposing to hypotension (such as dehydration, hypovolemia, and use of antihypertensives). Extreme caution should be used with elderly patients who are at risk for aspiration pneumonia, those who are concurrently taking hepatotoxic drugs, and those who should avoid anticholinergics (such as persons with benign prostatic hyperplasia). Elderly patients with dementia-related psychosis had a significantly higher incidence of cerebrovascular adverse events (e.g., stroke, TIA) and increased risk of mortality. It is unknown whether olanzapine crosses the placenta or is distributed in breast milk. The safety and efficacy of olanzapine have not been established in children less than 13 yr.

Drowsiness may occur but generally subsides with continued therapy. Tasks requiring mental alertness or motor skills should be avoided. Dehydration, particularly during exercise; exposure to extreme heat; and concurrent use of medications that cause dry mouth or other drying effects should also be avoided. A healthy diet and exercise program should be maintained to minimize weight gain. Notify the physician of extrapyramidal symptoms or excessive sedation. BP and therapeutic response should be assessed. Rapid postural changes should be avoided due to possible development of orthostatic hypotension.

Symptoms including sore tongue, problems eating or swallowing, fever, or infection need to be reported immediately.

Storage

Store at room temperature. Keep orally disintegrating tablets in blister until time of use. Unopened injection should be protected from light; do not freeze. Once constituted, drug is stable for 1 h at room temperature.

Administration

Take olanzapine without regard to food. Take as ordered and do not abruptly discontinue the drug or increase the dosage. Orally dissolving tablets may be dissolved on tongue without water.

Zyprexa IM is for IM use only. Dissolve vial contents with 2.1 mL of sterile water for injection (resulting solution is 5 mg/mL). Inject slowly, deep into muscle mass. Incompatible with diazepam, lorazepam, and haloperidol.

Zyprexa Relprevv injection suspension is for deep IM gluteal injection only; do not confuse the dosage form with the IM injection solution. NEVER give intravenously. Use the diluent provided to reconstitute. Use gloves when reconstituting, as Zyprexa Relprevv is irritating to the skin. Relprevv form MUST be administered in a health care facility with emergency equipment, and patient must be observed for 3 h following each dose.

Olmesartan Medoxomil

ohl-me-sar′tan med-ox′o-myl

Benicar Olmetec

CATEGORY AND SCHEDULE

Pregnancy Risk Category: C (D if used in second or third trimester)

Classification: Antihypertensive agents, angiotensin II receptor antagonists

MECHANISM OF ACTION

An angiotensin II receptor, type AT_1, antagonist that blocks the vasoconstrictor and aldosterone-secreting effects of angiotensin II, inhibiting the binding of angiotensin II to the AT_1 receptors. *Therapeutic Effect*: Causes vasodilation, decreases peripheral resistance, and decreases BP.

PHARMACOKINETICS

Rapidly and completely absorbed after PO administration. Hydroxylated in GI tract to active form. Metabolized in the GI tract. Recovered primarily in feces and, to a lesser extent, in urine. Not removed by hemodialysis. *Half-life:* 13 h.

AVAILABILITY

Tablets: 5 mg, 20 mg, 40 mg.

INDICATIONS AND DOSAGES

▸ Hypertension

PO

Adults, Elderly, Patients with mildly impaired hepatic or renal function. 20 mg once a day in patients who are not volume depleted. After 2 wks of therapy, if further reduction in BP is needed, may increase dosage to 40 mg/day.

Children 6 yr and older. Initially, 10 mg once per day for weight of 20-34 kg or 20 mg once per day for weight ≥ 35 kg. After 2 wks, the dose can increase to a maximum of 20 mg once daily for those < 35 kg or 40 mg once daily for those ≥ 35 kg.

CONTRAINDICATIONS

Hypersensitivity.

INTERACTIONS

Drug

Antihypertensives: Additive antihypertensive effect; ACE inhibitors may increase risk of hyperkalemia or renal effects.

NSAIDs: Possible diminished antihypertensive effect.

Herbal

None known.

Food

None known.

DIAGNOSTIC TEST EFFECTS

May increase blood hemoglobin and hematocrit levels.

SIDE EFFECTS

Occasional (3%)
Dizziness.
Rare (< 2%)
Headache, diarrhea, upper respiratory tract infection, hyperkalemia.

SERIOUS REACTIONS

- Overdosage may manifest as hypotension and tachycardia.
- Hypersensitivity.

PRECAUTIONS & CONSIDERATIONS

Caution is warranted in patients with hepatic and renal impairment and renal arterial stenosis. It is unknown whether olmesartan is distributed in breast milk. It may cause fetal or neonatal morbidity or mortality. Therefore, caution is warranted in lactation; discontinue use as soon as pregnancy is confirmed; assess patient for pregnancy before prescribing. Safety and efficacy of olmesartan have not been established in children under the age of 6 yr. No age-related precautions have been noted in elderly patients.

Dizziness may occur. Tasks that require mental alertness or motor skills should be avoided. Apical pulse and BP should be assessed immediately before each olmesartan dose and regularly throughout therapy. Be alert to fluctuations in apical pulse and BP. If an excessive reduction in BP occurs, place the patient in the supine position with feet slightly elevated and notify the physician. Diagnostic tests, such as hemoglobin and hematocrit levels and liver function tests, should be assessed. Maintain adequate hydration; exercising outside during hot weather should be avoided to decrease the risk of dehydration and hypotension. Caution is warranted when sedation or general anesthesia is required due to risk of hypotensive episode.

Storage
Store tablets at room temperature. The compounded oral suspension should be refrigerated and is stable up to 4 wks.

Administration
Take olmesartan without regard to meals. For children who cannot swallow tablets, the manufacturer supplies a recipe for a compounded suspension. Shake well before each use; measure dose with calibrated oral syringe.

Olopatadine

oh-loe-pa′ta-deen
★ Patanase, Patanol, Pataday
🍁 Patanol

CATEGORY AND SCHEDULE

Pregnancy Risk Category: C

Classification: Antihistamine; mast cell stabilizer, ophthalmic, nasal

MECHANISM OF ACTION

An antihistamine that inhibits histamine release from the mast cell. *Therapeutic Effect:* Inhibits symptoms associated with allergic conjunctivitis/allergic rhinitis.

PHARMACOKINETICS

The time to peak concentration is < 2 h and duration of action is 8 h. Minimal absorption after topical administration. Metabolized to inactive metabolites. Primarily excreted in urine. *Half-life:* 3-8 h.

AVAILABILITY

Nasal Spray Solution: 0.6%.

Ophthalmic Solution: 0.1%, 0.2%.

INDICATIONS AND DOSAGES

▸ **Allergic conjunctivitis**

OPHTHALMIC

Adults, Elderly, Children 3 yr and older. 0.1% solution: 1-2 drops in affected eye(s) twice daily q6-8h; 0.2% solution: 1 drop in affected eye(s) once daily.

▸ **Seasonal allergic rhinitis**

INTRANASAL

Adults, Elderly, Children 12 yr and older. 2 sprays per nostril once daily.

Children 6-11 yrs. 1 spray per nostril twice daily.

CONTRAINDICATIONS

Hypersensitivity to olopatadine hydrochloride or any other component of the formulation.

INTERACTIONS

Drug

Anticholinergics: Enhanced anticholinergic effects.

CNS depressants: Enhanced somnolence.

Herbal

None known.

Food

None known.

SIDE EFFECTS

Occasional

Ophthalmic use: Headache, weakness, cold syndrome, taste perversion, burning, stinging, dry eyes, foreign body sensation, hyperemia, keratitis, eyelid edema, itching, pharyngitis, rhinitis, sinusitis. Nasal spray: Bitter taste, nasal ulceration, epistaxis, pharyngolaryngeal pain, postnasal drip, cough, throat irritation, somnolence, dry mouth.

SERIOUS REACTIONS

- None reported.

PRECAUTIONS & CONSIDERATIONS

While rare, somnolence may occur with nasal use and may require caution with normal activities until effects of the drug are known. Use caution in pregnancy and lactation due to lack of data.

Storage

Store at room temperature.

Administration

Do not use ophthalmic olopatadine while wearing contacts. Wait 15 min after use before reinserting. To avoid contamination, do not touch the dropper tip to the eye area.

Prime nasal spray before initial use and when not used for more than 7 days. Avoid spraying in the eyes.

Olsalazine Sodium

ohl-sal′ah-zeen soo′dee-um

Dipentum

Do not confuse olsalazine with olanzapine.

CATEGORY AND SCHEDULE

Pregnancy Risk Category: C

Classification: Gastrointestinal, anti-inflammatory, 5-aminosalicylates

MECHANISM OF ACTION

A salicylic acid derivative that is converted to 5-aminosalicylic acid in the colon by bacterial action. Blocks prostaglandin production in bowel mucosa. *Therapeutic Effect:* Reduces colonic inflammation in inflammatory bowel disease.

PHARMACOKINETICS

PO: Partially absorbed; peak attained in 1.5 h. Excreted in urine as 5-aminosalicylic acid and metabolites; crosses placenta. *Half-life:* 5-10 h.

AVAILABILITY

Capsules: 250 mg.

INDICATIONS AND DOSAGES

▸ **Maintenance of controlled ulcerative colitis**

PO

Adults, Elderly. 1 g/day in 2 divided doses, preferably q12h.

OFF-LABEL USES

Treatment of Crohn disease.

CONTRAINDICATIONS

History of hypersensitivity to 5-aminosalicylates or other salicylates.

INTERACTIONS

Drug

Antacids: Do not administer olsalazine sodium with antacids.

Azithoprine, mercaptopurine: May increase side effects of these antineoplastics.

Warfarin, low-molecular-weight heparins: Possible increased risk for bleeding or excessive anticoagulation.

Herbal

None known.

Food

None known.

DIAGNOSTIC TEST EFFECTS

May increase AST (SGOT) and ALT (SGPT) levels.

SIDE EFFECTS

Frequent (5%-10%)

Headache, diarrhea (17%), abdominal pain or cramps, nausea.

Occasional (1%-5%)

Depression, fatigue, dyspepsia, upper respiratory tract infection, decreased appetite, rash, itching, arthralgia.

Rare (1%)

Dizziness, vomiting, stomatitis.

SERIOUS REACTIONS

- Sensitivity may occur in susceptible patients, manifested by cramping, headache, diarrhea, fever, rash, hives, itching, and wheezing. Discontinue drug immediately.
- Excessive diarrhea associated with extreme fatigue is noted rarely.
- Hepatotoxicity (rare).

PRECAUTIONS & CONSIDERATIONS

Caution is warranted with preexisting renal or hepatic disease. The drug should not be used during pregnancy or lactation. Safety and efficacy are not established in children. Serum alkaline phosphatase, AST, and ALT levels should be obtained before therapy. Adequate fluid intake should be maintained. Daily bowel activity and stool consistency and skin for rash should be assessed. Notify physician if persistent or increasing cramping, diarrhea, fever, pruritus, or rash occurs; olsalazine should be discontinued. Avoid adiminstration of any drug that could aggravate inflammatory colon disease; medical consultation is necessary for appropriate antibiotic selection.

Storage

Store at room temperature.

Administration

Take olsalazine with food in evenly divided doses.

Omalizumab

oh-mah-liz′uw-mab

★ 🍁 Xolair

Do not confuse with ofatumumab.

CATEGORY AND SCHEDULE

Pregnancy Risk Category: B

Classification: Anti-IgE monoclonal antibodies

MECHANISM OF ACTION

A monoclonal antibody that selectively binds to human immunoglobulin E (IgE), preventing it from binding to the surface of mast cells and basophiles. *Therapeutic Effect*: Prevents or reduces the number of asthmatic attacks because of allergens.

PHARMACOKINETICS

Absorbed slowly after SC administration, with peak concentration in 7-8 days. Excreted by the liver, reticuloendothelial system, and endothelial cells. *Half-life:* 26 days.

AVAILABILITY

Powder for Injection: 202.5 mg, provides 150 mg/1.2 mL after reconstitution.

INDICATIONS AND DOSAGES

▸ **Moderate to severe persistent asthma in patients who are reactive to a perennial allergen and whose asthma symptoms have been inadequately controlled with inhaled corticosteroids**

SC

Adults, Elderly, Children 12 yr and older. 150-375 mg every 2 or 4 wks; dose and dosing frequency are individualized based on weight and pretreatment immunoglobulin E (IgE) level (as shown below).

4-wk Dosing Table

Pretreatment Serum IgE Levels (units/mL)	Weight 30-60 kg	Weight 61-70 kg	Weight 71-90 kg	Weight 91-150 kg
30-100 mg	150 mg	150 mg	150 mg	300 mg
101-200 mg	300 mg	300 mg	300 mg	See next table
201-300 mg	300 mg	See next table	See next table	See next table

2-wk Dosing Table

Pretreatment Serum IgE Levels (units/mL)	Weight 30-60 kg	Weight 61-70 kg	Weight 71-90 kg	Weight 91-150 kg
101-200	See preceding table	See preceding table	See preceding table	225 mg
201-300	See preceding table	225 mg	225 mg	300 mg
301-400	225 mg	225 mg	300 mg	Do not dose
401-500	300 mg	300 mg	375 mg	Do not dose
501-600	300 mg	375 mg	Do not dose	Do not dose
601-700	375 mg	Do not dose	Do not dose	Do not dose

OFF-LABEL USES
Treatment of asthma resulting from food allergies.

CONTRAINDICATIONS
Hypersensitivity.

INTERACTIONS
Drug
None known.
Herbal
None known.
Food
None known.

DIAGNOSTIC TEST EFFECTS
May increase serum IgE levels.

SIDE EFFECTS
Frequent (11%-45%)
Injection site ecchymosis, redness, warmth, stinging, and urticaria; viral infections; sinusitis; headache; pharyngitis.
Occasional (3%-8%)
Arthralgia, leg pain, fatigue, dizziness.
Rare (2%)
Arm pain, earache, dermatitis, pruritus.

SERIOUS REACTIONS
- Anaphylaxis occurs within 2 h of the first dose or subsequent doses in 0.1% of patients.
- Malignant neoplasms occur in 0.5% of patients.

PRECAUTIONS & CONSIDERATIONS
Omalizumab is not intended to reverse acute bronchospasm or status asthmaticus. Because IgE is present in breast milk, omalizumab is also believed to be present in breast milk. Use omalizumab only if clearly needed. The safety and efficacy of omalizumab have not been established in children younger than 12 yr. No age-related precautions have been noted in elderly patients. Drink plenty of fluids to decrease the thickness of lung secretions.

Serum total IgE levels should be obtained before beginning omalizumab therapy because the drug dosage is based on these pretreatment levels. Pulse rate and quality as well as respiratory depth, rate, rhythm, and type should be monitored. Fingernails and lips should also be assessed for a blue or dusky color in light-skinned patients and a gray color in dark-skinned patients, which may be signs of hypoxemia. Rapidly acting sympathomimetic inhalants should be available for emergency use.

Storage
Store omalizumab in the refrigerator. The reconstituted solution is stable for 8 h if refrigerated or 4 h if stored at room temperature. Protect from direct sunlight.

Administration
! Expect to base omalizumab dosage on serum IgE levels obtained before beginning treatment. Do not use serum IgE levels obtained during treatment to determine omalizumab dosage because IgE levels remain elevated for up to 1 yr after the drug has been discontinued.

Use only clear or slightly opalescent solution; the solution is slightly viscous. Use only sterile water for injection to prepare for SC administration. Draw 1.4 mL sterile water for injection into a 3-mL syringe with a 1-inch, 18-gauge needle, and inject contents into the vial of powder. Swirl the vial for approximately 1 min; do not shake it. Then swirl the vial again for 5-10 seconds every 5 min until no gel-like particles appear in the solution. The drug takes 15-20 min to dissolve. Do not use the solution if the contents fail to dissolve completely in 40 min. Invert the vial for 15 seconds to allow the solution to drain toward the stopper. Using a new 3-mL syringe with a 1-inch, 18-gauge needle, withdraw the required 1.2-mL dose and replace the 18-gauge needle with a 25-gauge needle for SC administration. SC administration may take 5-10 seconds because of omalizumab's viscosity. Patients are usually observed in office for 2 h following a dose.

Omeprazole

om-eh-pray'zole

Prilosec, Prilosec OTC

Losec

Do not confuse Prilosec with prilocaine, Prinivil, Prozac, or Prevacid, or omeprazole with olmesartan. Do not confuse Losec with Lasix.

CATEGORY AND SCHEDULE

Pregnancy Risk Category: C

Classification: Gastrointestinal agents, antiulcer agents, antisecretory proton pump-inhibitors

MECHANISM OF ACTION

A benzimidazole that is converted to active metabolites that irreversibly bind to and inhibit hydrogen-potassium adenosine triphosphatase, an enzyme on the surface of gastric parietal cells. Inhibits hydrogen ion transport into gastric lumen. *Therapeutic Effect*: Increases gastric pH, reduces gastric acid production.

PHARMACOKINETICS

Route	Onset	Peak	Duration
PO	1 h	2 h	72 h

Rapidly absorbed from the GI tract. Protein binding: 95%. Primarily distributed into gastric parietal cells. Metabolized extensively in the liver. Primarily excreted in urine. Unknown whether removed by hemodialysis. *Half-life:* 0.5-1 h (increased in patients with hepatic impairment).

AVAILABILITY

Capsules (Delayed Release [Prilosec]): 10 mg, 20 mg, 40 mg.
Delayed-Release Tablets (Prilosec OTC): 20 mg.
Delayed-Release Granules for Oral Suspension: 2.5-mg, 10-mg packets.

INDICATIONS AND DOSAGES

▸ **Erosive esophagitis, poorly responsive gastroesophageal reflux disease (GERD), active duodenal ulcer, prevention and treatment of NSAID-induced ulcers**

PO

Adults, Elderly. 20 mg/day.

▸ **To maintain healing of erosive esophagitis**

PO

Adults, Elderly. 20 mg/day.

▸ **Pathologic hypersecretory conditions**

PO

Adults, Elderly. Initially, 60 mg/day up to 120 mg 3 times a day.

▸ **Duodenal ulcer caused by *Helicobacter pylori***

PO

Adults, Elderly. 20 mg twice a day for 10 days, with antibiotics.

▸ **Active benign gastric ulcer**

PO

Adults, Elderly. 40 mg/day for 4-8 wks.

▸ **Dyspepsia (OTC use)**

Adults. 20 mg once daily for no more than 14 days. Contact physician regarding long-term treatment if heartburn continues.

▸ **Usual pediatric dosage**

Children 1-16 yr and ≥ 20 kg. 20 mg once daily. See adult dosage if > 16 yr.

Children 1-16 yr and 10 to < 20 kg. 10 mg once daily.

Children 1-16 yr and 5 to < 10 kg. 5 mg/day.

OFF-LABEL USES
Prevention of NSAID-induced ulcers, stress-ulcer prophylaxis.

CONTRAINDICATIONS
Hypersensitivity to omeprazole or related drugs, including interstitial nephritis.

INTERACTIONS
Drug
Clopidogrel: Do not use omeprazole with clopidogrel. PPI may decrease the conversion of clopidogrel to its active metabolite, thereby reducing its effectiveness.
Diazepam, oral anticoagulants (warfarin), phenytoin: May increase the blood concentration of diazepam, oral anticoagulants, and phenytoin.
Ketoconazole: Decreases ketoconazole absorption.
Protease inhibitors: Reduces-absorption of many. Some contraindicate use of omeprazole concurrently.
Tacrolimus: May increase serum levels.
Herbal
None known.
Food
None known.

DIAGNOSTIC TEST EFFECTS
May increase serum alkaline phosphatase, AST (SGOT), and ALT (SGPT) levels. Rare decreases in platelet counts.

SIDE EFFECTS
Frequent (7%)
Headache.
Occasional (2%-3%)
Diarrhea, abdominal pain, nausea.
Rare (2%)
Dizziness, asthenia or loss of strength, vomiting, constipation, upper respiratory tract infection, back pain, rash, cough.

SERIOUS REACTIONS
- Anaphylaxis/angioedema.
- Interstitial nephritis.

PRECAUTIONS & CONSIDERATIONS
It is unknown whether omeprazole crosses the placenta; caution warranted in pregnancy. Omeprazole is excreted in human milk; a decision should be made whether to discontinue breastfeeding. Safety and efficacy have not been established in children under 1 yr. No age-related precautions have been noted in elderly patients. Consider dose reduction in chronic hepatic disease or Asian patients.

Notify the physician if headache, diarrhea, discomfort, or nausea occurs during omeprazole therapy. Serum chemistry laboratory values, particularly serum alkaline phosphatase, AST, and ALT levels should be obtained to assess liver function. Loose or soft stool may be noted early in the therapy protocol. Do not use Prilosec OTC for more than 2 wks without medical consultation.

Storage
Store at room temperature. Do not prepare granules ahead of time of administration.
Administration
Take omeprazole before meals. Do not crush capsules; swallow capsules whole. If patient has difficulty swallowing, capsule may be opened and contents sprinkled on a tablespoon of cool applesauce. Swallow without chewing and follow with a sip of water. The oral suspension is prepared

as follows: Mix 2.5- or 10-mg packet into 5 or 15 mL of water, respectively. Stir and allow to thicken 2-3 min. Stir and drink. Can also be given via nasogastric tube.

Onabotulinumtoxin A (formerly Botulinum Toxin Type A)

bot′yoo-lin-num toks′in type a

Botox, Botox Cosmetic

CATEGORY AND SCHEDULE

Pregnancy Risk Category: C

Classification: Miscellaneous skeletal muscle relaxants

O

MECHANISM OF ACTION

A neurotoxin that blocks neuromuscular conduction by binding to receptor sites on motor nerve endings and inhibiting the release of acetylcholine, resulting in muscle denervation. *Therapeutic Effect:* Reduces muscle activity.

AVAILABILITY

Injection: 50 units, 100 units, 200 units, per vial.

INDICATIONS AND DOSAGES

▸ Cervical dystonia in patients who have previously tolerated botulinum toxin type A

IM

Adults, Elderly. Mean dose of 236 units (range: 198-300 units) divided among the affected muscles, based on patient's head and neck position, localization of pain, muscle hypertrophy, patient response, and adverse reaction history.

▸ Cervical dystonia in patients who have not previously been treated with botulinum toxin type A

IM

Adults, Elderly. Administer at lower dosage than for patients who have previously tolerated the drug. Limit total dose injected into the sternocleidomastoid muscles to 100 units or less to decrease incidence of dysphagia.

▸ Strabismus

IM

Adults, Children older than 12 yr. 1.25-2.5 units into any one muscle.

Children 2 mo to 12 yr. 1-2.5 units into any one muscle.

▸ Blepharospasm

IM

Adults. Initially, 1.25-2.5 units. May increase up to 2.5-5.0 units at repeat treatments. Maximum: 5 units per injection or cumulative dose of 200 units over a 30-day period.

▸ Improvement of brow furrow/glabellar lines

IM

Adults 65 yr and younger. 20 units total dose injected over 5 sites.

▸ Axillary hyperhidrosis

INTRADERMAL

Adults. 50 units per axilla.

OFF-LABEL USES

Treatment of dynamic muscle contracture in children with cerebral palsy, focal task-specific dystonia, head and neck tremor unresponsive to drug therapy, hemifacial spasms, laryngeal dystonia, oromandibular dystonia, spasmodic torticollis, writer's cramp.

CONTRAINDICATIONS

Infection at proposed injection sites, hypersensitivity to albumin, botulinum toxin, or any component of the formulation.

INTERACTIONS

Drug

Aminoglycoside antibiotics, other drugs that interfere with neuromuscular transmission (such as curare-like compounds): May potentiate the effects of botulinum toxin type A.

Herbal

None known.

Food

None known.

DIAGNOSTIC TEST EFFECTS

None known.

SIDE EFFECTS

Frequent (11%-15%)

Localized pain, tenderness, or bruising at injection site; localized weakness in injected muscle; upper respiratory tract infection; neck pain; headache.

Occasional (2%-10%)

Increased cough, flu-like symptoms, back pain, rhinitis, dizziness, hypertonia, soreness at injection site, asthenia, dry mouth, nausea, somnolence.

Rare

Stiffness, numbness, diplopia, ptosis.

SERIOUS REACTIONS

- Mild to moderate dysphagia occurs in approximately 20% of patients.
- Arrhythmias and severe dysphagia (manifested as aspiration, pneumonia, and dyspnea) occur rarely but may cause death.
- Overdose produces systemic weakness and muscle paralysis, respiratory failure, death.

PRECAUTIONS & CONSIDERATIONS

Caution is warranted with neuromuscular junctional disorders, such as amyotrophic lateral sclerosis, Lambert-Eaton syndrome, motor neuropathy, and myasthenia gravis, because they may experience significant systemic effects, including respiratory compromise, and severe dysphagia. Be aware of signs of dysphagia and aspiration pneumonia, including fever, sputum production, and adventitious breath sounds after treatment. Safety and effectiveness are not established in children < 12 yr for blepharospasm or strabismus, < 16 yr for cervical dystonia, and < 18 yr for hyperhidrosis.

Clinical improvement should begin within 2 wks of the injection, but the drug's maximum benefit will appear approximately 6 wks after the injection. Resume normal activity slowly and carefully. Seek medical attention immediately if respiratory, speech, or swallowing difficulties occur.

Storage

Store drug vials in the refrigerator. The reconstituted solution may be refrigerated for up to 24 h. Administer the drug within 24 h after reconstitution. The solution normally appears as clear and colorless; discard the solution if particulate matter is present.

Administration

! Plan to have a physician inject the drug into the affected muscle.

Expect to administer the drug at the lowest effective dosage and at the longest effective dosing interval to avoid formation of neutralizing antibodies. Dilute drug with 0.9% NaCl. For a resulting dose of units/0.1 mL, draw up 1 mL of diluent to provide 10 units per 0.1 mL, 2 mL to provide 5 units per 0.1 mL, 2.5 mL to provide 4 units per 0.1 mL, 4 mL to provide 2.5 units per 0.1 mL, or 8 mL to provide 1.25 units per 0.1 mL. Slowly and gently inject the diluent

O

into the vial to avoid producing bubbles. Then rotate the vial gently to mix the drug. If a vacuum does not pull the diluent into the vial, discard it. For IM use, assist the physician, as necessary, while he or she injects the drug into the affected muscles using a 25-, 27-, or 30-gauge needle for superficial muscles and a 22-gauge needle for deeper muscles. For intradermal injection, inject each dose at a 45-degree angle to a depth of approximately 2 mm.

Ondansetron Hydrochloride

on-dan-seh'tron high-droh-klor'ide

Zofran, Zofran ODT, Zuplenz

Do not confuse Zofran with Zantac or Zosyn.

CATEGORY AND SCHEDULE

Pregnancy Risk Category: B

Classification: Antiemetics, selective 5-HT_3 serotonin receptor antagonists

MECHANISM OF ACTION

An antiemetic that blocks serotonin, both peripherally on vagal nerve terminals and centrally in the chemoreceptor trigger zone. *Therapeutic Effect*: Prevents nausea and vomiting.

PHARMACOKINETICS

Readily absorbed from the GI tract. Protein binding: 70%-76%. Metabolized in the liver. Primarily excreted in urine. Unknown whether removed by hemodialysis. All tablets are bioequivalently interchangeable. *Half-life:* 4 h.

AVAILABILITY

Oral Solution (Zofran): 4 mg/5 mL.
Orally Disintegrating Film, (Zuplenz): 4 mg, 8 mg.
Tablets (Zofran): 4 mg, 8 mg, 24 mg.
Tablets (Orally Disintegrating [Zofran ODT]): 4 mg, 8 mg.
Injection (Zofran): 2 mg/mL.
Injection (Premix): 32 mg/50 mL.

INDICATIONS AND DOSAGES

▸ Prevention of chemotherapy-induced nausea and vomiting

PO

Adults, Elderly, Children older than 11 yr. 24 mg as a single dose 30 min before starting chemotherapy, or 8 mg 30 min before chemotherapy and again 8 h after first dose; then q12h for 1-2 days.

Children 4-11 yr. 4 mg 30 min before chemotherapy and again 4 and 8 h after chemotherapy, then q8h for 1-2 days.

IV INFUSION

Adults, Elderly, Children 4-18 yr. 32 mg as a single dose, or 0.15 mg/kg/dose 30 min before chemotherapy, then 4 and 8 h after chemotherapy.

▸ Prevention of radiation-induced nausea and vomiting

PO

Adults, Elderly. 8 mg 1-2 h before radiation, followed by 8 mg 3 times a day, or if radiation is intermittent, 8-mg single dose 1-2 h before radiation.

▸ Prevention of postoperative nausea and vomiting

IV, IM

Adults, Elderly. 4 mg undiluted over 2-5 min.

Children weighing < 40 kg. 0.1 mg/kg.

Children weighing ≥ 40 kg. 4 mg.

PO

Adults, Elderly. 16 mg given as two 8-mg tablets 1 h before anesthesia.

OFF-LABEL USES

Hyperemesis gravidarum.

CONTRAINDICATIONS
Hypersensitivity to ondansetron or other selective 5-HT_3 receptor antagonists. Use with apomorphine.

INTERACTIONS
Drug
Apomorphine: Causes profound hypotension and loss of consciousness; contraindicated.
Phenytoin, carbamazepine, rifampicin: May decrease levels of ondansetron.
Tramadol: May increase patient-controlled administration of tramadol.
Herbal and Food
None known.

DIAGNOSTIC TEST EFFECTS
May transiently increase serum bilirubin, AST (SGOT), and ALT (SGPT) levels.

IV INCOMPATIBILITIES
Acyclovir (Zovirax), allopurinol (Aloprim), aminophylline, amphotericin B (Fungizone), amphotericin B complex (Abelcet, AmBisome, Amphotec), ampicillin (Polycillin), ampicillin and sulbactam (Unasyn), cefepime (Maxipime), cefoperazone (Cefobid), ertapenem, 5-fluorouracil, furosemide, insulin (regular), lansoprazole, lorazepam (Ativan), meropenem (Merrem IV), methylprednisolone (Solu-Medrol), micafungin, pantoprazole.

IV COMPATIBILITIES
Carboplatin (Paraplatin), cisplatin (Platinol), cyclophosphamide (Cytoxan), cytarabine (Cytosar), dacarbazine (DTIC-Dome), daunorubicin (Cerubidine), dexamethasone (Decadron), diphenhydramine (Benadryl), docetaxel (Taxotere), dopamine (Intropin), etoposide (VePesid), gemcitabine (Gemzar), heparin, hydromorphone (Dilaudid), ifosfamide (Ifex), magnesium, mannitol, mesna (Mesnex), methotrexate, metoclopramide (Reglan), mitomycin (Mutamycin), mitoxantrone (Novantrone), morphine, paclitaxel (Taxol), potassium chloride, teniposide (Vumon), topotecan (Hycamtin), vinblastine (Velban), vincristine (Oncovin), vinorelbine (Navelbine).

SIDE EFFECTS
Frequent (5%-13%)
Anxiety, dizziness, somnolence, headache, fatigue, constipation, diarrhea, hypoxia, urine retention.
Occasional (2%-4%)
Abdominal pain, xerostomia, fever, feeling of cold, redness and pain at injection site, paresthesia, asthenia.
Rare (1%)
Hypersensitivity reaction (including rash and pruritus), blurred vision.

O

SERIOUS REACTIONS
- Overdose may produce a combination of central nervous system (CNS) stimulant and depressant effects.
- Rare case of dystonic reactions.
- Rare cases of temporary vision loss, for a few minutes up to 48 h.
- Liver failure and death have been reported in patients with cancer receiving concurrent potentially hepatotoxic chemotherapy and antibiotics.

PRECAUTIONS & CONSIDERATIONS
Ondansetron is not a drug that stimulates gastric or intestinal peristalsis. It should not be used instead of nasogastric suction. Animal data have not indicated fetal harm. In humans, it is unknown whether ondansetron crosses the placenta or is distributed in breast milk. The safety and efficacy of ondansetron have

not been established in neonates. No age-related precautions have been noted in elderly patients. Alcohol, barbiturates, and tasks that require mental alertness or motor skills should be avoided.

Dizziness or drowsiness may occur. Pattern of daily bowel activity and stool consistency, hydration status, bilirubin, AST (SGOT), and ALT (SGPT) levels should be monitored. Onset of sudden blindness, which usually resolves in 2-3 h, should be immediately reported as it may indicate overdosage.

Storage

Store vials and oral products at room temperature. The infusion is stable for 48 h after dilution.

Administration

! Give all oral doses 30 min before chemotherapy and repeat at 8-h intervals, as prescribed.

Take ondansetron without regard to food. Orally disintegrating film or tablets may be dissolved on tongue without water.

For IV use, ondansetron may be given undiluted as an IV push over 2-5 min for doses up to 4 mg only. For IV infusion, dilute with 50 mL D5W or 0.9% NaCl before administration, and infuse over 15 min. May also give IM if dose is 4 mg or less.

Oprelvekin (Interleukin-11 [IL-11])

oh-prel′ve-kin

★ Neumega

Do not confuse Neumega with Neupogen. Do not confuse with interleukin-2.

CATEGORY AND SCHEDULE

Pregnancy Risk Category: C

Classification: Hematopoietic agents; platelet growth factor, interleukins.

MECHANISM OF ACTION

A hematopoietic recombinant version of human interleukin-11 (IL-11) that stimulates production of blood platelets, essential to the blood-clotting process. *Therapeutic Effect*: Increases platelet production.

PHARMACOKINETICS

Peak 1-6 h following single subcutaneous dose. Rapidly excreted by the kidneys. *Half-life:* 6.9 h.

AVAILABILITY

Injection: 5 mg.

INDICATIONS AND DOSAGES

▸ Prevention of thrombocytopenia as a result of chemotherapy

SC

Adults. 50 mcg/kg once a day, beginning 6-24 h after completion of chemotherapy, and usually for 10-21 days.

▸ Dosage in renal impairment

If CrCl < 30 mL/min, reduce to 25 mcg/kg once daily (i.e., a 50% dose reduction).

CONTRAINDICATIONS

Hypersensitivity.

INTERACTIONS

Drug

Platelet inhibitors, aspirin: Caution is warranted with NSAIDs and aspirin, which can affect platelet function.

Thiazide loop diuretics: Increase risk of hypokalemia.

Herbal

None known.

Food

None known.

DIAGNOSTIC TEST EFFECTS

May decrease albumin levels, hemoglobin and hematocrit (dilutional effect), usually within

3-5 days of initiation of therapy; reverses about 1 wk after therapy discontinued.

SIDE EFFECTS

Frequent

Nausea or vomiting (77%), fluid retention (59%), neutropenic fever (48%), diarrhea (43%), rhinitis (42%), headache (41%), dizziness (38%), fever (36%), insomnia (33%), cough (29%), rash or pharyngitis (25%), tachycardia (20%), vasodilation (19%).

SERIOUS REACTIONS

- Transient atrial fibrillation or flutter occurs in 10% of patients and may be caused by increased plasma volume; oprelvekin is not directly arrhythmogenic. Arrhythmias usually are brief and spontaneously convert to normal sinus rhythm.
- Papilledema, especially in children.
- Serious acute hypersensitivity.
- Congestive heart failure, dyspnea, pulmonary edema.

PRECAUTIONS & CONSIDERATIONS

Caution is warranted in patients with congestive heart failure (CHF), fluid retention, renal problems, stroke, or TIA and in those with a history of atrial arrhythmia. Although drug has been used in children, a safe and effective dose is not established; the effective dose often exceeds the maximum tolerated dose of 50 mcg/kg/day.

Notify the physician of palpitations or dyspnea. Fluid and electrolyte status should be closely monitored, particularly if the patient is receiving diuretic therapy. Fluid retention should be assessed as evidenced by dyspnea on exertion and peripheral edema; it generally occurs during the first week of therapy and continues for the duration of treatment. An ECG should be obtained. Platelet count should also be periodically assessed for therapeutic response. An electric razor and soft toothbrush should be uesd until platelet count is within normal range. CBC should be obtained before chemotherapy and at regular intervals thereafter.

Storage

Store in refrigerator. Once reconstituted, use within 3 h.

Administration

! Begin oprelvekin administration 6-24 h following completion of chemotherapy dose. Discontinue at least 48 h before starting next chemotherapy cycle.

For SC use, add 1 mL sterile water for injection to provide concentration of 5 mg/mL oprelvekin. Inject along inside surface of vial, and swirl contents gently to avoid excessive agitation. Discard unused portion. Give single injection in the abdomen, thigh, hip, or upper arm. Continue drug dosing until postnadir platelet count is > 50,000 cells/mcL. Expect drug to be discontinued at least 2 days before next planned chemotherapy cycle.

Orlistat

ohr'lih-stat

★ 🍁 Xenical, Alli (OTC)

Do not confuse Xenical with Xeloda.

CATEGORY AND SCHEDULE

Pregnancy Risk Category: B

OTC (Alli)

Classification: Gastrointestinals, obesity agents, lipase inhibitors

MECHANISM OF ACTION

A gastric and pancreatic lipase inhibitor that inhibits absorption of dietary fats by inactivating gastric and pancreatic enzymes. *Therapeutic Effect*: Resulting caloric deficit may positively affect weight control.

PHARMACOKINETICS

Minimal absorption after administration. Protein binding: 99%. Primarily eliminated unchanged in feces. Unknown if removed by hemodialysis.
Half-life: 1-2 h.

AVAILABILITY

Capsules: 120 mg (Rx).
Capsules: 60 mg (OTC).

INDICATIONS AND DOSAGES

▸ **Weight reduction in patients with body mass index of 27 kg/m² or over**

PO

Adults, Elderly, Children aged 12 yr and older. 120 mg 3 times a day (Xenical); 60 mg 3 times/day (Alli).

CONTRAINDICATIONS

Cholestasis, chronic malabsorption syndrome, hypersensitivity.

INTERACTIONS

Drug

Antidiabetic medications, insulin: Doses may require adjustment as glycemic control improves with weight loss.

Cyclosporine: Reduces cyclosporine absorption; do not coadminister. If necessary, give cyclosporine 2 h before or after orlistat.

Fat-soluble vitamins: Orlistat reduces absortion; take multivitamin supplement to ensure adequate nutrition. Take 2 h before or after orlistat, preferably at bedtime.

Levothyroxine: May decrease absorption of thyroid hormone. Administer at least 4 h apart.

Warfarin: May increase response to warfarin by limiting vitamin K absorption; monitor INR carefully.

Herbal and Food

None known.

DIAGNOSTIC TEST EFFECTS

Decreases blood glucose, total cholesterol, and serum LDL levels. Decreases absorption and levels of fat-soluble vitamins (A, D, E, K).

Rarely see increase in ALT and AST levels with prescription use.

SIDE EFFECTS

Frequent (20%-30%)

Headache, abdominal discomfort, flatulence, fecal urgency, fatty or oily stool.

Occasional (5%-14%)

Back pain, menstrual irregularity, nausea, fatigue, diarrhea, dizziness.

Rare (< 4%)

Anxiety, rash, myalgia, dry skin, vomiting.

SERIOUS REACTIONS

- Severe liver injury with hepatocellular necrosis or acute hepatic failure reported with prescription use (rare).
- Hyperoxaluria or calcium oxalate nephrolithiasis.

PRECAUTIONS & CONSIDERATIONS

Use with caution in patients with a history of pancreatitis or kidney stones. It is unknown whether orlistat is excreted in breast milk. Orlistat use is not recommended during pregnancy or in breastfeeding women. Safety and efficacy of orlistat have not been established in children under 12 yr; use in older children only under health professional supervision. No age-related precautions have been noted in elderly patients.

Unpleasant side effects, such as flatulence and fecal urgency, may occur but should diminish with time. Laboratory studies, such as blood glucose levels and lipid profile, should be obtained before and during therapy. Changes in coagulation parameters as well as height and weight should also be monitored. Monitor patients who are severely obese for diabetes or cardiovascular disease before beginning therapy.

Storage

Store at room temperature; protect from moisture.

Administration

Orlistat's side effects tend to be transient in nature, gradually diminishing during treatment as long as patient adheres to low-fat diet.

A nutritionally balanced, reduced-calorie diet should be maintained. Carbohydrates, fats, and protein should be distributed over three main meals. Give orlistat with each main meal or up to 1 h after such meals. If a meal is skipped, then skip that scheduled dose of orlistat. Weight loss will be most evident in the first 6 mo of use.

Orphenadrine

or-fen′a-dreen

Norflex

CATEGORY AND SCHEDULE

Pregnancy Risk Category: C

Classification: Skeletal muscle relaxants

MECHANISM OF ACTION

A skeletal muscle relaxant that is structurally related to diphenhydramine and may be thought to affect skeletal muscle indirectly by central atropine-like effects. *Therapeutic Effect*: Relieves musculoskeletal pain.

PHARMACOKINETICS

Well absorbed after PO and IM absorption. Protein binding: low. Metabolized in liver. Primarily excreted in urine and feces. *Half-life:* 14 h.

AVAILABILITY

Injection: 30 mg/mL (Norflex).
Tablets (Extended Release): 100 mg (Norflex).

INDICATIONS AND DOSAGES

▸ **Musculoskeletal pain**

IM/IV

Adults, Elderly. 60 mg 2 times/day. Switch to oral form for maintenance.

PO

Adults, Elderly. 100 mg 2 times/day.

OFF-LABEL USES

Drug-induced extrapyramidal reactions.

CONTRAINDICATIONS

Angle-closure glaucoma, myasthenia gravis, pyloric or duodenal obstruction, stenosing peptic ulcer, prostatic hypertrophy, obstruction of the bladder neck, achalasia, cardiospasm (megaesophagus), hypersensitivity to orphenadrine or any component of the formulation.

INTERACTIONS

Drug

Alcohol, central nervous system (CNS) depressants, propoxyphene: May increase CNS sedative effects.
Anticholinergics: May increase anticholinergic effects.
Propoxyphene: Reports of confusion, tremors, anxiety.

Herbal

St. John's wort, valerian, kava kava, gotu kola: May increase CNS depression.

Food

None known.

O

DIAGNOSTIC TEST EFFECTS
None known.

IV INCOMPATIBILITIES
None known.

IV COMPATIBILITIES
None known.

SIDE EFFECTS
Frequent
Drowsiness; dizziness; muscular weakness; hypotension; dry mouth, nose, throat, and lips; urinary retention; thickening of bronchial secretions.
Elderly, Frequent
Sedation, dizziness, hypotension.
Occasional
Flushing, visual or hearing disturbances, paresthesia, diaphoresis, chills, euphoria.

SERIOUS REACTIONS
- Hypersensitivity reaction, such as eczema, pruritus, rash, cardiac disturbances, and photosensitivity, may occur.
- Overdosage may vary from CNS depression, including sedation, apnea, hypotension, cardiovascular collapse, or death to severe paradoxical reaction, such as hallucinations, tremor, and seizures.

PRECAUTIONS & CONSIDERATIONS
Caution is warranted with tachycardia, cardiac decompensation, coronary insufficiency, cardiac arrhythmias, or urinary retention. It is unknown whether orphenadrine crosses the placenta or is distributed in breast milk; therefore, caution in lactation and pregnancy is warranted. Safety and efficacy of orphenadrine have not been established in children. Not a preferred drug for the elderly due to side effect risks.

Drowsiness and dizziness may occur but usually diminish with continued therapy. Avoid alcohol and tasks that require mental alertness or motor skills until the effects of the drug are known.

If bloody or tarry stools, continued weakness, diarrhea, fatigue, itching, nausea, or skin rash occurs, notify the physician.

Storage
Store oral and injection formulations at room temperature. Protect injection from light. Solution for injection normally appears clear, colorless; discard if cloudy or precipitate is present.

Administration
Do not crush extended-release product. Give without regard to food.

For IV, may administer undiluted. Give slowly over 5 min, with patient in the supine position. Keep patient supine for at least 10 min. IM is injected deeply into a large muscle, such as the deltoid.

Oseltamivir
ah-suhl-tahm′ah-veer
Tamiflu

CATEGORY AND SCHEDULE
Pregnancy Risk Category: C

Classification: Antivirals, neuraminidase inhibitors

MECHANISM OF ACTION
A selective inhibitor of influenza virus neuraminidase, an enzyme essential for viral replication. Acts against both influenza A and B viruses. *Therapeutic Effect*: Suppresses the spread of infection within the respiratory system and

reduces the duration of clinical symptoms.

PHARMACOKINETICS

Readily absorbed. Protein binding: 3%. Extensively converted to active drug in the liver. Primarily excreted in urine. *Half-life:* 6-10 h.

AVAILABILITY

Capsules: 30 mg, 45 mg, 75 mg.
Oral Suspension: 12 mg/mL.

INDICATIONS AND DOSAGES

NOTE: Because of the development of resistance, prescribers should consider available influenza susceptibility patterns when choosing appropriate treatments.

▸ **Influenza A or B infection**

PO

Adults, Elderly, Adolescents ≥ 13 yr and Children weighing > 40 kg. 75 mg twice a day for 5 days.
Children weighing 24-40 kg. 60 mg twice a day for 5 days.
Children weighing 16-23 kg. 45 mg twice a day for 5 days.
Children weighing ≤ 15 kg. 30 mg twice a day for 5 days. Not indicated in infants < 1 yr of age.

▸ **Prevention of influenza**

PO

Adults, Elderly, Adolescents ≥ 13 yr. 75 mg once a day for 10 days-6 weeks.
Children 1-12 yr. Children receive the usual weight based dose, but are given this dose just once per day for prevention. Do not give to infants.

▸ **Dosage in renal impairment**

PO

CrCL 10-30 mL/min or less.
Adult, Elderly. Decreased to 75 mg once a day for 5 days for active treatment. For prophylaxis, decrease to 75 mg every other day or 30 mg once daily. No data available for children. No data for CrCl < 10 mL/min.

OFF-LABEL USES

Use in swine flu (H1N1) treatment.

CONTRAINDICATIONS

Hypersensitivity to oseltamivir or any of its components, use in infants and neonates.

INTERACTIONS

Drug

Intranasal influenza vaccine: Do not give at same time; oseltamivir may interfere with response to vaccine. Give live vaccine 48 h after last oseltamivir dose whenever possible.

Herbal and Food

None known.

DIAGNOSTIC TEST EFFECTS

None known.

SIDE EFFECTS

Frequent (5%)

Nausea, vomiting, diarrhea.

Occasional (1%-4%)

Abdominal pain, bronchitis, dizziness, headache, cough, insomnia, fatigue, vertigo.

SERIOUS REACTIONS

- Colitis, pneumonia, and pyrexia occur rarely.

PRECAUTIONS & CONSIDERATIONS

Caution is warranted in patients with renal function impairment. Be aware that it is unknown whether oseltamivir is excreted in breast milk; therefore, caution in lactation is warranted. Oseltamivir is most suitable for treating influenza type A. Safety and efficacy of this drug have not been established in infants younger than 1 yr. No age-related precautions have been noted in elderly patients. Be aware that oseltamivir is not a substitute for a flu shot. Blood glucose should be monitored. Oseltamivir is on the

Centers for Disease Control and Prevention (CDC) list of approved medications for use in pandemic H5N1 flu (avian flu).

Storage

Store capsules at room temperature. After reconstitution, store suspension at room temperature for up to 10 days or may store refrigerated for up to 17 days. Do not freeze.

Administration

Give oseltamivir without regard to food. The drug should be started as soon as possible within the first 48 h of the first appearance of flu symptoms. The entire duration of therapy should be followed. Shake oral suspension well before each use.

If the oral suspension product is not available, the capsules may be opened and mixed with sweetened liquids such as regular or sugar-free chocolate syrup.

Oxacillin

ox-a-sill'in

CATEGORY AND SCHEDULE

Pregnancy Risk Category: B

Classification: Antibiotics, antistaphylococcal penicillins, penicillinase-resistant penicillin.

MECHANISM OF ACTION

A penicillin that binds to bacterial membranes. *Therapeutic Effect*: Bactericidal.

PHARMACOKINETICS

PO/IM: Peak 30-60 min; duration 4-6 h.

IV: Peak 5 min; duration 4-6 h. Metabolized in the liver; excreted in bile, urine, and breast milk; crosses the placenta. *Half-life:* 30-60 min.

AVAILABILITY

Powder for Injection: 1-g vials, 2-g vials.

Pre-mix IVPB Solution: 1 g/50 mL, 2 g/50 mL.

INDICATIONS AND DOSAGES

▸ **Upper respiratory tract, skin and skin-structure infections**

IV, IM

Adults, Elderly, Children weighing 40 kg or more. 250-500 mg q4-6h. Maximum: 12 g/day.

Children weighing < 40 kg. 50 mg/kg/day in divided doses q6h.

▸ **Lower respiratory tract and other serious infections**

IV, IM

Adults, Elderly, Children weighing ≥ 40 kg. 1 g q4-6h. Maximum: 12 g/day.

Children and Infants weighing < 40 kg. 100 mg/kg/day in divided doses q4-6 h. Neonates require extended dosage intervals and lower total daily dosage (e.g., 25-75 mg/kg/day).

CONTRAINDICATIONS

Hypersensitivity to any penicillin.

INTERACTIONS

Drug

Aminoglycosides: Infusions must be separated by 1 h due to physical incompatibility.

Erythromycin, lincosamides, tetracyclines: Possible decrease in antimicrobial effectiveness.

Methotrexate: Possible increase in methotrexate toxicity.

Oral contraceptives: May decrease effectiveness of these medications.

Probenecid: May increase oxacillin blood concentration and risk of toxicity.

Herbal and Food

None known.

DIAGNOSTIC TEST EFFECTS

May increase AST (SGOT) levels. May cause a positive Coombs' test.

IV INCOMPATIBILITIES

Amikacin, amphotericin B, caffeine, calcium chloride, calcium gluconate, diazepam, dobutamine, doxycycline, esmolol, gentamicin, haloperidol, hydralazine, inamrinone, phenytoin, promethazine, protamine, tobramycin.

SIDE EFFECTS

Frequent
Mild hypersensitivity reaction (fever, rash, pruritus), GI effects (nausea, vomiting, diarrhea).
Occasional
Phlebitis, thrombophlebitis (more common in elderly), hepatotoxicity (with high IV dosage).

SERIOUS REACTIONS

- Antibiotic-associated colitis and other superinfections may result from altered bacterial balance.
- A mild to severe hypersensitivity reaction may occur in those allergic to penicillins.

PRECAUTIONS & CONSIDERATIONS

Caution is warranted in patients with impaired renal function or a history of allergies, especially to cephalosporins. History of allergies, especially to cephalosporins or penicillins, should be determined before giving the drug. Withhold and promptly notify the physician if rash or diarrhea occurs. Severe diarrhea with abdominal pain, blood or mucus in stool, and fever may indicate antibiotic-associated colitis. Signs and symptoms of superinfection, including anal or genital pruritus, black hairy tongue, diarrhea, increased fever, sore throat, ulceration or changes of oral mucosa, and vomiting should be monitored. Intake and output, renal function tests, urinalysis, and the injection sites should be assessed.

For patients using oral contraceptives, there is a potential risk for decreased effectiveness; the patient should be advised to comply with the oral dosing schedule of contraceptives while taking this medication, as well as use an additional nonhormonal birth control method throughout the duration of treatment.

Storage
Store vials at room temperature. Once reconstituted, the solution remains stable for 3 days at room temperature or 7 days refrigerated. When further diluted with D5W or 0.9% NaCl, the solution is stable for 24 h.

Premix IVPB solution comes frozen. Thawed solution stable for 21 days under refrigeration or 48 h at room temperature.

Administration
For IV use add 5 mL to each 250-mg vial (concentration 50 mg/mL) or add 10 mL sterile water for injection to each 1-g vial to provide a concentration of 100 mg/mL. For piggyback administration, further dilute with 50-100 mL D5W or 0.9% NaCl. Administer IV piggyback over 30 min to 1h. Slower infusion time and IV concentrations of 20 mg/mL or less may help limit phlebitis. If needed, the drug may be given IV push slowly over 10 min after vial reconstitution.

For IM use, reconstitute each 1 g vial with 5.7 mL of sterile water for injection to provide a concentration of 250 mg/1.5 mL of oxacillin. Administer the injection deep into a large muscle mass within 1 h of preparation.

Oxaliplatin

ahks-al-eh-plah'tin

Eloxatin

CATEGORY AND SCHEDULE

Pregnancy Risk Category: D

Classification: Antineoplastic; platinum analogue

MECHANISM OF ACTION

A platinum-containing complex that cross-links with DNA strands, preventing cell division. Cell cycle-phase nonspecific. *Therapeutic Effect:* Inhibits DNA replication.

PHARMACOKINETICS

Rapidly distributed. Protein binding: 90%. Undergoes rapid, extensive nonenzymatic biotransformation. Excreted in urine. *Half-life:* 391 h (terminal).

AVAILABILITY

Injection Solution: 5 mg/mL.

INDICATIONS AND DOSAGES

▸ Metastatic colon or rectal cancer in patients whose disease has recurred or progressed during or within 6 mo of completing first-line therapy with bolus 5-fluorouracil (5-FU), leucovorin, and irinotecan

IV

Adults. Day 1: Oxaliplatin 85 mg/m² in 250-500 mL D5W and leucovorin 200 mg/m², both given simultaneously over more than 2 h in separate bags using a Y-line, followed by 5-FU 400 mg/m² IV bolus given over 2-4 min, followed by 5-FU 600 mg/m² in 500 mL D5W as a 22-h continuous IV infusion. Day 2: Leucovorin 200 mg/m² IV infusion given over more than 2 h, followed by 5-FU 400 mg/m² IV bolus given over 2-4 min, followed by 5-FU 600 mg/m² in 500 mL D5W as a 22-h continuous IV infusion.

▸ Dosage adjustments for neurotoxicity, gastrointestinal toxicity, or hematologic toxicity: Expect doses to be decreased or withheld depending on degree of toxicity and indication for use.

OFF-LABEL USES

Ovarian cancer, pancreatic cancer, non-Hodgkin lymphoma, breast cancer, lung cancer, prostate cancer, germ-cell carcinomas, and malignant mesothelioma.

CONTRAINDICATIONS

History of allergy to platinum compounds.

DRUG INTERACTIONS

Drug

None reported.

Herbal

None known.

Food

None known.

IV INCOMPATIBILITIES

Alkaline medications or solutions (e.g., 5-fluorouracil), aluminum needles or IV sets, sodium chloride solution or chloride-containing solutions, diazepam, cefepime.

SIDE EFFECTS

Frequent

Peripheral or sensory neuropathy (usually occurs in hands, feet, perioral area, and throat but may present as jaw spasm, abnormal tongue sensation, eye pain, chest pressure, or difficulty walking, swallowing, or writing), nausea, fatigue, diarrhea, vomiting, constipation, abdominal pain, fever, anorexia.

Occasional
Stomatitis, earache, insomnia, cough, difficulty breathing, backache, edema.
Rare
Dyspepsia, dizziness, rhinitis, flushing, alopecia.

SERIOUS REACTIONS

- Peripheral or sensory neuropathy can occur, sometimes precipitated or exacerbated by drinking or holding a glass of cold liquid during the IV infusion.
- Pulmonary fibrosis, characterized by a nonproductive cough, dyspnea, crackles, and radiologic pulmonary infiltrates, may require drug discontinuation.
- Hypersensitivity reaction (rash, urticaria, pruritus) occurs rarely.
- Hepatotoxicity.
- Extravasation necrosis.

PRECAUTIONS & CONSIDERATIONS

Use with caution in patients with renal function impairment. Dose adjustments may be necessary in patients with renal impairment, neurosensory toxicity, gastrointestinal toxicity, neutropenia, or thrombocytopenia. Premedication with antiemetics is recommended. Avoid mucositis prophylaxis with ice chips during oxaliplatin infusion. Elderly may be more sensitive to adverse effects. Safety and efficacy not established in children. Avoid use in pregnancy or breastfeeding.
Storage
Store at room temperature in original carton. Do not freeze; protect from light. After dilution, can be kept up to 6 h at room temperature or up to 24 h under refrigeration.
Administration
CAUTION: Observe and exercise appropriate precautions for handling, preparing, and administering cytotoxic drugs.
! Expect premedication with antiemetics, including 5-HT_3 blockers with or without a corticosteroid. Regimens do not require prehydration.

Must be diluted in D5W (usually 250 mL or 500 mL). Administer over 2-6 h. Flush infusion line with D5W before administration of any concomitant medications.

Oxandrolone

ox-an′droe-lone
★ Oxandrin
Do not confuse with testolactone or nandrolone, or oxymethalone

CATEGORY AND SCHEDULE

Pregnancy Risk Category: X
Controlled Substance Schedule: III

Classification: Androgenic anabolic steroid

MECHANISM OF ACTION

A synthetic testosterone derivative that promotes growth and development of male sex organs, maintains secondary sex characteristics in androgen-deficient males. *Therapeutic Effect:* Androgenic and anabolic actions.

PHARMACOKINETICS

Well absorbed from the GI tract. Protein binding: 94%-97%. Metabolized in liver. Primarily excreted in urine. Unknown whether removed by hemodialysis. *Half-life:* 5-13 h.

AVAILABILITY

Tablets: 2.5 mg, 10 mg (Oxandrin).

INDICATIONS AND DOSAGES

▸ **Cachexia**

Adults, Elderly. 2.5-20 mg in divided doses 2-4 times/day usually for 2-4 wks. Course of therapy is based on individual response. Repeat intermittently as needed.

Children. Total daily dose is less than or equal to 0.1 mg/kg. Repeat intermittently as needed.

OFF-LABEL USES

AIDS wasting syndrome, growth failure, Turner syndrome.

CONTRAINDICATIONS

Nephrosis, carcinoma of breast or prostate hypercalcemia, pregnancy, hypersensitivity to oxandrolone or any component of the formulation, nephrosis.

INTERACTIONS

Drug

Adrenocorticotropic hormone (ACTH), adrenal steroids: May increase the risk of edema and acne.

Adrenal steroids: May increase the effects of the adrenal steroids.

Insulin, oral hypoglycemic agents: May increase the effects of hypoglycemic agents.

Oral anticoagulants: May increase the effects of oral anticoagulants. Monitor INR.

Herbal

Chaparral: May increase liver enzymes.

Comfrey: May increase liver enzymes.

Eucalyptus: May increase risk of hepatotoxicity.

Germander: May increase liver enzymes.

Jin bu huan: May increase liver enzymes.

Kava kava: May increase liver enzymes.

Pennyroyal: May increase liver enzymes.

Skullcap: May increase the risk of liver damage.

Valerian: May increase risk of hepatotoxicity.

Food

None known.

DIAGNOSTIC TEST EFFECTS

May decrease levels of thyroxine-binding globulin, resulting in decreased total T_4 serum levels and increased resin uptake of T_3 and T_4. May increase PBI and radioactive iodine uptake.

May decrease HDL, increase LDL. May increase LFTs or cause suppression of clotting factors II, V, VII, and X, and an increase in PT.

SIDE EFFECTS

Frequent

Gynecomastia, acne, amenorrhea, other menstrual irregularities.

Females: Hirsutism, deepening of voice, clitoral enlargement that may not be reversible when drug is discontinued.

Occasional

Edema, nausea, insomnia, oligospermia, priapism, male pattern baldness, bladder irritability, hypercalcemia in immobilized patients or those with breast cancer, hypercholesterolemia.

Rare

Polycythemia with high dosage.

SERIOUS REACTIONS

- Peliosis hepatitis of the liver, spleen replaced with blood-filled cysts, hepatic neoplasms, and hepatocellular carcinoma have been associated with prolonged high-dosage, anaphylactic reactions.
- Children: compromised adult stature.
- Cholestatic jaundice.
- Priapism.

PRECAUTIONS & CONSIDERATIONS

Caution is warranted in patients with diabetes, epilepsy, and liver, cardiac, and renal disease. The drug is contraindicated during pregnancy. Oxandrolone use is contraindicated during lactation and is excreted in breast milk. Oxandrolone may accelerate bone maturation more rapidly than linear growth in children, and the effect may continue for 6 mo after the drug has been stopped. Its use in elderly patients may increase the risk of hyperplasia or stimulate growth of occult prostate carcinoma. Salt intake should be reduced.

Acne, nausea, pedal edema, or vomiting may occur. Women should report deepening of voice, hoarseness, and menstrual irregularities. Men should report difficulty urinating, frequent erections, and gynecomastia. Weight should be obtained each day. Weekly weight gains of more than 5 lb should be reported. Signs of anemia should be reported to health care provider. Avoid unnecessary activities that could result in unnecessary injury and bleeding.

Storage

Store oxandrolone at room temperature away from moisture, heat, and direct light.

Administration

Take oxandrolone with or without food. Take with a full glass of water. Duration of therapy will depend on the response of the patient.

Oxaprozin

ox-a-pro'zin

Daypro

Do not confuse oxaprozin with oxazepam.

CATEGORY AND SCHEDULE

Pregnancy Risk Category: C (D if used in third trimester or near delivery)

Classification: Analgesics, nonsteroidal anti-inflammatory drugs

MECHANISM OF ACTION

An NSAID that produces analgesic and anti-inflammatory effects by inhibiting prostaglandin synthesis. *Therapeutic Effect*: Reduces the inflammatory response and intensity of pain.

PHARMACOKINETICS

Well absorbed from the GI tract. Protein binding: 99%. Widely distributed. Metabolized in the liver. Primarily excreted in urine; partially eliminated in feces. Not removed by hemodialysis. *Half-life:* 42-50 h.

AVAILABILITY

Tablets: 600 mg.

INDICATIONS AND DOSAGES

▸ **Osteoarthritis**

PO

Adults, Elderly. 1200 mg once a day (600 mg in patients with low body weight or mild disease). Maximum: 1800 mg/day.

▸ **Rheumatoid arthritis**

PO

Adults, Elderly. 1200 mg once a day. Range: 600-1800 mg/day.

▸ **Juvenile rheumatoid arthritis (6 yr and older)**

Children weighing > 54 kg. 1200 mg/day.

Children weighing 32-54 kg.
900 mg/day.
Children weighing 22-31 kg.
600 mg/day.

▸ Dosage in renal impairment
For adults and elderly patients with renal impairment, the recommended initial dose is 600 mg/day; may be increased up to 1200 mg/day.

CONTRAINDICATIONS

Active peptic ulcer disease, chronic inflammation of GI tract, GI bleeding or ulceration, history of hypersensitivity to aspirin or NSAIDs, use within 10-14 days of coronary artery bypass graft (CABG).

INTERACTIONS

Drug
Antihypertensives: May decrease the effects of these drugs.
Aspirin, other salicylates, corticosteroids: May increase the risk of GI side effects such as bleeding. NSAIDs may negate cardioprotective effects of ASA.
Bone marrow depressants: May increase the risk of hematologic reactions.
Cyclosporine: May increase risk of decreased renal function.
Diuretics, β-adrenergic blockers, ACE inhibitors: May decrease antihypertensive effects.
First-time users of SSRIs also taking NSAIDs: May have a higher risk of GI effects.
Heparin, oral anticoagulants, thrombolytics: May increase the effects of these drugs.
Lithium: May increase the concentration and risk of toxicity of lithium.
Methotrexate: May increase the risk of methotrexate toxicity.
Probenecid: May increase the oxaprozin blood concentration.

Herbal
Feverfew: May decrease the effects of feverfew.
Ginkgo biloba: May increase the risk of bleeding.

Food
Alcohol: May increase the risk of dizziness or GI bleeding.

DIAGNOSTIC TEST EFFECTS

May increase BUN, serum creatinine, AST (SGOT), and ALT (SGPT) levels.

SIDE EFFECTS

Occasional (3%-9%)
Nausea, diarrhea, constipation, dyspepsia, edema.
Rare (< 3%)
Vomiting, abdominal cramps or pain, flatulence, anorexia, confusion, tinnitus, insomnia, somnolence.

SERIOUS REACTIONS

- Hypertension, acute renal failure, respiratory depression, GI bleeding, and coma occur rarely.

PRECAUTIONS & CONSIDERATIONS

Caution is warranted in patients with a history of GI tract disease, hepatic or renal impairment, and a predisposition to fluid retention. It is unknown whether oxaprozin is excreted in breast milk; therefore, caution is warranted in lactation. Oxaprozin should not be used during the third trimester of pregnancy because it may cause adverse effects in the fetus, such as premature closure of the ductus arteriosus. The safety and efficacy of oxaprozin have not been established in children. In elderly patients, GI bleeding or ulceration is more likely to cause serious complications, and age-related renal impairment may increase the risk of hepatotoxicity or renal toxicity; a decreased dosage is recommended. Cardiovascular event risk may be increased with duration of use or preexisting cardiovascular risk factors or disease. Use caution in patients with fluid retention, heart failure, or hypertension. Risk of myocardial infarction and stroke may be increased following CABG surgery. Do not administer within 4-6 half-lives before surgical procedures. Tasks that require mental alertness or motor skills should also be avoided until the drug's effects are known.

Notify the physician if bleeding, ecchymosis, edema, confusion, or weight gain occurs. BUN, serum alkaline phosphatase, bilirubin, creatinine, AST (SGOT), and ALT (SGPT) levels to assess hepatic and renal function should be assessed during therapy. Therapeutic response, such as decreased pain, stiffness, swelling, and tenderness; improved grip strength; and increased joint mobility, should be evaluated. Signs of blood dyscrasias including infection, poor circulation, bleeding, and poor healing should be reported to the health care provider immediately.

Storage

Store at room temperature tightly closed and protected from light.

Administration

Take oxaprozin with food, milk, or antacids if GI distress occurs.

Oxazepam

ox-a'ze-pam

Do not confuse oxazepam with oxaprozin.

CATEGORY AND SCHEDULE

Pregnancy Risk Category: D
Controlled Substance Schedule: IV

Classification: Anxiolytics, benzodiazepines

MECHANISM OF ACTION

A benzodiazepine that potentiates the effects of γ-aminobutyric acid by binding to specific receptors in the central nervous system. *Therapeutic Effect:* Produces anxiolytic effect and skeletal muscle relaxation.

PHARMACOKINETICS

Well absorbed from the GI tract. Protein binding: 97%. Metabolized in the liver. Primarily excreted in urine. Not removed by hemodialysis. *Half-life:* 5-20 h.

AVAILABILITY

Capsules: 10 mg, 15 mg, 30 mg.

INDICATIONS AND DOSAGES

▸ **Mild to moderate anxiety**

PO

Adults. 10-15 mg 3-4 times a day.

Elderly. Initially, 10 mg 3 times a day. May gradually increase up to 15 mg 3-4 times daily.

▸ **Severe anxiety**

PO

Adults. 15-30 mg 3-4 times a day.

▸ **Alcohol withdrawal**

PO

Adults. 15-30 mg 3-4 times a day.

CONTRAINDICATIONS

Hypersensitivity, psychoses, pregnancy.

INTERACTIONS

Drug

Alcohol, other CNS depressants, anticonvulsant medications: May potentiate CNS depression.

Herbal

Kava kava, valerian: May increase CNS depression.

Food

None known.

DIAGNOSTIC TEST EFFECTS

May elevate serum alkaline phosphatase, bilirubin, LDH, AST (SGOT), and ALT (SGPT) levels. May produce abnormal renal function test results.

SIDE EFFECTS

Frequent
Mild, transient somnolence at beginning of therapy.
Occasional
Dizziness, headache.
Rare
Paradoxical CNS reactions, such as hyperactivity or nervousness in children and excitement or restlessness in the elderly or debilitated (generally noted during the first 2 wks of therapy).

SERIOUS REACTIONS

- Abrupt or too-rapid withdrawal may result in pronounced restlessness, irritability, insomnia, hand tremor, abdominal or muscle cramps, diaphoresis, vomiting, and seizures.
- Overdose results in somnolence, confusion, diminished reflexes, and coma.

PRECAUTIONS & CONSIDERATIONS

Caution is warranted in patients with a history of drug dependence, CNS or respiratory depression, severe hepatic or renal impairment. Women on long-term therapy should use effective contraception during therapy and notify the physician if she becomes or may be pregnant. Alcohol and other CNS depressants should be avoided. While oxazepam has been used in children > 6 yr of age, absolute dosage has not been established.

Drowsiness and dizziness may occur. Tasks requiring mental alertness or motor skills should be avoided. CBC, blood chemistry, and hepatic and renal function should be monitored, especially during long-term therapy because of possible cardiovascular effects.

Psychological and physical dependence may occur with chronic administration. Elderly patients should be evaluated for adjustments in dosage. Abrupt withdrawal may result in pronounced irritability, restlessness, hand tremors, abdominal or muscle cramps, diaphoresis, vomiting, seizures.

Storage
Store at room temperature.
Administration
! Do not abruptly discontinue after long-term use. May give without regard to food.

Oxcarbazepine

oks-kar-bays′uh-peen
Trileptal
Do not confuse with carbamazepine.

CATEGORY AND SCHEDULE

Pregnancy Risk Category: C

Classification: Anticonvulsants

MECHANISM OF ACTION

An anticonvulsant that blocks sodium channels, resulting in stabilization of hyperexcited neural membranes, inhibition of repetitive neuronal firing, and diminishing synaptic impulses. *Therapeutic Effect*: Prevents seizures.

PHARMACOKINETICS

Completely absorbed from GI tract and extensively metabolized in the liver to active metabolite. Protein binding: 40%. Primarily excreted in urine. *Half-life:* 2 h; metabolite, 6-10 h.

AVAILABILITY

Oral Suspension: 300 mg/5 mL.
Tablets: 150 mg, 300 mg, 600 mg.

INDICATIONS AND DOSAGES

▸ **Adjunctive treatment of seizures**
PO
Adults, Elderly, and Children > 16 yr. Initially, 600 mg/day in 2 divided doses. May increase by up to 600 mg/day at weekly intervals. Recommended daily dose is 1200 mg/day.
Children aged 2-16 yr. 8-10 mg/kg/day initially, divided twice daily. Maximum: 600 mg/day, divided. Maintenance (based on weight); all daily doses divided and given twice daily: > 39 kg: 1800 mg/day; 29.1-39 kg: 1200 mg/day; 20-29 kg: 900 mg/day. If < 20 kg, then the maximum dose is 60 mg/kg/day, divided and given twice daily.

▸ **Conversion to monotherapy**
PO
Adults, Elderly. 600 mg/day in 2 divided doses (while decreasing concomitant anticonvulsant over 3-6 wks). May increase by 600 mg/day at weekly intervals up to 2400 mg/day.
Children age 4 yr and older. Initially, 8-10 mg/kg/day in 2 divided doses with simultaneous initial reduction of dose of concomitant antiepileptic.

▸ **Initiation of monotherapy**
PO
Adults, Elderly. 600 mg/day in 2 divided doses. May increase by 300 mg/day every 3 days up to 2400 mg/day.
Children age 4 yr and older. Initially, 8-10 mg/kg/day in 2 divided doses. Increase at 3-day intervals by 5 mg/kg/day to achieve maintenance dose by weight:
(70 kg): 1500-2100 mg/day;
(60-69 kg): 1200-2100 mg/day;
(50-59 kg): 1200-1800 mg/day;
(45-49 kg): 1200-1500 mg/day;
(35-44 kg): 900-1500 mg/day;
(25-34 kg): 900-1200 mg/day;
(20-24 kg): 600-900 mg/day.

▸ **Dosage in renal impairment**
For patients with creatinine clearance < 30 mL/min, give 50% of normal starting dose, then titrate slowly to desired dose.

OFF-LABEL USES

Bipolar disorder, trigeminal neuralgia.

CONTRAINDICATIONS

Hypersensitivity to this drug or to carbamazepine.

INTERACTIONS

Drug
All central nervous system (CNS) depressants, alcohol: May increase CNS depressive effects.
Calcium channel blockers: Oxcarbazepine may lower blood levels.
Carbamazepine, phenobarbital, phenytoin, valproic acid, verapamil: May decrease the blood concentration and effects of oxcarbazepine.
CYP450 3A4/5 enzyme inducers: May decrease plasma levels.
Oral contraceptives: May decrease the effectiveness of birth control.
Phenobarbital, phenytoin: May increase the blood concentration and risk of toxicity of these drugs.
Herbal
None known.
Food
None known.

DIAGNOSTIC TEST EFFECTS

May increase GGT level and other hepatic function test results. May increase or decrease blood glucose level. May decrease serum calcium, potassium, and sodium levels.

SIDE EFFECTS

Frequent (13%-22%)
Dizziness, nausea, headache, somnolence, fatigue, vertigo.
Occasional (5%-7%)
Vomiting, diarrhea, ataxia, nervousness, heartburn, indigestion, epigastric pain, constipation.
Rare (4%)
Tremor, rash, back pain, epistaxis, sinusitis, diplopia.

SERIOUS REACTIONS

- Clinically significant hyponatremia may occur.
- Serious hypersensitivity or rashes, including Stevens-Johnson syndrome and TENS.
- Aplastic anemia, agranulocytosis (rare).

PRECAUTIONS & CONSIDERATIONS

Caution is warranted in patients with renal impairment and a hypersensitivity to carbamazepine. Oxcarbazepine crosses the placenta and is distributed in breast milk. Oxcarbazepine is related to carbamazepine, considered to be teratogenic. No age-related precautions have been noted in children older than 4 yr. In elderly patients, age-related renal impairment may require dosage adjustment.

Drowsiness may occur, so alcohol and tasks requiring mental alertness or motor skills should be avoided. Notify the physician if dizziness, headache, nausea, and rash occur. Seizure disorder, including the onset, duration, frequency, intensity, and type of seizures, should be assessed before and during treatment. Serum sodium levels should be monitored; signs and symptoms of hyponatremia include confusion, headache, lethargy, malaise, and nausea.

Storage
Store all products at room temperature; keep suspension in original container. Use or discard suspension within 7 wks of first opening the bottle.
Administration
! If the patient must change to another anticonvulsant, plan to decrease the oxcarbazepine dose gradually as therapy begins with a low dose of the replacement drug. Do not abruptly discontinue.

May take without regard to food. Shake the oral suspension well. Do not administer it simultaneously with any other liquid medicine. Dosage may be mixed in a small glass of water if desired.

Oxiconazole

ox-i-con′a-zole
Oxistat
Do not confuse Oxistat with Nitrostat.

CATEGORY AND SCHEDULE

Pregnancy Risk Category: B

Classification: Antifungals, topical, dermatologics

MECHANISM OF ACTION

An imidazole antifungal agent that inhibits ergosterol synthesis. *Therapeutic Effect*: Destroys cytoplasmic membrane integrity of fungi. Fungicidal.

PHARMACOKINETICS

Low systemic absorption. Absorbed and distributed in each layer of the dermis. Excreted in the urine.

AVAILABILITY

Cream: 1% (Oxistat).
Lotion: 1% (Oxistat).

INDICATIONS AND DOSAGES

▸ **Tinea pedis**

TOPICAL

Adults, Elderly, Children aged 12 yr and older. Apply 1-2 times daily for 1 mo or until signs and symptoms significantly improve.

▸ **Tinea cruris, tinea corporis**

TOPICAL

Adults, Elderly, Children aged 12 yr and older. Apply 1-2 times daily for 2 wks or until signs and symptoms significantly improve.

CONTRAINDICATIONS

Hypersensitivity to oxiconazole.

INTERACTIONS

Drug

None known.

Herbal

None known.

Food

None known.

DIAGNOSTIC TEST EFFECTS

None known.

SIDE EFFECTS

Occasional

Itching, local irritation, stinging, dryness.

SERIOUS REACTIONS

• Hypersensitivity reactions characterized by rash, swelling, pruritus, maceration, and a sensation of warmth may occur.

PRECAUTIONS & CONSIDERATIONS

Caution should be used in patients with known hypersensitivity to other antifungal agents. It is unknown whether oxiconazole is distributed in breast milk; caution is warranted during lactation. Safety and efficacy of oxiconazole have not been established in children younger than 12 yr. No age-related precautions have been noted in elderly patients.

Signs and symptoms of a local reaction include blistering, burning, irritation, itching, oozing, redness, and swelling. Oxiconazole should be discontinued and the physician should be notified immediately. Hypersensitivity manifests as rash, swelling, pruritus, maceration, and sense of warmth and should be reported.

Storage

Store at room temperature.

Administration

Oxiconazole is for external use only. Shake lotion well before using. Apply and rub gently into the affected and surrounding area. Avoid contact with eyes, mouth, nose, or other mucous membranes. Topical therapy may be used for 2-4 wks. Area should not be covered with an occlusive dressing. Keep area clean and dry and wear light clothing to promote ventilation.

O

Oxybutynin

ox-i-byoo′ti-nin

★ Ditropan, Ditropan XL, Gelnique, Oxytrol 🍁 Ditropan XL, Oxytrol, Uromax

Do not confuse oxybutynin with Oxycontin, or Ditropan with diazepam.

CATEGORY AND SCHEDULE

Pregnancy Risk Category: B

Classification: Anticholinergics, urinary antispasmodic, urinary incontinence agents

MECHANISM OF ACTION

An anticholinergic that exerts antispasmodic (papaverine-like) and antimuscarinic (atropine-like)

action on the detrusor smooth muscle of the bladder. *Therapeutic Effect*: Increases bladder capacity and delays desire to void.

PHARMACOKINETICS

Route	Onset	Peak	Duration
PO	0.5-1 h	3-6 h	6-10 h

Rapidly absorbed from the GI tract. Metabolized in the liver. Primarily excreted in urine. Unknown if removed by hemodialysis. *Half-life:* 1-2.3 h.

AVAILABILITY

Syrup (Ditropan): 5 mg/5 mL.
Tablets (Ditropan): 5 mg.
Tablets (Extended Release [Ditropan XL]): 5 mg, 10 mg, 15 mg.
Transdermal (Oxytrol): 3.9 mg per 24 h.
Topical Gel (Gelnique): 10%; available in packets.

O

INDICATIONS AND DOSAGES

▸ Neurogenic bladder, overactive bladder

PO

Adults. 5 mg 2-3 times a day up to 5 mg 4 times a day.
Elderly. 2.5-5 mg twice a day. May increase by 2.5 mg/day every 1-2 days.
Children 5 yr and older. 5 mg twice a day up to 5 mg 3 times a day.

PO (EXTENDED RELEASE)

Adults. 5-10 mg once daily, up to 30 mg/day.
Children 6 yr and older. 5 mg once daily, up to 20 mg/day.

TRANSDERMAL

Adults. One patch (delivering 3.9 mg/24 h) applied twice a week. Apply every 3-4 days.

TOPICAL GEL

Adults. Apply 1 packet (100 mg) once daily.

CONTRAINDICATIONS

Hypersensitivity to oxybutynin or product components, urinary retention, gastric retention and other severe decreased GI motility conditions, uncontrolled narrow-angle glaucoma.

INTERACTIONS

Drug

Anticholinergics (such as antihistamines): May increase the anticholinergic effects of oxybutynin.
Alcohol, central nervous system (CNS) depressants: May increase CNS depressant effects.

Herbal

None known.

Food

None known.

DIAGNOSTIC TEST EFFECTS

None known.

SIDE EFFECTS

Frequent

Constipation, dry mouth, somnolence, decreased perspiration.

Occasional

Decreased lacrimation or salivation, impotence, urinary hesitancy and retention, suppressed lactation, blurred vision, mydriasis, nausea or vomiting, insomnia.

SERIOUS REACTIONS

• Overdose produces CNS excitation (including nervousness, restlessness, hallucinations, and irritability), hypotension or hypertension, confusion, tachycardia, facial flushing, and respiratory depression.

PRECAUTIONS & CONSIDERATIONS

Caution is warranted in patients with cardiovascular disease, glaucoma, suspected glaucoma, hypertension, hyperthyroidism, hepatic or renal impairment, neuropathy, benign prostatic hyperplasia, and reflux esophagitis. It is unknown whether oxybutynin crosses the placenta or is distributed in breast milk; therefore, caution in lactation is warranted. No age-related precautions have been noted in children older than 5 yr. Elderly patients may be more sensitive to the drug's anticholinergic effects, such as dry mouth and urine retention. Avoid alcohol and tasks that require mental alertness and motor skills until response to the drug is established.

Drowsiness and dizziness may occur. Intake and output, pattern of daily bowel activity and stool consistency, and symptomatic relief should be assessed. Overdose manifests as CNS excitation (restlessness, nervousness, hallucinations, irritability), hypotension or hypertension, confusion, tachycardia, facial flushing, and respiratory depression; these symptoms need to be reported to the health care provider immediately. The physician should be informed of xerostomic effects such as sore tongue, problems eating or swallowing, so that medication change can be evaluated.

Storage

Store at room temperature. Keep transdermal system in foil pouch until time of use. Gel is flammable; avoid excessive heat or flame.

Administration

Take oxybutynin without regard to food. Extended-release tablets should not be crushed or chewed.

Transdermal patch is applied to clear, dry skin of abdomen, hip, or buttock. Do not cut patch. Rotate application sites with each use. Remove patch prior to any MRI procedure to avoid burning.

Gently rub in gel on the abdomen, upper arms/shoulders, or thighs; the same site should not be used on consecutive days.

Oxycodone

ox-ee-koe'done

★ ETH-Oxydose, OxyContin, OxyFast, Roxicodone, Roxicodone Intensol 🍁 OxyContin, Oxy IR, Supeudol

Do not confuse oxycodone with hydrocodone or oxybutynin.

CATEGORY AND SCHEDULE

Pregnancy Risk Category: B (D if used for prolonged periods or at high dosages at term)

Controlled Substance Schedule: II

Classification: Analgesics, narcotic, synthetic opiate agonist.

O

MECHANISM OF ACTION

An opioid analgesic that binds with opioid receptors in the central nervous system (CNS). *Therapeutic Effect*: Alters the perception of and emotional response to pain.

PHARMACOKINETICS

Route	Onset	Peak	Duration
PO, immediate release	10-15 min	30-60 min	4-5 h
PO, controlled-release	NA	NA	12 h

Moderately absorbed from the GI tract. Protein binding: 38%-45%. Widely distributed. Metabolized in the liver. Excreted in urine. Unknown whether removed by hemodialysis.

Half-life: 2-3 h (3.2 h controlled release).

AVAILABILITY

Capsules (Immediate Release): 5 mg.
Oral Concentrate (Oxydose, OxyFast, Roxicodone Intensol): 20 mg/mL.
Oral Solution (Roxicodone): 5 mg/5 mL.
Tablets (Roxicodone): 5 mg, 15 mg, 30 mg.
Tablets (Extended Release [OxyContin]): 10 mg, 15 mg, 20 mg, 40 mg, 60 mg, 80 mg.

INDICATIONS AND DOSAGES

▸ Analgesia

PO (CONTROLLED RELEASE)
Adults, Elderly. Initially, 10 mg q12h. May increase every 1-2 days by 25%-50%.
PO (IMMEDIATE RELEASE)
Adults, Elderly. Initially, 5 mg q6h as needed. May increase up to 30 mg q4h. Usual: 10-30 mg q4h as needed.

O

CONTRAINDICATIONS

Hypersensitivity, narcotic addiction, severe respiratory depression in unmonitored setting, paralytic ileus.

INTERACTIONS

Drug
Alcohol, other CNS depressants, other narcotics, sedative-hypnotics, skeletal muscle relaxants, phenothiazines, benzodiazepines: May increase CNS or respiratory depression and hypotension.
Anticholinergics (e.g., antihistamines): May increase anticholinergic effects.
Potent CYP2D6 inhibitors: May increase oxycodone exposure.
Ritonavir: May cause a significant increase in oxycodone plasma concentrations.
Herbal
None known.
Food
None known.

DIAGNOSTIC TEST EFFECTS

May increase serum amylase and lipase levels.

SIDE EFFECTS

Frequent
Somnolence, dizziness, hypotension (including orthostatic hypotension), anorexia, constipation.
Occasional
Confusion, diaphoresis, facial flushing, urine retention, constipation, dry mouth, nausea, vomiting, headache, rash.
Rare
Allergic reaction, depression, paradoxical CNS hyperactivity or nervousness in children, paradoxical excitement and restlessness in elderly or debilitated patients.

SERIOUS REACTIONS

- Overdose results in respiratory depression, skeletal muscle flaccidity, cold or clammy skin, cyanosis, and extreme somnolence progressing to seizures, stupor, and coma.
- Hepatotoxicity may occur with overdose of the acetaminophen component of fixed-combination products.
- The patient who uses oxycodone repeatedly may develop a tolerance to the drug's analgesic effect and physical dependence.

PRECAUTIONS & CONSIDERATIONS

Extreme caution should be used in patients with acute alcoholism, anoxia, CNS depression, hypercapnia, respiratory depression or dysfunction, seizures, shock, or untreated myxedema. Caution is also warranted with acute abdominal conditions, Addison disease, chronic obstructive pulmonary disease (COPD), hypothyroidism, hepatic impairment, increased intracranial pressure, prostatic hypertrophy, and urethral stricture. Oxycodone readily crosses the placenta and is distributed in breast milk. Regular use of opioids during pregnancy may produce withdrawal symptoms in the neonate, including irritability, diarrhea, excessive crying, fever, hyperactive reflexes, seizures, sneezing, tremors, vomiting, and yawning. The neonate may develop respiratory depression if the mother receives oxycodone during labor. Children are more prone to experience paradoxical excitement. Children and elderly patients are more susceptible to the drug's respiratory depressant effects. Age-related renal impairment may increase the risk of urine retention in elderly patients.

Dizziness and drowsiness may occur, so change positions slowly and avoid alcohol, CNS depressants, and tasks that require mental alertness or motor skills until response to the drug is established. BP, respiratory rate, mental status, pattern of daily bowel activity, and clinical improvement should be monitored. The drug should be withheld and the physician should be notified if the respiratory rate is 12 breaths/min or less in an adult or 20 breaths/min or less in a child.

Overdose manifests as respiratory depression, skeletal muscle flaccidity, cold or clammy skin, cyanosis, and extreme somnolence progressing to seizures and stupor and need to be reported immediately. Hepatotoxicity may result from overdose of the acetaminophen component of fixed-combination products. Some predisposed patients may develop a tolerance to the drug's analgesic effect and physical dependence. Abrupt discontinuation of the drug may result in withdrawal effects.

Storage

Store products at room temperature. Protect oral solutions from light. Discard OxyFast solution 90 days after opening the bottle.

Administration

! Be aware that oxycodone's side effects are dependent on the dosage. Know that ambulatory patients and patients not in severe pain are more likely to experience dizziness, hypotension, nausea, and vomiting than those in the supine position or those in severe pain.

! Swallow controlled-release tablets (OxyContin) whole because crushing, breaking, or chewing them may lead to the rapid release and absorption of a potentially fatal dose. Be aware that OxyContin has a potential for abuse, and accidental overdose may result in death.

Take oral oxycodone without regard to food. Crush immediate-release tablets as needed.

Concentrated oral solution: Use care in measuring dose—highly concentrated. May add to 30 mL of liquid or semisolid food just before administration.

Oxymetholone

ox-ee-meth'oh-lone

★ Anadrol 🍁 Anapolon

Do not confuse with oxycodone or oxandrolone.

CATEGORY AND SCHEDULE

Pregnancy Risk Category: X

Controlled Substance Schedule: III

Classification: Androgenic-anabolic steroid.

MECHANISM OF ACTION
An androgenic-anabolic steroid that is a synthetic derivative of testosterone synthesized to accentuate anabolic as opposed to androgenic effects. *Therapeutic Effect*: Improves nitrogen balance in conditions of unfavorable protein metabolism with adequate caloric and protein intake, stimulates erythropoiesis, suppresses gonadotropic functions of pituitary, and may exert a direct effect upon the testes.

PHARMACOKINETICS
Metabolized in the liver via reduction and oxidation. Unchanged oxymetholone and its metabolites are excreted in urine. *Half-life:* Unknown.

AVAILABILITY
Tablets: 50 mg (Anadrol).

INDICATIONS AND DOSAGES
▸ **Anemia, chronic renal failure, acquired aplastic anemia, chemotherapy-induced myelosuppression, Fanconi anemia, red cell aplasia**

PO

Adults, Elderly, Children. 1-5 mg/kg/day. Response is not immediate, and a minimum of 3-6 mo should be given.

CONTRAINDICATIONS
Cardiac impairment, pregnancy, prostatic or breast cancer in males, metastatic breast cancer in women with active hypercalcemia, nephrosis or nephrotic phase of nephritis, severe liver disease, hypersensitivity to oxymetholone or any of its components.

INTERACTIONS
Drug

ACTH, adrenal steroids: May increase effects of adrenal steroids.

Hepatotoxic medications: May increase liver toxicity.

Insulin, oral hypoglycemics: May increase the effects of hypoglycemic agents.

Oral anticoagulants: May increase effects of oral anticoagulants.

Herbal

Chaparral, comfrey, germander, jin bu huan: May increase liver enzymes.

Eucalyptus, valerian: May increase risk of hepatotoxicity.

Kava kava, pennyroyal, skullcap: May increase risk of liver damage.

Food

None known.

DIAGNOSTIC TEST EFFECTS
May increase blood hemoglobin and hematocrit, LDL concentrations, serum alkaline phosphatase, bilirubin, calcium, potassium, SGOT (AST) levels, and sodium levels. May decrease HDL concentrations.

May cause suppression of clotting factors II, V, VII, and X, and an increase in PT.

SIDE EFFECTS
Frequent

Gynecomastia, acne.

Females: Hirsutism, deepening of voice, clitoral enlargement that may not be reversible when drug is discontinued, amenorrhea, menstrual irregularities.

Occasional

Edema, nausea, insomnia, oligospermia, male pattern baldness, bladder irritability, hypercalcemia in immobilized patients or those with breast cancer, hypercholesterolemia.

Rare

Liver damage, hypersensitivity.

SERIOUS REACTIONS
- Cholestatic jaundice, hepatic necrosis, and death occur rarely but have been reported in association with long-term androgenic-anabolic steroid use.
- Priapism.

PRECAUTIONS & CONSIDERATIONS

Caution is warranted in patients with diabetes, liver or renal impairment, congestive heart failure, hypertension, coronary artery disease, previous myocardial infarction, lipid-lipoprotein abnormalities, benign prostatic hyperplasia. Oxymetholone use is contraindicated during pregnancy and lactation and is excreted in breast milk. Safety and efficacy of oxymethalone have not been established in children and elderly patients. Adequate calories and protein should be consumed.

Acne, nausea, pedal edema, or vomiting may occur. Women should report deepening of voice, hoarseness, and menstrual irregularities. Men should report difficulty urinating, frequent erections, and gynecomastia. Weight should be obtained each day. Weekly weight gains of more than 5 lb should be reported.

Storage

Store at room temperature.

Administration

Dose should be individualized. Response is not often immediate and a minimum trial of 3-6 mo should be given. May give without regard to food.

Oxymorphone Hydrochloride

ox-ee-mor′fone high-droh-klor′ide

★ Numorphan, Opana, Opana ER

Do not confuse with morphine or hydromorphone.

CATEGORY AND SCHEDULE

Pregnancy Risk Category B (D if used for prolonged periods or at high dosages at term)

Controlled Substance Schedule: II

Classification: Analgesics, narcotic, opiate agonists

MECHANISM OF ACTION

An opioid agonist, similar to morphine, that binds at opiate receptor sites in the central nervous system (CNS). *Therapeutic Effect*: Reduces intensity of pain stimuli incoming from sensory nerve endings, altering pain perception and emotional response to pain; suppresses cough reflex.

PHARMACOKINETICS

Route	Onset (min)	Peak (min)	Duration (h)
SC	5-10	30-90	4-6
IM	5-10	30-60	3-6
IV	5-10	15-30	3-6

Well absorbed from the GI tract after oral administration. Widely distributed. Metabolized in liver via glucuronidation. Excreted in urine. *Half-life:* 1-2 h.

AVAILABILITY

Numorphan

Injection: 1 mg/mL, 1.5 mg/mL.

Opana

Tablet: 5 mg, 10 mg

Injection: 1 mg/mL

Opana ER

Tablets: 5 mg, 10 mg, 20 mg, 40 mg.

INDICATIONS AND DOSAGES

▸ **Analgesic, anxiety, preanesthesia**

IV

Adults, Elderly, Children 12 yr and older. Initially 0.5 mg.

SC/IM

Adults, Elderly, Children 12 yr and older. 1-1.5 mg IM or SC q4-6h as needed.

▸ **Acute or chronic moderate to severe pain**

PO

Adults, Elderly. 10-20 mg q4-6h (Opana) *or* 5 mg q12h, increasing by 5-10 mg q12h every 3-7 days (Opana

ER). NOTE: Opana ER is not for as-needed use and should be given only to patients needing continuous, around-the-clock pain relief.

▸ **Obstetric analgesic**

IM

Adults, Children 12 yr and older. 0.5-1 mg IM during labor.

OFF-LABEL USES

Cancer pain, intractable pain in narcotic-tolerant patients.

CONTRAINDICATIONS

Paralytic ileus, acute asthma attack, pulmonary edema secondary to chemical respiratory irritant, severe respiratory depression, upper airway obstruction, hypersensitivity.

INTERACTIONS

Drug

Anticholinergics: May increase urinary retention and severe constipation.

Alcohol, CNS depressants, tricyclic antidepressants: May increase CNS or respiratory depression, hypotension, profound sedation or coma. Alcohol increases maximum concentrations of oxymorphone.

Cimetidine: May increase activity of oxymorphone.

MAOIs: May produce severe, fatal reaction; plan to reduce dose to one-quarter usual dose.

Mixed antagonist/agonist opioid analgesics (buprenorphine, butorphanol, nalbuphine, pentazocine): May reduce oxymorphone effects and precipitate withdrawal.

Phenothiazines: May decrease effect of oxymorphone.

Propofol: May increase risk of bradycardia.

Herbal

Ginseng: May decrease opioid analgesic effectiveness.

Gotu kola, kava kava, valerian: May increase CNS or respiratory depression.

St. John's wort: May increase sedation.

Food

Alcohol: Alcohol administration with Opana ER can cause immediate release of high doses and potential fatal overdose.

DIAGNOSTIC TEST EFFECTS

May increase serum amylase levels and plasma lipase concentrations.

IV INCOMPATIBILITIES

No data available.

IV COMPATIBILITIES

Glycopyrrolate (Robinul), hydroxyzine (Vistaril), ranitidine (Zantac).

SIDE EFFECTS

Frequent

Drowsiness, dizziness, hypotension, decreased appetite, tolerance, constipation, or dependence.

Occasional

Confusion, diaphoresis, facial flushing, urinary retention, dry mouth, nausea, vomiting, headache, pain at injection site, abdominal cramps.

Rare

Allergic reaction, depression.

SERIOUS REACTIONS

- Hypotension, paralytic ileus, respiratory depression, and toxic megacolon rarely occur.
- Overdosage results in respiratory depression, skeletal muscle flaccidity, cold or clammy skin, cyanosis, extreme somnolence progressing to seizures, stupor, and coma.
- Tolerance to analgesic effect and physical dependence may occur with repeated use.
- Prolonged duration of action and cumulative effect may occur in

patients with impaired liver or renal function.

PRECAUTIONS & CONSIDERATIONS

Caution is warranted with acute alcoholism, anoxia, CNS depression, hypercapnia, respiratory depression or dysfunction, seizures, shock, untreated myxedema, acute abdominal conditions, Addison disease, chronic obstructive pulmonary disease (COPD), hypothyroidism, impaired liver function, increased intracranial pressure, and urethral stricture. Oxymorphone readily crosses the placenta, and it is unknown whether oxymorphone is distributed in breast milk. Its use may prolong labor if administered in the latent phase of the first stage of labor or before cervical dilation of 4-5 cm has occurred. Respiratory depression may occur in a neonate if the mother receives opiates during labor. Regular use of opiates during pregnancy may produce withdrawal symptoms in the neonate, including diarrhea, excessive crying, fever, hyperactive reflexes, irritability, seizures, sneezing, tremors, vomiting, and yawning. Safety and efficacy of oxymorphone have not been established in children younger than 12 yr. Elderly patients may be more susceptible to respiratory depression, and the drug may cause paradoxical excitement. Age-related prostatic hypertrophy or obstruction and renal impairment may increase the risk of urinary retention, and dosage adjustment is recommended in elderly patients. Alcohol and tasks that require mental alertness and motor skills should be avoided during therapy. Drug dependence and tolerance may occur with prolonged use at high dosages.

Excessive sedation or drowsiness, slow or shallow breathing, low BP, slow heart rate, and severe constipation should be reported to health care providers immediately.

Dizziness, hypotension, nausea, and vomiting may be experienced more frequently than those in supine position or having severe pain.

Storage

Store injection formulation at room temperature and protect from light. Slight yellow discoloration of parenteral form does not indicate a loss of potency. Oral dose forms are stored at room temperature.

Administration

! Oxymorphone's side effects depend on the dosage amount and route of administration but occur infrequently with oral antitussives. A high concentration injection should be used only in patients currently receiving high doses of another opiate agonist for severe, chronic pain caused by cancer or tolerance to opiate agonists.

May give undiluted as IV push or may give as IM or SC injection.

Extended-release or the immediate-release tablets should be given on an empty stomach either 1 h before or 2 h after eating. Opana ER: Do not crush, break, cut, or chew; swallow whole. Do not consume with alcohol.

Oxytocin

ox-ee-toe′sin

★ Pitocin

Do not confuse Pitocin with Pitressin.

CATEGORY AND SCHEDULE

Pregnancy Risk Category: C

Classification: Exogenous hormone

MECHANISM OF ACTION

An oxytocic that affects uterine myofibril activity and stimulates mammary smooth muscle. *Therapeutic Effect:* Contracts uterine smooth muscle. Enhances lactation.

PHARMACOKINETICS

Route	Onset	Peak	Duration
IV	Immediate	NA	1 h
IM	3-5 min	NA	2-3 h

Protein binding: 30%. Distributed in extracellular fluid. Metabolized in the liver and kidney. Primarily excreted in urine. *Half-life:* 1-6 min.

AVAILABILITY

Injection: 10 units/mL.

INDICATIONS AND DOSAGES

▸ Induction or stimulation of labor

IV

Adults. 0.5-1 milliunit/min. May gradually increase in increments of 1-2 milliunit/min. Rates of 9-10 milliunit/min are rarely required.

▸ Abortion, adjunct

IV

Adults. 10-20 milliunit/min.

Maximum: 30 units in any 12-h period.

▸ Control of postpartum bleeding

IV INFUSION

Adults. 10-40 units in 1 L IV fluid at a rate sufficient to control uterine atony.

IM

Adults. 10 units (total dose) after delivery.

O

CONTRAINDICATIONS

Adequate uterine activity that fails to progress, cephalopelvic disproportion, fetal distress without imminent delivery, grand multiparity, hyperactive or hypertonic uterus, obstetric emergencies that favor surgical intervention, prematurity, unengaged fetal head, unfavorable fetal position or presentation, when vaginal delivery is contraindicated (such as active genital herpes infection, placenta previa, or cord presentation, invasive cervical carcinoma), elective induction of labor.

INTERACTIONS

Drug

Caudal block anesthetics, vasopressors: May increase pressor effects.

Cyclopropane anesthetics: May cause maternal hypotension, bradycardia, abnormal AV rhythm.

Other oxytocics: May cause cervical lacerations, uterine hypertonus, or uterine rupture.

Herbal

None known.

Food

None known.

DIAGNOSTIC TEST EFFECTS

None known.

IV INCOMPATIBILITIES

Amphotericin B, diazepam, phenytoin, remifentanil.

IV COMPATIBILITIES

Heparin, insulin, multivitamins, potassium chloride, sodium bicarbonate, sodium bisulfite.

SIDE EFFECTS

Occasional

Tachycardia, premature ventricular contractions, hypotension, nausea, vomiting.

SERIOUS REACTIONS

- Hypertonicity may occur with tearing of the uterus, increased bleeding, abruptio placentae, and cervical and vaginal lacerations.
- In the fetus, bradycardia, CNS or brain damage, trauma due to rapid

propulsion, low Apgar score at 5 min, and retinal hemorrhage occur rarely.
• Prolonged IV infusion of oxytocin with excessive fluid volume has caused severe water intoxication with seizures, coma, and death.

PRECAUTIONS & CONSIDERATIONS

Induction of labor should be for medical, not elective, reasons. Oxytocin should be used as indicated and is not known to cause fetal abnormalities. Oxytocin is present in small amounts in breast milk. Oxytocin is not recommended for use in pregnant women because it may precipitate contractions and abortions. Oxytocin is contraindicated in elective induction of labor. Oxytocin is not used in children or elderly patients.

BP, pulse, respiration rates, intake and output, uterine contractions, including duration, frequency, and strength, and fetal heart rate should be monitored every 15 min. If uterine contractions last longer than 1 min, occur more frequently than every 2 min, or stop, notify the physician. Be alert to potential water intoxication and for unexpected or increased blood loss.

Storage

Store at room temperature.

Administration

Dilute 10-40 units (1-4 mL) in 1000 mL of 0.9% NaCl, lactated Ringer's solution, or D5W to provide a concentration of 10-40 milliunits/mL solution. Give by IV infusion and use an infusion device to control prescribed rate of flow.

Paclitaxel

pak-leh-tax'ell

Abraxane, Taxol

Do not confuse paclitaxel with Paxil, or Taxol with Taxotere.

NOTE: Abraxane should not be interchanged with Taxol; the two paclitaxel formulations are not equivalent.

CATEGORY AND SCHEDULE

Pregnancy Risk Category: D

Classification: Antineoplastic, taxanes

MECHANISM OF ACTION

An antineoplastic agent in the taxoid family that disrupts the microtubular cell network, which is essential for cellular function. Blocks cells in the late G2 phase and M phase of the cell. *Therapeutic Effect:* Inhibits cellular mitosis and replication.

PHARMACOKINETICS

Does not readily cross the blood-brain barrier. Protein binding: 89%-98%. Metabolized in the liver to active metabolites; eliminated by the bile. Not removed by hemodialysis. *Half-life:* 1.3-8.6 h.

AVAILABILITY

Injection. 6 mg/mL.
Injection, Protein-Bound (Abraxane). 100 mg.

INDICATIONS AND DOSAGES

▸ **Ovarian cancer**

IV (TAXOL)

Adults. 175 mg/m²/dose over 3 h or 135 mg/m²/dose over 24 h given q3wk. Follow with cisplatin 75 mg/m².

▸ **Breast carcinoma**

IV (TAXOL)

Adults, Elderly. 175 mg/m²/dose over 3 h q3wk or 135 mg/m² over 24 h.

IV (ABRAXANE)

Adults, Elderly. 260 mg/m² over 30 min q3wk.

▸ **Non–small cell lung carcinoma**

IV (TAXOL)

Adults, Elderly. 135 mg/m² over 24 h, followed by cisplatin 75 mg/m² q3wk.

▸ **Kaposi sarcoma**

IV (TAXOL)

Adults, Elderly. 135 mg/m²/dose over 3 h q3wk or 100 mg/m²/dose over 3 h q2wk.

▸ **Dosage in hepatic impairment**

Dosage adjustment may be needed based on liver enzymes, bilirubin levels, disease being treated, and product selected for use. See manufacturer information for details.

CONTRAINDICATIONS

History of hypersensitivity to paclitaxel or other drugs formulated in polyoxyethylated castor oil (Cremophor EL); patients with solid tumors who have baseline neutrophil counts < 1500 cells/mm³ or patients with AIDS-related Kaposi sarcoma who have baseline neutrophil counts < 1000 cells/mm³.

INTERACTIONS

Drugs

Strong CYP2C8 and CYP3A4 isoenzyme inhibitors (diazepam, ketoconazole, midazolam): Possible increase in action.

Herbal

St. John's wort: May decrease paclitaxel levels.

Food

None known.

IV INCOMPATIBILITIES

Polyvinylchloride (PVC) infusion sets (Taxol only). Abraxane is compatible with PVC.

SIDE EFFECTS

Expected

Diarrhea, alopecia, nausea, vomiting, neutropenia.

Frequent

Myalgia or arthralgia, peripheral neuropathy.

Occasional

Mucositis, hypotension during infusion, pain or redness at injection site, thrombocytopenia.

Rare

Bradycardia, severe hypotension, angioedema, generalized urticaria.

SERIOUS REACTIONS

- Severe hypersensitivity reactions, severe cardiac conduction abnormalities, severe peripheral neuropathy.
- Bone marrow suppression.

PRECAUTIONS & CONSIDERATIONS

Administer only under supervision of experienced cancer chemotherapy physician. Caution should be exercised in patients with bone marrow depression, AV block, hepatic impairment, recent myocardial infarction, angina pectoris, history of congestive heart failure, or currently using drug with effect on cardiac conduction system. Neutropenic nadir occurs at approximately day 11 of paclitaxel therapy. Elderly may have higher incidence of severe neuropathy, severe myelosuppression, or cardiovascular events. Avoid use in pregnant or breastfeeding patients. Safety and efficacy not established in children.

Storage

Store at room temperature in original package. Paclitaxel solutions for infusion stable at room temperature for up to 27 h. Paclitaxel protein-bound (Abraxane) solutions prepared for infusion are stable at room temperature up to 8 h.

Administration

CAUTION: Observe and exercise usual precautions for handling, preparing, and administering solutions of cytotoxic drugs.

Taxol: Premedicate with dexamethasone, diphenhydramine, and an H_2 antagonist. Use of an in-line filter of not greater than 0.22 micron is required during administration. Taxol is usually diluted in 0.9% NaCl, but other solutions are compatible (see manufacturer's info). Do not use PVC bags or tubing.

Abraxane: Protein-bound paclitaxel (Abraxane) is not interchangeable with conventional paclitaxel. Can be prepared and administered with PVC bags and infusion sets. Premedication is NOT required for Abraxane. Vials are reconstituted with 0.9% NaCl to form a suspension containing 5 mg/mL for infusion; the infusion solution is milky-white and homogeneous. Filtration is not recommended.

Palifermin

pal-ih-fur'min

★ 🍁 Kepivance

CATEGORY AND SCHEDULE

Pregnancy Risk Category: C

Classification: Keratinocyte growth factor

MECHANISM OF ACTION

An antineoplastic adjunct that binds to the keratinocyte growth factor receptor, present on epithelial cells of the buccal mucosa and tongue, resulting in the proliferation, differentiation,

P

and migration of epithelial cells. *Therapeutic Effect:* Reduces incidence and duration of severe oral mucositis.

PHARMACOKINETICS

Linear pharmacokinetics and extravascular distribution.
Total body clearance is twofold to fourfold higher in cancer patients than in healthy volunteers. *Half-life:* 3.3-5.7 h.

AVAILABILITY

Injection: 6.25-mg vials.

INDICATIONS AND DOSAGES

▸ **Prevention of oral mucositis**

IV

Adults, Elderly. The total regimen is 6 doses of 60 mcg/kg/day. Give the first 3 doses prior to myelotoxic therapy, for 3 consecutive days, with the third dose given 24-48 h before chemotherapy. The last 3 doses are given after myelotoxic therapy. The first of these are administered after, but on the same day of, hematopoietic stem cell infusion but at least 4 days after the most recent administration of palifermin.

CONTRAINDICATIONS

Patients allergic to *Escherichia coli*–derived proteins or any component of the product.

INTERACTIONS

Drug

Myelotoxic chemotherapy: Administration of palifermin during or within 24 h before or after myelotoxic chemotherapy results in increased severity and duration of oral mucositis.

Herbal

None known.

Food

None known.

DIAGNOSTIC TEST EFFECTS

May elevate serum lipase and serum amylase levels.

IV INCOMPATIBILITIES

Heparin, palifermin binds to heparin. No other data available.

SIDE EFFECTS

Frequent (28%-62%)

Rash, fever, pruritus, erythema, edema, pain at injection site.

Occasional (10%-17%)

Mouth and tongue thickness or discoloration, altered taste, dysesthesia (hyperesthesia, hypoesthesia, paresthesia), arthralgia.

SERIOUS REACTIONS

- Transient hypertension occurs occasionally.

PRECAUTIONS & CONSIDERATIONS

Use palifermin cautiously in women who are pregnant or breastfeeding. Excretion in breast milk is unknown. Safety and efficacy in children have not been established.

Storage

Store unopened vials in refrigerator. If not used immediately, the reconstituted solution may be stored in the refrigerator for 24 h. Protect from light. Warm to room temperature for up to 1 h before administration. Discard the solution if it is left at room temperature for longer than 1 h or if it becomes discolored or contains particles.

Administration

Reconstitute palifermin using aseptic technique. Slowly inject 1.2 mL of sterile water for injection to yield a final concentration of 5 mg/mL. Swirl gently to dissolve. Do not shake or agitate the solution. Dissolution takes < 3 min. Administer by IV bolus injection. If heparin is being used to maintain an IV line, use 0.9% NaCl to rinse the IV line before and after palifermin administration.

Paliperidone

pal-e-per'i-done

★ 🍁 Invega, Invega Sustenna

Do not confuse paliperidone with risperidone, or Invega with Invanz.

CATEGORY AND SCHEDULE

Pregnancy Risk Category: C

Classification: Antipsychotics, atypical

MECHANISM OF ACTION

A benzisoxazole derivative that is the active metabolite of risperidone. Activity is mediated through a combination of central dopamine type 2 (D2) and serotonin type 2 (5HT2A) receptor antagonism. Also active as an antagonist at α_1- and α_2-adrenergic receptors and H_1 histamine receptors. *Therapeutic Effect:* Suppresses psychotic behavior and stabilizes moods.

PHARMACOKINETICS

Oral form bioavailability roughly 28%; exposure increases when administered with food. Protein binding: 74%. Extensively metabolized in the liver. Excreted primarily in urine and feces. *Half-life,* Oral: 23 h (increased in those with renal impairment); Injection: 25-49 days.

AVAILABILITY

Tablets, Extended Release (Invega): 1.5 mg, 3 mg, 6 mg, 9 mg.

Injection, Extended-Release Suspension (Invega Sustenna): 39 mg, 78 mg, 117 mg, 156 mg, 234 mg.

INDICATIONS AND DOSAGES

▸ **Schizophrenia/schizoaffective disorder**

PO

Adults. 6 mg in the morning once daily. Initial dose titration is not required. If clinical assessment warrants, adjust up or down at increments of 3 mg/day no more than every 4-5 days. Maximum: 12 mg/day.

IM

Adults, Elderly. Give 234 mg on treatment day 1; 1 wk later, give 156 mg—both doses are given in deltoid muscle. The monthly maintenance dose is usually 117 mg IM (range of 39-234 mg). Monthly maintenance doses are given in either the deltoid or gluteal muscle.

▸ **Dosage in renal impairment (oral)**

CrCl 50-79 mL/min: No more than 3 mg/day initially; dosage is titrated slowly to desired effect. Maximum: 6 mg/day.

CrCl 10-49 mL/min: No more than 1.5 mg/day initially; dosage is titrated slowly to desired effect. Maximum: 3 mg/day.

▸ **Dosage in renal impairment (IM)**

CrCl 50-79 mL/min: Give 156 mg IM on treatment day 1; 1 wk later, give 117 mg IM—both doses are given in deltoid muscle. Monthly maintenance dose is 78 mg IM (range of 39-78 mg) in either the deltoid or gluteal muscle.

CrCl <50 mL/min: Do not use IM injection for dosing.

CONTRAINDICATIONS

Known hypersensitivity to either paliperidone or risperidone, or to any product excipients.

INTERACTIONS

Drug

Alcohol, other CNS depressants: May increase CNS depression.

Antihypertensives: Might increase risk of orthostasis.

Carbamazepine: May decrease the paliperidone blood concentration.

CYP2D6 inhibitors: May increase the levels/effects of paliperidone.

Dopamine agonists, levodopa: May decrease the effects of these drugs.

Valproic acid/divalproex: May increase the adverse effects/toxicity of paliperidone; raises levels up to 50%.

Herbal

St. John's wort: May lower paliperidone blood concentration.

Food

Ethanol: Avoid; may increase CNS depression.

DIAGNOSTIC TEST EFFECTS

May increase serum prolactin, blood glucose levels. May cause ECG changes. Occasionally lowers WBC.

SIDE EFFECTS

Frequent (≥ 5%)

Extrapyramidal symptoms, tachycardia, akathisia, somnolence, dyspepsia, constipation, increase in weight, nasopharyngitis, injection site reactions, dizziness.

Occasional (1%-5%)

Insomnia, headache, nausea, vomiting, rash, abdominal pain, dry skin.

Rare (< 1%)

Visual disturbances, fever, back pain, cough, arthralgia, angina, agitation or aggressive behavior, orthostatic hypotension, breast swelling.

SERIOUS REACTIONS

- Rare reactions include tardive dyskinesia (characterized by tongue protrusion, puffing of the cheeks, and chewing or puckering of the mouth) and neuroleptic malignant syndrome (marked by hyperpyrexia, muscle rigidity, change in mental status, irregular BP, tachycardia, or diaphoresis).
- Priapism.
- Neutropenia/agranulocytosis (rare).
- Seizures.
- New-onset diabetes mellitus.
- Orthostatic hypotension with IM dosing.

PRECAUTIONS & CONSIDERATIONS

Elderly patients with dementia-related psychosis had a significantly higher incidence of cerebrovascular adverse events (e.g., stroke, TIA) and increased risk of mortality. Caution is warranted in patients with breast cancer, hepatic or renal impairment, seizure disorders, recent MI, those at risk for aspiration pneumonia, suicidal tendencies. Paliperidone use should be avoided in combination with other drugs that are known to prolong the QT interval, in patients with congenital long QT syndrome, and in patients with a history of cardiac arrhythmias. Be aware that the drug may increase the risk of hyperglycemia or worsen diabetes mellitus. It is unknown whether paliperidone crosses the placenta or is excreted in breast milk. Breastfeeding is not recommended. The safety and efficacy of this drug have not been established in children. Elderly patients are more susceptible to orthostatic hypotension and may require a dosage adjustment because of age-related renal impairment.

Drowsiness and dizziness may occur but generally subside with continued therapy. Tasks requiring mental alertness or motor skills should be avoided. Notify the physician if altered gait, difficulty breathing, palpitations, pain or swelling in breasts, severe dizziness or fainting, trembling fingers, unusual movements, rash, fever, or visual changes occur. BP, heart rate, liver function test results, ECG, and weight should be assessed.

Storage

Store extended-release tablets and injection at room temperature. Protect tablets from moisture.

Administration

Swallow extended-release tablets whole with the aid of liquids. Do not chew, divide, or crush. The medication is contained within a nonabsorbable shell that will release the drug at a controlled rate. The tablet shell is eliminated from the body; patients should not be concerned if they occasionally notice something that looks like a tablet in their stool.

Give injection by the IM route only; do NOT administer intravenously. Initiate the first 2 doses in the deltoid muscle. Monthly maintenance doses can be administered in either the deltoid or gluteal muscle. Shake the syringe vigorously for a minimum of 10 seconds to ensure a homogeneous suspension. Use appropriate needle sizes. For deltoid injection, use a 1½-inch 22G needle for patients ≥ 90 kg (≥ 200 lb) and 1-inch 23G needle for patients < 90 kg (< 200 lb). For gluteal injection, use 1½-inch 22G needle regardless of patient weight.

Palonosetron

pal-oh-noe′seh-tron

★ Aloxi

CATEGORY AND SCHEDULE

Pregnancy Risk Category: B

Classification: Antiemetics, $5\text{-}HT_3$ serotonin receptor antagonist

MECHANISM OF ACTION

A $5\text{-}HT_3$ receptor antagonist that acts centrally in the chemoreceptor trigger zone and peripherally at the vagal nerve terminals. *Therapeutic Effect:* Prevents nausea and vomiting associated with chemotherapy.

PHARMACOKINETICS

Protein binding: 62%. Eliminated in urine. *Half-life:* 40 h.

AVAILABILITY

Injection: 0.25 mg/5 mL.
Capsules: 0.5 mg.

INDICATIONS AND DOSAGES

▸ **Chemotherapy-induced nausea and vomiting associated with moderately and highly emetogenic cancer chemotherapy**

IV

Adults, Elderly. 0.25 mg as a single dose 30 min before starting chemotherapy.

PO

Adults, Elderly. 0.5 mg as a single dose 60 min before starting chemotherapy.

▸ **Post-op nausea/vomiting prevention**

IV

Adults. 0.075 mg single dose, pre-anesthesia.

CONTRAINDICATIONS

Hypersensitivity.

INTERACTIONS

Drug, Herbal, and Food

None known.

DIAGNOSTIC TEST EFFECTS

None are well documented but may transiently increase serum bilirubin, AST (SGOT), and ALT (SGPT) levels.

P

IV INCOMPATIBILITIES

Do not mix palonosetron with any other drugs.

SIDE EFFECTS

Occasional (5%-9%)
Headache, constipation.
Rare (< 1%)
Diarrhea, dizziness, fatigue, abdominal pain, insomnia, anxiety, hyperkalemia, weakness.

SERIOUS REACTIONS

- Overdose may produce a combination of central nervous system (CNS) stimulant and depressant effects: Nonsustained tachycardia, bradycardia, hypotension.

PRECAUTIONS & CONSIDERATIONS

Caution is warranted in patients with history of cardiovascular disease. It is unknown whether palonosetron is excreted in breast milk. The safety and efficacy of palonosetron have not been established in children. No age-related precautions have been noted for elderly patients. Hypersensitivity may occur in patients who have exhibited hypersensitivity to other selective 5-HT_3 receptor antagonists.

Administer with caution in patients who have or may develop prolongation of cardiac conduction intervals, particularly QTc.

Alcohol, barbiturates, and tasks that require mental alertness or motor skills should be avoided until the effects of the drug are known.

Dizziness or drowsiness may occur. Pattern of daily bowel activity and stool consistency and hydration status should be monitored. Intolerable headache, persistent or intolerable constipation or diarrhea could be indicative of a serious reaction and should be reported immediately.

Storage
Store vials and capsules at room temperature. The solution normally appears clear and colorless.
Administration
Give the drug undiluted as an IV push over 30 seconds. Flush the IV line with 0.9% NaCl before and after administration.

Oral capsules may be taken without regard to food.

Pamidronate Disodium

pam-id′drow-nate
Aredia
Do not confuse Aredia with Adriamycin.

CATEGORY AND SCHEDULE

Pregnancy Risk Category: D

Classification: Bisphosphonates

MECHANISM OF ACTION

A bisphosphonate that binds to bone and inhibits osteoclast-mediated calcium resorption. *Therapeutic Effect:* Lowers serum calcium concentrations.

PHARMACOKINETICS

Route	Onset	Peak	Duration
IV	24-48 h	5-7 days	NA

After IV administration, rapidly absorbed by bone. Slowly excreted unchanged in urine. Unknown whether removed by hemodialysis. *Half-life:* bone, 300 days; unmetabolized, 2.5 h.

AVAILABILITY

Powder for Injection: 30 mg, 90 mg.

Injection Solution: 3 mg/mL, 6 mg/mL, 9 mg/mL.

INDICATIONS AND DOSAGES

▸ Hypercalcemia of malignancy

IV INFUSION

Adults, Elderly. Moderate hypercalcemia (corrected serum calcium level 12-13.5 mg/dL): 60-90 mg over 2-24 h. Severe hypercalcemia (corrected serum calcium level > 13.5 mg/dL): 90 mg over 2-24 h.

▸ Paget disease

IV INFUSION

Adults, Elderly. 30 mg/day over 4 h for 3 days.

▸ Osteolytic bone lesion

IV INFUSION

Adults, Elderly. 90 mg over 4 h once a month.

CONTRAINDICATIONS

Hypersensitivity to pamidronate or other bisphosphonates, such as etidronate, tiludronate, risedronate, and alendronate. For bone metastases, do not use pamidronate if CrCl is < 30 ml/min. In other indications, decide whether the potential benefit outweighs the potential risk.

INTERACTIONS

Drug

Calcium-containing medications, vitamin D, and antacids: Possible antagonism of pamidronate in treatment of hypercalcemia.

Use with other potentially nephrotoxic medications: May increase the risk of renal dysfunction.

Herbal and Food

None known.

DIAGNOSTIC TEST EFFECTS

May decrease serum phosphate, magnesium, calcium, and potassium levels.

IV INCOMPATIBILITIES

Calcium-containing IV fluids, including lactated Ringer's solutions.

SIDE EFFECTS

Frequent (> 10%)

Temperature elevation (at least 1° C) 24-48 h after administration; redness, swelling, induration, pain at catheter site in patients receiving 90 mg; anorexia, nausea, fatigue.

Occasional (1%-10%)

Constipation, rhinitis.

SERIOUS REACTIONS

- Hypophosphatemia, hypokalemia, hypomagnesemia, and hypocalcemia occur more frequently with higher dosages.
- Anemia, hypertension, tachycardia, atrial fibrillation, and somnolence occur more frequently with 90-mg doses.
- GI hemorrhage occurs rarely.
- Deterioration in renal function that may lead to renal failure.
- Osteonecrosis of the jaw.

PRECAUTIONS & CONSIDERATIONS

Dental implants are contraindicated for patients taking this drug. Caution is warranted with cardiac failure and renal impairment. Because no adequate and well-controlled studies have been conducted in pregnant women, it is unknown whether pamidronate causes fetal harm or is excreted in breast milk. Safety and efficacy of pamidronate have not been established in children. Elderly patients may become overhydrated and require careful monitoring of fluid and electrolytes. Dilute the drug in a smaller volume for elderly patients.

Hematocrit, hemoglobin, BUN, creatinine levels, and serum electrolyte levels, including serum calcium levels, should be established. If renal function deteriorates significantly, the use of further

P

doses must be carefully assessed. Pattern of daily bowel activity and stool consistency, BP, pulse, and temperature should also be monitored.

Storage

Store parenteral form at room temperature. The reconstituted vial is stable for 24 h when refrigerated; the IV solution is stable for 24 h after dilution.

Administration

Reconstitute each 30-mg vial with 10 mL sterile water for injection to provide concentration of 3 mg/mL. Allow the drug to dissolve before withdrawing. Further dilute with 1000 mL sterile 0.45% or 0.9% NaCl or D5W. Administer as IV infusion over 2-24 h for treatment of hypercalcemia and over 4 h for other indications. Adequate hydration is essential during pamidronate administration. Avoid overhydration in those with the potential for heart failure. Be alert for potential GI hemorrhage in those receiving a 90-mg dose.

P

Pancrelipase

pan-kre-li'pase

★ Creon, Pancreaze, Zenpep

CATEGORY AND SCHEDULE

Pregnancy Risk Category: C

Classification: Pancreatic enzymes

MECHANISM OF ACTION

Digestive enzymes that replace endogenous pancreatic enzymes. *Therapeutic Effect:* Assist in digestion of protein, starch, and fats.

AVAILABILITY

NOTE: These products are not considered bioequivalent by the FDA and cannot be interchanged.

Capsules (Delayed Release, Creon ONLY):

- 6000 units of lipase; 19,000 units of protease; 30,000 units of amylase.
- 12,000 units of lipase; 38,000 units of protease; 60,000 units of amylase.
- 24,000 units of lipase; 76,000 units of protease; 120,000 units of amylase.

Capsules (with Enteric-Coated Microspheres, Pancreaze ONLY):

- Pancreaze MT4: 4200 units of lipase; 10,000 units of protease; 17,500 units of amylase.
- Pancreaze MT10: 10,500 units of lipase; 25,000 units of protease; 43,750 units of amylase.
- Pancreaze MT16: 16,800 units of lipase; 40,000 USP units of protease; 70,000 units of amylase.
- Pancreaze MT20: 21,000 units of lipase; 37,000 units of protease; 61,000 units of amylase.

Capsules (Delayed Release. ZenPep ONLY):

- 5000 units of lipase; 17,000 units of protease; 27,000 units of amylase.
- 10,000 units of lipase; 34,000 units of protease; 55,000 units of amylase.
- 15,000 units of lipase; 51,000 units of protease; 82,000 units of amylase.
- 20,000 units of lipase; 68,000 units of protease; 109,000 units of amylase.

PHARMACOKINETICS

Pancreatic enzymes are not absorbed from the GI tract in any appreciable amount and are not systemically active. Enteric coatings or delayed release prevents inactivation by gastric acids.

INDICATIONS AND DOSAGES

▸ **Pancreatic enzyme replacement or supplement when enzymes are absent or deficient, such as with chronic pancreatitis, cystic fibrosis, or ductal obstruction from cancer of the pancreas or common bile duct; to reduce malabsorption; treatment of steatorrhea associated with**

bowel resection or postgastrectomy syndrome
PO
Adults, Children 4 yr and older. Initiate with 500 lipase units/kg per meal (maximum 2500 lipase units/kg per meal or a total of 10,000 lipase units/kg per day or less than 4000 lipase units/g fat ingested per day). Usually, half of the prescribed dose is given with each snack. The total daily dose should reflect roughly 3 meals plus 2-3 snacks per day.
Elderly. See adult dose. Enzyme doses expressed as lipase units/kg per meal should be decreased in older patients because they weigh more but tend to ingest less fat/kg in the diet.
Children 12 mo of age up to 4 yr. Initiate with 1000 lipase units/kg per meal (maximum 2500 lipase units/kg per meal or 10,000 lipase units/kg per day) or less than 4000 lipase units/g fat ingested per day. Usually, half of the prescribed dose is given with each snack. The total daily dose should reflect roughly 3 meals plus 2-3 snacks per day.
Infants (up to 12 mo). May give 2000-4000 lipase units per 120 mL of formula or per breastfeeding per day. Do not mix product contents directly into formula or breast milk.

▸ Dosage adjustments and limits
Dosing should not exceed the recommended maximum set forth by the Cystic Fibrosis Foundation Consensus Conferences Guidelines, as listed above. If steatorrhea persists, may increase cautiously. There is great inter-individual variation in response to enzymes. Changes in dosage may require an adjustment period of several days.

CONTRAINDICATIONS
None absolute. Rarely, patients allergic to pork might have severe hypersensitivity to porcine-derived pancreatic enzyme products.

INTERACTIONS
Drug
Acarbose, miglitol: May decrease the effects of these antidiabetic drugs.
Antacids: May decrease the effects of pancrelipase. Separate administration times.
Iron supplements: May decrease the absorption of iron supplements.
Herbal
None known.
Food
None known.

DIAGNOSTIC TEST EFFECTS
Porcine-derived products contain purines that may increase blood uric acid levels.

SIDE EFFECTS
Frequent
Diarrhea, abdominal pain, vomiting, constipation, flatulence, nausea, bloating and cramping.
Occasional
Perianal irritation.
Rare
Allergic reaction, mouth irritation, shortness of breath, wheezing.

SERIOUS REACTIONS
- Excessive dosage may produce nausea, vomiting, bloating, constipation, cramping, and diarrhea.
- Hyperuricosuria and hyperuricemia have occurred with extremely high dosages.
- Excessive dosage in children (e.g., > 6000 lipase units/kg/dose) may contribute to fibrosing colonopathy and colonic stricture.

PRECAUTIONS & CONSIDERATIONS
Products are not bioequivalent; drugs should not be changed or substituted without the advice of a medical practitioner. Pancrelipase should be used cautiously because

inhalation of the powder form may precipitate an asthma attack. It is unknown whether pancrelipase crosses the placenta or is distributed in breast milk. No age-related precautions have been noted in elderly patients.

Storage

Store at room temperature tightly closed. If exposed to moisture conditions > 70% for any period of time, the enzymes become inactive and should be discarded.

Administration

Take before or with meals or snacks. For infants, give immediately prior to each feeding. Contents of capsules may be mixed with a small amount of appleasauce, or other acidic food (pH of 4.5 or less; e.g., baby food bananas or pears). Contents may also be administered directly to the mouth. Follow administration with breast milk or formula. Do not mix directly into formula or breast milk. Do not crush, chew, or retain in the mouth to avoid oral mucosal irritation.

For children and other patients who are unable to swallow intact capsules, the capsules may be carefully opened and the contents sprinkled on small amounts of acidic soft food (pH 4.5 or less; commercial preparations of bananas, pears, applesauce). Swallow immediately. Do not crush or chew. Follow with water or juice. Do not retain drug in the mouth.

Panitumumab

Pan-ih-tu-mue'mab

★ 🍁 Vectibix

CATEGORY AND SCHEDULE

Pregnancy Risk Category: C.

Classification: Antineoplastic agent, monoclonal antibodies, signal transduction inhibitor

MECHANISM OF ACTION

An antineoplastic agent that binds specifically to epidermal growth factor receptor (EGFR) on normal and tumor cells and competitively inhibits the binding of ligands for EGFR. Blocks phosphorylation and activation of intracellular tyrosine kinases, resulting in inhibition of cell survival, growth, proliferation, and transformation. *Therapeutic Effect:* Inhibits growth and survival of selected human tumor cell lines expressing EGFR.

PHARMACOKINETICS

Pharmacokinetic parameters other than half-life have not been established. *Half-life:* 4-11 days.

AVAILABILITY

Injection Solution: 20 mg/mL.

INDICATIONS AND DOSAGES

▸ **EGFR-positive metastatic colorectal cancer**

IV

Adults. 6 mg/kg administered over 60 min every 14 days. Doses > 1000 mg should be administered over 90 min.

▸ **Dosing adjustments**

INFUSION REACTIONS

Infusion reactions, mild to moderate (grade 1 or 2): Reduce the infusion rate by 50% for the duration of infusion.

Infusion reactions, severe (grade 3 or 4): Immediately and permanently discontinue.

▸ **Dermatologic toxicity**

Dermatologic toxicity (grade 3 or 4): Withhold panitumumab if skin toxicity does not improve to grade 2 or lower within 1 mo; permanently discontinue.

Dermatologic toxicity (grade 2 or lower) and the patient is symptomatically improved after withholding no more than 2 doses of panitumumab. Treatment may be resumed at 50% the original dose. If toxicities recur, permanently discontinue drug. If toxicities do not recur, subsequent doses may be increased in increments of 25% of the original dose until the recommended dose of 6 mg/kg is obtained.

INTERACTIONS

Drug

Aspirin, NSAIDs: Increased GI irritation, nausea, vomiting.
Irinotecan: Increased frequency and severity of diarrhea.
Chemotherapy: Increased toxicity with combination chemotherapy.

Food and Herbal

None reported.

DIAGNOSTIC TEST EFFECTS

May decrease serum magnesium, calcium levels.

IV INCOMPATIBILITIES

Do not mix or infuse with other medications. Flush IV with 0.9% NaCl before and after administration.

SIDE EFFECTS

Frequent

Dermatologic toxicity, erythema, acneiform rash, pruritus, hypomagnesemia, fatigue, exfoliation, abdominal pain, paronychia, nausea, rash, diarrhea, constipation, fissures, vomiting, cough, acne, peripheral edema, dry skin.

Occasional

Nail disorder, stomatitis, mucositis, eyelash growth, conjunctivitis, ocular hyperemia, lacrimation increased.

Rare

Infusion reactions, eye/eyelid irritation.

SERIOUS REACTIONS

- Dermatologic toxicities, severe.
- Severe infusion reactions occur in 1%; fatal reactions reported in post-market experience.
- Pulmonary fibrosis.

PRECAUTIONS & CONSIDERATIONS

EGFR testing necessary to identify patients eligible for therapy. Use caution in patients with any hypersensitivities to panitumumab or its components. Sunlight may exacerbate skin reactions. Advise patients to wear sunscreen and protective clothing to limit sun exposure. Increased toxicity has been observed in patients receiving panitumumab in combination with chemotherapy. Safety and efficacy in children have not been established. Avoid use in pregnancy; use contraception during and for 6 mo after the last dose. Avoid breastfeeding during and for 2 mo after the last dose.

Monitor for severe infusion reactions during infusion. Monitor skin reactions; severe reactions require drug discontinuation permanently. Monitor daily serum electrolytes, as replacement therapy may be needed. Report any wheezing, progressive dyspnea, or other lung symptoms promptly.

Storage

Store vials in original cartons in refrigerator. Protect from light. Use diluted solution within 6 h of preparation if stored at room temperature or within 24 h if stored in the refrigerator.

Administration

Dilute solution with NS. Infuse over 60 min; doses over 1000 mg should be infused over 90 min. Administer with IV infusion pump using a low-protein binding 0.2- or 0.22-micrometer in-line filter. Flush line with NS before and after administration.

Pantoprazole

pan-toe-pra'zole

Protonix; Panto, Pantoloc

Do not confuse Protonix with Lotronex.

CATEGORY AND SCHEDULE

Pregnancy Risk Category: B

Classification: Gastrointestinals, proton-pump inhibitors (PPI)

MECHANISM OF ACTION

A benzimidazole that is converted to active metabolites that irreversibly bind to and inhibit hydrogen-potassium adenosine triphosphate, an enzyme on the surface of gastric parietal cells. Inhibits hydrogen ion transport into gastric lumen. *Therapeutic Effect:* Increases gastric pH and reduces gastric acid production.

PHARMACOKINETICS

Route	Onset	Peak	Duration
PO	NA	2.5 h	24 h

Rapidly absorbed from the GI tract. Protein binding: 98%. Primarily distributed into gastric parietal cells. Metabolized extensively in the liver. Excreted primarily in urine. Not removed by hemodialysis. *Half-life:* 1 h.

AVAILABILITY

Tablets (Delayed Release): 20 mg, 40 mg.
Powder for Injection: 40 mg.
Granules (Delayed Release) for Oral Suspension: 40 mg.

INDICATIONS AND DOSAGES

▸ **Erosive esophagitis**

PO

Adults, Elderly, Older Children ≥ 40 kg. 40 mg/day for up to 8 wks. If not healed after 8 wks, may continue an additional 8 wks.
Children ≥ 5yr and weighing 15 kg to < 40 kg. 20 mg once daily for up to 8 wks.

IV

Adults, Elderly. 40 mg/day for 7-10 days.

▸ **Hypersecretory conditions: Zollinger-Ellison syndrome**

PO

Adults, Elderly. Initially, 40 mg twice a day. May increase to 240 mg/day.

IV

Adults, Elderly. 80 mg twice a day. May increase to 80 mg q8h.

CONTRAINDICATIONS

Known hypersensitivity to any component of the formulation.

INTERACTIONS

Drug

Atazanavir, nelfinavir, delavirdine: Pantoprazole substantially decreases therapeutic effect.

Clopidogrel: When possible, do not give PPI with clopidogrel, as PPI will prevent activation of clopidogrel via CYP2C19.
Ketoconazole, ampicillin esters, dasatinib, iron salts: Pantoprazole may interfere with drug absorption.
Warfarin: Possible increases in INR and prothrombin time.
Herbal
None known.
Food
None known.

DIAGNOSTIC TEST EFFECTS
May increase serum creatinine, cholesterol, and uric acid levels.

IV INCOMPATIBILITIES
Do not mix with other medications. Flush IV with D5W, 0.9% NaCl, or lactated Ringer's solution before and after administration.

SIDE EFFECTS
Occasional
Diarrhea, headache, dizziness, pruritus, rash.

SERIOUS REACTIONS
- Hepatomegaly (rare).
- Serious hypersensitivity/dermatologic reactions (rare), such as angioedema, anaphylaxis, Stevens-Johnson syndrome.
- Neutropenia or thrombocytopenia.

PRECAUTIONS & CONSIDERATIONS
Caution is warranted in patients with a chronic or current hepatic disease. It is unknown whether pantoprazole crosses the placenta. The drug crosses into breast milk, and breastfeeding during use is not recommended. Safety and efficacy of pantoprazole have not been established in children under the age of 5 yr. No age-related precautions have been noted in elderly patients. Serum chemistry laboratory values, including serum creatinine and cholesterol levels, should be obtained before therapy.
Storage
Store oral forms at room temperature. Refrigerate vials and protect from light; do not freeze reconstituted vials. Once diluted, the drug is stable for 2 h at room temperature.
Administration
Take oral pantoprazole without regard to meals. Do not crush or split tablet; swallow tablet whole.

Granules should only be administered 30 min prior to a meal in apple juice or with a teaspoon of applesauce or give via NG tube in apple juice only. Granules will not dissolve and should not be chewed. Do not use any other liquids or foods to administer.

For IV use, mix 40-mg vial with 10 mL 0.9% NaCl injection. Infuse over 2 min. May also further dilute in 100 mL of D5W or 0.9% NaCl and infuse over 15 min. Do not administer by IV push or any other parenteral routes.

Paricalcitol
pare-i-cal′sih-tal
★ Zemplar

CATEGORY AND SCHEDULE
Pregnancy Risk Category: C

Classification: Vitamin D analogues, bone resorption inhibitors, renal agents

MECHANISM OF ACTION
A fat-soluble vitamin that is essential for absorption, utilization of calcium phosphate, and normal calcification

P

of bone. *Therapeutic Effect:* Stimulates calcium and phosphate absorption from the small intestine, promotes the secretion of calcium from bone to blood, promotes renal tubule phosphate resorption, acts on bone cells to stimulate skeletal growth and on parathyroid gland to suppress hormone synthesis and secretion.

PHARMACOKINETICS

Protein binding: More than 99%. Metabolized in the liver by multiple hepatic enzymes, including CYP3A4. Eliminated primarily in feces; minimal excretion in urine. Not removed by hemodialysis. *Half-life:* 13-17 h.

AVAILABILITY

Injection: 2 mcg/mL, 5 mcg/mL (Zemplar).
Capsules: 1 mcg, 2 mcg, 4 mcg (Zemplar).

P

INDICATIONS AND DOSAGES

▸ **Hyperparathyroidism and renal osteodystrophy**

Dosage is determined based on serum Ca, serum P, and plasma iPTH. Monitor at least q2wk for 3 mo, monthly for 3 mo, and then every 3 mo thereafter. In general, adjust no more frequently than q2-4 wk.

▸ **Predialysis Stage 3 or 4 chronic kidney disease**

PO

Adults with an iPTH ≤ 500 pg/mL. Initially, 1 mcg PO once daily or 2 mcg given 3 times per week given no more frequently than every other day. Adults with an iPTH > 500 pg/mL. Initially, 2 mcg PO once daily or 4 mcg PO 3 times per wk given no more than qod.
If Ca level or the Ca × P product elevated. Decrease or hold dose until normalized.
If iPTH concentrations are < 60 pg/mL or they decrease by > 60%. Decrease by 1 mcg/dose if given daily, or 2 mcg per dose if 3 times/wk. May further reduce or interrupt until normalized.
If iPTH decreases by ≥ 30% or ≤ 60%. Maintain same dose.
If iPTH decreases by < 30%, is the same, or is increasing. Increase by 1 mcg/dose for daily dosage or 2 mcg/dose for the 3 times/wk regimen.

▸ **Stage 5 ESRD on dialysis:**

PO

Adults. Initially calculate as follows: dose (mcgs) = baseline iPTH (pg/mL)/80. To avoid hypercalcemia, baseline serum Ca should be ≤ 9.5 mg/dL. Give calculated dose 3 times/wk, and no more frequently than every other day. Doses range from 1.6-24.7 mcg (mean 7-10 mcg per dose).
If Ca level or Ca × P elevated. Decrease recent dose by 2-4 mcg. May further reduce or interrupt until normalized.

IV

Adults. Initially, 0.04-0.1 mcg/kg IV bolus given no more than every other day; give at any time during dialysis. NOTE: Initial doses usually 2.5-5 mcg. Doses as high as 0.24 mcg/kg (total dose 16.8 mcg) have been administered.
If Ca level elevated, Ca × P product is > 75, or iPTH decreases by > 60%. Decrease or hold dose.
If iPTH decreases by < 30%, stays the same, or is increasing. Increase by 2-4 mcg/dose.
If iPTH decreases by > 30% or < 60% or is 1.5-3 times ULN. Maintain the same dose.

▸ **Usual pediatric dose for chronic kidney disease**

Children 5 yr and older. With iPTH < 500 pg/mL, initial dose 0.04 mcg/kg given 3 times/wk during dialysis.

If iPTH ≥ 500 pg/mL, initial dose 0.08 mcg/kg given 3 times/wk. Titrate dose by 0.04 mcg/kg based on lab values.

CONTRAINDICATIONS

Hypercalcemia, malabsorption syndrome, vitamin D toxicity, hypersensitivity to other vitamin D products or analogues.

INTERACTIONS

Drug

Aluminum-containing antacid (long-term use): May increase aluminum concentration and aluminum bone toxicity.
Calcium-containing preparations, thiazide diuretics: May increase the risk of hypercalcemia.
Cholestyramine and other fat-absorbing impairing drugs: May decrease absorption.
Digoxin: May increase the risk of digitalis toxicity.
Magnesium-containing antacids: May increase magnesium concentration.
Strong CYP3A4 inhibitors: Atazanavir, clarithromycin, indinavir, itraconazole, ketoconazole, nefazodone, nelfinavir, ritonavir, saquinavir, telithromycin, variconazole: increases risk of toxicity.

Herbal

None known.

Food

None known.

DIAGNOSTIC TEST EFFECTS

May decrease serum alkaline phosphatase.

SIDE EFFECTS

Occasional

Edema, nausea, vomiting, headache, dizziness.

Rare

Palpitations.

SERIOUS REACTIONS

- Early signs of overdosage are manifested as headache, somnolence, hypercalcemia, anorexia, nausea, vomiting, dry mouth, constipation, muscle and bone pain, and metallic taste sensation, weakness.
- Later signs of overdosage are evidenced by hypercalcemia, hypercalciuria, hyperphosphatemia, oversuppression of PTH, polyuria, polydipsia, anorexia, weight loss, nocturia, photophobia, rhinorrhea, pruritus, disorientation, hallucinations, hyperthermia, hypertension, and cardiac arrhythmias.
- Hypercalcemia occurs rarely.

PRECAUTIONS & CONSIDERATIONS

Caution is necessary in concomitant use of digoxin. It is unknown whether paricalcitol crosses the placenta or is distributed in breast milk. Safety and efficacy have not been established in children younger than 5 yr. No age-related precautions have been noted in elderly patients. Consume foods rich in vitamin D, including eggs, leafy vegetables, margarine, meats, milk, vegetable oils, and vegetable shortening.

Serum alkaline phosphatase, BUN, serum calcium, serum creatinine, serum magnesium, serum phosphate, and urinary calcium levels should be monitored monthly once therapeutic dosage is established for 3 mo, then every 3 mo thereafter. The therapeutic serum calcium level is 9-10 mg/dL.

Storage

Store at room temperature.

Administration

Give injection form as an IV bolus dose no more frequently than every other day, given at any time during dialysis. Capsules may be administered without regard to food. Discard any unused portion.

Paromomycin

par-oh-moe-mye′sin

Humatin

Do not confuse Humatin with Humira.

CATEGORY AND SCHEDULE

Pregnancy Risk Category: C

Classification: Amebicide: antibiotics, aminoglycosides, antiprotozoals

MECHANISM OF ACTION

An antibacterial agent that acts directly on amoebas and against normal and pathogenic organisms in the GI tract. Interferes with bacterial protein synthesis by binding to 30S ribosomal subunits. *Therapeutic Effect*: Produces amoebicidal effects. Suppresses intestinal flora, thus limiting ammonia production in patients with hepatic encephalopathy.

PHARMACOKINETICS

Poorly absorbed from the GI tract; most of the dose is eliminated unchanged in feces.

AVAILABILITY

Capsules: 250 mg.

INDICATIONS AND DOSAGES

▸ **Intestinal amebiasis**

PO

Adults, Elderly, Children. 25-35 mg/kg/day given in divided doses q8h for 5-10 days.

▸ **Hepatic coma**

PO

Adults, Elderly. 4 g/day given in divided doses q6-12h for 5-6 days.

OFF-LABEL USES

Cryptosporidiosis, giardiasis, leishmaniasis, microsporidiosis, mycobacterial infections, tapeworm infestation, trichomoniasis, typhoid carriers.

CONTRAINDICATIONS

Intestinal obstruction, hypersensitivity to paromomycin or any of its components.

INTERACTIONS

Drug

Digoxin: May decrease digoxin serum concentrations and efficacy.

Herbal

None known.

Food

Xylose, sucrose, fats: May cause decreased absorption of xylose, sucrose, and fats.

DIAGNOSTIC TEST EFFECTS

May increase LDH concentrations, SGOT (AST) and SGPT (ALT) levels.

SIDE EFFECTS

Occasional

Diarrhea, abdominal cramps, nausea, vomiting, heartburn.

Rare

Rash, pruritus, vertigo.

SERIOUS REACTIONS

• Nephrotoxicity (rare), ototoxicity (rare). Overdosage may result in nausea, vomiting, and diarrhea.

PRECAUTIONS & CONSIDERATIONS

Caution should be used in patients with proven ulcerative bowel disease. Liver and renal function tests should be performed before administering paromomycin. It is unknown whether paromomycin crosses the placenta and is distributed in breast milk. No precautions have been noted in children or elderly patients.

Sore throat, oral burning sensations, fever or fatigue, any or all can be indicative of superinfection and should be reported immediately. Impaired hearing should be reported immediately.

Storage

Store at room temperature; protect from moisture.

Administration

Give with meals. Take full course of therapy and do not skip doses.

Paroxetine Hydrochloride

par-ox'e-teen

Paxil, Paxil CR, Pexeva

Do not confuse paroxetine with pyridoxine, or Paxil with Doxil or Taxol.

CATEGORY AND SCHEDULE

Pregnancy Risk Category: D

Classification: Antidepressants, selective serotonin reuptake inhibitors

MECHANISM OF ACTION

An antidepressant, anxiolytic, and antiobsessional agent that selectively blocks uptake of the neurotransmitter serotonin at neuronal presynaptic membranes, thereby increasing its availability at postsynaptic receptor sites. *Therapeutic Effect:* Relieves depression, reduces obsessive-compulsive behavior, decreases anxiety.

PHARMACOKINETICS

Well absorbed from the GI tract. Protein binding: 95%. Widely distributed. Metabolized in the liver. Excreted in urine. Not removed by hemodialysis. *Half-life:* 15-20 h.

AVAILABILITY

Oral Suspension (Paxil): 10 mg/5 mL.

Tablets (Paxil, Pexeva): 10 mg, 20 mg, 30 mg, 40 mg.

Tablets (Controlled Release [Paxil CR]): 12.5 mg, 25 mg, 37.5 mg.

INDICATIONS AND DOSAGES

▸ **Major depressive disorder**

PO

Adults. Initially, 20 mg/day. May increase by 10 mg/day at intervals of more than 1 wk. Maximum: 50 mg/day.

PO (CONTROLLED RELEASE)

Adults. Initially, 25 mg/day. May increase by 12.5 mg/day at intervals of more than 1 wk. Maximum: 62.5 mg/day.

▸ **Generalized anxiety disorder**

PO

Adults. Initially, 20 mg/day. May increase by 10 mg/day at intervals of more than 1 wk. Range: 20-50 mg/day.

▸ **Obsessive compulsive disorder**

PO

Adults. Initially, 20 mg/day. May increase by 10 mg/day at intervals of more than 1 wk. Range: 20-60 mg/day.

▸ **Panic disorder**

PO

Adults. Initially, 10-20 mg/day. May increase by 10 mg/day at intervals of more than 1 wk. Range: 10-60 mg/day.

PO (CONTROLLED RELEASE)

Adults. Initially 12.5 mg/day. May increase by 12.5 mg/day at intervals of more than 1 wk. Maximum: 75 mg/day.

▸ **Social anxiety disorder**
PO
Adults. Initially 20 mg/day. May increase by 10 mg/day at intervals of > 1 wk. Range: 20-60 mg/day.
PO (CONTROLLED RELEASE)
Adults. Initially, 12.5 mg/day. May increase by 12.5 mg/day at intervals of more than 1 wk. Maximum: 37.5 mg/day.
▸ **Posttraumatic stress disorder**
PO
Adults. Initially, 20 mg/day. May increase by 10 mg/day at intervals of more than 1 wk. Range: 20-60 mg/day.
▸ **Premenstrual dysphoric disorder**
PO
Adults. (Paxil CR) Initially, 12.5 mg/day. May increase by 12.5 mg at weekly intervals to a maximum of 37.5 mg/day. May also give during luteal phase only.

CONTRAINDICATIONS

Use within 14 days of MAOIs. Hypersensitivity. Contraindicated for use with linezolid, pimozide, or thioridazine.

INTERACTIONS

Drug
Cimetidine: May increase paroxetine blood concentration.
Diazepam: Increased half-life of diazepam in the presence of paroxetine.
Drugs metabolized by CYP2D6 (e.g., risperidone, phenothiazines, TCAs, propafenone, flecainide): May increase risk of side effects due to inhibition of CYP2D6 by paroxetine.
MAOIs: May cause serotonin syndrome, marked by excitement, diaphoresis, rigidity, hyperthermia, autonomic hyperactivity, coma, and neuroleptic malignant syndrome. Contraindicated.
Phenobarbital, phenytoin: May decrease paroxetine blood concentration.
Pimozide and thioridazine: Contraindicated. May result in prolonged QT intervals.
Other antidepressants and alcohol: Possible increased side effects.
Sibutramine, serotonin agonists (triptants): Additive serotonin effects and increased risk serotonin syndrome.
Tamoxifen: Paroxetine may reduce efficacy due to CYP2D6 effects; choose different antidepressant.
Theophylline: Rare reports of increased theophylline levels. Monitor.
Warfarin: May increase effects of warfarin; monitor INR.
Herbal
St. John's wort: May increase paroxetine's pharmacologic effects and risk of toxicity.
Tryptophan: May cause headache, nausea, sweating, and dizziness similar to serotonin syndrome.
Food
None known.

DIAGNOSTIC TEST EFFECTS

May increase serum LFTs. May cause lowered serum sodium, may cause platelet dysfunction.

SIDE EFFECTS

Frequent
Nausea (26%); somnolence (23%); headache, dry mouth (18%); asthenia (15%); constipation (15%); dizziness, insomnia (13%); diarrhea (12%); diaphoresis (11%); tremor (8%).
Occasional
Decreased appetite, respiratory disturbance (such as increased cough) (6%); anxiety, nervousness (5%); flatulence, paresthesia,

yawning (4%); decreased libido, sexual dysfunction, abdominal discomfort (3%).
Rare
Palpitations, vomiting, blurred vision, altered taste, confusion.

SERIOUS REACTIONS

- Overdose may produce seizures, nausea, vomiting, agitation, and restlessness (serotonin syndrome).
- Bleeding with platelet dysfunction.
- Hyponatremia and SIADH in elderly especially.

PRECAUTIONS & CONSIDERATIONS

Caution is warranted in patients with suicidal tendency, cardiac disease, a history of seizures, impaired platelet aggregation, mania, hepatic and renal impairment, in volume-depleted patients, and in those using diuretics. Paroxetine use is not recommended in pregnancy due to a potential for teratogenic and nonteratogenic adverse effects and neonatal withdrawal. It is distributed in breast milk. The safety and efficacy of this drug have not been established in children. Antidepressants have been reported to increase the risk of suicidal thinking and behavior in children, adolescents, and young adults (18-24 yr of age) with major depressive disorder (MDD) and other psychiatric disorders. Patients should be closely monitored for clinical worsening, suicidality, or unusual changes in behavior, particularly during the initial 1-2 mo of therapy or following dosage adjustments. In elderly patients, age-related renal impairment may require dosage adjustment.

Alcohol and tasks that require mental alertness or motor skills should be avoided. CBC and liver and renal function tests should be performed before and periodically during therapy, especially with long-term use.

Storage
Store all products at room temperature.
Administration
! Make sure at least 14 days elapse between the use of MAOIs and paroxetine.

Take paroxetine as a single morning dose. Give it with food or milk if GI distress occurs. Scored tablets may be crushed or broken.

If discontinuing, expect tapering of dose to avoid withdrawal syndrome.

Pazopanib

pay-zoe'pan-ib
Votrient

CATEGORY AND SCHEDULE

Pregnancy Risk Category: D

Classification: Antineoplastics, biologic agents, signal transduction inhibitor.

P

MECHANISM OF ACTION

An oral multikinase inhibitor of angiogenesis. The drug inhibits vascular endothelial growth factor receptor (VEGFR)-1, VEGFR-2, VEGFR-3, platelet-derived growth factor receptor (PDGFR)-α and -β, fibroblast growth factor receptor (FGFR)-1 and -3, cytokine receptor (Kit), interleukin-2 receptor inducible T-cell kinase (Itk), leukocyte-specific protein tyrosine kinase (Lck), and transmembrane glycoprotein receptor tyrosine kinase (c-Fms). *Therapeutic Effect:* Inhibits tumor growth.

PHARMACOKINETICS

Well absorbed after oral administration of whole tablets; administration of crushed tablet greatly increases drug exposure and therefore tablets should not be crushed. Systemic exposure also increased when given with food, so the drug should be given on empty stomach. Protein binding: 99%. Substrate for P-glycoprotein and breast cancer resistant protein (BCRP). Hepatic metabolism via CYP3A4 (major), CYP1A2 (minor) and CYP2C8 (minor). Pazopanib inhibits most CYP450 isoenzymes, as well as UGT. Fecal excretion. *Half-life:* 30.9 h (increased in hepatic impairment or hyperbilirubinemia).

AVAILABILITY

Tablet: 200 mg.

INDICATIONS AND DOSAGES

▸ **Advanced renal cell cancer**

PO

Adults, Elderly. 800 mg once daily on an empty stomach.

▸ **Dosage adjustment for moderate hepatic impairment**

200 mg orally once daily. Not recommended in patients with severe hepatic impairment.

▸ **Dosage adjustment if strong CYP3A4 inhibitors used**

Reduce dosage to 400 mg once daily if interacting drug cannot be avoided.

CONTRAINDICATIONS

None absolute. Hypersensitivity, severe hepatic impairment potential contraindications.

INTERACTIONS

Drug

CYP3A4 Inhibitors (e.g., ketoconazole, nefazodone, clarithromycin, itraconazole, protease inhibitors for HIV): Pasopanib levels may increase. Consider reducing dose if alternate treatment not available.

CYP 3A4 inducers (e.g., rifampin, phenytoin, carbamazepine, phenobarbital): May increase metabolism of pazopanib and thus decrease levels. If inducer must be used, then pazopanib is not recommended.

Warfarin: Pazopanib has the potential to compete for CYP2C9 metabolism and could possible alter warfarin response; monitor INR.

Herbal

St. John's wort: Do not use with pazopanib as it will decrease pazopanib levels and efficacy.

Food

All food: Increased pazopanib exposure and risk of side effects; take on empty stomach.

Grapefruit juice: May increase pazopanib exposure; do not take with grapefruit juice.

DIAGNOSTIC TEST EFFECTS

Decreased WBC, platelets. Increased LFTs, TSH. Electrolyte abnormalities, disturbances of blood glucose. ECG changes.

SIDE EFFECTS

Frequent (> 20%)

Diarrhea, hypertension, hair color changes (depigmentation), nausea, anorexia, fatigue, and vomiting. May decrease magnesium and phosphorus levels, cause hyperglycemia.

Occasional

Alopecia, chest pain, dysgeusia (altered taste), dyspepsia, facial edema, hand-foot syndrome, proteinuria, rash, skin depigmentation, and weight loss.

Rare

Hypothyroidism.

SERIOUS REACTIONS

- Serious hypersensitivity reactions occur rarely, and may include angioedema.
- Leukopenia, thrombocytopenia.
- Severe and fatal hepatotoxicity.
- Serious bleeding (CNS, gastrointestinal, hemoptysis, etc.) or GI perforations.
- Arterial thrombosis.
- QT prolongation or arrhythmia, heart failure.
- Delayed wound healing.

PRECAUTIONS & CONSIDERATIONS

Use with caution in patients with hepatic disease, high blood pressure, cardiac disease, heart failure or arrhythmia, QT prolongation, a history of stroke, GI disease with GI bleeding in the past 6 months or a history of GI perforation or fistula, thyroid disease, had recent surgery or scheduled for surgery. Do not use in patients who are pregnant or planning to become pregnant; the drug can cause fetal harm. It is not known if pazopanib passes into breast milk; do not breastfeed while taking this medication. This drug has not been approved for use in children.

Storage

Store tablets at room temperature.

Administration

Give daily without food on an empty stomach (at least 1 h before or 2 h after a meal). Do not crush tablets. Do not take with grapefruit juice.

Pegaptanib

peg-ap'ta-nib

Macugen

CATEGORY AND SCHEDULE

Pregnancy Risk Category: B

Classification: Ophthalmics, biologic agents, vascular endothelial growth factor (VEGF) inhibitor.

MECHANISM OF ACTION

A biologic agent that binds to and inhibits vascular endothelial growth factor (VEGF). VEGFs induce angiogenesis and increase vascular permeability and inflammation, all of which contribute to the neovascular (wet) form of age-related macular degeneration (AMD). *Therapeutic Effect:* Inhibits progression of age-related macular degeneration.

PHARMACOKINETICS

Some systemic absorption after intraocular administration.
Any absorbed drug is primarily eliminated in the urine as parent drug and metabolites. Metabolized primarily by endo- and exonucleases. *Half-life:* 10 days (range, 6-14 days).

AVAILABILITY

Injection: 0.3-mg prefilled syringe.

INDICATIONS AND DOSAGES

▸ ***Wet age-related macular degeneration***

INTRAVITREOUS INJECTION

Adults, Elderly. 0.3 mg intravitreally, repeated every 6 wks.

CONTRAINDICATIONS

Ocular or periocular infections, hypersensitivity to pegaptanib.

INTERACTIONS

Drug

None known.

Herbal

None known.

Food

None known.

DIAGNOSTIC TEST EFFECTS

None known.

SIDE EFFECTS

Frequent

Temporary blurred vision, headache, dizziness.

Occasional
Burning sensation, eye pain, redness, light sensitivity, visual disturbances, increased intraocular pressure, corneal edema, eye discharge, vitreous floaters or opacities, keratitis.
Rare
Eye infection, cataract, allergic response, vision loss, nausea.

SERIOUS REACTIONS

- Serious hypersensitivity reactions occur rarely, and may include angioedema.
- Endophthalmitis, retinal detachment, traumatic cataract or other event due to eye injection.

PRECAUTIONS & CONSIDERATIONS

Caution is warranted in patients with severe renal insufficiency. Use in pregnancy only if clearly necessary; use caution during lactation. The safety and efficacy of pegaptanib have not been established in children. There are no specific age-related precautions for elderly patients.

Notify the physician if there is any sign of eye infection, eye pain, or visual loss. Report if the eye becomes red, sensitive to light, painful, or if there is a change in vision. Monitoring may consist of a check of intraocular pressure and also for perfusion of the optic nerve head immediately after the injection, within 30 min after the injection, and within the first week after the injection.
Storage
Refrigerate prefilled syringe. Do not freeze or shake.
Administration
Do NOT give intravenously. Only for use by ophthalmologists trained in these specialized intravitreal administration techniques. Do not mix with any other drugs or solutions. Adequate anesthesia and a broad-spectrum microbicide are necessary before injection. Prepare the syringe as directed. Use controlled aseptic conditions, which include the use of sterile gloves, a sterile drape, and a sterile eyelid speculum (or equivalent). Following the injection, monitor patient for elevation in intraocular pressure (IOP) and for endophthalmitis.

Pegaspargase

peg-as′par-jase
★ Oncaspar

CATEGORY AND SCHEDULE

Pregnancy Risk Category: C

Classification: Antineoplastics, natural and semisynthetic, asparaginase analogue

P

MECHANISM OF ACTION

An enzyme that breaks down extracellular supplies of the amino acid asparagine, which is necessary for the survival of leukemic cells. Binding to polyethylene glycol decreases the antigenicity of pegaspargase, making it less likely to cause a hypersensitivity reaction. Cell cycle–phase specific for G1 phase of cell division. *Therapeutic Effect*: Interferes with DNA, RNA, and protein synthesis in leukemic cells.

AVAILABILITY

Injection: 750 international units/mL.

INDICATIONS AND DOSAGES

▸ **Acute lymphocytic leukemia in combination with other chemotherapeutic agents**
IV, IM

Adults, Elderly, Children 1 yr and older. 2500 international units/m^2 every 14 days.

IV INCOMPATIBILITIES

Do not mix with other drugs at Y-site. Compatible only with dextrose 5% and 0.9% NaCl.

CONTRAINDICATIONS

Previous anaphylactic reaction or significant hemorrhagic event or thrombosis associated with L-asparaginase or pegaspargase therapy, pancreatitis (current or previous).

INTERACTIONS

Drug

Drug interactions are not well documented.

Antigout medications: May decrease the effects of these drugs.

Live-virus vaccine: May potentiate virus replication, increase vaccine side effects, and decrease the patient's antibody response to the vaccine.

Methotrexate: May block the effects of methotrexate. To avoid, give pegaspargase at least 10-14 days prior to MTX or shortly after MTX.

Steroids, vincristine: May increase hyperglycemia, risk of neuropathy, and disturbances of erythropoiesis.

Herbal

None known.

Food

None known.

DIAGNOSTIC TEST EFFECTS

May increase BUN, blood ammonia, and blood glucose levels; serum alkaline phosphatase, bilirubin, uric acid, AST (SGOT), and ALT (SGPT) levels; PT; and aPTT. May decrease blood clotting factors (including plasma fibrinogen, antithrombin, and plasminogen) as well as serum albumin, calcium, and cholesterol levels.

SIDE EFFECTS

Frequent

Allergic reaction (including rash, urticaria, arthralgia, facial edema, hypotension, and respiratory distress).

Occasional

Central nervous system (CNS) effects (including confusion, drowsiness, depression, nervousness, and fatigue), stomatitis, hypoalbuminemia, uric acid nephropathy (manifested as edema of the feet or lower legs), hyperglycemia.

Rare

Hyperthermia (fever or chills), CNS thrombosis.

SERIOUS REACTIONS

- The patient may have a hypersensitivity reaction, including anaphylaxis, during therapy.
- Pancreatitis, as evidenced by severe abdominal pain with nausea and vomiting, is a common reaction.
- Hepatotoxicity, as evidenced by jaundice and abnormal hepatic enzyme test results, may occur, especially in patients with preexisting hepatic impairment.
- An increased risk of hematologic toxicity and coagulation disorders occurs occasionally.
- Seizures occur rarely.

PRECAUTIONS & CONSIDERATIONS

Vaccinations and coming in contact with crowds and people with known infections should be avoided.

Any hypersensitivity reactions with L-asparginase therapy previously warrants careful consideration as to whether this drug should be used. Nausea may occur but will decrease during therapy. Notify the physician if fever, signs of local infection, or unusual bleeding from any site occurs. Antihistamines, epinephrine, and corticosteroids should be kept readily available before and during pegaspargase administration to ensure an adequate airway and treat any allergic reaction.

Adequate hydration should be maintained to protect against renal impairment. CBC, bone marrow tests, fibrinogen level, PT, aPTT, liver, pancreatic and renal function test results should be monitored before beginning therapy and whenever a week or longer has elapsed between drug doses.

Storage

Refrigerate—do not freeze—vials. Discard the solution if it is cloudy or contains a precipitate. Also discard it if it has been stored at room temperature for longer than 48 h or if the vial has been previously frozen because freezing destroys the drug's potency.

Administration

CAUTION: Observe and exercise usual cautions for handling and preparing solutions of cytotoxic drugs.

Avoid excessive agitation of the vial (do not shake). The IM administration route is preferred because it poses less risk of coagulopathy, hepatotoxicity, and GI or renal disorders than the IV route. Use one dose per vial; do not reenter the vial. Discard any unused portion.

Administer no more than 2 mL at any one IM site. Use multiple injection sites if more than 2 mL is being administered.

For IV, add dose to 100 mL 0.9% NaCl or D5W and administer the drug through IV infusion that is already running. Infuse over 1-2 h.

Observe patient for at least 1 h after each dose of pegaspargase.

Pegfilgrastim

pehg-phil-gras'tim

★ 🍁 Neulasta

Do not confuse Neulasta with Neumega.

CATEGORY AND SCHEDULE

Pregnancy Risk Category: C

Classification: Hematopoietic agents, colony-stimulating factors (CSF)

MECHANISM OF ACTION

A colony-stimulating factor that regulates the production of neutrophils within bone marrow. Also a glycoprotein that primarily affects neutrophil progenitor proliferation, differentiation, and selected end-cell functional activation. *Therapeutic Effect:* Increases phagocytic ability and antibody-dependent destruction; decreases incidence of infection.

PHARMACOKINETICS

Readily absorbed after subcutaneous administration. *Half-life:* 15-80 h.

AVAILABILITY

Solution for Injection: 6 mg/0.6 mL prefilled syringe.

INDICATIONS AND DOSAGES

▸ **To decrease the incidence of infection and febrile neutropenia during myelosuppressive chemotherapy for non-myeloid malignancies**

SC

Adults, Elderly > 45 kg. Give as a single 6-mg injection once per chemotherapy cycle.

CONTRAINDICATIONS

Hypersensitivity to *Escherichia coli*–derived proteins, pegfilgrastim, filgrastim, or any other components of the product. Do not use for peripheral blood progenitor cell mobilization.

INTERACTIONS

Drug

G-CSF, other exogenous growth factors: May result in development of antibodies causing immune-mediated neutropenia.

Lithium: May potentiate the release of neutrophils.

Herbal

None known.

Food

None known.

DIAGNOSTIC TEST EFFECTS

May increase LDH concentrations, leukocyte alkaline phosphatase scores, and serum alkaline phosphatase and uric acid levels.

SIDE EFFECTS

Frequent (15%-72%)

Bone pain, nausea, fatigue, alopecia, diarrhea, vomiting, constipation, anorexia, abdominal pain, arthralgia, generalized weakness, peripheral edema, dizziness, stomatitis, mucositis, neutropenic fever.

SERIOUS REACTIONS

- Allergic reactions, such as anaphylaxis, rash, and urticaria, occur rarely.
- Cytopenia resulting from an antibody response to growth factors occurs rarely.
- Splenomegaly occurs rarely; assess for left upper abdominal or shoulder pain.
- Adult respiratory distress syndrome (ARDS) may occur in patients with sepsis.

PRECAUTIONS & CONSIDERATIONS

Caution is warranted with concurrent use of medications with myeloid properties and in those with sickle cell disease. It is unknown whether pegfilgrastim crosses the placenta or is distributed in breast milk. Safety and efficacy of pegfilgrastim have not been established in children. The prefilled syringe should not be used in infants, children, and adolescents weighing < 45 kg. No age-related precautions have been noted in elderly patients.

CBC, hematocrit value, and platelet count should be obtained before initiation of pegfilgrastim therapy and routinely thereafter. Pattern of daily bowel activity and stool consistency should be assessed. Be aware of signs of peripheral edema, particularly behind the medial malleolus, which is usually the first area to show peripheral edema, and for evidence of mucositis (such as red mucous membranes, white patches, and extreme mouth soreness) and stomatitis.

Storage

Store in refrigerator in the carton until use but may warm to room temperature up to 48 h before use. Discard if left at room temperature for longer than 48 h. Protect from light. Avoid freezing, but if accidentally frozen, may allow to thaw in refrigerator before administration. Discard if freezing takes place a second time. Discard if discoloration or precipitate is present.

Administration

! Do not administer from 14 days before to 24 h after cytotoxic chemotherapy, as prescribed.

Do not shake prefilled syringe as this may disrupt the drug. If syringe is shaken, discard; do not use.

Pegfilgrastim should be injected subcutaneously. Compliance with pegfilgrastim regimen is important.

Peginterferon Alfa-2a

peg-inn-ter-fear'on

Pegasys

CATEGORY AND SCHEDULE

Pregnancy Risk Category: C

Classification: Biologic response modulators, interferons

MECHANISM OF ACTION

An immunomodulator that binds to specific membrane receptors on the cell surface, inhibiting viral replication in virus-infected cells, suppressing cell proliferation, and producing reversible decreases in leukocyte and platelet counts. *Therapeutic Effect:* Inhibits hepatitis C virus.

PHARMACOKINETICS

Readily absorbed after SC administration, with peak serum levels attained at 72-96 h. Excreted by the kidneys. *Half-life:* 80 h.

AVAILABILITY

Injection: 180 mcg/mL.

Prefilled Syringes for Injection: 180 mcg/0.5 mL.

INDICATIONS AND DOSAGES

▸ **Hepatitis C**

SC (AS MONOTHERAPY)

Adults 18 yr and older, Elderly. 180 mcg injected in abdomen or thigh once weekly for 48 wks.

SC (IN COMBINATION WITH RIBAVIRIN)

180 mcg once weekly plus ribavirin (800-1200 mg/day in 2 divided doses) for 24-48 wks.

▸ **Dosage in renal impairment**

For patients who require hemodialysis, dosage is 135 mcg injected in the abdomen or thigh once weekly for 48 wks.

▸ **Dosage in hepatic impairment**

For patients with progressive ALT (SGPT) increases above baseline values, dosage is 135 mcg injected in the abdomen or thigh once weekly for 48 wks.

▸ **Dosage adjustment for hematology parameters**

For patients with an absolute neutrophil count < 750 cells/mm^3, reduce dose to 135 mcg (0.75 mL). For those with an absolute neutrophil count < 500 cells/mm^3, discontinue treatment until the count returns to 1000 cells/mm^3. For those with a platelet count < 50,000 cells/mm^3, reduce dose to 90 mcg.

CONTRAINDICATIONS

Hypersensitivity to *E. coli,* protein, autoimmune hepatitis, decompensated hepatic disease, infants, neonates, benzyl alcohol hypersensitivity.

If used with ribavirin, also carefully review ribavirin contraindications.

INTERACTIONS

Drug

Bone marrow depressants: May increase myelosuppression.

Theophylline: May increase the serum level of theophylline.

Herbal

None known.

Food

None known.

DIAGNOSTIC TEST EFFECTS

May increase ALT (SGPT) level. May decrease the absolute neutrophil, platelet, and WBC counts. May cause a slight decrease in blood hemoglobin level and hematocrit.

SIDE EFFECTS

Frequent

Headache.

Occasional

Alopecia, nausea, insomnia, anorexia, dizziness, diarrhea, abdominal pain, flu-like symptoms, psychiatric reactions (depression, irritability, anxiety), injection site reaction, impaired concentration, diaphoresis, dry mouth, nausea, vomiting.

SERIOUS REACTIONS

- Serious, acute hypersensitivity reactions, such as urticaria, angioedema, bronchoconstriction, and anaphylaxis, may occur. Other rare reactions include pancreatitis, colitis, hyperthyroidism or hypothyroidism, endocrine disorders (e.g., diabetes mellitus), benzyl alcohol hypersensitivity, ophthalmologic disorders, and pulmonary disorders.
- Serious infections (bacterial, viral, fungal), some fatal, have been reported, especially if neutropenia occurs. Begin appropriate anti-infective therapy immediately and consider α interferon discontinuation.

PRECAUTIONS & CONSIDERATIONS

Monitor for new or exacerbation of the following serious events, some of which may become life threatening. Patients with persistently severe or worsening signs or symptoms should have their therapy withdrawn: Neuropsychiatric reactions, including severe depression. High/persistent fever may indicate serious infection, particularly in patients with neutropenia. Interferons suppress bone marrow function and may cause severe cytopenias or bleeding that will require dose reduction OR discontinuation. Those with HIV infection are most at risk. Watch for hypertension, supraventricular arrhythmias, chest pain, and myocardial infarction; administer with caution to those with preexisting or unstable cardiac disease. Ischemic and hemorrhagic cerebrovascular events have been observed. Patients with cirrhosis may be at risk of hepatic decompensation. Discontinue if Child-Pugh score ≥ 6 occurs. Hyperglycemia, hypoglycemia, and diabetes mellitus may worsen. Use with caution in patients with autoimmune disorders. Pulmonary disease, inflammatory bowel disease (colitis), and pancreatitis may be induced or aggravated. Use with caution in renal impairment (CrCl < 50 mL/min); note that ribavirin cotherapy must NOT be used if CrCl < 50 mL/min. May aggravate hypothroidism and hyperthyroidism. Peginterferon alfa-2a may cause spontaneous abortion. It is unknown whether peginterferon alfa-2a is distributed in breast milk. The safety and efficacy of peginterferon alfa-2a have not been established in children younger than 18 yr. Cardiac, central nervous system (CNS), and systemic effects may be more severe in elderly patients, particularly in those with renal impairment. Avoid performing tasks requiring mental alertness or motor skills until response to the drug has been established.

Flu-like symptoms may occur but usually diminish with continued therapy. Notify the physician of depression or suicidal thoughts. CBC, ECG, urinalysis, BUN level, and serum alkaline phosphatase, creatinine, AST (SGOT), and ALT (SGPT) levels should be obtained before and routinely during therapy. Chest radiographs should be assessed for pulmonary infiltrates.

Storage

Refrigerate vials and prefilled syringes; protect from light and freezing.

Administration

Inject the drug subcutaneously in the abdomen or thigh. The drug's therapeutic effect should appear in 1-3 mo.

Peginterferon Alfa-2b

peg-in-ter-feer'on

★ PEG-Intron 🍁 Unitron PEG

CATEGORY AND SCHEDULE

Pregnancy Risk Category: C

Classification: Biologic response modifier, interferons

MECHANISM OF ACTION

An immunomodulator that inhibits viral replication in virus-infected cells, suppresses cell proliferation, increases phagocytic action of macrophages, and augments specific cytotoxicity of lymphocytes for target cells. *Therapeutic Effect:* Inhibits hepatitis C virus.

AVAILABILITY

Injection Powder for Reconstitution: 50 mcg, 80 mcg, 120 mcg, 150 mcg.
Redipen Prefilled Syringes: 50 mcg/0.5 mL, 80 mcg/0.5 mL, 120 mcg/0.5 mL, 150 mcg/0.5 mL.

INDICATIONS AND DOSAGES

▸ **Chronic hepatitis C, monotherapy**

SC

Adults, Elderly. Administer appropriate dosage (see chart below) once weekly for 1 yr on the same day each week.

Vial(mcg/mL)	Weight (kg)	Strength mcg*	Strength mL*
100	37-45	40	0.4
160	46-56	50	0.5
240	57-72	64	0.4
300	73-88	80	0.5
	89-106	96	0.4
	107-136	120	0.5
	137-160	150	0.5

*Of peginterferon alpha-2b to administer.

▸ **Chronic hepatitis C**

SC

Adults. 1.5 mcg/kg/wk SC given with oral ribavirin (daily, see manufacturer literature). *Children 3-17 yr.* 60 mcg/kg/m^2 SC per wk, plus oral ribavirin (daily, weight-based).

CONTRAINDICATIONS

Hypersensitivity to *E. coli,* protein, autoimmune hepatitis, decompensated hepatic disease, infants, neonates. If used with ribavirin, also carefully review ribavirin contraindications.

INTERACTIONS

Drug

Bone marrow depressants: May increase myelosuppression.
Theophylline: May increase the serum level of theophylline.

Herbal

None known.

Food

None known.

DIAGNOSTIC TEST EFFECTS
May increase blood glucose and ALT (SGPT) levels. May decrease blood neutrophil and platelet counts.

SIDE EFFECTS
Frequent
Flu-like symptoms; inflammation, bruising, pruritus, and irritation at injection site.
Occasional
Psychiatric reactions (depression, anxiety, emotional lability, irritability), insomnia, alopecia, diarrhea.
Rare
Rash, diaphoresis, dry skin, dizziness, flushing, vomiting, dyspepsia.

SERIOUS REACTIONS
- Serious, acute hypersensitivity reactions (such as urticaria, angioedema, bronchoconstriction, and anaphylaxis), pulmonary disorders, endocrine disorders (e.g., diabetes mellitus), hypothyroidism, hyperthyroidism, and pancreatitis occur rarely.
- Ulcerative colitis may occur within 12 wks of starting treatment.

PRECAUTIONS & CONSIDERATIONS
Monitor for new or exacerbation of the following serious events, some of which may become life threatening. Patients with persistently severe or worsening signs or symptoms should have their therapy withdrawn. Neuropsychiatric reactions, including severe depression. High/persistent fever may indicate serious infection, particularly in patients with neutropenia. Interferons suppress bone marrow function and may cause severe cytopenias or bleeding that will require dose reduction OR discontinuation. Those with HIV infection are most at risk. Watch for hypertension, supraventricular arrhythmias, chest pain, and myocardial infarction; administer with caution to those with preexisting or unstable cardiac disease. Ischemic and hemorrhagic cerebrovascular events have been observed. Patients with cirrhosis may be at risk of hepatic decompensation. Discontinue if Child-Pugh score ≥ 6 occurs. Hyperglycemia, hypoglycemia, thyroid disease, and diabetes mellitus may worsen. Use with caution in patients with autoimmune disorders. Pulmonary disease, inflammatory bowel disease (colitis), and pancreatitis may be induced or aggravated. Use with caution in renal impairment (CrCl < 50 mL/min); note that ribavirin cotherapy must NOT be used if CrCl < 50 mL/min. Peginterferon alfa-2b may cause spontaneous abortion. It is unknown whether peginterferon alfa-2b is distributed in breast milk. The safety and efficacy of peginterferon alfa-2b have not been established in children younger than 3 yr.

Flu-like symptoms may occur but usually diminish with continued therapy. Notify the physician of bloody diarrhea, fever, persistent abdominal pain, depression, signs of infection, or unusual bruising or bleeding. CBC, ECG, urinalysis, BUN level, and serum alkaline phosphatase, creatinine, AST (SGOT), and ALT (SGPT) levels should be obtained before and routinely during therapy. Chest radiographs should be assessed for pulmonary infiltrates.

Storage
Store vials at room temperature. Use it immediately or after reconstitution or, if necessary, refrigerate it for up to 24 h.

Refrigerate prefilled syringes (Redipens); protect from light and

freezing. Once reconstituted, may store up to 24 h under refrigeration.
Administration
Administer subcutaneously (SC) on the same day of the week.

Reconstitute the drug vial by adding 0.7 mL sterile water for injection (the supplied diluent) to the vial. Administer as SC injection.

To reconstitute, hold the Redipen upright (dose button facing down) and press the 2 halves of the pen together until there is an audible click. Gently invert the pen to mix the solution. Do NOT shake.

Pegvisomant

peg-vis′oh-mant
Somavert
Do not confuse Somavert with somatrem or somatropin.

CATEGORY AND SCHEDULE

Pregnancy Risk Category: B

Classification: Acromegaly agent, growth hormone analogue

MECHANISM OF ACTION

A protein that selectively binds to growth hormone (GH) receptors on cell surfaces, blocking the binding of endogenous growth hormones and interfering with growth hormone signal transduction. *Therapeutic Effect:* Decreases serum concentrations of insulin-like growth factor 1 (IGF-1) and other GH-responsive serum proteins.

PHARMACOKINETICS

Not distributed extensively into tissues after SC administration. Less than 1% excreted in urine. *Half-life:* 6 days.

AVAILABILITY

Powder for Injection: 10-mg, 15-mg, 20-mg vials.

INDICATIONS AND DOSAGES

▸ Acromegaly
SC
Adults, Elderly. Initially, 40 mg as a loading dose, then 10 mg daily. After 4-6 wks, adjust dosage in 5-mg increments, up to 30 mg/day, based on serum IGF-1 concentrations.

CONTRAINDICATIONS

Latex allergy (stopper on vial contains latex), intravenous administration.

INTERACTIONS

Drug
Insulin, oral antidiabetics: May enhance the effects of these drugs, possibly resulting in hypoglycemia. Dosage should be decreased when initiating pegvisomant therapy.
Opioids: Decreased serum pegvisomant levels.
Herbal
None known.
Food
None known.

DIAGNOSTIC TEST EFFECTS

Interferes with measurement of serum growth hormone concentration. May markedly increase AST (SGOT), ALT (SGPT), and serum transaminase levels. Decreases effect of insulin on carbohydrate metabolism.

SIDE EFFECTS

Frequent
Infection (cold symptoms, upper respiratory tract infection, blister, ear infection).
Occasional
Back pain, dizziness, injection site reaction, peripheral edema, sinusitis, nausea.

Rare
Diarrhea, paresthesia.

SERIOUS REACTIONS

- Pegvisomant use may markedly elevate liver function test results, including serum transaminase levels.
- Substantial weight gain occurs rarely.

PRECAUTIONS & CONSIDERATIONS

Caution is warranted in patients with diabetes mellitus and in elderly patients. It is unknown whether pegvisomant is excreted in breast milk. The safety and efficacy of pegvisomant have not been established in children. In elderly patients, treatment should begin at the low end of the dosage range.

Notify the physician of yellowing of the skin or sclera of eyes or any other adverse effects. Serum alkaline phosphatase, bilirubin, AST (SGOT), and ALT (SGPT) levels should be monitored. Serum IGF-1 concentrations should be obtained 4-6 wks after therapy begins and periodically thereafter. The drug dosage should be adjusted based on these results, not on growth hormone assays. Progressive tumor growth with periodic imaging scans of the sella turcica should be monitored with tumors that secrete growth hormone. Diabetics should be assessed for hypoglycemia.

Storage
Store unreconstituted vials in the refrigerator. Administer the drug within 6 h of reconstitution.

Administration
The solution normally appears clear after reconstitution. Discard the solution if it appears cloudy or contains particles. Withdraw 1 mL sterile water for injection and inject it into the vial of pegvisomant, aiming the stream against the glass wall. Hold the vial between the palms of both hands and roll it gently to dissolve the powder; do not shake. Administer only one dose from each vial subcutaneously.

Pemetrexed

pem-eh-trex′ed
★ 🍁 Alimta
Do not confuse Pemetrexed with pralatrexate, or Alimta with Amitiza.

CATEGORY AND SCHEDULE

Pregnancy Risk Category: D

Classification: Antineoplastics, folic acid antagonist

MECHANISM OF ACTION

An antimetabolite that disrupts folate-dependent enzymes essential for cell replication. *Therapeutic Effect:* Inhibits the growth of malignant cell lines.

PHARMACOKINETICS

Protein binding: 81%. Most (70%-90%) of pemetrexed is eliminated in the urine as unchanged drug. Clearance is tied to glomerular filtration and tubular secretion. Not known if dialyzed. *Half-life:* 3.5 h (prolonged if CrCl < 90 mL/min)

AVAILABILITY

Powder for Injection: 500 mg.

INDICATIONS AND DOSAGES

! Pretreatment with corticosteroid (e.g., dexamethasone) the day before, day of, and 1 day after infusion, as prescribed, to reduce the incidence and severity of cutaneous reactions. To reduce toxicity, patients MUST take low-dose folic acid dose (usually

P

0.4-1 mg PO) or multivitamin with such folic acid every day. At least 5 daily doses MUST be taken during the 7-day period prior to the first dose; daily during the full course of therapy; and for 21days after the last dose. Also give vitamin B_{12} (1000 mcg IM) for 1 dose during the week preceding the first dose and for every 3 cycles thereafter; the maintenance doses may be given the same day as pemetrexed.

▸ **Malignant pleural mesothelioma, unresectable or nonsquamous non-small cell lung carcinoma**

IV

Adults, Elderly. 500 mg/m² infused over 10 min on day 1 of each 21-day cycle when used in combination with cisplatin 75 mg/m². Reductions in dosages are indicated as follows:

For absolute neutrophil count (ANC) < 500 mm³, nadir platelets equal to 50,000/mm³, grade 3 or grade 4 toxicities, diarrhea requiring hospitalization: Reduce IV dose to 75% of previous dose.

For nadir platelets < 50,000/mm³ regardless of nadir ANC or grades 3 or 4 mucositis: Reduce IV dose to 50% of previous dose.

For grades 3 or 4 neurotoxicities or any hematologic or nonhematologic grades 3 or 4 toxicity after 2 dose reductions: Discontinue drug.

CONTRAINDICATIONS

Hypersensitivity to pemetrexed, mannitol hypersensitivity.

INTERACTIONS

Drug

Cisplatin: Concomitant therapy may augment any adverse reactions.

Live vaccines: Avoid during treatment.

Nephrotoxic agents, probenecid: May delay pemetrexed clearance.

NSAIDs (short-acting, particularly ibuprofen, and long-acting, e.g., piroxicam): Increase the risk of myelosuppression and GI and renal toxicity. If the patient already has mild-moderate renal insufficiency, then short-acting NSAIDS (e.g., ibuprofen) should be discontinued 2 days before, the day of, and for 2 days after pemetrexed; long-acting NSAIDs (e.g., piroxicam) should be discontinued 5 days before, the day of, and for 2 days after pemetrexed.

Herbal

None known.

Food

None known.

DIAGNOSTIC TEST EFFECTS

May decrease platelet, RBC, and WBC counts.

IV INCOMPATIBILITIES

Use only 0.9% NaCl to reconstitute; flush the line before and after the infusion. Do not add any other medications to the IV line. Known to be incompatible with calcium-containing fluids, including lactated Ringer's injection and Ringer's injection.

SIDE EFFECTS

Frequent

Fatigue, nausea, vomiting, constipation, anorexia, stomatitis, pharyngitis, diarrhea, neutropenia, leukopenia, anemia, thrombocytopenia, chest pains, rash, desquamation, mood alteration or depression, dyspnea.

Occasional

Allergic reaction, hypersensitivity, dehydration, creatinine elevation, fever, infection without neutropenia, infection with grade 3 or 4 neutropenia, hypertension, thrombosis, embolism.

Rare
Febrile neutropenia, renal failure, esophagitis, odynophagia, dysphagia.

SERIOUS REACTIONS

- Myelosuppression, manifested as neutropenia, thrombocytopenia, or anemia, may occur.

PRECAUTIONS & CONSIDERATIONS

CBC with differential platelet count should be assessed before starting therapy and again on days 8 and 15 of each cycle and before starting a new cycle. New cycles should not be started with ANC < 1500 mm^3, platelet count ≤ 100,000 mm^3, and creatinine clearance less than 45 mL/min.

Caution is warranted with liver impairment as well as concurrent therapy with aspirin or other NSAIDs. Pemetrexed may be harmful to a fetus, and it is unknown whether pemetrexed is distributed in breast milk. Do not breastfeed once treatment has been initiated. Safety and efficacy of pemetrexed in children younger than 18 yr of age have not been established. Be aware that elderly patients may have higher incidence of fatigue, leukopenia, neutropenia, and thrombocytopenia.

Fastidious oral hygiene should be maintained. Do not have immunizations without physician's approval (drug lowers body's resistance). Crowds and those with infection should be avoided. Contraceptive measures should be used during therapy. Report fever, sore throat, signs of local infection, easy bruising, and unusual bleeding from any site immediately.

Storage
Store undiluted vial at room temperature. Reconstituted solution is stable for up to 24 h at room temperature or if refrigerated. Discard any reconstituted material after 24 h.

Administration
CAUTION: Observe and exercise usual cautions for handling, preparing, administering, and disposing of cytotoxic drugs.

Be aware that pretreatment with dexamethasone (or equivalent) will reduce the risk and incidence and severity of cutaneous reaction; treatment with folic acid and vitamin B_{12} will reduce risk of side effects.

Dilute 500-mg vial with 20 mL 0.9% NaCl to provide a concentration of 25 mg/mL. Gently swirl each vial until powder is completely dissolved. Solution appears clear and ranges in color from colorless to yellow or green-yellow. Further dilute prescribed amount of reconstituted solution to 100 mL with preservative-free sodium chloride (0.9% NaCl) and administer as IV infusion over 10 min.

P

Pemirolast Potassium

peh-meer′oh-last poe-tass′ee-um
★ Alamast

CATEGORY AND SCHEDULE

Pregnancy Risk Category: C

Classification: Ophthalmic, ophthalmic anti-inflammatory

MECHANISM OF ACTION

An antiallergic agent that prevents the activation and release of mediators of inflammation (e.g., mast cells). *Therapeutic Effect:* Reduces symptoms of allergic conjunctivitis.

PHARMACOKINETICS
Detected in plasma. Excreted in urine. *Half-life:* 4.5 h.

AVAILABILITY
Ophthalmic Solution: 0.1%.

INDICATIONS AND DOSAGES
▸ **Allergic conjunctivitis**
OPHTHALMIC
Adults, Elderly, Children 3 yr and older. 1-2 drops in affected eye(s) 4 times/day.

CONTRAINDICATIONS
Hypersensitivity to any component of the formulation.

INTERACTIONS
None reported.

SIDE EFFECTS
Ophthalmic: Transient ocular stinging, burning, itching, dry eye, foreign-body sensation, tearing.
Other: Headache, rhinitis, cold and flu symptoms, sinusitis, sneezing/nasal congestion.

SERIOUS REACTIONS
None reported.

PRECAUTIONS & CONSIDERATIONS
Safety and efficacy not established in children less than 3 yr of age. Caution if breastfeeding.
Storage
Store at room temperature.
Administration
Do not wear contact lens if eyes are red. If eyes are not red, remove contact lens before administration and wait 10 min before reinserting.

Wash your hands before use. Tilt head back slightly and pull lower eyelid down with index finger to form a pouch. To avoid contamination, do not touch tip of bottle to any surface. Instill the prescribed number of drops into the pouch. Close the eye gently for a few moments to spread the drops.

Penbutolol
pen-byoo-toh'lol
Levatol
Do not confuse with pindolol, Felbatol, or levobunolol.

CATEGORY AND SCHEDULE
Pregnancy Risk Category: C (D if used in the second or third trimester)

Classification:
Antihypertensives, nonspecific β-adrenergic blocking agent

MECHANISM OF ACTION
An antihypertensive that possesses nonselective β-blocking. Has moderate intrinsic sympathomimetic activity. *Therapeutic Effect:* Decreases heart rate, cardiac contractility, and BP; increases airway resistance, promoting bronchospasm, and decreases myocardial ischemia severity.

PHARMACOKINETICS
Rapidly and completely (100%) absorbed from the GI tract. Protein binding: 80%-98%. Metabolized in liver. 90% excreted in urine. *Half-life:* 17-26 h.

AVAILABILITY
Tablets: 20 mg (Levatol).

INDICATIONS AND DOSAGES
▸ **Hypertension**
PO
Adults, Elderly. Initially, 20 mg/day as a single dose. May increase to 40-80 mg/day.

CONTRAINDICATIONS

Cardiogenic shock, sinus bradycardia, second- or third-degree AV block, bronchial asthma, uncompensated overt cardiac failure, and those with known hypersensitivity to penbutolol.

INTERACTIONS

Drug

Calcium blockers: Increase risk of conduction disturbances.
Clonidine: May potentiate BP effects, especially upon withdrawal.
Cimetidine: May increase penbutolol concentrations.
Digoxin: Increases concentrations of this drug.
Diuretics, other hypotensives: May increase hypotensive effect.
Ergot derivatives: May cause peripheral ischemia.
Fentanyl: May cause severe hypotension.
Hydrocarbon inhalation anesthetics: May increase hypotension, myocardial depression.
Indomethacin, NSAIDs: May decrease antihypertensive effect.
Insulin, oral hypoglycemics: May mask symptoms of hypoglycemia and prolong hypoglycemic effect of these drugs.
Lidocaine: May prolong the elimination of lidocaine leading to toxicity.
Theophylline: May reduce elimination of theophylline; may reduce effects of both drugs by pharmacologic antagonism.
Verapamil: May increase risk of hypotension and bradycardia.
Sympathomimetics, xanthines: May mutually inhibit effects.

Herbal

Dong quai: May decrease BP.
St. John's wort, yohimbine: May decrease effectiveness of penbutolol.

Food

None known.

DIAGNOSTIC TEST EFFECTS

May increase ANA titer, SGOT (AST), SGPT (ALT), alkaline phosphatase, LDH, bilirubin, BUN, creatinine, potassium, uric acid, lipoproteins, triglycerides.

SIDE EFFECTS

Frequent

Decreased sexual ability, drowsiness, unusual tiredness or weakness, dizziness, fatigue, headache, insomnia, alteration of blood sugar levels, cough, bronchospasm.

Occasional

Diarrhea, bradycardia, depression, cold hands or feet, constipation, anxiety, nasal congestion, nausea, vomiting.

Rare

Altered taste; dry eyes; itching, numbness of fingers, toes, scalp; bradycardia; edema; AV block; worsening angina; adrenal insufficiency.

SERIOUS REACTIONS

- Abrupt withdrawal may result in sweating, palpitations, headache, and tremors.
- May cause insulin-induced hypoglycemia in patients with previously controlled diabetes.

PRECAUTIONS & CONSIDERATIONS

Caution is warranted in patients with inadequate cardiac function, impaired renal or hepatic function, diabetes mellitus, COPD, myasthenia gravis, peripheral vascular disease, hypotension, and hyperthyroidism. It is unknown whether penbutolol crosses the placenta or is distributed in breast milk. Safety and efficacy of penbutolol have not been established in children. In elderly patients, the incidence of dizziness may be increased.

Dizziness and drowsiness may be experienced during treatment. Avoid alcohol and tasks that require mental alertness or motor skills until the effects of the drug are known. In addition, avoid nasal decongestants and over-the-counter (OTC) cold preparations, especially those containing stimulants, without physician approval. Medication should not be taken when pulse is irregular or < 60 beats/min without advice of health care provider.

Abrupt withdrawal should be avoided, especially in hyperthyroidism, which could cause reactions similar to thyroid storm; rebound effects may produce angina or myocardial infarction (MI).

Storage

Store at room temperature. Keep tightly closed and protect from light.

Administration

May take without regard to food. The full antihypertensive effect of penbutolol should take 1-2 wks. Do not abruptly discontinue penbutolol but withdraw over a period of 1-2 wks.

Penciclovir Triphosphate

pen-sye'kloe-veer

Denavir

Do not confuse with acyclovir or indinavir.

CATEGORY AND SCHEDULE

Pregnancy Risk Category: B

Classification: Antivirals

MECHANISM OF ACTION

Penciclovir triphosphate selectively inhibits herpes simplex virus (HSV) polymerase competitively with deoxyguanosine triphosphate. Consequently, herpes viral DNA synthesis and, therefore, replication are selectively inhibited. *Therapeutic Effect:* An antiviral compound that has inhibitory activity against HSV-1 and HSV-2.

PHARMACOKINETICS

Measurable penciclovir concentrations were not detected in plasma or urine. The systemic absorption of penciclovir following topical administration has not been evaluated.

AVAILABILITY

Cream: 10 mg/g.

INDICATIONS AND DOSAGES

▸ Herpes labialis (cold sores)

TOPICAL

Adults, Elderly, Children 12 yr and over. Apply every 2 h during waking hours for a period of 4 days. Treatment should be started as early as possible (i.e., during the prodrome or when lesions appear).

OFF-LABEL USES

Topical adjunct to systemic treatment of herpes zoster.

CONTRAINDICATIONS

Hypersensitivity to penciclovir or any of its components or any related compound.

INTERACTIONS

Drug

OTC creams or ointments: May delay healing or increase risk of spreading the infection.

Herbal

None known.

Food
None known.

DIAGNOSTIC TEST EFFECTS
None known.

SIDE EFFECTS
Frequent
Headache.
Occasional
Change in sense of taste; decreased sensitivity of skin, particularly to touch; redness of the skin, skin rash (maculopapular, erythematous), local edema; skin discoloration; pruritus; hypoesthesia; parethesias; parosmia; urticaria; oral or pharyngeal edema.
Rare
Mild pain, burning, or stinging.

PRECAUTIONS & CONSIDERATIONS
Viral strains resistant to acyclovir are likely to be resistant to penciclovir. Also, effectiveness has not been established in immunocompromised patients.

It is unknown whether penciclovir crosses the placenta or is distributed into breast milk. Safety and efficacy have not been established in children under 12 yr of age. No age-related precautions have been noted in elderly patients. Do not apply near eyes, ears, or mucous membranes. Local irritation should be reported to the health care provider.
Storage
Store at room temperature.
Administration
Penciclovir is for external use only. Area of application should be clean and dry. Do not apply near the eyes. Apply every 2 h during waking hours for 4 days. Continue medication for the full time of treatment.

Penicillin G Benzathine
pen-i-sill′in G ben′za-theen
★ 🍁 Bicillin LA
Do not confuse with penicillin G potassium or penicillin G procaine.

CATEGORY AND SCHEDULE
Pregnancy Risk Category: B

Classification: Antibiotics, benzathine salt of natural penicillin G

MECHANISM OF ACTION
A penicillin that inhibits bacterial cell wall synthesis by binding to one or more of the penicillin-binding proteins of bacteria. Mostly used for gram-positive cocci *(Staphylococcus, S. pyogenes, S. viridans, S. faecalis, S. bovis, S. Pneumoniae),* spirochetes *(Treponema palladium). Therapeutic Effect:* Bactericidal.

PHARMACOKINETICS
IM
Very slow absorption; hydrolyzed to penicillin G. IM administration of 600,000 units to adults results in therapeutic blood levels of 0.03-0.05 units/mL for up to 10 days; similar levels for up to 14 days after 1.2 million units IM. Protein binding: Roughly 60%. Widely distributed throughout body tissues, with highest levels in the kidneys and lesser amounts in the liver, skin, and intestines. Penetrates into all other tissues and the spinal fluid to a lesser degree. Crosses placenta, excreted in breast milk. Drug is excreted rapidly by tubular excretion. Delayed in neonates and those with reduced kidney function. Duration 21-28 days. *Half-life:* 30-60 min.

AVAILABILITY

Injection Suspension (Prefilled Syringes [Bicillin LA]): 600,000 units/mL; 1.2 million units/2 mL; 2.4 million units/4 mL.

INDICATIONS AND DOSAGES

Treatment of respiratory infections, scarlet fever, erysipelas, otitis media, pneumonia, skin and soft tissue infections, bejel, pinta, yaws.

▸ **Group A streptococcal infections**

IM

Adults, Elderly. 1.2 million units as a single dose.

Older children > 27 kg. 900,000 units as a single dose.

Children ≤ 27 kg. 300,000 units-600,000 units as a single dose.

▸ **Prevention of rheumatic fever**

IM

Adults, Elderly. 1.2 million units every 3-4 wks or 600,000 units twice monthly.

Children. 25,000-50,000 units/kg every 3-4 wks.

▸ **Early syphilis**

IM

Adults, Elderly. 2.4 million units divided and administered in 2 separate injection sites.

▸ **Congenital syphilis**

IM

Children. 50,000 units/kg as single injection after a 10-day course of aqueous penicillin G.

▸ **Syphilis of more than 1-yr duration**

IM

Adults, Elderly. 2.4 million units divided and administered in 2 separate injection sites weekly for 3 wks.

Children. 50,000 units/kg weekly for 3 wks.

CONTRAINDICATIONS

Hypersensitivity to any penicillin.

INTERACTIONS

Drug

Erythromycin, lincomycins, tetracyclines: Possible decreased antimicrobial effect.

Methotrexate: Suspected increased risk of toxicity.

Probenecid, aspirin: Increases serum concentration of penicillin.

Oral contraceptives: Advise patient of a low risk for decreased contraception action, to maintain compliance with oral contraceptive use while taking antibiotics like penicillin, and to consider using additional nonhormonal-based contraceptions for the duration of therapy.

Herbal

None known.

Food

None known.

DIAGNOSTIC TEST EFFECTS

May cause a positive Coombs' test.

SERIOUS REACTIONS

- Hypersensitivity reactions, ranging from chills, fever, and rash to anaphylaxis, may occur.

SIDE EFFECTS

Occasional

Lethargy, fever, dizziness, rash, pain at injection site.

Rare

Seizures, interstitial nephritis.

PRECAUTIONS & CONSIDERATIONS

Caution is warranted with a hypersensitivity to cephalosporins, impaired cardiac or renal function, or seizure disorders. History of allergies, especially to cephalosporins or penicillins, should be determined before giving the drug. Signs and symptoms of superinfection, including anal or

P

genital pruritus, black hairy tongue, diarrhea, increased fever, sore throat, ulceration or changes of oral mucosa, and vomiting should be monitored. CBC, renal function test results, and urinalysis should be assessed.

Storage

Store prefilled syringes in the refrigerator. Do not freeze them.

Administration

Administer the drug undiluted by deep IM injection.

! Do not administer penicillin G benzathine IV, intra-arterially, or subcutaneously because doing so may cause heart attack, severe neurovascular damage, thrombosis, and death.

Penicillin G Potassium

pen-i-sill′in G

Pfizerpen

Do not confuse with penicillin G benzathine, penicillin G procaine.

CATEGORY AND SCHEDULE

Pregnancy Risk Category: B

Classification: Antibiotics, penicillins

MECHANISM OF ACTION

A penicillin that inhibits bacterial cell wall synthesis by binding to one or more of the penicillin-binding proteins of bacteria. *Therapeutic Effect:* Bactericidal.

PHARMACOKINETICS

Completely absorbed from IM injection sites. Peak blood levels reached rapidly after IV infusion. Bound primarily to albumin. Widely distributed but has limited penetration into cerebrospinal fluid unless meninges inflamed. 60% excreted within 5 h by kidney. *Half-life:* 20-30 min (prolonged in renal impairment).

AVAILABILITY

Injection, Lyophilized Powder: 5 million units.

Premixed Intravenous Piggyback (IVPB): 1 million units, 2 million units, 3 million units; all doses in 50 mL dextrose solution.

INDICATIONS AND DOSAGES

▸ **Sepsis, meningitis, pericarditis, endocarditis, pneumonia due to susceptible gram-positive organisms (not *Staphylococcus aureus*) and some gram-negative organisms**

NOTE: Total daily dose dependent on severity and type of infection.

IV, IM

Adults, Elderly. 2-24 million units/day in divided doses q4-6h.

Children. 100,000-400,000 units/kg/day in divided doses q4-6h.

▸ **Dosage in renal impairment**

Dosage interval is modified based on creatinine clearance.

Creatinine Clearance (mL/min)	Dosage Interval
10-50	Usual dose q8-12h
< 10	Usual dose q12-18h

CONTRAINDICATIONS

Hypersensitivity to any penicillin.

INTERACTIONS

Drug

Erythromycin, lincosamides, tetracyclines: May antagonize effects of penicillin.

Methotrexate: Increased or prolonged plasma levels of

P

methotrexate during high-dose penicillin treatment.
Oral contraceptives: Advise patient of a potential low risk for decreased contraceptive action, to maintain compliance with oral contraceptive while using antibiotics, and to consider using additional nonhormonal contraception for the duration of therapy.
Potassium-sparing agents: Consider potassium load during high-dose penicillin G potassium treatment.
Probenecid, aspirin: Increased or prolonged plasma levels of penicillin.
Typhoid vaccine: Potential decreased response; delay vaccine until penicillin treatment concluded.
Herbal
None known.
Food
None known.

DIAGNOSTIC TEST EFFECTS

May cause a positive Coombs' test.

IV INCOMPATIBILITIES

Include aminophylline, amphotericin B, dextran, diazepam, dobutamine, erythromycin, fat (lipid) emulsion, haloperidol, inamrinone, pentobarbital, phenytoin, protamine, quinidine.

IV COMPATIBILITIES

Include amiodarone, aztreonam, calcium gluconate, cimetidine, clindamycin, digoxin, dopamine, famotidine, furosemide, magnesium sulfate, metoclopramide, morphine, nitroglycerin, oxytocin.

SIDE EFFECTS

Occasional
Lethargy, fever, dizziness, rash, electrolyte imbalance, diarrhea, thrombophlebitis.
Rare
Seizures, interstitial nephritis.

SERIOUS REACTIONS

- Hypersensitivity reactions ranging from rash, fever, and chills to anaphylaxis.
- Antibiotic-associated colitis and other superinfections may result from altered bacterial balance.

PRECAUTIONS & CONSIDERATIONS

Caution is warranted in patients with a hypersensitivity to cephalosporins, impaired hepatic or renal function, a history of antibiotic-associated colitis, or seizure disorders. CBC, electrolyte levels, renal function test results, and urinalysis results should be monitored. Hypersensitivity to penicillin or cephalosporin should be established before beginning therapy. Any indications of superinfection, such as sore throat, oral burning sensation, fever, or fatigue, should be reported.
Storage
Thaw frozen premixed infusion bags at room temperature. The infusion is stable for 7 days if refrigerated and 24 hr at room temperature.
Administration
For IV use, follow the manufacturer's guidelines for dilution. After reconstitution, further dilute with 50-100 mL D5W or 0.9% NaCl to yield a final concentration of 100,000-500,000 units/mL (50,000 units/mL for infants and neonates). Infuse the solution over 1-2 hr for adults, 15-30 min for infants and children.

May be given IM if necessary. Dilute vial as directed to a usual concentration of 100,000 units/mL for IM use. In adults, the midlateral thigh or upper outer quadrant of the gluteus maximus may be used.

In children and infants use the midlateral muscles of the thigh.

Penicillin V Potassium

pen-i-sill'in V

Penicillin VK Apo-Pen VK, Novo-Pen VK, Nu-Pen VK

CATEGORY AND SCHEDULE

Pregnancy Risk Category: B

Classification: Antibiotics, penicillins

MECHANISM OF ACTION

A penicillin that inhibits cell wall synthesis by binding to bacterial cell membranes. *Therapeutic Effect:* Bactericidal.

PHARMACOKINETICS

Moderately absorbed from the GI tract. Protein binding: 80%. Widely distributed. Only a small amount of metabolism in the liver. Primarily excreted in urine. *Half-life:* 1 h (increased in impaired renal function).

AVAILABILITY

Tablets: 250 mg, 500 mg.
Powder for Oral Solution: 125 mg/5 mL, 250 mg/5 mL.

INDICATIONS AND DOSAGES

Effective for treatment of gram-positive cocci (*Staphylococcus aureus, S. viridans, S. faecalis, S. bovis, S. pneumoiae*), gram-negative cocci *(Neisseria gnorrhoeae, N. meningitis)*, gram-positive bacilli (*Bacillus anthracis, Clostridium perfrignens, C. tetani, C. dipththeriae*), gram-negative bacilli (*S. moniliformis*), spirochetes (*Treponema palladium*), *Actinomyces, Peptococcus,* and *Peptostreptococcus* spp.

▸ **Mild to moderate respiratory tract or skin or skin-structure infections, otitis media, necrotizing ulcerative gingivitis**

PO

Adults, Elderly, Children 12 yr and older. 125-500 mg q6-8h.
Children younger than 12 yr. 25-50 mg/kg/day in divided doses q6-8h. Maximum: 3 g/day.

▸ **Primary prevention of rheumatic fever**

PO

Adults, Elderly. 125-250 q6-8h for 10 days.
Children. 250 mg 2-3 times/day for 10 days.

CONTRAINDICATIONS

Hypersensitivity to any penicillin.

INTERACTIONS

Drug

Oral contraceptives: Advise patient of potential low risk for decreased contraceptive action, to maintain compliance with oral contraceptive use while taking antibiotics, and to consider using additional nonhormonal contraception during therapy.
Probenecid, aspirin: May increase penicillin blood concentration and risk of toxicity.
Tetracyclines, lincomycins, and erythromycin: Decreased antimicrobial effectiveness.

Herbal and Food

None known.

DIAGNOSTIC TEST EFFECTS

May cause a positive Coombs' test.

SIDE EFFECTS

Frequent

Mild hypersensitivity reaction (chills, fever, rash), nausea, vomiting, diarrhea.

Rare
Bleeding, allergic reaction, interstitial nephritis.

SERIOUS REACTIONS

• Severe hypersensitivity reactions, including anaphylaxis, may occur.
• Antibiotic-associated colitis and other superinfections may result from high dosages or prolonged therapy.

PRECAUTIONS & CONSIDERATIONS

Caution is warranted in patients with renal impairment, a history of seizures, or a history of allergies, particularly to cephalosporins. Penicillin V readily crosses the placenta, appears in cord blood and amniotic fluid, and is distributed in breast milk in low concentrations. Penicillin V may lead to allergic sensitization, candidiasis, diarrhea, and skin rash in infants. Use caution when giving to neonates and young infants because their immature renal function may delay renal excretion of the drug. Age-related renal impairment may require dosage adjustment in elderly patients.

History of allergies, especially to cephalosporins or penicillins, should be determined before giving the drug. Withhold and promptly notify the physician if rash or diarrhea occurs. Severe diarrhea with abdominal pain, blood or mucus in stool, and fever may indicate antibiotic-associated colitis. Signs of bleeding, including ecchymosis, overt bleeding, and swelling, should be assessed. Signs and symptoms of superinfection, including anal or genital pruritus, black hairy tongue, diarrhea, increased fever, sore throat, ulceration or changes of oral mucosa, and vomiting, should also be monitored. Intake and output, renal function tests, hemoglobin levels, and urinalysis should be obtained and reviewed. Possible superinfection evidenced by sore throat, oral burning sensation, fatigue, or fever should be reported immediately to the health care provider.

Storage
Store tablets at room temperature. After reconstitution, the oral solution is stable for 14 days if refrigerated.

Administration
Take the drug without regard to food. Space drug doses evenly around the clock.

Pentamidine Isethionate

pen-tam′i-deen ice-ethy-eye-oh-nate
★ NebuPent, Pentam-300

CATEGORY AND SCHEDULE

Pregnancy Risk Category: C

Classification: Antiprotozoals

MECHANISM OF ACTION

An anti-infective that interferes with nuclear metabolism and incorporation of nucleotides, inhibiting DNA, RNA, phospholipid, and protein synthesis. *Therapeutic Effect:* Produces antimicrobial and antiprotozoal effects.

PHARMACOKINETICS

Well absorbed after IM administration; minimally absorbed after inhalation. Widely distributed. Primarily excreted in urine. Minimally removed by hemodialysis. *Half-life:* 6.4 h (IV), 9.1-13.2 h (IM) (increased in impaired renal function).

AVAILABILITY

Injection (Pentam-300): 300 mg.

Powder for Nebulization (NebuPent): 300 mg.

INDICATIONS AND DOSAGES

▸ **Treatment of *Pneumocystis* infections in immunocompromised patients (injection); prevention in high-risk HIV-infected patients (inhalant)**

▸ ***Pneumocystis jaroveci* pneumonia (PCP)**

IV, IM

Adults, Elderly, Children. 4 mg/kg/day once a day for 14-21 days.

▸ **Prevention of PCP**

INHALATION

Adults, Elderly. 300 mg q4wk.
Children 5 yr and older. 300 mg q4wk.

OFF-LABEL USES

Treatment of African trypanosomiasis, cutaneous or visceral leishmaniasis.

CONTRAINDICATIONS

Hypersensitivity. NOTE: Concurrent use with some medications is not recommended (see Drug Interactions).

INTERACTIONS

Drug

Blood dyscrasia–producing medications, bone marrow depressants: May increase the abnormal hematologic effects of pentamidine.

Didanosine, zalcitabine: May increase the risk of pancreatitis. If IV pentamidine treatment is needed, temporarily interrupt treatment with these antivirals.

Foscarnet: May increase the risk of hypocalcemia, hypomagnesemia, and nephrotoxicity.

Nephrotoxic medications: May increase the risk of nephrotoxicity.

Herbal

None known.

Food

None known.

DIAGNOSTIC TEST EFFECTS

May increase BUN and serum alkaline phosphatase, bilirubin, creatinine, AST (SGOT), and ALT (SGPT) levels. May decrease serum calcium and magnesium levels. May alter blood glucose levels.

IV INCOMPATIBILITIES

Do not mix with other medications.

Do NOT reconstitute or infuse with saline solutions, as precipitates will form.

SIDE EFFECTS

Frequent

Injection (> 10%): Abscess, pain at injection site.

Inhalation (> 5%): Fatigue, metallic taste, shortness of breath, decreased appetite, dizziness, rash, cough, nausea, vomiting, chills.

Occasional

Injection (1%-10%): Nausea, decreased appetite, hypotension, fever, rash, altered taste, confusion.

Inhalation (1%-5%): Diarrhea, headache, anemia, muscle pain.

Rare

Injection (< 1%): Neuralgia, thrombocytopenia, phlebitis, dizziness.

SERIOUS REACTIONS

- Rare reactions include life-threatening or fatal hypotension, cardiac arrhythmias, hypoglycemia, leukopenia, nephrotoxicity or renal failure, anaphylactic shock, Stevens-Johnson syndrome, and toxic epidermal necrolysis are reported with IM and IV routes; monitor BP continuously throughout the infusion, and every 30 min for 2 h thereafter and every 4 h after that until BP stabilizes.
- Hyperglycemia and insulin-dependent diabetes mellitus (often

permanent) may occur even months after therapy has stopped.
• Pancreatitis (with systemic use).
• Severe or sudden hypotension with IV or IM use.
• IM use is painful and may result in sterile abscess.

PRECAUTIONS & CONSIDERATIONS

Caution is warranted in patients with diabetes mellitus, hypertension, hypotension, or renal or hepatic impairment. It is unknown whether pentamidine crosses the placenta or is distributed in breast milk. No age-related precautions have been noted in children, although safety and efficacy of the inhalation formulation are not established. No information is available regarding pentamidine use in elderly patients. Avoid alcohol.

Be sure to monitor blood pressure frequently, keeping patient supine, while giving IV or IM. Report any light-headedness, palpitations, shakiness or sweating, shortness of breath, cough, or fever. Drowsiness, decreased appetite, and increased thirst and urination may develop in the months following therapy, which may be indicative of drug-induced hyperglycemia. Adequate hydration should be maintained.

IV and IM sites should be evaluated for abscess development. Skin should be examined for rash. Hematology, liver, and renal function tests should be performed. Be alert for respiratory difficulty when administering pentamidine by inhalation.

Storage

Store vials at room temperature. After reconstitution, the IV solution is stable at room temperature for 48 h. Store the aerosol at room temperature for 48 h.

Administration

! Make sure the person is in the supine position during administration and has frequent BP checks until stable because of the risk of a life-threatening hypotensive reaction. Have resuscitative equipment readily available.

For intermittent IV infusion (piggyback), reconstitute each vial with 3-5 mL D5W or sterile water for injection. Withdraw the desired dose and further dilute with 50-250 mL D5W. Infuse the drug over 60 min. Discard any unused portion. Do not give the drug by IV injection or rapid IV infusion because this increases the risk of severe hypotension.

For IM use, reconstitute each 300-mg vial with 3 mL sterile water for injection to provide a concentration of 100 mg/mL.

For aerosol (nebulizer) use, reconstitute each 300-mg vial with 6 mL sterile water for injection. Avoid using 0.9% NaCl because it may cause a precipitate to form. Do not mix pentamidine with other medications in the nebulizer reservoir.

Pentazocine Hydrochloride

pen-tah-zoe'seen high-droh-klor'ide

Talwin

Combination Products:
With naloxone, a narcotic antagonist (oral) (Talwin NX); with acetaminophen (oral) (Talacen)

CATEGORY AND SCHEDULE

Pregnancy Category: C
Controlled Substance Schedule: C-IV (injection only)

Classification: Analgesics, narcotic mixed agonist-antagonist

MECHANISM OF ACTION

Narcotic antagonist and agonist that induces analgesia by stimulating the κ- and σ-receptors within the central nervous system (CNS). *Therapeutic Effect:* Alters processes affecting pain perception, emotional response to pain.

PHARMACOKINETICS

Well absorbed after administration. Widely distributed, including the cerebrospinal fluid (CSF). Metabolized in liver via oxidative and glucuronide conjugation pathways, extensive first-pass effect. Excreted in small amounts in the bile and feces as unchanged drug. *Half-life:* 2-3 h (prolonged with hepatic impairment).

AVAILABILITY

Tablets (Pentazocine + Naloxone [Talwin NX]): 50 mg pentazocine and 0.5 mg naloxone.
Tablets (Acetaminophen + Pentazocine [Talacen]): 25mg pentazocine with 650 mg acetaminophen.
Injection: 30 mg/mL (Talwin).

INDICATIONS AND DOSAGES

Treatment of moderate to severe pain alone or in combination with aspirin or acetaminophen.

▸ **Pain, analgesia, moderate to severe**

PO (TALWIN NX)

Adults, Elderly, Children 12 yr and older. 50 mg q3-4h. May increase to 100 mg q3-4h, if needed. Maximum: 600 mg/day.

IM/IV

Adults. 30 mg q3-4h. Do not exceed 30 mg IV or 60 mg IM per dose. Maximum: 360 mg/day.

▸ **Obstetric labor**

IM

Adults. 30 mg as a single dose.

IV

Adults. 20 mg when contractions are regular. May repeat 2-3 times q2-3h.

▸ **Pain, analgesia, mild to moderate**

PO (TALACEN)

Adults, Elderly, Children 12 yr and older. 1 tablet PO q4h, up to 6 tablets/day.

CONTRAINDICATIONS

Hypersensitivity to pentazocine or any component of the formulation such as acetaminophen, naloxone, or sulfites.

INTERACTIONS

Drug

Alcohol, central nervous system (CNS) depressants: May increase CNS or respiratory depression and hypotension.
Anticholinergics: Increased effect.
Fluoxetine: May cause hypertension, diaphoresis, ataxia, flushing, nausea, dizziness, and anxiety.
MAOIs: May produce serotonin syndrome.
Opioid analgesics: May increase withdrawal symptoms or cause additive effects.
Sibutramine: May increase risk of serotonin syndrome.
Tramadol: Potential seizure risk.

Herbal

Tobacco smoking: Increased pentazocine clearance.

Food

None known.

DIAGNOSTIC TEST EFFECTS

May increase amylase and lipase.

SIDE EFFECTS

Frequent

Drowsiness, euphoria, nausea, vomiting.

Occasional

Allergic reaction, histamine reaction (decreased BP, increased

P

sweating, flushing, wheezing), decreased urination, altered vision, constipation, dizziness, dry mouth, headache, hypotension, pain/burning at injection site.

SERIOUS REACTIONS

- Overdosage results in severe respiratory depression, skeletal muscle flaccidity, cyanosis, extreme somnolence progressing to convulsions, stupor, and coma.
- Abrupt withdrawal after prolonged use may produce symptoms of narcotic withdrawal (abdominal cramps, rhinorrhea, lacrimation, nausea, vomiting, restlessness, anxiety, increased temperature, piloerection).

PRECAUTIONS & CONSIDERATIONS

Caution is warranted in patients with head injury or increased intracranial pressure, respiratory disease, or respiratory depression before biliary tract surgery (produces spasm of spinchter of Oddi), acute myocardial infarction, severe heart disease, opioid dependence or abuse, addictive personality, impaired hepatic and renal function, acute abdominal conditions, Addison disease, prostatic hypertrophy, and patients taking other narcotics. It is unknown whether pentazocine crosses the placenta or is distributed in breast milk. Safety and efficacy have not been established in children less than 12 yr. Age-related renal or liver impairment may require decreased dosage. Use with caution in the elderly.

Pentazocine may cause withdrawal in patients currently dependent on narcotics. It may cause drowsiness and impaired judgment or coordination, so driving and tasks requiring alertness and coordination should be avoided. Alcohol should be avoided. Psychological and physical dependence may occur with chronic administration.

Storage

Store at room temperature.

Administration

Rotate injection site for IM use. SC route not recommended because of potential for severe local reactions. Avoid intra-arterial injection. Do not mix with barbiturates in solution or syringe.

May take oral pentazocine with food if GI upset occurs.

Pentobarbital

pen-toe-bar'bi-tal

★ Nembutal

Do not confuse with phenobarbital.

CATEGORY AND SCHEDULE

Pregnancy Risk Category: D

Controlled Substance Schedule: II

Classification: Anticonvulsants,, preanesthetics, sedative/hypnotic, barbiturates

MECHANISM OF ACTION

A barbiturate that binds at the γ-aminobutyric acid (GABA) receptor complex, enhancing GABA activity. *Therapeutic Effect:* Depresses central nervous system (CNS) activity and reticular activating system.

PHARMACOKINETICS

Well absorbed after PO, parenteral administration. Protein binding: 35%-55%. Rapidly, widely distributed. Metabolized in liver. Primarily excreted in urine. Removed by hemodialysis. *Half-life:* 15-48 h.

AVAILABILITY

Injection: 50 mg/mL.

INDICATIONS AND DOSAGES

▸ **Preanesthetic**

IM

Adults, Elderly. 150-200 mg.
Children. 2-6 mg/kg. Maximum: 100 mg/dose.

▸ **Hypnotic (historic use, not preferred)**

IM

Adults, Elderly. 150-200 mg at bedtime.
Children. 2-6 mg/kg. Maximum: 100 mg/dose at bedtime.

IV

Adults, Elderly. 100 mg initially then, after 1 min, may give additional small doses at 1-3 min intervals, up to 500 mg total.

▸ **Anticonvulsant**

! NOTE: IV infusion use is for mechanically ventilated patients only. EEG burst suppression generally occurs at levels of 20-50 mcg/mL.

IV

Adults. 10-15 mg/kg loading dose given slowly over 1-2 h. Additional doses of 5-10 mg/kg may be given (maximum total load dose = 30 mg/kg). Maintenance of 0.5-1 mg/kg/hr IV infusion. Titrate by 0.5 mg/kg/hr, as needed, based on serum levels and clinical response.

OFF-LABEL USES

For the reduction of increased intracranial pressure (ICP) in patients with head trauma (via coma induction if mechanically ventilated only). Sedative withdrawal.

CONTRAINDICATIONS

Porphyria, hypersensitivity to barbiturates.

INTERACTIONS

Drug

Alcohol, CNS depressants: May increase the depressive effects of pentobarbital.
Antihistamines, cold remedies (OTC): May have additive effect with any other CNS depressant ingredients.
Antiretroviral therapies for HIV: May decrease the effectiveness against HIV infection.
Barbiturates, chloral hydrate, opioid analgesics: May increase the risk of respiratory depression.
Carbamazepine: May increase metabolism.
Corticosteroids: May increase metabolism and decrease therapeutic effects.
Doxycycline: May decrease half-life.
Halogenated hydrocarbon anesthetics: May cause hepatotoxicity.
Metoprolol: May decrease effectiveness.
Procarbazine: May increase the risk of CNS depression.
Quetiapine: May decrease serum quetiapine concentrations.
Theophylline: May decrease theophylline effectiveness.
Tricyclic antidepressants and MAOIs: May increase metabolism and decrease effectiveness.
Warfarin and coumarin anticoagulants: May decrease anticoagulant effectiveness.

Herbal

Catnip oil: May increase risk of CNS depression.
Eucalyptol: May decrease effectiveness of barbiturates.
Kava kava, valerian: May increase CNS depression.
St. John's wort: May decrease CNS depressive effect of barbiturates.

Food

None known.

P

DIAGNOSTIC TEST EFFECTS

None known.

IV INCOMPATIBILITIES

In general, do not mix or infuse with other drugs. Pentobarbital easily precipitates with changes in pH. Amikacin (Amikin), aminophylline, atracurium (Tacrium), benzquinamide, butorphanol, cefazolin (Ancef), chlorpheniramine, clindamycin (Cleocin), codeine, cyclizine, diphenhydramine (Benadryl), droperidol (Inapsine), fenoldopam (Corlopam), fentanyl, glycopyrrolate (Robinul), hyaluronidase (Wydase), hydrocortisone (Solu-Cortef), hydromorphone (Dilaudid), insulin, kanamycin (Kantrex), levorphanol (Levo-Dromoran), lidocaine, meperidine (Demerol), metaraminol (Aramin), methadone, methyldopa (Aldomet), metocurine (Metubine), midazolam (Versed), nalbuphine (Nubain), neostigmine (Prostigmin), opium alkaloids, oxytetracycline, pancuronium (Pavulon), penicillin G (Pfizerpen), pentazocine (Talwin), perphenazine (Trilafon), prochlorperazine (Compazine), promazine, propofol (Diprivan), ranitidine (Zantac), scopolamine, sodium bicarbonate, sodium iodide, streptomycin, thiamine, thiopental (Pentothal), triflupromazine (Stelazine), tripelennamine (PBZ), vancomycin (Vancocin), verapamil.

SIDE EFFECTS

Occasional

Agitation, confusion, dizziness, somnolence.

Rare

Confusion, paradoxical CNS hyperactivity or nervousness in children, excitement or restlessness in elderly.

SERIOUS REACTIONS

- Agranulocytosis, megaloblastic anemia, apnea, hypoventilation, bradycardia, hypotension, syncope, hepatic damage, and Stevens-Johnson syndrome occur rarely.
- Abrupt withdrawal after prolonged therapy may produce effects ranging from markedly increased dreaming, nightmares or insomnia, tremor, sweating and vomiting, to hallucinations, delirium, seizures, and status epilepticus.
- Skin eruptions appear as hypersensitivity reactions.
- Overdosage produces cold or clammy skin, hypothermia, severe CNS depression, cyanosis, and rapid pulse.

PRECAUTIONS & CONSIDERATIONS

Caution is warranted in patients with liver or renal impairment, in elderly patients, or in patients with debilitated, suicidal tendencies, or a history of drug or alcohol abuse. Pentobarbital readily crosses the placenta and is distributed in breast milk. Barbiturates may cause fetal harm. Withdrawal symptoms may appear in neonates born to women receiving barbiturates during the last trimester of pregnancy. Its use may cause paradoxical excitement in children. Elderly patients taking pentobarbital may exhibit confusion, excitement, and mental depression. Alcohol consumption and caffeine should be avoided while taking pentobarbital. Tasks that require mental alertness or motor skills should be avoided because pentobarbital may cause dizziness and drowsiness. Drug should not be given if respirations drop to 10/min or less or pupils become dilated.

Storage

Store vials at room temperature.

P

Administration
Be aware that dosage must be individualized based on patient's age, weight, and condition.

Do not inject more than 5 mL in any one IM injection site because it produces tissue irritation. Inject IM dorsogluteally or into lateral aspect of thigh.

May give IV injection undiluted by slow IV push no faster than 50 mg/min. Pentobarbital infusions must be prepared right before use; use a 0.45-micron in-line filter during administration. Mix in D5W or 0.9% NaCl injection to a concentration no greater than 8 mg/mL to avoid precipitation. An infusion is stable for no more than 12-24 h.

Expect to hydrate adequately before and immediately after infusion to decrease the risk of adverse renal effects. Parenteral routes should be pursued only when oral administration is impossible or impractical. Beware that inadvertent intra-arterial injection may result in arterial spasm with severe pain and tissue necrosis. Also know that extravasation in SC tissue may produce redness, tenderness, and tissue necrosis. If either occurs, treat with 0.5% procaine solution injected into affected area and apply moist heat.

Pentosan Polysulfate

pen'toe-san poll'ee-sull'fate

★ 🍁 Elmiron

Do not confuse pentosan with pentostatin.

CATEGORY AND SCHEDULE

Pregnancy Risk Category: B

Classification: Urinary tract agents, anticoagulant

MECHANISM OF ACTION

A negatively charged synthetic sulfated polysaccharide with heparin-like properties that appears to adhere to bladder wall mucosal membrane; it may act as a buffering agent to control cell permeability, preventing irritating solutes in the urine. Has anticoagulant/fibrinolytic effects. *Therapeutic Effect:* Relieves bladder pain.

PHARMACOKINETICS

Poorly and erratically absorbed from the GI tract. Distributed in uroepithelium of the genitourinary tract, with lesser amount found in the liver, spleen, lung, skin, periosteum, and bone marrow. Metabolized in the liver and kidney (secondary). Eliminated in the urine. *Half-life:* 4.8 h.

AVAILABILITY

Capsules: 100 mg (Elmiron).

INDICATIONS AND DOSAGES

▸ **Interstitial cystitis**

PO

Adults, Elderly. 100 mg 3 times/day.

OFF-LABEL USES

Urolithiasis.

CONTRAINDICATIONS

Hypersensitivity to pentosan polysulfate sodium or structurally related compounds.

INTERACTIONS

Drug

Anticoagulants, high-dose aspirin: May increase risk of bleeding.

NSAIDs: May increase risk of bleeding and GI effects.

Herbal

Alfalfa, coenzyme Q, green tea: May decrease anticoagulant effectiveness.

Arnica, bilberry, black currant, bromelain, cat's claw, chamomile, clove oil, curcumin, dong quai, primrose oil, fenugreek, garlic, ginger, kava kava, licorice, red clover, skullcap, tan-shen : May increase risk of bleeding.
Chondroitin, ginseng: May increase INR serum values and increase anticoagulant effects.
Food
The effect of food on absorption of pentosan polysulfate sodium is not known.

DIAGNOSTIC TEST EFFECTS

May increase transaminase (ALT), alkaline phosphatase (SGOT), PTT, PT. May decrease WBC count, thrombocytes.

SIDE EFFECTS

Frequent
Alopecia areata (a single area on the scalp), diarrhea, nausea, headache, rash, abdominal pain, dyspepsia.
Occasional
Dizziness, depression, increased liver function tests.

SERIOUS REACTIONS

- Ecchymosis, epistaxis, gum hemorrhage have been reported (drug produces weak anticoagulant effect).
- Overdose may produce liver function abnormalities.

PRECAUTIONS & CONSIDERATIONS

Caution is warranted with GI ulcerations, polyps, diverticula, history of heparin-induced thrombocytopenia, hepatic or splenic function impairment, concurrent anticoagulant, thrombolytic, or antiplatelet therapy, and recent intracranial, intraspinal, or ophthalmologic surgery. It is unknown whether pentosan polysulfate sodium is distributed in breast milk. Safety and efficacy of pentosan polysulfate sodium have not been established in children younger than 16 yr. No age-related precautions have been noted in elderly patients.

The physician should be notified if any bleeding from gums or nose, bloody or black bowel movements, coughing up blood, bloody vomit or vomit that looks like coffee grounds, or severe stomach pain or diarrhea that does not stop occurs.
Storage
Store at room temperature.
Administration
Take with water on an empty stomach at least 1 h before or 2 h after meals.

Pentostatin

pen'toe-stat-in
★ Nipent
Do not confuse with pravastatin.

CATEGORY AND SCHEDULE

Pregnancy Risk Category: D

Classification: Antineoplastic, purine analogues

MECHANISM OF ACTION

An antimetabolite that inhibits the enzyme adenosine deaminase (ADA) (increases intracellular levels of adenine deoxynucleotide). Greatest activity in T cells of lymphoid system. Inhibits ADA and RNA synthesis. Produces DNA damage. *Therapeutic Effect:* Leads to tumor cell death.

PHARMACOKINETICS

After IV administration, rapidly distributed to body tissues (poorly distributed to cerebrospinal fluid).

Protein binding: 4%. Excreted primarily in urine unchanged or as active metabolite. *Half-life:* 5.7 h (2.6-10 h).

AVAILABILITY

Powder for Injection: 10 mg (Nipent), 2 mg/mL once reconstituted.

INDICATIONS AND DOSAGES

▸ **Hairy cell leukemia**

IV

Adults, Elderly. 4 mg/m^2 q2wk until complete response is attained (without any major toxicity). Discontinue if no response in 6 mo; partial response in 12 mo.

▸ **Dosage in renal impairment**

Only when benefits justify risks, give 2-3 mg/m^2 in patients with creatinine clearance of < 60 mL/min. Avoidance recommended if CrCl < 30 ml/min.

OFF-LABEL USES

Palliative therapy of chronic lymphocytic leukemia, prolymphocytic leukemia, cutaneous T-cell lymphoma.

CONTRAINDICATIONS

Pentostatin hypersensitivity.

INTERACTIONS

Drug

Allopurinol: May increase pentostatin toxicity.

Carmustine, cyclophosphamide, etoposide: Acute pulmonary edema, hypotension, and death when coadministered.

Fludarabine: Coadministration can cause severe pulmonary toxicity.

Vidarabine: May increase toxic effect of both drugs.

Herbal

None known.

Food

None known.

DIAGNOSTIC TEST EFFECTS

May elevate creatinine (3%-10%), hypercalcemia, hyponatremia (< 3%). Monitor CBC with differential and platelet count and renal function before each dose.

SIDE EFFECTS

Frequent

Nausea, vomiting, fever, fatigue, rash, pain, cough, upper respiratory tract infection, anorexia, diarrhea.

Occasional

Headache, pharyngitis, sinusitis, myalgia, chills, peripheral edema, anorexia, blurred vision, conjunctivitis, skin discoloration, sweating, anxiety, depression, dizziness, confusion.

SERIOUS REACTIONS

- Bone marrow depression is manifested as hematologic toxicity (principally leukopenia, anemia, thrombocytopenia). Doses higher than recommended (20-50 mg/m^2 in divided doses for more than 5 days) may produce severe renal, hepatic, pulmonary, or central nervous system (CNS) toxicity.

PRECAUTIONS &CONSIDERATIONS

Do not exceed recommended doses as nephrotoxicity, hepatoxicity, pulmonary and CNS toxicities have occurred at doses higher than recommended. Any of the following symptoms should be reported immediately: rash, hives, difficulty breathing, fever, chills; these symptoms can be indicators of possible infection: bleeding or unusual bruising, mouth sores, dark urine, yellowing of skin or eyes, pain, redness, swelling at injection site; persistent nausea, vomiting, diarrhea, appetite loss, or worsening general body weakness. Maintain adequate hydration during therapy to avoid developing hyperuricemia and urate precipitation. Rashes, occasionally severe, are common and may worsen with continued treatment; development of such rashes needs to be reported immediately because discontinuation of the drug therapy may be warranted.

Storage

Refrigerate unopened vials; use reconstituted solution or infusion within 8 h of reconstitution.

Administration

CAUTION: Observe and exercise appropriate precautions for handling, preparing, and administering cytotoxic drugs.

Administer only by IV; do not use intradermally, subcutaneously, intramuscularly, intra-arterially, or orally.

Reconstitute powder for injection with 5 mL sterile water for injection. Mix thoroughly to obtain complete dissolution to a 2 mg/mL concentration of pentostatin. Do not administer if particulate matter, cloudiness, or discoloration is noted. May administer reconstituted solution as a bolus injection given IV over 5 min, or may further dilute reconstituted solution with 25-50 mL of dextrose 5% in water or NaCl 0.9% injection for IV infusion over 20-30 min.

Pentoxifylline

pen-tox-iʹfih-lin

★ 🍁 Trental

Do not confuse Trental with Tegretol, Trandate.

CATEGORY AND SCHEDULE

Pregnancy Risk Category: C

Classification: Hemorrheologic agents, xanthine derivatives

MECHANISM OF ACTION

Synthetic dimethylxanthine derivative that is a blood viscosity-reducing agent that alters the flexibility of RBCs; inhibits production of tumor necrosis factor, neutrophil activation, and platelet aggregation. *Therapeutic Effect:* Reduces blood viscosity and improves blood flow.

PHARMACOKINETICS

Well absorbed after oral administration. Undergoes first-pass metabolism in the liver. Excreted primarily in urine. Unknown whether removed by hemodialysis. *Half-life:* 24-48 min; metabolite, 60-90 min.

AVAILABILITY

Tablets (Controlled Release [Trental]): 400 mg.

INDICATIONS AND DOSAGES

▸ **Intermittent claudication related to chronic occlusive arterial disease of the limbs**

PO

Adults, Elderly. 400 mg 3 times a day. Decrease to 400 mg twice a day if GI or CNS adverse effects occur. Continue for at least 8 wks.

CONTRAINDICATIONS

History of intolerance to xanthine derivatives, such as caffeine, theophylline, or theobromine; recent cerebral or retinal hemorrhage.

INTERACTIONS

Drug

Antihypertensives: Slight additive effect on blood pressure.

Aspirin, NSAIDs: May increase anticoagulant effects and risk of bleeding.

Warfarin, platelet aggregation inhibitors: Potential for additive risk of bleeding. Monitor.

Herbal
None known.
Food
None known.

DIAGNOSTIC TEST EFFECTS

Rare reports of prolonged prothrombin time.

SIDE EFFECTS

Occasional (2%-5%)
Dizziness, nausea, altered taste, dyspepsia, marked by heartburn, epigastric pain, and indigestion.
Rare (< 2%)
Rash, pruritus, anorexia, constipation, dry mouth, blurred vision, edema, nasal congestion, anxiety.

SERIOUS REACTIONS

- Angina and chest pain occur rarely and may be accompanied by palpitations, tachycardia, and arrhythmias.
- Signs and symptoms of overdose, such as flushing, hypotension, nervousness, agitation, hand tremor, fever, and somnolence, appear 4-5 h after ingestion and last for 12 h.
- Rare reports of bleeding; primarily in patients with other risk factors for bleeding.

PRECAUTIONS & CONSIDERATIONS

Caution is warranted in patients with chronic occlusive arterial disease, insulin-treated diabetes, hepatic or renal impairment, peptic ulcer disease, and recent surgery. It is unknown whether pentoxifylline crosses the placenta and is distributed in breast milk. Safety and efficacy of pentoxifylline have not been established in children. In elderly patients, age-related renal impairment may require cautious use. Caffeine should be limited and smoking should be avoided; smoking causes vasoconstriction and occlusion of peripheral blood vessels.

Dizziness may occur. Avoid tasks requiring mental alertness or motor skills until response to the drug has been established. Notify the physician of hand tremor. Notify the physician of red or dark urine, muscular pain or weakness, abdominal or back pain, gingival bleeding, black or red stool, coffee-ground vomitus, or blood-tinged mucus from cough. BP, heart rate and rhythm, pulse rate, serum creatinine (SCr), and AST (SGOT) levels should be monitored. Relief of signs and symptoms of intermittent claudication should be monitored; symptoms generally occur while walking or exercising or with weight bearing in the absence of walking or exercising. Patient's ability to tolerate stress should be considered as stress responses may compromise cardiovascular functions.
Storage
Store at room temperature.
Administration
Do not crush or break film-coated tablets. Take with meals to avoid GI upset. Therapeutic effect is generally noted in 2-4 wks.

Perindopril

per-in'doh-pril
★ Aceon 🍁 Coversyl

CATEGORY AND SCHEDULE

Pregnancy Risk Category: C (D if used in second or third trimester)

Classification: Angiotensin-converting enzyme (ACE) inhibitors

P

MECHANISM OF ACTION

An ACE inhibitor that suppresses the renin-angiotensin-aldosterone system and prevents conversion of angiotensin I to angiotensin II, a potent vasoconstrictor; may also inhibit angiotensin II at local vascular and renal sites. *Therapeutic Effect:* Reduces peripheral arterial resistance and BP.

AVAILABILITY

Tablets: 2 mg, 4 mg, 8 mg.

INDICATIONS AND DOSAGES

▸ Hypertension

PO

Adults, Elderly. 2-8 mg/day as single dose or in 2 divided doses. Initial dose is usually 4 mg once daily for 1-2 wks; then titrated. Maximum: 16 mg/day.

▸ Reduction of cardiac events and mortality in patients with CAD

PO

Adults. Initially, 4 mg once daily for 2 wk. Increase to 8 mg/day if tolerated.
Elderly. Initially, 2 mg once daily for 1 wk. Increase to 4 mg once daily, then 8 mg/day if tolerated.

OFF-LABEL USES

Management of heart failure.

CONTRAINDICATIONS

Hypersensitivity or history of angioedema from previous treatment with ACE inhibitors, idiopathic or hereditary angioedema, bilateral renal artery stenosis.

INTERACTIONS

Drug

Alcohol, antihypertensives, diuretics: May increase the effects of perindopril.
Lithium: May increase lithium blood concentration and risk of lithium toxicity.
NSAIDs, aspirin: May decrease hypotensive effects.
Potassium-sparing diuretics, drospirenone, eplerenone, potassium supplements: May cause hyperkalemia.

Herbal

None known.

Food

None known.

DIAGNOSTIC TEST EFFECTS

May increase BUN, serum alkaline phosphatase, serum bilirubin, serum creatinine, serum potassium, AST (SGOT), and ALT (SGPT) levels. May decrease serum sodium levels. May cause positive antinuclear antibody titer.

SIDE EFFECTS

Occasional (1%-5%)

Cough, back pain, sinusitis, upper extremity pain, dyspepsia, fever, palpitations, hypotension, dizziness, fatigue, syncope.

SERIOUS REACTIONS

- Excessive hypotension (first-dose syncope) may occur in patients with congestive heart failure (CHF) and in those who are severely salt or volume depleted.
- Angioedema (swelling of face and lips) and hyperkalemia occur rarely.
- Agranulocytosis and neutropenia may be noted in those with collagen vascular disease, including scleroderma and systemic lupus erythematosus, and impaired renal function.
- Nephrotic syndrome may be noted in those with history of renal disease.

PRECAUTIONS & CONSIDERATIONS

Caution is warranted with patients having a history of angioedema from previous treatment with ACE inhibitors, renal insufficiency, hypertension with CHF, renal artery stenosis, autoimmune disease, collagen vascular disease, pregnancy category C (first trimester), pregnancy category D (second and third trimesters), lactation. Perindopril crosses the placenta; it is unknown whether it is distributed in breast milk. Perindopril has caused fetal or neonatal morbidity or mortality. Safety and efficacy of perindopril have not been established in children. In elderly patients, age-related renal impairment may require cautious use of perindopril.

Dizziness may occur. Be alert to fluctuations in BP. If an excessive reduction in BP occurs, place the person in the supine position with legs elevated. CBC and blood chemistry should be obtained before beginning perindopril therapy, then every 2 wks for the next 3 mo, and periodically thereafter in patients with autoimmune disease, or renal impairment, and in those who are taking drugs that affect immune response or leukocyte count. BUN, serum creatinine, serum potassium, AST (SGOT), and ALT (SGPT) levels should also be monitored.

Storage

Store at room temperature; protect from moisture.

Administration

Take perindopril 1 h before meals. Do not skip doses or voluntarily discontinue the drug to avoid severe rebound hypertension.

Permethrin

per-meth′ren

★ A200 Lice, Acticin, Elimite, Nix, Pronto Plus, RID 🍁 Nix, Kwellada-P

CATEGORY AND SCHEDULE

Pregnancy Risk Category: B

Classification: Scabicides/pediculicides

MECHANISM OF ACTION

An antiparasitic agent that inhibits sodium influx through nerve cell membrane channels. *Therapeutic Effect:* Results in paralysis and death of parasites.

PHARMACOKINETICS

Less than 2% absorption after topical application. Detected in residual amounts on hair for ≥ 10 days following treatment. Metabolized by liver to inactive metabolites. Excreted in urine.

AVAILABILITY

Cream: 5% (Acticin, Elimite).
Creme Rinse, Topical: 1% (Nix).
Lice Control Sprays for furniture, bedding: 0.25% (Nix).
Shampoos or Hair Mouse/Gel Containing Piperonyl Butoxide, Pyrethrins in Combination (RID, A200 Lice, Pronto Plus): 4% with 0.33% pyrethrins.

INDICATIONS AND DOSAGES

▸ **Head lice**

SHAMPOO, GEL, MOUSSE, CREME RINSE (OTC)

Adults, Elderly, Children 2 mo and older. Shampoo hair, towel dry, apply to scalp, leave on for 10 min and rinse. Remove nits with nit comb. Repeat application if live lice are present 7 days after initial treatment.

▸ **Scabies**

TOPICAL CREAM (RX)

Adults, Elderly, Children 2 mo and older. Apply from head to feet, leave on for 8-14 h. Wash with soap and water. Repeat application if living mites are present 14 days after initial treatment.

OFF-LABEL USES

Demodicidosis, insect bite prophylaxis, leishmaniasis prophylaxis, malaria prophylaxis.

P

CONTRAINDICATIONS

Infants younger than 2 mo, hypersensitivity to pyrethyroid, pyrethrin, chrysanthemums, or any component of the formulation.

INTERACTIONS

Drug
None known.
Herbal
None known.
Food
None known.

DIAGNOSTIC TEST EFFECTS

None known.

SIDE EFFECTS

Occasional
Burning, pruritus, stinging, erythema, rash, swelling.

SERIOUS REACTIONS

• Shortness of breath and difficulty breathing have been reported.

PRECAUTIONS & CONSIDERATIONS

Caution should be used during pregnancy and in patients with asthma, pruritus, edema, and erythema. It is unknown whether permethrin is distributed in breast milk. No age-related precautions have been noted for suspension or topical use in children over 2 mo of age. Permethrin is not recommended for use in children 2 mo or younger. No age-related precautions have been noted in elderly patients.
Storage
Store all products at room temperature. Sprays are toxic to honeybees and fish and aquatic organisms. Take care to store away from children and pets.
Administration
Because scabies and lice are contagious, use caution to avoid spreading or infecting oneself. Use gloves when applying.

Shampoo hair, towel dry, apply rinse to scalp, leave on for 10 min then rinse. Remove nits with nit comb. Repeat application if live lice are present 7 days after initial treatment. If live lice are detected 14 days after the initial application of permethrin, retreatment is indicated. Also, in epidemic settings, a second application is recommended 2 wks after the first.

When using the topical formulation, apply and rub gently into the affected and surrounding area. Apply from head to feet and leave on for 8-14 h. Wash with soap and water. Repeat application if living mites are present 14 days after initial treatment.

Perphenazine

per-fen'a-zeen
Do not confuse with promazine.

CATEGORY AND SCHEDULE

Pregnancy Risk Category: C

Classification: Antipsychotics, phenothiazines

MECHANISM OF ACTION

An antipsychotic agent and antiemetic that blocks postsynaptic dopamine receptor sites in the brain. *Therapeutic Effect:* Suppresses behavioral response in psychosis and relieves nausea and vomiting.

AVAILABILITY

Tablets: 2 mg, 4 mg, 8 mg, 16 mg.

INDICATIONS AND DOSAGES

▸ **Treatment of psychotic disorders, schizophrenia**
▸ **Severe schizophrenia**
PO
Adults. 4-16 mg 2-4 times/day. Maximum: 64 mg/day.

Elderly. Initially, 2-4 mg/day. May increase at intervals of 4-7 days by 2-4 mg/day up to 32 mg/day.

▸ **Severe nausea and vomiting**

PO

Adults. 8-16 mg/day in divided doses up to 24 mg/day.

CONTRAINDICATIONS

Coma, myelosuppression, severe cardiovascular disease, hepatic damage, phenothiazine or sulfite hypersensitivity, severe central nervous system (CNS) depression, subcortical brain damage.

INTERACTIONS

Drug

Alcohol, other CNS depressants, barbiturate anesthetics, opioid analgesics: May increase hypotensive effects and CNS and respiratory depression.
Anticholinergics: May increase anticholinergic effects.
Antihypertensives: May increase the risk of hypotension.
Antithyroid agents: May increase the risk of agranulocytosis.
Epinephrine: May cause hypotension, tachycardia.
Haloperidol, droperidol, phenothiazines and related drugs, metoclopramide: May increase the severity and frequency of extrapyramidal symptoms.
Levodopa: May decrease the effects of this drug.
Lithium: May decrease perphenazine absorption and produce adverse neurologic effects.
MAOIs, tricyclic antidepressants: May increase anticholinergic and sedative effects.
Tetracyclines, fluoroquinolones, thiazide diuretics: Additive photosensitization.

Herbal

None known.

Food

None known.

DIAGNOSTIC TEST EFFECTS

May produce false-positive pregnancy and phenylketonuria test results. May produce ECG changes, including prolonged QT and QTc intervals and T-wave depression or inversion.

SIDE EFFECTS

Occasional

Marked photosensitivity, somnolence, dry mouth, blurred vision, lethargy, constipation or diarrhea, nasal congestion, peripheral edema, urine retention.

Rare

Ocular changes, altered skin pigmentation, hypotension, dizziness, syncope.

SERIOUS REACTIONS

- Extrapyramidal symptoms appear to be dose-related and are divided into 3 categories: akathisia (characterized by inability to sit still, tapping of feet), parkinsonian symptoms (including mask-like face, tremors, shuffling gait, hypersalivation), and acute dystonias (such as torticollis, opisthotonos, and oculogyric crisis).
- Tardive dyskinesia occurs rarely.
- Neuroleptic malignant syndrome (rare).
- Abrupt withdrawal after long-term therapy may precipitate nausea, vomiting, gastritis, dizziness, and tremors.

PRECAUTIONS & CONSIDERATIONS

Caution is warranted in patients with impaired respiratory, hepatic, renal, or cardiac function; alcohol withdrawal; history of seizures; urinary retention; glaucoma; prostatic hypertrophy; or hypocalcemia (increases susceptibility to dystonias). Be aware that perphenazine crosses the placenta and is distributed in breast milk. Be aware that children may develop extrapyramidal symptoms (EPS) or neuromuscular symptoms, especially dystonias. Elderly patients are more prone to anticholinergic effects, such as dry mouth, EPS, orthostatic hypotension, and sedation symptoms. Urine may darken. Drowsiness may occur. Alcohol and tasks that require mental alertness or motor skills should be avoided. Exposure to artificial light and sunlight should also be avoided during therapy. EPS, tardive dyskinesia, and potentially fatal, rare neuroleptic malignant syndrome, such as altered mental status, fever, irregular pulse or BP, and muscle rigidity should be monitored. Hydration status should also be assessed.

Notify health care provider if significant xerostomic side effects occur (sore tongue, problems eating or swallowing, difficulty wearing prosthesis) for possible medication change.

P

Storage

Store tablets at room temperature.

Administration

Therapeutic effect may take up to 6 wks to appear. Do not abruptly discontinue perphenazine. May administer tablets without regard to food.

Phenazopyridine Hydrochloride

fen-az′o-peer′i-deen high-droh-klor′ide

Azo-Gesic, Azo-Standard, Pyridium Phenazo, Pyridium

Do not confuse phenazopyridine with pyridoxine.

CATEGORY AND SCHEDULE

Pregnancy Risk Category: B

Classification: Urinary tract analgesic, nonnarcotic

MECHANISM OF ACTION

An agent that exerts topical analgesic effect on urinary tract mucosa. *Therapeutic Effect:* Relieves urinary pain, burning, urgency, and frequency.

PHARMACOKINETICS

Well absorbed from the GI tract. Partially metabolized in the liver. Primarily excreted in urine.

AVAILABILITY

Tablets (Azo-Gesic, Azo-Standard, OTC): 95 mg.
Tablets (Pyridium, Rx only): 100 mg, 200 mg.

INDICATIONS AND DOSAGES

▸ Treatment of urinary tract irritation from infection; urinary analgesic

PO

Adults. 190-200 mg 3 times a day. Use for 2 days when used with an antibacterial agent.

Children 6 yr and older. 12 mg/kg/day in 3 divided doses for 2 days. Use for 2 days when used with an antibacterial agent.

▸ Dosage in renal impairment

Dosage interval is modified based on creatinine clearance.

Creatinine Clearance (mL/min)	Dosage Interval
50-80	Usual dose q8-16h
< 50	Avoid use

CONTRAINDICATIONS

Hepatic or renal insufficiency, G6PD deficiency, hypersensitivity to phenazopyridine.

INTERACTIONS

Drug

None known.

Herbal
None known.
Food
None known.

DIAGNOSTIC TEST EFFECTS

May interfere with urinalysis tests based on color reactions, such as urinary glucose, ketones, protein, and 17-ketosteroids.

SIDE EFFECTS

Expected
Discoloration of urine (reddish-orange).
Occasional
Headache, GI disturbance, rash, pruritus.

SERIOUS REACTIONS

- Overdose may lead to hemolytic anemia, nephrotoxicity, or hepatotoxicity. Patients with renal impairment or severe hypersensitivity to the drug may also develop these reactions.
- A massive, acute overdose may result in methemoglobinemia.

PRECAUTIONS & CONSIDERATIONS

Caution is warranted in patients with hepatic or renal insufficiency or renal disease.

Notify the physician, and expect to discontinue the drug if skin or sclera turns yellow because this signifies impaired renal excretion. It is unknown whether phenazopyridine crosses the placenta or is distributed in breast milk. No age-related precautions have been noted in children older than 6 yr. Age-related renal impairment may increase the risk of toxicity in elderly patients.

Urine may turn a reddish-orange color and may permanently stain clothing. Irreversible staining of soft contact lenses has been reported.

Therapeutic response, including relief of urinary frequency, pain, and burning, should be assessed.
Storage
Store at room temperature.
Administration
Take phenazopyridine with food. Expect to discontinue the drug after 2 days as there is no evidence that it is effective after this period. Maintain hydration during treatment.

Phendimetrazine

fen-dye-me'tra-zeen
★ Adipost, Bontril PDM, Bontril Slow-Release, Melfiat, Prelu-2

CATEGORY AND SCHEDULE

Pregnancy Risk Category: C
Controlled Substance Schedule: III

Classification: Anorexiants, amphetamine-like central nervous system (CNS) stimulant

MECHANISM OF ACTION

A phenylalkylamine sympathomimetic agent with activity similar to amphetamines that stimulates the central nervous system CNS and elevates BP most likely mediated via norepinephrine and dopamine metabolism. Causes stimulation of the hypothalamus. *Therapeutic Effect:* Decreases appetite.

PHARMACOKINETICS

The pharmacokinetics of phendimetrazine tartrate has not been well established. Metabolized to active metabolite, phendimetrazine. Excreted in urine. *Half-life:* 2-4 h.

AVAILABILITY

Tablets: 35 mg (Bontril PDM).

Capsules (Extended Release): 105 mg (Adipost, Bontril Slow-Release, Melfiat, Prelu-2).

INDICATIONS AND DOSAGES

▸ **Obesity**

PO

Adults, Elderly. 105 mg/day in the morning or before the morning meal (sustained release); 35 mg 2-3 times/day (immediate release). Maximum: 70 mg 3 times/day.

CONTRAINDICATIONS

Advanced arteriosclerosis, agitated states, glaucoma, drug abuse, hyperthyroidism, moderate to severe hypertension or pulmonary hypertension, symptomatic cardiovascular disease, use within 14 days of a MAOI, hypersensitivity to phendimetrazine or sympathomimetics.

INTERACTIONS

Drug

Caffeine, caffeine-containing products: May increase risk of insomnia or dry mouth.

Guanethidine: May decrease hypotensive effect of guanethidine.

Hydrocarbon inhalants, general anesthetics: May increase risk of dysrhythmias.

Insulin, antidiabetic agents: May alter insulin or medication requirements as obesity is treated or diet changes.

MAOIs or within 14 days of MAOIs: May increase risk of hypertensive crisis.

Sibutramine: May increase risk of hypertension and tachycardia.

Tricyclic antidepressants, phenothiazines: May increase cardiovascular effects.

Herbal and Food

None known.

DIAGNOSTIC TEST EFFECTS

None known.

SIDE EFFECTS

Occasional

Constipation, nausea, diarrhea, dry mouth, dysuria, libido changes, flushing, hypertension, insomnia, nervousness, headache, dizziness, irritability, agitation, restlessness, palpitations, increased heart rate, sweating, tremor, urticaria.

SERIOUS REACTIONS

- Multivalvular heart disease, primary pulmonary hypertension, and arrhythmias occur rarely.
- Overdose may produce flushing, arrhythmias, and psychosis.
- Abrupt withdrawal following prolonged administration of high doses may produce extreme fatigue and depression.

PRECAUTIONS & CONSIDERATIONS

Caution is warranted in patients with diabetes mellitus or mild hypertension. Caution should be used with pregnancy. It is unknown whether phendimetrazine is excreted in breast milk. Be aware that safety and efficacy of this drug have not been established in children. No age-related precautions have been noted in elderly patients. Tasks that require mental alertness or motor skills should be avoided. Palpitations, dizziness, dry mouth, and pronounced nervousness should be reported.

Psychological and physical dependence may occur with chronic administration.

Storage

Store at room temperature.

Administration

Take extended-release capsule in the morning, 60 min before the morning meal. Do not chew, crush, or open the capsules. Take immediate-release tablets 1 h before meals.

Phenelzine Sulfate

fen'el-zeen sull'fate

Nardil

CATEGORY AND SCHEDULE

Pregnancy Risk Category: C

Classification: Antidepressant, monoamine oxidase inhibitors (MAOIs)

MECHANISM OF ACTION

An MAOI that inhibits the activity of the enzyme monoamine oxidase at central nervous system (CNS) storage sites, leading to increased levels of the neurotransmitters epinephrine, norepinephrine, serotonin, and dopamine at neuronal receptor sites. *Therapeutic Effect:* Relieves depression.

AVAILABILITY

Tablets: 15 mg.

INDICATIONS AND DOSAGES

▸ **Treatment of depression when uncontrolled by other means**

PO

Adults. 15 mg 3 times a day. May increase to 60-90 mg/day.

After effect achieved, lower dosage to lowest effective dose. Maintenance dose may be as low as 15 mg a day or every other day as long as required.

Elderly. Initially, 7.5 mg/day. May increase by 7.5-15 mg/day q3-4wk up to 60 mg/day in divided doses.

OFF-LABEL USES

Treatment of panic disorder, vascular or tension headaches.

CONTRAINDICATIONS

Hypersensitivity. Includes, but not limited to, cardiovascular or cerebrovascular disease, hepatic or renal impairment, pheochromocytoma.

Many drugs are contraindicated for concurrent use with an MAOI; review drug interactions carefully and follow appropriate wash-out periods before prescribing phenelzine. Specific contraindications include meperidine, sympathomimetics, L-dopa, COMT-inhibitors, dextromethorphan, other MAOIs, linezolid, buspirone, serotonin drugs (SSRIs, dexfenfluramine, sibutramine), tryptophan, bupropion, cocaine, surgical anesthetics, guanethedine; certain foods also forbidden.

INTERACTIONS

Drug

Alcohol, other CNS depressants: May increase CNS depression and sedative effects.

Amphetamine, ephedrine, indirect acting sympathomimetics: Increased pressor effects.

Buspirone: May increase BP.

Caffeine-containing medications: May increase the risk of cardiac arrhythmias and hypertension.

Carbamazepine, cyclobenzaprine, maprotiline, other MAOIs: May precipitate hypertensive crisis, convulsions, hyperpyretic crisis.

Dopamine, tryptophan: May cause sudden, severe hypertension.

Fluoxetine, trazodone, tricyclic antidepressants: May cause serotonin syndrome.

Insulin, oral antidiabetics: May increase the effects of these drugs.

Meperidine, other opioid analgesics: May produce diaphoresis, immediate excitation, rigidity, and severe hypertension or hypotension, sometimes leading to severe respiratory distress, vascular collapse, seizures, coma, and death.

Methylphenidate: May increase the CNS stimulant effects of methylphenidate.
Herbal
None known.
Food
Caffeine, chocolate, tyramine-containing foods (such as aged cheese): May cause sudden, severe hypertension.

DIAGNOSTIC TEST EFFECTS
None known.

SIDE EFFECTS
Frequent
Orthostatic hypotension, restlessness, GI upset, insomnia, dizziness, headache, lethargy, asthenia, dry mouth, peripheral edema.
Occasional
Flushing, diaphoresis, rash, urinary frequency, increased appetite, transient impotence.
Rare
Visual disturbances.

P

SERIOUS REACTIONS
- Hypertensive crisis occurs rarely and is marked by severe hypertension, occipital headache radiating frontally, neck stiffness or soreness, nausea, vomiting, diaphoresis, fever or chilliness, clammy skin, dilated pupils, palpitations, tachycardia or bradycardia, and constricting chest pain.
- Intracranial bleeding occurs rarely in cases of severe hypertension.

PRECAUTIONS & CONSIDERATIONS
Caution is warranted in patients with cardiac arrhythmias, frequent or severe headaches, hypertension, suicidal tendencies, and within several hours of ingestion of a contraindicated substance, such as tyramine-containing foods. Foods that require bacteria or molds for their preparation or preservation (such as yogurt and aged cheese), foods containing tyramine (including avocados, bananas, broad beans, figs, papayas, raisins, sour cream, soy sauce, beer, wine, yeast extracts, meat tenderizers, and smoked or pickled meats), and excessive amounts of caffeine-containing foods or beverages (such as chocolate, coffee, and tea) should be avoided during therapy.

Phenelzine sulfate is not recommended for use in children.

Alcohol and tasks that require mental alertness or motor skills should be avoided. Notify the physician if headache or neck soreness or stiffness occurs. If hypertensive crisis occurs, phentolamine 5-10 mg IV should be administered. Liver function tests should be performed before and periodically during therapy, especially with long-term use.
Storage
Store phenelzine tablets at room temperature. Do not freeze.
Administration
Take the drug with food or milk to alleviate GI symptoms. Depression may start to lift during the first week of therapy, but phenelzine's full therapeutic effect may require 2-6 wks of therapy.

Phenobarbital
fee-noe-bar′bi-tal
★ Luminal
Do not confuse phenobarbital with pentobarbital, or Luminal with Tuinal.

CATEGORY AND SCHEDULE
Pregnancy Risk Category: D
Controlled Substance Schedule: IV

Classification: Anticonvulsants, barbiturates, sedatives

MECHANISM OF ACTION

A barbiturate that enhances the activity of γ-aminobutyric acid (GABA) by binding to the GABA receptor complex. *Therapeutic Effect:* Depresses central nervous system (CNS) activity.

PHARMACOKINETICS

Route	Onset	Peak	Duration
PO	20-60 min	NA	6-10 h
IV	5 min	30 min	4-10 h

Well absorbed after PO or parenteral administration. Protein binding: 35%-50%. Rapidly and widely distributed. Metabolized in the liver. Excreted primarily in urine. Removed by hemodialysis. *Half-life:* 53-118 h.

AVAILABILITY

Elixir: 20 mg/5 mL.
Tablets: 15 mg, 30 mg, 60 mg, 100 mg.
Injection: 60 mg/mL, 130 mg/mL.

INDICATIONS AND DOSAGES

▸ Status epilepticus

IV

Adults, Elderly, Children, Neonates. Loading dose of 15-20 mg/kg as a single dose or in divided doses.

▸ Seizure control

PO, IV

Adults, Elderly, Children 12 yr and older. 1-3 mg/kg/day.
Children aged 6-12 yr. 3-6 mg/kg/day.
Children aged 1-5 yr. 6-8 mg/kg/day.
Children younger than 1 yr. 5-6 mg/kg/day.
Neonates. 3-4 mg/kg/day.

▸ Sedation

PO, IM

Adults, Elderly. 30-120 mg/day in 2-3 divided doses.
Children. 2 mg/kg 3 times a day.

▸ Hypnotic

PO, IV, IM, SC

Adults. 100-200 mg at bedtime.
Children. 3-5 mg/kg at bedtime.

OFF-LABEL USES

Prevention and treatment of hyperbilirubinemia, chronic cholestasis.

CONTRAINDICATIONS

Hypersensitivity to barbiturates, porphyria, marked hepatic impairment, or respiratory disease in which dyspnea or obstruction is evident.

INTERACTIONS

Drug

NOTE: Phenobarbital induces the metabolism of many important drugs.

Alcohol, other CNS depressant
May increase the effects of phenobarbital.

Antiretroviral protease inhibitors: May decrease PI blood concentrations, leading to loss of antiviral effect against HIV.

Carbamazepine: May increase the metabolism of carbamazepine.

Digoxin, glucocorticoids, metronidazole, quinidine, tricyclic antidepressants: May decrease the effects of these drugs.

Hormonal contraceptives: May decrease blood concentrations, leading to loss of contraceptive efficacy. Higher dose regimens or alternative or additional methods may be needed.

Phenytoin: Variable effects on serum concentrations; monitor closely.

Theophylline: May reduce theophylline concentrations.

Valproic acid: Increases the blood concentration and risk of toxicity of phenobarbital.

Warfarin: May reduce anticoagulant effect. Monitor INR.
Herbal
None known.
Food
None known.

DIAGNOSTIC TEST EFFECTS
May decrease serum bilirubin level. Therapeutic serum level is 10-40 mcg/mL; toxic serum level is > 50 mcg/mL.

IV INCOMPATIBILITIES
NOTE: In general, phenobarbital sodium injection is incompatible with many other injectable medications.

Amphotericin B complex (Abelcet, AmBisome, Amphotec), fentanyl (Sublimaze), fosphenytoin (cerebyx), hydrocortisone (Solu-Cortef), hydromorphone (Dilaudid), insulin, morphine.

SIDE EFFECTS
P
Occasional (1%-3%)
Somnolence.
Rare (< 1%)
Confusion; paradoxical CNS reactions, such as hyperactivity or nervousness in children and excitement or restlessness in elderly patients (generally noted during first 2 wks of therapy, particularly in the presence of uncontrolled pain).

SERIOUS REACTIONS
- Abrupt withdrawal after prolonged therapy may produce increased dreaming, nightmares, insomnia, tremor, diaphoresis, vomiting, hallucinations, delirium, seizures, and status epilepticus.
- Skin eruptions may be a sign of a hypersensitivity reaction.
- Blood dyscrasias, hepatic disease, and hypocalcemia occur rarely.
- Overdose produces cold or clammy skin, hypothermia, severe CNS depression, cyanosis, tachycardia, and Cheyne-Stokes respirations.
- Toxicity may result in severe renal impairment.

PRECAUTIONS & CONSIDERATIONS
Caution is warranted in patients with hepatic and renal impairment. Phenobarbital readily crosses the placenta and is distributed in breast milk. Phenobarbital use lowers serum bilirubin concentrations in neonates, produces respiratory depression in neonates during labor, and may increase the risk of maternal bleeding and neonatal hemorrhage during delivery. Neonates born to women who use barbiturates during the last trimester of pregnancy may experience withdrawal symptoms. Phenobarbital use may cause paradoxical excitement in children. Elderly patients taking phenobarbital may exhibit confusion, excitement, and mental depression.

Drowsiness and dizziness may occur, so alcohol and tasks requiring mental alertness or motor skills should be avoided. Notify the physician if headache, nausea, and rash occur. BP, heart rate, respiratory rate, CNS status, renal and hepatic function, and seizure activity should be monitored.
Storage
Store at room temperature.
Administration
PO
Take oral phenobarbital without regard to food. Crush tablets as needed. The elixir may be mixed with fruit juice, milk, or water.
IV, IM
Phenobarbital may be given undiluted or may be diluted with NaCl, D5W, or lactated Ringer's

solution. Expect to hydrate the patient adequately before and immediately after infusion to decrease the risk of adverse renal effects. Do not exceed an injection rate of 30 mg/min for children and 60 mg/min for adults. Injecting too rapidly may produce marked respiratory depression and severe hypotension. Be aware that inadvertent intra-arterial injection may result in arterial spasm with severe pain and tissue necrosis and that extravasation in subcutaneous tissue may produce redness, tenderness, and tissue necrosis. If either occurs, inject 0.5% procaine solution into the affected area and apply moist heat, as ordered.

For IM use, do not inject more than 5 mL in any one injection site because doing so may cause tissue irritation. Inject the drug deep intramuscularly.

Phenoxybenzamine

fen-ox-ee-ben'za-meen

★ Dibenzyline

CATEGORY AND SCHEDULE

Pregnancy Risk Category: C

Classification: Antihypertensives, sympatholytics, α-blocking agent

MECHANISM OF ACTION

An antihypertensive that produces long-lasting noncompetitive α-adrenergic blockade of postganglionic synapses in exocrine glands and smooth muscles. Relaxes urethra and increases opening of the bladder.
Therapeutic Effect: Controls hypertension.

PHARMACOKINETICS

Well absorbed from the GI tract. Distributed into fatty tissue. Metabolized in liver. Eliminated in urine and feces. Not removed by hemodialysis.
Half-life: 24 h.

AVAILABILITY

Tablets: 10 mg (Dibenzyline).

INDICATIONS AND DOSAGES

▸ **Treatment of hypertension caused by pheochromocytoma**

PO

Adults. Initially, 10 mg twice daily. May increase dose by 10 mg no more frequently than every other day to clinical response or a maximum of 20-40 mg 2-3 times/day.

OFF-LABEL USES

Prostatic obstruction, Raynaud disease, frostbite.

CONTRAINDICATIONS

Any condition compromised by hypotension, hypersensitivity to phenoxybenzamine or any component of the formulation.

INTERACTIONS

Drug

α-Adrenergic agonists: May decrease the effects of phenoxybenzamine

β-Blockers (used concurrently): May increase risk of toxicity (hypotension, tachycardia).

CNS depressants: May increase risk of CNS depression.

Ephedrine and OTC cold medicines containing ephedrine: May counteract hypotensive effects.

Hypotensive-producing medications: May increase the effects of phenoxybenzamine.

Herbal
Licorice, ma huang, yohimbine: May decrease the effects of phenoxybenzamine.
Food
None known.

DIAGNOSTIC TEST EFFECTS
None known.

SIDE EFFECTS
Frequent
Headache, nasal congestion, dizziness, drowsiness.
Occasional
Nausea, postural hypotension, syncope, dry mouth.
Rare
Palpitations, diarrhea, constipation, inhibition of ejaculation, weakness, altered vision, miosis, confusion.

SERIOUS REACTIONS
- Overdosage produces severe hypotension, irritability, lethargy, tachycardia, dizziness, and shock.

PRECAUTIONS & CONSIDERATIONS
Caution is warranted in patients with congestive heart failure, coronary artery disease, and renal function impairment. It is unknown whether phenoxybenzamine crosses the placenta or is distributed into breast milk. Safety and efficacy have not been established in children. Elderly patients may be more sensitive to hypotensive effects and may be at risk of developing phenoxybenzamine-induced hypothermia.

Dizziness and light-headedness may occur. Caution when driving and change positions slowly. Alcohol should be avoided.
Storage
Store at room temperature.
Administration
If GI irritation occurs, take with meals or milk.

Phentermine
fen′ter-meen
★ Adipex-P

CATEGORY AND SCHEDULE
Pregnancy Risk Category: C
Controlled Substance Schedule: IV

Classification: Anorexiants, Sympathomimetics

MECHANISM OF ACTION
A sympathomimetic amine structurally similar to dextroamphetamine and most likely mediated via norephinephrine and dopamine metabolism. Causes stimulation of the hypothalamus. *Therapeutic Effect:* Decreased appetite.

PHARMACOKINETICS
Well absorbed from the GI tract; resin absorbed slower. Excreted unchanged in urine. *Half-life:* 20 h.

AVAILABILITY
Capsules (as Hydrochloride): 37.5 mg (Adipex-P).
Tablets (as Hydrochloride): 37.5 mg (Adipex-P).

INDICATIONS AND DOSAGES
▸ **Obesity**
PO
Adults, Children older than 16 yr. Usually 1 capsule or tablet (37.5 mg) daily, administered before breakfast or 1-2 h after breakfast. Can adjust dose with tablets; for some, half-tablet (18.75 mg) daily is adequate.

CONTRAINDICATIONS

Advanced arteriosclerosis, agitated states, cardiovascular disease, anorexia nervosa, concurrent use or within 14 days of discontinuation of MAOI therapy, glaucoma, history of drug abuse, hypertension (moderate to severe), hyperthyroidism, hypersensitivity to phentermine or sympathomimetic amines.

INTERACTIONS

Drug

Caffeine and caffeine-containing products: Increased risk of insomnia.

Fenfluramine: May increase risk of pulmonary hypertension and valvular heart disease.

Hydrocarbon inhalants, general anesthetics: Increased risk of dysrhythmia.

MAOIs: May increase risk of hypertensive crisis (headache, hyperpyrexia, hypertension).

Sibutramine: May increase risk of hypertension and tachycardia.

Tricyclic antidepressants, ascorbic acid, phenothiazines: Decreased effect of phentermine.

Herbal

None known.

Food

None known.

DIAGNOSTIC TEST EFFECTS

May interfere and give false-positive amphetamine EMIT assay result.

SIDE EFFECTS

Occasional

Restlessness, insomnia, tremor, palpitations, tachycardia, elevation in BP, headache, dizziness, dry mouth, unpleasant taste, diarrhea or constipation, changes in libido.

SERIOUS REACTIONS

- Primary pulmonary hypertension (PPH), psychotic episodes, and valvular heart disease rarely occur.
- Anorectic agents have been associated with regurgitant multivalvular heart disease involving mitral, aortic, or tricuspid valves.
- Prolonged use may cause physical or psychological dependence.

PRECAUTIONS & CONSIDERATIONS

Caution is warranted in patients with cardiovascular disease, psychosis, diabetes, insomnia, porphyria, mild hypertension, Tourette syndrome, seizure disorders, and history of substance abuse. It is unknown whether phentermine is excreted in breast milk. Be aware that the safety and efficacy of this drug have not been established in children younger than 16 yr. Age-related liver or renal impairment may require decreased dosage in elderly patients. Phentermine may be habit forming, and it should not be abruptly discontinued.

Fast, pounding, or irregular heartbeat; chest pain; severe headache; trouble breathing; skin rash; blurred vision; confusion; or unexplained sore throat should be reported immediately.

Caution is warranted in patients having a history of drug abuse or addictive personality as prolonged use can cause physical or psychological dependence. Patients on chronic drug therapy may rarely have symptoms of blood dyscrasias, which include infection, bleeding, and poor healing.

Storage

Store at room temperature, tightly closed.

Administration

Do not take phentermine in the afternoon or evening because it can cause insomnia. May take before breakfast or 1-2 h after breakfast.

Phentolamine

fen-tole′a-meen

★ Rogitine

CATEGORY AND SCHEDULE

Pregnancy Risk Category: C

Classification: Sympatholytics, α-blocking

MECHANISM OF ACTION

An α-adrenergic blocking agent that produces peripheral vasodilation and cardiac stimulation. *Therapeutic Effect:* Decreases BP.

PHARMACOKINETICS

Poorly absorbed from the GI tract. Protein binding: 72%. Metabolized in liver. Eliminated in urine and feces. Not removed by hemodialysis. *Half-life:* 19 min.

P

AVAILABILITY

Injection: 5 mg/mL.

INDICATIONS AND DOSAGES

▸ **Extravasation—norepinephrine**

SC

Adults, Elderly. Infiltrate area with a small amount (1 mL) of solution (made by diluting 5-10 mg in 10 mL of NS) within 12 h of extravasation. Do not exceed 0.1-0.2 mg/kg or 10 mg total. If dose is effective, normal skin color should return to the blanched area within 1 h.

Children. Infiltrate area with a small amount (1 mL) of solution (made by diluting 5-10 mg in 10 mL of NS) within 12 h of extravasation. Do not exceed 0.1-0.2 mg/kg or 5 mg total.

▸ **Diagnosis of pheochromocytoma**

IM/IV

Adults, Elderly. 5 mg as a single dose.

Children. 0.05-0.1 mg/kg/dose. Maximum single dose: 5 mg.

▸ **Surgery for pheochromocytoma: Hypertension**

IM/IV

Adults, Elderly. 5 mg given 1-2 h before procedure and repeated as needed every 2-4 h.

Children. 0.05-0.1 mg/kg/dose given 1-2 h before procedure. Repeat as needed every 2-4 h until hypertension is controlled. Maximum single dose: 5 mg.

▸ **Hypertensive crisis**

IV

Adults, Elderly. 5-15 mg as a single dose.

OFF-LABEL USES

Treatment of pralidoxime-induced hypertension, erectile dysfunction (with papaverine for intracavernous injection), extravasation-dopamine, epinephrine, hyperhidrosis.

CONTRAINDICATIONS

Renal impairment, coronary or cerebral arteriosclerosis, hypersensitivity to phentolamine or related compounds.

INTERACTIONS

Drug

Alcohol: May increase the risk of disulfiram-type reactions.

β-Blockers: May exaggerate hypotensive effects.

Epinephrine, ephedrine: May decrease the effects of phentolamine; may cause tachycardia.

Sildenafil, tadalafil, vardenafil: May increase BP-lowering effects.

Herbal

None known.

Food

None known.

DIAGNOSTIC TEST EFFECTS
May increase liver function tests.

IV INCOMPATIBILITIES
Amphotericin B, cefazolin, cefoxitin, clindamycin, diazepam, furosemide, regular insulin, ketorolac, penicillin G, phenobarbital, phenytoin.

IV COMPATIBILITIES
Amiodarone (Cordarone), dobutamine (Dobutrex), dopamine, phenylephrine, norepinephrine (Levophed), papaverine, phenylephrine, verapamil.

SIDE EFFECTS
Occasional
Hypotension, tachycardia, arrhythmia, flushing, orthostatic hypotension, weakness, dizziness, nausea, vomiting, diarrhea, nasal congestion, pulmonary hypertension.

SERIOUS REACTIONS
- Symptoms of overdosage include tachycardia, shock, vomiting, and dizziness.
- Mixed agents, such as epinephrine, may cause more hypotension.

PRECAUTIONS & CONSIDERATIONS
Caution is warranted in patients with arrhythmias, cerebral vascular spasm or occlusion, hypotension, and tachycardia. Be aware that it is unknown whether phentolamine crosses the placenta or is distributed into breast milk. No age-related precautions have been noted in children or elderly patients.

Nasal congestion, increased heartbeat, palpitations, dizziness, headache, and hypotension are common side effects of phentolamine. BP should be monitored during its use. Symptoms including tachycardia, shock, vomiting, and dizziness may indicate overdosage and should be reported immediately.

Storage
Store at room temperature.

Administration
Phentolamine mesylate for injection is reconstituted for parenteral use by adding 1 mL of sterile water for injection to the vial, producing a solution containing 5 mg of phentolamine mesylate per milliliter. Discard any unused portion.

Phentolamine is sometimes added to peripheral pressor infusions to circumvent local tissue damage. The manufacturer indicates that admixing phentolamine at a concentration of 0.01 mg/mL with norepinephrine does not adversely affect the pressor action of norepinephrine.

Persons undergoing diagnostic testing for pheochromocytoma should be maintained in the supine position during phentolamine administration.

P

Phenylephrine (Systemic)

★ Neo-Synephrine, Pediacare Decongestant, Sudafed PE, Sudogest PE.
Do not confuse with pseudoephedrine, epinephrine.

CATEGORY AND SCHEDULE
Pregnancy Risk Category: C

Classification: Vasopressors, decongestants, sympathomimetic, α-adrenergic agonist

MECHANISM OF ACTION
Phenylephrine is a powerful postsynaptic α-receptor stimulant that acts on the α-adrenergic receptors of vascular smooth muscle,

with little effect on the β-receptors of the heart, lacking chronotropic and inotropic actions on the heart. Causes vasoconstriction of arterioles of nasal mucosa or conjunctiva, activates dilator muscles of the pupil to cause contraction, and produces systemic arterial vasoconstriction. *Therapeutic Effect:* Vasoconstriction, decreases heart rate, increases stroke output, increases blood pressure, decreases mucosal blood flow and relieves congestion, and increases systolic BP.

PHARMACOKINETICS

Phenylephrine is irregularly absorbed from and readily metabolized in the GI tract. After IV administration, a pressor effect occurs almost immediately and persists for 15-20 min. After IM administration, a pressor effect occurs within 10-15 min and persists for 50 min to 1 h. The pharmacologic effects of phenylephrine are terminated at least partially by the uptake of the drug into the tissues. Phenylephrine is metabolized in the liver and intestine by the enzyme monoamine oxidase (MAO). The metabolites and their route and rate of excretion have not been identified. *Half-life:* Up to 2.5 h, variable.

Route	Onset	Peak	Duration
IV	Immediate	NA	15-20 min
IM	10-15 min	NA	0.5-2 h
SC	10-15 min	NA	1 h

AVAILABILITY

Solution (Injection): 10 mg/mL.
Tablets, OTC (Sudafed PE, Sudogest PE): 10 mg.
Oral Solution (Sudafed PE, Pediacare Decongestant): 2.5 mg/5 mL.

INDICATIONS AND DOSAGES

Treatment of nasal congestion (temporary relief), mild to moderate hypotension, paroxysmal supraventricular tachycardia (PSVT), hypotensive prophylaxis during spinal anesthesia, vasoconstriction during anesthesia.

▸ **Paroxysmal supraventricular tachycardia (PSVT)**

Adults. The initial dose, given by rapid IV injection, should not exceed 0.5 mg. Subsequent doses may be increased in increments of 0.1-0.2 mg. Maximum single dose is 1 mg IV.
Children. 5-10 mcg/kg IV over 20-30 seconds.

▸ **Mild to moderate hypotension**

SC/IM
Adults. 2-5 mg IM or SC (range 1-10 mg), repeated no more than every 10-15 min. Maximum initial IM or SC dose is 5 mg.
Children. 0.1 mg/kg IM or SC every 1-2 h as needed. Maximum dose is 5 mg.
IV
Adults. 0.2 mg IV (range 0.1-0.5 mg), given no more frequently than every 10-15 min. Maximum initial IV dose is 0.5 mg.

▸ **Severe hypotension or shock**

IM, SC
Adults, Elderly. 2-5 mg/dose q1-2h.
Children. 0.1 mg/kg/dose q1-2h.
IV BOLUS
Adults, Elderly. 0.1-0.5 mg/dose q10-15min as needed.
Children. 5-20 mcg/kg/dose q10-15min.
IV INFUSION
Adults. Initially, 100-180 mcg/min IV infusion, with dose titration to the desired MAP and SVR. A maintenance infusion rate of 40-60 mcg/min IV is usually adequate after BP stabilizes.

Children. 5-20 mcg/kg IV bolus, followed by an initial IV infusion of 0.1-0.5 mcg/kg/min, titrated to desired effect. Titrate to achieve desired effect.

▸ **Hypotensive emergencies during spinal anesthesia**

IV

Adults. Initially, 0.2 mg IV. Subsequent doses should not exceed the previous dose by more than 0.1-0.2 mg. Maximum of 0.5 mg per dose.

▸ **Hypotension during spinal anesthesia in children**

IM/SC

Children. A dose of 0.044-0.088 mg/kg IM or SC is recommended by the manufacturer.

▸ **Hypotension prophylaxis during spinal anesthesia**

IM/SC

Adults. 2-3 mg SC or IM, 3 or 4 min before anesthesia. A dose of 2 mg SC or IM is usually adequate with low spinal anesthesia; 3 mg IM or SC may be necessary with high spinal anesthesia.

▸ **Vasoconstriction in regional anesthesia**

IV

Adults. The manufacturer states that the optimum concentration of phenylephrine HCl is 0.05 mg/mL (1:20,000). Solutions may be prepared for regional anesthesia by adding 1 mg of phenylephrine HCl to each 20 mL of local anesthesia solution. Some pressor response can be expected when at least 2 mg is injected.

▸ **Prolongation of spinal anesthesia**

IV

Adults. The addition of 2-5 mg to the anesthetic solution increases the duration of motor block by as much as 50% without an increase in the incidence of complications such as nausea, vomiting, or BP disturbances.

▸ **Nasal decongestion**

PO

Adults, Elderly, Children 13 yr and older. 10 mg q4-6h, up to 60 mg/day.
Children 6-12 yr. 5 mg q4-6h, up to 30 mg/day.
Children 4-5 yr. 2.5 mg q4-6h, up to 15 mg/day.

CONTRAINDICATIONS

Phenylephrine HCl injection should not be used with patients with severe hypertension, ventricular tachycardia or fibrillation, acute myocardial infarction (MI), atrial flutter or fibrillation, cardiac arrhythmias, cardiac disease, cardiomyopathy, closed-angle glaucoma, coronary artery disease, women who are in labor, during obstetric delivery, or in patients who have a known hypersensitivity to phenylephrine, sulfites, or to any one of its components.

INTERACTIONS

Drug

β-Adrenergic blockers: Risk of bradycardia with systemic absorption.
Halothane: Vasopressors may cause serious cardiac arrhythmias during halothane anesthesia and therefore should be used only with great caution or not at all.
MAO inhibitors: The pressor effect of sympathomimetic pressor amines and adrenergic agents is markedly potentiated in patients receiving MAO inhibitors.
Nitrous oxide/oxygen gas inhalation: May complicate nasal administration.
Oxytocics: The pressure effect of sympathomimetic pressor amines is potentiated.

P

Tricyclic antidepressants: Increased risk of dysrhythmias and hypertension.

Herbal

None known.

Food

None known.

DIAGNOSTIC TEST EFFECTS

None known.

SIDE EFFECTS

Frequent

Nasal: Rebound nasal congestion due to overuse, especially when used for more than 3 days.

Occasional

Mild central nervous system (CNS) stimulation (restlessness, nervousness, tremors, headache, insomnia), headache, reflex bradycardia, excitability, restlessness, and rarely arrhythmias.

Nasal: Stinging, burning, drying of nasal mucosa.

Ophthalmic: Transient burning or stinging, brow ache, blurred vision.

P

SERIOUS REACTIONS

- Overdose may induce ventricular extrasystoles and short paroxysms of ventricular tachycardia, a sensation of fullness in the head, and tingling of the extremities. If an excessive elevation of BP occurs, it can be immediately relieved by an α-adrenergic blocking agent (e.g., phentolamine).
- Peripheral vasoconstriction may lead to limb ischemia, gangrene.

PRECAUTIONS & CONSIDERATIONS

Caution is warranted in patients with metabolic acidosis, acute pancreatitis, heart disease, pheochromocytoma, severe hypertension, thrombosis, ventricular tachycardia, hypercapnia, phenylketonuria, hypoxia, atrial fibrillation, narrow-angle glaucoma, pulmonary hypertension, hypovolemia, mechanical obstruction such as severe valvular aortic stenosis, myocardial infarction, arterial embolism, atherosclerosis, Buerger disease, cold injury such as frostbite, diabetic endarteritis, Raynaud syndrome, and sensitivity to other sympathomimetics. It is unknown whether phenylephrine (systemic) crosses the placenta or is distributed into breast milk. Phenylephrine (systemic) should be used cautiously in children and elderly patients. Particular caution is warranted in children under 6 yr of age and in patients with diabetes, cardiovascular disease, hypertension, hyperthyroidism, increased intraocular pressure, prostatic hypertrophy, glaucoma, ischemic heart disease.

Storage

Store at room temperature.

Administration

To prepare a solution of phenylephrine for direct IV injection, 10 mg (1 mL) of phenylephrine hydrochloride injection should be diluted with 9 mL of sterile water for injection to provide a solution containing 1 mg of phenylephrine per milliliter. Infuse over 20-30 seconds into a large vein. Direct IV injection reserved for emergency administration.

To prepare a continuous IV infusion, final concentrations are usually 20-60 mcg/mL in either D5W or 0.9% NaCl. Whenever possible, infuse via central access. Infusion into very small veins can cause necrosis or gangrene.

Oral dose forms for nasal decongestant use may be given without regard to meals.

Phenytoin

fen'i-toyn

★ Dilantin, Dilantin Infatab, Dilantin-125 Suspension, Dilantin Kapseals, Phenytek

🍁 Dilantin, Dilantin Infatab, Dilantin-125 Suspension, Dilantin Kapseals

Do not confuse phenytoin with mephenytoin, or Dilantin with Dilaudid.

CATEGORY AND SCHEDULE

Pregnancy Risk Category: D

Classification: Anticonvulsants, hydantoins

MECHANISM OF ACTION

A hydantoin anticonvulsant that stabilizes neuronal membranes in the motor cortex by decreasing sodium and calcium ion influx into the neurons. Also acts as an antiarrhythmic agent by decreasing abnormal ventricular automaticity and shortening the refractory period, QT interval, and action potential duration. *Therapeutic Effect:* Limits the spread of seizure activity. Restores normal cardiac rhythm.

PHARMACOKINETICS

Slowly and variably absorbed after PO administration; slowly but completely absorbed after IM administration. Protein binding: 90%-95% (adults), 84% (neonates). Widely distributed; crosses the placenta and into breast milk. Metabolized in the liver. Phenytoin is one of only a few drugs in which metabolic capacity can be saturated at therapeutic levels. Below the saturation point, phenytoin is eliminated in a linear process. Above the saturation point, elimination is much slower and occurs via a zero-order process. Small increases in dose can produce large increases in plasma concentrations. Excreted primarily in urine. Not removed by hemodialysis. *Half-life:* 22 h (oral), 14 h (Infatabs).

AVAILABILITY

Chewable Tablets (Dilantin Infatabs): 50 mg.
Capsules (Extended Release [Dilantin]): 30 mg (27.6 mg phenytoin), 100 mg (92 mg phenytoin).
Capsules (Extended Release [Phenytek]): 200 mg, 300 mg.
Oral Suspension (Dilantin): 125 mg/5 mL.
Injection: 50 mg/mL.

INDICATIONS AND DOSAGES

▸ **Used in the treatment of status epilepticus of the grand mal type, prevention and treatment of seizures occurring during neurosurgery. Control of arrhythmias is common (off-label)**

▸ **Status epilepticus**

IV

Adults, Elderly, Children. 15-20 mg/kg by slow IV, followed by a maintenance dose of 100 mg every 6-8 h, PO or IV. Maintenance dose: 300 mg/day in 2-3 divided doses for adults and elderly; 6-7 mg/kg/day for children 10-16 yr; 7-8 mg/kg/day for children 7-9 yr; 7.5-9 mg/kg/day for children 4-6 yr; 8-10 mg/kg/day for children 6 mo to 3 yr. IV rate should not exceed 1-3 mg/kg/min.

Neonates. Loading dose: 15-20 mg/kg. Maintenance dose: 5-8 mg/kg/day.

▸ **Seizure control**

PO

Adults, Elderly. 100 mg or 125 mg suspension 3 times/day initially, followed by 300-400 mg/day, not to exceed 600 mg/day. Can administer 1 g loading dose in 3 divided doses (400 mg, 300 mg, 300 mg) given

P

at 2-h intervals. Once control is established, extended release 300 mg/day may be administered once daily.
Children 16 yr or younger. PO 5 mg/kg/day in 2-3 divided doses initially. Once control is established, follow with 4-8 mg/kg/day, not to exceed 300 mg/day.

▸ **Neurosurgery prophylaxis**
Adults. 10-20 mg/kg IV load. Maintenance: 4-6 mg/kg/day in 2 doses during surgery and postoperatively.

OFF-LABEL USES

Control of digoxin-induced arrhythmias, neuropathic pain/diabetic neuropathy, rare use for migraine prophylaxis.

CONTRAINDICATIONS

Hypersensitivity to hydantoins, seizures due to hypoglycemia.
IV: Adams-Stokes syndrome, second- and third-degree AV block, sinoatrial block, sinus bradycardia.

INTERACTIONS

NOTE: Many drugs may interact with phenytoin; closely review regimens. Commonly encountered interactions are listed.

Drug

Acetaminophen: May increase hepatotoxicity potential with chronic use.
Alcohol, other central nervous system (CNS) depressants: May increase CNS depression.
Amiodarone, cimetidine, disulfiram, felbamate, isoniazid, oxyphenbutazone, phenylbutazone, phenacemide, sulfonamides, trimethoprim: May increase phenytoin blood concentration, effects, and risk of toxicity.
Antacids, sucralfate: May decrease phenytoin absorption.
Antiretroviral protease inhibitors for HIV (PIs): Increases the metabolism of many PIs, decreasing efficacy. Many PIs inhibit phenytoin clearance, resulting in increased phenytoin levels.
Carbamazepine, rifampin, rifabutin: May decrease serum levels of phenytoin.
Corticosteroids, certain antineoplastics, coumarin anticoagulants, doxycycline, levodopa, felodipine, methadone, loop diuretics, hormonal contraceptives, quinidine: May reduce serum levels of these agents and reduce efficacy.
CNS depressants, alcohol: May increase depressant effects.
Cyclosporine: May reduce serum levels.
Disopyramide: May cause decreased bioavailability and serum concentrations; may enhance anticholinergic effect.
Fluconazole, ketoconazole, miconazole: May increase phenytoin blood concentration.
Folic acid: May cause folic acid deficiency.
Lidocaine: May increase cardiac depressant effects.
Metyrapone: May cause a subnormal response to metyrapone.
Mexiletine: May decrease cardiac effects and serum concentration.
Nondepolarizing muscle relaxants: May cause decreased effect or shorter duration of activity.
Phenobarbital, primidone, sodium valproate, valproic acid: May alter phenytoin levels, may increase phenobarbital levels, and decrease valproic acid levels.
Sympathomimetics (e.g., dopamine): May cause profound hypotension and cardiac arrest.
Theophylline: May decrease effects of both theophylline and phenytoin.

P

Valproic acid: May decrease the metabolism and increase the blood concentration of phenytoin.

Herbal

None known.

Food

Enteral nutrition therapy: May reduce serum concentrations of phenytoin. Hold enteral feedings 2 h prior to and after administration.

DIAGNOSTIC TEST EFFECTS

May increase blood glucose level and serum GGT and alkaline phosphatase levels. Therapeutic serum level is 10-20 mcg/mL; toxic serum level is > 25 mcg/mL.

IV INCOMPATIBILITIES

Do not mix with any other medications.

SIDE EFFECTS

Frequent

Drowsiness, lethargy, confusion, slurred speech, irritability, gingival hyperplasia, hypersensitivity reaction (including fever, rash, and lymphadenopathy), constipation, dizziness, nausea, vomiting, pink-colored urine.

Occasional

Headache, hirsutism, coarsening of facial features, insomnia, muscle twitching.

Rare

Dermatologic manifestations with fever: Scarlatiniform or morbiliform rashes.

SERIOUS REACTIONS

- Abrupt withdrawal may precipitate status epilepticus.
- Local irritation, inflammation, tenderness, necrosis and sloughing with or without extravasation at site of injection or IV infusion.
- Because of variances in bioavailability, brand interchange is not recommended and should be avoided.
- Blood dyscrasias, lymphadenopathy, and osteomalacia (caused by impaired vitamin D metabolism) may occur.
- Toxic phenytoin blood concentration (25 mcg/mL or more) may produce ataxia, nystagmus, or diplopia. As the level increases, extreme lethargy may lead to coma.
- There is no known antidote.
- Drug should not be given to anyone having a known sensitivity to phenytoin or any of its components.

PRECAUTIONS & CONSIDERATIONS

! Extreme caution should be used in patients with congestive heart failure (CHF), myocardial damage, myocardial infarction (MI), and respiratory depression. Caution is also warranted with hyperglycemia, hypotension, hepatic and renal impairment, and severe myocardial insufficiency, alcohol abuse, hypotension, acute intermittent porphyria. Phenytoin crosses the placenta and is distributed in small amounts in breast milk. Fetal hydantoin syndrome, marked by craniofacial abnormalities, digital or nail hypoplasia, and prenatal growth deficiency, has been reported. Pregnant women may experience more frequent seizures because of altered drug absorption and metabolism. Phenytoin use may increase the risk of neonatal hemorrhage and maternal bleeding during delivery. Children are more susceptible to coarsening of facial hair, hirsutism, and gingival hyperplasia. Lower dosages are recommended for elderly patients, although no age-related precautions have been noted for this age group.

Skin rash, nystagmus, ataxia, drowsiness, severe nausea or vomiting, gingival hyperplasia, or jaundice should be reported. Blood sugar levels may be affected by phenytoin, and changes in levels beyond normal should be reported.

Drowsiness, dizziness, and lethargy may occur, so alcohol and tasks that require mental alertness or motor skills should be avoided. Notify the physician if fever, swollen glands, sore throat, a skin reaction, or signs of hematologic toxicity (such as a bleeding tendency, bruising, fatigue, or fever) occur. History of the seizure disorder, including the duration, frequency, and intensity of seizures, should be assessed. CBC and blood chemistry tests should be performed to assess hepatic function before and periodically during phenytoin therapy. Repeat the CBC 2 wks after beginning phenytoin therapy and 2 wks after the phenytoin maintenance dose is established. CBC should be performed every month for 1 yr after the maintenance dose is established and every 3 mo thereafter.

Discontinuation of the drug abruptly should be avoided as this could precipitate seizures or status epilepticus. Dosages should be reduced or other anticonvulsant medication should be introduced gradually.

Storage

Oral dosage forms are stored at room temperature and protected from light and freezing. Injection should be stored in a cool, dry place at room temperature. For diluted infusions, prepare just prior to use and use within 1 h of preparation as the drug is poorly soluble and may precipitate.

Administration

Take oral phenytoin with food if GI distress occurs. Do not chew, open, or break capsules or take any discolored capsules. Tablets may be chewed. Shake the oral suspension well before each use. If administering with tube feedings, delay feeding 1-2 h before and after administration of phenytoin.

! Give phenytoin by IV push directly into a large vein through a large-gauge needle or IV catheter. Remember that the maintenance dose is usually given 12 h after the loading dose.

A slight yellow discoloration of the solution will not affect its potency. Phenytoin may be given undiluted or may be diluted with 0.9% NaCl. Dilute phenytoin dosage in NS to a final concentration of ≤ 6.7 mg/mL (e.g., 1000 mg would be diluted with NS to a minimum volume of 150 mL). Complete infusion within 1 h of preparation. MUST filter if diluted for IV infusion: Use 0.22- or a 0.45-micron final in-line filter between the IV catheter and IV tubing. Do not exceed an injection rate of 50 mg/min for adults to avoid cardiovascular collapse and severe hypotension. For elderly patients, administer 50 mg over 2-3 min. For neonates, do not exceed 0.5-1 mg/kg/min. To minimize pain from chemical irritation of the vein, flush the catheter with sterile saline solution after each bolus dose of phenytoin.

Phosphates, Potassium, Sodium, and Combinations

Poe-tass'eeum fos'fates

★ Fleet Enema, Fleet Phospho-Soda, K-Phos 500, K-Phos Neutral, Osmoprep, Visicol

CATEGORY AND SCHEDULE

Pregnancy Risk Category: C

Classification: Electrolyte replacement agents, minerals; gastrointestinal agents, laxatives

MECHANISM OF ACTION

Electrolytes that participate in bone deposition, calcium metabolism, and utilization of B complex vitamins and act as a buffer in maintaining acid-base balance. Also exert an osmotic effect in the small intestine, producing distention and promoting peristalsis. *Therapeutic Effect:* Correct hypophosphatemia, acidify urine in urinary tract infections, help to prevent calcium deposits in urinary tract (unapproved use), and promote evacuation of the bowel.

PHARMACOKINETICS

Following PO or IV use as a supplement, phosphate is absorbed via an active, energy-dependent process. Due to the formation of insoluble complexes, foods or drugs containing large amounts of calcium or aluminum decrease the amount of phosphate absorbed orally. Phosphorus is used in all energy-dependent body processes, where it is incorporated into molecules such as ATP. When used as a laxative or bowel evacuant, sodium phosphate salts act locally and quickly; no significant systemic distribution or metabolism is expected in most patients. Phosphate that is absorbed systemically is excreted almost exclusively by the kidneys. *Half-life:* Not available, but excretion is reduced in renal impairment.

AVAILABILITY

LAXATIVES
Oral Solution (Fleet Phospha-Soda): 4 mmol phosphate per mL.
Enema (Fleet Enema): 2.25 oz, 4.5 oz.
Tablets (Osmoprep): Total of 1.5 g of sodium phosphate per tablet.
Tablets (Visicol): Total of 1.5 g of sodium phosphate per tablet.

ELECTROLYTE REPLACEMENTS
Tablets (K-Phos 500): 500 mg phosphate (sodium-free).
Tablets (K-Phos Neutral): 250 mg (8 mmol) phosphate.
Injection (potassium phosphate): 3 mmol phosphate and 4.4 mEq potassium per mL.
Injection (sodium phosphate): 3 mmol phosphate and 4 mEq sodium per mL.

INDICATIONS AND DOSAGES

▸ **Hypophosphatemia**

PO (K-PHOS, K-PHOS NEUTRAL)
Adults, Elderly. 800 mg.
Children > 10 yr of age. 1200 mg.
Children 1-10 yr of age. 800 mg.
Children 6-12 mo of age. 360 mg.
Children up to 6 mo of age. 240 mg.
IV INFUSION
Adults, Elderly. 0.5 mmol/kg IV over 4-6 h.
Children. 0.25 mmol/kg over 4-6 h.

▸ **For bowel evacuation**

PO (OSMOPREP)
Adults, Elderly. 32 tablets (48 g) PO total, taken as follows: The evening before colonoscopy, 4 tablets are taken with 8 oz of clear liquids q15min for a total of 20 tablets. On the day of colonoscopy (starting 3-5 h before), 4 tablets are taken with 8 oz of clear liquids q15min for a total of 12 tablets. Do not repeat this regimen within 7 days.
PO (VISICOL)
Adults, Elderly. 40 tablets (60 g) PO total, taken as follows: The evening before colonoscopy, 3 tablets are taken with 8 oz of clear liquids q15min for a total of 20 tablets (last dose is 2 tablets). On the day of colonoscopy (starting 3-5 hours before), 3 tablets are taken with 8 oz of clear liquids q15min for a total of 20 tablets (the last dose is 2 tablets). Do not repeat this regimen within 7 days.

PO (FLEET PHOSPHO-SODA)
Adults, Elderly, Children 13 yr and older. 30 or 45 mL, taken as follows. Dilute the dose in one 8-oz glass of clear liquid. Drink, then follow with at least 3 full glasses of clear liquids. Do not exceed recommended dosage.
Children 5 to 12 yr. Reduction in the adult dose necessary. Consult physician.
RECTAL (FLEET ENEMA)
Adults, Elderly, Children 13 yr and older. 1 bottle (118 ml) per rectum.
RECTAL (FLEET ENEMA FOR CHILDREN)
Children 5 to 11 yr. 1 bottle (59 ml) per rectum.
Children 2-4 yr. ½ bottle (29.5 ml) per rectum; measured carefully by removing excess enema from bottle.

▸ **For constipation**

PO (FLEET PHOSPHO-SODA)
Adults, Elderly, Children 10 yr and older. 1 tbsp (15 mL); dilute the dose with 4 oz of cool water. Drink, then follow with at least one additional 8-oz glass of cool water.
Children 5 to 9 yr. ½ tbsp (7.5 mL); dilute the dose with 4 oz of cool water. Drink, then follow with at least one additional 8-oz glass of cool water.

▸ **Urine acidification**

PO
Adults, Elderly. 8 mmol (250 mg) 4 times a day.

OFF-LABEL USES

Prevention of calcium renal calculi.

CONTRAINDICATIONS

Abdominal pain or fecal impaction (rectal dosage form), CHF, hyperkalemia, hypernatremia, hyperphosphatemia, hypocalcemia, hypomagnesemia, phosphate renal calculi, severe renal impairment.

INTERACTIONS

Drug

Amiloride, ACE inhibitors, NSAIDs, potassium-containing medications, potassium-sparing diuretics, salt substitutes containing potassium phosphate: May increase potassium blood concentration.
Antacids: May decrease the absorption of phosphates.
Calcium-containing medications: May increase the risk of calcium deposition in soft tissues and decrease phosphate absorption.
Digoxin: May increase the risk of heart block caused by hyperkalemia when given with potassium phosphates.
Glucocorticoids: May cause edema when given with sodium phosphate.
Iron and iron-containing products: May inhibit absorption if taken within 2 h of phosphate dose.
Phosphate-containing medications: May increase the risk of hyperphosphatemia.
Sodium-containing medications: May increase the risk of edema when given with sodium phosphate.
Triamterine and other potassium-sparing diuretics: Concurrent use may increase the risk of hyperkalemia developing.

Herbal

None known.

Food

None known.

DIAGNOSTIC TEST EFFECTS

None known.

IV COMPATIBILITIES

Diltiazem (Cardizem), enalapril (Vasotec), famotidine (Pepcid), magnesium sulfate, metoclopramide (Reglan).

SIDE EFFECTS

Frequent

Mild laxative effect (in first few days of therapy), decrease in frequency and amount of urination.

Occasional

Diarrhea, nausea, abdominal pain, vomiting, slow or irregular heartbeat.

Rare

Headache, dizziness, confusion, heaviness of lower extremities, fatigue, muscle cramps, paresthesia, peripheral edema, arrhythmias, weight gain, thirst.

SERIOUS REACTIONS

- Hyperphosphatemia may produce extraskeletal calcification, headache, confusion, muscle cramps, paresthesia, arrhythmias.

PRECAUTIONS & CONSIDERATIONS

Caution is warranted in patients with adrenal insufficiency, cirrhosis, renal impairment, and concurrent use of potassium-sparing drugs. It is unknown whether phosphates cross the placenta or are distributed in breast milk. No age-related precautions have been noted in children or elderly patients.

Notify the physician of abdominal pain. Baseline phosphate levels and urinary pH should be obtained. Serum alkaline phosphatase, bilirubin, calcium, phosphorus, potassium, sodium, AST (SGOT), and ALT (SGPT) levels should be monitored throughout therapy. Pattern of daily bowel activity and stool consistency should also be assessed.

Injectible form contains aluminum, which may reach toxic levels with prolonged use; care is warranted in neonates.

Storage

Store all products at room temperature; protect oral tablets from moisture.

Administration

For oral use, dissolve tablets in a full glass of water. Give phosphates after meals or with food to decrease GI upset. Maintain high fluid intake to prevent renal calculi.

For IV use, dilute the drug before using. For peripheral lines, dilute at a concentration not to exceed 30 mmol per 500 mL. For central lines, may dilute 30 mmol in 250 mL. Generally, infuse over 4-6 h.

Phosphorated Carbohydrate Solution

fos'for-ate-ed kar-boe-hye'drate

★ Emetrol

CATEGORY AND SCHEDULE

Pregnancy Risk Category: NR

OTC

Classification: Gastrointestinal agents; antiemetics.

MECHANISM OF ACTION

An antiemetic whose mechanism of action has not been determined. Phosphorated carbohydrate solution consists of fructose, dextrose, and phosphoric acid, and it may directly act on the wall of the GI tract and reduce smooth muscle contraction and delays gastric emptying time through high osmotic pressure exerted by the solution of simple sugars. *Therapeutic Effect:* Relieves mild nausea and vomiting.

PHARMACOKINETICS

Fructose is slowly absorbed from the GI tract. Metabolized in liver by phosphorylation and partly converted to liver glycogen and glucose. Excreted in urine.

P

Dextrose is rapidly absorbed from GI tract. Distributed and stored throughout tissues. Metabolized in liver to carbon dioxide and water.

AVAILABILITY

Solution: 1.87 g fructose/1.87 g dextrose/21.5 mg phosphoric acid/ 5 mL (Emetrol).

INDICATIONS AND DOSAGES

▸ **Antiemetic**

PO

Adults, Elderly. 15-30 mL initially. May repeat dose every 15 min until distress subsides. Maximum: 5 doses in a 1-h period.

Children 2 yr and older. 5-10 mL initially. May repeat dose every 15 min until distress subsides. Maximum: 5 doses in a 1-h period.

Children under 2 yr. Do not use.

CONTRAINDICATIONS

Symptoms of appendicitis or inflamed bowel, hereditary fructose intolerance, hypersensitivity to any component of the formulation.

INTERACTIONS

Drug

None known.

Herbal

None known.

Food

None known.

DIAGNOSTIC TEST EFFECTS

May increase blood glucose concentrations.

SIDE EFFECTS

Frequent

Diarrhea, abdominal pain.

SERIOUS REACTIONS

• Fructose intolerance includes symptoms of fainting; swelling of face, arms, and legs; unusual bleeding; vomiting; weight loss; and yellow eyes and skin.

PRECAUTIONS & CONSIDERATIONS

Caution is warranted with diabetes mellitus because the condition may be aggravated because of the solution's high carbohydrate content as well as with children and elderly because of the risk of fluid and electrolyte loss as a result of vomiting. It is unknown whether phosphorated carbohydrate solution crosses the placenta or is distributed in breast milk. Safety and efficacy of phosphorated carbohydrate solution have not been established in children younger than 2 yr of age.

Storage

Store at room temperature tightly closed.

Administration

May repeat dose after 15 min if distress does not subside. Do not dilute phosphorated carbohydrate solution. Do not drink any other fluids immediately before or after taking this drug. Do not exceed more than 5 doses in 1-h period. If symptoms do not cease after 5 doses, contact the patient's health care provider.

Physostigmine

fi-zoe-stig′meen

Do not confuse physostigmine with Prostigmin or pyridostigmine.

CATEGORY AND SCHEDULE

Pregnancy Risk Category: C

Classification:

Parasympathomimetic, cholinesterase inhibitors

MECHANISM OF ACTION
A cholinergic that inhibits destruction of acetylcholine by enzyme acetylcholinesterase, thus enhancing impulse transmission across the myoneural junction.
Therapeutic Effect: Improves skeletal muscle tone, stimulates salivary and sweat gland secretions.

AVAILABILITY
Injection: 1 mg/mL.

INDICATIONS AND DOSAGES
▸ **To reverse central nervous system (CNS) effects of anticholinergic drugs and tricyclic antidepressants**
IV, IM
Adults, Elderly. Initially, 0.5-2 mg. If no response, repeat 10-30 min until response or adverse cholinergic effects occur. If initial response occurs, may give additional doses of 1-2 mg q30-60min as life-threatening signs, such as arrhythmias, seizures, and deep coma, recur.
Children. 0.01-0.03 mg/kg. May give additional doses q5-10min until response or adverse cholinergic effects occur or total dose of 2 mg is given.

OFF-LABEL USES
Treatment of hereditary ataxia.

CONTRAINDICATIONS
Hypersensitivity, mechanical intestinal (ileus) or urinary obstruction. Take care to differentiate between cholinergic crisis and myasthenic crisis prior to use.

INTERACTIONS
Drug
Atropine: Use care when giving to counteract cholinesterase inhibitor side effects, as cholinergic crisis may be induced.
Cholinesterase inhibitors: May increase the risk of toxicity.
Neuromuscular blockers: May prolong the action of succinylcholine and other related medicines.
Quinine: May antagonize the action of physostigmine.
Herbal
None known.
Food
None known.

DIAGNOSTIC TEST EFFECTS
None known.

IV INCOMPATIBILITIES
Do not mix with any other medications.

SIDE EFFECTS
Expected
Miosis, increased GI and skeletal muscle tone, bradycardia.
Occasional
Marked drop in BP (hypertensive patients).
Rare
Allergic reaction.

SERIOUS REACTIONS
• Parenteral overdose produces a cholinergic crisis manifested as abdominal discomfort or cramps, nausea, vomiting, diarrhea, flushing, facial warmth, excessive salivation, diaphoresis, urinary urgency, and blurred vision. Seizures and bradycardia may occur. If overdose occurs, stop all anticholinergic drugs and immediately administer 0.6-1.2 mg atropine sulfate IM or IV for adults or 0.01 mg/kg for infants and children younger than 12 yr.

PRECAUTIONS & CONSIDERATIONS
Caution is warranted in patients with bradycardia, bronchial asthma, epilepsy, GI disturbances, hypotension, parkinsonism, peptic ulcer disease,

and disorders that may be adversely affected by drug's vagotonic effects and in those who have recently had a myocardial infarction.Those with renal impairment may require reduced dosage. Use with caution during pregnancy and breastfeeding. The elderly may be more sensitive to the drug's effects.

Adverse effects usually subside after the first few days of therapy. Vital signs should be assessed immediately before and every 15-30 min after physostigmine administration. Cholinergic reactions, such as abdominal pain, dyspnea, hypotension, arrhythmias, muscle weakness, and diaphoresis, after drug administration should be assessed.

Storage

Store the injection at room temperature protected from light. Do not freeze.

Administration

For adults, administer at a rate not exceeding 1 mg/min. For children, administer at a rate not exceeding 0.5 mg/min.

During IM and especially IV administration, frequently monitor pulse, respiratory rate, blood pressure, and neurologic status.

Phytonadione

(vitamin K_1)

fye-toe-na-dye'own

★ Mephyton

CATEGORY AND SCHEDULE

Pregnancy Risk Category: C

Drug Class: Vitamins, fat soluble

MECHANISM OF ACTION

Needed for adequate blood clotting (factors II, VII, IX, X). *Therapeutic Effect:* Essential vitamin; reverses coagulopathy or coumarin toxicity.

PHARMACOKINETICS

PO/Injection: Readily absorbed from duodenum and requires bile salts, rapid hepatic metabolism, onset of action 6-12 h, normal PT in 12-24 h, crosses placenta, renal and biliary excretion; because of severe side effects, restrict IV route when other administration routes are not available.

AVAILABILITY

Tablets: 5 mg.

Injection: 1 mg/0.5 mL (neonatal), 10 mg/mL.

INDICATIONS AND DOSAGES

▸ **Hypoprothrombinemia caused by vitamin K malabsorption**

PO/IM

Adults. 2-25 mg; may repeat or increase to 50 mg.

Children, Infants. 2.5-5 mg as a single dose.

▸ **Prevention of hemorrhagic disease of the newborn**

SC/IM

Neonates. 0.5-1 mg after birth; repeat in 6-8 h if required.

▸ **Hypoprothrombinemia caused by oral anticoagulants**

PO/SC/IM

Adults. 2.5-10 mg; may repeat 12-48 h after PO dose or 6-8 h after subcutaneous/IM dose, based on PT.

NOTE: PO administration is preferred over parenteral use for a supratherapeutic INR when no significant bleeding is present (see warfarin monograph).

SIDE EFFECTS/ADVERSE REACTIONS

Occasional

Taste alterations, headache, cardiac irregularities (tachycardia), nausea, vomiting, hemoglobinuria, rash, urticaria, flushing, erythema, sweating, bronchospasms, dyspnea, cramp-like pain.

Rare
Hyperbilirubinemia.

CONTRAINDICATIONS

Hypersensitivity.

INTERACTIONS

Drug
Broad-spectrum antibiotics: Decreased action.
Mineral oil, orlistat, bile-acid sequestrants: Reduce oral absorption of vitamin K; separate administration times.
Warfarin and coumarin anticoagulants: Antagonist to coumarin anticoagulants.
Herbal
None known.
Food
Olestra: Those consuming regular olestra spreads may reduce vitamin K absorption.

SERIOUS REACTIONS

- Severe hypersensitivity reactions.

PRECAUTIONS & CONSIDERATIONS

Patients on chronic drug therapy may rarely have symptoms of blood dyscrasias, which can include infection, bleeding, and poor healing.
Storage
Protect tablets from light. Store all products at room temperature. Protect injection from light and freezing.
Administration
May give orally without regard to food. Do not administer orally at same time as orlistat.

Avoid IM administration in patients with coagulopathy. In neonates receiving prophylaxis at birth, the IM route is usually preferred. SC administration may result in erratic and delayed absorption. Dilute IV with normal saline or preservative-free D5W immediately before use if ordered doses exceed 1-2 mg. Protect from light. Infuse at a rate not to exceed 1 mg/min.

Pilocarpine Hydrochloride

pye-loe-kar′peen high-dro-clor′ide
🇺🇸 Isopto-Carpine, Pilopine-HS, Salagen 🇨🇦 Akarpine, Diocarpine

CATEGORY AND SCHEDULE

Pregnancy Risk Category: C

Classification: Cholinergic agonist

MECHANISM OF ACTION

A cholinergic that increases exocrine gland secretions by stimulating cholinergic receptors. *Therapeutic Effect:* Improves symptoms of dry mouth in patients with salivary gland hypofunction.

PHARMACOKINETICS

Route	Onset	Peak	Duration
PO	20 min	1 h	3-5 h

Absorption decreased if taken with a high-fat meal. Inactivation of pilocarpine thought to occur at neuronal synapses and probably in plasma. Excreted in urine. *Half-life:* 4-12 h.

AVAILABILITY

Tablets: 5 mg, 7.5 mg.
Ophthalmic Solution: 1%, 2%, 4%.
Ophthalmic Gel (Pilopine-HS): 4%.

INDICATIONS AND DOSAGES

▸ **Dry mouth associated with radiation treatment for head and neck cancer**
PO

Adults, Elderly. 5 mg 3 times a day. Range: 15-30 mg/day. Maximum: 2 tablets/dose.

▸ **Dry mouth associated with Sjögren syndrome**

PO

Adults, Elderly. 5 mg 4 times a day. Range: 10-30 mg/day.

▸ **Dosage in hepatic impairment**

Adults, Elderly. Dosage decreased to 5 mg twice a day for adults and elderly with hepatic impairment.

▸ **For glaucoma or ocular hypertension**

OPHTHALMIC SOLUTION

Adults and Children 2 yr and older. 1 drop into affected eye(s) up to 4 times per day. Start with lowest concentration of gtts.

Children and Infants < 2 yr. 1 drop of 1% solution into affected eye(s) 3 times per day.

OPHTHALMIC GEL

Adults. Apply a $\frac{1}{2}$-inch ribbon to lower conjunctival sac of the affected eye(s) once daily at bedtime.

▸ **For miosis induction**

OPHTHALMIC SOLUTION

Adults. Instill 1 drop (or 2 drops 5 min apart) of 1%, 2%, or 4% ophthalmic solution into the eye(s).

Infants, Children. Instill 1 drop of 1% or 2% ophthalmic solution into the eye(s) 15-60 min prior to surgery.

CONTRAINDICATIONS

Known hypersensitivity to pilocarpine; conditions in which miosis is undesirable, such as acute iritis and angle-closure glaucoma; uncontrolled asthma.

INTERACTIONS

Drug

Anticholinergics: May antagonize the effects of anticholinergics.

β-Blockers: May produce conduction disturbances.

Herbal

None known.

Food

High-fat meals: May decrease the absorption rate of pilocarpine.

DIAGNOSTIC TEST EFFECTS

None known.

SIDE EFFECTS

Frequent (29%)

Diaphoresis.

Occasional (5%-11%)

Headache, dizziness, urinary frequency, flushing, dyspepsia, nausea, asthenia, lacrimation, visual disturbances.

Rare (< 4%)

Diarrhea, abdominal pain, peripheral edema, chills.

SERIOUS REACTIONS

- Patients with diaphoresis who do not drink enough fluids may develop dehydration.

PRECAUTIONS & CONSIDERATIONS

Caution is warranted with hepatic impairment, pulmonary disease, and significant cardiovascular disease. Use with caution in pregnancy and lactation. The safety and efficacy of oral pilocarpine have not been established in children. Elderly patients have an increased incidence of diarrhea, dizziness, and urinary frequency. Adequate hydration should be maintained. Avoid tasks that require mental alertness or motor skills until response to the drug has been established.

Visual changes may occur, especially at night. Caution when driving at night or when performing hazardous activities in reduced lighting due to visual blurring. Pattern of daily bowel activity and stool consistency and urinary frequency should be assessed.

Storage

Store at room temperature; protect from excessive heat.

Administration

Take pilocarpine without regard to food. To avoid contamination, do not to touch the tip of the dropper or tube to any surface. Gently pull down lower eyelid to form a pouch in which to instill drops or ointment. Gently close eye(s). Compress lacrimal duct gently to limit systemic absorption. Blot excess away with clean tissue. If administering with other ophthalmic agents, allow at least 5 min between administration times.

Pimecrolimus

pim-e-kroe'li-mus

★ 🍁 Elidel

CATEGORY AND SCHEDULE

Pregnancy Risk Category: C

Classification: Dermatologics, immunosuppressives, topical anti-inflammatory

MECHANISM OF ACTION

An immunomodulator that inhibits release of cytokine, an enzyme that produces an inflammatory reaction. *Therapeutic Effect:* Produces anti-inflammatory activity.

PHARMACOKINETICS

Minimal systemic absorption with topical application. Metabolized in liver. Excreted in feces.

AVAILABILITY

Cream: 1% (Elidel).

INDICATIONS AND DOSAGES

▸ **Atopic dermatitis (eczema)**

TOPICAL

Adults, Elderly, Children 2-17 yr. Apply to affected area twice daily. Rub in gently and completely. Use as long as symptoms persist; discontinue if disease resolves. If persists > 6 wks, re-evaluate.

CONTRAINDICATIONS

Hypersensitivity to pimecrolimus or any component of the formulation, Netherton syndrome (potential for increased systemic absorption), application to active cutaneous viral infections.

INTERACTIONS

Drug

None known.

Herbal

None known.

Food

None known.

DIAGNOSTIC TEST EFFECTS

None known.

SIDE EFFECTS

Rare

Transient application-site sensation of burning or feeling of heat.

SERIOUS REACTIONS

- Lymphadenopathy and phototoxicity occur rarely.

PRECAUTIONS & CONSIDERATIONS

Only prescribed to those for whom other treatments have failed due to a possible risk of neoplastic disease (cancer), especially nonmelanoma skin cancer or lymphoma. Patients who have a new or changed skin lesion or lymphadenopathy should receive thorough examination. Caution should be used in immunocompromised patients and in those who are at an increased risk of varicella zoster virus infection, herpes simplex virus infection, or eczema herpeticum. Be aware that clinical infection at treatment sites should be cleared before commencing treatment. Consider discontinuing therapy if lymphadenopathy, or acute infections or if mononucleosis develops. It is unknown whether pimecrolimus is distributed in breast milk. Safety and efficacy of pimecrolimus have not been established in children younger than 2 yr of age. No age-related precautions have been noted in elderly patients.

Artificial sunlight or tanning beds should be avoided.

Storage

Store at room temperature. Do not freeze.

Administration

Gently cleanse area before application. Use occlusive dressings only as ordered. Apply sparingly and rub into area thoroughly. Do not use topical pimecrolimus on broken skin or in areas of infection, and do not apply to the face, inguinal areas, or wet skin.

P

Pimozide

pi'moe-zide

Orap

CATEGORY AND SCHEDULE

Pregnancy Risk Category: C

Classification: Antipsychotics

MECHANISM OF ACTION

A diphenylbutylpiperidine that blocks dopamine at postsynaptic receptor sites in the brain. *Therapeutic Effect:* Suppresses motor and phonic tics in those with Tourette syndrome.

PHARMACOKINETICS

PO: Onset erratic, peak 6-8 h. *Half-life:* 50-55 h. Metabolized in the liver, excreted in the urine, feces.

AVAILABILITY

Tablets: 1 mg, 2 mg (Orap).

INDICATIONS AND DOSAGES

▸ Tourette disorder

PO

Suppression of tics requires a slow and gradual introduction of the drug, balanced against the side effects.

Adults, Elderly. 1-2 mg/day in a single dose or divided doses 3 times/day. Maximum: 10 mg/day.

Children older than 12 yr. Initially, 0.05 mg/kg/day. Maximum: 10 mg/day.

OFF-LABEL USE

Delusions of parasitosis; refractory schizophrenia.

CONTRAINDICATIONS

Hypersensitivity. Other contraindications: patients taking drugs that may cause motor and phonic tics (e.g., pemoline, methylphenidate, and amphetamines). Congenital long QT syndrome, history of cardiac arrhythmias, patients taking other drugs that prolong the QT interval or reduce pimozide metabolism (see contraindicated drug list), untreated hypokalemia or hypomagnesemia, severe CNS depression, or coma. Drugs that are contraindicated due to effect on QT or drug metabolism: Mesoridazine, thioridazine, class IA or III antiarrhythmics, macrolide antibiotics (e.g., clarithromycin, erythromycin, azithromycin), SSRIs (e.g., citalopram, escitalopram, sertraline, fluvoxamine), systemic azole antifungals (e.g., itraconazole, ketoconazole), protease inhibitors (e.g., ritonavir, saquinovir, indinavir, and nelfinavir), nefazodone, zileuton. Any drug that potently inhibits CYP3A4 or prolongs the QT interval should be avoided.

INTERACTIONS

Drug

Alcohol, CNS depressants: May increase CNS and respiratory depression.
Aprepitant: May increase pimozide plasma concentrations.
Class IA and III antiarrhythmics: May increase risk for QT prolongation and cardiotoxicity.
Drugs that prolong QT interval: May increase risk for QT prolongation and cardiotoxicity.
Belladonna alkaloids: May increase anticholinergic effects.
Lithium: May increase extrapyramidal symptoms.
Phenylalanine: May increase incidence of tardive dyskinesia.
Sertraline: May increase plasma pimozide levels.
Tramadol: May increase risk of seizures.
Vitex: May decrease effectiveness of dopamine antagonists.

Herbal

Betel nut: May increase extrapyramidal side effects of pimozide.
Kava kava: May increase dopamine antagonist effects.

Food

Grapefruit juice: May inhibit metabolism of pimozide. Avoid.

DIAGNOSTIC TEST EFFECTS

None known.

SIDE EFFECTS

Occasional

Akathisia, dystonic extrapyramidal effects, parkinsonian extrapyramidal effects, tardive dyskinesia, blurred vision, ocular changes, constipation, decreased sweating, dry mouth, nasal congestion, dizziness, drowsiness, orthostatic hypotension, urinary retention, somnolence.

Rare

Rash, cholestatic jaundice, priapism.

SERIOUS REACTIONS

- Serious reactions such as blood dyscrasias, agranulocytosis, leukocytopenia, thrombocytopenia, cholestatic jaundice, neuroleptic malignant syndrome (NMS), constipation or paralytic ileus, priapism, QT prolongation and torsades de pointes, seizure, systemic lupus erythematosus-like syndrome, and temperature-regulation dysfunction (heatstroke or hypothermia) occur rarely.
- Abrupt withdrawal following long-term therapy may precipitate nausea, vomiting, gastritis, dizziness, and tremors.

PRECAUTIONS & CONSIDERATIONS

! Because of the significant risk for side effects, do not use for simple tics or tics other than those associated with Tourette disorder.

Caution is necessary with history of neuroleptic malignant syndrome, tardive dyskinesia, and impaired liver or kidney function. Caution is warranted with concomitant administration with inhibitors of cytochrome P450 1A2 and 3A4 enzymes as well as CNS depressants and fluoxetine. Safety and effectiveness have not been established in children under the age of 12 yr. Elderly and debilitated patients may require a lower initial dose.

History of drug-induced leukopenia/neutropenia is a risk factor for side effects. Monitor CBC frequently. Monitor for fever or other symptoms or signs of infection or neutropenia; treat promptly if such symptoms or signs occur. If absolute neutrophil count < 1000/mm^3, discontinue the drug until full recovery. Signs of tardive dyskinesia or akathisia should be immediately reported.

Storage

Store at room temperature.

Administration

May give without regard to food, but do not administer with grapefruit juice. Administration as a single dose at bedtime once titrated may improve tolerance.

Pindolol

pin'doe-loll

Visken

CATEGORY AND SCHEDULE

Pregnancy Risk Category: B (D if used in second or third trimester)

Classification:

Antihypertensives, nonselective β-adrenergic antagonist

MECHANISM OF ACTION

A nonselective β-blocker that blocks β_1- and β_2-adrenergic receptors. The partial agonist activity is greater for β_2- than β_1-receptors, making the drug a "vasodilatory" β-blocker, with intrinsic sympathomimetic actions. *Therapeutic Effect:* Slows heart rate, decreases cardiac output, decreases BP, and exhibits antiarrhythmic activity. Decreases myocardial ischemia severity by decreasing oxygen requirements.

PHARMACOKINETICS

Completely absorbed from GI tract. Metabolized in liver. Primarily excreted in urine. *Half-life:* 3-4 h (half-life increased with impaired renal function, elderly).

AVAILABILITY

Tablets: 5 mg, 10 mg.

INDICATIONS AND DOSAGES

▸ **Mild to moderate hypertension**

PO

Adults. Initially, 5 mg 2 times/day. Gradually increase dose by 10 mg/day at intervals of 2-4 wks. Maintenance: 10-30 mg/day in 2-3 divided doses. Maximum: 60 mg/day.

Elderly. Usual elderly dosage: Initially, 5 mg/day. May increase by 5 mg q3-4wk.

OFF-LABEL USES

Treatment of chronic angina pectoris.

CONTRAINDICATIONS

Hypersensitivity, bronchial asthma; overt cardiac failure; cardiogenic shock; second- and third-degree AV block; severe bradycardia.

INTERACTIONS

Drug

Anticholinergics, hydrocarbon inhalation anesthetics, fentanyl derivatives: May increase risk of hypotension.

Diuretics, other hypotensives: May increase hypotensive effect of pindolol.

Epinephrine, ephedrine: May cause hypertension or bradycardia.

Fluoxetine and other SSRI antidepressants: May increase antidepressant effect.

Indomethacin: May decrease antihypertensive effects.

Insulin and oral hypoglycemics: May mask symptoms of hypoglycemia and/or prolong hypoglycemic effect.
Lidocaine: May slow metabolism of drug.
Sympathomimetics, phenothiazines, xanthines: May mutually inhibit effects of pindolol.
Theophylline: May decrease bronchodilation effects.
Herbal
None known.
Food
None known.

DIAGNOSTIC TEST EFFECTS
May increase ANA titer, SGOT (AST), SGPT (ALT), alkaline phosphatase, LDH, bilirubin, BUN, creatinine, potassium, uric acid, lipoproteins, and triglycerides.

SIDE EFFECTS
Frequent
Decreased sexual ability, drowsiness, trouble sleeping, unusual tiredness or weakness.
Occasional
Bradycardia, depression, cold hands or feet, diarrhea, constipation, anxiety, nasal congestion, nausea, vomiting.
Rare
Altered taste; dry eyes; itching; numbness of fingers, toes, and scalp

SERIOUS REACTIONS
- Overdosage may produce profound bradycardia and hypotension.
- Abrupt withdrawal may result in sweating, palpitations, headache, and tremulousness.
- May precipitate CHF or myocardial infarction (MI) in patients with heart disease; thyroid storm in those with thyrotoxicosis; or peripheral ischemia in those with existing peripheral vascular disease.
- Hypoglycemia may occur in previously controlled diabetics.
- Signs of thrombocytopenia, such as unusual bleeding or bruising, occur rarely.

PRECAUTIONS & CONSIDERATIONS
Caution is warranted with bronchospastic disease, diabetes, hyperthyroidism, impaired renal or liver function, inadequate cardiac function, or peripheral vascular disease. Pindolol readily crosses the placenta and is distributed in breast milk. During delivery, pindolol may produce apnea, bradycardia, hypoglycemia, and hypothermia as well as low-birth-weight infants. Safety and efficacy have not been established in children. Caution should be used in elderly patients who may have age-related peripheral vascular disease. Nasal decongestants or over-the-counter (OTC) cold preparations (stimulants) should be avoided without physician approval. Excess salt and alcohol consumption should be limited.

Excessive fatigue, headache, prolonged dizziness, shortness of breath, or weight gain should be reported.
Storage
Store at room temperature, tightly closed and protected from light.
Administration
May be given with or without regard to meals. Tablets may be crushed. Do not abruptly discontinue the drug.

Pioglitazone
pye-oh-gli′ta-zone
★ 🍁 Actos

CATEGORY AND SCHEDULE
Pregnancy Risk Category: C

Classification: Antidiabetic agents, thiazolidinedione

MECHANISM OF ACTION

An antidiabetic that improves target-cell response to insulin without increasing pancreatic insulin secretion. Decreases hepatic glucose output and increases insulin-dependent glucose utilization in skeletal muscle. *Therapeutic Effect:* Lowers blood glucose concentration.

PHARMACOKINETICS

Rapidly absorbed. Highly protein bound (99%), primarily to albumin. Metabolized in the liver. Excreted in urine. Unknown whether removed by hemodialysis. *Half-life:* 16-24 h.

AVAILABILITY

Tablets: 15 mg, 30 mg, 45 mg.

INDICATIONS AND DOSAGES

▸ **Diabetes mellitus type 2, as monotherapy or in combination with other drugs**

PO

Adults, Elderly. With insulin: Initially, 15-30 mg once a day. Initially continue current insulin dosage; then decrease insulin dosage by 10%-25% if hypoglycemia occurs or plasma glucose level decreases to < 100 mg/dL. Maximum: 45 mg/day. *As monotherapy:* Monotherapy is not to be used if patient is well controlled with diet and exercise alone. Initially, 15-30 mg/day. May increase dosage in increments until 45 mg/day is reached. *With sulfonylureas:* Initially, 15-30 mg/day. Decrease sulfonylurea dosage if hypoglycemia occurs. *With metformin:* Initially, 15-30 mg/day.

CONTRAINDICATIONS

Active hepatic disease; diabetic ketoacidosis; increased serum transaminase levels, including ALT (SGPT) > 2.5 times normal serum level; type 1 diabetes mellitus; known NYHA class III or IV heart failure, hypersensitivity.

INTERACTIONS

Drug

Gemfibrozil: May increase the effect and toxicity of pioglitazone.
Ketoconazole: May significantly inhibit metabolism of pioglitazone.
Oral contraceptives: May alter the effects of oral contraceptives.
Rifampin: May decrease the effectiveness of pioglitazone.

Food

None known.

Herbal

None known.

DIAGNOSTIC TEST EFFECTS

May increase creatine kinase (CK) level. May decrease hemoglobin levels by 2%-4% and serum alkaline phosphatase, bilirubin, and transaminase ALT (SGOT) levels to 2.5 times normal serum levels. Fewer than 1% of patients experience ALT values 3 times the normal level.

SIDE EFFECTS

Frequent (9%-13%)

Headache, upper respiratory tract infection.

Occasional (5%-6%)

Sinusitis, myalgia, pharyngitis, aggravated diabetes mellitus.

SERIOUS REACTIONS

- Possible increased risk of myocardial ischemic events such as angina or MI; rosiglitazone more likely to cause.
- New onset or exacerbation of congestive heart failure.
- Macular edema (rare).
- Hepatic impairment and jaundice (rare).

PRECAUTIONS & CONSIDERATIONS

May cause or exacerbate heart failure in some patients. Patients should be monitored for signs and symptoms of heart failure, including excessive, rapid weight gain, dyspnea, or edema. Pioglitazone should not be used in patients with symptomatic heart failure or New York Heart Association (NYHA) class III or IV heart failure.

Caution is warranted with edema and hepatic impairment. It is unknown whether pioglitazone crosses the placenta or is distributed in breast milk. Pioglitazone use is not recommended in pregnant or breastfeeding women. Be aware that improvements in diabetic control may convert some anovulatory women to more regular ovulation; adequate contraception is advised. Safety and efficacy of pioglitazone have not been established in children. No age-related precautions have been noted in elderly patients. Avoid alcohol.

Food intake, blood glucose, and hemoglobin levels should be monitored before and during therapy. Hepatic enzyme levels should also be obtained before beginning pioglitazone therapy and periodically thereafter. Notify the physician of abdominal or chest pain, dark urine or light stool, hypoglycemic reactions, fever, nausea, palpitations, rash, vomiting, or yellowing of the eyes or skin. Be aware of signs and symptoms of hypoglycemia (anxiety, cool wet skin, diplopia, dizziness, headache, hunger, numbness in mouth, tachycardia, tremors) or hyperglycemia (deep rapid breathing, dim vision, fatigue, nausea, polydipsia, polyphagia, polyuria, vomiting); carry candy, sugar packets, or other sugar supplements for immediate response to hypoglycemia. Consult the physician when glucose demands are altered (such as with fever, heavy physical activity, infection, stress, trauma). Exercise, good personal hygiene (including foot care), not smoking, and weight control are essential parts of therapy.

Storage

Store tablets at room temperature.

Administration

Take pioglitazone without regard to meals.

Piperacillin/ Tazobactam

pi′per-a-sil-in/tay-zoe-bak′tam

★ Zosyn 🍁 Tazocin

Do not confuse Zosyn with Zofran or Zyvox.

CATEGORY AND SCHEDULE

Pregnancy Risk Category: B

Classification: Antibiotics, extended-spectrum penicillin and β-lactamase inhibitor

MECHANISM OF ACTION

Piperacillin inhibits cell wall synthesis by binding to bacterial cell membranes. Tazobactam inactivates bacterial β-lactamase. Active against gram-negative and anaerobic organisms, including *Pseudomonas* spp., as well as methicillin-sensitive gram positives. *Therapeutic Effect:* Bactericidal in susceptible organisms.

PHARMACOKINETICS

Protein binding: 16%-30%. Widely distributed. Primarily excreted unchanged in urine. Removed by hemodialysis. *Half-life:* 0.7-1.5 h (increased in hepatic cirrhosis and impaired renal function).

AVAILABILITY

! Piperacillin/tazobactam is a combination product in a ratio of piperacillin to tazobactam.

Powder for Injection: 2.25 g, 3.375 g, 4.5 g.

Premix IVPB Infusion: 2.25 g/50 mL, 3.375 g/50 mL, 4.5 g/100 mL.

INDICATIONS AND DOSAGES

▸ **Severe infections**

IV

Adults, Elderly, Children > 40 kg. 4.5 g q6-8h or 3.375 g q6h.

▸ **Moderate infections**

IV

Adults, Elderly, Children > 40 kg. 2.25 g q6-8h or 3.375 g q6h.

▸ **Dosage in renal impairment**

Dosage and frequency are modified based on creatinine clearance.

Creatinine Clearance (mL/min)	Dosage
20-40	3.375 g q6h for nosocomial pneumonia, 2.25 g IV q6h for all other indications.
< 20	2.25 g q8h for all indications except nosocomial pneumonia (2.25 g q6h)

▸ **Dosage in hemodialysis patients**

IV

Adults, Elderly. 2.25 g q8h with additional dose of 0.75 g after each dialysis session.

CONTRAINDICATIONS

Hypersensitivity to any penicillin or β-lactamase inhibitor.

INTERACTIONS

Drug

Hepatotoxic medications: May increase the risk of hepatotoxicity.

Probenecid: May increase piperacillin blood concentration and risk of toxicity.

Herbal

None known.

Food

None known.

DIAGNOSTIC TEST EFFECTS

May increase serum sodium, alkaline phosphatase, bilirubin, LDH, AST (SGOT), and ALT (SGPT) levels. May decrease serum potassium level. May cause a positive Coombs' test.

IV INCOMPATIBILITIES

Amiodarone, amphotericin B (Fungizone), amphocetiricin B complex (Abelcet, AmBisome, Amphotec), azithromycin (Zithromax), caspofungin (Cancidas), chlorpromazine (Thorazine), ciprofloxacin (Cipro), cisplatin, dacarbazine (DTIC), daunorubicin (Cerubidine), diltiazem, dobutamine (Dobutrex), doxorubicin (Adriamycin), doxorubicin liposomal (Doxil), droperidol (Inapsine), drotrecogin alfa, (Xigris), famotidine (Pepcid), haloperidol (Haldol), hydroxyzine (Vistaril), idarubicin (Idamycin), insulin regular, levofloxacin (Levaquin), midazolam (Versed), minocycline (Minocin), nalbuphine (Nubain), phenytoin, prochlorperazine (Compazine), promethazine (Phenergan), rocuronium, tobramycin, vancomycin (Vancocin).

IV COMPATIBILITIES

Aminophylline, bumetanide (Bumex), calcium gluconate, diphenhydramine (Benadryl), dopamine (Intropin), enalapril (Vasotec), furosemide (Lasix), granisetron (Kytril), heparin, hydrocortisone (Solu-Cortef), hydromorphone (Dilaudid), lorazepam (Ativan), magnesium sulfate, methylprednisolone (Solu-Medrol), metoclopramide (Reglan), morphine, ondansetron (Zofran), potassium chloride.

SIDE EFFECTS

Frequent

Diarrhea, headache, constipation, nausea, insomnia, rash.

Occasional

Vomiting, dyspepsia, pruritus, fever, agitation, candidiasis, dizziness, abdominal pain, edema, anxiety, dyspnea, rhinitis.

SERIOUS REACTIONS

- Antibiotic-associated colitis and other superinfections may result from altered bacterial balance.
- Seizures and other neurologic reactions are more likely to occur in patients with renal impairment and in those who have received an overdose.
- Severe hypersensitivity reactions, including anaphylaxis, occur rarely.

PRECAUTIONS & CONSIDERATIONS

Caution is warranted in patients with a history of allergies, especially to penicillin and cephalosporins, a preexisting seizure disorder, or renal impairment. Piperacillin readily crosses the placenta, appears in cord blood and amniotic fluid, and is distributed in breast milk in low concentrations. Piperacillin may lead to allergic sensitization, candidiasis, diarrhea, and skin rash in infants. The safety and efficacy of piperacillin have not been established in children younger than 12 yr. Age-related renal impairment may require dosage adjustment in elderly patients.

History of allergies, especially to cephalosporins or penicillins, should be determined before giving the drug. Withhold and promptly notify the physician if rash or diarrhea occurs. Severe diarrhea with abdominal pain, blood or mucus in stool, and fever may indicate antibiotic-associated colitis. Signs and symptoms of superinfection, including anal or genital pruritus, black hairy tongue, diarrhea, increased fever, sore throat, ulceration or changes of oral mucosa, and vomiting, should be monitored. Electrolytes (especially potassium), intake and output, renal function tests, urinalysis, and the injection sites should be assessed.

Storage

Store vials at room temperature before opening.

The reconstituted vial is stable for 24 h at room temperature and 48 h if refrigerated. Premix IVPBs arrive frozen; once thawed, they are stable for 24 h at room temperature or up to 14 days refrigerated.

Administration

For each gram of Zosyn, reconstitute with 5 mL D5W or 0.9% NaCl. Shake vigorously to dissolve. Further dilute with at least 50-100 mL D5W, 0.9% NaCl, dextrose 5% in 0.9% NaCl, or lactated Ringer's solution. Infuse the drug IV over 30 min.

P

Piroxicam

peer-ox'i-kam

★ Feldene 🍁 Nu-Pirox

Do not confuse Feldene with Seldane.

CATEGORY AND SCHEDULE

Pregnancy Risk Category: C (D if used in third trimester or near delivery)

Classification: Analgesics, nonsteroidal anti-inflammatory drug (NSAID)

MECHANISM OF ACTION

An NSAID that produces analgesic, antipyretic and anti-inflammatory effects by inhibiting the cyclo oxygenase pathway in prostaglandin synthesis. *Therapeutic Effect:* Reduces inflammatory response and intensity of pain.

PHARMACOKINETICS

Well absorbed orally. Protein binding: 99%. Metabolized in the liver; metabolites excreted in urine. *Half-life:* 3-3.5 h (increased in renal impairment).

AVAILABILITY

Capsules: 10 mg, 20 mg.

INDICATIONS AND DOSAGES

▸ **Acute or chronic rheumatoid arthritis and osteoarthritis**

PO

Adults, Elderly. Initially, 10-20 mg/day as a single dose or in divided doses. Some patients may require up to 30-40 mg/day.

P

OFF-LABEL USES

Treatment of acute gouty arthritis, ankylosing spondylitis.

CONTRAINDICATIONS

Active peptic ulcer disease, chronic inflammation of the GI tract, GI bleeding or ulceration, history of hypersensitivity to aspirin or NSAIDs, myocardial infarction, coronary artery bypass graft surgery.

INTERACTIONS

Drug

Antihypertensives, diuretics: May decrease the effects of antihypertensives and diuretics.
Aspirin, salicylates, corticosteroids: May increase the risk of GI bleeding and side effects. NSAIDs may negate the cardioprotective effect of ASA.
Cyclosporine: May increase risk of nephrotoxicity.
Heparin, oral anticoagulants, thrombolytics: May increase the effects of heparin, oral anticoagulants, and thrombolytics.
Lithium: May increase the blood concentration and risk of toxicity of lithium.
Methotrexate: May increase the risk of toxicity with methotrexate.

Herbal

Feverfew: May increase the risk of bleeding.
Ginkgo biloba: May increase the risk of bleeding.

Food

Alcohol: May increase risk of dizziness, GI bleeding.

DIAGNOSTIC TEST EFFECTS

May increase AST (SGOT) and ALT (SGPT) levels. May decrease serum uric acid levels.

SIDE EFFECTS

Frequent (4%-9%)
Dyspepsia, nausea, dizziness.
Occasional (1%-3%)
Diarrhea, constipation, abdominal cramps or pain, flatulence, stomatitis.
Rare (< 1%)
Hypertension, urticaria, dysuria, ecchymosis, blurred vision, insomnia, phototoxicity.

SERIOUS REACTIONS

• Rare reactions with long-term use include peptic ulcer disease, GI bleeding, gastritis, severe hepatic reaction (cholestasis, jaundice), nephrotoxicity (dysuria, hematuria, proteinuria, nephrotic syndrome), hematologic sensitivity (anemia, leukopenia, eosinophilia, thrombocytopenia), and a severe hypersensitivity reaction (fever, chills, bronchospasm).

PRECAUTIONS & CONSIDERATIONS

Cardiovascular event risk may be increased with duration of use or preexisting cardiovascular risk factors or disease. Use caution in patients with fluid retention, heart failure, or hypertension. Risk of myocardial infarction and stroke may be increased following CABG surgery. Do not administer within 4-6 half-lives before surgical procedures. Caution is warranted with GI disease, impaired hepatic function, and concurrent anticoagulant use. Notify the physician of pregnancy. Use with caution during lactation. This medicine is not approved for use in children. The elderly may be more susceptible to GI and CNS side effects. Tasks that require mental alertness or motor skills should also be avoided until drug effects are known.

CBC, hepatic and renal function test results, and pattern of daily bowel activity and stool consistency should be assessed before and during therapy. Therapeutic response, such as decreased pain, stiffness, swelling, and tenderness; improved grip strength; and increased joint mobility, should be evaluated.

Storage

Store at controlled room temperature; protect from moisture.

Administration

Do not crush or break capsules. Take piroxicam with food, milk, or antacids if GI distress occurs.

Pitavastatin

pit′a-vah′stat-in

★ Livalo

CATEGORY AND SCHEDULE

Pregnancy Risk Category: X

Classification:

Antihyperlipidemics, HMG-CoA reductase inhibitors

MECHANISM OF ACTION

An antihyperlipidemic "statin" that interferes with cholesterol biosynthesis by inhibiting the conversion of the enzyme HMG-CoA to mevalonate, a precursor to cholesterol. *Therapeutic Effect:* Decreases LDL cholesterol, VLDL, and plasma triglyceride levels, increases HDL concentration.

PHARMACOKINETICS

Well absorbed, even in presence of food. Protein binding: 99% protein bound in human plasma, mainly to albumin and α-1-acid glycoprotein. The principal route of pitavastatin metabolism is glucuronidation via liver UGTs with subsequent formation of pitavastatin lactone. There is only minimal metabolism by CYP2C9 and 2C8. Primarily eliminated in the feces; about 15% eliminated via the urine. *Half-life:* 12 h (increased in patients with severe renal dysfunction).

AVAILABILITY

Tablets: 1 mg, 2 mg, 4 mg.

INDICATIONS AND DOSAGES

▸ **Hyperlipidemia, dyslipidemia**

PO

Adults, Elderly. Initially 1-2 mg/day. With 1-mg adjustments based on lipid levels at intervals of 4 wks until desired level is achieved. Maximum: 4 mg/day.

▸ **Renal impairment (creatinine clearance < 30 mL/min)**

PO

Adults, Elderly. Patients with CrCl 30-59 mL/min and those with end-stage renal disease receiving hemodialysis should receive a starting dose of 1 mg once daily and a maximum dose of 2 mg/day. Do not use in those with severe renal impairment (CrCl < 30 mL/min) not yet on hemodialysis.

▸ **Concurrent erythromycin use**
PO
Adults, Elderly. Do not exceed 1 mg/day.
▸ **Concurrent rifampin use**
PO
Adults, Elderly. Do not exceed 2 mg/day.

CONTRAINDICATIONS

Hypersensitivity, active hepatic disease, breastfeeding, pregnancy, unexplained persistent elevations of serum transaminase levels; use with cyclosporine contraindicated; also do not use with protease inhibitors for HIV (not studied with these drugs) or in patients with CrCl < 30 mL/min not yet on hemodialysis.

INTERACTIONS

Drug
Cyclosporine or protease inhibitors: Increase the risk of myopathy. Do not give cyclosporine or protease inhibitors with pitavastatin.
Gemfibrozil, niacin: Increase the risk of myopathy. Use together with caution.
Erythromycin: Reduces pitavastatin clearance; reduce usual dose.
Rifampin: Increases pitavastatin exposure; reduce usual dose.
Warfarin: Enhances anticoagulant effect. Monitor INR.
Herbal
None known.
Food
Ethanol: Limit; may increase risk for hepatic effects.
Grapefruit juice: May increase exposure and increase risk for myopathy; manufacturer does not specifically recommend avoidance.

DIAGNOSTIC TEST EFFECTS

May increase serum creatinine kinase and liver transaminases.

SIDE EFFECTS

Generally well tolerated. Side effects are usually mild and transient.
Occasional (≥ 2%)
Myalgia, back pain, diarrhea, constipation, and pain in extremity.
Rare (< 2%)
Asthenia or unusual fatigue and weakness, headache, arthralgia, nasopharyngitis, urticaria, rash, pruritus.

SERIOUS REACTIONS

- Lens opacities may occur.
- Hypersensitivity reaction and hepatitis occur rarely.
- Myopathy and rhabdomyolysis (rare).

PRECAUTIONS & CONSIDERATIONS

Caution is warranted in patients with a history of hepatic disease, hypotension, severe acute infection; severe electrolyte, endocrine, metabolic imbalances or disorders; trauma; and uncontrolled seizures. Caution should also be used in those who consume a substantial amount of alcohol and those who have had recent major surgery. Pitavastatin use is contraindicated in pregnancy because the suppression of cholesterol biosynthesis may cause fetal toxicity. Also is contraindicated during lactation because it carries the risk of serious adverse reactions in breastfeeding infants. Safety and efficacy have not been established in children. No age-related precautions have been noted in elderly patients.

Notify the physician of headache, sore throat, muscle weakness and aches, severe gastric upset, or rash. Pattern of daily bowel activity and stool consistency should be assessed. Serum lipid cholesterol and triglyceride levels and hepatic function should be checked at baseline and periodically during treatment. At initiation of pitavastatin therapy, a standard cholesterol-lowering diet should be practiced and continued throughout therapy.

Storage

Store at room temperature and protect from light.

Administration

Take pitavastatin without regard to meals and at any time of day.

Podofilox

po-doe-fil′ox

★ Condyline, Condylox

CATEGORY AND SCHEDULE

Pregnancy Risk Category: C

Classification: Dermatologic, antimitotic agent

MECHANISM OF ACTION

An active component of podophyllin resin that binds to tubulin to prevent formation of microtubules, resulting in mitotic arrest. Many biological effects, such as it damages endothelium of small blood vessels, attenuates nucleoside transport, suppresses immune responses, inhibits macrophage metabolism, induces interleukin-1 and interleukin-2, decreases lymphocyte response to mitogens, and enhances macrophage growth. *Therapeutic Effect:* Removes genital warts.

PHARMACOKINETICS

Time to peak occurs in 1-2 h. Some degree of absorption. *Half-life:* 1-4.5 h.

AVAILABILITY

Gel: 0.5% (Condylox).
Solution: 0.5% (Condylox).

INDICATIONS AND DOSAGES

▸ **Anogenital warts**

TOPICAL

Adults. Apply 0.5% gel twice daily for 3 days, then withhold for 4 days. Repeat cycle up to 4 times.

▸ **Genital warts (condylomata acuminate)**

TOPICAL

Adults. Apply 0.5% solution or gel q12h in the morning and evening for 3 days, then withhold for 4 days. Repeat cycle up to 4 times.

OFF-LABEL USES

Common warts (nonbleeding) on the outside of skin.

CONTRAINDICATIONS

Hypersensitivity to podofilox or any component of its formulation.

INTERACTIONS

Drug

None known.

Herbal

None known.

Food

None known.

DIAGNOSTIC TEST EFFECTS

None known.

SIDE EFFECTS

Occasional

Erosion, inflammation, itching, pain, burning.

Rare

Nausea, vomiting.

SERIOUS REACTIONS

- Nausea and vomiting occur rarely and usually after cumulative doses.

PRECAUTIONS & CONSIDERATIONS

Caution is necessary with mucous membrane warts, bleeding warts, moles, birthmarks, or warts with hair; in patients with poor circulation or diabetes. Avoid use during prognancy; may be harmful to fetus. It is unknown whether podofilox is distributed in

P

breast milk. Safety and efficacy of podofilox have not been established in children or elderly. Nausea, vomiting, blood in urine, or dizziness should be reported immediately.

Genital warts are contagious. Make sure sexual partner has been examined. Condoms help protect spread. Patients should not engage in sexual activity during treatment.

Storage

Store at room temperature, tightly closed. Avoid excessive heat and do not freeze.

Administration

Apply on warts with supplied cotton-tip applicator. Allow to dry completely before putting legs together. Use no more than 10 cm^2/day and no more than 0.5 g/day of topical gel. Use no more than 10 cm^2/day and no more than 0.5 mL/day of topical solution. Remember that a treatment week cycle is twice a day for 3 days, then 4 days with no treatment. Can be used during menses.

P

Polycarbophil

polly-car'bow-fill

★ Fibercon, 🍁 Fiber-on-Tablet, Prodiem Bulk Fibre Therapy

CATEGORY AND SCHEDULE

Pregnancy Risk Category: C

Classification: OTC

MECHANISM OF ACTION

A bulk-forming laxative and antidiarrheal. As a laxative, retains water in the intestine and opposes dehydrating forces of the bowel. *Therapeutic Effect:* Promotes well-formed stools. As an antidiarrheal, absorbs fecal-free water, restores normal moisture level, and provides bulk. *Therapeutic Effect:* Forms gel and produces formed stool.

PHARMACOKINETICS

Route	Onset	Peak	Duration
PO	12-72 h	NA	NA

Acts in small and large intestines.

AVAILABILITY

Tablets: 500 mg, 625 mg.
Tablets (Chewable): 500 mg.

INDICATIONS AND DOSAGES

▸ **Constipation, diarrhea**

PO

Adults, Elderly, Children 12 yr and older. 1 g 1-4 times a day, or as needed. Maximum: 4 g/24 h.

Children aged 6-11 yr. 500 mg 1-4 times a day or as needed. Maximum: 2 g/24 h.

Children younger than 6 yr. Consult product labeling.

CONTRAINDICATIONS

Abdominal pain, dysphagia, nausea, partial bowel obstruction, symptoms of appendicitis, vomiting, hypercalcemia, hypercalciuria, esophageal stricture.

INTERACTIONS

Drug

Digoxin, oral anticoagulants, salicylates, tetracyclines: May decrease the effects of digoxin, salicylates, and tetracyclines.

Potassium-sparing diuretics, potassium supplements: May interfere with the effects of potassium-sparing diuretics and potassium supplements.

Herbal

None known.

Food

None known.

DIAGNOSTIC TEST EFFECTS

May increase blood glucose level.
May decrease serum potassium levels.

SIDE EFFECTS

Rare

Some degree of abdominal discomfort, nausea, mild cramps, griping, syncope or near syncope.

SERIOUS REACTIONS

• Esophageal or bowel obstruction may occur if administered with < 250 mL or 1 full glass of liquid.

PRECAUTIONS & CONSIDERATIONS

This drug may be used safely in pregnancy. Polycarbophil use is not recommended in children younger than 6 yr of age. No age-related precautions have been noted in elderly patients.

Pattern of daily bowel activity and stool consistency and serum electrolyte levels should be monitored. Adequate fluid intake should be maintained.

Administration

For severe diarrhea, give every half hour up to maximum daily dosage; for constipation, give with 8 oz liquid, as prescribed.

Drink 6-8 glasses of water a day to aid in stool softening. To promote defecation, increase fluid intake, exercise, and eat a high-fiber diet.

Polyethylene Glycol-Electrolyte Solution

pol-ee-eth′ill-een

★ GoLYTELY, MiraLax (OTC), Moviprep, NuLytely, TriLyte

🍁 Colyte, Klean-Prep

CATEGORY AND SCHEDULE

Pregnancy Risk Category: C

Classification: Laxatives, osmotic, stool softening, bowel evacuant

MECHANISM OF ACTION

A laxative that has an osmotic effect. *Therapeutic Effect:* Induces diarrhea and cleanses bowel without depleting electrolytes. OTC form for constipation acts as stool softener without inducing diarrhea.

PHARMACOKINETICS

Route	Onset	Peak	Duration
PO	1-2 h	NA	NA (bowel cleansing)
PO	2-4 days	NA	NA (constipation)

AVAILABILITY

Powder for Oral Solution.

Oral Solution.

INDICATIONS AND DOSAGES

▸ **Bowel cleansing**

PO

Adults, Elderly. Before GI examination: 240 mL (8 oz) q10min until 4 L consumed or rectal effluent clear. Nasogastric tube: 20-30 mL/min until 4 L given.

Children. 25 mL/kg/h until rectal effluent clear.

▸ **Constipation**

PO (MIRALAX)

Adults. 17 g or 1 heaping tbsp a day dissolved into water or juice.

CONTRAINDICATIONS

Bowel perforation, gastric retention, GI obstruction, megacolon, toxic colitis, toxic ileus.

INTERACTIONS

Drug

Oral medications: May decrease the absorption of oral medications if given within 1 h because they may be flushed from GI tract.

Herbal

None known.

Food

None known.

P

DIAGNOSTIC TEST EFFECTS

None known.

SIDE EFFECTS

Frequent (50%)
Some degree of abdominal fullness, nausea, bloating.
Occasional (1%-10%)
Abdominal cramping, vomiting, anal irritation.
Rare (< 1%)
Urticaria, rhinorrhea, dermatitis.

SERIOUS REACTIONS

- None known.

PRECAUTIONS & CONSIDERATIONS

Caution is warranted in patients with ulcerative colitis. It is unknown whether polyethylene glycol crosses the placenta or is distributed in breast milk. No age-related precautions have been noted in children or elderly patients.

Notify the physician if severe abdominal pain or bloating occurs. Blood glucose, BUN, serum electrolyte levels, urine osmolality, and pattern of daily bowel activity and stool consistency should be monitored.

Storage
Refrigerate reconstituted solutions; use within 48 h.

Administration
For bowel evacuant formulas: May use tap water to prepare solution. Shake vigorously for several minutes to ensure complete dissolution of powder. Take nothing by mouth 3 h or more before ingestion of solution. Give only clear liquids after administration. May give via nasogastric tube. Rapid drinking preferred. Chilled solution is more palatable.

For OTC formulas without electrolytes for constipation: Can be taken without regard to food. Mix dosage (17 g for adults) well in full glass (4-8 oz) of water, juice, soda, coffee, or tea prior to administration. Do not exceed recommended doses.

Polymyxin B

pol-i-mix′in B

★ Aerosporin

CATEGORY AND SCHEDULE

Pregnancy Risk Category: B

Classification: Antibiotics, polymyxins

MECHANISM OF ACTION

An antibiotic that alters cell membrane permeability in susceptible microorganisms. *Therapeutic Effect:* Bactericidal activity.

PHARMACOKINETICS

Most often administered topically; rarely administered IV. Does not penetrate into the CSF, synovial fluid, aqueous humor, or across the placenta. Minimal binding to plasma protein. Roughly 60% of a dose is excreted by the kidneys, but excretion is delayed with binding of the drug to phospholipids in kidney cells. Poor removal by hemodialysis. *Half-life:* 4-6 h (prolonged in renal impairment).

AVAILABILITY

Powder: 500,000 units (Aerosporin).

INDICATIONS AND DOSAGES

▸ **Mild to moderate infections**

IV

Adults, Elderly, Children 2 yr and older. 15,000-25,000 units/kg/day in divided doses q12hr.

Infants. 15,000-40,000 units/kg/day in divided doses q12h.

IM
Adults, Elderly, Children 2 yr and older. 25,000-30,000 units/kg/day in divided doses q4-6h.
Infants. 25,000-40,000 units/kg/day in divided doses q4-6h.

▸ **Usual irrigation dosage**
CONTINUOUS BLADDER IRRIGATION
Adults, Children > 2 yr of age. 200,000-400,000 units/day as a continuous bladder irrigation.

▸ **Usual ophthalmic dosage**
OPHTHALMIC
Adults, Elderly, Children. 1-3 drops containing 10,000-20,000 units/mL/hr until a favorable response occurs. Maximum: 25,000 units/kg/day or 2 million units/day.

IV INCOMPATIBILITIES
Cefoxitin, diazepam, cefoperazone, furosemide, heparin, hydrocortisone, regular insulin, oxacillin, pantoprazole, penicillin-class antibiotics.

CONTRAINDICATIONS
Hypersensitivity to polymyxin B or any component of the formulation, neuromuscular disease.

INTERACTIONS
Drug
Aminoglycosides, other nephrotoxic drugs: May increase nephrotoxicity.
Neuromuscular blocking agents or anesthetics: May produce muscle paralysis and prolonged or increased skeletal muscle relaxation. Watch for respiratory depression.
Herbal
None known.
Food
None known.

DIAGNOSTIC TEST EFFECTS
None known with topical use. With parenteral use, may increase serum creatinine and cause proteinuria.

Serum concentrations > 5 mcg/mL are toxic in adults.

SIDE EFFECTS
Frequent
Severe pain, irritation at IM injection sites, phlebitis, thrombophlebitis with IV administration.
Occasional
Fever, urticaria.

SERIOUS REACTIONS
- Nephrotoxicity, especially with concurrent/sequential use of other nephrotoxic drugs, renal impairment, concurrent/sequential use of muscle relaxants.
- Superinfection, especially with fungi, may occur.
- Neurotoxic reactions may be manifested by drowsiness, irritability, blurred vision, weakness, ataxia, and numbness of the extremities.
- Intrathecal administration may cause irritated meninges and meningitis-like symptoms.

PRECAUTIONS & CONSIDERATIONS
Caution should be used with impaired renal function. Safety and efficacy of polymyxin B have not been established in pregnant women or children younger than 2 yr. No age-related precautions have been noted in elderly patients.

Renal function should be carefully monitored. Neurotoxic reactions may be manifested by drowsiness, irritability, blurred vision, weakness, ataxia, and numbness of the extremities.

Storage
Store at room temperature before reconstitution and protect from light. After reconstitution, store under refrigeration. Discard any unused solution after 72 h.

Administration
For IV use, dissolve 500,000 units in 300-500 mL D5W for continuous IV infusion.

For IM injection, dissolve 500,000 units in 2 mL water for injection, 0.9% NaCl, or 1% procaine solution. IM injection is not routinely recommended because of severe pain at the injection sites.

For intrathecal administration, dissolve 500,000 units in 10 mL preservative-free 0.9% NaCl. Administer once daily for 3-4 days, then every other day for at least 2 wks after cerebrospinal fluid (CSF) cultures are negative.

For ophthalmic use, 500,000 units in 20-50 mL sterile water for injection or 0.9% NaCl. Instill drops and close the eye gently for 1-2 min. Remove excess solution around the eye with a tissue.

P

Polymyxin B Sulfate, Trimethoprim Sulfate

pol-i-mix′in B sul′fate, trye-meth′oh-prim sul′fate
Polytrim

CATEGORY AND SCHEDULE
Pregnancy Risk Category: C

Classification: Ophthalmics, anti-infectives

MECHANISM OF ACTION
Polymyxin B damages bacterial cytoplasmic membrane, which causes leakage of intracellular components. Trimethoprim is a folate antagonist that blocks bacterial biosynthesis of nucleic acids and proteins by interfering with metabolism of folinic acid. *Therapeutic Effect:* Produces antibacterial activity.

PHARMACOKINETICS
Absorption through intact skin and mucous membranes is insignificant.

AVAILABILITY
Ophthalmic Drops, Solution: 10,000 units/mL.

INDICATIONS AND DOSAGES
▸ Treatment of surface ocular bacterial conjunctivitis and blepharoconjunctivitis
OPHTHALMIC
Adults, Elderly, Children. Instill 1 drop in affected eye(s) every 3 h for 7–10 days. Maximum: 6 doses/day.

CONTRAINDICATIONS
Polymyxin or trimethoprim hypersensitivity.

INTERACTIONS
Drug
None reported.
Herbal
None known.
Food
None known.

SIDE EFFECTS
Occasional
Local irritation, redness, burning, stinging, itching.

SERIOUS REACTIONS
- Prolonged use may result in overgrowth of nonsusceptible organisms, including superinfection.
- Hypersensitivity reactions consisting of lid edema, itching, increased redness, tearing, and/or circumocular rash have been reported.
- Photosensitivity has been reported in patients taking oral trimethoprim.

PRECAUTIONS & CONSIDERATIONS
Avoid wearing contact lenses during treatment. Effectiveness and safety have not been established

in infants < 2 mo of age. Use with caution in pregnancy and lactation. Monitor patient for signs of ocular improvement; notify prescriber if eye inflammation or discharge increases, or eye is unusually reddened rather than improving.

Storage

Store at controlled room temperature and protect from light.

Administration

Wash hands before and after use. Tilt head back and pull lower eyelid down to form a pouch. Squeeze the prescribed number of drops into pouch and gently close eyes for 1-2 min.

Posaconazole

poe-sah-kone′ah-zole

★ Noxafil ★ Posanol

CATEGORY AND SCHEDULE

Pregnancy Risk Category: C

Classification: Antifungal, azole antifungals

MECHANISM OF ACTION

A tirazole antifungal that blocks the synthesis of ergosterol, a key component of fungal cell membrane, through the inhibition of the enzyme lanosterol 14α-demethylase and accumulation of methylated sterol precursors. *Therapeutic Effect:* Inhibits fungal cell membrane formation.

PHARMACOKINETICS

Food increases absorption; must take orally with food. Protein binding: > 98%. Not significantly metabolized; undergoes glucuronidation into metabolites. Primarily eliminated in feces (71%, 66% unchanged); partial excretion in urine (13%, < 0.2% unchanged). *Half-life:* 35 h.

AVAILABILITY

Oral Suspension: 40 mg/mL.

INDICATIONS AND DOSAGES

▸ **Prophylaxis of invasive Aspergillus and Candida fungal infections in patients who are severely immunocompromised**

PO

Adults, Children 13 yr and older. 200 mg (5 mL) 3 times/day.

▸ **Oropharyngeal candidiasis**

PO

Adults, Children 13 yr and older. 100 mg (2.5 mL) twice a day on the first day, then 100 mg (2.5 mL) once a day for 13 days.

▸ **Oropharyngeal candidiasis, refractory to itraconazole and/or fluconazole**

PO

Adults, Children 13 yr and older. 400 mg (10 mL) twice a day.

CONTRAINDICATIONS

Hypersensitivity to azole antifungals, posaconazole or its components; avoid coadministration with ergot alkaloids, sirolimus, simvastatin, or QTc-prolonging CYP3A4 substrates (pimozide, cisapride, quinidine).

INTERACTIONS

Drug

Atazanavir, ritonavir: Increased levels of posaconazole. Avoid if possible.

Calcium channel blockers: May increase the levels and effects of calcium channel blockers.

Cimetidine: May decrease the levels and effects of posaconazole; avoid concurrent use.

Cyclosporine: May increase the levels and effects of cyclosporine.

CYP3A4 substrates: May increase the levels and effects of CYP3A4 substrates. Contraindicated with

QTc-prolonging substrates (e.g., pimozide, cisapride, quinidine).
Ergot alkaloids: Contraindicated. May increase the levels and effects of ergot alkaloids.
HMG-CoA reductase inhibitors: May increase the levels and risk of myopathy; contraindicated with simvastatin.
Midazolam: May increase the levels and effects of midazolam.
Phenytoin: May increase the levels and effects of phenytoin; avoid concurrent use.
QT-prolonging agents: Increased risk of arrhythmia (torsades de pointes). Contraindicated.
Rifabutin: May increase the levels and effects of rifabutin; avoid concurrent use.
Sirolimus: May increase the levels and effects of these drugs.
Vinca alkaloids: May increase the levels and effects of vinca alkaloids.
Herbal
None known.
Food
Grapefruit juice: May increase posaconazole levels; avoid.

DIAGNOSTIC TEST EFFECTS

May decrease serum potassium. May increase LFTs, serum alkaline phosphatase, serum creatinine.

SIDE EFFECTS

Frequent
Diarrhea.
Occasional
Nausea, neutropenia, headache, vomiting, abdominal pain, flatulence, QTc prolongation, rash, hypokalemia, anemia, fever, dizziness, weakness, anorexia, fatigue, insomnia, mucositis, thrombocytopenia, myalgia, pruritus, dyspepsia, xerostoma.
Rare
Hypertension, blurred vision, tremor, hepatocellular damage, taste perversion, constipation, somnolence.

SERIOUS REACTIONS

- Hepatic dysfunction may occur.
- Arrhythmia (torsades de pointes) has been reported.

PRECAUTIONS & CONSIDERATIONS

Caution in patients with severe renal impairment, hepatic impairment, arrhythmia risk, electrolyte abnormalities, severe diarrhea or vomiting. Safety and efficacy not established in children less than 13 yr of age. No unique precautions in the elderly. Teratogenic in animal studies; use in pregnancy only if benefit to mother justifies risk to fetus. Do not breastfeed.
Storage
Store at room temperature.
Administration
Shake well before each use. Dose with a full meal or liquid nutritional supplement. If patients cannot tolerate PO nutrition, alternative antifungal therapy should be considered or closely monitor for lack of efficacy. Use dosing spoon provided with product. Rinse spoon with water after each use.

Potassium Iodide

poe-tas′ee-um eye′oh-dide
★ Losat, Lugol's solution, Pima, SSKI

CATEGORY AND SCHEDULE

Pregnancy Risk Category: D
OTC (tablets)

Classification: Antithyroid agents, hormones/hormone modifiers

MECHANISM OF ACTION

An agent that reduces viscosity of mucus by increasing respiratory tract secretions. Inhibits secretion of thyroid hormone, fosters colloid accumulation in thyroid follicles. *Therapeutic Effect:* Blocks thyroid radioiodine uptake.

PHARMACOKINETICS

Oral onset 24-48 h, peak 10-15 days, duration 6 wks. Primarily excreted in the urine.

AVAILABILITY

Solution: 1 mg/mL (SSKI), 100 mg/mL (Lugol's solution).
Syrup: 325/5 mL (Pima).
Tablets: 130 mg (Iosat).

INDICATIONS AND DOSAGES

▸ Expectorant

PO

Adults, Elderly, Children 3 yr and older. 325-650 mg q8h (Pima); 300-600 mg 3-4 times/day (SSKI).
Children younger than 3 yr. 162 mg q8h.

▸ Preoperative thyroidectomy

PO

Adults, Elderly, Children. 0.1-0.3 mL (3-5 drops of Lugol's solution) q8h or 50-250 mg (1-5 drops of SSKI) q8h. Administer 10 days before surgery.

▸ Radiation protectant to radioactive isotopes of iodine

PO

Adults, Elderly. 195 mg/day (Pima) for 10 days. Start 24 h before exposure.
Children more than 1 yr. 130 mg/day for 10 days. Start 24 h before exposure.
Children < 1 yr. 65 mg/day for 10 days. Start 24 h before exposure.

▸ Reduce risk of thyroid cancer following nuclear accident

PO

Adults, Elderly, Children weighing > 68 kg. 130 mg/day.
Children aged 3-18 yr. 65 mg/day.
Children aged 1 mo to 3 yr. 32 mg/day.
Children 1 mo and younger. 16 mg/day.

▸ Sporotrichosis

PO

Adults, Elderly. Initally, 5 drops (SSKI) q8h and increase to 40-50 drops q8h as tolerated for 3-6 mo.

▸ Thyrotoxic crisis

PO

Adults, Elderly. 300-500 mg (6-19 drops SSKI) q8h or 1 mL (Lugol's solution) q8h.

CONTRAINDICATIONS

Hypersensitivity to potassium, iodine compounds, or any of its components, pulmonary edema, hyperkalemia, impaired renal function, hyperthyroidism, iodine-induced goiter, pregnancy.

INTERACTIONS

Drug

ACE inhibitors: May increase risk of hyperkalemia, cardiac arrhythmias, or cardiac arrest.
Diuretics, potassium-sparing: May increase risk of hyperkalemia, cardiac arrhythmias, or cardiac arrest.
Lithium: May increase the hypothyroid effects.
Potassium (and potassium-containing products): May increase risk of hyperkalemia, cardiac arrhythmias, or cardiac arrest.

Herbal

None known.

Food

None known.

DIAGNOSTIC TEST EFFECTS

May alter thyroid function tests.

SIDE EFFECTS

Occasional

Irregular heartbeat, confusion, drowsiness, fever, rash, diarrhea, GI bleeding, metallic taste, nausea,

P

stomach pain, vomiting, numbness, tingling, weakness.
Rare
Goiter, salivary gland swelling and tenderness, thyroid adenoma, swelling of the throat and neck, myxedema, lymph node swelling.

SERIOUS REACTIONS

- Hypersensitivity symptoms include angioedema, muscle weakness, paralysis, peaked T-waves, flattened P-waves, prolongation of QRS complex, ventricular arrhythmias.

PRECAUTIONS & CONSIDERATIONS

Caution is warranted with congestive heart failure (CHF), hypertension, and pulmonary edema.

Potassium iodide crosses the placenta in amounts sufficient enough to cause fetal goiter and/or hypothyroidism. Prolonged use during pregnancy is not advised; is sometimes used short term to manage thyroid conditions in pregnancy. Excreted in breast milk; do not breastfeed while taking this drug.

CBC (particularly blood hematocrit and hemoglobin level), serum acid-base balance, and serum creatinine should be monitored. ECG and urinary pH should be assessed in those with cardiac disease.

Any indications of swelling in the throat or neck or salivary glands should be reported immediately.

Storage
Store at room temperature. Protect from light.

Administration
Take after meals with food or milk to minimize GI side effects. Mix SSKI dose in water, juice, milk, or broth.

Potassium Salts: Potassium Acetate/ Potassium Bicarbonate-Citrate/ Potassium Chloride/ Potassium Gluconate

poe-tah'see-um
Potassium acetate: No brands
Citric acid-Potassium bicarbonate: ★ Effer-K, Klor-Con/EF, K-Vescent
Potassium chloride: ★ K-Tab, Klor-Con, Micro-K 🍁 K-Dur, Slow-K
Potassium gluconate: No brands

CATEGORY AND SCHEDULE

Pregnancy Risk Category: C (A for potassium chloride)

Classification: Electrolyte replacements, minerals, potassium supplements

MECHANISM OF ACTION

An electrolyte that is necessary for multiple cellular metabolic processes. Primary action is intracellular. *Therapeutic Effect:* Is necessary for nerve impulse conduction and contraction of cardiac, skeletal, and smooth muscle; maintains normal renal function and acid-base balance.

PHARMACOKINETICS

Well absorbed from the GI tract. Enters cells by active transport from extracellular fluid. Primarily excreted in urine.

AVAILABILITY

Potassium Acetate
Injection: 2 mEq/mL.
Potassium Bicarbonate and Citric Acid
Tablet for Solution (Klor-Con/EF, Effer-K): 25 mEq.

Potassium Chloride
Capsules (Extended Release [Micro-K]): 8 mEq, 10 mEq.
Potassium Chloride Injection: 2 mEq/mL.
Premixed IVPB Infusion (central line only): 20 mEq/50 mL, 40 mEq/100mL.
Tablets (Extended Release [Klor-Con M10, Klor-Con M15, Klor-Con M20]): 10 mEq, 15 mEq, 20 mEq.
Tablets (Extended Release Wax-Matrix [K-Tab]): 8 mEq, 10 mEq.
Oral Solution: 20 mEq/15 mL, 40 mEq/15 mL.
Powder for Oral Solution: 20 mEq.
Potassium Gluconate
Tablets (Extended Release): 95 mg.

INDICATIONS AND DOSAGES

▸ **Prevention of hypokalemia (in patients on diuretic therapy)**
PO
Adults, Elderly. 20-40 mEq/day in 1-2 divided doses.
Children. 1-2 mEq/kg/day in 1-2 divided doses.

▸ **Treatment of hypokalemia**
PO
Adults, Elderly. 40-100 mEq/day given in 2-4 doses; further doses based on laboratory values.
Children. 2-5 mEq/day; further doses based on laboratory values.
IV
Adults, Elderly. For acute hypokalemia, usual IV dose is 20-40 mEq IVPB, followed by repeat laboratory monitoring. Maximum: 400 mEq/day.
Children. 2-5 mEq/kg/day usual rate 0.3-0.5 mEq 11g/hr. Maximum rate: 1 mEq/kg/hr.

CONTRAINDICATIONS

Concurrent use of potassium-sparing diuretics, digitalis toxicity, heat cramps, hyperkalemia, postoperative oliguria, severe burns, severe renal impairment, shock with dehydration or hemolytic reaction, untreated Addison disease.

INTERACTIONS

Drug
ACE inhibitors, β-adrenergic blockers, cyclosporine, drospirenone, eplerenone, heparin, NSAIDs, potassium-containing medications, potassium-sparing diuretics, salt substitutes: May increase potassium blood concentration.
Anticholinergics : May increase the risk of GI lesions or side effects from oral sustained-release potassium products.
Corticosteroids: May decrease potassium requirement.
Iodine and iodine-containing products: Do not use.
Herbal
None known.
Food
Iodine-containing shellfish: Contraindicated.

DIAGNOSTIC TEST EFFECTS

Increases serum potassium.

IV INCOMPATIBILITIES

NOTE: Incompatibilities depend on the salt form of potassium utilized. Consult specialized resources. Some incompatibilities for potassium chloride include amphotericin B complex (Abelcet, AmBisome, Amphotec), methylprednisolone (Solu-Medrol), phenytoin (Dilantin).

SIDE EFFECTS

Frequent
Skin rash.
Occasional
Nausea, vomiting, diarrhea, flatulence, abdominal discomfort with distention, phlebitis with IV administration (particularly when potassium concentration of > 40 mEq/L is infused).

Rare
Rash

SERIOUS REACTIONS

- Hyperkalemia (more common in elderly patients and those with impaired renal function) may be manifested as paresthesia, feeling of heaviness in the lower extremities, cold skin, grayish pallor, hypotension, confusion, irritability, flaccid paralysis, and cardiac arrhythmias.

PRECAUTIONS & CONSIDERATIONS

Caution is warranted with cardiac disease and concurrent use of potassium-sparing diuretics, digitalis toxicity, systemic acidosis, renal impairment, and tartrazine sensitivity (most common in those with aspirin hypersensitivity). It is unknown whether potassium crosses the placenta or is distributed in breast milk. No age-related precautions have been noted in children. Elderly patients may be at increased risk for hyperkalemia because of an impaired ability to excrete potassium. Consuming potassium-rich foods, including apricots, avocados, bananas, beans, beef, broccoli, brussels sprouts, cantaloupe, chicken, dates, fish, ham, lentils, milk, molasses, potatoes, prunes, raisins, spinach, turkey, watermelon, veal, and yams, is encouraged.

Notify the physician of a feeling of heaviness in the lower extremities and paresthesia. Serum potassium levels should be obtained before and throughout therapy. Intake and output, pattern of daily bowel activity, and stool consistency should also be monitored. Be alert for signs and symptoms of hyperkalemia, including cold skin, feeling of heaviness in lower extremities, paresthesia, and skin pallor.

Hypersensitivity to seafood, iodine, or iodine-containing products should be noted and if present, should not use this drug.

Storage
Store all products at room temperature.

Administration
! Potassium dosage must be individualized.

Give oral potassium with or after meals and with a full glass of water to decrease GI upset. Mix effervescent tablets, liquids, and powder with juice or water, and let them dissolve before administering. Swallow the tablets whole, and do not chew or crush them.

Dilute the drug to a concentration of no more than 40 mEq/L for peripheral lines, and mix it well before IV infusion. Do not add potassium to a hanging IV line. Usual infusion rate is 10 mEq/h. Rate should not exceed 1 mEq/min for adults. Maximum and recommended rates of infusion differ according to the institution and patient care setting (e.g., ICU vs. medical floor). Check the IV site closely during the infusion for evidence of phlebitis (hardness of vein; heat, pain, and red streaking of skin over vein) and extravasation (cool skin, little or no blood return, pain, and swelling).

Pralatrexate

pral′a-trex′ate
★ 🍁 Folotyn
Do not confuse with pralatrexate with pemetrexed, or Folotyn with Folacin, Follistim, or Foltrin.

CATEGORY AND SCHEDULE

Pregnancy Risk Category: D

Classification: Antineoplastics, folic acid antagonist

MECHANISM OF ACTION
An antimetabolite that disrupts folate-dependent enzymes essential for cell replication. *Therapeutic Effect:* Inhibits the growth of malignant cell lines.

PHARMACOKINETICS
Protein binding: 67%. Most (69%) of drug is eliminated in the urine as unchanged drug isomers. Clearance is tied to glomerular filtration. Not known if dialyzed. *Half-life:* 12-18 h (prolonged in renal impairment).

AVAILABILITY
Injection: 20 mg/mL, 40 mg/2 mL.

INDICATIONS AND DOSAGES
Patients should take low-dose (1-1.25 mg PO) folic acid daily beginning the 10 days preceding the first dose; during the full course of therapy; and for 30 days after the last dose. Also give vitamin B_{12} (1000 mcg IM single dose) no more than 10 wks prior to the first dose and q8-10wk thereafter; the maintenance doses may be given the same day as pralatrexate.

▸ **Refractory peripheral T-cell lymphoma**

IV

Adults. 30 mg/m^2 IV push once weekly for 6 wks in 7-wk cycles.

▸ **Dosage adjustment for toxicities**

Expect treatment interruption or dose reduction to 20 mg/m^2 to manage adverse drug reactions, such as stomatitis or neutropenia. See manufacturer recommendations for specific details.

CONTRAINDICATIONS
Hypersensitivity.

INTERACTIONS
Drug

Nephrotoxic agents, cisplatin, probenecid, sulfamethoxazole-trimethoprim: May delay pralatrexate clearance and increase risk of toxicity.

NSAIDs: Reduce renal clearance or pralatrexate and potential increase in GI, renal side effects.

Live vaccines: Avoid vaccination with live vaccines during treatment.

Herbal

None known.

Food

None known.

DIAGNOSTIC TEST EFFECTS
May decrease platelet, RBC, and WBC counts. May increase LFTs or serum creatinine.

IV INCOMPATIBILITIES
Use only 0.9% NaCl to reconstitute; flush the line before and after. Do not add any other medications to the IV solution. Known incompatibilities include calcium-containing solutions such as lactated Ringer's injection.

P

SIDE EFFECTS
Frequent

Mucositis/stomatitis, thrombocytopenia, nausea, and fatigue.

Occasional

Vomiting, constipation, anorexia, pharyngitis, diarrhea, neutropenia, leukopenia, anemia, rash, desquamation, mood alteration or depression, dyspnea.

Rare

Febrile neutropenia, renal failure, esophagitis, odynophagia, dysphagia, allergic reaction/hypersensitivity, dehydration, creatinine elevation, infection.

SERIOUS REACTIONS
- Expect stomatitis; may be severe and require dose adjustment or withholding treatment.

• Myelosuppression, manifested as neutropenia, thrombocytopenia, or anemia, may occur, with resultant risk of opportunistic or serious infection.
• Renal or liver dysfunction.
• Hypersensitivity, including toxic epidermal necrolysis (TEN).

PRECAUTIONS & CONSIDERATIONS

CBC with differential platelet count should be assessed before starting therapy and again during each cycle and before starting a new cycle. New cycles should not be started with ANC <1500 mm³, platelet count ≤ 100,000 mm³.

Caution is warranted with liver and renal impairment as well as concurrent therapy with NSAIDs. Pralatrexate may be harmful to a fetus, and it is unknown whether pralatrexate is distributed in breast milk. Do not breastfeed once treatment has been initiated. Contraceptive measures should be used during therapy. Safety and efficacy have not been established in children. Be aware that elderly patients may have higher incidence of fatigue, leukopenia, neutropenia, and thrombocytopenia.

Fastidious oral hygiene should be maintained. Do not have immunizations without physician's approval (drug lowers body's resistance). Crowds and those with infection should be avoided. Report fever, sore throat, signs of local infection, easy bruising, and unusual bleeding from any site immediately.

Storage

Store unopened injection vial refrigerated and protected from light in the original carton. Do not freeze. Unopened vial(s) are stable if in the original carton at room temperature for 72 h. Any vials left at room temperature for greater than 72 h should be discarded.

Administration

CAUTION: Observe and exercise usual cautions for handling, preparing, administering, and disposing of cytotoxic drugs.

Be aware that treatment with folic acid and vitamin B_{12} will help reduce risk of side effects.

For intravenous use only. Do not dilute the injection. Withdraw the required dose into the proper syringe and administer as IV push over 3-5 min via the side port of a free-flowing 0.9% NaCl injection.

Pralidoxime

pra-li-doks′eem

★ Protopam Chloride

CATEGORY AND SCHEDULE

Pregnancy Risk Category: C

Classification: Antidotes, cholinergic agonists

MECHANISM OF ACTION

Reactivates cholinesterase activity by 2-formyl-1-methylpyridinium ion. *Therapeutic Effect:* Restores cholinesterase activity following organophosphate anticholinesterase poisoning.

PHARMACOKINETICS

Onset of activity is 1 h and duration of action is short, which may require readministration. Not protein bound. Excreted in urine. *Half-life:* 1.2-2.6 h.

AVAILABILITY

Injection, Powder for Reconstitution: 1 g (Protopam Chloride).

P

INDICATIONS AND DOSAGES

▸ **Anticholinesterase overdosage**

IV

Adults, Elderly. 1-2 g initially, followed by increments of 250 mg q5min until response is observed.

▸ **Organophosphate poisoning**

IV

Adults, Elderly. 1-2 g initially in 100 mL 0.9% NaCl infused over 15-30 min or 5% solution in sterile water for injection over not < 5 min. Repeat 1-2 g in 1 h if muscle weakness persists.

Children. 25-50 mg/kg/dose. Repeat in 1-2 h if muscle weakness has not been relieved, then at 8-12 h intervals if cholinergic signs recur.

CONTRAINDICATIONS

Hypersensitivity to pralidoxime or any of its components.

INTERACTIONS

Drug

Aminophylline, caffeine, theophylline: May exacerbate effects of organophosphate poisoning; avoid use of these drugs when treating overdose.

Atropine: May decrease effects of pralidoxime.

Barbiturates: May increase effect of pralidoxime.

Reserpine, phenothiazines: May exacerbate effects of organophosphate poisoning.

Succinylcholine: May prolong respiratory paralysis due to organophosphate poisoning.

Thiamine: May delay excretion of pralidoxime due to competition at renal excretory site.

Herbal

None known.

Food

None known.

DIAGNOSTIC TEST EFFECTS

May increase SGOT (AST) and creatine kinase levels.

SIDE EFFECTS

Occasional

Blurred vision, dizziness, headache, laryngospasm, hyperventilation, nausea, tachycardia, hypertension, pain at injection site.

Rare

Rash, muscle rigidity, decreased renal function.

SERIOUS REACTIONS

• Excessive doses may cause blurred vision, nausea, tachycardia, and dizziness.

PRECAUTIONS & CONSIDERATIONS

NOTE: Pralidoxime is not effective in the treatment of poisoning due to phosphorus, inorganic phosphates, or organophosphates not having anticholinesterase activity. The drug is not indicated as an antidote for intoxication by pesticides of the carbamate class since it may increase the toxicity of carbaryl.

Caution is warranted with myasthenia gravis and renal impairment as well as in elderly patients. It is unknown whether pralidoxime crosses the placenta and is distributed in breast milk. Safety and efficacy of pralidoxime have not been established in children. Age-related renal impairment may require dosage adjustment in elderly patients. Avoid consuming an excessive amount of caffeine derivatives such as chocolate, cocoa, coffee, cola, or tea.

Resolution of clinical symptoms (muscle weakness, respiratory difficulty, muscarinic effects such as salivation, lacrimation, urination, and defecation) should be assessed.

Storage
Store vials for injection at room temperature.
Administration
Initiation of therapy must not be delayed until results of tests are available. Dilute 1 g with 20 mL of sterile water for injection. Solution may be further diluted and administered as 1-2 g in 100 mL 0.9% NaCl. Usually given over 15-30 min; rate should not exceed 200 mg/min. Slow IV infusion prevents tachycardia, laryngospasm, and muscle rigidity. Do not use if solution appears discolored or contains a precipitate. Expect concomitant use of atropine to treat the symptoms of overdose.

Pramipexole
pram-eh-pex′ol
Mirapex, Mirapex ER
Do not confuse Mirapex with Mifeprex or MiraLax.

CATEGORY AND SCHEDULE
Pregnancy Risk Category: C

Classification: Antiparkinsonian agents, dopaminergics

MECHANISM OF ACTION
An antiparkinsonian agent that stimulates dopamine receptors in the striatum. *Therapeutic Effect:* Relieves signs and symptoms of Parkinson disease.

PHARMACOKINETICS
Rapidly and extensively absorbed after PO administration. Protein binding: 15%. Widely distributed. Steady-state concentrations achieved within 2 days. Primarily eliminated in urine. Not removed by hemodialysis. *Half-life:* 8 h (12 h in patients older than 65 yr).

AVAILABILITY
Tablets: 0.125 mg, 0.25 mg, 0.5 mg, 1 mg, 1.5 mg.
Tablets, Extended Release: 0.375 mg, 0.75 mg, 1.5 mg, 3 mg, 4.5 mg.

INDICATIONS AND DOSAGES
▸ **Parkinson disease**
PO (IMMEDIATE RELEASE)
Adults, Elderly. Initially, 0.375 mg/day in 3 divided doses. Do not increase dosage more frequently than every 5-7 days. Maintenance: 1.5-4.5 mg/day in 3 equally divided doses.
PO (EXTENDED RELEASE)
Adults, Elderly. Initially, 0.375 mg once daily. Increase no more frequently than every 5-7 days. Maintenance: 1.5-4.5 mg/day.
▸ **Restless legs syndrome**
PO
Adults, Elderly. 0.125 mg once daily 2-3 h before bedtime. May increase after 4-7 days to 0.25 mg 2-3 h before bedtime if needed. Maximum of 0.5 mg 2-3 h before bedtime. Higher doses do not provide additional benefit. Slower titration if renally impaired.
▸ **Dosage in renal impairment**
Dosage and frequency of immediate-release tablets for Parkinson disease are modified based on creatinine clearance.

Creatinine Clearance (mL/min)	Initial Dose (mg/day)	Maximum Dose
> 60	0.125	1.5 mg 3×/day
35-59	0.125	1.5 mg 2×/day
15-34	0.125	1.5 mg 1×/day

Dosage of extended-release tablets also adjusted to CrCl:
CrCl 30-50 mL/min: 0.375 mg PO q48h; do not exceed 2.25 mg/day.

CrCl < 30 mL/min: Do not use extended release.

CONTRAINDICATIONS

History of hypersensitivity to pramipexole.

INTERACTIONS

Drug

Carbidopa and levodopa, levodopa: May increase plasma level of levodopa.
Cimetidine: Increases pramipexole plasma concentration and half-life.
Cimetidine, diltiazem, quinidine, quinine, ranitidine, triamterene, verapamil: May decrease pramipexole clearance.
Central nervous system (CNS) depressants: May increase CNS depressive effects.
Phenothiazines, butyrophenones, thioxanthenes, metoclopramide: May decrease effectiveness.

Herbal

None known.

Food

All foods: Delay peak drug plasma levels by 1 h but do not affect drug absorption.

DIAGNOSTIC TEST EFFECTS

None known.

SIDE EFFECTS

Frequent

Early Parkinson disease (10%-28%): Nausea, asthenia, dizziness, somnolence, insomnia, constipation.
Advanced Parkinson disease (17%-53%): Orthostatic hypotension, extrapyramidal reactions, insomnia, dizziness, hallucinations.

Occasional

Early Parkinson disease (2%-5%): Edema, malaise, confusion, amnesia, akathisia, anorexia, dysphagia, peripheral edema, vision changes, impotence.
Advanced Parkinson disease (7%-10%): Asthenia, somnolence, confusion, constipation, abnormal gait, dry mouth.

Rare

Advanced Parkinson disease (2%-6%): General edema, malaise, chest pain, amnesia, tremor, urinary frequency or incontinence, dyspnea, rhinitis, vision changes.

SERIOUS REACTIONS

- Excessive daytime drowsiness may result in falling asleep while engaged in activities, including the operation of motor vehicles, which sometimes results in accidents.
- Hallucinations; new or emergent compulsive actions (gambling, eating, shopping, etc.).
- Retroperitoneal fibrosis, pulmonary infiltrates, pleural effusion, pleural thickening, pericarditis, and cardiac valvulopathy have been reported with ergot-derived dopaminergic agents.

PRECAUTIONS & CONSIDERATIONS

Caution is warranted in patients with hallucinations, syncope, renal impairment, history of orthostatic hypotension, and in those using central nervous system (CNS) depressants concurrently. It is unknown whether pramipexole is distributed in breast milk. The safety and efficacy of pramipexole have not been established in children. Elderly patients are at increased risk for hallucinations.

Dizziness, drowsiness, light-headedness, and constipation may occur. Alcohol and tasks that require mental alertness or motor skills should be avoided. Change positions slowly to prevent orthostatic hypotension. Vital signs and renal function should be assessed at baseline. Relief of symptoms, such as improvement of mask-like facial expression, muscular rigidity, shuffling gait, and resting tremors of the hands and head, should be assessed during treatment.

Storage

Store at room temperature.

Administration

Take pramipexole without regard to food. Take with food if nausea is a problem. Do not abruptly discontinue pramipexole.

Pramlintide

pram'lin-tide

★ Symlin, SymlinPen

CATEGORY AND SCHEDULE

Pregnancy Risk Category: C

Classification: Antidiabetic agents, amylin analogues

P

MECHANISM OF ACTION

An analogue of amylin, a neuroendocrine hormone secreted by pancreatic β cells that works along with insulin to regulate postprandial glucose concentrations; endogenous amylin is stored with insulin in secretory granules and secreted with insulin. By acting as an amylinomimetic agent, pramlintide (1) slows gastric emptying, (2) prevents postprandial rise in plasma glucagon and lowering postprandial glucose, and (3) modulates centrally mediated appetite satiety leading to decreased caloric intake and potential weight loss. *Therapeutic Effect:* Lowers blood glucose concentration and HbA1C over time, improving diabetic control.

PHARMACOKINETICS

Bioavailability is 30%-40% after subcutaneous (SC) injection into the abdominal area. Maximum plasma concentration occurs 20 min after SC injection. Protein binding: 40%. Pramlintide is extensively metabolized by the kidneys; the primary metabolite has a similar half-life and is biologically active both in vitro and in vivo. *Half-life:* 48 min.

AVAILABILITY

Injection Pens (1000 mcg/mL): SymlinPen 60 allows for 15-, 30-, 45-, and 60-mcg doses; SymlinPen 120 allows for 60- and 120-mcg doses.

Vials: Contain 600 mcg/mL solution in 5-mL vial.

INDICATIONS AND DOSAGES

▸ **Diabetes mellitus for type 1 DM in patients who use mealtime insulin therapy**

SC

Adults. 15 mcg SC immediately prior to each major meal (≥ 250 kcal or 30 g of carbohydrates). Titrate upward in 15-mcg increments every 3 days to 60 mcg prior to each major meal; only if no significant nausea. If nausea or vomiting persists, reduce the dose. Reduce preprandial rapid or short-acting insulin and fixed-mix insulin dose by 50% when pramlintide is initiated. Adjust to achieve optimal glycemic control.

▸ **Diabetes mellitus for type 2 DM in patients who use mealtime insulin therapy with or without a sulfonylurea and/or metformin**

SC

Adults. 60 mcg SC immediately prior to each major meal (≥ 250 kcal or 30 g of carbohydrates); increase to 120 mcg prior to each major meal if no significant nausea for 3-7 days. If nausea or vomiting persists, reduce the dose. Reduce preprandial rapid or short-acting insulin or fixed-mix insulin dose by 50% when pramlintide is initiated. Adjust insulin to achieve optimal glycemic control.

CONTRAINDICATIONS

Hypersensitivity to pramlintide or product components, such as metacresol. Gastroparesis. Not for diabetic ketoacidosis. Not for patients with hypoglycemic unawareness.

INTERACTIONS

Drug

Insulin: While indicated to be coadministered with insulin therapy, pramlintide increases the risk of insulin-induced severe hypoglycemia, particularly in patients with type 1 diabetes and usually within the first 3 h following a pramlintide dose. Provide frequent pre- and post-meal glucose monitoring and an initial 50% reduction in pre-meal doses of short-acting insulin.

Acarbose, miglitol: Due to its effects on gastric emptying, pramlintide therapy should not be used with agents that slow the intestinal absorption of nutrients (e.g., α-glucosidase inhibitors).

Anticholinergics or prokinetic agents: Due to its effects on gastric emptying, do not use in patients taking these GI drugs due to lack of safety data.

β-Blockers: May mask signs of hypoglycemia.

Oral medications (e.g., oral contraceptives, antibiotics): Pramlintide slows GI transit times. For oral medications dependent on normal transit times efficacy, such as contraceptives and antibiotics, patients should be advised to take those drugs at least 1 h before pramlintide, or at a meal or snack when pramlintide is not administered.

Corticosteroids: May increase blood sugar.

Sulfonylureas: May increase risk of hypoglycemia; lower sulfonylurea dose may be needed.

Warfarin: May increase the effects of warfarin, resulting in increased INR. Monitor INR closely.

Herbal

Alfalfa, aloe, bilberry, bitter melon, burdock, celery, damiana, fenugreek, garcinia, garlic, ginger, ginseng (American), gymnema, marshmallow, stinging nettle: May enhance hypoglycemic effects.

Food

Alcohol: Hypoglycemia is more likely to occur if alcohol is ingested. High and chronic alcohol use may increase risk for pancreatitis.

DIAGNOSTIC TEST EFFECTS

Lowers blood sugar. May increase serum creatinine, amylase, or lipase.

SIDE EFFECTS

Frequent

Nausea is expected and can be reduced with slow titration. Decreased appetite, tiredness, dizziness, or indigestion. Nausea subsides with time.

Occasional

Hypoglycemia, stomach pain, vomiting, tiredness, diarrhea, dizziness, dyspepsia. Gastroesophageal reflux (GERD), asthenia, hyperhidrosis, headache.

Rare

Injection site reaction (redness, bruising) or lipodystrophy, eructation, flatulence, taste disturbance, pruritus, urticaria, rash.

SERIOUS REACTIONS

- Overdose may produce severe hypoglycemia, along with severe GI symptoms and vomiting.
- Rare reports of serious allergic reactions, including angioedema and rashes.

PRECAUTIONS & CONSIDERATIONS

Caution is warranted in patients with end-stage renal disease, hepatic dysfunction, and patients with significant GI disease where slowing of GI transit time may aggravate the condition. Be alert to conditions that alter blood glucose requirements or dietary intake, such as fever, increased activity, stress, or a surgical procedure. There are no data regarding pramlintide use during pregnancy. It is unknown whether the drug is distributed in breast milk; caution is recommended. The drug may alter the efficacy of oral hormonal contraceptives and the choice of an additional or alternate contraceptive may be desirable. Safety and efficacy of pramlintide have not been established in children. Hypoglycemia may be difficult to recognize in elderly patients.

Food intake and blood glucose should be monitored before and during therapy. Be aware of signs and symptoms of hypoglycemia (anxiety, cool wet skin, diplopia, dizziness, headache, hunger, numbness in the mouth, tachycardia, tremors) or hyperglycemia (deep rapid breathing, dim vision, fatigue, nausea, polydipsia, polyphagia, polyuria, vomiting); carry candy, sugar packets, or other sugar supplements for immediate response to hypoglycemia. Consult the physician when glucose demands are altered (such as with fever, heavy physical activity, infection, stress, trauma). Exercise, good personal hygiene (including foot care), not smoking, and weight control are essential parts of therapy.

Storage

Store unopened pens and vials in the original carton in a refrigerator. Do not freeze. Once opened and set up for first use, the pen or vial can be kept at a temperature not to exceed 86° F for up to 30 days; they may be kept refrigerated. Always protect from light and keep pen dry. Do not store the pen with the needle attached, as this will cause leakage from the pen and air bubbles may form in the cartridge.

Administration

Pramlintide and insulin should always be administered as separate injections and never be mixed.

For subcutaneous injection only; doses are given any time within the 60 min prior to the start of a main meal.

To administer from vials, use a U-100 insulin syringe (preferably a 0.3-mL size). If using a syringe calibrated for use with U-100 insulin using units, use the manufacturer's chart to convert the microgram dosage in unit increments.

If using pen, make sure you have prepared the pen for routine use. For routine use, wash hands. Check that the right pen is selected. Pull off pen cap. The cartridge liquid should be clear, colorless, and free of particles. Attach the needle and dial in the pen dose as the manufacturer directs. Inject the dose SC as directed in the upper thigh or abdomen; rotate injection sites with each use. After injection, reset the pen, remove and dispose of the used needle properly, and store the pen for next use by replacing the pen cap.

P

Prasugrel

pra'soo-grel

Effient

Do not confuse Effient with Effexor or prasugrel with pravachol.

CATEGORY AND SCHEDULE

Pregnancy Risk Category: B

Classification: Platelet aggregation inhibitor

MECHANISM OF ACTION

A thienopyridine derivative that inhibits binding of the enzyme adenosine phosphate (ADP) to its platelet receptor and subsequent ADP-mediated activation of platelet aggregation. *Therapeutic Effect:* Inhibits platelet aggregation and reduces thrombotic cardiovascular events (including stent thrombosis) in those with acute coronary syndromes managed with percutaneous coronary intervention (PCI).

PHARMACOKINETICS

Route	Onset	Peak	Duration
PO	1 h	30 min	> 3 days

Rapidly and well absorbed orally. Prasugrel is a prodrug and is quickly metabolized to a pharmacologically active metabolite via hydrolysis in the intestine to a thiolactone that is then actively converted in the liver by a single step, primarily by CYP3A4 and CYP2B6 and to a lesser extent by CYP2C9 and CYP2C19. The active metabolite is metabolized to 2 inactive compounds by S-methylation or conjugation with cysteine. Approximately 68% of the prasugrel dose is excreted in the urine and 27% in the feces as inactive metabolites. Active metabolite not dialyzable. *Half-life:* 7 h (mean half-life of active metabolite).

AVAILABILITY

Tablets: 5 mg, 10 mg.

INDICATIONS AND DOSAGES

▸ **Unstable angina; non-ST-elevation myocardial infarction (NSTEMI) or ST-elevation MI (STEMI) managed with PCI**

PO

Adults, Elderly < 75 yr of age. Initially 60 mg loading dose. Then, 10 mg once daily. Consider 5 mg once daily if weight < 60 kg. Patients should also take aspirin (75-325 mg) daily unless allergic.

CONTRAINDICATIONS

Hypersensitivity, active bleeding, prior transient ischemic attack or stroke.

INTERACTIONS

Drug

Anticoagulants (including warfarin and heparins); NSAIDS: May increase the risk of bleeding.

Herbal

Ginger, ginkgo biloba, white willow bark: May increase the risk of bleeding.

Food

None known.

DIAGNOSTIC TEST EFFECTS

Prolongs bleeding time. Be aware that abrupt discontinuation of prasugrel produces a return to normal aggregation of platelets within 5-9 days.

SIDE EFFECTS

Frequent (> 7%)

Bleeding, both minor (such as easy bruising or epistaxis) and major.

Occasional (3%-7%)

Headache, dizziness, arthralgia or back pain, nausea, dyspnea, cough, fatigue.

P

Infrequent (1%-3%)
Non-cardiac chest pain, leukopenia, rash, pyrexia, peripheral edema, pain in extremity, diarrhea.
Rare (< 1%)
Severe thrombocytopenia, anemia, abnormal hepatic function, allergic reactions.

SERIOUS REACTIONS

- Rare allergic reactions may include angioedema.
- Thrombotic thrombocytopenic purpura.
- Significant, sometimes fatal bleeding, such as GI hemorrhage or CNS bleeding.

PRECAUTIONS & CONSIDERATIONS

Caution is warranted with hematologic disorders, history of bleeding, hypertension, severe hepatic or renal impairment, and in preoperative persons. Do not use in patients with a history of transient ischemic attack or stroke. In elderly patients ≥ 75 yr of age, prasugrel is not recommended due to increased risk of serious bleeding and uncertain benefit, except in high-risk patients (diabetes or prior MI), where its benefit may be considered. Do not start prasugrel in patients likely to undergo urgent coronary artery bypass graft (CABG) surgery. When possible, discontinue at least 7 days prior to *any* surgery; abrupt discontinuation may increase clot and MI risk. Adult patients of low body weight (< 132 lb) may have a higher bleeding risk; use with caution and consider lower dosage. There are no data in human pregnancy, and it is not known if the drug is excreted in human milk. The safety and efficacy of prasugrel have not been established in children.

Be aware that it may take longer to stop bleeding during drug therapy. Notify the physician of unusual bleeding, particularly purple patches on the skin. Also, notify dentists and other physicians before surgery is scheduled or when new drugs are prescribed. Platelet count for thrombocytopenia, hemoglobin level, WBC count, and BUN, serum bilirubin, creatinine, AST (SGOT), and ALT (SGPT) levels should be monitored. Platelet count should be obtained before prasugrel therapy, every 2 days during the first week of treatment, and weekly thereafter until therapeutic maintenance dose is reached.

Storage
Store tablets at room temperature.
Administration
Take prasugrel without regard to food, at the same time each day. Do not crush coated tablets.

Inform patient of need for adherence to treatment. Those who have had PCI and have a stent and stop the drug too soon have a higher risk of blood clot, heart attack, and death.

Pravastatin

prav-i-sta′tin
★ 🍁 Pravachol
Do not confuse pravastatin with Prevacid, or Pravachol with propranolol.

CATEGORY AND SCHEDULE

Pregnancy Risk Category: X

Classification:
Antihyperlipidemics, HMG-CoA reductase inhibitors ("statins")

MECHANISM OF ACTION

An HMG-CoA reductase inhibitor that interferes with cholesterol biosynthesis by preventing the conversion of HMG-CoA reductase to mevalonate, a precursor to cholesterol. *Therapeutic Effect:* Lowers serum low density lipoprotein (LDL) and very low density lipoprotein (VLDL) cholesterol and plasma triglyceride levels; increases serum high density lipoprotein (HDL) concentration.

PHARMACOKINETICS

Poorly absorbed from the GI tract. Protein binding: 50%. Metabolized in the liver (minimal active metabolites). Primarily excreted in feces via the biliary system. Not removed by hemodialysis. *Half-life:* 2.7 h.

AVAILABILITY

Tablets: 10 mg, 20 mg, 40 mg, 80 mg.

INDICATIONS AND DOSAGES

▸ Hyperlipidemia, primary and secondary prevention of cardiovascular events in patient with elevated cholesterol levels

PO

Adults, Elderly. Initially, 40 mg/day. Titrate to desired response. Range: 10-80 mg/day.

Children 14-18 yr. 40 mg/day.

Children 8-13 yr. 20 mg/day.

▸ Dosage in hepatic and renal impairment

For adults, give 10 mg/day initially. Titrate to desired response.

CONTRAINDICATIONS

Hypersensitivity; active liver disease or unexplained, persistent elevations of serum transaminases; pregnancy; breastfeeding.

INTERACTIONS

Drug

Colchicine, cyclosporine, erythromycin, itraconazole: Increases the risk of acute renal failure and rhabdomyolysis or myopathy. Due to lack of CYP3A4 metabolism, these interactions are not as significant for pravastatin as with other "statins."

Herbal

None known.

Food

None known. Alcohol should be avoided during therapy.

DIAGNOSTIC TEST EFFECTS

May increase serum CK and transaminase concentrations. Transient increases in eosinophil counts. Rare decreases in platelets, WBC, and RBC indices.

SIDE EFFECTS

Pravastatin is generally well tolerated. Side effects are usually mild and transient.

Occasional (4%-7%)

Nausea, vomiting, diarrhea, constipation, abdominal pain, headache, rhinitis, rash, pruritus.

Rare (2%-3%)

Heartburn, myalgia, dizziness, cough, fatigue, flu-like symptoms.

SERIOUS REACTIONS

- Hypersensitivity occurs rarely.
- Rhabdomyolysis (rare).
- Hepatotoxicity (rare).
- Lens opacity may occur.

PRECAUTIONS & CONSIDERATIONS

Additional caution is warranted in patients with past liver disease; severe acute infection; trauma; severe metabolic or seizure disorders; severe electrolyte, endocrine, and metabolic disorders; and in any patient who consumes a substantial amount of alcohol. Withholding or discontinuing pravastatin may be necessary when the person is at risk for renal failure secondary to rhabdomyolysis. Pravastatin is contraindicated in pregnancy (category X) and may cause fetal harm. It is unknown whether pravastatin is distributed in breast milk; because there is risk of serious adverse reactions in breastfeeding infants, pravastatin is contraindicated during lactation. Safety and efficacy of pravastatin have not been established in children under 8 yr of age. No age-related precautions have been noted in elderly patients.

Dizziness and headache may occur. Tasks that require mental alertness or motor skills should be avoided until response to the drug is established. Notify the physician of muscle weakness, myalgia, severe gastric upset, or rash. Pattern of daily bowel activity and stool consistency should be assessed. Serum lipid cholesterol and triglyceride levels and hepatic function should be checked at baseline and periodically during treatment. Be aware that diet is an important part of treatment.

Storage

Store at room temperature.

Administration

May administer without regard to meals and may give at any time of day. Often given at bedtime.

P

Praziquantel

pray'zih-kwon'tel

★ 🍁 Biltricide

CATEGORY AND SCHEDULE

Pregnancy Risk Category: B

Classification: Antihelmintics

MECHANISM OF ACTION

An antihelmintic that increases cell permeability in susceptible helminths resulting in loss of intracellular calcium, massive contractions, and paralysis of their musculature, followed by attachment of phagocytes to the parasites.

Therapeutic Effect: Vermicidal. Dislodges the dead and dying worms.

PHARMACOKINETICS

Well absorbed from GI tract. Protein binding: 80%. Widely distributed, including cerebrospinal fluid (CSF). Metabolized in liver. Primarily excreted in urine. Not removed by hemodialysis. *Half-life:* 4-5 h.

AVAILABILITY

Tablets: 600 mg (Biltricide).

INDICATIONS AND DOSAGES

▸ **Schistosomiasis**

PO

Adults, Elderly, Children > 4 yr of age. 3 doses of 20 mg/kg as 1-day treatment. Do not give doses < 4 h or > 6 h apart.

▸ **Clonorchiasis/opisthorchiasis**

PO

Adults, Elderly, Children > 4 yr of age. 3 doses of 25 mg/kg as 1-day treatment.

CONTRAINDICATIONS

Ocular cysticercosis, hypersensitivity to praziquantel or any component of the formulation. Use with rifampin.

INTERACTIONS

Drug

Albendazole: May increase risk of albendazole adverse effects.

Carbamazepine, phenytoin, fosphenytoin: May decrease praziquantel effectiveness.

Cimetidine: May increase praziquantel concentrations.

Rifampin: Strong CYP450 inducers, such as rifampin, are contraindicated since therapeutically effective blood levels of praziquantel may not be achieved. Consider different drug for parasites. Stop rifampin 4 wks before use; may restart the day after treatment is complete.

Herbal

St. John's wort: Avoid. Effective blood levels of praziquantel may not be achieved.

Food

None known.

DIAGNOSTIC TEST EFFECTS

None known.

SIDE EFFECTS

Frequent

Headache, dizziness, malaise, abdominal pain.

Occasional

Anorexia, vomiting, diarrhea, severe cramping and abdominal pain may occur within 1 h of administration with fever, sweating, bloody stools.

Rare

Dizziness, urticaria.

SERIOUS REACTIONS

- Overdose should be treated with fast-acting laxative, as the drug can cause arrhythmia, convulsions, severe somnolence/coma.

PRECAUTIONS & CONSIDERATIONS

Caution should be used in patients with severe liver impairment and cardiac irregularities. It is unknown whether praziquantel is distributed in breast milk. Safety and efficacy have not been established in children. No age-related precautions have been noted in elderly patients. Symptoms of giddiness or urticaria may indicate a hypersensitivity reaction and should be reported.

Patients should be warned not to drive or perform hazardous tasks on the day of treatment and the following day.

Storage

Store at room temperature.

Administration

Doses should be spaced not < 4 h and not > 6 h apart. Tablets are scored and may be broken for dosage adjustment. If iron supplements are ordered, continue as directed, which may be up to 6 mo post therapy.

Prazosin Hydrochloride

pra'zoe-sin high-droh-klor'eyed

★ 🍁 Minipress

CATEGORY AND SCHEDULE

Pregnancy Risk Category: C

Classification: Antihypertensives, α-adrenergic antagonist

MECHANISM OF ACTION

An antidote, antihypertensive, and vasodilator that selectively blocks α_1-adrenergic receptors, decreasing peripheral vascular resistance. *Therapeutic Effect:* Produces vasodilation of veins and arterioles, decreases total peripheral resistance, and relaxes smooth muscle in bladder neck and prostate.

PHARMACOKINETICS

PO: Onset 2 h, peak 1-3 h, duration 6-12 h. *Half-life:* 2-4 h; metabolized in liver, excreted in bile, feces (> 90%), in urine (< 10%).

AVAILABILITY

Capsules: 1 mg, 2 mg, 5 mg.

INDICATIONS AND DOSAGES

▸ **Mild to moderate hypertension**

PO

Adults, Elderly. Initially, 1 mg 2-3 times a day. Maintenance: 6-15 mg/day in divided doses. Maximum: 20 mg/day.

P

OFF-LABEL USES

Treatment of urinary retention in benign prostatic hypertrophy, ergot alkaloid induced peripheral ischemia, pheochromocytoma, Raynaud phenomenon, treatment of hypertension in children.

CONTRAINDICATIONS

Hypersensitivity to prazosin or to quinazolines.

INTERACTIONS

Drug

Hypotension-producing medications, such as antihypertensives, phosphodiesterase-5 (PDE-5) inhibitors (e.g., vardenafil, sildenafil, tadalafil), and diuretics: May increase the effects of prazosin.

MAOIs: Additive hypotensive effect.

NSAIDs and sympathomimetics: May decrease the effects of prazosin.

Herbal

Licorice: Causes sodium and water retention and potassium loss.

Food

Alcohol: Additive hypotensive effect.

DIAGNOSTIC TEST EFFECTS

None known.

SIDE EFFECTS

Frequent (7%-10%)

Dizziness, somnolence, headache, asthenia (loss of strength, energy).

Occasional (4%-5%)

Palpitations, nausea, dry mouth, nervousness.

Rare (< 1%)

Angina, urinary urgency.

SERIOUS REACTIONS

- First-dose syncope (hypotension with sudden loss of consciousness) may occur 30-90 min following initial dose of more than 2 mg, a too-rapid increase in dosage, or addition of another antihypertensive agent to therapy. First-dose syncope may be preceded by tachycardia (pulse rate of 120-160 beats/min).
- Priapism (rare).
- Intraoperative floppy iris syndrome (IFIS) during cataract surgery (rare).

PRECAUTIONS & CONSIDERATIONS

Caution is warranted in patients with chronic renal failure. Caution should be used when driving or operating machinery. Tasks that require mental alertness or motor skills should be avoided until response to the drug is established. Use with caution in pregnancy; the drug is also excreted in breast milk in small amounts. Safety and efficacy not established in children. The elderly may be more sensitive to orthostasis.

Dizziness, light-headedness, and fainting may occur. Rise slowly from a lying to a sitting position, and permit legs to dangle momentarily before standing to avoid the hypotensive effect. Notify the physician if dizziness or palpitations become bothersome. BP and pulse should be obtained immediately before each dose, and every 15-30 min thereafter until BP is stabilized. Be alert for fluctuations in BP. Pattern of daily bowel activity and stool consistency should also be assessed.

Assess patient's tolerance to stress, which could compromise cardiovascular function.

Storage

Store at room temperature.

Administration

Take prazosin without regard to food. Take the first dose at bedtime to minimize the risk of fainting from first-dose syncope.

P

Prednisolone

pred-niss'oh-lone
Systemic: ★ Millipred, Orapred, Pediapred, Prednoral, Prelone
Ophthalmic: ★ Econopred, OmniPred, Pred Forte, Pred Mild
Do not confuse prednisolone with prednisone or Primidone.

CATEGORY AND SCHEDULE

Pregnancy Risk Category: C (D if used in first trimester)

Classification: Hormones and hormone modifiers, adrenal agents, corticosteroids, ophthalmic anti-inflammatory

MECHANISM OF ACTION

An adrenocortical steroid that inhibits accumulation of inflammatory cells at inflammation sites, phagocytosis, lysosomal enzyme release and synthesis, and release of mediators of inflammation. *Therapeutic Effect:* Prevents or suppresses cell-mediated immune reactions. Decreases or prevents tissue response to inflammatory process.

PHARMACOKINETICS

PO: Peak 1-2 h, duration 2 days.

AVAILABILITY

Oral Solution (Pediapred): 5 mg/5 mL.
Oral Solution (Orapred): 15 mg/5 mL.
Tablets: 5 mg.
Orally Disintegrating Tablets (Orapred ODT): 10 mg, 15 mg, 30 mg.
Syrup (Prelone): 15 mg/5 mL.
Ophthalmic Solution: 1%.
Ophthalmic Suspension (Pred Mild): 0.12%.
Ophthalmic Suspension (Pred Forte, Econopred, Omnipred): 1%.

INDICATIONS AND DOSAGES

▸ **Substitution therapy for deficiency states: acute or chronic adrenal insufficiency, congenital adrenal hyperplasia, and adrenal insufficiency secondary to pituitary insufficiency; nonendocrine disorders: arthritis; rheumatic carditis; allergic, collagen, intestinal tract, liver, ocular, renal, skin diseases; bronchial asthma; cerebral edema; malignancies**

PO
Adults, Elderly. 5-60 mg/day in divided doses.
Children. 0.1-2 mg/kg/day in 3-4 divided doses.

▸ **Treatment of conjuctivitis and corneal injury**

OPHTHALMIC
Adults, Elderly. 1-2 drops every hour during day and q2h during night. After response, decrease dosage to 1 drop q4h, then 1 drop 3-4 times a day.

CONTRAINDICATIONS

Hypersensitivity, acute superficial herpes simplex keratitis, systemic fungal infections, varicella, Cushing syndrome.

INTERACTIONS

Drug

Acetaminophen (chronic use or high dose, alone or in combination products): May increase risk of hepatotoxicity.
Alcohol, salicylates, NSAIDs: May increase GI side effects.
Amphotericin B, diuretics: May increase hypokalemia.
Barbiturates, rifampin, rifabutin: May result in decreased glucocorticoid activity.
Digoxin: May increase the risk of digoxin toxicity caused by hypokalemia.

P

Insulin, oral hypoglycemics: May decrease the effects of these drugs.
Ketoconazole, macrolide antibiotics (erythromycin, clarithromycin): May result in increased glucocorticoid activity.
Live-virus vaccines: May decrease the patient's antibody response to vaccine, increase vaccine side effects, and potentiate virus replication.

Herbal
None known.

Food
None known.

DIAGNOSTIC TEST EFFECTS

May increase blood glucose and serum lipid, amylase, and sodium levels. May decrease serum calcium, potassium, and thyroxine levels.

May decrease response to antigenic skin tests.

SIDE EFFECTS

Frequent
Insomnia, heartburn, nervousness, abdominal distention, increased sweating, acne, mood swings, increased appetite, facial flushing, delayed wound healing, increased susceptibility to infection, diarrhea or constipation.

Occasional
Headache, edema, change in skin color, frequent urination.

Rare
Tachycardia, allergic reaction (such as rash and hives), psychological changes, hallucinations, depression. Ophthalmic: Stinging or burning, posterior subcapsular cataracts.

SERIOUS REACTIONS

- Long-term therapy may cause hypocalcemia, hypokalemia, muscle wasting (especially in the arms and legs), osteoporosis, spontaneous fractures, amenorrhea, cataracts, glaucoma, peptic ulcer disease, and congestive heart failure (CHF).
- Hypothalamic-pituitary adrenal (HPA) axis suppression and potential glucocorticosteroid insufficiency after withdrawal of treatment.
- Prolonged therapy in children may retard bone growth.
- Abruptly withdrawing the drug after long-term therapy may cause anorexia, nausea, fever, headache, severe or sudden joint pain, rebound inflammation, fatigue, weakness, lethargy, dizziness, and orthostatic hypotension.
- Suddenly discontinuing prednisolone may be fatal.

PRECAUTIONS & CONSIDERATIONS

Caution is warranted in patients with cirrhosis, CHF, diabetes mellitus, hypertension, hypothyroidism, myasthenia gravis, ocular herpes simplex, osteoporosis, peptic ulcer disease, thromboembolic disorders, and ulcerative colitis. Monitor the growth and development of children receiving long-term steroid therapy. Avoid alcohol and limit caffeine intake during therapy.

May cause changes in blood glucose levels; levels should be monitored closely during therapy.

Mood swings, ranging from euphoria to depression, may occur. Notify the physician of fever, muscle aches, sore throat, and sudden weight gain or swelling. The mouth should be assessed daily for signs and symptoms of candidal infection, such as white patches and painful mucous membranes and tongue. Blood glucose level, intake and output, BP, serum electrolyte levels, pattern of daily bowel activity, height, and weight should be monitored before and during therapy. Be alert to signs and symptoms of infection caused by reduced immune response, including fever, sore throat, and vague symptoms, as normal infection symptoms may be masked.

Storage
Store ophthalmic upright. Store all products at room temperature; do not freeze. Protect ODT form from moisture.

Administration
Shake ophthalmic preparation well before using. Instill drops into conjunctival sac, as prescribed. Avoid touching the applicator tip to any surface to avoid contamination. Do not abruptly discontinue the drug without physician approval.

Oral medication doses should be taken with a light meal or milk. For oral solution, confirm correct product selection against close ordered due to various concentrations available. For ODT form, keep in original package until time of use; remove with dry hands. Let dissolve on tongue, with or without water.

Prednisone

pred'ni-sone

★ Prednisone Intensol, Deltasone, Sterapred 🍁 Winpred

Do not confuse prednisone with prednisolone or Primidone.

CATEGORY AND SCHEDULE

Pregnancy Risk Category: C (D if used in first trimester)

Classification: Hormones/hormone modifiers, adrenal agents, corticosteroids, anti-inflammatory

MECHANISM OF ACTION

An adrenocortical steroid that inhibits accumulation of inflammatory cells at inflammation sites, phagocytosis, lysosomal enzyme release and synthesis, and release of mediators of inflammation. *Therapeutic Effect:* Prevents or suppresses cell-mediated immune reactions. Decreases or prevents tissue response to inflammatory process.

PHARMACOKINETICS

Well absorbed from the GI tract. Protein binding: 70%-90%. Widely distributed. Metabolized in the liver and converted to prednisolone. Conversion to prednisolone impaired in severe liver disease. Excreted primarily in urine. Not removed by hemodialysis. *Half-life:* 3.4-3.8 h.

AVAILABILITY

Oral Concentrate (Prednisone Intensol): 5 mg/mL.
Oral Solution: 5 mg/5 mL.
Tablets: 1 mg, 2.5 mg, 5 mg, 10 mg, 20 mg, 50 mg.

INDICATIONS AND DOSAGES

▸ **Substitution therapy in deficiency states: acute or chronic adrenal insufficiency, congenital adrenal hyperplasia, and adrenal insufficiency secondary to pituitary insufficiency; nonendocrine disorders: arthritis; rheumatic carditis; allergic, collagen, intestinal tract, liver, ocular, renal, skin diseases; bronchial asthma; cerebral edema; malignancies**

PO
Adults, Elderly. 5-60 mg/day in divided doses.
Children. 0.05-2 mg/kg/day in 1-4 divided doses.

▸ **Immunosuppression or anti-inflammation**

PO
Adults, Elderly. 5-60 mg/day divided into 1-4 doses.

CONTRAINDICATIONS

Hypersensitivity, acute superficial herpes simplex keratitis, systemic fungal infections, varicella.

INTERACTIONS

Drug

Acetaminophen (chronic long-term or high-dose, alone or in combination products): May increase risk of hepatotoxicity.

Alcohol, salicylates, NSAIDs: May cause increased GI side effects.

Amphotericin B diuretics: May increase hypokalemia.

Barbiturates, rifampin, rifabutin: May decrease glucocorticoid activity.

Digoxin: May increase the risk of digoxin toxicity caused by hypokalemia.

Insulin, oral hypoglycemics: May decrease the effects of these drugs.

Ketoconazole, macrolide antibiotics (erythromycin, clarithromycin): May increase glucocorticoid activity.

Live-virus vaccines: May decrease the patient's antibody response to vaccine, increase vaccine side effects, and potentiate virus replication.

Herbal

None known.

Food

None known.

DIAGNOSTIC TEST EFFECTS

May increase blood glucose and serum lipid, amylase, and sodium levels. May decrease serum calcium, potassium, and thyroxine levels.

May decrease response to antigenic skin tests.

SIDE EFFECTS

Frequent

Insomnia, heartburn, nervousness, abdominal distention, increased sweating, acne, mood swings, increased appetite, facial flushing, delayed wound healing, increased susceptibility to infection, diarrhea or constipation; pain at injection site.

Occasional

Headache, edema, change in skin color, frequent urination.

Rare

Tachycardia, allergic reaction (including rash and hives), psychological changes, hallucinations, depression.

SERIOUS REACTIONS

- Long-term therapy may cause muscle wasting in the arms and legs, osteoporosis, spontaneous fractures, amenorrhea, cataracts, glaucoma, peptic ulcer disease, and CHF.
- Hypothalamic-pituitary adrenal (HPA) axis suppression and potential glucocorticosteriod insufficiency after withdrawal of treatment.
- Prolonged therapy in children may retard bone growth.
- Abruptly withdrawing the drug following long-term therapy may cause anorexia, nausea, fever, headache, sudden or severe joint pain, rebound inflammation, fatigue, weakness, lethargy, dizziness, and orthostatic hypotension.
- Suddenly discontinuing prednisone may be fatal.

PRECAUTIONS & CONSIDERATIONS

Prednisone therapy is contraindicated in cases of acute superficial herpes simplex keratitis, systemic fungal infections, varicella. Caution is warranted in patients with CHF, cirrhosis, diabetes mellitus, glaucoma, hypertension, hyperthyroidism, myasthenia gravis, ocular herpes simplex, osteoporosis, renal disease, and esophagitis. Prednisone crosses the placenta and is distributed in breast milk. Prolonged prednisone use in the first trimester of pregnancy causes cleft palate in the neonate.

Prolonged treatment or high dosages may decrease the cortisol secretion and short-term growth rate in children. Elderly patients may be more susceptible to developing hypertension or osteoporosis. Never give prednisone with live-virus vaccines, such as smallpox vaccine; avoid exposure to chickenpox or measles. A dentist or other physician should be informed of prednisone therapy if taken within the past 12 mo. May cause changes in blood glucose levels and levels should be monitored closely during therapy.

Mood swings, ranging from euphoria to depression, may occur. Notify the physician of fever, muscle aches, sore throat, and sudden weight gain or swelling. Initially, tuberculosis skin test, radiographs, and ECG should be checked. Blood glucose level, intake and output, BP, serum electrolyte levels, height, and weight should be monitored before and during therapy. Be alert to signs and symptoms of infection caused by reduced immune response, including fever, sore throat, and vague symptoms. The mouth should be assessed daily for signs and symptoms of candidal infection, such as white patches and painful mucous membranes and tongue.

Storage

Store at room temperature. Do not freeze oral solutions.

Administration

Take prednisone without regard to meals; give with food if GI upset occurs. Take single doses before 9:00 AM; give multiple doses at evenly spaced intervals. Do not abruptly discontinue prednisone without physician approval.

Pregabalin

pre-gab′a-lyn

Lyrica

Do not confuse Lyrica with Cymbalta or pregabalin with gabapentin.

CATEGORY AND SCHEDULE

Pregnancy Risk Category: C

Controlled Substance Schedule: V

Classification: Neurologic agents, anticonvulsant

MECHANISM OF ACTION

Exact mechanism of pregabalin's antinociceptive and antiseizure action is unknown. Effects may be related to high-affinity binding to α_2-delta site, an auxiliary subunit of voltage-gated calcium channels in CNS tissue. *Therapeutic Effect:* Alleviation of fibromyalgia, postherpetic neuralgia, and partial-onset seizure symptoms.

PHARMACOLOGY

Well absorbed after oral administration; bioavailability is more than 90%. Steady state achieved within 24-48 h. Distributed across the blood-brain barrier; negligible metabolism. Largely eliminated through renal excretion, 90% unchanged. *Half-life:* 6 h. In renal impairment, clearance is proportional to CrCl.

AVAILABILITY

Capsules: 25 mg, 50 mg, 75 mg, 100 mg, 150 mg, 200 mg, 225 mg, 300 mg.

INDICATIONS AND DOSAGES

▸ **Neuropathic pain associated with diabetic peripheral neuropathy**

PO

Adults, Elderly. Initially, 50 mg 3 times/day increasing to 100 mg 3 times/day within 1 wk based on efficacy and tolerability. Do not exceed 300 mg/day.

▸ **Partial-onset seizures**

PO

Adults, Elderly. Initially, 75 mg 2 times/day or 50 mg 3 times/day increased to a maximum dose of 300 mg 2 times/day or 200 mg 3 times/day.

▸ **Postherpetic neuralgia**

PO

Adults, Elderly. Initially, 75 mg 2 times/day or 50 mg 3 times/day, increasing to 300 mg/day within 1 wk based on efficacy and tolerability. Dosage may be increased to 300 mg 2 times/day or 200 mg 3 times/day not to exceed 600 mg/day.

▸ **Fibromyalgia**

PO

Adults, Elderly. Initially, 75 mg 2 times/day increasing to 150 mg 2 times/day within 1 wk based on efficacy and tolerability. May further increase dose to 225 mg 2 times/day not to exceed 450 mg/day.

▸ **Dosage adjustment for renal function impairment adults**

PO

CrCl 30-60 mL/min: 75-300 mg/day PO given in 2 or 3 divided doses.
CrCl 15-30 mL/min: 25-150 mg/day PO given in 1 or 2 divided doses.
CrCl < 15 mL/min: 25-75 mg PO once daily.

▸ **Treatment for patients on hemodialysis**

PO

Adults, Elderly. Maintenance based on CrCl as recommended plus supplemental posthemodialysis dose administered after each 4 h of hemodialysis as follows:
If maintenance dose is 25 mg/day, postdialysis dose is 25-50 mg.
If maintenance dose is 25-50 mg/day, postdialysis dose is 50-75 mg.
If maintenance dose is 50-75 mg/day, postdialysis dose is 75-100 mg.
If maintenance dose is 75 mg/day, postdialysis dose is 100-150 mg.

OFF-LABEL USES

Treatment of generalized anxiety disorder.

CONTRAINDICATIONS

Alcohol, hypersensitivity to pregabalin or any of its components.

INTERACTIONS

Drug

ACE inhibitors: May increase risk of angioedema.
All CNS depressants, alcohol, lorazepam, oxycodone, and other opiates: May have additive cognitive and gross motor function effects; may increase CNS depressant effects.
Immunosuppressants: May increase risk of infection developing.
Thiazolidinedione antidiabetic agents: May cause peripheral edema; use caution in concurrent use.

Herbal

None known.

Food

Alcohol: Increases sedative effects.

DIAGNOSTIC TEST EFFECTS

May increase creatinine kinase levels; significant decreases in platelet counts (20% below baseline or < 150×10^3/mcL) have been documented in about 2-3% of patients. PR interval of the ECG may be prolonged by about 3-6 msec.

SIDE EFFECTS

Frequent

Dizziness, somnolence, ataxia, headache, tremor, blurred vision, peripheral edema, weight gain.

Occasional
Abnormal gait, fatigue, asthenia, confusion, euphoria, increased appetite, speech disorder, vertigo, myoclonus, anxiety, depression, disorientation, lethargy, nervousness, dry mouth, constipation, increased appetite, GI effects.
Other
Reductions in visual acuity, visual field changes, and funduscopic changes are sometimes noted.

SERIOUS REACTIONS

- Unexplained muscle pain, tenderness, weakness, especially if accompanied by general body discomfort or fever.
- A severe hypersensitivity reaction, including anaphylaxis, occurs rarely.

PRECAUTIONS & CONSIDERATIONS

No gender- or race-related precautions have been noted.

It is unknown whether pregabalin crosses the placenta or is excreted in breast milk; caution in pregnancy and lactation is warranted. Many anticonvulsants can cause fetal harm. Males should also use adequate contraception, as male-mediated teratogenicity may occur. Safety and efficacy are not established in children. Because of possible renal function impairment, dosage adjustment may be needed in the elderly. Caution warranted in patients with New York Heart Association class III or IV cardiac status.

Drug may cause drowsiness and dizziness; use caution when driving or performing other activities that require mental or physical acuity.

Symptoms of unexplained muscle pain, tenderness, or weakness, especially if accompanied by general body discomfort or fever, should be reported immediately.

Storage
Store at room temperature.
Administration
Drug may be taken without regard to food; however, if GI effects occur, it can be taken with a meal. Advise the patient to take medication as directed; if medication needs to be discontinued, it should be tapered over a 1-wk period unless safety concerns (hypersensitivity, rash) dictate a more rapid withdrawal. Patients taking antiepileptic medications should continue to take these medications unless otherwise advised by their healthcare practitioner.

Primaquine

prim′a-kween
Do not confuse with primidone.

CATEGORY AND SCHEDULE

Pregnancy Risk Category: C

Classification: Antiprotozoals

MECHANISM OF ACTION

An antimalarial and antirheumatic that eliminates tissue exoerythrocytic forms of *Plasmodium falciparum*. Disrupts mitochondria and binds to DNA. *Therapeutic Effect:* Inhibits parasite growth.

PHARMACOKINETICS

Well absorbed. Metabolized in the liver to the active metabolite, carboxyprimaquine. Excreted in the urine in small amounts as unchanged drug. *Half-life:* 4-6 h.

AVAILABILITY

Tablets: 26.3 mg (primaquine phosphate).

P

INDICATIONS AND DOSAGES

▸ **Treatment of malaria (caused by *Plasmodium vivax*)**

PO

Adults, Elderly. 15-mg base daily for 14 days.

Children. 0.5-0.6 mg base/kg/day once daily for 14 days.

▸ **Malaria prophylaxis (off-label use)**

Adults, Elderly. 30-mg base daily. Begin 1 day before departure and continue for 7 days after leaving malarious area.

OFF-LABEL USES

With clindamycin in treatment of *Pneumocystis carinii* in AIDS.

CONTRAINDICATIONS

Concomitant medications that cause bone marrow suppression, rheumatoid arthritis, lupus erythematosus, glucose-6-phosphate dehydrogenase (G6PD) deficiency, pregnancy, hypersensitivity to primaquine or any of its components.

Use with quinacrine or recent use of quinacrine.

INTERACTIONS

Drug

Aurothioglucose: May increase risk of blood dyscrasias.

Levomethadyl: May increase risk of cardiotoxicity (QT prolongation, torsades de pointes, cardiac arrest).

Quinacrine: Potentiates toxicities of primaquine; contraindicated for use together.

Herbal

None known.

Food

Grapefruit juice: May increase primaquine exposure; avoid if possible.

DIAGNOSTIC TEST EFFECTS

None known.

SIDE EFFECTS

Frequent

Abdominal pain, nausea, vomiting.

Rare

Leukopenia, hemolytic anemia, methemoglobinemia.

SERIOUS REACTIONS

- Leukopenia, hemolytic anemia, methemoglobinemia occur rarely.
- Overdosage includes symptoms of abdominal cramps, vomiting, burning epigastric distress, central nervous system and cardiovascular disturbances, cyanosis, methemoglobinemia, moderate leukocytosis or leukopenia, and anemia.
- Acute hemolysis occurs, but patients recover completely if the dosage is discontinued.

PRECAUTIONS & CONSIDERATIONS

Caution is warranted with erythrocytic G6PD deficiency or nicotinamide adenine dinucleotide (NADH) methemoglobin reductase deficiency, a family personal history of favism, and a previous idiosyncrasy to primaquine phosphate (as manifested by hemolytic anemia, methemoglobinemia, or leukopenia). Primaquine crosses the placenta, but it is unknown whether it is distributed in breast milk. In general, primaquine use is avoided during pregnancy. Children are especially susceptible to primaquine's fatal effects.

Signs suggestive of hemolytic anemia such as darkening of urine, marked fall of hemoglobin or erythrocytic count, should be reported and primaquine should be discontinued promptly.

Storage

Store at room temperature.

P

Administration
26.3 mg primaquine = 15 mg base. The adult dose of 1 tablet (15 mg base) daily for 14 days should not be exceeded. Take dose with food.

Primidone

pri′mi-done
★ Mysoline
Do not confuse primidone with prednisone.

CATEGORY AND SCHEDULE

Pregnancy Risk Category: D

Classification: Anticonvulsant, barbiturate derivative

MECHANISM OF ACTION

A barbiturate that decreases motor activity from electrical and chemical stimulation and stabilizes the seizure threshold against hyperexcitability. *Therapeutic Effect:* Reduces seizure activity.

PHARMACOKINETICS

Extensive distribution after oral administration. Metabolism of primidone in the liver produces phenobarbital (15%-25%) and PEMA. Phenobarbital and primidone induce hepatic enzymes (e.g., UGT, CYP2C, CYP3A, and CYP1A2). Excretion is primarily renal, roughly 40%-60% as primidone, with smaller amounts as PEMA and phenobarbital. Phenobarbital is inactivated by the liver before renal excretion of the metabolites. *Half-life:* 10-12 h (primidone), 53-118 h (phenobarbital).

AVAILABILITY

Tablets: 50 mg, 250 mg.

INDICATIONS AND DOSAGES

▸ **Seizure control (general tonic-clonic [grand mal], complex partial psychomotor seizures)**

PO

Adults, Elderly, Children 8 yr and older. 125-250 mg/day at bedtime. May increase by 125-250 mg/day every 3-7 days. Maximum: 2 g/day.
Children younger than 8 yr. Initially, 50-125 mg/day at bedtime. May increase by 50-125 mg/day every 3-7 days. Usual dose: 10-25 mg/kg/day in divided doses. Maximum: 1 g/day.
Neonates. 12-20 mg/kg/day in divided doses.

OFF-LABEL USES

Treatment of essential tremor.

CONTRAINDICATIONS

Porphyria, hypersensitivity to primidone or phenobarbital.

INTERACTIONS

Drug

NOTE: Primidone and metabolites induce the metabolism of many important drugs.
Acetaminophen, corticosteroids: May decrease effects of these drugs.
Alcohol, other central nervous system (CNS) depressants: May increase the effects of primidone.
Antiretroviral protease inhibitors: May decrease PI blood concentrations, leading to loss of antiviral effect against HIV.
Carbamazepine: May increase the metabolism of carbamazepine causing lower blood concentration.
Digoxin, glucocorticoids, metronidazole, quinidine, tricyclic antidepressants: May decrease the effects of these drugs.
Halothane, halogenated hydrocarbon inhalation anesthetics, haloperidol, phenothiazines: May cause

increased metabolism and hepatotoxicity.
Hormonal contraceptives: May decrease blood concentrations, leading to loss of contraceptive efficacy. Higher-dose regimens or alternative or additional methods may be needed.
Phenobarbital: May raise serum levels and risk of toxicity.
Phenytoin: Variable effects on serum concentrations; monitor closely.
Theophylline: May reduce theophylline concentrations.
Valproic acid: Increases the blood concentration and risk of toxicity of primidone.
Warfarin: May reduce anticoagulant effect. Monitor INR.

Herbal
None known.

Food
None known.

DIAGNOSTIC TEST EFFECTS

May decrease serum bilirubin level. Therapeutic serum level is 5-12 mcg/mL; toxic serum level is > 12 mcg/mL.

SIDE EFFECTS

Frequent
Ataxia, dizziness.

Occasional
Anorexia, drowsiness, mental changes, nausea, vomiting, paradoxical excitement.

Rare
Rash.

SERIOUS REACTIONS

- Abrupt withdrawal after prolonged therapy may produce effects ranging from increased dreaming, nightmares, insomnia, tremor, diaphoresis, and vomiting to hallucinations, delirium, seizures, and status epilepticus.
- Skin eruptions or mouth sores may be a sign of a hypersensitivity reaction.
- Blood dyscrasias, hepatic disease, or hypocalcemia occur rarely.
- Overdose produces cold or clammy skin, hypothermia, and severe CNS depression, followed by high fever and coma.

PRECAUTIONS & CONSIDERATIONS

Caution is warranted in patients with hepatic and renal impairment. Antiepileptic drugs (AEDs) may increase the risk of suicidal thoughts or behavior in patients taking these drugs for any indication. Monitor for the emergence or worsening of depression, suicidal thoughts, and any unusual changes in mood or behavior. Primidone and metabolites readily cross the placenta and are distributed in breast milk. May cause fetal harm during pregnancy. Produces respiratory depression in neonates during labor, and may increase the risk of maternal bleeding and neonatal hemorrhage during delivery. Neonates may also experience withdrawal symptoms. Primidone use may cause paradoxical excitement in children. Elderly patients may exhibit confusion, excitement, and mental depression.

Dizziness may occur, so change positions slowly—from recumbent to sitting position before standing. Alcohol and tasks requiring mental alertness or motor skills should be avoided. CBC, neurologic status (including duration, frequency, and severity of seizures), and serum concentrations of primidone should be assessed before and during treatment.

Storage
Store at room temperature in a well-closed container protected from light.

Administration
Administer primidone at the same time each day. Do not abruptly discontinue primidone after long-term use because this may precipitate seizures. Strict maintenance of drug therapy is essential for seizure control. May take with food. For patients with difficulty swallowing, the tablets may be crushed and mixed with foods or fluids prior to administration.

Probenecid

proe-ben′e-sid
★ 🍁 Benuryl
Do not confuse probenecid with procainamide.

CATEGORY AND SCHEDULE
Pregnancy Risk Category: C

Classification: Antigout agents, uricosurics

MECHANISM OF ACTION
A uricosuric that competitively inhibits reabsorption of uric acid at the proximal convoluted tubule. Also inhibits renal tubular secretion of weak organic acids, such as penicillins. *Therapeutic Effect:* Promotes uric acid excretion, reduces serum uric acid level, and increases plasma levels of penicillins and cephalosporins.

AVAILABILITY
Tablets: 500 mg.

INDICATIONS AND DOSAGES
▸ **Gout**
PO
Adults, Elderly. Initially, 250 mg twice a day for 1 wk; then 500 mg twice a day. May increase by 500 mg q4wk. Maximum: 2 g/day. Maintenance: Dosage that maintains normal uric acid level.

▸ **As an adjunct to penicillin or cephalosporin therapy to prolong antibiotic plasma levels**
PO
Adults, Elderly. 2 g/day in divided doses.
Children weighing >50 kg. Receive adult dosage.
Children aged 2-14 yr. Initially, 25 mg/kg. Maintenance: 40 mg/kg/day in 4 divided doses.

▸ **Gonorrhea**
PO
Adults, Elderly. 1 g 30 min before procaine, penicillin G, ampicillin, amoxicillin, or cefoxitin.

CONTRAINDICATIONS
Hypersensitivity to probenecid, children under 2 yr of age, known blood dyscrasias, uric acid kidney stones. Not recommended in severe renal impairment as efficacy is lost due to mechanism of action. Do not use probenecid until an acute gouty attack has subsided. Use of salicylates is contraindicated because they antagonize the uricosuric action of probenecid.

INTERACTIONS
Drug
Alcohol, salicylates and pyrazinamide: May increase serum urate level, decrease uricosuric activity. Salicylates are contraindicated, no matter if low or high dose.
Antineoplastics: May increase the risk of uric acid nephropathy. May prolong the levels of cisplatin.
Cephalosporins and penicillins: Increased levels and prolongation of antibiotics used for therapeutic

effect. Monitor for CNS reactions.
Heparin: May increase and prolong the effects of heparin.
Ketorolac, other NSAIDs: May result in increased toxicity. Do not use ketorolac with probenecid due to bleeding risk if levels increase.
Methotrexate: Increases plasma concentrations of methotrexate and toxicity risk. Reduce dose of methotrexate and monitor serum levels.
Sulfonamides: Significant increase in total sulfonamide plasma levels and decreases the renal excretion of conjugated sulfonamides.
Sulfonylureas: Reduced clearance and increased antidiabetic effects; may require dose reduction.
Thiopental, ketamine: Prolongs anesthetic effects.
Topiramate: May alter topiramate concentrations and efficacy.
Zalcitabine: May increase antiviral concentrations and toxicity; may need reduced dose.

Herbal
None known.

Food
None known.

DIAGNOSTIC TEST EFFECTS

Falsely high readings for theophylline using the Schack and Waxler technique on human plasma. Also, a reducing substance may appear in the urine and will disappear on discontinuation. Suspected glycosuria should be confirmed by using a test specific for glucose.

SIDE EFFECTS

Frequent (6%-10%)
Headache, anorexia, nausea, vomiting.

Occasional (1%-5%)
Lower back or side pain, rash, hives, itching, dizziness, flushed face, frequent urge to urinate, gingivitis.

SERIOUS REACTIONS

- Severe hypersensitivity reactions, including anaphylaxis, occur rarely and usually within a few hours after administration following previous use. If severe hypersensitivity reactions develop, discontinue the drug immediately and contact the physician.
- Pruritic maculopapular rash, possibly accompanied by malaise, fever, chills, arthralgia, nausea, vomiting, leukopenia, and aplastic anemias, should be considered a toxic reaction.

PRECAUTIONS & CONSIDERATIONS

Caution is warranted in patients with hematuria, peptic ulcer disease, and renal colic. Avoid alcohol and large doses of aspirin or other salicylates. Limit intake of high purine foods, such as fish and organ meats.

High fluid intake (3000 mL/day) should be encouraged; intake and output should be monitored; output should be at least 2000 mL/day. CBC, serum uric acid level, and urine for cloudiness, odor, and unusual color should also be monitored. Signs and symptoms of a therapeutic response, including improved joint range of motion and reduced joint tenderness, redness, and swelling, should be evaluated.

Storage
Store at room temperature.

Administration
! Do not start giving probenecid until acute gouty attack has subsided; continue drug if acute attack occurs during therapy.

Give probenecid orally with or immediately after meals or milk.

Drink at least 6-8 eight-oz. glasses of fluid each day to prevent renal calculi. Some patients will receive alkalization of the urine concurrently (e.g., potassium citrate) to limit nephropathy. It may take more than 1 wk for the full therapeutic effect of the drug to be evident.

Procainamide Hydrochloride

proe-kane'a-mide

Procan SR

Do not confuse procainamide with procaine.

CATEGORY AND SCHEDULE

Pregnancy Risk Category: C

Classification: Antiarrhythmics, Group IA

MECHANISM OF ACTION

Increases the effective refractory period of atria, bundle of His-Purkinje system and ventricles of the heart. *Therapeutic Effect:* Reduces conduction velocity in the atria and resolves ventricular arrhythmia.

PHARMACOKINETICS

IV administration produces therapeutic level within minutes. Distributes widely throughout the body. Protein binding: 15%-20%. Undergoes acetylation in the liver to N-acetylprocainamide (NAPA), which is also cardioactive. Metabolic clearance is greater in patients who are rapid acetylators. Significant amounts of both unchanged procainamide and N-acetylprocainamide (NAPA) are eliminated renally by glomerular filtration and active tubular secretion. Removed by hemodialysis. *Half-life:* 3 h (increased in congestive heart failure, hepatic impairment, and renal dysfunction).

AVAILABILITY

Injection Solution: 100 mg/mL, 500 mg/mL.

INDICATIONS AND DOSAGES

▸ **Treat ventricular arrhythmias**

IV

Adults. 15-17 mg/kg at a rate or 20-30 mg/min load. Or 100 mg IV q5min by slow IV push until arrhythmia resolves, up to 1000 mg.

Children. 3-6 mg/kg over 5 min. Do not exceed 100 mg as a single dose. May repeat q5-10min to a maximum dose of 15 mg/kg.

IV INCOMPATIBILITIES

Include acyclovir, ceftizoxime, diazepam, hydralazine, imipenem-cilastatin (Primaxin), lansoprazole (Prevacid), metronidazole (Flagyl), milrinone, phenytoin.

CONTRAINDICATIONS

Complete heart block due to possible asystole, idiosyncratic hypersensitivity to procainamide or sulfites, lupus erythromatosus, torsades de pointes.

Contraindicated for use with many medications, including but not limited to, cisapride, dofetilide, dronedarone, pimozide, propafenone, saquinavir boosted with ritonavir, thioridazine, due to proarrhythmic effects.

INTERACTIONS

Drug

Astemizole, cisapride, dofetilide, phenothiazines, type 5 photodiesterase inhibitors (e.g., sildenafil, vardenafil), terfenadine, ziprasidone, and other drugs that increase QT interval: Many are contraindicated

P

for concurrent use. May cause potent vasodilation, increased irregular heartbeat, and increased side effects.
Cimetidine, ranitidine, trimethoprim: Reduce tubular secretion of procainamide and NAPA.
Diltiazem, verapamil: Additive effects on heart conduction.
Macrolide antibiotics (erythromycin, clarithromycin, azithromycin), ketolide antibiotics (telithromycin): May increase side effects and risk of irregular heartbeat.
Quinidine: Additive effects on heart conduction; quinidine raises procainamide concentrations.
Succinylcholine and neuromuscular blockers: Potential for prolonged neuromuscular blockade.
Herbal
None known.
Food
None known.

P

DIAGNOSTIC TEST EFFECTS

Therapeutic serum level is up to 10 mcg/mL; toxic serum level is >12 mcg/mL. Monitoring of NAPA levels is indicated with impaired renal function. Do not exceed combined total concentrations of 25 mcg/mL (NAPA + PA). May cause positive antinuclear antibody (ANA) test. Elevated liver enzymes, alkaline phosphatase (ALT, SGOT), and bilirubin.

SIDE EFFECTS

Frequent
Ataxia, dizziness. GI effects also common (anorexia, nausea, vomiting, abdominal pain, diarrhea, or bitter taste).
Occasional
Dizziness, giddiness, weakness, mental depression, psychosis with hallucinations.
Rare
Neutropenia, thrombocytopenia, hemolytic anemia.

SERIOUS REACTIONS

- Neutropenia, thrombocytopenia, and hemolytic anemia may develop over time; usually reverses upon discontinuation of drug therapy.
- Skin eruptions may be a sign of a hypersensitivity reaction.
- Blood dyscrasias, hepatic disease, and hypocalcemia occur rarely.
- Particularly with IV administration, proarrhythmia, QT prolongation, AV block, and torsades de pointes. Watch for excessive hypotension.
- Lupus-like syndrome.

PRECAUTIONS & CONSIDERATIONS

Caution is warranted in patients with myasthenia gravis, bundle-branch block, congestive heart failure (CHF), liver and renal impairment, marked AV-conduction disturbances, severe digoxin toxicity, and supraventricular tachyarrhythmias. Be aware that procainamide crosses the placenta and that procainamide is distributed in breast milk. No age-related precautions have been noted in children. Elderly patients are more susceptible to the drug's hypotensive effect. In elderly patients, age-related renal impairment may require dosage adjustment.

GI upset, headache, dizziness, and joint pain may occur. Notify the physician if fever, joint pain or stiffness, and signs of upper respiratory infection occur. ECG for cardiac changes, particularly widening of QRS and prolongation of PR and QT intervals, should be monitored. Pulse, pattern of daily bowel activity and stool consistency, skin for hypertensive reaction, intake and output, serum electrolyte levels, and BP should be assessed during therapy.

Driving, operating machinery, and engaging in exercises requiring mental acuity or alertness should be avoided until the patient knows how he/she reacts to the drug.

Most hematologic events occur during the first 12 wks of therapy; monitor CBC at weekly intervals for the first 3 mo of therapy, and periodically thereafter. Report any signs of infection (such as fever, chills, sore throat, or stomatitis), bruising, or bleeding. Blood counts usually return to normal within 1 mo of discontinuation.

Storage

Store unopened vials at room temperature.

When diluted with D5W, solution is stable for up to 24 h at room temperature or for 7 days if refrigerated. Solutions darker than light amber in color should be discarded.

Administration:

! Know that procainamide dosage and the interval of administration are individualized based on age, clinical response, renal function, and underlying myocardial disease.

May give procainamide by IM injection, IV push, or IV infusion. IM injection may be painful and is rarely used. For IV push, dilute with 5-10 mL D5W. For IV push, with patient in the supine position, administer at a rate not exceeding 25-50 mg/min. For initial loading IV infusion, add 1 g to 50 mL D5W to provide a concentration of 20 mg/mL. For IV infusion, add 1 g to 250-500 mL D5W to provide concentration of 2-4 mg/mL. Know that the maximum concentration is 4 g/250 mL. For initial loading infusion, infuse 1 mL/min for up to 25-30 min. For maintenance IV infusion, infuse at 2-6 mg/min. If a fall in BP exceeds 15 mm Hg, discontinue drug and contact physician. Continuously monitor BP and ECG during IV administration.

Procarbazine Hydrochloride

pro-kar'ba-zeen

★ ✿ Matulane

Do not confuse procarbazine with dacarbazine.

CATEGORY AND SCHEDULE

Pregnancy Risk Category: D

Classification: Antineoplastics, alkylating agents

MECHANISM OF ACTION

A methylhydrazine derivative that inhibits DNA, RNA, and protein synthesis. May also directly damage DNA. Cell cycle-phase specific for S phase of cell division. Has weak MAO-inhibiting activity. *Therapeutic Effect:* Causes cell death.

PHARMACOKINETICS

PO: Peak levels 1 h; concentrates in liver, kidney, skin; metabolized in liver, excreted in urine.

AVAILABILITY

Capsules: 50 mg.

INDICATIONS AND DOSAGES

▸ **Advanced Hodgkin disease**

PO

Adults, Elderly. Initially, 2-4 mg/kg/day as a single dose or in divided doses for 1 wk, then 4-6 mg/kg/day. Continue until maximum response occurs, leukocyte

count falls below 4000/mm^3, or platelet count falls below 100,000/mm^3.
Maintenance: 1-2 mg/kg/day.
Children. 50-100 mg/m^2/day for 10-14 days of a 28-day cycle.
Maintenance: 50 mg/m^2/day.

OFF-LABEL USES

Treatment of lung carcinoma, malignant melanoma, multiple myeloma, non-Hodgkin lymphoma, polycythemia vera, primary brain tumors.

CONTRAINDICATIONS

Known hypersensitivity to the drug. Myelosuppression, breastfeeding, MAOI therapy.

INTERACTIONS

Drug

Alcohol: May cause a disulfiram-like reaction.

Antihistamines, barbiturates, narcotics: May increase CNS depressive effects.

Bone marrow depressants: May increase myelosuppression.

Insulin, oral antidiabetics: May increase the effects of these drugs.

Linezolid, other MAOIs, sympathomimetic drugs, tricyclic antidepressants: Should be avoided due to the MAO-inhibiting activity of procarbazine; could result in significant hypertension, or tyramine, pressor, or serotonin-type reactions.

Herbal

Tobacco: Use associated with a risk of secondary lung cancer. Stop smoking.

Food

Foods with high tyramine content (e.g., wine, yogurt, ripe cheese, and bananas), as well as excessive caffeine: Avoid and limit due to potential MAOI activity of procarbazine.

P

DIAGNOSTIC TEST EFFECTS

Decreased WBC, platelets, RBC indices.

SIDE EFFECTS

Frequent

Severe nausea, vomiting, respiratory disorders (cough, effusion), myalgia, arthralgia, drowsiness, nervousness, insomnia, nightmares, diaphoresis, hallucinations, seizures.

Occasional

Hoarseness, tachycardia, nystagmus, retinal hemorrhage, photophobia, photosensitivity, urinary frequency, nocturia, hypotension, diarrhea, stomatitis, paresthesia, unsteadiness, confusion, decreased reflexes, foot drop. Azoospermia and infertility.

Rare

Hypersensitivity reaction (dermatitis, pruritus, rash, urticaria), hyperpigmentation, alopecia.

SERIOUS REACTIONS

- Procarbazine's major toxic effects are myelosuppression manifested as hematologic toxicity (mainly leukopenia, thrombocytopenia, and anemia) and hepatotoxicity manifested as jaundice and ascites.
- Infections may occur secondary to leukopenia.
- Bleeding (e.g., purpura, petechiae, epistaxis, hemoptysis).

PRECAUTIONS & CONSIDERATIONS

Caution is warranted in patients with hepatic and renal impairment. Alcohol should be avoided. Procarbazine is a known teratogen and carcinogen and should not be used during pregnancy or breastfeeding.

Caution is warranted if general anesthesia or sedation is required because of the increased risk for hypotensive episode.

Notify the physician if bleeding, easy bruising, fever, or sore throat occurs. CBC with differential, bone marrow test, urinalysis, BUN level, and LFTs should be monitored periodically. Good oral hygiene should be practiced. Procarbazine should be discontinued if stomatitis, diarrhea, paresthesia, neuropathy, confusion, or a hypersensitivity reaction occurs.

Storage
Store at room temperature.

Administration
Administer procarbazine with food or fluids if the patient has severe GI side effects or difficulty swallowing.

Prochlorperazine

proe-klor-per'a-zeen

Compazine, Compro

Nu-Prochlor

Do not confuse prochlorperazine with chlorpromazine, or Compazine with Copaxone.

CATEGORY AND SCHEDULE

Pregnancy Risk Category: C

Classification: Antiemetics, phenothiazines

MECHANISM OF ACTION

A phenothiazine that acts centrally to inhibit or block dopamine receptors in the chemoreceptor trigger zone and peripherally to block the vagus nerve in the GI tract. *Therapeutic Effect:* Relieves nausea and vomiting and improves psychotic conditions.

PHARMACOKINETICS

Route	Onset* (min)	Peak	Duration (h)
Tablets, oral solution	30-40	NA	3-4
Capsules (extended release)	30-40	NA	10-12
Rectal	60	NA	3-4

*As an antiemetic.

Variably absorbed after PO administration. Widely distributed. Metabolized in the liver and GI mucosa. Excreted primarily in urine. Unknown whether removed by hemodialysis. *Half-life:* 23 h.

AVAILABILITY

Tablets: 5 mg, 10 mg.
Suppositories (Compro): 25 mg.
Injection: 5 mg/mL.

INDICATIONS AND DOSAGES

▸ **Nausea and vomiting**

PO

Adults, Elderly. 5-10 mg 3-4 times a day.
Children weighing 18-39 kg. 2.5 mg 3 times/day or 5 mg 2 times/day.
Children weighing 14-17 kg. 2.5 mg 2-3 times/day.
Children weighing 9-13 kg. 2.5 mg 1-2 times/day.

IM or IV

Adults, Elderly. 5-10 mg. May repeat q3-4h.
Children. 0.132 mg/kg/dose q6-8h.

RECTAL

Adults, Elderly. 25 mg twice a day.

▸ **Psychosis**

PO

Adults, Elderly. 5-10 mg 3-4 times a day. Maximum: 150 mg/day.
Children. 2.5 mg 2-3 times a day. Maximum: 25 mg for children aged 6-12 yr; 20 mg for children aged 2-5 yr.

P

CONTRAINDICATIONS

Hypersensitivity to phenothiazines. Do not use in comatose states or in the presence of large amounts of CNS depressants (alcohol, barbiturates, narcotics, etc.). Do not use in children < 2 yr or < 9 kg, or during pediatric surgery.

INTERACTIONS

Drug

Alcohol, other CNS depressants, barbiturate anesthetics, opioid analgesics: May increase CNS and respiratory depression and the hypotensive effects of prochlorperazine.
Anticholinergics: May increase anticholinergic effects.
Antihypertensives: May increase hypotension.
Antithyroid agents: May increase the risk of agranulocytosis.
Epinephrine: Possible risk of hypotension, tachycardia.
Levodopa: May decrease the effects of levodopa.
Lithium: May decrease the absorption of prochlorperazine and produce adverse neurologic effects.
MAOIs, tricyclic antidepressants: May increase the anticholinergic and sedative effects of prochlorperazine.
Phenothiazines and related drugs (haloperidol, droperidol), metoclopramide: May increase extrapyramidal symptoms.
Tetracyclines: Possible additive photosensitization.

Herbal

None known.

Food

None known.

DIAGNOSTIC TEST EFFECTS

May elevate prolactin levels. May cause false-positive phenylketonuria (PKU) test results.

IV INCOMPATIBILITIES

Manufacturer recommends that drug not be mixed with other agents in the syringe. For IV infusion, the drug is incompatible with many drugs; refer to specialty references to check compatibilities.

SIDE EFFECTS

Frequent

Somnolence, hypotension, dizziness, fainting (commonly occurring after first dose, occasionally after subsequent doses, and rarely with oral form).

Occasional

Dry mouth, blurred vision, lethargy, constipation, diarrhea, myalgia, nasal congestion, peripheral edema, urine retention.

SERIOUS REACTIONS

- Extrapyramidal symptoms appear to be dose-related and are divided into three categories: akathisia (marked by inability to sit still, tapping of feet), parkinsonian symptoms (including mask-like face, tremors, shuffling gait, hypersalivation), and acute dystonias (such as torticollis, opisthotonos, and oculogyric crisis). A dystonic reaction may also produce diaphoresis or pallor.
- Tardive dyskinesia, manifested as tongue protrusion, puffing of the cheeks, and puckering of the mouth, is a rare reaction that may be irreversible.
- Abrupt withdrawal after long-term therapy may precipitate nausea, vomiting, gastritis, dizziness, and tremors.
- Blood dyscrasias, particularly agranulocytosis and mild leukopenia, may occur.
- Prochlorperazine use may lower the seizure threshold.

PRECAUTIONS & CONSIDERATIONS

Caution is warranted in patients with Parkinson disease or seizures.

Prochlorperazine crosses the placenta and is distributed in breast milk. The safety and efficacy of this drug have not been established in children younger than 2 yr or weighing < 9 kg. A decreased prochlorperazine dosage is recommended for elderly patients, who are more susceptible to the drug's sedative, anticholinergic, extrapyramidal, and hypotensive effects. Alcohol, barbiturates, and tasks that require mental alertness or motor skills should be avoided until the drug's effects are known. Orthostatic hypotension may occur; avoid rapid postural changes.

BP, CBC for blood dyscrasias, and hydration status should be monitored. Be alert for extrapyramidal symptoms such as rapid tongue movement.

Signs of tardive dyskinesia or akathisia need to be immediately reported to the health care provider.

Storage

Store prochlorperazine at room temperature and protect from light. Solution should be clear or slightly yellow. Store tablets at room temperature. Store suppositories in a cool place at room temperature.

Administration

Take oral prochlorperazine without regard to food. Avoid skin contact with prochlorperazine oral solution because it may cause contact dermatitis.

For IV use, keep the person recumbent—head low and legs raised—for 30-60 min after drug administration to minimize the drug's hypotensive effect. May give by IV push slowly over 5-10 min. May give by IV infusion over 30 min after proper dilution in 0.9% NaCl injection. IM injection should be made deeply into the dorsogluteal muscle.

For rectal use, moisten the suppository with cold water before inserting it well into the rectum.

Progesterone

proe-jess'ter-one

★ Crinone, Endometrin, First-Progesterone VGS, Prochieve, Prometrium 🍁 Crinone, Evometrin, Prometrium

CATEGORY AND SCHEDULE

Pregnancy Risk Category: D

Classification: Hormones, progestins, fertility agents

MECHANISM OF ACTION

A natural steroid hormone that promotes mammary gland development and relaxes uterine smooth muscle. *Therapeutic Effect:* Decreases abnormal uterine bleeding; transforms endometrium from proliferative to secretory in an estrogen-primed endometrium, supports early pregnancy during reproductive assistance.

PHARMACOKINETICS

IM, rectal, vaginal: Duration 24 h; excreted in urine, feces; metabolized in liver.

AVAILABILITY

Capsules (Prometrium): 100 mg, 200 mg.
Injection in Oil: 50 mg/mL.
Vaginal Gel (Crinone, Prochieve): 4% (45 mg), 8% (90 mg).
Vaginal Insert (Endometrin): 100 mg.
Vaginal Suppository (First-Progesterone, Compounded): 25 mg, 100 mg.

P

INDICATIONS AND DOSAGES

▸ Amenorrhea

PO

Adults. 400 mg daily in evening for 10 days.

IM

Adults. 5-10 mg for 6-8 days. Withdrawal bleeding expected in 48-72 h if ovarian activity produced proliferative endometrium.

VAGINAL

Adults. Apply 45 mg (4% gel) every other day for 6 or fewer doses.

▸ Abnormal uterine bleeding

IM

Adults. 5-10 mg for 6 days. When estrogen given concomitantly, begin progesterone after 2 wks of estrogen therapy; discontinue when menstrual flow begins.

▸ Prevention of endometrial hyperplasia

PO

Adults. 200 mg in evening for 12 days per 28-day cycle in combination with daily conjugated estrogen.

▸ Infertility

VAGINAL

Adults. 90 mg (8% gel) once a day (twice a day in women with partial or complete ovarian failure).

OFF-LABEL USES

Premenstrual syndrome, preterm delivery prophylaxis.

CONTRAINDICATIONS

Breast cancer; history of active cerebral apoplexy; thromboembolic disorders or thrombophlebitis; missed abortion; severe hepatic dysfunction; undiagnosed vaginal bleeding; use as a pregnancy test. Assess for allergy to peanuts and sesame seed as some formulations (Prometrium, Injection in Oil) include these oils and should be avoided in hypersensitive individuals.

INTERACTIONS

Drug

Bromocriptine: May interfere with the effects of bromocriptine.

Herbal

None known.

Food

None known.

DIAGNOSTIC TEST EFFECTS

May increase serum LDL and serum alkaline phosphatase levels. May decrease glucose tolerance and HDL concentrations. May cause abnormal serum thyroid, metapyrone, hepatic, and endocrine function test results.

SIDE EFFECTS

Frequent

Breakthrough bleeding or spotting at beginning of therapy, amenorrhea, change in menstrual flow, breast tenderness.

Gel: drowsiness.

Occasional

Edema, weight gain or loss, rash, pruritus, photosensitivity, skin pigmentation.

Rare

Pain or swelling at injection site, acne, depression, alopecia, hirsutism.

SERIOUS REACTIONS

• Thrombophlebitis, cerebrovascular disorders, retinal thrombosis, and pulmonary embolism occur rarely.

PRECAUTIONS & CONSIDERATIONS

Caution is warranted in patients with conditions aggravated by fluid retention, diabetes mellitus, and history of depression. Use with caution in those with a history of hormonally responsive cancers. Progesterone use should be avoided during pregnancy. Progesterone is distributed in breast milk. Safety and efficacy of progesterone have not been established in children. No age-related precautions have been noted in elderly patients. Women using progesterone vaginal gel form should avoid performing tasks that require mental alertness or motor skills until response to the drug has been established. Use sunscreen and wear protective clothing until tolerance to sunlight and ultraviolet light has been determined. Avoid smoking because of the increased risk of blood clot formation and myocardial infarction (MI). Some patients experience drowsiness; do not drive or perform other tasks requiring mental alertness.

Notify the physician of chest pain, migraine headache, peripheral paresthesia, sudden decrease in vision, sudden shortness of breath, pain, redness, swelling, warmth in the calf, abnormal vaginal bleeding, or other symptoms. BP and weight should be monitored.

Storage

Store progesterone at room temperature. Avoid exposure to high heat.

Administration

Take the daily dose of oral progesterone in the evening to minimize the effects of dizziness and drowsiness. May take with food.

Insert vaginal forms as directed; if patient is at high altitude, there are special instructions for the use of the gel applicators.

Shake vial well before withdrawing dose. Administer deep IM injection only in the upper arm or outer quadrant of gluteal muscle. Rarely, a residual lump, change in skin color, or sterile abscess occurs at the injection site. Rotate injection sites. NEVER give intravenously.

Promethazine Hydrochloride

proe-meth'a-zeen high-droh-clor'ide

★ Phenadoz, Phenergan 🍁 Histanil

Do not confuse promethazine with promazine.

CATEGORY AND SCHEDULE

Pregnancy Risk Category: C

Classification: Antiemetics/antivertigo, antihistamines, H_1 receptor antagonist, phenothiazines

MECHANISM OF ACTION

A phenothiazine that acts as an antihistamine, antiemetic, and sedative-hypnotic. As an antihistamine, inhibits histamine at histamine receptor sites. As an antiemetic, diminishes vestibular stimulation, depresses labyrinth function, and acts on the chemoreceptor trigger zone. As a sedative-hypnotic, produces central nervous system (CNS) depression by decreasing stimulation to the brain stem reticular formation. *Therapeutic Effect:* Prevents allergic responses mediated by histamine, such as rhinitis, urticaria, and pruritus. Prevents and relieves nausea and vomiting.

PHARMACOKINETICS

Route	Onset (min)	Peak	Duration (h)
PO	20	NA	2-8
IV	3-5	NA	2-8
IM	20	NA	2-8
Rectal	20	NA	2-8

Well absorbed from the GI tract after IM administration. Widely distributed. Metabolized in the liver. Excreted primarily in urine. Not removed by hemodialysis. *Half-life:* 16-19 h.

P

AVAILABILITY

Syrup: 6.25 mg/mL.
Tablets: 12.5 mg, 25 mg, 50 mg.
Injection: 25 mg/mL, 50 mg/mL.
Suppositories: 12.5 mg, 25 mg, 50 mg.
Suppositories (Phenadoz): 12.5 mg, 25 mg.

INDICATIONS AND DOSAGES

▸ **Allergic symptoms**
PO
Adults, Elderly. 12.5 mg 3 times a day and at bedtime.
Children ≥ 2 yr. 6.25-12.5 mg 3 times/day as needed.
IV, IM
Adults, Elderly. 25 mg. May repeat in 2 h.

▸ **Motion sickness**
PO
Adults, Elderly. 25 mg 30-60 min before departure; may repeat q12h as needed.
Children ≥ 2 yr. 12.5-25 mg twice daily as needed, with first dose given 30-60 min before departure.

P

▸ **Prevention of nausea and vomiting**
PO, IV, IM, RECTAL
Adults, Elderly. 12.5-25 mg q4-6h as needed.
Children ≥ 2 yr. 0.5 mg/lb every 4-6h as needed.

▸ **Preoperative and postoperative sedation; adjunct to analgesics**
IV, IM
Adults, Elderly. 25-50 mg as a single dose.
Children ≥ 2 yr. 0.25-0.5 mg/lb mg as a single dose.

▸ **Sedative**
PO, IV, IM, RECTAL
Adults, Elderly. 25-50 mg at bedtime.
Children ≥ 2 yr. 0.5 mg/lb at bedtime. Maximum: 25 mg/dose.

CONTRAINDICATIONS

Comatose states, hypersensitive or idiosyncratic reaction to promethazine or other phenothiazines. Do not use for lower respiratory tract symptoms of asthma. Not for children < 2 yr of age.

INTERACTIONS

Drug
Alcohol, other CNS depressants: May increase CNS depressant effects.
Anticholinergics: May increase anticholinergic effects.
General anesthetics: May cause hypotensive effects.
MAOIs: May intensify and prolong the anticholinergic and CNS depressant effects of promethazine.
Herbal
None known.
Food
None known.

DIAGNOSTIC TEST EFFECTS

May suppress wheal and flare reactions to antigen skin testing unless the drug is discontinued 4 days before testing.

IV INCOMPATIBILITIES

Allopurinol (Aloprim), amphotericin B complex (Abelcet, AmBisome, Amphotec), most cephalosporins, clindamycin, dexamethasone, diazepam, ertapenem (Invanz), furosemide, heparin, ketorolac (Toradol), lansoprazole (Prevacid), methylprednisolone (Solu-Medrol), nalbuphine (Nubain), pantoprazole (Protonix), phenobarbital, phenytoin, piperacillin and tazobactam (Zosyn), sodium bicarbonate.

IV COMPATIBILITIES

Atropine, diphenhydramine (Benadryl), glycopyrrolate (Robinul), hydromorphone (Dilaudid), hydroxyzine (Vistaril), meperidine (Demerol), midazolam (Versed), morphine, nalbuphine (Nubain), prochlorperazine (Compazine).

SIDE EFFECTS

Expected
Somnolence, disorientation; in elderly, hypotension, confusion, syncope.

Frequent
Dry mouth, nose, or throat; urine retention; thickening of bronchial secretions.

Occasional
Epigastric distress, flushing, visual disturbances, hearing disturbances, wheezing, paresthesia, diaphoresis, chills.

Rare
Dizziness, urticaria, photosensitivity, nightmares.

SERIOUS REACTIONS

• Children may experience paradoxical reactions, such as excitation, nervousness, tremor, hallucinations, hyperactive reflexes, and seizures. Infants and young children have experienced CNS depression manifested as respiratory depression, sleep apnea, and sudden infant death syndrome.
• Long-term therapy may produce extrapyramidal symptoms, such as dystonia (abnormal movements), pronounced motor restlessness (most frequently in children), and parkinsonism (elderly patients).
• Blood dyscrasias, particularly agranulocytosis, occur rarely.
• Cholestatic jaundice is considered a hypersensitivity reaction.

PRECAUTIONS & CONSIDERATIONS

Caution is warranted in patients with asthma, history of seizures, cardiovascular disease, hepatic impairment, sleep apnea, and possible Reye syndrome. Use with caution in narrow-angle glaucoma, prostatic hypertrophy, stenosing peptic ulcer, pyloric obstruction, and bladder-neck obstruction due to anticholinergic effects. Promethazine readily crosses the placenta and may produce extrapyramidal symptoms and jaundice in neonates if taken during pregnancy. It is unknown whether the drug is excreted in breast milk. Children are more likely to experience adverse reactions. Promethazine is not recommended for children younger than 2 yr. Elderly patients are more sensitive to the drug's anticholinergic effects, such as dry mouth, confusion, dizziness, hypotension, syncope, and sedation. Avoid CNS depressants, drinking alcoholic beverages, and tasks that require alertness or motor skills until response to the drug is established.

Drowsiness and dry mouth may occur. Pulse rate, electrolytes, BP, and therapeutic response should be monitored. Assess vital signs 30 min after dosing if used as a sedative.

Storage
Store most products at room temperature. Refrigerate rectal suppositories.

Administration
Take promethazine without regard to food. Crush scored tablets as needed.

For IV use, promethazine may be given undiluted or diluted with 0.9% NaCl; final dilution should not exceed 25 mg/mL. Inject the drug at a rate of 25 mg/min through the tubing of an infusing IV solution, as prescribed. Injecting the drug too rapidly may cause a transient drop in BP, resulting in orthostatic hypotension and reflex tachycardia.

! Avoid giving subcutaneously because significant tissue necrosis may occur. Inject the drug carefully because inadvertent intra-arterial injection may produce severe arteriospasm, possibly resulting in gangrene.

The IM route is preferred for injection because IV may cause chemical irritation or tissue damage. For IM use, inject deep into a large muscle mass.

For rectal use, unwrap and moisten the suppository with cold water before inserting it well into the rectum.

Propafenone Hydrochloride

proe-pa-fen′one high-droh-clor′ide

Rythmol, Rythmol SR

CATEGORY AND SCHEDULE

Pregnancy Risk Category: C

Classification: Antiarrhythmics, class IC

MECHANISM OF ACTION

An antiarrhythmic that decreases the fast sodium current in Purkinje or myocardial cells. Decreases excitability and automaticity; prolongs conduction velocity and the refractory period. *Therapeutic Effect:* Suppresses arrhythmias.

PHARMACOKINETICS

Peak 3-5 h. *Half-life:* 2-10 h. Metabolized in liver; excreted in urine (metabolite).

AVAILABILITY

Tablets (Rythmol): 150 mg, 225 mg, 300 mg.
Capsules (Extended Release [Rythmol SR]): 225 mg, 325 mg, 425 mg.

INDICATIONS AND DOSAGES

▸ **Maintenance of sinus rhythm for refractory paroxysmal or chronic AFib AND documented life-threatening ventricular arrhythmias, such as sustained ventricular tachycardia**

PO (PROMPT RELEASE)
Adults, Elderly. Initially, 150 mg q8h; may increase at 3- to 4-day intervals to 225 mg q8h, then to 300 mg q8h. Maximum: 900 mg/day.
PO (EXTENDED RELEASE)
Adults, Elderly. Initially, 225 mg q12h. May increase at 5-day intervals. Maximum: 425 mg q12h.

Dose adjustment, moderate to severe hepatic impairment
Give approximately 20%-30% of the usual dose (immediate release). Do not use extended release form for dosing.

OFF-LABEL USES

Treatment of supraventricular arrhythmias. Wolff-Parkinson-White syndrome.

CONTRAINDICATIONS

Known hypersensitivity; bradycardia; bronchospastic disorders; cardiogenic shock; electrolyte imbalance; sinoatrial, AV, and intraventricular impulse generation or conduction disorders, such as sick sinus syndrome or AV block, without the presence of a pacemaker; uncontrolled congestive heart failure (CHF).

INTERACTIONS

Drug

Cyclosporine: Cyclosporine levels may increase.
Digoxin: Propafenone produces dose-related increases in serum digoxin levels. Digoxin dosage should be reduced by roughly 50%; monitor closely.
Local anesthetics: Potentiated effects.
Propranolol: Propafenone increases propranolol concentrations.
QT-prolonging drugs: May have additive effect on QT interval.
Quinidine, procainamide: Should not be used at the same time as propafenone.

Rifampin: Induces propafenone metabolism.
Theophylline: Propafenone increases theophylline levels. Monitor closely.
Warfarin: Propafenone increases warfarin levels. Monitor INR closely.
Herbal
None known.
Food
None known.

DIAGNOSTIC TEST EFFECTS

Therapeutic serum level is generally in the range of 0.5-2 mcg/mL but clinical level monitoring is rarely used. May cause ECG changes, such as QRS widening and PR interval prolongation, and positive ANA titers.

SIDE EFFECTS

Frequent (7%-13%)
Dizziness, nausea, vomiting, altered taste, constipation.
Occasional (3%-6%)
Headache, dyspnea, blurred vision, dyspepsia (heartburn, indigestion, epigastric pain).
Rare (< 2%)
Rash, weakness, dry mouth, diarrhea, edema, hot flashes.

SERIOUS REACTIONS

- Propafenone may produce or worsen existing arrhythmias.
- Overdose may produce hypotension, somnolence, bradycardia, and atrioventricular conduction disturbances.
- Agranulocytosis (fever, chills, weakness, and neutropenia). Generally, occurs in the first 2 mo and will normalize with discontinuation.

PRECAUTIONS & CONSIDERATIONS

Caution is warranted with CHF, conduction disturbances, impaired hepatic or renal function, and recent MI.

Notify the physician if blurred vision, GI upset, dizziness, or headache occurs. Tasks that require mental alertness or motor skills should be avoided until response to the drug has been established. Electrolyte imbalances should be corrected before beginning propafenone therapy. Pulse rate for quality and irregularity, pattern of daily bowel activity and stool consistency, serum electrolyte levels, and hepatic enzymes should be assessed. Patient should be assessed for stress responses that can have adverse cardiovascular effects.
Storage
Store at room temperature.
Administration
Take without regard to meals. Do not skip doses. Extended-release capsules may also be taken without regard to food. Do not crush or divide.

Propantheline

proe-pan'the-leen

CATEGORY AND SCHEDULE

Pregnancy Risk Category: C

Classification: Anticholinergics

MECHANISM OF ACTION

A quaternary ammonium compound that has anticholinergic properties and that inhibits action of acetylcholine at postganglionic parasympathetic sites. *Therapeutic Effect:* Reduces gastric secretions and urinary frequency, urgency, and urge incontinence.

PHARMACOKINETICS

Onset occurs within 90 min but < 50% is absorbed from the GI tract. Extensive hepatic metabolism. Excreted in the urine and feces. *Half-life:* 2.9 h.

AVAILABILITY

Tablets: 7.5 mg, 15 mg.

INDICATIONS AND DOSAGES

▸ **Peptic ulcer (historic use)**

PO

Adults, Elderly. 15 mg 3 times/day 30 min before meals and 30 mg at bedtime.

Children. 1-2 mg/kg/day in 3-4 divided doses.

OFF-LABEL USES

For neurogenic bladder and related urinary incontinence.

CONTRAINDICATIONS

GI or genitourinary (GU) obstruction, myasthenia gravis, narrow-angle glaucoma, autonomic neuropathy, toxic megacolon, severe ulcerative colitis, unstable cardiovascular adjustment in acute hemorrhage, hypersensitivity to propantheline or other anticholinergics.

P

INTERACTIONS

Drug

Digoxin: May increase serum digoxin levels by increasing absorption due to decreased gastrointestinal motility.

Herbal

None known.

Food

None known.

SIDE EFFECTS

Frequent

Dry mouth, decreased sweating, constipation.

Occasional

Blurred vision, intolerance to light, urinary hesitancy, drowsiness, agitation, excitement.

Rare

Confusion, increased intraocular pressure, orthostatic hypotension, tachycardia.

SERIOUS REACTIONS

- Overdosage may produce temporary paralysis of ciliary muscle, pupillary dilation, tachycardia, palpitations, hot, dry, or flushed skin, absence of bowel sounds, hyperthermia, increased respiratory rate, ECG abnormalities, nausea, vomiting, rash over face or upper trunk, central nervous system stimulation, and psychosis, marked by agitation, restlessness, rambling speech, visual hallucinations, paranoid behavior, and delusions, followed by depression.

PRECAUTIONS & CONSIDERATIONS

Caution is warranted with chronic obstructive pulmonary disease (COPD), CHF, coronary artery disease, esophageal reflux or hiatal hernia associated with reflux esophagitis, gastric ulcer, hyperthyroidism, hypertension, liver or renal disease, tachyarrhythmias, autonomic neuropathy, prostatic hypertrophy, glaucoma, diarrhea, known or suspected GI infections, and mild to moderate ulcerative colitis. It is unknown whether propantheline crosses the placenta or is distributed in breast milk. Infants and young children are more susceptible to the drug's toxic effects. Propantheline use in elderly patients may cause agitation, confusion, drowsiness, or excitement. Hot baths and saunas should be avoided.

Tasks that require mental alertness or motor skills should be avoided until effects of the drug are known.

Dry mouth may be experienced during therapy. Good oral hygiene should be practiced. Physicians should be alerted to any significant xerostomic side effects such as increased caries, sore tongue, problems eating or swallowing, difficulty wearing prosthesis, as a medication change may need to be considered.

Storage
Store at room temperature.
Administration
Give propantheline 30 min before meals and at bedtime.

Propofol

pro'poe-fall
Diprivan, Fresenius Propoven

CATEGORY AND SCHEDULE
Pregnancy Risk Category: B

Classification: Anesthetics, general

MECHANISM OF ACTION
A rapidly acting general anesthetic that inhibits sympathetic vasoconstrictor nerve activity and decreases vascular resistance.
Therapeutic Effect: Produces hypnosis rapidly.

PHARMACOKINETICS

Route	Onset	Peak	Duration
IV	40 seconds	N/A	3-10 min

Rapidly and extensively distributed. Protein binding: 97%-99%. Metabolized in the liver. Excreted primarily in urine. Unknown whether removed by hemodialysis.
Half-life: 3-12 h.

AVAILABILITY
Injection: 10 mg/mL.

INDICATIONS AND DOSAGES
▸ Intensive care unit sedation
IV
Adults, Elderly. Initially, 0.3 mg/kg/h. May increase by 0.3-0.6 mg/kg/h q5-10min until desired effect is obtained. Maintenance: 0.3-3 mg/kg/h.

▸ Anesthesia
IV
Adults, American Society of Anesthesiologists (ASA) I and II patients. 2-2.5 mg/kg (about 40 mg q10 seconds until onset of anesthesia). Maintenance: 0.1-0.2 mg/kg/min.
Elderly, Debilitated, Hypovolemic, ASA III or IV patients. 1-1.5 mg/kg (about 20 mg q10 seconds until onset of anesthesia). Maintenance: 0.05-0.1 mg/kg/min.
Children aged 3 yr and older, ASA I or II patients. 2.5-3.5 mg/kg (lower dosage for ASA III or IV patients).
Children aged 2 mo to 16 yr. Maintenance dose: 0.125-0.3 mg/kg/min.

CONTRAINDICATIONS
Known hypersensitivity to propofol emulsion or any of its components, including allergies to eggs, egg products, soybeans, or soy products.

INTERACTIONS
Drug
Alcohol, narcotics, sedative-hypnotics, antipsychotics, skeletal muscle relaxants, inhalational anesthetics, other CNS depressants: May increase hypotensive and CNS and respiratory depressant effects of propofol.
Herbal
None known.
Food
None known.

DIAGNOSTIC TEST EFFECTS
Increased triglycerides.

IV INCOMPATIBILITIES
Amikacin (Amikin), amphotericin B complex (Abelcet, AmBisome, Amphotec), bretylium (Bretylol), calcium chloride, ciprofloxacin

P

(Cipro), diazepam (Valium), digoxin (Lanoxin), doxorubicin (Adriamycin), gentamicin (Garamycin), methylprednisolone (Solu-Medrol), minocycline (Minocin), phenytoin (Dilantin), tobramycin (Nebcin), verapamil (Isoptin).

IV COMPATIBILITIES

Acyclovir (Zovirax), bumetanide (Bumex), calcium gluconate, ceftazidime (Fortaz), dobutamine (Dobutrex), dopamine (Intropin), enalapril (Vasotec), fentanyl, heparin, insulin, labetalol (Normodyne, Trandate), lidocaine, lorazepam (Ativan), magnesium, milrinone (Primacor), nitroglycerin, norepinephrine (Levophed), potassium chloride, vancomycin (Vancocin).

SIDE EFFECTS

Frequent

Involuntary muscle movements, apnea (common during induction; lasts longer than 60 seconds), hypotension, nausea, vomiting, IV site burning or stinging or phlebitis.

Occasional

Twitching, bucking, jerking, thrashing, headache, dizziness, bradycardia, hypertension, fever, abdominal cramps, paresthesia, coldness, cough, hiccups, facial flushing, greenish-colored urine.

Rare

Rash, dry mouth, agitation, confusion, myalgia, thrombophlebitis.

SERIOUS REACTIONS

- Propofol infusion syndrome, may result in death (severe metabolic acidosis, hyperkalemia, lipemia, rhabdomyolysis, hepatomegaly, cardiac and renal failure). Associated with prolonged high-dose infusions.
- Pancreatitis.
- Too-rapid infusion in those with increased intracranial pressure/ neurosurgical needs may cause hypotension and sudden drops in intracranial perfusion. Avoid.
- Too-rapid IV administration may produce severe hypotension, respiratory depression, and involuntary muscle movements.
- The patient may experience an acute allergic reaction, characterized by abdominal pain, anxiety, restlessness, dyspnea, erythema, hypotension, pruritus, rhinitis, and urticaria.

PRECAUTIONS & CONSIDERATIONS

Caution is warranted in patients with circulatory, hepatic, lipid metabolism, renal, or respiratory disorder, history of pancreatitis, history of epilepsy, and in debilitated patients. Propofol crosses the placenta and is not recommended for obstetric use. Propofol is distributed in breast milk and is not recommended for breastfeeding women. The safety and efficacy of propofol have not been established in children. However, the Food and Drug Administration has approved the drug for use in children older than 3 yr. Lower propofol dosages are recommended for elderly patients.

Drug should be administered only by qualified personnel trained in anesthesia; resuscitative equipment should be available. Changes in PVC, PAC, ST segment may be evidenced; frequent monitoring of ECG is recommended. Physician should be notified if patient's respirations are < 10/min for possible CNS changes or respiratory dysfunction.

Be aware that urine may turn green. Vital signs should be obtained before propofol administration. ABG levels, BP, heart and respiratory rates, oxygen saturation, depth of sedation, and lipid and triglyceride levels should be monitored if propofol is given for longer than 24 h.

Overdosage is treated by discontinuing the drug, using artificial ventilation, vasopressor agents, or anticholinergics.

Storage

Store propofol at room temperature at or below 77° F. Do not freeze. Do not use propofol if the emulsion separates.

Administration

! Don't give propofol through the same IV line as blood or plasma.

Shake well before using. Propofol may be given undiluted, or it may be diluted only with D5W to a concentration of no < 2 mg/mL (4 mL D5W to 1 mL propofol yields 2 mg/mL). Discard any unused portions of the drug. Too-rapid IV administration of propofol may produce irregular muscle movements, respiratory depression, and severe hypotension. Observe for signs of inadvertent intra-arterial injection, such as delayed onset of drug action, pain or discolored skin near the injection site, or blue or white discoloration of the hand if a hand or arm IV site is used.

Use controlled infusion pump for prolonged infusions. To limit infection risk, administration must be completed within 12 h of spiking the vial; discard tubing and any unused portion after 12 h.

Propranolol Hydrochloride

proe-pran'oh-lole
high-droh-chlor'ride

★ Inderal, Inderal LA, InnoPran XL 🍁 Inderal LA

Do not confuse Inderal with Adderall, or Isordil or Indocin or propranolol with Pravachol.

CATEGORY AND SCHEDULE

Pregnancy Risk Category: C (D if used in second or third trimester)

Classification: Nonselective β-adrenergic antagonist, class II

MECHANISM OF ACTION

An antihypertensive, antianginal, antiarrhythmic, and antimigraine agent that blocks β_1- and β_2-adrenergic receptors. Decreases oxygen requirements. Slows AV conduction and increases refractory period in AV node. Large doses increase airway resistance. *Therapeutic Effect:* Slows sinus heart rate; decreases cardiac output, BP, and myocardial ischemia severity. Exhibits antiarrhythmic activity.

PHARMACOKINETICS

Route	Onset	Peak	Duration
PO	1-2 h	N/A	6 h

Well absorbed from the GI tract. Protein binding: 93%. Widely distributed. Metabolized in the liver. Primarily excreted in urine. Not removed by hemodialysis. *Half-life:* 3-5 h.

AVAILABILITY

Tablets (Inderal): 10 mg, 20 mg, 60 mg, 80 mg.

Capsules (Extended Release [Inderal LA]): 60 mg, 80 mg, 120 mg, 160 mg.
Capsules (Extended Release [InnoPran XL]): 80 mg, 120 mg.
Oral Solution (Inderal): 20 mg/5 mL, 40 mg/5 mL.
Injection (Inderal): 1 mg/mL.

INDICATIONS AND DOSAGES

▸ **Hypertension**
PO
Adults, Elderly. Initially, 40 mg twice a day. May increase dose every 3-7 days. Range: Up to 480 mg/day in divided doses. Maximum: 640 mg/day.
Children. Initially, 0.5-1 mg/kg/day in 4 divided doses. Usual dose: 1-5 mg/kg/day. Maximum: 8 mg/kg/day.

▸ **Angina**
PO
Adults, Elderly. Initially, 10-20 mg 2-4 times per day. Titrate to 160-320 mg/day in divided doses. (Long acting): Initially, 80 mg/day. Maximum: 320 mg/day.

▸ **Arrhythmias**
IV
Adults, Elderly. Usual dose is 1-3 mg IV. Second dose can be give after 2-3 min if needed. Subsequent doses can be given every 4-6 h if needed.
PO
Adults, Elderly. Initially, 10-30 mg q6-8h. May gradually increase dose. Range: 80-320 mg/day.

▸ **Life-threatening arrhythmias**
IV
Adults, Elderly. Usual dose is 1-3 mg IV. Second dose can be give after 2-3 min if needed. Subsequent doses can be given every 4-6 h if needed.

▸ **Hypertrophic subaortic stenosis**
IV
Adults, Elderly. Usual dose is 1-3 mg IV. Second dose can be give after 2-3 min if needed. Subsequent doses can be given every 4-6 h if needed.

▸ **Adjunct to α-blocking agents to treat pheochromocytoma**
PO
Adults, Elderly. 60 mg/day in divided doses with α-blocker for 3 days before surgery. Maintenance (inoperable tumor): 30 mg/day with α-blocker.

▸ **Migraine headache prophylaxis**
PO
Adults, Elderly. 80 mg/day in divided doses. Or 80 mg once daily as extended-release capsule. Increase up to 160-240 mg/day in divided doses.

▸ **Reduction of cardiovascular mortality and reinfarction in patients with previous myocardial infarction (MI)**
PO
Adults, Elderly. 180-240 mg/day in divided doses.

▸ **Essential tremor**
PO
Adults, Elderly. Initially, 40 mg twice a day increased up to 120-320 mg/day in 2-3 divided doses.

OFF-LABEL USES

Treatment adjunct for anxiety, mitral valve prolapse syndrome, thyrotoxicosis, acute myocardial infarction, esophageal varices, hemangioma, portal hypertension, scleroderma renal crisis, unstable aneurysm, variceal bleeding prophylaxis.

CONTRAINDICATIONS

Asthma, bradycardia, cardiogenic shock, heart block, uncompensated congestive heart failure (CHF) known hypersensitivity to propranolol.

INTERACTIONS

Drug
Didanosine: Possible decreased hypotensive effects.
Diphenhydramine: Suspected plasma level increases.

Diuretics, other antihypertensives: May increase hypotensive effect.
Epinephrine, ephedrine, OTC and Rx combination cold products, other sympathomimetics: Possible hypertensive effects or bradycardia.
Halogen, hydrocarbon inhalation anesthetics: May increase hypotensive effects and risk of myocardial depression.
Indomethacin, NSAIDs: May decrease hypotensive effect.
Insulin, oral hypoglycemics: May mask symptoms of hypoglycemia and prolong the hypoglycemic effect of insulin and oral hypoglycemics.
IV phenytoin: May increase cardiac depressant effect.
Lidocaine: Possible slower metabolism of lidocaine.
NSAIDs: May decrease antihypertensive effect.

Herbal
None known.

Food
None known.

DIAGNOSTIC TEST EFFECTS

May increase serum antinuclear antibody titer and BUN, serum LDH, serum lipoprotein, serum alkaline phosphatase, serum bilirubin, serum creatinine, serum potassium, serum uric acid, AST (SGOT), ALT (SGPT), and serum triglyceride levels.

IV INCOMPATIBILITIES

Amphotericin B complex (Abelcet, AmBisome, Amphotec).

IV COMPATIBILITIES

Alteplase (Activase), heparin, milrinone (Primacor), potassium chloride, propofol (Diprivan).

SIDE EFFECTS

Frequent
Diminished sexual ability, drowsiness, difficulty sleeping, unusual fatigue or weakness.

Occasional
Bradycardia, depression, sensation of coldness in extremities, diarrhea, constipation, anxiety, nasal congestion, nausea, vomiting.

Rare
Altered taste, dry eyes, pruritus, paresthesia.

SERIOUS REACTIONS

- Overdose may produce profound bradycardia and hypotension.
- Abrupt withdrawal may result in sweating, palpitations, headache, and tremors.
- Propranolol administration may precipitate CHF and myocardial infarction (MI) in patients with cardiac disease; thyroid storm in those with thyrotoxicosis; and peripheral ischemia in those with existing peripheral vascular disease.
- Hypoglycemia may occur in patients with previously controlled diabetes.

PRECAUTIONS & CONSIDERATIONS

Caution is warranted with diabetes and hepatic and renal impairment. Propranolol crosses the placenta and is distributed in breast milk. Propranolol use should be avoided in pregnant women after the first trimester because it may result in low-birth-weight infants. The drug may also produce apnea, bradycardia, hypoglycemia, hypothermia during childbirth. No age-related precautions have been noted in children. In elderly patients, age-related peripheral vascular disease may increase susceptibility to decreased peripheral circulation. Be aware that salt and alcohol intake should be restricted. Nasal decongestants or OTC cold preparations (stimulants) should not be used without physician approval. Tasks that require mental alertness or motor skills should be avoided.

Notify the physician of behavioral changes, fatigue, rash, dizziness, excessively slow pulse rate (< 60 beats/min), or peripheral numbness. BP for hypotension; respiratory status for shortness of breath; pattern of daily bowel activity and stool consistency, ECG for arrhythmias, and pulse for quality, rate, and rhythm should be monitored during treatment. If pulse rate is 60 beats/min or lower or systolic BP is < 90 mm Hg, withhold the medication and contact the physician. In those receiving propranolol for treatment of angina, the onset, type (sharp, dull, squeezing), radiation, location, intensity, and duration of anginal pain and its precipitating factors, including exertion and emotional stress, should be recorded. Signs and symptoms of CHF, such as decreased urine output, distended neck veins, dyspnea (particularly on exertion or lying down), night cough, peripheral edema, and weight gain should also be assessed.

P

Abrupt withdrawal is contraindicated because it can result in palpitations, headache, tremors, and sweating. Blood glucose levels should be monitored regularly after initiating therapy in patients with diabetes mellitus because propranolol can cause hyperglycemic effects. Rapid postural changes should be avoided because orthostatic hypotensive effects may occur.

Storage

Store at room temperature.

Administration

For oral use, crush scored tablets if necessary. Take at same time each day. Do not abruptly discontinue the drug. Compliance with the therapy regimen is essential to control anginal pain, arrhythmias, and hypertension. Take extended-release capsules once daily (InnoPran XL is designed for bedtime administration). Do not crush, chew, or divide.

For IV use, give undiluted for IV push. For IV infusion, may dilute each 1 mg in 10 mL D5W. Do not exceed 1 mg/min injection rate. For IV infusion, give 1 mg over 10-15 min.

Propylthiouracil

proe-pill-thye-oh-yoor′a-sill

★ PTU

CATEGORY AND SCHEDULE

Pregnancy Risk Category: D

Classification: Thyroid hormone antagonist

MECHANISM OF ACTION

A thiourea derivative that blocks oxidation of iodine in the thyroid gland and blocks synthesis of thyroxine and tri-iodothyronine. *Therapeutic Effect:* Inhibits synthesis of thyroid hormone.

PHARMACOKINETICS

Onset 30-40 min, duration 2-4 h. *Half-life:* 1-2 h; excreted in urine, bile, and breast milk; crosses placental barrier.

AVAILABILITY

Tablets: 50 mg.

INDICATIONS AND DOSAGES

▸ **Hyperthyroidism**

PO

Adults, Elderly. Initially, 300-450 mg/day in divided doses q8h. Maintenance: 100-150 mg/day in divided doses q8-12h.

Children 6 yr and older. When no other options available. Initially, 50 mg/day PO divided q8h. For children 6-10 yr, the usual doses are 50-150 mg/day in divided doses.

For 10 yr and over, initially 150-300 mg/day, divided. Titrate up or down based on clinical response and TSH and free T4 levels.
Neonates. 5-10 mg/kg/day in divided doses q8h.

CONTRAINDICATIONS

Hypersensitivity to the drug; use in breastfeeding.

INTERACTIONS

Drug
Amiodarone, iodinated glycerol, iodine, potassium iodide: May decrease response of propylthiouracil.
Anticholinergics, sympathomimetics: May increase side effects in uncontrolled patients.
Central nervous ystem (CNS) depressants: May be more responsive to depressant effects in uncontrolled hypothyroidism.
Digoxin: May increase digoxin blood concentration as patient becomes euthyroid.
I^{131}: May decrease thyroid uptake of I^{131}.
Oral anticoagulants: May decrease the effects of oral anticoagulants.
Vasoconstrictors: May increase risk in patients with uncontrolled hypothyroidism.
Herbal
None known.
Food
None known.

DIAGNOSTIC TEST EFFECTS

May increase LDH, serum alkaline phosphatase, bilirubin, AST (SGOT), and ALT (SGPT) levels and prothrombin time.

SIDE EFFECTS

Frequent
Urticaria, rash, pruritus, nausea, skin pigmentation, hair loss, headache, paresthesia.
Occasional
Somnolence, lymphadenopathy, vertigo.
Rare
Drug fever, lupus-like syndrome.

SERIOUS REACTIONS

- Agranulocytosis as long as 4 mo after therapy, pancytopenia, and fatal hepatitis have occurred.

PRECAUTIONS & CONSIDERATIONS

Caution is warranted with concurrent use of other agranulocytosis-inducing drugs and in persons older than 40 yr. Propylthiouracil crosses the placenta and should be avoided during pregnancy. Breastfeeding is contraindicated because the drug readily crosses to breast milk. Use cautiously in children because of the risk of hepatic dysfunction. Safety and effectiveness in children below the age of 6 have not been established. Restrict the consumption of iodine products and seafood.

Notify the physician of somnolence, jaundice, nausea, vomiting, illness, unusual bleeding or bruising, rash, itching, swollen lymph glands, or a pulse rate < 60 beats/min. Weight, pulse, prothrombin time, LDH, serum alkaline phosphatase, bilirubin, AST, and ALT levels should be monitored. Prolonged therapy may cause blood dyscrasias, evidenced by bleeding, infection, and poor healing.

Report immediately any evidence of sore throat, skin eruptions, fever, headache, or general malaise.

Storage
Store at room temperature. Keep tightly closed and protected from light.
Administration
Space doses evenly around the clock. Give consistently with regard to food.

Protamine Sulfate

proe′ta-meen sull′fate

Do not confuse protamine with ProAmatine, Protopam, or Protropin.

CATEGORY AND SCHEDULE

Pregnancy Risk Category: C

Classification: Heparin antagonist

MECHANISM OF ACTION

A protein that complexes with heparin to form a stable salt. *Therapeutic Effect:* Reduces anticoagulant activity of heparin.

PHARMACOKINETICS

IV: Onset 5 min; duration 2 h.

AVAILABILITY

Injection: 10 mg/mL.

P

INDICATIONS AND DOSAGES

▸ **Heparin overdose (antidote and treatment), hemorrhage**

IV

Adults, Elderly. 1 mg protamine sulfate neutralizes 90-115 units of heparin. Heparin disappears rapidly from circulation, reducing the dosage demand for protamine as time elapses.

▸ **For LMWH toxicity/hemorrhage with enoxaparin**

IV

Adults. If enoxaparin was in previous 8 h, give 1 mg IV for every 1 mg of enoxaparin. If it has been > 8 h since enoxaparin or if a second dose needed, give 0.5 mg IV for every 1 mg of enoxaparin. May give another dose if the aPTT measured at 2-4 h after the initial infusion remains prolonged. In all cases, the anti-Xa activity is never completely neutralized (maximum 60%-75%).

▸ **For LMWH toxicity/hemorrhage with dalteparin or tinzaparin**

IV

Adults. 1 mg IV for every 100 anti-Xa international units of dalteparin or tinzaparin. A second dose (0.5 mg IV for every 100 anti-Xa international units) may be administered if the aPTT measured at 2-4 h after the initial infusion remains prolonged. In all cases, the anti-Xa activity is never completely neutralized (maximum 60%-75%).

CONTRAINDICATIONS

None known.

INTERACTIONS

Drug

Oral anticoagulants, including aspirin and NSAIDs: May increase anticoagulant effects, possible hemorrhage and should be avoided.

Herbal

None known.

Food

None known.

DIAGNOSTIC TEST EFFECTS

None known. Assessment of PPT, PT or INR, CBC, should be performed periodically to assess effectiveness.

SIDE EFFECTS

Frequent

Decreased BP, dyspnea.

Occasional

Hypersensitivity reaction (urticaria, angioedema); nausea and vomiting, which generally occur in those sensitive to fish and seafood, vasectomized men, infertile men, those on isophane (NPH) insulin, or those previously on protamine therapy.

Rare

Back pain.

SERIOUS REACTIONS

- Too-rapid IV administration may produce acute hypotension, bradycardia, pulmonary hypertension, dyspnea, transient flushing, and feeling of warmth.
- Heparin rebound may occur several hours after heparin has been neutralized (usually 8-9 h after protamine administration). Heparin rebound occurs most often after arterial or cardiac surgery.

PRECAUTIONS & CONSIDERATIONS

This drug is intended for use only in acute care situations in hospitals and emergency rooms. Caution is warranted with a history of allergy to fish and seafood, in those previously on protamine therapy because of a propensity to hypersensitivity reaction, and in infertile or vasectomized men and those on isophane (NPH) or insulin therapy. An electric razor or soft toothbrush should be used to prevent bleeding until coagulation studies normalize.

Notify the physician of black or red stool, coffee-ground vomitus, dark or red urine, or red-speckled mucus from cough. Activated clotting time, aPTT, BP, cardiac function, and other coagulation tests should be monitored.

Storage

Store vials at room temperature.

Administration

May give intravenously (IV) undiluted over 10 min or may further dilute in 0.9% NaCl or D5W injection prior to IV infusion. Solutions are stable for 24 h when refrigerated. Do not exceed 5 mg/min or 50 mg in any 10-min period. Make sure the patient is supine while protamine is being administered to prevent injury from a hypotensive episode or other complication.

Protriptyline

proe-trip'ti-leen

★ Vivactil

CATEGORY AND SCHEDULE

Pregnancy Risk Category: C

Classification: Antidepressants, tricyclic

MECHANISM OF ACTION

A tricyclic antidepressant that increases synaptic concentration of norepinephrine and serotonin by inhibiting their reuptake by presynaptic membranes. *Therapeutic Effect:* Produces antidepressant effect.

PHARMACOKINETICS

Well absorbed from the GI tract. Protein binding: 92%. Widely distributed. Extensively metabolized in liver. Excreted in urine. Not removed by hemodialysis. *Half-life:* 54-92 h.

AVAILABILITY

Tablets: 5 mg, 10 mg (Vivactil).

INDICATIONS AND DOSAGES

▸ **Depression**

PO

Adults. 15-40 mg/day divided into 3-4 doses/day. Maximum: 60 mg/day.
Elderly. 5 mg 3 times/day. May increase gradually. Maximum: 30 mg/day.

OFF-LABEL USES

Narcolepsy, sleep apnea.

CONTRAINDICATIONS

Acute recovery period after myocardial infarction, coadministration with cisapride, use of MAOIs within 14 days, hypersensitivity to protriptyline or any component of the formulation, QT prolongation.

INTERACTIONS

Drug

Alcohol, barbiturates, benzodiazepines and other central nervous system (CNS) depressants: May increase CNS and respiratory depression and the hypotensive effects of protriptyline.

Cimetidine, quinidine, and inhibitors of CYP2D6 (e.g., phenothiazines, fluoxetine, sertraline, paroxetine, propafenone, and flecainide): May increase protriptyline blood concentration and risk of toxicity.

Clonidine, guanadrel, guanethidine: May decrease the effects of clonidine and guanadrel.

Direct-acting sympathomimetics, epinephrine, levonordefrin: Possible increased cardiac sympathomimetic effects.

MAOIs: May increase the risk of hyperpyrexia, hypertensive crisis, and seizures.

Phenothiazines, muscarinic blockers, antihistamines: May increase the anticholinergic and sedative effects of protriptyline.

Phenytoin: May decrease protriptyline blood concentration.

Tramadol: May increase seizure risk.

Herbal

St. John's wort: May have additive effects.

Food

None known.

DIAGNOSTIC TEST EFFECTS

Therapeutic serum level for protriptyline is 70-250 ng/mL. However, plasma levels should not guide management of the patient.

SIDE EFFECTS

Frequent

Drowsiness, weight gain, fatigue, dry mouth, blurred vision, constipation, delayed micturition, postural hypotension, diaphoresis, disturbed concentration, increased appetite, urinary retention.

Occasional

GI disturbances, such as nausea, diarrhea, GI distress, metallic taste sensation.

Rare

Paradoxical reaction, marked by agitation, restlessness, nightmares, insomnia, extrapyramidal symptoms, particularly fine hand tremor.

SERIOUS REACTIONS

- High dosage may produce confusion, seizures, severe drowsiness, arrhythmias, fever, hallucinations, agitation, shortness of breath, vomiting, and unusual tiredness or weakness.
- Abrupt withdrawal from prolonged therapy may produce severe headache, malaise, nausea, vomiting, and vivid dreams.
- ECG changes, including QT prolongation.
- Agranulocytosis (rare).

PRECAUTIONS & CONSIDERATIONS

Caution is warranted in patients with increased intraocular pressure, overactive or agitated patients, seizure disorder, bipolar disorder, suicidal ideation, cardiovascular disease, hyperthyroidism, urinary retention, and concurrent use of guanethidine or other peripherally acting antihypertensives. Be aware that protriptyline crosses the placenta and is minimally distributed in breast milk. Safety and efficacy have not been established in children. Antidepressants have been reported to increase the risk of suicidal thinking and behavior in children, adolescents, and young adults (18-24 yr of age) with major depressive disorder (MDD) and other psychiatric disorders. Patients should be closely monitored for clinical worsening, suicidality, or unusual changes in behavior, particularly during the initial 1-2 mo of therapy or following dosage adjustments. Expect to use lower dosages in elderly patients. Higher dosages are not tolerated well and increase the risk of toxicity in elderly patients.

Significant xerostomic side effects such as sore tongue or problems eating or swallowing should be reported as medication change may be needed.

Anticholinergic, sedative effects and postural hypotension usually develop during early therapy. Avoid unnecessary exposure to sunlight.

Storage

Store at room temperature.

Administration

May be taken with food to decrease GI distress. Dose increases should occur during the morning dose. Avoid taking the last dose of the day in the evening, as protriptyline is more stimulating than other TCAs.

Pseudoephedrine

soo-doe-e-fed′rin

★ 🍁 Sudafed Children's, Sudafed Congestion, Sudogest, Sudogest Children's, Wal-phed

CATEGORY AND SCHEDULE

Pregnancy Risk Category: C

Restricted OTC due to U.S. Combat Methamphetamine Epidemic Act of 2005. Products are kept behind counters prior to purchase, logs are maintained of product purchases, amounts, and consumer IDs, ensuring daily and monthly allowable limits are not exceeded.

Classification: Direct-acting α-adrenergic and β-adrenergic sympathomimetic, decongestant

MECHANISM OF ACTION

A sympathomimetic that directly stimulates α-adrenergic and β-adrenergic receptors. *Therapeutic Effect:* Produces vasoconstriction of respiratory tract mucosa; shrinks nasal mucous membranes; reduces edema, and nasal congestion.

PHARMACOKINETICS

Route	Onset	Peak	Duration (h)
PO	15-30 min	NA	4-6 (tablets, syrup)
PO	NA	NA	8-12 (extended release)

Well absorbed from the GI tract. Partially metabolized in the liver. Primarily excreted in urine. Not removed by hemodialysis. *Half-life:* 9-16 h (children, 3.1 h).

AVAILABILITY

Tablets: 30 mg.

Oral Solution: 15 mg/5mL, 30 mg/5mL

INDICATIONS AND DOSAGES

▸ **Decongestant**

PO

Adults, Children 12 yr and older. 60 mg q4-6h. Maximum: 240 mg/day.

Children aged 6-11 yr. 30 mg q4-6h. Maximum: 120 mg/day.

Children 2-5 yr. 15 mg q4-6h. Maximum: 60 mg/day.

Children younger than 2 yr. Safety and effective use have not been established.

Elderly. 30-60 mg q6h as needed.

PO (EXTENDED RELEASE)

Adults, Children 12 yr and older. 120 mg q12h.

CONTRAINDICATIONS

Breastfeeding women, coronary artery disease, severe hypertension, acute recovery phase of MI, use within 14 days of MAOIs.

P

INTERACTIONS

Drug

Antihypertensive, β-blockers, diuretics: May decrease the effects of these drugs.
Hydrocarbon inhalation anesthetics: May cause dysrhythmias.
MAOIs: May increase cardiac stimulant and vasopressor effects.
Sympathomimetics: Possible increased CNS, cardiovascular effects.

Herbal

None known.

Food

None known.

DIAGNOSTIC TEST EFFECTS

None known.

SIDE EFFECTS

Occasional (5%-10%)

Nervousness, restlessness, insomnia, tremor, headache.

Rare (1%-4%)

Diaphoresis, weakness.

P

SERIOUS REACTIONS

- Large doses may produce tachycardia, palpitations (particularly in patients with cardiac disease), light-headedness, nausea, and vomiting.
- Overdose in patients older than 60 yr may result in hallucinations, CNS depression, and seizures.

PRECAUTIONS & CONSIDERATIONS

Caution is warranted with diabetes, heart disease, hyperthyroidism, benign prostatic hyperplasia, and in elderly patients. Pseudoephedrine crosses the placenta and is distributed in breast milk. The safety and efficacy of pseudoephedrine have not been established in children younger than 2 yr. Age-related benign prostatic hyperplasia may require a dosage adjustment in elderly patients.

BP should be monitored for increases.

Storage

Store products at room temperature.

Administration

Do not crush extended-release tablets; swallow them whole. Discontinue therapy and notify the physician if dizziness, insomnia, irregular or rapid heartbeat, tremors, or other side effects occur.

Psyllium

sill'ee-yum

★ Hydrocil, Metamucil, Reguloid

CATEGORY AND SCHEDULE

Pregnancy Risk Category: B
OTC

Classification: Laxative, natural fiber, bulk forming.

MECHANISM OF ACTION

A bulk-forming laxative that dissolves and swells in water providing increased bulk and moisture content in stool.
Therapeutic Effect: Promotes peristalsis and bowel motility.

PHARMACOKINETICS

Route	Onset	Peak	Duration
PO	12-24 h	2-3 days	NA

Acts in small and large intestines.

AVAILABILITY

Powder (Hydrocil, Metamucil).
Wafer (Metamucil): 3.4 g/dose.
Capsules (Metamucil): 0.52 g.

INDICATIONS AND DOSAGES

▸ **Constipation, irritable bowel syndrome**

PO

! 3.4 g powder equals 1 rounded tsp, 1 packet, or 1 wafer.

Adults, Elderly. 2-5 capsules/dose 1-3 times a day. 1 rounded tsp or 1 tbsp of powder 1-3 times a day. 2 wafers 1-3 times a day.

Children 6-11 yr. ½-1 tsp powder in water 1-3 times a day.

CONTRAINDICATIONS

Fecal impaction, GI obstruction, appendicitis, dysphagia.

INTERACTIONS

Drug

Digoxin, oral anticoagulants, salicylates: May decrease the effects of digoxin, oral anticoagulants, and salicylates by decreasing absorption.

Potassium-sparing diuretics, potassium supplements: May interfere with the effects of potassium-sparing diuretics and potassium supplements.

Herbal

None known.

Food

None known.

DIAGNOSTIC TEST EFFECTS

May increase blood glucose level. May decrease serum potassium level.

SIDE EFFECTS

Rare

Some degree of abdominal discomfort, nausea, mild abdominal cramps, griping, faintness.

SERIOUS REACTIONS

- Esophageal or bowel obstruction may occur if administered < 250 mL of liquid.

PRECAUTIONS & CONSIDERATIONS

Caution is warranted with esophageal strictures, intestinal adhesions, stenosis, and ulcers. This drug may be used safely in pregnancy. Safety and efficacy of psyllium have not been established in children younger than 6 yr of age. No age-related precautions have been noted in elderly patients.

Pattern of daily bowel activity and stool consistency and serum electrolyte levels should be monitored. Adequate fluid intake should be maintained.

Storage

Store products at room tempeature. Keep tightly closed to protect from moisture.

Administration

Administer at least 2 h before or after other medication administration. Drink 6-8 glasses of water a day to aid in stool softening. Powder should not be swallowed in dry form but should be mixed with at least 1 full glass (8 oz) of liquid and then followed by 8 oz of liquid; inadequate amount of fluid may cause GI obstruction. To promote defecation, increase fluid intake, exercise, and eat a high-fiber diet.

Pyrantel Pamoate

pi-ran′tel pam′oh-ate

★ Pin-X, Reese's Pinworm, Pronto Plus Pinworm

🍁 Combantrin Suspension

CATEGORY AND SCHEDULE

Pregnancy Risk Category: C

OTC

Classification: Pyrimidine derivative, antihelmintic

P

MECHANISM OF ACTION

A depolarizing neuromuscular blocking agent that causes the release of acetylcholine and inhibits cholinesterase. *Therapeutic Effect:* Results in a spastic paralysis of the worm and consequent expulsion from the host's intestinal tract.

PHARMACOKINETICS

Poorly absorbed through GI tract. Time to peak occurs in 1-3 h. Partially metabolized in liver. Primarily excreted in feces; minimal elimination in urine.

AVAILABILITY

Caplets: 180 mg (62.5 mg pyrantel base) (Reese's Pinworm Caplets).
Oral Liquid or Suspension: 50 mg/mL of pyrantel base (Pronto Plus Pinworm, Pin-X, Reese's Pinworm Liquid)

INDICATIONS AND DOSAGES

▸ ***Enterobiasis vermicularis* (pinworm)**

PO

Adults, Elderly, Children older than 2 yr. 11 mg base/kg once. Repeat in 2 wks. Maximum: 1 g/day.

▸ **Weight-based liquid dosage (taken as a single dose of 50 mg/mL base solution)**

Less than 25 1b or under 2 yr old: Do not use unless directed by doctor

Weight (lb)	Dosage
25-37	½ tsp (2.5 mL)
38-62	1 tsp (5 mL)
63-87	1½ tsp (7.5 mL)
88-112	2 tsp (10 mL)
113-137	2½ tsp (12.5 mL)
138-162	3 tsp (15 mL)
163-187	3½ tsp (17.5 mL)
188	over 4 tsp (20 mL)

CONTRAINDICATIONS

Hypersensitivity to pyrantel or any of its components.

INTERACTIONS

Drug

Piperazine: May decrease effects of pyrantel.

Herbal

None known.

Food

None known.

DIAGNOSTIC TEST EFFECTS

None known.

SIDE EFFECTS

Occasional

Nausea, vomiting, headache, dizziness, drowsiness, GI distress, weakness.

SERIOUS REACTIONS

• Overdosage includes symptoms of anorexia, nausea, abdominal cramps, vomiting, diarrhea, and ataxia.

PRECAUTIONS & CONSIDERATIONS

Caution is necessary in pregnancy and in patients with liver disease. Pyrantel should not be used concurrently with piperazines. It is unknown whether pyrantel is distributed in breast milk. No age-related precautions have been noted in children or elderly. The entire family should be treated for pinworms. Wash bedding and clothes in hot, soapy water to avoid being reinfected. Tactful discussion regarding proper toileting techniques should be discussed to avoid transmission of infection or reinfection.

Storage

Store all products at room temperature.

Administration

May be taken with or without food. Shake suspension well before using.

Pyrazinamide

pye-ra-zin'a-mide

Tebrazid

CATEGORY AND SCHEDULE

Pregnancy Risk Category: C

Classification: Antitubercular agent

MECHANISM OF ACTION

An antitubercular whose exact mechanism of action is unknown. *Therapeutic Effect:* Either bacteriostatic or bactericidal, depending on the drug's concentration at the infection site and the susceptibility of infecting bacteria.

PHARMACOKINETICS

PO: Peak 2 h. *Half-life:* 9-10 h. Metabolized in liver, excreted in urine (metabolites and unchanged drug).

AVAILABILITY

Tablets: 500 mg.

INDICATIONS AND DOSAGES

▸ **Tuberculosis (in combination with other antituberculars)**

PO

Adults. 15-30 mg/kg/daily. Maximum: 3 g/day.

Children. 15-30 mg/kg/day. Maximum: 3 g/day.

▸ **Twice-weekly regimen**

PO

Adults, Children. 50-75 mg/kg twice weekly based on lean body weight. (Doses may exceed maximum 3 g/day dose. However, these higher doses have been well tolerated when given only twice per week). Twice weekly regimen not for HIV patients with low CD4 counts.

CONTRAINDICATIONS

Severe hepatic dysfunction, hypersensitivity, acute gout.

INTERACTIONS

Drug

Allopurinol, colchicine, probenecid, sulfinpyrazone: May decrease the effects of these drugs.

Herbal

None known.

Food

None known.

DIAGNOSTIC TEST EFFECTS

May increase AST (SGOT), ALT (SGPT), and serum uric acid concentrations.

SIDE EFFECTS

Frequent

Arthralgia, myalgia (usually mild and self-limiting).

Rare

Hypersensitivity reaction (rash, pruritus, urticaria), photosensitivity, gouty arthritis.

SERIOUS REACTIONS

- Hepatotoxicity, gouty arthritis, thrombocytopenia, and anemia occur rarely.

PRECAUTIONS & CONSIDERATIONS

Caution is warranted in patients with diabetes mellitus, a history of gout, and renal impairment. Caution should be used with possible cross-sensitivity to ethionamide, isoniazid, and niacin. Use with caution in pregnancy as there are not adequate data. Small amounts of pyrazinamide are excreted into breast milk. There are no particular cautions in children. Liver function test results should be monitored. Side effects such as anorexia, fever, jaundice, liver tenderness, malaise, nausea, and vomiting may occur. If any liver reactions occur, stop the drug and notify the physician promptly. Serum uric acid levels should be monitored and signs and symptoms of gout, such as hot, painful, swollen joints, especially the ankle, big toe, or knee, should be assessed. Blood glucose levels should be evaluated, especially in persons with diabetes mellitus, because pyrazinamide administration may make diabetic management difficult. Skin should be assessed for rash or eruptions.

It is important to test for noninfectious status by ensuring that compliance with anti-TB for 3 wks or longer has occurred; that culture has confirmed TB susceptiblity to anti-infectives; patient has 3 consecutive negative sputum smears; and patient is not coughing.

Storage

Store at room temperature, well closed.

Administration

Take pyrazinamide with food to reduce GI upset.

P

Pyridostigmine Bromide

peer-id-oh-stig′meen brom′ide

★ Mestinon, Mestinon Timespan

🍁 Mestinon, Mestinon-SR

Do not confuse pyridostigmine with physostigmine or Mesitonin with Mesantoin or Metatensin.

CATEGORY AND SCHEDULE

Pregnancy Risk Category: C

Classification: Cholinergic, cholinesterase inhibitor.

MECHANISM OF ACTION

A cholinergic that prevents destruction of acetylcholine by inhibiting the enzyme acetylcholinesterase, thus enhancing impulse transmission across the myoneural junction. *Therapeutic Effect:* Produces miosis; increases tone of intestinal, skeletal muscle tone; stimulates salivary and sweat gland secretions.

PHARMACOKINETICS

PO: Onset 20-30 min, duration 3-6 h.
IV/IM/SC: Onset 2-15 min, duration 2.5-4 h.
Metabolized in liver, excreted in urine.

AVAILABILITY

Syrup (Mestinon): 60 mg/5 mL.
Tablets (Mestinon): 60 mg.
Tablets (Extended Release [Mestinon Timespan]): 180 mg.
Injection (Mestinon): 5 mg/mL.

INDICATIONS AND DOSAGES

▸ **Myasthenia gravis**

PO

Adults, Elderly. Initially, 60 mg 3 times a day. Dosage increased at 48-h intervals. Maintenance: 60 mg to 1.5 g a day.

PO (EXTENDED RELEASE)

Adults, Elderly. 180-540 mg once or twice a day with at least a 6-h interval between doses.

IV, IM

Adults, Elderly. 2 mg q2-3h.
Children, Neonates. 0.05-0.15 mg/kg/dose. Maximum single dose: 10 mg.

▸ **Reversal of nondepolarizing neuromuscular blockade**

IV

Adults, Elderly. 0.1-0.25 mg/kg with, or shortly after, 0.6-1.2 mg atropine sulfate or an equipotent dose of glycopyrrolate.
Children. 0.25 mg/kg.

CONTRAINDICATIONS

Mechanical GI or urinary tract obstruction, cholinesterase inhibitor toxicity.

INTERACTIONS

Drug

Atropine and other anticholinergics: Counteract effects of cholinesterase inhibitors. Use care when giving to counteract cholinesterase inhibitor side effects, as cholinergic crisis may be induced.

Cholinesterase inhibitors: May increase the risk of toxicity.

Neuromuscular blockers: May prolong the action of succinylcholine and other related medicines.

Quinine: May antagonize the action of pyridostigmine.

Herbal

None known.

Food

None known.

DIAGNOSTIC TEST EFFECTS

None known.

IV INCOMPATIBILITIES

Do not mix pyridostigmine with any other medications.

SIDE EFFECTS

Frequent

Miosis, increased GI and skeletal muscle tone, bradycardia, constriction of bronchi and ureters, diaphoresis, increased salivation.

Occasional

Headache, rash, temporary decrease in diastolic BP with mild reflex tachycardia, short periods of atrial fibrillation (in hyperthyroid patients), marked drop in BP (in hypertensive patients).

SERIOUS REACTIONS

• Overdose may produce a cholinergic crisis, manifested as increasingly severe muscle weakness that appears first in muscles involving chewing and swallowing and is followed by muscle weakness of the shoulder girdle and upper extremities, respiratory muscle paralysis, and pelvis girdle and leg muscle paralysis. If overdose occurs, stop all cholinergic drugs and immediately administer 1-4 mg atropine sulfate IV for adults or 0.01 mg/kg for infants and children younger than 12 yr.

PRECAUTIONS & CONSIDERATIONS

Caution is warranted in patients with bradycardia, bronchial asthma, cardiac arrhythmias, epilepsy, hyperthyroidism, peptic ulcer disease, recent coronary occlusion, and vagotonia. Keep a log of energy level and muscle strength to help guide drug dosing.

Notify the physician of diarrhea, difficulty breathing, profuse salivation or sweating, irregular heartbeat, muscle weakness, severe abdominal pain, or nausea and vomiting. Therapeutic response to the drug, such as decreased fatigue, improved chewing and swallowing, and increased muscle strength, should be monitored. Respirations should be closely assessed.

Caution is warranted with postural changes because of possible orthostatic hypotensive effects.

Storage

Store products at room temperature, tightly closed and protected from light. Keep silica gel pack in with all tablets in original container.

Administration

! Drug dosage and frequency of administration are dependent on the daily clinical response, including exacerbations, physical and emotional stress, and remissions.

Crush tablets as needed. Take larger doses at times of increased fatigue, for example 30-45 min before meals. May break extended-release tablets but do not chew or crush them.

For IV and IM use, give large doses concurrently with 0.6-1.2 mg atropine sulfate IV, as prescribed, to minimize side effects.

Pyridoxine Hydrochloride (Vitamin B_6)

peer-i-dox′een high-droh-chlor′ride

★ Neuro-K 500

Do not confuse pyridoxine with paroxetine, pralidoxime, or Pyridium.

CATEGORY AND SCHEDULE

Pregnancy Risk Category: A
OTC (tablets, capsules), Rx (injectible)

Classification: Vitamins, water soluble, vitamin B_6

MECHANISM OF ACTION

Acts as a coenzyme for various metabolic functions, including metabolism of proteins, carbohydrates, and fats. Aids in the breakdown of glycogen and in the synthesis of γ-aminobutyric acid in the central nervous system (CNS). *Therapeutic Effect:* Prevents pyridoxine deficiency. Protects against neurotoxicity of certain drugs that are pyridoxine antagonists.

PHARMACOKINETICS

Readily absorbed primarily in jejunum. Stored in the liver, muscle, and brain. Metabolized in the liver. Primarily excreted in urine. Removed by hemodialysis. *Half-life:* 15-20 days.

AVAILABILITY

Tablets: 20 mg, 25 mg, 50 mg, 100 mg, 250 mg, 500 mg.
Injection: 100 mg/mL.

INDICATIONS AND DOSAGES

▸ **Pyridoxine deficiency**

PO

Adults, Elderly. Initially, 2.5-10 mg/day; then 2-5 mg/day when clinical signs are corrected.

Children. Initially, 5-25 mg/day for 3 wks, then 1.5-2.5 mg/day.

▸ **Pyridoxine-dependent seizures**

PO, IV, IM

Infants. Initially, 10-100 mg/day. Maintenance: PO: 50-100 mg/day.

▸ **Drug-induced neuritis**

PO (TREATMENT)

Adults, Elderly. 100-200 mg/day in divided doses.

Children. 10-50 mg/day.

PO (PROPHYLAXIS)

Adults, Elderly. 25-100 mg/day.

Children. 1-2 mg/kg/day.

CONTRAINDICATIONS

Hypersensitivity to pyridoxine or any of its components.

INTERACTIONS

Drug

Immunosuppressants, isoniazid, penicillamine: May antagonize pyridoxine, causing anemia or peripheral neuritis.

Levodopa: Reverses the effects of levodopa.

Herbal

None known.

Food

None known.

DIAGNOSTIC TEST EFFECTS

None known.

IV INCOMPATIBILITIES

Consult current compatibility resources for known incompatibilities.

SIDE EFFECTS

Occasional

Stinging at IM injection site.

Rare
Headache, nausea, somnolence; sensory neuropathy (paresthesia, unstable gait, clumsiness of hands) with high doses.

SERIOUS REACTIONS

- Long-term megadoses (2-6 g over > 2 mo) may produce sensory neuropathy (reduced deep tendon reflexes, profound impairment of sense of position in distal limbs, gradual sensory ataxia). Toxic symptoms subside when drug is discontinued.
- Seizures have occurred after IV megadoses.

PRECAUTIONS & CONSIDERATIONS

Pyridoxine crosses the placenta and is excreted in breast milk. High doses of pyridoxine in pregnancy may produce seizures in neonates. No age-related precautions have been noted in children or elderly patients. Foods rich in pyridoxine, including avocados, bananas, bran, carrots, eggs, organ meats, tuna, shrimp, hazelnuts, legumes, soybeans, sunflower seeds, and wheat germ, are encouraged.

Improvement of deficiency symptoms, including CNS abnormalities (anxiety, depression, insomnia, motor difficulty, paresthesia, and tremors) and skin lesions (glossitis, seborrhea-like lesions around eyes, mouth, nose), should be monitored.

Storage
Store vials for parenteral use and oral forms at room temperature. Use the solution immediately if reconstituted.

Administration
Scored tablets may be crushed.

! Give pyridoxine orally unless malabsorption, nausea, or vomiting occurs. Avoid IV use in cardiac patients.

Take extended-release capsules and tablets whole without crushing or breaking them. Have the patient avoid chewing the capsule or tablet.

For IV use, pyridoxine may be given undiluted or may be added to IV solutions and given as an infusion.

IM injections may cause discomfort.

Pyrimethamine

pye-ri-meth'a-meen
Daraprim
Do not confuse Daraprim with Dantrium, Daranide.

CATEGORY AND SCHEDULE

Pregnancy Risk Category: C

Classification: Antiprotozoals, antimalarial

MECHANISM OF ACTION

An antiprotozoal with blood and some tissue schizonticidal activity. Inhibits tetrahydrofolic acid synthesis. *Therapeutic Effect:* Highly selective activity against plasmodia and *Toxoplasma gondii* infections.

PHARMACOKINETICS

Well absorbed, peak levels occurring between 2 and 6 h following administration. Protein binding: 87%. Eliminated slowly. *Half-life:* Approximately 96 h.

AVAILABILITY

Tablets: 25 mg (Daraprim).

INDICATIONS AND DOSAGES

▸ Toxoplasmosis

PO

Adults. Initially, 50-75 mg daily, with 1-4 g daily of a sulfonamide of the sulfapyrimidine type (e.g., sulfadoxine). Continue for 1-3 wks, depending on response and tolerance, then reduce dose to one-half that

previously given for each drug and continue for additional 4-5 wks.
Children. 1 mg/kg/day divided into 2 equal daily doses; after 2-4 days reduce to one-half and continue for approximately 1 mo. The usual pediatric sulfonamide dosage is used.

▸ **Acute malaria**

PO

Adults (in combination with sulfonamide). 25 mg daily for 2 days.
Adults (without concomitant sulfonamide). 50 mg daily for 2 days.
Children aged 4-10 yr. 25 mg daily for 2 days.

▸ **Chemoprophylaxis of malaria**

PO

Adults and Children > 10 yr. 25 mg once weekly.
Children aged 4-10 yr. 12.5 mg once weekly.
Infants and Children under 4 yr. 6.25 mg once weekly.

P

OFF-LABEL USES

Prophylaxis for *Pneumocystis* pneumonia (PCP) and *Toxoplasma gondii* in HIV-infected patients.

CONTRAINDICATIONS

Hypersensitivity to pyrimethamine, megaloblastic anemia due to folate deficiency, monotherapy for treatment of acute malaria, breastfeeding.

INTERACTIONS

Drug

Antifolic drugs: Pyrimethamine may be used with sulfonamides, quinine, and other antimalarials, and with other antibiotics. However, concomitant may increase the risk of bone marrow suppression.
Benzodiazepines: Mild hepatotoxicity has been reported with lorazepam.

Herbal and Food

None known.

DIAGNOSTIC TEST EFFECTS

None known.

SIDE EFFECTS

Frequent

Anorexia, vomiting.

Occasional

Atrophic glossitis, hematuria, lowered blood counts.

Rare

Pulmonary eosinophilia, cardiac rhythm changes.

SERIOUS REACTIONS

- Megaloblastic anemia, leukopenia, thrombocytopenia, pancytopenia. May be severe and require leucovorin rescue or prophylaxis, depending on the indication for use.
- Pulmonary eosinphilia (rare).
- Serious hypersensitivity, Stevens-Johnson syndrome and other serious skin reactions.

PRECAUTIONS & CONSIDERATIONS

Caution is warranted in patients with megaloblastic anemia resulting from folate deficiency, seizures or epilepsy, kidney disease, and liver disease. It is unknown whether pyrimethamine crosses the placenta. It passes through the breast milk and may be harmful to the infant. No age-related precautions have been noted in elderly patients.

Storage

Store at room temperature away from heat and moisture.

Administration

Take with food and a full glass of water to decrease stomach upset.

Quazepam

kwaz'ze-pam

★ Doral

CATEGORY AND SCHEDULE

Pregnancy Risk Category: X

Controlled Substance Schedule: IV

Classification: Benzodiazepines, sedatives/hypnotics

MECHANISM OF ACTION

BZ-1 receptor-selective benzodiazepine with sedative properties. *Therapeutic Effect:* Produces sedative effect from its central nervous system (CNS) depressant action.

PHARMACOKINETICS

Rapidly absorbed from GI tract. Protein binding: 95%. Extensively metabolized in liver. Excreted in urine and feces. Unknown whether removed by hemodialysis. *Half-life:* 39-73 h (terminal).

AVAILABILITY

Tablets: 7.5 mg, 15 mg (Doral).

INDICATIONS AND DOSAGES

▸ **Insomnia**

PO

Adults. Initially, 15 mg at bedtime. Adjust from 7.5 mg to 15 mg at bedtime, depending on initial response. Optimal effective dose is thought to be 15 mg.

Elderly, debilitated, liver disease. Initially, 7.5 mg at bedtime. If needed, can increase to 15 mg if lower dose not effective after 1-2 nights.

CONTRAINDICATIONS

Pregnancy, sleep apnea, hypersensitivity to quazepam or any component of the formulation.

INTERACTIONS

Drug

Alcohol, CNS depressants, antihistamines, psychotropic medications: Potentiate effects of quazepam.

Azole antifungals: May inhibit liver metabolism and increase quazepam blood serum concentrations.

CYP2B5 substrate (e.g., efavirenz, bupropion): Quazepam is a CYP2B6 inhibitor and may increase plasma concentrations of these drugs; monitor.

Theophylline: May decrease quazepam effectiveness.

Herbal

Dong quai, kava kava, magnolia, passionflower, skullcap, tan-shen, valerian: May increase CNS-depressant effect of quazepam.

Food

Caffeine: May decrease sedative and anxiolytic effects of quazepam.

DIAGNOSTIC TEST EFFECTS

None known.

SIDE EFFECTS

Frequent

Headache, mild daytime drowsiness most common. Muscular incoordination (ataxia), light-headedness, slurred speech (particularly in elderly or debilitated patients).

Occasional

Confusion, blurred vision, dry mouth, dyspepsia.

Rare

Behavioral problems such as anger, impaired memory, paradoxical reactions such as insomnia, nervousness, or irritability.

SERIOUS REACTIONS

- Anaphylaxis or angioedema.
- Abrupt or too-rapid withdrawal may result in pronounced

restlessness, irritability, insomnia, hand tremors, abdominal and muscle cramps, sweating, vomiting, and seizures.
• Overdosage results in somnolence, confusion, diminished reflexes, and coma.
• "Sleep driving" and other complex behaviors reported while not fully awake, with no memory of event. If such an event reported, discontinue drug.

PRECAUTIONS & CONSIDERATIONS

Caution should be used in patients with impaired renal or hepatic function, and smaller initial doses should be used. Quazepam crosses the placenta and is distributed in breast milk. Chronic ingestion of quazepam during pregnancy may produce withdrawal symptoms in women and CNS depression in neonates; therefore, the benefit of taking in patients who desire to become pregnant should be weighed against the risk to the fetus and neonate. Safety and efficacy of quazepam have not been established in children. In elderly patients, use small initial doses and gradually increase them to avoid excessive sedation or ataxia as evidenced by muscular incoordination.

Drowsiness and dizziness are expected side effects. Avoid tasks that require mental alertness or motor skills. Concomitant use with alcohol should also be avoided.

Storage

Store at room temperature.

Administration

Best taken on an empty stomach. Take quazepam at bedtime. Tablets may be crushed. Do not abruptly stop quazepam.

Quetiapine

kwe-tye′a-peen

★ 🍁 Seroquel, Seroquel XR

Do not confuse Seroquel with Serzone.

CATEGORY AND SCHEDULE

Pregnancy Risk Category: C

Classification: Antipsychotics, atypical

MECHANISM OF ACTION

A dibenzepine derivative that antagonizes dopamine, serotonin, histamine, and α_1-adrenergic receptors. *Therapeutic Effect:* Diminishes manifestations of psychotic disorders. Produces moderate sedation, few extrapyramidal effects, and no anticholinergic effects.

PHARMACOKINETICS

Well absorbed after PO administration. Protein binding: 83%. Widely distributed in tissues; central nervous system (CNS) concentration exceeds plasma concentration. Undergoes extensive first-pass metabolism in the liver. Primarily excreted in urine. *Half-life:* 6-7 h.

AVAILABILITY

Tablets: 25 mg, 50 mg, 100 mg, 200 mg, 300 mg, 400 mg.
Extended-Release Tablets: 50 mg, 150 mg, 200 mg, 300 mg, 400 mg.

INDICATIONS AND DOSAGES

▸ **Management of manifestations of psychotic disorders and schizophrenia**

PO (IMMEDIATE RELEASE)

Adults, Elderly. Initially, 25 mg twice a day, then 25-50 mg 2-3 times a day on the second and third days, up to 300-400 mg/day in divided doses 2-3 times a day by the fourth day. Further adjustments of 25-50 mg twice a day may be made at intervals of 2 days of longer. *Maintenance:* 300-800 mg/day administered in 2-3 divided doses (adults).

PO (EXTENDED RELEASE)

Adults. Initially, 300 mg once daily, increasing by up to 300 mg/day. *Maintenance:* 400-800 mg/day as one daily dose.

Elderly. Initially, 50 mg once daily, increasing by up to 50 mg/day. *Maintenance:* 50-200 mg/day as one daily dose.

▸ **Adjunctive treatment to antidepressants for depression**

PO (EXTENDED-RELEASE TABLETS)

Adults. Initially, 50 mg once per day in evening; increase on day 3 up to 150 mg/day. Effective range 150-300 mg/day.

▸ **Bipolar mania**

PO (EXTENDED-RELEASE TABLETS)

Adults. Initially, 300 mg once per day in evening; increase to 600 mg/day on day 2. Effective maintenance range 400-800 mg/day. Used as monotherapy or adjunct to lithium or divalproex.

▸ **Depressive episodes associated with bipolar disorder**

PO (EXTENDED-RELEASE TABLETS)

Adults. Initially, 50 mg once per day in evening; titrate to reach 300 mg/day by day 4. Effective maintenance range 400-800 mg/day.

▸ **Dosage in hepatic impairment, elderly or debilitated patients, and those predisposed to hypotensive reactions**

These patients should receive a lower initial dose and lower dosage increases.

CONTRAINDICATIONS

Hypersensitivity to quetiapine.

INTERACTIONS

Drug

Alcohol, other central nervous system (CNS) depressants: May increase CNS depression.

Antihypertensives: May increase the hypotensive effects of these drugs.

Hepatic enzyme inducers (such as carbamazepine, rifampin phenytoin): May increase quetiapine clearance.

Strong CYP3A4 inhibitors (e.g., ketoconazole, clarithromycin, nefazodone, protease inhibitors): May decrease the clearance of quetiapine. Lower doses of quetiapine may be required.

Herbal

None known.

Food

High-fat meals: Increase the effects of quetiapine.

DIAGNOSTIC TEST EFFECTS

May decrease serum total and free thyroxine (T_4) serum levels. May increase serum cholesterol, triglyceride, AST (SGOT), and ALT (SGPT) levels. May produce a false-positive pregnancy test result.

SIDE EFFECTS

Frequent (10%-19%)

Headache, somnolence, dizziness.

Occasional (3%-9%)

Constipation, orthostatic hypotension, tachycardia, dry mouth, dyspepsia, rash, asthenia, abdominal pain, rhinitis.

Rare (2%)

Back pain, fever, weight gain.

SERIOUS REACTIONS

• Overdosage may produce heart block, hypotension, hypokalemia, and tachycardia.

PRECAUTIONS & CONSIDERATIONS

Elderly patients with dementia-related psychosis have an increased risk of death when treated with atypical antipsychotics vs. placebo. Caution is warranted with Alzheimer disease, cardiovascular disease (such as congestive heart failure or history of myocardial infarction), cerebrovascular disease, diabetes mellitus, seizures, hepatic impairment, dehydration, hypothyroidism, hypovolemia, a history of breast cancer, and a history of drug abuse or dependence. It is unknown whether quetiapine is distributed in breast milk. However, this drug is not recommended for breastfeeding women. The safety and efficacy of quetiapine have not been established in children. As with other drugs used for mood disorders, this drug may increase the risk of suicidal thinking and behavior in children, adolescents, and young adults (18-24 yr) with major depressive disorder and other psychiatric disorders. All patients should be monitored for suicidal thoughts, mood changes, or unusual behaviors. For elderly patients, lower initial and target dosages may be necessary.

Drowsiness and dizziness may occur but generally subside with continued therapy. Tasks requiring mental alertness or motor skills should be avoided. Dehydration, particularly during exercise, exposure to extreme heat, and concurrent use of medications that cause dry mouth or other drying effects, should also be avoided. BP, pulse rate, weight, pattern of daily bowel activity, and stool consistency should be assessed.

Storage

Store at room temperature.

Administration

Take quetiapine without food or with a light meal. With immediate-release quetiapine, dosage adjustments should occur at 2-day intervals. With extended-release quetiapine, do not crush, cut, or chew; dosage adjustments may occur daily. When restarting therapy for persons who have been off quetiapine for longer than 1 wk, follow the initial titration schedule, as prescribed. When restarting therapy for persons who have been off quetiapine for < 1 wk, titration is not required and the maintenance dose can be reinstituted. Do not abruptly discontinue.

Quinapril

kwin'a-pril

★ 🍁 Accupril

Do not confuse Accupril with Accolate or Accutane.

CATEGORY AND SCHEDULE

Pregnancy Risk Category: C (D if used in second or third trimester)

Classification:

Antihypertensives, angiotensin-converting enzyme (ACE) inhibitors

MECHANISM OF ACTION

An ACE inhibitor that suppresses the renin-angiotensin-aldosterone system and prevents the conversion of angiotensin I to angiotensin II, a potent vasoconstrictor; may also inhibit angiotensin II at local vascular and renal sites. *Therapeutic Effect:* Reduces peripheral arterial resistance, BP, and pulmonary capillary wedge pressure; improves cardiac output.

PHARMACOKINETICS

Route	Onset	Peak	Duration
PO	1 h	2 h	24 h

Readily absorbed from the GI tract. Protein binding: 97%. Metabolized in the liver, GI tract, and extravascular tissue to active metabolite. Excreted primarily in urine. Minimal removal by hemodialysis. *Half-life:* 1-2 h; metabolite, 3 h (increased in those with impaired renal function).

AVAILABILITY

Tablets: 5 mg, 10 mg, 20 mg, 40 mg.

INDICATIONS AND DOSAGES

▸ **Hypertension (monotherapy)**
PO
Adults. Initially, 10-20 mg/day. May adjust dosage at intervals of at least 2 wks or longer. Maintenance: 20-80 mg/day as single dose or 2 divided doses. Maximum: 80 mg/day.
Elderly. Initially, 10 mg/day. May increase by 2.5-5 mg q1-2wk.

▸ **Hypertension (combination therapy)**
PO
Adults. Initially, 5 mg/day titrated to patient's needs.
Elderly. Initially, 5 mg/day. May increase by 2.5-5 mg q1-2wk.

▸ **Adjunct to manage heart failure**
PO
Adults, Elderly. Initially, 5 mg twice a day. Range: 20-40 mg/day divided into 2 doses.

Dosage in renal impairment
Dosage is titrated to the patient's clinical response after the following initial doses:

Creatinine Clearance (mL/min)	Initial Dose (mg)
> 60	10
30-60	5
10-29	2.5

OFF-LABEL USES

Treatment of hypertension and renal crisis in scleroderma, diabetic nephropathy, valvular regurgitation.

CONTRAINDICATIONS

Bilateral renal artery stenosis; angioedema related to this or another ACE inhibitor or hereditary angioedema.

INTERACTIONS

Drug
Alcohol, antihypertensives, diuretics: May increase the effects of quinapril.
Lithium: May increase lithium blood concentration and risk of lithium toxicity.
NSAIDs: May decrease the effects of quinapril.
Potassium-sparing diuretics, drospirenone, potassium supplements: Increased risk of hyperkalemia.
Tetracycline, quinolones: May reduce the absorption of these medications due to magnesium content in quinapril tablets.

Herbal
Garlic: May increase antihypertensive effect.
Ginseng, yohimbe: May worsen hypertension.

Food
High-fat meals: Decrease absorption moderately.

DIAGNOSTIC TEST EFFECTS

May increase BUN, serum alkaline phosphatase, serum bilirubin, serum creatinine, serum potassium, AST (SGOT), and ALT (SGPT) levels. May decrease serum sodium levels. May cause positive antinuclear antibody titer.

SIDE EFFECTS

Frequent (5%-7%)
Headache, dizziness.

Occasional (3%-4%)
Fatigue, vomiting, nausea, hypotension, chest pain, dry cough, syncope, hyperkalemia.
Rare (< 2%)
Diarrhea, dyspnea, rash, palpitations, impotence, insomnia, malaise.

SERIOUS REACTIONS

- Excessive hypotension (first-dose syncope) may occur in patients with congestive heart failure (CHF) and in those who are severely salt or volume depleted.
- Angioedema occurs rarely.
- Agranulocytosis and neutropenia may be noted in those with collagen vascular disease, including scleroderma and systemic lupus erythematosus, and impaired renal function.
- Nephrotic syndrome may be noted in those with history of renal disease.

PRECAUTIONS & CONSIDERATIONS

Caution is warranted with CHF, collagen vascular disease, hyperkalemia, hypovolemia, renal impairment, and renal stenosis. Quinapril crosses the placenta, and it is unknown whether it is distributed in breast milk. Quinapril may cause fetal or neonatal morbidity or mortality, so it should be avoided in pregnancy. Safety and efficacy of quinapril have not been established in children. Elderly patients may be more sensitive to the hypotensive effect of quinapril.

Be alert to fluctuations in BP. If an excessive reduction in BP occurs, place the patient in the supine position with legs elevated. CBC and blood chemistry should be obtained before beginning quinapril therapy, then every 2 wks for the next 3 mo, and periodically thereafter in patients with autoimmune disease, or renal impairment, and in those who are taking drugs that affect immune response or leukocyte count. BUN, serum creatinine, serum potassium levels are important indicators.
Storage
Store at room temperature; protect from light.
Administration
Take quinapril without regard to food. Crush tablets as desired.

Quinidine

kwin'i-deen
Do not confuse quinidine with clonidine or quinine.

CATEGORY AND SCHEDULE

Pregnancy Risk Category: C

Classification: Antiarrhythmics, class IA, antiprotozoals

MECHANISM OF ACTION

An antiarrhythmic that decreases sodium influx during depolarization, decreases potassium efflux during repolarization, and reduces calcium transport across the myocardial cell membrane. Decreases myocardial excitability, conduction velocity, and contractility. *Therapeutic Effect:* Suppresses arrhythmias.

AVAILABILITY

Injection: 80 mg/mL.
Tablets: 200 mg, 300 mg.
Tablets (Extended Release): 300 mg.
Tablets (Extended Release): 324 mg.

INDICATIONS AND DOSAGES

▸ **Conversion and reduction of relapse for atrial fib/flutter and suppression of ventricular arrhythmias**
PO
Adults, Elderly. 200-600 mg q6-8h (long acting): 324-648 mg q8-12h.

Children. 15-60 mg/kg/day in divided doses q6h.
IV INFUSION
Adults, Elderly. 5-10 mg/kg as a slow IV infusion as a single dose. Most respond at ≤ 5 mg/kg; discontinue use if no response after 10 mg/kg total.

▸ **Treatment of severe malaria (rare)**
Adults. See manufacturer's prescribing information for the use of IV and PO quinidine for the treatment of susceptible *P. falciparum* malaria.

CONTRAINDICATIONS

Complete AV block, intraventricular conduction defects (widening of QRS complex). Known quinidine allergy or a history of thrombocytopenia or thrombocytic purpura during quinidine or quinine therapy. In patients adversely affected by an anticholinergic agent (e.g., myasthenia gravis).

INTERACTIONS

Drug
Antimyasthenics: May decrease effects of these drugs on skeletal muscle.
Digoxin: May increase digoxin serum concentration.
Drugs metabolized by CYP2D6: Quinidine inhibits metabolism (e.g., mexilitene, phenothiazines, tricyclic antidepressants) or active conversion (e.g., codeine) of these drugs.
Haloperidol: Serum levels increased when quinidine coadministered.
Neuromuscular blockers, oral anticoagulants: May increase effects of these drugs.
Other antiarrhythmics, pimozide, and other drugs prolonging QT interval: May increase cardiac effects.
Urinary alkalizers such as antacids: May decrease quinidine renal excretion.
Verapamil: Decreases quinidine clearance and raises serum levels.
Herbal
None known.
Food
None known.

DIAGNOSTIC TEST EFFECTS

Therapeutic serum level is 2-5 mcg/mL; toxic serum level is > 5 mcg/mL.

IV INCOMPATIBILITIES

Acyclovir, aminophylline, amphotericin B, ampicillin, ampicillin-sulbactam (Unasyn), azathioprine (Imuran), aztreonam (Azactam), bretylium, cephalosporin class antibiotics, clindamycin (Cleocin), dexamethasone, diazepam, ertapenem (Invanz), furosemide (Lasix), heparin, inamrinone, insulin, methylprednisolone (Solu-Medrol), penicillin antibiotics, nitroprusside, pantoprazole (Protonix), phenobarbital, phenytoin, sodium bicarbonate.

IV COMPATIBILITIES

Milrinone (Primacor).

SIDE EFFECTS

Frequent
Abdominal pain and cramps, nausea, diarrhea, vomiting (can be immediate, intense).
Occasional
Mild cinchonism (ringing in ears, blurred vision, hearing loss) or severe cinchonism (headache, vertigo, diaphoresis, lightheadedness, photophobia, confusion, delirium).
Rare
Hypotension (particularly with IV administration), hypersensitivity

reaction (fever, anaphylaxis, photosensitivity reaction), syncope.

SERIOUS REACTIONS

- Cardiotoxic effects occur most commonly with IV administration and are observed as conduction changes (50% widening of QRS complex, prolonged QT interval, flattened T waves, and disappearance of P wave), ventricular tachycardia or flutter, frequent premature ventricular contractions (PVCs), or complete AV block.
- Quinidine-induced syncope and hypotension may occur with the usual dosage.
- Patients with atrial flutter and fibrillation may experience a paradoxical, extremely rapid ventricular rate that may be prevented by prior digitalization.
- Hepatotoxicity with jaundice due to drug hypersensitivity may occur.

PRECAUTIONS & CONSIDERATIONS

Caution is warranted in patients with digoxin toxicity, incomplete AV block, hepatic and renal impairment, myasthenia gravis, myocardial depression, and sick sinus syndrome. Direct sunlight and artificial light should be avoided.

Monitor BP and pulse rate before giving quinidine unless the person is on a continuous cardiac monitor. Notify the physician if fever, ringing in the ears, or visual disturbances occur. CBC; BUN; serum alkaline phosphatase, bilirubin, creatinine, AST (SGOT), and ALT (SGPT) levels; intake and output; pattern of bowel activity and stool consistency; and serum potassium should be monitored in those receiving long-term therapy. ECG for cardiac changes, particularly prolongation of PR or QT interval and widening of the QRS complex, should also be assessed; notify the physician of significant ECG changes.

Storage

Store oral forms and unopened vials at room temperature.

Diluted infusion is stable for 24 h at room temperature when diluted with D5W.

Administration

Do not crush or chew sustained-release tablets. Take quinidine with food to reduce GI upset.

! Continuously monitor BP and ECG during IV administration; adjust the rate of the infusion as appropriate and as ordered to minimize arrhythmias and hypotension.

For IV infusion, dilute 800 mg with 50 mL D5W to provide concentration of 16 mg/mL. Give at rate of 1 mL (16 mg)/min or less because a rapid rate may markedly decrease arterial pressure. Administer with patient in supine position.

Quinine

kwye′nine

★ Qualaquin

Do not confuse with quinidine.

CATEGORY AND SCHEDULE

Pregnancy Risk Category: C

Classification: Antiprotozoals

MECHANISM OF ACTION

A cinchona alkaloid that relaxes skeletal muscle by increasing the refractory period, decreasing excitability of motor endplates (curare-like), and affecting distribution of calcium with muscle fiber. Antimalaria: Depresses oxygen uptake and carbohydrate metabolism, elevates pH in intracellular organelles of parasites. *Therapeutic Effect:* Relaxes skeletal muscle; produces parasite death.

PHARMACOKINETICS

Rapidly absorbed mainly from upper small intestine. Protein binding: 70%-95%. Metabolized in liver. Excreted in feces, saliva, and urine. *Half-life:* 8-14 h (adults), 6-12 h (children).

AVAILABILITY

Capsules: 324 mg (Qualaquin).

INDICATIONS AND DOSAGES

▸ Treatment of malaria

PO

Adults, Elderly, Children ≥ 16 yr. 648 mg PO q8h for 7 days.

▸ Dosage in renal impairment

In patients with severe chronic renal failure, the following modified dosage is recommended: Give 1 dose of 648 mg; then 12 h after, begin maintenance dose of 324 mg q12h for 7 days.

CONTRAINDICATIONS

Known hypersensitivity to quinine or to mefloquine or quinidine because of cross-sensitivity, reactions include thrombocytopenia, thrombotic thrombocytopenic purpura or hemolytic uremic syndrome; prolonged QT intervals, G6PD deficiency; myasthenia gravis, blackwater fever, optic neuritis.

INTERACTIONS

Drug

Alkalinizing agents, cimetidine, ranitidine: May increase quinine serum concentrations.

Antacids: Decrease quinine absorption; do not give concomitantly.

CYP3A4 inhibitors: Decrease quinine metabolism.

Digoxin: May increase blood concentration of digoxin.

Drugs metabolized by CYP3A4 and CYP2D6: Quinine inhibits these enzymes.

Halofantrine, mefloquine: May increase risk of seizures and ECG abnormalities. Avoid concomitant use.

Neuromuscular blockers: May increase effects of these drugs.

Phenobarbital, phenytoin, rifampin: May decrease quinine serum concentrations.

Warfarin: May increase anticoagulant effect.

Herbal

St. John's wort: May decrease quinine levels.

Food

None known.

DIAGNOSTIC TEST EFFECTS

May interfere with 17-OH steroid determinations. May result in positive Coombs' test.

SIDE EFFECTS

Frequent

A cluster of symptoms occur to some degree in almost all patients: headache, vasodilation and sweating, nausea, tinnitus, vertigo or dizziness, blurred vision, disturbance in color perception, vomiting, diarrhea, abdominal pain (mild cinchonism). May cause hypoglycemia.

Occasional

Extreme flushing of skin with intense generalized pruritus is most typical hypersensitivity reaction; also rash, wheezing, dyspnea. Prolonged therapy: cardiac conduction disturbances, decreased hearing, optic neuritis.

SERIOUS REACTIONS

- Overdosage (severe cinchonism) may result in cardiovascular effects, severe headache, intestinal cramps with vomiting and diarrhea, apprehension, confusion, seizures, blindness, deafness, and respiratory depression.
- Serious hypersensitivity reactions: anaphylactoid reactions, serious skin rashes, Stevens-Johnson syndrome and TENS, angioedema, bronchospasm, thrombotic or immune thrombocytopenic purpura (TTP or ITP) and hemolytic-uremic syndrome (HUS), thrombocytopenia, blackwater fever, granulomatous hepatitis, and acute interstitial nephritis.
- Cardiotoxic effects (widening of QRS complex, prolonged QT interval), ventricular tachycardia.

PRECAUTIONS & CONSIDERATIONS

Though once widely used off-label, quinine is not approved to treat nocturnal leg cramps due to lack of data for efficacy, and potential risk of serious and potentially life-threatening reactions. Caution is warranted in patients with cardiovascular disease, myasthenia gravis, and asthma. Be aware that quinine is contraindicated in pregnant women. Quinine readily crosses the placenta and is distributed in breast milk. Be aware that quinine may cause congenital malformations such as deafness, limb abnormalities, visceral defects, visual changes, and stillbirths. Reliable contraception should be used. Safety and efficacy not established in children < 16 yr. In elderly patients, age-related renal impairment may require dosage adjustment.

Fasting blood sugar should be checked. Watch for signs of hypoglycemia such as cold sweating, tremors, tachycardia, hunger, and anxiety. Visual or hearing difficulties, shortness of breath, rash, itching, and nausea should be reported.

Storage

Store at room temperature.

Administration

Take quinine with food. Do not crush to avoid bitter taste. Do not administer with aluminum- or magnesium-containing antacids.

Quinupristin/ Dalfopristin

quin-u′pris-tin; dal-foe′pris-tin

★ 🍁 Synercid

CATEGORY AND SCHEDULE

Pregnancy Risk Category: B

Classification: Anti-infective, streptogramins

MECHANISM OF ACTION

The site of action is the bacterial ribosome. Dalfopristin inhibits the early phase of protein synthesis and quinupristin inhibits the late phase of protein synthesis. The actions are synergistic. Active against gram-positive aerobic organisms. *Therapeutic Effect:* Bacteriostatic against *Enterococcus faecium* (including vancomycin-resistant strains) and bactericidal against strains of methicillin-susceptible staphylococci (e.g., MSSA) and *Streptococcus pyogenes*.

PHARMACOKINETICS

Maximum concentration for dalfopristin is roughly 8 mcg/mL and for quinupristin roughly 3 mcg/mL after q8h dosing. Drugs penetrate well into blister fluid. Primary route

Q

of elimination is biliary and fecal excretion, accounting for roughly 80% of a dose. *Elimination half-life:* Less than 1 h for both components; however, action at infection much longer due to post-antibiotic effect.

AVAILABILITY

Powder for Injection: 500-mg vials (containing 150 mg quinupristin with 350 mg dalfopristin).

INDICATIONS AND DOSAGES

▸ **Serious or life-threatening infections (e.g., bacteremia, endocarditis) associated with vancomycin-resistant *E. faecium* (VREF)**

IV

Adults, Children ≥ 16 yr.
7.5 mg/kg q8h.

▸ **Complicated skin or skin-structure infections due to methicillin-sensitive *Staph aureus* or *Strep pyogenes***

IV

Adults, Children ≥ 16 yr.
7.5 mg/kg q12h.

▸ **Pediatric dosage (emergency use)**

IV

Children under 15 yr. Limited numbers of children treated with a dose of 7.5 mg/kg q8h or q12h has been used under emergency conditions.

CONTRAINDICATIONS

Known hypersensitivity to the drug, or prior hypersensitivity to other streptogramins (e.g., pristinamycin or virginiamycin).

INTERACTIONS

Drug

Drugs metabolized by CYP3A4: Quinupristin/dalfopristin inhibits CYP3A4 significantly and can decrease metabolism of these drugs. Medications include protease inhibitors, cisapride, diltiazem, midazolam, vinca alkaloids, taxanes, cyclosporine, HMG-CoA reductase inhibitors (statins), nifedipine, tacrolimus, quinidine, verapamil, and many others. Use particular caution with those narrow therapeutic index drugs metabolized by CYP3A4.

DIAGNOSTIC TEST EFFECTS

May increase total and conjugated bilirubin levels.

IV INCOMPATIBILITIES

NaCl (saline) solutions (e.g., NS injection) or any drugs mixed in a saline solution.

IV COMPATIBILITIES

NOTE: Only compatible with the following if mixed in dextrose solutions; if any of these IV drugs are mixed in saline solutions, they will not be compatible.
Aztreonam (Azactam), ciprofloxacin (Cipro), haloperidol, metoclopramide, potassium chloride.

SIDE EFFECTS

Frequent (> 10%)
Venous irritation, hyperbilirubinemia, erythema, edema, infusion site reactions (edema, inflammation, pain).
Occasional (2%-5%)
Nausea, diarrhea, vomiting, headache, pruritus, thrombophlebitis.
Rare
Maculopapular rash, sweating, urticaria, arthralgia, myalgia.

SERIOUS REACTIONS

- Rare reactions include hypersensitivity reactions such as angioedema and anaphylaxis.
- Possible risk for pseudomembranous colitis and superinfection.

- If myalgia or arthralgias are severe, decreasing medication frequency to q12h may alleviate.
- Hyperbilirubinemia, jaundice, hemolysis or hemolytic anemia, pancytopenia, hepatitis, tachycardia, syncope, tremor, ventricular arrhythmia have also been rarely reported.

PRECAUTIONS & CONSIDERATIONS

Venous irritation is common; use suggested techniques to reduce risk (see Administration). Episodes of arthralgia and myalgia, some severe, have been reported; use caution in patients taking other medications that may cause myalgia. Should superinfection occur during therapy, appropriate measures should be taken. The drug may compete with bilirubin for excretion; use with caution in patients with diseases that may be exacerbated if bilirubin levels increase. Use with caution in pregnancy and lactation; there are no adequate data in pregnancy and it is not know if the drug is excreted in breast milk. While the drug's safety and efficacy is not established in children < 16 yr of age, emergency protocols have utilized the drug in limited numbers of pediatric patients (see Dosage).

Sometimes after starting treatment with antibiotics, patients can develop watery and bloody stools (with or without stomach cramps and fever) even as late as two or more months after having taken the last dose of the antibiotic. If this occurs, patients should contact their physician as soon as possible.

Storage

Refrigerate unopened vials. Do not freeze. Reconstituted, diluted product is stable up to 5 h at room temperature or up to 54 h if stored under refrigeration.

Administration

For IV infusion use only. Reconstitute the 500-mg single-dose vial by slowly adding 5 mL of D5W or SWI. Do NOT use saline solutions. Gently swirl; do not shake. Allow foam to disappear. The resulting solution should be clear and will have a concentration of 100 mg/mL. Dilute further before infusion. Add proper weight-based dose to 250 mL of D5W. An infusion volume of 100 mL may be used for central line infusions. If moderate to severe venous irritation occurs following peripheral administration of a 250-mL dilution, consider increasing the dilution volume to 500 or 750 mL, changing the infusion site, or infusing by a peripherally inserted central catheter (PICC) or a central venous catheter. Administer by IV infusion over 60 min.

! Following completion of a peripheral infusion, the vein should be flushed with D5W to minimize venous irritation. Do NOT Flush with saline or heparin because of incompatibility concerns.

Rabeprazole

rah-bep'rah-zole

★ Aciphex

Do not confuse Aciphex with Accupril or Aricept.

CATEGORY AND SCHEDULE

Pregnancy Risk Category: B

Classification: Gastrointestinals, proton-pump inhibitors

MECHANISM OF ACTION

A proton-pump inhibitor that converts to active metabolites that irreversibly bind to and inhibit hydrogen-potassium adenosine triphosphate, an enzyme on the surface of gastric parietal cells. Actively secretes hydrogen ions for potassium ions, resulting in an accumulation of hydrogen ions in gastric lumen. *Therapeutic Effect:* Increases gastric pH, reducing gastric acid production.

PHARMACOKINETICS

Rapidly absorbed from the GI tract after passing through the stomach relatively intact. Protein binding: 96%. Metabolized extensively in the liver to inactive metabolites. Excreted primarily in urine. Unknown whether removed by hemodialysis. *Half-life:* 1-2 h is dose-dependent (increased with hepatic impairment).

AVAILABILITY

Tablets (Delayed Release): 20 mg.

INDICATIONS AND DOSAGES

▸ **Erosive/ulcerative or symptomatic gastroesophageal reflux disease (GERD)**

PO

Adults, Elderly. 20 mg/day for 4-8 wks. Maintenance: 20 mg/day.

Children 12 yr and older. 20 mg/day for up to 8 wks.

▸ **Duodenal ulcer**

PO

Adults, Elderly. 20 mg/day before morning meal for 4 wks. Some patients may require an additional 4 wks of therapy.

▸ **Pathologic hypersecretory conditions, including Zollinger-Ellison syndrome**

PO

Adults, Elderly. Initially, 60 mg once a day. May increase to 100 mg once a day or 60 mg twice a day. Continue as long as necessary.

▸ ***Helicobacter pylori* infection**

PO

Adults, Elderly. 20 mg twice a day for 7 days administered with amoxicillin 1000 mg twice daily for 7 days and clarithromycin 500 mg twice daily for 7 days.

CONTRAINDICATIONS

Hypersensitivity to rabeprazole or any other proton-pump inhibitor. If treating *H. pylori,* then must consider contraindications to other medications in the eradication regimen.

INTERACTIONS

Drug

Atazanavir, nelfinavir, delavirdine: Avoid coadministration due to decreased concentrations.

Clopidogrel: Avoid use of PPI with clopidogrel, as PPI may prevent formation of active moiety by inhibiting CYP2C19, negating efficacy of clopidogrel.

Cyclosporine: May increase plasma level of cyclosporine. Monitor.

Dasatinib, gefitinib: Decreases antineoplastic absorption. Avoid.

Digoxin: May increase the plasma concentration of digoxin.

Ethanol: Avoid because of increased GI irritation.
Iron salts: May interfere with absorption of iron salts.
Ketoconazole, itraconazole: May decrease the blood concentration of ketoconazole and itraconazole.
Warfarin: May increase effect of warfarin. Monitor PT/INR closely.
Herbal
St. John's wort: May decrease the levels of rabeprazole.
Food
None significant.

DIAGNOSTIC TEST EFFECTS

May increase serum alkaline phosphatase, AST (SGOT), and ALT (SGPT) levels.

SIDE EFFECTS

Rare (< 2%)
Headache, nausea, dizziness, rash, diarrhea, malaise.

SERIOUS REACTIONS

- Hyperglycemia, hypokalemia, hyponatremia, and hyperlipidemia occur rarely.

R

PRECAUTIONS & CONSIDERATIONS

Caution is warranted in patients with severely impaired hepatic function. It is unknown whether rabeprazole crosses the placenta or is distributed in breast milk. Safety and efficacy of rabeprazole have been established in children 12 yr and older. No age-related precautions have been noted in elderly patients.

Notify the physician if diarrhea, GI discomfort, headache, nausea, or skin rash occurs. Laboratory values, especially serum chemistries and liver function test results, should be assessed before therapy.

Administration
Take rabeprazole without regard to meals. Do not crush, chew, or split tablet; swallow it whole.

Raloxifene

ra-lox'i-feen
★ 🍁 Evista
Do not confuse raloxifene with propoxyphene or Avinza.

CATEGORY AND SCHEDULE

Pregnancy Risk Category: X

Classification: Estrogen-receptor modulators, selective, hormones/hormone modifiers

MECHANISM OF ACTION

A selective estrogen receptor modulator that affects some receptors like estrogen. *Therapeutic Effect:* Like estrogen, prevents bone loss and improves lipid profiles, reduces breast cancer risk in postmenopausal women.

PHARMACOKINETICS

Rapidly absorbed after PO administration. Highly bound to plasma proteins (95%) and albumin. Undergoes extensive first-pass metabolism in liver. Excreted mainly in feces and, to a lesser extent, in urine. Unknown whether removed by hemodialysis. *Half-life:* 28-33 h.

AVAILABILITY

Tablets: 60 mg.

INDICATIONS AND DOSAGES

▸ **Prevention or treatment of osteoporosis**
PO
Adults, Elderly. 60 mg a day.

▸ **For invasive breast cancer prophylaxis in postmenopausal women with osteoporosis or in postmenopausal women who are at high risk for developing the disease**
PO
Adults, Elderly. 60 mg a day.

CONTRAINDICATIONS
Active or history of venous thromboembolic events, such as deep vein thrombosis, pulmonary embolism, and retinal vein thrombosis; women who are at risk for stroke; women who are or may become pregnant or are breastfeeding.

INTERACTIONS
Drug
Cholestyramine: Reduces raloxifene absorption and enterohepatic recycling; do not use together.
Drugs highly protein-bound (i.e., diazepam, lidocaine): Use with caution because raloxifene may affect protein binding of other drugs.
Hormone replacement therapy, systemic estrogen: Do not use raloxifene concurrently with these drugs.
Levothyroxine: May decrease levothyroxine's absorption.
Warfarin: May decrease INR and the effects of warfarin.
Herbal
None known.
Food
None known.

DIAGNOSTIC TEST EFFECTS
Lowers serum total cholesterol and LDL levels but does not affect HDL or triglyceride levels. Slightly decreases platelet count and serum inorganic phosphate, albumin, calcium, and protein levels.

SIDE EFFECTS
Frequent (10%-25%)
Hot flashes, flu-like symptoms, arthralgia, sinusitis. Hot flashes subside with time.
Occasional (5%-9%)
Weight gain, nausea, myalgia, pharyngitis, cough, dyspepsia, leg cramps, rash, depression.
Rare (3%-4%)
Vaginitis, urinary tract infection, peripheral edema, flatulence, vomiting, fever, migraine, diaphoresis.

SERIOUS REACTIONS
• Deep vein thrombosis (DVT), pulmonary embolism, coronary events or stroke.

PRECAUTIONS & CONSIDERATIONS
Caution is warranted in patients with cardiovascular disease, hypertriglyceridemia, unexplained uterine bleeding, hepatic or renal impairment, and a history of cervical or uterine cancer. It is unknown whether raloxifene is distributed in breast milk; however, this drug is not recommended for breastfeeding women. Raloxifene may cause fetal harm and is contraindicated during pregnancy. Raloxifene is not used in children. No age-related precautions have been noted in elderly patients. Avoid alcohol consumption and cigarette smoking during raloxifene therapy. Also avoid prolonged immobility during travel because limited movement increases the risk of venous thromboembolic events. Discontinue use 72 h prior to and during any prolonged immobilization (such as postsurgical recovery). Exercise is encouraged.

Bone mineral density, platelet count, serum levels of inorganic phosphate, calcium, total and LDL cholesterol, and protein should be monitored.

Storage
Store at room temperature.
Administration
Take raloxifene without regard to food at any time of day.
Take supplemental calcium and vitamin D if daily dietary intake is inadequate.

Raltegravir

ral-teg'ra-vir

Isentress

CATEGORY AND SCHEDULE

Pregnancy Risk Category: C

Classification: Antiretrovirals, HIV integrase strand transfer inhibitors

MECHANISM OF ACTION

An integrase strand transfer inhibitor that inhibits catalytic activity of HIV integrase, an HIV encoded enzyme needed for viral replication. Directly impacts the formation of the HIV provirus, which is needed for viral progeny. *Therapeutic Effect:* Impairs HIV replication, slowing the progression of HIV infection.

PHARMACOKINETICS

Efficacy not affected by food. Protein binding: 83%. Eliminated mainly by metabolism via a UGT1A1-mediated glucuronidation pathway. There is biliary secretion. Excreted mostly in urine (32%, raltegravir and metabolites) and feces (51%, mostly as raltegravir). Unknown if removed by hemodialysis. *Half-life:* 9 h.

AVAILABILITY

Tablets (Isentress): 400 mg.

INDICATIONS AND DOSAGES

▸ HIV infection (in combination with other antiretrovirals)

PO

Adults, Elderly. 400 mg twice daily. During coadministration with rifampin, dose should be 800 mg twice daily.

▸ Dosage in renal and hepatic impairment

No dosage adjustments recommended for renal impairment or for mild-moderate hepatic disease; use normal dose even in end-stage renal disease. There is no experience in severe hepatic disease.

CONTRAINDICATIONS

Hypersensitivity.

INTERACTIONS

Drug

HMG-CoA reductase inhibitors ("statins"): Use caution; increased risk for myopathy and rhabdomyolysis.

Strong inducers of UGT1A1 (rifampin, phenobarbital, phenytoin): May result in reduced plasma concentrations of raltegravir. When given with rifampin, an increased dose of raltegravir is necessary.

Mild UGT1A1 inducers (e.g., efavirenz, etravirine, tipranavir): Decreases the concentration of raltegravir, but no dose adjustment has been recommended.

Strong UGT1A1 inhibitors (e.g., atazanavir): Increases the concentration of raltegravir, but no dose adjustment has been recommended.

Omeprazole and other PPIs: Increases the concentration of raltegravir due to increased solubility at higher stomach acid pH, but no dose adjustment recommended.

Herbal

St. John's wort: Decreases the concentration of antiretroviral medications and may lead to loss of efficacy. Avoid.

Food

None known. High-fat food increases absorption slightly but does not affect final efficacy.

R

DIAGNOSTIC TEST EFFECTS

May elevate AST (SGOT) and ALT (SGPT) levels. Increased serum cholesterol and triglycerides. May increase serum amylase, blood glucose. May decrease blood hemoglobin levels, platelet count, and WBC count. May cause elevations in creatine phosphokinase.

SIDE EFFECTS

Frequent (≥ 2%)
Insomnia, headache.
Occasional (< 2%)
Asthenia, fatigue, dizziness, depression (particularly in subjects with a preexisting history of psychiatric illness), changes in mood or behavior, abdominal pain, gastritis, dyspepsia, vomiting, nausea, myalgia, reactivation of herpes zoster or herpes simplex.
Rare
Lowered blood counts, altered fat distribution, nephrolithiasis, anxiety, paranoia, depression, suicidal ideation, or unusual behaviors.

SERIOUS REACTIONS

- Hepatotoxicity; hepatitis.
- Neutropenia, thrombocytopenia, and anemia may increase risk of bleeding or opportunistic infection.
- Rhabdomyolysis.
- Hypersensitivity reactions; Stevens-Johnson syndrome has been reported.
- Cardiovascular events including myocardial ischemia and/or infarction have been reported.
- Nephrotoxicity; including renal tubular necrosis, oliguria, renal failure.

PRECAUTIONS & CONSIDERATIONS

Caution is warranted in patients with liver function impairment and in those coinfected with hepatitis B, as well as those with a history of depression or mood disorders. Carefully screen for drug interactions. There are no adequate data in human pregnancy. Breastfeeding is not recommended in this patient population because of the possibility of HIV transmission. Be aware that safety and efficacy have not been established in children. No age-related precautions have been noted in elderly patients. During initial treatment, patients responding to antiretroviral therapy may develop an inflammatory response to indolent or residual opportunistic infections (an immune reconstitution syndrome), which may necessitate further evaluation and treatment.

Raltegravir is not a cure for HIV infection, nor does it reduce risk of transmission to others. Expect to obtain baseline laboratory testing, especially CBC, liver function, and renal function before starting therapy and at periodic intervals. Assess for hypersensitivity reaction, skin reactions, fatigue or nausea, myalgia, unusual changes in moods or behavior. Have patient report sore throat, fever, and other signs of infection promptly.

Storage
Store at room temperature.
Administration
Tablets may be taken without regard to food or meals; give with a full glass of liquid.

Ramelteon
rah-mel'tee-on
★ Rozerem

CATEGORY AND SCHEDULE
Pregnancy Risk Category: C

Classification: Sedatives/hypnotics, melatonin receptor agonist

MECHANISM OF ACTION
A nonbenzodiazepine that binds to melatonin receptors in the CNS, which helps regulate circardian rhythm and normal sleep/wake cycles. *Therapeutic Effect:* Induces sleep in those with difficulty with sleep onset.

PHARMACOKINETICS
Total absorption of ramelteon is around 84%, but absolute oral bioavailability is only 1.8% due to extensive first-pass metabolism. Protein binding: 82%; extensive tissue distribution. Metabolism to metabolites via CYP1A2 (major) and the CYP2C and CYP3A4 families (minor). Overall mean systemic exposure of M-II, one of the metabolites, is approximately 20- to 100-fold higher than that of the parent drug. Elimination of metabolites occurs 84% in urine and only 4% in feces. Less than 0.1% excreted as the parent compound. Not removed by hemodialysis. *Half-life:* 1-2.6 h; M-II metabolite: 2-6 h.

AVAILABILITY
Tablet: 8 mg.

INDICATIONS AND DOSAGES
▸ **Insomnia**
PO
Adults, Elderly. 8 mg within 30 min of bedtime.

▸ **Hepatic impairment**
Do not use in severe hepatic impairment due to increased concentrations.

CONTRAINDICATIONS
Hypersensitivity (angioedema); use with fluvoxamine.

INTERACTIONS
Drug
Alcohol: May lead to increased risk of abnormal behaviors and amnesia. Avoid.
CYP1A2 inhibitors (e.g., fluvoxamine, atazanavir, mexiletine, norfloxacin, tacrine, zileuton): May increase the blood level and effects of ramelteon. Contraindicated with fluvoxamine due to large increases in ramelteon exposure and maximum concentration.
Ketoconazole, fluconazole, and other CYP3A4 or 2C9 inhibitors: May increase ramelteon exposure and adverse effects, especially strong CYP2C9 inhibitors.
CYP1A2 inducers (e.g., rifampin): May decrease the blood level and effects of ramelteon.
Herbal
Melatonin: Duplication of treatment; do not take together due to increased risk of side effects.
Valerian, kava kava: Potential for additive CNS effects.
Food
Heavy meals: May reduce onset of ramelteon action if taken with or immediately after a heavy meal.

DIAGNOSTIC TEST EFFECTS
May reduce blood cortisol levels. May decrease testosterone levels and increase prolactin levels.

SIDE EFFECTS
Frequent
Drowsiness, dizziness, fatigue.

Occasional (4%-10%)
Somnolence, dry mouth, dyspepsia, nausea.
Rare (2%-3%)
Hallucinations, anxiety, confusion, abnormal dreams, mood changes, neuralgia, dysmenorrhea, gynecomastia, amenorrhea, galactorrhea, decreased libido, or problems with fertility.

SERIOUS REACTIONS

- Severe allergic reactions (e.g., angioedema) occur occasionally, usually with first doses.
- Hallucinations, bizarre behaviors, "sleep driving" (i.e., driving while not fully awake after ingestion of a hypnotic) and other complex behaviors with amnesia are possible with hypnotic use.

PRECAUTIONS & CONSIDERATIONS

Caution is warranted in patients with clinical depression or other psychiatric illness, mild-moderate hepatic impairment, and compromised respiratory function, such as sleep apnea or COPD. Use cautiously in elderly patients. Safety and efficacy have not been evaluated in children. Be aware that melatonin is involved in hormonal regulation, which may have complex effects on fertility and other hormonal processes. The drug is likely excreted in breast milk. Use during pregnancy and lactation is not recommended.

Do not ingest alcohol as this may increase the risk of unusual behaviors. Only take ramelteon when going to bed; otherwise, may be at risk if hazardous tasks such as driving are performed. Confine any activities to those necessary to prepare for sleep. Be aware that allergic reactions are most likely to occur with the first several drug doses. Monitor for dyspnea, throat closing, swelling of the tongue, nausea, vomiting. Notify prescriber if insomnia not responsive within 1 wk, as further evaluation is necessary.

Storage
Keep tightly closed at cool room temperature.
Administration
Take within the 30 min prior to bedtime, at approximately the same time each night. Do not take with, or immediately following, a high-fat meal. Do not crush or break tablets. Patients should be able to devote time for a full night's rest.

Ramipril

ram'i-pril
Altace
Do not confuse Altace with Alteplase or Artane.

CATEGORY AND SCHEDULE

Pregnancy Risk Category: C (D if used in second or third trimester)

Classification: Antihypertensives, angiotensin-converting enzyme (ACE) inhibitors

MECHANISM OF ACTION

An ACE inhibitor that suppresses the renin-angiotensin-aldosterone system. Decreases plasma angiotensin II, increases plasma renin activity, and decreases aldosterone secretion. *Therapeutic Effect:* Reduces peripheral arterial resistance and BP.

PHARMACOKINETICS

Route	Onset	Peak	Duration
PO	1-2 h	3-6 h	24 h

Well absorbed from the GI tract. Protein binding: 73%. Metabolized in the liver to active metabolite. Primarily excreted in urine (60%). Not removed by hemodialysis. *Half-life:* 2-17 h.

AVAILABILITY

Capsules: 1.25 mg, 2.5 mg, 5 mg, 10 mg.

INDICATIONS AND DOSAGES

▸ **Hypertension (monotherapy)**

PO

Adults, Elderly. Initially, 2.5 mg/day. Maintenance: 2.5-20 mg/day as single dose or in 2 divided doses.

▸ **Hypertension (in combination with other antihypertensives)**

PO

Adults, Elderly. Initially, 1.25-5 mg/day titrated to patient's needs.

▸ **Congestive heart failure (CHF) post-myocardial infarction (MI)**

PO

Adults, Elderly. Initially, 1.25-2.5 mg twice a day. Maximum: 5 mg twice a day; doses should be increased about 3 wks apart.

▸ **Risk reduction for MI, stroke, and death from cardiovascular causes**

PO

Adults, Elderly. Initially, 2.5 mg twice a day. If hypotensive, decrease to 1.25 mg twice a day, and after 1 wk at starting dose, dose can be titrated to 5 mg twice a day.

▸ **Dosage in renal impairment**

Creatinine clearance ≤ 40 mL/min. 25% of normal dose.

Renal failure and hypertension. Initially, 1.25 mg/day titrated upward to a maximum daily dose of 5 mg.

Renal failure and CHF. Initially, 1.25 mg/day, titrated up to 2.5 mg twice a day.

OFF-LABEL USES

Treatment of hypertension and renal crisis in scleroderma, diabetic nephropathy.

CONTRAINDICATIONS

Hypersensitivity or history of angioedema from previous treatment with ACE inhibitors, idiopathic or hereditary angioedema, bilateral renal artery stenosis.

INTERACTIONS

Drug

Alcohol, antihypertensives, diuretics: May increase the effects of ramipril.

Angiotensin II receptor blockers, potassium-sparing diuretics drospirenone, eplerenone, salt substitutes, potassium supplements: May cause hyperkalemia.

Lithium: May increase lithium blood concentration and risk of lithium toxicity.

NSAIDs: May decrease the effects of ramipril and decrease renal function.

Herbal

Garlic: May increase antihypertensive effect.

Ephedra, ginseng, yohimbe: May worsen hypertension.

Food

None known.

DIAGNOSTIC TEST EFFECTS

May increase BUN, serum alkaline phosphatase, serum bilirubin, serum creatinine, serum potassium, AST (SGOT), and ALT (SGPT) levels. May decrease serum sodium levels. May cause positive antinuclear antibody titer.

SIDE EFFECTS

Frequent (5%-12%)

Cough, headache.

Occasional (2%-4%)

Dizziness, fatigue, nausea, asthenia (loss of strength).

Rare (< 2%)

Palpitations, insomnia, nervousness, malaise, abdominal pain, myalgia, hyperkalemia.

R

SERIOUS REACTIONS

- Excessive hypotension (first-dose syncope) may occur in patients with CHF and in those who are severely salt or volume depleted.
- Angioedema occurs rarely.
- Agranulocytosis and neutropenia may be noted in those with collagen vascular disease, including scleroderma and systemic lupus erythematosus, and impaired renal function.
- Nephrotic syndrome may be noted in those with history of renal disease.
- Hyperkalemia may occur, especially with concomitant potassium-sparing agents.
- Cholestatic jaundice, which may progress to hepatic necrosis. Discontinue if abnormal liver function tests.
- Renal dysfunction may occur. Increases in serum creatinine may occur after initiation of therapy. Monitor serum creatinine and discontinue if progressive or severe decline in function.

PRECAUTIONS & CONSIDERATIONS

Caution is warranted in patients with CHF, collagen vascular disease, hyperkalemia, hypovolemia, renal impairment, and renal artery stenosis. Ramipril crosses the placenta, is distributed in breast milk, and may cause fetal or neonatal morbidity or mortality. If pregnancy is detected, ramipril should be discontinued as soon as possible. Safety and efficacy of ramipril have not been established in children. Elderly patients may be more sensitive to the hypotensive effect of ramipril.

Dizziness and light-headedness may occur. Tasks that require mental alertness or motor skills should be avoided until effects of drug are known. Notify the physician if chest pain, cough, or palpitations occur. Be alert to fluctuations in BP. If an excessive reduction in BP occurs, place the patient in the supine position with legs elevated. CBC and blood chemistry, including BUN and serum creatinine, should be obtained before beginning ramipril therapy, then every 2 wks for the next 3 mo, and periodically thereafter in patients with autoimmune disease or renal impairment and in those who are taking drugs that affect immune response or leukocyte count. BUN, serum creatinine, serum potassium levels, and WBC count should also be monitored. Crackles and wheezing should be assessed in persons with CHF.

Storage

Store at room temperature.

Administration

Take ramipril without regard to food. Swallow the capsules whole, and do not chew or break them. The capsule can be opened and the contents sprinkled on a small amount (about 4 oz) of applesauce or mixed in 120 mL of water or apple juice if needed. Be sure to have patient consume entire dose.

Ranitidine

ra-ni'ti-deen

Zantac, Zantac 75, Zantac 150, Zantac EFFERdose

Do not confuse Zantac with Xanax, Zarontin, Ziac, Zofran, or Zyrtec.

CATEGORY AND SCHEDULE

Pregnancy Risk Category: B

OTC (tablets, 75 mg, 150 mg)

Classification: Antihistamines, H_2, gastrointestinals

MECHANISM OF ACTION

An antiulcer agent that inhibits histamine action at H_2 receptors of gastric parietal cells. *Therapeutic Effect:* Inhibits gastric acid secretion when fasting, at night, or when stimulated by food, caffeine, or insulin. Reduces volume and hydrogen ion concentration of gastric acid.

PHARMACOKINETICS

Rapidly absorbed from the GI tract. Protein binding: 15%. Widely distributed. Metabolized in the liver. Excreted primarily in urine. Not removed by hemodialysis. *Half-life:* 2.5 h (increased with impaired renal function).

AVAILABILITY

Tablets (Effervescent [Zantac EFFERdose]): 25 mg.
Granules (Zantac EFFERdose): 150 mg.
Syrup (Zantac): 15 mg/mL.
Tablets (Zantac 75): 75 mg (OTC).
Tablets (Zantac 150): 150 mg (OTC).
Tablets (Zantac): 150 mg, 300 mg.
Infusion, Premixed: 50 mL (Zantac 50 mg).
Injection (Zantac): 25 mg/mL.

INDICATIONS AND DOSAGES

▸ **Duodenal ulcers, gastric ulcers, gastroesophageal reflux disease (GERD)**

PO

Adults, Elderly. 150 mg twice a day or 300 mg after evening meal or at bedtime. Maintenance: 150 mg at bedtime.

Children aged 1 mo to 16 yr. 2-4 mg/kg/day in divided doses twice a day. Maximum: 300 mg/day. Maintenance for children: 150 mg/day.

▸ **Erosive esophagitis**

PO

Adults, Elderly. 150 mg 4 times a day. Maintenance: 150 mg 2 times/day or 300 mg at bedtime.

Children. 5-10 mg/kg/day in 2 divided doses.

▸ **Hypersecretory conditions**

PO

Adults, Elderly. 150 mg twice a day. May increase up to 6 g/day.

▸ **Usual parenteral dosage**

IV, IM

Adults, Elderly. 50 mg/dose q6-8h. Maximum: 400 mg/day.

Children. 2-4 mg/kg/day in divided doses q6-8h. Maximum: 200 mg/day.

▸ ***Helicobacter pylori* eradication**

PO

Adults, Elderly. 150 mg twice daily in combination with antibiotics. Used as alternative to PPIs.

▸ **Prevention of heartburn**

PO

Adults, Elderly. 75-150 mg before meals that cause heartburn. Maximum: 150 mg/day. Do not use more than 14 days.

Children older than 12 yr. 75 mg before meals that cause heartburn. Maximum: 150 mg/day. Do not use more than 14 days.

▸ **Usual neonatal dosage**

PO

Neonates. 2 mg/kg/day in divided doses q12-24h.

IV

Neonates. Initially, 1.5 mg/kg/dose; then 1.5-2 mg/kg/day in divided doses q12-24h.

▸ **Dosage in renal impairment**

For patients with creatinine clearance < 50 mL/min, give 150 mg PO q24h or 50 mg IV or IM q18-24h.

OFF-LABEL USES

Stress gastritis prophylaxis in critically ill patients.

R

CONTRAINDICATIONS

Hypersensitivity or history of acute porphyria.

INTERACTIONS

Drug

Antacids: May decrease the absorption of ranitidine.
Atazanavir, cyanocobalamin: Ranitidine may decrease absorption of these medications.
Cefuroxime, cefpodoxime: Rantidine may decrease the absorption so separate administration by 2 h.
Cyclosporine: Increased effect/toxicity of cyclosporine.
Ketoconazole: May decrease the absorption of ketoconazole.
Ethanol: Avoid since may worsen gastric irritation.
Warfarin: Variable effects on warfarin require monitoring of PT/INR.

Herbal

None known.

Food

None known.

DIAGNOSTIC TEST EFFECTS

Interferes with skin tests using allergen extracts. May increase hepatic function enzyme, γ-glutamyl transpeptidase, and serum creatinine levels.

IV INCOMPATIBILITIES

Amphotericin B (Abelcet, AmBisome, Amphotec) caspofungin, diazepam, lansoprazole, pantoprazole, phenytoin.

IV COMPATIBILITIES

Diltiazem (Cardizem), dobutamine, dopamine, heparin, hydromorphone (Dilaudid), insulin, lidocaine, lorazepam (Ativan), morphine, norepinephrine (Levophed), potassium chloride, propofol (Diprivan).

SIDE EFFECTS

Occasional (2%)

Diarrhea.

Rare (1%)

Constipation, headache (may be severe).

SERIOUS REACTIONS

- Reversible hepatitis and blood dyscrasias occur rarely.

PRECAUTIONS & CONSIDERATIONS

Caution is warranted in patients with impaired hepatic or renal function and in elderly patients. Ranitidine does cross the placenta and is distributed in breast milk; use with caution. No age-related precautions have been noted in children. Elderly patients are more likely to experience confusion, especially those with hepatic or renal impairment. Smoking should be avoided. Also avoid alcohol, aspirin, and coffee, all of which may cause GI distress, during ranitidine therapy.

Notify the physician if headache occurs. Blood chemistry laboratory test results, including BUN, serum alkaline phosphatase, bilirubin, creatinine, AST (SGOT), and ALT (SGPT) levels to assess hepatic and renal function, should be obtained before and during therapy.

Storage

Store all products at room temperature. Protect injection from light. IV infusion (piggyback) is stable for 48 h at room temperature. Discard if discolored or precipitate forms.

Administration

Take oral ranitidine without regard to meals; however, it is best given after meals or at bedtime. Give 2 h after ketoconazole, cefuroxime, or cefpodoxime administration.

Effervescent dose should be dissolved in at least 5 mL (1 tsp of water) and administered once completely dissolved. Effervescent dose should not be chewed, swallowed whole, or dissolved on the tongue.

IV solutions normally appear clear and are colorless to yellow; slight darkening does not affect potency. For IV push, dilute each 50 mg with 20 mL 0.9% NaCl or D5W. For intermittent IV infusion (piggyback), dilute each 50 mg with 50 mL 0.9% NaCl or D5W. For IV infusion, dilute with 250-1000 mL 0.9% NaCl or D5W. Administer IV push over minimum of 5 min to prevent arrhythmias and hypotension. Infuse IV piggyback over 15-20 min. May give as continuous IV infusion over 24 h.

For IM use, ranitidine may be given undiluted. Give deep IM into large muscle mass, such as the gluteus maximus.

Ranolazine

rah-nole'a-zine

Ranexa

CATEGORY AND SCHEDULE

Pregnancy Risk Category: C

Classification: Cardiovascular agents, antianginals

MECHANISM OF ACTION

A piperazine compound that belongs in a group known as partial fatty-acid oxidation (PFox) inhibitors. The exact mechanism of action is not clear. The drug may inhibit the late sodium current and reduce intracellular sodium and calcium overload in ischemic cardiac myocytes. No negative chronotropic or inotropic effects; minimal effects on heart rate and blood pressure. May prolong QT interval. *Therapeutic Effect:* Stabilizes angina, reducing pain and improving exercise tolerance. May be used with other antianginal agents.

PHARMACOKINETICS

Variable absorption. Protein binding: 62%. Extensively metabolized in the liver by CYP3A4 and CYP2D6; drug and metabolites primarily (75%) excreted in the urine, excretion in feces (25%). Not known if removed by hemodialysis. *Half-life:* 7 h (prolonged in severe hepatic impairment).

AVAILABILITY

Tablets, Extended Release: 500 mg, 1000 mg.

INDICATIONS AND DOSAGES

▸ **Chronic stable angina**

PO

Adults, Elderly. 500 mg twice daily. May increase to 1000 mg twice daily based on clinical response.

▸ **Use with moderate inhibitors of CYP3A4**

Limit maximal dose to 500 mg PO twice daily.

▸ **Hepatic impairment**

Do not use in severe hepatic impairment.

▸ **Severe renal impairment**

Avoid use.

CONTRAINDICATIONS

Hypersensitivity to ranolazine, concurrent use of strong inhibitors or inducers of CYP3A4, severe hepatic disease.

INTERACTIONS

Drug

Alcohol: May lead to decreased psychomotor function.

Digoxin: Ranolazine causes an increase in digoxin concentrations; digoxin dose may need adjustment. Monitor.

Strong CYP3A4 inducers (e.g., rifampin, rifabutin, rifapentine, phenobarbital, phenytoin, carbamazepine): May decrease the blood level and effects of ranolazine. Contraindicated.
Strong CYP3A4 inhibitors (ketoconazole, itraconazole, clarithromycin, nefazodone, most protease inhibitors): Contraindicated. Likely to increase the blood level and effects of ranolazine and risk of QT prolongation.
Moderate CYP3A4 inhibitors (cyclosporine, diltiazem, verapamil, aprepitant, erythromycin, fluconazole): May increase the blood level and effects of ranolazine and risk of QT prolongation; use lower dose of ranolazine.
CYP2D6 substrates (e.g., phenothiazines, TCAs): Ranolazine may decrease metabolism of these drugs.
Drugs that prolong QTc interval: May have additive effects on EKG.
Herbal
St. John's wort: May decrease the blood level and effects of ranolazine. Contraindicated.
Food
Grapefruit juice: May increase ranolazine exposure. Avoid.

DIAGNOSTIC TEST EFFECTS

Small reductions in hemoglobin A1c, but not efficacious for diabetes. Increases serum creatinine by 0.1 mg/dL, regardless of previous renal function; the increases in creatinine stabilize and do not progress.

SIDE EFFECTS

Frequent (> 4%)
Dizziness, headache, constipation, and nausea.
Occasional (0.5%-2%)
Asthenia, bradycardia, palpitations, tinnitus, vertigo, abdominal pain, dry mouth, vomiting, peripheral edema, dyspnea, hypotension.
Rare (< 0.5%)
Renal failure, eosinophilia, blurred vision, confusion, hematuria, hypoesthesia, paresthesia, tremor, pulmonary fibrosis, thrombocytopenia, leukopenia, and pancytopenia.

SERIOUS REACTIONS

- Severe allergic reactions (e.g., angioedema) occur occasionally.
- QT prolongation and proarrhythmia.

PRECAUTIONS & CONSIDERATIONS

There is no role for ranolazine in treating acute coronary syndromes; the drug is no more effective than placebo for these conditions. Caution is warranted in patients with a history of familial QT prolongation or with risks for QT interval prolongation, such as taking other drugs that may prolong the QT interval. Electrolyte imbalances should be corrected before use. Use cautiously in patients with mild to moderate hepatic or renal disease. Use in pregnancy only when clearly needed; no data. It is not known if the drug is excreted in breast milk. Safety and efficacy have not been evaluated in children. Use cautiously in elderly patients.

Ranolazine may cause dizziness, so patients should avoid hazardous tasks until the effects of the drug are known. Patients should check with prescriber prior to OTC medication use. Compliance is important to avoid angina. Assess therapeutic response, including BP, regularity of pulse, decrease in anginal pain, and improvement in exercise tolerance.

Storage
Keep tightly closed at cool room temperature.
Administration
May take ranolazine without regard to meals. Do not administer with grapefruit juice. Swallow whole; do not break, crush, or chew extended-release tablets. Commonly used with drugs like beta-blockers, nitrates, calcium channel blockers, anti-platelet therapy, lipid-lowering therapy, ACE inhibitors, or angiotensin receptor blockers.

Rasagiline

ra-sa'ji-leen
Azilect
Do not confuse rasagiline with selegiline.

CATEGORY AND SCHEDULE

Pregnancy Risk Category: C

Classification: Antiparkinsonian agents, dopaminergics, selective MAO-B inhibitors

R

MECHANISM OF ACTION

An antiparkinsonian agent that irreversibly and selectively inhibits the activity of monoamine oxidase type B, the enzyme that breaks down dopamine, thereby increasing dopaminergic action in the brain. *Therapeutic Effect:* Relieves signs and symptoms of Parkinson disease.

PHARMACOKINETICS

Rapidly absorbed from the GI tract; AUC not significantly affected by food; bioavailability 36%. Crosses the blood-brain barrier. Metabolized in the liver, primarily by CYP1A2, prior to excretion. Excreted primarily in urine (62%) and feces (7%) as metabolites. *Half-life:* 3 h; little correlation between half-life and duration of MAO-B inhibition.

AVAILABILITY

Tablets: 0.5 mg, 1 mg.

INDICATIONS AND DOSAGES

▸ **Monotherapy for Parkinson disease**
PO
Adults, Elderly. 1 mg once daily.
▸ **Parkinson disease with levodopa/carbidopa therapy**
PO
Adults, Elderly. Initially, 0.5 mg once daily. If sufficient response not attained, may increase to 1 mg once daily.
▸ **Patients taking concomitant CYP1A2 inhibitors or with mild hepatic impairment**
PO
Adults, Elderly. Do not exceed 0.5 mg once daily.

CONTRAINDICATIONS

Hypersensitivity to rasagiline. Concomitant use of meperidine, dextromethorphan, tramadol, methadone, or propoxyphene. Also, do not give with linezolid, selegiline, and other MAOIs (whether selective or nonselective) within 14 days, as well as cyclobenzaprine or St. John's wort.

INTERACTIONS

Drug
CYP1A2 inhibitors (e.g., ciprofloxacin, amiodarone, mexiletine, norfloxacin, tacrine, tizanidine, zileuton): Use lower dose of rasagiline since metabolism is decreased.
Buspirone: Manufacturer of buspirone contraindicates use of MAOIs.

SSRIs, SNRIs, other antidepressants: May cause serotonin syndrome. Fluoxetine and fluvoxamine should not be used concurrently. Manufacturer recommends 14 days of wash-out between use of any antidepressant and use of rasagiline.
Dextromethorphan: Psychosis and bizarre behavior reported. Contraindicated.
Meperidine, tramadol, propoxyphene, methadone: May cause diaphoresis, excitation, hypertension or hypotension, coma, and even death. Contraindicated.
Linezolid, selegiline, and other MAOIs (selective or nonselective): May cause additive MAOI effects and hypertensive crisis. Contraindicated.
Sympathomimetic medications (e.g., pseudoephedrine): May cause hypertensive crisis; use not recommended.
Herbal
Ma huang: Contains ephedra (see sympathomimetic interactions). Avoid.
St. John's wort: Contraindicated; may cause serotonin syndrome or hypertensive crisis.
Tryptophan: May cause hypertensive crisis. Avoid.
Food
Tyramine-rich foods: Dietary tyramine restriction is not ordinarily required. However, certain foods (e.g., aged cheeses, such as Stilton cheese, or certain wines) may contain very high amounts (i.e., > 150 mg) of tyramine and could potentially cause a hypertensive "cheese" reaction.

DIAGNOSTIC TEST EFFECTS

None known.

SIDE EFFECTS

Frequent (> 3%)
Dyskinesia, weight loss, orthostatic hypotension, vomiting, anorexia, arthralgia, abdominal pain, nausea, dyspepsia, constipation, dry mouth, rash, abnormal dreams, falls/accidents.
Occasional (2%-3%)
Depression, confusion, fever, gastroenteritis, arthritis, ecchymosis, malaise, paresthesia, vertigo.
Rare (1%)
Headache, myalgia, anxiety, hallucinations, diarrhea, insomnia, increased libido.

SERIOUS REACTIONS

- Symptoms of overdose may vary from CNS depression, characterized by sedation, apnea, cardiovascular collapse, and death, to severe paradoxical reactions, such as hallucinations, tremor, and seizures.
- Other serious effects may include involuntary movements, psychosis, delusions, and hostility.
- Syndrome of hyperpyrexia similar to neuroleptic malignant syndrome.
- Impulse control problems, such as hypersexuality, pathological gambling, shopping, or other compulsive behaviors.
- Increased rate of melanoma in Parkinson patients, cause unknown.

PRECAUTIONS & CONSIDERATIONS

Caution is warranted in patients with cardiac disease, hypertension, dementia, history of peptic ulcer disease, profound tremor, psychosis, and tardive dyskinesia. It is unknown whether rasagiline crosses the placenta or is distributed in breast milk. The safety and efficacy of rasagiline have not been established in children. No age-related precautions have been noted in elderly patients. Monitor for melanomas on a regular basis.

Dizziness, drowsiness, lightheadedness, and dry mouth are common side effects of the drug but will diminish or disappear with continued treatment. Alcohol and tasks that require mental alertness or motor skills should be avoided. Change positions slowly to prevent orthostatic hypotension. Notify the physician if agitation, headache, increased BP, hyperpyrexia, lethargy, or confusion occurs. Baseline vital signs should be assessed. Relief of symptoms, such as improvement of mask-like facial expression, muscular rigidity, shuffling gait, and resting tremors of the hands and head, should be assessed during treatment.

Storage

Store at room temperature.

Administration

May administer with or without food. Be aware that tyramine-rich foods, such as certain alcoholic beverages and aged cheese, should be limited to prevent a hypertensive reaction.

R

Rasburicase

rass-bur′e-case

★ Elitek 🍁 Fasturtec

CATEGORY AND SCHEDULE

Pregnancy Risk Category: C

Classification:

Antihyperuricemic, enzyme

MECHANISM OF ACTION

A recombinant form of urate oxidase, an enzyme not endogenous to humans that catalyzes enzymatic oxidation of uric acid into a readily excreted metabolite, allantoin, thus lowering high serum uric acid levels. *Therapeutic Effect:* Reduces uric acid concentrations in both serum and urine.

PHARMACOKINETICS

No significant accumulation occurs over 5 days of IV infusion dosing. The enzyme is cleared metabolically. Pharmacokinetic parameters are similar in adult and pediatric patients. *Half-life:* 16-20 h.

AVAILABILITY

Powder for Injection (Elitek): 1.5 mg, 7.5 mg.

INDICATIONS AND DOSAGES

▸ To prevent uric acid nephropathy during chemotherapy

IV INFUSION

Adults and Children 2 yr and older. 0.2 mg/kg IV over 30 min given once daily for up to 5 days. Only a single course is given.

CONTRAINDICATIONS

History of the following reactions to rasburicase: anaphylaxis, severe hypersensitivity, hemolysis, methemoglobinemia. Mannitol hypersensitivity. Glucose-6-phosphate dehydrogenase (G6PD) deficiency.

INTERACTIONS

Drug

Allopurinol: Rasburicase cannot break down xanthine and hypoxanthine, and the increased renal load can result in xanthine nephropathy and renal calculi.

Herbal

None known.

Food

None known.

DIAGNOSTIC TEST EFFECTS

! Interference with uric acid measurements: Rasburicase enzymatically degrades uric acid in blood samples left at room temperature. Collect blood sample in a prechilled tube containing heparin and immediately immerse and maintain sample in an ice water bath. Assay plasma sample within 4 h of collection. These directions are important since treatment is based on uric acid measurements.

Rasburicase may cause methemoglobinemia, hemolysis, or lowered WBC count.

IV INCOMPATIBILITIES

Do not mix or infuse rasburicase with any other medications.

SIDE EFFECTS

Frequent

Vomiting, nausea, pyrexia, peripheral edema, anxiety, headache, abdominal pain, constipation, and diarrhea.

Occasional

Rash, inflammation of mucous membranes.

SERIOUS REACTIONS

- Severe hypersensitivity, including anaphylaxis.
- Methemoglobinemia.
- Hemolysis or neutropenia (rare).

PRECAUTIONS & CONSIDERATIONS

Hydrogen peroxide, one of the by-products of breakdown of uric acid to allantoin, can induce hemolytic anemia or methemoglobinemia, especially in patients with G6PD deficiency or methemoglobin reductase deficiency. Appropriate patient monitoring and support measures such as transfusions or methylene-blue administration in the case of methemoglobinemia should be initiated. Use with caution in bone marrow suppression or neutropenia. Pregnant women should receive rasburicase only if clearly needed. It is unknown whether rasburicase crosses the placenta. Rasburicase is excreted in breast milk; use with caution in nursing women. No age-related precautions have been noted in children or in elderly patients. Children < 2 yr were more likely not to achieve target uric acid concentrations at 48 h. There are insufficient data to determine the efficacy and safety of rasburicase in neonates and infants; only seven infants between 1 and 6 mo of age were included in clinical trials. Young children may be more susceptible to side effects.

High fluid intake (3000 mL/day) should be encouraged; intake and output should be monitored. Urine output should be at least 2000 mL/day; check urine for cloudiness and unusual color and odor. CBC, hepatic enzyme test results, and serum uric acid levels should also be assessed. Be sure to follow recommended methods for samples and processing. The drug should be discontinued if rash or other evidence of allergic reaction appears. Avoid tasks that require mental alertness or motor skills until response to the drug has been established.

Storage

Refrigerate unreconstituted vials, protect from light, and do not freeze. Once diluted as an infusion, may refrigerate and use within 24 h of preparation. Do not use if precipitate forms or solution is discolored.

Administration

For intravenous (IV) infusion use only. Reconstitute only with the diluent provided. Reconstitute with 1 mL of diluent (1.5 mg vial) or 5 mL of diluent (7.5 mg vial). Gently swirl

R

the vial to mix; do not shake. Must be further diluted. Withdraw the needed dosage and mix with 0.9% NaCl for injection to achieve a final volume of 50 mL.

Infuse IV over 30 min. No filters should be used for the infusion. Use a different line than the one used for other medications. If use of a separate line is not possible, the line should be flushed with at least 15 mL of 0.9% NaCl prior to and after infusion with rasburicase.

Repaglinide

re-pag'lih-nide

★ Prandin 🍁 GlucoNorm

CATEGORY AND SCHEDULE

Pregnancy Risk Category: C

Classification: Antidiabetic agents, meglitinides

MECHANISM OF ACTION

An antihyperglycemic that stimulates release of insulin from β-cells of the pancreas by depolarizing β-cells, leading to an opening of calcium channels. Resulting calcium influx induces insulin secretion. *Therapeutic Effect:* Lowers blood glucose concentration.

PHARMACOKINETICS

Rapidly, completely absorbed from the GI tract. Protein binding: > 98%. Metabolized in the liver to inactive metabolites. Excreted primarily in feces with a small amount in urine. Unknown whether removed by hemodialysis. *Half-life:* 1 h.

AVAILABILITY

Tablets: 0.5 mg, 1 mg, 2 mg.

INDICATIONS AND DOSAGES

▸ **Diabetes mellitus type 2**

PO

Adults, Elderly. 0.5-4 mg with each meal, up to 4 times/day. Maximum: 16 mg/day. NOTE: The starting dose for patients not previously treated or with HbA1c < 8% is 0.5 mg taken with meals. For patients previously treated or with HbA1c ≥ 8.0%, the initial dose is 1-2 mg taken with each meal.

If patient has CrCl < 40 mL/min, begin with the 0.5 mg dose and carefully titrate.

CONTRAINDICATIONS

Diabetic ketoacidosis, type 1 diabetes mellitus, coadministration of gemfibrozil, known hypersensitivity.

INTERACTIONS

Drug

Agents inhibiting CYP2C8 (e.g., gemfibrozil, montelukast, trimethoprim): Increase repaglinide concentrations. Dose adjustment of repaglinide may be necessary. Gemfibrozil is contraindicated.

Agents inhibiting CYP3A4 (e.g., azole antifungals, macrolide antibiotics, nefazodone, protease inhibitors): May increase the effects of repaglinide. Dose adjustment of repaglinide may be necessary.

β-Blockers, MAOIs, NSAIDs, probenecid, salicylates, sulfonamides, warfarin: May promote hypoglycemia β-blockers; may additionally mask signs of hypoglycemia.

Carbamazepine, phenobarbital, phenytoin, rifampin, nevirapine, rifamycins: May decrease the effects of repaglinide.

Corticosteroids, estrogens, phenothiazines, and others: May promote hyperglycemia.

Herbal

Gymenma, garlic: May cause hypoglycemia.

St. John's wort: May decrease repaglinide levels.

DIAGNOSTIC TEST EFFECTS

Expect lowered blood glucose and also lowered HbAlc over time. Rarely, increases in liver enzymes occur.

SIDE EFFECTS

Frequent (6%-16%)
Upper respiratory tract infection, headache, rhinitis, bronchitis, back pain.
Occasional (3%-5%)
Diarrhea, dyspepsia, sinusitis, nausea, arthralgia, urinary tract infection.
Rare (2%)
Constipation, vomiting, paresthesia, allergy.

SERIOUS REACTIONS

- Hypoglycemia occurs in 16% to 31% of patients.
- Chest pain occurs rarely, but risk of myocardial ischemia may increase with use with NPH insulin. Avoid.
- Other rare serious reactions have included pancreatitis, Stevens-Johnson syndrome, and jaundice with hepatitis.

PRECAUTIONS & CONSIDERATIONS

Repaglinide is not indicated for use in combination with NPH insulin (increases risk of myocardial ischemia), but may be used along with metformin or a thiazolidinedione. There have been no clinical studies establishing conclusive evidence of macrovascular risk reduction. Caution is warranted in patients with hepatic or moderate to severe renal impairment. It is unknown whether repaglinide is distributed in breast milk. The safety of repaglinide use during prenancy or lactation has not been established. Safety and efficacy of repaglinide have not been established in children. No age-related precautions have been noted in the elderly, but hypoglycemia may be more difficult to recognize in this patient population.

Food intake and blood glucose should be monitored before and during therapy. Be aware of the signs and symptoms of hypoglycemia (anxiety, cool wet skin, diplopia, dizziness, headache, hunger, numbness in mouth, tachycardia, tremors) or hyperglycemia (deep rapid breathing, dim vision, fatigue, nausea, polydipsia, polyphagia, polyuria, vomiting); carry candy, sugar packets, or other sugar supplements for immediate response to hypoglycemia. Consult the physician when glucose demands are altered (such as with fever, heavy physical activity, infection, stress, trauma). Exercise, good personal hygiene (including foot care), not smoking, and weight control are essential parts of therapy.

Storage
Store tablets at room temperature.

Administration
Ideally, take repaglinide within 15 min of a meal 2-4 times/day; however, it may be taken immediately or as long as 30 min before a meal. Allow at least 1 wk to elapse to assess response to the drug before new dosage adjustment is made.

Reserpine

reh-zer'peen

Do not confuse with Risperdal, risperidone.

CATEGORY AND SCHEDULE

Pregnancy Risk Category: C

Classification:

Antihypertensives, Rauwolfia alkaloid, antiadrenergics, peripheral

R

MECHANISM OF ACTION

An antihypertensive that depletes stores of catecholamines and 5-hydroxytryptamine in many organs, including the brain and adrenal medulla. Depression of sympathetic nerve function results in a decreased heart rate and a lowering of arterial BP. Depletion of catecholamines and 5-hydroxytryptamine from the brain is thought to be the mechanism of the sedative and tranquilizing properties. *Therapeutic Effects:* Decrease BP and heart rate; sedation.

PHARMACOKINETICS

Characterized by slow onset of action and sustained effects. Both cardiovascular and central nervous system (CNS) effects may persist for a period following withdrawal of the drug. Mean maximum plasma levels attained after a median of 3.5 h. Bioavailability approximately 50% of that of a corresponding intravenous dose. Protein binding: 96%. *Half life:* 33 h.

R

AVAILABILITY

Tablets: 0.25 mg, 0.1 mg.

INDICATIONS AND DOSAGES

▸ **Hypertension**

PO

Adults. Usual initial dosage 0.5 mg daily for 1 or 2 wks. For maintenance, reduce to 0.1-0.25 mg daily.

Children. Reserpine is not recommended for use in children.

▸ **Psychiatric disorders**

PO

Adults. Initial dosage, 0.5 mg daily; may range from 0.1 to 1 mg. Adjust dosage upward (in increments of 0.1-0.25 mg) or downward according to response.

CONTRAINDICATIONS

Hypersensitivity, mental depression or history of mental depression (especially with suicidal tendencies), active peptic ulcer, ulcerative colitis, patients receiving electroconvulsive therapy.

INTERACTIONS

Drug

β-Blockers: Reserpine may increase effect.

CNS depressants/ethanol: Reserpine may increase CNS effects.

Levodopa, quinidine, procainamide, digitalis glycosides: Reserpine may increase effects/toxicity, causing cardiac rhythm disturbance. Use caution.

MAO inhibitors: May cause hypertensive reactions. Avoid.

Sympathomimetics: Action of direct-acting amines (epinephrine, isoproterenol, phenylephrine, metaraminol) is prolonged and action of indirect-acting amines (ephedrine, tyramine, amphetamines) is inhibited.

Tricyclic antidepressants: May increase antihypertensive effects.

Herbal

Ephedra/yohimbe: May worsen hypertension.

Valerian, St. John's wort, kava kava, gotu kola: May increase CNS depression.

Garlic: May have increased antihypertensive effects.

Food

Ethanol: May increase CNS depression.

DIAGNOSTIC TEST EFFECTS

None known.

SIDE EFFECTS

Occasional

Burning in the stomach, nausea, vomiting, diarrhea, dry mouth, nosebleed, stuffy nose, dizziness, headache, nervousness, nightmares, drowsiness, muscle aches, weight gain, redness of the eyes.

Rare

Difficulty breathing, swelling, gynecomastia, decreased libido.

SERIOUS REACTIONS

- Irregular heartbeat.
- Heart problems.
- Feeling faint.
- Severe mental depression.

PRECAUTIONS & CONSIDERATIONS

Caution is warranted in patients with a history of peptic ulcer, ulcerative colitis, or gallstones (biliary colic may be precipitated and GI secretions and motility increased). Use caution in renal impairment since reserpine can lower glomerular filtration. If patient will receive surgery, preoperative withdrawal of reserpine does not ensure against circulatory instability; alert anesthesiologist of hypotensive risk. Anticholinergic and/or adrenergic drugs (e.g., metaraminol, norepinephrine) have been employed to treat adverse effects. Be aware that reserpine is excreted in the breast milk. Not a drug of choice in children, as they are susceptible to the side effects; usually last-line treatment; see manufacturer information. Elderly patients may be more susceptible to the hypotensive effects of reserpine. A low-salt diet should be followed. Change positions slowly to avoid orthostatic hypotension.

Dizziness, loss of appetite, diarrhea, upset stomach, vomiting, headache, dry mouth, and decreased sexual ability may occur. Notify physician immediately if depression, nightmares, fainting, slow heartbeat, chest pain, or swollen ankles and feet occur. Watch for the emergence of depressive symptoms, and alert physician for evaluation if they occur.

Storage

Store at room temperature.

Administration

Take with food or milk to avoid GI irritation. Take at the same time each day.

Respiratory Syncytial Immune Globulin

res′purr-ah-tore-ee sin-sish′ee-al ih-mewn′ glah′byew-lin

★ RespiGam

CATEGORY AND SCHEDULE

Pregnancy Risk Category: C

Classification: Immune globulins

MECHANISM OF ACTION

An immune serum with a high concentration of neutralizing and protective antibodies specific for respiratory syncytial virus (RSV). *Therapeutic Effect:* Provides protection against RSV infection and decreases the severity of existing infection.

AVAILABILITY

Injection: 2500 mcg RSV immune globulin.

INDICATIONS AND DOSAGES

▸ **Prevention of RSV in children with bronchopulmonary dysplasia and history of premature birth**

IV

Children younger than 24 mo. 750 mg/kg (15 mL/kg). Give prior to the beginning of RSV season and continue monthly throughout the season. RSV season typically begins

R

in November and continues through April. Administer at a rate of 1.5 mL/kg/h for the first 15 min. If tolerated, increase the rate to 3 mL/kg/h for 15 min, then to a maximum rate of 6 mL/kg/h until infusion is complete. Do not exceed maximum infusion rate.

IV INCOMPATIBILITIES

Manufacturer states do not mix or infuse with any other medications.

CONTRAINDICATIONS

IgA deficiency.

INTERACTIONS

Drug

Live-virus vaccines: May decrease immune response to live-virus vaccines.

Herbal

None known.

Food

None known.

DIAGNOSTIC TEST EFFECTS

None known.

SIDE EFFECTS

Occasional (2%-6%)

Fever, vomiting, wheezing.

Rare (< 1%)

Diarrhea, rash, tachycardia, hypertension, hypoxia, injection-site inflammation.

SERIOUS REACTIONS

- Hypersensitivity reactions, characterized by dizziness, flushing, anxiety, palpitations, pruritus, myalgia, and arthralgia, occur rarely.

PRECAUTIONS & CONSIDERATIONS

Caution is warranted in patients with pulmonary disease. ABG, blood chemistry, serum osmolality electrolyte, and total protein levels should be monitored. Cardiopulmonary status and vital signs should be assessed before giving the drug, before each dosage or rate increase, every 30 min during the infusion, and 30 min after the infusion is completed. Child's body weight should be recorded. Baseline pulmonary assessment, including breath sounds, the presence of intercostal retractions, and respiratory rate, should be performed.

Storage

Refrigerate vials. Do not freeze.

Administration

Do not shake the vials. Start the infusion within 6 h and complete it within 12 h of opening the vial.

Retapamulin

Re-tap'a-muel'in

★ ALTABAX

Do not confuse ALTABAX with Bactroban.

CATEGORY AND SCHEDULE

Pregnancy Risk Category: B

Classification: Topical anti-infective, pleuromutilin

MECHANISM OF ACTION

A pleuromutilin antibacterial agent that selectively inhibits bacterial protein synthesis by interacting at a site on the 50S subunit of the bacterial ribosome through an interaction that is different from that of other antibiotics. Effective against *Staphylococcus aureus* (only methicillin-susceptible strains) or *Streptococcus pyogenes*. *Therapeutic Effect:* Prevents bacterial growth and replication.

PHARMACOKINETICS

Systemic exposure through intact and abraded skin is low. Roughly 11% of patients will have a measurable level just above the lower limit of quantitation 0.5 ng/mL. The liver metabolizes any drug absorbed, via CYP3A4. Excretion pathways have not been determined due to low clinical significance of absorption.

AVAILABILITY

Ointment: 1% (ALTABAX).

INDICATIONS AND DOSAGES

▸ **Impetigo due to susceptible isolates**

TOPICAL

Adults, Elderly, Children over 9 mo. Apply a thin layer to the affected area (up to 100 cm^2 in adults or 2% total BSA in children) twice daily for 5 days.

OFF-LABEL USES

Treatment of infected eczema, folliculitis, minor bacterial skin infections.

CONTRAINDICATIONS

Severe sensitivity to retapamulin.

INTERACTIONS

Drug, Herbal, and Food

None known.

DIAGNOSTIC TEST EFFECTS

None known.

SIDE EFFECTS

Frequent

None.

Occasional

Application site irritation.

Rare

Rash, contact dermatitis. Epistaxis if inadvertently applied to nasal mucosa.

SERIOUS REACTIONS

• Superinfection may result in bacterial or fungal infections, especially with prolonged or repeated therapy.

• Discontinue in the event of sensitization or severe local irritation (rare).

PRECAUTIONS & CONSIDERATIONS

It is unknown whether retapamulin crosses the placenta or is distributed in breast milk. No age-related precautions have been noted in children over 9 mo of age or elderly patients. Isolation precautions should be in effect for those with highly communicable conditions or resistant organisms.

Keep linens and clothing clean and dry; change frequently. Avoid contact of personal items with others. Watch for improvement in lesions (size of area affected, number of lesions, drying of lesions) and improvements in skin symptoms (e.g., itching).

Storage

Store at room temperature.

Administration

For external use on the skin only. Impetigo is spread by direct contact with moist discharges. Apply to affected areas; glove and gown if facility requires. Cover affected areas with gauze dressing if desired. Concurrent use of other topical products on the same application site has not been studied and is not recommended.

Reteplase

reh'te-place

★🍁 Retavase

Do not confuse reteplase or Retavase with Restasis.

CATEGORY AND SCHEDULE

Pregnancy Risk Category: C

Classification: Thrombolytics

R

MECHANISM OF ACTION

A tissue plasminogen activator that activates the fibrinolytic system by directly cleaving plasminogen to generate plasmin, an enzyme that degrades the fibrin of the thrombus. *Therapeutic Effect:* Exerts thrombolytic action.

PHARMACOKINETICS

Rapidly cleared from plasma. Eliminated primarily in the feces and urine. *Half-life:* 13-16 min.

AVAILABILITY

Powder for Injection: 10.4 units (18.1 mg).

INDICATIONS AND DOSAGES

▸ **Acute myocardial infarction (MI)**

IV BOLUS

Adults, Elderly. 10 units over 2 min; repeat in 30 min.

CONTRAINDICATIONS

Active internal bleeding, AV malformation or aneurysm, bleeding diathesis, history of cerebrovascular accident, intracranial neoplasm, recent intracranial or intraspinal surgery, or trauma, severe uncontrolled hypertension.

INTERACTIONS

Drug

Aminocaproic acid: May decrease the effectiveness of reteplase.

Clopidogrel, heparin, low-molecular-weight heparin, nonsteroidal anti-inflammatory agents (NSAIDs), platelet aggregation antagonists (such as abciximab, aspirin, dipyridamole), ticlopidine, warfarin: Increase the risk of bleeding.

Herbal

Ginkgo biloba: May increase the risk of bleeding.

Food

None known.

DIAGNOSTIC TEST EFFECTS

May decrease fibrinogen and serum plasminogen levels.

IV INCOMPATIBILITIES

Do not mix with other medications.

SIDE EFFECTS

Frequent

Bleeding at superficial sites, such as venous injection sites, catheter insertion sites, venous cutdowns, arterial punctures, and sites of recent surgical procedures, gingival bleeding.

SERIOUS REACTIONS

- Bleeding at internal sites may occur, including intracranial, retroperitoneal, GI, genitourinary, and respiratory sites.
- Lysis or coronary thrombi may produce atrial or ventricular arrhythmias and stroke.

PRECAUTIONS & CONSIDERATIONS

Caution is warranted with recent (within past 10 days) major surgery or GI bleeding, organ biopsy, trauma, cerebrovascular disease, cardiopulmonary resuscitation, diabetic retinopathy, endocarditis, left heart thrombus, occluded AV cannula at infected site, severe hepatic or renal disease, thrombophlebitis, in elderly patients, and in pregnant women or within the first 10 postpartum days. It is unknown whether reteplase is distributed in breast milk. Safety and efficacy of reteplase have not been established in children. Elderly patients are more susceptible to bleeding. Use reteplase cautiously in this population. An electric razor and a

R

soft toothbrush should be used to reduce the risk of bleeding.

Notify the physician of black or red stool, coffee-ground vomitus, dark or red urine, red-speckled mucus from cough, chest pain, headache, palpitations, or shortness of breath. Continuous cardiac monitoring should be performed. BP and pulse and respiration rates should be checked every 15 min until stable; then check hourly. Serum creatine kinase (CK), and CK-MB concentrations, 12-lead ECG, electrolyte levels, hematocrit, platelet count, aTT, aPTT, PT, and fibrinogen level should be evaluated before therapy starts.

Storage

Unopened kits are stored at room temperature in original carton sealed to protect from light.

Use within 4 h of reconstitution. Discard any unused portion.

Administration

Reconstitute only with sterile water for injection immediately before use. Reconstituted solution contains 1 unit/mL. Do not shake the vial. Slight foaming may occur; let stand for a few minutes to allow bubbles to dissipate. Give through a dedicated IV line. If injected through an IV line containing heparin, use a 0.9% NaCL or D5W solution flush prior to and following the reteplase injection. Give as a 10-unit plus 10-unit double bolus, with each IV bolus administered over 2 min. Give the second bolus 30 min after the first bolus injection. Do not add other medications to the bolus injection solution. Do not give second IV bolus if serious bleeding occurs after first bolus.

Ribavirin

rye-ba-vye′rin

★ Copegus, Rebetol, RibaPak, Ribasphere, Virazole

🍁 Virazole

Do not confuse ribavirin with riboflavin.

CATEGORY AND SCHEDULE

Pregnancy Risk Category: X

Classification: Antivirals

MECHANISM OF ACTION

A synthetic nucleoside that inhibits replication of RNA and DNA viruses, inhibits influenza virus RNA polymerase activity, and interferes with expression of messenger RNA. *Therapeutic Effect:* Inhibits viral protein synthesis and replication of viral RNA and DNA.

PHARMACOKINETICS

Readily absorbed from the respiratory tract or GI tract. Protein binding: None. Widely distributed into erythrocytes. Metabolized in the liver and intracellularly. Excreted in urine and feces. Unknown whether removed by hemodialysis. *Half-life:* Inhalation 6.5-11 h (children), oral capsules 44-298 h, oral tablets 120-170 h.

AVAILABILITY

Capsules (Rebetol, Ribasphere): 200 mg.

Tablets (Copegus): 200 mg.

Tablet (dose pack) (RibaPak): 400 mg, 600 mg and RibaPak 400/600: 400 mg, 600 mg.

Powder for Nebulizer Solution (Aerosol [Virazole]): 6 g.

Oral Solution (Rebetol): 40 mg/mL.

R

INDICATIONS AND DOSAGES

▸ **Chronic hepatitis C**

NOTE: Dose based on weight and genotype status. See prescribing information for details.

PO (COPEGUS WITH PEGASYS)

Adults. Monoinfection, genotype 1,4: < 75 kg: 1000 mg/day in 2 divided doses, ≥ 75 kg: 1200 mg/day in 2 divided doses; Monoinfection, genotype 2, 3: 800 mg/day in 2 divided doses; Coinfection with HIV: 800 mg/day.

PO (REBETROL WITH INTRONA)

Adults ≤ 75 kg. 400 mg in AM, 600 mg in PM.

Adults > 75 kg. 600 mg in AM, 600 mg in PM.

PO (REBETROL WITH PEGINTRON)

Adults. Range is 800-1400 mg/day (given in divided doses AM and PM). Exact daily amount is based on body weight. See manufacturer's prescribing literature.

USUAL PEDIATRIC DOSE (REBETROL WITH PEGINTRON OR INTRON A)

Children 3-17 years and ≤ 61 kg. 15 mg/kg/day (divided doses AM and PM). See adult Rebetrol dose if > 61 kg.

▸ **Severe lower respiratory tract infection caused by respiratory syncytial virus (RSV)**

INHALATION

Children, Infants. Use with Viratek small-particle aerosol generator at a concentration of 20 mg/mL (6 g reconstituted with 300 mL sterile water) over 12-18 h/day for 3-7 days.

OFF-LABEL USES

Treatment of influenza A or B and West Nile virus, IV available from CDC for severe acute respiratory syndrome (SARS).

CONTRAINDICATIONS

Pregnant women and men whose female partners are pregnant; known hypersensitivity reactions to ribavirin; autoimmune hepatitis; hemoglobinopathies; renal impairment with CrCl < 50 mL/min; significant uncompensated cardiac disease; active pancreatitis; coadministration with didanosine. Monotherapy with ribavirin is NOT effective for chronic hepatitis C; must use with interferon. Do not use at all in cirrhotic chronic hepatitis C with hepatic decompensation (Child-Pugh score > 6) before or during treatment, or in cirrhotic patients coinfected with HIV.

INTERACTIONS

Drug

Didanosine: May increase the risk of pancreatitis and peripheral neuropathy and decrease the effects of didanosine.

Interferons, alpha: May increase the risk of hemolytic anemia.

Live influenza vaccine: May diminish the effects of the vaccine.

Nucleoside analogues (including adefovir, didanosine, emtricitabine, entecavir, lamivudine, stavudine, zalcitabine, zidovudine): May increase the risk of lactic acidosis.

Stavudine: May decrease effect of stavudine.

Herbal

None known.

Food

None known.

DIAGNOSTIC TEST EFFECTS

None known.

SIDE EFFECTS

Frequent (> 10%)

Dizziness, headache, fatigue, fever, insomnia, irritability, depression, emotional lability, impaired concentration, alopecia,

rash, pruritus, nausea, anorexia, dyspepsia, vomiting, decreased hemoglobin, hemolysis, arthralgia, musculoskeletal pain, dyspnea, sinusitis, flu-like symptoms.
Occasional (10%-1%)
Nervousness, altered taste, weakness.

SERIOUS REACTIONS

- Cardiac arrest, apnea, ventilator dependence, bacterial pneumonia, pneumonia, and pneumothorax occur rarely.
- Anemia usually occurs in 1-2 wks of starting treatment.
- When used with interferon: severe depression and suicidal ideation, hemolytic anemia, bone marrow suppression, autoimmune and infectious disorders, pulmonary dysfunction, pancreatitis, and diabetes.

PRECAUTIONS & CONSIDERATIONS

Use inhaled ribavirin cautiously with asthma, chronic obstructive pulmonary disease (COPD), and those requiring mechanical ventilation. Caution should be used with oral ribavirin in the elderly and with cardiac or pulmonary disease, renal impairment, or a history of psychiatric disorders.

Report any difficulty breathing or itching, redness, or swelling of the eyes. Respiratory tract secretions should be obtained for diagnostic testing before giving the first dose of ribavirin or at least during the first 24 h of therapy. Complete blood count (CBC) with differential should be obtained. Pretreat and test women of childbearing age monthly for pregnancy. Adequate contraception must be practiced by males and females during treatment. Hematology reports should be assessed for anemia at wks 2 and 4 and periodically thereafter as needed.

Storage
Nebulizer solution is stable for 24 h at room temperature. Discard solution for nebulization after 24 h. Discard solution if discolored or cloudy.Oral solution may be stored at room temperature or refrigerated. Capsules and tablets are stored at room temperature.

Administration
! Ribavirin may be given via nasal or oral inhalation. Add 50-100 mL sterile water for injection or inhalation to 6-g vial. Transfer to a flask, serving as reservoir for aerosol generator. Further dilute to final volume of 300 mL, giving a solution concentration of 20 mg/mL. Use only aerosol generator available from the drug manufacturer. Do not give at the same time with other drug solutions for nebulization. Discard reservoir solution when fluid levels are low and at least every 24 h. Be aware that there is controversy over the safety of administering ribavirin to ventilator-dependent patients; only experienced personnel should administer the drug.
! Health care workers who are pregnant or trying to get pregnant should avoid contact with aerosolized ribavirin.

Capsules should not be opened, crushed, chewed, or broken. Capsules or oral solution may be taken without regard to food. Tablets should be given with food.

Rifabutin

rif'a-byoo'ten
Mycobutin
Do not confuse rifabutin with rifampin.

CATEGORY AND SCHEDULE

Pregnancy Risk Category: B

Classification:
Antimycobacterials

MECHANISM OF ACTION

An antitubercular agent that inhibits DNA-dependent RNA polymerase. Broad spectrum of antimicrobial activity, including activity against mycobacteria such as *Mycobacterium avium* complex (MAC). *Therapeutic Effect:* Prevents MAC disease.

PHARMACOKINETICS

Readily absorbed from the GI tract (high-fat meals delay absorption). Protein binding: 85%. Widely distributed. Crosses the blood-brain barrier. Extensive intracellular tissue uptake. Metabolized in the liver to active and inactive metabolites. Excreted in urine; eliminated in feces. Unknown if removed by hemodialysis. *Half-life:* 16-69 h.

AVAILABILITY

Capsules: 150 mg.

INDICATIONS AND DOSAGES

▸ **Prevention of MAC disease (first episode or recurrent episodes) in HIV-infected patients with < 50 CD4+ cells/mm³**

PO

Adults, Elderly. 300 mg once daily or in 2 divided doses if GI upset occurs.

Children ≥ 6 yr of age: 5 mg/kg (maximum: 300 mg) once daily per CDC.

▸ **Dosage in renal impairment**

Dosage is modified based on creatinine clearance. If creatinine clearance is < 30 mL/min, reduce dosage by 50%.

OFF LABEL USES

Alternative treatment for tuberculosis or active MAC infection in adults and children.

CONTRAINDICATIONS

Active tuberculosis; hypersensitivity to other rifamycins, including rifampin.

INTERACTIONS

NOTE: Rifabutin may decrease the effects of numerous drugs, including CYP3A4 substrates.

Drug

Antiretroviral protease inhibitors for HIV: May increase rifabutin concentrations and many labels suggest rifabutin dosage decrease with concurrent use.

Clarithromycin, itraconazole, fluconazole: May increase rifabutin concentrations.

Clopidogrel: May increase therapeutic effect of clopidogrel.

CYP3A4 inducers (carbamazepines, phenobarbital, phenytoin): May decrease effects of rifabutin.

Isoniazid: May increase the risk of hepatotoxicity.

Oral contraceptives: May decrease contraceptive effectiveness.

Zidovudine: May decrease blood concentration of zidovudine but does not affect the drug's inhibition of HIV.

Herbal

None known.

Food

High-fat meals: May decrease the rate of absorption.

DIAGNOSTIC TEST EFFECTS

May increase serum alkaline phosphatase, AST (SGOT), and ALT (SGPT) levels.

SIDE EFFECTS

Frequent (30%)

Red-orange or red-brown discoloration of urine, feces, saliva, skin, sputum, sweat, or tears. Soft contact lenses may be permanently stained.

Occasional (3%-11%)
Rash, nausea, abdominal pain, diarrhea, dyspepsia, belching, headache, altered taste, uveitis, corneal deposits.
Rare (< 2%)
Anorexia, flatulence, fever, myalgia, vomiting, insomnia.

SERIOUS REACTIONS

- Hepatitis and thrombocytopenia occur rarely. Anemia and neutropenia may also occur.
- Uveitis may cause visual impairment.
- Potential for superinfection, such as *Clostridium difficile*–associated diarrhea.

PRECAUTIONS & CONSIDERATIONS

Caution should be used with liver or renal impairment. The safety of this drug for use in children is not established. Be aware that it is unknown whether rifabutin crosses the placenta or is excreted in breast milk. No age-related precautions have been noted in elderly patients. Avoid crowds and those with known infection.

Feces, perspiration, saliva, skin, sputum, tears, and urine may be discolored red-brown or red-orange during drug therapy. Soft contact lenses may be permanently discolored. Rifabutin may decrease the effectiveness of oral contraceptives. Alternative methods of contraception should be used. Expect to perform a biopsy of suspicious nodes, if present. Also, expect to obtain blood or sputum cultures and a chest x-ray to rule out active tuberculosis. If ordered, obtain baseline complete blood count (CBC) and liver function test results.

Storage
Store at room temperature.

Administration
Should take on an empty stomach. Take with food if GI irritation occurs. May mix capsule contents with applesauce if unable to swallow capsules whole.

Rifampin

rye′fam-pin
Rifadin Rofact
Do not confuse rifampin with rifabutin, Rifamate, rifapentine, or Ritalin.

CATEGORY AND SCHEDULE

Pregnancy Risk Category: C

Classification:
Antimycobacterials

MECHANISM OF ACTION

An antitubercular agent that interferes with bacterial RNA synthesis by binding to DNA-dependent RNA polymerase, thus preventing its attachment to DNA and blocking RNA transcription. *Therapeutic Effect:* Bactericidal in susceptible microorganisms.

PHARMACOKINETICS

Well absorbed from the GI tract (food delays absorption). Protein binding: 80%. Widely distributed. Metabolized in the liver to active metabolite. Eliminated primarily by the biliary system. Not removed by hemodialysis. *Half-life:* 3-4 h (increased in hepatic impairment).

AVAILABILITY

Capsules (Rifadin): 150 mg, 300 mg.
Injection, Powder for Reconstitution (Rifadin): 600 mg.

INDICATIONS AND DOSAGES

▸ **Tuberculosis**

PO, IV

Adults, Elderly. 10 mg/kg/day in divided doses q12-24h. Maximum: 600 mg/day.

Children. 10-20 mg/kg/day in divided doses q12-24h.

▸ **Prevention of meningococcal infections**

PO, IV

Adults, Elderly. 600 mg q12h for 2 days.

Children 1 mo and older. 10 mg/kg given q12h for 2 days. Maximum: 600 mg/dose.

Infants younger than 1 mo. 10 mg/kg/day in divided doses q12h for 2 days.

▸ **Staphylococcal infections**

PO, IV

Adults, Elderly. 600 mg once a day.

Children. 15 mg/kg/day in divided doses q12h.

▸ ***Staphylococcus aureus* infections (in combination with other anti-infectives)**

PO

Adults, Elderly. 300-600 mg twice a day.

▸ **Prevention of *Haemophilus influenzae* infection**

PO

Adults, Elderly. 600 mg/day for 4 days.

Children 1 mo and older. 20 mg/kg/day in divided doses q12h for 5-10 days.

Children younger than 1 mo. 10 mg/kg/day in divided doses q12h for 2 days.

OFF-LABEL USES

Treatment of atypical mycobacterial infection, select cases of endocarditis, refractory sinusitis, leprosy, Legionnaires' disease.

CONTRAINDICATIONS

Concomitant therapy with fosamprenavir, saquinavir, hypersensitivity to rifampin or any other rifamycins.

INTERACTIONS

NOTE: Rifampin may decrease the effects of numerous drugs, including CYP1A2, 2A6, 2B6, 2C8, 2C9, 2C19, 3A4 substrates.

Drug

Alcohol, hepatotoxic medications: May increase the risk of hepatotoxicity.

Aminophylline, theophylline: May increase clearance of these drugs.

Amiodarone, chloramphenicol, digoxin, disopyramide, fluconazole, methadone, mexiletine, oral anticoagulants, oral antidiabetics, phenytoin, quinidine, tocainide, verapamil: May decrease the effects of these drugs.

Antacids: Reduce the absorption of rifampin. Give rifampin at least 1 h before an antacid.

Antiretroviral protease inhibitors (PIs): Markedly decreased PI concentrations; HIV treatment failure and resistance expected. Saquinavir or fosamprenavir contraindicate use of rifampin. Other HIV medicines are not recommended; choose alternative to rifampin when possible.

Clopidogrel: May increase the therapeutic effects.

Macrolide antibiotics: May increase levels/toxicity of rifampin.

Oral contraceptives: May decrease oral contraceptive effectiveness.

Herbal

St. John's wort: May decrease rifampin levels.

Food

All foods: Food may decrease rifampin concentrations.

DIAGNOSTIC TEST EFFECTS

May increase serum alkaline phosphatase, bilirubin, uric acid, AST (SGOT), and ALT (SGPT) levels. Cross-reactivity and false-positive urine screening tests for opiates using the KIMS method. Inhibits standard microbiological assays for serum folate and vitamin B_{12}; use alternate assays. Reduced biliary excretion of contrast media used for visualization of the gallbladder; perform before the morning dose of rifampin.

IV INCOMPATIBILITIES

Diltiazem (Cardizem), amiodarone, minocycline, tramadol.

SIDE EFFECTS

Expected

Red-orange or red-brown discoloration of urine, feces, saliva, skin, sputum, sweat, or tears.

Occasional (2%-5%)

Hypersensitivity reaction (such as flushing, pruritus, or rash).

Rare (1%-2%)

Diarrhea, dyspepsia, nausea, candida as evidenced by sore mouth or tongue.

SERIOUS REACTIONS

- Rare reactions include hepatotoxicity (risk is increased when rifampin is taken with isoniazid), hepatitis, blood dyscrasias, Stevens-Johnson syndrome, and antibiotic-associated colitis.

PRECAUTIONS & CONSIDERATIONS

Caution is warranted with active alcoholism, a history of alcohol abuse, or liver dysfunction. May exacerbate porphyria. Be aware that rifampin crosses the placenta and is distributed in breast milk. No age-related precautions have been noted or in children or in elderly patients. Avoid alcohol and any other medications, including antacids, without consulting with the physician. The reliability of oral contraceptives may be affected by rifampin, so alternative methods of contraception should be used.

Feces, sputum, sweat, tears, or urine may become red-orange or red-brown, and soft contact lenses may be permanently stained. Notify the physician of any new symptoms or if fatigue, fever, flu, nausea, unusual bleeding or bruising, vomiting, weakness, or yellow eyes and skin occurs. CBC results should be evaluated for blood dyscrasias, and bleeding, bruising, infection manifested as a fever or sore throat, and unusual tiredness and weakness should be assessed.

Storage

Store capsules and unopened vials at room temperature. Extemporaneous oral suspension stable for 4 wks at room temperature or refrigerated.

Reconstituted vial is stable for 24 h. Once the reconstituted vial is further diluted, it is stable for 4 h in D5W or 24 h in 0.9% NaCl.

Administration

Preferably give oral rifampin 1 h before or 2 h after meals with 8 oz of water. Rifampin may be given with food to decrease GI upset, but this will delay the drug's absorption. For those unable to swallow capsules, rifampin's contents may be mixed with applesauce or jelly. Alternatively, the manufacturer provides instruction for compounding a suspension; shake well before each use. Give rifampin at least 1 h before administering antacids.

! Administer rifampin by IV infusion only. Avoid IM and SC administration. Reconstitute

600-mg vial with 10 mL sterile water for injection to provide a concentration of 60 mg/mL. Withdraw the desired dose and further dilute with 500 mL D5W. Evaluate periodically for extravasation as evidenced by local inflammation and irritation. Infuse over 3 h (may dilute with 100 mL D5W and infuse over 30 min).

Rifapentine

rif-a-pen'teen

★ Priftin

Do not confuse with rifampin or rifabutin.

CATEGORY AND SCHEDULE

Pregnancy Risk Category: C

Classification:
Antimycobacterials

MECHANISM OF ACTION

An antitubercular agent that inhibits bacterial RNA synthesis by binding to DNA-dependent RNA polymerase in *Mycobacterium tuberculosis.* This action prevents the enzyme from attaching to DNA, thereby blocking RNA transcription. *Therapeutic Effect:* Bactericidal.

AVAILABILITY

Tablets: 150 mg.

INDICATIONS AND DOSAGES

▸ **Tuberculosis (in combination with at least one other antituberculosis agent)**

PO

Adults, Elderly. Intensive phase: 600 mg twice weekly for 2 mo (interval between doses not < 3 days). Continuation phase: 600 mg weekly for 4 mo.

CONTRAINDICATIONS

Hypersensitivity to rifapentine, rifampin, rifabutin.

INTERACTIONS

NOTE: Rifapentine may decrease the effects of numerous drugs, including CYP2C8, 2C9, and 3A4 substrates.

Drug

Amiodarone, chloramphenicol, digoxin, disopyramide, fluconazole, methadone, mexiletine, oral anticoagulants, oral antidiabetics, phenytoin, quinidine, tocainide, verapamil: May decrease the effects of these drugs.

Antiretrovial protease inhibitors (PIs): Markedly decreased PI concentrations; HIV treatment failure and resistance expected. Saquinavir or fosamprenavir contraindicate use of rifapentine. Other HIV medicines are not recommended; choose alternative to rifapentine when possible.

Clopidogrel: May increase the therapeutic effects.

Isoniazid: May increase the risk of hepatoxocity.

Herbal

None known.

Food

All foods: Increases maximum serum concentrations.

DIAGNOSTIC TEST EFFECTS

May increase serum AST (SGOT), ALT (SGPT), and bilirubin levels. May inhibit standard microbiological assays for serum folate and vitamin B_{12}; choose alternative methods.

SIDE EFFECTS

Rare (< 4%)

Red-orange or red-brown discoloration of urine, feces, saliva, skin, sputum, sweat, or tears; arthralgia, pain, nausea, vomiting, headache, dyspepsia, hypertension, dizziness, diarrhea.

R

SERIOUS REACTIONS

• Hyperuricemia, neutropenia, proteinuria, hematuria, antibiotic associated colitis, and hepatitis occur rarely.

PRECAUTIONS & CONSIDERATIONS

Caution is warranted in alcoholic patients and in those with liver function impairment. May exacerbate porphyria. Feces, sputum, sweat, tears, and urine may become red-orange or red-brown, and soft contact lenses may be permanently stained. The reliability of oral contraceptives may be affected by rifapentine, so alternative methods of contraception should be used. Initial complete blood count (CBC) and liver function test results should be evaluated. Evaluate for diarrhea, GI upset, nausea, or vomiting as well as pattern of daily bowel activity and stool consistency.

Storage

Store at room temperature protected from heat and humidity.

Administration

May give with or without food; administration with food reduces GI irritation. Be aware that rifapentine is used only in combination with another antituberculosis agent.

Rifaximin

rye-faks′eh-men

★ 🍁 Xifaxan

CATEGORY AND SCHEDULE

Pregnancy Risk Category: C

Classification: Antibiotics, miscellaneous

MECHANISM OF ACTION

An anti-infective that inhibits bacterial RNA synthesis by binding to a subunit of bacterial DNA-dependent RNA polymerase. *Therapeutic Effect:* Bactericidal.

PHARMACOKINETICS

< 0.4% absorbed after PO administration. Widely distributed in the GI tract. *Half-life:* 6 h. Excreted primarily in feces as unchanged drug.

AVAILABILITY

Tablets: 200 mg, 550 mg.

INDICATIONS AND DOSAGES

▸ **Reduce recurrence of hepatic encephalopathy**

PO

Adults, Elderly. 550 mg twice per day.

▸ **Traveler's diarrhea**

PO

Adults, Elderly, Children 12 yr and older. 200 mg 3 times a day for 3 days.

CONTRAINDICATIONS

Hypersensitivity to rifaximin or other rifamycin antibiotics or diarrhea with fever or blood in the stool.

INTERACTIONS

Drug

None known.

Herbal

None known.

Food

None known.

DIAGNOSTIC TEST EFFECTS

None known.

SIDE EFFECTS

Occasional (5%-11%)

Flatulence, headache, abdominal discomfort, rectal tenesmus, defecation urgency, nausea.

Rare (2%-4%)
Constipation, fever, vomiting.

SERIOUS REACTIONS

- Hypersensitivity reactions, including dermatitis, angioneurotic edema, pruritus, rash, and urticaria, may occur.
- Superinfection occurs rarely.

PRECAUTIONS & CONSIDERATIONS

Caution should be used with diarrhea complicated by fever and/or blood in the stool, or diarrhea due to pathogens other than *Escherichia coli.* Due to lack of efficacy, do not use where *Campylobacter jejuni, Shigella* spp., or *Salmonella* spp. are suspected as causative pathogens. Caution should be used with severe hepatic impairment (Child-Pugh class C). It is unknown if rifaximin is distributed in breast milk. Safety and efficacy of rifaximin have not been established in children younger than 12 yr. In elderly patients with normal renal function, no age-related precautions are noted.

Notify physician if diarrhea worsens within 48 h, fever develops, or blood is in stool.

Storage
Store tablets at room temperature.

Administration
Take rifaximin with or without food. Do not break or crush film-coated tablets.

Riluzole

rye'loo-zole
★ 🍁 Rilutek

CATEGORY AND SCHEDULE

Pregnancy Risk Category: C

Classification: Neuroprotectives, glutamate inhibitor

MECHANISM OF ACTION

An amyotrophic lateral sclerosis (ALS) agent that inhibits presynaptic glutamate release in the central nervous system (CNS) and interferes postsynaptically with the effects of excitatory amino acids. *Therapeutic Effect:* Extends survival of ALS patients.

PHARMACOKINETICS

Well absorbed from the GI tract (high-fat meal decreases absorption). Protein binding: 96%. Metabolized extensively in the liver to major and minor metabolites via CYP1A2. Primarily eliminated in the urine as metabolites. *Half-life:* 12 h.

AVAILABILITY

Tablets: 50 mg.

INDICATIONS AND DOSAGES

▸ ALS

PO
Adults, Elderly. 50 mg q12h.

CONTRAINDICATIONS

Severe hypersensitivity reactions to riluzole.

INTERACTIONS

Drug
Amiodarone, amitriptyline, fluvoxamine, ketoconazole, quinolones, theophylline: May increase the effects and risk of toxicity of riluzole.
Carbamazepine, omeprazole, phenobarbital, rifampin, tobacco smoking: May decrease the effects of riluzole.

Herbal
None known.

Food
Alcohol: May increase CNS depression.
Caffeine: May increase the effects and risk of toxicity of riluzole.

High-fat meals: May decrease the absorption and effects of riluzole.

DIAGNOSTIC TEST EFFECTS

May increase liver function test results. May decrease WBC count.

SIDE EFFECTS

Frequent (> 10%)

Nausea, asthenia, reduced respiratory function.

Occasional (1%-10%)

Edema, tachycardia, headache, dizziness, somnolence, depression, vertigo, tremor, pruritus, alopecia, abdominal pain, diarrhea, anorexia, dyspepsia, vomiting, stomatitis, increased cough.

SERIOUS REACTIONS

- Hepatic insufficiency and potential for hepatic failure.
- Marked neutropenia and resultant opportunistic infection risk.
- Hypersensitivity pneumonitis and interstitial lung disease.

PRECAUTIONS & CONSIDERATIONS

Caution is warranted in patients with renal or hepatic impairment. Alcohol should be avoided as well as tasks requiring mental alertness or motor skills until response to the medication has been established.

Notify the physician of fever. Blood chemistry tests to evaluate hepatic function should be obtained before and during therapy. The drug should be discontinued if the ALT level exceeds 10 times the upper normal limit.

Storage

Store at room temperature protected from bright light.

Administration

Take riluzole at least 1 h before or 2 h after a meal at the same time each day.

Rimabotulinumtoxin B (formerly Botulinum Toxin Type B)

bot'yoo-lin-num toks'in type b

★ Myobloc

CATEGORY AND SCHEDULE

Pregnancy Risk Category: C

Classification: Miscellaneous skeletal muscle relaxants

MECHANISM OF ACTION

A neurotoxin that inhibits acetylcholine release at the neuromuscular junction. *Therapeutic Effect:* Produces flaccid paralysis.

AVAILABILITY

Injection: 2500 units/0.5 mL, 5000 units/mL, 10,000 units/2 mL.

INDICATIONS AND DOSAGES

▸ **To reduce the severity of symptoms in patients with cervical dystonia who have previously tolerated rimabotulinumtoxin B**

IM

Adults, Elderly. 2500-5000 units divided among the affected muscles.

▸ **To reduce the severity of symptoms in patients with cervical dystonia who have not previously been treated with rimabotulinumtoxin B**

IM

Adults, Elderly. Administer at lower dosage than for patients who have previously tolerated the drug.

CONTRAINDICATIONS

Infection at proposed injection site, hypersensitivity to albumin, any botulinum toxin or any component of the formulation.

R

INTERACTIONS

Drug

Aminoglycoside antibiotics, other drugs that interfere with neuromuscular transmission (such as curare-like compounds): May potentiate the effects of rimabotulinumtoxin B.

Herbal

None known.

Food

None known.

DIAGNOSTIC TEST EFFECTS

None known.

SIDE EFFECTS

Frequent (12%-19%)

Infection, neck pain, headache, injection site pain, dry mouth.

Occasional (4%-10%)

Flu-like symptoms, generalized pain, increased cough, back pain, myasthenia.

Rare

Dizziness, nausea, rhinitis, headache, vomiting, edema, allergic reaction.

SERIOUS REACTIONS

- Mild to moderate dysphagia occurs in approximately 10% of patients.
- Arrhythmias and severe dysphagia (manifested as aspiration, pneumonia, and dyspnea) occur rarely, but may cause death.
- Overdose produces systemic weakness and muscle paralysis, respiratory failure, death.

PRECAUTIONS & CONSIDERATIONS

Caution is warranted for persons with neuromuscular junctional disorders, such as amyotrophic lateral sclerosis, Lambert-Eaton syndrome, motor neuropathy, and myasthenia gravis, because they may experience significant systemic effects, including respiratory compromise and severe dysphagia. Be aware of signs of dysphagia and aspiration pneumonia, including fever, sputum production, and adventitious breath sounds after treatment. Safety and effectiveness have not been established for use in children.

Resume normal activity slowly and carefully. Seek medical attention immediately if respiratory, speech, or swallowing difficulties occur.

Storage

Store unopened vials under refrigeration. Do not freeze. Do not shake. May be diluted with 0.9% NaCl for use. If diluted, the product must be used within 4 h.

Administration

! Plan to have a physician inject the drug into the affected muscle.

Dilute drug with 0.9% NaCl. Slowly and gently inject the diluent into the vial to avoid producing bubbles. Then rotate the vial gently to mix the drug. If a vacuum does not pull the diluent into the vial, discard it. For IM use, assist the physician as necessary while he or she injects the drug into the affected muscles using a 25-, 27-, or 30-gauge needle for superficial muscles and a 22-gauge needle for deeper muscles. Know that drug's effect lasts for 12-16 wks at doses of 5000 or 10,000 units.

Risedronate

rye-se-droe′nate

★ 🍁 Actonel, Atelvia

Do not confuse Actonel with Actos, or Altevia with Altoprev.

CATEGORY AND SCHEDULE

Pregnancy Risk Category: C

Classification: Bisphosphonates

MECHANISM OF ACTION

A bisphosphonate that binds to bone hydroxyapatite and inhibits osteoclasts. *Therapeutic Effect:* Reduces bone turnover (the number of sites at which bone is remodeled) and bone resorption.

AVAILABILITY

Tablets: 5 mg, 30 mg (Actonel)
Once-Weekly Tablet, Immediate Release: 35 mg (Actonel)
Once-Weekly Tablet, Delayed Release: 35 mg (Atelvia).
Once-Monthly Tablet: 150 mg (Actonel)

INDICATIONS AND DOSAGES

▸ **Paget disease**

PO

Adults, Elderly. 30 mg/day for 2 mo. Retreatment may occur after for 2-mo post-treatment observation period.

▸ **Prevention and treatment of postmenopausal osteoporosis**

PO

Adults, Elderly. 5 mg/day or 35 mg once weekly or 150 mg once monthly on the same day each month.

▸ **Glucocorticoid-induced osteoporosis**

PO

Adults, Elderly. 5 mg/day.

▸ **Treatment of male osteoporosis.**

PO

Adults, Elderly. 35 mg once weekly.

CONTRAINDICATIONS

Hypersensitivity to other bisphosphonates, including etidronate, ibandronate, tiludronate, risedronate, and alendronate; hypocalcemia; inability to stand or sit upright for at least 30 min; renal impairment when serum creatinine clearance is < 30 mL/min, or esophageal abnormality delaying emptying (e.g., stricture).

INTERACTIONS

Drug

Antacids or supplements containing aluminum, calcium, magnesium; oral calcium, iron, and magnesium salts; vitamin D: May decrease the absorption of risedronate. Separate administration by at least 2 h.

NSAIDs: May enhance GI toxic effects.

Phosphate supplements: May enhance hypocalcemic effects.

Herbal

None known.

Food

All Food: Reduces absorption.

DIAGNOSTIC TEST EFFECTS

May interfere with diagnostic imaging, technetium-99m-diphosphonate in bone scans.

SIDE EFFECTS

Frequent (30%)

Arthralgia.

Occasional (8%-12%)

Rash, flu-like symptoms, peripheral edema.

Rare (3%-5%)

Bone pain, sinusitis, asthenia, dry eye, tinnitus.

SERIOUS REACTIONS

- Overdose causes hypocalcemia, hypophosphatemia, and significant GI disturbances.
- Esophageal irritation occurs if administration instructions are not followed.
- Osteonecrosis of the jaw.
- Atypical femur fractures.

PRECAUTIONS & CONSIDERATIONS

Caution is warranted in patients with cardiac failure or renal impairment. Because there are no adequate and well-controlled studies in pregnant women, it is unknown whether risedronate causes fetal harm or is excreted in breast milk. Safety and efficacy have not been established in children. Elderly patients require careful monitoring of fluid and electrolytes. Consider beginning weight-bearing exercises and modifying behavioral factors.

Hypocalcemia and vitamin D deficiency, if present, should be corrected before beginning risedronate therapy. Monitor serum eletrolytes and renal function before and during treatment. Thigh or groin pain should be investigated.

Because of concern about osteonecrosis, preventive dental care is important, and invasive dental procedures should be avoided while on therapy.

Administration

For all immediate-release products: Take the drug with a full glass (6-8 oz) of plain water first thing in the morning and at least 30 min before first beverage, food, or medication of the day. Taking risedronate with other beverages, including coffee, mineral water, and orange juice, significantly reduces the absorption of the drug. Avoid lying down or bending over for at least 30 min after taking risedronate to potentiate delivery to the stomach and reduce the risk of esophageal irritation. Do not crush or chew the tablet.

For delayed-release tablets (Atelvia): Administer immediately after breakfast with at least 4 oz of plain water. Swallow tablets whole; do not chew, cut, or crush. Avoid lying down for at least 30 min after taking this medicine.

R

Risperidone

ris-per'i-done

Risperdal, Risperdal Consta, Risperdal M-Tabs

Do not confuse risperidone with reserpine, or Risperdal with Restoril.

CATEGORY AND SCHEDULE

Pregnancy Risk Category: C

Classification: Antipsychotics, atypical

MECHANISM OF ACTION

A benzisoxazole derivative that may antagonize dopamine and serotonin receptors. *Therapeutic Effect:* Suppresses psychotic behavior.

PHARMACOKINETICS

Oral form is well absorbed from the GI tract; unaffected by food. Protein binding: 90%. Extensively metabolized in the liver to active metabolite. Excreted primarily in urine. *Half-life:* Oral, 3-20 h; metabolite, 21-30 h (increased in elderly); injection, 3-6 days. Excreted primarily in urine and feces.

AVAILABILITY

Oral Solution (Risperdal): 1 mg/mL.
Tablets (Risperdal): 0.25 mg, 0.5 mg, 1 mg, 2 mg, 3 mg, 4 mg.
Tablets (Orally Disintegrating [Risperdal M-Tabs]): 0.5 mg, 1 mg, 2 mg, 3 mg, 4 mg.
Injection Long-Acting (Risperdal Consta): 12.5 mg, 25 mg, 37.5 mg, 50 mg.

INDICATIONS AND DOSAGES

▸ **Schizophrenia**

PO

Adults. Initially, 1 mg twice a day. May increase dosage slowly, 1-2 mg/day on a weekly basis. Maintenance range: 2-8 mg/day.
Elderly. Initially, 0.5 mg twice a day. May increase dosage slowly. Range: 2-6 mg/day.
Adolescents aged 13-17 yr. Initially, 0.5 mg once a day, adjusted in increments of 0.5-1 mg/day. Range: 1-6 mg/day, but doses > 3 mg/day do not yield additional benefits.
IM
Adults, Elderly. 25 mg q2wk. Maximum: 50 mg q2wk.

▸ **Mania, bipolar**
PO
Adults, Elderly. Initially, 2-3 mg as a single daily dose. May increase at 24-h intervals of 1 mg/day. Range: 1-6 mg/day.
Children aged 10-17 yr. Initially 0.5 mg/day. May increase at 24-h intervals of 0.5-1 mg/day, up to a maximum of 2.5 mg/day.
IM
Adults, Elderly. 25 mg q2wk. Maximum: 50 mg q2wk.

▸ **Irritability associated with autistic disorder**
PO
Children 5 yr and older. < 15 kg, use with caution; < 20 kg, 0.25 mg/day. After 4 days, may increase to 0.5 mg/day. Maintain dose for at least 14 days, then increase dose by 0.25 mg/day q2wk. Clinical response peaks at 1 mg/day; > 20 kg, 0.5 mg/day. After 4 days, may increase to 1 mg/day. Maintain dose for at least 14 days, then increase dose by 0.5 mg/day q2wk. Clinical response peaks at 2.5 mg/day.

▸ **Dosage in renal impairment**
Initial oral dosage for adults and elderly patients is 0.25-0.5 mg twice a day. Dosage is titrated slowly to desired effect.

OFF-LABEL USES

Behavioral symptoms associated with dementia, pervasive developmental disorder, Tourette disorder.

CONTRAINDICATIONS

Known hypersensitivity to risperidone.

INTERACTIONS

Drug
Alcohol, other CNS depressants: May increase CNS depression.
Carbamazepine: May decrease the risperidone blood concentration.
Clozapine: May increase the risperidone blood concentration.
CYP2D6 inhibitors: May increase the levels/effects of risperidone.
Dopamine agonists, levodopa: May decrease the effects of these drugs.
Fluoxetine, paroxetine: May increase the risperidone blood concentration and the risk of extrapyramidal symptoms.
Valproic acid: May increase the adverse effects/toxicity of risperidone.
Verapamil, SSRIs, and lithium: May increase the levels/effects of risperidone.
Herbal
Kava kava, gotu kola, St. John's wort, valerian: May increase central nervous system (CNS) depression.
Food
Ethanol: Avoid; may increase CNS depression.

DIAGNOSTIC TEST EFFECTS

May increase serum prolactin, creatinine, alkaline phosphatase, uric acid, AST (SGOT), ALT (SGPT), and triglyceride levels. May decrease blood glucose and serum potassium, protein, and sodium levels. May cause ECG changes.

SIDE EFFECTS

Frequent (13%-26%)
Agitation, anxiety, insomnia, headache, constipation.
Occasional (4%-10%)
Dyspepsia, rhinitis, somnolence, dizziness, nausea, vomiting, rash, abdominal pain, dry skin, tachycardia.
Rare (2%-3%)
Visual disturbances, fever, back pain, pharyngitis, cough, arthralgia, angina, aggressive behavior, orthostatic hypotension, breast swelling, weight gain.

SERIOUS REACTIONS

- Rare reactions include tardive dyskinesia (characterized by tongue protrusion, puffing of the cheeks, and chewing or puckering of the mouth) and neuroleptic malignant syndrome (marked by hyperpyrexia, muscle rigidity, change in mental status, irregular pulse or BP, tachycardia, diaphoresis, cardiac arrhythmias, rhabdomyolysis, and acute renal failure).
- Priapism.
- Neutropenia/agranulocytosis (rare).
- Seizures or heart arrhythmias (rare).
- New-onset diabetes mellitus.

R

PRECAUTIONS & CONSIDERATIONS

Caution is warranted in patients with cardiac disease, diabetes, breast cancer, hepatic or renal impairment, seizure disorders, recent MI, those at risk for aspiration pneumonia, suicidal tendencies.

Be aware that risperidone may increase the risk of hyperglycemia. It is unknown whether risperidone crosses the placenta or is excreted in breast milk. Breastfeeding is not recommended for patients taking this drug. Elderly patients are more susceptible to orthostatic hypotension and may require a dosage adjustment because of age-related renal or hepatic impairment. Elderly patients with dementia-related psychosis have a significantly higher incidence of cerebrovascular adverse events (e.g., stroke, TIA) and increased risk of mortality.

Drowsiness and dizziness may occur but generally subside with continued therapy. Tasks requiring mental alertness or motor skills should be avoided. Notify the physician if altered gait, difficulty breathing, palpitations, pain or swelling in breasts, severe dizziness or fainting, trembling fingers, unusual movements, rash, fever, or visual changes occur. BP, heart rate, liver function test results, ECG, and weight should be assessed.

Storage
Store tablets at room temperature; protect M-Tabs from moisture and keep in blister pack until time of use. The IM injection may be given up to 6 h after reconstitution, but immediate administration is recommended. If 2 min pass before the injection, reconstitute the solution by shaking the upright vial vigorously back and forth for as long as it takes to resuspend the microspheres. Store the drug below 77° F (25° C) once it is in suspension.

Administration
Take risperidone without regard to food. Mix the oral solution with water, orange juice, coffee, or low-fat milk, but not with cola or tea.

For M-Tabs, once removed from blister pack, place immediately on tongue. Do not split or chew tablet because it will dissolve within seconds and may be swallowed with or without liquid.

For IM administration, use only the diluent and needle supplied in the dose pack. All the components in the dose pack will be required for administration. Do not substitute any components. Prepare the suspension according to the manufacturer's directions. Inject the drug intramuscularly into the upper outer quadrant of the gluteus maximus. Do not administer the drug by the IV route.

Ritonavir

ri-tone'a-veer

Norvir

Do not confuse ritonavir with, Retrovir, or Norvir with Norvasc.

CATEGORY AND SCHEDULE

Pregnancy Risk Category: B

Classification: Antiretrovirals, protease inhibitors

MECHANISM OF ACTION

Inhibits HIV-1 and HIV-2 proteases, rendering these enzymes incapable of processing the polypeptide precursors; this results in the production of noninfectious, immature HIV particles. *Therapeutic Effect:* Impedes HIV replication, slowing the progression of HIV infection.

PHARMACOKINETICS

Well absorbed after PO administration (absorption increased with food). Protein binding: 98%-99%. Extensively metabolized in the liver to active metabolite. Eliminated primarily in feces. Unknown whether removed by hemodialysis. *Half-life:* 3-5 h.

AVAILABILITY

Oral Solution: 80 mg/mL.
Soft Gelatin Capsules: 100 mg.
Tablets: 100 mg.

INDICATIONS AND DOSAGES

▸ **HIV infection**

PO

Adults, Children 12 yr and older. 600 mg twice a day. If nausea occurs at this dosage, give 300 mg twice a day for 1 day, 400 mg twice a day for 2 days, 500 mg twice a day for 1 day, then 600 mg twice a day thereafter. *Children younger than 12 yr.* Initially, 250 mg/m^2 twice a day. Increase by 50 mg/m^2 up to 400 mg/m^2. Maximum: 600 mg twice a day.

CONTRAINDICATIONS

Known hypersensitivity to ritonavir or any of its ingredients. Ritonavir is contraindicated with many drugs (see Drug Interactions) because ritonavir-mediated CYP3A inhibition can result in serious and/or life-threatening reactions, or there is reduced efficacy of ritonavir or the interacting drug when given together.

INTERACTIONS

NOTE: Please see detailed manufacturer's information for management of drug interactions. In some cases, dosage adjustment for the agent or choice of an alternate agent is recommended.

Drug

Alfuzosin, cisapride, pimozide, voriconazole: Ritonavir increases levels and risk of cardiovascular adverse outcomes. Contraindicated.

Antacids, buffered didanosine: Reduce ritonavir absorption, separate administration times.

Antiarrhythmics (i.e., amiodarone, flecainide, propafenone, quinidine): Ritonavir increases levels and risk of proarrhythmia. Contraindicated.

Antidepressants: May increase the blood concentration of these drugs.

Cyclosporine, other immunosuppressants: Ritonavir may increase blood concentrations; monitor closely.

Disulfiram, drugs causing disulfiram-like reaction (such as metronidazole): May produce a disulfiram-like reaction.

Enzyme inducers (including carbamazepine, dexamethasone, nevirapine, phenobarbital, phenytoin, rifabutin, rifampin): May increase the metabolism and decrease the efficacy of ritonavir. Consider alternative to rifampin; increases liver toxicity risk if taken with saquinavir-ritonavir.
Ergot derivatives (e.g., dihydroergotamine, ergonovine, ergotamine, methylergonovine): Ritonavir increases levels and risk of ergot toxicity. Contraindicated.
Lovastatin, simvastatin: Ritonavir increases levels and risk of myopathy and rhabdomyolysis. Contraindicated.
Oral contraceptives, theophylline: May decrease the effectiveness of these drugs.
Oral midazolam, triazolam: Ritonavir increases levels causing benzodiazepine toxicity and respiratory depression risk.
Phosphodiesterase-5 inhibitors (e.g., sildenafil, vardenafil, tadalafil): Increases PDE-5 inhibitor blood levels and risk of hypotension. Contraindicated for use with sildenafil for pulmonary HTN.
Herbal
St. John's wort: May decrease the blood concentration and effect of ritonavir. Contraindicated.
Food
All Food: Enhances absorption; take with food.

DIAGNOSTIC TEST EFFECTS

May alter serum CK, GGT, triglyceride, uric acid, AST (SGOT), and ALT (SGPT) levels as well as creatinine clearance.

SIDE EFFECTS

Frequent
GI disturbances (abdominal pain, anorexia, diarrhea, nausea, vomiting), circumoral and peripheral paresthesias, altered taste, headache, dizziness, fatigue, asthenia.
Occasional
Allergic reaction, flu-like symptoms, hypotension.
Rare
Diabetes mellitus, hyperglycemia.

SERIOUS REACTIONS

- Serious hypersensitivity reactions have included erythema multiforme, Stevens-Johnson Syndrome, or anaphylactoid reactions.
- Hepatitis.
- Pancreatitis.
- Spontaneous bleeding in patients with hemophilia.
- PR interval prolongation.

PRECAUTIONS & CONSIDERATIONS

Caution should be used in patients with impaired hepatic function. Be aware that breastfeeding is not recommended in this population because of the possibility of HIV transmission. No age-related precautions have been noted in children older than 2 yr. There are no known effects of this drug's use in elderly patients.

When beginning combination therapy with ritonavir and nucleosides, it may promote GI tolerance by first beginning ritonavir alone and then by adding nucleosides before completing 2 wks of ritonavir monotherapy. Check baseline laboratory test results, if ordered, especially liver function tests and serum triglycerides, before beginning ritonavir therapy and at periodic intervals during therapy. Monitor for signs and symptoms of GI disturbances or neurologic abnormalities, particularly paresthesias.

When used as "booster" in combination with other protease inhibitors, be sure to consult specific dosage recommendations of both agents.

Storage

Store capsules or solution in the refrigerator, always in the original container. Protect the drug from light. Refrigerate the oral solution unless it is used within 30 days and stored below 77° F.

Administration

Administer with food. May improve the taste of the oral solution by mixing it with Advera, chocolate milk, or Ensure within 1 h of dosing. Continue therapy for the full length of treatment, and evenly space drug doses around the clock. Separate administration from buffered didanosine or antacids by 2.5 h.

Rituximab

rye-tuck'ih-mab

Rituxan

Do not confuse Rituxan with Remicade or rituximab with infliximab.

CATEGORY AND SCHEDULE

Pregnancy Risk Category: C

Classification: Antineoplastics, disease-modifying antirheumatic drugs (DMARDs), monoclonal antibodies

MECHANISM OF ACTION

Binds to CD20, the antigen found on the surface of B lymphocytes and B-cell non-Hodgkin lymphomas. *Therapeutic Effect:* Produces cytotoxicity, reducing tumor size. Immunomodulatory activity reduces joint destruction in RA.

PHARMACOKINETICS

Rapidly depletes B cells. Excretion: uncertain. *Half-life* proportional to dose: 3.2 days after first infusion and 8.6 days after fourth infusion.

AVAILABILITY

Injection: 10 mg/mL.

INDICATIONS AND DOSAGES

▸ **Non-Hodgkin lymphoma: different treatment protocols depending on type**

IV INFUSION

Adults. 375 mg/m^2 once weekly for 4 wks. May administer a second 4-wk course; refer to specific protocol utilized.

▸ **CD20+ chronic lymphocytic leukemia**

IV INFUSION

Adults. 375 mg/m^2 on day 1 in cycle 1 and 500 mg/m^2 in cycles 2-6, used in combination with cyclophosphamide/fludarabine, administered q 28 days. NOTE: PCP prophylaxis and herpes viral prophylaxis are recommended during treatment and for up to 12 mo following as appropriate.

▸ **Rheumatoid arthritis**

IV INFUSION

Adults. 1000 mg on days 1 and 15 in combination with methotrexate. Give q24 wk or based on response, but not sooner than q16 wk.

CONTRAINDICATIONS

Hypersensitivity to murine proteins. Hold use in severe, active infections.

INTERACTIONS

Drug

Antihypertensives: May intensify hypotensive effects; hold for 12 h prior to treatment.

Cisplatin: May increase risk of renal toxicity.

Live-virus vaccines: May have reduced response to vaccination; immunosuppression may increase risk of viral disease. Avoid use of such vaccines.

Herbal and Food

None known.

DIAGNOSTIC TEST EFFECTS

Reduces lymphocyte, WBC, RBC, platelet counts.

IV INCOMPATIBILITIES

Do not mix rituximab with any other medications. Specific incompatibilities include aldesleukin, amphotericin B, ciprofloxacin, cyclosporine, daunorubicin, doxorubicin, furosemide, levofloxacin, ondansetron, quinupristin-dalfopristin, sodium bicarbonate, topotecan, vancomycin.

SIDE EFFECTS

Frequent

Fever (49%), chills (32%), asthenia (16%), headache (14%), angioedema (13%), hypotension (10%), nausea (18%), rash or pruritus (10%).

Occasional (< 10%)

Myalgia, dizziness, abdominal pain, throat irritation, vomiting, neutropenia, rhinitis, bronchospasm, urticaria.

SERIOUS REACTIONS

- Arrhythmias may occur, particularly in those with a history of preexisting cardiac conditions.
- Progressive multifocal leukoencephalopathy (PML) due to latent JC virus has been reported with use; can be fatal.
- Tumor lysis syndrome leading to acute renal failure requiring dialysis may occur 12-24 h following a dose.
- Severe, sometimes fatal mucocutaneous reactions have been reported.
- A hypersensitivity reaction marked by hypotension, bronchopasm, and angioedema may occur. Fatal infusion reactions with 24 h of infusion; 80% of these occur with the first infusion.
- Resultant immunosuppression may place at risk for serious opportunistic infections or reactivation of hepatitis B with fulminant hepatitis.
- Bowel obstruction and perforation.

PRECAUTIONS & CONSIDERATIONS

Caution is warranted in patients with a history of cardiac disease and the elderly. Be aware that rituximab may cause fetal B-cell depletion. Women with childbearing potential should use reliable contraceptive methods during treatment and for up to 12 mo afterward. It is unknown whether rituximab is distributed in breast milk. The safety and efficacy of rituximab have not been established in children.

Administer aggressive intravenous hydration, antihyperuricemic agents, and monitor renal function if hyperuricemia and tumor lysis syndrome occur. Monitor neurologic function. Monitor cardiac function and BP and evaluate complaints of chest or abdominal pain promptly. Obtain CBC with differential prior to each dose and at regular intervals. Patients should avoid crowds, persons with illness, and vaccinations during treatment. Report any signs of infection promptly. Treat and withhold rituximab if serious infection occurs.

Infusion-related reactions, including chills, fever, hypotension, and rigors, which usually occur 30 min to 2 h after beginning the first rituximab infusion, should be monitored; slowing the infusion resolves these symptoms. CBC should be obtained before and regularly during therapy.

Storage
Refrigerate unopened vials. The diluted solution is stable for up to 24 h if refrigerated and at room temperature for an additional 24 hr.

Administration
! Expect to pretreat the patient with acetaminophen and diphenhydramine before each infusion to help minimize infusion-related reactions. With rheumatoid arthritis, pretreat with a corticosteoid before each rituximab dose. Do not give rituximab by IV push or bolus.

For IV infusion only. Withdraw the needed amount into an infusion bag, and dilute it with 0.9% NaCl or D5W to a final concentration of 1-4 mg/mL. For the initial infusion, infuse the drug at 50 mg/h. The infusion rate may be increased, as necessary, in increments of 50 mg/h every 30 min to a maximum rate of 400 mg/h. For subsequent infusions, the drug may be administered initially at 100 mg/h and increased in increments of 100 mg/h every 30 min to a maximum rate of 400 mg/h.

Always carefully monitor for serious infusion reactions.

Rivastigmine

riv'a-stig'mine
Exelon

CATEGORY AND SCHEDULE

Pregnancy Risk Category: B

Classification: Alzheimer agents, cholinesterase inhibitors

MECHANISM OF ACTION

A carbamate cholinesterase inhibitor that inhibits the enzyme acetylcholinesterase, thus increasing the concentration of acetylcholine (ACh) at cholinergic synapses and enhancing cholinergic function in the central nervous system (CNS). *Therapeutic Effect:* Slows the progression of Alzheimer disease and Parkinson dementia.

PHARMACOKINETICS

Well absorbed after PO and transdermal administration. Rapidly and extensively metabolized at CNS receptor sites via cholinesterase, which mediates hydrolysis to the decarbamylated phenolic metabolite. The metabolite is metabolized in the liver, but is of no therapeutic consequence. No interactions with CYP450 are observed. The metabolite is 90% excreted in the urine in 24 h post-dose. *Half-life:* Plasma: 1-2 h; however, CNS cholinesterase inhibition lasts much longer (~ 10 h). A carbamate moiety remains at the CNS acetylcholinesterase receptor for up to 10 h, preventing the hydrolysis of ACh.

AVAILABILITY

Capsules: 1.5 mg, 3 mg, 4.5 mg, 6 mg.
Oral Solution: 2 mg/mL.
Transdermal Patch: 4.6 mg/24 h, 9.5 mg/24 h.

INDICATIONS AND DOSAGES

▸ **Alzheimer disease or Parkinson dementia**

PO

Adults, Elderly. Initially, 1.5 mg twice daily with food. After 2 wks (Alzheimer disease) or 4 wks (Parkinson dementia), may increase to 3 mg twice daily if tolerated. Subsequently, increase dose by 1.5 mg twice daily, at intervals of 2 wks (Alzheimer disease) or 4 wks (Parkinson dementia) or more.

Maximum: 6 mg twice daily. If GI adverse effects occur, discontinue for several doses, and then restart at lower dose. If interrupted for several days, reinitiate with the lowest daily dose (1.5 mg twice daily) and slowly retitrate.
TRANSDERMAL
Adults, Elderly. Initially, one 4.6 mg/24 h patch applied once daily. After 4 wks, may increase to the 9.5 mg/24 h patch if tolerated. If treatment is interrupted for > 3 days, begin with initial titration. To switch from oral to patch: For patients receiving less than 6 mg/day of oral rivastigmine, use the 4.6 mg/24 h patch. For patients receiving 6-12 mg/day of oral rivastigmine, use the 9.5 mg/24 h patch. Apply the first patch on the day following the last oral dose.

CONTRAINDICATIONS

History of hypersensitivity to rivastigmine or carbamate derivatives, acute jaundice, active GI bleeding.

INTERACTIONS

Drug
Anticholinergics: May decrease the effect of rivastigmine.
Cholinergic agonists, neuromuscular blockers, succinylcholine: May increase cholinergic effects.
NSAIDs: Increase GI irritation. Monitor for GI bleeding.
Herbal
Tobacco smoking: May decrease cholinergic effects.
Food
None known.

DIAGNOSTIC TEST EFFECTS

Infrequent increased liver function enzymes.

SIDE EFFECTS

Frequent
Significant nausea and weight loss; slow titration improves GI tolerance. Dizziness and diarrhea are also common.
Occasional
Insomnia, urinary tract infection, vomiting, abdominal pain, fatigue.
Rare
Asthenia, flu-like symptoms, hypertension, anxiety, hallucinations, increase in aggression, rhinitis, somnolence, syncope, dyspepsia, constipation, flatulence. Parkinson tremor may be worsened.

SERIOUS REACTIONS

- Vagotonic effects may include bradycardia, heart block, and syncopal episodes.
- May induce extrapyramidal symptoms.
- GI ulcer or bleeding; pancreatitis (rare).
- Overdose may result in cholinergic crisis, characterized by severe nausea, increased salivation, diaphoresis, bradycardia, hypotension, flushed skin, abdominal pain, respiratory depression, seizures, and cardiorespiratory collapse. Increasing muscle weakness may result in death if respiratory muscles are involved.

The antidote is 1-2 mg IV atropine sulfate with subsequent doses based on therapeutic response.

PRECAUTIONS & CONSIDERATIONS

Caution is warranted with asthma; bladder outflow obstruction; prostatic hypertrophy; asthma or chronic obstructive pulmonary disease (COPD); peptic ulcer disease; history of seizures, sick sinus syndrome, or other supraventricular conduction disturbances (bradycardia); and concurrent use of NSAIDs. There is no role for rivastigmine during pregnancy or lactation. Rivastigmine is not prescribed for children. Be aware that rivastigmine is not a cure for dementia but may slow the progression of its symptoms.

Notify the physician if abdominal pain, diarrhea, excessive sweating or salivation, dizziness, or nausea and vomiting occur or if hypertension is present. Baseline vital signs should be assessed. Cholinergic reactions, such as diaphoresis, dizziness, excessive salivation, facial warmth, abdominal cramps or discomfort, lacrimation, pallor, and urinary urgency, should be monitored.

Storage

Store at room temperature. Keep patch in original closed foil pouch until time of use.

Administration

Take oral rivastigmine with food to increase GI tolerance.

Measure oral solution with the supplied oral syringe. Give undiluted, or it may be diluted in a small glass of water, cold fruit juice, or soda; stir well. Patient should drink entire glass to ensure proper dose. Stable for up to 4 h mixed with these beverages.

Apply transdermal patch once daily to clean, dry, hairless, intact healthy skin in an area not rubbed by tight clothing or elastic. Application to the upper or lower back may be preferable to avoid removal by the patient; however, the chest or upper arm may also be used. Do not apply to red, irritated, or damaged skin. Do not use on areas with recent application of lotions, creams, or powder. Rotate application sites daily. Do not apply to the same site more than once every 14 days. Always remove the old patch before applying a new patch so that overdose does not occur.

Rizatriptan

rize-a-trip'tan

★ Maxalt, Maxalt-MLT

CATEGORY AND SCHEDULE

Pregnancy Risk Category: C

Classification: Antimigraine agent; $5HT_1$-receptor agonist; serotonin receptor agonists

MECHANISM OF ACTION

A serotonin receptor agonist that binds selectively to vascular receptors, producing a vasoconstrictive effect on cranial blood vessels. *Therapeutic Effect:* Relieves migraine headache.

PHARMACOKINETICS

Well absorbed after PO administration. Protein binding: 14%. Crosses the blood-brain barrier. Metabolized by the liver to inactive metabolite. Eliminated primarily in urine and, to a lesser extent, in feces. *Half-life:* 2-3 h.

AVAILABILITY

Tablets (Maxalt): 5 mg, 10 mg.
Oral Disintegrating Tablets (Maxalt-MLT): 5 mg, 10 mg.

INDICATIONS AND DOSAGES

▸ **Acute migraine attack**

PO (TABLETS OR ODT)

Adults, Elderly. 5-10 mg. If headache improves, but then returns, dose may be repeated after 2 h. Maximum: 30 mg/24 h.

CONTRAINDICATIONS

Basilar or hemiplegic migraine, coronary artery disease, ischemic heart disease (including angina pectoris, history of myocardial infarction [MI], silent ischemia, and

Prinzmetal angina), uncontrolled hypertension, use within 24 h of ergotamine-containing preparations or another serotonin receptor agonist; use within 14 days of MAOIs, hypersensitivity to rizatriptan.

INTERACTIONS

Drug

Dextromethorphan, fluoxetine, fluvoxamine, paroxetine, sertraline, tramadol: May produce hyperreflexia, incoordination, and weakness.

Selective 5-HT_1 antagonist, ergotamine-containing medications: May produce a vasospastic reaction.

MAOIs: Increase plasma concentration of rizatriptan, and increase risk of serotonergic crisis.

Propranolol: Increases rizatriptan levels. Maximum rizatriptan 5 mg/dose and 15 mg/24 h.

Herbal

None known.

Food

All foods: Delays peak drug concentration by 1 h.

R

DIAGNOSTIC TEST EFFECTS

None known.

SIDE EFFECTS

Frequent (7%-9%)

Dizziness, somnolence, paresthesia, fatigue.

Occasional (3%-6%)

Nausea, chest pressure, dry mouth.

Rare (2%)

Headache; neck, throat, or jaw pressure; photosensitivity.

SERIOUS REACTIONS

- Cardiac reactions (such as ischemia, coronary artery vasospasm, and MI) and noncardiac vasospasm-related reactions (including hemorrhage and cerebrovascular accident) occur rarely, particularly in patients with hypertension, diabetes, or a strong family history of coronary artery disease; obese patients; smokers; males older than 40 yr; and postmenopausal women.

PRECAUTIONS & CONSIDERATIONS

Caution is warranted in patients with mild to moderate hepatic or renal impairment and cardiovascular risk factors. It is unknown whether rizatriptan is excreted in breast milk. The safety and efficacy of rizatriptan have not been established in children. Rizatriptan is not recommended for elderly patients. Smoking, exposure to sunlight and ultraviolet rays, and tasks that require mental alertness or motor skills should be avoided.

Dizziness may occur. Notify the physician immediately if anxiety, chest pain, palpitations, or tightness in the throat occurs. BUN level and serum alkaline phosphatase, bilirubin, creatinine AST (SGOT), and ALT (SGPT) levels should be obtained before treatment to assess renal and hepatic function. ECG should also be obtained at baseline. Migraines and associated symptoms, including nausea and vomiting, photophobia, and phonophobia (sound sensitivity), should be assessed before and during treatment.

Storage

Store tablets at room temperature. ODT form should be kept in original sealed blister pack until time of use; protect from moisture.

Administration

Do not crush, chew, or split tablets. Preferably take without food. Do not remove the orally disintegrating tablet from the blister pack until just before taking it. Open packet with dry hands, and place ODT on the tongue to dissolve. Then swallow it. Do not administer ODT with water.

Ropinirole

ro-pin'i-role

Requip, Requip XL

CATEGORY AND SCHEDULE

Pregnancy Risk Category: C

Classification: Antiparkinsonian agents, dopaminergics

MECHANISM OF ACTION

An antiparkinsonian agent that stimulates dopamine receptors in the striatum. *Therapeutic Effect:* Relieves signs and symptoms of Parkinson disease.

Reduces uncomfortable leg sensations, movement, and sleep disturbance in restless leg syndrome (RLS).

PHARMACOKINETICS

Rapidly absorbed after PO administration. Food does not alter efficacy. Protein binding: 40%. Extensively distributed throughout the body. Extensively metabolized. Steady-state concentrations achieved within 2 days. Eliminated in urine. Unknown whether removed by hemodialysis. *Half-life:* 6 h.

AVAILABILITY

Tablets: 0.25 mg, 0.5 mg, 1 mg, 2 mg, 3 mg, 4 mg, 5 mg.
Extended Release Tablets: 2 mg, 4 mg, 6 mg, 8 mg, 12 mg.

INDICATIONS AND DOSAGES

▸ **Parkinson disease**

PO (IMMEDIATE-RELEASE TABLETS)

Adults, Elderly. Initially, 0.25 mg 3 times a day. May increase dosage every 7 days. Titrate gradually, as follows: wk 2, 0.5 mg 3 times a day; wk 3, 0.75 mg 3 times a day. After wk 4, dosage may be increased every week, if needed, by 1.5-3 mg/day to a maximum dose of 24 mg/day.

PO (EXTENDED RELEASE)

Adults, Elderly. Initially, 2 mg once daily for 1-2 wks, followed by increases of 2 mg/day at 1 wk or longer intervals as appropriate. Maximum: 24 mg/day.

▸ **Restless legs syndrome**

PO

Adults, Elderly. Initially, 0.25 mg daily 1-3 h before bedtime. May increase dosage after 2 days to 0.5 mg daily then 1 mg daily after 7 days. May titrate dose 0.5 mg/wk every 7 days. Maximum: 4 mg/day.

CONTRAINDICATIONS

Hypersensitivity to ropinirole.

INTERACTIONS

Drug

Antipsychotics, butyrophenones, carbamazepine, cigarette smoking, phenobarbibital, metoclopramide, phenothiazines, rifampin, thioxanthenes: Decrease the effectiveness of ropinirole.

Central nervous system (CNS) depressants: May increase CNS depressant effects.

Cimetidine, diltiazem, enoxacin, erythromycin, fluvoxamine, mexiletine, norfloxacin, tacrine: Increase ropinirole blood concentration.

Estrogens: Reduce the clearance of ropinirole.

Levodopa: Increases the blood concentration of levodopa.

Quinolones: Increase ropinirole blood concentration.

Herbal

Kava kava, gotu kola, valerian, St. John's wort: May increase CNS depression.

R

Food
Ethanol: May increase CNS depression.

DIAGNOSTIC TEST EFFECTS

May increase serum alkaline phosphatase level.

SIDE EFFECTS

Frequent (40%-60%)
Nausea, dizziness, somnolence.
Occasional (4%-12%)
Syncope, vomiting, fatigue, viral infection, dyspepsia, diaphoresis, asthenia, orthostatic hypotension, abdominal discomfort, pharyngitis, abnormal vision, dry mouth, hypertension, hallucinations, confusion.
Rare (< 4%)
Anorexia, peripheral edema, memory loss, rhinitis, sinusitis, palpitations, impotence.

SERIOUS REACTIONS

- Excessive daytime drowsiness may result in falling asleep while engaged in activities, including the operation of motor vehicles.
- Hallucinations; new or emergent compulsive actions (gambling, eating, shopping, etc.).
- Retroperitoneal fibrosis, pulmonary infiltrates, pleural effusion, pleural thickening, pericarditis, and cardiac valvulopathy have been reported with ergot-derived dopaminergic agents.

PRECAUTIONS & CONSIDERATIONS

Caution is warranted in patients with hallucinations (especially elderly), renal or hepatic impairment, syncope, history of orthostatic hypotension, and those who take CNS depressants concurrently. Because ropinirole is distributed in breast milk, it may cause drug-related effects in the breastfeeding infant. The safety and efficacy of ropinirole have not been established in children. No age-related precautions have been noted in elderly patients, but they are more likely than other age groups to experience hallucinations.

Dizziness, drowsiness, and orthostatic hypotension are common initial responses to the drug. Alcohol and tasks that require mental alertness or motor skills should be avoided until the effects of the drug are known. Change positions slowly to prevent orthostatic hypotension. Vital signs and serum alkaline phosphatase levels should be assessed at baseline. Relief of symptoms, such as improvement of mask-like facial expression, muscular rigidity, shuffling gait, and resting tremors of the hands and head, should be assessed during treatment.

Storage
Store at controlled room temperature.

Administration
Taking ropinirole with food may decrease risk of nausea. Extended-release tablets should be swallowed whole; do not cut, crush, or chew. Patients taking the drug for RLS should take it within 1-3 h of their expected bedtime.

For Parkinson disease, plan to discontinue the drug gradually at 7-day intervals, as follows: first decrease the frequency from 3 times a day to twice a day for 4 days; for the remaining 3 days, decrease the frequency to once a day before complete withdrawal, as prescribed. For restless legs syndrome, doses up to 4 mg/day may be discontinued without tapering.

Rosiglitazone

roz-ih-gli'ta-zone

Avandia

Do not confuse Avandia with Avalide, Avinza, Coumadin, or Prandin.

CATEGORY AND SCHEDULE

Pregnancy Risk Category: C

Classification: Antidiabetic agents, thiazolidinediones

MECHANISM OF ACTION

Thiazolidinedione that improves target-cell response to insulin without increasing pancreatic insulin secretion. Decreases hepatic glucose output and increases insulin-dependent glucose utilization in skeletal muscle. *Therapeutic Effect:* Lowers blood glucose concentration.

PHARMACOKINETICS

Rapidly absorbed. Protein binding: 99.8%. Metabolized in the liver. Excreted primarily in urine, with a lesser amount in feces. Not removed by hemodialysis. *Half-life:* 3-4 h.

AVAILABILITY

Tablets: 2 mg, 4 mg, 8 mg.

INDICATIONS AND DOSAGES

NOTE: In September 2010, the FDA placed rosiglitazone in a restricted access program due to CV events. Only those currently treated with rosiglitazone and benefiting are to continue treatment. New patients receive ONLY if not achieving control with other drugs and unable to take pioglitazone (Actos).

▸ **Diabetes mellitus type 2, monotherapy, or combination therapy**

PO

Adults, Elderly. Initially, 4 mg as single daily dose or in divided doses twice a day. May increase to 8 mg/day after 12 wks of therapy if fasting glucose level is not adequately controlled.

CONTRAINDICATIONS

Hypersensitivity to rosiglitazone, active hepatic disease, diabetic ketoacidosis, increased serum transaminase levels, including ALT (SGPT) > 2.5 times the normal serum level, type 1 diabetes mellitus, New York Heart Association (NYHA) class III/IV heart failure before initiation. Should not be used in any patient with symptomatic heart failure.

INTERACTIONS

Drug

Amiodarone, paclitaxel, pioglitazone, repaglinide: May have increased levels.

Atazanavir, gemfibrozil, ritonovir, trimethoprim: Levels and effects of rosiglitazone may be increased.

Bile acide sequestrants, carbamazepine, corticosteroids, lutenizing hormone-releasing hormone, phenobarbital, phenytoin, rifampin, rifapentine: Levels and effects of rosiglitazone may be decreased.

Insulin, pregabalin: May exacerbate fluid retention.

Herbal

Hypoglycemic herbs (alfalfa, bilberry, bitter melon, burdock, celery, daminana, fenugreek, garcinia, garlic, ginger, ginseng, symnema, marshmallow, and stinging nettle: May enhance hypoglycemic effects.

Food

Ethanol: Avoid; may cause hypoglycemia.

R

DIAGNOSTIC TEST EFFECTS

May decrease hematocrit and hemoglobin and serum alkaline phosphatase, bilirubin, and AST (SGOT) levels. < 1% of patients experience ALT values that are 3 times the normal level.

SIDE EFFECTS

Frequent (9%)
Upper respiratory tract infection.
Occasional (2%-4%)
Headache, edema, back pain, fatigue, sinusitis, diarrhea.

SERIOUS REACTIONS

- Increase risk of myocardial ischemic events such as angina or MI.
- New onset or exacerbation of congestive heart failure.
- Macular edema (rare).
- Hepatic impairment and jaundice (rare).

PRECAUTIONS & CONSIDERATIONS

Caution is warranted with mild CHF, edema, hepatic impairment, and coronary artery disease or other cardiac disease. May cause or exacerbate heart failure or cause ischemic heart events in some patients (see Contraindications). Monitor for signs and symptoms of heart failure, including excessive, rapid weight gain; dyspnea; or edema. It is unknown whether rosiglitazone crosses the placenta or is distributed in breast milk. Rosiglitazone use is not recommended in pregnant or breastfeeding women. Rosiglitazone use may result in ovulation in some previously anovulatory women, increasing pregnancy risk. Reliable contraception is recommended. Safety and efficacy of rosiglitazone have not been established in children. No age-related precautions have been noted in elderly patients.

Food intake, blood glucose, and hemoglobin A1c should be monitored before and during therapy. Hepatic enzyme levels should also be obtained before beginning rosiglitazone therapy and periodically thereafter. Notify the physician of abdominal or chest pain, dark urine or light stool, hypoglycemic reactions, fever, nausea, palpitations, rash, vomiting, or yellowing of the eyes or skin. Be aware of signs and symptoms of hypoglycemia (anxiety, cool wet skin, diplopia, dizziness, headache, hunger, numbness in mouth, tachycardia, tremors) or hyperglycemia (deep rapid breathing, dim vision, fatigue, nausea, polydipsia, polyphagia, polyuria, vomiting); carry candy, sugar packets, or other sugar supplements for immediate response to hypoglycemia. Consult the physician when glucose demands are altered (such as with fever, heavy physical activity, infection, stress, trauma). Exercise, good personal hygiene (including foot care), not smoking, and weight control are essential parts of therapy.

Storage
Store at room temperature.
Administration
Take rosiglitazone without regard to meals.

Rosuvastatin

row-soo-vah-stah'tin
★ 🍁 Crestor

CATEGORY AND SCHEDULE

Pregnancy Risk Category: X

Classification: Antihyperlipidemics, HMG-CoA reductase inhibitors ("statins")

MECHANISM OF ACTION

An antihyperlipidemic that interferes with cholesterol biosynthesis by inhibiting the conversion of the enzyme HMG-CoA to mevalonate, a precursor to cholesterol. *Therapeutic Effect:* Decreases LDL cholesterol, VLDL, and plasma triglyceride levels, increases HDL concentration.

PHARMACOKINETICS

Protein binding: 88%. Minimal hepatic metabolism. Primarily eliminated in the feces. *Half-life:* 19 h (increased in patients with severe renal dysfunction).

AVAILABILITY

Tablets: 5 mg, 10 mg, 20 mg, 40 mg.

INDICATIONS AND DOSAGES

▸ **Hyperlipidemia, dyslipidemia**

PO

Adults, Elderly. 5-40 mg/day. Consider lower initial dose of 5 mg/day if of Asian descent. Usual starting dosage is 10 mg/day, with adjustments based on lipid levels at intervals of 2-4 wks until desired level is achieved. Doses may be increased by 5-10 mg once daily. Maximum: 40 mg/day.

Children 10 yr and older. 5-20 mg/day.

▸ **Renal impairment (creatinine clearance < 30 mL/min)**

PO

Adults, Elderly. 5 mg/day; do not exceed 10 mg/day.

▸ **Concurrent lopinavir-ritonavir use**

PO

Adults, Elderly. 10 mg/day.

▸ **Concurrent cyclosporine use**

PO

Adults, Elderly. 5 mg/day.

▸ **Concurrent lipid-lowering therapy**

PO

Adults, Elderly. 10 mg/day.

CONTRAINDICATIONS

Active hepatic disease; breastfeeding; pregnancy; unexplained, persistent elevations of serum transaminase levels.

INTERACTIONS

Drug

Antiretroviral protease inhibitors (e.g., fosamprenavir, ritonavir, nelfinavir, darunavir, others), colchicine: Decrease rosuvastatin clearance, increasing levels. Use lowest effective dose of rosuvastatin to avoid myopathy. Do not exceed 10 mg/day.

Cyclosporine, gemfibrozil, niacin: Increase the risk of myopathy. Use lowest effective dose of rosuvastatin to avoid myopathy. Do not exceed 5 mg/day in those taking cyclosporine.

Erythromycin: Reduces the plasma concentration of rosuvastatin slightly; relevance unknown.

Ethinyl estradiol, norgestrel: Increase the plasma concentrations of ethinyl estradiol and norgestrel.

Warfarin: Enhances anticoagulant effect. Monitor INR.

Herbal

None known.

Food

Ethanol: Avoid; may increase hepatic effects.

DIAGNOSTIC TEST EFFECTS

May increase serum creatine phosphokinase and transaminase concentrations. May produce hematuria and proteinuria.

SIDE EFFECTS

Rosuvastatin is generally well tolerated. Side effects are usually mild and transient.

Occasional (3%-9%)

Pharyngitis; headache; diarrhea; dyspepsia, including heartburn and epigastric distress; nausea.

Rare (< 3%)
Myalgia, asthenia or unusual fatigue and weakness, back pain.

SERIOUS REACTIONS

- Lens opacities may occur.
- Hypersensitivity reaction and hepatitis occur rarely.
- Severe myopathy and rhabdomyolysis.
- Rare cases of hepatic impairment, jaundice, or pancreatitis.

PRECAUTIONS & CONSIDERATIONS

Caution is warranted in patients with a history of hepatic disease, hypotension, severe acute infection; severe electrolyte, endocrine, metabolic imbalances or disorders; trauma; and uncontrolled seizures. Caution should also be used in those who consume a substantial amount of alcohol and those who have had recent major surgery. Rosuvastatin use is contraindicated in pregnancy because the suppression of cholesterol biosynthesis may cause fetal toxicity. Rosuvastatin is contraindicated during lactation because it carries the risk of serious adverse reactions in breastfeeding infants. Safety and efficacy of rosuvastatin have not been established in children < 10 yr. No age-related precautions have been noted in elderly patients.

Notify the physician of headache, sore throat, muscle weakness and aches, severe gastric upset, or rash. Pattern of daily bowel activity and stool consistency should be assessed. Serum lipid cholesterol and triglyceride levels and hepatic function should be checked at baseline and periodically during treatment. At initiation of rosuvastatin therapy, a standard cholesterol-lowering diet should be practiced and continued throughout rosuvastatin therapy.

Storage
Store at room temperature.

Administration
Take rosuvastatin without regard to meals and administer at any time of day.

Rufinamide

roo-fin'a-mide
★ Banzel

CATEGORY AND SCHEDULE

Pregnancy Risk Category: C

Classification: Anticonvulsants

MECHANISM OF ACTION

A unique anticonvulsant whose exact mechanism is unknown. Data suggest modulation of sodium channels, primarily through prolongation of the inactive state of the channel. Slows sodium channel recovery and limits sustained repetitive firing of sodium-dependent action potentials. Reduces the QTc interval of the EKG. *Therapeutic Effect:* Reduces seizure frequency.

PHARMACOKINETICS

Well absorbed after PO administration with food. Protein binding: 34%. Extensively metabolized in the liver, primarily to an inactive carboxylic acid metabolite produced via enzymatic hydrolysis. Rufinamide is not metabolized through CYP450; however, it is a weak inhibitor of CYP2E1 and a weak inducer of CYP3A4. Most of the metabolites are excreted in the urine. Some removal by hemodialysis. *Half-life:* 6-10 h.

AVAILABILITY

Tablets: 200 mg, 400 mg.

INDICATIONS AND DOSAGES

▸ Lennox-Gaustaut syndrome

PO

Adults, Elderly. Initially, 400-800 mg/day given in 2 equally divided doses. Increase by 400-800 mg/day every 2 days until the target and maximum daily dose of 3200 mg/day, given in 2 equally divided doses, is reached.

Children 4 yr and older. Initially, approximately 10 mg/kg/day given in 2 equally divided doses. Increase dose by approximately 10-mg/kg increments every other day to a target dose of 45 mg/kg/day or 3200 mg/day, whichever is less, given in 2 equally divided doses.

▸ Dosage in hepatic impairment

Use caution in mild to moderate impairment, do not use if severe impairment.

CONTRAINDICATIONS

History of hypersensitivity to rufinamide, familial short QT syndrome.

INTERACTIONS

Drug

Divalproex or valproic acid: Increases rufinamide levels. Patients stabilized on rufinamide before prescribed valproate should begin valproate therapy at a low dose, and titrate. Similarly, patients on valproate should begin rufinamide at a dose lower than 400 mg, then titrate.

Oral and other hormonal contraceptives: May decrease contraceptive levels and efficacy.

Mexilitene: Additive effect on QTc interval on EKG.

Phenytoin or phenobarbital: May decrease rufinamide levels.

Herbal

None known.

Food

All food: Increases absorption; take with food.

DIAGNOSTIC TEST EFFECTS

Decreased WBC or platelet counts, shortening of QTc interval of EKG.

SIDE EFFECTS

Frequent

Somnolence is most common. Others include headache, fatigue, nausea, gait disturbance, dizziness, ataxia.

Occasional

Diplopia, nasopharyngitis, tremor, nystagmus, blurred vision, and vomiting.

Rare

Flu-like symptoms, bronchitis, psychomotor hyperactivity, aggression, inattention, ear infection, pruritus, rash.

SERIOUS REACTIONS

- Cardiac effects may include bradycardia, heart block, and syncopal episodes (infrequent).
- New-onset convulsions.
- Neutropenia, thrombocytopenia (infrequent).
- Multiorgan hypersensitivity syndrome (rash, urticaria, facial edema, fever, eosinophilia, stuporous state, and severe hepatitis).

PRECAUTIONS & CONSIDERATIONS

Antiepileptic drugs increase the risk of suicidal thoughts or behavior in patients taking these drugs for any indication. Monitor for depression, suicidal thoughts, or any unusual changes in mood or behavior. Caution should be used with other drugs that shorten the QT interval, or in patients with known cardiac arrhythmias. Use caution in hepatic impairment. It is not known if the drug crosses the placenta or is excreted in breast milk. Rufinamide reduces the efficacy of hormonal contraceptives; alternative methods of reliable contraception are advised. Safety and efficacy not established in children under 4 yr of age.

Notify the physician if rash associated with fever occurs, as this could be indicative of a serious hypersensitivity reaction. Baseline vital signs should be assessed. Notify physician if change in heart rate or regularity occurs. Monitor for change in frequency of seizure activity.

Storage

Store at room temperature. Protect from moisture.

Administration

Rufinamide tablets are scored on both sides and can be cut in half for dosing flexibility. Tablets can be administered whole, as half-tablets, or crushed. The tablets should be given with food.

As with all antiepileptic drugs, rufinamide dosage should be gradually tapered to minimize the risk of precipitating seizures, seizure exacerbation, or status epilepticus.

R

Salicylic Acid

sal-i-sill'ik as'id

★ Clearasil, Compound W, Compound W One Step, Dr. Scholl's Clear Away, Dermarest, DuoFilm, Gordofilm, Ionil Plus Shampoo, Keralyt, Mosco Corn and Callus Remover, Neutrogena Acne Wash, Neutrogena On The Spot Acne Patch, Salac, Salactic, Salvax, Stridex, Tinamed, Trans-Ver-Sal

CATEGORY AND SCHEDULE

Pregnancy Risk Category: C
OTC, Rx

Classification: Antipsoriatics, dermatologics, keratolytics, salicylates

MECHANISM OF ACTION

A keratolytic agent that produces desquamation of hyperkeratotic epithelium by dissolution of intercellular cement and causes the cornified tissue to swell, soften, macerate, and desquamate. *Therapeutic Effect:* Decreases acne, psoriasis, and promotes wart removal.

PHARMACOKINETICS

Minimal systemic absorption. Protein binding: 50%-80%. Bound to serum albumin. Metabolized to salicylate glucoronides and salicyluric acid. Excreted in urine.

AVAILABILITY

Salicylic acid is available in a variety of branded products OTC. The following list represents commonly found products:

Products for acne or psoriasis treatment
Cream: 2% (Clearasil).
Gel: 2% (Clearasil), 3% (Keralyt), 6% (Keralyt).
Topical Foam: 2% (Neutrogena Acne Wash, Salac, Clearasil Foaming Cleanser), 6% (Salvax).
Topical Lotion: 2%, 3%, 6% (Dermarest Psoriasis).
Scalp Solution: 3% (Dermarest Scalp).
Shampoos: 2 % (Ionil Plus Therapeutic Shampoo).
Patch: 2% (Neutrogena On The Spot Acne Patch).
Products for wart or callus removal:
Liquid: 17% (Compound W, DuoFilm, Gordoflm, Mosco Corn and Callus Remover, Salactic, Tinamed).
Patch: 15% (Trans-Ver-Sal Plantar Wart Removal Patch, Compound W One Step Pads; Dr Scholl's Clear Away)

INDICATIONS AND DOSAGES

▸ **Acne**

TOPICAL

Adults, Elderly, Children. Apply cream, foam, gel, liquid, pads, patch, or soap 1-3 times/day.

▸ **Callus, corn, wart removal**

TOPICAL

Adults, Elderly, Children. Apply gel, liquid, plaster, or patch to wart 1-2 times/day.

▸ **Dandruff, psoriasis, seborrheic dermatitis**

TOPICAL

Adults, Elderly, Children. Apply cream, ointment, or shampoo 3-4 times/day.

CONTRAINDICATIONS

Children younger than 2 yr, diabetes, impaired circulation, hypersensitivity to salicylic acid or any of its components.

INTERACTIONS

Drug

Ammonium sulfate: May increase plasma salicylate levels.
Corticosteroids: May decrease plasma salicylate levels.
Heparin: May decrease platelet adhesiveness and interfere with hemostasis in heparin-treated patients.
Methotrexate: May increase risk of methotrexate toxicity.
Pyranzinamide: May inhibit pyrazinamide-induced hyperuricemia.
Tolbutamide: May increase risk of hypoglycemia.
Uricosuric agents: May decrease the effects of probenecid, sulfinpyrazone, and phenylbutazone.
Varicella virus vaccine: May increase risk of developing Reye syndrome.

Herbal

Tamarind: May increase risk of salicylate toxicity.

Food

None known.

DIAGNOSTIC TEST EFFECTS

None expected with usual topical use. Elevated salicylate level from topical use occurs rarely.

SIDE EFFECTS

Occasional

Burning, erythema, irritation, pruritus, stinging.

Rare

Dizziness, nausea, vomiting, diarrhea, hypoglycemia.

SERIOUS REACTIONS

• Symptoms of salicylate toxicity include lethargy, hyperpnea, diarrhea, and psychic disturbances.

PRECAUTIONS & CONSIDERATIONS

Salicylic acid should not be applied to areas that are irritated, infected, or reddened; birthmarks; genital or facial warts; or mucous membranes. It is unknown whether salicylic acid crosses the placenta or is distributed in breast milk. Salicylic acid is not recommended for use in children younger than 2 yr. Some products are not approved for use in children. No age-related precautions have been noted in elderly patients. Use of abrasive soaps and cleansers, alcohol-containing preparations, other topical acne preparations, cosmetic soaps that dry skin, and medicated cosmetics should be avoided.

Administration

Use cream, pads, foam, or liquid cleansers for acne by cleansing the skin 1-2 times/day. Massage gently into skin, work into lather, and rinse thoroughly. Pads should be wet with water before using and disposed of after use. Do not flush pads.

Use gel for acne by applying a small amount to clean, dry skin on the face in the morning or evening. If peeling or drying occurs, use every other day. Some products may be used up to 3-4 times/day.

Use patches for acne by washing face, and allow skin to dry for at least 5 min. Apply patch directly over pimple being treated at bedtime. Remove in the morning.

When using shower/bath gels or soap (2%), use once daily in shower or bath. Massage over skin prone to acne. Rinse well.

Use gel or liquid (17%) for callus, corns, or warts by cleaning and drying the area. Apply to each wart and allow to dry. Repeat 1-2 times/day for up to 12 wks as needed.

Use patch (15%) for callus, corns, or warts by applying directly over affected area at bedtime. Leave in place overnight and remove in the morning. Repeat daily for up to 12 wks as needed. May trim patch to fit area.

Use cream for dandruff, psoriasis, or seborrheic dermatitis by cleaning and drying skin. Apply to affected area 3-4 times/day. Apply to clean, dry skin. Some products may remain overnight.

Massage shampoo (1.8%-3%) for dandruff, psoriasis, or seborrheic dermatitis into wet hair. Leave in place for several minutes and rinse thoroughly. Some products may be used 2-3 times/wk.

Salmeterol

sal-me′te-rol

Serevent Diskus (Canada) Serevent Diskhaler, Serevent Diskus

Do not confuse Serevent with Serentil.

CATEGORY AND SCHEDULE

Pregnancy Risk Category: C

Classification: Respiratory agents, bronchodilators, long-acting β-agonists

MECHANISM OF ACTION

An adrenergic agonist that stimulates β_2-adrenergic receptors in the lungs, resulting in relaxation of bronchial smooth muscle. *Therapeutic Effect:* Relieves bronchospasm and reduces airway resistance.

PHARMACOKINETICS

Route	Onset	Peak	Duration
Inhalation	30-48 min	2-4 h	12 h

Low systemic absorption; acts primarily in the lungs. Protein binding: 96%. Metabolized by hydroxylation. Primarily eliminated in feces. *Half-life:* 5.5 h.

AVAILABILITY

Powder for Oral Inhalation (Serevent Diskus): 50 mcg/actuation.

INDICATIONS AND DOSAGES

▸ **Prevention and maintenance treatment of asthma**

INHALATION (DISKUS)

Adults, Elderly, Children 4 yr and older. 1 inhalation (50 mcg) q12h.

▸ **Prevention of exercise-induced bronchospasm**

INHALATION (DISKUS)

Adults, Elderly, Children 4 yr and older. 1 inhalation (50 mcg) at least 30 min before exercise. Not for patients already on 12 h dosing.

▸ **Chronic obstructive pulmonary disease (COPD)**

INHALATION

Adults, Elderly. 1 inhalation q12h.

CONTRAINDICATIONS

History of hypersensitivity to salmeterol; not to be used as monotherapy for asthma; not for acute bronchospasm treatment.

INTERACTIONS

Drug

β-Blockers: May decrease the effects of β-blockers.

Nonselective β-blockers: May decrease the effects of salmeterol.

MAOIs, tricyclic antidepressants: May potentiate cardiovascular effects.

Sympathomimetics: May increase the adverse effects of salmeterol.

Herbal

None known.

Food

None known.

DIAGNOSTIC TEST EFFECTS

May decrease serum potassium level.

SIDE EFFECTS

Frequent (28%)

Headache.

S

Occasional (3%-7%)
Cough, tremor, dizziness, vertigo, throat dryness or irritation, pharyngitis.
Rare (3%)
Palpitations, tachycardia, tremors, nausea, heartburn, GI distress, diarrhea.

SERIOUS REACTIONS

- At high doses, salmeterol may prolong the QT interval, which may precipitate ventricular arrhythmias.
- Hypokalemia and hyperglycemia may occur.

SERIOUS REACTIONS

- Long-acting β_2-agonists may increase the risk of asthma-related deaths.

PRECAUTIONS & CONSIDERATIONS

Caution is warranted in patients with cardiovascular disorders (such as coronary insufficiency, arrhythmias, and hypertension), seizure disorders, and thyrotoxicosis. Salmeterol is not for acute asthma symptoms and may cause paradoxical bronchospasm. It is unknown whether salmeterol is excreted in breast milk. No age-related precautions have been noted in children older than 4 yr. Elderly patients may require a lower dosage because of increased sensitivity to sympathomimetics and increased susceptibility to tachycardia and tremors. Avoid excessive use of caffeinated products, such as chocolate, cocoa, cola, coffee, and tea.

Notify the physician of chest pain or dizziness. Pulse rate and quality; respiratory rate, depth, rhythm, and type; BP; and serum potassium levels should be monitored. Evidence of cyanosis, a blue or a dusky color in light-skinned patients or a gray color in dark-skinned patients, should also be assessed.

NOTE: This drug is not for the relief of acute attacks.
Storage
Keep the drug canister at room temperature because cold decreases the drug's effects.
Administration
Instruct the patient to open and prepare mouthpiece of Diskus device and slide device lever to activate the first dose (see package instructions). Do not advance the lever more than once at any one time as this will release further doses that will be wasted. Holding the Diskus mouthpiece level to, but away from, the mouth, exhale. Then, put the mouthpiece to the lips and breathe in the dose deeply and slowly. Remove the Diskus from the mouth, hold breath for at least 10 sec, and then exhale slowly. Instruct patient to close the Diskus, which will also reset the dose lever for the next scheduled dose. After administration, instruct patient to rinse mouth with water to minimize dry mouth. The Diskus device and mouthpiece should be kept dry; do not wash.

To prevent exercise-induced bronchospasm, administer the dose at least 30-60 min before exercising.

Sapropterin

sap'rop-ter'in
Kuvan

CATEGORY AND SCHEDULE

Pregnancy Risk Category: C

Classification: Metabolic agents, enzyme adjunct

MECHANISM OF ACTION

A synthetic form of BH4, the cofactor for the enzyme phenylalanine hydroxylase (PAH).

PAH hydroxylates phenylalanine (Phe) through an oxidative reaction to form tyrosine. In patients with PKU, PAH activity is absent or deficient. Treatment with BH4 activates the PAH enzyme, improves oxidative metabolism of Phe, and decreases Phe levels. *Therapeutic Effect*: Diminishes manifestations of phenylketonuria. Blood Phe levels decrease within 24 h after a single administration, although maximal effect may take up to a month.

PHARMACOKINETICS

Best absorption occurs when taken with food. Eliminated via normal metabolic processes for BH4. Half-life: Roughly 6.7 h.

AVAILABILITY

Tablets (Kuvan): 100 mg.

INDICATIONS AND DOSAGES

▸ Phenylketonuria

PO

Adults, Children 4 yr and older. Initially, give 10 mg/kg once daily. Adjust as needed. Range 5-20 mg/kg once daily. Blood Phe must be monitored regularly.

CONTRAINDICATIONS

None.

INTERACTIONS

Drug

Levodopa: May increase irritability, overstimulation, or convulsions.

Methotrexate and other folate antagonists: These drugs can decrease BH4 levels by inhibiting the enzyme dihydropteridine reductase (DHPR).

PDE-5 inhibitors (sildenafil, vardenafil, tadalafil): May cause excessive hypotension.

Herbal

None known.

Food

All foods: Food increases drug absorption for maximal effectiveness.

DIAGNOSTIC TEST EFFECTS

Expected to reduce phenylalanine (PHE) levels.

SIDE EFFECTS

Frequent (≥ 4%)

Headache, diarrhea, abdominal pain, upper respiratory tract infection, pharyngolaryngeal pain, vomiting, and nausea.

Occasional (3%)

Rhinorrhea, nasal congestion, dizziness.

Rare (≤ 2%)

Increased catabolism, leukopenia, potential for rash or allergy.

SERIOUS REACTIONS

- Overstimulation and other neurologic changes.
- Seizures occur rarely.
- Bleeding or gastritis.

PRECAUTIONS & CONSIDERATIONS

Some patients may not respond adequately to treatment. Response to treatment cannot be predetermined by laboratory testing (e.g., genetic testing) and can only be determined by a therapeutic trial of the drug. Caution is warranted with hepatic or renal impairment, history of seizures or conditions that may lower the seizure threshold. It is unknown whether the drug crosses the placenta or is excreted in breast milk. The safety and efficacy have not been established in children less than 4 yr of age. No age-related precautions are known for other age groups.

Growth, blood pressure, adherence to low phenylalanine diet, and compliance should be assessed regularly during treatment. Monitor

S

Phe levels at baseline, after 1 wk, and periodically for up to 1 mo, and during continued treatment. Monitor for signs of allergy or intolerance. Symptoms including sore tongue, convulsions, problems eating or swallowing, fever, or infection need to be reported immediately.

Storage

Store at room temperature. Keep tightly closed and protect from moisture until time of use.

Administration

To be used in conjunction with a Phe-restricted diet. Take orally with food to increase absorption. Dissolve tablets in 4-8 oz (120-240 mL) of water or apple juice and take within 15 min. Full dissolution may not occur. Patient may swallow any small tablet fragments that do not dissolve. If fragments remain in dose cup, rinse and have patient swallow remnants to ensure entire dose taken.

Saquinavir

sa-kwin′a-veer

Invirase

Do not confuse saquinavir with Sinequan.

CATEGORY AND SCHEDULE

Pregnancy Risk Category: B

Classification: Antiretrovirals, protease inhibitors

MECHANISM OF ACTION

Inhibits HIV protease, rendering the enzyme incapable of processing the polyprotein precursors needed to generate functional proteins in HIV-infected cells. *Therapeutic Effect:* Intereferes with HIV replication, slowing the progression of HIV infection.

PHARMACOKINETICS

Poorly absorbed after PO administration (absorption increased with high-calorie and high-fat meals). Protein binding: 98%. Metabolized in the liver to inactive metabolite. Eliminated primarily in feces. Unknown whether removed by hemodialysis. *Half-life:* 13 h.

AVAILABILITY

Capsules: 200 mg.
Tablet: 500 mg.

INDICATIONS AND DOSAGES

▸ HIV infection in combination with other antiretrovirals

PO

Adults, Elderly. 1000 mg twice a day within 2 h after a full meal. Should be given only in combination with ritonavir 100 mg twice a day.

▸ Dosage for severe hepatic impairment

The use of saquinavir "boosted" with ritonavir is contraindicated. Use saquinavir without ritonavir.

▸ Dosage adjustments when given in combination therapy

Lopinavir/ritonavir. 1000 mg 2 times a day.

CONTRAINDICATIONS

Significant hypersensitivity to saquinavir, ritonavir, severe hepatic impairment or use with rifampin due to the risk of severe hepatotoxicity; congential or documented QT prolongation, refractory hypokalemia or hypomagnesemia, those treated with QT-prolonging medications; complete AV block without pacemaker or those at high risk of complete AV block. Coadministration with CYP3A substrates for which increased plasma levels may result in serious of life-threatening reactions (see Drug Interactions for contraindicated drugs).

INTERACTIONS

Drug

NOTE: Please see detailed manufacturer's information for management of additional drug interactions other than those listed. In some cases, dosage adjustment for the agent or choice of an alternate agent is recommended.

Alfuzosin, cisapride, pimozide, trazodone: Increases levels of these drugs and risk of cardiovascular adverse outcomes. Contraindicated.

Antiarrhythmics, (e.g., class 1A and class III agents, amiodarone, flecainide, propafenone, quinidine), certain macrolides, phenothiazines, certain atypical neuroleptics, and other QT-prolonging drugs: Increases levels and risk of proarrhythmia. Contraindicated.

Carbamazepine, dexamethasone, phenobarbital, phenytoin: May reduce saquinavir plasma concentration.

Colchicine: Increased risk of colchicine toxicity.

Cyclosporine, fluticasone, other immunosuppressants: May increase immunosuppressant blood concentrations; monitor closely.

Digoxin, calcium channel blockers, ibutilide, sotalol: Increased heart med concentrations. Monitor.

Ergot derivatives (e.g., dihydroergotamine, ergonovine, ergotamine, methylergonovine): Increases levels and risk of ergot toxicity. Contraindicated

Lovastatin, simvastatin: Increases levels and risk of myopathy and rhabdomyolysis. Contraindicated.

Omeprazole: Increases saquinavir concentrations. Avoid.

Oral midazolam, triazolam: Ritonavir increases levels causing benzodiazepine toxicity and respiratory depression risk.

Phosphodiesterase-5 inhibitors (e.g., sildenafil, vardenafil, tadalafil): Increases PDE-5 inhibitor blood levels and risk of hypotension. Contraindicated for use with sildenafil for pulmonary HTN.

Rifampin: Decreases antiretroviral effective concentrations and increases risk of hepatotoxicity. Contraindicated.

Warfarin: May increase warfarin levels. Monitor INR.

Herbal

Garlic, St. John's wort: May decrease the plasma concentration and effect of saquinavir.

Food

High-fat meal: Maximally increases saquinavir's bioavailability.

Grapefruit juice: May increase saquinavir plasma concentration.

DIAGNOSTIC TEST EFFECTS

May alter serum CK levels, elevate liver function test results and blood glucose levels.

SIDE EFFECTS

Frequent (≥ 5%)

Appetite loss, headaches, malaise, diarrhea, nausea, vomiting; usually improve over time.

Occasional

Abdominal discomfort and pain; photosensitivity; stomatitis; accumulation of fat in waist, abdomen, or back of neck.

Rare

Confusion, ataxia, asthenia, rash, hyperglycemia.

SERIOUS REACTIONS

- Pancreatitis.
- Stevens-Johnson syndrome and other serious skin rashes.
- Hepatitis/liver failure.
- Reports of bleeding in patients with hemophilia.
- New-onset diabetes mellitus.

PRECAUTIONS & CONSIDERATIONS

Caution is warranted in patients with diabetes mellitus or liver impairment. Breastfeeding is not recommended in this population because of the possibility of HIV transmission. Be aware that the safety and efficacy of saquinavir have not been established in children. There is no information on the effects of this drug's use in elderly patients, so it should be used with caution. Avoid exposure to sunlight. Saquinavir is not a cure for HIV infection, nor does it reduce the risk of transmission to others; illnesses associated with advanced HIV infection may occur.

Check the baseline laboratory and diagnostic test results, especially liver function test results, if ordered, before beginning saquinavir therapy and at periodic intervals during therapy. Closely monitor for signs and symptoms of GI discomfort.

Assess the patient's pattern of daily bowel activity and stool consistency. Inspect the mouth for signs of mucosal ulceration. Notify the physician if nausea, numbness, persistent abdominal pain, tingling, or vomiting occurs.

Storage
Store at room temperature.

Administration
Give within 2 h after a full meal. Keep in mind that if saquinavir is taken on an empty stomach, the drug might not produce antiviral activity. When used with ritonavir, saquinavir should be administered at the same time. Continue therapy for the full length of treatment and evenly space drug doses around the clock.

Sargramostim (Granulocyte Macrophage Colony-Stimulating Factor, GM-CSF)

sar-gram'oh-stim

★🍁 Leukine

Do not confuse Leukine with Leukeran.

CATEGORY AND SCHEDULE

Pregnancy Risk Category: C

Classification: Hematopoietic agents, recombinant DNA origin, colony-stimulating factors

MECHANISM OF ACTION

A colony-stimulating factor that stimulates proliferation and differentiation of hematopoietic cells to activate mature granulocytes and macrophages. *Therapeutic Effect:* Assists bone marrow in making new WBCs and increases their chemotactic, antifungal, and antiparasitic activity. Increases cytoneoplastic cells and activates neutrophils to inhibit tumor cell growth.

PHARMACOKINETICS

Effect	Onset	Peak	Duration
Increase WBCs	7-14 days	NA	1 wk

Detected in serum within 15 min after SC administration. *Half-life:* IV, 1 h; SC, 2.7 h.

AVAILABILITY

Injection Solution: 500 mcg/mL.
Injection Powder for Reconstitution: 250 mcg.

INDICATIONS AND DOSAGES

▸ **Myeloid recovery following bone marrow transplant (BMT)**

IV INFUSION

Adults, Elderly. Usual parenteral dosage: 250 mcg/m²/day (as 2-h infusion) beginning 2-4 h after autologous bone marrow infusion and not < 24 h after the last dose of chemotherapy or radiation treatment. Discontinue if blast cells appear or underlying disease progresses.

▸ **Bone marrow transplant failure, engraftment delay**

IV INFUSION

Adults, Elderly. 250 mcg/m²/day for 14 days. Infuse over 2 h. May repeat after 7 days off therapy if engraftment has not occurred with 500 mcg/m²/day for 14 days. Then, if needed, a third course of 500 mcg/m²/day for 14 days may be tried after 7 days off treatment. If still no improvement, unlikely to have benefit from further dosing.

▸ **Stem cell transplant**

IV, SC

Adults. 250 mcg/m²/day.

▸ **Mobilization of peripheral blood progenitor cells (PBPCs)**

IV, SC

Adults. 250 mcg/m²/day IV over 24 h or SC once daily continued through the period of PBPCs, according to protocol.

▸ **Postperipheral blood progenitor cell transplantation**

IV, SC

Adults. 250 mcg/m²/day IV over 24 h or SC once daily, continuing until ANC > 1500 cells/mm³ for 3 consecutive days.

▸ **Neutrophil recovery following chemotherapy in acute myelogenic leukemia (AML)**

IV

Adults. 250 mcg/m²/day IV over 4 h starting 4 days after completion of induction chemotherapy, continuing until ANC > 1500 cells/mm³ for 3 consecutive days. Maximum: 42 days.

OFF-LABEL USES

Treatment of AIDS-related neutropenia; chronic, severe neutropenia; drug-induced neutropenia; myelodysplastic syndrome.

CONTRAINDICATIONS

Within the 24 h before or after chemotherapy or radiotherapy; excessive leukemic myeloid blasts in bone marrow or peripheral blood (> 10%); known hypersensitivity to GM-CSF, yeast-derived products, or components of drug.

INTERACTIONS

Drug

Lithium, steroids: May increase the effects of sargramostim.

Herbal

None known.

Food

None known.

DIAGNOSTIC TEST EFFECTS

Increased WBC (expected). May increase serum bilirubin, creatinine, and hepatic enzyme levels.

IV INCOMPATIBILITIES

Acyclovir, amphotericin B complex (Abelcet, AmBisome, Amphotec), ampicillin, ampicillin-sulbactam (Unasyn), ganciclovir, haloperidol, hydrocortisone (Solu-Cortef), hydromorphone (Dilaudid), hydroxyzine, imipenem-cilastatin (Primaxin), lorazepam (Ativan), methylprednisolone (Solu-Medrol), morphine, sodium bicarbonate, tobramycin.

IV COMPATIBILITIES

Calcium gluconate, dopamine, heparin, magnesium, potassium chloride.

SIDE EFFECTS

Frequent

GI disturbances, including nausea, diarrhea, vomiting, stomatitis, anorexia, and abdominal pain; arthralgia or myalgia; headache; malaise; rash; pruritus.

Occasional

Peripheral edema, hypertension, weight gain, dyspnea, asthenia, fever, leukocytosis, capillary leak syndrome (such as fluid retention, irritation at local injection site, and peripheral edema).

Rare

Rapid or irregular heartbeat, thrombophlebitis.

SERIOUS REACTIONS

- Pleural or pericardial effusion occurs rarely after infusion.
- Rare anaphylactoid reactions.

PRECAUTIONS & CONSIDERATIONS

Caution is warranted with congestive heart failure (CHF), hypoxia, impaired hepatic or renal function, preexisting cardiac disease, preexisting fluid retention, and pulmonary infiltrates. It is unknown whether sargramostim crosses the placenta or is distributed in breast milk. Safety and efficacy of this drug have not been established in children. Neonates should not receive the drug reconstituted with preservatives such as benzyl alcohol, which may cause a gasping syndrome. No age-related precautions have been noted in elderly patients. Avoid situations that might place risk for contracting an infectious disease such as influenza.

Notify the physician of chest pain, chills, fever, palpitations, or dyspnea. Follow-up blood tests should be maintained to evaluate the effectiveness of drug therapy. CBC, pulmonary, liver, and kidney function test results, platelet count, vital signs, and weight should be monitored.

Storage

Refrigerate powder, reconstituted solution, and diluted solution for injection. Do not shake. Do not use past expiration date. Reconstituted solution is normally clear and colorless. Use reconstituted solution within 6 h; discard unused portion. Use one dose/vial; do not reenter vial.

Administration

The subcutaneous (SC) route is preferred, as it allows for increased exposure of sargramostim to hematopoietic cells. When given SC, rotate injection sites.

For IV use, to reconstitute, add 1 mL preservative-free sterile water for injection to 250-mcg vial. Direct sterile water for injection to side of vial, and gently swirl contents to avoid foaming. Do not shake or vigorously agitate. After reconstitution, further dilute with 0.9% NaCl. If final concentration is < 10 mcg/mL, add 1 mg albumin per mL 0.9% NaCl to provide a final albumin concentration of 0.1%.

! Albumin is added before sargramostim to prevent drug adsorption to components of drug delivery system. Give each single dose over 2, 4, or 24 h, as directed by physician. Consider administration with analgesics and antipyretics.

Expect to discontinue or decrease dose by 50% if a rapid increase in blood counts occurs.

Saxagliptin

sax'a-glip'tin

Onglyza

Do not confuse with sitagliptin.

CATEGORY AND SCHEDULE

Pregnancy Risk Category: B

Classification: Antidiabetic agents, dipeptidyl peptidase-4 (DPP-4) inhibitor

MECHANISM OF ACTION

A "gliptin," or dipeptidyl peptidase-4 inhibitor (DPP-4), that decreases the breakdown of glucagon-like peptide-1 (GLP-1), resulting in more prompt and appropriate secretion of insulin and suppression of glucagon in response to blood sugar increases following meals or snacks, improving glucose tolerance. *Therapeutic Effect:* Inhibits DPP-4 enzyme activity for a 24-h period. Lowers blood glucose concentration and also HbA1C over time.

PHARMACOKINETICS

May administer with or without food. Protein binding is negligible. Median time to maximal plasma concentration occurs 2 h (saxagliptin) and 4 h (active metabolite) after dosing. Liver metabolism is mediated by CYP3A4/5. The major metabolite is also a DPP-4 inhibitor, which is 50% as potent as saxagliptin. Strong CYP3A4/5 inhibitors and inducers will alter the pharmacokinetics of both. Renal (60%) and fecal (22%) excretion. Removed by hemodialysis. *Half-life:* 2.5 h (saxagliptin); 3 h (active metabolite).

AVAILABILITY

Tablets: 2.5 mg, 5 mg.

INDICATIONS AND DOSAGES

▸ **Type 2 diabetes mellitus**

PO

Adults, Elderly. 2.5 mg or 5 mg once daily. May be given with sulfonylureas, metformin, or a thiazolidinedione.

▸ **Dosage in renal impairment (CrCl < 50 mL/min) or taking strong CYP3A4 inhibitors**

Recommend no more than 2.5 mg once daily. If on hemodialysis, give the daily dose after dialysis.

CONTRAINDICATIONS

Hypersensitivity to saxagliptin. Not for type 1 diabetes mellitus or diabetic ketoacidosis. Not studied with insulin.

INTERACTIONS

Drug

β-Blockers: May mask signs of hypoglycemia.
Strong CYP3A4/5 inhibitors (e.g., ketoconazole, protease inhibitors for HIV, clarithromycin, itraconazole, nefazodone, and telithromycin): Increase saxagliptin levels. Lower dose recommended.
Rifampin, other CYP3A4 inducers: May reduce saxagliptin levels.
Corticosteroids: May increase blood sugar.
Sulfonylureas: May increase risk of hypoglycemia; lower sulfonylurea dose may be needed.
Warfarin: May increase the effects of warfarin, resulting in increased INR. Monitor INR closely.

Herbal

Alfalfa, aloe, bilberry, bitter melon, burdock, celery, damiana, fenugreek, garcinia, garlic, ginger, ginseng (American), gymnema, marshmallow, stinging nettle: May enhance hypoglycemic effects.
St. John's wort: May reduce saxagliptin levels.

Food

Grapefruit juice: May increase saxagliptin levels. Do not significantly alter intake.

DIAGNOSTIC TEST EFFECTS

Lowers blood sugar. May reduce lymphocyte count.

SIDE EFFECTS

Frequent

Headache, nasopharyngitis, hypoglycemia.

Occasional
Decreased appetite, nausea, abdominal pain.
Rare
Hypoglycemia. Peripheral edema when used with thiazolidinedione.

SERIOUS REACTIONS

- Overdose may produce severe hypoglycemia.
- Rare reports of serious allergic reactions, including angioedema and exfoliative skin rashes, such as Stevens-Johnson syndrome.

PRECAUTIONS & CONSIDERATIONS

There have been no clinical studies establishing conclusive evidence of macrovascular risk reduction with saxagliptin. Caution is warranted in patients with impaired renal function or who are taking potentially interacting medications. Be alert to conditions that alter blood glucose requirements or dietary intake, such as fever, increased activity, stress, or a surgical procedure. There are no data regarding saxagliptin use during pregnancy. It is unknown whether the drug is distributed in breast milk; caution is recommended. Safety and efficacy of saxagliptin have not been established in children. Hypoglycemia may be difficult to recognize in elderly patients.

Food intake and blood glucose should be monitored before and during therapy. Be aware of signs and symptoms of hypoglycemia (anxiety, cool wet skin, diplopia, dizziness, headache, hunger, numbness in the mouth, tachycardia, tremors) or hyperglycemia (deep rapid breathing, dim vision, fatigue, nausea, polydipsia, polyphagia, polyuria, vomiting); carry candy, sugar packets, or other sugar supplements for immediate response to hypoglycemia.

Consult the physician when glucose demands are altered (such as with fever, heavy physical activity, infection, stress, trauma). Exercise, good personal hygiene (including foot care), not smoking, and weight control are essential parts of therapy.
Storage
Store tablets at room temperature.
Administration
May take orally without regard to food or the timing of meals or snacks.

Scopolamine

skoe-pol'a-meen
★ Isopto Hyoscine, Maldemar, Trans-Derm Scop, Scopace

CATEGORY AND SCHEDULE

Pregnancy Risk Category: C

Classification: Anticholinergics, antiemetics/antivertigo, cycloplegics, gastrointestinals, mydriatics, ophthalmics, preanesthetics, sedatives/hypnotics

MECHANISM OF ACTION

An anticholinergic that reduces excitability of labyrinthine receptors, depressing conduction in the vestibular cerebellar pathway. *Therapeutic Effect:* Prevents motion-induced nausea and vomiting.

AVAILABILITY

Tablet: 0.4 mg.
Transdermal System: 1.5 mg.
Ophthalmic Solution: 0.25%.
Injection: 0.4 mg/mL.

INDICATIONS AND DOSAGES

▸ **Postoperative nausea or vomiting**
TRANSDERMAL
Adults, Elderly. 1 patch no sooner than 1 h before surgery and removed 24 h after surgery.

▸ **Motion sickness**
Adults, Elderly. 1 patch at least 4 h (ideally 12 h) before exposure, reapplying every 3 days as needed.
▸ **Excessive motility of the GI tract**
PO
Adults. 0.4-0.8 mg every 8 h.
▸ **Aspiration prophylaxis, sedation induction prior to intubation or for bradycardia during surgery**
SUBCUTANEOUS/IV/IM
Adults. 0.3-0.6 mg as a single dose.
▸ **For cycloplegia or mydriasis induction during eye examination**
OPHTHALMIC
Adults. Instill 1-2 drops in eye(s) 1 h before refraction.
Children. Instill 1 drop in eye(s) 1 h before refraction.
▸ **For iritis or uveitis**
OPHTHALMIC
Adults. Instill 1-2 drops in affected eye(s) up to 4 times daily.
Children. Instill 1 drop in affected eye(s) 1, 2, or 3 times daily.

CONTRAINDICATIONS

Hypersensitivity to scopolamine or other belladonna alkaloids. Angle-closure glaucoma, GI or genitourinary obstruction, myasthenia gravis, paralytic ileus, tachycardia, thyrotoxicosis.

INTERACTIONS

Drug
Antihistamines, tricyclic antidepressants: May increase the anticholinergic effects of scopolamine.
Central nervous system (CNS) depressants: May increase CNS depression.
Pramlintide: May enhance GI effects of scopolamine.
Herbal
None known.
Food
Ethanol: May increase CNS depression.

DIAGNOSTIC TEST EFFECTS

May interfere with gastric secretion test.

SIDE EFFECTS

Frequent (> 15%)
Dry mouth, somnolence, blurred vision.
Rare (1%-5%)
Dizziness, restlessness, hallucinations, confusion, difficulty urinating, rash.

SERIOUS REACTIONS

- Rare hypersensitivity reactions.
- Idiosyncratic psychiatric reactions, such as confusion, agitation, hallucinations, or delirium.
- Overdose: lethargy, coma, confusion, hallucinations, convulsion, vision changes, dry flushed skin, decreased bowel sounds, urinary retention, tachycardia, hypertension, and supraventricular arrhythmias.

PRECAUTIONS & CONSIDERATIONS

Caution is warranted in patients with cardiac disease, renal or hepatic impairment, glaucoma, bladder obstruction, prostatic hypertrophy, or risk for GI ileus, psychoses, and seizures. Tasks that require mental alertness or motor skills should be avoided. Children and the elderly are more susceptible to the anticholinergic effects. Scopolamine is not used in pregnancy except for obstetric delivery by C-section.

Scopolamine is excreted in breast milk.

Patients who participate in underwater sports should be aware of the potentially disorienting effects.

Storage
Store all products at room temperature. Keep patches in protective foil until time of use.

S

Administration
Wash hands. Apply transdermal patch to the hairless area behind one ear. Replace the patch after 72 h or if it becomes dislodged. Wash hands after applying the patch. Use only one patch at a time and do not cut it.

If patient will undergo MRI procedure, remove patch prior to the MRI to avoid burns.

For oral use, it is most common to administer scopolamine on an empty stomach, 30 min before meals and at bedtime.

The injection may be administered subcutaneously, intramuscularly, or intravenously. For IV use, dilute injection with an equal volume of sterile water for injection. Inject slowly IV over 2-3 min.

For ophthalmic use, instill the dosage of eyedrops, then apply gentle pressure to the lacrimal sac for 1-2 min to limit systemic absorption. To avoid contamination, do not touch the dropper tip to any surface.

Secobarbital

see-koe-bar′bi-tal

★ Seconal

CATEGORY AND SCHEDULE

Pregnancy Risk Category: D
Controlled Substance Schedule: II

Classification: Barbiturates, preanesthetics, sedatives/hypnotics

MECHANISM OF ACTION

A barbiturate that depresses the central nervous system (CNS) activity by binding to barbiturate site at the GABA-receptor complex enhancing GABA activity and depressing reticular activity system. *Therapeutic Effect:* Produces hypnotic effect as a result of central nervous system (CNS) depression.

PHARMACOKINETICS

Well absorbed from the GI tract. Protein binding: 52%-57%. Crosses blood-brain barrier. Widely distributed. Metabolized in liver by microsomal enzyme system to inactive and active metabolites. Excreted primarily in urine. Not removed by hemodialysis. *Half-life:* 15-40 h.

AVAILABILITY

Capsules: 100 mg (Seconal sodium).

INDICATIONS AND DOSAGES

▸ **Insomnia**

PO

Adults. 100 mg at bedtime, range 100-200 mg.

▸ **Preoperative sedation**

PO

Adults. 100-300 mg 1-2 h before procedure.

Children. 2-6 mg/kg 1-2 h before procedure. Maximum: 100 mg/dose.

CONTRAINDICATIONS

History of manifest or latent porphyria, marked liver dysfunction, marked respiratory disease in which dyspnea or obstruction is evident, and hypersensitivity to secobarbital or barbiturates.

INTERACTIONS

Drug

Alcohol, CNS depressants: May increase the CNS depressant effects.

Anticoagulants: May decrease anticoagulant activity.

Corticosteroids: May increase metabolism of corticosteroids.

Doxycycline: May shorten the half-life of doxycycline.
Griseofulvin: May decrease levels of griseofulvin by interfering with its metabolism.
Estradiol, estrone, progesterone, other steroidal hormones: May decrease the effect of these hormones by increasing their metabolism.
MAOIs: May prolong the effects of secobarbital by inhibiting its metabolism.
Phenytoin, sodium valproate, valproic acid: May decrease the metabolism and increase the concentration and risk of toxicity with secobarbital.
Herbal
St. John's wort, kava kava, gotu kola, valerian: May increase CNS depressant effects.
Food
None known.

DIAGNOSTIC TEST EFFECTS

None known.

SIDE EFFECTS

Frequent
Somnolence.
Occasional
Agitation, confusion, hyperkinesia, ataxia, CNS depression, nightmares, nervousness, psychiatric disturbance, hallucinations, insomnia, anxiety, dizziness, abnormality in thinking, hypoventilation, apnea, bradycardia, hypotension, syncope, nausea, vomiting, constipation, headache.
Rare
Hypersensitivity reactions, fever, liver damage, megaloblastic anemia.

SERIOUS REACTIONS

- Agranulocytosis, megaloblastic anemia, apnea, hypoventilation, bradycardia, hypotension, syncope, hepatic damage, and Stevens-Johnson syndrome rarely occur.
- Tolerance and physical dependence may occur with repeated use.

PRECAUTIONS & CONSIDERATIONS

Secobarbital crosses the placenta and is distributed in breast milk. Its use may cause paradoxical excitement in children. Elderly patients taking secobarbital may exhibit confusion, excitement, and mental depression. Alcohol consumption and caffeine intake should be limited while taking secobarbital. Avoid tasks that require mental alertness or motor skills because this drug may cause dizziness and drowsiness.
Storage
Store at controlled room temperature, tightly closed.
Administration
Give secobarbital without regard to meals.

As a hypnotic, administer at bedtime. Preoperatively, given 1 to 2 h before surgery.

Selegiline

seh-leg′ill-ene
Eldepryl, Emsam, Zelapar
Apo-Selegiline
Do not confuse selegiline with Stelazine, or Eldepryl with enalapril.

CATEGORY AND SCHEDULE

Pregnancy Risk Category: C

Classification: Antiparkinsonian agents, dopaminergics

MECHANISM OF ACTION

An antiparkinsonian agent that irreversibly inhibits the activity of monoamine oxidase type B, the enzyme that breaks down dopamine, thereby increasing dopaminergic action. *Therapeutic Effect:* Relieves signs and symptoms of Parkinson disease.

PHARMACOKINETICS

Rapidly absorbed from the GI tract. Crosses the blood-brain barrier. Metabolized in the liver to the active metabolites. Excreted primarily in urine. *Half-life:* 17 h (amphetamine), 20 h (methamphetamine).

AVAILABILITY

Capsules: 5 mg.
Tablets: 5 mg.
Tablets, Oral Disintegrating (Zelapar): 1.25 mg.
Transdermal System (Emsam): 6 mg, 9 mg, 12 mg per 24 h patch.

INDICATIONS AND DOSAGES

▸ **Adjunctive treatment for parkinsonism**

PO

Adults. 10 mg/day in divided doses, such as 5 mg at breakfast and lunch, given concomitantly with each dose of carbidopa and levodopa.

Elderly. Initially, 5 mg in the morning. May increase up to 10 mg/day.

ORAL DISINTEGRATING TABLETS

Adults. Initially, 1.25 mg daily for 6 wks. May increase to 2.5 mg daily.

▸ **Depression**

TRANSDERMAL

Adults. Initially 6 mg/24 h applied once a day. May increase by 3 mg/day every 2 wks. Maximum of 12 mg/24 h.

Elderly. 6 mg/24 h.

CONTRAINDICATIONS

Hypersensitivity to selegiline. Pheochromocytoma. Concomitant use of dextromethorphan, meperidine, methadone, propoxyphene, tramadol, other MAOIs. Other drugs that should be avoided include carbamazepine and oxcarbazepine, sympathomimetic amines, general anesthesia, cocaine, sympathomimetic vasoconstrictors, SSRIs, SNRIs, and tricyclic antidepressants. Hypertensive crises caused by the ingestion of foods containing high amounts of tyramine are possible at higher daily doses of selegiline.

INTERACTIONS

Drug

Amphetamine, ephedrine, sympathomimetics, methylphenidate, cocaine: Increased pressor effects.
Buspirone: May increase BP.
Caffeine-containing medications: May increase the risk of cardiac arrhythmias and hypertension.
Carbamazepine, cyclobenzaprine, maprotiline, other MAOIs: May precipitate hypertensive crisis, convulsions, hyperpyretic crisis.
Fluoxetine, other SSRIs, SNRIs, trazodone, tricyclic antidepressants: May cause serotonin syndrome.
Insulin, oral antidiabetics: May increase the effects of these drugs.
Meperidine, other opioid analgesics: May produce diaphoresis, immediate excitation, rigidity, and severe hypertension or hypotension, sometimes leading to severe respiratory distress, vascular collapse, seizures, coma, and death.

Herbal

Trytophan: May cause sudden, severe hypertension.
St. John's wort: May cause serotonin syndrome.

Food

Tyramine-rich foods: May produce a severe hypertensive reaction.

DIAGNOSTIC TEST EFFECTS

None known.

SIDE EFFECTS

Frequent (4%-10%)
Nausea, dizziness, light-headedness, syncope, abdominal discomfort.
Occasional (2%-3%)
Confusion, hallucinations, dry mouth, vivid dreams, dyskinesia.
Rare (1%)
Headache, myalgia, anxiety, diarrhea, insomnia.

SERIOUS REACTIONS

- Symptoms of overdose may vary from CNS depression, characterized by sedation, apnea, cardiovascular collapse, and death, to severe paradoxical reactions, such as hallucinations, tremor, and seizures.
- Other serious effects may include involuntary movements, impaired motor coordination, loss of balance, blepharospasm, facial grimaces, feeling of heaviness in the lower extremities, depression, nightmares, delusions, overstimulation, sleep disturbance, and anger.

PRECAUTIONS & CONSIDERATIONS

Caution is warranted in patients with cardiac arrhythmias, dementia, history of peptic ulcer disease, profound tremor, psychosis, and tardive dyskinesia. It is unknown whether selegiline crosses the placenta or is distributed in breast milk. The safety and efficacy of selegiline have not been established in children. Antidepressants increase the risk of suicidal thinking and behavior in children, adolescents, and young adults (aged 18-24 yr) with major depressive disorder and other psychiatric disorders. Monitor any patient closely for suicidal thoughts, mood changes, or unusual behaviors. Selegiline is not approved for treating bipolar depression. No age-related precautions have been noted in elderly patients. Be aware that tyramine-rich foods, such as wine and aged cheese, should be avoided to prevent a hypertensive reaction.

Dizziness, drowsiness, light-headedness, and dry mouth are common side effects of the drug but will diminish or disappear with continued treatment. Alcohol and tasks that require mental alertness or motor skills should be avoided. Change positions slowly to prevent orthostatic hypotension. Notify the physician if agitation, headache, lethargy, or confusion occurs. Baseline vital signs should be assessed. Relief of symptoms, such as improvement of mask-like facial expression, muscular rigidity, shuffling gait, and resting tremors of the hands and head, should be assessed during treatment.

Administration
Keep in mind that therapy should begin with the lowest dosage, then increase gradually over 3-4 wks. With oral disintegrating tablets, administer in the morning before breakfast allowing tablet to dissolve. Food or drink should be avoided 5 min before and after administration.

Transdermal patches should be applied to clean, dry, hairless area of skin on upper torso, thigh, or arm at the same time every day. Application area should not be exposed to heat. Application sites should be rotated. Hands should be washed before and after patch application.

Senna

sen'na

★ Black Draught, Fletchers Laxative Liquid, Ex-Lax, Ex-Lax Maximum Strength, Perdiem, SennaGen, SenaLax, Senexon, Senokot, Senosol, Senosol-X

CATEGORY AND SCHEDULE

Pregnancy Risk Category: C
OTC

Classification: Laxatives, stimulant, anthraquinone derivative

MECHANISM OF ACTION

A GI stimulant that has a direct effect on intestinal smooth musculature by stimulating the intramural nerve plexi. *Therapeutic Effect:* Increases peristalsis and promotes laxative effect.

PHARMACOKINETICS

Route	Onset	Peak	Duration
PO	6-12 h	NA	NA
Rectal	0.5-2 h	NA	NA

Minimal absorption after oral administration. Hydrolyzed to active form by enzymes of colonic flora. Absorbed drug metabolized in the liver. Eliminated in feces via biliary system.

AVAILABILITY

(Dosage expressed in sennosides)
Granules (Senokot): 15 mg/tsp.
Liquid: 8.8 mg/5 mL
Tablets: 8.6 mg, 10 mg, 15 mg, 17 mg, 25 mg.

INDICATIONS AND DOSAGES

▸ Constipation

PO (TABLETS)

Adults, Elderly. 2 tablets at bedtime. Maximum: 4 tablets (34.4 mg sennosides) twice a day.
Children >27 kg. 1 tablet at bedtime. Maximum: 17.2 mg sennosides twice a day.

SYRUP

Adults, Elderly. 10-15 mL at bedtime. Maximum: 15 mL twice a day.
Children aged 5-15 yr. 5-10 mL at bedtime. Maximum: 10 mL twice a day.
Children aged 1-5 yr. 2.5-5 mL at bedtime. Maximum: 1 tsp twice a day.
Infants 1-12 mo > 27 kg. 1.25-2.5 mL at bedtime. Maximum: 2.5 mL twice daily.

PO (GRANULES)

Adults, Elderly. 1 tsp at bedtime. Maximum: 2 tsp twice a day.
Children weighing > 27 kg. Half (½) teaspoon at bedtime up to 1 tsp twice/day.

▸ Bowel evacuation

PO

Adults, Elderly. 1-2 tablets or 1-2 tsp 12-14 hr before examination. 75 mL between 2:00 and 4:00 PM on day before procedure.

CONTRAINDICATIONS

Abdominal pain, appendicitis, intestinal obstruction, nausea, vomiting.

INTERACTIONS

Drug

Oral medications: May decrease transit time of concurrently administered oral medications.

Herbal

None known.

Food

None known.

DIAGNOSTIC TEST EFFECTS

May increase blood glucose level. May decrease serum potassium level.

S

SIDE EFFECTS

Frequent

Pink-red, red-violet, red-brown, or yellow-brown discoloration of urine.

Occasional

Some degree of abdominal discomfort, nausea, mild cramps, griping, faintness.

SERIOUS REACTIONS

- Long-term use may result in laxative dependence, chronic constipation, and loss of normal bowel function.
- Prolonged use or overdose may result in electrolyte and metabolic disturbances (such as hypokalemia, hypocalcemia, and metabolic acidosis or alkalosis), vomiting, muscle weakness, persistent diarrhea, malabsorption, and weight loss.

PRECAUTIONS & CONSIDERATIONS

Senna should be used cautiously for extended periods (> 1 wk). It is unknown whether senna is distributed in breast milk. Not a first-line agent for constipation in pregnancy; stimulant laxatives may induce premature labor. Safety and efficacy of senna have not been established in children younger than 2 yr. No age-related precautions have been noted in elderly patients, but this population should be monitored for signs and symptoms of dehydration and electrolyte loss.

Pattern of daily bowel activity and stool consistency and serum electrolyte levels should be monitored. Adequate fluid intake should be maintained.

Storage

Store at room temperature. Keep granules tightly closed. Protect chocolate chews from high temperatures.

Administration

Take senna on an empty stomach for faster results. Drink at least 6-8 glasses of water a day to aid in stool softening. Avoid giving within 1 h of other oral medications because drug absorption is decreased. To promote defecation, increase fluid intake, exercise, and eat a high-fiber diet. Oral senna generally produces a laxative effect in 6-12 h, but it can take 24 h.

Sertaconazole

sir-tah-con′ah-zole

★ Ertaczo

CATEGORY AND SCHEDULE

Pregnancy Risk Category: C

Classification: Antifungals, topical, dermatologics

MECHANISM OF ACTION

An imidazole derivative that inhibits synthesis of ergosterol, a vital component of fungal cell formation. *Therapeutic Effect:* Damages the fungal cell membrane, altering its function.

AVAILABILITY

Cream: 2%.

INDICATIONS AND DOSAGES

▸ **Tinea pedis**

TOPICAL

Adults, Elderly, Children 12 yr and older. Apply to affected area twice a day for 4 wks.

CONTRAINDICATIONS

Known sensitivity to sertaconazole nitrate or any of its components or to other imidazoles.

INTERACTIONS

Drug
None known.
Herbal
None known.
Food
None known.

DIAGNOSTIC TEST EFFECTS

None known.

SIDE EFFECTS

Rare (2%)
Burning, tenderness, erythema, dryness, pruritus, hyperpigmentation, and contact dermatitis at application site.

SERIOUS REACTIONS

- None known.

PRECAUTIONS & CONSIDERATIONS

It is unknown whether sertaconazole is excreted in breast milk. No age-related precautions have been noted. Skin should be assessed for dermatitis, dryness, erythema, hyperpigmentation, burning sensation, or pruritus.
Storage
Store at room temperature.
Administration
Rub gently into affected, surrounding areas. Avoid contact with eyes, nose, and mouth. Keep the affected area clean and dry. Continue sertaconazole treatment for the full length of therapy.

S

Sertraline

sir'trall-een
Zoloft Apo-Sertraline, Novo-Sertraline, PMS-Sertraline, Zoloft
Do not confuse sertraline with Serentil.

CATEGORY AND SCHEDULE

Pregnancy Risk Category: C

Classification: Antidepressants, serotonin selective reuptake inhibitors

MECHANISM OF ACTION

An antidepressant, anxiolytic, and obsessive-compulsive disorder agent that blocks the reuptake of the neurotransmitter serotonin at central nervous system (CNS) neuronal presynaptic membranes, increasing its availability at postsynaptic receptor sites. *Therapeutic Effect:* Relieves depression, reduces obsessive-compulsive behavior, decreases anxiety.

PHARMACOKINETICS

Incompletely and slowly absorbed from the GI tract; food increases absorption. Protein binding: 98%. Widely distributed. Undergoes extensive first-pass metabolism in the liver to active compound. Excreted in urine and feces. Not removed by hemodialysis. *Half-life:* 26 h.

AVAILABILITY

Oral Concentrate: 20 mg/mL.
Tablets: 25 mg, 50 mg, 100 mg.

INDICATIONS AND DOSAGES

▸ **Depression, obsessive-compulsive disorder (OCD)**
PO
Adults, Children aged 13-17 yr. Initially, 50 mg/day with morning

or evening meal. May increase by 50 mg/day at 7-day intervals.
Elderly, Children 6-12 yr. Initially, 25 mg/day. May increase by 25-50 mg/day at 7-day intervals. Maximum: 200 mg/day.

▸ **Panic disorder, posttraumatic stress disorder, social anxiety disorder**

PO

Adults, Elderly. Initially, 25 mg/day. May increase by 50 mg/day at 7-day intervals. Range: 50-200 mg/day. Maximum: 200 mg/day.

▸ **Premenstrual dysphoric disorder**

PO

Adults. Initially, 50 mg/day either every day or during the luteal phase of menstrual cycle. May increase up to 100-150 mg/day in 50-mg increments.

OFF-LABEL USES

Hot flashes, cholestatic pruritus.

CONTRAINDICATIONS

Hypersensitivity; use within 14 days of MAOIs; concurrent use of pimozide. The oral concentrate is contraindicated with disulfiram due to the alcohol content of the concentrate.

INTERACTIONS

Drug

CY2D6 substrates (benzodiazepines, phenothiazines, β-blockers, TCAs, bupropion): Sertraline may increase blood levels and risk of side effects.

Disulfiram, metronidazole: May interact with alcohol in oral concentrate. Avoid.

Highly protein-bound medications (such as digoxin and warfarin): May increase the blood concentration and risk of toxicity of these drugs.

MAOIs, amphetamines, busipirone, meperidine, nefazodone, sumatriptan, ritonavir, tramadol, venlafaxine: May cause serotonin syndrome, hypertensive crisis, hyperpyrexia, seizures, and serotonin syndrome (marked by diaphoresis, diarrhea, fever, mental changes, restlessness, and shivering). MAOIs contraindicated.

NSAIDS, aspirin, other drugs affecting coagulation: May increase bleeding risk.

Pimozide: Increased pimozide levels may increase risk of serious ventricular arrhythmias. Contraindicated.

Thioridazine, mesoridazine: May increase risk of serious ventricular arrhythmias.

Herbal

Gotu kola, kava kava, St. John's wort, valerian: May increase CNS depression.

Food

Ethanol: May increase CNS depression.

DIAGNOSTIC TEST EFFECTS

May increase serum total cholesterol, triglyceride, AST (SGOT), and ALT (SGPT) levels. May decrease serum uric acid level.

SIDE EFFECTS

Frequent (12%-26%)

Headache, nausea, diarrhea, insomnia, somnolence, dizziness, fatigue, rash, dry mouth.

Occasional (4%-6%)

Anxiety, nervousness, agitation, tremor, dyspepsia, diaphoresis, vomiting, constipation, abnormal ejaculation, visual disturbances, altered taste.

Rare (< 3%)

Flatulence, urinary frequency, paresthesia, hot flashes, chills.

SERIOUS REACTIONS

• Overdose (serotonin syndrome) symptoms may include nausea, vomiting, sedation, dizziness,

S

sweating, facial flushing, mental status changes, myoclonia, restlessness, shivering, and hypertension.

- SIADH and hyponatremia have been reported rarely, most commonly in elderly patients.
- Bleeding from platelet dysfunction.

PRECAUTIONS & CONSIDERATIONS

Caution is warranted in patients with cardiac disease, hepatic impairment, seizure disorders, those who have had a recent myocardial infarction (MI), and in those with suicidal tendency. Sertraline is not recommended in pregnancy due to a potential for teratogenic and nonteratogenic adverse effects and neonatal withdrawal. It is unknown whether sertraline is distributed in breast milk. Notify the physician if pregnancy occurs. Sertraline is not approved for use in children with major depressive disorder but is approved for the treatment of OCD in children aged 6 yr and older. Antidepressants increase the risk of suicidal thinking and behavior in children, adolescents, and young adults (18-24 yr) with major depressive disorder and other psychiatric disorders. All patients should be monitored for suicidal thoughts, mood changes, or unusual behaviors. Sertraline is not approved for treating bipolar depression. Lower initial sertraline dosages are recommended for elderly patients, although no age-related precautions have been noted in this age group.

Dizziness may occur, so alcohol and tasks that require mental alertness or motor skills should be avoided. Notify the physician if fatigue, headache, sexual dysfunction, or tremor occurs. CBC and liver and renal function tests should be performed before and periodically during therapy, especially with long-term use.

Storage

Store at room temperature.

Administration

! Make sure at least 14 days elapse between the use of MAOIs and sertraline.

Take sertraline with food or milk if GI distress occurs. Oral solution must be diluted immediately before use with 4 oz of *only* water, orange juice, ginger ale, lemon/lime soda, or lemonade. Solution may appear hazy. Once diluted the oral solution must be taken immediately.

Sevelamer

seh-vel′a-mer

Renagel, Renvela

Do not confuse Renagel with Reglan or Regonol.

CATEGORY AND SCHEDULE

Pregnancy Risk Category: C

Classification: Metabolics

MECHANISM OF ACTION

An antihyperphosphatemia agent that binds with dietary phosphorus in the GI tract, thus allowing phosphorus to be eliminated through the normal digestive process and decreasing the serum phosphorus level. *Therapeutic Effect:* Decreases incidence of hypercalcemic episodes in patients receiving calcium acetate treatment. Decreases serum phosphate in patients with end-stage renal disease without the risk of increasing serum calcium levels.

PHARMACOKINETICS

Not absorbed systemically. Unknown whether removed by hemodialysis. Excreted in feces.

S

AVAILABILITY

Tablets: 400 mg, 800 mg.
Powder for Oral Suspension: 0.8 g, 2.4 g.

INDICATIONS AND DOSAGES

▸ Hyperphosphatemia

PO

Adults, Elderly. 800-1600 mg with each meal, depending on severity of hyperphosphatemia. Maintenance dose is based on goal of lowering serum phosphate to < 5.5 mg/dL.

CONTRAINDICATIONS

Hypersensitivity to any ingredients, bowel obstruction, hypophosphatemia.

INTERACTIONS

Drug

Ciprofloxacin, antiarrhythmics, antiseizure medications, thyroid horomones, mycophenolate: Binding may result in decreased absorption.Administer these drugs at least 1 h before or 3 h after sevelamer.

Herbal and Food

None known.

DIAGNOSTIC TEST EFFECTS

None known.

SIDE EFFECTS

Frequent (11%-20%)

Infection, pain, hypotension, diarrhea, dyspepsia, nausea, vomiting.

Occasional (1%-10%)

Headache, constipation, hypertension, thrombosis, increased cough.

SERIOUS REACTIONS

• Fecal impaction, ileus (rare), bowel obstruction or perforation (rare) have been reported.

PRECAUTIONS & CONSIDERATIONS

Caution is warranted in patients with dysphagia, severe GI tract motility disorders, swallowing disorders, and in those who have undergone major GI tract surgery. Sevelamer is not distributed in breast milk. The safety and efficacy of sevelamer have not been established in children. No age-related precautions have been noted in elderly patients.

Serum bicarbonate, chloride, calcium, and phosphorus levels should be monitored. Notify the physician of diarrhea, signs of hypotension (such as light-headedness), nausea or vomiting, or a persistent headache.

Storage

Store at room temperature; protect from moisture.

Administration

Take sevelamer with food. Do not break, crush, or chew tablets because the contents expand in water. Take other medications at least 1 h before or 3 h after sevelamer.

For the oral suspension powder, each 0.8 g powder should be mixed in 30 mL of water. Each 2.4 g should be mixed in 60 mL of water. Stir vigorously right before administration, as the powder does not dissolve.

Sildenafil

sill-den'a-fill

★ 🍁 Revatio, Viagra

Do not confuse Viagra with Vaniqa.

CATEGORY AND SCHEDULE

Pregnancy Risk Category: B

Classification: Erectile dysfunction agents, pulmonary vasodilators, phosphodiesterase-5 enzyme inhibitors

MECHANISM OF ACTION
An agent that inhibits phosphodiesterase type 5, the enzyme responsible for degrading cyclic guanosine monophosphate (cGMP) in the corpus cavernosum of the penis or the smooth muscle of pulmonary vasculature, resulting in smooth muscle relaxation and increased blood flow. *Therapeutic Effect:* Facilitates an erection in ED. In PAH, results in vasodilation in pulmonary vasculature.

AVAILABILITY
Tablets (Viagra): 25 mg, 50 mg, 100 mg.
Tablets (Revatio): 20 mg.
Injection Solution (Revatio): 10 mg/12.5 mL.

INDICATIONS AND DOSAGES
▸ **Erectile dysfunction**
PO
Adults. 50 mg (30 min-4 h before sexual activity). Range: 25-100 mg. Maximum dosing frequency is once daily.
Elderly (> 65 yr). Consider starting dose of 25 mg.
▸ **Pulmonary arterial hypertension (PAH)**
PO (REVATIO)
Adults, Elderly. 20 mg 3 times daily, administered 4-6 h apart.
IV (REVATIO)
Adults, Elderly. 10 mg 3 times daily, administered 4-6 h apart.

OFF-LABEL USES
Treatment of sexual dysfunction associated with the use of selective serotonin reuptake inhibitors (SSRIs), Raynaud phenomenon, PAH in children.

CONTRAINDICATIONS
Concurrent use of nitrates in any form, known hypersensitivity; use in PAH contraindicated with certain protease inhibitors for HIV.

INTERACTIONS
Drug
α-Blockers, nitrates: Potentiates the hypotensive effects of nitrates. Sildenafil contraindicated in patients receiving nitrates.
Azole antifungals, cimetidine, erythromycin, itraconazole, ketoconazole, protease inhibitors, other CYP3A4 inhibitors: May increase the effects of sildenafil. Select drugs (e.g., ritonavir) are not recommended for use with sildenafil.
Herbal
St. John's wort: May decrease sildenafil levels.
Food
Grapefruit juice: May increase sildenafil levels.
High-fat meals: Delay drug's maximum effectiveness by 1 h.

DIAGNOSTIC TEST EFFECTS
None known.

SIDE EFFECTS
Frequent
Headache (16%), flushing (10%).
Occasional (3%-7%)
Dyspepsia, nasal congestion, UTI, abnormal vision, diarrhea.
Rare (2%)
Dizziness, rash.

SERIOUS REACTIONS
- Severe or sudden hypotension.
- Prolonged erections (lasting over 4 h) and priapism (painful erections lasting > 6 h) occur rarely.
- Decreased eyesight or loss of sight.
- Sudden decrease or loss of hearing.
- Heart attack, stroke, irregular heartbeats.

PRECAUTIONS & CONSIDERATIONS
Caution is warranted with an anatomic deformity of the penis; cardiac, hepatic, or renal impairment; and conditions that increase the risk of priapism, including leukemia,

multiple myeloma, and sickle cell anemia. Seek treatment immediately if an erection lasts longer than 4 h.

Storage

Store at room temperature.

Administration

Sildenafil is usually taken 1 h before sexual activity, but it may be taken anywhere from 4 h to 30 min beforehand.

When sildenafil (Revatio) is used for PAH, administer doses at least 4-6 h apart. High-fat meals may affect the drug's absorption rate and effectiveness.

Given IV as an IV bolus injection.

Silodosin

sil'oh-doe'sin

Rapaflo

Do not confuse Rapaflo with Rapamune.

CATEGORY AND SCHEDULE

Pregnancy Risk Category: B (Not indicated for use in women)

Classification:

Urinary tract agents, antiadrenergics, specific peripheral α-blockers

MECHANISM OF ACTION

A selective antagonist of postsynaptic adrenergic α-1 receptors of subtype 1-A, which are located in the human prostate, bladder base, bladder neck, prostatic capsule, and prostatic urethra. *Therapeutic Effect:* Causes smooth muscle in these tissues to relax, resulting in an improvement in urine flow and a reduction in BPH symptoms.

PHARMACOKINETICS

Well absorbed when taken with a meal, and widely distributed. Protein binding: 94%-99%. Extensive metabolism via glucuronidation, alcohol and aldehyde dehydrogenase, and CYP3A4. Metabolites excreted in the urine and feces. Unknown whether it is removed by hemodialysis. *Half-life:* Mean 13.3 h (increased in renal impairment).

AVAILABILITY

Hard Gelatin Capsules: 4 mg, 8 mg.

INDICATIONS AND DOSAGES

▸ **Benign prostatic hyperplasia**

PO

Adults, Elderly. 8 mg once a day with the same meal each day.

▸ **Dosage for renal impairment**

CrCl 30-50 mL/min: limit dosage to 4 mg once daily.

CrCl < 30 mL/min: contraindicated.

▸ **Severe hepatic impairment**

Contraindicated with severe hepatic impairment (Child-Pugh score ≥10).

OFF-LABEL USES

Adjunct to medical management of kidney stones, to assist passage.

CONTRAINDICATIONS

History of sensitivity to silodosin. Severe renal or hepatic impairment. Concomitant administration with strong CYP3A4 inhibitors (e.g., ketoconazole, clarithromycin, itraconazole, ritonavir).

INTERACTIONS

Drug

Antihypertensive agents, nitrates: Increased potential for hypotension.

CYP3A4 inducers: May reduce silodosin levels, decrease effect.

CYP3A4 inhibitors: May increase silodosin levels and increase side effects such as hypotension risk; potent inhibitors (e.g., itraconazole, ketoconazole, ritonavir) are contraindicated.

Cyclosporine and other strong Pg-inhibitors: Increase silodosin exposure. Avoid.

S

Other α-blockers, such as alfuzosin, doxazosin, prazosin, tamsulosin, and terazosin: May increase the α-blockade effects of both drugs.
Phosphodiesterase (PDE5) Inhibitors (e.g., sildenafil, vardenafil, tadalafil): May result in symptomatic hypotension; use caution.
Herbal
None known.
Food
Grapefruit juice: May increase silodosin exposure. Avoid increases in intake.

DIAGNOSTIC TEST EFFECTS

None expected.

SIDE EFFECTS

Frequent (≥ 3%)
Dizziness, retrograde ejaculation.
Occasional (1%-3%)
Diarrhea, headache, orthostatic hypotension.
Rare (< 1%)
Nasal congestion, pharyngitis, rhinitis, abdominal pain, asthenia, nausea, vertigo, impotence.

SERIOUS REACTIONS

- Severe orthostatic hypotension with syncope may be preceded by tachycardia and usually occurs with increased exposure.
- Rare reports of jaundice, impaired hepatic function, and increased transaminases.
- α-blockers associated with intraoperative floppy iris syndrome during cataract surgery.
- Priapism (very rare).
- Toxic skin eruptions (very rare).

PRECAUTIONS & CONSIDERATIONS

Caution is warranted in patients with renal impairment or moderate hepatic impairment, and in those taking antihypertensive therapy. Silodosin is not indicated for use in women or children. No age-related precautions have been noted in elderly patients.

Dizziness and light-headedness may occur. Tasks that require mental alertness or motor skills should be avoided until response to the drug is established. Caution should be used when getting up from a sitting or lying position. BP and renal function should be monitored. Fully evaluate prostate symptoms to rule out carcinoma. If a patient will have eye surgery, inform the ophthalmologist of the use of this drug.
Storage
Store capsules at room temperature; protect from light and moisture.
Administration
Take silodosin with the same meal each day. Do not crush or chew capsules.

Silver Sulfadiazine

sil′ver sul-fa-dye′a-zeen
★ SSD, SSD AF, Silvadene, Thermazene 🍁 Dermazin, Flamazine

CATEGORY AND SCHEDULE

Pregnancy Risk Category: B (D, if near-term pregnancy)

Classification: Anti-infectives, topical, dermatologics

MECHANISM OF ACTION

An anti-infective that acts on cell wall and cell membrane. Releases silver slowly in concentrations selectively toxic to bacteria. *Therapeutic Effect:* Produces bactericidal effect.

PHARMACOKINETICS

Variably absorbed. Significant systemic absorption may occur if applied to extensive burns. Absorbed medication excreted unchanged in urine. *Half-life:* 10 h (half-life increased with impaired renal function).

AVAILABILITY

Cream: 1% (Silvadene, SSD, SSD AF).

INDICATIONS AND DOSAGES

▸ **Burns**

TOPICAL

Adults, Elderly, Children. Apply topically to a thickness of approximately 1.66 mu (1/16 inch) 2 times daily.

OFF-LABEL USES

Treatment of minor bacterial skin infection, dermal ulcer.

CONTRAINDICATIONS

Hypersensitivity to silver sulfadiazine, sulfonamides, or any component of the formulation; do not use in infants < 2 mo of age.

INTERACTIONS

Drug

Collagenase, papain, sutilains: May be inactivated.

Herbal and Food

None known.

DIAGNOSTIC TEST EFFECTS

None known.

SIDE EFFECTS

Side effects characteristic of all sulfonamides may occur when systemically absorbed such as with extensive burn areas, anorexia, nausea, vomiting, headache, diarrhea, dizziness, photosensitivity, joint pain.

Frequent

Burning feeling at treatment site.

Occasional

Brown-gray skin discoloration, rash, itching.

Rare

Increased sensitivity of skin to sunlight.

SERIOUS REACTIONS

- If significant systemic absorption occurs, serious reactions such as hemolytic anemia, hypoglycemia, diuresis, peripheral neuropathy, Stevens-Johnson syndrome, agranulocytosis, disseminated lupus erythematosus, anaphylaxis, hepatitis, and toxic nephrosis may occur.
- Fungal superinfections may occur.
- Interstitial nephritis occurs rarely.

PRECAUTIONS & CONSIDERATIONS

Caution is warranted in patients with impaired renal or hepatic function or G6PD deficiency. Be aware that silver sulfadiazine is not recommended during pregnancy unless burn area is > 20% of body surface. Be aware that it is unknown whether silver sulfadiazine is distributed in breast milk. There is a risk of kernicterus in neonates; do not use in infants younger than 2 mo. No age-related precautions have been noted in children or elderly patients.

Skin should be assessed for burns, surrounding areas for pain, burning, itching, and rash. Antihistamines may provide relief. Silver sulfadiazine therapy should continue unless reactions are severe.

Storage

Store at room temperature. Cream will occasionally darken either in the jar or after application to the skin. This color change results from a light-catalyzed reaction, which is a common characteristic of all silver salts. The antimicrobial activity of the product is not substantially diminished because the color change reaction involves such a small amount of the active drug.

Administration

Apply topical preparation to cleansed and debrided burns using sterile glove. Keep burn areas covered with silver sulfadiazine cream at all times. Reapply to areas where removed by activity. Dressings may be ordered on individual basis.

Simethicone

si-meth'i-kone

★ Alka-Seltzer Gas Relief, Gas-X, Genasym, Infants' Mylicon, Mylanta Gas, Phazyme 🍁 Gax-X, Infacol, Ovol, Pediacol, Phazyme

CATEGORY AND SCHEDULE

Pregnancy Risk Category: C
OTC

Classification: Siloxane polymer, antiflatulent

MECHANISM OF ACTION

An antiflatulent that changes surface tension of gas bubbles, allowing easier elimination of gas. *Therapeutic Effect:* Drug dispersal, prevents formation of gas pockets in the GI tract.

PHARMACOKINETICS

Does not appear to be absorbed from GI tract. Excreted unchanged in feces.

AVAILABILITY

Oral Drops (Infants' Mylicon): 40 mg/0.6 mL.
Softgel (Alka-Seltzer Gas Relief, Gas-X, Mylanta Gas): 125 mg.
Softgel (Phazyme): 180 mg.
Tablets (Chewable [Gas-X, Mylanta Gas]): 80 mg, 125 mg.

INDICATIONS AND DOSAGES

▸ **Antiflatulent**

PO

Adults, Elderly, Children 12 yr and older. 40-360 mg after meals and at bedtime. Maximum: 500 mg/day.
Children aged 2-11 yr. 40 mg 4 times a day.
Children younger than 2 yr. 20 mg 4 times a day.

OFF-LABEL USES

Adjunct to bowel radiography and gastroscopy.

CONTRAINDICATIONS

None known.

INTERACTIONS

Drug

None known.

Herbal

None known.

Food

None known.

DIAGNOSTIC TEST EFFECTS

None known.

SIDE EFFECTS

None known.

SERIOUS REACTIONS

• None known.

PRECAUTIONS & CONSIDERATIONS

It is unknown whether simethicone crosses the placenta or is distributed in breast milk. Simethicone may be used safely in children and elderly patients. Before simethicone administration, the abdomen should be assessed for signs of tenderness, rigidity, and the presence of bowel sounds. Do not give if bowel obstruction or perforation is suspected. Avoid carbonated beverages during simethicone therapy.

Storage

Store at room temperature; protect chewable tablets from moisture.

Administration

Take simethicone after meals and at bedtime, as needed. Chew tablets thoroughly before swallowing. Shake suspension well before using.

Simvastatin

sim'va-sta-tin

Zocor Apo-Simvastatin, Zocor

Do not confuse Zocor with Cozaar.

CATEGORY AND SCHEDULE

Pregnancy Risk Category: X

Classification:

Antihyperlipidemics, HMG-CoA reductase inhibitors, "statins"

MECHANISM OF ACTION

An HMG-CoA reductase inhibitor that interferes with cholesterol biosynthesis by inhibiting the conversion of the enzyme HMG-CoA to mevalonate. *Therapeutic Effect:* Decreases serum LDL, cholesterol, VLDL, and plasma triglyceride levels; slightly increases serum HDL concentration.

PHARMACOKINETICS

Well absorbed from the GI tract. Protein binding: 95%. Undergoes extensive first-pass metabolism. Hydrolyzed to active metabolite. Eliminated primarily in feces. Unknown whether removed by hemodialysis. *Half-life:* < 3 h.

AVAILABILITY

Tablets: 5 mg, 10 mg, 20 mg, 40 mg, 80 mg.

INDICATIONS AND DOSAGES

▸ **To decrease elevated total and LDL cholesterol in hypercholesterolemia (types IIa and IIb), lower triglyceride levels, and increase HDL levels; to reduce the risk of death and prevent myocardial infarction (MI) in patients with heart disease and elevated cholesterol level; to reduce risk of revascularization procedures; to decrease risk of stroke or transient ischemic attack; to prevent cardiovascular events**

PO

Adults. Initially, 10-40 mg/day in evening. Dosage adjusted at 4-wk intervals. Range: 5-80 mg/day. Maximum: 80 mg/day.

Elderly. Initially, 10 mg/day in evening. May increase by 5-10 mg/day q4wk. Range: 5-80 mg/day. Maximum: 80 mg/day.

Children aged 10-17 yr. 10 mg/day in evening. Range: 10-40 mg/day. Maximum: 40 mg/day.

▸ **Dose adjustments for adults taking select drugs concurrently**

With gemfibrozil, danazol, or cyclosporine. Initially, 5 mg once daily in the evening. Maximum: 10 mg/day.

With amiodarone or verapamil. 5-20 mg PO once daily in the evening. Maximum: 20 mg/day.

With diltiazem. 5-40 mg PO once daily in the evening. Maximum: 40 mg/day.

▸ **Dosage in renal impairment (adults)**

If CrCl < 20 mL/min: Initiate with 5 mg/day and monitor closely.

CONTRAINDICATIONS

Hypersensitivity, active hepatic disease or unexplained, persistent elevations of liver function test results, pregnancy, breastfeeding. Also, avoid use with strong CYP3A4 inhibitors, such as itraconazole, ketoconazole, erythromycin, clarithromycin, telithromycin, HIV protease inhibitors (e.g., ritonavir), nefazodone.

INTERACTIONS

Drug

Amiodarone, verapamil: May increase simvastatin levels, limit dose to 20 mg/day.

Cyclosporine, danazol, gemfibrozil: May increase simvastatin levels, limit dose to 10 mg/day.

Erythromycin, immunosuppressants, niacin: Increases the risk of acute renal failure and rhabdomyolysis.

Itraconazole, ketoconazole: May increase simvastatin blood concentration and cause muscle inflammation, myalgia, or weakness.

Warfarin: May increase anticoagulant effects.

Herbal

St. John's wort: May reduce simvastatin levels.

Food

Grapefruit juice: Avoid large changes in intake, as can increase simvastatin levels.

DIAGNOSTIC TEST EFFECTS

May increase serum CK and serum transaminase concentrations.

SIDE EFFECTS

Simvastatin is generally well tolerated. Side effects are usually mild and transient.

Occasional (2%-3%)

Headache, abdominal pain or cramps, constipation, upper respiratory tract infection.

Rare (< 2%)

Diarrhea, flatulence, asthenia (loss of strength and energy), nausea, or vomiting.

SERIOUS REACTIONS

- Lens opacities may occur.
- Hypersensitivity reaction occurs rarely.
- Severe myopathy and rhabdomyolysis.
- Rare cases of hepatic impairment, jaundice, or pancreatitis.

PRECAUTIONS & CONSIDERATIONS

Caution is warranted in patients with hepatic disease; severe electrolyte, endocrine, or metabolic disorders; and who consume substantial amounts of alcohol or who are of Asian descent. Withholding or discontinuing simvastatin may be necessary when the person is at risk for renal failure secondary to rhabdomyolysis. Simvastatin use is contraindicated in pregnancy because suppression of cholesterol biosynthesis may cause fetal toxicity. Simvastatin is contraindicated in lactation because there is a risk of serious adverse reactions in breastfeeding infants. Safety and efficacy of simvastatin have not been established in children less than 10 yr of age. No age-related precautions have been noted in elderly patients.

Notify the physician of headache or muscle weakness and aches. Pattern of daily bowel activity and stool consistency should be assessed. Serum lipid cholesterol and triglyceride levels and hepatic function should be checked at baseline and periodically during treatment. Before beginning therapy, a standard cholesterol-lowering diet for a minimum of 3-6 mo should be practiced and then continued throughout simvastatin therapy.

Storage

Store at room temperature.

Administration

Take simvastatin without regard to meals and administer in the evening.

Sirolimus

sir-oh-leem′us

Rapamune

CATEGORY AND SCHEDULE

Pregnancy Risk Category: C

Classification:

Immunosuppressives

MECHANISM OF ACTION

An immunosuppressant that inhibits T-lymphocyte proliferation induced by stimulation of cell-surface receptors, mitogens, alloantigens, and lymphokines. Prevents activation of the enzyme target of rapamycin, a key regulatory kinase in cell-cycle progression. *Therapeutic Effect:* Inhibits proliferation of T and B cells, essential components of the immune response; prevents organ transplant rejection.

AVAILABILITY

Oral Solution: 1 mg/mL.
Tablets: 1 mg, 2 mg.

INDICATIONS AND DOSAGES

NOTE: Dosing is by body weight and depends on whether patient is low-moderate risk or high risk.

▸ **Prevention of organ transplant rejection**

PO

Adults and Children ≥ 13 yr and ≥ 40 kg. Loading dose: 6 mg. Maintenance: 2 mg/day.

Children 13 yr and older weighing < 40 kg. Loading dose: 3 mg/m^2. Maintenance: 1 mg/m^2/day.

▸ **Dosage in hepatic impairment**

Expect reductions (33%-50%) in dose in accordance with degree of impairment.

CONTRAINDICATIONS

Hypersensitivity to sirolimus, malignancy.

INTERACTIONS

Drug

Strong CYP3A4 inhibitors (e.g., cyclosporine, diltiazem, ketoconazole, protease inhibitors, quinidine, verapamil): May increase the blood concentration and risk of toxicity of sirolimus.

Strong CYP3A4 inducers (e.g., carbamazepine, phenobarbital, phenytoin, rifampin): May decrease the blood concentration and effects of sirolimus.

Herbal

St. John's wort: Avoid, as may lower sirolimus concentrations and increase risk of rejection.

Food

Grapefruit, grapefruit juice: May decrease the metabolism of sirolimus. Avoid.

DIAGNOSTIC TEST EFFECTS

May decrease blood hemoglobin level, hematocrit, and platelet count. May increase serum cholesterol, creatinine, and triglyceride levels.

Following cyclosporine withdrawal, target sirolimus trough concentrations are 16-24 ng/mL the first year after

S

transplantation. Then, the target troughs should be 12-20 ng/mL.

SIDE EFFECTS

Occasional

Hypercholesterolemia, hyperlipidemia, hypertension, rash; with high doses (5 mg/day): anemia, arthralgia, diarrhea, hypokalemia, and thrombocytopenia.

SERIOUS REACTIONS

- Angioedema.
- Sirolimus increases the risk of infection and may be associated with the development of lymphoma.

PRECAUTIONS & CONSIDERATIONS

Caution is warranted in patients with chickenpox, herpes zoster, hepatic impairment, and infection. Also, avoid coming in contact with people with colds or other infections. Liver function tests, CBCs, and sirolimus levels should be monitored.

Storage

Store tablets at room temperature, tightly closed and protected from light. The oral solution should be refrigerated; do not freeze and protect from light. Once opened, a bottle is stable for only 30 days. After oral solution is drawn into oral syringe, may keep a maximum of 24 h at room temperature or under refrigeration.

Administration

Take the drug at the same time each day. Notify the physician if a dose is missed.

Administer consistently with or without food. Administer 4 h after cyclosporine. Do not administer with grapefruit juice.

Do not crush, chew, or split sirolimus tablets.

Sirolimus oral solution may develop a slight haze when refrigerated. Allow the product to stand at room temperature and shake gently until the haze disappears. The presence of a haze does not affect the product quality. Assemble the bottle with the adapter for the oral syringe as directed. Always keep the bottle upright. Use the supplied amber oral syringe to withdraw the dosage. Empty into a glass or plastic container holding at least 2 oz (60 mL) of water or orange juice. Do not dilute in any other juice, especially not grapefruit juice. Use only plastic or glass containers. Stir vigorously for 1 min and drink at once. Refill the container with 120 mL of water or orange juice, stir vigorously, and drink at once. Be careful not to get the solution on the skin, as it is irritating.

Sitagliptin

si'ta-glip-tin

Januvia

Do not confuse sitagliptin with saxagliptin, or Januvia with Jantoven or Janumet.

CATEGORY AND SCHEDULE

Pregnancy Risk Category: B

Classification:

Antidiabetic agents, dipeptidyl peptidase-4 (DPP-4) inhibitor

MECHANISM OF ACTION

A "gliptin," or dipeptidyl peptidase-4 inhibitor (DPP-4), that decreases the breakdown of glucagon-like peptide-1 (GLP-1), resulting in more prompt and appropriate secretion of insulin and suppression of glucagon in response to blood sugar increases following meals or snacks, improving glucose tolerance. *Therapeutic Effect:* Inhibits DPP-4 enzyme activity for a 24-h period. Lowers blood glucose concentration and also HbA1C over time; works well with other antidiabetic medications.

PHARMACOKINETICS

Rapidly and well absorbed. May administer with or without food. Protein binding: Low, 38%. Median time to maximal plasma concentration occurs 2 h after dosing. Roughly 79% of sitagliptin is excreted unchanged in the urine with metabolism being a minor pathway. Metabolites are excreted in the urine and feces. *Half-life:* 12.4 h (increased in renal insufficiency).

AVAILABILITY

Tablets: 25 mg, 50 mg, 100 mg.

INDICATIONS AND DOSAGES

▸ **Type 2 diabetes mellitus**

PO

Adults, Elderly. 100 mg once daily. May be given with sulfonylureas or insulin.

▸ **Dosage in renal impairment**

CrCl 30-49 mL/min: 50 mg once daily.

CrCl < 30 mL/min: 25 mg once daily. If on hemodialysis, give the daily dose after dialysis.

CONTRAINDICATIONS

Hypersensitivity to sitagliptin. Not for type 1 diabetes mellitus or diabetic ketoacidosis. Not studied or recommended in patients with a history of pancreatitis.

INTERACTIONS

Drug

β-Blockers: May mask signs of hypoglycemia.

Digoxin: Slight increase in digoxin exposure; monitor clinically.

Corticosteroids: May increase blood sugar.

Sulfonylureas or insulin: May increase risk of hypoglycemia; lower sulfonylurea or insulin dose may be needed.

Herbal

Alfalfa, aloe, bilberry, bitter melon, burdock, celery, damiana, fenugreek, garcinia, garlic, ginger, ginseng (American), gymnema, marshmallow, stinging nettle: May enhance hypoglycemic effects.

Food

None significant known.

DIAGNOSTIC TEST EFFECTS

Lowers blood sugar. Slight increases in serum creatinine or WBC count. Elevations in hepatic enzymes or serum amylase may occur.

SIDE EFFECTS

Frequent

Headache, nasopharyngitis, upper respiratory tract infection, hypoglycemia.

Occasional

Decreased appetite, nausea, constipation, abdominal pain, peripheral edema.

Rare

Rash, vasculitis.

SERIOUS REACTIONS

- Overdose may produce severe hypoglycemia.
- Pancreatitis, including fatal hemorrhagic and nonhemorrhagic and necrotizing.
- Rare reports of serious allergic reactions, including anaphylaxis, angioedema, and serious rashes (Stevens Johnson syndrome).

PRECAUTIONS & CONSIDERATIONS

There have been no clinical studies establishing conclusive evidence of macrovascular risk reduction with sitagliptin. Caution is warranted in patients with impaired renal function. Be alert to conditions that alter blood glucose requirements or dietary intake, such as fever, increased activity, stress, or a surgical procedure. There are no data regarding sitagliptin use during pregnancy. It is unknown whether the drug is distributed in breast milk; caution is recommended. Safety and efficacy of sitagliptin have not been established in children. Hypoglycemia may be difficult to recognize in elderly patients.

Food intake and blood glucose should be monitored before and during therapy. Be aware of signs and symptoms of hypoglycemia (anxiety, cool wet skin, diplopia, dizziness, headache, hunger, numbness in the mouth, tachycardia, tremors) or hyperglycemia (deep rapid breathing, dim vision, fatigue, nausea, polydipsia, polyphagia, polyuria, vomiting); carry candy, sugar packets, or other sugar supplements for immediate response to hypoglycemia.

Consult the physician when glucose demands are altered (such as with fever, heavy physical activity, infection, stress, trauma). Exercise, good personal hygiene (including foot care), not smoking, and weight control are essential parts of therapy.

S

Storage
Store tablets at room temperature.

Administration
May take orally without regard to food or the timing of meals or snacks.

Sodium Bicarbonate

so′dee-um by-car′bon-ate

CATEGORY AND SCHEDULE

Pregnancy Risk Category: C

Classification: Alkalinizing agents, electrolyte replacements

MECHANISM OF ACTION

An alkalinizing agent that dissociates to provide bicarbonate ion.
Therapeutic Effect: Neutralizes hydrogen ion concentration, raises blood and urinary pH.

PHARMACOKINETICS

Route	Onset	Peak	Duration
PO	15 min	NA	1-3 h
IV	Immediate	NA	8-10 min

After administration, sodium bicarbonate dissociates to sodium and bicarbonate ions. With increased hydrogen ion concentrations, bicarbonate ions combine with hydrogen ions to form carbonic acid, which then dissociates to CO_2, which is excreted by the lungs.

AVAILABILITY

Tablets: 325 mg, 650 mg.
Injection: 0.5 mEq/mL (4.2%), 0.6 mEq/mL (5%), 0.9 mEq/mL (7.5%), 1 mEq/mL (8.4%).

INDICATIONS AND DOSAGES

▸ **Cardiac arrest**

IV

Adults, Elderly. Initially, 1 mEq/kg (as 7.5%-8.4% solution). May repeat with 0.5 mEq/kg q10min during continued cardiopulmonary arrest. Use in the postresuscitation phase is based on arterial blood pH, partial pressure of carbon dioxide in arterial blood ($Paco_2$), and base deficit calculation.

Children, Infants. Initially, 1 mEq/kg. To limit the risk of hypernatremia and serious adverse events, the rate of administration in children and infants under the age of 2 yr should therefore be limited to no more than 8 mEq/kg/day. A 4.2% solution may be preferred for such slow administration.

▸ **Metabolic acidosis (not severe)**
IV
Adults, Elderly, Children. 2-5 mEq/kg over 4-8 h. May repeat based on laboratory values.
▸ **Metabolic acidosis (associated with chronic renal failure)**
PO
Adults, Elderly. Initially, 20-36 mEq/day in divided doses.
▸ **Renal tubular acidosis (distal)**
PO
Adults, Elderly. 0.5-2 mEq/kg/day in 4-5 divided doses.
Children. 2-3 mEq/kg/day in 4-5 divided doses.
▸ **Renal tubular acidosis (proximal)**
PO
Adults, Elderly, Children. 5-10 mEq/kg/day in 4-5 divided doses.
▸ **Urine alkalinization**
PO
Adults, Elderly. Initially, 4 g, then 1-2 g q4h. Maximum: 16 g/day.
Children. 84-840 mg/kg/day in 4-6 divided doses.
▸ **Antacid**
PO
Adults, Elderly. 300 mg-2 g 1-4 times a day.
▸ **Hyperkalemia**
IV
Adults, Elderly. 44.6-50 mEq over 5 min.

CONTRAINDICATIONS

Excessive chloride loss due to diarrhea, vomiting, or GI suctioning; hypocalcemia; metabolic or respiratory alkalosis.

INTERACTIONS

Drug
Calcium-containing products: May result in milk-alkali syndrome.
Corticosteroids: May cause edema and hypertension.
Lithium, salicylates: May increase the excretion of these drugs.
Methenamine: May decrease the effects of methenamine.
Herbal
None known.
Food
Milk, other dairy products: May result in milk-alkali syndrome.

DIAGNOSTIC TEST EFFECTS

May increase serum and urinary pH.

IV INCOMPATIBILITIES

NOTE: Many injectable drugs and infusions are incompatible with sodium bicarbonate, due to the alkaline pH. Always refer to specialized references when checking compatibility. Some incompatibilities include ascorbic acid, diltiazem (Cardizem), dobutamine (Dobutrex), dopamine (Intropin), hydromorphone (Dilaudid), magnesium sulfate, midazolam (Versed), morphine, norepinephrine (Levophed).

IV COMPATIBILITIES

Aminophylline, furosemide (Lasix), heparin, insulin, mannitol, milrinone (Primacor), phenylephrine (Neo-Synephrine), potassium chloride, propofol (Diprivan).

SIDE EFFECTS

Frequent
Abdominal distention, flatulence, belching.

SERIOUS REACTIONS

• Excessive or chronic use may produce metabolic alkalosis (characterized by irritability, twitching, paresthesias, cyanosis, slow or shallow respirations, headache, thirst, and nausea).
• Fluid overload results in headache, weakness, blurred vision, behavioral changes, incoordination, muscle twitching, elevated BP, bradycardia,

S

tachypnea, wheezing, coughing, and distended neck veins.

• Extravasation may occur at the IV site, resulting in tissue necrosis and ulceration.

PRECAUTIONS & CONSIDERATIONS

Caution is warranted with congestive heart failure (CHF), renal insufficiency, edema, and concurrent corticosteroid therapy. Sodium bicarbonate use may produce hypernatremia and increased deep tendon reflexes in the neonate or fetus whose mother is administered chronically high doses. Sodium bicarbonate may be distributed in breast milk. No age-related precautions have been noted in children; however, sodium bicarbonate should not be used as an antacid in children younger than 6 yr. In elderly patients, age-related renal impairment may require cautious use. Check with the physician before taking any OTC drugs because they may contain sodium.

Serum calcium, phosphate and uric acid levels, blood and urinary pH, $Paco_2$ and CO_2, plasma bicarbonate, and serum electrolyte levels should be monitored. Pattern of daily bowel activity and stool consistency and clinical improvement of metabolic acidosis, including relief from disorientation, hyperventilation, and weakness, should also be assessed.

Storage

Store vials at room temperature.

Administration

! Sodium bicarbonate may be given by IV push, IV infusion, or orally. Dosage is individualized based on age, weight, clinical conditions, and laboratory values and on the severity of acidosis. Metabolic alkalosis may result if the bicarbonate deficit is fully corrected during the first 24 h.

Take oral sodium bicarbonate 1-3 h after meals. Do not take other oral drugs within 2 h of sodium bicarbonate administration.

Sodium bicarbonate may be given undiluted. For IV push, give up to 1 mEq/kg over 1-3 min for cardiac arrest. Do not exceed an infusion rate of 1 mEq/kg/h.

Sodium Chloride

so′dee-um klor′ide

★ Muro 128, Nasal Mist, Nasal Moist, Ocean, SalineX, SeaMist, Slo-Salt

CATEGORY AND SCHEDULE

Pregnancy Risk Category: C

OTC (tablets, nasal solution, ophthalmic solution, ophthalmic ointment)

Classification: Electrolyte replacements, vitamins/minerals

MECHANISM OF ACTION

Sodium is a major cation of extracellular fluid that controls water distribution, fluid and electrolyte balance, and osmotic pressure of body fluids; it also maintains acid-base balance.

PHARMACOKINETICS

Well absorbed from the GI tract. Widely distributed. Excreted primarily in urine.

AVAILABILITY

Tablets: 1 g.

Injection (Concentrate): 23.4% (4 mEq/mL).

Injection, infusions: 0.45%, 0.9%, 3%.

Irrigation: 0.45%, 0.9%.

Nasal Gel (Nasal Moist): 0.65%.

Nasal Solution (OTC [SalineX]): 0.4%.
Nasal Solution (OTC [Nasal Moist, SeaMist]): 0.65%.
Ophthalmic Solution (OTC [Muro 128]): 5%.
Ophthalmic Ointment (OTC [Muro 128]): 5%.

INDICATIONS AND DOSAGES

▸ **Prevention and treatment of sodium and chloride deficiencies; source of hydration**
IV
Adults, Elderly. 1-2 L/day 0.9% or 0.45%. Assess serum electrolyte levels before giving additional fluid.

▸ **Prevention of heat prostration and muscle cramps from excessive perspiration**
PO
Adults, Elderly. 1-2 g 3 times a day.

▸ **Relief of dry and inflamed nasal membranes**
INTRANASAL
Adults, Elderly. Use as needed.

▸ **Diagnostic aid in ophthalmoscopic exam, treatment of corneal edema**
OPHTHALMIC SOLUTION
Adults, Elderly. Apply 1-2 drops q3-4h.
OPHTHALMIC OINTMENT
Adults, Elderly. Apply once a day or as directed.

CONTRAINDICATIONS

Fluid retention, hypernatremia.

INTERACTIONS

Drug
Corticosteroids: May increase fluid retention.
Herbal
None known.
Food
None known.

DIAGNOSTIC TEST EFFECTS

None known.

SIDE EFFECTS

Frequent
Facial flushing.
Occasional
Fever; irritation, phlebitis, or extravasation at injection site. Ophthalmic: Temporary burning or irritation.

SERIOUS REACTIONS

- Too-rapid administration may produce peripheral edema, congestive heart failure (CHF), and pulmonary edema.
- Excessive dosage may cause hypokalemia, hypervolemia, and hypernatremia.
- Too-rapid correction of hyponatremia with hypertonic saline (e.g., 3%) may produce cerebral edema.

PRECAUTIONS & CONSIDERATIONS

Caution is warranted with cirrhosis, CHF, hypertension, and renal impairment. Do not administer sodium and chloride preserved with benzyl alcohol to neonates. No age-related precautions have been noted in children or elderly patients.

Notify the physician of acute redness of eyes, floating spots, severe eye pain or pain on exposure to light, a rapid change in vision (side and straight ahead), or headache after ophthalmic administration. Fluid balance, weight, acid-base balance, BP, and serum electrolyte levels should be monitored. Be alert for signs and symptoms of hypernatremia (edema, hypertension, and weight gain) and hyponatremia (dry mucous membranes, muscle cramps, nausea, and vomiting).

Storage
Store vials at room temperature.

Administration
! Dosage is based on acid-base status, age, weight, clinical condition, and fluid and electrolyte status.

Do not crush or break enteric-coated or slow-release tablets. Take tablets with a full glass of water.

For IV use, administer hypertonic solutions (3% or 5%) through a large vein at a rate not exceeding 1 mEq/kg/h. Avoid infiltration. Dilute vials containing 2.5-4 mEq/mL (concentrated NaCl) with D5W or $D_{10}W$ before administration.

For nasal use, inhale slowly just before releasing the drug into nose. Then release air gently through the mouth. Continue this technique for 20-30 seconds.

For ophthalmic use, place a finger on the lower eyelid, and pull it out until a pocket is formed between the eye and lower lid. Hold the dropper above the pocket and instill the prescribed number of drops (or apply a thin strip of ointment) in the pocket. Close the eyes gently so that the drug is not squeezed out of the sac. After administering the solution, apply gentle finger pressure to the lacrimal sac for 1-2 min to reduce systemic absorption.

Sodium Ferric Gluconate Complex

so′dee-um fer′ick glue′koe-nate calm′plex

★ 🍁 Ferrlecit

CATEGORY AND SCHEDULE

Pregnancy Risk Category: B

Classification: Hematinics, minerals, iron replacements

MECHANISM OF ACTION

A trace element that repletes total iron content in body. Replaces iron found in hemoglobin, myoglobin, and specific enzymes; allows oxygen transport via hemoglobin. *Therapeutic Effect:* Prevents and corrects iron deficiency.

AVAILABILITY

Solution for Injection: 12.5 mg/mL elemental iron.

INDICATIONS AND DOSAGES

▸ **Iron deficiency anemia**

IV INFUSION

Adults, Elderly. 125 mg in 100 mL 0.9% NaCl infused over 1 h. May administer undiluted, at a rate 12.5 mg/min. Minimum cumulative dose 1 g elemental iron given over 8 sessions at sequential dialysis treatments. May be given during dialysis session.

Children older than 6 yr. 1.5 mg/kg elemental iron diluted in 25 mL 0.9% NaCl infused over 1 h. Maximum 125 mg/dose given over 8 sessions at sequential dialysis treatments. May be given during dialysis session.

CONTRAINDICATIONS

Hypersensitivity, evidence of iron overload, and all anemias not associated with iron deficiency.

INTERACTIONS

Drug

ACE inhibitors: May increase risk of infusion/sensitivity infusion reactions.

Iron preparations: Do not give concurrently with oral iron or other injectable irons because excessive iron intake may produce excessive iron storage (hemosiderosis).

Herbal

None known.

Food

None known.

DIAGNOSTIC TEST EFFECTS

Expect increases in hemoglobin, hematocrit, and other indices of RBC production.

IV INCOMPATIBILITIES

Do not mix with other medications.

SIDE EFFECTS

Frequent (> 3%)
Flushing, hypotension, hypersensitivity reaction.
Occasional (1%-3%)
Injection-site reaction, headache, abdominal pain, chills, flu-like syndrome, dizziness, leg cramps, dyspnea, nausea, vomiting, diarrhea, myalgia, pruritus, edema.

SERIOUS REACTIONS

- A potentially fatal hypersensitivity reaction occurs rarely, characterized by cardiovascular collapse, cardiac arrest, dyspnea, bronchospasm, angioedema, and urticaria.
- Rapid administration may cause hypotension associated with flushing, light-headedness, fatigue, weakness, or severe pain in the chest, back, or groin.

PRECAUTIONS & CONSIDERATIONS

Caution is warranted in patients with asthma, hepatic impairment, rheumatoid arthritis, and significant allergies. It is unknown whether sodium ferric gluconate complex is distributed in breast milk. No age-related precautions have been noted in elderly patients. However, lower initial dosages of sodium ferric gluconate complex are recommended in elderly patients. Safety and efficacy are not established in children less than 6 yr of age.

Stools may become black during iron therapy, but this effect is harmless unless accompanied by abdominal cramping or pain and red streaking and sticky consistency of stool. Notify the physician of abdominal cramping or pain or red streaking or sticky consistency of stool. Laboratory test results, especially CBC, serum iron concentrations, and vital signs, should be monitored. Test results may not be meaningful for 3 wks after beginning sodium ferric gluconate complex therapy. Patients with rheumatoid arthritis or iron deficiency anemia should be assessed for acute exacerbation of joint pain and swelling.

Storage
Store at room temperature. If diluted in 0.9% NaCl, use infusion immediately after preparation.

Administration
! May give undiluted as slow IV injection or IV infusion without test dose. Administration as an infusion may limit the risk of significant hypotension.

The standard recommended dilution is 125 mg (10 mL) diluted with 100 mL 0.9% NaCl. Infuse over 1 h. The drug may be administered during dialysis treatments.

Sodium Oxybate

sew-dee′um ox′ee-bate
★ 🍁 Xyrem

CATEGORY AND SCHEDULE

Pregnancy Risk Category: B
Controlled Substance Schedule: III

Classification: Depressants, central nervous system (CNS)

MECHANISM OF ACTION

A naturally occurring inhibitory neurotransmitter that binds to γ-aminobutyric acid (GABA)-B receptors and sodium oxybate specific receptors with its highest concentrations in the basal ganglia, which meditates sleep cycles, temperature regulation, cerebral glucose metabolism and blood flow, memory, and emotion control. *Therapeutic Effect:* Reduces the number of sleep episodes.

S

PHARMACOKINETICS
Rapidly and incompletely absorbed. Absorption is delayed and decreased by a high-fat meal. Protein binding: < 1%. Widely distributed, including cerebrospinal fluid (CSF). Metabolized in liver. Excretion is < 5% in the urine and negligible in feces. Unknown whether removed by hemodialysis. *Half-life:* 20-53 min.

AVAILABILITY
Oral Solution: 500 mg/mL (Xyrem).

INDICATIONS AND DOSAGES
▸ **Cataplexy of narcolepsy**

PO

Adults, Elderly, Children aged 16 yr or older. 4.5 g/day in 2 equal doses of 2.25 g, the first taken at bedtime while in bed and the second 2.5-4 h later. Maximum: 9 g/day in 2-wk increments of 1.5 g/day. Maximum dose: 9 g/day.

CONTRAINDICATIONS
Metabolic/respiratory alkalosis, current treatment with sedative hypnotics, succinic semialdehyde dehydrogenase deficient, history of substance abuse including active alcoholism, hypersensitivity to sodium oxybate or any component of the formulation.

S

INTERACTIONS
Drug

Alcohol, barbiturates, benzodiazepines, centrally acting muscle relaxants, opioid analgesics: May increase CNS and respiratory depressant effects. Do not use with other sedatives or hypnotics.

Methamphetamine: May increase risk of unconsciousness and seizure-like tremor.

Herbal

None known.

Food

None known.

DIAGNOSTIC TEST EFFECTS
May increase sodium and glucose level. May cause positive antinuclear antibody (ANA) test (without symptoms).

SIDE EFFECTS
Frequent

Mild bradycardia.

Occasional

Headache, vertigo, dizziness, restless legs, abdominal pain, muscle weakness.

Rare

Dream-like state of confusion.

SERIOUS REACTIONS
- Agitation, excitation, increased BP, and insomnia may occur on abrupt discontinuation of sodium oxybate.
- Abuse potential. Abuse of drug may cause seizure, respiratory depression, and profound decreases in level of consciousness, possible coma, and death. Other neuropsychiatric events: psychosis, paranoia, hallucinations, and agitation.
- Sleepwalking with amnesia and unusual behaviors, including participating in hazardous activities (e.g., smoking, driving). If occurs, discontinue the drug.

PRECAUTIONS & CONSIDERATIONS
Only available through the Xyrem Success Program to ensure proper use and monitoring of risks. Patients and prescribers must enroll, then the drug is sent to the patient. Caution is warranted in patients with a history of depression, hypertension, pregnancy, concurrent ingestion of alcohol, other CNS depressants, and renal or liver impairment. It is unknown whether sodium oxybate is excreted in breast milk. Use caution if giving sodium oxybate to pregnant women. Safety and efficacy of this drug have not been established in children or the

elderly. Age-related liver or renal impairment may require decreased dosage in elderly patients. High-fat meals should be avoided because they will delay absorption of the drug.

Dizziness and light-headedness may occur. Avoid alcohol and tasks that require mental alertness or motor skills. Notify physician of signs of metabolic alkalosis or irritability, twitching, numbness or tingling of extremities, cyanosis, slow or shallow respiration, headache, thirst, nausea.

Storage

Store at room temperature. The diluted oral solution should be consumed within 24 h.

Administration

Be aware that sodium oxybate is available only through restricted distribution. Food significantly reduces bioavailability, so allow at least 2 h after eating before giving the first dose of sodium oxybate. Mix this medicine with 2 oz (¼ cup) of water before using. Mix both doses of medicine before going to bed, and store the second dose close to the bed. Take the second dose 2½ to 4 h after taking the first dose. Set an alarm clock to wake up to take the second dose on time.

Sodium Polystyrene Sulfonate

so′dee-um pol-ee-stye′reen sul′foe-nate

★ Kayexalate, Kionex, Marlexate, SPS 🍁 Kayexylate, PMS-Sodium Polystyrene Sulfonate

CATEGORY AND SCHEDULE

Pregnancy Risk Category: C

Classification: Resins

MECHANISM OF ACTION

An ion exchange resin that releases sodium ions in exchange primarily for potassium ions. *Therapeutic Effect:* Moves potassium from the blood into the intestine so it can be expelled from the body.

PHARMACOKINETICS

Onset 2-24 h. Not absorbed. Excreted in feces.

AVAILABILITY

Suspension (SPS): 15 g/60 mL.
Powder for Suspension (Kayexalate, Kionex): 15 g/60 mL.

INDICATIONS AND DOSAGES

▸ **Hyperkalemia**

PO

Adults, Elderly. 60 mL (15 g) 1-4 times a day.
Children. 1 g/kg/dose q6h.

RECTAL

Adults, Elderly. 30-50 g q1-2h initially, as needed to correct hyperkalemia, then q6h.
Children. 1 g/kg q2-6h.

CONTRAINDICATIONS

Hypokalemia, hypocalcemia, intestinal obstruction, or perforation.

Do not give orally in neonates; do not use in neonates with reduced gut motility.

INTERACTIONS

Drug

Cation-donating antacids, laxatives (such as magnesium hydroxide): May decrease effect of sodium polystyrene sulfonate and cause systemic alkalosis in patients with renal impairment.

Herbal

None known.

Food

None known.

S

DIAGNOSTIC TEST EFFECTS

May decrease serum calcium and magnesium levels.

SIDE EFFECTS

Frequent

High dosage: Anorexia, nausea, vomiting, constipation.

High dosage in elderly: Fecal impaction characterized by severe stomach pain with nausea or vomiting.

Occasional

Diarrhea, sodium retention marked by decreased urination, peripheral edema, and increased weight.

SERIOUS REACTIONS

• Potassium deficiency may occur. Early signs of hypokalemia include confusion, delayed thought processes, extreme weakness, irritability, and ECG changes (including prolonged QT interval; widening, flattening, or inversion of T wave; and prominent U waves).

• Hypocalcemia, manifested by abdominal or muscle cramps, occurs occasionally.

• Arrhythmias and severe muscle weakness may be noted.

• Resin impaction, possible colonic necrosis, colitis or perforation.

S

PRECAUTIONS & CONSIDERATIONS

Caution is warranted in patients with edema, hypertension, and severe CHF. It is unknown whether sodium polystyrene sulfonate crosses the placenta or is distributed in breast milk. Use caution in neonates, and only give rectally. Rectal administration may cause impaction in young infants/neonates. Elderly patients may be at increased risk for fecal impaction. Foods rich in potassium should be consumed.

Because sodium polystyrene sulfonate does not rapidly correct severe hyperkalemia (it may take hours to days), consider other measures, such as dialysis, IV glucose and insulin, IV calcium, and IV sodium bicarbonate to correct severe hyperkalemia in a medical emergency. Serum potassium levels, calcium and magnesium, and pattern of daily bowel activity and stool consistency should be assessed. Clinical condition and ECG are valuable in determining when treatment should be discontinued.

Storage

Store at room temperature. Once suspension is prepared, use within 24 h.

Administration

Once suspension is prepared, shake suspension well prior to use. Give oral sodium polystyrene sulfonate with 20-100 mL of water to aid in potassium removal, facilitate passage of resin through the intestinal tract, and prevent constipation. The amount of fluid needed may be simply determined by allowing 3 mL to 4 mL per g of resin. Do not mix this drug with foods or liquids containing potassium. Drink the entire amount of the resin for best results. Chilling oral suspension will help improve the taste.

For rectal use, after initial cleansing enema, insert large rubber tube well into sigmoid colon and tape in place. Introduce suspension with 100 mL sorbitol or water by gravity. Flush with 50-100 mL fluid and clamp. Retain for several hours, if possible. Irrigate colon with a non–sodium-containing solution to remove resin.

Solifenacin

sohl-e-fen'ah-sin

VESIcare

Do not confuse VESIcare with Viscol.

CATEGORY AND SCHEDULE

Pregnancy Risk Category: C

Classification: Anticholinergics, urinary incontinence agents, bladder antispasmodics.

MECHANISM OF ACTION

A urinary antispasmodic that acts as a direct antagonist at muscarinic acetylcholine receptors in cholinergically innervated organs. Reduces tonus (elastic tension) of smooth muscle in the bladder and slows parasympathetic contractions. *Therapeutic Effect:* Decreases urinary bladder contractions, increases residual urine volume, and decreases detrusor muscle pressure.

PHARMACOKINETICS

Well absorbed. Protein binding: 99%. Solifenacin is extensively metabolized in the liver by CYP3A4; but alternate metabolic pathways exist. Excreted mostly in urine (69%) and some in feces. *Half-life:* 45-68 h (increased in renal and liver dysfunction).

AVAILABILITY

Tablets: 5 mg, 10 mg.

INDICATIONS AND DOSAGES

▸ **Overactive bladder**

PO

Adults, Elderly. 5 mg/day; if tolerated, may increase to 10 mg/day.

▸ **Dosage in renal or hepatic impairment or taking CYP3A4 inhibitors**

For patients with severe renal impairment, moderate hepatic impairment, or concomitant use of CYP3A4 inhibitors, maximum dosage is 5 mg/day.

CONTRAINDICATIONS

GI or gastrourinary obstruction, paralytic ileus, severe hepatic impairment, uncontrolled angle-closure glaucoma, urinary retention.

INTERACTIONS

Drug

Aminoglutethimide, carbamazepine, nafcillin, nevirapine, phenobarbital, phenytoin: May decrease the effects and serum level of solifenacin.

Azole antifungals, potent CYP3A4 inhibitors (e.g., clarithromycin, erythromycin, imatinib, isoniazid, nefazodone, protease inhibitors, verapamil): May increase the effects and serum level of solifenacin. Maximum dose 5 mg daily with potent CYP3A4 inhibitors.

Herbal

St. John's wort: May decrease the effects and serum level of solifenacin.

Food

Grapefruit, grapefruit juice: May increase the effects and serum level of solifenacin.

DIAGNOSTIC TEST EFFECTS

None known.

SIDE EFFECTS

Frequent (5%-11%)

Dry mouth, constipation, blurred vision.

Occasional (3%-5%)

Urinary tract infection, dyspepsia, nausea.

Rare (1%-2%)

Dizziness, dry eyes, fatigue, depression, edema, hypertension, upper abdominal pain, vomiting, urinary retention.

SERIOUS REACTIONS

- GI obstruction occurs rarely.
- Overdose can result in severe central anticholinergic effects.
- Acute urinary retention requiring treatment.
- Rare cases of hypersensitivity, such as angioedema.

PRECAUTIONS & CONSIDERATIONS

Caution is warranted with bladder outflow obstruction, congenital or acquired prolonged QT interval, controlled angle-closure glaucoma, decreased GI motility, GI obstructive disorders, hepatic or renal impairment, and in pregnant women.

Storage

Store at room temperature; protect from light.

Administration

Take solifenacin without regard to food but with liquid; swallow tablets whole.

Sorafenib

sore-a-fen′ib

★ 🍁 Nexavar

Do not confuse sorafenib with sunitinib.

CATEGORY AND SCHEDULE

Pregnancy Risk Category: D

Classification: Antineoplastics, biologic agents, signal transduction inhibitor

MECHANISM OF ACTION

An oral multikinase inhibitor. The drug inhibits multiple intracellular (CRAF, BRAF, and mutant BRAF) and cell surface kinases (KIT, FLT-3, RET, VEGFR-1, VEGFR-2, VEGFR-3, and PDGFR-β). Several of these kinases are thought to be involved in tumor cell signaling, angiogenesis, and apoptosis. *Therapeutic Effect:* Inhibits tumor growth.

PHARMACOKINETICS

Food decreases oral absorption. Protein binding: 99.5%. Sorafenib is metabolized in the liver by oxidative metabolism, mediated by CYP 3A4, and UGT1A9 mediates glucuronidation. A total of 8 metabolites have been identified. The major active metabolite, pyridine N-oxide, shows in vitro potency similar to that of sorafenib. Most of the dose was recovered within 14 days, with 77% excreted in the feces and 19% excreted in the urine as glucuronidated metabolites. Unchanged sorafenib is found in the feces but not in the urine. *Half-life:* 25-48 h.

AVAILABILITY

Tablet: 200 mg.

INDICATIONS AND DOSAGES

▸ **Advanced renal cell or hepatocellular cancer**

PO

Adults, Elderly. 400 mg twice daily on an empty stomach.

▸ **Dosage adjustment if strong CYP3A4 inducers used**

May consider dose increase, with caution.

▸ **Dosage adjustment for toxicity**

Management of side effects may require temporary interruption and/or dose reduction. Dose may be reduced to 400 mg once daily or to 400 mg every other day. See manufacturer's information for full recommendations.

CONTRAINDICATIONS

Hypersensitivity. Do not use with carboplatin and paclitaxel for squamous cell lung cancer, due to an increase in mortality with the addition of sorafenib.

INTERACTIONS

Drug

Carboplatin and paclitaxel: Increased mortality in patients with squamous cell lung cancer. Do not use sorafenib.

UGT1A1 and UGT1A9 substrates (e.g., irinotecan): Sorafenib inhibits UGT and may increase toxicity of these drugs.

Docetaxel: Sorafenib increases docetaxel exposure.

Doxorubicin: Increase in doxorubicin exposure.

Fluorouracil: Both increases and decreases in the AUC of fluorouracil were observed.

CYP2B6 and CYP2C8 substrates: Sorafenib inhibits these enzymes; use caution with drugs such as bupropion.

Strong CYP inducers (e.g., rifampin, phenytoin, carbamazepine, phenobarbital, dexamethasone): May increase metabolism of sorafenib and thus decrease sorafenib concentrations; may need dose increase.

Warfarin: Sorafenib is a competitive inhibitor of CYP2C9 and could possibly alter warfarin response; also independently increases INR; monitor INR.

Herbal

St. John's wort: May increase metabolism of sorafenib and thus decrease sorafenib concentrations; avoid.

Food

All foods: Decreases absorption; administer on empty stomach.

DIAGNOSTIC TEST EFFECTS

Decreased WBC, platelets. Increased INR, liver enzymes, serum amylase, lipase. Hypoalbuminemia. Electrolyte abnormalities (hypophosphatemia).

SIDE EFFECTS

Frequent (> 20%)

Fatigue, weight loss, rash/skin desquamation, hand-foot syndrome, alopecia, diarrhea, anorexia, nausea, hypophosphatemia, and abdominal pain.

Occasional

Chest pain, hypertension, dysgeusia (altered taste), dyspepsia, mouth ulcers, facial edema, proteinuria, arthralgia or myalgia, depression, hoarseness, skin erythema.

Rare

Difficult wound healing, renal impairment, erectile dysfunction, tinnitus.

SERIOUS REACTIONS

- Serious hypersensitivity reactions occur rarely, and may include angioedema.
- Leukopenia, thrombocytopenia.
- Severe and fatal hepatotoxicity, or pancreatitis.
- Serious bleeding (CNS, gastrointestinal, hemoptysis, etc.) or GI perforations.
- Chest pain may indicate cardiac ischemia or infarction and requires prompt evaluation.

PRECAUTIONS & CONSIDERATIONS

Use with caution in patients with hepatic disease, high blood pressure, cardiac disease, heart failure or arrhythmia, a history of stroke, GI disease with GI bleeding in the past 6 months or a history of GI perforation or fistula, thyroid disease, had recent surgery or scheduled for surgery. Do not use in patients who are pregnant or planning to become pregnant; the drug can cause fetal harm. Women of childbearing potential should be advised to avoid becoming pregnant, and both males and females should use adequate birth control during treatment. It is not known if sorafenib passes into breast milk; do not breastfeed while taking this medication. This drug has not been approved for use in children.

Storage

Store tablets at room temperature; protect from moisture.

Administration

Administer sorafenib orally without food (at least 1 h before or 2 h after a meal). Treatment is continued until clinical benefit no longer realized, or unacceptable toxicity occurs.

Sotalol

soe'ta-lole

★ Betapace, Betapace AF, Sorine

Do not confuse sotalol with Stadol.

CATEGORY AND SCHEDULE

Pregnancy Risk Category: B (D if used in second or third trimester)

Classification: Cardiovascular agents; antiarrhythmics, class III; adrenergic β-blockers

S

MECHANISM OF ACTION

A β-adrenergic blocking agent that prolongs action potential, effective refractory period, and QT interval. Decreases heart rate and AV node conduction; increases AV node refractoriness. *Therapeutic Effect:* Produces antiarrhythmic activity.

PHARMACOKINETICS

Well absorbed from the GI tract. Protein binding: None. Widely distributed. Excreted primarily unchanged in urine. Removed by hemodialysis. *Half-life:* 12 h (increased in elderly patients and in patients with impaired renal function).

AVAILABILITY

Tablets (Betapace, Sorine): 80 mg, 120 mg, 160 mg, 240 mg.
Tablets (Betapace AF): 80 mg, 120 mg, 160 mg.
Solution for Injection: 150 mg/10 mL.

INDICATIONS AND DOSAGES

▸ **Documented, life-threatening ventricular arrhythmias**

PO

Adults, Elderly. Initially, 80 mg twice a day. May increase gradually at 2- to 3-day intervals. Range: 240-320 mg/day in 2 divided doses.

Children, Infants. The manufacturer provides detailed dosing instructions based on BSA to individualize dosing.

▸ **Maintenance (delay in time to recurrence) for A Fib/A Flutter currently in sinus rhythm**

PO (BETAPACE AF)

Adults, Elderly. Initially, 80 mg twice a day. This dose may be all that is needed in many patients. If needed, may increase up to 120 mg twice daily after 3 days. Maximum: 160 mg twice daily.

▸ **Conversion from oral to IV dosing if needed**

IV

Adult, Elderly.

PO Dose	IV Dose
80 mg	75 mg
120 mg	112.5 mg
160 mg	150 mg

▸ **Dosage in renal impairment**

Dosage interval is modified based on creatinine clearance and formulation used. See manufacturer specific recommendations.

Creatinine Clearance (mL/min)	Dosage Interval
30-59	24 h
10-29*	36-48 h
< 10	Individualized

* If afib, do not use if < 40 mL/min

OFF-LABEL USES

Maintenance of normal heart rhythm in chronic or recurring atrial fibrillation or flutter.

CONTRAINDICATIONS

Hypersensitivity, sinus bradycardia (< 50 bpm), sick sinus syndrome or 2nd- and 3rd-degree AV block (unless functioning pacemaker present), congenital or acquired long QT syndrome, QT interval > 450 msec, cardiogenic shock, uncontrolled CHF, hypokalemia (< 4 mEq/L), bronchial asthma.

INTERACTIONS

Drug

Calcium channel blockers: May increase effect on AV conduction and BP.

Clonidine: May potentiate rebound hypertension after clonidine is discontinued.

Digoxin: May increase risk of proarrhythmias.

Insulin, oral hypoglycemics: May mask signs of hypoglycemia and prolong the effects of insulin and oral hypoglycemics.

Other β-blockers: Additive effects on cardiac conduction; avoid.

QT-prolonging agents (e.g., Class IA and Class III antiarrhythmics (amiodarone, flecainide, propafenone) previously mentioned, alfuzosin, cisapride, clarithromycin, droperidol, erythromycin, haloperidol, methadone, certain phenothiazines (chlorpromazine, mesoridazine, and thioridazine), pimozide, tricyclic antidepressants, ziprasidone): Additive QT effects; some drugs are contraindicated.

Sympathomimetics: May inhibit the effects of sympathomimetics.

Herbal

Ephedra: May worsen arrhythmias.

Food

None known.

DIAGNOSTIC TEST EFFECTS

May increase blood glucose, serum alkaline phosphatase, serum LDH, serum lipoprotein, AST (SGOT), ALT (SGPT), and serum triglyceride levels.

SIDE EFFECTS

Frequent

Diminished sexual function, drowsiness, insomnia, unusual fatigue or weakness.

Occasional

Depression, cold hands or feet, diarrhea, constipation, anxiety, nasal congestion, nausea, vomiting.

Rare

Altered taste; dry eyes; itching; numbness of fingers, toes, or scalp.

SERIOUS REACTIONS

• Bradycardia, congestive heart failure (CHF), hypotension, bronchospasm, hypoglycemia, prolonged QT interval, torsades de pointes, ventricular tachycardia, and premature ventricular complexes may occur.

PRECAUTIONS & CONSIDERATIONS

Note the differences in indications and usage of Betapace and Sorine versus Betapace AF.

Caution is warranted with cardiomegaly, CHF, diabetes mellitus, history of ventricular tachycardia, hypokalemia, hypomagnesemia, severe and prolonged diarrhea, and those at risk for developing thyrotoxicosis. Sotalol crosses the placenta and is excreted in breast milk. The safety and efficacy of sotalol have not been established in children with organ dysfunction. In elderly patients, age-related peripheral vascular disease may increase susceptibility to decreased peripheral circulation. Tasks that require mental alertness or motor skills should be avoided.

Monitor BP for hypotension and pulse for bradycardia during treatment. If pulse rate is 55 beats/min or lower or systolic BP is < 90 mm Hg, withhold the medication and contact the physician. Continuous cardiac monitoring should be performed when beginning sotalol therapy. Signs and symptoms of CHF should also be assessed.

Storage

Store tablets at room temperature protected from humidity. The compounded oral solution is stable for 3 mo when stored at controlled room temperature.

Administration

Take sotalol without regard to food. Do not abruptly discontinue the drug.

The manufacturer provides for an oral solution that may be extemporaneously prepared. Shake well prior to each use.

For IV use, see manufacturer's literature. Must dilute as an IV infusion and dose is infused using an infusion pump over 5 h.

S

Spironolactone

speer-on-oh-lak'tone

★ Aldactone 🍁 Novo-Spiroton

Do not confuse Aldactone with Aldactazide.

CATEGORY AND SCHEDULE

Pregnancy Risk Category: C (D if used in pregnancy-induced hypertension)

Classification: Diuretics, potassium sparing

MECHANISM OF ACTION

A potassium-sparing diuretic that interferes with sodium reabsorption by competitively inhibiting the action of aldosterone in the distal tubule, thus promoting sodium and water excretion and increasing potassium retention. *Therapeutic Effect:* Produces diuresis; lowers BP; diagnostic aid for primary aldosteronism.

PHARMACOKINETICS

Route	Onset	Peak	Duration
PO	24-48 h	48-72 h	48-72 h

Well absorbed from the GI tract (absorption increased with food). Protein binding: 91%-98%. Metabolized in the liver to active metabolite. Excreted primarily in urine. Unknown whether removed by hemodialysis. *Half-life:* 1.3-2 h (metabolite, 10-35 h).

AVAILABILITY

Tablets: 25 mg, 50 mg, 100 mg.

INDICATIONS AND DOSAGES

▸ **Edema or the treatment of ascites due to cirrhosis**

PO

Adults, Elderly. 25-200 mg/day as a single dose or in 2 divided doses.

Children (unlabeled use). 1.5-3.3 mg/kg/day once daily or in 2-4 divided doses.

Neonates (unlabeled use). 1-3 mg/kg/day in 1-2 divided doses once daily or in 2-4 divided doses.

▸ **CHF, severe with ACEI and loop diuretic**

Adults. 12.5-25 mg/day. Maximum: 50 mg/day.

▸ **Hypertension**

PO

Adults, Elderly. 50-100 mg/day in 1-2 doses/day. After 2 wks, may be

titrated to 200 mg/day in 2-4 divided doses.
Children. 1.5-3.3 mg/kg/day in divided doses.

▸ **Hypokalemia**
PO
Adults, Elderly. 25-100 mg/day as a single dose or in 2 divided doses.

▸ **Primary aldosteronism**
PO
Adults, Elderly. 100-400 mg/day as a single dose or in 2 divided doses.

▸ **Dosage in renal impairment**
Dosage interval is modified based on creatinine clearance.

Creatinine Clearance (mL/min)	Dosage Interval
10-50	Usual dose q24h
< 10	Avoid use

OFF-LABEL USES
Treatment of female hirsutism, polycystic ovary disease, indications in children.

CONTRAINDICATIONS
Acute renal insufficiency, anuria, BUN and serum creatinine levels more than twice normal values, hyperkalemia.

INTERACTIONS
Drug
ACE inhibitors (such as captopril), drospirenone, eplerenone, potassium-containing medications, potassium supplements: May increase the risk of hyperkalemia.
Anticoagulants, heparin: May decrease the effects of these drugs.
Digoxin: May increase the half-life of digoxin.
Lithium: May decrease the clearance and increase the risk of toxicity of lithium.
NSAIDs: May decrease the antihypertensive effect of spironolactone.
Herbal
Natural licorice: May increase mineralocorticoid effects of spironolactone.
Food
Salt substitutes or diet rich in potassium should normally be avoided.

DIAGNOSTIC TEST EFFECTS
May increase urinary calcium excretion; BUN and blood glucose levels; serum creatinine, magnesium, potassium, and uric acid levels. May decrease serum sodium level.

Sporadic reports of interference with some digoxin assays.

SIDE EFFECTS
Frequent
Hyperkalemia (in patients with renal insufficiency and those taking potassium supplements), dehydration, hyponatremia, lethargy.
Occasional
Nausea, vomiting, anorexia, abdominal cramps, diarrhea, headache, ataxia, somnolence, confusion, fever.
Male: Gynecomastia, impotence, decreased libido.
Female: Menstrual irregularities (including amenorrhea and postmenopausal bleeding), breast tenderness.
Rare
Rash, urticaria, hirsutism.

SERIOUS REACTIONS
- Severe hyperkalemia may produce arrhythmias, bradycardia, and ECG changes (tented T waves, widening QRS complex, and ST segment depression). These may proceed to cardiac standstill or ventricular fibrillation.
- Cirrhosis patients are at risk for hepatic decompensation if dehydration or hyponatremia occurs.
- Patients with primary aldosteronism may experience rapid

S

weight loss and severe fatigue during high-dose therapy.

PRECAUTIONS & CONSIDERATIONS

Caution is warranted in patients with hyponatremia, hepatic or renal impairment, dehydration, and concurrent use of potassium supplements. An active metabolite of spironolactone is excreted in breast milk. Breastfeeding is not recommended for patients taking this drug. Safety and efficacy not established in children. Elderly patients may be more susceptible to hyperkalemia. In addition, age-related renal impairment may require cautious use in this age group. Avoid foods high in potassium, such as apricots, bananas, legumes, meat, orange juice, raisins, whole grains, including cereals, and white and sweet potatoes. Also, avoid performing tasks that require mental alertness or motor skills until response to the drug has been established.

An increase in the frequency and volume of urination may occur. Notify the physician of an irregular heartbeat, diarrhea, muscle twitching, cold and clammy skin, confusion, drowsiness, dry mouth, or excessive thirst. BP, vital signs, electrolytes, and intake and output should be monitored before and during treatment. Be especially alert for evidence of hyperkalemia, such as arrhythmias, colic, diarrhea, and muscle twitching, followed by paralysis and weakness. Also be aware signs of hyponatremia may result in cold and clammy skin, confusion, and thirst.

Storage

Store tablets at room temperature.

Administration

Take spironolactone with food to enhance its absorption. Crush scored tablets as needed. The drug's therapeutic effect takes several days to begin and can last for several days once the drug is discontinued.

S

Stavudine (d4T)

stav'yoo-deen

★ 🍁 Zerit

CATEGORY AND SCHEDULE

Pregnancy Risk Category: C

Classification: Antiretrovirals, nucleoside reverse transcriptase inhibitors

MECHANISM OF ACTION

Inhibits HIV reverse transcriptase by terminating the viral DNA chain. Also inhibits RNA- and DNA-dependent DNA polymerase, an enzyme necessary for HIV replication. *Therapeutic Effect:* Impedes HIV replication, slowing the progression of HIV infection.

PHARMACOKINETICS

Rapidly and completely absorbed after PO administration. Undergoes minimal metabolism. Excreted in urine. *Half-life:* 1.2-1.6 h (increased in renal impairment).

AVAILABILITY

Capsules: 15 mg, 20 mg, 30 mg, 40 mg.

Oral Solution: 1 mg/mL.

INDICATIONS AND DOSAGES

▸ **HIV infection (in combination with other antiretrovirals)**

PO

Adults, Children weighing ≥ 60 kg. 40 mg twice a day.

Adults weighing < 60 kg. 30 mg twice a day.

Children weighing ≥ 30-60 kg. 30 mg twice a day.

Children weighing < 30 kg. 1 mg/kg twice a day.

Neonates (< 14 days old). 0.5 mg/kg every 12 h.

▸ **HIV infection in patients with a recent history and complete resolution of peripheral neuropathy or elevated liver function test results (50% of recommended dose)**

Adults weighing ≥ 60 kg. 20 mg twice a day.

Adults weighing < 60 kg. 15 mg twice a day.

▸ **Dosage in renal impairment**

Dosage and frequency are modified based on creatinine clearance and patient weight.

Creatinine Clearance (mL/min)	Weight ≥ 60 kg	Weight < 60 kg
> 50	40 mg q12h	30 mg q12h
26-50	20 mg q12h	15 mg q12h
10-25	20 mg q24h	15 mg q24h Note: Administer after hemodialysis dose on day of dialysis

CONTRAINDICATIONS

Hypersensitivity to the drug. Do not give with didanosine due to increase in toxicity, such as serious and potentially fatal pancreatitis.

INTERACTIONS

Drug

Ethambutol, isoniazid, lithium, phenytoin, zalcitabine: May increase the risk of peripheral neuropathy development.

Hydroxyurea: May increase the risk of hepatotoxicity.

Doxorubicin, zidovudine: May have antagonistic antiviral effect.

Herbal

None known.

Food

None known.

DIAGNOSTIC TEST EFFECTS

Commonly increases AST (SGOT) and ALT (SGPT) levels. May decrease neutrophil count.

SIDE EFFECTS

Frequent

Headache (55%), diarrhea (50%), chills and fever (38%), nausea and vomiting, myalgia (35%), rash (33%), asthenia (28%), insomnia, abdominal pain (26%), anxiety (22%), arthralgia (18%), back pain (20%), diaphoresis (19%), malaise (17%), depression (14%).

Occasional

Anorexia, weight loss, nervousness, dizziness, conjunctivitis, dyspepsia, dyspnea, redistribution/accumulation of body fat, including "buffalo hump."

Rare

Constipation, vasodilation, confusion, migraine, urticaria, abnormal vision.

SERIOUS REACTIONS

- Peripheral neuropathy (numbness, tingling, or pain in the hands and feet) occurs in 15%-21% of patients.
- Ulcerative stomatitis (erythema or ulcers of oral mucosa, glossitis, gingivitis), pneumonia, and benign skin neoplasms occur occasionally.
- Pancreatitis and lactic acidosis occur rarely, as does hepatic steatosis, but all may result in hospitalization or death.

PRECAUTIONS & CONSIDERATIONS

Caution is warranted in patients with a history of peripheral neuropathy or liver or renal impairment, especially those with chronic active hepatitis. Breastfeeding is not recommended in this population because of the possibility of HIV transmission. No age-related precautions have been noted in children. There is no information on the effects of this drug's use in elderly patients. Avoid taking any medications, including over-the-counter (OTC) drugs, without first notifying the physician. Stavudine is not a cure for HIV infection, nor does it reduce risk of transmission to others, and illnesses, including opportunistic infections, may develop.

Check baseline laboratory test results, if ordered, especially liver function test results, before beginning stavudine therapy and at periodic intervals during therapy. Monitor for signs and symptoms of peripheral neuropathy, which is characterized by numbness, pain, or tingling in the feet or hands. Be aware that peripheral neuropathy symptoms resolve promptly if stavudine therapy is discontinued. Also, know that symptoms may worsen temporarily after the drug is withdrawn. If symptoms resolve completely, expect to resume drug therapy at a reduced dosage. Assess for dizziness, headache, muscle or joint aches, myalgia, weight loss, conjunctivitis, nausea, and vomiting. Monitor for evidence of a rash and signs of chills or a fever. Determine sleep pattern and pattern of daily bowel activity and stool consistency.

Storage

Store capsules at room temperature. Reconstitute and dispense the oral solution in original container and keep tightly closed in a refrigerator; do not freeze. Discard any unused portion after 30 days.

Administration

Take without regard to meals. If oral solution is used, it should be shaken vigorously before use. Continue stavudine therapy for the full length of treatment and evenly space doses around the clock.

S

Streptomycin

strep-toe-mye'sin

CATEGORY AND SCHEDULE

Pregnancy Risk Category: D

Classification: Antibiotics, aminoglycosides, antimycobacterials

MECHANISM OF ACTION

An aminoglycoside that binds directly to the 30S ribosomal subunits causing a faulty peptide sequence to form in the protein chain. *Therapeutic effect:* Inhibits bacterial protein synthesis.

AVAILABILITY

Injection: 1 g.

INDICATIONS AND DOSAGES

▸ **Tuberculosis**

IM

Adults. 15 mg/kg/day. Maximum: 1 g/day.

Elderly. 10 mg/kg/day. Maximum: 750 mg/day.

Children. 20-40 mg/kg/day. Maximum: 1 g/day.

NOTE: May also give as directly observed therapy 2-3 times/wk.

Other indications for adults: Brucellosis, endocarditis, *Mycobacterium avium* complex, plague, tularemia, given every 12 h; dose and duration depends on indication.

▸ **Dosage in renal impairment**

Creatinine Clearance (mL/min)	Dosage Interval
10-50	q24-72h
< 10	q72-96h

OFF-LABEL USES

Plague, tularemia, resistant enterococcal endocarditis.

CONTRAINDICATIONS

Hypersensitivity to streptomycin; clinically significant hypersensitivity to other aminoglycosides may contraindicate use due to cross-sensitivity.

INTERACTIONS

Drug

Amphotericin, loop diuretics: May increase the nephrotoxicity of streptomycin.

Neuromuscular blockers: May increase the effects of streptomycin.

Herbal and Food

None known.

DIAGNOSTIC TEST EFFECTS

Increased BUN and serum creatinine may occur.

SIDE EFFECTS

Occasional

Hypotension, drowsiness, headache, drug fever, paresthesia, rash, nausea, vomiting, anemia, arthralgia, weakness, tremor.

SERIOUS REACTIONS

- Nephrotoxicity (as evidenced by increased BUN and serum creatinine levels and decreased creatinine clearance) may be reversible if the drug is stopped at the first sign of nephrotoxic symptoms.
- Irreversible ototoxicity (manifested as tinnitus, dizziness, ringing or roaring in the ears, and impaired hearing) and neurotoxicity (as evidenced by headache, dizziness, lethargy, tremor, and visual disturbances) occur occasionally.

PRECAUTIONS & CONSIDERATIONS

Caution is warranted in patients with tinnitus, vertigo, neuromuscular disorders, and renal impairment. Before giving streptomycin, determine whether hypersensitive to aminoglycosides, pregnant, or being treated for other medical conditions such as myasthenia gravis or parkinsonism. Streptomycin can cause fetal harm (ototoxicity) when administered to a pregnant woman and readily crosses the placental barrier. Discontinuation of breastfeeding is recommended during use. Hearing, renal function, and serum concentrations of streptomycin should be monitored. If symptoms of hearing loss, dizziness, or fullness or roaring in the ears occur, notify the physician.

Storage

Store unopened vials at room temperature protected from light. Reconstituted infusions should also be protected from light.

Administration

For IM use, inject streptomycin deep into a large muscle mass. Be aware that for patients who are unable to tolerate IM injections, streptomycin may be given as an IV infusion over 30-60 min. (Dilute desired dose in at least 100 mL NS.)

Succimer

sux'sim-mer

★ Chemet

CATEGORY AND SCHEDULE

Pregnancy Risk Category: C

Classification: Antidotes, chelators

MECHANISM OF ACTION

An analogue of dimercaprol that forms water-soluble chelates with heavy metals, which are excreted renally. *Therapeutic Effect:* Treats lead intoxication in children.

PHARMACOKINETICS
Rapidly absorbed from the GI tract. Extensively metabolized. Excreted in feces (39%), urine (9%-25%), and lungs (1%). Removed by hemodialysis. *Half-life:* 2 h-2 days.

AVAILABILITY
Capsules: 100 mg (Chemet).

INDICATIONS AND DOSAGES
▸ **Lead poisoning, in pediatric patients with blood lead levels about 45 mcg/dL**

PO

Children 12 mo and older. 10 mg/kg q8h for 5 days, then 10 mg/kg q12h for 14 days. Maximum: 500 mg/dose. Repeat treatment may be needed. Wait 2 wks between courses.

OFF-LABEL USES
Lead poisoning in adults, arsenic intoxication, mercury intoxication.

CONTRAINDICATIONS
Hypersensitivity to succimer or any component of its formulation.

INTERACTIONS
Drug

None known.

Herbal

None known.

Food

None known.

DIAGNOSTIC TEST EFFECTS
May decrease serum creatine phosphokinase and serum uric acid measurements. May cause false-positive results for urinary ketones using nitroprusside reagents such as Ketostix.

SIDE EFFECTS
Occasional

Anorexia, diarrhea, nausea, vomiting, rash, odor to breath and urine, increased liver function tests.

Rare

Neutropenia.

SERIOUS REACTIONS
- Elevated blood lead levels and symptoms of intoxication may occur after succimer therapy because of redistribution of lead from bone to soft tissues and blood.
- Elevated liver function tests have been reported.

PRECAUTIONS & CONSIDERATIONS
Do not use for lead-induced encephalopathy. Use caution in hepatic or renal impairment. It is unknown whether succimer is distributed in breast milk. Safety and efficacy have not been established in children younger than 12 mo. Plasma lead levels should be monitored and kept < 15 mcg/dL.

Sulfurous odor to breath and urine may occur but will subside when succimer is discontinued.

Storage

Store at controlled room temperature and avoid excessive heat.

Administration

Keep in mind that succimer is not a substitute for effective abatement of lead exposure. Capsules may be opened and contents sprinkled onto soft food. Make sure all food is eaten. Capsule contents may also be placed on a spoon and followed by a fruit drink.

Sucralfate
soo-kral'fate

★ Carafate 🍁 Apo-Sucralate, Novo-Sucralate, Sulcrate

Do not confuse Carafate with Cafergot.

CATEGORY AND SCHEDULE
Pregnancy Risk Category: B

Classification: Gastrointestinals, mucosal protectants

S

MECHANISM OF ACTION

An antiulcer agent that forms an ulcer-adherent complex with proteinaceous exudate, such as albumin, at the ulcer site. Also forms a viscous, adhesive barrier on the surface of intact mucosa of the stomach or duodenum. *Therapeutic Effect:* Protects damaged mucosa from further destruction by absorbing gastric acid, pepsin, and bile salts.

PHARMACOKINETICS

Minimally absorbed from the GI tract. Eliminated in feces, with small amount excreted in urine. Not removed by hemodialysis.

AVAILABILITY

Oral Suspension: 500 mg/5 mL.
Tablets: 1 g.

INDICATIONS AND DOSAGES

▸ **Active duodenal ulcers**

PO

Adults, Elderly. 1 g 4 times a day (before meals and at bedtime) for up to 8 wks.

▸ **Maintenance therapy after healing of acute duodenal ulcers**

PO

Adults, Elderly. 1 g twice a day.

OFF-LABEL USES

Prevention and treatment of stress-related mucosal damage, especially in acutely or critically ill patients; treatment of gastric ulcer and treatment of gastroesophageal reflux disease.

CONTRAINDICATIONS

Hypersensitivity.

INTERACTIONS

Drug

Antacids: May interfere with binding of sucralfate.

Tetracyclines, thyroid hormone replacements, digoxin, phenytoin, quinolones, such as ciprofloxacin, theophylline: May decrease the absorption of these drugs. Separate times of administration by at least 2-3 h to avoid interactions.

Herbal

None known.

Food

None known.

DIAGNOSTIC TEST EFFECTS

None known.

SIDE EFFECTS

Frequent (2%)

Constipation.

Occasional (< 2%)

Dry mouth, backache, diarrhea, dizziness, somnolence, nausea, indigestion, rash, hives, itching, abdominal discomfort.

Reports of hyperglycemia with suspension use.

SERIOUS REACTIONS

- Esophageal or intestinal bezoar (very rare).

PRECAUTIONS & CONSIDERATIONS

It is unknown whether sucralfate crosses the placenta or is distributed in breast milk. Safety and efficacy of sucralfate have not been established in children. No age-related precautions have been noted in elderly patients.

Dry mouth may occur, so take sips of tepid water or suck on sour hard candy to relieve it. Before sucralfate administration, the abdomen should be assessed for signs of tenderness, rigidity, and the presence of bowel sounds. Pattern of daily bowel activity and stool consistency should be monitored throughout therapy.

Storage
Store at room temperature; protect tablets from moisture to avoid crumbling.
Administration
! 1 g equals 10 mL suspension.
Shake suspension well before each use.
Take 1 h before meals on an empty stomach and at bedtime. Tablets may be crushed or dissolved in water. Do not take antacids within 30 min of sucralfate.

Sulfacetamide

sul-fa-see′ta-mide
★ Bleph-10, Carmol, Klaron, Mexar, Ovace 🍁 Ak-Sulf, Bleph-10, Diosulf, Sodium Sulamyd

CATEGORY AND SCHEDULE

Pregnancy Risk Category: C

Classification: Anti-infectives, ophthalmics, antibiotics, sulfonamides

MECHANISM OF ACTION

Interferes with synthesis of folic acid that bacteria require for growth. *Therapeutic Effect:* Prevents further bacterial growth. Bacteriostatic.

PHARMACOKINETICS

Small amounts may be absorbed into the cornea. Excreted rapidly in urine. *Half-life:* 7-13 h.

AVAILABILITY

Lotion: 10% (Carmol, Klaron, Ovace).
Ophthalmic Ointment: 10%.
Ophthalmic Solution: 10% (Bleph-10).
Shampoo, Topical Gel, Topical Foam, Topical Solutions, Soaps: 10%.

INDICATIONS AND DOSAGES

▸ **Treatment of corneal ulcers, conjunctivitis, and other superficial infections of the eye, prophylaxis after injuries to the eye/removal of foreign bodies, adjunctive therapy for trachoma and inclusion conjunctivitis**
OPHTHALMIC
Adults, Elderly. Ointment: Apply small amount in lower conjunctival sac 1-4 times/day and at bedtime. Solution: 1-3 drops to lower conjunctival sac q2-3h.
▸ **Seborrheic dermatitis, seborrheic sicca (dandruff), secondary bacterial skin infections**
TOPICAL
Adults, Elderly. Apply 1-4 times/day.

OFF-LABEL USES

Treatment of bacterial blepharitis, blepharoconjunctivitis, bacterial keratitis, keratoconjunctivitis.

CONTRAINDICATIONS

Hypersensitivity to sulfonamides or any component of preparation (some products contain sulfite), use in combination with silver-containing products.

INTERACTIONS

Drug
Silver-containing preparations: These products are incompatible together.
Herbal
None known.
Food
None known.

DIAGNOSTIC TEST EFFECTS

None known.

SIDE EFFECTS

Frequent
Transient ophthalmic burning, stinging. Eye ointment causes temporary blurred vision.

Occasional
Headache.
Rare
Hypersensitivity (erythema, rash, itching, swelling, photosensitivity).

SERIOUS REACTIONS

- Superinfection, drug-induced lupus erythematosus, Stevens-Johnson syndrome occur rarely; nephrotoxicity with high systemic absorption (very rare).

PRECAUTIONS & CONSIDERATIONS

Caution should be used with extremely dry eye. It is unknown if whether sulfacetamide crosses the placenta or is distributed in breast milk. Do not use sulfacetamide during the third trimester of pregnancy. Safety and efficacy of sulfacetamide have not been established in children 2 mo or younger. No age-related precautions have been noted in elderly patients. Be aware that sulfacetamide application of lotion to large infected, denuded, or debrided areas should be avoided.

Sulfacetamide may cause sensitivity to light. Sunglasses should be worn and avoid bright light.

Storage
Store at room temperature and protect from light. Discolored solution should not be used.

Administration
For ophthalmic use, tilt the head back. Place solution in conjunctival sac. Close eyes, and then press gently on the lacrimal sac for 1 min. Wait at least 10 min before using another eye preparation.

For topical treatment, cleanse area before application to ensure direct contact with affected area. Apply at bedtime and allow to remain overnight.

Sulfasalazine

sul-fa-sal′a-zeen
★ Azulfidine, Azulfidine EN-tabs, Sulfazine EC 🍁 Salazopyrin, Salazopyrin EN-Tabs
Do not confuse Azulfidine with azathioprine, sulfasalazine with sulfadiazine, or sulfisoxazole.

CATEGORY AND SCHEDULE

Pregnancy Risk Category: B (D if given near term)

Classification: Disease-modifying antirheumatic drugs, gastrointestinals, 5-aminosalicylates

MECHANISM OF ACTION

A sulfonamide that inhibits prostaglandin synthesis, acting locally in the colon. *Therapeutic Effect:* Decreases inflammatory response, interferes with GI secretion.

PHARMACOKINETICS

Poorly absorbed from the GI tract. Cleaved in colon by intestinal bacteria, forming sulfapyridine and mesalamine (5-ASA). Absorbed in colon. Widely distributed. Metabolized in the liver. Primarily excreted in urine. *Half-life:* sulfapyridine, 6-14 h; 5-ASA, 0.6-1.4 h.

AVAILABILITY

Tablets (Azulfidine): 500 mg.
Tablets (Delayed Release [Azulfidine EN-tabs, Sulfazine EC]): 500 mg.

INDICATIONS AND DOSAGES

▸ **Ulcerative colitis**
PO
Adults, Elderly. 1 g 3-4 times a day in divided doses q6-8h.

Maintenance: 2 g/day in divided doses q6-8h. Maximum: 4 g/day.
Children > 6 yr. 40-60 mg/kg/day in divided doses q4-6h. Maintenance: 30 mg/kg/day in divided doses q6h. Maximum: 2 g/day.

▸ **Rheumatoid arthritis**

PO

Adults, Elderly. Initially, 0.5-1 g/day for 1 wk. Increase by 0.5 g/wk, up to 2 g/day in divided doses.

▸ **Juvenile rheumatoid arthritis**

PO

Children > 6 yr. Initially, 10 mg/kg/day. May increase by 10 mg/kg/day at weekly intervals. Range: 30-50 mg/kg/day. Maximum: 2 g/day.

OFF-LABEL USES

Treatment of ankylosing spondylitis, Crohn disease with colonic involvement.

CONTRAINDICATIONS

Intestinal or urinary obstruction; porphyria; hypersensitivity to sulfasalazine, its metabolites, other 5-aminosalicylates, sulfonamides, or salicylates.

INTERACTIONS

Drug

Anticonvulsants, methotrexate, oral anticoagulants, oral antidiabetics: May increase the effects of these drugs.

Hemolytics: May increase the toxicity of sulfasalazine.

Hepatotoxic medications: May increase the risk of hepatotoxicity.

Thioguanine or 6-mercaptopurine: 5-Aminosalicylates may increase sensitivity to myelosuppressive effects.

Herbal

None known.

Food

None known.

DIAGNOSTIC TEST EFFECTS

None known.

SIDE EFFECTS

Frequent (33%)

Anorexia, nausea, vomiting, headache, oligospermia (generally reversed by withdrawal of drug).

Occasional (3%)

Hypersensitivity reaction (rash, urticaria, pruritus, fever, anemia).

Rare (< 1%)

Tinnitus, hypoglycemia, diuresis, photosensitivity.

SERIOUS REACTIONS

- Anaphylaxis, Stevens-Johnson syndrome, hematologic toxicity (leukopenia, agranulocytosis), hepatotoxicity, and nephrotoxicity occur rarely.

PRECAUTIONS & CONSIDERATIONS

Caution is warranted with bronchial asthma, G6PD deficiency, blood dyscrasia, impaired hepatic or renal function, or severe allergies. Sulfasalazine may produce infertility and oligospermia in men. Sulfasalazine readily crosses the placenta and is excreted in breast milk. Lactating patients should not breastfeed premature infants or those with hyperbilirubinemia or G6PD deficiency. If given near term, sulfasalazine may produce hemolytic anemia, jaundice, and kernicterus in the newborn. No age-related precautions have been noted in children older than 6 yr or elderly patients. Avoid the sun and ultraviolet light; photosensitivity may last for months after the last dose of sulfasalazine.

Adequate hydration should be maintained (minimum output 1500 mL/24 h) and to prevent nephrotoxicity. Skin should be examined for rash; withhold the drug at the first sign of a rash. Pattern of daily bowel activity and stool consistency should be monitored; drug dosage may need to be increased if disease symptoms are not controlled. Report hematologic effects such as bleeding, ecchymosis, fever, jaundice, pallor, purpura, pharyngitis, and weakness.

Storage

Store at room temperature; avoid excessive heat exposure.

Administration

Space drug doses evenly at intervals not to exceed 8 h. Administer sulfasalazine after meals, if possible, to prolong intestinal passage. Swallow delayed-release tablets whole without chewing or crushing them. Take the drug with 8 oz of water.

Sulindac

sul-in'dak

★ Clinoril 🍁 Apo-Sulin, Novo Sundac

Do not confuse Clinoril with Clozaril.

CATEGORY AND SCHEDULE

Pregnancy Risk Category: C (D if used in third trimester or near delivery)

Classification: Analgesics, nonsteroidal anti-inflammatory drugs (NSAID)

MECHANISM OF ACTION

An NSAID that produces analgesic and anti-inflammatory effects by inhibiting prostaglandin synthesis. *Therapeutic Effect:* Reduces inflammatory response and intensity of pain.

PHARMACOKINETICS

Route	Onset	Peak	Duration
PO (antirheumatic)	7 days	2-3 wks	NA

Well absorbed from the GI tract. Metabolized in liver to active metabolite. Primarily excreted in urine. Not removed by hemodialysis. *Half-life:* 7.8 h; metabolite: 16.4 h.

AVAILABILITY

Tablets: 150 mg, 200 mg.

INDICATIONS AND DOSAGES

▸ **Rheumatoid arthritis, osteoarthritis, ankylosing spondylitis**

PO

Adults, Elderly. Initially, 150 mg twice a day; may increase up to maximum 400 mg/day.

▸ **Acute shoulder pain, gouty arthritis, bursitis, tendinitis**

PO

Adults, Elderly. 200 mg twice a day. Usually 7-14 days.

CONTRAINDICATIONS

Active peptic ulcer disease, chronic inflammation of the GI tract, GI bleeding or ulceration, history of hypersensitivity to aspirin or NSAIDs, within 14 days of coronary artery bypass graft (CABG) surgery.

INTERACTIONS

Drug

Antihypertensives, diuretics: May decrease the effects of antihypertensives and diuretics.

Aspirin, salicylates, corticosteroids: May increase the risk of GI bleeding and side effects. NSAIDs may negate the cardioprotective effect of ASA.

Cyclosporine: May increase risk of nephrotoxicity.

Heparin, oral anticoagulants, thrombolytics: May increase the effects of heparin, oral anticoagulants, and thrombolytics.
Lithium: May increase the blood concentration and risk of toxicity of lithium.
Methotrexate, pemetrexed: May increase the risk of toxicity with methotrexate or pemetrexed.
Herbal
Feverfew: May increase the risk of bleeding.
Ginkgo biloba: May increase the risk of bleeding.
Food
Alcohol: May increase risk of dizziness, GI bleeding.

DIAGNOSTIC TEST EFFECTS

May increase liver function test results and serum alkaline phosphatase level.

SIDE EFFECTS

Frequent (4%-9%)
Diarrhea or constipation, indigestion, nausea, maculopapular rash, dermatitis, dizziness, headache.
Occasional (1%-3%)
Anorexia, abdominal cramps, flatulence.

SERIOUS REACTIONS

- NSAID-induced peptic ulcer, GI bleeding, gastritis.
- Rare reactions include cholestatis, jaundice, nephrotoxicity, hematologic sensitivity (e.g., leukopenia).
- Severe hypersensitivity reaction (bronchopasm) possible.

PRECAUTIONS & CONSIDERATIONS

Cardiovascular event risk may be increased with duration of use of preexisting cardiovascular risk factors or disease. Use caution in patients with fluid retention, heart failure, or hypertension. Risk of myocardial infarction and stroke may be increased following CABG surgery. Do not administer within 4-6 half-lives before surgical procedures.

Caution is warranted in patients with a history of GI tract disease, hepatic or renal impairment, a predisposition to fluid retention, and concurrent use of anticoagulant therapy. It is unknown whether sulindac is excreted in breast milk. Sulindac should not be used during the third trimester of pregnancy because it might cause adverse effects in the fetus, such as premature closure of the ductus arteriosus. Use with caution during lactation. This medicine is not approved for use in children. The elderly may be more susceptible to GI and CNS side effects. Alertness or motor skills should also be avoided until effects are known.

CBC, especially platelet count, skin for rash, and liver and renal function test results should be assessed before and periodically during therapy. Therapeutic response, such as decreased pain, stiffness, swelling, and tenderness; improved grip strength; and increased joint mobility, should be evaluated.
Storage
Store tablets at room temperature.
Administration
Take sulindac orally with food, milk, or antacids if GI distress occurs. Therapeutic antiarthritic effect will occur 1-3 wks after therapy begins.

Sumatriptan

soo-ma-trip′tan

★ Alsuma Autoinjector, Imitrex

🍁 Imitrex, Imitrex DF

Do not confuse sumatriptan with somatropin.

CATEGORY AND SCHEDULE

Pregnancy Risk Category: C

Classification: Migraine agents, serotonin receptor agonists

MECHANISM OF ACTION

A serotonin receptor agonist that binds selectively to vascular receptors, producing a vasoconstrictive effect on cranial blood vessels. *Therapeutic Effect:* Relieves migraine headache.

PHARMACOKINETICS

Route	Onset (min)	Peak (h)	Duration (h)
Nasal	15-30	NA	24-48
PO	30	2	24-48
SC	10	1	24-48

Rapidly absorbed after SC administration. Absorption after PO administration is incomplete, with significant amounts undergoing hepatic metabolism, resulting in low bioavailability (about 14%). Protein binding: 10%-21%. Widely distributed. Undergoes first-pass metabolism in the liver. Excreted in urine. *Half-life:* 2 h.

AVAILABILITY

Tablets: 25 mg, 50 mg, 100 mg.
Injection: 6 mg/0.5 mL.
Nasal Spray: 5 mg/spray, 20 mg/spray.

INDICATIONS AND DOSAGES

▸ **Acute migraine attack**

PO

Adults. 25-100 mg. Dose may be repeated after at least 2 h. Maximum: 100 mg/single dose;
200 mg/24 h.

SC

Adults. 6 mg. Maximum: Two 6-mg injections/24 h (separated by at least 1 h).

INTRANASAL

Adults. 5 or 10 mg (1 or 2 sprays) into 1 nostril as a single dose or 20 mg into 1 nostril as a single dose. Maximum: 40 mg/24 h.

CONTRAINDICATIONS

Basilar or hemiplegic migraine, cerebrovascular accident, ischemic heart disease (including angina pectoris, history of myocardial infarction [MI], silent ischemia, and Prinzmetal angina), severe hepatic impairment, transient ischemic attack, peripheral vascular disease, uncontrolled hypertension, use within 14 days of MAOIs, use within 24 h of ergotamine preparations or other "triptans."

INTERACTIONS

Drug

Ergotamine-containing medications: May produce vasospastic reaction.

MAOIs: May increase sumatriptan blood concentration and half-life. Contraindicated.

Serotonin agonists, linezolid, SSRI, or SNRI antidepressants: May increase risk of serotonin syndrome. Do not use other "triptans" or ergot preparations within 24 h.

Herbal

St. John's wort: May increase serotonergic effects. Avoid.

Food

None known.

DIAGNOSTIC TEST EFFECTS

None known.

S

SIDE EFFECTS

Frequent

Oral (5%-10%): Tingling, nasal discomfort.

SC (> 10%): Injection site reactions, tingling, warm or hot sensation, dizziness, vertigo.

Nasal (> 10%): Bad or unusual taste, nausea, vomiting.

Occasional

Oral (1%-5%): Flushing, asthenia, visual disturbances.

Subcutaneous (2%-10%): Burning sensation, numbness, chest discomfort, drowsiness, asthenia.

Nasal (1%-5%): Nasopharyngeal discomfort, dizziness.

Rare

Oral (< 1%): Agitation, eye irritation, dysuria.

Subcutaneous (< 2%): Anxiety, fatigue, diaphoresis, muscle cramps, myalgia.

Nasal (< 1%): Burning sensation.

SERIOUS REACTIONS

- Excessive dosage may produce tremor, red extremities, reduced respirations, cyanosis, seizures, and paralysis.
- Peripheral vascular ischemia, colonic ischemia, or ocular ischemia with transient or significant partial vision loss occurs rarely.
- Hypertensive crisis.
- Rare serious hypersensitivity reactions.
- Serious arrhythmias occur rarely, especially in patients with hypertension, diabetes, or a strong family history of coronary artery disease; obese patients; and smokers.

PRECAUTIONS & CONSIDERATIONS

Caution is warranted in patients with epilepsy, a hypersensitivity to sumatriptan, and hepatic or renal impairment. Use in pregnancy not recommended unless benefits outweigh risks. It is unknown whether sumatriptan is distributed in breast milk. The safety and efficacy of sumatriptan have not been established in children. Use in the elderly not recommended.

Dizziness may occur. Notify the physician immediately if palpitations, a rash, wheezing, pain or tightness in the chest or throat, or facial edema occurs. ECG should be obtained at baseline. Migraines and associated symptoms, including nausea and vomiting, photophobia, and phonophobia (sound sensitivity), should be assessed before and during treatment.

Storage

Store tablets, nasal spray, injections at room temperature and protect from light. Do not refrigerate injection or nasal spray.

Administration

Swallow oral tablets whole with a full glass of water.

Expect to administer first SC dosage in physician's office if patient has identifiable cardiovascular risk factors. Never give intravenously because this drug may precipitate coronary vasospasm. Patients using autoinjector should be thoroughly instructed in autoinjection technique.

For SC use, follow the manufacturer's instructions for using the autoinjection device. Inject the drug into an area with adequate SC tissue because the needle will penetrate the skin and adipose tissue as deeply as 6 mm. Do not administer more than 2 SC injections during any 24-h period and allow at least 1 h between injections. After injecting the medication, discard the syringe.

For nasal use, each unit contains only one spray, so do not test the spray before use. Blow the nose gently to clear nasal passages. With the head upright, close one of the nostrils with an index finger and breathe gently through the mouth. Insert the nozzle about ½ inch into the open nostril. Close mouth, then breathe through the nose while depressing the blue plunger and releasing the spray. Remove the nozzle from the nose, and gently breathe in through the nose and out through the mouth for 10-20 seconds. Do not breathe in deeply.

Sunitinib

sue-ni'ti-nib

Sutent

Do not confuse with sorafenib.

CATEGORY AND SCHEDULE

Pregnancy Risk Category: D

Classification:

Antineoplastics, biologic agents, signal transduction inhibitor

MECHANISM OF ACTION

An oral multikinase inhibitor. The drug inhibits platelet-derived growth factor receptors (PDGFR-α and PDGFR-β), vascular endothelial growth factor receptors (VEGFR-1, VEGFR-2 and VEGFR-3), stem cell factor receptor (Kit), Fms-like tyrosine kinase-3 (FLT-3), colony-stimulating factor receptor Type 1 (CSF-1R), and the glial cell-line derived neurotrophic factor receptor (RET). Several of these kinases are thought to be involved in tumor cell signaling, angiogenesis, and apoptosis. *Therapeutic Effect:* Inhibits tumor growth.

PHARMACOKINETICS

Food decreases oral absorption. Protein binding: 95%. Sunitinib is metabolized in the liver by CYP 3A4. The active metabolite is also metabolized by CYP3A4. Most (61%) of the dose is excreted in the feces and 16% excreted in the urine. *Half-life:* 40-60 h (parent); 80-110 h (metabolite).

AVAILABILITY

Capsules: 12.5 mg, 25 mg, 50 mg.

INDICATIONS AND DOSAGES

▸ **Advanced renal cell cancer or gastrointestinal stromal tumor (GIST)**

PO

Adults, Elderly. 50 mg once daily for 4 wks on treatment, followed by 2 wks off.

▸ **Dosage adjustment if strong CYP3A4 inhibitors used**

Reduce dose to 37.5 mg once daily if an alternate to the CYP3A4 inhibitor cannot be chosen.

▸ **Dosage adjustment for toxicity**

Management of side effects may require temporary interruption and/or dose reduction. Dose may be adjusted by 12.5 mg up or down as required and tolerated.

CONTRAINDICATIONS

Hypersensitivity.

INTERACTIONS

Drug

CYP3A4 inhibitors (e.g., ketoconazole, nefazodone, clarithromycin, itraconazole, protease inhibitors for HIV): Sunitinib levels may increase. Reduce dose if alternate treatment not available.

CYP3A4 inducers (e.g., rifampin, phenytoin, carbamazepine, phenobarbital): May increase metabolism of sunitinib and thus decrease sunitinib concentrations; may need dose increase. A maximum of 87.5 mg daily of sunitinib should be considered; the patient

S

should be monitored carefully for toxicity.
QT-prolonging agents (e.g., class Ia and III antiarrhythmics): May have additive effects on QT interval; use caution.
Warfarin: Sunitinib is a competitive inhibitor of CYP2C9 and could possibly alter warfarin response; also independently increases INR; monitor INR.
Herbal
St. John's wort: May increase metabolism of sunitinib and thus decrease sunitinib concentrations; avoid.
Food
Grapefruit juice: Might increase sunitinib levels; avoid.

DIAGNOSTIC TEST EFFECTS

Decreased WBC, platelets. Increased INR, liver enzymes, serum creatinine, amylase, or lipase. Changes in TSH. Electrolyte abnormalities, QT prolongation (rare).

SIDE EFFECTS

Frequent (> 20%)
Fatigue, asthenia, fever, diarrhea, nausea, mucositis/stomatitis, vomiting, dyspepsia, abdominal pain, constipation, hypertension, peripheral edema, rash, hand-foot syndrome, skin discoloration, dry skin, hair color changes, hypothyroidism, altered taste, headache, back pain, arthralgia, extremity pain, cough, dyspnea, anorexia, and bleeding.
Occasional
Chest pain, proteinuria, myalgia, depression, hoarseness, skin erythema or peeling.
Rare
Hypertension, difficult wound healing.

SERIOUS REACTIONS

• Serious hypersensitivity reactions occur rarely, and may include angioedema.
• Leukopenia, thrombocytopenia.
• Severe and fatal hepatotoxicity.
• Adrenal toxicity.
• Serious bleeding (CNS, gastrointestinal, hemoptysis, etc.) or GI perforations.
• Chest pain may indicate cardiac ischemia or infarction and requires prompt evaluation.
• Heart failure and QT prolongation are other potentially serious cardiac effects.

PRECAUTIONS & CONSIDERATIONS

Use with caution in patients with hepatic disease, high blood pressure, cardiac disease, heart failure or arrhythmia, a history of stroke, GI disease with GI bleeding in the past 6 months or a history of GI perforation or fistula, thyroid disease, had recent surgery or scheduled for surgery. Do not use in patients who are pregnant or planning to become pregnant; the drug can cause fetal harm. Women of childbearing potential should be advised to avoid becoming pregnant, and both males and females should use adequate birth control during treatment. It is not known if sunitinib passes into breast milk; do not breastfeed while taking this medication. This drug has not been approved for use in children.
Storage
Store at room temperature; protect from moisture.
Administration
Administer sunitinib orally without regard to food or timing of meals. Do not take with grapefruit juice. Treatment is continued until clinical benefit no longer realized, or unacceptable toxicity occurs.

Tacrolimus

tak-roe-leem'us

★ Prograf, Protopic 🍁 Advagraf, Prograf, Protopic

Do not confuse Protopic with Protonix, Protopam, Protopin.

CATEGORY AND SCHEDULE

Pregnancy Risk Category: C

Classification:

Immunosuppressives, organ transplant agents, topical dermatologics

MECHANISM OF ACTION

An immunologic agent that inhibits T-lymphocyte activation by binding to intracellular proteins, forming a complex, and inhibiting phosphatase activity. *Therapeutic Effect:* Suppresses the immunologically mediated inflammatory response; prevents organ transplant rejection and controls inflammatory skin disorders.

PHARMACOKINETICS

Variably absorbed after PO administration (food reduces absorption). There is some systemic absorption with topical use, but the drug does not accumulate. Protein binding: 75%-97%. Extensively metabolized in the liver. Excreted in urine. Not removed by hemodialysis. *Half-life:* 11.7 h.

AVAILABILITY

Capsules (Prograf): 0.5 mg, 1 mg, 5 mg.
Injection (Prograf): 5 mg/mL.
Ointment (Protopic): 0.03%, 0.1%.

INDICATIONS AND DOSAGES

▸ **Prevention of liver transplant rejection**

PO

Adults, Elderly. 0.1-0.15 mg/kg/day in 2 divided doses 12 h apart.
Children. 0.15-0.2 mg/kg/day in 2 divided doses 12 h apart.

IV

Adults, Elderly, Children. 0.03-0.05 mg/kg/day as a continuous infusion.

▸ **Prevention of kidney transplant rejection**

PO

Adults, Elderly. 0.2 mg/kg/day in 2 divided doses 12 h apart.

IV

Adults, Elderly. 0.03-0.05 mg/kg/day as continuous infusion.

▸ **Atopic dermatitis**

TOPICAL

Adults, Elderly, Children 2 yr and older. Apply 0.03% ointment to affected area twice a day; 0.1% ointment may be used in adolescents >15 yr, adults, and elderly patients. Continue until 1 wk after symptoms have cleared.

OFF-LABEL USES

Prevention of organ rejection in patients receiving allogeneic bone marrow, heart, pancreas, pancreatic island cell, or small-bowel transplant; treatment of autoimmune disease; severe recalcitrant psoriasis.

CONTRAINDICATIONS

Concurrent use with cyclosporine (increases the risk of nephrotoxicity), hypersensitivity to HCO-60 polyoxyl 60 hydrogenated castor oil (used in solution for injection), hypersensitivity to tacrolimus.

INTERACTIONS

Drug

Aminoglycosides, amphotericin B, cisplatin: Increase the risk of renal dysfunction.
Antacids: Decrease the absorption of tacrolimus.

Antifungals, bromocriptine, calcium channel blockers, cimetidine, clarithromycin, cyclosporine, danazol, diltiazem, erythromycin, methylprednisolone, metoclopramide, voriconazole: Increase tacrolimus blood concentration.
Carbamazepine, phenobarbital, phenytoin, rifamycin: Decrease tacrolimus blood concentration.
Cyclosporine: Increases the risk of nephrotoxicity. Do not use within 24 h of each other.
Live-virus vaccines: May potentiate virus replication, increase vaccine side effects, and decrease the patient's antibody response to the vaccine.
Other immunosuppressants: May increase the risk of infection or lymphomas.
Herbal
St. John's wort, echinacea: May decrease the effects of tacrolimus.
Food
Grapefruit, grapefruit juice: May alter the effects of the drug.
High-fat food: May decrease the absorption.

DIAGNOSTIC TEST EFFECTS
May increase blood glucose, BUN, and serum creatinine levels, as well as WBC count. May decrease serum magnesium level and RBC and thrombocyte counts. May alter serum potassium level.

IV INCOMPATIBILITIES
Do not mix tacrolimus with other medications.

IV COMPATIBILITIES
Calcium gluconate, dexamethasone (Decadron), diphenhydramine (Benadryl), dobutamine (Dobutrex), dopamine (Intropin), furosemide (Lasix), heparin, hydromorphone (Dilaudid), insulin, leucovorin, lorazepam (Ativan), morphine, nitroglycerin, potassium chloride.

SIDE EFFECTS
Frequent (> 30%)
Headache, tremor, insomnia, paresthesia, diarrhea, nausea, constipation, vomiting, abdominal pain, hypertension.
Occasional (10%-29%)
Rash, pruritus, anorexia, asthenia, peripheral edema, photosensitivity.

SERIOUS REACTIONS
- Nephrotoxicity (characterized by increased serum creatinine level and decreased urine output), neurotoxicity (including tremor, headache, and mental status changes), and pleural effusion are common adverse reactions.
- Thrombocytopenia, leukocytosis, anemia, atelectasis, sepsis, and infection occur occasionally.
- Rare cases of malignancy (e.g., nonmelanoma skin cancers and lymphoma) have been reported, even with topical use.
- Post-transplant diabetes mellitus.

PRECAUTIONS & CONSIDERATIONS
Caution is warranted in patients with immunosuppression and hepatic or renal impairment. Tacrolimus crosses the placenta and is distributed in breast milk. Women taking this drug should not breastfeed. Hyperkalemia and renal dysfunction have been noted in neonates. Post-transplant lymphoproliferative disorder is more common in children, especially children younger than 3 yr. Do not use topical form in children under 2 yr of age. Age-related renal impairment may require a dosage adjustment in elderly patients. Avoid crowds and

people with infection. Also avoid exposure to sunlight and artificial light because these may cause a photosensitivity reaction.

Notify the physician of change in mental status, chest pain, dizziness, headache, decreased urination, rash, respiratory infection, or unusual bleeding or bruising. CBC should be monitored weekly during the first month of therapy, twice monthly during the second and third months of treatment, then monthly for the rest of the first year. Liver function test results and serum creatinine and potassium levels should also be assessed.

Storage

Store capsules and unopened vials at room temperature. Avoid exposure of all products to extremes of heat or cold; do not freeze.

Store the diluted infusion in a glass or polyethylene containers and discard after 24 h. Do not store it in a polyvinyl chloride container because the container may absorb the drug or affect its stability.

Administration

! If unable to take capsules, initiate therapy with IV infusion. Give oral dose 8-12 h after discontinuing IV infusion. Titrate dosage based on clinical assessments of rejection and tolerance. With hepatic or renal impairment, give the lowest IV and oral doses, as prescribed. Plan to delay administration for 48 h or longer with postoperative oliguria.

Take oral tacrolimus on an empty stomach at the same time each day. If GI intolerance occurs, be consistent with taking oral tacrolimus with regard to timing and type of meal. Notify the physician if a dose is missed. Do not give this drug with grapefruit or grapefruit juice or within 2 h of antacids.

Keep oxygen and an aqueous solution of epinephrine 1:1000 available at the bedside before beginning the IV infusion. Dilute the drug with 250-1000 mL 0.9% NaCl or D5W, depending on the desired dose, to provide a concentration of 4-20 mcg/mL. Administer tacrolimus as a continuous IV infusion. Monitor continuously for the first 30 min of the infusion and at frequent intervals thereafter. Stop the infusion immediately at the first sign of a hypersensitivity reaction.

Tacrolimus ointment is for external use only. Rub the ointment gently and completely into clean, dry skin. Do not cover the treated area with an occlusive dressing.

Tadalafil

ta-dal'a-fil

★ 🍁 Adcirca, Cialis

CATEGORY AND SCHEDULE

Pregnancy Risk Category: B

Classification: Erectile dysfunction agents, pulmonary vasodialtors, phosphodiesterase-5 enzyme inhibitors

MECHANISM OF ACTION

An agent that inhibits phosphodiesterase type 5, the enzyme responsible for degrading cyclic guanosine monophosphate (cGMP) in the corpus cavernosum of the penis or the smooth muscle of pulmonary vasculature, resulting in smooth muscle relaxation and increased blood flow. *Therapeutic Effect:* Facilitates an erection in ED. In PAH, results in vasodilation in pulmonary vasculature.

PHARMACOKINETICS

Route	Onset	Peak	Duration
PO	16 min	2 h	36 h

Rapidly absorbed after PO administration. Drug has no effect on penile blood flow without sexual stimulation. Metabolized in liver to inactive metabolites. *Half-life:* 17.5 h. Excreted in feces and urine.

AVAILABILITY

Tablets (Cialis): 2.5 mg, 5 mg, 10 mg.
Tablets (Adcirca): 20 mg.

INDICATIONS AND DOSAGES

▸ **Erectile dysfunction**

PO

Adults, Elderly. 10 mg 30 min before sexual activity. Dose may be increased to 20 mg or decreased to 5 mg, based on patient tolerance. Daily treatment as 2.5 mg once daily is also an option. Dose may be increased to 5 mg based on patient tolerance. Maximum dosing frequency is once daily.

▸ **Dosage for ED in renal impairment**

CrCl 31-50 mL/min: Initially, 5 mg before sexual activity once a day. Maximum is 10 mg no more frequently than once q48h. CrCl ≤ 30 mL/min: 5 mg before sexual activity given not more than q72h.

▸ **Dosage for ED in mild or moderate hepatic impairment (Child-Pugh class A or B)**

Limit dose to 10 mg once a day.

▸ **Dosage for ED (only) with concurrent inhibitors of CYP3A4**

PO

Adults. For use "as needed": Maximum recommended dose is 10 mg given once q 72 h.
For once daily use: Do not exceed 2.5 mg once daily.

▸ **Pulmonary arterial hypertension (PAH)**

PO (ADCIRCA)

Adults, Elderly. 40 mg (two 20-mg tablets) once daily.

▸ **Dosage for PAH in renal impairment**

CrCl 31-80 mL/min: 20 mg/day initially, and cautiously increase to 40 mg/day if needed/tolerated. CrCl of ≤ 30 mL/min: Avoid use for PAH.

▸ **Dosage for PAH in mild or moderate hepatic impairment (Child-Pugh class A or B)**

Limit dose to 20 mg once a day.

CONTRAINDICATIONS

Hypersensitivity to tadalafil, concurrent use of sodium nitroprusside or nitrates in any form, severe hepatic impairment.

INTERACTIONS

Drug

α-Adrenergic blockers, nitrates: Potentiate the hypotensive effects of these drugs. Tadalafil contraindicated in patients receiving nitrates.
α-Blockers (e.g., doxazosin): May produce additive hypotensive effects.
Strong CY3A4 inhibitors (apenavir, atazanavir, azole antifungals, clarithromycin, delavirdine, fosamprenavir, indinavir, isoniazid, nefazodone, nelfinavir, ritonavir, troleandomycin): May increase tadalafil blood concentration. Use requires dose adjustments for ED; do not use strong inhibitors with tadalafil for PAH.
Strong CY3A4 inducers (e.g., rifampin): Lowers tadalafil levels. Avoid use when tadalafil prescribed for PAH.

Herbal

St. John's wort: May decrease tadalafil levels.

Food

Alcohol: Increases the risk of orthostatic hypotension.

DIAGNOSTIC TEST EFFECTS
None known.

SIDE EFFECTS
Frequent
The most common effect is headache.
Occasional
Dyspepsia, back pain, myalgia, nasal congestion, flushing.
Rare
Dizziness, rash.

SERIOUS REACTIONS
- Prolonged erections (lasting over 4 h) and priapism (painful erections lasting over 6 h) occur rarely.
- Decreased eyesight or loss of sight.
- Sudden decrease or loss of hearing.
- Heart attack, stroke, irregular heartbeats.

PRECAUTIONS & CONSIDERATIONS
Caution is warranted in patients with an anatomic deformity of the penis; cardiac, hepatic, or renal impairment; and conditions that increase the risk of priapism, including leukemia, multiple myeloma, and sickle cell anemia. Certain underlying conditions (e.g., cardiovascular disease, impaired autonomic control of blood pressure, aortic stenosis) could be adversely affected by vasodilatory effects of tadalafil. Not recommended in patients with pulmonary venoocclusive disease. No age-related precautions have been noted in elderly patients. This drug is not indicated for use in women and children. Seek treatment immediately if an erection lasts longer than 4 h.
Storage
Store tablets at room temperature.
Administration
Take tadalafil without regard to food. When used as needed for ED, take at least 30 min before sexual activity. When taken on a daily basis, tadalafil should be taken at the same time every day without regard to sexual activity.

When tadalafil (Adcirca) is used for PAH, administer doses once daily; do not divide dosing.

Talc Powder, Sterile
★ Sclerosol

CATEGORY AND SCHEDULE
Pregnancy Risk Category: B

Classification: Sclerosing agents

MECHANISM OF ACTION
A sclerosing agent that induces inflammatory reaction. *Therapeutic Effect:* Obliterates the pleural space and prevents reaccumulation of pleural fluid.

PHARMACOKINETICS
Systemic absorption after intrapleural administration has not been studied.

AVAILABILITY
Aerosol Spray, Intrapleural: 4 g (Sclerosol).

INDICATIONS AND DOSAGES
▸ **Pleural effusions**
AEROSOL
Adults. 4-8 g as single treatment.

CONTRAINDICATIONS
Sensitivity to talc powder or any component of the formulation.

INTERACTIONS
Drug
None known.
Herbal
None known.

Food
None known.

DIAGNOSTIC TEST EFFECTS
None known.

SIDE EFFECTS
Rare
Pain.

SERIOUS REACTIONS
- Atrial arrhythmias, hypotension, cardiac arrest, chest pain, tachycardia, hypovolemia, asystolic arrest, myocardial infarction, and respiratory complications have been reported.

PRECAUTIONS & CONSIDERATIONS
Be aware that pulmonary complications can occur with talc use. It is unknown whether talc crosses the placenta or is distributed in breast milk. Safety and efficacy have not been established in children. No age-related precautions have been noted in elderly patients.
Storage
Store aerosol at room temperature. Protect from direct sunlight.
Administration
Shake canister well, remove protective cap, and securely attach the actuator button with the selected delivery tube (either 15 or 25 cm long) to the valve stem. The total dose should be administered in several short bursts, given with the delivery tube pointing in different directions. Delivery depends on the extent and duration of manual compression of the actuator button. The canister should be kept in an upright position during administration. The spray valve delivers talc at a rate of approximately 0.4 g/s, but the medication is not delivered as a metered dose.

Tamoxifen
ta-mox'i-fen
Nolvadex Novo-Tamoxifen, Tamofen

CATEGORY AND SCHEDULE
Pregnancy Risk Category: D

Classification: Antineoplastics, antiestrogens, selective estrogen receptor modulator (SERM)

MECHANISM OF ACTION
A nonsteroidal antiestrogen that competes with estradiol for estrogen-receptor binding sites in the breasts, uterus, and vagina. The expression of estrogen-dependent genes (RNA transcription) is altered, mostly in the G2 phase of the cell cycle. Also decreases insulin-like growth factor type 1 (associated with cancer cell growth) and induces transforming growth factor β (TGF-β), which inhibits the activity of breast cancer cells. Induces the reexpression of the tumor suppressor gene maspin in breast cancer tissue. *Therapeutic Effect:* Cytostatic. Decreases breast cancer risk and breast cancer recurrence.

PHARMACOKINETICS
Well absorbed from the GI tract. Protein binding: 99%. Extensively metabolized in the liver by CYP 3A (major), 2C9, and 2D6. Inhibits P-glycoprotein. The main metabolite found in plasma is N-desmethyl tamoxifen, which is active. Drug undergoes some enterohepatic circulation. Parent drug and metabolites are excreted primarily in the feces by the biliary tract, largely as conjugates. *Half-life:* Biphasic elimination 7-14 h (initial) and 5-7 days (terminal). Half-life of main metabolite is about 14 days.

AVAILABILITY
Tablets: 10 mg, 20 mg.

INDICATIONS AND DOSAGES
▸ **Adjunctive treatment of breast cancer**

PO

Adults, Elderly. 20-40 mg/day in divided doses twice daily.

▸ **Metastatic breast cancer (males and females)**

PO

Adults, Elderly. 20-40 mg/day in divided doses twice daily.

▸ **Prevention of breast cancer in high-risk women**

PO

Adults, Elderly. 20 mg/day.

▸ **Ductal carcinoma in situ (DCIS)**

PO

Adults, Elderly. 20 mg/day for 5 yr.

OFF-LABEL USES
Induction of ovulation.

CONTRAINDICATIONS
Hypersensitivity to tamoxifen, pregnancy, concurrent warfarin therapy, history of deep vein thrombosis or pulmonary embolism.

INTERACTIONS
Drug

Anastrozole, letrozole: May decrease the effects of anastrozole. Do not use together.

Bromocriptine: Elevates levels of tamoxifen and active metabolite.

Carbamazepine, phenobarbital, phenytoin, rifampin: May decrease tamoxifen concentrations.

CYP2D6 inhibitors: May decrease tamoxifen effectiveness; use with caution.

Estrogens: Antagonize effects of tamoxifen.

Other cytotoxic agents: May increase thromboembolic risk.

Warfarin: May enhance the anticoagulant effects of warfarin.

Herbal

Black cohosh, dong quai: May increase effects in estrogen-dependent tumors.

St. John's wort: May decrease effects of tamoxifen.

Food

None known.

DIAGNOSTIC TEST EFFECTS
May increase serum cholesterol, calcium, and triglyceride levels. Rarely will cause decreases in platelets or WBC count. T4 elevations due to increases in thyroid-binding globulin, with no clinical hyperthyroidism. Variations in usual vaginal smears and Pap smears are infrequently seen.

SIDE EFFECTS
Frequent

Women (> 10%): Hot flashes, nausea, vomiting, amenorrhea or changes in menstruation.

Occasional

Women (≤ 1%): Genital itching, vaginal discharge, endometrial hyperplasia or polyps.

Men: Impotence, decreased libido.

Men and women: Headache, nausea, vomiting, rash, bone pain, confusion, weakness, somnolence, fluid retention, weight loss, skin changes.

SERIOUS REACTIONS
- Retinopathy, corneal opacity, and decreased visual acuity.
- Very rare reports of serious hypersensitivity (erythema multiforme, Stevens-Johnson syndrome, bullous rash, interstitial pneumonitis, or angioedema).
- Rare reports of pancreatitis associated with increased lipid levels.

T

• Deep venous thrombosis, pulmonary thrombosis, stroke, or cardiac thrombus.
• Potential increased risk of endometrial cancer or uterine sarcoma.

PRECAUTIONS & CONSIDERATIONS

Caution is warranted in patients with leukopenia and thrombocytopenia. Tamoxifen use should be avoided during pregnancy, especially during the first trimester, because it can cause fetal harm. Nonhormonal contraception should be used during treatment. It is unknown whether tamoxifen is distributed in breast milk; however, breastfeeding is not recommended. Tamoxifen use has been studied in girls aged 2-10 yr with McCune-Albright syndrome and precocious puberty. No age-related precautions have been noted in elderly patients.

Initially, an increase in bone and tumor pain may occur, which indicates a good tumor response to tamoxifen. Notify the physician if nausea and vomiting, leg cramps, weakness, weight gain, or vaginal bleeding, itching, or discharge develops. Intake and output, weight, CBC, and serum calcium levels should be monitored before and periodically during tamoxifen therapy. An estrogen receptor assay test should be performed before beginning treatment. Signs and symptoms for hypercalcemia, including constipation, deep bone or flank pain, excessive thirst, hypotonicity of muscles, increased urine output, nausea and vomiting, and renal calculi, should be assessed.

Storage

Store at room temperature. Keep tightly closed.

Administration

Take oral tamoxifen without regard to food.

Tamsulosin

tam-sool'o-sin

★ 🍁 Flomax

Do not confuse Flomax with Fosamax or Volmax.

CATEGORY AND SCHEDULE

Pregnancy Risk Category: B (not indicated for use in women.)

Classification: Urinary tract agents, antiadrenergics, specific peripheral α-blockers

MECHANISM OF ACTION

An α_1 antagonist that targets receptors around the bladder neck and prostate capsule. *Therapeutic Effect:* Relaxes smooth muscle and improves urinary flow and symptoms of prostatic hyperplasia.

PHARMACOKINETICS

Well absorbed and widely distributed. Protein binding: 94%-99%. Metabolized in the liver primarily by CYP3A4 and CYP2D6. Excreted primarily in urine. Unknown whether it is removed by hemodialysis. *Half-life:* 9-13 h.

AVAILABILITY

Capsules: 0.4 mg.

INDICATIONS AND DOSAGES

▸ **Benign prostatic hyperplasia**

PO

Adults. 0.4 mg once a day, approximately 30 min after same meal each day. May increase dosage to 0.8 mg if inadequate response in 2-4 wks.

▸ **Dosage with strong CYP3A4 inhibitors**

Limit dosage to 0.4 mg once daily.

▸ **Severe hepatic impairment**

Do not use.

CONTRAINDICATIONS
History of sensitivity to tamsulosin.

INTERACTIONS
Drug
α-Adrenergic blocking agents (such as doxazosin, prazosin, terazosin): May increase the α-blockade effects of both drugs.
β-Blockers, calcium channel blockers, phosphodiesterase-5 inhibitors: May increase the potential for hypotension.
CYP3A4 inducers: May reduce tamsulosin levels, decrease effect.
CYP3A4 inhibitlors: May increase tamsulosin levels and increase side effects such as hypotension risk; tamsulosin dose adjustment required with strong inhibitors.
Warfarin: May alter the effects of warfarin.
Herbal
Herbs with hypotensive properties (black cohosh, coleus, golden seal, hawthorn, mistletoe, periwinkle, quinine): May increase the potential for hypotension.
Saw palmetto: Unknown whether it will interact but it is recommended to avoid use.
St. John's wort: May decrease tamsulosin's effects.
Food
None known.

DIAGNOSTIC TEST EFFECTS
None known.

SIDE EFFECTS
Frequent (7%-9%)
Dizziness, somnolence.
Occasional (3%-5%)
Headache, anxiety, insomnia, orthostatic hypotension.
Rare (< 2%)
Nasal congestion, pharyngitis, rhinitis, nausea, vertigo, impotence.

SERIOUS REACTIONS
- Severe orthostatic hypotension with syncope may be preceded by tachycardia.
- Rare reports of jaundice, impaired hepatic function, and increased transaminases.
- α-blockers associated with intraoperative floppy iris syndrome during cataract surgery.
- Priapism (very rare).
- Toxic skin eruptions (very rare).

PRECAUTIONS & CONSIDERATIONS
Caution is warranted in patients with hepatic impairment. Tamsulosin is not indicated for use in women or children. No age-related precautions have been noted in elderly patients.

Dizziness and light-headedness may occur. Tasks that require mental alertness or motor skills should be avoided until response to the drug is established. Caution should be used when getting up from a sitting or lying position. BP should be monitored.
Storage
Store capsules at room temperature.
Administration
Take at the same time each day, 30 min after the same meal. Do not crush or open capsule.

T

Tapentadol
ta-pen'ta-dol
Nucynta
Do not confuse tapentadol with Toradol or tramadol.

CATEGORY AND SCHEDULE
Pregnancy Risk Category: C
Controlled Substance Schedule: II

Classification: Analgesics, opioid-like, centrally acting

MECHANISM OF ACTION

A potent centrally acting analgesic that binds to μ-opioid receptors, inhibiting ascending pain pathways. Also inhibits reuptake of norepinephrine and serotonin. Reduces the intensity of pain stimuli reaching sensory nerve endings. *Therapeutic Effect:* Alters the perception of and emotional response to pain.

PHARMACOKINETICS

Route	Onset	Peak	Duration
PO	< 1 h	1.25 h	4-6 h

Good absorption after PO administration. Protein binding: Low, 20%. Extensively metabolized in the liver. The major metabolic pathway is conjugation to produce glucuronides. Roughly 70% of the dose is excreted in urine in the conjugated form. A total of 3% of drug excreted in urine as unchanged drug. No metabolites contribute to analgesic activity. Tapentadol and its metabolites are excreted almost exclusively (99%) via the kidneys. *Half-life:* 4 h.

AVAILABILITY

Tablets: 50 mg, 75 mg, 100 mg.

T

INDICATIONS AND DOSAGES

▸ Moderate to moderately severe pain

PO (IMMEDIATE RELEASE)

Adults. Initially, 50 mg, 75 mg, or 100 mg every 4-6 h adjusted to pain intensity. On the first day, the 2nd dose may be given as soon as 1 h after the first dose, if adequate pain relief is not attained. Subsequent dosing is 50-100 mg every 4-6 h and adjusted to adequate analgesia/tolerability. Maximum daily limits: 700 mg total on the first day, and 600 mg/day total on subsequent days.

▸ Dosage in hepatic impairment

In moderate impairment, initially do not exceed 50 mg q8h, with a maximum of 3 doses in 24 h. If needed and tolerated, may give q6h. Increase interval if more frequent dosing not tolerated. Not recommended if hepatic impairment is severe.

CONTRAINDICATIONS

Significant respiratory depression, acute or severe bronchial asthma or hypercapnia in unmonitored settings or the absence of resuscitative equipment, paralytic ileus; use with MAOIs or within 14 days of MAOIs.

INTERACTIONS

Drug

Alcohol, other central nervous system (CNS) depressants: May increase CNS or respiratory depression and hypotension. Avoid.
MAOIs: Additive effects on norepinephrine levels, which may lead to hypertensive crisis; contraindicated.
Serotonin agonists, SSRIs, SNRIs: Possible additive effects on serotonergic actions; use caution.

Herbal

None known.

Food

None known.

DIAGNOSTIC TEST EFFECTS

May increase GGT, AST (SGOT), and ALT (SGPT) levels.

SIDE EFFECTS

Frequent (> 5%)

Dizziness, nausea, vomiting, somnolence, constipation.

Occasional (2%-5%)

Fatigue, dry mouth, dyspepsia, feeling hot, decreased appetite, insomnia, pruritis, sweating.

Rare (< 2%)
Rash, hot flush, CNS stimulation (such as nervousness, headache, anxiety, agitation, tremor, euphoria, mood swings, and hallucinations), blurred vision, urticaria, urinary retention.

SERIOUS REACTIONS

- Hypersensitivity.
- Respiratory or CNS depression.
- Seizures.
- Serotonin syndrome (rare).
- Increased intracranial pressure in at-risk patients (rare).

PRECAUTIONS & CONSIDERATIONS

Extreme caution should be used with acute abdominal conditions, biliary tract disease, severe hepatic or renal impairment (not recommended for use), increased intracranial pressure or head injury, seizure disorders, and those with potential risk for respiratory depression (e.g., hypoxia, hypercapnia, or upper airway obstruction). Opioid dependence is possible. There is a potential for drug abuse. Monitor patients closely for signs of abuse and addiction. Tapentadol crosses the placenta and may cause withdrawal in the neonate. The drug is distributed in breast milk. The safety and efficacy of this drug have not been established in children. The elderly may be more susceptible to side effects, so care should be used in initial dosing.

Blurred vision, dizziness, and drowsiness may occur, so tasks requiring mental alertness or motor skills should be avoided until the drug effects are known. Notify the physician of any chest pain, difficulty breathing, excessive sedation, muscle weakness, palpitations, seizures, severe constipation, or tremors. Liver and renal function studies should be obtained before therapy. BP, pulse rate, pattern of daily bowel activity and stool consistency, bladder for urine retention, and therapeutic response should be monitored.

Storage
Store the tablets at room temperature.

Administration
Take tapentadol orally without regard to food. Do not abruptly discontinue; tapering is recommended.

Tazarotene

ta-zare'oh-teen

★ 🍁 Tazorac, Avage

CATEGORY AND SCHEDULE

Pregnancy Risk Category: X

Classification: Dermatologics, retinoids

MECHANISM OF ACTION

Modulates differentiation and proliferation of epithelial tissue, binds selectively to retinoic acid receptors. *Therapeutic Effect:* Restores normal differentiation of the epidermis and reduces epidermal inflammation.

PHARMACOKINETICS

Minimal systemic absorption occurs through the skin. Binding to plasma proteins is > 99%. Metabolism is in the skin and liver. Elimination occurs through the fecal and renal pathways. *Half-life:* 18 h.

AVAILABILITY

Gel: 0.05%, 0.1% (Tazorac).
Cream: 0.05% (Tazorac), 0.1% (Avage, Tazorac).

INDICATIONS AND DOSAGES

▸ **Psoriasis**
TOPICAL

T

Adults, adolescents, children older than 12 yr. Thin film applied once daily in the evening; only cover the lesions, and area should be dry before application.

▸ **Acne vulgaris**

TOPICAL

Adults, adolescents, children older than 12 yr. Thin film applied to affected areas once daily in the evening after the face is gently cleansed and dried.

▸ **Fine facial wrinkles, facial mottled hyperpigmentation (liver spots), hypopigmentation associated with photoaging**

TOPICAL

Adults, children older than 17 yr. Thin film applied to affected areas once daily in the evening, after face is gently cleansed and dried.

CONTRAINDICATIONS

Should not be used in pregnant women, patients with hypersensitivity to tazarotene, benzyl alcohol, any one of its components, or other retinoid or vitamin A derivatives.

INTERACTIONS

Drug

Ethanol, benzoyl peroxide, resorcinol, salicylic acid, sulfur: Increases the drying effect.

Quinolones, phenothiazines, sulfonamides, sulfonylureas, tetracyclines, thiazide diuretics: Increase the risk of photosensitivity.

Herbal

None known.

Food

None known.

DIAGNOSTIC TEST EFFECTS

None known.

SIDE EFFECTS

Frequent

Desquamation, burning or stinging, dry skin, itching, erythema, worsening of psoriasis, irritation, skin pain, pruritis, xerosis, photosensitivity.

Occasional

Irritation, skin pain, fissuring, localized edema, skin discoloration, rash, desquamation, contact dermatitis, skin inflammation, bleeding, dry skin, hypertriglyceridemia, peripheral edema, acne vulgaris, cheilitis.

PRECAUTIONS & CONSIDERATIONS

Caution is warranted in patients with other skin conditions such as eczema, sunburn, and undiagnosed skin lesions. Tazarotene is contraindicated during pregnancy. It is unknown whether it enters the breast milk. Safety and efficacy have not been established in children or elderly patients.

Burning or stinging after application, dryness, itching, peeling, or redness of the skin may occur during tazarotene therapy. Avoid direct exposure to UV light.

Storage

Store at room temperature away from heat and direct light.

Administration

Tazarotene is for external use only. Apply only on face, once daily at bedtime, or as directed by physician. Remove any makeup, gently wash face with a mild cleanser, and pat skin dry. Wait at least 20 min to make sure face is dry before applying a small, pea-sized amount (about ¼-inch wide) of medication. Apply in a thin layer over wrinkles and discolored spots, avoiding eye and mouth areas. Wash hands after using the medication. In the morning, apply a moisturizing sunscreen with SPF 15 or greater.

T

Telavancin

tel'a-van'sin

Vibativ

Do not confuse with vancomycin, Vibramycin, or vigabatrin.

CATEGORY AND SCHEDULE

Pregnancy Risk Category: C

Classification: Antibiotics, glycopeptides

MECHANISM OF ACTION

Telavancin is a semisynthetic glycopeptide antibiotic that is a derivative of vancomycin. Binds to bacterial cell walls of gram-positive bacteria only, disrupting and altering cell membrane integrity and permeability and inhibiting RNA synthesis. Effective against methicillin-resistant *Staph aureus* (MRSA). *Therapeutic Effect:* Bactericidal.

PHARMACOKINETICS

Poorly absorbed from the GI tract, so must be given intravenously by infusion. Widely distributed. Protein binding: 93%. Metabolized to 3 hydroxylated metabolites, but metabolic pathways not mediated by CYP450 system. Primarily excreted in the urine. Minimally (5%-6%) removed by hemodialysis. *Half-life:* 8-9 h (increased in impaired renal function).

AVAILABILITY

Powder for Injection: 250 mg, 750 mg.

INDICATIONS AND DOSAGES

▸ **Treatment of skin and soft-tissue infections**

▸ **IV INFUSION**

Adults, Elderly. 10 mg/kg once every 24 h for 7-14 days.

▸ **Dosage for renal impairment**

CrCl > 50 mL/min: No dosage adjustment needed.

CrCl 30-50 mL/min: 7.5 mg/kg IV q24h.

CrCl 10-29 mL/min: 10 mg/kg IV q48h.

CrCl < 10 mL/min: Insufficient evidence for dose recommendations, including those with end-stage renal disease or on hemodialysis. Use is not recommended.

OFF-LABEL USES

Nosocomial pneumonia.

CONTRAINDICATIONS

Hypersensitivity.

INTERACTIONS

Drug

Anticoagulants, including heparins and warfarin: Telavancin interferes with certain coagulation assays, which may cause confusion in monitoring anticoagulation. Interference is limited if blood samples are collected as close as possible prior to a patient's next dose of telavancin.

Drugs with nephrotoxic or ototoxic potential, such as aminoglycosides, amphotericin B, cisplatin, cyclosporine, foscarnet: May increase the risk of toxicity of telavancin.

QT-prolonging drugs (e.g., class 1A and III antiarrhythmics, ranolazine, some antipsychotics, some quinolones): Use with caution since effect of telavancin on QT interval may be additive.

Herbal

None known.

Food

None known.

DIAGNOSTIC TEST EFFECTS

May increase BUN or serum creatinine level, proteinuria.

T

Telavancin interferes with certain coagulation assays (e.g., PT, INR, aPTT, and ACT, and heparin anti-Xa). The effects dissipate over time, as plasma concentrations of telavancin decrease. Telavancin also interferes with urine qualitative dipstick protein assays and quantitative dye methods (e.g., pyrogallol red-molybdate). Microalbumin assay methods are not affected.

IV INCOMPATIBILITIES

Do not mix with or administer other medications simultaneously through the same IV line.

SIDE EFFECTS

Frequent (≥ 10%)
Taste disturbance, nausea, vomiting, increased serum creatinine, and foamy urine.
Occasional (4%-7%)
Dizziness, diarrhea, pruritus, rash, rigors, pain at infusion site.
Rare (3% or less)
Decreased appetite, abdominal pain, phlebitis, thrombophlebitis, vertigo, tinnitus, extravasation.

SERIOUS REACTIONS

- *Clostridium difficile*-associated diarrhea (CDAD), including pseudomembranous colitis.
- Superinfection.
- Nephrotoxicity and ototoxicity.
- Infusion reactions similar to the "red man" syndrome of vancomycin (redness on face, neck, arms, and back; chills; fever; tachycardia; pruritus; rash) may result from too-rapid infusion.
- QT prolongation (rare).
- Serious hypersensitivity.

PRECAUTIONS & CONSIDERATIONS

Caution is warranted in patients with preexisting hearing impairment or renal dysfunction and in those taking other ototoxic or nephrotoxic medications concurrently. Also use with caution in patients with electrolyte disturbances or other known risks for QT prolongation. Lower clinical cure rates have been observed in patients with renal impairment. Telavancin crosses the placenta and has potential to cause fetal harm. Women of childbearing potential should have a serum pregnancy test prior to administration and should use effective contraception during treatment. It is unknown whether it is distributed in breast milk. Age-related renal impairment may increase the risk of toxicity in elderly patients. Careful dose selection is recommended.

Notify the physician if rash, tinnitus, or signs and symptoms of nephrotoxicity occur. Laboratory tests are an important part of therapy. Assess skin for rash, infusion rate tolerance, intake and output, renal function, balance, and hearing acuity; assess IV site during telavancin therapy.

Storage
Store unopened vials in a refrigerator; do not freeze. After reconstitution, the total time in the vial plus the time in the infusion bag should not exceed 4 h at room temperature or 72 h under refrigeration.

Administration
Telavancin is for IV infusion use only after dilution. For reconstitution add 15 mL to the 250-mg vial or 45 mL to the 750-mg vial, respectively, using D5W, sterile water for injection, or 0.9% NaCl injection. Mix thoroughly to reconstitute; usually reconstitution takes < 2 min, but can take up to 20 min. Aseptically remove the required dose from the vial for further dilution.

T

For doses ranging from 150-800 mg, further dilute the appropriate volume of reconstituted solution with 100-250 mL of D5W, 0.9% NaCl, or lactated Ringer's injection. For other doses, dilute to a final concentration of 0.6-8 mg/mL with the mentioned compatible fluids.

Administer slowly via intravenous infusion over 60 min. Too-rapid IV administration can lead to infusion-related reactions such as red man syndrome. If the same IV line is used for sequential administration of other medications, flush the line before and after each telavancin dose with D5W, 0.9% NaCl, or lactated Ringer's injection.

Telbivudine

tell-biv′yoo-deen

Tyzeka Sebivo

Do not confuse telbivudine with lamivudine, or Tyzeka with Tykosyn or Tasigna.

CATEGORY AND SCHEDULE

Pregnancy Risk Category: B

Classification:

Antiretrovirals, nucleoside reverse transcriptase inhibitors

MECHANISM OF ACTION

An antiviral that inhibits hepatitis B virus (HBV) DNA polymerase, an enzyme necessary for HBV replication. *Therapeutic Effect:* Interrupts HBV replication, slowing the progression of hepatitis B infection.

PHARMACOKINETICS

Rapidly and completely absorbed from the GI tract; efficacy not influenced by food. Protein binding: Low, 3.3%. Widely distributed. Primarily excreted unchanged in urine. Removed by hemodialysis (23%). *Half-life:* 15 h (increased in impaired renal function).

AVAILABILITY

Tablets (Tyzeka): 600 mg.
Oral Solution (Tyzeka): 100 mg/5 mL.

INDICATIONS AND DOSAGES

▸ **Chronic hepatitis B**

PO

Adults, Children 16 yr and older. 600 mg once per day.

▸ **Dosage in renal impairment (adult and adolescent)**

Dosage and frequency are modified based on creatinine clearance.

CrCl	Tablet Dosage	Oral Solution Dosage
≥ 50 mL/min	No adjustment	No adjustment
30-49 mL/min	600 mg q48h	400 mg once daily
< 30 mL/min not on hemodialysis	600 mg q72h	200 mg once daily
Hemodialysis (HD) or peritoneal dialysis (CAPD)	600 mg q96h (given after HD)	Not established

CONTRAINDICATIONS

Hypersensitivity.

INTERACTIONS

Drug

Cyclosporine, tacrolimus, and other transplant medications: Closely monitor renal function and transplant status.

HMG-CoA reductase inhibitors ("statins"): Potential for increased

serious myopathy; use together with caution. Others drugs that require caution include corticosteroids, chloroquine, hydroxychloroquine, fibric acid derivatives, penicillamine, zidovudine, cyclosporine, erythromycin, niacin, and certain azole antifungals.
Interferons: May increase risk of peripheral neuropathy.
Metformin, cotrimoxazole: Use caution since these and other medications, like telbivudine, are substantially dependent on renal excretion and increase risk of lactic acidosis.
Herbal
None known.
Food
None known.

DIAGNOSTIC TEST EFFECTS

May increase serum amylase, AST (SGOT), and ALT (SGPT) levels. May increase creatine kinase (CK). Rarely lowers platelet, WBC, or RBC counts.

SIDE EFFECTS

Frequent (≥ 3%)
Fatigue, increased creatine kinase (CK), headache, cough, diarrhea, abdominal pain, nausea, pharyngolaryngeal pain, flu-like illness, arthralgia, fever, rash, back pain, dizziness, myalgia, increased liver function tests, dyspepsia, insomnia, and abdominal distention.
Occasional (1%-2%)
Diarrhea, myopathy, pruritus.
Rare (< 1%)
Paresthesia, hypoesthesia, serious reactions (see below).

SERIOUS REACTIONS

- Myopathy with rhabdomyolysis.
- Peripheral neuropathy.
- Lactic acidosis.
- Severe hepatomegaly with steatosis.

PRECAUTIONS & CONSIDERATIONS

Lactic acidosis and severe hepatomegaly with steatosis, including fatal cases, have been reported. Severe acute exacerbations of hepatitis B may occur if treatment is discontinued. Closely monitor patients who discontinue therapy. Caution is warranted in patients with impaired renal function, a history of peripheral neuropathy. Be aware that telbivudine crosses the placenta, and it is unknown whether telbivudine is distributed in breast milk. Breastfeeding is not recommended. Be aware that the safety and efficacy of this drug have not been established in children. In elderly patients, age-related renal impairment may require dosage adjustment. The oral solution contains sodium that may need to be taken into account in patients on a low-sodium diet. This drug is not a cure for hepatitis B infection and does not reduce the risk of transmission of HBV to others.

Before starting drug therapy, check the baseline lab values, especially renal function. Expect to monitor the serum amylase, BUN, and serum creatinine levels. Monitor for unusual weakness or fatigue, trouble breathing, or irregular pulse, which could indicate lactic acidosis. Assess for altered sleep patterns, cough, dizziness, headache, nausea, and pattern of daily bowel activity and stool consistency. Avoid activities that require mental acuity if dizziness occurs. Closely monitor for symptoms of peripheral neuropathy (tingling or burning sensations of extremities) or myopathy (muscle weakness or pain).
Storage
Store tablets and oral solution in the original containers at room

T

temperature. Do not store in a damp place and do not freeze the oral solution. Oral solution expires 2 mo after opening the bottle. Keep tightly closed.

Administration

Give telbivudine without regard to meals, at roughly the same time each day. Take for the full length of treatment and evenly space drug doses. Use supplied dose cup for the oral solution. Do not abruptly or prematurely discontinue, as rebound, serious hepatitis may result.

Telithromycin

tell-ith'roe-my-sin

Ketek

CATEGORY AND SCHEDULE

Pregnancy Risk Category: C

Classification: Antibiotics, ketolides

MECHANISM OF ACTION

A ketolide that blocks protein synthesis by binding to ribosomal receptor sites on the bacterial cell wall. *Therapeutic Effect:* Bactericidal.

PHARMACOKINETICS

Protein binding: 60%-70%. More of drug is concentrated in WBCs than in plasma, and drug is eliminated more slowly from WBCs than from plasma. Partially metabolized by the liver, 50% of metabolism is dependent on CYP3A4. Minimally excreted in feces and urine. *Half-life:* 10 h.

AVAILABILITY

Tablets: 300 mg, 400 mg.

INDICATIONS AND DOSAGES

▸ **Community-acquired pneumonia**

PO

Adults, Elderly. 800 mg once a day for 7-10 days.

▸ **Dosage for severe renal impairment**

For CrCl < 30 mL/min: Reduce dose to 600 mg once daily. In those on hemodialysis, give after dialysis session on dialysis days.

▸ **Dosage for multiple insufficiency**

For severe renal (CrCl < 30 mL/min) PLUS coexisting hepatic impairment, reduce to 400 mg once daily.

CONTRAINDICATIONS

Hypersensitivity to telithromycin or to any macrolides, including hepatic dysfunction, concurrent use of cisapride or pimozide, myasthenia gravis, congenital QT prolongation.

INTERACTIONS

Drug

Antiarrhythmics: May result in additive effects, even resulting in serious arrhythmias.

Atorvastatin, colchicine, digoxin, lovastatin, metoprolol, simvastatin, midazolam, triazolam, theophylline: May increase the blood concentration and toxicity of these drugs. Simvastatin, lovastatin, or atorvastatin should be stopped during telithromycin treatment.

Carbamazepine, phenobarbital, phenytoin, rifampin: May decrease the blood concentration of telithromycin.

Cisapride and pimozide: Increases blood concentration resulting in significantly increased QT interval.

Itraconazole, ketoconazole: May increase the blood concentration of telithromycin.

Sotalol: Decreases the blood concentration of sotalol.

T

Herbal
None known.
Food
None known.

DIAGNOSTIC TEST EFFECTS
May increase platelet count and AST (SGOT) and ALT (SGPT) levels.

SIDE EFFECTS
Occasional (4%-11%)
Diarrhea, nausea, headache, dizziness.
Rare (2%-3%)
Vomiting, loose stools, altered taste, dry mouth, flatulence, visual disturbances.

SERIOUS REACTIONS
- Hepatic dysfunction, severe hypersensitivity reaction, and QT prolongation arrhythmias occur rarely.
- Myasthenia gravis with life-threatening and fatal respiratory depression occurs rarely.
- Antibiotic-associated colitis and other superinfections may result from altered bacterial balance.
- Vagal symptoms with loss of conciousness.

PRECAUTIONS & CONSIDERATIONS
Caution is warranted in patients with uncorrected hypokalemia, hypomagnesemia, bradycardia, concomitant use of class IA or III antiarrhythmics, and patients with significant renal impairment. It is unknown whether telithromycin is distributed in breast milk. Use during pregnancy and lactation only if benefits outweight risks. Safety and efficacy of telithromycin have not been established in children. In elderly patients with normal renal function, no age-related precautions have been noted.

Be aware that there is a potential for visual disturbances or decreased cognition during treatment; minimize hazardous tasks during treatment.
Storage
Store at room temperature.
Administration
May administer without regard to meals. Do not break or crush film-coated tablets.

Telmisartan
tel-meh-sar'tan
★ 🍁 Micardis

CATEGORY AND SCHEDULE
Pregnancy Risk Category: C (D if used in second or third trimester)

Classification: Antihypertensives, angiotensin II receptor antagonists

MECHANISM OF ACTION
An angiotensin II receptor, type AT_1, antagonist that blocks vasoconstrictor and aldosterone-secreting effects of angiotensin II, inhibiting the binding of angiotensin II to the AT_1 receptors. *Therapeutic Effect:* Causes vasodilation, decreases peripheral resistance, and decreases BP.

PHARMACOKINETICS
Rapidly and completely absorbed after PO administration. Protein binding: > 99.5%. Undergoes metabolism in the liver to inactive metabolite. Excreted in feces. Unknown whether removed by hemodialysis. *Half-life:* 24 h.

AVAILABILITY
Tablets: 20 mg, 40 mg, 80 mg.

INDICATIONS AND DOSAGES
▸ **Hypertension**
PO

Adults, Elderly. 40 mg once a day. Range: 20-80 mg/day.

▸ **Cardiovascular risk reduction**

PO

Adults, Elderly 55 yr and older. Titrate to target dose of 80 mg once a day. It is not known if lower doses are effective.

OFF-LABEL USES

Treatment of congestive heart failure (CHF).

CONTRAINDICATIONS

Hypersensitivity to telmisartan.

INTERACTIONS

Drug

Digoxin: Increases digoxin plasma concentration.

Potassium supplements, potassium-sparing diuretics, ACE inhibitors, drospirenone, eplerenone: May increase risk of hyperkalemia.

Warfarin: Slightly decreases warfarin plasma concentration.

Herbal

Dong quai, garlic: May increase antihypertensive effect.

Ephedra, ginseng, yohimbe: May decrease antihypertensive effect.

Food

None known.

DIAGNOSTIC TEST EFFECTS

May increase serum creatinine and potassium levels. May decrease blood hemoglobin and hematocrit levels.

SIDE EFFECTS

Occasional (3%-7%)

Upper respiratory tract infection, sinusitis, back or leg pain, diarrhea, skin ulcer.

Rare (1%)

Dizziness, headache, fatigue, nausea, heartburn, myalgia, cough, peripheral edema, hyperkalemia.

SERIOUS REACTIONS

- Overdosage may manifest as hypotension and tachycardia. Bradycardia occurs less often.
- Renal dysfunction (rare).
- Liver problems (rare).
- Hypersensitivity reactions.

PRECAUTIONS & CONSIDERATIONS

Caution is warranted in patients with hepatic and renal impairment, renal artery stenosis (bilateral or unilateral), and volume depletion. It is unknown whether telmisartan is excreted in breast milk; it may cause fetal harm. Avoid fetal or neonatal exposure; breastfeeding is not recommended. Safety and efficacy of telmisartan have not been established in children. No age-related precautions have been noted in elderly patients.

Dizziness may occur. Tasks that require mental alertness or motor skills should be avoided. Notify the physician if fever or sore throat occurs. Apical pulse and BP should be assessed immediately before each dose and regularly throughout therapy. Be alert to fluctuations in apical pulse and BP. If an excessive reduction in BP occurs, place the patient in the supine position with feet slightly elevated and notify the physician. Pulse rate and BUN, serum creatinine, and serum electrolyte levels should be assessed. Maintain adequate hydration; exercising outside during hot weather should be avoided in order to decrease the risk of dehydration and hypotension.

Storage

Store at room temperature. Do not remove from packaging until right before administration.

Administration
May be given concurrently with other antihypertensives. If BP is not controlled by telmisartan alone, a diuretic may be added.

Take telmisartan without regard to meals.

Temazepam

te-maz′e-pam
★ Restoril 🍁 Apo-Temazepam, Novo-Temazepam, PMS-Temazepam, Restoril
Do not confuse Restoril with Vistaril or Zestril.

CATEGORY AND SCHEDULE

Pregnancy Risk Category: X
Controlled Substance Schedule: IV

Classification: Benzodiazepines, sedatives/hypnotics

MECHANISM OF ACTION

A benzodiazepine that enhances the action of the inhibitory neurotransmitter γ-aminobutyric acid, resulting in central nervous system (CNS) depression. *Therapeutic Effect:* Induces sleep.

PHARMACOKINETICS

Well absorbed from the GI tract. Protein binding: 96%. Widely distributed. Crosses the blood-brain barrier. Metabolized in the liver. Primarily excreted in urine. Not removed by hemodialysis. *Half-life:* 4-18 h.

AVAILABILITY

Capsules: 7.5 mg, 15 mg, 22.5 mg, 30 mg.

INDICATIONS AND DOSAGES

▸ **Insomnia**
PO
Adults, Children 18 yr and older. 15-30 mg at bedtime.
Elderly, Debilitated. 7.5-15 mg at bedtime.

CONTRAINDICATIONS

Hypersensitivity to temazepam, pregnancy.

INTERACTIONS

Drug
Alcohol, other CNS depressants: May increase CNS depression.
Herbal
Kava kava, valerian: May increase CNS depression.
Food
None known.

DIAGNOSTIC TEST EFFECTS

None known.

SIDE EFFECTS

Frequent
Somnolence, sedation, rebound insomnia (may occur for 1-2 nights after drug is discontinued), dizziness, confusion, euphoria.
Occasional
Asthenia, anorexia, diarrhea.
Rare
Paradoxical CNS excitement or restlessness (particularly in elderly or debilitated patients).

SERIOUS REACTIONS

- Abrupt or too-rapid withdrawal may result in pronounced restlessness, irritability, insomnia, hand tremor, abdominal or muscle cramps, vomiting, diaphoresis, and seizures.
- Overdose results in somnolence, confusion, diminished reflexes, respiratory depression, and coma.

PRECAUTIONS & CONSIDERATIONS

Caution is warranted in patients with mental impairment and the potential for drug dependence.

Temazepam is pregnancy risk category X and crosses the placenta and may be distributed in breast milk. Long-term use of temazepam during pregnancy may produce withdrawal symptoms and CNS depression in neonates. Temazepam use is not recommended for children younger than 18 yr. To avoid ataxia or excessive sedation in elderly patients, plan to administer small doses initially and to increase dosage gradually.

Avoid alcohol, CNS depressants, and tasks that require mental alertness and motor skills. BP, pulse rate, respiratory rate, rhythm, and depth should be assessed before administering temazepam. Cardiovascular, mental, and respiratory status should be monitored throughout therapy.

Storage

Store at room temperature.

Administration

If desired, open temazepam capsules and mix the contents with food. Take temazepam 30 min before bedtime.

Temozolomide

tem-oh-zohl'oh-mide

Temodar Temodal

CATEGORY AND SCHEDULE

Pregnancy Risk Category: D

Classification: Antineoplastics, alkylating agents

MECHANISM OF ACTION

An imidazotetrazine derivative that acts as a prodrug and is converted to a highly active cytotoxic metabolite. Its cytotoxic effect is associated with methylation of DNA. *Therapeutic Effect:* Inhibits DNA replication, causing cell death.

PHARMACOKINETICS

Rapidly and completely absorbed after PO administration. Protein binding: 15%. Peak plasma concentration occurs in 1 h. Penetrates the blood-brain barrier. Eliminated primarily in urine and, to a much lesser extent, in feces. *Half-life:* 1.6-1.8 h.

AVAILABILITY

Capsules: 5 mg, 20 mg, 100 mg, 140 mg, 180 mg, 250 mg.
Powder for Injection: 100 mg.

INDICATIONS AND DOSAGES

▸ **Newly diagnosed glioblastoma multiforme**

PO OR INFUSION

Adults. 75 mg/m^2 daily for 42 days concomitant with focal radiotherapy; then, 150 mg/m^2 once daily for days 1-5 of a 28-day cycle for the first maintenance cycle. Usually 6 cycles total, but dose can be escalated in cycle 2-6 up to 200 mg/m^2; doses are based on tolerance and ANC and platelet counts.

▸ **Anaplastic astrocytoma**

PO OR IV INFUSION

Adults, Elderly. Initially, 150 mg/m^2/day on days 1-5 of a 28-day treatment cycle. Subsequent doses based on platelet count and absolute neurophil count. Maintenance: May be escalated up to a maximum of 200 mg/m^2/day for 5 days q4wk. Continue until disease progression. Minimum: 100 mg/m^2/day for 5 days for subsequent cycle.

CONTRAINDICATIONS

Hypersensitivity to temozolomide or to DTIC, also known as dacarbazine.

INTERACTIONS

Drug

Live-virus vaccines: May potentiate virus replication, increase vaccine side effects, and decrease the patient's antibody response to the vaccine.

Valproic acid: Decreases the clearance of temozolomide.

Herbal

None known.

Food

All foods: Decrease the rate of drug absorption.

IV INCOMPATIBILITIES

Do not infuse with any other medications simultaneously.

DIAGNOSTIC TEST EFFECTS

May decrease blood hemoglobin levels and neutrophil, platelet, and WBC counts.

SIDE EFFECTS

Frequent (33%-53%)

Nausea, vomiting, headache, fatigue, constipation.

Occasional (10%-16%)

Diarrhea, asthenia, fever, dizziness, peripheral edema, incoordination, insomnia.

Rare (5%-7%)

Paresthesia, drowsiness, anorexia, urinary incontinence, anxiety, pharyngitis, cough.

SERIOUS REACTIONS

- Elderly patients and women are at increased risk for developing severe myelosuppression, characterized by neutropenia and thrombocytopenia and usually occurring within the first few cycles. Neutrophil and platelet counts reach their nadirs approximately 26-28 days after administration and recover within 14 days of the nadir.
- Serious allergic reactions are rare.

PRECAUTIONS & CONSIDERATIONS

Caution is warranted in patients with severe hepatic or renal impairment. Temozolomide use should be avoided during pregnancy because the drug may cause fetal harm. Although it is unknown whether temozolomide is excreted in breast milk, women taking this drug should avoid breastfeeding. The safety and efficacy of temozolomide have not been established in children. Elderly patients (i.e., older than 70 yr) have a higher risk of developing grade 4 neutropenia and grade 4 thrombocytopenia. Vaccinations and coming in contact with crowds and people with known infections should be avoided.

Notify the physician if the patient experiences easy bruising, fever, signs of local infection, sore throat, or unusual bleeding from any site. Before administration, ANC must be > 1500/mm^3 and the platelet count must be > 100,000/mm^3. To control nausea and vomiting, antiemetics should be administered. A CBC on day 22 (21 days after the first dose) or within 48 h of that day and then weekly until the ANC is > 1500/mm^3 and the platelet count is > 100,000/mm^3 should be ordered.

Storage

Store capsules at room temperature. Unopened injection vials are stored in the refrigerator and protected from light; do not freeze. Reconstituted product must be used within 14 h, including infusion time.

Administration

CAUTION: Observe and exercise usual cautions for handling, preparing, and administering solutions of cytotoxic drugs. Avoid exposure to capsule contents.

Administer temozolomide on an empty stomach because food reduces the rate and extent of drug absorption and increases the risk of nausea and vomiting. For best results, take temozolomide at bedtime. Swallow the capsule whole with a glass of water. If the patient cannot swallow, open the capsule and mix the contents with applesauce or apple juice.

The injection is for IV infusion only. Bring the vial to room temperature prior to reconstitution. Reconstitute each vial with 41 mL sterile water for injection; the final concentration will be 2.5 mg/mL. Gently swirl; do not shake. Withdraw the appropriate dose and transfer into an empty 250-mL PVC infusion bag. Infuse IV using a pump over a period of exactly 90 min. Flush the lines before and after each infusion.

Temsirolimus

tem′sir-oh′li-mus

Torisel

CATEGORY AND SCHEDULE

Pregnancy Risk Category: D

Classification:

Antineoplastics, biologic response modifiers

MECHANISM OF ACTION

Prevents activation of the enzyme target of rapamycin (mTOR), a key regulatory kinase in cell-cycle progression. Results in G1 growth arrest of tumor cells. *Therapeutic Effect:* Inhibits proliferation of tumor cells.

PHARMACOKINETICS

Extensively metabolized in the liver primarily by CYP3A4. Five temsirolimus metabolites are formed, but sirolimus is the principal and active metabolite. Temsirolimus and metabolites are primarily eliminated via the feces, and the drug exhibits a bi-exponential decline in whole blood concentrations. *Half-life:* Mean 17.3 hours (temsirolimus), and mean 54.6 h (sirolimus).

AVAILABILITY

Injection: 25 mg/mL.

INDICATIONS AND DOSAGES

▸ Advanced renal cell cancer

IV INFUSION

Adults. 25 mg as IV infusion once weekly.

▸ Dosage adjustments for toxicity

Expect to withhold treatment if significant neutropenia or thrombocytopenia occurs. Expect new dosage once restarted to decrease, but that a dosage will not go below 15 mg/wk.

▸ Dosage adjustments for mild hepatic impairment

Reduce to 15 mg IV infusion once weekly.

▸ Dosage for co-use of strong CYP3A4 inhibitor

12.5 mg as IV infusion once weekly is suggested.

▸ Dosage for co-use of strong CYP3A4 inducer

Consider dose increase up to 50 mg/wk. Monitor closely.

CONTRAINDICATIONS

Hypersensitivity to temsirolimus; bilirubin > 1.5 × ULN.

INTERACTIONS

Drug

Itraconazole, ketoconazole, clarithromycin, erythromycin, protease inhibitors, nefazodone, verapamil: May increase the blood concentration and risk of toxicity of temsirolimus.

Carbamazepine, phenobarbital, phenytoin, rifampin: May decrease the blood concentration and effects of temsirolimus.
Live vaccines: Avoid during treatment.
Herbal
St. John's wort: Avoid, as may lower temsirolimus concentrations.
Food
Grapefruit juice: May increase temsirolimus and sirolimus exposure; avoid.

IV INCOMPATIBILITIES
Do not mix or infuse with other medications.

DIAGNOSTIC TEST EFFECTS
May decrease blood hemoglobin level, hematocrit, WBC, and platelet count. May increase blood glucose, serum cholesterol, creatinine, and triglyceride levels, as well as liver enzymes.

SIDE EFFECTS
Frequent (≥ 20%)
Rash, asthenia, mucositis, nausea, edema, and anorexia. Anemia, hyperglycemia, hyperlipemia, hypertriglyceridemia, lymphopenia, hypophosphatemia, thrombocytopenia, leukopenia, elevated hepatic enzymes.
Occasional (10%-20%)
Diarrhea, cough, abdominal pain, infection or sore throat, vomiting, weight loss, chest pain, headache, nail disorder/thinning, insomnia, epistaxis, dry skin.
Less Common
Hypertension, arthralgia, hypokalemia.

SERIOUS REACTIONS
- Increases the risk of infection and may be associated with the development of secondary malignancy.
- Worsening of, or new, hepatic impairment.
- Hypersensitivity reactions may be extensive.
- Interstitial lung disease.
- Renal failure.
- Bowel perforations or poor wound healing.
- Bleeding, including intracerebral bleeding.

PRECAUTIONS & CONSIDERATIONS
Caution is warranted in patients with chickenpox, herpes zoster, hepatic impairment, and infection. Temsirolimus can cause fetal harm. Women of childbearing potential should be advised to avoid becoming pregnant throughout treatment and for 3 mo after therapy has stopped. Men with partners of childbearing potential should use reliable contraception throughout treatment and are recommended to continue this for 3 mo after the last dose. Breastfeeding is not recommended. This drug is not approved for use in children.

Avoid coming in contact with people with colds or other infections. Liver function tests, CBC should be monitored regularly. Report rash, signs or symptoms of infection, dyspnea, or any other unusual symptoms promptly for evaluation.
Storage
Store unopened injection kits refrigerated; do not freeze and protect from light. Once diluted, the vial solution is stable for up to 24 h at room temperature. After further dilution for infusion, complete infusion within 6 h of preparation.
Administration
CAUTION: Observe and exercise usual precautions for handling, preparing, and administering solutions of cytotoxic drugs. Notify the physician if a dose is missed.

▸ **Premedicate with IV diphenhydramine (25-50 mg, or similar antihistamine) roughly 30 min before the start of each infusion.**
Use only diluent provided; inject 1.8 mL into the vial. The concentration will be 10 mg/mL. Must be further diluted. Withdraw the required dosage and inject rapidly into a 250-mL container (glass, polyolefin, or polyethylene) of 0.9% NaCl injection. Mix by gentle inversion. Avoid excessive shaking as this may cause foaming.

Use an administration set of non-DEHP tubing. An in-line polyethersulfone filter with a pore size of not greater than 5 microns is recommended. Infuse IV over a 30-60 min period once a week. The use of an infusion pump is preferred.

Tenofovir

ten-oh′foh-veer

★ 🍁 Viread

CATEGORY AND SCHEDULE

Pregnancy Risk Category: B

Classification: Antiretrovirals, nucleotide reverse transcriptase inhibitors

MECHANISM OF ACTION

A nucleotide analogue that inhibits viral reverse transcriptase by being incorporated into viral DNA, resulting in DNA chain termination. *Therapeutic Effect:* Slows HIV replication and reduces HIV RNA levels (viral load). Slows hepatitis B replication and progression of hepatitis B disease.

PHARMACOKINETICS

Well absorbed orally. Protein binding: Negligible. Intracellularly phosphorylated to the active metabolite tenofovir diphosphate. Prolonged intravellular half-life (15-50 h). Roughly 70%-80% of the dose is recovered in the urine as unchanged drug. Dependent on glomerular filtration and active renal tubular secretion. *Half-life:* 17 h.

AVAILABILITY

Tablets: 300 mg.

INDICATIONS AND DOSAGES

▸ **HIV infection (in combination with other antiretrovirals)**
PO
Adults, Elderly, Children 12 yr and older and weight ≥ 35 kg. 300 mg once a day.

▸ **Chronic hepatitis B infection**
PO
Adults, Elderly. 300 mg once a day.

▸ **Dosage adjustment for renal impairment (adults)**
CrCl 30-49 mL/min: 300 mg q48h.
CrCl 10-29 mL/min: 300 mg q72-96h.
Hemodialysis: 300 mg every 7 days or after roughly 12 h of dialysis.

CONTRAINDICATIONS

Hypersensitivity to tenofovir, concurrent use of tenofovir-containing combinations.

INTERACTIONS

Drug
Acyclovir, cidofovir, ganciclovir, valacyclovir, valganciclovir: May increase the blood concentrations of tenofovir.
Adefovir: May compete for tubular secretion; avoid use together.
Atazanavir, lopinavir, ritonavir: May increase tenofovir blood concentrations, decreases atazanavir concentrations.

T

Didanosine: May increase didanosine blood concentration.
Potentially nephrotoxic drugs (e.g., aminoglycosides, cisplatin, vancomycin, others): May increase risk for neprotoxicity; use caution.
Herbal
None known.
Food
High-fat food: Increases tenofovir bioavailability.

DIAGNOSTIC TEST EFFECTS

May elevate liver function test results. May alter serum CK, GGT, uric acid, AST (SGOT), ALT (SGPT), and triglyceride levels as well as creatinine clearance.

SIDE EFFECTS

Frequent
Rash, diarrhea, headache, pain, depression, asthenia, nausea.
Occasional
Insomnia, fever, dizziness, myalgia, sweating.

SERIOUS REACTIONS

- Lactic acidosis and hepatomegaly with steatosis (rare).
- Renal dysfunction, renal tubular acidosis.

PRECAUTIONS & CONSIDERATIONS

Caution should be used with impaired liver or renal function. Use with caution during pregnancy; use is not recommended during lactation due to the risk of transmittal of the HIV virus. There is no experience in children less than 12 yr of age. Check baseline laboratory test results, if ordered, especially liver function test results and serum triglyceride levels before beginning tenofovir therapy and at periodic intervals during therapy. Tenofovir is not a cure for HIV or HBV infection, nor does it reduce risk of transmission to others.

Monitor CD4 cell count, complete blood count (CBC), hemoglobin levels, HIV RNA plasma levels, liver function test results, and reticulocyte count. Assess pattern of daily bowel activity and stool consistency. Notify the physician if nausea, persistent abdominal pain, or vomiting occurs.
Storage
Store at controlled room temperature.
Administration
May be taken without regard to food. Continue drug therapy for the full length of treatment.

Terazosin

ter-a'zoe-sin
Apo-Terazosin, Hytrin, Novo-Terazosin

CATEGORY AND SCHEDULE

Pregnancy Risk Category: C

Classification: Antiadrenergics, α-blocking, peripheral

MECHANISM OF ACTION

An antihypertensive and benign prostatic hyperplasia agent that blocks α-adrenergic receptors. Produces vasodilation, decreases peripheral resistance, and targets receptors around bladder neck and prostate. *Therapeutic Effect:* In hypertension, decreases BP. In benign prostatic hyperplasia, relaxes smooth muscle and improves urine flow.

PHARMACOKINETICS

Route	Onset	Peak	Duration
PO	15 min	1-2 h	12-24 h

Rapidly, completely absorbed from the GI tract. Protein binding: 90%-94%. Metabolized in the liver to active metabolite. Eliminated primarily in feces via the biliary system; excreted in urine. Not removed by hemodialysis. *Half-life:* 9.2-12 h.

AVAILABILITY

Capsules: 1 mg, 2 mg, 5 mg, 10 mg.

INDICATIONS AND DOSAGES

▸ Mild to moderate hypertension

PO

Adults, Elderly. Initially, 1 mg at bedtime. Slowly increase dosage to desired levels. Range: 1-5 mg/day as single or 2 divided doses. Maximum: 20 mg.

▸ Benign prostatic hyperplasia

PO

Adults, Elderly. Initially, 1 mg at bedtime. May increase up to 10 mg/day. Maximum: 20 mg/day.

CONTRAINDICATIONS

Hypersensitivity to terazosin or other α_1-blockers. Concurrent use with phosphodiesterase-5 inhibitors.

INTERACTIONS

Drug

Estrogen, NSAIDs, other sympathomimetics: May decrease the effects of terazosin.

Hypotension-producing medications, such as antihypertensives and diuretics: May increase the effects of terazosin.

Phosphodiesterase-5 inhibitors (e.g., sildenafil, tadalafil, vardenafil): May increase the hypotensive effects. Use is contraindicated.

Herbal

Dong quai, ginseng, garlic, yohimbe: May decrease the effects of terazosin.

Saw palmetto: May interfere with effects of terazosin.

Food

None known.

DIAGNOSTIC TEST EFFECTS

May decrease blood hemoglobin and hematocrit levels, serum albumin level, total serum protein level, and WBC count.

SIDE EFFECTS

Frequent (5%-9%)

Dizziness, headache, unusual tiredness.

Rare (< 2%)

Peripheral edema, orthostatic hypotension, myalgia, arthralgia, blurred vision, nausea, vomiting, nasal congestion, somnolence.

SERIOUS REACTIONS

- Severe orthostatic hypotension with syncope may be preceded by tachycardia and usually occurs with increased exposure or first dose.
- Rare reports of jaundice, impaired hepatic function, and increased transaminases.
- α-blockers assocoiated with intraoperative floppy iris syndrome during cataract surgery.
- Priapism (very rare).
- Toxic skin eruptions (very rare).

PRECAUTIONS & CONSIDERATIONS

Caution is warranted in patients with confirmed or suspected coronary artery disease. It is unknown whether terazosin crosses the placenta or is distributed in breast milk. The safety and efficacy of terazosin have not been established in children. No age-related precautions have been noted in elderly patients, but this age group may be more sensitive to the drug's hypotensive effects. Caution should be used when driving or operating machinery. Tasks that require mental alertness or motor skills should be avoided until response to the drug is established.

Nasal congestion, dizziness, light-headedness, and fainting may occur. Rise slowly from a lying to a sitting position, and permit legs to dangle momentarily before standing to avoid the hypotensive effect. BP and pulse should be obtained immediately before each dose, and every 15-30 min thereafter until BP is stabilized. Be alert for fluctuations in BP. Genitourinary symptoms and peripheral edema should also be assessed.

Storage

Store at room temperature.

Administration

! If terazosin is discontinued for several days, restart therapy with a 1-mg dose at bedtime.

Take terazosin without regard to food. Administer first dose at bedtime to minimize the risk of fainting at the first dose.

Terbinafine

ter-been'a-feen

Lamisil, Lamisil AT

Apo-Terbinafine, Lamisil, Novo-Terbinafine

Do not confuse terbinafine with terbutaline, or Lamisil with Lamictal.

OTC (topical forms)

Rx (tablets)

CATEGORY AND SCHEDULE

Pregnancy Risk Category: B

Classification: Antifungals, topical, dermatologics

MECHANISM OF ACTION

A fungicidal antifungal that inhibits the enzyme squalene epoxidase, thereby interfering with fungal biosynthesis. *Therapeutic Effect:* Results in death of fungal cells.

AVAILABILITY

Tablets (Lamisil): 250 mg.
Gel or Cream (Lamisil AT): 1%.
Granules (Lamisil): 125 mg/packet, 187.5 mg/packet
Topical Solution (Lamisil, Lamisil AT): 1%.

INDICATIONS AND DOSAGES

▸ **Tinea pedis**

TOPICAL

Adults, Elderly, Children 12 yr and older. Apply twice a day until signs and symptoms significantly improve.

▸ **Tinea cruris, tinea corporis**

TOPICAL

Adults, Elderly, Children 12 yr and older. Apply twice a day until signs and symptoms significantly improve.

▸ **Onychomycosis**

PO

Adults, Elderly, Children 12 yr and older. 250 mg/day for 6 wks (fingernails) or 12 wks (toenails).

▸ **Tinea versicolor**

TOPICAL SOLUTION

Adults, Elderly. Apply to the affected area twice a day at least 7 days and no longer than 4 wks.

CONTRAINDICATIONS

Hypersensitivity to terbinafine. Not recommended for patients with active or chronic liver disease.

INTERACTIONS

Drug

Alcohol, other hepatotoxic medications: May increase the risk of hepatotoxicity.

Hepatic enzyme inducers, including rifampin: May increase terbinafine clearance.

Hepatic enzyme inhibitors, including cimetidine: May decrease terbinafine clearance.

Herbal

None known.

Food

None known.

DIAGNOSTIC TEST EFFECTS
May increase SGOT (AST) and SGPT (ALT) levels. Rare decreases in lymphocyte and WBC counts.

SIDE EFFECTS
Frequent (13%)
Oral: Headache.
Occasional (3%-6%)
Oral: Diarrhea, rash, dyspepsia, pruritus, taste disturbance, nausea.
Rare
Oral: Abdominal pain, flatulence, urticaria, depressed mood, visual disturbance.
Topical: Irritation, burning, pruritus, dryness.

SERIOUS REACTIONS
- Hepatobiliary dysfunction (including cholestatic hepatitis), serious skin reactions, and severe neutropenia occur rarely.
- Ocular lens and retinal changes have been noted.
- Lupus-like syndrome with systemic treatment (rare).

PRECAUTIONS & CONSIDERATIONS
As appropriate, monitor liver function when receiving treatment for longer than 6 wks. Use with caution in renal impairment due to lack of sufficient data.

Topical therapy may be used for a minimum of 1 wk and is not to exceed 4 wks. Discontinue the medication and notify the physician if a local reaction occurs. Separate personal items that come in contact with affected areas.

Storage
Store oral and topical products at room temperature.

Administration
Rub the topical form well into the affected and surrounding area. Keep affected areas clean and dry and wear light clothing to promote ventilation. Avoid contact with eyes, mouth, nose, or other mucous membranes. The treated area should not be covered with an occlusive dressing.

When taking terbinafine tablets, take without regard to food. Granules may be sprinkled on a spoonful of nonacidic food that should be swallowed without chewing.

Terbutaline
ter-byoo′te-leen
Bricanyl
Do not confuse terbutaline with tolbutamide or terbinafine.

CATEGORY AND SCHEDULE
Pregnancy Risk Category: B

Classification: Adrenergic agonists, bronchodilators, short-acting β-agonist

MECHANISM OF ACTION
An adrenergic agonist that stimulates β_2-adrenergic receptors, resulting in relaxation of uterine and bronchial smooth muscle. *Therapeutic Effect:* Relieves bronchospasm and reduces airway resistance. Also inhibits uterine contractions.

PHARMACOKINETICS
Small amounts distributed across the placenta. Partial metabolism in the liver and excretion in the urine, about 60% as unchanged drug and the rest as metabolites, with a small amount excreted via the bile in the feces. *Half-life:* 3.4 h.

AVAILABILITY
Tablets: 2.5 mg, 5 mg.
Injection: 1 mg/mL.

INDICATIONS AND DOSAGES

▸ **Bronchospasm**

PO

Adults, Elderly, Children 15 yr and older. Initially, 2.5 mg 3-4 times a day. Maintenance: 2.5-5 mg 3 times a day q6h while awake. Maximum: 15 mg/day.

Children aged 12-14 yr. 2.5 mg 3 times a day. Maximum: 7.5 mg/day.

Children 6-11 yr. Initially, 0.05 mg/kg/dose q8h. May increase up to 0.15 mg/kg/dose. Maximum: 5 mg/day.

SC

Adults, Children 12 yr and older. Initially, 0.25 mg. Repeat in 15-30 min if substantial improvement does not occur. Maximum: 0.5 mg/4 h.

Children younger than 12 yr. 0.005-0.01 mg/kg/dose to a maximum of 0.25 mg q15-20min for 3 doses.

OFF-LABEL USES

Inhibition of uterine contractions from premature labor.

CONTRAINDICATIONS

History of hypersensitivity to sympathomimetics.

INTERACTIONS

Drug

β-Blockers: May decrease the effects of β-blockers.

Digoxin, sympathomimetics: May increase the risk of arrhythmias.

MAOIs: May increase the risk of hypertensive crisis.

Tricyclic antidepressants: May increase cardiovascular effects.

Herbal

Ephedra, yohimbe: May increase central nervous system (CNS) stimulation.

Food

None known.

DIAGNOSTIC TEST EFFECTS

May decrease serum potassium level.

SIDE EFFECTS

Frequent (18%-23%)

Tremor, anxiety.

Occasional (10%-11%)

Somnolence, headache, nausea, heartburn, dizziness.

Rare (1%-3%)

Flushing, asthenia, mouth and throat dryness or irritation (with inhalation therapy).

SERIOUS REACTIONS

- Too-frequent or excessive use may lead to decreased drug effectiveness and severe, paradoxical bronchoconstriction.
- Excessive sympathomimetic stimulation may cause palpitations, extrasystoles, tachycardia, chest pain, a slight increase in BP followed by a substantial decrease, chills, diaphoresis, and blanching of skin.

PRECAUTIONS & CONSIDERATIONS

Caution is warranted in patients with cardiovascular disorders, hypertension, diabetes mellitus, a history of seizures, and hyperthyroidism. Avoid excessive use of caffeinated products, such as chocolate, cocoa, cola, coffee, and tea.

Anxiety, nervousness, and shakiness may occur. Notify the physician of chest pain, difficulty breathing, dizziness, flushing, headache, muscle tremors, or palpitations. Pulse rate and quality, respiratory rate, depth, rhythm, and type, BP, ABG levels, and serum potassium levels should be monitored. Fingernails and lips should be assessed for a blue or dusky color in light-skinned patients and a gray color in dark-skinned patients, which are signs of hypoxemia.

Storage

Store tablets and injection at room temperature. Protect injection from light.

T

Administration
Take terbutaline with food if the patient experiences GI upset. Crush tablets as needed.

The drug may be injected subcutaneously into the lateral deltoid region. Do not use solution if it appears discolored.

Terconazole

ter-kon'a-zole

★ 🍁 Terazol 3, Terazol 7, Zazole

CATEGORY AND SCHEDULE

Pregnancy Risk Category: C

Classification: Antifungals, topical, dermatologics

MECHANISM OF ACTION

An antifungal that disrupts fungal cell membrane permeability.
Therapeutic Effect: Produces antifungal activity.

PHARMACOKINETICS

Extent of systemic absorption varies 5%-8% in women who have had a hysterectomy versus 12%-16% in women with a uterus.

AVAILABILITY

Suppository: 80 mg (Terazol 3, Zazole).
Cream: 0.4% (Terazol 7, Zazole), 0.8% (Terazol 3, Zazole).

INDICATIONS AND DOSAGES

▸ **Vulvovaginal candidiasis**

INTRAVAGINAL

Adults, Elderly. 1 suppository vaginally at bedtime for 3 days.
Adults, Elderly. One applicatorful at bedtime for 7 days (0.4% cream) or for 3 days (0.8% cream).

CONTRAINDICATIONS

Hypersensitivity to terconazole or any component of the formulation.

INTERACTIONS

Drug
Spermicides (e.g., nonoxynol-9): Spermicide inactiviated; may lead to contraceptive failure.
Herbal
None known.
Food
None known.

DIAGNOSTIC TEST EFFECTS

None known.

SIDE EFFECTS

Frequent
Headache, vulvovaginal burning.
Occasional
Dysmenorrhea, pain in female genitalia, abdominal pain, fever, itching.
Rare
Chills.

SERIOUS REACTIONS

- Flu-like syndrome has been reported.

PRECAUTIONS & CONSIDERATIONS

Caution should be used in the first trimester of pregnancy. It is unknown whether terconazole crosses the placenta or is distributed in breast milk. Safety and efficacy of terconazole have not been established in children. No age-related precautions have been noted in elderly patients.

Storage
Store at room temperature.

Administration
Insert suppository or administer cream vaginally at bedtime. Complete full course of therapy. Contact physician if burning or irritation occurs.

Teriparatide

ter-i-par′a-tide

★ 🍁 Forteo

CATEGORY AND SCHEDULE

Pregnancy Risk Category: C

Classification: Hormones/hormone modifiers, parathyroid hormone analogue

MECHANISM OF ACTION

A synthetic polypeptide hormone that acts on bone to mobilize calcium; also acts on kidney to reduce calcium clearance, increase phosphate excretion. *Therapeutic Effect:* Promotes an increased rate of release of calcium from bone into blood, stimulates new bone formation.

PHARMACOKINETICS

Bioavailability following subcutaneous use about 95%. Peak serum concentrations occur 30 min after administration and decline to nonqualifiable within 3 h. There is hepatic and extra-hepatic clearance. Peripheral metabolism of teriparatide is believed to occur by nonspecific liver enzymes followed by excretion via the kidneys. *Half-life:* 1 h after SC administration.

AVAILABILITY

Injection: 2.4-mL prefilled pen containing 600 mcg teriparatide (Forteo).

INDICATIONS AND DOSAGES

▸ **Osteoporosis**

SC

Adults, Elderly. 20 mcg once daily into the thigh or abdominal wall.

CONTRAINDICATIONS

Serum calcium above normal level, those at increased risk for osteosarcoma (Paget disease, unexplained elevations of alkaline phosphatase, open epiphyses, prior radiation therapy that includes the skeleton), hypercalcemic disorder (e.g., hyperparathyroidism), hypersensitivity to teriparatide or any of the components of the formulation.

INTERACTIONS

Drug

Digoxin: May increase serum digoxin concentration.

Herbal

None known.

Food

None known.

DIAGNOSTIC TEST EFFECTS

May increase serum calcium.

SIDE EFFECTS

Occasional

Leg cramps, nausea, dizziness, headache, orthostatic hypotension, increased heart rate.

SERIOUS REACTIONS

• In animal studies, teriparatide has been associated with an increase in osteosarcoma.

PRECAUTIONS & CONSIDERATIONS

Caution is warranted in patients with bone metastases, cardiovascular disease, history of skeletal malignancies, metabolic bone diseases other than osteoporosis, and concurrent therapy with digoxin. Be aware that teriparatide use for more than 2 yr is not recommended. Teriparatide should be used in women who have passed menopause and cannot become pregnant or breastfeed.

Teriparatide is not indicated for children. Teriparatide may cause fast heartbeat, dizziness, light-headedness, and fainting. Avoid alcohol and tasks that require mental alertness and change positions slowly. Signs of toxicity are rash, nausea, dizziness, and leg cramps.

Storage

Refrigerate and minimize the time out of the refrigerator. Do not freeze. Each pen can be used for up to 28 days after the first injection. After 28 days, discard.

Administration

Administer SC injection into the thigh or abdominal wall. Administration sites should be rotated. For the first administration, patients should sit or lie down to minimize hypotension.

Testosterone

tess-toss′ter-one

Androderm, AndroGel, Delatestryl, Depo-Testosterone, First Testosterone, Striant, Testim, Testopel

Do not confuse testosterone with testolactone.

CATEGORY AND SCHEDULE

Pregnancy Risk Category: X

Controlled Substance Schedule: III

Classification: Androgens, hormones/hormone modifiers

MECHANISM OF ACTION

A primary endogenous androgen that promotes growth and development of male sex organs and maintains secondary sex characteristics in androgen-deficient males. *Therapeutic Effect:* Helps relieve androgen deficiency.

PHARMACOKINETICS

Well absorbed after IM administration. Protein binding: 98%. Undergoes first-pass metabolism in the liver. Excreted primarily in urine. Unknown whether removed by hemodialysis. *Half-life:* 10-100 min.

AVAILABILITY

Cypionate Injection (Depo-Testosterone): 100 mg/mL, 200 mg/mL.

Ethanate Injection (Delatestryl): 200 mg/mL.

Kit (Prescription Compounding) (First Testosterone): 100 mg/mL mixed to cream or gel.

Subcutaneous Pellets (Testopel): 75 mg.

Topical Gel (AndroGel): 25 mg/2.5 g, 50 mg/5 g.

Topical Gel (Testim): 50 mg/5 g.

Transdermal Patch (Androderm): 2.5 mg/day, 5 mg/day.

Buccal (Striant): 30 mg.

INDICATIONS AND DOSAGES

▸ **Male hypogonadism**

IM

Adults. 50-400 mg q2-4wk.

Adolescents. Initially 40-50 mg/m^2/dose monthly until growth rate falls to prepubertal levels. 100 mg/m^2/dose until growth ceases. Maintanence virilizing dose: 100 mg/m^2/dose twice a month.

SC (PELLETS)

Adults, Adolescents. 150-450 mg q3-6mo.

TRANDERMAL (PATCH [ANDRODERM])

Adults, Elderly. Start therapy with 5 mg/day patch applied at night. Apply patch to abdomen, back, thighs, or upper arms.

TRANSDERMAL (GEL [ANDROGEL])

Adults, Elderly. Initial dose of 5 mg of 1% gel delivers 50 mg testosterone and is applied once daily to the abdomen, shoulders, or upper arms. May increase to 7.5 g, then to 10 g, if necessary.

TRANSDERMAL (GEL [TESTIM])

Adults, Elderly. Initial dose of 5 g delivers 50 mg testosterone and is applied once a day to the shoulders or upper arms. May increase to 10 g per day.

BUCCAL SYSTEM (STRIANT)

Adults, Elderly. 30 mg q12h.

▸ **Delayed puberty**

IM

Adults. 50-200 mg q2-4wk.

Adolescents. 40-50 mg/m^2/dose every month for 6 mo.

SC (PELLETS)

Adults, Adolescents. 150-450 mg q3-6mo.

▸ **Breast carcinoma**

IM (CYPIONATE OR ETHANATE)

Adults. 200-400 mg q2-4wk.

CONTRAINDICATIONS

Cardiac impairment, hypercalcemia, pregnancy, prostate or breast cancer in males, severe hepatic or renal disease.

INTERACTIONS

Drug

Hepatotoxic medications: May increase the risk of hepatotoxicity.

Oral anticoagulants: May increase the effects of oral anticoagulants.

Herbal

None known.

Food

None known.

DIAGNOSTIC TEST EFFECTS

May increase blood hemoglobin level and hematocrit, as well as serum LDL, alkaline phosphatase, bilirubin, calcium, potassium, sodium, and AST (SGOT) levels. May decrease serum HDL level.

SIDE EFFECTS

Frequent

Gynecomastia, acne.

Females: Hirsutism, amenorrhea or other menstrual irregularities, deepening of voice, clitoral enlargement that may not be reversible when drug is discontinued.

Occasional

Edema, nausea, insomnia, oligospermia, priapism, male pattern baldness, bladder irritability, hypercalcemia (in immobilized patients or those with breast cancer), hypercholesterolemia, inflammation and pain at IM injection site.

Transdermal: Pruritus, erythema, skin irritation.

Rare

Polycythemia (with high dosage), hypersensitivity.

SERIOUS REACTIONS

- Peliosis hepatitis (presence of blood-filled cysts in parenchyma of liver), hepatic neoplasms, and hepatocellular carcinoma have been associated with prolonged high-dose therapy.
- Anaphylactic reactions occur rarely.

PRECAUTIONS & CONSIDERATIONS

Caution is warranted in patients with diabetes and hepatic or renal impairment. Testosterone use is contraindicated during breastfeeding. Use testosterone with caution in children because its safety and efficacy have not been established. Testosterone use in elderly patients may increase the risk of hyperplasia or stimulate growth of occult prostate carcinoma. Avoid taking any other medications, including OTC drugs, without first consulting the physician. Consume a diet high in calories and protein; food may be better tolerated if small, frequent meals are eaten.

Notify the physician of weight gain of ≥ 5 lb/wk, acne, nausea, vomiting, or foot swelling. Females should report deepening of voice, hoarseness, or menstrual irregularities; males should report difficulty urinating, frequent erections, or gynecomastia. Blood hemoglobin and hematocrit, BP, intake and output, weight, serum cholesterol, electrolyte levels, and liver function tests should be monitored. Hand or wrist radiographs should be obtained when using the drug in prepubertal children.

Storage

IM formulations should be kept refrigerated. Other formulations may be kept at room temperature. Topical gels are typically flammable; therefore, avoid fire, flame, and smoking.

Administration

Do not give testosterone IV. For IM use, inject testosterone deep into the gluteal muscle. Warming and shaking redissolves crystals that may form in long-acting preparations. A wet needle may cause the solution to become cloudy; this does not affect potency.

Apply Androderm to clean, dry skin on the back, abdomen, upper arms, or thighs. Do not apply it to the scrotum, bony prominences, such as the shoulder; or oily, damaged, or irritated skin. Do not apply Androderm to the same site for 7 days.

Apply the transdermal gel to clean, dry, intact skin of shoulder or upper arm, preferably in the morning. Androgel may also be applied to the abdomen. Open the packet, squeeze the entire contents into the palm of the hand, and apply at once to the affected site. Allow the gel to dry. Do not apply the gel to the genital areas.

Apply Striant to the gum area above the incisor tooth, alternating sides of the mouth with each application. Striant is not affected by consumption of alcohol or food, gum chewing, or tooth brushing. Remove Striant product before placing the new one.

Tetrabenazine

tet'ra-ben'a-zine

★ Xenazine 🍁 Nitoman

Do not confuse Xenazine with Xenadrine or Xenical, or tetrabenazine with phenoxybenzamine.

CATEGORY AND SCHEDULE

Pregnancy Risk Category: C

Classification: Neurologic agents; monoamine depletor; adrenergic inhibitor

MECHANISM OF ACTION

A selective, reversible, centrally acting dopamine-depleting drug that works by inhibiting vesicular monoamine transporter 2 (VMAT2). Tetrabenazine depletes presynaptic dopamine, norepinephrine, and serotonin storage and antagonizes postsynaptic dopamine receptors. Weak binding affinity at the dopamine-2 receptor. *Therapeutic Effect:* Improves symptoms associated with hyperkinetic movement disorders such as Huntington disease.

PHARMACOKINETICS

Absorption at least 75% of PO dose. Protein binding: 85%. Nineteen identified metabolites; the major liver enzyme involved is CYP2D6. Peak plasma concentrations reached within 1.5 h. Primarily excreted in urine (major) and feces (minor) as metabolites. *Half-life:* 4-8 h (increased in hepatic impairment).

AVAILABILITY

Tablets: 12.5 mg, 25 mg.

INDICATIONS AND DOSAGES

▸ **For Huntington chorea**

PO

Adults. Initially,12.5 mg PO each morning. After 1 wk, increase to 12.5 mg PO twice daily. May increase by 12.5 mg each week. The maximum recommended single dose is 25 mg.

Those needing > 50 mg/day should be genotyped for CYP2D6 expression first. *For CYP2D6 Extensive and Intermediate Metabolizers (patients who express CYP2D6):* At doses above 50 mg per day, titrate up slowly at weekly intervals by 12.5 mg. Doses above 50 mg/day should be divided and given in a three times a day regimen. The maximum recommended total daily dose is 100 mg and the maximum recommended single dose is 37.5 mg. Reduce dose if not tolerated. *For CYP2D6 Poor Metabolizers (patients who do not express CYP2D6:* In patients who are CYP2D6 poor metabolizers, dosing is similar except that the recommended maximum single dose is 25 mg, and the maximum recommended daily dose is 50 mg/day.

▸ **Dosage adjustment if receiving strong CYP2D6 inhibitors**

The daily dose of tetrabenazine should be halved in patients newly receiving strong CYP2D6 inhibitors. In patients on a stable dose of a strong CYP2D6 inhibitor, follow the same dosing guidelines as those for poor metabolizers of CYP2D6.

▸ **Dose adjustment for adverse events**

If adverse events such as akathisia, restlessness, parkinsonism, depression, insomnia, anxiety, or intolerable sedation occur, reduce the dose. If the adverse event does not resolve, consider discontinuing. Tetrabenazine may be abruptly discontinued, but chorea may occur 12-18 h after the last dose. If tetrabenazine therapy is interrupted for ≥ 5 days, retitrate the dose.

CONTRAINDICATIONS

Hypersensitivity, hepatic impairment, inadequately treated depression or current suicidality, use with MAOIs or within 14 days of MAOIs, use with reserpine or within 20 days of reserpine.

INTERACTIONS

Drug

Alcohol or other CNS depressants: May have additive sedative effects.

Any strong CYP2D6 inhibitor (e.g., fluoxetine, paroxetine, quinidine): Decreases tetrabenazine elimination, and may require reduction in tetrabenazine dosage.

MAOIs: Contraindicated because the MAOI activity directly inhibits the action of tetrabenazine.

QT-prolonging agents (e.g., class IA and III antiarrhythmics, cisapride, pimozide, etc.): Increase the risk of QT prolongation. Avoid.

Reserpine: Binds irreversibly to VMAT2 with a duration of several days. Using tetrabenazine concurrently may cause overdosage and major depletion of serotonin and norepinephrine in the CNS. At least 20 days should elapse after stopping reserpine before starting tetrabenazine. Contraindicated.

Herbal and Food
None known.

DIAGNOSTIC TEST EFFECTS
Hyperprolactinemia. Before patients are given a daily dose > 50 mg, they should be tested for the CYP2D6 gene to determine whether they are poor metabolizers (PMs).

SIDE EFFECTS
Frequent
Common adverse effects such as depression, dysphagia, nausea, fatigue, insomnia, sedation/somnolence, parkinsonism, and akathisia/restlessness may be dose-dependent and may resolve or lessen with dosage adjustment or specific treatment.
Occasional
Anxiety, irritability, change in appetite, shortness of breath, headache, unsteady gait, anxiety, ecchymosis, dysuria.
Rare
See Serious Reactions.

SERIOUS REACTIONS
- Neuroleptic malignant syndrome (NMS) (rare).
- Dysphagia interfering with oral intake.
- Increase in QT interval.
- Tardive dyskinesia or akathisia.

PRECAUTIONS & CONSIDERATIONS
NOTE: Tetrabenazine is available only from a Specialty Pharmacy Network; the physician and patient must complete and sign the Xenazine Treatment Form to enroll.

This drug can increase the risk of depression and suicidal thoughts and behavior (suicidality). Close observation of patients should accompany therapy. Report unusual or worsening behaviors of concern promptly to the treating physician. Use with caution in those with a history of breast cancer, with cardiac disease such as heart failure, recent heart attack or arrhythmia, orthostasis, or electrolyte imbalances. It is not known if the drug crosses the placenta, and it is unknown if tetrabenazine is distributed in breast milk. Breastfeeding is not recommended. Be aware that the safety and efficacy of this drug have not been established in children.

Before starting drug therapy, check baseline lab values, especially hepatic function. Expect to monitor for unusual movements, behaviors, difficulty swallowing or speaking, excessive sedation, dizziness, nausea, and pattern of daily activity. Avoid activities that require mental acuity if dizziness or sedation occurs.
Storage
Store tablets at room temperature.
Administration
Give tetrabenazine without regard to meals, at roughly the same times each day.

Tetracycline
tet-ra-sye′kleen
🍁 Apo-Tetra, Nu-Tetra

CATEGORY AND SCHEDULE
Pregnancy Risk Category: D

Classification: Anti-infectives, tetracyclines

MECHANISM OF ACTION
A tetracycline antibiotic that inhibits bacterial protein synthesis by binding to ribosomes. *Therapeutic Effect:* Bacteriostatic.

PHARMACOKINETICS

Readily absorbed from the GI tract. Protein binding: 30%-60%. Widely distributed. Excreted in urine; eliminated in feces through biliary system. Not removed by hemodialysis. *Half-life:* 6-11 h (increased in impaired renal function).

AVAILABILITY

Capsules: 250 mg, 500 mg.

INDICATIONS AND DOSAGES

▸ **Inflammatory acne vulgaris, Lyme disease, mycoplasmal disease, *Legionella* infections, Rocky Mountain spotted fever, chlamydial infections in patients with gonorrhea**

PO

Adults, Elderly. 250-500 mg q6-12h. Duration of therapy and exact dose is based on indication.

Children 8 yr and older. 25-50 mg/kg/day in 4 divided doses. Maximum: 3 g/day.

▸ ***Helicobacter pylori* infections**

PO

Adults, Elderly. 500 mg 2-4 times a day (in combination with another antibiotic and acid suppressant therapy).

▸ **Dosage in renal impairment**

Dosage interval is modified based on creatinine clearance.

Creatinine Clearance (mL/min)	Dosage Interval
50-80	Usual dose q8-12h
10-50	Usual dose q12-24h
< 10	Usual dose q24h

CONTRAINDICATIONS

Children 8 yr and younger, hypersensitivity to tetracyclines or sulfites.

INTERACTIONS

Drug

Aluminum-, calcium-, or magnesium-containing antacids, iron, zinc, sodium bicarbonate, sucralfate, didanosine, quinapril: May decrease tetracycline absorption.

Retinoic acid derivatives: May enhance retinoic acid's adverse effects.

Carbamazepine, phenobarbital, phenytoin, rifamycin: May decrease tetracycline blood concentration.

Cholestyramine, colestipol: May decrease tetracycline absorption.

Oral contraceptives: May decrease the efficacy of oral contraceptives.

Warfarin: May increase warfarin's anticoagulant effects.

Herbal

Dong quai, St. John's wort: May increase the risk of photosensitivity.

Food

Dairy products: Inhibit tetracycline absorption.

DIAGNOSTIC TEST EFFECTS

May increase BUN and serum alkaline phosphatase, amylase, bilirubin, AST (SGOT), and ALT (SGPT) levels.

SIDE EFFECTS

Frequent

Dizziness, light-headedness, diarrhea, nausea, vomiting, abdominal cramps, possibly severe photosensitivity.

Occasional

Pigmentation of skin or mucous membranes, rectal or genital pruritus, stomatitis.

SERIOUS REACTIONS

- Superinfection (especially fungal) may occur.

T

- Bulging fontanelles occur rarely in infants.
- Pseudotumor cerebri and increased intracranial pressure.
- Hepatotoxicity (rare).
- Hypersensitivity.

PRECAUTIONS & CONSIDERATIONS

Caution is warranted with those who cannot avoid the sun or ultraviolet exposure because such exposure can produce a severe photosensitivity reaction. Tetracycline readily crosses the placenta and is distributed in breast milk. Women in the last half of pregnancy should avoid using tetracycline because it may inhibit skeletal growth of the fetus. Tetracycline use is not recommended for children 8 yr and younger because it may cause permanent discoloration of teeth or enamel hypoplasia and may inhibit skeletal growth. No age-related precautions have been noted in elderly patients.

History of allergies, especially to tetracyclines, should be determined before drug therapy. Pattern of daily bowel activity, stool consistency, food intake and tolerance, and skin for rash should be assessed. Be alert for signs and symptoms of superinfection, such as anal or genital pruritus, diarrhea, and ulceration or changes of the oral mucosa or tongue. BP and level of consciousness should be monitored because of the potential for increased intracranial pressure.

Storage

Store at room temperature protected from moisture; do not keep past expiration date.

Administration

Space drug doses evenly around the clock. Take capsules with a full glass of water 1 h before or 2 h after a meal. Doses should be separated from antacids; administer 1-2 h before or 4 h after.

! Never use expired tetracycline, as toxic alterations occur.

Thalidomide

thal-lid′oh-mide

★ 🍁 Thalomid

CATEGORY AND SCHEDULE

Pregnancy Risk Category: X

Classification: Immunomodulators, tumor necrosis factor modulators

MECHANISM OF ACTION

An immunomodulator whose exact mechanism is unknown. Has sedative, anti-inflammatory, and immunosuppressive activity, which may be due to selective inhibition of the production of tumor necrosis factor-α. Also is an inhibitor of angiogenesis. *Therapeutic Effect:* Improves muscle wasting in HIV patients; treats a variety of cancer syndromes.

AVAILABILITY

Capsules: 50 mg, 100 mg, 150 mg, 200 mg.

INDICATIONS AND DOSAGES

▸ **AIDS-related muscle wasting (unlabeled)**

PO

Adults. 100-200 mg a day.

▸ **Leprosy**

PO

Adults, Elderly. Initially, 100-300 mg/day as single bedtime dose, at least 1 h after the evening meal. Continue until active reaction subsides, then reduce dose q2-4wk in 50-mg increments.

▸ **Multiple myeloma**

PO

Adults. 200 mg a day (as a single bedtime dose, at least 1 h after the evening meal in combination with dexamethasone on specified days as determined by regimen).

OFF-LABEL USES

Behçet syndrome, discoid lupus erythematosus, treatment of Crohn disease, recurrent aphthous ulcers in HIV patients, wasting syndrome associated with HIV or cancer.

CONTRAINDICATIONS

Pregnancy, neutropenia, peripheral neuropathy; sensitivity to thalidomide.

INTERACTIONS

Drug

Alcohol, other CNS depressants: May increase sedative effects.

Medications associated with peripheral neuropathy (such as isoniazid, lithium, metronidazole, phenytoin): May increase peripheral neuropathy.

Medications that decrease effectiveness of hormonal contraceptives (such as carbamazepine, protease inhibitors, rifampin): May decrease the effectiveness of the contraceptive; patient must use two other methods of contraception.

Herbal

Cat's claw, echinacea: May intensify thalidomide's immunosuppressant effects.

Food

None known.

DIAGNOSTIC TEST EFFECTS

None known.

SIDE EFFECTS

Frequent

Somnolence, dizziness, mood changes, constipation, dry mouth, peripheral neuropathy.

Occasional

Increased appetite, weight gain, headache, loss of libido, edema of face and limbs, nausea, alopecia, dry skin, rash, hypothyroidism.

SERIOUS REACTIONS

- Neutropenia, peripheral neuropathy, severe skin rash, and thromboembolism occur rarely.
- Highly teratogenic, causing limb malformations, etc.

PRECAUTIONS & CONSIDERATIONS

Only available to practitioners and patients enrolled in the STEPS Program, to ensure appropriate prescribing and monitoring to avoid pregnancy exposure. Because thromboembolic events have been reported, patients should be monitored closely, and prophylactic anticoagulation may be considered. Risk may be greater with concomitant dexamethasone use. Caution is warranted with history of seizures, renal or hepatic impairment, cardiac disease, or constipation.

! Thalidomide is contraindicated in pregnant women. Women of childbearing age should perform a pregnancy test within 24 h before beginning thalidomide therapy and then every 2-4 wks.

! Because thalidomide is a known teratogen, contraception must be used by both men and women taking the drug 4 wks before, during treatment, and 4 wks following discontinuation.

Avoid consuming alcohol or using other drugs that cause drowsiness during thalidomide therapy. Also avoid tasks that require mental alertness or motor skills until response to the drug has been established. Notify the physician if symptoms of peripheral neuropathy occur. HIV viral load, nerve conduction studies, and WBC count should be monitored.

Storage

Store capsules at room temperature. Protect from light.

Administration

Administer thalidomide with water at least 1 h after the evening meal and, if possible, at bedtime because of the risk of developing somnolence.

Theophylline

thee-off'i-lin

★ Elixophyllin, Theo-24, Theochron, Uniphyl

🍁 Apo-Theo-LA, Novo-Theophyl, Pulmophylline, Theolair, Uniphyl

CATEGORY AND SCHEDULE

Pregnancy Risk Category: C

Classification: Bronchodilators, methylxanthines

MECHANISM OF ACTION

A methylxanthine derivative with two distinct actions in the airways of patients with reversible obstruction: smooth muscle relaxation and suppression of the response of airways to stimuli. Mechanisms of action are not known with certainty. Theophylline is known to increase the force of contraction of diaphragmatic muscles by enhancing calcium uptake through adenosine-mediated channels. *Therapeutic Effect:* Causes bronchodilation.

PHARMACOKINETICS

The pharmacokinetics of theophylline vary widely among similar patients and cannot be predicted by age, sex, body weight, or other demographic characteristics. Rapidly and completely absorbed after oral administration in solution or immediate-release solid oral dosage form. Distributed freely into fat-free tissues. Extensively metabolized in liver. *Half-life:* 4-8 h.

AVAILABILITY

Elixir: 80 mg/15 mL (Elixophyllin).
Premixed IV Infusion Solution: 80 mg/100 mL, 200 mg/100 mL, 400 mg/100 mL, 800 mg/100 mL.
Tablet, Extended Release (BID dosing, Theocron): 100 mg, 200 mg, 300 mg.
24-hr Controlled Release Tablet (Uniphyl): 400 mg.
24-hr Extended Release Capsule (Theo-24): 100 mg, 200 mg, 300 mg, 400 mg.

INDICATIONS AND DOSAGES

▸ **Chronic lung diseases**

PO

Adults, Adolescents, Children. Acute symptoms: 5 mg/kg using immediate-release product.

▸ **Maintenance therapy**

Adults, Children weighing > 45 kg. 10 mg/kg/day (maximum 300 mg/day) divided q6-8h. After 3 days, increase to 400 mg/day divided q6-8h. After 3 more days, increase to 600 mg/day. Maximum: 800 mg.

IV

5 mg/kg load over 20 min, maintenance 0.25 mg/kg/h (CHF, elderly), 0.4 mg/kg/h (nonsmokers), 0.7 mg/kg/h (young adult smokers). Slow titration: Initial dose 16 mg/kg/day or 400 mg daily, whichever is less, doses divided every 6-8 h.

▸ **Dosage adjustment after serum theophylline measurement:**

Serum level 5-10 mcg/mL if symptoms not controlled, increase dose by 25% and recheck in 3 days. Serum level 10-20 mcg/mL, maintain dosage if tolerated, recheck level every 6-12 mo. Serum level 20-25 mcg/mL, decrease dose by 25%, recheck level in 3 days. Serum level 25-30 mcg/mL, skip next dose, decrease dose by 25%, recheck level in 3 days. Serum level > 30 mcg/mL, skip next 2 doses, decrease dose by 50%, recheck level in 3 days.

OFF-LABEL USES

Apnea of prematurity.

CONTRAINDICATIONS

Hypersensitivity to theophylline or any component of the formulation.

INTERACTIONS

Drug

Adenosine: May decrease the effects of adenosine.
Cimetidine, ciprofloxacin, erythromycin, fluvoxamine, norfloxacin, tacrine: May increase theophylline blood concentration and risk of theophylline toxicity.
Phenytoin, primidone, rifampin: May increase theophylline metabolism.
Smoking: May decrease theophylline blood concentration.

Herbal

St. John's wort: May increase metabolism of theophylline.

Food

Charcoal-broiled foods; high-protein, low-carbohydrate diet: May decrease the theophylline blood level.
High-fat meal: May cause "dose dumping" of Theo-24 product. Avoid.

DIAGNOSTIC TEST EFFECTS

None known. Measure serum theophylline level to guide all dosage adjustments.

IV INCOMPATIBILITIES

Amphotericin B, cefepime (Maxipime), diazepam, hetastarch, inamrinone, lansoprazole (Prevacid), phenytoin.

SIDE EFFECTS

Anxiety, dizziness, headache, insomnia, light-headedness, muscle twitching, restlessness, seizures, dysrhythmias, fluid retention with tachycardia, hypotension, palpitations, pounding heartbeat, sinus tachycardia, anorexia, bitter taste, diarrhea, dyspepsia, gastroesophageal reflux, nausea, vomiting, urinary frequency, increased respiratory rate, flushing, urticaria.

SERIOUS REACTIONS

- Overdose may result in seizures, cardiac arrhythmias, severe vomiting.

PRECAUTIONS & CONSIDERATIONS

Caution is warranted in patients with peptic ulcer, hyperthyroidism, seizure disorders, hypertension, and cardiac arrhythmias (excluding bradyarrhythmias). Be aware that dose adjustments must be made for smokers. Be aware that theophylline crosses the placenta and is distributed in breast milk. A dose reduction should be used when starting theophylline in elderly patients. Avoid excessive amounts of caffeine as well as extremes in dietary protein and carbohydrates. Charbroiled foods may increase elimination and reduce the half-life.

Nervousness, restlessness, and increased heart rate may occur during theophylline therapy. Signs and symptoms of theophylline toxicity are persistent; serum theophylline level should be drawn and dose should be withheld.

Storage

Store oral products at room temperature. Premixed infusion should be kept in protective overwrap until time of use; do not freeze.

Administration

Take this medication with a full glass of water on an empty stomach, at least 1 h before or 2 h after a meal.

Do not chew or crush the extended-release tablets; swallow them whole. Extended-release capsules may be swallowed whole or opened and the contents mixed with soft food and swallowed without chewing.

For intravenous use, use a controlled-rate infusion pump. Loading doses should not exceed 20 mg/min IV rate. Maximal concentration for infusion is 0.8 mg/mL. Measure theophylline concentrations every 12-24 h during infusion therapy.

Thiamine (Vitamin B_1)

thy'a-min

🍁 Betaxin

CATEGORY AND SCHEDULE

Pregnancy Risk Category: A (C if used in doses above recommended daily allowance)

OTC (tablets)

Classification: Vitamins, water soluble; B-vitamins

MECHANISM OF ACTION

A water-soluble vitamin that combines with adenosine triphosphate in the liver, kidneys, and leukocytes to form thiamine diphosphate, a coenzyme that is necessary for carbohydrate metabolism. *Therapeutic Effect:* Prevents and reverses thiamine deficiency.

PHARMACOKINETICS

Readily absorbed from the GI tract, primarily in duodenum, after IM administration. Widely distributed. Metabolized in the liver. Primarily excreted in urine.

AVAILABILITY

Tablets: 50 mg, 100 mg, 250 mg, 500 mg.
Injection: 100 mg/mL.

INDICATIONS AND DOSAGES

▸ **Dietary supplement**

PO

Adults, Elderly. 1-2 mg/day.
Children. 0.5-1 mg/day.
Infants. 0.2-0.3 mg/day.

▸ **Thiamine deficiency**

PO

Adults, Elderly. 5-30 mg/day, as a single dose or in 3 divided doses, for 1 mo.
Children. 10-50 mg/day in 3 divided doses for 1 mo.

▸ **Thiamine deficiency in patients who are critically ill or have malabsorption syndrome**

IV, IM

Adults, Elderly. 5-30 mg, 3 times a day for 1 mo.
Children. 10-25 mg/day for 1 mo.

▸ **Treatment of Wernicke-Korsakoff syndrome**

IV

Adults, Elderly. Initially, 100 mg, followed by 50-100 mg/day until normal dietary intake of thiamine is established.

CONTRAINDICATIONS

Sensitivity to thiamine or components of formulation.

INTERACTIONS

Drug
None known.
Herbal
None known.
Food
Alcohol: Can deplete thiamine from body.

DIAGNOSTIC TEST EFFECTS

None known.

T

IV INCOMPATIBILITIES

Aminophylline, hydrocortisone (Solu-Cortef), furosemide, imipenem/cilastatin (Primaxin IV), methylprednisolone (Solu-Medrol), phenobarbital, phenytoin, sodium bicarbonate.

IV COMPATIBILITIES

Famotidine (Pepcid), multivitamins.

SIDE EFFECTS

Frequent

Pain, induration, and tenderness at IM injection site.

SERIOUS REACTIONS

• IV administration may result in a rare, severe hypersensitivity reaction marked by a feeling of warmth, pruritus, urticaria, weakness, diaphoresis, nausea, restlessness, tightness in throat, angioedema, cyanosis, pulmonary edema, GI tract bleeding, and cardiovascular collapse.

PRECAUTIONS & CONSIDERATIONS

Caution is warranted with Wernicke encephalopathy. Thiamine crosses the placenta; it is unknown whether it is excreted in breast milk. No age-related precautions have been noted in children or elderly patients. Consuming foods rich in thiamine, including legumes, nuts, organ meats, pork, rice bran, seeds, wheat germ, whole-grain and enriched cereals, and yeast, is encouraged.

Urine may appear bright yellow during therapy. Before and during treatment, signs and symptoms of thiamine deficiency, including peripheral neuropathy, ataxia, hyporeflexia, muscle weakness, nystagmus, ophthalmoplegia, confusion, peripheral edema, bounding arterial pulse, and tachycardia, should be assessed.

Storage

Store tablets and unopened vials at room temperature. Once diluted for infusion, use within 24 h.

Administration

IM and IV administration routes are used only in acutely ill patients and in those who are unresponsive to the PO route, such as those with malabsorption syndrome. The IM route is preferred over the IV route. The solution may be given by IV push or may be added to most IV solutions and given as an IV infusion.

IM injection may cause discomfort. Discomfort may be reduced by applying cool compresses.

Thioridazine

thye-or-rid′a-zeen

Do not confuse thioridazine with thiothixene or Thorazine.

CATEGORY AND SCHEDULE

Pregnancy Risk Category: C

Classification: Antipsychotics, phenothiazines

MECHANISM OF ACTION

A phenothiazine that blocks dopamine at postsynaptic receptor sites. Possesses strong anticholinergic and sedative effects. *Therapeutic Effect:* Suppresses behavioral response in psychosis; reduces locomotor activity and aggressiveness.

AVAILABILITY

Tablets: 10 mg, 25 mg, 50 mg, 100 mg.

INDICATIONS AND DOSAGES

▸ **Psychosis**

PO

Adults, Elderly, Children 12 yr and older. Initially, 10-50 mg 3 times a day; dosage increased gradually q4-7 days. Maximum: 300 mg/day. *Children aged 2-11 yr.* Initially, 0.5 mg/kg/day in 2-3 divided doses. Maximum: 3 mg/kg/day.

OFF-LABEL USES

Treatment of behavioral problems in children, dementia, depressive neurosis.

CONTRAINDICATIONS

Hypersensitivity; use with drugs known to prolong the QTc interval or congenital long QT syndrome or cardiac arrhythmias; CNS depression or comatose states; heart disease of extreme degree. Do not use with CYP2D6 inhibitors or in poor metabolizers (genetically) of CYP2D6.

INTERACTIONS

Drug

Alcohol, other CNS depressants: May increase respiratory depression and the hypotensive effects of thioridazine.

Antithyroid agents: May increase the risk of agranulocytosis.

CYP2D6 inhibitors (e.g., fluvoxamine, fluoxetine, paroxetine, pindolol, propranolol, others): Increase the risk of QT prolongation by decreasing thioridazine metabolism; contraindicated.

Extrapyramidal symptom–producing medications: May increase the risk of extrapyramidal symptoms.

Hypotension-producing agents: May increase hypotension.

Levodopa: May decrease the effects of levodopa.

Lithium: May decrease the absorption of thioridazine and produce adverse neurologic effects.

MAOIs: May increase the anticholinergic and sedative effects of thioridazine.

QT-prolonging agents (e.g., class 1A and III antiarrhythmics, cisapride, pimozide, select quinolone antibiotics, tricyclic antidepressants, macrolides, etc.): Increase the risk of QT prolongation, contraindicated.

Herbal

None known.

Food

None known.

DIAGNOSTIC TEST EFFECTS

May cause ECG changes. Elevation of prolactin. May lower WBC count. Rare elevations in hepatic enzymes.

SIDE EFFECTS

Occasional

Drowsiness during early therapy, dry mouth, blurred vision, lethargy, constipation or diarrhea, nasal congestion, peripheral edema, urine retention.

Rare

Ocular changes, altered skin pigmentation (in those taking high doses for prolonged periods), photosensitivity, darkening of urine.

SERIOUS REACTIONS

- Prolonged QT interval may produce torsades de pointes, a form of ventricular tachycardia, and sudden death.
- Leukopenia, agranulocytosis occur rarely.
- Hepatotoxicity with jaundice and biliary stasis (rare).
- Extrapyramidal movement disorders.
- Neuroleptic malignant syndrome.

PRECAUTIONS & CONSIDERATIONS

Caution is warranted in patients with benign prostatic hypertrophy, decreased GI motility, seizures, urinary retention, and visual problems. Urine may darken and drowsiness and dizziness may occur but generally subside with continued therapy. Alcohol, tasks requiring mental alertness or motor skills, and exposure to artificial light and sunlight should be avoided. BP, CBC, ECG, serum potassium level, and liver function test results, including serum alkaline phosphatase, bilirubin, AST (SGOT), and ALT (SGPT) levels, should be monitored. Extrapyramidal symptoms should be assessed.

Storage

Store tablets at room temperature.

Administration

Full therapeutic effect may take up to 6 wks to appear. Do not abruptly discontinue the drug after long-term use. May take tablets without regard to food.

Thiothixene

thye-oh-thix'een

★ 🍁 Navane

Do not confuse thiothixene with thioridazine.

CATEGORY AND SCHEDULE

Pregnancy Risk Category: C

Classification: Antipsychotics

T

MECHANISM OF ACTION

An antipsychotic that blocks postsynaptic dopamine receptor sites in brain. Has α-adrenergic blocking effects and depresses the release of hypothalamic and hypophyseal hormones. *Therapeutic Effect:* Suppresses psychotic behavior.

PHARMACOKINETICS

Well absorbed from the GI tract after PO administration. Widely distributed. Metabolized in the liver. Excreted primarily in urine. Unknown whether removed by hemodialysis. *Half-life:* Biphasic, 3.4 h (initial); 34 h (terminal).

AVAILABILITY

Capsules: 1 mg, 2 mg, 5 mg, 10 mg, 20 mg.

INDICATIONS AND DOSAGES

▸ **Psychosis**

PO

Adults, Elderly, Children older than 12 yr. Initially, 2 mg 3 times a day or 5 mg twice daily. Maximum: 60 mg/day.

CONTRAINDICATIONS

Blood dyscrasias, circulatory collapse, central nervous system (CNS) depression, coma, history of seizures.

Hypersensitivity to thiothixene; sensitivity to phenothiazines due to potential cross-sensitivity.

INTERACTIONS

Drug

Alcohol, other CNS depressants: May increase CNS and respiratory depression and the hypotensive effects of thiothixene.

Extrapyramidal symptom–producing medications: May increase the risk of extrapyramidal symptoms.

Levodopa: May inhibit the effects of levodopa.

QT-prolonging medications: May increase cardiac effects.

Herbal

Kava kava, St. John's wort, valerian: May increase CNS depression.

Food

None known.

DIAGNOSTIC TEST EFFECTS

Elevation of prolactin. May lower WBC count. Rare elevations in hepatic enzymes (usually transient) or prolongation of QT interval.

SIDE EFFECTS

Expected
Hypotension, dizziness, syncope (occur frequently after first injection, occasionally after subsequent injections, and rarely with oral form).
Frequent
Transient drowsiness, dry mouth, constipation, blurred vision, nasal congestion.
Occasional
Diarrhea, peripheral edema, urine retention, nausea.
Rare
Ocular changes, altered skin pigmentation (in those taking high doses for prolonged periods), photosensitivity.

SERIOUS REACTIONS

- The most common extrapyramidal reaction is akathisia, characterized by motor restlessness and anxiety. Akinesia, marked by rigidity, tremor, increased salivation, mask-like facial expression, and reduced voluntary movements, occurs less frequently. Dystonias, including torticollis, opisthotonos, and oculogyric crisis, occur rarely.
- Tardive dyskinesia, characterized by tongue protrusion, puffing of the cheeks, and chewing or puckering of the mouth, occurs rarely but may be irreversible. Elderly women have a greater risk of developing this reaction.
- Neuroleptic malignant syndrome occurs rarely.
- Rare cases of leukopenia.

PRECAUTIONS & CONSIDERATIONS

Caution is warranted in patients with alcohol withdrawal, dementia-related psychosis, severe cardiovascular disorders, glaucoma, benign prostatic hyperplasia, and exposure to extreme heat. Thiothixene crosses the placenta and is distributed in breast milk. Children are more prone to develop extrapyramidal and neuromuscular symptoms, especially dystonias. Safety and efficacy not established in children under 12 yr of age. Elderly patients are more prone to anticholinergic effects (such as dry mouth), extrapyramidal symptoms, orthostatic hypotension, and increased sedation.

Drowsiness and dizziness may occur but generally subside with continued therapy. Alcohol, tasks requiring mental alertness or motor skills, and exposure to artificial light and sunlight should be avoided. Notify the physician if fluid retention, fever, or visual disturbances occur. Pattern of daily bowel activity and stool consistency, BP, and signs of extrapyramidal reactions should be assessed.
Storage
Store tablets at room temperature.
Administration
Take thiothixene without regard to food. The drug's full therapeutic effect may take up to 6 wks to appear.

Thyroid

thye′roid
★ Armour Thyroid, Bio-Throid, Nature-Thyroid NT, NP-Thyroid

CATEGORY AND SCHEDULE

Pregnancy Risk Category: A

Classification: Hormones/hormone modifiers, thyroid agents

MECHANISM OF ACTION

A natural hormone derived from animal sources, usually beef or pork, that is involved in normal metabolism, growth, and development, especially the central nervous system (CNS) of infants. Possesses catabolic and anabolic effects. Provides both levothyroxine and liothyronine hormones.
Therapeutic Effect: Increases basal metabolic rate, enhances gluconeogenesis, stimulates protein synthesis.

PHARMACOKINETICS

Partially absorbed from the GI tract. Protein binding: 99%. Widely distributed. Metabolized in liver to active liothyronine (T_3) and inactive, reverse triiodothyronine (rT_3) metabolites. Eliminated by biliary excretion. *Half-life:* 2-7 days.

AVAILABILITY

Capsules: 15 mg, 30 mg, 60 mg, 90 mg, 120 mg, 180 mg, 240 mg (Bio-Throid).
Tablets: 15 mg, 30 mg, 60 mg, 90 mg, 120 mg, 180 mg, 240 mg, 300 mg (Armour Thyroid). 32.5 mg, 65 mg, 130 mg, 195 mg (Nature-Thyroid NT).

INDICATIONS AND DOSAGES

▸ **Hypothyroidism**

PO

Adults, Elderly. Initially, 15-30 mg. May increase by 15 mg increments q2-4wk. Maintenance: 60-120 mg/day. Use 15 mg initially in patients with cardiovascular disease or myxedema.
Children 12 yr and older. 90 mg/day.
Children 6-12 yr. 60-90 mg/day.
Children 1-5 yr. 45-60 mg/day.
Children older than 6-12 mo. 30-45 mg/day.
Children 3 mo and younger. 15-30 mg/day.

CONTRAINDICATIONS

Uncontrolled adrenal cortical insufficiency, untreated thyrotoxicosis, treatment of obesity, uncontrolled angina, uncontrolled hypertension, uncontrolled myocardial infarction, and hypersensitivity to any component of the formulations.

INTERACTIONS

Drug

Antidiabetic drugs: As thyroid replacement ensues, antidiabetic requirements may change; monitor.
Cholestyramine, colestipol: May decrease absorption of thyroid hormones.
Digoxin: May alter digoxin dose requirements as thyroid function corrected due to increased metabolic rate; monitor.
Enteral feedings, antacids, calcium and iron supplements: May decrease the absorption of thyroid hormones.
Estrogens, oral contraceptives: May decrease effects of thyroid hormones.
Oral anticoagulants: May increase hypoprothrombinemic effects of oral anticoagulants

Herbal

Bugleweed: May decrease effects of thyroid hormones.

Food

Coffee, dairy foods, soybean flour (infant formula), cotton seed meal, walnuts, and dietary fiber: May decrease absorption of thyroid hormones.

DIAGNOSTIC TEST EFFECTS

Dose is adjusted based on monitoring of TSH resopnse. Changes in TBG levels must be considered when interpreting T4 and T3 values.

SIDE EFFECTS

Rare

Dry skin, GI intolerance, skin rash, hives, severe headache.

SERIOUS REACTIONS

- Excessive dosage produces signs and symptoms of hyperthyroidism, including weight loss, palpitations, increased appetite, tremors, nervousness, tachycardia, hypertension, headache, insomnia, and menstrual irregularities.
- Cardiac arrhythmias occur rarely.

PRECAUTIONS & CONSIDERATIONS

Caution is warranted in patients with angina pectoris, hypertension, or other cardiovascular disease as well as adrenal insufficiency, coronary artery disease, and diabetes mellitus. Thyroid hormone does not cross the placenta and is minimally excreted in breast milk. No age-related precautions have been noted in children. Elderly patients may be more sensitive to thyroid effects. Individualized dosages are recommended for this population.

Reversible hair loss can occur during the first few months of therapy. Notify the physician of chest pain, edema of feet or ankles, insomnia, nervousness, tremors, weight loss, or a pulse rate of 100 beats/min or more. Weight and vital signs, especially pulse rate and rhythm, should be monitored.

Storage

Store tablets at room temperature; protect from moisture.

Administration

Begin therapy with small doses and increase the dosage gradually, as prescribed. Take at the same time each day to maintain hormone levels. Take on an empty stomach.

Replacement therapy for hypothyroidism is lifelong.

Tiagabine

ti-ah-ga′bean

★ Gabitril

CATEGORY AND SCHEDULE

Pregnancy Risk Category: C

Classification: Anticonvulsants

MECHANISM OF ACTION

An anticonvulsant that enhances the activity of γ-aminobutyric acid, the major inhibitory neurotransmitter in the central nervous system (CNS). *Therapeutic Effect:* Inhibits seizures.

PHARMACOKINETICS

Rapid and nearly complete (90%-95%) absorption orally. Meals do not change the extent of absorption. Steady state occurs in 2 days. Protein binding: 96%. Two metabolic pathways exist: (1) oxidation via the liver (forms inactive 5-oxo-tiagabine) and (2) glucuronidation. Only 2% excreted unchanged, the rest is excreted into the urine and feces as metabolites. *Half-life:* 7 to 9 h (healthy controls). Decreaed by 50%- 65% in hepatic enzyme-induced patients compared to uninduced patients (half-life increases in hepatic disease).

AVAILABILITY

Tablets: 2 mg, 4 mg, 12 mg, 16 mg.

INDICATIONS AND DOSAGES

▸ **Adjunctive treatment of partial seizures**

PO

Adults, Elderly. Initially, 4 mg once a day. May increase by 4-8 mg/day at weekly intervals. Maximum: 56 mg/day.
Children aged 12-18 yr. Initially, 4 mg once a day. May increase by 4 mg at week 2 and by 4-8 mg at weekly intervals thereafter. Maximum: 32 mg/day.

CONTRAINDICATIONS

Hypersensitivity to tiagabine.

INTERACTIONS

Drug

Carbamazepine, phenobarbital, phenytoin: May increase tiagabine clearance; however, dose titration for tiagabine usually assumes patient is treated with enzyme-inducing drugs.

Valproic acid: May increase free tiagabine concentration. Tiagabine decreases (~ 10%) steady-state valproic acid levels. Monitor for any needed adjustments.

Herbal

None known.

Food

None known.

DIAGNOSTIC TEST EFFECTS

A therapeutic range is not definitively established. Effective trough plasma concentrations ranged from < 1 ng/mL to 234 ng/mL (median, 23.7 ng/mL). In some instances, measurement of levels is helpful to gauge treatment.

SIDE EFFECTS

Frequent (20%-34%)

Dizziness, asthenia, somnolence, nervousness, confusion, headache, infection, tremor.

Occasional

Nausea, diarrhea, abdominal pain, impaired concentration.

SERIOUS REACTIONS

- Overdose is characterized by agitation, confusion, hostility, and weakness. Full recovery occurs within 24 h.

PRECAUTIONS & CONSIDERATIONS

Antiepileptic drugs (AEDs) increase the risk of suicidal thoughts or behavior in patients taking these drugs for any indication. Monitor for the emergence or worsening of depression, suicidal thoughts, and/or any unusual changes in mood or behavior. Use during pregnancy and lactation only when benefits outweigh potential risks. Use in children below 12 yr has not been established. Caution is warranted in patients with hepatic impairment and in those who take other CNS depressants concurrently.

Dizziness may occur, so change positions slowly—from recumbent to sitting position before standing—and alcohol and tasks requiring mental alertness or motor skills should be avoided. History of the seizure disorder, including the duration, frequency, and intensity of seizures, should be reviewed before and during therapy. CBCs and blood chemistry tests to assess hepatic and renal function should be performed before and during treatment.

Storage

Store tablets at room temperature. Protect from light and moisture.

Administration

Tiagabine should be taken with food.

Do not abruptly discontinue the drug. Be aware that in patients without epilepsy, tiagibine is associated with new onset seizure risk.

T

Ticarcillin Disodium/ Clavulanate Potassium

tyekar-sill'in/klav'yoo-la-nate

Timentin

CATEGORY AND SCHEDULE

Pregnancy Risk Category: B

Classification: Antibiotics, penicillins, extended-spectrum penicillin and β-lactamase inhibitor

MECHANISM OF ACTION

Ticarcillin binds to bacterial cell walls, inhibiting cell wall synthesis. Clavulanate inhibits the action of bacterial β-lactamase. Good activity against gram-negative and anaerobic organisms, including *Pseudomonas* spp., as well as methicillin-sensitive gram positives. *Therapeutic Effect:* Bactericidal.

PHARMACOKINETICS

Widely distributed. Protein binding: ticarcillin 45%-60%, clavulanate 9%-30%. Minimally metabolized in the liver. Primarily excreted unchanged in urine. Removed by hemodialysis. *Half-life:* 1-1.2 h (increased in impaired renal function).

AVAILABILITY

Powder for Injection: 3.1 g.
Premixed Solution for Infusion: 3.1 g/100 mL.

INDICATIONS AND DOSAGES

▸ **Skin and skin-structure, bone, joint, and lower respiratory tract infections; septicemia; endometriosis; urinary tract infection**

IV

Adults, Elderly ≥ *60 kg.* 3.1 g (3 g ticarcillin) q4-6h. Maximum: 18-24 g/day.
Adults, Elderly < *60 kg.* 200-300 mg/kg/day divided q4-6h.
Children 3 mo and older. Mild to moderate infections, 200 mg/kg/day (based on ticarcillin content) divided q6h; severe infections, 300 mg/kg/day (based on ticarcillin content) divided q4-6h. Maximum 18-24 g/day.

▸ **Dosage in renal impairment**

Dosage interval is modified based on creatinine clearance.
Adult CrCl 30-60 mL/min: loading dose of 3.1 g, then 2 g q4h or 3.1 g q8h.
Adult CrCl 10-30 mL/min: loading dose of 3.1 g, then 2 g IV q8h or 3.1 g q12h.
Adult CrCl < 10 mL/min: loading dose of 3.1 g, then 2 g IV q12h.
Adult CrCl < 10 mL/min with hepatic impairment: 3.1 g IV, then 2 g IV q24h.

CONTRAINDICATIONS

Hypersensitivity to any penicillin.

INTERACTIONS

Drug

Anticoagulants, heparin, NSAIDs, thrombolytics: May increase the risk of hemorrhage with high dosages of ticarcillin.
Probenecid: May increase ticarcillin blood concentration and risk of toxicity.

Herbal and Food

None known.

DIAGNOSTIC TEST EFFECTS

May increase serum sodium, alkaline phosphatase, bilirubin, LDH, AST (SGOT), and ALT (SGPT) levels. May decrease serum potassium level. May cause a positive Coombs' test.

IV INCOMPATIBILITIES

Amphotericin B complex (Abelcet, AmBisome, Amphotec), azithromycin, caspofungin, cefamandole, diazepam, dobutamine. drotrecogin alfa (Xigris), erythromycin, ganciclovir, haloperiodol, inamrinone, lansoprazole (Prevacid IV), phenytoin, promethazine, quinupristin-dalfopristin (Synercid), vancomycin (Vancocin).

IV COMPATIBILITIES

Diltiazem (Cardizem), heparin, insulin, morphine, propofol (Diprivan).

SIDE EFFECTS

Frequent
Phlebitis or thrombophlebitis (with IV dose), rash, urticaria, pruritus, altered smell or taste.
Occasional
Nausea, diarrhea, vomiting.
Rare
Headache, fatigue, hallucinations, bleeding, or ecchymosis.

SERIOUS REACTIONS

- Overdosage may produce seizures and other neurologic reactions.
- Antibiotic-associated colitis and other superinfections may result from bacterial imbalance.
- Severe hypersensitivity reactions, including anaphylaxis, occur rarely.

PRECAUTIONS & CONSIDERATIONS

Caution is warranted in patients with renal impairment. Sodium load may require caution in some patients. Ticarcillin readily crosses the placenta, appears in cord blood and amniotic fluid, and is distributed in breast milk in low concentrations. Ticarcillin may lead to allergic sensitization, candidiasis, diarrhea, and skin rash in infants. The safety and efficacy of ticarcillin have not been established in children younger than 3 mo. Age-related renal impairment may require dosage adjustment in elderly patients.

History of allergies, especially to cephalosporins or penicillins, should be determined before giving the drug. Withhold and promptly notify the physician if rash or diarrhea occurs. Severe diarrhea with abdominal pain, blood or mucus in stool, and fever may indicate antibiotic-associated colitis. Signs and symptoms of superinfection, including anal or genital pruritus, black hairy tongue, diarrhea, increased fever, sore throat, ulceration or changes of oral mucosa, and vomiting should be monitored. Food tolerance, intake and output, renal function tests, urinalysis, and the injection sites should be assessed.

Storage
The solution normally appears colorless to pale yellow; a darker color indicates a loss of potency. The reconstituted IV infusion (piggyback) is stable for 6 h at room temperature and 3 days if refrigerated. Premixed infusion arrives frozen, and thawed solution is stable for 24 h at room temperature, or 7 days if refrigerated.

Administration
This drug is available in ready-to-use containers. For IV infusion (piggyback), reconstitute each 3.1-g vial with 13 mL sterile water for injection or 0.9% NaCl to provide a concentration of 200 mg ticarcillin and 6.7 mg clavulanic acid per milliliter. Shake the vial to assist reconstitution. Further dilute with D5W or 0.9% NaCl to a concentration between 10 and 100 mg/mL. Infuse the drug over 30 min. Because of the potential for hypersensitivity reactions such as anaphylaxis, start the initial dose at a few drops per minute, and then increase it slowly to the ordered rate. Stay with the patient for the first

10-15 min during the initial dose; then check every 10 min during the infusion for signs and symptoms of hypersensitivity or anaphylaxis.

Ticlopidine

tye-klo′pa-deen

CATEGORY AND SCHEDULE

Pregnancy Risk Category: B

Classification: Platelet inhibitors

MECHANISM OF ACTION

An aggregation inhibitor that inhibits the release of adenosine diphosphate from activated platelets, which prevents fibrinogen from binding to glycoprotein IIb/IIIa receptors on the surface of activated platelets. *Therapeutic Effect:* Inhibits platelet aggregation and thrombus formation.

AVAILABILITY

Tablets: 250 mg.

INDICATIONS AND DOSAGES

▸ **Prevention of stroke**

PO

Adults, Elderly. 250 mg twice a day.

OFF-LABEL USES

Treatment of intermittent claudication, sickle cell disease.

CONTRAINDICATIONS

Active pathologic bleeding, such as bleeding peptic ulcer and intracranial bleeding; hematopoietic disorders, including neutropenia and thrombocytopenia; presence of hemostatic disorder; severe hepatic impairment; hypersensitivity to ticlopidine.

INTERACTIONS

Drug

Aspirin, heparin, oral anticoagulants, thrombolytics: May increase the risk of bleeding with these drugs.

Herbal

None known.

Food

None known.

DIAGNOSTIC TEST EFFECTS

May increase serum cholesterol, serum alkaline phosphatase, bilirubin, triglyceride, AST (SGOT), and ALT (SGPT) levels. May prolong bleeding time. May decrease neutrophil and platelet counts.

SIDE EFFECTS

Frequent (5%-13%)

Diarrhea, nausea, dyspepsia, including heartburn, indigestion, GI discomfort, and bloating.

Rare (1%-2%)

Vomiting, flatulence, pruritus, dizziness.

SERIOUS REACTIONS

- Neutropenia occurs in approximately 2% of patients.
- Thrombotic thrombocytopenia purpura, agranulocytosis, hepatitis, cholestatic jaundice, and tinnitus occur rarely.

PRECAUTIONS & CONSIDERATIONS

Caution is warranted in patients with an increased risk of bleeding and severe hepatic or renal disease. There are no adequate data regarding use during pregnancy or breastfeeding. Safety and efficacy of ticlopidine in children have not been established. No age-related precautions have been noted in elderly patients.

Ticlopidine should be discontinued 10-14 days before surgery if antiplatelet effect is not desired.

Laboratory studies, particularly hepatic enzyme tests and CBC, should be obtained. Pattern of daily bowel activity and stool consistency, BP for hypotension, and skin for rash should be monitored.

Administration

Take ticlopidine with food or just after meals to increase bioavailability and decrease GI discomfort.

Tigecycline

tye-gi-sye′kleen

★ 🍁 Tygacil

CATEGORY AND SCHEDULE

Pregnancy Risk Category: D

Classification:

Anti-infectives, glycylcycline

MECHANISM OF ACTION

A glycylcycline antibiotic that is a derivative of minocycline, which inhibits bacterial protein synthesis by binding to the 30S ribosomal subunit. *Therapeutic Effects:* Bacteriostatic.

PHARMACOKINETICS

Peak 2-3 h. Protein binding: 71%-89%. Widely distributed. Excreted in breast milk; crosses placenta. Not extensively metabolized. Overall, the primary route of elimination for tigecycline is biliary excretion of unchanged drug and its metabolites. Glucuronidation and renal excretion of unchanged tigecycline are secondary routes. Not removed by hemodialysis. *Half-life:* 27-42 h (increased in hepatic impairment).

AVAILABILITY

Powder for Injection: 50 mg.

INDICATIONS AND DOSAGES

▸ **Community-acquired pneumonia, complicated skin and skin-structure infections, complicated intra-abdominal infections**

IV INFUSION

Adults, Elderly. Initially, 100 mg IV loading dose, then 50 mg every 12 h.

▸ **Dosage adjustment for hepatic impairment**

No dosage adjustment for mild to moderate hepatic impairment (Child-Pugh A or Child-Pugh B). For those with severe hepatic impairment (Child Pugh C), initially 100 mg IV, then 25 mg every 12 h. Monitor closely.

CONTRAINDICATIONS

Children younger than 18 yr, hypersensitivity to tigecycline, last half of pregnancy. Not recommended for use with systemic retinoids.

INTERACTIONS

Drug

Isotretinoin: Contraindicated use.

Hormonal contraceptives: May decrease the effects of hormonal contraceptives.

Warfarin: May increase anticoagulant response; monitor INR.

Herbal

St. John's wort: May increase the risk of photosensitivity.

Food

None known.

IV INCOMPATIBILITIES

Amiodarone, amphotericin B (all forms), diazepam, esomeprazole (Nexium), hydralazine, methylprednisolone (Solu-Medrol), nicardipine, pantoprazole (Protonix), phenytoin, quinupristin/dalfopristin (Synercid), verapamil, voriconazole (Vfend).

T

IV COMPATIBILITIES

Amikacin, dobutamine, dopamine, gentamicin, haloperidol, lidocaine, metoclopramide, morphine, norepinephrine, piperacillin/tazobactam (Zosyn), potassium chloride, propofol, ranitidine, theophylline, tobramycin.

DIAGNOSTIC TEST EFFECTS

May increase serum amylase, total bilirubin, AST (SGOT), and ALT (SGPT), as well as prothrombin time.

SIDE EFFECTS

Frequent

Nausea, vomiting, diarrhea, abdominal pain, headache, and increased ALT.

Occasional

Dizziness, possibly severe photosensitivity, drowsiness, vertigo, vaginal candidiasis, injection site pain or phlebitis.

Rare

Stomatitis, increased creatinine.

SERIOUS REACTIONS

- Hypersensitivity may include anaphylaxis.
- Superinfection (especially fungal) may occur.
- Tinnitus and hearing loss have been reported.
- Benign increased intracranial pressure (pseudotumor cerebri).
- Interstitial nephritis, azotemia, metabolic acidosis, acute renal failure.
- Rare cases of acute pancreatitis, hepatitis with jaundice, eosinophilia.
- Tooth discoloration and enamel hypoplasia in children and during fetal development.
- Pseudomembranous colitis from *Clostridium difficile* infection may occur during treatment or at any time several months after therapy is discontinued.

PRECAUTIONS & CONSIDERATIONS

History of allergies, especially to tetracyclines, should be determined before drug therapy, as cross-sensitivity may occur.

Not considered efficacious at decreasing mortality in patients with hospital-associated pneumonia. Caution is warranted in patients with renal impairment and in those who cannot avoid sun or ultraviolet exposure because such exposure may produce a severe photosensitivity reaction. Safe and effective use not established in children < 18 yr. Do not use in children under 8 yr or in pregnancy because of the likelihood of permanent intrinsic staining in erupted permanent teeth. Caution is recommended for use during lactation.

Dizziness, drowsiness, and vertigo may occur. Avoid tasks that require mental alertness or motor skills until response to the drug is established. Pattern of daily bowel activity, stool consistency, food intake and tolerance, renal function, skin for rash should be assessed. Be alert for signs and symptoms of superinfection, such as anal or genital pruritus, diarrhea, sore tongue, fever, fatigue, and ulceration or changes of the oral mucosa or tongue; report symptoms to health care provider immediately. BP and level of consciousness should be monitored because of the potential for increased intracranial pressure. Advise patient to report any signs or symptoms associated with frequent loose stools or bloody diarrhea. Advise patient to maintain compliance with hormonal contraceptive medications while using an additional nonhormonal form of contraception throughout the duration of therapy.

Storage
Store unopened vials at room temperature. Once reconstituted for infusion, may keep up to 24 h.
Administration
Tigecycline is given by slow IV infusion only after dilution. Reconstitute each vial with 5.3 mL 0.9% NaCl, D5W, or lactated Ringer's to a concentration of 10 mg/mL. Withdraw the appropriate dose (25 mg, 50 mg, or 100 mg) and add to a 100-mL intravenous bag for infusion of either 0.9% NaCl, D5W, or lactated Ringer's. The maximum concentration in the intravenous bag should be 1 mg/mL. The reconstituted solution should be yellow to orange in color; if not, the solution should be discarded. Infuse over 30-60 min.

Tiludronate Disodium

ti-loo'dro-nate
★ Skelid

CATEGORY AND SCHEDULE

Pregnancy Risk Category: C

Classification: Bisphosphonates

T

MECHANISM OF ACTION

A calcium regulator that inhibits functioning osteoclasts through disruption of cytoskeletal ring structure and inhibition of osteoclastic proton pump. *Therapeutic Effect:* Inhibits bone resorption.

PHARMACOKINETICS

Poorly absorbed after oral administration; oral bioavailability < 6%. Rapidly taken into bone, with uptake greatest at sites of active bone turnover. Excreted in urine. Half-life: 150 h from plasma (a longer terminal half-life reflects release from skeleton as bone is resorbed).

AVAILABILITY

Tablets: 200 mg.

INDICATIONS AND DOSAGES

▸ Paget disease

PO

Adults, Elderly. 400 mg once a day for 3 mo.

CONTRAINDICATIONS

GI disease, such as dysphagia and gastric ulcer, biphosphonate hypersensitivity, renal impairment (CrCl < 30 mL/min).

INTERACTIONS

Drug
Antacids containing aluminum or magnesium, calcium: May interfere with the absorption of tiludronate.
Herbal
None known.
Food
Beverages other than plain water, dietary supplements, food: May interfere with absorption.

DIAGNOSTIC TEST EFFECTS

Reduces serum calcium and serum phosphate concentrations. Significantly decreases serum alkaline phosphatase level in patients with Paget disease.

SIDE EFFECTS

Frequent (6%-9%)
Nausea, diarrhea, generalized body pain, back pain, headache.
Occasional
Rash, dyspepsia, vomiting, rhinitis, sinusitis, dizziness.

SERIOUS REACTIONS

• Overdose causes hypocalcemia, hypophosphatemia, and significant GI disturbances.

- Esophageal irritation occurs if not given with 6-8 oz of plain water or if the patient lies down within 30 min of drug administration.
- Severe and occasionally debilitating bone, joint, or muscle pain.
- Osteonecrosis of the jaw.

PRECAUTIONS & CONSIDERATIONS

Caution is warranted in patients with hyperparathyroidism, hypocalcemia, and vitamin D deficiency. Because there are no adequate and well-controlled studies in pregnant women, it is unknown whether tiludronate causes fetal harm or is excreted in breast milk. Safety and efficacy of tiludronate have not been established in children. No age-related precautions have been noted in elderly patients.

Consider beginning weight-bearing exercises and modifying behavioral factors, such as reducing alcohol consumption and stopping cigarette smoking. Plan to correct hypocalcemia and vitamin D deficiency, if present, before starting therapy. All patients must have adequate calcium and vitamin D intake daily. Serum electrolytes, including serum alkaline phosphatase and serum calcium levels, should be monitored.

Storage

Store tablets at room temperature.

Administration

! Give at least 2 h before the first food, beverage, or medication of the day. Expected benefits occur only when tiludronate is taken with a full glass (6-8 oz) of plain water first thing in the morning.

Taking with beverages other than plain water, including mineral water, orange juice, and coffee, significantly reduces absorption of the medication.

! Do not lie down for at least 30 min after taking the medication. Remaining upright helps the drug move quickly to the stomach and reduces the risk of esophageal irritation.

Timolol

tim'oh-lole

★ Betimol, Blocadren, Istalol, Timoptic, Timoptic OcuDose, Timoptic-XE, Timoptic OcuMeter

★ Apo-Timop, Tim-AK, Timoptic, Timoptic XE

Do not confuse timolol with atenolol, or Timoptic with Viroptic.

CATEGORY AND SCHEDULE

Pregnancy Risk Category: C (D if used in second or third trimester)

Classification: Antihypertensives, antiadrenergics, β-blocking

MECHANISM OF ACTION

An antihypertensive, antimigraine, and antiglaucoma agent that blocks β_1- and β_2-adrenergic receptors. *Therapeutic Effect:* Reduces intraocular pressure (IOP) by reducing aqueous humor production, lowers BP, slows the heart rate, and decreases myocardial contractility.

PHARMACOKINETICS

Route	Onset	Peak	Duration
PO	15-45 min	0.5-2.5 h	4 h
Ophthalmic	30 min	1-2 h	12-24 h

Well absorbed from the GI tract. Protein binding: 10%. Minimal

T

absorption after ophthalmic administration. Metabolized in the liver. Excreted primarily in urine. Not removed by hemodialysis. *Half-life:* 4 h. Systemic absorption may occur with ophthalmic administration.

AVAILABILITY

Tablets (Blocadren): 5 mg, 10 mg, 20 mg.
Ophthalmic Gel-forming Solution (Timoptic-XE): 0.25%, 0.5%.
Ophthalmic Solution (Betimol, Istalol, Timoptic, Timoptic OccuDose): 0.25%, 0.5%.

INDICATIONS AND DOSAGES

▸ **Mild to moderate hypertension**
PO
Adults, Elderly. Initially, 10 mg twice a day, alone or in combination with other therapy. Gradually increase at intervals of not < 1 wk. Usual dose is 10-20 mg twice daily. Maximum: 60 mg.
▸ **Reduction of cardiovascular mortality in definite or suspected acute myocardial infarction (MI)**
PO
Adults, Elderly. 10 mg twice a day, beginning 1-4 wks after MI.
▸ **Migraine prevention**
PO
Adults, Elderly. Initially, 10 mg twice a day. Range: 10-30 mg/day.
▸ **Reduction of IOP in open-angle glaucoma, aphakic glaucoma, ocular hypertension, and secondary glaucoma**
OPHTHALMIC
Adults, Elderly, Children. 1 drop of 0.25% solution in affected eye(s) twice a day. May be increased to 1 drop of 0.5% solution in affected eye(s) twice a day. When IOP is controlled, dosage may be reduced to 1 drop once a day. If patient is switched to timolol from another antiglaucoma agent, administer concurrently for 1 day. Discontinue other agent on following day.
OPHTHALMIC GEL SOLUTION (TIMOPTIC XE)
Adults, Elderly. 1 drop of 0.25% or 0.5% solution in affected eye(s) once a day.

OFF-LABEL USES

Systemic: Treatment of chronic angina pectoris, hypertrophic cardiomyopathy, pheochromocytoma, thyrotoxicosis, tremors.

CONTRAINDICATIONS

History of bronchial asthma or severe chronic obstructive pulmonary disease (COPD); sinus bradycardia; second-and third-degree heart block; overt cardiac failure; cardiogenic shock; hypersensitivity to timolol.

INTERACTIONS

Drug
Diuretics, other antihypertensives: May increase hypotensive effect.
Insulin, oral hypoglycemics: May mask symptoms of hypoglycemia and prolong hypoglycemic effects of these drugs.
NSAIDs: May decrease antihypertensive effect.
Sympathomimetics, xanthines: May mutually inhibit effects.
Herbal
None known.
Food
None known.

DIAGNOSTIC TEST EFFECTS

May increase serum antinuclear antibody titer and BUN, glucose, serum creatinine, potassium, lipoprotein, triglyceride, and uric acid levels.

SIDE EFFECTS

Frequent

Diminished sexual function, drowsiness, difficulty sleeping, unusual tiredness or weakness. Ophthalmic: Eye irritation, visual disturbances.

Occasional

Depression, cold hands or feet, diarrhea, constipation, anxiety, nasal congestion, nausea, vomiting, bradycardia, bronchospasm.

Rare

Altered taste; dry eyes; itching; numbness of fingers, toes, or scalp.

SERIOUS REACTIONS

- Overdose may produce profound bradycardia, hypotension, and bronchospasm.
- Abrupt withdrawal may result in diaphoresis, palpitations, headache, and tremors.
- Timolol administration may precipitate CHF and MI in patients with cardiac disease; thyroid storm in those with thyrotoxicosis; and peripheral ischemia in those with existing peripheral vascular disease.
- Hypoglycemia may occur in patients with previously controlled diabetes.
- Ophthalmic overdose may produce bradycardia, hypotension, bronchospasm, and acute cardiac failure.

PRECAUTIONS & CONSIDERATIONS

Caution is warranted with hyperthyroidism, impaired hepatic or renal function, and inadequate cardiac function. Precautions apply to both oral and ophthalmic administration because of the possible systemic absorption of ophthalmic timolol. Timolol is distributed in breast milk and is not for use in breastfeeding women because of the potential for serious adverse effects in the breastfed infant. Timolol use should be avoided in pregnant women after the first trimester because it may result in low-birth-weight infants. The drug may also produce apnea, bradycardia, hypoglycemia, or hypothermia during childbirth. The safety and efficacy of oral timolol have not been established in children. In elderly patients, age-related peripheral vascular disease increases susceptibility to decreased peripheral circulation. Be aware that salt and alcohol intake should be restricted. Nasal decongestants or OTC cold preparations (stimulants) should not be used without physician approval. Tasks that require mental alertness or motor skills should be avoided.

Notify the physician of excessive fatigue, prolonged dizziness or headache, or shortness of breath. Pattern of daily bowel activity and stool consistency, ECG for arrhythmias (particularly premature ventricular contractions), BP, heart rate, IOP (with ophthalmic preparation), and liver and renal function test results should be monitored during treatment. If pulse rate is 60 beats/min or lower or systolic BP is < 90 mm Hg, withhold the medication and contact the physician.

Storage

Store tablets at room temperature. Store ophthalmic products upright and protected from light at room temperature.

Administration

Take timolol without regard to meals. Tablets may be crushed. Do not abruptly discontinue timolol. Compliance is essential to control angina, arrhythmias, glaucoma, and hypertension.

! When administering ophthalmic gel, invert container and shake once before each use.

T

For ophthalmic administration, place a finger on the lower eyelid and pull it out until pocket is formed between the eye and lower lid. Hold the dropper above the pocket and place the prescribed number of drops or amount of prescribed gel into pocket. Close eyes gently so that medication will not be squeezed out of the sac. Apply gentle digital pressure to the lacrimal sac at the inner canthus for 1 min after installation to lessen the risk of systemic absorption.

Tinidazole

ty-ni′da-zole

Tindamax Fasigyn

CATEGORY AND SCHEDULE

Pregnancy Risk Category: C (X for first trimester)

Classification: Antiprotozoals

MECHANISM OF ACTION

A nitroimidazole derivative that is converted to the active metabolite by reduction of cell extracts of *Trichomonas.* The active metabolite causes DNA damage in pathogens. *Therapeutic Effect:* Produces antiprotozoal effect.

PHARMACOKINETICS

Rapidly and completely absorbed. Protein binding: 12%. Distributed in all body tissues and fluids; crosses blood-brain barrier. Significantly metabolized. Excreted primarily in urine; partially eliminated in feces. *Half-life:* 12-14 h.

AVAILABILITY

Tablets: 250 mg, 500 mg.

INDICATIONS AND DOSAGES

▸ **Intestinal amebiasis**

PO

Adults, Elderly. 2 g/day for 3 days.
Children 3 yr and older. 50 mg/kg/day (up to 2 g) for 3 days.

▸ **Amebic hepatic abscess**

PO

Adults, Elderly. 2 g/day for 3-5 days.
Children 3 yr and older. 50 mg/kg/day (up to 2 g) for 3-5 days.

▸ **Giardiasis**

PO

Adults, Elderly. 2 g as a single dose.
Children 3 yr and older. 50 mg/kg (up to 2 g) as a single dose.

▸ **Trichomoniasis**

PO

Adults, Elderly. 2 g as a single dose.

▸ **Bacterial vaginosis**

PO

Adults (nonpregnant). 2 g once daily for 2 days; or 1 g taken once daily for 5 days.

▸ **Patients on hemodialysis**

These patients should receive an extra half-dose after the end of dialysis.

CONTRAINDICATIONS

First trimester of pregnancy, hypersensitivity to nitroimidazole derivatives or to tinidazole; do not breastfeed during, and for 3 days following, last dose.

INTERACTIONS

Drug

Alcohol: May cause a disulfiram-type reaction.
Cholestyramine, oxytetracycline: May decrease the effectiveness of tinidazole; separate dosage times.
Cimetidine, ketoconazole: Decrease the metabolism of tinidazole.
Cyclosporine, fluorouracil, lithium, phenytoin, tacrolimus: May increase blood levels of these drugs.

T

Disulfiram: May increase the risk of psychotic reactions (separate dose by 2 wks).
Warfarin: Increase the risk of bleeding. Monitor INR closely, during and for up to a week following, end of treatment.
Herbal
None known.
Food
None known.

DIAGNOSTIC TEST EFFECTS

May increase serum LDH, triglyceride, AST (SGOT), and ALT (SGPT) levels. May lower WBC counts.

SIDE EFFECTS

Occasional (2%-4%)
Metallic or bitter taste, nausea, weakness, fatigue, or malaise.
Rare (< 2%)
Epigastric distress, anorexia, vomiting, headache, dizziness, red-brown or darkened urine, vaginal candidiasis.

SERIOUS REACTIONS

- Peripheral neuropathy, characterized by paresthesia, is usually reversible if tinidazole treatment is stopped as soon as neurologic symptoms appear.
- Superinfection, hypersensitivity reaction, and seizures occur rarely.
- Blood dyscrasias are rare but are part of hypersensitivity reactions.

PRECAUTIONS & CONSIDERATIONS

Caution is warranted in patients with blood dyscrasia, candidiasis (may present more prominent symptoms during tinidazole therapy), central nervous system disease (risk of seizure or peripheral neuropathy), liver impairment, and concurrent treatment with related agents such as metronidazole. Tinidazole crosses the placenta and is distributed in breast milk. Contraindicated in the first trimester of pregnancy, and breastfeeding should be avoided during and up to 72 h after the last dose of treatment. Safety and efficacy of tinidazole have not established in children younger than 3 yr. No age-related precautions have been noted in elderly patients. Avoid alcohol while taking tinidazole and for at least 3 days after discontinuing the medication.
Storage
Store at room temperature. Extemporaneously prepared oral suspension is stable for 7 days at room temperature.
Administration
Scored tablets may be crushed. Take with meals or snack to minimize GI irritation. Do not miss a dose; complete the full length of treatment.

The manufacturer gives instructions for preparing an oral suspension, if needed. Shake well before each use.

Tinzaparin

tin-za-pair'in
★ 🍁 Innohep

CATEGORY AND SCHEDULE

Pregnancy Risk Category: B

Classification: Anticoagulants, low-molecular-weight heparin (LMWH)

MECHANISM OF ACTION

A low-molecular-weight heparin that inhibits factor Xa. Causes less inactivation of thrombin, inhibition of platelets, and bleeding than standard heparin. Does not significantly influence bleeding time, PT, aPTT. *Therapeutic Effect:* Produces anticoagulation.

PHARMACOKINETICS

Well absorbed after SC administration. Eliminated primarily in urine. *Half-life:* 3-4 h.

AVAILABILITY

Injection: 20,000 anti-Xa international units/mL.

INDICATIONS AND DOSAGES

▸ Deep vein thrombosis

SC

Adults, Elderly. 175 anti-Xa international units/kg once a day. Continue for at least 6 days and until patient is sufficiently anticoagulated with warfarin (international normalizing ratio [INR] of 2 or more for 2 consecutive days).

CONTRAINDICATIONS

Elderly with renal insufficiency; active major bleeding; concurrent heparin therapy, hypersensitivity to heparin, sulfite, benzyl alcohol, or pork products; thrombocytopenia associated with positive in vitro test for antiplatelet antibody.

INTERACTIONS

Drug

Anticoagulants, platelet inhibitors: May increase the risk of bleeding.

Herbal

Ginkgo biloba: May increase the risk of bleeding.

Food

None known.

DIAGNOSTIC TEST EFFECTS

Increases (reversible) LDH, serum alkaline phosphatase, AST (SGOT), and ALT (SGPT) levels.

SIDE EFFECTS

Frequent (16%)

Injection site reaction, such as inflammation, oozing, nodules, and skin necrosis.

Rare (< 2%)

Nausea, asthenia, constipation, epistaxis.

SERIOUS REACTIONS

• Overdose may lead to bleeding complications ranging from local ecchymoses to major hemorrhage. Antidote: Dose of protamine sulfate (1% solution) should be equal to dose of tinzaparin injected. 1 mg protamine sulfate neutralizes 100 anti-Xa international units (IU) of tinzaparin. A second dose of 0.5 mg protamine per 100 anti-Xa IU of tinzaparin may be given if aPTT tested 2-4 h after the initial infusion remains prolonged.

PRECAUTIONS & CONSIDERATIONS

Caution is warranted in patients with conditions associated with increased risk of hemorrhage, history of recent GI ulceration and hemorrhage, history of heparin-induced thrombocytopenia, impaired renal function, uncontrolled arterial hypertension, and in elderly patients. Patients should be monitored closely for bleeding and neurologic status if tinzaparin is administered during or immediately after lumbar puncture, spinal anesthesia, or epidural anesthesia. Tinzaparin should be used with caution in pregnant women, particularly during the last trimester and immediately postpartum because it increases the risk of maternal hemorrhage. It is unknown whether tinzaparin is excreted in breast milk. Safety and efficacy of tinzaparin have not been established in children. Elderly patients may be more susceptible to bleeding.

Notify the physician of chest pain, injection site reaction, such as inflammation, nodules, oozing, numbness, pain, swelling or tingling of joints, unusual bleeding, or bruising. PT, INR, and CBC, including platelet count, should be monitored before and during therapy. Be aware of signs of bleeding, including bleeding at injection or surgical sites or from gums, blood in stool, bruising, hematuria, and petechiae.

Storage

Store at room temperature.

Administration

! Do not mix with other injections or infusions. Do not give intramuscularly. Administer tinzaparin by subcutaneous route only.

Patient should be supine or sitting down before administering by SC injection into the abdominal wall as directed. Do not rub the injection site after administration. Rotate injection site daily.

Tioconazole

tyo-con'a-zole

★ Vagistat-1

CATEGORY AND SCHEDULE

Pregnancy Risk Category: C

Classification: Antifungals, vaginal

MECHANISM OF ACTION

An imidazole derivative that inhibits synthesis of ergosterol (vital component of fungal cell formation). *Therapeutic Effect:* Damaging fungal cell membrane. Fungistatic.

PHARMOCOKINETICS

Negligible absorption from vaginal application.

AVAILABILITY

Vaginal Ointment: 6.5% (Vagistat-1).

INDICATIONS AND DOSAGES

▸ **Vulvovaginal candidiasis**

INTRAVAGINAL. *Adults, Elderly.* 1 applicatorful just before bedtime as a single dose.

CONTRAINDICATIONS

Hypersensitivity to tioconazole or other imidazole antifungal agents.

INTERACTIONS

Drug

Spermicides (e.g., nonoxynol-9): Spermicide inactivated; may lead to contraceptive failure.

Herbal

None known.

Food

None known.

DIAGNOSTIC TEST EFFECTS

None known.

SIDE EFFECTS

Frequent (25%)

Headache.

Occasional (1%-6%)

Burning, itching.

Rare (< 1%)

Irritation, vaginal pain, dysuria, dryness of vaginal secretions, vulvar edema/swelling.

SERIOUS REACTIONS

- None reported.

PRECAUTIONS & CONSIDERATIONS

Caution is warranted in patients with diabetes and HIV or AIDS infection. It is unknown whether tioconazole is distributed in breast milk. Safety and efficacy have not

T

been established in children. No age-related precautions have been noted in elderly patients. Separate personal items that come in contact with affected areas.

Storage

Store at room temperature.

Administration

Insert applicatorful high into vagina just before bedtime. Contact physician if itching or burning continues. Be aware that tioconazole base may interact with latex or rubber. Condoms or diaphragms should not be used within 72 h of administration.

Tiotropium

ty-oh'tro-pee-um

★ 🍁 Spiriva

CATEGORY AND SCHEDULE

Pregnancy Risk Category: C

Classification: Respiratory agents, anticholinergics, bronchodilators

MECHANISM OF ACTION

An anticholinergic that binds to recombinant human muscarinic receptors at the smooth muscle, resulting in long-acting bronchial smooth-muscle relaxation. *Therapeutic Effect:* Relieves bronchospasm.

PHARMACOKINETICS

Route	Onset	Peak	Duration
Inhalation	NA	NA	24-36 h

Binds extensively to tissue. Protein binding: 72%. Metabolized by oxidation. Excreted in urine. *Half-life:* 5-6 days.

AVAILABILITY

Powder for Inhalation: 18 mcg/capsule (in blister packs containing 6 capsules with inhaler).

INDICATIONS AND DOSAGES

▸ **Chronic obstructive pulmonary disease (COPD)**

INHALATION

Adults, Elderly. 18 mcg (1 capsule)/day via HandiHaler inhalation device.

CONTRAINDICATIONS

History of hypersensitivity to atropine or its derivatives, including ipratropium.

INTERACTIONS

Drug

Ipratropium: Concurrent administration not recommended.

Herbal

None known.

Food

None known.

DIAGNOSTIC TEST EFFECTS

None known.

SIDE EFFECTS

Frequent (6%-16%)

Dry mouth, sinusitis, pharyngitis, dyspepsia, urinary tract infection, rhinitis.

Occasional (4%-5%)

Abdominal pain, peripheral edema, constipation, epistaxis, vomiting, myalgia, rash, oral candidiasis.

SERIOUS REACTIONS

- Angina pectoris, angiodema or hypersensitivity, paradoxical bronchospasm, and flu-like symptoms occur rarely.
- Inadvertent oral swallowing of capsule may cause more pronounced anticholinergic effects.

PRECAUTIONS & CONSIDERATIONS

This is not a rescue medication. Caution is warranted with angle-closure glaucoma, benign prostatic hyperplasia, and bladder neck obstruction. There are no adequate data regarding use in pregnancy. It is unknown whether tiotropium is distributed in breast milk. The safety and efficacy of tiotropium have not been established in children. Elderly patients are more likely to experience constipation, dry mouth, and urinary tract infection. Drink plenty of fluids to decrease the thickness of lung secretions. Avoid excessive use of caffeinated products, such as chocolate, cocoa, cola, coffee, and tea.

Pulse rate and quality; respiratory rate, depth, rhythm, and type; ABG levels; and clinical improvement should be monitored. Fingernails and lips should be assessed for cyanosis, including a blue or dusky color in light-skinned patients and a gray color in dark-skinned patients, which are signs of hypoxemia.

Storage

Store tiotropium capsules at room temperature. Protect them from extreme temperatures and moisture. Do not store capsules in the HandiHaler device.

Administration

! Do not swallow capsules orally.

For inhalation, open the HandiHaler dustcap by pulling it up; then open the mouthpiece. Place the capsule in the center chamber and firmly close the mouthpiece until you hear a click, leaving the dustcap open. Use only 1 capsule for inhalation at a time. Holding the HandiHaler device with the mouthpiece up, press the piercing button completely once and then release it. Exhale completely before inhaling slowly and deeply, at a rate sufficient to hear the capsule vibrate. Hold breath for as long as is comfortable and then exhale slowly. Repeat this process a second time to ensure the full dose is received. Rinse mouth with water immediately after inhalation to prevent mouth and throat dryness and oral candidiasis.

Tipranavir

tip-ran'ah-veer

★ 🍁 Aptivus

CATEGORY AND SCHEDULE

Pregnancy Risk Category: C

Classification:

Antiretrovirals, protease inhibitors

MECHANISM OF ACTION

A nonpeptidic protease inhibitor that suppresses HIV protease, an enzyme necessary for splitting viral polyprotein precursors into mature and infectious viral particles. *Therapeutic Effect:* Interrupts HIV replication, slowing the progression of HIV infection; effective against some resistant strains due to chemical structure.

PHARMACOKINETICS

Coadministration with ritonavir (100 mg twice daily) increases bioavailability and thus the drug must be given with ritonavir to attain efficacy. Roughly 99% bound to plasma proteins. Primarily metabolized in liver via CYP3A4. Most of the drug is eliminated as parent and metabolites via fecal excretion. *Half-life:* 15 h (increased in impaired hepatic function).

AVAILABILITY

Capsules: 250 mg.
Oral Solution: 100 mg/mL.

INDICATIONS AND DOSAGES

▸ **HIV infection (in combination with other antiretrovirals)**

PO

Adults. Treatment-experienced: 500 mg tipranavir (with ritonavir 200 mg) twice daily with food.

Children 2 to < 18 yr. 14 mg/kg tipranavir with 6 mg/kg ritonavir (or 375 mg/m^2 coadministered with ritonavir 150 mg/m^2) taken twice daily not to exceed the adult dose. If intolerant, consider decreasing to 12 mg/kg tipranavir with 5 mg/kg ritonavir (or tipranavir 290 mg/ m^2 coadministered with 115 mg/m^2 ritonavir) taken twice daily provided virus is not multidrug resistant.

CONTRAINDICATIONS

Hypersensitivity to tipranavir; moderate or severe (Child-Pugh class B or C, respectively) hepatic impairment; and coadministration with alfuzosin, ergot alkaloids, cisapride, pimozide, oral midazolam, triazolam, St. John's Wort, lovastatin, simvastatin, rifampin, sildenafil, amiodarone, flecainide, propafenone, quinidine. Also, since this drug is boosted with ritonavir, review ritonavir contraindications.

T

INTERACTIONS

NOTE: Please see detailed manufacturer's information for management of additional drug interactions other than those listed. In some cases, dosage adjustment for the agent or choice of an alternate agent is recommended.

Drug

Alfuzosin: May increase alfuzosin levels. Contraindicated.

Amiodarone, flecainide, propafenone, quinidine: Potential for serious and/or life-threatening cardiac arrhythmias from increased plasma concentrations. Contraindicated.

Antifungal agents, delavirdine, NNRTIs: May increase levels of tipranavir.

Calcium channel blockers: Tipranavir may increase concentrations of calcium channel blockers.

Clarithromycin: May increase levels of clarithromycin.

CYP3A4 inducers: May decrease effects of tipranavir.

CYP3A4 inhibitors: May increase effects of tipranavir.

CYP3A4 substrates: Levels of CYP3A4 substrates may be increased by tipranavir. Contraindicated with cisapride and pimozide.

Ergot alkaloids: Effects of ergot alkaloids may be increased. Contraindicated.

HMG-CoA reductase inhibitors: Tipranavir may increase side effects. Use contraindicated with lovastatin, simvastatin.

Sildenafil (when given routinely for pulmonary HTN): Levels may be increased by tipranavir. Contraindicated.

Triazolam, oral midazolam: Increases the risk of prolonged sedation. Contraindicated.

Rifamycins: Decrease tipranavir concentrations. Avoid.

Vitamin E: If taking tipranavir oral solution, avoid additional vitamin E, as the oral solution contains amount higher than recommended daily intake (RDI).

Warfarin: Increased anticoagulant effect. Monitor INR.

Herbal

St. John's wort: May decrease tipranavir blood concentration and effect. Contraindicated.

Food

All food: Enhances tipranavir blood concentration; give with food.

DIAGNOSTIC TEST EFFECTS

May increase serum AST (SGOT) and ALT (SGPT), serum amylase, lipase, triglyceride, or cholesterol levels, blood glucose. May decrease WBC.

SIDE EFFECTS

Frequent (≥ 5%)
Diarrhea, nausea, pyrexia, vomiting, fatigue, headache, and abdominal pain. Rash is more common in children.
Occasional
Insomnia; accumulation of fat in waist, abdomen, or back of neck ("buffalo hump"), hyperlipidemia.
Rare
Abnormal taste sensation, heartburn, hyperglycemia.

SERIOUS REACTIONS

- Intracranial hemorrhage.
- Stevens-Johnson syndrome and other serious skin rashes.
- Hepatitis/liver failure.
- Reports of bleeding in patients with hemophilia.
- New-onset diabetes or exacerbations of diabetes.

PRECAUTIONS & CONSIDERATIONS

Tipranavir contains a sulfonamide moiety. Use with caution in patients with a known sulfonamide allergy. Caution is warranted in patients with liver function impairment, hemophilia, diabetes, or heart disease. Be aware that it is unknown if tipranavir is excreted in breast milk. Breastfeeding is not recommended in this population because of the possibility of HIV transmission. Use with caution during pregnancy due to lack of data. The safety and efficacy of this drug have not been established in children under the age of 2 yr.

Establish baseline lab values and monitor hepatic function before and during therapy. Assess the pattern of GI side effects and stool consistency. Evaluate for abdominal discomfort or headache.

Storage
Capsules should be stored in a refrigerator prior to opening the bottle. After opening may store at room temperature; use within 60 days after first opening the bottle. The oral solution should be stored at room temperature; do not refrigerate or freeze. The solution must be used within 60 days after first opening the bottle.

Administration
Take tipranavir with food and with ritonavir twice daily. If a dose is missed, take the next dose at the regularly scheduled time; do not double the dose.

Tirofiban

tye-roe-fye′ban
★ 🍁 Aggrastat
Do not confuse Aggrastat with Aggrenox.

CATEGORY AND SCHEDULE

Pregnancy Risk Category: B

Classification: Platelet inhibitors, platelet glycoprotein IIb/IIIa inhibitors

MECHANISM OF ACTION

An antiplatelet and antithrombotic agent that binds to platelet receptor glycoprotein IIb/IIIa, preventing binding of fibrinogen. *Therapeutic Effect:* Inhibits platelet aggregation and thrombus formation.

PHARMACOKINETICS

Poorly bound to plasma proteins; unbound fraction in plasma: 35%.

Limited metabolism. Eliminated primarily in the urine (65%) and, to a lesser amount, in the feces. Removed by hemodialysis. *Half-life:* 2 h. Clearance is significantly decreased in severe renal impairment (creatinine clearance < 30 mL/min).

AVAILABILITY

Injection Premix: 12.5 mg/250 mL, 5 mg/100 mL.

INDICATIONS AND DOSAGES

▸ **Acute coronary syndrome (unstable angina or non-STEMI) with intervention**

IV

Adults, Elderly. Initially, 0.4 mcg/kg/min for 30 min; then continue at 0.1 mcg/kg/min through procedure and for 12-24 h after procedure. In clinical trials, tirofiban was administered with heparin for 48-108 h.

▸ **Severe renal insufficiency (creatinine clearance < 30 mL/min)**

Adults, Elderly. Half the usual rate of infusion.

CONTRAINDICATIONS

Active internal bleeding or a history of bleeding diathesis within previous 30 days, arteriovenous malformation or aneurysm, coagulopathy, hemophilia, pericarditis, stroke, trauma, history of intracranial hemorrhage, history of thrombocytopenia or hypersensitivity after prior exposure to tirofiban, intracranial neoplasm, major surgical procedure within previous 30 days, severe hypertension.

INTERACTIONS

Drug

Drugs that affect hemostasis (such as aspirin, heparin, NSAIDs, and warfarin): May increase the risk of bleeding. Do not give with another GP-IIb/IIIa inhibitor.

Herbal and Food

None known.

DIAGNOSTIC TEST EFFECTS

Decreases hematocrit, hemoglobin, and platelet count.

IV INCOMPATIBILITIES

Do not mix with other medications. Only heparin can go through the same IV catheter.

SIDE EFFECTS

Occasional (3%-6%)

Pelvic pain, bradycardia, dizziness, leg pain.

Rare (1%-2%)

Edema and swelling, vasovagal reaction, diaphoresis, nausea, fever, headache.

SERIOUS REACTIONS

- Signs and symptoms of overdose include generally minor mucocutaneous bleeding and bleeding at the femoral artery access site. However, major bleeding may occur at any site.
- Thrombocytopenia occurs rarely.

PRECAUTIONS & CONSIDERATIONS

Caution is warranted in patients with hemorrhagic retinopathy, platelet counts < 150,000/mm^3, renal impairment, and those who are also receiving drugs affecting hemostasis, such as warfarin. There are no data regarding use in pregnancy. It is unknown whether tirofiban is distributed in breast milk. Safety and efficacy of tirofiban have not been established in children. There is an increased risk of bleeding in elderly patients. Be aware that it may take longer to stop bleeding during tirofiban therapy.

Notify the physician of any unusual bleeding or before a surgery or new drugs are prescribed. aPTT should be monitored 6 h after the beginning of the heparin infusion. Heparin dosage should be adjusted to maintain aPTT at approximately twice control. Nasogastric tube and urinary catheter should be avoided, if possible.

Storage

Store premixed infusion at room temperature and protect from light. Do not freeze. Use only clear solution. Discard unused solution 24 h after start of infusion.

Administration

! Heparin and tirofiban can be administered through the same IV line.

For the premixed infusion, tear off the dust cover to open the IntraVia container. Check the IntraVia container for leaks. Do not use plastic containers in series connections because doing so may result in air embolism caused by drawing air from the first container that holds no solution. For loading dose, give 0.4 mcg/kg/min for 30 min. For continuous maintenance infusion, give 0.1 mcg/kg/min.

Tizanidine

tye-zan'i-deen

Zanaflex

CATEGORY AND SCHEDULE

Pregnancy Risk Category: C

Classification: Relaxants, skeletal muscle

MECHANISM OF ACTION

A skeletal muscle relaxant that increases presynaptic inhibition of spinal motor neurons mediated by α_2-adrenergic agonists, reducing facilitation to postsynaptic motor neurons. *Therapeutic Effect:* Reduces muscle spasticity.

PHARMACOKINETICS

Route	Onset	Peak	Duration
PO	NA	1-2 h	3-6 h

Metabolized in the liver. *Half-life:* 4-8 h.

AVAILABILITY

Capsules: 2 mg, 4 mg, 6 mg.
Tablets: 2 mg, 4 mg.

INDICATIONS AND DOSAGES

▸ **Muscle spasticity**

PO

Adults, Elderly. Initially 2-4 mg, gradually increased in 2- to 4-mg increments and repeated q6-8h. Maximum: 3 doses/day or 36 mg/24 h.

OFF-LABEL USES

Spasticity associated with multiple sclerosis or spinal cord injury.

CONTRAINDICATIONS

Hypersensitivity to tizanidine; co-use with fluvoxamine or ciprofloxacin, or other potent inhibitors of CYP1A2 is contraindicated.

INTERACTIONS

Drug

Alcohol, other central nervous system (CNS) depressants: May increase CNS depressant effects.

Antihypertensives: May increase tizanidine's hypotensive potential.

CYP1A2 potent inhibitors (e.g., fluvoxamine, ciprofloxacin): Contraindicated due to decreased tizanidine elimination and side effect risk. Other inhibitors (e.g., zileuton, other quinolone antibiotics, mexilitene, amiodarone, cimetidine, acyclovir) should be avoided if possible.

Oral contraceptives: May reduce tizanidine clearance.

T

Phenytoin: May increase serum levels and risk of toxicity of phenytoin.
Herbal
None known.
Food
None known.

DIAGNOSTIC TEST EFFECTS
May increase serum alkaline phosphatase, AST (SGOT), and ALT (SGPT) levels.

SIDE EFFECTS
Frequent (41%-49%)
Dry mouth, somnolence, asthenia.
Occasional (4%-16%)
Dizziness, urinary tract infection, constipation.
Rare (3%)
Nervousness, amblyopia, pharyngitis, rhinitis, vomiting, urinary frequency.

SERIOUS REACTIONS
- Hypotension (a reduction in either diastolic or systolic BP) may be associated with bradycardia, orthostatic hypotension, and rarely syncope. The risk of hypotension increases as dosage increases; BP may decrease within 1 h after administration.
- Hepatocellular liver injury, jaundice, hepatic failure (rare).
- Rare reports of psychosis or hallucinations.

PRECAUTIONS & CONSIDERATIONS
Caution is warranted in patients with hypotension and cardiac, hepatic, or renal disease. There are no data in pregnancy or lactation. The safety and efficacy of tizanidine have not been established in children. In elderly patients, drug clearance is reduced and warrants cautious use.

Low BP, impaired coordination, and sedation may occur. Avoid alcohol, CNS depressants, and tasks that require mental alertness or motor skills until drug effects are known. Baseline liver function tests should be obtained, and periodic monitoring, particularly in the first 6 mo of treatment, is recommended. Therapeutic response, such as decreased stiffness, tenderness, and intensity of skeletal muscle pain and improved mobility, should be assessed.
Storage
Store capsules and tablets at room temperature; protect from moisture.
Administration
Do not abruptly discontinue the medication.

Tobramycin Sulfate
toe-bra-mye'sin
★ AK-Tob, Nebcin, PMS-Tobramycin, TOBI, Tobrex
🍁 Apo-Tobramycin, PMS-Tobramycin, TOBI, Tobrex

CATEGORY AND SCHEDULE
Pregnancy Risk Category: D

Classification: Antibiotics, aminoglycosides

MECHANISM OF ACTION
An aminoglycoside antibiotic that irreversibly binds to protein on bacterial ribosomes. *Therapeutic Effect:* Interferes with protein synthesis of susceptible microorganisms.

PHARMACOKINETICS
Rapid, complete absorption after IM administration. Protein binding: 30%. Widely distributed (does not cross the blood-brain barrier; low concentrations in cerebrospinal

fluid). Inhaled tobramycin acts locally in lungs. Excreted unchanged in urine. Removed by hemodialysis. *Half-life:* 2-4 h (increased in impaired renal function and neonates; decreased in cystic fibrosis and febrile or burn patients).

AVAILABILITY

Injection Solution (Nebcin): 10 mg/mL, 40 mg/mL.
Premix Infusion: 60 mg/50 mL, 80 mg/50 mL.
Ophthalmic Ointment (Tobrex): 0.3%.
Ophthalmic Solution (AK-Tob, Tobrex): 0.3%.
Nebulization Solution (TOBI): 60 mg/mL.

INDICATIONS AND DOSAGES

▸ **Skin and skin-structure, bone, joint, respiratory tract, postoperative, intra-abdominal, and burn wound infections; complicated urinary tract infection; septicemia; meningitis**
IV, IM
Adults, Elderly. 3-6 mg/kg/day in 2-3 divided doses or 5-7 mg/kg once a day.
Children 5-12 yr. Usual dosage 2-2.5 mg/kg/dose q8h.
Children < 5 yr. Usual dosage, 2.5 mg/kg/dose q8h.

▸ **Superficial eye infections, including blepharitis, conjunctivitis, keratitis, and corneal ulcers**
OPHTHALMIC OINTMENT
Adults, Elderly. Apply a thin strip to conjunctiva q8-12h (q3-4h for severe infections).
OPHTHALMIC SOLUTION
Adults, Elderly. 1-2 drops in affected eye q4h (2 drops/h for severe infections).

▸ **Bronchopulmonary infections in patients with cystic fibrosis**
INHALATION SOLUTION (TOBI)
Adults, Children ≥ 6 yr. 300 mg (1 ampule) twice a day for 28 days, then off for 28 days.

▸ **Dosage in renal impairment (adults)**
Dosage and frequency are modified based on the degree of renal impairment and the serum drug concentration.
For traditional dosing regimens.
CrCl 40-60 mL/min. Dosage interval q12h.
CrCl 20-40 mL/min. Dosage interval q24h.
CrCl < 20 mL/min. Monitor levels to determine dosage interval.

CONTRAINDICATIONS

Hypersensitivity to tobramycin, other aminoglycosides (cross-sensitivity), and their components.

INTERACTIONS

Drug

Nephrotoxic medications, other aminoglycosides, ototoxic medications: May increase the risk of nephrotoxicity and ototoxicity.
Neuromuscular blockers and botulinum toxins: May increase neuromuscular blockade.

Herbal and Food

None known.

DIAGNOSTIC TEST EFFECTS

May increase serum bilirubin, BUN, serum creatinine, serum LDH, SGOT (AST), and SGPT (ALT) levels. May decrease serum calcium, magnesium, potassium, and sodium concentrations. In traditional dose regimens, the therapeutic peak serum level is 4-12 mcg/mL and trough is 0.5-2 mcg/mL; peaks up to 20 mcg/mL may be required for some infections. For all regimens, toxic trough levels is > 2 mcg/mL.

IV INCOMPATIBILITIES

Amphotericin B complex (Abelcet, AmBisome, Amphotec), heparin, hetastarch (Hespan), indomethacin

(Indocin), propofol (Diprivan), sargramostim (Leukine, Prokine).

IV COMPATIBILITIES

Amiodarone (Cordarone), calcium gluconate, diltiazem (Cardizem), hydromorphone (Dilaudid), magnesium sulfate, midazolam (Versed), morphine, theophylline.

SIDE EFFECTS

Occasional
IM: Pain, induration.
IV: Phlebitis, thrombophlebitis.
Topical: Hypersensitivity reaction (fever, pruritus, rash, urticaria).
Ophthalmic: Tearing, itching, redness, eyelid swelling.
Rare
Hypotension, nausea, vomiting.

SERIOUS REACTIONS

- Nephrotoxicity (as evidenced by increased BUN and serum creatinine levels and decreased creatinine clearance) may be reversible if the drug is stopped at the first sign of nephrotoxic symptoms.
- Irreversible ototoxicity (manifested as tinnitus, dizziness, ringing or roaring in ears, and hearing loss) and neurotoxicity (manifested as headache, dizziness, lethargy, tremor, and visual disturbances) occur occasionally. The risk of these reactions increases with higher dosages or prolonged therapy.
- Superinfections, particularly fungal infections, may result from bacterial imbalance with any administration route.
- Anaphylaxis may occur.

PRECAUTIONS & CONSIDERATIONS

Caution is warranted in patients with concomitant use of neuromuscular blockers and in those with impaired renal function or auditory or vestibular impairment. Tobramycin readily crosses the placenta and is distributed in breast milk. Tobramycin may cause fetal nephrotoxicity. The ophthalmic form should not be used in breastfeeding mothers and only when specifically indicated in pregnant women. Immature renal function in neonates and premature infants may increase the risk of toxicity. Age-related renal impairment may require a dosage adjustment in elderly patients.

Determine the patient's history of allergies, especially to aminoglycosides, sulfites, and parabens (for topical and ophthalmic routes), before giving the drug. Intake and output and urinalysis results, as appropriate, should be monitored. To maintain adequate hydration, encourage the patient to drink fluids. Monitor urinalysis results for casts, RBCs, WBCs, and decreased specific gravity. Be alert for ototoxic and neurotoxic side effects. If giving ophthalmic tobramycin, monitor the patient's eye for burning, itching, redness, eyelid swelling, and tearing. If giving topical tobramycin, monitor for itching and redness. Be alert for signs and symptoms of superinfection, particularly changes in the oral mucosa, diarrhea, and genital or anal pruritus. Monitor peak and trough serum drug levels.

Storage
Store ophthalmic preparation and solution vials for injection at room temperature. Solutions may be discolored by light or air, but discoloration does not affect drug potency.

Administration
! Space parenteral doses evenly around the clock. Be aware that dosages are based on ideal body weight. Expect to monitor serum drug levels.

For IV use, dilute with 50-100 mL of D5W or 0.9% NaCl. The amount of diluent for infant and children dosages depends on individual needs. Infuse over 20-60 min.

For IM use, to minimize injection site discomfort, administer the IM injection slowly and deep into the gluteus maximus rather than the lateral aspect of the thigh.

For ophthalmic use, place a gloved finger on the lower eyelid, and pull it out until a pocket is formed between the eye and lower lid. Hold the dropper above the pocket and place the correct number of drops (or ¼-½ inch of ointment) into the pocket. Close the eye gently. After administering ophthalmic solution, apply digital pressure to the lacrimal sac for 1-2 min to minimize drainage into the nose and throat, thereby reducing the risk of systemic effects. After applying ophthalmic ointment, close the eye for 1-2 min. Roll the eyeball to increase the drug's contact with the eye. Use a tissue to remove excess solution or ointment around the eye.

Nebulization doses should be inhaled as close to 12 h apart as possible and not < 6 h apart. Do not mix with dornase alfa (Pulmozyme) in the nebulizer. If taking several medications, use them in the following order: bronchodilator first, then chest therapy, then other inhaled medications and, finally, nebulized tobramycin.

Tolcapone

toll'ka-pone

★ Tasmar

CATEGORY AND SCHEDULE

Pregnancy Risk Category: C

Classification: Antiparkinsonian agents, COMT inhibitors

MECHANISM OF ACTION

An antiparkinsonian agent that inhibits the enzyme catechol-O-methyltransferase (COMT), potentiating dopamine activity and increasing the duration of action of levodopa. *Therapeutic Effect:* Relieves signs and symptoms of Parkinson disease.

PHARMACOKINETICS

Rapidly absorbed after PO administration. Protein binding: 99%. Metabolized in the liver. Eliminated primarily in urine (60%) and, to a lesser extent, in feces (40%). Unknown whether removed by hemodialysis. *Half-life:* 2-3 h.

AVAILABILITY

Tablets: 100 mg, 200 mg.

INDICATIONS AND DOSAGES

▸ Adjunctive treatment of Parkinson disease

PO

Adults, Elderly. Initially, 100 mg 3 times a day concomitantly with each dose of carbidopa and levodopa. May increase dose to 200 mg 3 times/day if benefit outweighs risk of hepatotoxicity. Maximum: 600 mg/day.

CONTRAINDICATIONS

Hypersensitivity (including hepatocellular injury or rhabdomyolysis or pyrexia); use within 14 days of nonselective MAOIs; hepatic disease.

INTERACTIONS

Drug

Dobutamine, dopamine, epinephrine, isoetharine, isoproterenol, epinephrine, methyldopa, norepinephrine: May increase the risk of arrhythmias and changes in BP.

T

Nonselective MAOIs (including phenelzine): May inhibit catecholamine metabolism and increase risk of cardiovascular side effects such as hypertensive crisis. Containdicated.
Other central nervous system (CNS) depressants: May increase CNS depression.
Herbal
None known.
Food
None significant.

DIAGNOSTIC TEST EFFECTS

May increase AST (SGOT) and ALT (SGPT) levels.

SIDE EFFECTS

! Frequency of side effects increases with dosage. The following effects are based on a 200-mg dose.
Frequent (16%-35%)
Nausea, insomnia, somnolence, anorexia, diarrhea, muscle cramps, orthostatic hypotension, excessive dreaming.
Occasional (4%-11%)
Headache, vomiting, confusion, hallucinations, constipation, diaphoresis, bright yellow urine, dry eyes, abdominal pain, dizziness, flatulence.
Rare (2%-3%)
Dyspepsia, neck pain, hypotension, fatigue, chest discomfort.

SERIOUS REACTIONS

- Rare reports of loss of impulse control, such as urge to gamble excessively or unusual sexual urges.
- Too-rapid withdrawal from therapy may produce withdrawal-emergent hyperpyrexia, characterized by fever, muscular rigidity, and altered level of consciousness.
- Dyskinesia and dystonia occur frequently.
- Hallucinations.
- Orthostatic hypotension.
- Hepatocellular injury.

PRECAUTIONS & CONSIDERATIONS

Caution is warranted in patients with baseline hypotension, renal impairment, a history of hallucinations, and orthostatic hypotension. Because of a risk of acute fulminant liver failure, tolcapone should be reserved for patients not responding to other therapies. Notify the physician if a female patient is planning to become pregnant. It is unknown whether tolcapone is distributed in breast milk. Tolcapone is not used in children. Elderly patients are at increased risk for hallucinations. Typically, hallucinations in elderly patients occur within the first 2 wks of therapy.

Dizziness, drowsiness, and nausea may occur initially but will diminish or disappear with continued treatment. Alcohol and tasks that require mental alertness or motor skills should be avoided until the effects of the drug are fully known. Change positions slowly to prevent orthostatic hypotension. Also, urine may turn bright yellow. Notify the physician if dark urine, falls, fatigue, itching, loss of appetite, persistent nausea, yellowing of the skin and sclera of the eyes, or abnormal contractions of the head, neck, or trunk occur. Baseline vital signs should be assessed. AST (SGOT) and ALT (SGPT) levels should be monitored before increasing dose and then q2-4 wks for next 6 mo. Relief of symptoms, such as improvement of mask-like facial expression, muscular rigidity, shuffling gait, and resting tremors of the hands and head, should also be assessed during treatment.

Storage
Store tablets at room temperature.
Administration
! Always administer tolcapone with carbidopa and levodopa.

Take tolcapone without regard to food.

Tolmetin

tole′met-in

CATEGORY AND SCHEDULE

Pregnancy Risk Category: C (D if used in third trimester or near delivery)

Classification: Analgesics, nonsteroidal anti-inflammatory drugs

MECHANISM OF ACTION

A nonsteroidal anti-inflammatory (NSAID) that produces analgesic and anti-inflammatory effect by inhibiting prostaglandin synthesis. *Therapeutic Effect:* Reduces inflammatory response and intensity of pain stimulus reaching sensory nerve endings.

PHARMACOKINETICS

Rapidly absorbed from the GI tract. Metabolized in liver. Excreted in urine. Minimally removed by hemodialysis. *Half-life:* 5 h.

AVAILABILITY

Tablets: 200 mg, 600 mg.
Capsules: 400 mg.

INDICATIONS AND DOSAGES

▸ **Rheumatoid arthritis, osteoarthritis**

PO

Adults, Elderly. Initially, 400 mg 3 times/day (including 1 dose upon arising, 1 dose at bedtime). Adjust dose at intervals of 1-2 wks. Maintenance: 600-1800 mg/day in 3-4 divided doses.

▸ **Juvenile rheumatoid arthritis**

PO

Children older than 2 yr. Initially, 20 mg/kg/day in 3-4 divided doses. Maintenance: 15-30 mg/kg/day in 3-4 divided doses.

OFF-LABEL USES

Treatment of ankylosing spondylitis, psoriatic arthritis.

CONTRAINDICATIONS

Hypersensitivity to aspirin or other NSAIDs. Use within 14 days of CABG.

INTERACTIONS

Drug
Antihypertensive, diuretics: May decrease the effects of antihypertensives and diuretics.
Aspirin salicylates, corticosteroids: May increase the risk of GI bleeding and side effects. NSAIDs may negate the cardioprotective effect of ASA.
Cyclosporine: May increase risk of nephrotoxicity.
Heparain, oral anticoagulants, thrombolytics: May increase the effects of heparin, oral anticoagulants, and thrombolytics.
Lithium: May increase the blood concenration and risk of toxicity of lithium.
Methotrexate, pemetrexed: May increase the risk of toxicity with methotrexate or premetrexed.
Herbal
Feverfew: May increase the risk of bleeding.
Ginkgo biloba: May increase the risk of bleeding.
Food
Alcohol: May increase risk of dizziness, GI bleeding.

DIAGNOSTIC TEST EFFECTS
May increase BUN, potassium, liver function tests. May decrease hemoglobin, hematocrit. May prolong bleeding time.

SIDE EFFECTS
Occasional
Nausea, vomiting, diarrhea, abdominal cramping, dyspepsia (heartburn, indigestion, epigastric pain), flatulence, dizziness, visual disturbances, headache, weight decrease or increase.
Rare
Constipation, anorexia, rash, pruritus.

SERIOUS REACTIONS
- NSAID-induced peptic ulcer, GI bleeding, gastritis.
- Rare reactions include cholestasis, jaundice, nephrotoxicity, hematologic sensitivity (e.g., leukopenia).
- Severe hypersensitivity reaction (bronchopasm) possible.

PRECAUTIONS & CONSIDERATIONS
Caution is warranted in patients with impaired renal function, coagulation disorders, and history of upper GI disease. Cardiovascular event risk may be increased with duration of use or preexisting cardiovascular risk factors or disease. Use caution in patients with fluid retention, heart failure, or hypertension. Risk of myocardial infarction and stroke may be increased following CABG surgery. Do not administer within 4-6 half-lives before surgical procedures. Tolmetin should not be administered to patients with MI or in the setting of coronary artery bypass graft surgery. Tolmetin crosses the placenta. Tolmetin use should be avoided during the last trimester of pregnancy as the drug may adversely affect the fetal cardiovascular system causing premature closure of ductus arteriosus. Tolmetin is distributed to breast milk; breastfeeding is not recommended. Safety and efficacy of tolmetin have not been established in children younger than 2 yr. GI bleeding or ulceration is more likely to cause serious adverse effects in elderly patients.
Storage
Store at room temperature.
Administration
Take with food, milk, or antacids if GI distress occurs. Therapeutic effect is noted in 1-3 wks.

T

Tolnaftate
tole-naf'tate
Absorbine Jr., Antifungal Jock Itch, Fungi-Guard, Lamisil AF Spray, Q-Naftate, Termin8, Tinactin Antifungal, Tinaderm
Dr. Scholl's Athlete's Foot, Fungicure

CATEGORY AND SCHEDULE
Pregnancy Risk Category: B
OTC

Classification: Antifungals, topical

MECHANISM OF ACTION
An antifungal that distorts hyphae and stunts mycelial growth in susceptible fungi. *Therapeutic Effect:* Fungicidal.

AVAILABILITY
Aerosol, Liquid, Topical: 1% (Tinactin Antifungal).
Aerosol, Powder, Topical: 1% (Tinactin Antifungal, Tinactin Antifungal Jock Itch).

Cream: 1% (Fungi-Guard, Tinactin Antifungal, Tinactin Antifungal Jock Itch).
Gel: 1% (Absorbine Jr.).
Powder: 1% (Tinactin Antifungal).
Solution, Topical: 1% (Absorbine Jr. Tinaderm).

INDICATIONS AND DOSAGES

▸ **Tinea pedis, tinea cruris, tinea corporis**

TOPICAL

Adults, Elderly, Children 2 yr and older. Spray aerosol or apply 1-3 drops of solution or a small amount of cream, gel, or powder 2 times daily for 2-4 wks.

CONTRAINDICATIONS

Nail and scalp infections, hypersensitivity to tolnaftate or any component of its formulation.

INTERACTIONS

Drug
None known.
Herbal
None known.
Food
None known.

DIAGNOSTIC TEST EFFECTS

None known.

SIDE EFFECTS

Rare
Irritation, burning, pruritus, contact dermatitis.

SERIOUS REACTIONS

• None known.

PRECAUTIONS & CONSIDERATIONS

It is unknown whether tolnaftate is excreted in breast milk. No age-related precautions have been noted in children. Age-related renal impairment may require dosage adjustment in elderly patients.

Affected areas should be kept clean and dry. Light clothing should be worn to promote ventilation as well as ventilated shoes. Shoes and socks should be changed at least once a day.
Storage
Store at room temperature.
Sprays are flammable and under pressure; do not store or use near heat, flame, or smoking.
Administration
Apply and rub gently into the affected and surrounding area. Wash hands before and after applying tolnaftate to the skin.

Tolterodine

tol-tare'oh-deen

★ 🍁 Detrol, Detrol LA

CATEGORY AND SCHEDULE

Pregnancy Risk Category: C

Classification: Anticholinergics, urinary antispasmodic, urinary incontinence agents

MECHANISM OF ACTION

An antispasmodic that exhibits potent antimuscarinic activity by interceding via cholinergic muscarinic receptors, thereby inhibiting urinary bladder contraction. *Therapeutic Effect:* Decreases urinary frequency, urgency.

PHARMACOKINETICS

Rapidly and well absorbed after PO administration. Protein binding: 96%. Extensively metabolized in the liver to active metabolite. Excreted primarily in urine. Unknown whether removed by hemodialysis. *Half-life:* 1.9-3.7 h.

AVAILABILITY

Tablets (Detrol): 1 mg, 2 mg.
Capsules (Extended Release [Detrol LA]): 2 mg, 4 mg.

INDICATIONS AND DOSAGES

▸ **Overactive bladder**
PO (EXTENDED RELEASE)
Adults, Elderly. 4 mg once a day.
PO (IMMEDIATE RELEASE)
Adults, Elderly. 1-2 mg twice a day.
▸ **Dosage in severe renal or hepatic impairment or if taking potent inhibitors of CYP3A4**
PO (IMMEDIATE RELEASE)
Adults, Elderly. 1 mg twice a day.
PO (EXTENDED RELEASE)
Adults, Elderly. 2 mg once a day.

CONTRAINDICATIONS

Hypersensitivity to tolterodine, urinary retention, gastric retention and other severe decreased GI motility conditions, uncontrolled narrow-angle glaucoma.

INTERACTIONS

Drug
Anticholinergics (such as antihistamines): May increase the anticholinergic effects.
Alcohol, central nervous system (CNS) depressants: May increase CNS depressant effects.
Clarithromycin, erythromycin, itraconazole, ketoconazole, miconazole: May increase tolterodine blood concentration.
Fluoxetine: May inhibit tolterodine metabolism.
Herbal and Food
None known.

DIAGNOSTIC TEST EFFECTS

None known.

SIDE EFFECTS

Frequent (40%)
Dry mouth.
Occasional (4%-11%)
Headache, dizziness, fatigue, constipation, dyspepsia (heartburn, indigestion, epigastric discomfort), upper respiratory tract infection, urinary track infection, dry eyes, abnormal vision (accommodation problems), nausea, diarrhea.
Rare (3%)
Somnolence, chest or back pain, arthralgia, rash, weight gain, dry skin.

SERIOUS REACTIONS

• Overdose can result in severe anticholinergic effects, including abdominal cramps, facial warmth, excessive salivation or lacrimation, diaphoresis, pallor, urinary urgency, blurred vision, and prolonged QT interval.

PRECAUTIONS & CONSIDERATIONS

Caution is warranted in patients with renal impairment, clinically significant bladder outflow obstruction (increases risk of urine retention), GI obstructive disorders such as pyloric stenosis, myasthenia gravis, and treated angle-closure glaucoma. It is unknown whether tolterodine is distributed in breast milk. However, breastfeeding is not recommended. The safety and efficacy of this drug have not been established in children. No age-related precautions have been noted in elderly patients.

Blurred vision, GI upset, constipation, and dry eyes and mouth may occur. Notify the physician of a change in vision. Incontinence and residual urine in the bladder should be determined.

Storage
Store at room temperature.
Administration
Take tolterodine without regard to food. Swallow extended-release

capsules whole; do not open, crush, or chew.

Tolvaptan

toll-vap'tan

★ Samsca

CATEGORY AND SCHEDULE

Pregnancy Risk Category: C

Classification: Vasopressin antagonist

MECHANISM OF ACTION

A selective vasopressin V_2-receptor antagonist with an affinity for the V_2-receptor that is 1.8 times that of native arginine vasopressin (AVP). Tolvaptan affinity for the V_2-receptor is 29 times greater than for the V_{1a}-receptor. Causes an increase in urine water excretion that increases free water clearance (aquaresis), decreases urine osmolality, and increases serum sodium. Urinary excretion of sodium and potassium is not significantly changed. *Therapeutic Effect:* Restores normal fluid and electrolyte status.

PHARMACOKINETICS

Peak 2-4 h after oral administration; food does not influence. Protein binding: 99%. Tolvaptan is a substrate and inhibitor of P-glycoprotein (P-gp). Metabolized in liver, tolvaptan is eliminated entirely by nonrenal routes and mainly, if not exclusively, metabolized by CYP3A. Metabolites are not active. *Half-life:* 12 h.

AVAILABILITY

Tablets: 15 mg, 30 mg.

INDICATIONS AND DOSAGES

▸ **Hyponatremia**

PO

Adults. Initially, 15 mg once daily. May increase at 24-h intervals to 30 mg once daily, and to a maximum of 60 mg once daily as needed to raise serum sodium. Monitor serum sodium and volume status closely.

▸ **Renal impairment**

Dose adjustments not necessary in those with CrCl > 10 mL/min. If CrCl < 10 mL/min, use is not recommended. Contraindicated in anuria.

CONTRAINDICATIONS

Known allergy to tolvaptan; anuria (no benefit can be expected); use with strong CYP3A4 inhibitors (see Interactions); hypovolemic hyponatremia. Not for those requiring urgent intervention to raise serum sodium acutely or in those unable to sense or to respond appropriately to thirst.

INTERACTIONS

Drug

CYP3A4 inducers: May decrease the levels and effects of tolvaptan. If cannot be avoided, dose increase of tolvaptan may be necessary.

CYP3A4 inhibitors (e.g., erythromycin): May increase the levels and effects of tolvaptan. Reduce tolvaptan dose with use of moderate inhibitors (e.g., erythromycin, diltiazem, verapamil). Use with strong CYP3A4 inhibitors is contraindicated, including ketoconazole, itraconazole, clarithromycin, nefazodone, ritonavir, and indinavir.

CYP3A4 substrates: Tolvaptan may increase the levels and effects of CYP3A4 substrates, including midazolam and amlodipine, simvastatin, and other "statins."

T

Avoid use of these agents during and for 1 wk after conclusion of treatment.
Cyclosporine and other P-gp inhibitors: May increase exposure to tolvaptan; dose reduction of tolvaptan may be needed.
Digoxin: May increase the levels of digoxin by inhibiting P-gp.
Potassium-sparing drugs: May increase serum potassium additively; monitor.
Herbal
St. John's wort: May reduce tolvaptan levels. Avoid.
Food
Grapefruit juice: May increase tolvaptan exposure. Avoid.

DIAGNOSTIC TEST EFFECTS

Increased sodium levels (serum Na^+); may increase serum potassium.

SIDE EFFECTS

Frequent
Thirst, dry mouth, asthenia, constipation, polyuria, and hyperglycemia.
Occasional to Rare
Hyperkalemia, vomiting, diarrhea, orthostatic hypotension, fever, confusion, dehydration, diabetic ketoacidosis, ischemic colitis, thrombosis.

T

SERIOUS REACTIONS

- Worsening of heart failure.
- Dehydration.
- Increased risk of GI bleeding, especially in cirrhotic patients.

PRECAUTIONS & CONSIDERATIONS

Use with caution in patients with hyponatremia with underlying congestive heart failure or cirrhosis. Avoid use with hypertonic saline. Because of the potential increased risk of gastrointestinal bleeding in patients with cirrhosis, use in patients with cirrhosis only when the need to treat outweighs this risk. Based on animal data, tolvaptan may cause fetal harm and should be given in pregnancy only when benefits outweigh risks. Breastfeeding is not recommended during therapy. There are no adequate data in children of any age.

Monitor neurologic status closely to avoid overly rapid correction of serum Na^+ concentration (> 12 mEq/L over 24 h) during treatment. Monitor for signs of heart decompensation, orthostatic hypotension, and dehydration. Follow all instructions for fluid intake. Fluid restriction may be needed as the dose of tolvaptan is decreased.
Storage
Store tablets at room temperature.
Administration
! Only given in settings where serum Na^+ concentrations, volume status, and blood pressure can be monitored closely.

Give at the same time daily, with or without food. Do not administer with grapefruit juice.

Topiramate

toe-peer'a-mate
Topamax
Do not confuse with Toprol XL.

CATEGORY AND SCHEDULE

Pregnancy Risk Category: C

Classification: Anticonvulsants

MECHANISM OF ACTION

An anticonvulsant that blocks repetitive, sustained firing of neurons by enhancing the ability of γ-aminobutyric acid to induce an influx of chloride ions into the neurons; may also block sodium channels. *Therapeutic Effect:* Decreases seizure activity.

PHARMACOKINETICS

Rapidly absorbed after PO administration. Protein binding: 15%-41%. Not extensively metabolized. Excreted primarily unchanged in urine. Removed by hemodialysis. *Half-life:* 21 h.

AVAILABILITY

Capsules (Sprinkle): 15 mg, 25 mg.
Tablets: 25 mg, 50 mg, 100 mg, 200 mg.

INDICATIONS AND DOSAGES

▸ Initial monotherapy epilepsy
Adults, Children > 10 yr. Initiate therapy at 50 mg/day in 2 divided doses. Increase by 50 mg/day (in divided doses) weekly to a recommended maintenance dose of 400 mg/day in 2 divided doses.

▸ Adjunctive treatment of partial seizures, Lennox-Gastaut syndrome, generalized tonic-clonic seizures
PO
Adults, Elderly, Children older than 16 yr. Initially, 25-50 mg/day for 1 wk. May increase by 25-50 mg/day at weekly intervals. Maintenance dose is individualized. Usual range: 200-400 mg/day in 2 divided doses, dependent on seizure type. Maximum: 1600 mg/day.
Children 2-16 yr. Initially, 1-3 mg/kg/day (maximum 25 mg); initial dose given nightly. May increase by 1-3 mg/kg/day at weekly intervals. Maintenance: 5-9 mg/kg/day in 2 divided doses.

▸ Migraine prevention
PO
Adults, Elderly. 25 mg/day for 1 wk, followed by titration of 25 mg/wk to a target of 100 mg/day in 2 divided doses.

▸ Dosage in renal impairment
For adults, expect to reduce drug dosage by 50% if CrCl < 70 mL/min. A supplemental dose may be required if on hemodialysis.

OFF-LABEL USES

Treatment of alcohol dependence.

CONTRAINDICATIONS

Hypersensitivity to topiramate or other carbonic anhydrase inhibitors.

INTERACTIONS

Drug
Alcohol, other central nervous system (CNS) depressants: May increase CNS depression.
Carbamazepine, phenytoin, valproic acid: May decrease topiramate blood concentration.
Carbonic anhydrase inhibitors: May increase the risk of renal calculi.
Metformin: Possible reduced clearance of metformin. Monitor.
Oral contraceptives: May decrease the effectiveness of oral contraceptives.
Herbal and Food
None known.

DIAGNOSTIC TEST EFFECTS

None known.

SIDE EFFECTS

Frequent (10%-30%)
Somnolence, dizziness, ataxia, nervousness, nystagmus, diplopia, paresthesia, nausea, tremor.
Occasional (3%-9%)
Confusion, breast pain, dysmenorrhea, dyspepsia, depression, asthenia, pharyngitis, weight loss, anorexia, rash, musculoskeletal pain, abdominal pain, difficulty with coordination,

T

sinusitis, agitation, flu-like symptoms.

Rare (2%-3%)

Mood disturbances, such as irritability and depression; dry mouth; aggressive behavior; kidney stones.

SERIOUS REACTIONS

- Psychomotor slowing, impaired concentration, language problems (such as word-finding difficulties), and memory disturbances occur occasionally. May be mild, or may require drug discontinuation.
- Serious and potentially fatal exfoliative dermatologic reactions.
- Metabolic acidosis (rare); may also lead to kidney stones.
- Oligohydrosis and hyperthermia (rare).

PRECAUTIONS & CONSIDERATIONS

Antiepileptic drugs (AEDs) increase the risk of suicidal thoughts or behavior in patients taking these drugs for any indication. Monitor for the emergence or worsening of depression, suicidal thoughts, or unusual changes in behavior or mood. Caution is warranted in patients with impaired hepatic and renal function, a predisposition to renal calculi, and hypersensitivity to topiramate. It is unknown whether topiramate is distributed in breast milk. Be aware that topiramate decreases oral contraceptive effectiveness, and an alternative means of contraception should be used during therapy. No age-related precautions have been noted in children older than 2 yr. In elderly patients, age-related renal impairment may require dosage adjustment.

Drowsiness and dizziness may occur, so alcohol and tasks requiring mental alertness or motor skills should be avoided. Notify the physician of blurred vision or other visual changes. Seizure disorder, including the onset, duration, frequency, intensity, and type of seizures, should be assessed before and during treatment. Renal function, including BUN and serum creatinine levels, should also be monitored. Adequate hydration should be maintained to decrease the risk of kidney stones.

Storage

Store at room temperature. Protect all proudcts from moisture.

Administration

Do not break tablets because they have a bitter taste. Take topiramate without regard to food. Capsules may be swallowed whole or contents sprinkled on a teaspoonful of soft food and swallowed immediately. They should not be chewed. Do not abruptly discontinue topiramate because this may precipitate seizures. Strict maintenance of drug therapy is essential for seizure control.

Topotecan

toe-poe-tee'kan

Hycamtin

CATEGORY AND SCHEDULE

Pregnancy Risk Category: D

Classification: Antineoplastics, topoisomerase inhibitors

MECHANISM OF ACTION

A DNA topoisomerase inhibitor that interacts with topoisomerase I, an enzyme that allows DNA replication by producing reversible single-strand breaks in DNA that relieve torsional strain. Topotecan prevents religation of the DNA strand, resulting in damage to double-strand DNA and cell death.

Therapeutic Effect: Destroys cancer cells.

PHARMACOKINETICS

Hydrolyzed to active form after IV administration. Protein binding: 35%. Excreted in urine. *Half-life:* 2-3 h (increased in impaired renal function).

AVAILABILITY

Powder for Injection: 4 mg (single-dose vial).
Capsules: 0.25 mg, 1 mg.

INDICATIONS AND DOSAGES

▸ **Ovarian carcinoma, small cell lung carcinoma (SCLC)**

IV

Adults, Elderly. 1.5 mg/m^2/day over 30 min for 5 consecutive days, beginning on day 1 of a 21-day course. Minimum of 4 courses is recommended. If severe neutropenia (neutrophil count < 1500/mm^2) or if platelet count < 25,000 mm^3 occurs during treatment, reduce dose for subsequent courses by 0.25 mg/m^2, or administer filgrastim (G-CSF) no sooner than 24 h after the last dose of topotecan.

PO (FOR SCLC ONLY)

Adults, Elderly. 2.3 mg/m^2/day for 5 consecutive days, beginning on day 1 of a 21-day course. Round dose to nearest combination of capsule strengths, using the minimal number of capsules possible.

▸ **For stage IV-B cervical cancer**

IV INFUSION

Adults, Elderly. 0.75 mg/m^2 on days 1-3 in combination with cisplatin (50 mg/m^2 IV on day 1 only) given every 3 wks.

▸ **Dosage in renal impairment**

For moderate renal impairment (CrCl 20-39 mL/min), dose adjustment of oral or IV dosing is required for ovarian and SCLC (see manufacturer recommendations); for cervical cancer, do not use.

▸ **Dosage for toxicities**

Expect to withhold doses and/or decrease dosage if significant toxicities occur.

OFF-LABEL USES

Treatment of solid tumors including osteosarcoma, neuroblastoma, pediatric leukemia, rhabdomyosarcoma.

CONTRAINDICATIONS

Baseline neutrophil count < 1500 cells/mm^3, breastfeeding, pregnancy, severe myelosuppression.

INTERACTIONS

Drug

Cisplatin: May increase the severity of myelosuppression.
Live-virus vaccines: May potentiate virus replication, increase vaccine side effects, and decrease the patient's antibody response to the vaccine.
Other bone marrow depressants: May increase the risk of myelosuppression.

Herbal and Food

None known.

DIAGNOSTIC TEST EFFECTS

May increase serum bilirubin, AST (SGOT), and ALT (SGPT) levels. May decrease RBC, leukocyte, neutrophil, and platelet counts.

IV INCOMPATIBILITIES

Dexamethasone (Decadron), 5-fluorouracil, mitomycin (Mutamycin).

IV COMPATIBILITIES

Carboplatin (Paraplatin), cisplatin (Platinol AQ), cyclophosphamide (Cytoxan), doxorubicin (Adriamycin), etoposide (VePesid), gemcitabine (Gemzar), granisetron (Kytril), ondansetron (Zofran), paclitaxel (Taxol), vincristine (Oncovin).

SIDE EFFECTS

Frequent
Nausea (77%), vomiting (58%), diarrhea and total alopecia (42%), headache (21%), dyspnea (21%).
Occasional
Paresthesia (9%), constipation and abdominal pain (3%).
Rare
Anorexia, malaise, arthralgia, asthenia, myalgia.

SERIOUS REACTIONS

- Severe neutropenia (neutrophil count < 500 cells/mm^3) occurs in 60% of patients, usually during the first course of therapy. The neutrophil nadir usually occurs at a median of 11 days after starting therapy.
- Thrombocytopenia (platelet count < 25,000/mm^3) occurs in 26% of patients, and severe anemia (RBC count < 8 g/dL) occurs in 40% of patients. The platelet and RBC nadirs usually occur at a median of 15 days after starting the first course of therapy.

T

PRECAUTIONS & CONSIDERATIONS

Caution is warranted with hepatic and renal impairment and mild myelosuppression.

Because of the risk of fetal harm, pregnant women should not take topotecan, especially in the first trimester. It is unknown whether topotecan is distributed in breast milk; however, breastfeeding is not recommended. The safety and efficacy of topotecan have not been established in children. In elderly patients, age-related renal impairment may require dosage adjustment. Vaccinations and coming in contact with crowds and people with known infections should be avoided.

CBC, especially blood hemoglobin levels, and platelet count, should be assessed before each topotecan dose. Myelosuppression may precipitate life-threatening anemia, hemorrhage, and infection. If platelet count drops, minimize trauma (for example, by avoiding IM or rectal drug administration and by gently repositioning the person). Premedicate with antiemetics, if ordered, on the day of treatment, starting at least 30 min before topotecan administration. Electrolyte levels, hydration status, and intake and output should also be monitored because diarrhea and vomiting are common side effects of topotecan.
Storage
Store vials at room temperature in original cartons. Reconstituted vials diluted for infusion are stable at room temperature in ambient lighting for up to 24 h.
Administration
CAUTION: Observe and exercise appropriate precautions for handling, preparing, and administering cytotoxic drugs. As prescribed, do not give topotecan if baseline neutrophil count is < 1500 cells/mm^3 and platelet count is < 100,000/mm^3.

Reconstitute each 4-mg vial with 4 mL sterile water for injection. Further dilute with 50-100 mL 0.9% NaCl or D5W. Administer the drug by IV infusion over 30 min. Be aware that extravasation is associated with only mild local reactions, such as ecchymosis and erythema.

The oral capsules may be taken without regard to food. Do not open, divide, or crush the capsules. Swallow intact.

Toremifene

tore'em-i-feen

★ Fareston

CATEGORY AND SCHEDULE

Pregnancy Risk Category: D

Classification: Antineoplastics, antiestrogens, selective estrogen receptor modulator (SERM)

MECHANISM OF ACTION

A nonsteroidal antiestrogen and antineoplastic agent that binds to estrogen receptors on tumors, producing a complex that decreases DNA synthesis and inhibits estrogen effects. *Therapeutic Effect:* Blocks growth-stimulating effects of estrogen in breast cancer.

PHARMACOKINETICS

Well absorbed after PO administration. Metabolized in the liver. Eliminated in feces. *Half-life:* Approximately 5 days.

AVAILABILITY

Tablets: 60 mg.

INDICATIONS AND DOSAGES

▸ **Breast cancer**

PO

Adults. 60 mg/day until disease progression is observed.

OFF-LABEL USES

Treatment of desmoid tumors, endometrial carcinoma.

CONTRAINDICATIONS

Hypersensitivity, pregnancy, history of thromboembolic disease.

INTERACTIONS

Drug

Carbamazepine, phenobarbital, phenytoin: May decrease toremifene blood concentration.

Thiazide diuretics: May increase risk of hypercalcemia.

Warfarin: May increase PT.

Herbal

None known.

Food

None known.

DIAGNOSTIC TEST EFFECTS

May increase serum alkaline phosphatase, bilirubin, calcium, and AST (SGOT) levels. Rarely lowers WBC or platelet counts.

SIDE EFFECTS

Frequent

Hot flashes (35%); diaphoresis (20%); nausea (14%); vaginal discharge (13%); dizziness, dry eyes (9%).

Occasional (2%-5%)

Edema, vomiting, vaginal bleeding.

Rare

Fatigue, depression, lethargy, anorexia.

SERIOUS REACTIONS

- Ocular toxicity (cataracts, glaucoma, decreased visual acuity) and hypercalcemia may occur.
- Very rare reports of serious hypersensitivity (erythema multiforme, Stevens-Johnson syndrome, bullous rash, interstitial pneumonitis, or angioedema).
- Deep venous thrombosis, pulmonary thrombosis, stroke, or cardiac thrombus.
- Potential increased risk of endometrial hyperplasia.

PRECAUTIONS & CONSIDERATIONS

Caution is warranted in patients with preexisting endometrial hyperplasia, leukopenia, and thrombocytopenia.

Toremifene use should be avoided during pregnancy because this drug may cause fetal harm. Nonhormonal methods of contraception should be used during treatment. It is unknown whether toremifene is distributed in breast milk; however, breastfeeding is not recommended. Toremifene is not prescribed for children; the safety and efficacy of this drug in children have not been established. No age-related precautions have been noted in elderly patients.

Initial flare-up of symptoms, including bone pain and hot flashes, may occur but will subside with continued therapy. Notify the physician if nausea and vomiting, leg cramps, shortness of breath, weakness, weight gain, or vaginal bleeding, discharge, or itching occurs. Estrogen receptor assay test should be performed before starting therapy. CBC and serum calcium levels should be monitored before and periodically during toremifene therapy. Be aware of signs and symptoms of hypercalcemia, including constipation, deep bone or flank pain, excessive thirst, hypotonicity of muscles, increased urine output, nausea and vomiting, and renal calculi.

Storage

Store tablets at room temperature.

Administration

Take oral toremifene without regard to food.

T

Torsemide

tor′se-mide

★ Demadex

Do not confuse torsemide with furosemide.

CATEGORY AND SCHEDULE

Pregnancy Risk Category: B

Classification: Diuretics, loop

MECHANISM OF ACTION

A loop diuretic that enhances the excretion of sodium, chloride, potassium, and water at the ascending limb of the loop of Henle; also reduces plasma and extracellular fluid volume. *Therapeutic Effect:* Produces diuresis; lowers BP.

PHARMACOKINETICS

Route	Onset	Peak	Duration
PO	1 h	1-2 h	6-8 h
IV	10 min	1 h	6-8 h

Rapidly and well absorbed from the GI tract. Protein binding: 97%-99%. Metabolized in the liver. Primarily excreted in urine. Not removed by hemodialysis. *Half-life:* 3.3 h.

AVAILABILITY

Tablets: 5 mg, 10 mg, 20 mg, 100 mg.

Injection: 10 mg/mL.

INDICATIONS AND DOSAGES

▸ **Hypertension**

PO

Adults, Elderly. Initially, 5 mg/day. May increase to 10 mg/day if no response in 4-6 wks. Usual range: 2.5-10 mg/day. If no response, additional antihypertensive added.

▸ **Edema associated with congestive heart failure (CHF)**

PO, IV

Adults, Elderly. Initially, 10-20 mg/day. May increase by approximately doubling dose until desired therapeutic effect is attained. Doses > 200 mg have not been adequately studied.

▸ **Edema associated with chronic renal failure**

PO, IV

Adults, Elderly. Initially, 20 mg/day. May increase by approximately doubling dose until desired therapeutic effect is attained. Doses

> 200 mg have not been adequately studied.

▸ **Hepatic cirrhosis**

PO, IV

Adults, Elderly. Initially, 5 mg/day given with aldosterone antagonist or potassium-sparing diuretic. May increase by approximately doubling dose until desired therapeutic effect is attained. Doses > 40 mg have not been adequately studied.

CONTRAINDICATIONS

Anuria, hepatic coma, severe electrolyte depletion.

INTERACTIONS

Drug

Amphotericin B, nephrotoxic medications, ototoxic medications: May increase the risk of nephrotoxicity and ototoxicity.

Digoxin: May increase the risk of digoxin toxicity associated with torsemide-induced hypokalemia.

Lithium: May increase the risk of lithium toxicity.

NSAIDs, probenecid: May decrease the diuretic effect of torsemide.

Other antihypertensives: May increase the risk of hypotension.

Other hypokalemia-causing medications: May increase the risk of hypokalemia.

Herbal and Food

None known.

DIAGNOSTIC TEST EFFECTS

May increase BUN, serum creatinine, and serum uric acid levels. May decrease serum calcium, chloride, magnesium, potassium, and sodium levels.

IV INCOMPATIBILITIES

There are few data with other medications.

IV COMPATIBILITIES

Milrinone (Primacor), nesiritide (Natrecor).

SIDE EFFECTS

Frequent (10%-40%)

Headache, dizziness, rhinitis.

Occasional (1%-3%)

Asthenia, insomnia, nervousness, diarrhea, constipation, nausea, dyspepsia, edema, ECG changes, pharyngitis, cough, arthralgia, myalgia.

Rare (< 1%)

Syncope, hypotension, arrhythmias.

SERIOUS REACTIONS

• Ototoxicity may occur with high doses or a too-rapid IV administration.

• Overdose produces acute, profound water loss; volume and electrolyte depletion; dehydration; decreased blood volume; and circulatory collapse.

PRECAUTIONS & CONSIDERATIONS

Caution is warranted in patients with ascites, hepatic cirrhosis, renal impairment, systemic lupus erythematosus, history of ventricular arrhythmias, hypersensitivity to sulfonamides, with cardiac patients and elderly patients. It is unknown whether torsemide is excreted in breast milk. The safety and efficacy of this drug have not been established in children. No age-related precautions have been noted in elderly patients. Consuming foods high in potassium, such as apricots, bananas, legumes, meat, orange juice, raisins, whole grains, including cereals, and white and sweet potatoes, is encouraged. Avoid taking other medications, including OTC drugs, without first consulting the physician.

An increase in the frequency and volume of urination may occur. Notify the physician of cramps, dizziness, an irregular heartbeat, muscle weakness, nausea, or hearing abnormalities. BP, vital signs, electrolytes, intake and output, and weight should be monitored before and during treatment. Be aware of signs of electrolyte disturbances such as hypokalemia or hyponatremia. Hypokalemia may cause arrhythmias, altered mental status, muscle cramps, asthenia, and tremor. Less potassium is lost with torsemide than with furosemide.

Storage

Store torsemide at room temperature.

Administration

Take torsemide with food to avoid GI upset, preferably with breakfast to prevent nocturia.

! Flush IV line with 0.9% NaCl before and after torsemide administration.

Torsemide may be given undiluted as IV push over 2 min. For continuous IV infusion, dilute with 0.9% or 0.45% NaCl or D5W and infuse over 24 h. Administer IV push slowly because too-rapid administration may cause ototoxicity.

T

Tramadol

tray'mah-doal

★ Rybix, Ryzolt, Ultram, Ultram ER 🍁 Ralivia, Tridural, Ultram, Zytram XL

Do not confuse tramadol with Toradol, or Ultram with Ultane, or Rybix with Zydis.

CATEGORY AND SCHEDULE

Pregnancy Risk Category: C

Classification: Analgesics, opioid-like, centrally acting

MECHANISM OF ACTION

An analgesic that binds to μ-opioid receptors and inhibits reuptake of norepinephrine and serotonin. Reduces the intensity of pain stimuli reaching sensory nerve endings. *Therapeutic Effect:* Alters the perception of and emotional response to pain.

PHARMACOKINETICS

Route	Onset	Peak	Duration
PO	< 1 h	2-3 h	4-6 h

Rapidly and almost completely absorbed after PO administration. Protein binding: 20%. Extensively metabolized in the liver to active metabolite (reduced in patients with advanced cirrhosis). Primarily excreted in urine. Minimally removed by hemodialysis. *Half-life:* 6-7 h.

AVAILABILITY

Oral Disintegrating Tablets (Rybix): 50 mg.

Tablets (Ultram): 50 mg.

Extend-Release Tablets (Ryzolt, Ultram ER): 100 mg, 200 mg, 300 mg.

INDICATIONS AND DOSAGES

▸ **Moderate to moderately severe pain**

PO (IMMEDIATE RELEASE)

Adults, Elderly. 50-100 mg q4-6h. Maximum: 400 mg/day for patients younger than 75 yr; 300 mg/day for patients older than 75 yr.

PO (EXTENDED RELEASE, ULTRAM ER)

Adults, Elderly. Initially, 100 mg once daily; titrate in 100 mg increments every 5 days. Maximum: 300 mg/day.

PO (EXTENDED RELEASE, RYZOLT)

Adults, Elderly. Initially, 100 mg once daily; titrate in 100 mg increments every 2-3 days. Maximum: 300 mg/day.

▸ Dosage in renal impairment

For patients with creatinine clearance of < 30 mL/min, increase dosing interval to q12h. Do not use extended-release tablets. Maximum: 200 mg/day.

▸ Dosage in hepatic impairment

Dosage is decreased to 50 mg q12h. Do not use extended-release tablets.

CONTRAINDICATIONS

Opiate agonist hypersensitivity, acute alcohol intoxication; concurrent use of centrally acting analgesics, hypnotics, opioids, or psychotropic drugs.

INTERACTIONS

Drug

Alcohol, other central nervous system (CNS) depressants: May increase CNS or respiratory depression and hypotension.

Carbamazepine: Decreases tramadol blood concentration.

MAOIs: Increase tramadol blood concentration.

Herbal and Food

None known.

DIAGNOSTIC TEST EFFECTS

May increase GGT, AST (SGOT), and ALT (SGPT) levels.

SIDE EFFECTS

Frequent (5%-15%)

Dizziness or vertigo, nausea, constipation, headache, somnolence.

Occasional (5%-10%)

Vomiting, pruritus, CNS stimulation (such as nervousness, anxiety, agitation, tremor, euphoria, mood swings, and hallucinations), asthenia, diaphoresis, dyspepsia, dry mouth, diarrhea.

Rare (< 5%)

Malaise, vasodilation, anorexia, flatulence, rash, blurred vision, urine retention or urinary frequency, menopausal symptoms.

SERIOUS REACTIONS

- Hypersensitivity.
- Respiratory or CNS depression.
- Seizures.
- Serotonin syndrome (rate).
- Increased intracranial pressure in at-risk patients (rare).

PRECAUTIONS & CONSIDERATIONS

Extreme caution should be used with acute abdominal conditions, hepatic or renal impairment, increased intracranial pressure, opioid dependence, and a sensitivity to opioids. Tramadol crosses the placenta and is distributed in breast milk. The safety and efficacy of tramadol have not been established in children. Age-related renal impairment may require a dosage adjustment in elderly patients. Alcohol and OTC drugs, such as analgesics and sedatives, should be avoided.

Blurred vision, dizziness, and drowsiness may occur, so tasks requiring mental alertness or motor skills should be avoided. Notify the physician of any chest pain, difficulty breathing, excessive sedation, muscle weakness, palpitations, seizures, severe constipation, or tremors. Liver and renal function studies should be obtained before therapy. BP, pulse rate, pattern of daily bowel activity and stool consistency, bladder for urine retention, and therapeutic response should be monitored during tramadol use.

Storage

Store at room temperature. Keep ODT form in blister pack until time of use and protected from moisture; remove with dry hands.

Administration
Take tramadol without regard to food.
Do not abruptly discontiue; tapering is recommended. Extended-release tablets should not be cut, chewed, or crushed. ODT tablets may be administered with or without water; let dissolve on tongue (do not chew).

Trandolapril

tran-doe′la-pril
Mavik
Do not confuse with tramadol.

CATEGORY AND SCHEDULE
Pregnancy Risk Category: C (D if used in second or third trimester)

Classification: Antihypertensives, angiotensin-converting enzyme (ACE) inhibitors

MECHANISM OF ACTION
An ACE inhibitor that suppresses the renin-angiotensin-aldosterone system and prevents the conversion of angiotensin I to angiotensin II, a potent vasoconstrictor; may also inhibit angiotensin II at local vascular and renal sites. Decreases plasma angiotensin II, increases plasma renin activity, and decreases aldosterone secretion. *Therapeutic Effect:* Reduces peripheral arterial resistance and pulmonary capillary wedge pressure; improves cardiac output and exercise tolerance.

PHARMACOKINETICS
Slowly absorbed from the GI tract. Protein binding: 80%. Metabolized in the liver and GI mucosa to active metabolite. Primarily excreted in urine. Removed by hemodialysis. *Half-life:* 24 h.

AVAILABILITY
Tablets: 1 mg, 2 mg, 4 mg.

INDICATIONS AND DOSAGES
▸ **Hypertension (without diuretic)**
PO
Adults, Elderly. Initially, 1 mg once a day in nonblack patients, 2 mg once a day in black patients. Adjust dosage at least at 7-day intervals. Maintenance: 2-4 mg/day. Maximum: 8 mg/day.
▸ **Heart failure post-MI**
PO
Adults, Elderly. Initially, 0.5-1 mg, titrated to target dose of 4 mg/day.

CONTRAINDICATIONS
Hypersensitivity or history of angioedema from previous treatment with ACE inhibitors, idiopathic or hereditary angioedema, bilateral renal artery stenosis.

INTERACTIONS
Drug
Alcohol, antihypertensives, diuretics: May increase the effects of trandolapril.
Lithium: May increase lithium blood concentration and risk of lithium toxicity.
NSAIDs: May decrease the effects of trandolapril.
Potassium-sparing diuretics, drospirenone, eplerenone, potassium supplements: May cause hyperkalemia.
Herbal
None known.
Food
None known.

DIAGNOSTIC TEST EFFECTS
May increase BUN, serum alkaline phosphatase, serum bilirubin, serum creatinine, serum potassium, AST (SGOT), and ALT (SGPT)

levels. May decrease serum sodium levels. May cause positive antinuclear antibody titer or decreased WBC.

SIDE EFFECTS

Frequent (23%-35%)
Dizziness, cough.
Occasional (3%-11%)
Hypotension, dyspepsia (heartburn, epigastric pain, indigestion), syncope, asthenia (loss of strength), tinnitus.
Rare (< 1%)
Palpitations, insomnia, drowsiness, nausea, vomiting, constipation, flushed skin, hyperkalemia.

SERIOUS REACTIONS

- Excessive hypotension (first-dose syncope) may occur in patients with CHF and in those who are severely salt or volume depleted.
- Angioedema occurs rarely.
- Agranulocytosis and neutropenia may be noted in those with collagen vascular disease including scleroderma and systemic lupus erythematosus.
- Cholestatic jaundice, which may progress to hepatic necrosis. Discontinue if abnormal liver function tests.
- Renal dysfunction may occur. Increases in serum creatinine may occur after initiation of therapy. Monitor serum creatinine and discontinue if progressive or severe decline in function.

PRECAUTIONS & CONSIDERATIONS

Caution is warranted in patients with CHF, collagen vascular disease, hyperkalemia, hypovolemia, renal impairment, and renal stenosis. Trandolapril crosses the placenta, is distributed in breast milk, and may cause fetal or neonatal morbidity or mortality. Discontinue as soon as pregnancy is detected. Safety and efficacy of trandolapril have not been established in children. No age-related precautions have been noted in elderly patients.

Dizziness and light-headedness may occur. Tasks that require mental alertness or motor skills should be avoided. Notify the physician of chest pain, cough, diarrhea, difficulty swallowing, fever, palpitations, sore throat, swelling of the face, or vomiting. Be alert to fluctuations in BP. If an excessive reduction in BP occurs, place the person in the supine position with legs elevated. CBC and blood chemistry should be obtained before beginning trandolapril therapy, then every 2 wks for the next 3 mo, and periodically thereafter. Crackles and wheezing should be assessed in persons with CHF. BUN, serum creatinine, and serum potassium levels, WBC count, urinalysis, intake and output, and pattern of daily bowel activity and stool consistency should also be monitored.

Storage
Store tablets at room temperature.
Administration
Take trandolapril without regard to food. Crush tablets as necessary.

Tranylcypromine

tran-ill-sip'roe-meen
Parnate

CATEGORY AND SCHEDULE

Pregnancy Risk Category: C

Classification: Antidepressants, monoamine oxidase inhibitors (MAOIs).

MECHANISM OF ACTION

An MAOI that inhibits the activity of the enzyme monoamine oxidase at central nervous system (CNS) storage sites, leading to increased levels of the neurotransmitters epinephrine, norepinephrine, serotonin, and dopamine at neuronal receptor sites. *Therapeutic Effect:* Relieves depression.

AVAILABILITY

Tablets: 10 mg.

INDICATIONS AND DOSAGES

▸ **Depression refractory to or intolerant of other therapy**

PO

Adults, Elderly. Initially, 10 mg twice a day. May increase by 10 mg/day at 1- to 3-wk intervals up to 60 mg/day in divided doses.

CONTRAINDICATIONS

Hypersensitivity, cerebrovascular defects or cardiovascular disorders, coma, pheochromocytoma, elective surgery, alcohol use, liver disease. Many drugs are contraindicated for concurrent use with an MAOI; review drug interactions carefully and follow appropriate wash-out periods before prescribing tranylcypromine. Specific contraindications include other MAOIs, linezolid, COMT inhibitors, tricyclic antidepressants, cyclobenzaprine, bupropion, SSRI or SNRI antidepressants, buspirone, sympathomimetics, meperidine, dextromethorphan, foods with a high tyramine content, and caffeine.

INTERACTIONS

Drug

Alcohol, other CNS depressants: May increase CNS depressant effects.

Buspirone: May increase BP.

Caffeine-containing medications: May increase the risk of cardiac arrhythmias and hypertension.

Carbamazepine, cyclobenzaprine, linezolid, maprotiline, other MAOIs: May precipitate hypertensive crisis.

Dopamine, tryptophan: May cause sudden, severe hypertension.

Fluoxetine, trazodone, tricyclic antidepressants: May cause serotonin syndrome and neuroleptic malignant syndrome.

Insulin, oral antidiabetics: May increase the effects of these drugs.

Meperidine, other opioid analgesics: May produce diaphoresis, immediate excitation, rigidity, and severe hypertension or hypotension, sometimes leading to severe respiratory distress, vascular collapse, seizures, coma, and death.

SSRI: May cause serotonin syndrome.

Herbal

St. John's wort: Possible risk of serotonin syndrome. Contraindicated.

Food

Caffeine, chocolate, tyramine-containing foods (such as aged cheese): May cause sudden, severe hypertension.

DIAGNOSTIC TEST EFFECTS

None known.

SIDE EFFECTS

Frequent

Orthostatic hypotension, restlessness, GI upset, insomnia, dizziness, lethargy, weakness, dry mouth, peripheral edema.

Occasional

Flushing, diaphoresis, rash, urinary frequency, increased appetite, transient impotence.

Rare

Visual disturbances, syncope.

SERIOUS REACTIONS

• Hypertensive crisis occurs rarely and is marked by severe hypertension, occipital headache radiating frontally, neck stiffness or soreness, nausea, vomiting, diaphoresis, fever or chills, clammy skin, dilated pupils, palpitations, tachycardia or bradycardia, and constricting chest pain.

• Intracranial bleeding occurs rarely in cases of severe hypertension.

PRECAUTIONS & CONSIDERATIONS

Caution is warranted in patients with cardiac arrhythmias, epilepsy, frequent or severe headaches, hypertension, suicidal tendencies, and within several hours of ingestion of contraindicated substances, such as tyramine-containing food. Foods that require bacteria or molds for their preparation or preservation (such as yogurt and aged cheese), foods containing tyramine (such as avocados, bananas, broad beans, meat tenderizers, liver, smoked or pickled meats and fish, papayas, figs, raisins, sour cream, soy sauce, beer, wine, and yeast extracts), and excessive amounts of caffeine-containing foods or beverages (including chocolate, coffee, and tea) should be avoided.

This drug is not approved for use in children. Antidepressants increase the risk of suicidal thinking and behavior in children, adolescents, and young adults (18-24 yr) with depression. All patients should be monitored for suicidal thoughts, mood changes, or unusual behaviors.

Dizziness may occur, so change positions slowly, and alcohol and tasks that require mental alertness or motor skills should be avoided. Notify the physician if headache or neck soreness or stiffness occurs.

If hypertensive crisis occurs, phentolamine 5-10 mg IV should be administered. BP, temperature, and weight should be assessed.

Storage

Store at room temperature.

Administration

! Make sure at least 14 days elapse between the use of tranylcypromine and a selective serotonin reuptake inhibitor (5 wks for fluoxetine).

Take the second daily dose no later than 4:00 PM to avoid insomnia. Depression may start to lift during the first week of therapy and the drug's full therapeutic benefit will occur within 3 wks.

Trastuzumab

tras-too'-ze-mab

★ 🍁 Herceptin

CATEGORY AND SCHEDULE

Pregnancy Risk Category: D

Classification: Antineoplastics, monoclonal antibodies, targeted signal transduction inhibitor

MECHANISM OF ACTION

Binds to the HER-2 protein, which is overexpressed in 25%-30% of primary breast cancers, and certain gastric cancers, thereby inhibiting proliferation of tumor cells. *Therapeutic Effect:* Inhibits the growth of tumor cells and mediates antibody-dependent cellular cytotoxicity.

PHARMACOKINETICS

Half-life: 5.8 days (range: 1-32 days).

AVAILABILITY

Injection, Powder for Reconstitution: 440 mg.

INDICATIONS AND DOSAGES

NOTE: Regimens may vary with cancer type and combination chemotherapies used. The most common doses are listed below.

▸ **Breast cancer**

IV INFUSION

Adults, Elderly. Initially, 4 mg/kg as an infusion of 90 min on wk 1 then 2 mg/kg weekly as at least a 30-min infusion.

▸ **Adjuvant treatment of HER-2 overexpressing breast cancer**

IV INFUSION

Adults, Elderly. Initial dose of 4 mg/kg over 90 min, then 2 mg/kg over 30 min weekly for 52 wks; OR, give initial dose of 8 mg/kg over 90 min, then 6 mg/kg over 30-90 min q3wk for 52 wks.

▸ **Metastatic HER-2 overexpressing gastric cancer**

IV INFUSION

Adults, Elderly. Initial dose of 8 mg/kg over 90 min, then 6 mg/kg over 30-90 min q3wk.

CONTRAINDICATIONS

Preexisting cardiac disease.

INTERACTIONS

Drug

Cyclophosphamide, doxorubicin, epirubicin: May increase the risk of cardiac dysfunction.

Herbal

None known.

Food

None known.

DIAGNOSTIC TEST EFFECTS

None known.

IV INCOMPATIBILITIES

Do not mix trastuzumab with any other medications or with D5W.

SIDE EFFECTS

Frequent (> 20%)

Pain, asthenia, fever, chills, headache, abdominal pain, back pain, infection, nausea, diarrhea, vomiting, cough, dyspnea.

Occasional (5%-15%)

Tachycardia, CHF, flu-like symptoms, anorexia, edema, bone pain, arthralgia, insomnia, dizziness, paresthesia, depression, rhinitis, pharyngitis, sinusitis.

Rare (< 5%)

Allergic reaction, anemia, leukopenia, neuropathy, herpes simplex.

SERIOUS REACTIONS

- Cardiomyopathy, ventricular dysfunction, and CHF occur rarely.
- Pulmonary toxicity, including dyspnea, interstitial pneumonitis, pulmonary edema, hypoxia, acute respiratory distress syndrome, and pulmonary fibrosis.
- Exacerbation of chemotherapy-induced neutropenia may lead to opportunistic infection risk.
- Infusion reactions may be severe (fever and chills, nausea, vomiting, pain [in some cases at tumor sites], headache, dizziness, dyspnea, hypotension, rash, and asthenia).

PRECAUTIONS & CONSIDERATIONS

Caution should be used in those who have previously received cardiotoxic drug therapy or radiation therapy to the chest wall. Trastuzumab may cause fetal harm and should be avoided in pregnancy. Breastfeeding during treatment is not recommended. The safety and efficacy of trastuzumab have not been established in children. Age-related cardiac dysfunction may require cautious use in elderly patients.

Vaccinations and coming in contact with crowds, people with known infections, and anyone who has recently received an oral polio vaccine should be avoided.

Notify the physician of nausea and vomiting, abdominal pain, back pain, chills, and fever. Left ventricular function and baseline ECG and multigated acquisition (MUGA) scan should be obtained before starting therapy. CBC should be monitored before and periodically during therapy. Signs and symptoms of deteriorating cardiac or lung function should also be assessed.

Storage

Refrigerate unopened vials. After reconstitution of the vial with bacteriostatic water for injection, the solution is stable for 28 days if refrigerated. After reconstitution of the vial with sterile water for injection without a preservative, use the solution immediately; discard unused portions.

Administration

! Do not give trastuzumab by IV push or IV bolus. Do not use dextrose solutions for reconstitution.

Reconstitute the vial with 20 mL bacteriostatic water for injection (with benzyl alcohol) to yield a concentration of 21 mg/mL. If the patient is hypersensitive to benzyl alcohol, use sterile water for injection. Add the calculated dose from the vial to an IV solution of 250 mL 0.9% NaCl (do not use D5W). Gently mix contents in bag. The reconstituted IV solution normally appears colorless to pale yellow. IV solution reconstituted in 0.9% NaCl is stable for up to 24 h if refrigerated. Give loading dose (4 mg/kg) over 90 min. If tolerated, give maintenance infusion (2 mg/kg) over 30 min.

Travoprost

tra′voh-prost

Travatan-Z

Do not confuse Travatan-Z with Xalatan.

CATEGORY AND SCHEDULE

Pregnancy Risk Category: C

Classification:

Ophthalmic agents, prostaglandin analogues, antiglaucoma agents

MECHANISM OF ACTION

A synthetic analogue of prostaglandin with ocular hypotensive activity.
Therapeutic Effect: Reduces intraocular pressure (IOP) by increasing the outflow of aqueous humor.

PHARMACOKINETICS

Absorbed through the cornea and hydrolyzed to the active free acid form. Peak aqueous humor concentrations occur roughly 2 h after administration. Reduction in IOP starts approximately 2 h after administration and effectiveness peaks around 12 h. Plasma levels only detectable in first hour of administration. Any absorbed drug metabolized by liver and metabolites excreted primarily by the kidney.
Half-life: 45 min.

AVAILABILITY

Ophthalmic Solution: 0.004%.

INDICATIONS AND DOSAGES

▸ **Glaucoma, ocular hypertension**

OPHTHALMIC

Adults, Elderly. 1 drop in affected eye(s) once daily, in the evening.

CONTRAINDICATIONS

Hypersensitivity to travoprost or any component of the formulation.

DIAGNOSTIC TEST EFFECTS
None known.

SIDE EFFECTS
Frequent
Conjunctival hyperemia, growth of eyelashes, increased iris pigmentation, and ocular pruritus.
Occasional
Ocular dryness, visual disturbance, foreign body sensation, eye pain, pigmentation of the periocular skin, blepharitis, cataract, superficial punctate keratitis, eyelid erythema, ocular irritation, and eyelash darkening.
Rare
Intraocular inflammation (iritis).

SERIOUS REACTIONS
• Systemic adverse events, including infections (colds and upper respiratory tract infections), headaches, skin rash/allergic reactions, have been reported.

PRECAUTIONS & CONSIDERATIONS
May permanently increase pigmentation in iris and eyelid and produce changes in eye color and changes in eyelashes (color, length, shape). Use with caution in patients with uveitis or risk factors for macular edema. Effects in pregnancy and lactation not known; use with caution and only if clearly needed in women who are pregnant or breastfeeding. Safety and effectiveness have not been established in children. Remove contact lenses to apply; wait 15 min after administration to reinsert.
Storage
Store bottle at room temperature.
Administration
If more than 1 topical ophthalmic agent is being used, wait at least 5 min between administration of each. Tilt the head back slightly and pull the lower eyelid down with the index finger to form a pouch. Instill drop(s) and gently close the eyes for 1-2 min. Do not blink. Do not touch the tip of the dropper to any surface to avoid contamination.

Trazodone
tray'zoe-done
★ Desyrel, Oleptro 🍁 Apo-Trazodone, Novo-Trazodone, PMS-Trazodone, Trazorel
Do not confuse Desyrel with Delsym or Zestril.

CATEGORY AND SCHEDULE
Pregnancy Risk Category: C

Classification: Antidepressants, miscellaneous

MECHANISM OF ACTION
An antidepressant that blocks the reuptake of serotonin at neuronal presynaptic membranes, increasing its availability at postsynaptic receptor sites. *Therapeutic Effect:* Relieves depression.

PHARMACOKINETICS
Well absorbed from the GI tract. Protein binding: 85%-95%. Metabolized in the liver. Excreted primarily in urine. Unknown whether removed by hemodialysis. *Half-life:* 5-9 h.

AVAILABILITY
Tablets: 50 mg, 100 mg, 150 mg, 300 mg.
Extented-Release Tablets (Oleptro): 150 mg, 300 mg.

INDICATIONS AND DOSAGES
▸ **Depression**
PO

Adults. Initially, 150 mg/day in equally divided doses. Increase by 50 mg/day at 3- to 4-day intervals until therapeutic response is achieved. Maximum: 600 mg/day.
Elderly. Initially, 25-50 mg at bedtime. May increase by 25-50 mg every 3-7 days. Range: 75-150 mg/day.
Children 6-18 yr. Initially, 1.5-2 mg/kg/day in divided doses. May increase gradually to 6 mg/kg/day in 3 divided doses. Maximum: 400 mg/day.

OFF-LABEL USES

Treatment of neurogenic pain.

CONTRAINDICATIONS

Hypersensitivity; do not use within 14 days of MAOIs.

INTERACTIONS

Drug
Alcohol, CNS depression-producing medications: May increase CNS depression.
CYP3A4 inducers (e.g., carbamazepine, rifampin): May necessitate higher dose of trazodone.
CYP3A4 inhibitors (e.g., ketoconazole, itraconazole, Clarithromycin, protease inhibitors): May necessitate lower dose of trazodone.
Digoxin or phenytoin: Monitor for increased serum levels of these drugs.
MAOIs: Risk of serotonin syndrome; avoid.
NSAIDs, aspirin: Potential for increased risk of bleeding.
Serotonergic medications: Serotonin syndrome may occur.
Warfarin: Monitor for increased or decreased INR.
Herbal
St. John's wort: May increase the adverse effects of trazodone.
Food
None known.

DIAGNOSTIC TEST EFFECTS

May decrease WBC counts.

SIDE EFFECTS

Frequent (3%-9%)
Somnolence, dry mouth, light-headedness, dizziness, headache, blurred vision, nausea, vomiting.
Occasional (1%-3%)
Nervousness, fatigue, constipation, generalized aches and pains, mild hypotension.
Rare
Photosensitivity reaction.

SERIOUS REACTIONS

- Priapism, diminished or improved libido, retrograde ejaculation, and impotence occur rarely.
- Trazodone appears to be less cardiotoxic than other antidepressants, although arrhythmias may occur in patients with preexisting cardiac disease.
- Serotonin syndrome or neuroleptic malignant syndrome-like reactions (rare).
- Platelet dysfunction and bleeding risk (GI, etc.).

PRECAUTIONS & CONSIDERATIONS

Caution is warranted with arrhythmias and cardiac disease. Trazodone crosses the placenta and is minimally distributed in breast milk. The use of trazodone in children is not FDA approved. Antidepressants increase the risk of suicidal thinking and behavior in children, adolescents, and young adults (18-24 yr) with major depressive disorder and other psychiatric disorders. All patients should be monitored for suicidal thoughts, mood changes, or unusual behaviors. Lower dosages are recommended for elderly patients, who are more likely to experience hypotensive or sedative effects.

Anticholinergic and sedative effects may occur, so avoid alcohol and tasks that require mental alertness or motor skills. Tolerance usually develops to these side effects. Notify the physician if a painful, prolonged penile erection occurs. CBC, neutrophil and WBC counts, and liver and renal function tests should be assessed during therapy. ECG should also be obtained to assess for arrhythmias.

Storage

Store at room temperature.

Administration

Take trazodone shortly after a meal or snack to reduce the risk of dizziness or light-headedness. Crush immediate-release tablets as needed.

Take extended-release tablets at the same time every day in the late evening, preferably at bedtime, on an empty stomach. Swallow whole or break in half along the score line, and do not chew or crush.

When discontinued, gradual dose reduction is recommended.

Treprostinil

treh-prost′in-ill

★ 🍁 Remodulin, Tyvaso

CATEGORY AND SCHEDULE

Pregnancy Risk Category: B

Classification: Platelet inhibitors, prostaglandins, vasodilators

MECHANISM OF ACTION

An antiplatelet that directly dilates pulmonary and systemic arterial vascular beds, inhibiting platelet aggregation. *Therapeutic Effect:* Reduces symptoms of pulmonary arterial hypertension associated with exercise.

PHARMACOKINETICS

Rapidly, completely absorbed after subcutaneous infusion; 91% bound to plasma protein. Metabolized by the liver. Excreted mainly in the urine with a lesser amount eliminated in the feces. *Half-life:* 2-4 h.

AVAILABILITY

Injection: 1 mg/mL, 2.5 mg/mL, 5 mg/mL, 10 mg/mL.
Nebulizer Solution: 1.74 mg/2.9 mL.

INDICATIONS AND DOSAGES

▸ **Pulmonary arterial hypertension**

CONTINUOUS SC OR IV INFUSION

Adults, Elderly. Initially, 1.25 ng/kg/min. Reduce infusion rate to 0.625 ng/kg/min if initial dose cannot be tolerated. Increase infusion rate in increments of no more than 1.25 ng/kg/min weekly for the first 4 wks and then no more than 2.5 ng/kg/min per week for the duration of infusion.

▸ **Hepatic impairment (mild to moderate)**

Adults, Elderly. Decrease the initial dose to 0.625 ng/kg/min based on ideal body weight and increase cautiously.

▸ **Inhaled Dose for PAH**

NEBULIZER

Adults. Intially, 3 breaths (18 mcg) 4 times per day. May increase by 3 breaths q1-2wk to target of 9 breaths/dose. May reduce dose as low as 1-2 breaths/dose if needed.

CONTRAINDICATIONS

Hypersensitivity to treprostinil.

INTERACTIONS

Drug

Anticoagulants, aspirin, heparin, thrombolytics: May increase the risk of bleeding.

Drugs that alter BP, including antihypertensive agents, diuretics, vasodilators: Reduced BP caused by treprostinil may be exacerbated by these drugs.

Herbal

None known.

Food

None known.

DIAGNOSTIC TEST EFFECTS

None known.

SIDE EFFECTS

Frequent

Infusion site pain, erythema, induration, rash.

Occasional

Headache, diarrhea, jaw pain, vasodilation, nausea.

Rare

Dizziness, hypotension, pruritus, edema.

SERIOUS REACTIONS

- Abrupt withdrawal or sudden large reductions in dosage may result in worsening of pulmonary arterial hypertension symptoms.

PRECAUTIONS & CONSIDERATIONS

Caution is warranted in patients with liver or renal impairment and in elderly patients. It is unknown whether treprostinil is distributed in breast milk. Safety and efficacy of treprostinil have not been established in children. In elderly patients, age-related decreased cardiac, hepatic, and renal function as well as concurrent disease or other drug therapy may require dosage adjustment. Consider dosage selection carefully in elderly patients because of the increased incidence of diminished organ function. Notify the physician of signs of increased pulmonary artery pressure, such as dyspnea, cough, or chest pain.

Storage

Store at room temperature and administer without further dilution. Do not use a single vial for longer than 30 days after initial use.

Administration

Give as a continuous SC infusion via SC catheter, using an infusion pump designed for SC drug delivery. Calculate the infusion rate using the following formula: Infusion rate (mL/h) = Dose (ng/kg/min) multiplied by Weight (kg) multiplied by (0.00006/treprostinil dosage strength concentration [mg/mL]). To avoid potential interruptions in drug delivery, provide the patient with immediate access to a backup infusion pump and spare subcutaneous infusion sets. Abrupt withdrawal or sudden large reductions in dosage may result in worsening of pulmonary arterial hypertension symptoms.

For nebullizer use, see manufacturer's instructions for the Tyvaso inhalation system.

Tretinoin

tret'i-noyn

★ Altinac, Avita, Refissa, Renova, Retin-A, Retin-A Micro, Tretin-X

🍁 Rejuva-A, Stieva-A, Vesanoid

CATEGORY AND SCHEDULE

Pregnancy Risk Category: D (oral), C (topical)

Classification: Antineoplastics, retinoids, dermatologics, keratolytics

MECHANISM OF ACTION

A retinoid that decreases cohesiveness of follicular epithelial cells. Increases turnover of follicular epithelial cells. Bacterial skincounts are not altered. Transdermal: Exerts its effects on growth and differentiation of epithelial cells. Antineoplastic: Induces maturation, decreases proliferation of acute promyelocytic leukemia (APL) cells. *Therapeutic Effect:* Causes expulsion of blackheads; alleviates fine wrinkles, hyperpigmentation; causes repopulation of bone marrow and blood by normal hematopoietic cells.

PHARMACOKINETICS

Topical: Minimally absorbed.
Oral: Well absorbed following oral administration. Protein binding: 95%. Metabolized in liver. Primarily excreted in urine, minimal excretion in feces. *Half-life:* 0.5-2 h.

AVAILABILITY

Capsules: 10 mg.
Cream: 0.025% (Altinac, Avita, Retin-A), 0.02% (Renova), 0.05% (Altinac, Renova, Retin-A), 0.1% (Altinac, Retin-A).
Gel: 0.01% (Retin-A), 0.025% (Avita, Retin-A), 0.04% (Retin-A Micro), 0.1% (Retin-A Micro).
Topical Liquid: 0.05% (Retin-A).

INDICATIONS AND DOSAGES

▸ Acne
TOPICAL
Adults. Apply once daily at bedtime.

▸ Palliation of fine facial wrinkles, hyperpigmentation, and roughness due to photoaging
TOPICAL
Adults. Apply a pea-sized amount of 0.02% or 0.05% product to affected area once daily before bedtime for 24-48 wks.

▸ Acute promyelocytic leukemia
PO
Adults, Children > 1 yr. 45 mg/m²/day given as 2 evenly divided doses until complete remission is documented. Discontinue therapy 30 days after complete remission or after 90 days of treatment, whichever comes first.

CONTRAINDICATIONS

Sensitivity to retinoids or parabens (used as preservative in gelatin capsule).

INTERACTIONS

Drug
TOPICAL
Keratolytic agents (e.g., sulfur, benzoyl peroxide, salicylic acid), medicated soaps, shampoos, astringents, spice or lime cologne, permanent wave solutions, hair depilatories: May increase skin irritation.
Photosensitive medication (thiazides, tetracyclines, fluoroquinolones, phenothiazines, sulfonamides): May augment phototoxicity.
PO
Ketoconazole: May increase tretinoin concentration.
Herbal
Vitamin A: May increase risk of vitamin A toxicity.
Food
None known.

DIAGNOSTIC TEST EFFECTS

PO
Leukocytosis occurs commonly (40%). May elevate liver function tests, cholesterol, triglycerides.

SIDE EFFECTS

Expected
TOPICAL
Temporary change in pigmentation, photosensitivity, local inflammatory reactions (peeling, dry skin, stinging, erythema, pruritus) are to be expected and are reversible with discontinuation of tretinoin.

Frequent
PO
Headache, fever, dry skin/oral mucosa, bone pain, nausea, vomiting, rash.
Occasional
PO
Mucositis, earache or feeling of fullness in ears, flushing, pruritus, increased sweating, visual disturbances, hypo/hypertension, dizziness, anxiety, insomnia, alopecia, skin changes.
Rare
PO
Change in visual acuity, temporary hearing loss.

SERIOUS REACTIONS

PO
- Retinoic acid syndrome (fever, dyspnea, weight gain, abnormal chest auscultatory findings, episodic hypotension) occurs commonly as does leukocytosis. Syndrome generally occurs during first month of therapy (sometimes occurs following first dose).
- Pseudo tumor cerebri may be noted, especially in children (headache, nausea, vomiting, visual disturbances).
- Possible tumorigenic potential when combined with ultraviolet radiation.

TOPICAL
- Possible tumorigenic potential when combined with ultraviolet radiation.

PRECAUTIONS & CONSIDERATIONS

Caution should be used in patients with elevated cholesterol and/or triglycerides and considerable sun exposure in their occupation or hypersensitivity to sun. Be aware that tretinoin should be avoided in pregnant women. Be aware that it is unknown whether tretinoin is distributed in breast milk; exercise caution in nursing mother. Tretinoin may have a teratogenic and embryotoxic effect.

All women of childbearing potential should be warned of risk to fetus if pregnancy occurs. Two reliable forms of contraceptives should be used concurrently during therapy and for 1 mo after discontinuation of therapy, even in infertile, premenopausal women. A pregnancy test should be obtained within 1 wk before institution of therapy. Liver function tests and cholesterol and triglyceride levels should be monitored before and during therapy.

Avoid exposure to sunlight or sunbeds; sunscreens and protective clothing should be used. Affected areas should also be protected from wind, cold. If skin is already sunburned, do not use until fully recovered. Keep tretinoin away from eyes, mouth, angles of nose, and mucous membranes. Do not use medicated, drying, or abrasive soaps; wash face no more than 2-3 times daily with mild soap. Avoid use of preparations containing alcohol, menthol, spice, or lime such as shaving lotions, astringents, and perfume. Mild redness, peeling are expected; decrease frequency or discontinue medication if excessive reaction occurs. Nonmedicated cosmetics may be used; however, cosmetics must be removed before tretinoin application.

Storage
Store at room temperature.

Administration
Take oral tretinoin with food. Do not crush or break capsule.

For topical administration, thoroughly cleanse area before applying tretinoin. Lightly cover only the affected area. Liquid may be applied with fingertip, gauze, or cotton, taking care to avoid running onto unaffected skin. Keep medication away from eyes, mouth, angles of nose, mucous membranes. Wash hands immediately after application. Improvement noted during first 24 wks of therapy. Therapeutic results noted in 2-3 wks; optimal results in 6 wks.

Triamcinolone

tri-am-sin'oh-lone

★ Nasacort AQ, Kenalog, Aristospan, Oralone, Triderm, Pediaderm TA 🍁 Oracort, Triderm

CATEGORY AND SCHEDULE

Pregnancy Risk Category: C

Classification: Corticosteroids, systemic, topical, nasal, dermatologic anti-inflammatory agents

MECHANISM OF ACTION

A corticosteroid that controls the rate of protein synthesis, depresses migration of polymorphonuclear leukocytes, reverses capillary permeability, and stabilizes lysosomal membranes. *Therapeutic Effect:* Prevents or controls inflammation.

T

PHARMACOKINETICS

Intranasal or local injection: Low overall systemic absorption. Protein binding: 91%. Undergoes extensive metabolism in liver. Excreted in urine. Topical: Mostly metabolized locally in the skin. Amount systemically absorbed depends on affected area and skin condition (absorption increased with fever, hydration, inflamed or denuded skin). Use of occlusive dressings may increase percutaneous absorption.

AVAILABILITY

Oral Dental Paste (Oralone): 0.1%.
Nasal Spray (Nasacort AQ): 55 mcg/actuation.
Triamcinolone Acetonide Injection Suspension (Kenalog): 10 mg/mL, 40 mg/mL.
Triamcinolone Hexacetonide Injection Suspension (Aristospan): 5 mg/mL, 20 mg/mL.
Topical Cream: 0.1%, 0.5%, 0.025%.
Topical Lotion: 0.025%, 0.1%.
Topical Ointment: 0.025%, 0.1%.
Topical Spray: 0.147 mg/g.

INDICATIONS AND DOSAGES

▸ **Corticosteroid-responsive dermatoses**

TOPICAL (OINTMENT, CREAM, LOTION, SPRAY)

Adults, Elderly. Apply 2-4 times per day.

▸ **For the treatment of symptoms of seasonal and perennial allergic rhinitis**

NASAL (NASACORT AQ)

Adults, Elderly, Children ≥ 12 yr. 2 sprays into each nostril once daily. Once controlled, reduce to lowest effective dose.

Children 6-11 yr. 1 spray into each nostril once daily. May give up to 2 sprays in each nostril once daily if needed. Once controlled, reduce to lowest effective dose.

Children 2-5 yr: No more than 1 spray into each nostril once daily.

▸ **For ulcerative or inflammatory oral lesions**

TOPICAL DENTAL PASTE

Adults, Elderly. Apply 2-3 times per day after meals and at bedtime.

▸ **For the relief of joint inflammation associated with osteoarthritis or rheumatoid arthritis, or the relief of bursitis**

INTRA-ARTICULAR (ACETONIDE SUSPENSION)

Adults, Elderly, Children ≥ 6 yr. 2.5-15 mg at appropriate site. Repeat as needed.
INTRA-ARTICULAR (HEXACECETONIDE SUSPENSION)
Adults. 2-20 mg at appropriate site. Repeat at intervals of 3-4 wks as needed.

CONTRAINDICATIONS

Hypersensitivity to triamcinolone or other corticosteroids. Untreated localized infection of nasal mucosa (nasal form).

INTERACTIONS

Drug, Herbal, and Food
None known.

DIAGNOSTIC TEST EFFECTS

None known.

SIDE EFFECTS

Frequent
Intranasal: Mild nasopharyngeal irritation; nasal burning, stinging, or dryness; rhinorrhea; change in taste.
Topical or injectable use: Burning, dryness, stinging.
Occasional
Intranasal: Pharyngeal candidiasis, headache.
Topical: Pruritus.
Rare
Topical: Allergic contact dermatitis, purpura or blood-containing blisters, thinning of skin with easy bruising, telangiectasis or raised dark red spots on skin.

SERIOUS REACTIONS

- Anaphylaxis, hypersensitivity reactions, and increased intraocular pressure occur rarely with use.
- Nasal septal perforation with prolonged innappropriate use of nasal form.
- Excessive use or overdosage may lead to systemic hypercorticism and adrenal suppression (HPA axis suppression).

PRECAUTIONS & CONSIDERATIONS

Caution is warranted with active or quiescent tuberculosis, or other untreated systemic infections (including fungal, bacterial, or viral). It is unknown whether triamcinolone crosses the placenta and is distributed in breast milk, but the drug is probably excreted in breast milk in low quantities. Be aware that the safety and efficacy of most of these products have not been established in children younger than 2-6 yr, dependent on the product prescribed. Be aware that children may absorb larger amounts of topical corticosteroids, which should be used sparingly. No age-related precautions have been noted in elderly patients. HPA axis suppression should be monitored by urinary free cortisol tests and an ACTH stimulation test.
Storage
Store at room temperature. Store nasal spray upright.
Administration
Topical: Gently cleanse area before topical application. Use occlusive dressings only as ordered. Apply sparingly, and rub into area thoroughly.
Nasal: Prime nasal spray as manufacturer directs before first use. Tilt head slightly forward. Insert spray tip up into the nostril, pointing away from nasal septum. Spray the drug into the nostril while holding the other nostril closed, and at the same time inhale through the nose.
Injection: Injection suspension products are not to be given intravenously. May be given intralesionally or intra-articularly. Shake well before each use. Use of specialized injection techniques, by experienced physician, is required.

Triamterene

try-am'ter-een

Dyrenium

Do not confuse triamterene with trimipramine.

CATEGORY AND SCHEDULE

Pregnancy Risk Category: C (D if used in pregnancy-induced hypertension)

Classification: Diuretics, potassium sparing

MECHANISM OF ACTION

A potassium-sparing diuretic that inhibits sodium, potassium, ATPase. Interferes with sodium and potassium exchange in distal tubule, cortical collecting tubule, and collecting duct. Increases sodium and decreases potassium excretion. Also increases magnesium, decreases calcium loss. *Therapeutic Effect:* Produces diuresis and lowers BP.

PHARMACOKINETICS

Route	Onset	Peak	Duration
PO	2-4 h	NA	7-9 h

Incompletely absorbed from the GI tract. Widely distributed. Metabolized to at least one active metabolite. About 50% of a dose is excreted in the urine. Roughly 21% is eliminated as unchanged drug. The remainder is eliminated via biliary/fecal routes. *Half-life:* 1.5-2.5 h (increased in renal impairment).

AVAILABILITY

Capsules: 50 mg, 100 mg.

INDICATIONS AND DOSAGES

▸ **Edema, hypertension**

PO

Adults, Elderly. 50-100 mg/day as a single dose or in 2 divided doses. Maximum: 300 mg/day.

OFF-LABEL USES

Prevention and treatment of hypokalemia.

CONTRAINDICATIONS

Hypersensitivity, diabetic neuropathy, drug-induced or preexisting hyperkalemia, progressive or severe renal disease, anuria, severe hepatic disease.

INTERACTIONS

Drug

ACE inhibitors (such as captopril), eplerenone, drospirenone, spironolactone, potassium-containing medications, potassium supplements: May increase the risk of hyperkalemia.

Dofetilide: Avoid use with dofetilide since triamterene may compete for renal elimination.

Lithium: May decrease the clearance and increase the risk of toxicity of lithium.

Metformin: May increase risk of lactic acidosis by competing for renal secretion.

NSAIDs: May decrease the antihypertensive effect of triamterene.

Herbal

None known.

Food

None known.

DIAGNOSTIC TEST EFFECTS

May increase urinary calcium excretion; BUN and blood glucose levels; and serum calcium, creatinine, potassium, magnesium, and uric acid levels. May decrease serum sodium levels.

T

SIDE EFFECTS

Occasional

Fatigue, nausea, diarrhea, abdominal pain, leg cramps, headache.

Rare

Anorexia, asthenia, rash, dizziness.

SERIOUS REACTIONS

- Triamterene use may result in hyponatremia (somnolence, dry mouth, increased thirst, lack of energy) or severe hyperkalemia (irritability, anxiety, heaviness of legs, paresthesia, hypotension, bradycardia, ECG changes [tented T waves, widening QRS complex, ST segment depression]).
- Agranulocytosis, nephrolithiasis, and thrombocytopenia occur rarely.

PRECAUTIONS & CONSIDERATIONS

Caution is warranted in patients with diabetes mellitus, history of renal calculi, hepatic or renal impairment, and concurrent use of potassium-sparing diuretics or potassium supplements. Triamterene crosses the placenta and is distributed in breast milk. Breastfeeding is not recommended for patients taking this drug. The safety and efficacy of this drug have not been established in children. Elderly patients may be at increased risk for developing hyperkalemia. Avoid consuming salt substitutes and foods high in potassium.

An increase in the frequency and volume of urination may occur. Notify the physician of dry mouth, fever, headache, nausea and vomiting, persistent or severe weakness, sore throat, or unusual bleeding or bruising. Blood pressure (BP), vital signs, electrolytes, intake and output, and weight should be monitored before and during treatment. Be aware of signs of electrolyte disturbances such as hypokalemia or hyponatremia. Hypokalemia may cause arrhythmias, altered mental status, muscle cramps, asthenia, and tremor.

Storage

Store at room temperature.

Administration

Take triamterene with food if GI disturbances occur. Do not crush or break capsules. Therapeutic effect takes several days to begin and can last for several days after the drug is discontinued.

Triazolam

trye-ay'zoe-lam

★ Halcion

🍁 Apo-Triazo

Do not confuse Halcion with Haldol or Healon.

CATEGORY AND SCHEDULE

Pregnancy Risk Category: X

Controlled Substance Schedule: IV

Classification: Benzodiazepines, sedatives/hypnotics

MECHANISM OF ACTION

A benzodiazepine that enhances the action of the inhibitory neurotransmitter γ-aminobutyric acid, resulting in central nervous system (CNS) depression.

Therapeutic Effect: Induces sleep.

AVAILABILITY

Tablets: 0.125 mg, 0.25 mg.

INDICATIONS AND DOSAGES

▸ **Insomnia**

PO

Adults, Children older than 18 yr. Typically, 0.25 mg at bedtime, 0.125 mg may be sufficient for some patients. Maximum: 0.5 mg.

Elderly. 0.125-0.25 mg at bedtime. Maximum: 0.25 mg.

CONTRAINDICATIONS

Angle-closure glaucoma; CNS depression; pregnancy or breastfeeding; severe, uncontrolled pain; sleep apnea; ethanol intoxication. Triazolam is contraindicated with ketoconazole, itraconazole, nefazodone, and other medications that potentially impair CYP3A4 metabolism.

INTERACTIONS

Drug

Alcohol, other CNS depressants: May increase CNS depression.

Protease inhibitors for HIV, ketoconazole, itraconazole, nefazodone: Increase triazolam concentrations, resulting in clinically significant potentiation of sedation. Contraindicated.

Herbal

Kava kava, valerian: May increase CNS depression.

Food

Grapefruit, grapefruit juice: May alter the absorption of triazolam.

DIAGNOSTIC TEST EFFECTS

None known.

T

SIDE EFFECTS

Frequent

Somnolence, sedation, dry mouth, headache, dizziness, nervousness, light-headedness, incoordination, nausea, rebound insomnia (may occur for 1-2 nights after drug is discontinued).

Occasional

Euphoria, tachycardia, abdominal cramps, visual disturbances.

Rare

Paradoxical CNS excitement or restlessness (particularly in elderly or debilitated patients).

SERIOUS REACTIONS

• Abrupt or too-rapid withdrawal may result in pronounced restlessness, irritability, insomnia, hand tremors, abdominal or muscle cramps, vomiting, diaphoresis, and seizures.
• Overdose results in somnolence, confusion, diminished reflexes, respiratory depression, and coma.

PRECAUTIONS & CONSIDERATIONS

Caution is warranted in persons with a potential for drug abuse and in hepatic or renal impairment. Pregnancy should be determined before therapy begins. Do not give during pregnancy or breastfeeding. Drowsiness may occur. Avoid alcohol, CNS depressants, and tasks that require mental alertness or motor skills. Cardiovascular, mental, and respiratory status and hepatic function should be monitored throughout therapy.

Administration

Take triazolam without regard to food. Crush tablets as needed. Do not administer the drug with grapefruit juice.

Trifluridine

trye-flure'i-deen

★ 🍁 Viroptic

Do not confuse with Zostrix.

CATEGORY AND SCHEDULE

Pregnancy Risk Category: C

Classification: Antivirals, ophthalmics

MECHANISM OF ACTION

An antiviral agent that incorporates into DNA causing increased rate of mutation and errors in protein formation. *Therapeutic Effect:* Prevents viral replication.

PHARMACOKINETICS
Intraocular solution is undetectable in serum. *Half-life:* 12 min.

AVAILABILITY
Ophthalmic Solution: 1% (Viroptic).

INDICATIONS AND DOSAGES
▸ **Herpes simplex virus ocular infections**

OPHTHALMIC

Adults, Elderly, Children older than 6 yr. 1 drop into affected eye q2h while awake. Maximum: 9 drops/day. Continue until corneal ulcer has completely reepithelialized; then, 1 drop q4h while awake (minimum: 5 drops/day) for an additional 7 days.

CONTRAINDICATIONS
Hypersensitivity to trifluridine or any component of the formulation.

INTERACTIONS
Drug
None known.
Herbal
None known.
Food
None known.

DIAGNOSTIC TEST EFFECTS
None known.

SIDE EFFECTS
Frequent
Transient stinging or burning with instillation.
Occasional
Edema of eyelid.
Rare
Hypersensitivity reaction.

SERIOUS REACTIONS
• Ocular toxicity may occur if used longer than 21 days.

PRECAUTIONS & CONSIDERATIONS
Be aware that trifluridine use should not exceed 21 days because of the potential for ocular toxicity. It may cause transient irritation of the conjunctiva and cornea. Be aware that trifluridine is not recommended during pregnancy or lactation because of its mutagenic effects in vitro. Safety and efficacy have not been established in children younger than 6 yr. No age-related precautions have been noted in elderly patients.

If no improvement occurs after 7 days or complete healing after 14, contact the physician. Report any itching, swelling, redness, or increased irritation.

Storage
Refrigerate trifluridine; avoid freezing.
Administration
For ophthalmic use, do not touch applicator tip to any surface. Place finger on lower eyelid and pull out until pocket is formed between eye and lower lid. Hold dropper above pocket and place prescribed number of drops in pocket. Close eyes gently so medication will not be squeezed out of sac. Apply gentle finger pressure to the lacrimal sac at inner canthus for 1 min following instillation (lessens risk of systemic absorption). If more than 1 ophthalmic drug is being used, separate administration by at least 5-10 min.

Trihexyphenidyl
trye-hex-ee-fen′i-dill

CATEGORY AND SCHEDULE
Pregnancy Risk Category: C

Classification: Anticholinergics, antiparkinsonian agents

MECHANISM OF ACTION

An anticholinergic agent that blocks central cholinergic receptors (aids in balancing cholinergic and dopaminergic activity). *Therapeutic Effect:* Decreases salivation, relaxes smooth muscle.

PHARMACOKINETICS

Well absorbed from GI tract. Primarily excreted in urine. *Half-life:* 3.3-4.1 h.

AVAILABILITY

Elixer: 2 mg/5 mL.
Tablets: 2 mg, 5 mg.

INDICATIONS AND DOSAGES

▸ **Parkinsonism**

PO

Adults, Elderly. Initially, 1 mg on first day. May increase by 2 mg/day at intervals of 3-5 days up to 6-10 mg/day (12-15 mg/day in patients with postencephalitic parkinsonism).

▸ **Drug-induced extrapyramidal symptoms**

PO

Adults, Elderly. Initially, 1 mg/day. Range: 5-15 mg/day.

CONTRAINDICATIONS

Angle-closure glaucoma, GI obstruction, paralytic ileus, intestinal atony, severe ulcerative colitis, prostatic hypertrophy, myasthenia gravis, megacolon, hypersensitivity to trihexyphenidyl or any component of the formulation.

INTERACTIONS

Drug

Alcohol, central nervous system (CNS) depressants: May increase sedative effect.

Amantadine, anticholinergics, MAOIs: May increase anticholinergic effects.

Antacids, antidiarrheals: May decrease absorption and effects of trihexyphenidyl.

Herbal

None known.

Food

None known.

DIAGNOSTIC TEST EFFECTS

None known.

SIDE EFFECTS

Elderly (older than 60 yr) tend to develop mental confusion, disorientation, agitation, psychotic-like symptoms.

Frequent

Drowsiness, dry mouth.

Occasional

Blurred vision, urinary retention, constipation, dizziness, headache, muscle cramps.

Rare

Seizures, depression, rash.

SERIOUS REACTIONS

- Hypersensitivity reaction (eczema, pruritus, rash, cardiac disturbances, photosensitivity) may occur.
- Overdosage may vary from CNS depression (sedation, apnea, cardiovascular collapse, death) to severe paradoxical reaction (hallucinations, tremor, seizures).

PRECAUTIONS & CONSIDERATIONS

Caution is warranted in patients with treated open-angle glaucoma, autonomic neuropathy, pulmonary disease, esophageal reflux, hiatal hernia, heart disease, hyperthyroidism, and hypertension. It is unknown whether trihexyphenidyl crosses the placenta or is distributed in breast milk. Safety and efficacy have not been established in children. Elderly patients are more sensitive to the effects of trihexyphenidyl as well as anxiety, confusion, and nervousness.

Dry mouth, drowsiness, and dizziness are expected side effects of this drug. Avoid alcohol and do not drive, use machinery, or engage in other activities that require mental acuity if dizziness or blurred vision occurs.

Storage

Store at room temperature.

Administration

Be aware not to use sustained-release capsules for initial therapy. Once stabilized, may switch, on mg-for-mg basis, giving in 2 daily doses and with food. High doses may be divided into 4 doses, at mealtimes, and at bedtime.

Trimethobenzamide

trye-meth-oh-ben′za-mide

★ Tigan

CATEGORY AND SCHEDULE

Pregnancy Risk Category: C

Classification: Antiemetics

MECHANISM OF ACTION

Trimethobenzamide acts at the medullary chemoreceptor trigger zone by centrally blocking dopamine receptors (D2 subtype). May be a weak 5-HT3 receptor antagonist. *Therapeutic Effect:* Relieves nausea and vomiting.

PHARMACOKINETICS

Route	Onset	Duration
PO	10-40 min	3-4 h
IM	15-30 min	2-3 h

Partially absorbed from the GI tract. Distributed primarily to the liver. Metabolic fate unknown. Excreted in urine. *Half-life:* 7-9 h.

AVAILABILITY

Capsules: 300 mg.
Injection: 100 mg/mL.

INDICATIONS AND DOSAGES

▸ **Nausea and vomiting**

PO

Adults, Elderly. 300 mg 3-4 times a day.

Children weighing 30-100 lb. 100-200 mg 3-4 times a day.

IM

Adults, Elderly. 200 mg 3-4 times a day.

CONTRAINDICATIONS

Hypersensitivity to trimethobenzamide; agranulocytosis; use of parenteral form in children.

INTERACTIONS

Drug

CNS depressants: May increase CNS depression.

Herbal

None known.

Food

None known.

DIAGNOSTIC TEST EFFECTS

None known.

SIDE EFFECTS

Frequent

Somnolence.

Occasional

Blurred vision, diarrhea, dizziness, headache, muscle cramps.

Rare

Rash, seizures, depression, opisthotonos, parkinsonian syndrome, Reye syndrome (marked by vomiting, seizures).

SERIOUS REACTIONS

- Extrapyramidal symptoms such as muscle rigidity and allergic skin reactions, occurs rarely.
- Children may experience paradoxical reactions, marked by restlessness, insomnia, euphoria, nervousness, and tremor.
- Overdose may produce CNS depression (manifested as sedation,

apnea, cardiovascular collapse, and death) or severe paradoxical reactions (such as hallucinations, tremor, and seizures).

PRECAUTIONS & CONSIDERATIONS

Caution is warranted with dehydration, electrolyte imbalances, high fever, and the debilitated or elderly. It is unknown whether trimethobenzamide crosses the placenta or is distributed in breast milk. No age-related precautions have been noted in elderly patients. Do not administer the parenteral form to children. Tasks that require mental alertness or motor skills should be avoided until response to the drug has been established.

Drowsiness may occur. Notify the physician of headache, visual disturbances, restlessness, or involuntary muscle movements. BP, intake and output, vomitus, and skin for hydration status should be assessed.

Administration

! Do not administer trimethobenzamide by the IV route because it produces severe hypotension.

Take oral trimethobenzamide without regard to food. Don't crush, open, or break the capsules.

For IM use, inject the drug deep into a large muscle mass, usually the upper outer gluteus maximus.

T

Trimethoprim

trye-meth'oh-prim

Primsol, Proloprim

CATEGORY AND SCHEDULE

Pregnancy Risk Category: C

Classification: Antibiotics, folate antagonists

MECHANISM OF ACTION

A folate antagonist that blocks bacterial biosynthesis of nucleic acids and proteins by interfering with the metabolism of folinic acid. *Therapeutic Effect:* Bacteriostatic.

PHARMACOKINETICS

Rapidly and completely absorbed from the GI tract. Protein binding: 42%-46%. Widely distributed, including to the cerebrospinal fluid (CSF). Metabolized in the liver. Primarily excreted in urine. Moderately removed by hemodialysis. *Half-life:* 8-10 h (increased in impaired renal function and newborns; decreased in children).

AVAILABILITY

Oral Solution (Primsol): 50 mg/5 mL.

Tablets (Proloprim): 100 mg, 200 mg.

INDICATIONS AND DOSAGES

▸ Acute, uncomplicated urinary tract infection

PO

Adults, Elderly, Children 12 yr and older. 100 mg q12hr or 200 mg once a day for 10-14 days.

Children younger than 12 yr. 4-6 mg/kg/day in 2 divided doses for 10 days.

▸ Dosage in renal impairment

Dosage and frequency are modified based on creatinine clearance.

Creatinine Clearance (mL/min)	Dosage Interval
> 30	No change
15-29	Reduce dose by 50%

OFF-LABEL USES

Prevention of bacterial urinary tract infection, treatment of pneumonia caused by *Pneumocystis carinii.*

CONTRAINDICATIONS

Hypersensitivity, infants younger than 2 mo, megaloblastic anemia caused by folic acid deficiency.

INTERACTIONS

Drug

ACE inhibitors, potassium-sparing agents: Increased risk of hyperkalemia.

Folate antagonists (including methotrexate): May increase the risk of megaloblastic anemia.

Herbal

None known.

Food

None known.

DIAGNOSTIC TEST EFFECTS

May increase BUN and serum bilirubin, creatinine, AST (SGOT), and ALT (SGPT) levels.

SIDE EFFECTS

Occasional

Nausea, vomiting, diarrhea, decreased appetite, abdominal cramps, headache.

Rare

Hypersensitivity reaction (pruritus, rash), methemoglobinemia (bluish fingernails, lips, or skin; fever; pale skin; sore throat; unusual tiredness), photosensitivity.

SERIOUS REACTIONS

- Stevens-Johnson syndrome, erythema multiforme, exfoliative dermatitis, and anaphylaxis occur rarely.
- Hematologic toxicity (thrombocytopenia, neutropenia, leukopenia, megaloblastic anemia) is more likely to occur in elderly, debilitated, or alcoholic patients; in patients with impaired renal function; and in those receiving prolonged high dosage.

PRECAUTIONS & CONSIDERATIONS

Caution is warranted in patients with impaired hepatic or renal function or folic acid deficiency. Trimethoprim readily crosses the placenta and is distributed in breast milk. No age-related precautions have been noted in elderly patients, but they may have an increased incidence of thrombocytopenia. Avoid sun and ultraviolet light.

Report bleeding, bruising, skin discoloration, fever, pallor, rash, sore throat, and tiredness. Hematology and renal function tests should be assessed before and during therapy.

Storage

Store at room temperature.

Administration

Take trimethoprim without regard to food (or with food if stomach upset occurs). Space drug doses evenly around the clock and complete the full course of trimethoprim therapy, which usually lasts 10-14 days.

Trimipramine

trye-mih-prah'meen

★ Surmontil

🍁 Novo-Tripramine

Do not confuse with desipramine or triamterene.

CATEGORY AND SCHEDULE

Pregnancy Risk Category: C

Classification: Antidepressants, tricyclic

MECHANISM OF ACTION

A tricyclic antibulimic, anticataplectic, antidepressant, antinarcoleptic, antineuralgic, antineuritic, and antipanic agent that blocks the reuptake of neurotransmitters, such as norepinephrine and serotonin, at presynaptic membranes, increasing their concentration at postsynaptic receptor sites. May demonstrate less autonomic toxicity than other tricyclic antidepressants. *Therapeutic Effect:* Results in antidepressant effect. Anticholinergic effect controls nocturnal enuresis.

PHARMACOKINETICS

Rapidly, completely absorbed after PO administration and not affected by food. Protein binding: 95%. Metabolized in liver (significant first-pass effect). Primarily excreted in urine. Not removed by hemodialysis. *Half-life:* 16-40 h.

AVAILABILITY

Capsules: 25 mg, 50 mg, 100 mg (Surmontil).

INDICATIONS AND DOSAGES

▸ **Depression**

PO

Adults. 50-150 mg/day at bedtime. Maximum: 200 mg/day for outpatients, 300 mg/day for inpatients.

Elderly. Initially, 25 mg/day at bedtime. May increase by 25 mg q3-7 days. Maximum: 100 mg/day.

CONTRAINDICATIONS

Acute recovery period after myocardial infarction (MI), cardiac conduction defects, within 14 days of MAOI ingestion, hypersensitivity to trimipramine or any component of the formulation.

INTERACTIONS

Drug

Alcohol, central nervous system (CNS) depressants: May increase CNS and respiratory depression and the hypotensive effects of trimipramine.

Anticoagulants: May increase risk of bleeding.

Antipsychotics (haloperidol, risperidone, quetiapine): May increase the cardiac effects (QT prolongation, torsades de pointes, cardiac arrest).

Antithyroid agents: May increase the risk of agranulocytosis.

Amprenavir, atazanavir: May increase serum concentrations and risk of toxicity of trimipramine.

Atomoxetine: May increase plasma concentrations of atomoxetine.

Barbiturates: May decrease trimipramine serum concentrations and possible additive adverse effects.

Baclofen: May increase the risk of memory loss and/or muscle tone.

Cimetidine: May increase trimipramine blood concentration and risk of toxicity.

Class 1, 1A, and III antiarrhythmic agents; cisapride; cotrimoxazole; fluconazole; gatifloxacin; gemifloxacin; grepafloxacin; sparfloxacin; telithromycin; halofantrine; halothane; sympathomimetics; vasopressin; zolmitriptan: May increase the cardiac effects.

Clonidine, guanadrel: May decrease the effects of clonidine and guanadrel.

Duloxetine, fluoxetine, paroxetine, sertraline: May increase serum concentrations and risk of toxicity.

Estrogens: May increase the antidepressant effectiveness and risk of tricyclic toxicity.

MAOIs: May increase the risk of hyperpyrexia, hypertensive crisis, and seizures.

Phenothiazines: May increase anticholinergic and sedative effects of trimipramine.

Phenytoin: May decrease trimipramine blood concentration.

Quinidine: May increase the risk of trimipramine toxicity.

Herbal
Ginkgo biloba: May decrease seizure threshold.
St. John's wort: May have additive effect.

DIAGNOSTIC TEST EFFECTS

May alter blood glucose levels and ECG readings.

SIDE EFFECTS

Frequent
Drowsiness, fatigue, dry mouth, blurred vision, constipation, delayed micturition, postural hypotension, diaphoresis, disturbed concentration, increased appetite, urinary retention, photosensitivity.
Occasional
GI disturbances, such as nausea, and a metallic taste sensation.
Rare
Paradoxical reaction, marked by agitation, restlessness, nightmares, insomnia, extrapyramidal symptoms, particularly fine hand tremors.

SERIOUS REACTIONS

- High dosage may produce cardiovascular effects, such as severe postural hypotension, dizziness, tachycardia, palpitations, arrhythmias, and seizures. High dosage may also result in altered temperature regulation, including hyperpyrexia or hypothermia.
- Abrupt withdrawal from prolonged therapy may produce headache, malaise, nausea, vomiting, and vivid dreams.

PRECAUTIONS & CONSIDERATIONS

Caution is warranted in patients with cardiac disease, diabetes mellitus, glaucoma, hiatal hernia, history of seizures, history of urinary obstruction or retention, hyperthyroidism, increased intraocular pressure (IOP) decreased GI motility, liver disease, prostatic hypertrophy, renal disease, and schizophrenia. It is unknown whether trimipramine crosses the placenta or is distributed in breast milk. Be aware that trimipramine is not recommended in children younger than 18 yr. Antidepressants increase the risk of suicidal thinking and behavior in children, adolescents, and young adults (18-24 yr) with major depressive disorder and other psychiatric disorders. All patients should be monitored for suicidal thoughts, mood changes, or unusual behaviors. Dose reduction may be required in elderly patients.

Tolerance usually develops to anticholinergic effects, postural hypotension, and sedative effects during therapy. Avoid tasks that require mental alertness or motor skills until response to trimipramine is established.

Administration
Take with food or milk if GI distress occurs.

Triptorelin Pamoate

trip'toe-rel-in
★ 🍁 Trelstar Depot, Trelstar LA

CATEGORY AND SCHEDULE

Pregnancy Risk Category: X

Classification: Antineoplastics, hormones/hormone modifiers, gonadotropin-releasing hormone analogues.

MECHANISM OF ACTION

A gonadotropin-releasing hormone (GnRH) analogue and antineoplastic agent that inhibits gonadotropin hormone secretion through a negative feedback mechanism. Circulating levels of luteinizing hormone, follicle-stimulating hormone, testosterone, and estradiol rise initially, then subside with continued therapy. *Therapeutic Effect:* Suppresses growth of abnormal prostate tissue.

AVAILABILITY

Powder for Injection (Trelstar Depot): 3.75 mg.
Powder for Injection (Trelstar LA): 11.25 mg.
Powder for Injection (Trelstar LA): 22.5 mg.

INDICATIONS AND DOSAGES

▸ **Prostate cancer**

IM

Adults, Elderly. 3.75 mg once q28 days (Trelstar Depot). 11.25 mg q12wk (Trelstar LA); 22.5 mg q24wk (Trelstar LA).

CONTRAINDICATIONS

Hypersensitivity to luteinizing hormone-releasing hormone (LHRH) or LHRH agonists, pregnancy.

INTERACTIONS

Drug

Hyperprolactinemic drugs: Reduce the number of pituitary gonadotropin-releasing hormone (GnRH) receptors.

Herbal

None known.

Food

None known.

DIAGNOSTIC TEST EFFECTS

May alter serum pituitary-gonadal function test results. May cause transient increase in serum testosterone levels, usually during first week of treatment. May increase blood sugar.

SIDE EFFECTS

Frequent (> 5%)

Hot flashes, skeletal pain, headache, impotence.

Occasional (2%-5%)

Insomnia, vomiting, leg pain, fatigue.

Rare (< 2%)

Dizziness, emotional lability, diarrhea, urinary retention, urinary tract infection, anemia, pruritus.

SERIOUS REACTIONS

- Bladder outlet obstruction, skeletal pain, hematuria, and spinal cord compression (with weakness or paralysis of the lower extremities) may occur.
- Risk for osteoporosis with long-term use.
- Rare serious hypersensitivity (anaphylaxis).
- New-onset diabetes mellitus and associated health risks.

PRECAUTIONS & CONSIDERATIONS

Women who are or might be pregnant should not use this drug. Pregnancy should be determined before beginning triptorelin therapy. It is unknown whether triptorelin is excreted in breast milk. The safety and efficacy of triptorelin have not been established in children. No age-related precautions have been noted in elderly patients.

Blood in urine, increased skeletal pain, and urine retention may occur initially, but these symptoms usually subside within 1 wk. Notify the physician if difficulty breathing, infection at the injection site, numbness of the arms or legs, breast pain or swelling, persistent nausea or vomiting, or rapid heartbeat develop. Prostatic acid phosphatase (PAP), prostate-specific antigen (PSA), and serum testosterone levels should be obtained periodically during therapy. Serum testosterone and PAP levels should increase during the first week of therapy. The testosterone level should then decrease to baseline level or less within 2 wks, and the PAP level should decrease within 4 wks.

A worsening of signs and symptoms of prostatic cancer, especially during the first week of therapy, because of a transient increase in testosterone level should be carefully assessed.

Storage

Store injection kits at room temperature; do not freeze.

Administration

Administer under the supervision of a physician. Do not miss injections. For intramuscular (IM) use only; never give intravenously. The product should be reconstituted with sterile water only. Using a syringe fitted with a 21-gauge needle, withdraw 2 mL sterile water, and inject into the vial. Shake well to thoroughly disperse particles to obtain a uniform suspension. The suspension will appear milky. Withdraw the entire contents of the vial into the syringe and use immediately. Inject IM into either buttock. IM injection sites should be alternated.

Trospium

trose'pee-um

★ 🍁 Sanctura, Sanctura XR

CATEGORY AND SCHEDULE

Pregnancy Risk Category: C

Classification: Anticholinergics, urinary antispasmodic, urinary incontinence agents

MECHANISM OF ACTION

An anticholinergic that antagonizes the effect of acetylcholine on muscarinic receptors, producing parasympatholytic action.

Therapeutic Effect: Reduces smooth muscle tone in the bladder.

PHARMACOKINETICS

Minimally absorbed after PO administration. Protein binding: 50%-85%. Distributed in plasma. Excreted mainly in feces and, to a lesser extent, in urine. *Half life:* 20 h.

AVAILABILITY

Tablets: 20 mg.

Extended-Release Capsules: 60 mg.

INDICATIONS AND DOSAGES

▸ **Overactive bladder**

PO (IMMEDIATE RELEASE)

Adults. 20 mg 2 times/day.

Elderly (75 yr and older). Initially, 20 mg 2 times/day. Titrate dosage down to 20 mg once a day, based on tolerance.

PO (EXTENDED RELEASE)

Adults. 60 mg once per day in the morning.

▸ **Dosage in renal impairment**

For patients with creatinine clearance < 30 mL/min, dosage reduced to 20 mg once a day at bedtime. Do not use XR form.

CONTRAINDICATIONS

Hypersensitivity, urinary retention, gastric retention, or uncontrolled narrow-angle glaucoma or patients at risk for these conditions.

INTERACTIONS

Drug

Other anticholinergic agents: Increases the severity and frequency of side effects and may alter the absorption of other drugs because of anticholinergic effects on GI motility.

Digoxin, metformin, morphine, pancuronium, procainamide, tenofovir, vancomycin: May increase trospium blood concentration.

Herbal
None known.
Food
High-fat meal: May reduce trospium absorption.
Alcohol: May increase risk of anticholinergic effects of extended release dose form.

DIAGNOSTIC TEST EFFECTS
None known.

SIDE EFFECTS
Frequent (20%)
Dry mouth.
Occasional (≤ 4%)
Constipation, headache.
Rare (< 2%)
Fatigue, upper abdominal pain, dyspepsia, flatulence, dry eyes, urine retention.

SERIOUS REACTIONS
- Overdose may result in severe anticholinergic effects, such as abdominal pain, nausea and vomiting, confusion, depression, diaphoresis, facial flushing, hypertension, hypotension, respiratory depression, irritability, nervousness, and restlessness.
- Supraventricular tachycardia and hallucinations occur rarely.

PRECAUTIONS & CONSIDERATIONS
Caution is warranted with renal or hepatic impairment, intestinal atony, obstructive GI disorders, significant bladder obstruction, ulcerative colitis, myasthenia gravis, and angle-closure glaucoma. It is unknown whether trospium crosses the placenta or is distributed in breast milk. The safety and efficacy of trospium have not been established in children. Elderly patients (age 75 and older) have a higher incidence of constipation, dry mouth, dyspepsia, urine retention, and urinary tract infection.

Notify the physician of increased salivation or sweating, an irregular heartbeat, nausea and vomiting, or severe abdominal pain. Intake and output, pattern of daily bowel activity and stool consistency, and symptomatic relief should be assessed.
Storage
Store trospium at room temperature.
Administration
Do not break or crush the tablets. Take the drug at least 1 h before meals or on an empty stomach. Do not take trospium with high-fat meals because it may reduce absorption.

Do not crush, cut, or chew extended-release capsules. Dose with water on an empty stomach, at least 1 h before a meal. Alcohol should not be consumed within 2 h of extended-release administration.

Ursodiol

your-soo'dee-ol

★ Actigall, Urso 250, Urso Forte

🍁 DOM-Ursodiol C, PHL-Ursodiol C, PMS-Ursodiol C

CATEGORY AND SCHEDULE

Pregnancy Risk Category: B

Classification: Gallstone dissolution agent

MECHANISM OF ACTION

A gallstone-solubilizing agent that suppresses the hepatic synthesis and secretion of cholesterol; inhibits the intestinal absorption of cholesterol. *Therapeutic Effect:* Changes the bile of patients with gallstones from precipitating (capable of forming crystals) to cholesterol solubilizing (capable of being dissolved).

AVAILABILITY

Capsules: 300 mg.
Tablets: 250 mg, 500 mg.

PHARMACOKINETICS

With oral dosing, 90% is absorbed in the small bowel. Undergo hepatic extraction; also distributed in bile and small intestine. Steady-state concentrations are reached in ~ 3 wks. Metabolized in the colon and excreted as metabolites in the feces.

INDICATIONS AND DOSAGES

▸ **Dissolution of radiolucent, noncalcified gallstones when cholecystectomy is not recommended**

PO

Adults, Elderly. 8-10 mg/kg/day in 2-3 divided doses. Treatment may require months. Obtain ultrasound image of gallbladder at 6-mo intervals for first year. If gallstones have dissolved, continue therapy and repeat ultrasound within 1-3 mo.

▸ **Primary biliary cirrhosis**

PO

Adults, Elderly. 13-15 mg/kg/day in 2-4 divided doses with food.

▸ **Prevention of gallstones**

PO

Adults, Elderly. 300 mg twice a day.

OFF-LABEL USES

Treatment of alcoholic cirrhosis, biliary atresia, biliary cirrhosis, cystic fibrosis, cholestatic jaundice syndrome, chronic hepatitis, congenital dilation of lobar intrahepatic duct, gallstone formation, sclerosing cholangitis, prophylaxis of liver transplant rejection.

CONTRAINDICATIONS

Hypersensitivity to the drug or any other bile acid agents. Patients with cholelithiasis or biliary tract disease and compelling reasons for cholecystectomy, including unremitting acute cholesystitis, cholangitis, biliary obstruction, gallstone pancreatitis, or biliary-GI fistula, are NOT candidates for gallstone dissolution via use of ursodiol. The drug will not dissolve calcified cholesterol stones, radiopaque stones, or radiolucent bile pigment stones.

INTERACTIONS

Drug

Aluminum-based antacids, cholestyramine: May decrease the absorption and effects of ursodiol.
Estrogens, oral contraceptives: May decrease the effects of ursodiol.

Herbal

None known.

Food

None known.

DIAGNOSTIC TEST EFFECTS

May improve liver function test results as the drug improves the patient's clinical condition.

SIDE EFFECTS

All were similar to placebo.

Frequent

Abdominal pain, diarrhea, dyspepsia, flatulence, nausea.

Common

Cholecystitis, constipation, gastrointestinal disorder, vomiting.

SERIOUS REACTIONS

- None significant.

PRECAUTIONS & CONSIDERATIONS

Patients with ascites, hepatic encephalopathy, variceal bleeding, or in need of liver transplant should be treated for those specific causes. There have been no adequate and well-controlled studies of the use of ursodiol in pregnant women. It is not known if the drug is excreted in breast milk; use caution during lactation. The safety and effectiveness of ursodiol have not been established in children.

Blood serum chemistry values, including BUN, serum alkaline phosphatase, bilirubin, creatinine, AST (SGOT), and ALT (SGPT) levels, should be obtained before the start of ursodiol therapy, 1 and 3 mo after therapy begins, and every 6 mo thereafter to assess response to ursodiol treatment.

Storage

Store at room temperature.

Administration

Take with meals or a snack because the drug dissolves more readily in the presence of bile acid and pancreatic juice. Avoid taking antacids 1 h before or 2 h after taking ursodiol. Therapy with ursodiol is usually for several months.

U

Ustekinumab

us'te-kin'you-mab

★ 🍁 Stelara

CATEGORY AND SCHEDULE

Pregnancy Risk Category: B

Classification:

Immunomodulators, monoclonal antibodies, antipsoriatic agents

MECHANISM OF ACTION

A monoclonal antibody that binds specifically to p40 protein subunit of interleukins 12 and 23; inhibiting the interleukins' activity, decreasing inflammation and immune responses. *Therapeutic Effect:* Reduces inflammation, redness, and scaling of psoriatic plaques, improving symptoms.

PHARMACOKINETICS

Time to peak serum concentration 7 days (90 mg) or 13.5 days (45 mg); steady state reached at roughly day 28 of treatment. *Half-life:* 15-46 days or longer.

AVAILABILITY

Injection: 45 mg/0.5 mL, 90 mg/mL; in single-use vials or prefilled syringes.

INDICATIONS AND DOSAGES

▸ **Moderate to severe plaque psoriasis**

SC

Adults ≤ 100 kg. 45 mg initially, then 45 mg 4 wks later, then 45 mg q12wk.

Adults > 100 kg. 90 mg initially, then 90 mg 4 wks later, then 90 mg q12wk.

CONTRAINDICATIONS

None. Withhold in any patient with a clinically important, active, serious infection, especially active TB.

INTERACTIONS

Drug

Other biologics for psoriasis and traditional immunosuppressives: Concomitant use has not been evaluated. There may be an increased risk of serious infections with combined use.
Narrow therapeutic index drugs metabolized via CYP450 enzymes: Ustekinumab may alter metabolism; monitor such drugs closely.
Vaccines, live: Avoid use. Altered immune response and increased risk of secondary transmission of infection from vaccine. Must NOT receive BCG vaccine for up to 1 yr after ustekinumab discontinued.

DIAGNOSTIC TEST EFFECTS

None known.

SIDE EFFECTS

Frequent (3%-10%)
Headache, fatigue, nasopharyngitis, mild upper respiratory infections.
Occasional (1%-2%)
Injection site erythema.
Rare (<1%)
Cellulitis, certain injection site reactions (pain, swelling, pruritus, induration, hemorrhage, bruising, and irritation). See Serious Reactions.

SERIOUS REACTIONS

- Rare reactions include hypersensitivity reactions, risk for malignancies (e.g., nonmelanoma skin malignancy), neurologic events, and serious infections (such as pneumonia, tuberculosis).
- Reversible posterior leukoencephalopathy syndrome (RPLS) is a rare serious neurologic disorder; can present with seizures, headache, confusion, and visual disturbances; if suspected, discontinue drug. Rarely can be fatal.

PRECAUTIONS & CONSIDERATIONS

Serious infections, sepsis, tuberculosis, and opportunistic infections have occurred during therapy. Patients should be screened for active or recent infection, tuberculosis risk factors, and latent tuberculosis infection before initiating therapy. Closely monitor patients developing infection during therapy. Caution is warranted with neurologic disease, history of sensitivity to monoclonal antibodies, preexisting or recent onset of CNS disturbances, in elderly patients. Due to potential risk of malignancy, use with caution in those with past malignancy. There are no clinical data in pregnant women; animal studies do not show teratogenic effects. It is unknown if the drug is excreted in breast milk. The safety and efficacy of ustekinumab have not been established in children. Cautious use in the elderly is necessary because they may be at increased risk for serious infection and malignancy. Avoid receiving live vaccines during treatment. The needle cover on the prefilled syringe contains latex and the cover should not be handled by those with latex allergy.
Storage
Refrigerate. Do not freeze. Protect from light; store in original carton until administration.
Administration
For subcutaneous use, rotate injection sites. The solution should be colorless to slightly yellow and may contain a few small translucent/white particles. Do not use if discolored, cloudy. Do not shake. Use a 27-gauge, 0.5-inch needle if dosing from the vial. Injection sites include the front middle thigh, gluteal or abdominal region, and the outer area of upper arm. Do not inject within 2 inches of the navel. Do not administer intralesionally, or where skin is tender, bruised, red, or indurated. Discard any unused portion. Injection site reactions generally occur in the first month of treatment and decrease with continued therapy.

Valacyclovir

val-a-sye′kloe-veer

★ 🍁 Valtrex

Do not confuse valacyclovir with valganciclovir.

CATEGORY AND SCHEDULE

Pregnancy Risk Category: B

Classification: Antivirals

MECHANISM OF ACTION

A virustatic antiviral that is converted to acyclovir triphosphate, becoming part of the viral DNA chain. *Therapeutic Effect:* Interferes with DNA synthesis and replication of herpes simplex virus and varicella zoster virus.

PHARMACOKINETICS

Rapidly absorbed after PO administration. Protein binding: 13%-18%. Rapidly converted by hydrolysis to the active compound acyclovir. Widely distributed to tissues and body fluids (including cerebrospinal fluid [CSF]). Eliminated primarily in urine. Removed by hemodialysis. *Half-life:* 2.5-3.3 h (increased in impaired renal function).

AVAILABILITY

Caplets: 500 mg, 1000 mg.

INDICATIONS AND DOSAGES

▸ **Herpes zoster (shingles)**

PO

Adults, Elderly. 1 g 3 times a day for 7 days.

▸ **Herpes labialis (cold sores)**

PO

Adults, Elderly, Children 12 yr and older. 2 g twice a day for 2 doses starting at the first sign of symptom of lesions.

▸ **Initial episode of genital herpes**

PO

Adults, Elderly. 1 g twice a day for 10 days.

▸ **Recurrent episodes of genital herpes**

PO

Adults, Elderly. 500 mg twice a day for 3 days.

▸ **Prevention of genital herpes**

PO

Adults, Elderly. 500-1000 mg/day. In immunocompetent heterosexuals, this dose also reduces risk of partner transmission. If HIV-infected, the suppressive dose is 500 mg twice a day.

▸ **Varicella (chickenpox in immunocompetent patients)**

PO

Children 2 to < 18 yr. 20 mg/kg/dose 3 times per day for 5 days (maximum 1 g 3 times per day). Start at first sign/symptom, preferably within 24 h of rash onset.

▸ **Dosage in renal impairment (adults)**

Dosage and frequency are modified based on creatinine clearance.

Creatinine Clearance (mL/min)	Herpes Zoster	Genital Herpes (recurrence)
30-49	1 g q12h	500 mg q12h
10-29	1 g q24h	500 mg q24h
< 10	500 mg q24h	500 mg q24h

No data available for use in children with CrCl < 50 mL/min.

CONTRAINDICATIONS

Hypersensitivity to or intolerance of acyclovir, valacyclovir, or their components.

INTERACTIONS

Drug

Cimetidine, probenecid: May increase acyclovir blood concentration.

Entecavir, tenofovir: May increase blood concentration of these medicines by reducing renal elimination.
Herbal
None known.
Food
None known.

DIAGNOSTIC TEST EFFECTS

None known.

SIDE EFFECTS

Frequent
Herpes zoster (10%-17%): Nausea, headache.
Genital herpes (17%): Headache.
Occasional
Herpes zoster (3%-7%): Vomiting, diarrhea, constipation (50 yr or older), asthenia, dizziness (50 yr or older).
Genital herpes (3%-8%): Nausea, diarrhea, dizziness.
Rare
Herpes zoster (1%-3%): Abdominal pain, anorexia.
Genital herpes (1%-3%): Asthenia, abdominal pain.

SERIOUS REACTIONS

- Thrombotic thrombocytopenic purpura/hemolytic uremic syndrome.
- Dehydration may contribute to decreased urination and renal dysfunction.
- Rare serious hypersensitivity reactions.

PRECAUTIONS & CONSIDERATIONS

Caution is warranted in patients with advanced HIV infection, bone marrow or renal transplantation, concurrent use of nephrotoxic agents, dehydration, fluid or electrolyte imbalance, neurologic abnormalities, and renal or liver impairment. Be aware that valacyclovir may cross the placenta and be distributed in breast milk. Safety and efficacy have not been established in children less than 2 yr of age. In elderly patients, age-related renal impairment may require dosage adjustment. Do not touch lesions with fingers to avoid spreading infection to new sites. Avoid sexual intercourse during the duration of lesions to prevent infecting partner.

Tissue cultures should be obtained from those with herpes simplex and herpes zoster before giving the first dose of valacyclovir. Therapy may proceed before test results are known. Complete blood count (CBC), liver or renal function tests, fluid intake, and urinalysis should be monitored. Maintain adequate fluids. Fingernails should be kept short and hands clean. Pap smears should be done at least annually because of increased risk of cervical cancer in women with genital herpes.
Storage
Store tablets at room temperature. Store compounded oral suspension refrigerated for up to 28 days.
Administration
Give oral valacyclovir without regard to meals. Do not crush or break tablets. Continue therapy for the full length of treatment, and evenly space doses around the clock.

The manufacturer provides for an oral suspension that may be compounded for children. Shake well before each use.

Adequate hydration is important to reduce risk of crystallization within kidneys.

Valganciclovir

val-gan-sye'kloh-veer
★ 🍁 Valcyte
Do not confuse valganciclovir with valacyclovir.

CATEGORY AND SCHEDULE

Pregnancy Risk Category: C

Classification: Antivirals

MECHANISM OF ACTION

A synthetic nucleoside that competes with viral DNA esterases and is incorporated directly into growing viral DNA chains. *Therapeutic Effect:* Interferes with DNA synthesis and viral replication.

PHARMACOKINETICS

Well absorbed and rapidly converted to ganciclovir by intestinal and hepatic enzymes. Widely distributed. Slowly metabolized intracellularly. Excreted primarily unchanged in urine. Removed by hemodialysis. *Half-life:* 18 h (increased in impaired renal function).

AVAILABILITY

Tablets: 450 mg.
Oral Solution: 50 mg/mL.

INDICATIONS AND DOSAGES

▸ Cytomegalovirus (CMV) retinitis in patients with normal renal function

PO

Adults. Initially, 900 mg (two 450-mg tablets) twice a day for 21 days. Maintenance: 900 mg once a day.

▸ Prevention of CMV after kidney, heart, or kidney-pancreas transplant

PO

Adults, Elderly. 900 mg once a day beginning within 10 days of transplant and continuing until 100 days post-transplant (heart or kidney-pancreas transplant) or for 200 days (kidney transplant).

Children 4 mo to 16 yr. See calculation. Dose is given once daily starting within 10 days of transplant and continuing until 100 days post-transplant (kidney or heart): Pediatric dose (mg) = 7 × BSA × CrCl (calculated using a modified Schwartz formula). If Schwartz CrCl > 150 mL/min/1.73 m^2, then a maximum value of 150 mL/min/1.73 m^2 is used in the dose equation. The dose equation accounts for renal impairment and may be used to calculate dose in renal dysfunction in pediatrics.

▸ Dosage in renal impairment (adults)

Dosage and frequency are modified based on creatinine clearance.

Creatinine Clearance (mL/min)	Induction Dosage (mg)	Maintenance Dosage
40-59	450 twice/ day	450 mg once/ day
25-39	450 once/ day	450 mg once q2 days
10-24	450 q2 days	450 mg twice/ week
< 10	Not recommended	

CONTRAINDICATIONS

Hypersensitivity to acyclovir, ganciclovir, or valganciclovir.

INTERACTIONS

Drug

Amphotericin B, cyclosporine: May increase the risk of nephrotoxicity.
Bone marrow depressants: May increase bone marrow depression.
Didanosine (DDI): May increase didanosine concentrations and related toxicity.
Imipenem and cilastatin: May increase the risk of seizures.
Mycophenolate: May increase serum concentration of valganciclovir and mycophenolate metabolites; monitor for toxicity. Interaction only occurs in presence of renal impairment.
Probenecid: Decreases renal clearance of valganciclovir.
Tenofovir: May decrease excretion of tenofovir.
Zidovudine (AZT): May increase the risk of hematologic toxicity.

V

Herbal
None known.
Food
All foods: Maximize drug bioavailability.

DIAGNOSTIC TEST EFFECTS
May decrease blood hematocrit and hemoglobin levels, platelet count, and WBC count.

SIDE EFFECTS
Frequent (9%-41%)
Diarrhea, neutropenia, headache, fever, insomnia, nausea, vomiting, abdominal pain, anemia, tremor.
Occasional (3%-8%)
Thrombocytopenia, paresthesia.
Rare (1%-3%)
Abdominal pain, anesthenia.

SERIOUS REACTIONS
- Hematologic toxicity, including severe neutropenia (most common), anemia, and thrombocytopenia may occur.
- Retinal detachment occurs rarely.
- An overdose or dehydration may result in renal toxicity.
- Valganciclovir may decrease sperm production and fertility.

PRECAUTIONS & CONSIDERATIONS
Valganciclovir has not been indicated for use in patients with liver transplant. Caution should be used in patients with a history of cytopenic reactions to other drugs, preexisting cytopenias, and renal impairment and in elderly patients, who are at a greater risk of renal impairment. Patients on dialysis should not use this drug. Valganciclovir should not be used during pregnancy, and effective contraception should be used during therapy because of the mutagenic and teratogenic potential of valganciclovir. Women taking valganciclovir should avoid breastfeeding. Breastfeeding may be resumed no sooner than 72 h after the last dose of valganciclovir. Men must also use barrier contraception during and for 90 days after use of the drug. Use with caution in children because the long-term effects on fertility or carcinogenesis ara not known. There is no experience in infants < 4 mo of age. In elderly patients, age-related renal impairment may require dosage adjustment.

Blood chemistry, hematologic baselines, and serum creatinine levels should be evaluated. Intake and output should be monitored, and ensure that the patient maintains adequate hydration. Ophthalmologic examinations should be obtained every 4-6 wks during treatment. Valganciclovir may temporarily or permanently inhibit sperm production in men; valganciclovir may temporarily or permanently suppress fertility in women.

Storage
Store tablets at room temperature. Store the compounded oral solution refrigerated for up to 49 days. Do not freeze.

Administration
CAUTION: Because ganciclovir shares some of the properties of antitumor agents (i.e., carcinogenicity and mutagenicity), handle and dispose according to guidelines issued for cytotoxic drugs. Do not break or crush the tablets. Avoid contact of tablets or oral solution with skin or eyes: Wash your skin well with soap and water or rinse your eyes in contact occurs.

Give valganciclovir with food. Cannot be substituted for ganciclovir on a one-to-one basis.

The manufacturer provides for an oral solution that may be

compounded for children. Adults should not be dosed with the solution.

Maintain adequate hydration to reduce risk of renal cystallization.

Valproic Acid/ Valproate Sodium/ Divalproex Sodium

val-pro′ick

Valproic acid:

Depakene, Stavzor

Valproate sodium:

Depacon

Divalproex sodium:

Depakote, Depakote ER, Depakote Sprinkle Epival

CATEGORY AND SCHEDULE

Pregnancy Risk Category: D

Classification: Anticonvulsants

MECHANISM OF ACTION

An anticonvulsant, mood-stabilizing, and antimigraine agent that directly increases concentration of the inhibitory neurotransmitter γ-aminobutyric acid. *Therapeutic Effect:* Reduces seizure activity.

PHARMACOKINETICS

Well absorbed from the GI tract. Protein binding: 80%-90%. Metabolized in the liver. Excreted primarily in urine. Not removed by hemodialysis. *Half-life:* 6-16 h (may be increased in patients with hepatic impairment, elderly patients, and children younger than 18 mo).

AVAILABILITY

Valproic Acid

Syrup (Depakene): 250 mg/5 mL.
Capsules (Depakene): 250 mg.
Capsules (Delayed Release [Stavzor]): 125 mg, 250 mg, 500 mg.

Valproate Sodium

Injection (Depacon): 100 mg/mL.

Divalproex Sodium

Tablets (Delayed Release [Depakote]): 125 mg, 250 mg, 500 mg.
Tablets (Extended Release [Depakote ER]): 250 mg, 500 mg.
Capsules Sprinkles (Depakote Sprinkle): 125 mg.

INDICATIONS AND DOSAGES

▸ **Seizures**

PO

Adults, Elderly, Children 10 yr and older. Initially, 10-15 mg/kg/day in 2-3 divided doses. May increase by 5-10 mg/kg/day at weekly intervals up to 30-60 mg/kg/day. Usual adult dosage: 1000-2500 mg/day.

IV

Adults, Elderly, Children. Same as oral dose but given q6h.

PO (EXTENDED-RELEASE TABLETS)

Adults, Elderly, Children. Initially, 10-15 mg/kg/day given once daily. Maximum 60 mg/kg/day.

PO (DELAYED-RELEASE TABLETS, DELAYED-RELEASE CAPSULES)

Adults, Elderly, Children. Initially, 10-15 mg/kg/day divided twice daily. Maximum 60 mg/kg/day.

▸ **Manic episodes**

PO

Adults, Elderly. Initially, 750 mg/day in divided doses twice daily. Maximum: 60 mg/kg/day.

▸ **Prevention of migraine headaches**

PO (EXTENDED-RELEASE TABLETS)

Adults, Elderly. Initially, 500 mg/day for 7 days. May increase up to 1000 mg/day.

PO (DELAYED-RELEASE TABLETS, DELAYED-RELEASE CAPSULES)

Adults, Elderly. Initially, 250 mg twice a day. May increase up to 1000 mg/day.

OFF-LABEL USES

Treatment of myoclonic, simple partial, bipolar disorder/mania, and tonic-clonic seizures.

CONTRAINDICATIONS

Active hepatic disease or significant hepatic function impairment; hypersensitivity to the drug; known urea cycle disorders.

INTERACTIONS

Drug

Alcohol, other central nervous system (CNS) depressants: May increase CNS depressant effects.
Amitriptyline, primidone: May increase the blood concentration of these drugs.
Anticoagulants, heparin, platelet aggregation inhibitors, thrombolytics: May increase the risk of bleeding.
Carbamazepine: May decrease valproic acid blood concentration.
Carbapenem antibiotics (ertapenem, imipenem, meropenem): May reduce serum valproic acid concentrations to subtherapeutic levels.
Felbamate: May increase valproic acid concentration.
Hepatotoxic medications: May increase the risk of hepatotoxicity.
Phenytoin: May increase the risk of phenytoin toxicity and decrease the effects of valproic acid.
Topiramate: Increased risk of hyperammonemia.

Herbal

None known.

Food

None known.

DIAGNOSTIC TEST EFFECTS

May increase serum LDH, bilirubin, AST (SGOT), and ALT (SGPT) levels, pancreatic enzymes, or ammonia levels. May alter thyroid function tests. Therapeutic serum level is 50-100 mcg/mL; toxic serum level is > 100 mcg/mL. May cause false-positive urine ketone test.

IV INCOMPATIBILITIES

Do not mix valproic acid with any other medications; few compatibility data are available.

SIDE EFFECTS

Frequent

Abdominal pain, irregular menses, diarrhea, transient alopecia, indigestion, nausea, vomiting, tremors, weight gain or loss.

Occasional

Constipation, dizziness, drowsiness, headache, skin rash, unusual excitement, restlessness, asthenia.

Rare

Mood changes, diplopia, nystagmus, spots before eyes, unusual bleeding or ecchymosis.

SERIOUS REACTIONS

- Hepatotoxicity may occur, particularly in the first 6 mo of valproic acid therapy. It may be preceded by loss of seizure control, malaise, weakness, lethargy, anorexia, and vomiting rather than by abnormal serum liver function test results.
- Blood dyscrasias may occur.
- Life-threatening pancreatitis.
- Hyperammonemia and encephalopathy.
- Multiorgan hypersensitivity reaction.
- Hypothermia has been reported.

PRECAUTIONS & CONSIDERATIONS

Caution is warranted in patients with bleeding abnormalities and a history of hepatic disease. Antiepileptic drugs (AEDs) may increase the risk of suicidal thoughts or behavior. Monitor for the emergence or worsening of depression, suicidal thoughts or behavior, and/or any unusual changes in mood or behavior. Valproic acid crosses the placenta and is distributed in breast milk. Children younger than 2 yr are at increased risk for hepatotoxicity. Lower dosages are recommended for elderly patients, although no age-related precautions have been noted for this age group. Congenital malformations have been associated with valproate exposure during pregnancy; administer to women of childbearing potential only if essential for seizure management.

Drowsiness and dizziness may occur, so alcohol and tasks requiring mental alertness or motor skills should be avoided. Notify the physician of abdominal pain, altered mental status, bleeding, easy bruising, lethargy, loss of appetite, nausea, vomiting, weakness, or yellowing of skin. Seizure disorder, including the onset, duration, frequency, intensity, and type of seizures, should be assessed before and during treatment. CBC and serum alkaline phosphatase, ammonia, bilirubin, AST (SGOT), and ALT (SGPT) levels should also be monitored. CBC and platelet count should be obtained before beginning valproic acid therapy, 2 wks later, and again 2 wks after the maintenance dose has been established.

Storage

Store oral dosage forms and injection vials at room temperature. Diluted infusions are stable for 24 h; discard unused portion.

Administration

Take oral valproic acid without regard to food. Do not take it with carbonated drinks. Sprinkle-cap contents may be sprinkled on semisolid food (e.g., applesauce, pudding) and given immediately; however, do not break, chew, or crush the sprinkle beads. Give delayed-release or extended-release tablets and capsules whole. Do not abruptly discontinue valproic acid after long-term use because this may precipitate seizure. Strict maintenance of drug therapy is essential for seizure control.

For IV use, dilute each single dose with at least 50 mL D5W, 0.9% NaCl, or lactated Ringer's solution. Infuse dose over 60 min and not to exceed 20 mg/min. Faster infusion rates of up to 15 mg/kg over 5-10 min (1.5-3 mg/kg/min) have been used; however, the incidence of adverse events may be higher.

Valrubicin

val-rue'bih-sin

★ Valstar 🍁 Valtaxin

Do not confuse valrubicin with valsartan.

CATEGORY AND SCHEDULE

Pregnancy Risk Category: C

Classification: Antineoplastic, anthracyclines

MECHANISM OF ACTION

An anthracycline that inhibits incorporation of nucleosides into nucleic acids. *Therapeutic Effect:* Causes chromosomal damage, arresting cells in the G_2 phase of cell division, and interfering with DNA synthesis.

PHARMACOKINETICS

Due to intravesical administration, drug is concentrated in bladder wall; minimal absorption into circulation. Voided with urine.

V

AVAILABILITY
Concentrate Solution: 40 mg/mL for intravesical instillation.

INDICATIONS AND DOSAGES
▸ **Bladder cancer**
INTRAVESICAL
Adults, Elderly. 800 mg once weekly for 6 wks.

CONTRAINDICATIONS
Perforated bladder; sensitivity to valrubicin, anthracyclines, or polyoxyl castor oil; urinary tract infection.

INTERACTIONS
Drug
None known.
Herbal
None known.
Food
None known.

DIAGNOSTIC TEST EFFECTS
None known.

SIDE EFFECTS
Expected
Red-colored urine.
Frequent
Local intravesical reaction: Local bladder symptoms, urinary frequency or urgency, dysuria, hematuria, bladder pain, cystitis, bladder spasms.
Systemic: Abdominal pain, nausea, urinary tract infection.
Occasional
Local intravesical reaction: Nocturia, local burning, urethral pain, pelvic pain, gross hematuria.
Systemic: Diarrhea, vomiting, urine retention, microscopic hematuria, asthenia, headache, malaise, back pain, chest pain, dizziness, rash, anemia, fever, vasodilation.
Rare
Systemic: Flatus, peripheral edema, hyperglycemia, pneumonia, myalgia.

SERIOUS REACTIONS
Serious systemic toxicity if bladder wall is perforated.

PRECAUTIONS & CONSIDERATIONS
Evaluate bladder status before administration; delay administration in patients with perforated bladder or compromised mucosal integrity. Avoid in patients with a small bladder capacity (i.e., those who cannot tolerate a 75-mL instillation) and use cautiously in patients with irritable bladder symptoms (e.g., neurogenic bladder) as an increased incidence of bladder spasm and spontaneous discharge of the intravesical instillate may occur. All patients of reproductive age should be advised to use an effective contraceptive method during the treatment period. Monitor for disease recurrence or progression by using cystoscopy, biopsy, and urine cytology every 3 mo.
Storage
Unopened vials should be stored under refrigeration in the carton; diluted solution is stable for 12 h at temperatures up to 25° C (77° F).
Administration
CAUTION: Observe and exercise appropriate precautions for handling, preparing, and administering cytotoxic drugs.

Use of gloves during dose preparation and administration is recommended; avoid skin contact. Prepare and store instillation solution in glass, polypropylene, or polyolefin containers. Non-DEHP-containing administration sets are recommended for administration. For each instillation, contents of four 200 mg/5 mL vials should be allowed to warm to room temperature. 20 mL should be withdrawn from the four vials and diluted with 55 mL NaCl 0.9%

injection, providing 75 mL diluted valrubicin solution. The diluted solution should be instilled in the bladder slowly via gravity flow over several minutes. Drug should be retained in the bladder for 2 h before voiding. Clamping of the urinary catheter is not advised. At the end of 2 h, patients should void. Instillation solution is red; advise patients that red-tinged urine is typical for the first 24 h after administration.

Valsartan

val-sar'tan

Diovan

Do not confuse valsartan with Valstan.

CATEGORY AND SCHEDULE

Pregnancy Risk Category: C (D if used in second or third trimester)

Classification:

Antihypertensives, angiotensin II receptor antagonists

MECHANISM OF ACTION

An angiotensin II receptor, type AT_1, antagonist that blocks vasoconstrictor and aldosterone-secreting effects of angiotensin II, inhibiting the binding of angiotensin II to the AT_1 receptors. *Therapeutic Effect:* Causes vasodilation, decreases peripheral resistance, and decreases BP.

PHARMACOKINETICS

Poorly absorbed after PO administration. Food decreases peak plasma concentration. Protein binding: 95%. Metabolized in the liver. Recovered primarily in feces and, to a lesser extent, in urine. Unknown whether removed by hemodialysis. *Half-life:* 6 h.

AVAILABILITY

Tablets: 40 mg, 80 mg, 160 mg, 320 mg.

INDICATIONS AND DOSAGES

▸ **Hypertension**

PO

Adults, Elderly. Initially, 80-160 mg/day in patients who are not volume depleted, up to a maximum of 320 mg/day.

Children 6 to 16 yr. Initially, 1.3 mg/kg once daily (up to 40 mg/day). Adjust to clinical response. Doses > 2.7 mg/kg (160 mg/day) PO have not been studied. Not for use if CrCl < 30 mL/min/1.73m^2.

▸ **Congestive heart failure (CHF)**

PO

Adults, Elderly. Initially, 40 mg twice a day. May increase up to 160 mg twice a day. Maximum: 320 mg/day.

▸ **Post-myocardial infarction (MI)**

PO

Adults, Elderly. May be initiated as early as 12 h after an MI. Initially 20 mg twice daily. Titrate to target dose of 160 mg twice daily, as tolerated.

CONTRAINDICATIONS

Hypersensitivity to the drug.

INTERACTIONS

Drug

Cyclosporine, rifampin, ritonavir: May increase valsartan systemic exposure.

Diuretics: Produces additive hypotensive effects.

Eplerenone, drospirenone, potassium-sparing diuretics, potassium supplements: Increased serum potassium.

Lithium: Elevated lithium concentrations and risk of toxic effects.

Herbal

None known.

V

Food
Decreases peak plasma concentration of valsartan.

DIAGNOSTIC TEST EFFECTS
May increase AST (SGOT), ALT (SGPT), and serum bilirubin, creatinine, and potassium levels. May decrease blood hemoglobin and hematocrit levels.

SIDE EFFECTS
Common
Headache, dizziness, viral infection, fatigue, and abdominal pain.
Less frequent (1%-2%)
Insomnia, heartburn, diarrhea, nausea, vomiting, arthralgia, edema, cough, increases in serum creatinine, hyperkalemia.

SERIOUS REACTIONS
- Overdosage may manifest as hypotension and tachycardia. Bradycardia occurs less often.
- Anaphylactoid reactions, angioedema (rare).

PRECAUTIONS & CONSIDERATIONS
Caution is warranted in patients with coronary artery disease, mild to moderate hepatic impairment, renal impairment, and renal artery stenosis and in those receiving potassium-sparing diuretics or potassium supplements. For those with severe CHF, signs and symptoms of impaired renal function, which may develop during valsartan therapy, should be monitored. It is unknown whether valsartan is distributed in breast milk; it may cause fetal harm. Women should avoid valsartan during the second and third trimester of pregnancy. Safety and efficacy of valsartan have not been established in children under 6 yr. No age-related precautions have been noted in elderly patients.

Dizziness may occur. Tasks that require mental alertness or motor skills should be avoided. Notify the physician if fever or sore throat occurs. Apical pulse and BP should be assessed immediately before each valsartan dose and regularly throughout therapy. Be alert to fluctuations in apical pulse and BP. If an excessive reduction in BP occurs, place the person in the supine position with feet slightly elevated and notify the physician. Serum electrolyte levels, liver and renal function tests, urinalysis, and pulse rate should be assessed. Maintain adequate hydration; exercising outside during hot weather should be avoided to decrease the risk of dehydration and hypotension.
Storage
Store at room temperature, tightly closed. Protect from moisure. An oral suspension may be compounded and stored for 30 days at room temperature or 75 days refrigerated in a glass bottle.
Administration
Valsartan may be given concurrently with other antihypertensives.

Take valsartan without regard to meals.

For children, the manufacturer provides directions for supplying a compounded suspension. It is more bioavailable than the tablets, so dose adjustment may be needed. Shake well before each use.

Vancomycin
van-koe-mye'sin
★ 🍁 Vancocin

CATEGORY AND SCHEDULE
Pregnancy Risk Category: B

Classification: Antibiotics, glycopeptides

MECHANISM OF ACTION

A tricyclic glycopeptide antibiotic that binds to bacterial cell walls, altering cell membrane permeability and inhibiting RNA synthesis. *Therapeutic Effect:* Bactericidal.

PHARMACOKINETICS

PO: Poorly absorbed from the GI tract. Some patients with enterocolitis may absorb effectively. Orally administered drug is primarily eliminated in feces. Parenteral: Widely distributed. Protein binding: 55%. Primarily excreted unchanged in urine. Not removed by hemodialysis. *Half-life:* 4-11 h (increased in impaired renal function).

AVAILABILITY

Capsules: 125 mg, 250 mg.
Powder for Injection: 500 mg, 1 g, 5 g, 10 g.
Infusion (Premix): 500 mg/100 mL, 1 g/200 mL.

INDICATIONS AND DOSAGES

▸ **Treatment of bone, respiratory tract, skin, and soft-tissue infections, endocarditis, peritonitis, and septicemia; prevention of bacterial endocarditis in those at risk (if penicillin is contraindicated) when undergoing biliary, dental, GI, genitourinary, or respiratory surgery or invasive procedures**

IV

Adults, Elderly. 15-18 mg/kg or 1 g q12h.

Children older than 1 mo. 40 mg/kg/day in divided doses q6-8h.

Neonates. Initially, 10-15 mg/kg q8-12h.

▸ **Staphylococcal enterocolitis, antibiotic-associated pseudomembranous colitis caused by *Clostridium difficile***

PO

NOTE: Oral vancomycin is not effective for systemic infection.

Adults, Elderly. 125-500 mg q6h for 7-10 days.

Children. 40 mg/kg/day in divided doses q6h for 7-10 days. Maximum: 2 g/day.

▸ **Dosage in renal impairment**

After a loading dose, subsequent dosages and frequency are modified based on creatinine clearance, the severity of the infection, and the serum concentration of the drug.

OFF-LABEL USES

Treatment of brain abscess, perioperative infections, staphylococcal or streptococcal meningitis.

CONTRAINDICATIONS

Hypersensitivity.

INTERACTIONS

Drug

Aminoglycosides, amphotericin B, aspirin, bumetanide, carmustine, cisplatin, cyclosporine, ethacrynic acid, furosemide, streptozocin: May increase the risk of ototoxicity and nephrotoxicity of parenteral vancomycin.

Cholestyramine, colestipol: May decrease the effects of oral vancomycin.

Herbal

None known.

Food

None known.

DIAGNOSTIC TEST EFFECTS

May increase serum creatinine, BUN. Therapeutic peak serum level is 20-40 mcg/mL; therapeutic trough serum level is 10-20 mcg/mL. Toxic peak serum level is > 80 mcg/mL; toxic trough serum level is > 20 mcg/mL.

IV INCOMPATIBILITIES

Albumin, amphotericin B complex (Abelcet, AmBisome, Amphotec), aztreonam (Azactam), cefazolin (Ancef), cefepime (Maxipime), cefotaxime (Claforan), cefotetan (Cefotan), cefoxitin (Mefoxin), ceftazidime (Fortaz), ceftriaxone (Rocephin), cefuroxime (Zinacef), foscarnet (Foscavir), heparin, idarubicin (Idamycin), nafcillin (Nafcil), piperacillin and tazobactam (Zosyn), propofol (Diprivan), ticarcillin and clavulanate (Timentin).

IV COMPATIBILITIES

Amiodarone (Cordarone), calcium gluconate, diltiazem (Cardizem), hydromorphone (Dilaudid), insulin, lorazepam (Ativan), magnesium sulfate, midazolam (Versed), morphine, potassium chloride.

SIDE EFFECTS

Frequent

PO: Bitter or unpleasant taste, nausea, vomiting, mouth irritation (with oral solution).

Rare

Parenteral: Phlebitis, thrombophlebitis, or pain at peripheral IV site; dizziness; vertigo; tinnitus; chills; fever; rash; necrosis with extravasation.

PO: Rash.

SERIOUS REACTIONS

- Nephrotoxicity and ototoxicity may occur.
- "Red man" syndrome (redness on face, neck, arms, and back; chills; fever; tachycardia; nausea or vomiting; pruritus; rash; unpleasant taste) may result from too-rapid infusion.
- Neutropenia.

PRECAUTIONS & CONSIDERATIONS

Caution is warranted in patients with preexisting hearing impairment or renal dysfunction and in those taking other ototoxic or nephrotoxic medications concurrently. Vancomycin crosses the placenta; it is unknown whether it is distributed in breast milk. Close monitoring of serum drug levels is recommended in premature neonates and young infants. Age-related renal impairment may increase the risk of ototoxicity and nephrotoxicity in elderly patients. Dosage adjustment is recommended.

Notify the physician if rash, tinnitus, or signs and symptoms of nephrotoxicity occur. Laboratory tests are an important part of therapy. Assess skin for rash, intake and output, renal function, balance, and hearing acuity; assess IV site during vancomycin therapy.

Storage

Store capsules and unopened vials at room temperature. Once diluted for infusion, the infusions from the vials are stable for 7 days under refrigeration. Keep premix infusions frozen until time of thawing; once thawed, they are stable for 72 h at room temperature or up to 30 days refrigerated.

Administration

Oral capsules may be administered without regard to food; swallow whole.

! Give vancomycin by intermittent IV infusion (piggyback). Do not give by IV push, because this may result in exaggerated hypotension. For intermittent IV infusion (piggyback), reconstitute each 500-mg or 1-g vial with 10 mL or 20 mL, respectively, of sterile water for injection to provide a concentration of 50 mg/mL. Further dilute to a final concentration of

V

no more than 5 mg/mL. Discard the solution if a precipitate forms. Administer the solution over 60 min or longer. Monitor the patient's BP closely during the infusion. Infusion rate of no more than 10-15 mg/min is recommended in adults.

Vardenafil

van-den'a-fil

★ 🍁 Levitra, Staxyn

Do not confuse Levitra with Lexiva.

CATEGORY AND SCHEDULE

Pregnancy Risk Category: B

Classification: Impotence agents, phosphodiesterase inhibitors

MECHANISM OF ACTION

An erectile dysfunction agent that inhibits phosphodiesterase type 5, the enzyme responsible for degrading cyclic guanosine monophosphate in the corpus cavernosum of the penis, resulting in smooth muscle relaxation and increased blood flow. *Therapeutic Effect:* Facilitates an erection.

PHARMACOKINETICS

Rapidly absorbed after PO administration. Extensive tissue distribution. Protein binding: 95%. Metabolized in the liver. Excreted primarily in feces; a lesser amount eliminated in urine. Drug has no effect on penile blood flow without sexual stimulation. *Half-life:* 4-5 h.

AVAILABILITY

Tablets: 2.5 mg, 5 mg, 10 mg, 20 mg.
Orally Disintegrating Tablets (Staxyn): 10 mg.

INDICATIONS AND DOSAGES

▸ **Erectile dysfunction**

PO (LEVITRA)

Adults. 10 mg approximately 1 h before sexual activity. Dose may be increased to 20 mg or decreased to 5 mg, based on patient tolerance. Maximum dosing frequency is once daily.

Elderly (older than 65 yr). 5 mg.

PO (STAXYN)

NOTE: Staxyn is not interchangeable with Levitra.

Adults. 10 mg approximately 1 h before sexual activity. Maximum dose frequency is once daily. If lower dose is needed, choose a different product.

▸ **Dosage in moderate hepatic impairment**

PO

For patients with Child-Pugh class B hepatic impairment, dosage is 5 mg 60 min before sexual activity.

▸ **Dosage with concurrent ritonavir**

PO

Adults. 2.5 mg in a 72-h period.

▸ **Dosage with concurrent ketoconazole or itraconazole (at 400 mg/day), indinavir, atazanavir, saquinavir, clarithromycin, ketoconazole, or itraconazole (400 mg/day)**

PO

Adults. 2.5 mg in a 24-h period.

▸ **Dosage with concurrent ketoconazole or itraconazole (at 200 mg/day) or erythromycin**

PO

Adults. 5 mg in a 24-h period.

▸ **Stable α-adrenergic blocker therapy**

PO

Adults. 5-mg in a 24-h period.

OFF-LABEL USES

Raynaud phenomenon.

CONTRAINDICATIONS
Concurrent use of sodium nitroprusside, or nitrates in any form.

INTERACTIONS
Drug

α-Adrenergic blockers, nitrates: Potentiates the hypotensive effects of these drugs. Use of vardenafil with nitrates is contraindicated.

Erythromycin, indinavir, itraconazole, ketoconazole, ritonavir: May increase vardenafil blood concentration.

Herbal

None known.

Food

High-fat meals: Delay drug's maximum effectiveness.

DIAGNOSTIC TEST EFFECTS
None known.

SIDE EFFECTS
Occasional

Headache, flushing, rhinitis, indigestion, nausea, sinusitis.

Rare (< 2%)

Dizziness, changes in color vision, blurred vision.

SERIOUS REACTIONS
- Prolonged erections (lasting over 4 h) and priapism (painful erections lasting > 6 h) occur rarely.
- Hypotension.
- Vision or hearing loss.

PRECAUTIONS & CONSIDERATIONS
Caution is warranted in patients with an anatomic deformity of the penis; cardiac, hepatic, or renal impairment; and conditions that increase the risk of priapism, including leukemia, multiple myeloma, and sickle cell anemia. No age-related precautions have been noted in elderly patients, but their initial dose should be 5 mg. The drug currently has no indications in females or children. Be aware that vardenafil is not effective without sexual stimulation. Seek treatment immediately if an erection lasts longer than 4 h.

Storage

Store at room temperature. ODT form should remain in original blister pack until just prior to use. Protect from moisture.

Administration

Take vardenafil approximately 1 h before sexual activity. Do not crush or break film-coated tablets. High-fat meals delay the drug's maximum effectiveness.

Do not remove ODT from packaging until immediately before use. Place the ODT form (Staxyn) on the tongue, where it will disintegrate. Take without liquid. May be taken with or without food.

Varenicline
var-en'i-kleen

Chantix

Champix

CATEGORY AND SCHEDULE
Pregnancy Risk Category: C

Classification: Smoking deterrent

MECHANISM OF ACTION
Selectively binds $\alpha_4\beta_2$ neuronal nicotinic acetylcholine receptors; possesses agonist activity at lower level than nicotine while blocking nicotine binding to receptors, thus blocking ability of nicotine to stimulate central nervous mesolimbic dopamine system.

PHARMACOKINETICS
Extensively absorbed, peak concentration within 3-4 h of oral administration. Minimal metabolism;

92% excreted unchanged in the urine. Removed by hemodialysis. *Half-life:* 24 h (increased in renal impairment).

AVAILABILITY

Tablets: 0.5 mg, 1 mg.

INDICATIONS AND DOSAGES

▸ Smoking cessation aid

PO

Adults, Elderly. Days 1-3: 0.5 mg once daily; days 4-7: 0.5 mg twice daily; day 8–end of treatment: 1 mg twice daily. Administer for 12 wks; additional 12 wks may increase likelihood of long-term abstinence. If patient has considerable nausea with recommended doses, consider reduction.

▸ Dosage in renal impairment

CrCl < 30 mL/min: Titrate from 0.5 mg once daily to maximum dose of 0.5 mg twice daily.

End-stage renal disease. Maximum dose 0.5 mg once daily.

CONTRAINDICATIONS

History of serious hypersensitivity reactions or skin reactions to the drug.

INTERACTIONS

Drug

NOTE: Physiological changes resulting from smoking cessation (regardless of treatment) may alter the levels or response to certain drugs (e.g., theophylline, warfarin, insulin) for which dosage adjustment may be necessary.

Nicotine replacement: When used with nicotine, the incidence of nausea, headache, vomiting, dizziness, dyspepsia, and fatigue was greater for the combination than for using nicotine alone.

Cimetidine: Increases varenicline blood concentration.

Herbal

None known.

Food

None known.

DIAGNOSTIC TEST EFFECTS

Abnormal liver function test results reported.

SIDE EFFECTS

Frequent (> 10%)

Nausea, insomnia, headache, abnormal dreams. Effects are usually transient and attenuate after titration.

Occasional (5%-10%)

Constipation, flatulence, vomiting.

SERIOUS REACTIONS

- Depressed mood, suicidal ideation, suicidal behavior.
- Serious hypersensitivity, angioedema, and serious skin rashes.

PRECAUTIONS & CONSIDERATIONS

All patients should be monitored for neuropsychiatric symptoms, such as changes in behavior, agitation, depressed mood, suicidal ideation, and suicidal behavior, and worsening of preexisting psychiatric illness; varenicline therapy should be discontinued in the presence of such symptoms. Varenicline has not been studied in pregnant women. May be excreted in human milk; use in nursing mothers is not recommended. While some pharmacokinetic studies have been performed in children 12 yr and older, no data are available regarding clinical use.

In some cases, the patients reported somnolence, dizziness, loss of consciousness, or difficulty concentrating that resulted in impairment, or concern about potential impairment, in driving or operating machinery. Use caution driving or operating machinery until the effects of the drug are known. Nicotine withdrawal symptoms may still occur.

Inform patient that the benefits of smoking cessation on health are immediate and substantial; watch for changes in mood or skin rashes.

Storage

Store at room temperature.

Administration

Start varenicline 1 wk before date set to stop smoking. Take after eating with a full glass of water.

Vasopressin

vay-soe-press'in

Pitressin Pressyn

Do not confuse Pitressin with Pitocin.

CATEGORY AND SCHEDULE

Pregnancy Risk Category: C

Classification: Hormones/ hormone modifiers, pituitary hormones, antidiuretic hormone (ADH)

MECHANISM OF ACTION

A posterior pituitary hormone that increases reabsorption of water by the renal tubules. Increases water permeability at the distal tubule and collecting duct. Directly stimulates smooth muscle in the GI tract. *Therapeutic Effect:* Promotes water retention and restoration of sodium/ water balance; increases peripheral vascular resistance to restore BP; causes peristalsis of the GI tract; and vasoconstricts vascular bed, especially the capillaries, small arterioles, and venules.

PHARMACOKINETICS

Route	Onset	Peak	Duration
IV	NA	NA	0.5-1 h
IM/SC	1-2 h	NA	2-8 h

Distributed throughout extracellular fluid. Metabolized and rapidly destroyed in the liver and kidneys. Roughly 5% excreted in urine unchanged. *Half-life:* 10-20 min.

AVAILABILITY

Injection: 20 units/mL.

INDICATIONS AND DOSAGES

▸ **Cardiac arrest**

IV

Adults, Elderly. 40 units as a one-time bolus.

▸ **Diabetes insipidus**

IV INFUSION

Adults, Children. 0.5 milliunits/ kg/h. May double dose q30min. Maximum: 10 milliunits/kg/h.

IM, SC

Adults, Elderly. 5-10 units 2-4 times a day. Range: 5-60 units/day.

Children. 2.5-10 units, 2-4 times a day.

▸ **Abdominal distention, postoperative**

IM, SC

Adults, Elderly. Initially, 5 units. Subsequent doses, 10 units q3-4h.

▸ **GI hemorrhage**

IV INFUSION

Adults, Elderly. Initially, 0.2-0.4 unit/min may titrate to maximum of 0.8 unit/min.

Children. 0.002-0.005 unit/kg/min. Titrate as needed. Maximum: 0.01 unit/kg/min.

▸ **Vasodilatory shock**

IV INFUSION

Adults, Elderly. Initially, 0.01-0.04 units/min. Titrate to desired effect.

OFF-LABEL USES

Treatment of esophageal variceal bleeding or GI hemorrhage due to ulceration; vasodilatory/cardiogenic shock.

CONTRAINDICATIONS

Hypersensitivity.

INTERACTIONS

Drug

Alcohol, demeclocycline, lithium, norepinephrine: May decrease the effects of vasopressin.

Carbamazepine, chlorpropamide, clofibrate: May increase the effects of vasopressin.

Tricyclic antidepressants: May increase the effects of vasopressin; concurrent use not recommended.

Herbal

None known.

Food

None known.

DIAGNOSTIC TEST EFFECTS

None known.

IV INCOMPATIBILITIES

Amphotericin B complex (Abelcet, AmBisome, Amphotec), diazepam (Valium), etomidate (Amidate), furosemide (Lasix), regular insulin, phenytoin, thiopentothal.

IV COMPATIBILITIES

Dobutamine (Dobutrex), dopamine (Intropin), heparin, lorazepam (Ativan), midazolam (Versed), milrinone (Primacor), verapamil (Calan, Isoptin).

SIDE EFFECTS

Frequent

Pain at injection site (with vasopressin tannate).

Occasional

Abdominal cramps, nausea, vomiting, diarrhea, dizziness, diaphoresis, pale skin, circumoral pallor, tremors, headache, eructation, flatulence.

Rare

Chest pain; confusion; allergic reaction, including rash or hives, pruritus, wheezing or difficulty breathing, facial and peripheral edema; sterile abscess (with vasopressin tannate).

SERIOUS REACTIONS

- Anaphylaxis, MI, and water intoxication have occurred.
- Water intoxication may be treated with water restriction and discontinuing vasopressin until polyuria occurs. Severe symptoms may require osmotic diuresis or with loop diuretics.

PRECAUTIONS & CONSIDERATIONS

Caution is warranted in patients with arteriosclerosis, asthma, cardiac disease, goiter with cardiac complications, migraine, nephritis, renal disease, seizures, and vascular disease. Vasopressin should be used cautiously in breastfeeding women. Vasopressin should be used cautiously in children and in elderly patients because of the risk of water intoxication and hyponatremia in these age groups.

Notify the physician of chest pain, headache, shortness of breath, or other symptoms. BP, serum electrolyte levels, pulse rate, urine specific gravity, intake and output, and weight should be monitored before and during therapy. Be alert for early signs of water intoxication, such as somnolence, headache, and listlessness.

Storage

Store at room temperature.

IV infusions generally stable for 24 h at room temperature. Discard any unused solution.

Administration

For diabetes insipidus, may give intranasally on cotton pledgets or by nasal spray; individualize dosage.

For IV use, dilute with D5W or 0.9% NaCl to concentration of 0.1-1 unit/mL. Give as IV infusion.

For resuscitation only, may give by bolus IV injection into a peripheral vein, followed by an injection of 20 mL IV fluid. Elevate the extremity to facilitate drug delivery to the central circulation.

For IM or SC, give with 1-2 glasses of water to reduce side effects.

Venlafaxine

ven-la-fax'een

Effexor, Effexor XR

CATEGORY AND SCHEDULE

Pregnancy Risk Category: C

Classification: Antidepressants, serotonin and norepinephrine reuptake inhibitors

MECHANISM OF ACTION

A phenethylamine derivative that potentiates central nervous system (CNS) neurotransmitter activity by inhibiting the reuptake of serotonin, norepinephrine, and, to a lesser degree, dopamine. *Therapeutic Effect:* Relieves depression and anxiety.

PHARMACOKINETICS

Well absorbed from the GI tract. Protein binding: 25%-30%. Metabolized in the liver to active metabolite. Excreted primarily in urine. Not removed by hemodialysis. *Half-life:* 3-7 h; metabolite, 9-13 h (increased in hepatic or renal impairment).

AVAILABILITY

Capsules (Extended Release [Effexor XR]): 37.5 mg, 75 mg, 150 mg.
Tablets (Effexor): 25 mg, 37.5 mg, 50 mg, 75 mg, 100 mg.

INDICATIONS AND DOSAGES

▸ **Depression**

PO

Adults, Elderly. Initially, 75 mg/day in 2-3 divided doses with food. May increase by 75 mg/day at intervals of 4 days or longer. Maximum: 375 mg/day in 3 divided doses.

PO (EXTENDED RELEASE)

Adults, Elderly. 75 mg/day as a single dose with food. May increase by 75 mg/day at intervals of 4 days or longer. Maximum: 225 mg/day.

▸ **Anxiety disorder, panic disorder**

PO (EXTENDED RELEASE)

Adults. Initially, 37.5-75 mg/day. Dosage may be increased by 75 mg/day at intervals ≥ 4 days. Maximum: 225 mg/day.

▸ **Dosage in renal and hepatic impairment**

Expect to decrease venlafaxine dosage by 50% in patients with moderate hepatic impairment, 25% in patients with mild to moderate renal impairment, and 50% in patients on dialysis (withhold dose until completion of dialysis).

OFF-LABEL USES

Diabetic neuropathy and other neuropathic pain, premenstrual dysphoric disorder (PMDD), hot flashes, fibromyalgia.

CONTRAINDICATIONS

Hypersensitivity; use within 14 days of MAOIs.

INTERACTIONS

Drug

MAOIs, serotonergic agents, linezolid, SSRIs, triptans: May cause neuroleptic malignant syndrome, autonomic instability (including rapid fluctuations of vital signs), extreme agitation, hyperthermia, mental status changes, myoclonus, rigidity, and coma. MAOI use contraindicated. Allow at least 14 days to elapse before switching from an MAOI to venlafaxine and at least 7 days switching venlafaxine to an MAOI.

V

Do not give with desvenlafaxine or other SNRIs.
Thioridazine: Use contraindicated. Venlafaxine raises serum concentrations of thioridazine via inhibition of CYP2D6.
Herbal
St. John's wort: May increase risk of serotonin syndrome.
Food
None known.

DIAGNOSTIC TEST EFFECTS

May increase BUN level and serum alkaline phosphatase, bilirubin, cholesterol, uric acid, AST (SGOT), and ALT (SGPT) levels. May decrease serum phosphate and sodium levels. May alter blood glucose and serum potassium levels.

SIDE EFFECTS

Frequent (> 20%)
Nausea, somnolence, headache, dry mouth.
Occasional (10%-20%)
Dizziness, insomnia, constipation, diaphoresis, nervousness, asthenia, ejaculatory disturbance, anorexia.
Rare (< 10%)
Anxiety, blurred vision, diarrhea, vomiting, tremor, abnormal dreams, impotence, weight loss.

SERIOUS REACTIONS

- A sustained increase in diastolic BP of 10-15 mm Hg occurs occasionally.
- Serotonin syndrome.

PRECAUTIONS & CONSIDERATIONS

Caution is warranted in patients with suicidal tendencies and those with abnormal platelet function, congestive heart failure, volume depletion, hyperthyroidism, mania, angle-closure glaucoma, hepatic and renal impairment, and seizure disorder. Notify the physician if pregnant or planning to become pregnant. Complications have been observed in neonates exposed to venlafaxine in the third trimester; consider tapering in the third trimester. It is unknown whether venlafaxine is excreted in breast milk. The safety and efficacy of venlafaxine have not been established in children. Antidepressants have been reported to increase the risk of suicidal thinking and behavior in children, adolescents, and young adults (18-24 yr of age) with major depressive disorder (MDD) and other psychiatric disorders. No age-related precautions have been noted in elderly patients.

Drowsiness, dizziness, and lightheadedness may occur, so avoid alcohol and tasks that require mental alertness or motor skills. Monitor for clinical worsening, suicidality, and unusual changes in behavior. BP, pulse rate, and weight should be assessed during therapy.
Storage
Store at room temperature.
Administration
! When discontinuing venlafaxine, plan to taper the dosage slowly over 2 wks.

Take venlafaxine with food or milk if the patient experiences GI distress. Crush scored tablets if needed. Extended-release (ER) capsules and tablets should be administered with food at approximately the same time each day. Swallow whole with fluid and do not divide, crush, chew, or place in water. If needed, the ER capsules may be carefully opened and contents sprinkled on a spoonful of applesauce. Swallow immediately without chewing, and follow with a glass of water.

Verapamil

ver-ap'a-mill

Calan, Calan SR, Covera-HS, Isoptin SR, Verelan, Verelan PM

Apo-Verap, Apo-Verap SR, Isoptin, Isoptin SR, Nu-Verap, Nu-Verap SR

Do not confuse Isoptin with Intropin, or Verelan with Virilon, Vivarin, or Voltaren.

CATEGORY AND SCHEDULE

Pregnancy Risk Category: C

Classification: Antiarrhythmics, class IV, calcium channel blockers

MECHANISM OF ACTION

A calcium channel blocker and antianginal, antiarrhythmic, and antihypertensive agent that inhibits calcium ion entry across cardiac and vascular smooth-muscle cell membranes. This action causes the dilation of coronary arteries, peripheral arteries, and arterioles. *Therapeutic Effect:* Decreases heart rate and myocardial contractility and slows SA and AV conduction. Decreases total peripheral vascular resistance by vasodilation.

PHARMACOKINETICS

Route	Onset	Peak	Duration
PO	30 min	1-2 h	6-8 h
PO (extended release)	30 min	NA	NA
IV	1-2 min	3-5 min	10-60 min

Well absorbed from the GI tract. Protein binding: 90% (60% in neonates). Undergoes first-pass metabolism in the liver to active metabolite. Primarily excreted in urine. Not removed by hemodialysis. *Half-life:* 2-8 h.

AVAILABILITY

Capsules (Modified Release [Verelan PM]): 100 mg, 200 mg, 300 mg.
Capsules (Extended Release [Verelan]): 120 mg, 180 mg, 240 mg, 360 mg.
Tablets (Calan): 40 mg, 80 mg, 120 mg.
Tablets (Sustained Release [Calan SR, Isoptin SR]): 120 mg, 180 mg, 240 mg.
Tablets (Modified Release [Covera-HS]): 180 mg, 240 mg.
Injection: 2.5 mg/mL.

INDICATIONS AND DOSAGES

▸ **Supraventricular tachyarrhythmias, temporary control of rapid ventricular rate with atrial fibrillation or flutter**

IV

Adults, Elderly. Initially, 5-10 mg; repeat in 30 min with 10-mg dose.
Children 1-15 yr. 0.1 mg/kg (up to 5-mg maximum single dose). May repeat in 30 min up to a maximum second dose of 10 mg. Not recommended in children younger than 1 yr.

▸ **Arrhythmias, including prevention of recurrent paroxysmal supraventricular tachycardia and control of ventricular resting rate in chronic atrial fibrillation or flutter**

PO

Adults, Elderly. 240-480 mg/day in 3-4 divided doses.

▸ **Vasospastic angina (Prinzmetal variant), unstable (crescendo or preinfarction) angina, chronic stable (effort-associated) angina**

PO

Adults. Initially, 80-120 mg 3 times a day. For elderly patients and those with hepatic dysfunction, 40 mg 3 times a day. Titrate to optimal dose. Maintenance: 240-480 mg/day in 3-4 divided doses.

PO (COVERA-HS)

Adults, Elderly. 180-480 mg/day at bedtime.

▸ **Hypertension**
PO
Adults, Elderly. Initially, 40-80 mg 3 times a day. Maintenance: 480 mg or less a day, in divided doses.
PO (SUSTAINED RELEASE)
Adults, Elderly. Initially, 120 or 180 mg PO once daily in the morning. May increase to 240 mg PO twice per day.
PO (COVERA-HS)
Adults, Elderly. 180-480 mg/day at bedtime.
PO (EXTENDED RELEASE)
Adults, Elderly. 120-240 mg/day. Usually given once per day in morning. Maximum: 480 mg/day.
PO (VERELAN PM)
Adults, Elderly. Initially, 200 mg/day at bedtime. Dosage may be increased by 100 mg/day up to 400 mg/day.
▸ **Dosage in hepatic impairment**
Verapamil clearance is reduced. Where possible (based on the dosage form/strength), reduce initial verapamil oral dosage. Titrate based on clinical goals.

OFF-LABEL USES

Treatment of hypertrophic cardiomyopathy, vascular headaches.

CONTRAINDICATIONS

Atrial fibrillation or flutter and an accessory bypass tract, cardiogenic shock, heart block, sinus bradycardia, ventricular tachycardia; hypersensitivity.

INTERACTIONS

Drug
Amiodarone: Monitor closely for cardiotoxicity with bradycardia and decreased cardiac output.
β-Blockers: May have additive effect.
Colchicine: May increase risk of colchicine toxicity.
Cyclosporine: May increase cyclosporine concentration.
Digoxin: May increase digoxin blood concentration.
Disopyramide: May increase negative inotropic effect.
Dofetilide: Use contraindicated; significantly increases dofetilide concentrations.
Eletriptan: Increases eletriptan concentrations; do not use within 72 h of verapamil.
Procainamide, quinidine: May increase risk of QT-interval prolongation. Verapamil raises quinidine concentrations.
Statins (atorvastatin, lovastatin, simvastatin): Statin levels may be increased.
Strong inhibitors of CYP3A4 isoenzymes (erythromycin, clarithromycin, fluconazole, itraconazole, ketoconazole, metronidazole): Increase concentrations of verapamil.
Herbal
None known.
Food
Alcohol: Verapamil inhibits ethanol elimination and may prolong the intoxicating effects.
Grapefruit, grapefruit juice: May increase verapamil blood concentration.

DIAGNOSTIC TEST EFFECTS

ECG waveform may show increased PR interval.

IV INCOMPATIBILITIES

Amphotericin B complex (Abelcet, AmBisome, Amphotec), albumin, ceftazidime (Fortaz), diazepam, ertapenem (Invanz), furosemide, hydralazine, lansoprazole (Prevacid IV), nafcillin (Nafcil), pantoprazole (Protonix), phenobarbital, phenytoin, piperacillin-tazobactam (Zosyn), propofol (Diprivan), sodium bicarbonote, sodium lactate injection, sulfamethoxazole-trimethoprim, tigecycline (Tygacil).

IV COMPATIBILITIES

Amiodarone (Cordarone), calcium chloride, calcium gluconate, dexamethasone (Decadron), digoxin (Lanoxin), dobutamine (Dobutrex), dopamine (Intropin), heparin, hydromorphone (Dilaudid), lidocaine, magnesium sulfate, metoclopramide (Reglan), milrinone (Primacor), morphine, multivitamins, nitroglycerin, norepinephrine (Levophed), potassium chloride, potassium phosphate, procainamide (Pronestyl), propranolol (Inderal).

SIDE EFFECTS

Frequent (7%)
Constipation.
Occasional (2%-4%)
Dizziness, light-headedness, headache, asthenia, nausea, peripheral edema, hypotension, gingival hyperplasia.
Rare (< 1%)
Bradycardia, dermatitis or rash.

SERIOUS REACTIONS

- Rapid ventricular rate in atrial flutter or fibrillation, marked hypotension, extreme bradycardia, congestive heart failure (CHF), asystole, and second- and third-degree AV block occur rarely.

PRECAUTIONS & CONSIDERATIONS

Caution is warranted in patients with CHF, hepatic or renal impairment, and sick sinus syndrome and in those concurrently receiving β-blockers or digoxin. Verapamil crosses the placenta and is distributed in breast milk. Breastfeeding is not recommended for patients taking this drug. No age-related precautions have been noted in children. In elderly patients, age-related renal impairment may require cautious use. Alcohol and tasks that require alertness and motor skills should also be avoided until the drug effects are known.

Be aware that ECG should be monitored for changes, particularly PR-interval prolongation. Notify the physician of significant PR interval or other ECG changes. BP, pulse, and stool consistency and frequency should be assessed. The onset, type (sharp, dull, or squeezing), radiation, location, intensity, and duration of anginal pain and its precipitating factors, such as exertion and emotional stress, should be recorded. Be aware that concurrent administration of sublingual nitroglycerin therapy may be used for relief of anginal pain.

Storage
Store at room temperature. Protect from moisture.

Administration
Most dosage forms may be taken without regard to food; however, it is recommended to take sustained-release tablets with food. Swallow extended-release or sustained-released preparations whole and without chewing or crushing. If needed, open extended-release capsules and sprinkle contents on applesauce. Swallow the applesauce immediately, without chewing. Do not abruptly discontinue verapamil. Compliance is essential to control anginal pain.

For IV use, give undiluted, if desired. Administer IV push over more than 2 min for adults and children and over > 3 min for elderly patients. Continuous ECG monitoring during IV injection is required for children and recommended for adults.

Monitor ECG for asystole, extreme bradycardia, heart block, PR-interval prolongation, and rapid ventricular rates. Notify the physician of significant ECG changes. Monitor BP every 5-10 min or as ordered. Keep the patient in a recumbent position for at least 1 h after IV administration.

Vigabatrin

vi-ga'ba-trin

Sabril

CATEGORY AND SCHEDULE

Pregnancy Risk Category: C

Classification: Anticonvulsants

MECHANISM OF ACTION

An anticonvulsant that enhances the activity of γ-aminobutyric acid (GABA), the major inhibitory neurotransmitter in the central nervous system (CNS). Gaba-transaminase is irreversibly inhibited to increase levels of GABA in the brain. *Therapeutic Effect:* Inhibits seizures.

PHARMACOKINETICS

Well absorbed orally. Does not bind to plasma proteins. Not metabolized by liver. Primarily eliminated through the kidney. *Half-life:* 7.5 h (in adults). Shorter in children, and increased in renal impairment and the elderly.

V

AVAILABILITY

Tablets: 500 mg.
Powder for Oral Solution: 50 mg/mL after reconstitution.

INDICATIONS AND DOSAGES

▸ **Adjunctive treatment of refractory partial seizures**

PO

Adults, Elderly. Initially, 500 mg twice per day. May increase by 500 mg/day at weekly intervals. Recommended target dose 1.5 g twice daily.

▸ **Monotherapy for infantile spasms (IS) where benefits outweigh risks**

PO

Infants and Children aged 1 mo to 2 yr. Initially, 50 mg/kg/day divided and given twice per day. May titrate by 25 to 50 mg/kg/day every 3 days. Maximum of 150 mg/kg/day.

▸ **Dosage in renal impairment (adults)**

CrCl 51-80 mL/min: Decrease dose by 25%.
CrCl 31-50 mL/min: Decrease dose by 50%.
CrCl 11-30 mL/min: Decrease dose by 75%.
Hemodialysis: Effect of dialysis on the drug not adequately studied.

CONTRAINDICATIONS

None known.

INTERACTIONS

Drug

Alcohol, other central nervous system (CNS) depressants: May increase CNS-depressant effects.
Clonazepam: Increased clonazepam levels have been reported; monitor for toxicity.
Phenytoin: Decreased phenytoin levels have been reported; may need to adjust phenytoin dose.

Herbal

None known.

Food

None known.

DIAGNOSTIC TEST EFFECTS

May decrease hemoglobin, hematocrit, or alter RBC indices. Decreases ALT and AST in up to 90% of patients. In some patients, these enzyme levels become undetectable. The suppression of ALT and AST activity may preclude the use of these markers, especially

ALT, to detect early hepatic injury. May increase the amount of amino acids in the urine, possibly leading to a false-positive test for certain rare genetic metabolic diseases (e.g., α aminoadipic aciduria).

SIDE EFFECTS

Frequent

Visual changes and vision loss, dizziness, headache, anemia, somnolence, fatigue, edema, weight gain, peripheral neuropathy.

Occasional

Diarrhea, nasopharyngitis, asthenia, nausea, rash, vomiting, nystagmus, fever, dysmenorrhea, arthralgia.

SERIOUS REACTIONS

- Causes progressive and permanent bilateral concentric visual field constriction in a high percentage (30% or more) of patients. May also reduce visual acuity. Risk increases with total dose and duration of use, but no exposure is known that is free of risk of vision loss.
- Neurotoxicity: Vacuolization, MRI changes (infants and young children), neuromotor impairment, peripheral neuropathy.
- Angioedema or other serious hypersenstivity reactions, associated with fevere, rash and lymphadenopathy.

PRECAUTIONS & CONSIDERATIONS

Because of the risk of permanent vision loss, the drug is available only through a special restricted distribution called the SHARE program; prescribers and pharmacies must be registered to prescribe and distribute the drug; patients must be enrolled and meet criteria for use. Periodic vision testing is required for patients, but cannot reliably prevent vision damage; the onset of visual loss is unpredictable.

Caution is warranted in patients with renal impairment and in those who take other CNS depressants concurrently. Antiepileptic drugs (AEDs), including Sabril, increase the risk of suicidal thoughts or behavior in patients taking these drugs for any indication. Patients treated with any AED for any indication should be monitored for the emergence or worsening of depression, suicidal thoughts or behavior, and/or any unusual changes in mood or behavior. The drug may cause harm in pregnancy, and it is recommended that breastfeeding be avoided, due to risk to vision and neurologic health in an infant if exposed to the drug.

Patients should not perform hazardous tasks until the effects of the drug are known. Alcohol should be avoided. Somnolence and dizziness may occur, so change positions slowly—from recumbent to sitting position before standing. History of seizure disorders, including the duration, frequency, and intensity of seizures, should be reviewed before and during therapy. CBC and blood chemistry tests to assess hepatic and renal function should be performed before and during treatment.

Storage

Store at room temperature.

Administration

May be taken without regard to food. For the oral solution, each packet contains vigabatrin 500 mg. Reconstitute dose immediately before administration. Empty the entire contents of the appropriate number of packets into an empty clean cup. For each packet, dissolve the powder with 10 mL cold or room temperature water. The final solution concentration will be 50 mg/mL. Do not use any other liquid to reconstitute. Using a clean spoon or stirring device, carefully stir the contents of the cup until all of the powder has dissolved, producing a clear solution. Measure the appropriate dose using a calibrated oral syringe, and administer immediately. For infants and small children, place the tip of the oral syringe between the cheek and gum and administer slowly in small increments. Discard any unused solution. Each dose must be reconstituted immediately before administration. As with all anticonvulsants, do not abruptly discontinue the drug.

Vinblastine Sulfate

vin-blass′teen sul′fate

Do not confuse vinblastine with vincristine or vinorelbine.

CATEGORY AND SCHEDULE

Pregnancy Risk Category: D

Classification: Antineoplastic, vinca alkaloids

MECHANISM OF ACTION

A vinca alkaloid that binds to microtubular protein of mitotic spindle, causing metaphase arrest. *Therapeutic Effect:* Inhibits cell division.

PHARMACOKINETICS

Highly bound to blood cells and tissues; widely distributed. Does not cross the blood-brain barrier. Protein binding: 75%. Metabolized in the liver via CYP3A4. There is an active metabolite, desacetyl-vinblastine. Eliminated through the bile and faces. *Half-life:* Elimination is triphasic. The α half-life is < 5 min, β half-life is 50-155 min, and the final elimination half-life is 23-85 h.

AVAILABILITY

Powder for Injection: 10 mg.
Injection: 1 mg/mL.

INDICATIONS AND DOSAGES

NOTE: The dosing of vinblastine varies widely depending upon the protocol being used. Check doses carefully. For example, the AVBD regimen for Hodgkin disease is 6 mg/m^2 IV on days 1 and 15 every 28 days along with doxorubicin, bleomycin, and dacarbazine.

▸ **Remission induction in advanced testicular carcinoma, advanced mycosis fungoides, breast carcinoma, choriocarcinoma, disseminated Hodgkin disease, non-Hodgkin lymphoma, Kaposi sarcoma (KS), or Letterer-Siwe disease**

IV

Adults, Elderly. Initially, 3.7 mg/m^2 as a single dose. Increase dose by about 1.8 mg/m^2 at weekly intervals until desired therapeutic response is attained, WBC count falls below 3000/mm^3, or maximum weekly dose of 18.5 mg/m^2 is reached. For most, the weekly dosage is in the range of 5.5-7.4 mg/m^2.

Children. Initially, 2.5 mg/m^2 as a single dose. Increase dose by about 1.25 mg/m^2 at weekly intervals until desired therapeutic response is attained, WBC count falls below 3000/mm^3, or maximum weekly dose of 7.5-12.5 mg/m^2 is reached.

▸ **Maintenance dose for treatment**

IV

Adults, Elderly, Children. Administer one increment less than dose required to produce WBC count of 3000/mm^3. Each subsequent dose given only when WBC count returns to 4000/mm^3 and at least 7 days have elapsed since previous dose. In some cases, oncolytic activity occurs before leukopenic effect and there is no need to alter the size of subsequent doses.

V

▸ **Dose in hepatic impairment**

IV

Reduce dose by 50% if total bilirubin is 1.5-3 mg/dL. Reduce dose by 75% if total bilirubin > 3 mg/dL. If total bilirubin is > 5 mg/dL, do not administer.

OFF-LABEL USES

Non–small cell lung carcinoma, bladder cancer.

CONTRAINDICATIONS

Bacterial infection, severe leukopenia, significant granulocytopenia (unless it stems from disease being treated); intrathecal administration.

INTERACTIONS

Drug

Strong inhibitors of CYP3A4 isoenzymes (erythromycin, clarithromycin, fluconazole, itraconazole, ketoconazole, metronidazole): Increase concentrations of vinblastine.

Phenytoin: Vinblastine may decrease phenytoin concentration and induce seizure activity.

Herbal

None known.

Food

None known.

DIAGNOSTIC TEST EFFECTS

Decreases WBC.

IV INCOMPATIBILITIES

Do not mix with other medications.

SIDE EFFECTS

Frequent

Nausea, vomiting, alopecia.

Occasional

Constipation or diarrhea, rectal bleeding, headache, paresthesia (occur 4-6 h after administration and persist for 2-10 h); malaise; asthenia; dizziness; pain at tumor site; jaw or face pain; depression; dry mouth.

Rare

Dermatitis, stomatitis, phototoxicity, hyperuricemia.

SERIOUS REACTIONS

- Hematologic toxicity is manifested as leukopenia and, less commonly, anemia. The WBC count reaches its nadir 4-10 days after initial therapy and recovers within 7-14 days (21 days with high vinblastine dosages).
- Thrombocytopenia is usually mild and transient, with recovery occurring in a few days.
- Hepatic insufficiency may increase the risk of toxic drug effects.
- Acute shortness of breath or bronchospasm may occur, particularly when vinblastine is administered concurrently with mitomycin.
- Universally fatal if given intrathecally.
- Extravasation may cause cellulitis and phlebitis. Sloughing may occur.

PRECAUTIONS & CONSIDERATIONS

Leukopenia is common; may be more severe in older patients. Toxicity may be greater in patients with hepatic impairment.

Use with caution in patients with poor cardiac reserve or cachexia. Acute shortness of breath and severe bronchospasm have been reported following the administration of vinca alkaloids. Progressive dyspnea may require chronic therapy and the vinca should not be readministered if it occcurs. Vinblastine can cause fetal harm; females of childbearing potential should be advised to avoid becoming pregnant. Breastfeeding is not advised. Men may have alterations in sperm production or quality. A CBC should be done before each dose, and care should be taken to administer the dose according to recommended schedules and no more often than every 7 days. Patients should report mouth sores, sore throat, fevers, and other effects of neutropenia.

Storage
Refrigerate unopened vials. Nonpreserved solutions should be used immediately. Preservative-containing solutions made with 0.9% NaCl may be stored refrigerated for up to 28 days.

Administration
CAUTION: Observe and excercise appropriate precautions for handling, preparing, and administering cytotoxic drugs. Label products as follows: "DO NOT REMOVE COVERING UNTIL MOMENT OF INJECTION. FATAL IF GIVEN INTRATHECALLY. FOR INTRAVENOUS USE ONLY."

Reconstitute powder for injection with 10 mL NS injection (with or without preservative) to a concentration of 1 mg/mL. Inject into tubing of a running IV infusion or directly into a vein over 1 min. Do not dilute in large volumes or infuse over a prolonged period to reduce risk of vein irritation and extravasation. Carefully position IV to avoid extravasation. Rinsing the syringe and needle with venous blood before withdrawal has been suggested. If extravasation occurs, discontinue immediately and give any remaining portion of the dose into another vein. Use of hyaluronidase and applying moderate heat to the area may help disperse drug and minimize discomfort.

Vincristine Sulfate

vin-cris'teen sul'fate

★ Vincasar PFS

Do not confuse vincristine with vinblastine

CATEGORY AND SCHEDULE

Pregnancy Risk Category: D

Classification: Antineoplastic, vinca alkaloids

MECHANISM OF ACTION

A vinca alkaloid that binds to microtubular protein of mitotic spindle, causing metaphase arrest. *Therapeutic Effect:* Inhibits cell division.

PHARMACOKINETICS

Within 15-30 min of injection, most of the drug is distributed to tissues, where it is tightly bound. Does not cross the blood-brain barrier. Protein binding: 75%. Metabolized in the liver. Primarily eliminated in feces by biliary system. *Half-life:* 10-37 h.

AVAILABILITY

Injection: 1 mg/mL.

INDICATIONS AND DOSAGES

NOTE: Dosing varies widely with protocol being used. Check doses carefully. The dose in children and adults does not usually exceed 2 mg/wk. Lower doses are used in patients with hepatic disease or underlying neurologic problems. For example, the MOPP regimen for Hodgkin disease uses vincristine 1.4 mg/m^2 on days 1 and 8 with mechlorethamine, procarbazine, and prednisone; cycle repeats every 28 days.

▸ **Acute leukemia, advanced non-Hodgkin lymphoma, disseminated**

Hodgkin disease, neuroblastoma, rhabdomyosarcoma, Wilms tumor

IV

Adults, Elderly. 0.4-1.4 mg/m^2 once a week.

Children. 1-2 mg/m^2 once a week during induction phase.

Children weighing < 10 kg or with a body surface area < 1 m^2. 0.05 mg/kg once a week during induction phase. Maximum: 2 mg.

▸ **Dosage in hepatic impairment**

Reduce dosage by 50% if total bilirubin concentration is 1.5-3 mg/dL.

Reduce dosage by 75% if total bilirubin concentration > 3 mg/dL.

Hold dose if bilirubin is > 5 mg/dL.

OFF-LABEL USES

Idiopathic thrombocytopenic purpura (ITP), small lung cell carcinoma.

CONTRAINDICATIONS

Patients receiving radiation therapy through ports that include the liver; patients with demyelinating form of Charcot-Marie-Tooth syndrome; intrathecal administration.

INTERACTIONS

Drug

Strong inhibitors of CYP3A4 isoenzymes (erythromycin, clarithromycin, itraconazole): Increase concentrations of vincristine significantly and may cause neurotoxicity.

L-aspariginase or pegaspargase: Give vincristine 12-24 h before these drugs; giving these drugs before vincristine reduces hepatic clearance and increases toxicity of vincristine.

Mitomycin: Increased risk of pulmonary reactions.

Phenytoin: May decrease phenytoin concentration.

Herbal

None known.

Food

None known.

DIAGNOSTIC TEST EFFECTS

Increased serum uric acid. Decreased WBC and platelets.

IV INCOMPATIBILITIES

Do not mix with other medications.

SIDE EFFECTS

Expected

Peripheral neuropathy (occurs in nearly every patient; first clinical sign is depression of Achilles tendon reflex). Alopecia.

Frequent

Peripheral paresthesia, constipation or obstipation (upper colon impaction with empty rectum), abdominal cramps, headache, jaw pain, hoarseness, diplopia, ptosis or drooping of eyelid, urinary tract disturbances.

Occasional

Nausea, vomiting, diarrhea, abdominal distention, stomatitis, fever.

Rare

Mild leukopenia, mild anemia, thrombocytopenia.

SERIOUS REACTIONS

- Universally fatal if given intrathecally. There are only a few cases documented of survival.
- Extravasation may cause cellulitis and phlebitis. Sloughing may occur.
- Acute shortness of breath and bronchospasm may occur, especially when vincristine is administered concurrently with mitomycin.
- Prolonged or high-dose therapy may produce foot or wrist drop, difficulty walking, slapping gait, ataxia, and muscle wasting.
- Neurotoxicity is dose-limiting, presents as sensory impairment and paresthesias in "stocking-glove" distribution. Cranial nerves and

hearing and vision may be affected in severe cases.

• Acute uric acid nephropathy may occur.

PRECAUTIONS & CONSIDERATIONS

If CNS leukemia is diagnosed, additional agents are required because vincristine does not penetrate in adequate amounts. Patients with preexisting neuromuscular disease or on other neurotoxic drugs may be more susceptible to neurologic toxicities. Acute shortness of breath and severe bronchospasm have been reported following the administration of vinca alkaloids. Progressive dyspnea may require chronic therapy and the vinca should not be readministered. Take care to avoid contamination of the eye as severe irritation (or corneal ulceration) may result. Vincristine sulfate can cause fetal harm; females of childbearing potential should be advised to avoid becoming pregnant. Breastfeeding is not advised. Men may have alterations in sperm production or quality. A CBC should be done before each dose, and serum uric acid should be determined frequently during early treatment.

Storage

Store unopened vials under refrigeration. Protect from light; do not freeze. Diluted solution stable for 7 days under refrigeration or 2 days at room temperature. In ambulatory pumps, solution is stable for 7-10 days at room temperature.

Administration

CAUTION: Observe and excercise appropriate precautions for handling, preparing, and administering cytotoxic drugs. Label products: "DO NOT REMOVE COVERING UNTIL MOMENT OF INJECTION. FATAL IF GIVEN INTRATHECALLY. FOR INTRAVENOUS USE ONLY."

May be diluted with normal saline or D5W. Inject into tubing of a running IV infusion or directly into a vein. May be injected over about 1 min. Carefully position IV to avoid extravasation. If extravasation occurs, discontinue immediately and give any remaining portion of the dose into another vein. Use of hyaluronidase and applying moderate heat to the area may help disperse drug and minimize discomfort.

Vinorelbine

vin-oh-rel′bean

★ 🍁 Navelbine

Do not confuse vinorelbine with vinblastine.

CATEGORY AND SCHEDULE

Pregnancy Risk Category: D

Classification: Antineoplastic, vinca alkaloids

MECHANISM OF ACTION

A semisynthetic vinca alkaloid that interferes with mitotic microtubule assembly. *Therapeutic Effect:* Prevents cell division.

PHARMACOKINETICS

Widely distributed after IV administration. Protein binding: 80%-90%. Metabolized in the liver. Active metabolite. Primarily eliminated in feces by biliary system. *Half-life:* 28-43 h.

AVAILABILITY

Injection: 10 mg/mL.

INDICATIONS AND DOSAGES

▸ **Unresectable, advanced non–small cell lung carcinoma (as monotherapy)**

IV

Adults, Elderly. 30 mg/m² administered q 7 days over 6-10 min.

▸ **Advanced non–small-cell lung carcinoma (in combination with cisplatin)**

IV

Adults, Elderly. 25 mg/m² given q 7 days, in combination with cisplatin (100 mg/m² given q4wk)

▸ **Dosage adjustment guidelines**

Dosage adjustments should be based on granulocyte count obtained on the day of treatment, as follows:

Granulocyte Count (cells/mm³) on Day of Treatment	% of Starting Dose
> 1500	100%
1000-1499	50%
< 1000	Do not administer

Additional dosage adjustments are required for patients experiencing fever or sepsis during granulocytopenia or patients who had two consecutive doses withheld because of granulocytopenia:

Granulocyte Count (cells/mm³) on Day of Treatment	% of Starting Dose
> 1500	75%
1000-1499	37.5%
< 1000	Do not administer

Dosage adjustments based on total bilirubin:

Total Bilirubin (mg/dL)	% of Starting Dose
≤ 2	100%
2.1-3	50%
> 3	25%

▸ **Dose adjustments for neurotoxicity**

If Grade ≥ 2 neurotoxicity occurs, discontinue the drug.

OFF LABEL USES

Breast cancer, cervical cancer.

CONTRAINDICATIONS

Pretreatment granulocyte counts < 1000 cells/mm³. Intrathecal administration.

INTERACTIONS

Drug

Cisplatin: Increased risk of granulocytopenia.

Drugs that are potent CYP3A4 inhibitors: May reduce metabolism and increase risk of toxicity.

Mitomycin: Increased risk of pulmonary toxicity.

Paclitaxel: Increased risk of neurotoxicity.

Herbal

None known.

Food

None known.

DIAGNOSTIC TEST EFFECTS

Decreased WBC. Increased AST, bilirubin.

IV INCOMPATIBILITIES

Do not mix with other medications.

SIDE EFFECTS

Frequent

Asthenia; mild or moderate nausea; constipation; erythema, pain, or vein discoloration at injection site; fatigue; peripheral neuropathy manifested as paresthesia and hyperesthesia; diarrhea; alopecia.

Occasional

Phlebitis, dyspnea, loss of deep tendon reflexes.

Rare

Chest pain, jaw pain, myalgia, arthralgia, rash.

SERIOUS REACTIONS

• Dose-limiting toxicity: Bone marrow depression is manifested mainly as granulocytopenia, which may be severe. Other hematologic toxicities, including neutropenia, thrombocytopenia, leukopenia, and anemia, increase the risk of infection and bleeding.

- Acute shortness of breath and severe bronchospasm occur infrequently, particularly in patients with preexisting pulmonary dysfunction and in those receiving mitomycin concurrently. Fatal interstitial pulmonary changes and acute respiratory distress syndrome have occurred.
- Severe, sometimes fatal, constipation, paralytic ileus, intestinal obstruction, necrosis, or perforation.
- Expected to be universally fatal if given intrathecally.
- Extravasation may cause cellulitis and phlebitis. Sloughing may occur.

PRECAUTIONS & CONSIDERATIONS

Granulocyte count before treatment should be at least 1000 cells/mm^3. Obtain complete blood count with differentials on the day of treatment. Caution if bone marrow reserve is compromised by previous radiation therapy or chemotherapy. Use with caution in hepatic impairment.

Patients with preexisting neuropathy disease or on other neurotoxic drugs may be more susceptible to such toxicities. Acute shortness of breath and severe bronchospasm have been reported following the administration of vinca alkaloids. Take care to avoid contamination of the eye as severe irritation (or corneal ulceration) may result. Vinorelbine can cause fetal harm; females of child-bearing potential should be advised to avoid becoming pregnant. Breastfeeding is not advised. Men may have alterations in sperm production or quality. Patients receiving radiation therapy may be more likely to have radiation recall type events. Patients should report mouth sores, sore throat, fevers, and other effects of neutropenia.

Storage

Store unopened vials in cartons under refrigeration. Protect from light; do not freeze. Unopened vials are stable at temperatures up to 25° C (77° F) for up to 72 h. Diluted solution may be used for up to 24 h under normal room light when stored in polypropylene syringes or polyvinyl chloride bags under refrigeration or at room temperature.

Administration

CAUTION: Observe and excercise appropriate precautions for handling, preparing, and administering cytotoxic drugs. Label syringes: "DO NOT REMOVE COVERING UNTIL MOMENT OF INJECTION. FATAL IF GIVEN INTRATHECALLY. FOR INTRAVENOUS USE ONLY."

Dilute injection solution in the syringe or IV bag. Doses in a syringe should be diluted to 1.5-3 mg/mL with D5W or normal saline (NS). Doses diluted in an IV bag should be diluted to 0.5-2 mg/mL with D5W, normal saline (NS), 0.45% NaCl injection, 5% dextrose with 0.45% NaCl injection, Ringer's injection, or lactated Ringer's injection. Diluted solution should be administered over 6-10 min into the side port of a free-flowing IV closest to the IV bag, followed by flushing with at least 75-125 mL of a recommended dilution solution. Carefully position IV needle to minimize extravasation risk. If extravasation occurs, discontinue immediately and give any remaining portion of the dose into another vein. Use of hyaluronidase and applying moderate heat to the area may help disperse drug and minimize discomfort.

Vitamin A

vight'ah-myn A

★ Aquasol A, Dofsol-A

Do not confuse Aquasol A with Anusol.

CATEGORY AND SCHEDULE

Pregnancy Risk Category: A (X if used in doses above recommended daily allowance; also, injectable form is category X)

OTC, Rx

Classification: Vitamin, fat-soluble vitamin

MECHANISM OF ACTION

A fat-soluble vitamin that may act as a cofactor in biochemical reactions. *Therapeutic Effect:* Essential for normal function of retina, visual adaptation to darkness, bone growth, testicular and ovarian function, and embryonic development; preserves integrity of epithelial cells.

PHARMACOKINETICS

Rapidly absorbed from the GI tract if bile salts, pancreatic lipase, protein, and dietary fat are present. Transported in blood to the liver, where it is metabolized; stored in parenchymal hepatic cells, then transported in plasma as retinol, as needed. Excreted primarily in bile and, to a lesser extent, in urine.

AVAILABILITY

Soft-Gel Capsules, OTC: 8000 units, 10,000 units, 15,000 units, 25,000 units.

Capsules, Rx (Dofsol-A): 50,000 units.

Injection (Aquasol A): 50,000 units/mL.

INDICATIONS AND DOSAGES

▸ **Severe vitamin A deficiency**

PO

Adults, Elderly, Children 8 yr and older. 100,000 units/day for 3 days, then 50,000 units/day for 14 days, then 10,000-20,000 units/day for 2 mo.

Children 1-8 yr. 10,000 units/kg/day for 5 days, then 5000-10,000 units/day for 2 mo.

Children younger than 1 yr. 10,000 units/day for 5 days, then 7500-15,000 units for 10 days.

IM

Adults, Elderly, Children 8 yr and older. 100,000 units/day for 3 days; then 50,000 units/day for 14 days, followed by 10,000-20,000 units/day PO for 2 mo.

Children aged 1-8 yr. 17,500-35,000 units/day for 10 days.

Children younger than 1 yr. 7500-15,000 units/day.

▸ **Malabsorption syndrome**

PO

Adults, Elderly, Children 8 yr and older. 10,000-50,000 units/day.

▸ **Dietary supplement**

Females ≥ 14 yr. 2333 international units/day.

Males ≥ 14 yr. 3000 international units/day.

Pregnant Adolescent Females aged 14-18 yr. 2500 international units/day.

Pregnant Adult Female. 2566 international units/day.

Lactating Adolescent Females aged 14-18 yr. 4000 international units/day during first 6 mo of breastfeeding.

Lactating Adult Female. 4333 internationl units during first 6 mo of breastfeeding.

Children aged 9-13 yr. 2000 international units/day.

Children aged 4-8 yr. 1333 international units/day.

V

Children aged 1-3 yr. 1000 international units/day.
Infants (term) aged 7-12 mo. 1666 international units/day, based on dietary intake of breast milk, formula, or other food sources.
Infants (term) aged birth-6 mo. 1333 international units/day, based on dietary intake of human breast milk.

CONTRAINDICATIONS

Hypervitaminosis A; oral use in malabsorption syndrome; hypersensitivity, IV administration.

INTERACTIONS

Drug

Cholestyramine, colestipol, mineral oil: May decrease the absorption of vitamin A.
Isotretinoin: May increase the risk of toxicity.
Oral contraceptives: Increase plasma vitamin A levels.
Orlistat: May decrease oral vitamin A absorption.
Retinoids: Vitamin A should not be used concurrently in patients receiving systemic retinoids as may cause vitamin A toxicity.

Herbal and Food

None known.

DIAGNOSTIC TEST EFFECTS

May increase BUN and serum cholesterol, calcium, and triglyceride levels. May decrease blood erythrocyte and leukocyte counts.

SIDE EFFECTS

Occasional (1%-10%)

Fever, headache, irritability, lethargy, malaise, vertigo, drying or cracking of the skin, hypercalcemia, weight loss, visual changes, hypervitaminosis A.

SERIOUS REACTIONS

- Chronic overdosage produces malaise, nausea, vomiting, drying or cracking of skin or lips, inflammation of tongue or gums, irritability, alopecia, and night sweats.
- Bulging fontanelles have occurred in infants.
- Excessive dryness of eyes may lead to corneal irritation.

PRECAUTIONS & CONSIDERATIONS

Caution is warranted in patients with renal impairment. Vitamin A crosses the placenta and is distributed in breast milk. The RDA in pregnancy is usually < 3000 units/day. Safety of amounts > 6000 units/day not established for any female of childbearing potential. Use caution when administering high doses of vitamin A to children and elderly patients. Consuming foods rich in vitamin A, including cod, halibut, tuna, and shark, is encouraged; naturally occurring vitamin A is found only in animal sources. Avoid taking cholestyramine (Questran), colestipol, and mineral oil during vitamin A therapy.

Before and during treatment, assess for signs and symptoms of vitamin A deficiency, including night blindness, dry and brittle nails, alopecia, and drying of corneas. Be alert for symptoms of overdose when receiving prolonged administration of > 25,000 units/day. The therapeutic serum vitamin A level is 80-300 units/mL.

Storage

Store oral capsules and solution in a cool place. Store injection in refrigerator and protect from light; do not freeze.

Administration

! IM administration is used only in acutely ill patients or patients unresponsive to the oral route, such as those with malabsorption syndrome. For adults, an IM injection dose of 1 mL (50,000 units) may be given in the deltoid muscle; a dose > 1 mL should be given in a large muscle mass, such as the gluteus maximus muscle. The anterolateral thigh is the preferred site for infants younger than 7 mo. Do not administer intravenously.

Do not crush, open, or break capsules. Take vitamin A without regard to food.

Vitamin D (Cholecalciferol, Vitamin D_3; Ergocalciferol, Vitamin D_2)

vight′ah-myn D

★ Calcidol, Calciferol, Drisdol

CATEGORY AND SCHEDULE

Pregnancy Risk Category: A (D if used in doses above recommended daily allowance)

Classification: Vitamin; fat-soluble vitamin

MECHANISM OF ACTION

A fat-soluble vitamin that stimulates calcium and phosphate absorption from small intestine, promotes secretion of calcium from bone to blood, and promotes resorption of phosphate in renal tubules; also acts on bone cells to stimulate skeletal growth and on parathyroid gland to suppress hormone synthesis and secretion. *Therapeutic Effect:* Essential for absorption and utilization of calcium and phosphate and normal bone calcification. Reduces parathyroid hormone level. Improves phosphorus and calcium homeostasis in chronic renal failure.

PHARMACOKINETICS

Readily absorbed from small intestine; vitamin D_3 may be absorbed more rapidly and more completely than vitamin D_2. Concentrated primarily in liver and fat deposits. Activated in the liver and kidneys. Eliminated by biliary system; excreted in urine. *Half-life:* 14 h for cholecalciferol; 19-48 h for ergocalciferol.

AVAILABILITY

Capsules (Ergocalciferol, Drisdol): 50,000 units (1.25 mg).

Oral Liquid Drops (Calcidol, Calciferol, Drisdol): 8000 units/mL.

Tablets (Cholecalciferol, Vitamin D_3): 400 units, 1000 units.

Capsules (Cholecalciferol, Vitamin D_3): 10,000 units.

INDICATIONS AND DOSAGES

▸ **Dietary supplement**

PO

Adults, Elderly. 10 mcg (400 units)/day.

Children. 5 mcg.

Infants. 5 mcg (400-800 units)/day.

▸ **Renal failure**

PO

Adults, Elderly. 0.5 mg/day.

Children. 0.1-1 mg/day.

▸ **Hypoparathyroidism**

PO

Adults, Elderly. 1250-5000 mcg/day (with calcium supplements).

Children. 1250-5000 mcg/day (with calcium supplements).

V

▸ **Nutritional rickets, osteomalacia**
PO
Adults, Elderly, Children. 25-125 mcg/day for 8-12 wks.
Adults, Elderly (with malabsorption syndrome). 250-7500 mcg/day.
Children (with malabsorption syndrome). 250-625 mcg/day.
▸ **Vitamin D–dependent rickets**
PO
Adults, Elderly. 250 mcg to 1.5 mg/day.
Children. 75-125 mcg/day.
Maximum: 1500 mcg/day.
▸ **Vitamin D–resistant rickets**
PO
Adults, Elderly. 250-1500 mcg/day (with phosphate supplements).
Children. Initially 1000-2000 mcg/day (with phosphate supplements). May increase in 250- to 600-mcg increments q3-4mo.

CONTRAINDICATIONS

Hypercalcemia, malabsorption syndrome, vitamin D toxicity. Drisdol capsules contain tartrazine; don't use if tartrazine allergic (use caution if aspirin allergic).

INTERACTIONS

Drug
Aluminum-containing antacids (long-term use): May increase aluminum blood concentration and risk of aluminum bone toxicity.
Calcium-containing preparations, thiazide diuretics: May increase the risk of hypercalcemia.
Magnesium-containing antacids: May increase magnesium blood concentration.
Mineral oil: Excessive use of mineral oil decreases vitamin D absorption.
Orlistat: Decreases vitamin D absorption.
Herbal
None known.
Food
None known.

DIAGNOSTIC TEST EFFECTS

May increase serum cholesterol, calcium, magnesium, and phosphate levels. May decrease serum alkaline phosphatase level.

SIDE EFFECTS

None known.

SERIOUS REACTIONS

- Early signs and symptoms of overdose are weakness, headache, somnolence, nausea, vomiting, dry mouth, constipation, muscle and bone pain, and metallic taste.
- Later signs and symptoms of overdose include polyuria, polydipsia, anorexia, weight loss, nocturia, photophobia, rhinorrhea, pruritus, disorientation, hallucinations, hyperthermia, hypertension, and cardiac arrhythmias.

PRECAUTIONS & CONSIDERATIONS

Caution is warranted in patients with coronary artery disease, renal calculi, and renal impairment. It is unknown whether vitamin D crosses the placenta or is distributed in breast milk. Children may be more sensitive to the effects of vitamin D. No age-related precautions have been noted in elderly patients. Those receiving chronic renal dialysis should not take magnesium-containing antacids during vitamin D therapy. Consuming foods rich in vitamin D, including milk, eggs, leafy vegetables, margarine, meats, and vegetable oils and shortening, is encouraged.

BUN, serum alkaline phosphatase, calcium, creatinine, magnesium, and phosphate levels, and urinary calcium levels should be monitored.

Depending on condition, serial bone radiographs may help assess response to treatment.

Storage
Store at room temperature in a cool place. Do not freeze.
Administration
! Be aware that 1 mcg of vitamin D = 40 international units.
Begin vitamin D therapy at the lowest possible dosage. Take vitamin D without regard to food. Swallow the capsules whole and avoid crushing, chewing, or opening them.

Vitamin E

vight'ah-myn E
★ Aquasol E
Do not confuse Aquasol E with Anusol.

CATEGORY AND SCHEDULE

Pregnancy Risk Category: A (C if used in doses above recommended daily allowance)
OTC

Classification: Vitamins; fat-soluble vitamin

MECHANISM OF ACTION

An antioxidant that prevents oxidation of vitamins A and C, protects fatty acids from attack by free radicals, and protects RBCs from hemolysis by oxidizing agents. *Therapeutic Effect:* Prevents and treats vitamin E deficiency.

PHARMACOKINETICS

Variably absorbed from the GI tract (requires bile salts, dietary fat, and normal pancreatic function). Concentrated primarily in adipose tissue. Metabolized in the liver. Eliminated primarily by the biliary system.

AVAILABILITY

Oral Drops (Aquasol-E): 15 units/0.3 mL.
Topical Oil: 933 IU/mL.

INDICATIONS AND DOSAGES

▸ **Vitamin E deficiency**
PO
Adults, Elderly. 60-75 units/day. Adults with malabsorption may require 100-400 IU/day. Maximum tolerable limit considered 1000 IU/day.
Children. 1 unit/kg/day.
▸ **To moisturize the skin**
TOPICAL
Adults: Apply to affected area of the skin as needed.

OFF-LABEL USES

To decrease the severity of tardive dyskinesia, mastalgia associated with premenstrual syndrome.

CONTRAINDICATIONS

None known.

INTERACTIONS

Drug
Cholestyramine, colestipol, mineral oil: May decrease the absorption of vitamin E.
Iron (large doses): May increase vitamin E requirements.
Oral anticoagulants: Increased anticoagulant effects with vitamin E doses exceeding 400 units/day.
Orlistat: Decreases vitamin E absorption.
Herbal
None known.
Food
None known.

DIAGNOSTIC TEST EFFECTS

None known.

SIDE EFFECTS

None known.

SERIOUS REACTIONS

• Chronic overdose may produce fatigue, weakness, nausea, headache, blurred vision, flatulence, and diarrhea.

PRECAUTIONS & CONSIDERATIONS

Vitamin E use may impair the hematologic response with iron deficiency anemia. It is unknown whether vitamin E crosses the placenta or is distributed in breast milk. No age-related precautions have been noted with normal dosages in children or in elderly patients. Consuming foods high in vitamin E, including eggs, meats, milk, leafy vegetables, margarine, and vegetable oils and shortening, is encouraged.

Notify the physician of signs and symptoms of toxicity, including blurred vision, diarrhea, nausea, dizziness, flu-like symptoms, or headache.

Storage

Store in a cool, dry place at room temperature.

Administration

Do not crush, open, or break capsule. Take vitamin E without regard to food. Vitamin E drops may be dropped directly into the mouth or mixed with fruit juice, cereal, or other food. Topical oil is for external use only; do not ingest; gently massage into skin, avoiding eyes and mucous membranes.

V

Voriconazole

vohr-ee-con′ah-zole

★ 🍁 Vfend, Vfend IV

CATEGORY AND SCHEDULE

Pregnancy Risk Category: D

Classification: Antifungals, azole antifungals

MECHANISM OF ACTION

A triazole derivative that inhibits the synthesis of ergosterol, a vital component of fungal cell wall formation. *Therapeutic Effect:* Damages fungal cell wall membrane.

PHARMACOKINETICS

Rapidly and completely absorbed after PO administration. Widely distributed. Protein binding: 58%. Metabolized in the liver. Primarily excreted as a metabolite in urine. Removed by hemodialysis. *Half-life:* 6 h.

AVAILABILITY

Tablets: 50 mg, 200 mg.
Injection Powder for Reconstitution: 200 mg.
Powder for Oral Suspension: 200 mg/5 mL.

INDICATIONS AND DOSAGES

▸ **Invasive aspergillosis, other serious fungal infections caused by *Scedosporium apiospermum* and *Fusarium* spp**

PO

Adults, Elderly, Children > 12 yr weighing ≥ 40 kg. Initially, 400 mg q12h for 2 doses on day 1. Maintenance: 200 mg q12h (may increase to 300 mg q12h).
Adults, Elderly, Children > 12 yr weighing < 40 kg. Initially, 200 mg q12h for 2 doses on day 1. Maintenance: 100 mg q12h (may increase to 150 mg q12h).

▸ **Usual parenteral dosage**

IV

Adults, Elderly, Children over 12 yr. Initially, 6 mg/kg/dose q12h for 2 doses, then 4 mg/kg/dose q12h (may decrease to 3 mg/kg/dose if patient is unable to tolerate 4 mg/kg/dose).

▸ **Candidemia in nonneutropenic patients; deep tissue *Candida* infections**

PO
Adults, Elderly, Children > 12 yr weighing ≥ 40 kg. After initial IV loading dose, 200 mg q12h.
Adults, Elderly, Children > 12 yr weighing < 40 kg. After initial IV loading dose, 100 mg q12h.
IV
Adults, Elderly, Children > 12 yr Initially, 6 mg/kg/dose q12h for 2 doses, then 3-4 mg/kg/dose q12h.

▸ **Esophageal candidiasis**
PO
Adults, Elderly, Children > 12 yr weighing ≥ 40 kg. 200 mg q12h for minimum of 14 days, then at least 7 days following resolution of symptoms.
Adults, Elderly, Children > 12 yr weighing < 40 kg. 100 mg q12h for minimum 14 days, then at least 7 days following resolution of symptoms.
Adults. Elderly, Children > 12 yr. Initially, 6 mg/kg/dose q12h for 2 doses, then 3 mg/kg/dose q12h.

▸ **Dosage in hepatic insufficiency**
Give standard loading dose but reduce maintenance dose by 50% if mild to moderate hepatic cirrhosis (Child-Pugh class A, B). Not studied in patients with severe hepatic disease.

CONTRAINDICATIONS

Hypersensitivity to voriconazole. Many medications are contraindicated for use with Vfend. See Drug Interactions.

INTERACTIONS

Drug
Drugs that are substrates for CY3A4 (e.g., cyclosporine, methadone, protease inhibitors, NNRTIs, benzodiazepines, "statins," tacrolimus, vinca alkaloids) or CYP2C9 (warfarin, sulfonylureas): Risk of augmented effects/side effects of these drugs increased as voriconazole reduces their metabolism. Increased monitoring required.
Efavirenz, fosphenytoin, phenytoin: Decrease voriconazole concentrations and dose increase recommended (see manufacturer's information).
Ergot alkaloids, cisapride, pimozide, quinidine, sirolimus: Contraindicated. Voriconazole significantly increases the levels of these drugs, resulting in risk of serious toxicity.
Rifampin, rifabutin, ritonavir, carbamazepine, phenobarbital, primidone: Contraindicated. Significantly reduce voriconazole levels. Also, rifabutin levels significantly increased.
Herbal
St. John's wort: Contraindicated. Significantly reduces voriconazole concentrations.
Food
Absorption reduced with high-fat meal.

DIAGNOSTIC TEST EFFECTS

May increase serum alkaline phosphatase and SGPT (ALT) levels.

IV INCOMPATIBILITIES

Must not be infused with any blood product or with concentrated electrolytes or with sodium bicarbonate solutions, even if in separate IV lines (or cannulas). IV solutions containing (nonconcentrated) electrolytes or TPN solutions can be infused at the same time, but must be through a separate line. If infused via a multiple-lumen catheter, TPN needs to be administered using a different port from Vend IV. Consult specialized resources for other Y-site incompatibility information.

V

SIDE EFFECTS

Frequent (5%-20%)
Abnormal vision, fever, nausea, rash, vomiting.
Occasional (2%-5%)
Headache, chills, hallucinations, photophobia, tachycardia, hypertension.

SERIOUS REACTIONS

- Hepatotoxicity occurs rarely.
- Optic neuritis, papilledema, especially with prolonged treatment.
- Rare cases of QT prolongation or arrhythmias.
- Anaphylactoid-like reactions during infusion.

PRECAUTIONS & CONSIDERATIONS

Caution should be used in patients with hypersensitivity to other azole antifungal agents, impaired renal or liver function, or proarrhythmic conditions. Correct hypocalemia, hypokalemia, and hypomagnesemia before initiating voriconazole. Be aware that voriconazole may cause fetal harm. Use effective contraception during voriconazole treatment. Breastfeeding is not recommended during treatment. Be aware that the safety and efficacy of voriconazole have not been established in children younger than 12 yr. No age-related precautions have been noted in elderly patients. Oral suspension contains sucrose. Tablets contain lactose; do not use in those with hereditary intolerance or enzyme deficiency.

Expect to monitor liver and renal function test results. Evaluate and monitor visual function, including color perception, visual acuity, and visual field, for drug therapy lasting longer than 28 days. Avoid driving at night because voriconazole may cause visual changes, such as blurred vision or photophobia. Avoid performing hazardous tasks if changes in vision occur. Avoid direct sunlight.

Storage
Store powder for injection at room temperature. Use reconstituted solution immediately. If not used immediately, infusion expires in 24 h under refrigeration.

Powder for oral suspension should be stored in refrigerator until reconstituted. Reconstituted oral suspension stable for 14 days at room temperature. Do not refrigerate or freeze once reconstituted.
Administration
Give oral voriconazole 1 h before or 1 h after a meal. Shake suspension well prior to each use; use calibrated dispenser provided to measure dose.

Injection is for IV infusion only. Reconstitute 200-mg vial with 19 mL sterile water for injection to provide a concentration of 10 mg/mL. Further dilute with 0.9% NaCl or D5W to provide a concentration not < 0.5 mg/mL or > 5 mg/mL. Infuse over 1-2 h at a rate not to exceed 3 mg/kg/h.

Vorinostat

vor-in'o-stat
Zolinza

CATEGORY AND SCHEDULE

Pregnancy Risk Category: D

Classification: Antineoplastic

MECHANISM OF ACTION

Inhibits histone deacetylase enzymes HDAC1, HDAC2, HDAC3, and HDAC6. In many different malignant cell lines, HDAC inhibitors inhibit the cell cycle and induce apoptosis. They may also stimulate the immune system and block angiogenesis.

PHARMACOKINETICS

Well absorbed orally; 71% bound to plasma proteins. Major pathways of metabolism involve glucuronidation and hydrolysis, then β-oxidation. Metabolites are not active. Roughly 53% of inactive drug plus metabolites excreted in urine. *Half-life:* 2 h.

AVAILABILITY

Capsules: 100 mg.

INDICATIONS AND DOSAGES

▸ Cutaneous T-cell lymphoma

PO

Adults, Elderly. 400 mg once daily; if not tolerated, may reduce to 300 mg once daily or 300 mg once daily 5 days/wk.

CONTRAINDICATIONS

None known.

INTERACTIONS

Drug

Valproic acid (other HDAC inhibitors): Severe thrombocytopenia and GI bleeding.

Warfarin: Prolonged INR.

Herbal and Food

None significant.

DIAGNOSTIC TEST EFFECTS

Increased serum glucose, serum creatinine. May lower platelet count.

SIDE EFFECTS

Frequent (> 20%)

Fatigue, anorexia, diarrhea, dysgeusia, nausea, thrombocytopenia, anemia, weight loss.

Occasional (10%-20%)

Dizziness, headache, alopecia, pruritus, constipation, decreased appetite, dry mouth, vomiting, anemia, muscle spasms, cough, upper respiratory tract infection, increased serum creatinine, chills, peripheral edema, pyrexia, hyperglycemia.

SERIOUS REACTIONS

- Pulmonary embolism, deep vein thrombosis.
- Squamous cell carcinoma.
- Severe thrombocytopenia with GI bleeding.
- QT prolongation.
- Angioneurotic edema, exfoliative skin rashes, and other serious allergic events (rare).

PRECAUTIONS & CONSIDERATIONS

Vorinostat is not available in most pharmacies; patients must be registered in the ACT program to receive the drug. Use caution in patients with hepatic or renal impairment, with diabetes, or with fluid and electrolyte disturbances. Hypokalemia or hypomagnesemia should be corrected prior to use. Vorinostat may cause fetal harm; women of childbearing potential are encouraged to use adequate contraception. It is not known if the drug is excreted in breast milk. Safety and efficacy are not established in children. Monitor for signs and symptoms of thromboembolic disease; monitor glucose, electrolytes, CBC, serum creatinine. ECG is required at baseline and periodically during treatment. Antiemetics, antidiarrheals, and fluid and electrolyte replacement may be necessary. Patients should be instructed to drink at least 2 L of fluid per day to prevent dehydration.

Storage

Store at room temperature.

Administration

CAUTION: Observe and exercise appropriate precautions for handling cytotoxic drugs.

Take with food. Swallow capsules whole. Do not open or crush capsules; avoid contact with powder.

Warfarin Sodium

war'far-in soe'dee-um

★ Coumadin, Jantoven

🍁 Apo-Warfarin, Coumadin, Mylan-Warfarin, Taro-Warfarin

CATEGORY AND SCHEDULE

Pregnancy Risk Category: X

Classification: Oral anticoagulant (Coumarin type)

MECHANISM OF ACTION

A coumarin derivative that interferes with hepatic synthesis of vitamin K–dependent clotting factors, resulting in depletion of coagulation factors II, VII, IX, and X. *Therapeutic Effect:* Prevents further extension of formed existing clot; prevents new clot formation.

PHARMACOKINETICS

Route	Onset	Peak	Duration
PO	1.5-3 days	5-7 days	2-5 days

Well absorbed from the GI tract. Metabolized in the liver. Not removed by hemodialysis. *Half-life:* 1-2.5 days, but highly variable among individuals.

AVAILABILITY

Tablets (Coumadin, Jantoven): 1 mg, 2 mg, 2.5 mg, 3 mg, 4 mg, 5 mg, 6 mg, 7.5 mg, 10 mg.
Injection (Coumadin): 5-mg vial.

INDICATIONS AND DOSAGES

▸ **Anticoagulant**

PO, IV

Adults, Elderly. Initially, 5-10 mg/day for 2-5 days PO (or 2-5 mg initially IV); then adjust based on international normalized ratio (INR). Maintenance: 2-10 mg/day.
Children. Initially, 0.1-0.2 mg/kg (maximum 10 mg). Maintenance: 0.05-0.34 mg/kg/day.

▸ **Usual elderly dosage (maintenance)**

PO, IV

Elderly. 2-5 mg/day, carefully adjust per INR.

CONTRAINDICATIONS

Known hypersensitivity to warfarin. Anticoagulation is contraindicated in any circumstance in which the risk of hemorrhage is greater than the potential benefit of anticoagulation such as (1) pregnancy; (2) hemorrhagic tendencies or blood dyscrasias; (3) recent or contemplated surgery of the eye, CNS, or major trauma; (4) bleeding tendencies associated with active ulceration or overt bleeding of the GI, GU, or respiratory tracts; cerebral aneurysms, dissecting aorta; or pericarditis or pericardial effusions, and bacterial endocarditis; (5) threatened abortion, eclampsia, and preeclampsia; (6) inadequate laboratory facilities to monitor the patient; (7) unsupervised patients with senility, alcoholism, or psychosis or other lack of patient cooperation; (8) spinal puncture and other diagnostic or therapeutic procedures with potential for uncontrollable bleeding; (9) miscellaneous: including major regional or lumbar block anesthesia, malignant hypertension; alcoholism; elderly; any disease state where an increased risk of bleeding would be detrimental.

INTERACTIONS

Drug

NOTE: Many drug products can interfere with warfarin, so caution should be used.

Alcohol: Acute alcohol use (binge drinking) may increase PT/INR. Chronic alcohol use may decrease PT/INR.
Acetaminophen, celecoxib: Possible increase in anticoagulant effects; monitor INR.
Amiodarone, chloral hydrate, cimetidine, ciprofloxacin, clarithromycin, diflunisal, erythromycin, fluconazole, fluoroquinolones, gemfibrozil, HMG-CoA reductase inhibitors, indomethacin, itraconazole, ketoconazole, levofloxacin, metronidazole, NSAIDs, oral hypoglycemics, orlistat, phenytoin, propoxyphene, proton-pump inhibitors, salicylates, SSRIs, sulfamethoxazole/trimethoprim, sulfonamides, systemic corticosteroids, tetracyclines, thyroid products, vitamin E: Possible increase in anticoagulant effects; monitor INR.
Argatroban: Increases INR and PT, so increased monitoring is needed if warfarin is also given.
Barbiturates, carbamazepine, cholestyramine, estrogens, griseofulvin, primidone, rifampin, vitamin K: Decreased warfarin action.
NSAIDs, salicylates: If NSAIDs must be used, monitor patient (avoid aspirin).
Herbal
Herbal products (American ginseng, coenzyme Q_{10}, St. John's wort): May decrease the effectiveness of warfarin.
Cranberry, dong quai, evening primrose oil, feverfew, garlic, ginger, ginkgo, glucosamine, green tea, omega-3-acids, SAM-e: May increase the risk of bleeding by potentiating action of warfarin.
Many herbal products: *Can interfere with warfarin, so caution should be used.*
Food
Foods with a high vitamin K content: Decreased effect (decreased PT/INR).
Cranberry juice: Increased effect (increased PT/INR).

DIAGNOSTIC TEST EFFECTS

Warfarin increases the PT and INR. Goal INR for most patients is 2.0-3.0.

SIDE EFFECTS

Occasional
GI distress, such as nausea, anorexia, abdominal cramps, diarrhea.
Rare
Hypersensitivity reaction, including dermatitis and urticaria, especially in those sensitive to aspirin. Purple toe syndrome and necrosis; risk factors include known or suspected deficiency in protein C– mediated anticoagulant response.

SERIOUS REACTIONS

- Bleeding complications ranging from local ecchymoses to major hemorrhage: the treatment depends on INR and type or presence of bleeding. Drug should be held and/or vitamin K or phytonadione administered.

Recommendations are as follows:
- *Adults with INR < 5 and exceeding therapeutic range but NO significant bleeding.* Lower or omit a warfarin dose; monitor INR; lower warfarin dosage once reach target INR.
- *Adults with INR ≥ 5 and < 9 and NO significant bleeding.* Omit next 1 or 2 warfarin doses; monitor INR. Lower dosage once target INR reached. Alternatively, omit warfarin dose and give 1-2.5 mg PO of vitamin K1. If more rapid

W

reversal required (e.g, surgery) give ≤ 5 mg PO of vitamin K1; INR should decrease in 24 h. If INR still elevated, give additional 1-2 mg PO vitamin K1.

• *Adults with INR ≥ 9 in the absence of significant bleeding.* Hold warfarin. Give 2.5-5 mg PO vitamin K1. Monitor INR. If the INR is still elevated, may give additional vitamin K1. Lower warfarin dosage once reach target INR.

• *Adults with serious bleeding at any elevation of INR.* Hold warfarin. Give vitamin K1 10 mg IV slow infusion, supplemented with fresh frozen plasma or prothrombin complex concentrate, depending on urgency. Recombinant factor VIIa may be considered. Vitamin K1 can be repeated q12h. *Adults with life-threatening bleeding.* Hold warfarin. Give prothrombin complex concentrate supplemented with vitamin K1 10 mg IV slow infusion. Recombinant factor VIIa may be considered. Repeat steps as needed to reduce INR.

• Hepatotoxicity, blood dyscrasias, necrosis, vasculitis, and local thrombosis occur rarely.

PRECAUTIONS & CONSIDERATIONS

Identification of risk factors for bleeding and certain genetic variations (CYP2C9 and VKORC1 metabolism) in a patient warrants frequent INR monitoring and the use of lower warfarin doses. Caution is warranted in patients at risk for hemorrhage and in those with active tuberculosis, diabetes, gangrene, heparin-induced thrombocytopenia, or necrosis. Warfarin use may cause teratogenic effect or fetal bleeding. Warfarin crosses the placenta and is distributed in breast milk. In elderly patients, a lower dose of warfarin is recommended. Other nonessential medications, including OTC drugs, should be avoided. An electric razor and soft toothbrush should be used. Avoid alcohol, drastic dietary changes, dangerous recreational sports, and salicylates.

Notify the physician before having dental work or surgery. INR should be determined before administration and daily after therapy begins until INR stabilizes. Once INR is stabilized, INR determinations should be followed every 4-6 wks. Monitor clinically for signs of bleeding. Carefully assess for new medicines (prescription and OTC), as well as supplement use, at every appointment.

Storage

Store at room temperature and protect from light. For injection, use reconstituted solution within 4 h; discard unused portion.

Administration

Remember that warfarin dosage is highly individualized based on PT, INR, and genetics.

Split scored tablets as needed. Give oral warfarin without regard to food. Take warfarin exactly as prescribed at the same time each day. Do not change from one brand of warfarin to another.

For IV use, to reconstitute, add 2.7 mL sterile water for injection to 5-mg vial to produce a final concentration of 2 mg/mL. Administer dose as a bolus injection slowly over 1-2 min, but do not administer intramuscularly.

Yohimbine

yoe-him'been

Erex, Yocon, Yohimbe

CATEGORY AND SCHEDULE

Pregnancy Risk Category: NA

Do not use during pregnancy.

Classification: Antiadrenergics, α-blocking, impotence agents

MECHANISM OF ACTION

An herb that produces genital blood vessel dilation, improves nerve impulse transmission to genital area. Increases penile blood flow, central sympathetic excitation impulses to genital tissues. *Therapeutic Effect:* Improves sexual vigor, affects impotence; clinical studies show may not always be effective.

PHARMACOKINETICS

Rapidly absorbed. Extensive metabolism in liver and kidneys. Minimal excretion in urine as unchanged drug. *Half-life:* < 30 min.

AVAILABILITY

Tablets: 5.4 mg (Yocon).

INDICATIONS AND DOSAGES

NOTE: There are no FDA-approved indications for Yohimbe, which is regulated as a dietary supplement, and not as a drug.

▸ **Erectile dysfunction impotence**

PO (YOCON, Rx ONLY)

Adults, Elderly. 5.4 mg 3 times/day. Reduce dose if side effects occur. May reduce to half-tablet 3 times daily followed by gradual increases to 1 tablet 3 times daily as tolerated.

OFF-LABEL USES

Treatment of SSRI-induced sexual dysfunction, raise blood pressure in autonomic failure.

CONTRAINDICATIONS

Renal disease, hypersensitivity to yohimbine or any component of the formulation.

INTERACTIONS

Drug

Antidiabetics, antihypertensives: May interfere with the effects of these drugs.

Clonidine: May antagonize the effects of clonidine.

MAOIs, linezolid, sympathomimetics, tricyclic antidepressants: Has additive effects with these drugs.

Use with MAOIs is not recommended due to additive effect of yohimbine on MAO.

Herbal

Ephedra: May increase the risk of hypertensive crises.

Ginkgo biloba, St. John's wort: May have additive therapeutic and adverse effects.

Food

Caffeine-containing products (such as coffee, tea, and chocolate) and tyramine-containing foods (such as aged cheese and Chianti wine): May increase the risk of hypertensive crises.

DIAGNOSTIC TEST EFFECTS

None known.

SIDE EFFECTS

Excitement, tremors, insomnia, anxiety, hypertension, tachycardia, dizziness, headache, irritability, salivation, dilated pupils, nausea, vomiting, hypersensitivity reaction.

SERIOUS REACTIONS

- Seizures, severe hypotension, irregular heartbeats, and renal failure may occur.
- Overdose can be fatal.

PRECAUTIONS & CONSIDERATIONS

Caution is warranted in patients with anxiety, heart disease, hepatic disease, diabetes mellitus, hypertension, posttraumatic stress disorder, and schizophrenia. Yohimbine is generally not used in females. Its use is contraindicated in breastfeeding and pregnant women. Safety and efficacy of yohimbine have not been established in children. Age-related liver and renal impairment may require discontinuation of yohimbine in elderly patients. Over-the-counter drugs should be avoided without first consulting with the prescriber.

Storage

Store at room temperature.

Administration

May administer without regard to meals.

Y

Zafirlukast

za-feer'loo-kast

Accolate

Do not confuse Accolate with Accupril or Aclovate.

CATEGORY AND SCHEDULE

Pregnancy Risk Category: B

Classification: Selective leukotriene receptor antagonist

MECHANISM OF ACTION

Antiasthmatic that binds to leukotriene receptors, inhibiting bronchoconstriction caused by sulfur dioxide, cold air, and specific antigens, such as grass, cat dander, and ragweed. *Therapeutic Effect:* Reduces airway edema and smooth muscle constriction; alters cellular activity associated with the inflammatory process.

PHARMACOKINETICS

Rapidly absorbed after PO administration (food reduces absorption). Protein binding: 99%. Extensively metabolized in the liver. Primarily excreted in feces. Unknown if removed by hemodialysis. *Half-life:* 10 h (terminal).

AVAILABILITY

Tablets: 10 mg, 20 mg.

INDICATIONS AND DOSAGES

▸ **For the prevention and chronic treatment of asthma**

PO

Adults, Elderly, Children 12 yr and older. 20 mg twice a day.

Children aged 5-11 yr. 10 mg twice a day.

▸ **Dosage in hepatic impairment**

Zafirlukast clearance decreased 60%; not studied in patients with hepatitis or cirrhosis.

CONTRAINDICATIONS

Known hypersensitivity.

INTERACTIONS

Drug

Aspirin: Increased plasma levels of zafirlukast.

Erythromycin: Reduced plasma levels of zafirlukast.

Drugs metabolized by CYP2C9 and CYP3A4 isoenzymes (carbamazepine, erythromycin, fluoxetine, glimepiride, glipizide, nateglinide, phenobarbital, rifampin, rifapentine, phenytoin): Inhibits CYP2C9 and CYP3A4 isoenzymes and may increase plasma concentrations of these drugs.

Theophylline: Rare reports of increased theophylline levels; mechanism unknown.

Warfarin: Increased PT/INR; zafirlukast inhibits warfarin metabolism.

Herbal

None known.

Food

None known.

DIAGNOSTIC TEST EFFECTS

May increase ALT (SGPT) level.

SIDE EFFECTS

Frequent

Headache.

Occasional

Nausea, diarrhea, dizziness, fever, infection, myalgia, pain, vomiting, weakness, increased ALT.

Rare

Agranulocytosis, bleeding, eosinophilia, hepatic failure, hepatitis, vasculitis with clinical features of Churg-Strauss syndrome.

SERIOUS REACTIONS

- See rare reactions; also rare serious allergic reactions, including angioedema.
- Concurrent administration of inhaled corticosteroids may increase the risk of upper respiratory tract infections in patients greater than 55 yr of age.

PRECAUTIONS & CONSIDERATIONS

Caution is warranted in patients with impaired hepatic function, whether from prior use of zafirlukast or not. Zafirlukast is pregnancy category B and is distributed in breast milk. It is not recommended for breastfeeding women. The safety and efficacy of this drug have not been established in children younger than 5 yr. Although no specific age-related precautions have been noted in elderly patients, they may be more at risk for infection and zafirlukast exposure is increased. Be aware that zafirlukast is not intended to treat acute asthma episodes. Drink plenty of fluids to decrease the thickness of lung secretions.

Liver function, pulse rate and quality, as well as respiratory depth, rate, rhythm, and type should be monitored. Fingernails and lips should be assessed for cyanosis, manifested as a blue or dusky color in light-skinned patients and a gray color in dark-skinned patients. Notify the physician of any abdominal pain, nausea, flu-like symptoms, jaundice, or worsening of asthma.

Storage

Store at room temperature. Protect from light and moisture.

Administration

Take zafirlukast 1 h before or 2 h after meals. Do not crush or break tablets. Take zafirlukast as prescribed, even during symptom-free periods. Do not alter the dosage or abruptly discontinue other asthma medications.

Zaleplon

zal′eh-plon

Sonata Stamoc

CATEGORY AND SCHEDULE

Pregnancy Risk Category: C

Controlled Substance Schedule: IV

Classification: Hypnotic, nonbenzodiazepine

MECHANISM OF ACTION

A nonbenzodiazepine that enhances the action of the inhibitory neurotransmitter γ-aminobutyric acid. *Therapeutic Effect:* Induces sleep.

AVAILABILITY

Capsules: 5 mg, 10 mg.

PHARMACOKINETICS

PO: Rapid absorption, but heavy, high-fat meals delay absorption; peak plasma levels in 1 h; wide tissue distribution; rapid hepatic metabolism (CYP3A4 minor pathway); excretion in urine.

INDICATIONS AND DOSAGES

▸ Insomnia

PO

Adults. 10 mg at bedtime. Range: 5-20 mg.

Elderly. 5 mg at bedtime, with a recommended maximum of 10 mg.

▸ Dosage in hepatic impairment (adults)

PO
5 mg at bedtime in mild to moderate impairment. Not recommended if impairment severe.

CONTRAINDICATIONS

Known hypersensitivity to zaleplon.

INTERACTIONS

Drug
All CNS-depressant drugs (anticonvulsants, antipsychotics, barbiturates, benzodiazepines, opioid agonists) and alcohol: Central nervous system (CNS) depression.
Cimetidine, erythromycin, and strong CYP3A4 inhibitors: Increased concentration of zaleplon. If taking cimetidine, decrease dose of zalepon to 5 mg.
Flumazenil: Suggested to antagonize effects of zaleplon.
Rifampin and rifamycin derivatives: Decreased effects of zaleplon.
Herbal
None known.
Food
Heavy, high-fat meals: Onset of sleep may be delayed by approximately 2 h.

SIDE EFFECTS

Expected
Somnolence, sedation, mild rebound insomnia (on first night after drug is discontinued).
Frequent
Nausea, headache, myalgia, dizziness, weakness.
Occasional
Amnesia, abdominal pain, asthenia, dysmenorrhea, dyspepsia, eye pain, paresthesia, somnolence.
Rare
Anaphylaxis, angioedema, bundle-branch block, cerebral ischemia, intestinal obstruction, tremors, amnesia, hyperacusis (acute sense of hearing), fever, glaucoma, abnormal liver function tests, pericardial effusion, pulmonary embolus, ventricular tachycardia, ventricular extrasystoles.

SERIOUS REACTIONS

- Zaleplon may produce altered concentration, behavior changes, and impaired memory.
- Taking the drug while up and about may result in adverse CNS effects, such as hallucinations, impaired coordination, dizziness, and light-headedness. There is a possibility that performance of hazardous tasks, like driving, may be affected the day after taking a hypnotic.
- Overdosage results in somnolence, confusion, diminished reflexes, and coma.

PRECAUTIONS & CONSIDERATIONS

Use is contraindicated in patients with hypersensitivity to zaleplon. Caution is warranted in patients with mild to moderate hepatic impairment, signs or symptoms of depression, and a hypersensitivity to aspirin (it may cause an allergic-type reaction). Use is not recommended in pregnancy. Do not use during breastfeeding because zaleplon enters the breast milk. Drowsiness may occur. Avoid alcohol, CNS depressants, and tasks that require mental alertness or motor skills. Zaleplon should be administered with caution in elderly or smaller patients or those with compromised respiratory, hepatic, or renal function. Safety and efficacy in children have not been established. Disturbed sleep may occur for 1 or 2 nights after discontinuing the drug.
Administration
For best effect, avoid administering following a heavy or high-fat meal.

Best taken on empty stomach or with light snack only. Can be taken at bedtime, or later if the patient is in bed and cannot fall asleep.

Zanamivir

za-na'mi-veer

★ 🍁 Relenza

CATEGORY AND SCHEDULE

Pregnancy Risk Category: B

Classification: Antiviral, neuraminidase inhibitor

MECHANISM OF ACTION

An antiviral that appears to inhibit the influenza virus enzyme neuraminidase, which is essential for viral replication. *Therapeutic Effect:* Affects viral release from infected cells.

AVAILABILITY

Powder for Inhalation: 5 mg/blister.

PHARMACOKINETICS

Inhalation: 4%-17% of inhaled dose is absorbed, peak serum levels 1-2 h, low plasma protein binding (< 10%), excreted unchanged in urine.

INDICATIONS AND DOSAGES

Influenza virus infection

INHALATION

Adults, Elderly, Children aged 7 yr and older. 2 inhalations (one 5-mg blister per inhalation for a total dose of 10 mg) twice a day (about 12 h apart) for 5 days.

▸ **Prevention of influenza virus infection**

INHALATION

Adults, Elderly, Children aged 5 yr and older. 2 inhalations once a day for 10 days (household settings) or for 28 days (community outbreak).

CONTRAINDICATIONS

Do not use in those with allergy history to any ingredient of product, including lactose (contains milk proteins).

INTERACTIONS

Drug

Influenza nasal vaccine, live: Decreased effect of zanamivir: Use of zanamivir is not recommended 48 h before and up to 2 wks after the administration of the live, attentuated influenza vaccine (e.g., FluMist, H1N1 nasal vaccine).

Herbal

None known.

Food

None known.

DIAGNOSTIC TEST EFFECTS

May increase serum creatine kinase level and liver function test results.

SIDE EFFECTS

Frequent

More with prophylaxis: Headache, throat or tonsil discomfort and pain, nasal signs and symptoms, cough, viral infections.

Occasional

Diarrhea, sinusitis, nausea, bronchitis, cough, dizziness, headache, vomiting, infection, sinusitis.

More with prophylaxis: Fever or chills, cough, fatigue, malaise, anorexia or an increased or decreased appetite, muscle pain, musculoskeletal pain.

SERIOUS REACTIONS

Allergic or allergic-like reaction, arrhythmia, bronchospasm if a history of chronic obstructive pulmonary disease (COPD) or asthma, central nervous system (CNS) effects (confusion, delusions, altered consciousness, delirium, delusions, hallucinations), hemorrhage, serious cutaneous rash, seizure.

PRECAUTIONS & CONSIDERATIONS

Use with caution in patients with a history of hypersensitivity. Caution should be used in patients with asthma or COPD; these patients should still be given the influenza vaccine. Be aware that persons requiring an inhaled bronchodilator at the same time as zanamivir should receive the bronchodilator before zanamivir. Dizziness may occur. Avoid contact with those who are at high risk for influenza. Use in pregnancy has not been well established. Use with caution in breastfeeding patients. Safety has not been established for prophylaxis in children younger than 5 yr and in treatment of patients younger than 7 yr. One concern about children is their ability to use the Diskhaler.

Storage

Store at controlled room temperature, in provided packaging. Do not have Diskhaler puncture blister until time of use.

Administration

Using the Diskhaler device provided, exhale completely; then put the white mouthpiece to the lips and breathe in the dose deeply and slowly. Remove mouthpiece from mouth, hold breath for at least 10 seconds, and exhale slowly. Continue treatment for the full 5-day course, and evenly space doses around the clock (~12 h apart). For prophylactic therapy, patients should use therapy once daily for 10 or 28 days. Patients should be made aware that they should immediately report any signs or symptoms of bronchospasm or respiratory distress.

Zidovudine

zyde-oh'vue-deen

★ Retrovir, AZT (synonym)

🍁 Apo-Zidovudine, Novo-AZT, Retrovir

Do not confuse Retrovir with ritonavir.

CATEGORY AND SCHEDULE

Pregnancy Risk Category: C

Classification: Antiretroviral, nucleoside reverse transcriptase inhibitor

MECHANISM OF ACTION

A nucleoside reverse transcriptase inhibitor that interferes with viral RNA-dependent DNA polymerase, an enzyme necessary for viral HIV replication. *Therapeutic Effect:* Interferes with HIV replication, slowing the progression of HIV infection.

PHARMACOKINETICS

Rapidly and completely absorbed from the GI tract. Protein binding: 25%-38%. Undergoes first-pass metabolism in the liver. Crosses the blood-brain barrier and is widely distributed, including to cerebrospinal fluid. Excreted primarily in urine. Minimal removal by hemodialysis. *Half-life:* 0.8-1.2 h (increased in impaired renal function).

AVAILABILITY

Injection: 10 mg/mL.
Capsule: 100 mg.
Tablet: 300 mg.
Oral Solution: 50 mg/5 mL.

INDICATIONS AND DOSAGES

▸ **HIV infection**

PO
Adults, Elderly. 300 mg twice daily OR 200 mg three times per day.
IV
Adults, Elderly. 1 mg/kg/dose q4h.

▸ **Reducing maternal-fetal HIV transmission**
PO AND IV REGIMEN
Pregnant women at > 14 wks of pregnancy. 100 mg PO 5 times per day until the start of labor. During labor and delivery, give 2 mg/kg (total body weight) IV (over 1 h) followed by an IV infusion of 1 mg/kg/h (total body weight) until clamping of the umbilical cord.

▸ **Dose for neonate once delivered**
PO
Neonates. 2 mg/kg q6h starting within 12 h after birth and continuing through 6 wks of age. If unable to take PO, may give 1.5 mg/kg IV (infused over 30 min) q6h. Preterm neonates require special care–see manufacturer's literature.

▸ **Usual dose, pediatrics with HIV infection (non-neonatal)**
PO
Adolescents, Children, and Infants > 4 wks. 240 mg/m^2 twice daily OR 160 mg/m^2 three times per day. See manufacturer information for complete details.

▸ **Renal failure**
Dosage adjustments recommended for all patients maintained on hemodialysis or peritoneal dialysis, or those with CrCl < 15 mL/min (see manufacturer's literature).

CONTRAINDICATIONS

Potentially life-threatening reactions (e.g., anaphylaxis, Stevens-Johnson syndrome) to the drug or formulations.

INTERACTIONS

Drug
Acetaminophen, clarithromycin: Decreased blood levels of zidovudine.
Bone marrow suppressive agents: Additive hermatologic effects.
Fluconazole, atovaquone, methadone, probenecid, valproic acid: Increased serum levels of zidovudine; consider dose reduction.
Phenytoin: Alterations in oral clearance of zidovudine.
Stavudine, ribavirin, or doxorubicin: Antagonize zidovudine action. Avoid combination.

IV INCOMPATIBILITIES

Lansoprazole, biologic or colloidal fluids.

SIDE EFFECTS

Expected
Nausea, headache, malaise.
Frequent
Abdominal pain, asthenia, rash, fever, acne, anorexia.
Occasional
Diarrhea, myalgia, somnolence.
Rare
Dizziness, paresthesia, vomiting, insomnia, dyspnea, altered taste.

SERIOUS REACTIONS

- Serious reactions include anemia, which occurs most commonly after 4-6 wks of therapy, and granulocytopenia; both effects are more likely to occur in patients who have a low hemoglobin level or granulocyte count before beginning therapy.
- Neurotoxicity (as evidenced by ataxia, fatigue, lethargy, nystagmus, and seizures) may occur.
- Precipitation (particularly IV use) in renal tubules may occur when the solubility (2.5 mg/mL) is exceeded

in the intratubular fluid. Adequate hydration can prevent.

PRECAUTIONS & CONSIDERATIONS

! May cause severe neutropenia or anemia; be alert for granulocyte count < 1000/mm³ or hemoglobin < 9.5 g/dL. Dose reduction recommended for those with severe renal disease. Severe hepatic dysfunction may result from lactic acidosis with hepatomegaly and steatosis. Zidovudine is excreted in breast milk, and use during lactation not recommended due to drug excretion and risk of HIV transmission.

Storage

Store oral products and injection at room temperature; protect from moisture. Protect injection from light. The diluted infusion is stable for 24 h at room temperature and 48 h if refrigerated.

Administration

Oral doses may be taken without regard to meals; give with adequate fluids.

Injection is administered as IV infusion; avoid rapid/bolus injection. Do not give IM. Withdraw appropriate dose from injection solution vial and dilute in D5W to a concentration not to exceed 4 mg/mL; infuse over at least 60 min.

Zinc Oxide/Zinc Sulfate

zink ox'ide/zink sul'fate

★ zinc oxide, topical: Balmex, Desitin; zinc sulfate, oral: Zincate

CATEGORY AND SCHEDULE

Pregnancy Risk Category: C

Classification: Mineral

MECHANISM OF ACTION

A mineral that acts as a cofactor for enzymes that are important for protein and carbohydrate metabolism. *Therapeutic Effect:* Zinc oxide acts as a mild astringent and skin protectant. Zinc sulfate helps maintain normal growth and tissue repair, as well as skin hydration.

INDICATIONS AND DOSAGES

▸ **Mild skin irritations and abrasions (such as chapped skin, diaper rash)**

TOPICAL (ZINC OXIDE)

Adults, Elderly, Children. Apply as needed.

▸ **Treatment and prevention of zinc deficiency, wound healing**

PO (ZINC SULFATE)

Adults, Elderly. 220 mg 3 times a day.

INTERACTIONS

Drug

Tetracyclines, fluoroquinolones: Oral zinc can decrease absorption of these antibiotics; separate administration times by 2 h or more.

SIDE EFFECTS

Altered taste with oral use, may cause mild GI upset. With topical use, dry skin may occur.

SERIOUS REACTIONS

• None known.

Ziprasidone

zye-pray'za-done

★ Geodon 🍁 Zeldox

CATEGORY AND SCHEDULE

Pregnancy Risk Category: C

Classification: Antipsychotic, atypical

MECHANISM OF ACTION

A piperazine derivative that antagonizes α-adrenergic, dopamine, histamine, and serotonin receptors; also inhibits reuptake of serotonin and norepinephrine. *Therapeutic Effect:* Diminishes symptoms of schizophrenia and depression.

AVAILABILITY

Injection: 20 mg/mL.
Capsule: 20 mg, 40 mg, 60 mg, 80 mg.

PHARMACOKINETICS

Well absorbed after PO administration. Food increases bioavailability. Protein binding: 99%. Extensively metabolized in the liver. Not removed by hemodialysis. *Half-life:* 7 h.

INDICATIONS AND DOSAGES

▸ Schizophrenia

PO

Adults, Elderly. Initially, 20 mg twice a day with food. Titrate at intervals of no < 2 days. Maximum: 80 mg twice a day.

IM (ACUTE AGITATION)

Adults, Elderly. 10 mg q2h OR 20 mg q4h. Maximum: 40 mg/day. Convert to oral therapy as soon as possible.

▸ Bipolar mania

PO

Adults, Elderly. Initially, 40 mg twice a day; may increase to 60 mg twice a day after a few days if needed; maximum 80 mg twice a day.

▸ Dosage in renal impairment

No adjustments needed for oral dosing. For IM dosing, the cyclodextrin excipient is cleared renally; use with caution in patients with impaired renal function.

CONTRAINDICATIONS

Known hypersensitivity to ziprasidone, cardiac conduction defects, or a known history of QT prolongation (e.g., AV block, congenital long QT syndrome); uncompensated heart failure or recent acute myocardial infarction, significant untreated electrolyte imbalance, do not give IM injection intravenously.

INTERACTIONS

Drug

Carbamazepine: Reduced plasma levels.
Central nervous system (CNS) depressants: Increased risk of CNS depressant effects; use caution.
Drugs that lower blood pressure: Increased risk of hypotension.
Drugs that prolong the QT interval: Avoid use of these drugs in combination with ziprasidone.
Ketoconazole and other strong inhibitors of CYP3A4 isoenzymes: Increased plasma levels of ziprasidone.
Phenothiazines and related drugs (haloperidol, droperidol), metoclopramide: Increased extrapyramidal effects.

SIDE EFFECTS

Frequent

Headache, somnolence, dizziness.

Occasional

Rash, orthostatic hypotension, weight gain, restlessness, constipation, dyspepsia, hyperglycemia, onset of diabetes mellitus.

SERIOUS REACTIONS

- Prolongation of QT interval may produce torsades de pointes, a form of ventricular tachycardia. Patients with bradycardia, hypokalemia, or hypomagnesemia are at increased risk.

PRECAUTIONS & CONSIDERATIONS

May antagonize levodopa, dopamine agonists. QT prolongation and risk of sudden death; bradycardia; hypokalemia; hypomagnesemia; electrolyte depletion caused by diarrhea, diuretics, or vomiting; neuromalignant syndrome; tardive dyskinesia; seizures; suicide; lactation; children; dementia-related psychosis in the elderly.

Storage

Store at room temperature; protect from light. After reconstitution, the IM injection may be stored between 58-86° F for up to 24 h if protected from light.

Administration

Administer oral capsules with food, at consistent times daily. Injection should ONLY be administered IM; do not give intravenously. Do not give intravenously. Do not mix with any other drugs. Add 1.2 mL of SWI to the vial; shake vigorously until dissolved. To administer a 10-mg dose, draw up 0.5 mL. To administer 20 mg, draw up 1 mL. Discard any unused portion. Inject dose slowly and deeply into a large muscle (e.g., upper outer quadrant of the gluteus maximus or lateral thigh). If possible, keep patient recumbent for 30 min to minimize risk of hypotension.

Zoledronic Acid

zole-eh-drone′ick ass′id

(US) Reclast, Zometa (CAN) Aclasta, Zometa

Do not confuse Zometa with Reclast; these two products have different indications and dosage regimens.

CATEGORY AND SCHEDULE

Pregnancy Risk Category: D

Classification: Osteoporosis therapy adjunct, bisphosphonate

MECHANISM OF ACTION

A bisphosphonate that inhibits the resorption of mineralized bone and cartilage; inhibits increased osteoclastic activity and skeletal calcium release induced by stimulatory factors produced by tumors. *Therapeutic Effect:* Increases urinary calcium and phosphorus excretion; decreases serum calcium and phosphorus levels, inhibits bone resorption.

PHARMACOKINETICS

IV INFUSION

Shows triphasic half-life; plasma protein binding 22%; little to no metabolism; excreted mainly in urine; a high percentage of the dose remains bound to bone.

AVAILABILITY

Zometa Injection: 4 mg/5 mL concentrate for further dilution.
Reclast Infusion: 5 mg/100 mL solution for IV infusion.

INDICATIONS AND DOSAGES

▸ **Hypercalcemia**

IV INFUSION (ZOMETA)

Adults, Elderly. 4 mg IV infusion given over not < 15 min. Retreatment may be considered, but at least 7 days should elapse to allow for full response to initial dose.

▸ **Multiple myeloma**

IV INFUSION (ZOMETA)

Adults, Elderly. 4 mg IV infusion over a minimum of 15 min. May retreat at 7 days or more if needed for hypercalcemia of malignancy.

▸ **Dose adjustment for Zometa for renal impairment**

CrCl 50-60 ml/min: Reduce dose to 3.5 mg.
CrCl 40-49 ml/min: Reduce dose to 3.3 mg.

CrCl 30-39 ml/min: Reduce dose to 3 mg.
CrCl < 30 ml/min: Do not use.

▸ **Osteoporosis, Paget disease**
IV INFUSION (RECLAST)
Adults. 5 mg IV once yearly.

▸ **Dose adjustment for once-yearly Reclast for renal impairment**
CrCl 35 ml/min or over: No dosage adjustment needed.
CrCl < 35 ml/min: Not recommended due to lack of clinical data. Zoledronic acid is usually contraindicated when SCr > 4.5 mg/dL.

CONTRAINDICATIONS

Hypersensitivity to the drug or other bisphosphonates, hypocalcemia, pregnancy, severe renal impairment.

INTERACTIONS

Drug

Loop diuretics: May increase risk of hypocalcemia.
Nephrotoxic drugs: Use with caution due to additive renal effects; aminoglycosides may also have additive effect to lower serum calcium.
Thalidomide: Combination use for multiple myeloma may increase risk of renal dysfunction.

IV INCOMPATIBILITIES

Calcium-containing IV products and infusions (e.g., lactacted Ringer's injection). Do not mix or infuse with any other medications.

SIDE EFFECTS

Frequent
Fever, nausea, vomiting, constipation.
Occasional
Hypotension, anxiety, insomnia, flu-like symptoms (fever, chills, bone pain, myalgia, and arthralgia).
Rare
Conjunctivitis; incapacitating joint, muscle, or bone pain.

SERIOUS REACTIONS

- Renal toxicity may occur if IV infusion is administered in < 15 min.
- Osteonecrosis of the jaw.

PRECAUTIONS & CONSIDERATIONS

Avoid invasive dental procedures, such as dental implants.

Data for use in children are not available; monitor hypercalcemic parameters, ensure good hydration; requires dose adjustment in renal impairment; bronchospasm in aspirin-sensitive asthmatic patients; hypocalcemia; hypoparathyroidism; do not use during lactation; may cause fetal harm so do not use during pregnancy.

Storage
Store unopened vials or bottles of solution at room temperature. For Reclast, once the bottle is opened, the solution may be stored in the refrigerator for 24 h, but let warm up to room temperature before use.

Administration
For *Reclast*, give as a 5-mg infusion over no less than 15 min. For *Zometa*, must dilute the IV concentrate, in the appropriate dose, immediately with either 100 mL of 0.9% NaCl injection or dextrose 5% for injection. Do not inject the concentrate directly. Infuse the diluted drug over at least 15 min. When treating hypercalcemia, patient should be well hydrated to maintain urine output of 2 L/day.

For all uses: Patients must receive adequate calcium and vitamin D supplementation; recommendations vary with indication for use. Also, infuse via separate vented infusion line; do not allow contact with any calcium-containing large-volume parenterals or other IV medications. Renal function must be carefully monitored during treatment and before retreatment.

Zolmitriptan

zohl-mih-trip′tan

Zomig, Zomig-ZMT,

Zomig Rapimelt

CATEGORY AND SCHEDULE

Pregnancy Risk Category: C

Classification: Migraine agents, serotonin receptor agonists

MECHANISM OF ACTION

A serotonin receptor agonist that binds selectively to vascular receptors, producing a vasoconstrictive effect on cranial blood vessels. *Therapeutic Effect:* Relieves migraine headache.

PHARMACOKINETICS

Rapidly but incompletely absorbed after PO administration. Protein binding: 15%. Undergoes first-pass metabolism in the liver to active metabolite. Eliminated primarily in urine (60%) and, to a lesser extent, in feces (30%). *Half-life:* 3 h.

AVAILABILITY

Nasal Spray: 5 mg/actuation device.
Tablets: 2.5 mg, 5 mg.
Orally Dissolving Tablets (ODT): 2.5 mg, 5 mg.

CONTRAINDICATIONS

Known ischemic or vasospastic heart disease (angina, coronary vasospasm, MI) or other significant CV disease (e.g., uncontrolled HTN, stroke, TIA, and peripheral vascular disease, including ischemic bowel disease). Do not use within 24 h of use of other 5-HT1 agonists or an ergot-type drug. Not for use in hemiplegic or basilar migraine. Do not use during or within 2 wks of MAOI therapy. Hypersensitivity to zolmitriptan.

INDICATIONS AND DOSAGES

▸ Acute migraine attack

PO

Adults, Elderly. Initially, 2.5 mg or less. If headache returns, may repeat dose in 2 h. Maximum: 10 mg/24 h.

INTRANASAL

Adults, Elderly. 5 mg (1 spray) into 1 nostril. May repeat in 2 h. Maximum: 10 mg/24 h.

INTERACTIONS

Drug

Selective serotonin reuptake inhibitors, ergot-containing drugs (avoid use within 24 h of taking this drug): Potential serotonin crises.
Cimetidine: Decreased plasma levels of zolmitriptan.

SIDE EFFECTS

Frequent

Oral: Dizziness; tingling; neck, throat, or jaw pressure; somnolence.
Nasal: Altered taste, paresthesia.

Occasional

Oral: Warm or hot sensation, asthenia, chest pressure.
Nasal: Nausea, somnolence, nasal discomfort, dizziness, asthenia, dry mouth.

Rare

Diaphoresis, myalgia, paresthesia.

SERIOUS REACTIONS

Cardiac reactions (including ischemia, coronary artery vasospasm, and myocardial infarction [MI]) and noncardiac vasospasm-related reactions (such as hemorrhage and cerebrovascular accident) occur rarely, particularly in patients with hypertension, diabetes, or a strong family history of coronary artery disease; obese patients; smokers; men older than 40 yr; and postmenopausal women.

PRECAUTIONS & CONSIDERATIONS

Arrhythmias associated with conduction disorders. Renal or hepatic impairment; drug may cause coronary vasospasm Phenylketonuric patients should be informed that ODT form contains phenylalanine (a component of aspartame); caution should be used in lactating patients, elderly patients, and children.

Storage

Store at room temperature. Keep ODT form in original blister package until time of use; protect from light and moisture.

Administration

Administer tablets with a sip of water. For ODT form, place on the tongue, where it will dissolve and be swallowed with the saliva; no need to administer with liquid. For the nasal spray, follow manufacturer's instructions for use; each device contains a single dose.

Zolpidem Tartrate

zole-pi′dem tar′trate

★ Ambien CR, Edluar

Do not confuse Ambien with Amen.

CATEGORY AND SCHEDULE

Pregnancy Risk Category: C

Controlled Substance Schedule: IV

Classification: Nonbarbiturate, nonbenzodiazepine sedative-hypnotic

MECHANISM OF ACTION

A nonbenzodiazepine that enhances the action of the inhibitory neurotransmitter γ-aminobutyric acid. *Therapeutic Effect:* Induces sleep and improves sleep quality.

PHARMACOKINETICS

Route	Onset	Peak	Duration
PO	30 min	NA	6-8 h

Rapidly absorbed from the GI tract. Protein binding: 92%. Metabolized in the liver; excreted in urine. Not removed by hemodialysis. *Half-life:* 1.4-4.5 h (increased in hepatic impairment).

AVAILABILITY

Tablets: 5 mg, 10 mg.
Controlled-Release Tablets: 6.25 mg, 12.5 mg (Ambien CR).
Sublingual Tablets: 5 mg, 10 mg (Edluar).

CONTRAINDICATIONS

Hypersensitivity, including angiodema or anaphylaxis.

INDICATIONS AND DOSAGES

▸ **Insomnia**

PO (IMMEDIATE-RELEASE TABLETS)
Adults. 10 mg at bedtime.
Elderly, Debilitated, Hepatic insufficiency. 5 mg at bedtime.
PO (AMBIEN CR)
Adults. 12.5 mg at bedtime.
Elderly, Debiliated, or Hepatic insufficiency. 6.25 mg at bedtime.
SL (EDLUAR)
Adults. 10 mg at bedtime.
Elderly, Debiliated, or Hepatic insufficiency. 5 mg at bedtime.

INTERACTIONS

Drug

▸ **Alcohol, all CNS depressants**

Increased central nervous system (CNS) depression.

▸ **Ketoconazole and other CYP3A inhibitors**

Increase exposure to zolpidem; consider lower zolpidem dose.

SIDE EFFECTS

Occasional

Headache.

Rare

Dizziness, nausea, diarrhea, muscle pain.

SERIOUS REACTIONS

- Overdosage may produce severe ataxia, bradycardia, altered vision (such as diplopia), severe drowsiness, nausea and vomiting, difficulty breathing, and unconsciousness.
- Abrupt withdrawal of the drug after long-term use may produce asthenia, facial flushing, diaphoresis, vomiting, and tremor.
- Drug tolerance or dependence may occur with prolonged, high-dose therapy.
- Complex behaviors such "sleep driving" (i.e., driving while not fully awake, with amnesia for the event) have been reported; these can cause risk to patient or community.

PRECAUTIONS & CONSIDERATIONS

May cause abnormal thinking and complex behavior; use with caution in elderly, depression, hepatic disease, COPD, and sleep apnea.

Storage

Store at room temperature. Keep sublingual tablets in original blister package until time of use; protect from light and moisture.

Administration

The effect of the drug may be slowed by ingestion with or immediately after a meal. Administer immediately before bedtime. Swallow extended-release tablets whole; do not divide, crush, or chew. Sublingual tablets are placed under the tongue and allowed to disintegrate; do not swallow and do not take with water.

Zonisamide

zoh-nis'ah-mide

Zonegran

CATEGORY AND SCHEDULE

Pregnancy Risk Category: C

Classification: Anticonvulsant (sulfonamide derivative)

MECHANISM OF ACTION

A succinimide that may stabilize neuronal membranes and suppress neuronal hypersynchronization by blocking sodium and calcium channels. *Therapeutic Effect:* Reduces seizure activity.

PHARMACOKINETICS

Well absorbed after PO administration. Extensively bound to RBCs. Protein binding: 40%. Primarily excreted in urine. *Half-life:* 63 h (plasma), 105 h (RBCs).

AVAILABILITY

Capsules: 25 mg, 50 mg, 100 mg.

INDICATIONS AND DOSAGES

▸ **Partial seizures**

PO

Adults, Elderly, Children older than 16 yr. Initially, 100 mg/day for 2 wks. May increase by 100 mg/day at intervals of 2 wks or longer. Range: 100-600 mg/day.

CONTRAINDICATIONS

Hypersensitivity to zonisamide or sulfonamides.

INTERACTIONS

Drug

It has been proposed that drugs that inhibit CYP3A4 enzymes might alter zonisamide serum levels.

Carbamazepine, phenytoin, and other hepatic enzyme inducing medications: Increase metabolism and clearance of zonisamide.

SIDE EFFECTS

Frequent

Somnolence, dizziness, anorexia, headache, agitation, irritability, nausea.

Occasional

Fatigue, ataxia, confusion, depression, impaired memory or concentration, insomnia, abdominal pain, diplopia, diarrhea, speech difficulty.

Rare

Paresthesia, nystagmus, anxiety, rash, dyspepsia, weight loss, kidney stones, psychosis or depression, pancreatitis, CPK elevation.

SERIOUS REACTIONS

- Overdose is characterized by bradycardia, hypotension, respiratory depression, and coma.
- Leukopenia, anemia, and thrombocytopenia occur rarely.
- Kidney stones (rare).

PRECAUTIONS & CONSIDERATIONS

There is an increased risk of suicidal behavior in patients receiving anticonvulsants (AEDS). Monitor patients for emerging or worsening depression, suicidal thoughts, or unusual moods or behaviors. Use with caution in hepatic disease, dehydration, and renal impairment and in those predisposed to kidney stones. As a carbonic anhydrase inhibitor, zonisamide may cause metabolic acidosis; this risk may be higher in children. Zonisamide should be used in pregnancy only if the benefits outweigh the risks. Zonisamide is excreted in human breast milk, and breastfeeding during treatment is not recommended. The safe and effective use of Zonisamide in infants and children under age 16 has not been established. Cases of oligohidrosis, hyperthermia, and heat stroke have been reported (mainly in children) during clinical trials.

All patients with dehydration, hypovolemia, or other predisposing factors to heat intolerance should have their condition corrected before treatment. Limit exposure to temperature extremes and medications that might aggravate temperature regulation. Somnolence, fatigue, dizziness, and difficulty with concentration may occur, particularly in the first month of therapy. Avoid driving or operating machinery, or performing other tasks that require mental alertness until drug effects are known. Periodically monitor hydration status and serum chemistry.

As with all anticonvulsants, do not abruptly discontinue the drug.

Storage

Store at room temperature in a dry place protected from light.

Administration

May be taken without regard to food.

Swallow capsules whole. Maintain good hydration to help reduce risk of kidney stones.

APPENDIX A
FDA Pregnancy Categories

! Medications should be used during pregnancy only if clearly needed.

A: Adequate and well-controlled studies have failed to show a risk to the fetus in the first trimester of pregnancy (also, no evidence of risk has been seen in later trimesters). Possibility of fetal harm appears remote.

B: Animal reproduction studies have failed to show a risk to the fetus, no adequate and well-controlled studies have been done in pregnant women.

C: Animal reproduction studies have shown an adverse effect on the fetus, and no adequate and well-controlled studies have been done in humans. However, the benefits may warrant use of the drug in pregnant women despite potential risks.

D: Positive evidence has been found of human fetal risk based on data from investigational or marketing experience or from studies in humans, but the potential benefits may warrant use of the drug despite potential risks (e.g., use in life-threatening situations in which other medications cannot be used or are ineffective).

X: Animal or human studies have shown fetal abnormalities, and/or there is evidence of human fetal risk based on adverse reaction data from investigational or marketing experience where the risks in using the medication clearly outweigh potential benefits.

APPENDIX B
Normal Laboratory Values

HEMATOLOGY/COAGULATION

Test	Normal Range
Activated partial thromboplastin time (aPTT)	25-35 seconds
Erythrocyte count (RBC count)	M: 4.3-5.7 million cells/mm^3 F: 3.8-5.1 million cells/mm^3
Hematocrit (HCT, Hct)	M: 39%-49%, F: 35%-45%
Hemoglobin (Hb, Hgb)	M: 13.5-17.5 g/dL, F: 12.0-16.0 g/dL
Leukocyte count (WBC count)	4.5-11.0 thousand cells/mm^3
Leukocyte differential count	
Basophils	0%-0.75%
Eosinophils	1%-3%
Lymphocytes	23%-33%
Monocytes	3%-7%
Neutrophils—bands	3%-5%
Neutrophils—segmented	54%-62%
Mean corpuscular hemoglobin (MCH)	26-34 pg/cell
Mean corpuscular hemoglobin concentration (MCHC)	31%-37% Hb/cell
Mean corpuscular volume (MCV)	80-100 fL
Partial thromboplastin time (PTT)	60-85 seconds
Platelet count (thrombocyte count)	150-450 thousand/mm^3
Prothrombin time (PT)	11-13.5 seconds
RBC count (see Erythrocyte count)	

CLINICAL CHEMISTRY (SERUM PLASMA/URINE)

Test	Normal Range
Alanine animotransferase (ALT, SGPT)	0-55 units/L
Albumin	3.5-5 g/dL
Alkaline phosphatase	M: 53-128 units/L, F: 42-98 units/L
Anion gap	5-14 mEq/L
Aspartate aminotransferase (AST, SGOT)	0-50 units/L
Bilirubin (conjugated direct)	0-0.4 mg/dL
Bilirubin (total)	0.2-1.2 mg/dL
Calcium (total)	8.4-10.2 mg/dL
Carbon dioxide (CO_2) total	20-34 mEq/L
Chloride	96-112 mEq/L
Cholesterol (total)	Less than 200 mg/dL
C-reactive protein	68-8200 ng/mL
Creatine kinase (CK)	M: 38-174 units/L, F: 26-140 units/L
Creatine kinase isoenzymes	Fraction of total: Less than 0.04-0.06
Creatinine	M: 0.7-1.3 mg/dL, F: 0.6-1.1 mg/dL
Creatinine clearance	M: 90-139 mL/min/1.73 m^2 F: 80-125 mL/min/1.73 m^2

Test	Normal Range
Free thyroxine index (FTI)	
Glucose	Adults: 70-105 mg/dL Older than 60 yr: 80-115 mg/dL
Hemoglobin A_{1c}	5.6%-7.5% of total Hgb
Homovanillic acid (HVA)	1.4-8.8 mg/day
17-Hydroxycorticosteroids (17-OHCS)	M: 3-10 mg/day, F: 2-8 mg/day
Iron	M: 65-175 mcg/dL F: 50-170 mcg/dL
Iron-binding capacity, total (TIBC)	250-450 mcg/dL
Lactate dehydrogenase (LDH)	0-250 units/L
Magnesium	1.3-2.3 mg/dL
Oxygen (PO_2)	83-100 mm Hg
Oxygen saturation	95%-98%
pH	7.35-7.45
Phosphorus, inorganic	2.7-4.5 mg/dL
Potassium	3.5-5.1 mEq/L
Protein (total)	6-8.5 g/dL
Sodium	136-146 mEq/L
Specific gravity	1.002-1.030
Thyrotropin (TSH)	0.5 to 5 mIU/mL
Thyroxine (T_4) total	5-12 mcg/dL
Triglycerides (TG)	20-190 mg/dL
Tri-iodothyronine resin uptake test (TxRU)	22%-37%
Urea nitrogen	7-25 mg/dL
Urea nitrogen/creatinine ratio	10:1 to 20:1
Uric acid	M: 3.5-7.2 mg/dL F: 2.6-6 mg/dL
Vanillylmandelic acid (VMA)	2-7 mg/day

Modified from *Saunders Nursing Drug Handbook 2011*. St. Louis, 2011, Saunders.

APPENDIX C
English-to-Spanish Drug Phrases Translator

TAKING THE MEDICATION HISTORY

English	Spanish	Pronunciation
Are you allergic to any medications? (If yes:)	¿ Es alérgico a algún medicamento? (sì:)	(Ehs ah-lehr-hee-koh ah ahl-goon meh-dee-kah-mehn-toh) (see:)
Which medications are you allergic to?	¿A cuál medicamento es alérgico?	(ah koo-ahl meh-dee-kah-mehn-toh ehs ah-lehr-hee-koh)
What happens when you develop an allergic reaction?	¿Qué le pasa cuando desarrolla una reacción alérgica?	(Keh leh pah-sah koo-ahn-doh deh-sah-roh-yah oo-nah reh-ahk-see-ohn ah-lehr-hee-kah)
What did you do to relieve or stop the allergic reaction?	¿Qué hizo para aliviar o detener la reacción alérgica?	(Keh ee-soh pah-rah ah-lee-bee-ahr oh deh-teh-nehr lah reh-ahk-see-ohn ah-lehr-hee-kah)
Do you take any over-the-counter, prescription, or herbal medications? (If yes:)	¿Toma medicamentos sin receta, con receta, o naturistas (hierbas medicinales)? (sì:)	(Toh-mah meh-dee-kah-mehn-tohs seen reh-seh-tah, kohn reh-seh-tah, oh nah-too-rees-tahs [ee-ehr-bahs meh-dee-see-nah-lehs]) (see:)
Why do you take each medication?	¿Porqué toma cada medicamento?	(Pohr-keh toh-mah kah-dah meh-dee-kah-mehn-toh)
What is the dosage for each medication?	¿Cuál es la dosis de cada medicamento?	(Koo-ahl ehs lah doh-sees deh kah-dah meh-dee-kah-mehn-toh)
How often do you take each medication?	¿Con qué frequencia toma cada medicamento?	(Kohn keh freh-koo-ehn-see-ah toh-mah kah-dah meh-dee-kah-mehn-toh)
Once a day?	¿Una vez por dìa; diariamente?	(Oo-nah behs pohr dee-ah; dee-ah-ree-ah-mehn-teh)
Twice a day?	¿Dos veces por dìa?	(dohs beh-sehs pohr dee-ah)
Three times a day?	¿Tres veces por dìa?	(Trehs beh-sehs pohr dee-ah)
Four times a day?	¿Cuatro veces por dìa?	(Koo-ah-troh beh-sehs pohr-dee-ah)
Every other day?	¿Cada tercer dìa?	(Kah-dah tehr-sehr dee-ah)
Once a week?	¿Una vez por semana?	(Oo-nah behs pohr seh-mah-nah)
How does each medication make you feel?	¿Como le hace sentir cada medicamento?	(Koh-moh leh ah-seh sehn-teer kah-dah meh-dee-kah-mehn-toh)
Does the medication make you feel better?	¿Le hace sentir mejor el medicamento?	(Leh ah-seh sehn-teer meh-hohr ehl meh-dee-kah-mehn-toh)
Does the medication make you feel the same or unchanged?	¿Le hace sentir igual o sin cambio el medicamento?	(Leh ah-seh sehn-teer ee-goo-ahl oh seen kam-bee-oh ehl meh-dee-kah-mehn-toh)

Does the medication make you feel worse?	¿Se siente peor con el medicamento?	(Seh see-ehn teh peh-ohr kohn ehl meh-dee-kah-mehn-toh)
(If yes:)	(si:)	(see:)
What do you do to make yourself feel better?	¿Qué hace para sentirse mejor?	(Keh ah-seh pah-rah sehn-teer-seh meh-hohr)

PREPARING FOR A REGIMEN OF MEDICATION

Medication Purpose

English	Spanish	Pronunciation
This medication will help relieve:	Este medicamento le ayudará a aliviar:	(Ehs-teh meh-dee-kah-mehn-toh leh ah-yoo-dah-rah ah ah-lee-bee-ahr)
—abdominal gas	gases intestinales	(gah-sehs een-tehs-tee-nah-lehs)
—abdominal pain	dolor intestinal; dolor en el abdomen	(doh-lohr een-tehs-tee-nahl; doh-lohr ehn ehl ahb-doh-mehn)
—chest congestion	congestión del pecho	(kohn-hehs-tee-ohn dehl peh-choh)
—chest pain	dolor del pecho	(doh-lohr dehl peh-choh)
—constipation	constipación; estreñimiento	(kohns-tee-pah-see-ohn; ehs-treh-nyee-mee-ehn-toh)
—cough	tos	(tohs)
—headache	dolor de cabeza	(doh-lohr-deh kah-beh-sah)
—muscle aches and pains	achaques musculares y dolores	(ah-chah-kehs moos-koo-lah-rehs ee doh-loh-rehs)
—pain	dolor	(doh-lohr)
This medication will prevent:	Este medicamento prevendrá:	(Ehs-teh meh-dee-kah-mehn-toh preh-behn-drah)
—blood clots	coágulos de sangre	(koh-ah-goo-lohs deh sahn-greh)
—constipation	constipación; estreñimiento	(kohns-tee-pah-see-ohn; ehs-treh-nyee-mee-ehn-toh)
—contraception	contracepción; embarazo	(kohn-trah-sehp-see-ohn; ehm-bah-rah-soh)
—diarrhea	diarrea	(dee-ah-reh-ah)
—infection	infección	(een-fehk-see-ohn)
—seizures	convulciónes; ataque epiléptico	(kohn-bool-see-ohn-ehs; ah-tah-keh eh-pee-lehp-tee-koh)
—shortness of breath	respiración corta; falta de aliento	(rehs-pee-rah-see-ohn kohr-tah; fahl-tah deh ah-lee-ehn-toh)
—wheezing	el resollar; la respiración ruidosa, sibilante	(ehl reh-soh-yahr; lah rehs-pee-rah-see-ohn roo-ee-doh-sah, see-bee-lahn-teh)

Continued

English	Spanish	Pronunciation
This medication will increase your:	Este medicamento aumentará su:	(Ehs-teh meh-dee-kah-mehn-toh ah-oo-mehn-tah-rah soo:)
—ability to fight infections	habilidad a combatir infecciones	(ah-bee-lee-dahd ah kohm-bah-teer een-fehk-see-oh-nehs)
—appetite	apetito	(ah-peh-tee-toh)
—blood iron levels	nivel de hierro en la sangre	(nee-behl deh ee-eh-roh ehn lah sahn-greh)
—blood sugar	azúcar en la sangre	(ah-soo-kahr ehn lah sahn-greh)
—heart rate	pulso; latido	(pool-soh; lah-tee-doh)
—red blood cell count	cuenta de células rojas	(koo-ehn-tah deh seh-loo-lahs roh-hahs)
—thyroid hormone levels	niveles de hormona tiroide	(nee-beh-lehs deh ohr-moh-nah tee-roh-ee-deh)
—urine volume	volumen de orina	(boh-loo-mehn deh oh-ree-nah)
This medication will decrease your:	Este medicamento reducirá su:	(Ehs-teh meh-dee-kah-mehn-toh reh-doo-see-rah soo:)
—anxiety	ansiedad	(ahn-see-eh-dahd)
—blood cholesterol level	nivel de colesterol en la sangre	(nee-behl deh koh-lehs-teh-rohl ehn lah sahn-greh)
—blood lipid level	nivel de lìpido en la sangre	(nee-behl deh lee-pee-doh ehn lah sahn-greh)
—blood pressure	presión arterial; de sangre	(preh-see-ohn ahr teh-ree-ahl; deh sahn-greh)
—blood sugar level	nivel de azúcar en la sangre	(nee-behl deh ah-soo-kahr ehn lah sahn-greh)
—heart rate	pulso; latido	(pool-soh; lah-tee-doh)
—stomach acid	ácido en el estómago	(ah-see-doh ehn ehl ehs-toh-mah-goh)
—thyroid hormone levels	niveles de hormona tiroide	(nee-beh-lehs deh ohr-moh-nah tee-roh-ee-deh)
—weight	peso	(peh-soh)
This medication will treat:	Este medicamento sirve para:	(Ehs-teh meh-dee-kah-mehn-toh seer-beh pah-rah)
—cancer of your ________	cancer de su ________	(kahn-sehr deh soo)
—depression	depression	(deh-preh-see-ohn)
—HIV infection	infección de VIH	(een-fehk-see-ohn deh beh ee ah-cheh)
—inflammation	inflamación	(een-flah-mah-see-ohn)
—swelling	hinchazon	(een-chah-sohn)
—the infection in your ________	la infección en su ________	(lah een-fehk-see-ohn ehn soo)
—your abnormal heart rhythm	su ritmo anormal de corazón	(soo reet-moh ah-nohr-mahl deh koh-rah-sohn)
—your allergy to ________	su alergia a ________	(soo eh-lehr-hee-ah ah)
—your rash	su erupción; sarpullido	(soo eh-roop-see-ohn; sahr-poo-yee-doh)

Compiled from Skidmore-Roth L: *Mosby's Drug Guide for Nurses,* ed. 9. St. Louis, 2011, Mosby.

INDEX

Trade names are in **bold.**

INDEX

INDEX

INDEX

INDEX

INDEX

INDEX

INDEX

INDEX

INDEX